10TH EDITION

MANUAL OF
CLINICAL
MICROBIOLOGY

10TH EDITION

MANUAL OF CLINICAL MICROBIOLOGY

EDITOR IN CHIEF

JAMES VERSALOVIC

Department of Pathology, Texas Children's Hospital, and Department of Pathology
and Immunology, Baylor College of Medicine, Houston, Texas

EDITORS

KAREN C. CARROLL
Division of Medical Microbiology
Department of Pathology
The Johns Hopkins University School of Medicine
Baltimore, Maryland

GUIDO FUNKE
Department of Medical Microbiology and Hygiene
Gärtner & Colleagues Laboratories
Ravensburg, Germany

JAMES H. JORGENSEN
Department of Pathology
University of Texas Health Science Center
San Antonio, Texas

MARIE LOUISE LANDRY
Department of Laboratory Medicine
Yale University School of Medicine
New Haven, Connecticut

DAVID W. WARNOCK
National Center for Emerging and
Zoonotic Infectious Diseases
Centers for Disease Control and Prevention
Atlanta, Georgia

Volume 2

ASM
PRESS

Washington, DC

Address editorial correspondence to ASM Press, 1752 N St. NW,
Washington, DC 20036-2904, USA

Send orders to ASM Press, P.O. Box 605, Herndon, VA 20172, USA
Phone: (800) 546-2416 or (703) 661-1593
Fax: (703) 661-1501
E-mail: books@asmusa.org
Online: estore.asm.org

Library of Congress Cataloging-in-Publication Data
Manual of clinical microbiology / editor in chief, James Versalovic ; editors, Karen C. Carroll ...
[et al.].—10th ed.
p. ; cm.
Clinical microbiology
Includes bibliographical references and indexes.
ISBN 978-1-55581-463-2 (hardcover)
1. Medical microbiology—Handbooks, manuals, etc. 2. Diagnostic microbiology—Handbooks,
manuals, etc. I. Versalovic, James. II. American Society for Microbiology. III. Title: Clinical
microbiology.
[DNLM: 1. Microbiology. 2. Microbiological Techniques. QW 4]
QR46.M425 2011
616.9'041—dc22
2010035191

10 9 8 7 6 5 4 3 2 1

ISBN 978-1-55581-463-2 (print edition), 978-1-55581-678-0 (print/e-book bundle)

CONTENTS

Volume 2

section IV

VIROLOGY / 1262

VOLUME EDITOR: MARIE LOUISE LANDRY
SECTION EDITORS: ANGELA M. CALIENDO,
CHRISTINE C. GINOCCHIO, YI-WEI TANG, AND
ALEXANDRA VALSAMAKIS

GENERAL

RNA VIRUSES

DNA VIRUSES

EDITORIAL BOARD

CONTRIBUTORS

SHARON L. ABBOTT
Microbial Diseases Laboratory, California Department of
Public Health, 850 Marina Bay Parkway, E-164,
Richmond, CA 94804

STEPHAN W. ABERLE
Department of Virology, Medical University of Vienna,
Kinderspitalgasse 15, A-1095 Vienna, Austria

ADRIANO AGUZZI
Institute of Neuropathology, University Hospital Zürich,
Schmelzbergstrasse 12, CH-8091 Zürich, Switzerland

ABDALLA O. A. AHMED
Department of Medical Microbiology, Faculty of Medicine,
Umm Al-Qura University, P.O. Box 7607, 21955 Makkah Al
Mukarramah, Saudi Arabia

AFSAR ALI
Emerging Pathogens Institute, University of Florida at
Gainesville, Gainesville, FL 32610

DAVID A. ANDERSON
Macfarlane Burnet Institute for Medical Research and Public
Health, AMREP, 85 Commercial Road, Melbourne,
Victoria 3004, Australia

GEORGE F. ARAJ
Department of Pathology and Laboratory Medicine, American
University of Beirut Medical Center, PO Box 11-0236,
Beirut 1107-2020, Lebanon

MAX Q. ARENS
Department of Pediatrics, Washington University School of
Medicine, 660 S. Euclid Avenue, Box 8237,
St. Louis, MO 63110

RONALD M. ATLAS
Department of Biology, University of Louisville,
Louisville, KY 40202

ROBERT L. ATMAR
Department of Medicine and Department of Molecular
Virology and Microbiology, Baylor College of Medicine,
1 Baylor Plaza, MS BCM280, Houston, TX 77030

S. ARUNMOZHI BALAJEE
Mycotic Diseases Branch, Division of Foodborne, Waterborne,
and Environmental Diseases, National Center for Emerging
and Zoonotic Infectious Diseases, Centers for Disease
Control and Prevention, Atlanta, GA 30333

ELLEN JO BARON
Department of Pathology, Stanford University School of
Medicine, Stanford, CA 94305, and Cepheid, 904 Caribbean
Drive, Sunnyvale, CA 94089

KARSTEN BECKER
Institute of Medical Microbiology, University Hospital of
Münster, 48149 Münster, Germany

WILLIAM J. BELLINI
Measles, Mumps, Rubella, and Herpesvirus Branch, Division
of Viral Diseases, National Center for Immunization and
Respiratory Diseases, Centers for Disease Control and
Prevention, Atlanta, GA 30333

ANJA BERGER
Bayerisches Landesamt für Gesundheit und
Lebensmittelsicherheit, Dienststelle Oberschleißheim,
Veterinärstraße 2, D-85764 Oberschleißheim, Germany

KATHRYN A. BERNARD
National Microbiology Laboratory, Public Health Agency of
Canada, Winnipeg, Manitoba R3E 3R2, Canada

BEVERLEY-ANN BIGGS
Victorian Infectious Diseases Service, Royal Melbourne
Hospital, Parkville, Victoria 3050, and Department of
Medicine, University of Melbourne, Parkville, Victoria 3050,
Australia

ROBERT A. BONOMO
Medical Service, Louis Stokes Cleveland VA Medical
Center, and Department of Medicine, Case Western Reserve
University, Cleveland, OH 44106

CHERYL A. BOPP
Enteric Diseases Laboratory Branch, Division of Foodborne,
Waterborne, and Environmental Diseases, National Center
for Emerging and Zoonotic Infectious Diseases, Centers for
Disease Control and Prevention, Atlanta, GA 30333

DONALD H. BOUYER
Department of Pathology, University of Texas Medical
Branch, Galveston, TX 77555-0609

MICHAEL D. BOWEN
Gastroenteritis and Respiratory Viruses Laboratory Branch,
Division of Viral Diseases, National Center for Immunization
and Respiratory Diseases, Centers for Disease Control and
Prevention, Atlanta, GA 30333

CLAUDIA BRANDT
Institute of Medical Microbiology, Johann Wolfgang Goethe
University, Paul Ehrlich Strasse 40, 60596 Frankfurt,
Germany

MARY E. BRANDT
Mycotic Diseases Branch, Division of Foodborne, Waterborne,
and Environmental Diseases, National Center for Emerging
and Zoonotic Infectious Diseases, Centers for Disease
Control and Prevention, Atlanta, GA 30333

EDWARD B. BREITSCHWERDT
Department of Clinical Sciences and Center for Comparative
Medicine and Translational Research, College of Veterinary
Medicine, North Carolina State University, Raleigh,
NC 27606

BARBARA A. BROWN-ELLIOTT
Department of Microbiology, University of Texas Health
Center at Tyler, Tyler, TX 75708

DAVID A. BRUCKNER
Department of Pathology and Laboratory Medicine, David
Geffen School of Medicine at UCLA, P.O. Box 951713,
Los Angeles, CA 90095-1713

AMY E. BRYANT
Infectious Diseases Section, VA Medical Center, 500 W. Fort
Street (Building 45), Boise, ID 83702-7221

RICHARD S. BULLER
Department of Pediatrics, Washington University School of
Medicine, St. Louis, MO 63110

ANGELA M. CALIENDO
Department of Pathology and Laboratory Medicine, Emory
University School of Medicine, Atlanta, GA 30322

VITALIANO CAMA
Division of Parasitic Diseases, Centers for Disease Control and
Prevention, Atlanta, GA 30341

SHELDON CAMPBELL
Department of Laboratory Medicine, Yale University School
of Medicine, New Haven, CT 06520, and VA Connecticut
Healthcare System, West Haven, CT 06516

A. BETTS CARPENTER
Molecular Microbiology and Cytology Laboratories, LabCorp,
Charleston, WV 25312, and Department of Pathology,
Joan C. Edwards School of Medicine, Marshall University,
Huntington, WV 25704

KAREN C. CARROLL
Division of Medical Microbiology, Department of Pathology,
The Johns Hopkins University School of Medicine, Baltimore,
MD 21287

MARIA da GLÓRIA SIQUEIRA CARVALHO
Respiratory Diseases Branch, National Center for
Immunization and Respiratory Diseases, Centers for Disease
Control and Prevention, Atlanta, GA 30333

BRUNO B. CHOMEL
Department of Population Health and Reproduction, School of
Veterinary Medicine, University of California, Davis, CA 95616

SUNWEN CHOU
Department of Medicine, Oregon Health and Sciences
University, Portland, OR 97239

DIANE M. CITRON
R. M. Alden Research Laboratory, Culver City, CA 90230

TOM COENYE
Laboratory of Pharmaceutical Microbiology, Ghent University,
B-9000 Gent, Belgium

PATRICIA S. CONVILLE
Microbiology Service, Department of Laboratory Medicine,
Warren Grant Magnuson Clinical Center, National Institutes
of Health, 10 Center Drive, MSC 1508, Bethesda,
MD 20892-1508

NATALIE A. COUNIHAN
Section of Microbial Pathogenesis, Yale University School of
Medicine, 295 Congress Avenue, New Haven,
CT 06519-1418

ELLIOT P. COWAN
Center for Biologics Evaluation and Research, U.S. Food and
Drug Administration, Rockville, MD 20852

DAVID L. COX
Laboratory Reference and Research Branch, Division of STD
Prevention, National Center for HIV/AIDS, Viral Hepatitis,
STD and TB Prevention, Centers for Disease Control and
Prevention, Atlanta, GA 30333

FRANCIS E. G. COX
Department of Infectious and Tropical Diseases, London
School of Hygiene and Tropical Medicine, London WC1E
7HT, United Kingdom

JAMES E. CROWE, JR.
Department of Pediatrics and Department of Microbiology and Immunology, Vanderbilt University School of Medicine, Nashville, TN 37232

BART J. CURRIE
Menzies School of Health Research and Northern Territory Clinical School, Royal Darwin Hospital, Darwin, Northern Territory 0811, Australia

MELANIE T. CUSHION
Division of Infectious Diseases, Department of Internal Medicine, University of Cincinnati College of Medicine, Cincinnati, OH 45267-0560

INGER K. DAMON
Poxvirus and Rabies Branch, Division of High-Consequence Pathogens and Pathology, National Center for Emerging and Zoonotic Infectious Diseases, Centers for Disease Control and Prevention, Atlanta, GA 30333

ERIC DANNAOUI
Unité Mycologie Moléculaire, CNRS URA3012, Centre National de Référence Mycologie et Antifongiques, Institut Pasteur, 75724 Paris Cedex 15, France

G. SYBREN DE HOOG
Centraalbureau voor Schimmelcultures, P.O. Box 85167, NL-3508 AD Utrecht, The Netherlands

PETER DEPLAZES
Institute of Parasitology, University of Zurich, Winterthurerstrasse 266a, CH-8057 Zurich, Switzerland

EDWARD P. DESMOND
Mycobacteriology and Mycology Section, Microbial Diseases Laboratory, California Department of Public Health, 850 Marina Bay Parkway, Richmond, CA 94804

CHARLENE S. DEZZUTTI
Department of Obstetrics, Gynecology, and Reproductive Sciences, Magee-Womens Research Institute, University of Pittsburgh, Pittsburgh, PA 15213

DANIEL J. DIEKEMA
Division of Infectious Diseases, Department of Internal Medicine, and Division of Medical Microbiology, Department of Pathology, University of Iowa College of Medicine, Iowa City, IA 52242

LENIE DIJKSHOORN
Department of Infectious Diseases, Leiden University Medical Center, 2300 RC Leiden, The Netherlands

GARY V. DOERN
Department of Pathology, University of Iowa Carver College of Medicine, Iowa City, IA 52242

FRANÇOISE DROMER
Unité Mycologie Moléculaire, CNRS URA3012, Centre National de Référence Mycologie et Antifongiques, Institut Pasteur, 75724 Paris Cedex 15, France

J. STEPHEN DUMLER
Division of Medical Microbiology, Department of Pathology, The Johns Hopkins University School of Medicine, 720 Rutland Avenue, Ross 624, Baltimore, MD 21205

MARCELA ECHAVARRIA
Clinical Virology Laboratory, Center for Medical Education and Clinical Research, University Hospital, Buenos Aires C1431FWO, Argentina

PAUL H. EDELSTEIN
University of Pennsylvania Medical Center, Philadelphia, PA 19104-4283

JOHANNES ELIAS
Institute for Hygiene and Microbiology, University of Würzburg, 97080 Würzburg, Germany

HERMES ESCALANTE
Department of Microbiology, School of Biological Sciences, Universidad Nacional de Trujillo, Avenida Juan Pablo II S/N, Ciudad Universitaria, Trujillo, Peru

ANA V. ESPINEL-INGROFF
Medical Mycology Research Laboratory, Infectious Diseases/ Internal Medicine, Virginia Commonwealth University, Richmond, VA 23298-0049

ANDREAS ESSIG
Institute of Medical Microbiology and Hygiene, University of Ulm, Albert-Einstein Allee 23, D-89079 Ulm, Germany

RICHARD R. FACKLAM (RETIRED)
Respiratory Diseases Branch, National Center for Immunization and Respiratory Diseases, Centers for Disease Control and Prevention, Atlanta, GA 30333

J. J. FARMER III (RETIRED)
United States Public Health Service, Stone Mountain, GA 30087

MARY JANE FERRARO
Clinical Microbiology Laboratory, Massachusetts General Hospital and Harvard Medical School, Boston, MA 02114

PATRICIA I. FIELDS
Enteric Diseases Laboratory Branch, Division of Foodborne, Waterborne, and Environmental Diseases, National Center for Emerging and Zoonotic Infectious Diseases, Centers for Disease Control and Prevention, Atlanta, GA 30333

SYDNEY M. FINEGOLD
Infectious Diseases Section, VA Medical Center, and Department of Medicine and Department of Microbiology, Immunology, and Molecular Genetics, University of California at Los Angeles School of Medicine, Los Angeles, CA 90073

DORAN L. FINK
Laboratory of Parasitic Diseases, National Institute of Allergy and Infectious Diseases, National Institutes of Health, Bethesda, MD 20892

COLLETTE FITZGERALD
Enteric Diseases Laboratory Branch, Division of Foodborne,
Waterborne, and Environmental Diseases, National Center
for Emerging and Zoonotic Infectious Diseases, Centers for
Disease Control and Prevention, Atlanta, GA 30333

MICHAEL S. FORMAN
Division of Medical Microbiology, Department of Pathology,
The Johns Hopkins Medical Institutions, Baltimore,
MD 21287

JULIE D. FOX
Provincial Laboratory for Public Health and Department of
Microbiology and Infectious Diseases, University of Calgary,
3030 Hospital Drive NW, Calgary, Alberta T2N 4W4, Canada

RENO FREI
Clinical Microbiology, University Hospital Basel, 4031 Basel,
Switzerland

MATTHIAS FROSCH
Institute for Hygiene and Microbiology, University of
Würzburg, 97080 Würzburg, Germany

CHARLES F. FULHORST
Department of Pathology and Department of Microbiology
and Immunology, University of Texas Medical Branch,
301 University Boulevard, Route 0609, Galveston,
TX 77555-0609

GUIDO FUNKE
Department of Medical Microbiology and Hygiene, Gärtner &
Colleagues Laboratories, D-88212 Ravensburg, Germany

HECTOR H. GARCIA
Department of Microbiology, Universidad Peruana Cayetano
Heredia, and Cysticercosis Unit, Instituto de Ciencias
Neurológicas, Lima, Peru

LYNNE S. GARCIA
LSG & Associates, 512 12th Street, Santa Monica,
CA 90402-2908

DEA GARCIA-HERMOSO
Unité Mycologie Moléculaire, CNRS URA3012, Centre
National de Référence Mycologie et Antifongiques, Institut
Pasteur, 75724 Paris Cedex 15, France

BARBARA C. GÄRTNER
Institute for Virology, University of the Saarland, D-66421
Homburg/Saar, Germany

CHARLOTTE A. GAYDOS
Division of Infectious Diseases, Department of Medicine,
Johns Hopkins University, 530 Rangos Building, 855 North
Wolfe Street, Baltimore, MD 21205

ANNE M. GAYNOR
Department of Molecular Microbiology, Washington
University School of Medicine, St. Louis, MO 63110

PETER GERNER-SMIDT
Enteric Diseases Laboratory Branch, Division of Foodborne,
Waterborne, and Environmental Diseases, National Center
for Emerging and Zoonotic Infectious Diseases, Centers for
Disease Control and Prevention, Atlanta, GA 30333

ANTOINE GESSAIN
EPVO Unit, Department of Virology, Institut Pasteur, 75015
Paris, France

MAHMOUD A. GHANNOUM
Center for Medical Mycology, Department of Dermatology,
University Hospitals/Case Western Reserve University, 11100
Euclid Avenue, Cleveland, OH 44106

CHRISTINE C. GINOCCHIO
Department of Pathology and Laboratory Medicine, North
Shore-LIJ Health System Laboratories, and Department of
Molecular Medicine, The Feinstein Institute for Medical
Research, Hofstra North Shore-LIJ School of Medicine,
Lake Success, NY 11042

MARKUS GLATZEL
Institute of Neuropathology, Universitätsklinikum Hamburg-
Eppendorf, Martinistraβe 52, D-20246 Hamburg, Germany

BEATRIZ L. GOMEZ
Corporación para Investigaciones Biológicas, Medellín,
Colombia

STEPHEN R. GRAVES
Hunter Area Pathology Service and Australian Rickettsial
Reference Laboratory, Locked Bag 1, Hunter Region Mail
Centre, NSW 2310, Australia

PATTI E. GRAVITT
Department of Epidemiology and Department of Molecular
Microbiology and Immunology, Johns Hopkins Bloomberg
School of Public Health, Baltimore, MD 21205

BRIGITTE P. GRIFFITH
Department of Laboratory Medicine, Yale University School
of Medicine, New Haven, CT 06520

FELIX GRIMM
Institute of Parasitology, University of Zurich,
Winterthurerstrasse 266a, CH-8057 Zurich, Switzerland

JOSEP GUARRO
Facultat de Medicina, Universitat Rovira i Virgili, Sant
Llorenç, 21, 43201 Reus, Spain

WILLIAM J. HALSALL
Center for Medical Mycology, Department of Dermatology,
University Hospitals/Case Western Reserve University, 11100
Euclid Avenue, Cleveland, OH 44106

PATRICIA C. HARRIS
Quidel Corporation—Diagnostic Hybrids, 1055 E. State
Street, Suite 100, Athens, OH 45701

KEVIN C. HAZEN
Clinical Microbiology and Molecular Diagnostics (Infectious Diseases), Department of Pathology, University of Virginia Health System, Charlottesville, VA 22908-0904

DAVID W. HECHT
Department of Medicine, Loyola University Medical Center, Maywood, IL 60153

DEBORAH A. HENRY
University of British Columbia, Vancouver, British Columbia, Canada

SARAH K. HIGHLANDER
Department of Molecular Virology and Microbiology and Human Genome Sequencing Center, Baylor College of Medicine, Houston, TX 77030

JANET A. HINDLER
Department of Pathology and Laboratory Medicine, UCLA Medical Center, Los Angeles, CA 90095-1713

RICHARD L. HODINKA
Departments of Pediatrics and Pathology and Clinical Virology Laboratory, Children's Hospital of Philadelphia and University of Pennsylvania School of Medicine, Philadelphia, PA 19104

ALEX R. HOFFMASTER
Bacterial Special Pathogens Branch, Division of High-Consequence Pathogens and Pathology, National Center for Emerging and Zoonotic Infectious Diseases, Centers for Disease Control and Prevention, Atlanta, GA 30333

SAMANTHA J. HOOT
Seattle Biomedical Research Institute and Program in Pathobiology, Department of Global Health, University of Washington, Seattle, WA 98109-5219

AMY J. HORNEMAN
Pathology and Laboratory Service, VA Maryland Health Care System, Baltimore, MD 21201

REBECCA T. HORVAT
Department of Pathology and Laboratory Medicine, University of Kansas School of Medicine, Kansas City, KS 66160

SUSAN A. HOWELL
Mycology, St. Johns Institute of Dermatology, GSTS Pathology, London SE1 7EH, United Kingdom

EIJA HYYTIÄ-TREES
Enteric Diseases Laboratory Branch, Division of Foodborne, Waterborne, and Environmental Diseases, National Center for Emerging and Zoonotic Infectious Diseases, Centers for Disease Control and Prevention, Atlanta, GA 30333

JOSEPH P. ICENOGLE
Measles, Mumps, Rubella, and Herpesvirus Branch, Division of Viral Diseases, National Center for Immunization and Respiratory Diseases, Centers for Disease Control and Prevention, Atlanta, GA 30333

NANCY C. ISHAM
Center for Medical Mycology, Department of Dermatology, University Hospitals/Case Western Reserve University, 11100 Euclid Avenue, Cleveland, OH 44106

J. MICHAEL JANDA
Microbial Diseases Laboratory, California Department of Public Health, 850 Marina Bay Parkway, E-164, Richmond, CA 94804

KEITH R. JEROME
Department of Laboratory Medicine, University of Washington, and Vaccine and Infectious Disease Division, Fred Hutchinson Cancer Research Center, 1100 Fairview Avenue N., D3-100, Seattle, WA 98109

XI JIANG
Cincinnati Children's Hospital Medical Center, University of Cincinnati College of Medicine, Cincinnati, OH 45229-3039

JUAN A. JIMENEZ
Cysticercosis Unit, Instituto de Ciencias Neurológicas, Lima, Peru

ELIZABETH M. JOHNSON
Mycology Reference Laboratory, Health Protection Agency, South West Laboratory, Myrtle Road, Kingsdown, Bristol BS2 8EL, United Kingdom

JEFFREY L. JONES
Parasitic Diseases Branch, Division of Parasitic Diseases and Malaria, Center for Global Health, Centers for Disease Control and Prevention, Atlanta, GA 30333

MALCOLM K. JONES
School of Veterinary Sciences, The University of Queensland, Brisbane, Queensland 4072, and Queensland Institute of Medical Research, 300 Herston Road, Herston, Queensland 4006, Australia

TIMOTHY F. JONES
Communicable and Environmental Disease Services, Tennessee Department of Health, Nashville, TN 37243

JEANNE A. JORDAN
Epidemiology and Biostatistics, School of Public Health and Health Services, The George Washington University, 231 Ross Hall, 2300 I Street NW, Washington, DC 20037

JAMES H. JORGENSEN
Department of Pathology, The University of Texas Health Science Center, 7703 Floyd Curl Drive, San Antonio, TX 78229-3700

PETER KÄMPFER
Institut für Angewandte Mikrobiologie, Justus-Liebig-Universität Giessen, D-35392 Giessen, Germany

JAMES B. KAPER
Department of Microbiology and Immunology, University of Maryland School of Medicine, Baltimore, MD 21201

WILLIAM E. KEENE
Oregon Public Health Division, Portland, OR 97232-2162

JENNIFER KEISER
Department of Medical Parasitology and Infection Biology,
Swiss Tropical and Public Health Institute, CH-4002 Basel,
Switzerland

VOLKHARD A. J. KEMPF
Institute for Medical Microbiology and Infection Control,
University Hospital of the Johann Wolfgang Goethe
University, Paul Ehrlich-Strasse 40, D-60596 Frankfurt am
Main, Germany

EIJA KÖNÖNEN
Institute of Dentistry, University of Turku, FI-20520 Turku,
and Department of Infectious Disease Surveillance and
Control, National Institute for Health and Welfare (THL),
FI-00271 Helsinki, Finland

THOMAS G. KSIAZEK
Galveston National Laboratory, Pathology Department,
University of Texas Medical Branch, Galveston, TX 77555

JAIME A. LABARCA
Department of Medicine, Facultad de Medicina, Pontificia
Universidad Católica de Chile, Lira 63, Santiago, Chile

RENU B. LAL
Viral Surveillance and Diagnostic Branch, Influenza Division,
National Center for Immunization and Respiratory Diseases,
Centers for Disease Control and Prevention, Atlanta,
GA 30333

DARYL M. LAMSON
Division of Infectious Diseases, Wadsworth Center, Albany,
NY 12201

ROBERT S. LANCIOTTI
Arboviral Diseases Branch, Division of Vector-Borne Diseases,
National Center for Emerging and Zoonotic Infectious
Diseases, Centers for Disease Control and Prevention,
Fort Collins, CO 80521

MARIE LOUISE LANDRY
Department of Laboratory Medicine, Yale University School
of Medicine, New Haven, CT 06520-8035

MARK T. LaROCCO
St. Luke's Episcopal Hospital, 6720 Bertner Avenue, Houston,
TX 77030

ANDREW J. LAWSON
Gastrointestinal, Emerging and Zoonotic Infections
Department, Health Protection Agency, Centre for Infections,
London NW9 5HT, United Kingdom

AMY L. LEBER
Clinical/Molecular Microbiology, Virology, Immunoserology,
Department of Laboratory Medicine, Nationwide Children's
Hospital, Building C, Room 1868, 700 Children's Drive,
Columbus, OH 43205

JACQUES LE BRAS
Laboratoire de Parasitologie, Hôpital Bichat and Université
Paris Descartes, 46 rue Henri Huchard, 75018 Paris, France

NATHAN A. LEDEBOER
Clinical Microbiology and Molecular Diagnostics, Dynacare
Laboratories and Froedtert Memorial Lutheran Hospital, and
Department of Pathology, Medical College of Wisconsin,
Milwaukee, WI 53226

KARIN LEDER
Infectious Disease Epidemiology Unit, Department of
Epidemiology and Preventive Medicine, Monash University,
Prahran, Victoria 3181, Australia

ELLIOT J. LEFKOWITZ
Department of Microbiology, The University of Alabama at
Birmingham, Birmingham, AL 35294

DIANE S. LELAND
Department of Pathology and Laboratory Medicine, Indiana
University School of Medicine, Indianapolis, IN 46202

PAUL N. LEVETT
Saskatchewan Disease Control Laboratory, Regina,
Saskatchewan, Canada

SHOU-YEAN GRACE LIN
Mycobacteriology and Mycology Section, Microbial Diseases
Laboratory, California Department of Public Health, 850
Marina Bay Parkway, Richmond, CA 94804

DAVID S. LINDSAY
Center for Molecular Medicine and Infectious Diseases,
Department of Biomedical Sciences and Pathobiology,
Virginia-Maryland Regional College of Veterinary Medicine,
Virginia Tech, 1410 Prices Fork Road, Blacksburg,
VA 24061-0342

STEPHEN E. LINDSTROM
Viral Surveillance and Diagnostic Branch, Influenza Division,
National Center for Immunization and Respiratory Diseases,
Centers for Disease Control and Prevention, Atlanta,
GA 30333

ANDREA J. LINSCOTT
Department of Pathology, Ochsner Medical Center,
1514 Jefferson Highway, New Orleans, LA 70121

JOHN J. LiPUMA
Department of Pediatrics and Communicable Diseases,
University of Michigan Medical School, Ann Arbor,
MI 48109

MIKE LOEFFELHOLZ
Department of Pathology, University of Texas Medical
Branch, 301 University Blvd., Galveston, TX 77555

NIALL A. LOGAN
Department of Biological and Biomedical Sciences, School of
Life Sciences, Glasgow Caledonian University, Cowcaddens
Road, Glasgow G4 0BA, United Kingdom

OLIVIER LORTHOLARY
Unité Mycologie Moléculaire, CNRS URA3012, Centre
National de Référence Mycologie et Antifongiques, Institut
Pasteur, 75724 Paris Cedex 15, France

NELL S. LURAIN
Department of Immunology/Microbiology, Rush University
Medical Center, Chicago, IL 60612

RICARDO G. MAGGI
Department of Clinical Sciences and Center for Comparative
Medicine and Translational Research, College of Veterinary
Medicine, North Carolina State University, Raleigh,
NC 27606

THOMAS MARTH
Division of Internal Medicine, Krankenhaus Maria Hilf, Maria
Hilf Strasse 2, 54550 Daun, Germany

ROBERT F. MASSUNG
Rickettsial Zoonoses Branch, Division of Vector-Borne
Diseases, National Center for Emerging and Zoonotic
Infectious Diseases, Centers for Disease Control and
Prevention, Atlanta, GA 30333

ALEXANDER MATHIS
Institute of Parasitology, University of Zurich, CH-8057
Zurich, Switzerland

JAMES B. McAULEY
Rush University Medical Center, 1653 W. Congress Parkway,
Chicago, IL 60612

KARIN L. McGOWAN
Clinical Microbiology Laboratory, Children's Hospital of
Philadelphia, Departments of Pathology and Laboratory
Medicine, Pediatrics, and Microbiology, University of
Pennsylvania School of Medicine, Philadelphia, PA 19104

DONALD P. McMANUS
Queensland Institute of Medical Research, 300 Herston Road,
Herston, Queensland 4006, Australia

LEONEL MENDOZA
Biomedical Laboratory Diagnostics and Department of
Microbiology and Molecular Genetics, Michigan State
University, East Lansing, MI 48824-1031

ROBERT C. MOELLERING, JR.
Department of Medicine, Beth Israel Deaconess Medical
Center and Harvard Medical School, 110 Francis Street, Suite
6A, Boston, MA 02215

RHODA ASHLEY MORROW
Department of Laboratory Medicine, University of Washington,
1616 Eastlake Avenue E., Room 5186, Seattle, WA 98109

IRVING NACHAMKIN
Department of Pathology and Laboratory Medicine,
University of Pennsylvania School of Medicine, 3400 Spruce
Street, Philadelphia, PA 19104-4283

ISABEL NAJERA
Department of Medicine, Stanford University, Stanford, CA,
94305, and Roche Palo Alto LLC, 3431 Hillview Avenue,
Palo Alto, CA 94304

JAMES P. NATARO
Department of Pediatrics, University of Virginia School of
Medicine, Charlottesville, VA 22908

RONALD C. NEAFIE
Parasitic Infections Branch, Armed Forces Institute of
Pathology, 6825 16th Street NW, Washington, DC 20306

ALEXANDR NEMEC
Laboratory for Bacterial Genetics, National Institute of Public
Health, 10042 Prague, Czech Republic

STUART T. NICHOL
Viral Special Pathogens Branch, Division of High-
Consequence Pathogens and Pathology, National Center
for Emerging and Zoonotic Infectious Diseases, Centers for
Disease Control and Prevention, Atlanta, GA 30333

MICHAEL A. NOBLE
Department of Pathology and Laboratory Medicine,
University of British Columbia, Room 366, 2733 Heather
Street, Vancouver, British Columbia V5Z 1M9, Canada

FREDERICK S. NOLTE
Department of Pathology and Laboratory Medicine, Medical
University of South Carolina, Charleston, SC 29425

SUSAN NOVAK-WEEKLEY
SCPMG Regional Reference Laboratories, 1668 Sherman
Way, North Hollywood, CA 91605

THOMAS B. NUTMAN
Laboratory of Parasitic Diseases, National Institute of Allergy
and Infectious Diseases, National Institutes of Health,
Bethesda, MD 20892

LILLIAN A. ORCIARI
Poxvirus and Rabies Branch, Division of High-Consequence
Pathogens and Pathology, National Center for Emerging and
Zoonotic Infectious Diseases, Centers for Disease Control and
Prevention, Atlanta, GA 30333

S. MICHELE OWEN
Laboratory Branch, Division of HIV/AIDS Prevention,
National Center for HIV/AIDS, Viral Hepatitis, STD and
TB Prevention, Centers for Disease Control and Prevention,
Atlanta, GA 30333

KANTI PABBARAJU
Provincial Laboratory for Public Health, 3030 Hospital Drive
NW, Calgary, Alberta T2N 4W4, Canada

FRANTISKA PALICOVA
Department of Medical Microbiology, Center for Laboratory
Medicine, Kantonsspital Luzern, CH-6000 Lucerne 16,
Switzerland

GRAEME P. PALTRIDGE
Bacteriology and Parasitology Laboratory, Canterbury Health
Laboratories, Christchurch, New Zealand

XIAOLI PANG
Provincial Laboratory for Public Health and Department of
Laboratory Medicine and Pathology, University of Alberta,
Edmonton, Alberta T6G 2J2, Canada

JEAN B. PATEL
Clinical and Environmental Microbiology Branch, Division of
Healthcare Quality Promotion, National Center for Emerging
and Zoonotic Infectious Diseases, Centers for Disease Control
and Prevention, Atlanta, GA 30333

SHARON J. PEACOCK
Department of Medicine, University of Cambridge,
Addenbrooke's Hospital, Cambridge CB2 0QQ,
United Kingdom

PHILIP E. PELLETT
Department of Immunology and Microbiology, Wayne State
University School of Medicine, Detroit, MI 48201

JEANNINE M. PETERSEN
Bacterial Diseases Branch, Division of Vector-Borne Diseases,
National Center for Emerging and Zoonotic Infectious
Diseases, Centers for Disease Control and Prevention,
Fort Collins, CO 80521

JOSEPH F. PETROSINO
Department of Molecular Virology and Microbiology and
Human Genome Sequencing Center, Baylor College of
Medicine, Houston, TX 77030

CATHY A. PETTI
Department of Medicine, Stanford University School of
Medicine, Stanford, CA 94305

MICHAEL A. PFALLER
Department of Pathology, University of Iowa College of
Medicine, 200 Hawkins Drive, Iowa City, IA 52242-1009

GABY E. PFYFFER
Department of Medical Microbiology, Center for Laboratory
Medicine, Kantonsspital Luzern, CH-6000 Lucerne 16,
Switzerland

ALLAN PILLAY
Laboratory Reference and Research Branch, Division of STD
Prevention, National Center for HIV/AIDS, Viral Hepatitis,
STD and TB Prevention, Centers for Disease Control and
Prevention, Atlanta, GA 30333

GARY W. PROCOP
Department of Molecular Pathology, Pathology and
Laboratory Medicine Institute/L11, Cleveland Clinic, 9500
Euclid Avenue, Cleveland, OH 44195

ELISABETH PUCHHAMMER-STÖCKL
Department of Virology, Medical University of Vienna,
Kinderspitalgasse 15, A-1095 Vienna, Austria

JUSTIN D. RADOLF
Departments of Medicine and of Genetics and Developmental
Biology, University of Connecticut Health Center,
Farmington, CT 06030

J. KAMILE RASHEED
Clinical and Environmental Microbiology Branch, Division of
Healthcare Quality Promotion, National Center for Emerging
and Zoonotic Infectious Diseases, Centers for Disease Control
and Prevention, Atlanta, GA 30333

MEGAN E. RELLER
Division of Medical Microbiology, Department of Pathology,
The Johns Hopkins University School of Medicine, 720
Rutland Avenue, Ross 628, Baltimore, MD 21205

LOUIS B. RICE
Department of Medicine, Alpert Medical School, Brown
University, Providence, RI 02903

ELVIRA RICHTER
National Reference Center for Mycobacteria, Research Center
Borstel, 23845 Borstel, Germany

SANDRA S. RICHTER
Department of Clinical Pathology, Cleveland Clinic, 9500
Euclid Avenue, L40, Cleveland, OH 44195

MARION RIFFELMANN
HELIOS Klinikum Krefeld, D-47805 Krefeld, Germany

CHRISTINE ROBINSON
Department of Pathology, The Children's Hospital, Aurora,
CO 80045

WILLIAM O. ROGERS
Naval Medical Research Unit 2, Phnom Penh, Cambodia

PIERRE E. ROLLIN
Viral Special Pathogens Branch, Division of High-
Consequence Pathogens and Pathology, National Center
for Emerging and Zoonotic Infectious Diseases, Centers for
Disease Control and Prevention, Atlanta, GA 30333

JOSÉ R. ROMERO
Pediatrics, Arkansas Children's Hospital, Little Rock,
AR 72202-3591

PAUL A. ROTA
Measles, Mumps, Rubella, and Herpesvirus Branch, Division
of Viral Diseases, National Center for Immunization and
Respiratory Diseases, Centers for Disease Control and
Prevention, Atlanta, GA 30333

KATHRYN L. RUOFF
Department of Pathology, Dartmouth Hitchcock Medical
Center, Lebanon, NH 03756

CHARLES E. RUPPRECHT
Poxvirus and Rabies Branch, Division of High-Consequence
Pathogens and Pathology, National Center for Emerging and
Zoonotic Infectious Diseases, Centers for Disease Control and
Prevention, Atlanta, GA 30333

MARTIN E. SCHRIEFER
Bacterial Diseases Branch, Division of Vector-Borne Diseases,
National Center for Emerging and Zoonotic Infectious
Diseases, Centers for Disease Control and Prevention, Fort
Collins, CO 80521

W. EVAN SECOR
Parasitic Diseases Branch, Division of Parasitic Diseases
and Malaria, Center for Global Health, Centers for Disease
Control and Prevention, Atlanta, GA 30333

SEAN V. SHADOMY
Bacterial Special Pathogens Branch, Division of High-
Consequence Pathogens and Pathology, National Center
for Emerging and Zoonotic Infectious Diseases, Centers for
Disease Control and Prevention, Atlanta, GA 30333

ROBERT W. SHAFER
Departments of Medicine and Pathology, Stanford University,
Stanford, CA 94305

SUSAN E. SHARP
Kaiser Permanente and Oregon Health Sciences University,
Portland, OR 97230

YVONNE R. SHEA
Microbiology Service, Department of Laboratory Medicine,
Clinical Center, National Institutes of Health, Building 10,
Room 2C325, 10 Center Drive, MSC 1508, Bethesda,
MD 20892

HARSHA SHEOREY
Department of Microbiology, St. Vincent's Hospital
Melbourne, Fitzroy, Victoria 3065, Australia

PATRICIA LYNN SHEWMAKER
Respiratory Diseases Branch, National Center for
Immunization and Respiratory Diseases, Centers for Disease
Control and Prevention, Atlanta, GA 30333

ROBYN Y. SHIMIZU
Department of Pathology and Laboratory Medicine, UCLA
Health System, Los Angeles, CA 90095-1713

KAMALJIT SINGH
Rush University Medical Center, 1653 W. Congress Parkway,
Chicago, IL 60612

JAMES W. SNYDER
Department of Pathology and Laboratory Medicine,
University of Louisville School of Medicine and Hospital,
530 S. Jackson Street, Louisville, KY 40202

YULI SONG
Oral Care, R&D, Procter & Gamble, Mason, OH 45040

DAVID P. SPEERT
University of British Columbia, Vancouver, British Columbia,
Canada

BARBARA SPELLERBERG
Institute of Medical Microbiology and Hygiene, University of
Ulm, Albert Einstein Allee 11, 89081 Ulm, Germany

KENDRA E. STAUFFER
Bacterial Special Pathogens Branch, Division of High-
Consequence Pathogens and Pathology, National Center
for Emerging and Zoonotic Infectious Diseases, Centers for
Disease Control and Prevention, Atlanta, GA 30333

KATHLEEN A. STELLRECHT
Department of Pathology and Laboratory Medicine, Albany
Medical Center, Albany, NY 12208

DENNIS L. STEVENS
Infectious Diseases Section, VA Medical Center, 500 W. Fort
Street (Building 45), Boise, ID 83702-7221

NANCY A. STROCKBINE
Enteric Diseases Laboratory Branch, Division of Foodborne,
Waterborne, and Environmental Diseases, National Center
for Emerging and Zoonotic Infectious Diseases, Centers for
Disease Control and Prevention, Atlanta, GA 30333

RICHARD C. SUMMERBELL
Sporometrics Inc. and Dalla Lana School of Public Health,
University of Toronto, Toronto, Ontario, Canada

DEANNA A. SUTTON
Department of Pathology, University of Texas Health Science
Center at San Antonio, San Antonio, TX 78229-3900

JANA M. SWENSON
Clinical and Environmental Microbiology Branch, Division of
Healthcare Quality Promotion, National Center for Emerging
and Zoonotic Infectious Diseases, Centers for Disease Control
and Prevention, Atlanta, GA 30333

ELLA M. SWIERKOSZ
Department of Pathology, Saint Louis University School of
Medicine, St. Louis, MO 63104

YI-WEI TANG
Department of Pathology and Department of Medicine,
Vanderbilt University School of Medicine, Nashville, TN
37232

DAVID TAYLOR-ROBINSON
Department of Medicine, Imperial College London, St. Mary's
Campus, London, United Kingdom

GARY E. TEGTMEIER
Community Blood Center of Greater Kansas City, Kansas
City, MO 64111

LÚCIA MARTINS TEIXEIRA
Instituto de Microbiologia, Universidade Federal do Rio de
Janeiro, Rio de Janeiro, RJ 21941, Brazil

SAM R. TELFORD III
Cummings School of Veterinary Medicine, Tufts University,
200 Westboro Road, North Grafton, MA 01536

FRED C. TENOVER
Cepheid, 904 Caribbean Drive, Sunnyvale, CA 94089

KENNETH D. THOMPSON
Department of Pathology, The University of Chicago Medical
Center, Chicago, IL 60637

RICHARD B. THOMSON, JR.
Clinical Microbiology Laboratories, Department of Pathology
and Laboratory Medicine, Evanston Hospital and NorthShore
University HealthSystem, 2650 Ridge Avenue, Evanston,
IL 60201

GRAHAM TIPPLES
National Microbiology Laboratory, Public Health Agency of
Canada, 1015 Arlington Street, Winnipeg, Manitoba R3E
3R2, Canada

PETER TRAYNOR
Oxoid Australia Pty Limited, Thermo Fisher Scientific,
Adelaide, South Australia 5031, Australia

THEODORE F. TSAI
Novartis Vaccines, 350 Massachusetts Avenue, Cambridge,
MA 02139

JOHN D. TURNIDGE
SA Pathology at Women's and Children's Hospital, 72 King
William Road, North Adelaide, South Australia 5006, Australia

STEVE J. UPTON
Division of Biology, Ackert Hall, Kansas State University,
Manhattan, KS 66506-4901

ALEXANDRA VALSAMAKIS
Division of Medical Microbiology, Department of Pathology,
The Johns Hopkins Medical Institutions, Baltimore,
MD 21287

PETER A. R. VANDAMME
Laboratorium voor Microbiologie, Faculteit Wetenschappen,
Universiteit Gent, Ledeganckstraat 35, B-9000 Gent, Belgium

MARIO VANEECHOUTTE
Laboratory Bacteriology Research, Department of Clinical
Chemistry, Microbiology, and Immunology, University of
Ghent, B-9000 Ghent, Belgium

JAMES VERSALOVIC
Department of Pathology, Texas Children's Hospital, Feigin
Center, Suite 830, 1102 Bates Avenue, and Department of
Pathology and Immunology, Baylor College of Medicine,
Houston, TX 77030

RAQUEL VILELA
Biomedical Laboratory Diagnostics, Michigan State
University, East Lansing, MI 48824-1031

GOVINDA S. VISVESVARA
Waterborne Diseases Prevention Branch, Division of
Foodborne, Waterborne, and Environmental Diseases,
National Center for Emerging and Zoonotic Infectious
Diseases, Centers for Disease Control and Prevention,
Atlanta, GA 30333

ULRICH VOGEL
Institute for Hygiene and Microbiology, University of
Würzburg, 97080 Würzburg, Germany

CHRISTOPH von EICHEL-STREIBER
Institut für Medizinische Mikrobiologie und Hygiene,
Johannes Gutenberg-Universität Mainz, Hochhaus am
Augustaplatz, D-55131 Mainz, Germany

CHRISTOF von EIFF
Pfizer Pharma GmbH, 10785 Berlin, Germany

ALEXANDER von GRAEVENITZ
Institute of Medical Microbiology, University of Zurich,
Gloriastrasse 32, CH-8006 Zurich, Switzerland

WILLIAM G. WADE
Department of Microbiology, King's College London, Guy's
Campus, London SE1 9RT, United Kingdom

KEN B. WAITES
Department of Pathology, University of Alabama at
Birmingham, Birmingham, AL 35249

DAVID H. WALKER
Department of Pathology and Center for Biodefense and
Emerging Infectious Diseases, University of Texas Medical
Branch, Galveston, TX 77555-0609

RICHARD J. WALLACE, JR.
Department of Microbiology, University of Texas Health
Center at Tyler, Tyler, TX 75708

DAVID WANG
Department of Molecular Microbiology and Department of
Pathology and Immunology, Washington University School of
Medicine, St. Louis, MO 63110

DAVID W. WARNOCK
National Center for Emerging and Zoonotic Infectious
Diseases, Centers for Disease Control and Prevention,
Atlanta, GA 30333

GEORGES WAUTERS
Department of Microbiology, Université catholique de
Louvain, B-1200 Brussels, Belgium

RAINER WEBER
Division of Infectious Diseases and Hospital Epidemiology,
Department of Internal Medicine, University Hospital,
CH-8091 Zurich, Switzerland

MELVIN P. WEINSTEIN
Departments of Medicine and Pathology, Robert Wood
Johnson Medical School, 1 Robert Wood Johnson Place,
MEB 364, New Brunswick, NJ 08903-0019

LOUIS M. WEISS
Albert Einstein College of Medicine, 1300 Morris Park
Avenue, Room 504 Forchheimer Building, Bronx, NY 10461

PETER F. WELLER
Department of Medicine, Harvard Medical School, and
Division of Infectious Diseases and Allergy and Inflammation
Division, Beth Israel Deaconess Medical Center, Boston,
MA 02215

NELE WELLINGHAUSEN
Department of Medical Microbiology and Hygiene, Gärtner &
Colleagues Laboratories, D-88212 Ravensburg, Germany

THEODORE C. WHITE
Seattle Biomedical Research Institute and Program in
Pathobiology, Department of Global Health, University of
Washington, Seattle, WA 98109-5219

ANDREAS F. WIDMER
Infection Control and Hospital Epidemiology, University
Hospital Basel, 4031 Basel, Switzerland

DANNY L. WIEDBRAUK
Virology and Molecular Biology, Warde Medical Laboratory,
300 W. Textile Road, Ann Arbor, MI 48108

CARL-HEINZ WIRSING von KÖNIG
HELIOS Klinikum Krefeld, D-47805 Krefeld, Germany

FRANK G. WITEBSKY
Microbiology Service, Department of Laboratory Medicine,
Warren Grant Magnuson Clinical Center, National Institutes
of Health, 10 Center Drive, MSC 1508, Bethesda,
MD 20892-1508

GAIL L. WOODS
Pathology and Laboratory Medicine Service (LR/113),
Central Arkansas Veterans Healthcare System, 4300 W. 7th
Street, Little Rock, AR 72205-5484

LIHUA XIAO
Waterborne Diseases Prevention Branch, Division of
Foodborne, Waterborne, and Environmental Diseases,
National Center for Emerging and Zoonotic Infectious
Diseases, Centers for Disease Control and Prevention,
Atlanta, GA 30333

JOSEPH D. C. YAO
Division of Clinical Microbiology, Department of Laboratory
Medicine and Pathology, College of Medicine, Mayo Clinic,
Rochester, MN 55905

SHERIF ZAKI
Infectious Diseases Pathology Branch, Division of High-
Consequence Pathogens and Pathology, National Center
for Emerging and Zoonotic Infectious Diseases, Centers for
Disease Control and Prevention, Atlanta, GA 30333

REINHARD ZBINDEN
Institute of Medical Microbiology, University of Zurich,
Gloriastrasse 32, CH-8006 Zurich, Switzerland

Acknowledgment of Previous Contributors
The *Manual of Clinical Microbiology* is by its nature a continuously revised work which
refines and extends the contributions of previous editions. Since its first edition in
1970, many eminent scientists have contributed to this important reference work. The
American Society for Microbiology and its Publications Board gratefully acknowledge the
contributions of all of these generous authors over the life of this *Manual*.

PREFACE

The *Manual of Clinical Microbiology* (MCM) is the most authoritative reference in the field of diagnostic microbiology, and a team of 22 editors and 267 authors worked closely together with a group of several individuals at ASM Press (including eight freelance copy editors) to deliver the 10th edition in its prescribed 4-year publication cycle. As a profession, we are proud members of the American Society for Microbiology, and its book publishing arm, ASM Press, remains steadfastly committed to the utmost quality that the MCM readership has come to expect. As a new editor in chief, a chapter author, and a former section editor, I am proud that this commitment to excellence by everyone associated with the production of the *Manual* has always been apparent.

As in so many professional endeavors, our work rests on the shoulders of giants who preceded us. I must thank Patrick Murray, who initially asked me to succeed him as the fourth editor in chief of the *Manual*. Clearly, I had extremely large shoes to fill, as Pat had elevated the *Manual* to an unprecedented level in terms of scope and quality. My job was made immensely easier by Pat's guidance and his generosity in sharing his cumulative experience from past editions. No editor in chief could ask for more support than I received from Pat. Another prior editor of the *Manual*, Ellen Jo Baron, who served as a volume editor for several editions, provided many lessons on the "how" of editing as well as inspiration in aiming for superior quality with every chapter of the *Manual*. As a section editor working under Ellen, I immersed myself in the *Manual* and grasped its essence. In this spirit of appreciation, I must also convey a special thanks to the team at ASM Press. Ken April has served as an extremely capable and committed production editor, as we both navigated role transitions. His predecessor, Susan Birch, was a pillar working closely with Pat Murray on multiple prior editions of the *Manual*, and her expertise benefited this edition when we requested her advice. Ken kept us on track with a tight production timeline while juggling several other book projects for ASM Press in parallel. With a deep sense of gratitude, I thank Jeff Holtmeier, director of ASM Press throughout much of the planning and publication process of MCM10, who believed in me and gave me the opportunity to serve as editor in chief of the 10th edition. I know that Jeff viewed this editorship as a keystone position at ASM Press, and I am profoundly grateful for the privilege of guiding the *Manual* through the publication of the current edition.

This edition of the *Manual* will be the first to have a full-scale, Web-based HTML electronic edition. In addition to the complete contents of the printed edition, the electronic edition will contain an image library consisting of all the figures from the printed edition and more than 400 supplementary figures generously contributed by Pat Murray from his laboratory collection and the collections of a few chapter authors.

In conclusion, I want to make a few comments about our profession. Clinical microbiology will be challenged by new developments in molecular diagnostics, microbial genomics, and metagenomics. Novel viruses may require the development of targeted assays relying on newly generated nucleic acid sequencing data. The recently emerging field of human microbiome research is already upsetting the apple cart and challenging notions of single-agent or polymicrobial infections. Can microbial communities or dysbiosis predispose to or result in infectious diseases? In spite of all of the rapid changes in molecular microbiology and metagenomics, the field of clinical microbiology must sustain its core practices of culture, microscopic visualization, direct antigen detection, serology, biochemical or phenotypic characterization, and antimicrobial susceptibility testing. The *Manual of Clinical Microbiology* continues to represent the glue that binds clinical microbiology by describing its core practices and approaches while disseminating old and new knowledge to generations of practitioners around the globe.

JAMES VERSALOVIC

Author and Editor Conflicts of Interest

The authors and editors of this *Manual* have disclosed any potentially relevant conflicts of interest below, including relationships that might detract from an author's objectivity in presentation of information and interests whose value would be enhanced by the data presented.

David A. Anderson (chapter 88) is a coinventor of reagents licensed from the Burnet Institute to MP Biomedicals Asia Pacific for use in hepatitis E virus diagnostics (HEV IgM ELISA 3.0, HEV sandwich ELISA 4.0, and Assure rapid HEV IgM).

Ellen Jo Baron (chapters 16 and 47) is an employee of Cepheid, a molecular diagnostics company. She has received royalties, honoraria, or consulting income from OpGen, bioMérieux, Merck, MorphDesign, Hardy Diagnostics, and Elsevier. She is a member of product/scientific advisory boards of MicroPhage, Key Scientific Products, NanoMR, OpGen, and Immunosciences, Inc.

Karsten Becker (chapter 19) is a member of advisory boards and has received travel and research grant support and lecture fees from several companies in the pharmaceutical and diagnostic industry.

Edward B. Breitschwerdt (chapter 46) holds U.S. patent 7,115,385 (Media and Methods for Cultivation of Cultivation of Microorganisms, issued 3 October 2006) in conjunction with Sushama Sontakke and North Carolina State University. He is the chief scientific officer of Galaxy Diagnostics, a company that provides diagnostic testing for the detection of *Bartonella* species infection in animals and in human patient samples.

Angela M. Caliendo (section editor; coauthor of chapters 4, 78, and 79) has served on the scientific advisory boards of Roche Diagnostics, Idaho Technologies, Quidel, Abbott Molecular, and GenProbe; has participated in clinical trials with Roche and Qiagen; and has been a consultant to DiaSorin/Biotrin.

Karen C. Carroll (volume editor; coauthor of chapters 3 and 9) has served on the scientific advisory boards of OpGen, Inc., NanoMR, and Quidel Corp. She has received research support from Akonni Biosystems, BD Diagnostics, Great Basin Scientific, Ibis Biosciences, MicroPhage, Inc., and ProDesse, Inc.

David L. Cox (chapter 57) has worked with four companies to evaluate their tests: SpanSpirolipin, ChemBio DPP Syphilis, Bio-Rad BioPlex, and DiaSorin Liaison. He has published papers on the first two assays, the Bio-Rad manuscript is "in progress," and the DiaSorin project is in its final stages.

Mary Jane Ferraro (chapters 67 and 69) has been a member of the Becton Dickinson Worldwide Microbiology Advisory Committee and the bioMérieux Microbiology Advisory Committee.

Barbara Gärtner (chapter 99) has received lecture fees from DiaSorin, Biotest, Roche, GlaxoSmithKline, Siemens, and Merz in the past. She has also conducted research sponsored by DiaSorin, Virion, Medac, Abbott, Roche, Novitech, Bio-Rad, Kenta-Biotech, Genzyme-Virotech, Euroimmun, Wyeth, and Dako.

Christine C. Ginocchio (section editor; coauthor of chapters 77, 78, and 102) has received research funding from, is a member of the scientific advisory boards of, and has participated in clinical trials sponsored by Gen-Probe and Luminex Molecular Diagnostics. She has received consulting fees from Abbott and Nanosphere and research funding from Hologic and Diagnostic Hybrids (Quidel), and she has received honoraria from and participated in clinical trials sponsored by bioMérieux and BD Diagnostics.

Patti E. Gravitt (chapter 102) is a member of the Women's Health Scientific Advisory Board of Qiagen Corp. and has consulted for Roche.

VIROLOGY

VOLUME EDITOR: MARIE LOUISE LANDRY
SECTION EDITORS: ANGELA M. CALIENDO, CHRISTINE C. GINOCCHIO, YI-WEI TANG, AND ALEXANDRA VALSAMAKIS

Taxonomy and Classification of Viruses

ELLIOT J. LEFKOWITZ

75

INTRODUCTION

Taxonomy

Taxonomy at its most basic level involves the classification and naming of objects. Living objects have been grouped for hundreds of years according the Linnaean system (33), a classification scheme that places living things hierarchically into groups of species followed by groupings into higher-level taxa (from genera to families, orders, classes, phyla, kingdoms, and domains, including a number of now-recognized intervening ranks) dependent on common shared characteristics. Taxonomic assignments were originally based on visible structural similarities between organisms. Assignments now also include molecular and genetic information.

Taxonomy functions beyond mere categorization. By having information about, and an understanding of, a few of the organisms in a group of closely related taxa, it is often possible to extend that knowledge to other organisms in related taxa for which much less biological information may be available. For viruses, this process of comparative analysis plays a critical role in increasing our overall knowledge of the molecular biology, pathogenesis, epidemiology, and evolution of poorly understood or newly isolated viruses. This knowledge enhances our ability to respond to new threats by supporting the development of diagnostics, vaccines, and other antiviral therapies.

Viruses

Viruses are not easily placed on the evolutionary tree of life (24, 35, 43). They are not accurately represented by side branches sprouting off from the main branches or by their own single branch growing out from the base of the tree. In fact, it is likely that viruses have multiple independent evolutionary origins (14, 25) that cannot be easily or completely separated from the evolution of their hosts, as they cannot reproduce or evolve separately from their hosts (18, 26). Indeed, the host represents one the most important characteristics of a virus that must be considered when making taxonomic assignments. Therefore, viruses might be better represented as individual twigs arising from branches spread throughout the rest of the tree.

In addition to distinct evolutionary histories, viruses differ from other domains of life in the variety of possible coding molecules they utilize to store their genetic programs (3, 17). Every other domain of life has, as the basic reservoir of its genetic program, double-stranded DNA (dsDNA). Virus genomes may be composed of dsDNA, single-stranded DNA (ssDNA), dsRNA, or ssRNA (which may be positive or negative sense with respect to the mRNA coding strand). In addition, reverse transcription may be a part of their molecular programs. Genome topology (linear, circular, single segment, or multiple segments) also varies between different viruses. All of these unique features, as well as numerous other criteria, are taken into account when classifying viruses and making taxonomic assignments.

VIRAL TAXONOMY

ICTV Classification of Viruses

The process of making taxonomic assignments is the responsibility of a number of different organizations that have the internationally recognized authority to oversee or contribute to the process by defining the rules, methods, and nomenclature to be used in making assignments for particular domains or subdomains of life (21, 28, 37). For viruses, the Virology Division of the International Union of Microbiological Societies has charged the International Committee on Taxonomy of Viruses (ICTV) with the task of developing, refining, and maintaining a universal viral taxonomy (16, 40).

The ICTV currently recognizes five hierarchical ranks that are used to define the universal viral taxonomy: the order, family, subfamily, genus, and species. The 2009 ICTV viral taxonomy comprises 6 orders, 87 families, 19 subfamilies, 348 genera, and 2,290 species. The official viral taxonomy is published on the ICTV website (http://www.ictvonline.org) and in the ICTV reports (16). The first report of the ICTV was based on deliberations made at and after the 1968 (Helsinki) International Congress of Virology (22). Subsequent reports have been published at regular intervals, authored by numerous and collaborating virologists, with the most recent report, the eighth, published in 2005. A ninth report is in production. These reports provide a history of the efforts and the logic used in forming taxa, term definitions, the official taxonomy, and a description of higher-level taxa.

Initially, the ICTV only recognized and made assignments to ranks at the genus level and above. In 1991, the rank of species was added (23). A viral species is defined as "a polythetic class of viruses that constitute a replicating lineage and occupy a particular ecological niche." The term "polythetic class" refers to a grouping of viruses (in this case, species) whose members share a set of common characteristics but do not necessarily all have in common any one single defining characteristic. This definition of a viral species is therefore different from that of higher-level taxa, which are defined by a universal shared set of characteristics that must be present in all members of any one taxon. Note that, in general, every species is a member of a genus, which in turn is a member of a family. A few families are also members of one of the six orders that are currently recognized, but the majority of viral families do not belong to an order. Some species are not yet assigned to a genus (but may be assigned to a family), and a few genera are not yet assigned to a family; additional biological information must become available before these assignments can be made. Subfamily and order assignments are optional and therefore not necessary to complete a taxonomic hierarchy.

The ICTV is governed by a series of statutes and follows rules and definitions provided by the International Code of Virus Classification and Nomenclature (16) to make taxonomic assignments and name virus taxa. Any modifications or additions to the official ICTV taxonomic classification and names, as well as changes to the statutes or code, must be approved by the voting membership of the ICTV. Any individual can submit proposals to the ICTV for the modification of existing taxa or the creation of new taxa.

In addition to defining the process and rules for virus classification, the ICTV Code also defines the rules to be followed for name assignment. Higher-level taxon names are composed of a single word ending with a suffix that is dependent on taxon rank. The suffix "-virales" identifies an order. Families are identified by the suffix "-viridae", subfamilies are identified by the suffix "-virinae", and genera are identified by the suffix "-virus". Species names should be as concise as possible but normally comprise two or more words. It is common for a species name to end with the word "virus" or have "-virus" as a suffix, but this is not required. When written, names of taxa are italicized, and the first letter of the name is capitalized. (As a part of a species name, the first letter of any proper noun, such as a geographic location, is also capitalized.) It is often difficult to determine in a particular context if a species name should

be written in the formal italicized manner, since species names often coincide with the common names used to refer to a virus. Taxa are abstract concepts that do not physically exist. As an example, when referring to the species *Variola virus* that belongs to the genus *Orthopoxvirus* and the family *Poxviridae*, all names refer to abstract taxa and are therefore written in the formal italicized manner. However, when referring to variola virus, the physical entity that causes smallpox, the name is neither capitalized nor italicized.

It is important to note that the ICTV is only concerned with making taxonomic assignments at the species level and higher, although many viral isolates assigned to one particular species can be further subdivided into categories based on sequence phylogeny, immune reactivity, or other properties. In many cases, these subspecies-level assignments are made on an ad hoc basis by an individual investigator and reported in a journal article. In other instances, a more organized effort may have been made to subdivide a species into a series of "types" based on a defined set of demarcation criteria. Examples of viruses for which subspecies-level assignments have been made include hepatitis C virus (42), dengue virus (20), and human immunodeficiency virus (39).

CRITERIA FOR TAXONOMIC CLASSIFICATION

Character-Based Descriptors

Taxonomic classification is accomplished by comparing and contrasting sets of characters that can be used to define the properties of any particular taxon. Any aspect of viral biology can be defined by a set of characters. These characters may have values represented by quantitative measures, such as the triangulation (T) number used to categorize icosahedral virion capsid structure, or they may be purely qualitative descriptors, such as the presence or absence of a host-derived lipid envelope.

Viruses are described by choosing a set of appropriate characters and then assigning values to these characters as necessary. The ICTVdb species and isolate database (described in more detail below) provides one example of a comprehensive character list for describing viruses (8, 9). This list is summarized in Table 1. Over 2,500 different

TABLE 1 ICTVdb character list

Major category(ies)	No. of available characters	Character examples
Classification	31	Name; NCBI taxon ID; ICTVdb decimal code; synonyms
Taxonomic structure	13	Order; family; subfamily; genus; species
Isolate information	77	Location; date; host; tissues; method of isolation
Virion properties	1,050	Morphology (size, envelope, capsid); physicochemical and physical properties; nucleic acid (genome type and configuration); proteins
Genome organization and replication	462	Attachment; penetration; transcription; translation; protein processing; genome replication; assembly
Biological properties	954	Host range; transmission; disease; pathology
Antigenicity	75	Antigenic determinants; epitopes; serological relationships; immunity; variation; diagnostics; vaccines
Comments, references, and contributors	35	Publication; database; website; contact

characters are available for use, and many of these have multiple values that might be associated with any one viral taxon or isolate. For example, a particular isolate may be described by the location and date of its isolation, each of which would be associated with the appropriate value (e.g., country and year). Characters describing a particular species may include its host range and a list of diseases associated with viruses belonging to that species. Over 40,000 different descriptors or values can be associated with the character set of the ICTVdb.

There is no one master character list utilized by the ICTV for classifying viruses. This is because every taxon is unique and characters useful for describing one taxon may be entirely inappropriate for describing another. The ICTVdb character list may be useful in providing a list of potential characters that might be used for any particular classification, but significant research still needs to be performed to determine the most appropriate set of choices. Character

selection and character value assignment can only be performed by investigators with relevant expertise. Therefore, the research scientists who comprise the ICTV study groups that are responsible for making taxonomic assignments for each viral family set the rules of classification for the viruses that fall under their areas of expertise (12, 16, 31).

The rules for taxonomic classification are defined by a set of demarcation criteria specific to each rank of every taxonomic hierarchy. These demarcation criteria can then be used by research scientists either to determine that a newly isolated virus belongs to an existing species (and therefore there is no need for it to be further classified) or to submit a proposal to the appropriate study group for the creation of a new species (or higher-level taxon) if the isolate, based on the demarcation criteria, is sufficiently different from other viruses that it warrants the creation of a new taxon. Demarcation criteria are provided in each chapter of the ICTV reports describing any particular taxon. Table 2

TABLE 2 Criteria for taxonomic classification

Order: *Picornavirales*
  Virion
    Nonenveloped, icosahedral particles
    Capsid proteins composed of three distantly related jelly roll domains forming particles with pseudo-T=3 symmetry
  Genome
    Positive-sense ssRNA
    1 or 2 monocistronic genome segments
    5′-bound VPg protein
    Genome serves as the mRNA
    Genome typically contains a 3′ poly(A) tail
  Protein
    Primary polyprotein translation product proteolytically cleaved into mature proteins by 1 or more virus-encoded proteinases
    Functional domains include a superfamily III helicase (Hel), cysteine protease (Pro), and RNA-dependent RNA polymerase (Pol)
    Nonstructural proteins are arranged as Hel-VPg-Pro-Pol

Family: *Picornaviridae*
  Genome
    Single monocistronic genome segment
  Protein
    Conserved genome organization
    Conserved set of functional mature proteins
    Protein sequence conservation (protease-polymerase region)

Genus: *Enterovirus*
  Protein
    At least 50% amino acid identity over the length of the polyprotein
    VPg sequence conservation
    Lacks an L protein
    Possesses a type 1 internal ribosomal entry site
  Host
    Virus replication primarily in (but not limited to) the gastrointestinal tract

Species: *Human Enterovirus C*
  Host range
    Human
  Genome
    Conserved genome map (organization of protein functional domains)
    Common polyprotein proteolytic processing program
    Within-species genetic recombination
  Sequence similarity
    Amino acid identity: 70% in the P1 structural proteins
    Amino acid identity: 70% in the 2C + 3CD nonstructural proteins
    Similar base G+C composition (within 2.5%)
  Phylogeny
    Monophyletic

provides examples of some of the specific criteria utilized to define a species and its upper-level taxa for the species *Human enterovirus C* (polioviruses were recently reclassified as belonging to this species) (31). Different sets of characters are utilized at each level in the taxonomic hierarchy to describe the viruses that would be assigned to that level and below. The order-, family-, and genus-level characters are universal and must be present in all viruses assigned to that taxon, while the species-level characters are polythetic and therefore do not necessarily need to be present in all members of the species.

Sequence-Based Characters

Characters that describe virus morphology and structure have always been important classification criteria. With the advent of genome sequencing, sequence-based comparison has assumed an increasingly important role in classification. Table 2 provides a number of different sequence-based criteria at each rank that are used to define the important characteristics of that rank. There are conserved functional amino acid domains present in all members of the order *Picornavirales*. Conserved protease and polymerase protein sequences help define the family. A specific level of amino acid conservation across the whole polyprotein is required to place a virus within the *Enterovirus* genus. An even higher level of sequence identity is required for members of a particular species. Classification based on sequence comparison is now one of the major defining characteristics of all viral taxa. How these comparisons are made, how the relationships are measured, and the extent to which they are included in the taxon demarcation criteria varies significantly from taxon to taxon. This is understandable given the inherent differences in mutability between viruses, especially between viruses of different genomic composition. Viruses with dsDNA genomes show much less variability at the sequence level than RNA viruses. This difference is a direct consequence of the error rates of their DNA and RNA polymerases (14). Therefore, the measures used (as defined by each ICTV study group) to define specific sequence-based demarcation criteria will also vary from one taxon to another.

Sequence-based comparisons can be measured using a variety of different techniques. The most basic involve pairwise comparisons in which two sequences are aligned and the number of nucleotide or amino acid differences between each aligned position are counted. When comparing multiple sequences, a table of distances is then compiled that provides the percent similarity between every possible pairwise comparison in the set. Depending on the particular taxon and hierarchical rank under study, nucleotide or amino acid sequences can be compared and alignments of complete viral genomes,

a portion of the genome, or individual genes can be utilized. By examining these sequence distance tables, a study group can set specific similarity levels that define the demarcation criteria for classification of viruses into different taxa.

More sophisticated analyses based on pairwise sequence comparisons can be utilized to provide alternative methods for visualizing differences, choosing cutoffs, and making assignments. One method used in recent years is the pairwise analysis of sequence conservation (PASC) (4). PASC utilizes pairwise sequence alignments of either whole genomic nucleotide sequences or individual gene nucleotide or amino acid sequences. A pairwise alignment is constructed between every possible pair of available sequences. Once all pairwise alignments have been constructed, the percent identity is calculated for each aligned pair and then plotted versus the number of aligned pairs producing similar identities. Figure 1A provides an example of a PASC plot using amino acid alignments of the DNA polymerase gene of all virus isolates that belong to the family *Poxviridae* (30). As can be seen, several distinct peaks are produced, each of which corresponds to comparisons between viruses classified into particular ranks of the *Poxviridae* taxonomic hierarchy. The lowest percent identity (20 to 30%) corresponds to comparisons between viruses from different subfamilies. Genus-level comparisons produce multiple peaks from 45 to 75% identity. Peaks for interspecies comparisons vary between 80 and 98% identity, with the most prominent interspecies peaks occurring at 97 and 98% identity. Intraspecies comparisons (comparisons between strains of the same species) show very high levels of identity (99% and greater). Figure 1B shows how these taxa are arrayed on the *Poxviridae* phylogenetic tree. By utilizing PASC, a new virus isolate can be compared to all existing isolates, and by plotting its similarity to isolates already assigned to a known taxon, a determination can be made as to whether the new isolate can be assigned to an existing taxon or if a proposal for creation of a new taxon should be considered. It is interesting that, from a biological point of view, the distinct patterns of conservation that are exhibited by the peaks present in the PASC graph suggest that the evolutionary history of the protein being analyzed (in this case, poxvirus DNA polymerase) has selected for protein sequences that exhibit distinct peaks of fitness. PASC is now utilized by a number of ICTV study groups for making taxonomic assignments (1, 2).

One final sequence-based analysis that is extensively utilized as a demarcation criterion for making taxonomic assignments is phylogenetic analysis (19, 31). Phylogenetic analysis utilizes a multiple-sequence alignment constructed from the nucleotide or amino acid sequence of a whole

FIGURE 1 Taxonomic demarcation via sequence similarity. (A) PASC was carried out on the viral DNA-dependent DNA polymerase gene (the vaccinia virus E9L gene homolog) for every completely sequenced poxvirus genome. Each protein was aligned to every other protein, and the percent identity of each pairwise comparison was then included in a histogram plot of all possible comparisons. Peaks are identified across the top of the figure according to the taxa represented by particular pairwise sequence comparisons. (B) Phylogenetic reconstruction of the *Poxviridae* family of viruses based on their DNA polymerase protein sequences. Subfamily and genera demarcations are identified. Terminal nodes are labeled according to genus. Sequences belonging to one of the genera labeled either group A or B coincide with the A and B comparison peaks at the top of panel A. (C) Phylogenetic prediction based on the multiple nucleic acid sequence alignment of the core genomic region of each representative orthopoxvirus species or strain. BR, strain Brighton Red; GRI, strain GRI-90. Reprinted with modification from *Virus Research* (30) with permission of the publisher.

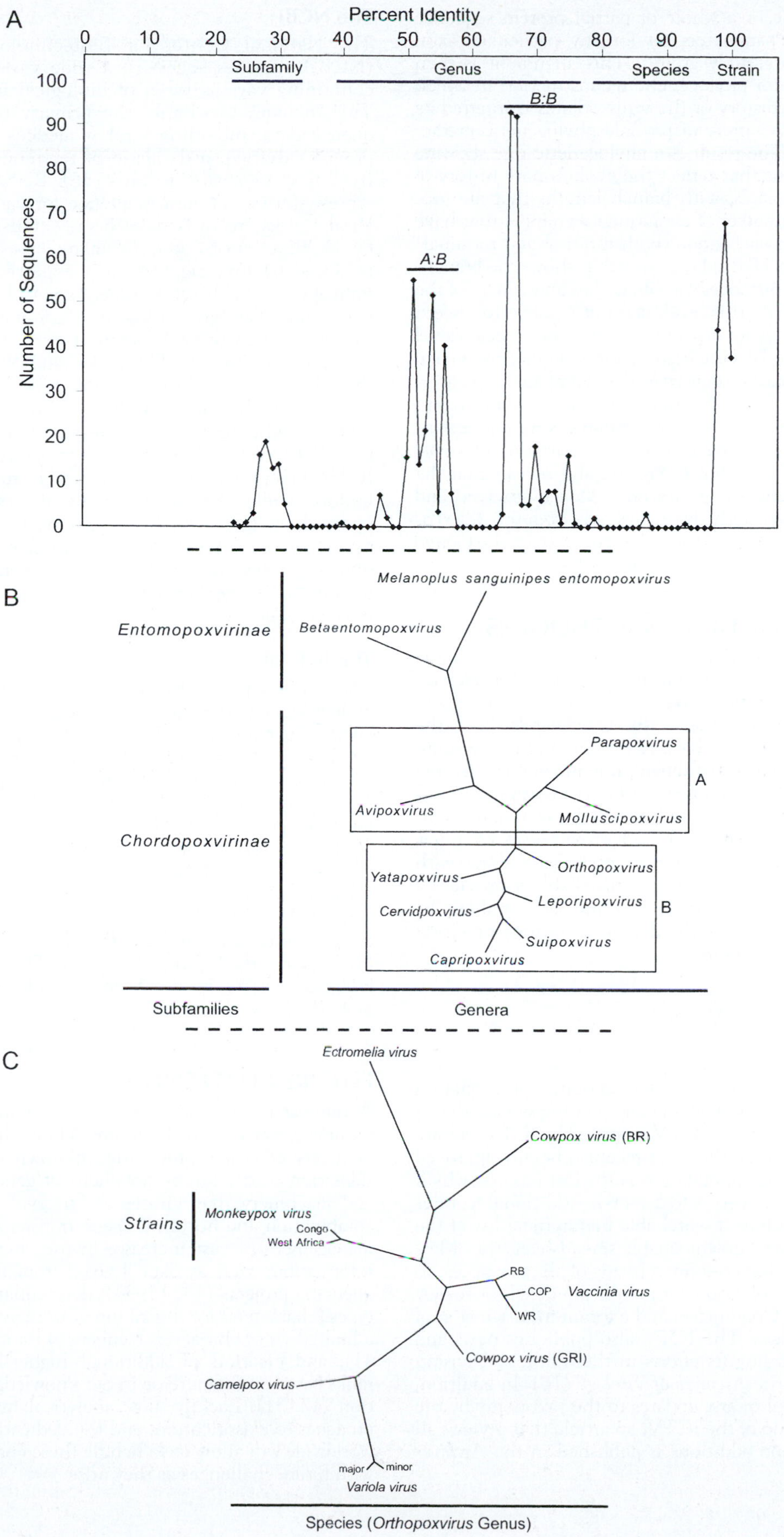
A
Percent Identity
0 10 20 30 40 50 60 70 80 90 100
Subfamily
Genus
Species
Strain
B:B
A:B
Number of Sequences
100 90 80 70 60 50 40 30 20 10 0
B
Melanoplus sanguinipes entomopoxvirus
Entomopoxvirinae
Betaentomopoxvirus
Parapoxvirus
A
Avipoxvirus
Molluscipoxvirus
Chordopoxvirinae
Orthopoxvirus
Yatapoxvirus
Leporipoxvirus
B
Cervidpoxvirus
Suipoxvirus
Capripoxvirus
Subfamilies
Genera
C
Ectromelia virus
Cowpox virus (BR)
Strains
Monkeypox virus
Congo
West Africa
RB
COP
Vaccinia virus
WR
Cowpox virus (GRI)
Camelpox virus
major
minor
Variola virus
Species (Orthopoxvirus Genus)

or partial genome or a whole or partial protein sequence (with the exact parameters set for any particular taxon by the appropriate study group). This alignment is then used as the basis for phylogenetic reconstruction in which the evolutionary history of the virus isolates is inferred by applying one of a variety of possible phylogenetic prediction algorithms. The result is a phylogenetic tree showing branching patterns that reflect the evolutionary history of the individual isolates, with branch lengths that are proportional to the number of evolutionary changes that have occurred between each node (both internal and terminal) of the tree. Figure 1B displays a tree that shows the branching topology and distances for subfamilies and genera of the family *Poxviridae*. At this level, it is not possible to discern the species topology for any of the genera, but species-level arrangements can be visualized if, for example, individual species for the genus *Orthopoxvirus* are compared separately (Fig. 1C) (30). A newly described virus can be compared to any isolate on these trees to determine taxonomic assignment in a manner similar to PASC (and in a more robust manner). Close inspection of Fig. 1C also reveals that the differentiation between species (e.g., *Monkeypox virus* and *Ectromelia virus*) is clearly distinguishable from the differentiation between isolates of the same species (e.g., the Congo and West African monkeypox virus clades).

TAXONOMY OF HUMAN PATHOGENS

As categorized according to the 2009 ICTV taxonomy, viruses that infect humans fall into 4 orders: the *Herpesvirales*, *Mononegavirales*, *Nidovirales*, and *Picornavirales*. (The other existing orders, the *Caudovirales* and the *Tymovirales* contain only bacteriophage and plant viruses, respectively.) Human pathogens are further subdivided into 25 families (not all of which belong to an order), 13 subfamilies, and 66 genera (with each genus usually comprising multiple species). Table 3 provides an overview of the taxa that contain human pathogens along with representative species for each genus. Table 4 provides a few of the structural features that define each viral family. Finally, Fig. 2 displays stylized representations of virion morphology for each family.

TAXONOMY DATABASES

The ICTV

The ICTV produces an extensive amount of information during the process of classifying and naming viruses that is published regularly in the ICTV reports. The ICTV website provides a database of the most recent officially approved viral taxonomy since publication of the last reports (which occurs, on average, every 4 to 5 years). Additional features of the website include a searchable hierarchical list of the current taxonomy; a downloadable spreadsheet, the "Master Species List," that contains a listing of all taxa; access to past and present taxonomy proposals submitted for review to the Executive Committee; and a forum for discussion of ICTV-related issues. The ICTV also publicizes news and information regarding its efforts in the Virology Division News section of the *Archives of Virology* (10). In addition, following approval of any updates to the taxonomy by the voting membership of the ICTV, an article that reviews all of the changes and additions is published in the *Archives of Virology* (11).

The NCBI

The National Center for Biotechnology Information (NCBI) provides access to a wide variety of databases containing various types of biological information (5). This includes GenBank, the primary repository of sequence data, including viral sequences (6). NCBI also provides RefSeq, a database of reference sequences derived from GenBank records (38). RefSeq contains one representative genomic sequence for each viral species. Viral RefSeq records have been extensively annotated by NCBI curators, and in many cases, they are also reviewed by investigators with expertise on individual viral species. Each viral sequence is linked to the NCBI taxonomic database using a taxonomy identification that is assigned to each taxon at every rank of the viral taxonomic hierarchy. The ICTV and NCBI taxonomies should be completely congruent; however, this has not always been the case. The ICTV and NCBI have therefore worked extensively in the past few years to update the NCBI viral taxonomy so that it reflects the official ICTV taxonomy, and this effort is mostly complete. Unfortunately, NCBI taxonomy is not automatically updated when new ICTV taxonomy is approved. A lag period of several months, therefore, exists before any officially approved ICTV taxonomy is fully represented in the NCBI taxonomy that is linked to GenBank and RefSeq sequence records.

The ICTVdb

The ICTV reports provide extensive descriptions of the biological properties of viral taxa at the level of genera, families/subfamilies, and orders. For species, the ICTV reports provide only a list of approved species and the demarcation criteria used to differentiate species belonging to any one genus. No descriptive information is provided for each species, and no information on subspecies levels of classification are provided. The ICTVdb was created to alleviate this gap. It serves as the viral species index, the isolate database, and the repository for species information generated by the ICTV (8, 9). It also provides information on individual viral isolates that have been provided by investigators throughout the world. The ICTVdb was established in 1987 and has been available on the Web since 1998 (http://www.ictvdb.org).

FUTURE CHALLENGES

A number of challenges will impact viral taxonomic assignment now and in the future. These challenges include discovery of novel, previously unknown viruses (7); consideration of the full complement of genetic mechanisms and machinery that viruses use to evolve, including recombination and horizontal gene transfer (29, 32, 36, 44); management of vast increases in the amount of available information, such as data derived from metagenomic sequencing projects (13, 15, 34); determination of new data types (characters) for describing viruses; availability of only a limited set of characters (sequence) for classification (27, 41); and creation of additional higher-level taxonomic ranks based on an increase in our knowledge of viral evolution (12, 31). Luckily, new analytical methods, new approaches to classification, and the dedication of virologists worldwide will allow us to handle these challenges and deal with future challenges as they arise.

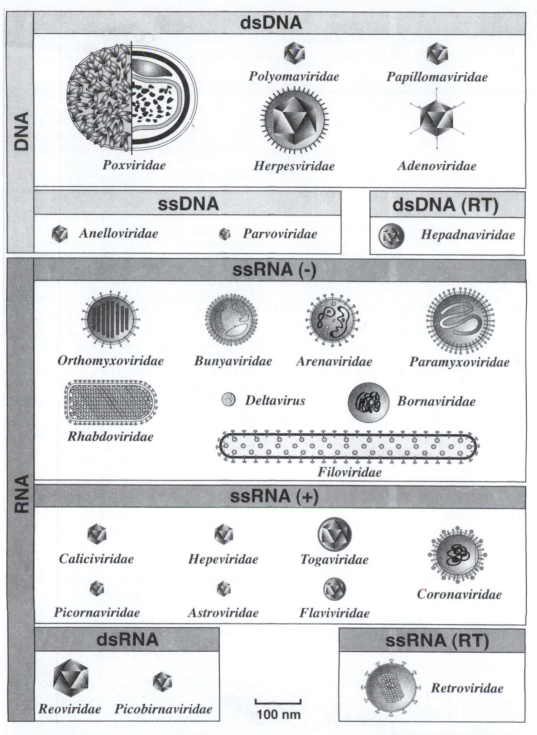

FIGURE 2 Virion morphology. Depiction of the shapes and sizes of viruses of families that include animal, zoonotic, and human pathogens. The virions are drawn to scale, but artistic license
has been used in representing their structure. In some, the cross-sectional structure of capsid and
envelope are shown, with a representation of the genome; with the very small virions, only their
size and symmetry are depicted. RT, reverse transcribing; +, positive-sense genome; −, negative-
sense genome. Reprinted with modification from *Virus Taxonomy. Eighth Report of the International
Committee on Taxonomy of Viruses* (16) with permission of the publisher.

TABLE 3 Taxonomic classification of viruses infecting humans

Genome composition and order	Family	Subfamily	Genus	Species (ICTV type species or common examples)
dsDNA, linear				
Herpesvirales	*Herpesviridae*	*Alphaherpesvirinae*	*Simplexvirus*	*Human herpesvirus 1* (herpes simplex virus type 1); *Human herpesvirus 2* (herpes simplex virus type 2); *Macacine herpesvirus 1* (B virus)
			Varicellovirus	*Human herpesvirus 3* (varicella-zoster virus)
		Betaherpesvirinae	*Cytomegalovirus*	*Human herpesvirus 5* (human cytomegalovirus)
			Roseolovirus	*Human herpesvirus 6 and 7*
		Gammaherpesvirinae	*Lymphocryptovirus*	*Human herpesvirus 4* (Epstein-Barr virus)
			Rhadinovirus	*Human herpesvirus 8* (Kaposi's sarcoma-associated herpesvirus)
Unassigned	*Adenoviridae*		*Mastadenovirus*	*Human adenovirus A to G*
Unassigned	*Poxviridae*	*Chordopoxvirinae*	*Molluscipoxvirus*	*Molluscum contagiosum virus*
			Orthopoxvirus	*Cowpox virus; Monkeypox virus; Vaccinia virus; Variola virus*
			Parapoxvirus	*Orf virus*
			Yatapoxvirus	*Yaba monkey tumor virus*
dsDNA, circular				
Unassigned	*Papillomaviridae*		*Alphapapillomavirus*	*Human papillomavirus 32*
			Betapapillomavirus	*Human papillomavirus 5*
			Gammapapillomavirus	*Human papillomavirus 4*
			Mupapillomavirus	*Human papillomavirus 1*
			Nupapillomavirus	*Human papillomavirus 41*
Unassigned	*Polyomaviridae*		*Polyomavirus*	*BK polyomavirus; JC polyomavirus*
ssDNA, linear				
Unassigned	*Parvoviridae*	*Parvovirinae*	*Bocavirus*	Not classified (human bocavirus)
			Dependovirus	*Adeno-associated virus 1 to 5*
			Erythrovirus	*Human parvovirus B19*
ssDNA, circular				
Unassigned	*Anelloviridae*		*Alphatorquevirus*	*Torque teno virus 1* (torque tenovirus)
dsDNA, reverse transcribing circular				
Unassigned	*Hepadnaviridae*		*Orthohepadnavirus*	*Hepatitis B virus*
ssRNA, linear, negative sense				
Mononegavirales	*Bornaviridae*		*Bornavirus*	*Borna disease virus*
	Filoviridae		*Ebolavirus*	*Cote d'Ivoire ebolavirus; Sudan ebolavirus; Zaire ebolavirus*
			Marburgvirus	*Lake Victoria marburgvirus*
	Paramyxoviridae	*Paramyxovirinae*	*Henipavirus*	*Hendra virus; Nipah virus*
			Morbillivirus	*Measles virus*
			Respirovirus	*Human parainfluenza virus 1 and 3*
			Rubulavirus	*Human parainfluenza virus 2 and 4; Mumps virus*
		Pneumovirinae	*Metapneumovirus*	*Human metapneumovirus*
			Pneumovirus	*Human respiratory syncytial virus*
	Rhabdoviridae		*Lyssavirus*	*Rabies virus*
ssRNA, linear, negative sense, segmented				
Unassigned	*Orthomyxoviridae*		*Influenzavirus A*	*Influenza A virus*
			Influenzavirus B	*Influenza B virus*
			Influenzavirus C	*Influenza C virus*
ssRNA, linear, positive sense				
Nidovirales	*Coronaviridae*	*Coronavirinae*	*Alphacoronavirus*	*Human coronavirus 229E; Human coronavirus NL63*
			Betacoronavirus	*Betacoronavirus 1; Human coronavirus HKU1; Severe acute respiratory syndrome-related coronavirus*
		Torovirinae	*Torovirus*	*Human torovirus*

(Continued on next page)

TABLE 3 *(Continued)*

Genome composition and order	Family	Subfamily	Genus	Species (ICTV type species or common examples)
Picornavirales	*Picornaviridae*		*Aphthovirus*	*Foot-and-mouth disease virus*
			Enterovirus	*Human enterovirus A* (human coxsackievirus A2; human enterovirus 71); *Human enterovirus B* (human coxsackievirus B1; human echovirus); *Human enterovirus C* (human poliovirus 1 to 3; human coxsackievirus A1); *Human enterovirus D* (human enterovirus 68, 70, and 94)
				Human rhinovirus A, B, C
			Hepatovirus	*Hepatitis A virus*
			Parechovirus	*Human parechovirus*
Unassigned	*Astroviridae*		*Mamastrovirus*	*Human astrovirus*
Unassigned	*Caliciviridae*		*Norovirus*	*Norwalk virus*
			Sapovirus	*Sapporo virus*
Unassigned	*Flaviviridae*		*Flavivirus*	*Dengue virus; Japanese encephalitis virus; Kyasanur Forest disease virus; Langat virus; Louping ill virus; Murray Valley encephalitis virus; Omsk hemorrhagic fever virus; Powassan virus; St. Louis encephalitis virus; Tick-borne encephalitis virus; Wesselsbron virus; West Nile virus; Yellow fever virus; Zika virus*
			Hepacivirus	*Hepatitis C virus*
Unassigned	*Hepeviridae*		*Hepevirus*	*Hepatitis E virus*
Unassigned	*Togaviridae*		*Alphavirus*	*Barmah Forest virus; Chikungunya virus; Eastern equine encephalitis virus; Mayaro virus; O'nyong-nyong virus; Ross River virus; Semliki Forest virus; Sindbis virus; Venezuelan equine encephalitis virus; Western equine encephalitis virus*
ssRNA, linear, ambisense, segmented				
Unassigned	*Arenaviridae*		*Arenavirus*	*Guanarito virus; Junín virus; Lassa virus; Lymphocytic choriomeningitis virus; Machupo virus; Sabiá virus*
Unassigned	*Bunyaviridae*		*Hantavirus*	*Hantaan virus; Puumala virus; Sin Nombre virus; Thottapalayam virus;* multiple other species
			Nairovirus	*Crimean-Congo hemorrhagic fever virus; Dugbe virus*
			Orthobunyavirus	*Bunyamwera virus; Bwamba virus; California encephalitis virus; Guama virus; Madrid virus; Nyando virus; Oropouche virus; Tacaiuma virus*
			Phlebovirus	*Punta Toro virus; Rift Valley fever virus; Sandfly fever Naples virus*
dsRNA, linear, segmented				
Unassigned	*Picobirnaviridae*		*Picobirnavirus*	*Human picobirnavirus*
Unassigned	*Reoviridae*	*Sedoreovirinae*	*Orbivirus*	*Changuinola virus; Corriparta virus; Great Island virus; Lebombo virus; Orungo virus*
			Rotavirus	Rotavirus A, B, and C
			Seadornavirus	*Banna virus*
		Spinareovirinae	*Coltivirus*	*Colorado tick fever virus*
			Orthoreovirus	*Mammalian orthoreovirus*
ssRNA, linear, dimer, reverse transcribing				
Unassigned	*Retroviridae*	*Orthoretrovirinae*	*Deltaretrovirus*	*Primate T-lymphotropic virus 1 and 2*
			Lentivirus	*Human immunodeficiency virus 1 and 2*
		Spumaretrovirinae	*Spumavirus*	*Simian foamy virus*
ssRNA, circular, negative sense				
Unassigned	Unassigned		*Deltavirus*	*Hepatitis delta virus*

TABLE 4 Summary of important characteristics used to differentiate families of viruses infecting humans

Classification (family)	Virus properties						
	Virion					Genome	
	Envelope	Shape	Size (nm)	Nucleocapsid symmetry	Molecule[a]	Structure	Size (kb or kbp)
Adenoviridae	–	Isometric	70–90	Icosahedral	dsDNA, linear	Monopartite, inverted terminal repeats, 5′ ends covalently linked to terminal protein	26–45
Anelloviridae	–	Isometric	30	Icosahedral	ssDNA (–), circular	Monopartite	2.6–3.9
Arenaviridae	+	Spherical	110–130	Helical	ssRNA, circular	2 ambisense (±) segments	10.6 (total)
Astroviridae	–	Isometric	28–30	Icosahedral	ssRNA (+), linear	Monopartite	6.4–7.4
Bornaviridae	+	Spherical	90	Helical	ssRNA (–), linear	Monopartite	8.9
Bunyaviridae	+	Spherical, pleomorphic	80–120	Helical	ssRNA, linear	3 negative or ambisense segments	11–19 (total)
Caliciviridae	–	Isometric	27–40	Icosahedral	ssRNA (+), linear	Monopartite, 5′-end covalently linked protein (VPg)	7.4–8.5
Coronaviridae	+	Spherical, pleomorphic	120–160	Helical	ssRNA (+), linear	Monopartite	27–32
Deltavirus[b]	+	Spherical	36–43	Helical	ssRNA (–), circular	Monopartite, requires hepatitis B virus for replication	1.7
Filoviridae	+	Filamentous pleomorphic	800 long (variable) by 80 diam	Helical	ssRNA (–), linear	Monopartite	19
Flaviviridae	+	Spherical	40–60	Icosahedral	ssRNA (+), linear	Monopartite	9.3–12.6
Hepadnaviridae	+	Spherical	42–50	Icosahedral	dsDNA, circular	Monopartite, reverse transcribing	3.0–3.3
Hepeviridae	–	Isometric	27–34	Icosahedral	ssRNA (+), linear	Monopartite	7.2
Herpesviridae	+	Spherical	120–260	Icosahedral	dsDNA, linear	Monopartite, terminal and internal repeats, multiple isomeric forms	110–240
Orthomyxoviridae	+	Pleomorphic	80–120	Helical	ssRNA (–), linear	6–8 segments, depending on genus	10–14.6 (total)
Papillomaviridae	–	Isometric	55	Icosahedral	dsDNA, circular	Monopartite, supercoiled	6.8–8.4
Paramyxoviridae	+	Pleomorphic	150–300	Helical	ssRNA (–), linear	Monopartite	13–20
Parvoviridae	–	Isometric	18–26	Icosahedral	ssDNA, linear	Monopartite	4–6
Picobirnaviridae	–	Isometric	30–40	Icosahedral	dsRNA, linear	2 segments	4.2 (total)
Picornaviridae	–	Isometric	30	Icosahedral	ssRNA (+), linear	Monopartite, 5′-end covalently linked protein (VPg)	7.2–8.8
Polyomaviridae	–	Isometric	40–45	Icosahedral	dsDNA, circular	Monopartite, supercoiled	4.7–5.4
Poxviridae	+	Brick shaped or oval	220–450 long by 140–260 diam	Complex	dsDNA, linear	Monopartite, inverted terminal repeats, both ends covalently closed	135–360
Reoviridae	–	Isometric	60–80	Icosahedral	dsRNA, linear	10–12 segments, depending on genus	16–29 (total)
Retroviridae	+	Spherical	80–100	Icosahedral	ssRNA (+), linear	Monopartite, diploid, reverse transcribing	7–11
Rhabdoviridae	+	Bullet shaped	180 long by 75 diam	Helical	ssRNA (–), linear	Monopartite	11–12
Togaviridae	+	Spherical	70	Icosahedral	ssRNA (+), linear	Monopartite	9.8–11.9
Prions[c]	NA[d]	Rods	Protein PrP^{SC}	NA	NA	No nucleic acid; self-replicating infectious prion protein (PrP) with a mol wt of 33,000–35,000	NA

[a] +: positive sense; –: negative sense.
[b] Genus (unassigned family).
[c] Not classified by the ICTV.
[d] NA, not applicable.

REFERENCES

1. Adams, M. J., J. F. Antoniw, M. Bar-Joseph, A. A. Brunt, T. Candresse, G. D. Foster, G. P. Martelli, R. G. Milne, S. K. Zavriev, and C. M. Fauquet. 2004. The new plant virus family Flexiviridae and assessment of molecular criteria for species demarcation. *Arch. Virol.* **149:**1045–1060.

2. Adams, M. J., J. F. Antoniw, and C. M. Fauquet. 2005. Molecular criteria for genus and species discrimination within the family Potyviridae. *Arch. Virol.* **150:**459–479.

3. Baltimore, D. 1971. Expression of animal virus genomes. *Bacteriol. Rev.* **35:**235–241.

4. Bao, Y., Y. Kapustin, and T. Tatusova. 2008. Virus classification by pairwise sequence comparison (PASC), p. 342–348. *In* B. W. J. Mahy and M. H. V. Van Regenmortel (ed.), *Encyclopedia of Virology.* Elsevier, Boston, MA.

5. Baxevanis, A. D. 2008. Searching NCBI databases using Entrez. *Curr. Protoc. Bioinformatics* **1:**1.3.

6. Benson, D. A., I. Karsch-Mizrachi, D. J. Lipman, J. Ostell, and E. W. Sayers. 2009. GenBank. *Nucleic Acids Res.* **37:**D26–D31.

7. Briese, T., J. T. Paweska, L. K. McMullan, S. K. Hutchison, C. Street, G. Palacios, M. L. Khristova, J. Weyer, R. Swanepoel, M. Egholm, S. T. Nichol, and W. I. Lipkin. 2009. Genetic detection and characterization of Lujo virus, a new hemorrhagic fever-associated arenavirus from southern Africa. *PLoS Pathog.* **5:**e1000455.

8. Buchen-Osmond, C. 1997. Further progress in ICTVdB, a universal virus database. *Arch. Virol.* **142:**1734–1739.

9. Buechen-Osmond, C., and M. Dallwitz. 1996. Towards a universal virus database—progress in the ICTVdB. *Arch. Virol.* **141:**392–399.

10. Carstens, E. B. 2009. Report from the 40th meeting of the Executive Committee of the International Committee of Taxonomy of Viruses. *Arch. Virol.* **155:**133–146.

11. Carstens, E. B., and L. A. Ball. 2009. Ratification vote on taxonomic proposals to the International Committee on Taxonomy of Viruses (2008). *Arch. Virol.* **154:**1181–1188.

12. Davison, A. J., R. Eberle, B. Ehlers, G. S. Hayward, D. J. McGeoch, A. C. Minson, P. E. Pellett, B. Roizman, M. J. Studdert, and E. Thiry. 2009. The order Herpesvirales. *Arch. Virol.* **154:**171–177.

13. Delwart, E. L. 2007. Viral metagenomics. *Rev. Med. Virol.* **17:**115–131.

14. Domingo, E., C. R. Parrish, and J. J. Holland. 2008. *Origin and Evolution of Viruses,* 2nd ed. Academic Press, San Diego, CA.

15. Edwards, R. A., and F. Rohwer. 2005. Viral metagenomics. *Nat. Rev. Microbiol.* **3:**504–510.

16. Fauquet, C. M., M. A. Mayo, J. Maniloff, U. Desselberger, and L. A. Ball (ed.). 2005. *Virus Taxonomy. Eighth Report of the International Committee on Taxonomy of Viruses.* Academic Press, San Diego, CA.

17. Fields, B. N., D. M. Knipe, and P. M. Howley. 2007. *Fields Virology,* 5th ed. Wolters Kluwer Health/Lippincott Williams & Wilkins, Philadelphia, PA.

18. Gibbs, A. J., C. H. Calisher, and F. Garcia-Arenal. 1995. *Molecular Basis of Virus Evolution.* Cambridge University Press, Cambridge, England.

19. Gorbalenya, A. E., L. Enjuanes, J. Ziebuhr, and E. J. Snijder. 2006. Nidovirales: evolving the largest RNA virus genome. *Virus Res.* **117:**17–37.

20. Henchal, E. A., and J. R. Putnak. 1990. The dengue viruses. *Clin. Microbiol. Rev.* **3:**376–396.

21. International Commission on Zoological Nomenclature. 1999. *International Code of Zoological Nomenclature (Code International de Nomenclature Zoologique),* 4th ed. International Trust for Zoological Nomenclature, London, United Kingdom.

22. International Committee on Nomenclature of Viruses, and P. Wildy. 1971. *Classification and Nomenclature of Viruses. First Report of the International Committee on Nomenclature of Viruses.* S. Karger, Basel, Switzerland.

23. International Committee on Taxonomy of Viruses, M. H. V. Van Regenmortel, and International Union of Microbiological Societies, Virology Division. 2000. *Virus Taxonomy: Classification and Nomenclature of Viruses. Seventh Report of the International Committee on Taxonomy of Viruses.* Academic Press, San Diego, CA.

24. Koonin, E. V., T. G. Senkevich, and V. V. Dolja. 2009. Compelling reasons why viruses are relevant for the origin of cells. *Nat. Rev. Microbiol.* **7:**615. (Author's reply, **7:**615.)

25. Koonin, E. V., T. G. Senkevich, and V. V. Dolja. 2006. The ancient virus world and evolution of cells. *Biol. Direct.* **1:**29.

26. Koonin, E. V., Y. I. Wolf, K. Nagasaki, and V. V. Dolja. 2008. The Big Bang of picorna-like virus evolution antedates the radiation of eukaryotic supergroups. *Nat. Rev. Microbiol.* **6:**925–939.

27. Labonte, J. M., K. E. Reid, and C. A. Suttle. 2009. Phylogenetic analysis indicates evolutionary diversity and environmental segregation of marine podovirus DNA polymerase gene sequences. *Appl. Environ. Microbiol.* **75:**3634–3640.

28. Lapage, S. P., P. H. A. Sneath, E. F. Lessel, V. B. D. Skerman, H. P. R. Seeliger, and W. A. Clark (ed.). 1992. *International Code of Nomenclature of Bacteria.* American Society for Microbiology, Washington, DC.

29. Lavigne, R., D. Seto, P. Mahadevan, H. W. Ackermann, and A. M. Kropinski. 2008. Unifying classical and molecular taxonomic classification: analysis of the Podoviridae using BLASTP-based tools. *Res. Microbiol.* **159:**406–414.

30. Lefkowitz, E. J., C. Wang, and C. Upton. 2006. Poxviruses: past, present and future. *Virus Res.* **117:**105–118.

31. Le Gall, O., P. Christian, C. M. Fauquet, A. M. King, N. J. Knowles, N. Nakashima, G. Stanway, and A. E. Gorbalenya. 2008. Picornavirales, a proposed order of positive-sense single-stranded RNA viruses with a pseudo-T=3 virion architecture. *Arch. Virol.* **153:**715–727.

32. Lima-Mendez, G., J. Van Helden, A. Toussaint, and R. Leplae. 2008. Reticulate representation of evolutionary and functional relationships between phage genomes. *Mol. Biol. Evol.* **25:**762–777.

33. Linné, C. V., M. S. J. Engel-Ledeboer, and H. Engel. 1964. *Carolus Linnaeus Systema Naturae, 1735.* B. de Graff, Nieuwkoop, The Netherlands.

34. Monier, A., J. M. Claverie, and H. Ogata. 2008. Taxonomic distribution of large DNA viruses in the sea. *Genome Biol.* **9:**R106.

35. Mushegian, A. 2008. Gene content of LUCA, the last universal common ancestor. *Front. Biosci.* **13:**4657–4666.

36. Odom, M. R., R. C. Hendrickson, and E. J. Lefkowitz. 2009. Poxvirus protein evolution: family wide assessment of possible horizontal gene transfer events. *Virus Res.* **144:**233–249.

37. Polaszek, A. 2005. A universal register for animal names. *Nature* **437:**477.

38. Pruitt, K. D., T. Tatusova, and D. R. Maglott. 2007. NCBI reference sequences (RefSeq): a curated non-redundant sequence database of genomes, transcripts and proteins. *Nucleic Acids Res.* **35:**D61–D65.

39. Robertson, D. L., J. P. Anderson, J. A. Bradac, J. K. Carr, B. Foley, R. K. Funkhouser, F. Gao, B. H. Hahn, M. L. Kalish, C. Kuiken, G. H. Learn, T. Leitner, F. McCutchan, S. Osmanov, M. Peeters, D. Pieniazek, M. Salminen, P. M. Sharp, S. Wolinsky, and B. Korber. 2000. HIV-1 nomenclature proposal. *Science* **288:**55–56.

40. Schleifer, K. H. 2008. The International Union of Microbiological Societies, IUMS. *Res. Microbiol.* **159:**45–48.

41. Schoenfeld, T., M. Patterson, P. M. Richardson, K. E. Wommack, M. Young, and D. Mead. 2008. Assembly of viral metagenomes from yellowstone hot springs. *Appl. Environ. Microbiol.* **74:**4164–4174.

42. Simmonds, P., J. Bukh, C. Combet, G. Deleage, N. Enomoto, S. Feinstone, P. Halfon, G. Inchauspe, C. Kuiken, G. Maertens, M. Mizokami, D. G. Murphy, H. Okamoto, J. M. Pawlotsky, F. Penin, E. Sablon, I. T. Shin, L. J. Stuyver, H. J. Thiel, S. Viazov, A. J. Weiner, and A. Widell. 2005. Consensus proposals for a unified system of nomenclature of hepatitis C virus genotypes. *Hepatology* **42:**962–973.

43. Villarreal, L. P. 2005. *Viruses and the Evolution of Life.* ASM Press, Washington, DC.

44. Walsh, D. A., and A. K. Sharma. 2009. Molecular phylogenetics: testing evolutionary hypotheses. *Methods Mol. Biol.* **502:**131–168.

Specimen Collection, Transport, and Processing: Virology

MICHAEL S. FORMAN AND ALEXANDRA VALSAMAKIS

76

In recent years, there have been many advances in diagnostic virology, including improvements in cell culture methods and the development of viral antigen (Ag) and nucleic acid (NA) assays. The test(s) of choice vary by virus and by syndrome (synopsized in Table 1 and in chapter 78). Regardless of the detection method chosen, accurate test results rely on preanalytical steps, including specimen selection, collection, transport, and processing, that are described in this chapter. General guidelines for these procedures are described. Collection and processing of specific specimen types are then discussed in detail. A final section on specimen transport containing general information and selected topics of importance is included.

SPECIMEN SELECTION, COLLECTION, AND PROCESSING: GENERAL GUIDELINES

Specimen Selection

Different clinical specimens are suitable for the diagnosis of specific diseases through virologic testing (Table 2). Clinical symptoms often indicate the target organ(s) involved and, in combination with an understanding of viral pathogenesis, help to determine the most appropriate specimen(s) to collect. Viral infections can be detected by sampling the affected organ, where the highest levels of viral replication occur, or by testing suitable alternate specimens that serve as indicators of replication in the target organ (such as plasma as a surrogate for end organ replication in infections such as those caused by cytomegalovirus [CMV], hepatitis B virus, hepatitis C virus, and BK virus, or stool or respiratory specimens to implicate enteroviruses as a potential cause of meningitis).

Specimen Collection

Specimen collection is guided by the diagnostic test best suited to establish a particular diagnosis (17). Important specimen collection variables that can affect result accuracy are time of procurement relative to symptom onset and collection method (inclusive of containers and transport medium). Most acute presentations of virus infection can be divided temporally into the period prior to symptom onset, when shedding typically begins; the acute phase of illness, when shedding decreases and immunoglobulin M (IgM) becomes detectable; and the symptom resolution phase, when shedding ceases and IgG is detected. The level and duration of virus shedding depend on the virus, infected organ or organ system, and host factors such as age and immune status. For assays designed to detect virus growth or viral macromolecules, specimens with high concentrations of viral particles, viral Ags, or viral NA molecules will improve the laboratory's ability to make an accurate diagnosis. Optimal specimens (guided by the differential diagnosis list and test method) should therefore be collected as soon as possible after symptom onset (within 1 to 3 days). For serologic diagnosis, the timing of serum collection and the type of antibody detected vary for specific viruses (Table 3). If a virus-specific IgM assay is available, an acute-phase serum specimen from the first few days of illness should be obtained. For IgG assays, sera from the acute and convalescent phases (2 to 4 weeks after symptom resolution) should be obtained to demonstrate a rise in antibody concentration.

Collection methods can have profound effects on detection rates. Specimens should be collected only with validated devices and containers. For specimens collected on swabs, particular attention should be paid to swab type. Acceptable swabs include polyester, Dacron, and rayon with plastic or aluminum shafts. Wooden-shaft swabs may contain formaldehyde and other compounds that are toxic to cultured cells and therefore are not suitable for virus recovery. Calcium alginate-aluminum shaft swabs should not be used, as they impair recovery of many enveloped viruses, may interfere with fluorescent-antibody tests, and are inhibitory to PCR (40, 61).

The use of viral transport medium (VTM) during specimen collection is highly dependent on specimen source. In general, liquid specimens such as blood, cerebrospinal fluid (CSF), urine, and bronchoalveolar lavage (BAL) fluid do not require VTM; therefore, these specimens should be transported and processed with particular attention to optimal temperature and storage times to ensure accurate test results. A more detailed discussion

TABLE 1 Methods used for detection of viruses

Source	Disease(s)	Virus(es)[a]	Detection method(s)[b]
Cardiac	Myocarditis, pericarditis	Adenoviruses	Culture, histology, NA
		Enteroviruses	Culture, NA
		Influenza viruses	Culture, serology
		Human metapneumovirus	NA
Central nervous system	Encephalitis	Arboviruses	NA, serology
		CMV	NA
		EBV	NA
		Hemorrhagic fever viruses[c]	Culture, EM, IA, serology
		HSV	NA
		HIV	NA
		Measles virus	NA, histology
		Mumps virus	Culture, NA
		Parechoviruses	Culture, NA
		Rabies	Histology, IA
		VZV	NA
	Meningitis	Arboviruses	NA, serology
		Enteroviruses	Culture, NA
		HSV	NA
		LCMV	Serology
		Mumps virus	Culture, NA
		Parechoviruses	Culture, NA
	PML[d]	JCV	Histology, NA
Cutaneous	Maculopapular rash	Adenoviruses	Culture
		Enteroviruses	Culture, NA
		HHV-6	NA
		Measles virus	Culture, serology
		Parvovirus B19	NA, serology
		Rubella virus	Culture, serology
	Vesicular rash	Enteroviruses	Culture, NA
		HSV	Culture, IA, NA
		Poxviruses[c]	Culture, EM, histology
		VZV	Culture, IA, NA
Fetal, newborn		CMV	Culture, NA
		HBV	NA, serology
		HIV	NA, serology
		Parechovirus type 3	Culture, NA
		Parvovirus B19	NA, serology
		Rubella virus	Culture, serology
Gastrointestinal	Parotitis	Adenoviruses	Culture, IA, NA
		CMV	Culture, NA
		Enteroviruses	Culture, NA
		EBV	Serology
		HHV-6	NA, serology
		HIV-1	Serology
		Mumps virus	Culture, NA
		Parainfluenza viruses	Culture, IA, NA
	Diarrhea	Adenoviruses 40 and 41	IA, NA
		Astrovirus	NA
		CMV	Culture, histology, NA
		Norovirus	NA
		Parechoviruses	Culture, NA
		Rotaviruses	IA
	Hepatitis	Adenoviruses	Culture, NA
		CMV	Culture, histology, NA
		EBV	NA, serology
		HAV	Serology
		HBV	IA, NA, serology
		HCV	NA, serology
		HDV	Serology
		HEV	Serology

(Continued on next page)

TABLE 1 Methods used for detection of viruses (*Continued*)

Source	Disease(s)	Virus(es)[a]	Detection method(s)[b]
Hematopoietic	Lymphoid disorders[e]	EBV	Histology, NA
		HIV	NA, serology
		HTLV-1	NA, serology
	Erythroid disorders	Parvovirus B19	NA, serology
Ocular	Chorioretinitis	CMV	NA
		HSV	NA
		VZV	NA
	Conjunctivitis	Adenoviruses	Culture, IA
		Enteroviruses	Culture, NA
	Keratoconjunctivitis	Adenoviruses	Culture, IA
		HSV	Culture, IA
		VZV	Culture, IA
Respiratory	Bronchiolitis	Adenoviruses	Culture, IA, NA
		Enteroviruses	Culture, NA
		Human coronaviruses	NA, serology
		Human metapneumovirus	NA
		Influenza viruses	Culture, EA, IA, NA
		Parainfluenza viruses	Culture, IA, NA
		RSV	Culture, IA, NA
		Rhinoviruses	Culture, NA
	Croup	Human metapneumovirus	Culture, NA
		Influenza viruses	Culture, EA, IA, NA
		Parainfluenza viruses	Culture, IA, NA
		Rhinoviruses	Culture, NA
		RSV	Culture, IA, NA
	Pharyngitis	Adenoviruses	Culture, IA, NA
		CMV	Serology
		EBV	Serology
		Enteroviruses	Culture, NA
		HSV	Culture, NA
		Human coronaviruses	NA, serology
		RSV	Culture, IA, NA
	Pneumonia	Adenoviruses	Culture, IA, NA
		CMV	Culture, histology, IA, NA
		Hantavirus	EM, NA, serology
		HSV	Culture, IA, NA
		Human coronaviruses	NA, serology
		Human metapneumovirus	NA
		Influenza viruses	Culture, EA, IA, NA
		Parainfluenza viruses	Culture, IA, NA
		Rhinoviruses	Culture, NA
		RSV	Culture, IA, NA
		VZV	Culture, NA
	Rhinitis, coryza	Adenoviruses	Culture, IA, NA
		Coronaviruses	EM, NA
		Enteroviruses	Culture, NA
		Human coronaviruses	NA, serology
		Human metapnuemovirus	NA
		Influenza viruses	Culture, EA, IA, NA
		Parainfluenza viruses	Culture, IA, NA
		Rhinoviruses	Culture, NA
		RSV	Culture, IA, NA
Urogenital	Hemorrhagic cystitis	Adenovirus (type 11)	Culture, NA
		BK virus	NA
	Urethritis, genital herpes	HSV	Culture, IA, NA
		VZV	Culture, IA, NA
	Genital warts, carcinoma	HPV	Histology, NA
	Molluscum contagiosum	Molluscum contagiosum virus	Histology
	Cervicitis	Adenoviruses	Culture
		HSV	Culture, NA

[a]Refer to specific chapters for individual viruses; only major viral pathogens, not including rare causes of disease. LCMV, lymphocytic choriomeningitis virus; JCV, JC virus; HHV-6, human herpesvirus 6; HBV, hepatitis B virus; HTLV-1, human T-cell lymphotropic virus 1.

[b]Most common detection methods used. NA assays include hybrid capture, NA sequence-based assays, and PCR. IA, immunoassay (includes immunofluorescent-antibody assay, enzyme-linked immunosorbent assay, and immunochromatographic tests. EM, electron microscopy; EA, enzyme (neuraminidase) assay.

[c]Hemorrhagic fever viruses and smallpox virus processing in BSL 4 facilities.

[d]PML, progressive multifocal leukoencephalopathy.

[e]Includes posttransplant lymphomas, immunoblastic B-cell lymphomas, and adult T-cell leukemia/lymphoma.

TABLE 2 Specimens for viral diagnostic tests

Virus(es)	Bone marrow	Blood[a]	CSF	Feces	Respiratory[b]	Skin	Genital	Oral	Urine	Eye[c]	Tissue	Amniotic fluid	Pericardial fluid
Adenoviruses		+	+	+	+		+	+	+	+	+		
Arboviruses		+	+								+		
Arenaviruses		+	+		+				+				
Astrovirus				+									
Calicivirus				+									
Coronavirus		+		+	+						+		
Cytomegalovirus	+	+	+	+	+		+	+	+	+	+	+	
Enteroviruses		+	+	+	+	+		+	+	+	+		+
Epstein-Barr virus	+	+	+								+		
Filoviruses		+		+	+				+				
Hepatitis A virus		+		+									
Hepatitis B virus[d]		+											
Hepatitis C virus		+									+		
Hepatitis D virus		+											
Hepatitis E virus		+		+									
Herpes simplex virus		+	+	+[c]	+	+	+	+		+	+	+	
Human herpesvirus 6	+	+	+								+		
Human herpesvirus 8		+				+		+					
Human metapneumovirus					+						+		
Influenza viruses					+						+		+
Measles virus					+				+		+		
Mumps virus			+					+	+		+		
Papillomaviruses							+				+		
Parainfluenza viruses					+			+			+		
Parvovirus	+	+			+						+	+	
Parechoviruses			+	+	+								
Polyomaviruses			+						+		+		
Poxviruses						+		+					
Rabies virus			+			+		+			+		
Respiratory syncytial virus					+						+		
Retroviruses		+	+		+		+				+		
Rhinoviruses					+						+		
Rotaviruses				+[e]									
Rubella virus	+	+			+			+	+		+	+	
Varicella-zoster virus	+	+			+	+				+	+		

[a] Includes direct virus detection tests such as culture, Ag detection, and NA detection. Serology is considered separately (see Table 3).
[b] Includes throat swabs and nasal wash and nasal swabs, nasopharyngeal aspirate, and BAL specimens.
[c] Includes conjunctiva, cornea, and aqueous and vitreous fluids.
[d] Similar specimen types for distantly related GBV virus C (also referred to as hepatitis G virus).
[e] Neonatal infections.

TABLE 3 Serology as a primary diagnostic tool: timing of serum collection and antibody testing for relevant viruses[a]

Antibody testing at presentation	Antibody testing 4–10 days after presentation	Antibody testing 2–4 wk after presentation[b]
Arboviruses (IgM)		
EBV (IgM)	HEV (IgM)	Arboviruses
Hantavirus (IgM, IgG)	Arboviruses (IgM)[c]	Human coronaviruses (SARS-CoV)
HAV (IgM)		Measles virus
HBV (IgM, IgG)		Mumps virus
HCV (IgG)		Rubella virus
HDV (IgM, IgG)		
HIV (IgG)		
HTLV (IgG)		
LCMV (IgM)		
Parvovirus B19 (IgM)		

[a]HAV, hepatitis A virus; HTLV, human T-cell lymphotropic virus; LCMV, lymphocytic choriomeningitis virus.
[b]Convalescent-phase antibody; includes IgG and total antibody (IgG and IgM).
[c]CSF IgM also useful.

of different available transport media can be found in "Specimen Transport" below.

Specimen Processing

Specimen Acceptance Criteria

The virology laboratory is responsible for establishing specimen acceptance and rejection criteria. Upon arrival in the laboratory, the specimen and information provided with the test request should be examined to ensure that all criteria have been fulfilled. Specimens should be rejected if (i) they are unlabeled or mislabeled, (ii) improper specimen collection devices or containers have been utilized, (iii) specimen containers are broken and/or leaking, (iv) transport time has exceeded maximum limits, or (v) duplicate specimens have been collected within a time period that is clinically not useful. Important specimen information that should be provided includes patient data (name, hospital number, sex, birth date, and location), ordering physician, specimen source, specific viruses suspected, time and date of specimen collection, and specific diagnostic tests requested. Specimen source and suspected viruses can dictate the choice of specific cell culture lines and Ag and NA assays. Time of sample collection is important, since delays can affect viral recovery and macromolecule stability. A care provider must be contacted immediately regarding rejected specimens or incomplete patient information. Although failure to detect a virus may occur as a consequence of inappropriate specimen handling, there are instances when a given specimen must be processed even though quality has been compromised (specimens collected by surgical procedures, the patient is no longer accessible, or the sample is unique and another cannot be collected). The final report should include a comment stating that the sample integrity was compromised, that negative results must be interpreted with caution, and that the sample should be resubmitted if clinically indicated.

Safety Issues during Processing

Most specimens encountered in the diagnostic virology laboratory contain viruses that are classified as BSL 2 agents. They are of moderate potential hazard to personnel and the environment and should be processed in a biological safety cabinet to protect laboratory personnel from laboratory-acquired infection, to protect the specimen from environmental contamination, and to prevent cross-contamination between samples. Viruses such as arboviruses, arenaviruses, filoviruses, variola virus, severe acute respiratory syndrome coronavirus (SAR-CoV), avian influenza virus, and rabies virus pose a high risk of serious or life-threatening disease. These are BSL 3 and 4 agents that require the highest level of precautions and should not be cultured in routine clinical laboratories. They are associated with specific clinical histories and presentations and are diagnosed by laboratories specifically designed to work with them. Testing for these viruses can be referred to the Centers for Disease Control and Prevention (CDC; Atlanta, GA) or the CDC's Division of Vector-Borne Infectious Diseases (Fort Collins, CO).

At times, laboratory workers may unknowingly work with specimens that contain BSL 3 and BSL 4 viruses. All specimens should be handled with standard precautions, and specific procedures should be in place when the laboratory is requested to handle BSL 3 and 4 agents. CDC biosafety guidelines for SARS-CoV state that handling and processing of specimens can be performed in a BSL 2 facility, with the exception of propagation in cell culture and characterization of viral agents recovered in cultures of specimens from patients suspected to have SARS. Avian influenza virus H5N1 guidelines state that specimens to be tested by reverse transcription PCR can have NA extraction lysis buffer added prior to being shipped to a public health laboratory. Of note, NA extraction reagents TRIzol and a viral lysis buffer, AVL (Qiagen), have been shown to inactivate infectivity of alphaviruses, flaviviruses, filoviruses, and bunyaviruses (6). Many NA extraction methods employ both heat and detergents during lysis; however, comprehensive studies to determine their effect on virus infectivity have not been described.

Samples from patients with transmissible spongiform encephalopathies with the highest infectivity include brain, spinal cord, and eye samples. CSF and other tissue may also be infectious. Standard precautions should be followed when working with these samples. Specific decontamination procedures for residual sample and waste can be found in the *WHO Infection Control Guidelines for Transmissible Spongiform Encephalopathies* (66).

General Processing Procedures

Upon receipt in the laboratory, specimens should be assessed for sufficiency, taking into account all tests that have been requested. The ordering physician should be contacted to set priorities if the specimen volume is insufficient for all tests ordered. Additional specimen can be retrieved from other laboratories with the caveat that contamination from inappropriate handling, improper storage conditions, or delay in processing can affect both culture and NA testing. Excess specimen should be saved at −70°C in case additional tests are needed or repeat testing is required. Detailed specimen processing protocols for different test methodologies have been described previously (25).

COLLECTION AND PROCESSING OF SELECTED SPECIMENS

Blood

Detection and quantification of viremia have many uses, depending upon the virus infection. It can function as a marker of disseminated disease, an indicator of end organ disease, and a marker of disease activity in chronic infections. In infections where viremia precedes symptom onset, detection of virus in blood can be used to preempt disease through the early initiation of treatment. Finally, quantification of viremia can be used to monitor therapeutic efficacy. Accordingly, blood has become a suitable specimen for many different virologic assays, including a growing number of commercial assays for virus detection and quantification, and it should therefore be processed following the instructions dictated by the specific test method.

Blood samples are collected in 3- to 5-ml vacuum tube collection systems. Detection of viruses in plasma or leukocyte fractions requires the use of anticoagulant tubes. The most commonly used anticoagulants are EDTA, heparin,

and acid-citrate-dextrose. Heparinized blood is useful primarily for virus recovery from whole blood, although it can impair the infectivity of human immunodeficiency virus type 1 (HIV-1) (3, 29). EDTA is the preferred anticoagulant for obtaining plasma for NA testing, as heparin inhibits many NA amplification enzymes and because improved NA stability in frozen, stored specimens has been observed with EDTA compared to heparin (14, 20).

Whole blood used for NA amplification must be processed to remove inhibitors of DNA polymerases such as heme and metabolic precursors of heme. Many different extraction protocols are used in both commercial and laboratory-developed amplification tests to remove inhibitors and concentrate NA. For any type of specimen derived from whole blood, special care should be taken to adhere to blood collection, processing, and storage requirements specified by the assay's manufacturer, since any deviation may affect test performance. Assay performance must be verified by the individual laboratory prior to implementing any change in preanalytical steps described in the manufacturer's package insert (Table 4).

TABLE 4 Plasma processing and storage conditions for selected NA tests

Test (manufacturer)[a]	Interval between collection and separation	Storage conditions	Maximum no. of freeze-thaw cycles
Aptima HCV RNA Qualitative Assay (Gen-Probe, FDA approved)	≤24 h	2–8°C, ≤48 h, or −20°C	3
Aptima HIV-1 RNA Qualitative Assay (Gen-Probe, FDA approved)	≤24 h	2–8°C, ≤5 days, or −20°C[c]	3
COBAS Amplicor CMV Monitor Test (Roche, RUO)	24 h	15–30°C, ≤24 h 2–8°C, ≤5 days, or −20 to −80°C	3
COBAS Amplicor HBV Monitor Test[b] (Roche, RUO)	24 h	15–30°C, ≤3 days 2–8°C, ≤7 days, or −20 to −80°C, ≤6 wk	4
COBAS TaqMan HBV Test[b] (Roche, FDA approved)	24 h	15–30°C, ≤3 days 2–8°C, ≤7 days, or −20 to −80°C, ≤6 wk	5
COBAS AMPLICOR HCV MONITOR Test, version 2.0[b] (Roche, RUO)	6 h	2–8°C, ≤3 days, or ≥−70°C	2
COBAS AmpliPrep/COBAS TaqMan HCV Test[b] (Roche, FDA approved)	6 h	2–8°C ≤3 days, or ≥−70°C, ≤6 wk	5
AMPLICOR or COBAS AMPLICOR HIV-1 Monitor Test, version 1.5 (Roche, FDA approved)	6 h	2–8°C ≤5 days, or −70°C	3
COBAS AmpliPrep/COBAS TaqMan HIV-1 Test[b] (Roche, FDA approved)	6 h	18–30°C, ≤24 h 2–8°C, ≤5 days, or −20 to −80°C	5
RealTime HBV[b] (Abbott, CE IVD, FDA approved)	≤6 h, 2–30°C	15–30°C, ≤24 h 2–8°C, ≤3 days, or ≤−70°C	1[e]
RealTime HCV[b, d] (Abbott, CE IVD)	≤6 h, 2–30°C	15–30°C, ≤24 h 2–8°C, ≤3 days, or ≤−70°C	1[e]
RealTime HIV-1 (Abbott, FDA approved)	≤6 h, 15–30°C ≤24 h, 2–8°C	15–30°C, ≤24 h 2–8°C, ≤5 days, or ≤−70°C, >5 days	3
Versant HBV bDNA 3.0[b] (Siemens, RUO)	4 h, EDTA or ACD[f] 2 h, PPT	2–8 or ≤−20°C, ≤5 days −60 to −80°C, >5 days	4
Versant HCV RNA 3.0 (Siemens, FDA approved)	4 h, EDTA or ACD 2 h, PPT	2–8°C, ≤48 h −20°C, ≤3 days, or −60 to −80°C	4
Versant HIV-1 RNA 3.0 (Siemens, FDA approved)	4 h, EDTA or ACD 2 h, PPT	2–8°C, ≤48 h[g] 18–30°C, ≤24 h (PPT only) or frozen at −60 to −80°C	3

[a]RUO, research use only; CE IVD, Conformité Européenne mark for in vitro diagnostics.
[b]Test also verified for serum. Storage conditions apply to HighPure and AmpliPrep extraction.
[c]Long-term storage of serum has not been evaluated.
[d]Not available in the United States.
[e]Once thawed, specimen may be stored at 2–8°C for ≤6 h.
[f]ACD, acid-citrate-dextrose.
[g]If viral pellets are prepared within 30 min of plasma separation.

Plasma is obtained by centrifuging blood collected in tubes containing spray-dried anticoagulant (EDTA) at $1,500 \times g$ for 20 min at 25°C. Plasma Preparation Tubes (PPT; BD, Franklin Lakes, NJ) have spray-dried EDTA and a gel barrier that results in physical separation of plasma and cellular constituents, eliminating the need for decanting plasma. These tubes decrease the incidence of errors that occur when processing multiple specimens simultaneously (i.e., plasma is decanted into a tube labeled with another patient's name). However, falsely elevated HIV-1 RNA levels were observed from centrifuged PPT that were stored frozen or for prolonged periods at ~4°C (24, 36, 48, 51); therefore, these tubes are no longer recommended for use in quantitative HIV-1 tests. No decline in hepatitis C virus RNA levels was observed in blood stored in PPT at 4°C for 72 h (22). Plasma processing and storage conditions for various plasma-based NA tests are shown in Table 4.

Serum is used for serologic testing and for NA assays. Serum specimens are separated from clotted blood by centrifugation at $1,000 \times g$ for 10 min and refrigerated (4°C) for short-term storage (24 to 48 h) or frozen (<-20°C) for longer periods. Barrier tubes similar to plasma partitioning tubes are also available to separate serum from other blood constituents (SST; BD Diagnostic Systems). Similar to the case with PPT tubes, their suitability should be demonstrated in NA detection and quantification assays prior to implementation.

Leukocytes can be fractionated from whole blood, and they are particularly useful in the diagnosis of CMV and Epstein-Barr virus (EBV) infections. Isolated leukocytes can be cocultured with human diploid fibroblasts such as MRC-5 cells (conventional or shell vial culture [53]), directly stained with fluorescence-labeled antibody to detect the CMV viral protein pp65 in leukocyte nuclei (CMV antigenemia assay [57]), or extracted to detect CMV and EBV genomes by molecular techniques. Quantifying leukocyte input is essential for optimizing assay performance (41). Leukocytes can be separated by gradient sedimentation from 3 to 5 ml of blood anticoagulated with EDTA, sodium citrate, or heparin using several methods. Media such as Ficoll-Paque PLUS (Amersham Biosciences Corp., Piscataway, NJ), Cell Preparation Tubes (BD), and Lymphosep lymphocyte separation medium (MP Biomedicals, LLC, Irvine, CA) can be used to separate lymphocytes. Mono-Poly resolving medium (MP Biomedicals, LLC) and Polymorphprep (Technoclone, Vienna, Austria) enable the resolution of both mononuclear and polymorphonuclear leukocytes into two distinct bands. Histopaque-1077 (Sigma Diagnostics, St. Louis, MO) is used for isolation of mononuclear cells, and Zeptogel (ZeptoMetrix, Buffalo, NY) is used for isolation of the total leukocyte fraction. For optimal results, leukocytes should be fractionated as soon as possible after collection.

Bone Marrow

Bone marrow can be used to identify viral etiologies of aplastic anemia, congenital anemia, chronic red cell aplasia, and hemophagocytic lymphohistiocytosis (27, 67). Aspirated bone marrow is placed in tubes containing EDTA. The same processing considerations with respect to timing, anticoagulants, and removal of inhibitors apply to bone marrow as to blood.

Cerebrospinal Fluid

Depending upon the virus, NA detection, culture, or serology performed on CSF can be useful in detecting viral central nervous system infections (Table 1, chapter 78). CSF is collected using sterile technique, by inserting a spinal needle into the L4-L5 interspace, located in the midline between the left and right iliac crest. CSF should not be collected in VTM, as specimen dilution can impair virus detection. For molecular assays, NAs should be extracted prior to testing since CSF contains globulins, cell-derived proteins, and other uncharacterized substances that inhibit the activity of thermostable polymerases used in PCR (23, 47). A detailed discussion of NA extraction methods can be found in chapter 4. No processing is required for conventional methods.

Amniotic Fluid

Although rare, viruses can infect the fetus. Amniotic fluid is the specimen source of choice for the detection of viruses in utero. NA tests are the most commonly used. Amniotic fluid is collected by amniocentesis and sent to the laboratory in a sterile container without VTM.

Respiratory (Oropharyngeal, Nasopharyngeal Swab, Nasopharyngeal Aspirate, Nasal Wash, Throat, and BAL Fluid)

Viral respiratory diseases can be identified by testing a variety of respiratory specimens. Respiratory viruses can be detected by conventional techniques such as direct Ag detection methods (enzyme immunoassay, immunochromatographic assays, and immunofluorescence-labeled-antibody staining), culture, and NA tests (Table 1, chapter 78).

Many respiratory viruses infect ciliated epithelial cells that line the posterior nasopharynx. The posterior nasopharynx can be sampled with nasopharyngeal swabs, aspirates, and washes. Nasopharyngeal swabs are generally collected from older children and adults. Nasopharyngeal aspirates have been the specimen of choice for infants and younger children (2, 38); however, this practice may change with the introduction of next-generation swabs (discussed below). Results of studies comparing the efficacies of conventional rayon nasopharyngeal swabs and aspirates in respiratory virus tests are highly variable. Nasal wash specimens typically do not contain a large number of virus-infected cells; however, they are often collected from adults, particularly thrombocytopenic patients in whom nasopharyngeal aspiration is contraindicated. BAL and bronchial specimens are useful in the diagnosis of lower respiratory tract infections and offer a less invasive alternative to open lung biopsy. Nose and throat specimens have not traditionally been acceptable for respiratory virus detection due to the fact that many viruses are present at low levels in these sites. However, these specimens may be suitable for use in highly sensitive NA detection tests. For children, the sensitivities of influenza A virus and respiratory syncytial virus (RSV) detection in combined nose and throat specimens by real-time PCR were 92 and 93%, respectively, compared to nasopharyngeal aspirates (37). Whether nose and throat specimens are suitable for adults, who typically shed smaller amounts of virus than children, is unknown.

Nasopharyngeal swab samples are collected by inserting a flexible, fine-shafted swab deep into the nares, approximately half the distance between the angles of the nares and pinna. The swab is rotated three times, removed, and placed in VTM. Two new swab types designed for optimum specimen absorption and release are now available. One swab (Sigma-Swab; Medical Wire and Equipment Co.) has an open-cell foam bud construction, and the other (flocked swabs; Copan Diagnostics, Inc.) is made from nylon fiber using a proprietary spray-on technology. Several studies have demonstrated that flocked swabs are a viable option for obtaining respiratory samples. Enhanced cell recovery has been observed with flocked swabs compared to rayon (13). Flocked swabs performed comparably to rayon swabs for the detection of influenza A virus by NA test (16). At this time, it is not possible to make a definitive statement regarding the performance of flocked nasopharyngeal swabs and nasopharyngeal aspirates, since the data comparing the two specimen types are conflicting, with one study reporting equivalent detection of multiple viruses by fluorescent antibody (FA) (1) and another reporting comparability that varied by virus (62). Flocked swabs were equivalent to nasopharyngeal aspirates for influenza A virus detection by PCR, but nasopharyngeal aspirates were superior for influenza A virus detection by FA and RSV detection by FA and PCR (10).

Aspirates are collected by passage of an appropriately sized tube or catheter into the nasopharynx and suctioning material with a syringe or vacuum device. Suction traps are typically rinsed with VTM to remove residual sample remaining within the aspirate apparatus. Aspirates therefore usually contain VTM. Nasal wash specimens are obtained by instilling several milliliters of sterile saline into each nostril while the patient's head is tilted back slightly; the head is then brought forward, and the saline is allowed to flow into a small container held beneath the nose (8). BAL specimens are collected by inserting a fiber-optic bronchoscope into the involved segment of the lung, instilling saline, and applying suction to remove the lavage specimen.

All respiratory specimens are acceptable for culture (2, 34, 42, 55, 56). Respiratory specimens are often contaminated with antibiotic-resistant bacteria that can overgrow cultures and prevent virus detection. Removal of most microbial contaminants by centrifugation (3,000 × g for 20 min) or filtration of the specimen (0.2-μm pore size) is advantageous; however, these procedures also remove virus-infected cells, resulting in reduced viral titers. Centrifuged or filtered specimens are not suitable for Ag or NA detection. These assays should not be affected by bacteria, the loss of host cells during processing may compromise Ag test sensitivity, and NA tests have not been approved for use with acellular specimens.

Mucus in respiratory specimens can significantly affect Ag detection. In FA tests, mucus can inhibit adherence of cells to slides and can cause nonspecific fluorescence. It also prevents penetration of the sample into filtration devices. To prevent these complications, mucus threads can be broken by repeated aspiration through a small-bore pipette.

Oral

The different types of oral specimens include oral mucosal cells (including lesions), whole saliva, glandular duct saliva (from parotid, sublingual, and submandibular glands), and oral mucosal transudates. Oral mucosal cells are suitable for virus isolation and NA detection. Cells are dislodged with a swab or plastic spatula; the collection device is then placed in VTM for transport to the laboratory. Saliva is a heterogenous specimen with multiple constituents, including cells (epithelial cells and leukocytes), microorganisms (bacteria and fungi), antibodies (IgA and low levels of IgG), digestive enzymes, mucin, and foreign particles. It is suitable for virus isolation and NA detection. It is collected by initially tilting the head forward and catching fluid from the lower lip into a collection container and then by catching residual, expectorated fluid after 5 min. Parotid gland saliva is particularly useful for diagnosing parotitis. It is collected with a swab approximately 30 s after massaging the area between the cheek and teeth at the level of the ear. Transudates obtained from capillaries in the buccal mucosa and the base of pocket between the teeth and gums (gingival crevice) contain high levels of IgG and IgM. These oral mucosal transudates (also called gingival crevicular fluid, crevicular fluid saliva, or crevicular fluid) are acceptable, noninvasive samples for use in serologic assays for a variety of viruses, including HIV, measles virus, and rubella virus. A number of collection devices are commercially available; the collection method for each device is slightly different (reviewed in reference 28).

Urine

Viruses can be detected in urine using molecular techniques or culture. To collect urine specimens, the external genitalia are cleaned with a detergent-impregnated towelette. A volume of 5 to 10 ml of midstream-voided urine is collected in a sterile container. Urine must be processed for use in virus detection assays. Its acidic pH and the presence of microbial contaminants can inhibit virus growth. Urine also contains substances that inhibit PCR (4, 35). To improve virus recovery, pH can be neutralized with sodium bicarbonate (7.5% solution) and bacteria can be removed by filtration (0.2-μm pore size) prior to culture. Attempts to improve virus recovery by culturing cell pellets versus supernatant after centrifugation have yielded variable results (5). For molecular assays, NAs can be extracted from urine or urine dried onto filter disks using a variety of extraction methods (44, 58).

Feces (Rectal Swab)

Many viruses that cause gastroenteritis are noncultivable and require Ag or NA tests for detection (11, 45, 60). Enteroviruses can be detected by NA detection or fecal culture, but care must be taken in the interpretation of a positive result since asymptomatic shedding can occur in feces. Fecal samples (2 to 4 g) are placed into a clean, dry, leakproof container or by inserting a swab 4 to 6 cm into the rectum and rotating the swab against the mucosa. The swab is removed and placed in VTM. Fecal samples are preferred over rectal swabs since swabs often collect insufficient quantities of specimen.

Eye

Viral causes of conjunctival, corneal, and retinal disease can be detected by collection of samples from the eye. Conjunctival swabs are collected from the lower conjunctiva with a flexible, fine-shafted Dacron or rayon swab moistened with sterile saline and placed in VTM. The RPS Adeno Detector (RPS, Inc., Sarasota, FL), a lateral-flow immunochromatographic cartridge test for the detection of ocular adenovirus infections, uses a built-in sampling pad to touch the eye and collect fluid from the conjunctiva. Scrapings of the cornea should be collected by an ophthalmologist or by other adequately trained personnel. Retinal pathogens are detected in the aqueous and vitreous fluids by molecular techniques, since they are not easily cultivated from these samples. These fluids have been shown to inhibit PCR (64); therefore, the original specimen must be extracted to remove inhibitors. Vitreous and aqueous fluids are obtained from the eye during ocular surgery.

Tissue (Biopsy or Autopsy)

Lung tissue is an ideal source for detecting lower respiratory tract viral infections. Other tissues that may yield positive viral results include liver, spleen, kidney, lymph node, and brain. Methods such as culture, histology, Ag detection (immunohistochemical stains), and NA detection can be used to identify viruses in tissue. The major drawback of tissue specimens is the invasive nature of biopsy. However, for certain patients, biopsy is the only option. An attempt should be made to excise the specimen from areas directly adjacent to the affected tissue.

Fresh tissue specimens for NA detection are weighed (25 mg is optimal for most tissues), minced, treated with proteolytic enzymes, and extracted. NAs can also be obtained from formalin-fixed, paraffin-embedded tissues after deparaffinization and extraction; however, fresh tissue is superior for NA recovery. Tissue specimens for culture are ground with a sterile mortar and pestle or a tissue grinder and resuspended in VTM. The tissue specimen is centrifuged (1,000 × g for 15 min at 4°C) to remove cell debris that may be toxic to cell culture, and the supernatant is inoculated onto cell monolayers.

Genital

The most common viral causes of genital lesions are herpes simplex viruses (HSVs) that are easily detected by direct Ag and NA methods or culture. Additionally, human papillomavirus (HPV) genotypes associated with a high risk of developing cervical cancer (genotypes 16, 18, 31, 33, 35, 39, 45, 51, 52, 56, 58, 59, 66, and 68) can be detected in cervical specimens using molecular tests.

Genital ulcers should be swabbed; specimens destined for culture should be submitted in VTM. Dry swabs that are placed into solution during processing should be suitable for NA detection. Cervical specimens are collected with swabs or brushes. Prior to collection, mucus should be removed from the cervical os with a cleaning swab and discarded. Endocervical specimens are collected by inserting a swab to a depth of 1 cm into the cervical canal and rotating it for 5 s. Endocervical cells can also be obtained using a Cytobrush. Cervical samples collected in manufacturer-specific formats or as liquid-based cytology specimens are appropriate for detection of HPV high-risk genotypes (46). Cervical brush specimens in standard transport medium for the hc2 High-Risk HPV DNA Test (Qiagen) may be stored for up to 2 weeks at room temperature, after which specimens can be stored for an additional week at 2 to 8°C. If testing is to be performed more than 3 weeks from collection, specimens should be placed at −20°C for up to 3 months. Cervical biopsy specimens must be placed into 1 ml of standard transport medium and stored frozen at −20°C. Specimens in PreservCyt (Hologic) liquid-based cytology medium may be held for up to 3 weeks at temperatures between 4 and 37°C prior to hc2 testing and up to 18 weeks at 20 to 30°C prior to Cervista (Hologic) testing. PreservCyt specimens cannot be frozen prior to testing for high-risk HPV.

Skin

Viruses can cause rashes with many different appearances, including maculopapular, petechial, and vesicular. Recovery of viruses from maculopapular and petechial rashes requires biopsy of skin, which is not routinely assayed by most clinical laboratories. Viral causes of disseminated diseases manifested by maculopapular and petechial rashes are usually identified by testing peripheral blood rather than skin.

Vesicular lesions are commonly caused by HSV, varicella-zoster virus (VZV), and enteroviruses. Fresh vesicles should be sampled for optimal virus detection. Vesicles can rupture and ulcerate. Ulcers that have crusted may not contain viable virus or viral Ags. Samples are obtained by disrupting the surface of the lesion and collecting fluid with a swab or by aspiration with a 26- or 27-gauge needle attached to a tuberculin syringe (18). Specimens should be collected gently, without causing bleeding, since the presence of neutralizing antibody in blood can impair recovery. The base of the lesion should be scraped to collect cellular material for Ag detection assays using direct immunofluorescence (HSV and VZV). Smears may be prepared at bedside. Swabs should be placed in VTM if the specimen will be tested by NA amplification assays, certain Ag detection formats (such as immunofluorescent-antibody staining), and/or culture.

SPECIMEN TRANSPORT

Once a clinical specimen has been collected, it should be transported to the laboratory as soon as possible, since virus viability decreases with time (some clinically important viruses are more labile than others). Overall diagnostic yield improves when specimens are expeditiously processed for viral culture. Viability is not required for Ag or NA detection techniques; therefore, transport time is not as much of an issue for these assays, unless degradation of the viral RNA or DNA is a consideration. However, for timely diagnosis, delay should be avoided during transport of these specimens to the laboratory.

Transport Conditions

Several steps may be taken to help preserve viruses during specimen transport to the laboratory, including (i) transport of nonblood specimens at 4°C with wet ice or cold packs, especially if transit time is greater than 1 h; (ii) use of VTM if appropriate, as described below; and (iii) avoiding freezing unless a delay of 24 h is anticipated (65). If processing delay is unavoidable, specimens should be frozen at −60°C (dry ice). It should be noted that freezing can significantly compromise recovery of RSV, CMV, and VZV.

Storage and transport conditions may vary somewhat based on the stability characteristics of specific viruses or viral NAs. RSV is thermolabile; 90% of infectivity is lost after 24 h at 37°C and 4 days at 4°C (26). A study to determine the feasibility of shipping adenovirus samples in M4RT showed that the virus is stable for up to 5 days at ambient temperatures (50). SARS-CoV infectivity is maintained in serum, sputum, and feces for 96 h and in urine for 72 h (15). CMV infectious titers in blood were decreased by up to 91% after storage at 4°C for 24 h (43). The data on CMV DNA quantification after storage are conflicting, with some studies reporting no decline in CMV DNA levels after 24 h (43) and 72 h (49), while another showed increased levels in blood stored at room temperature or at 4°C prior to plasma separation from lymphocytes (52). The increased levels of CMV DNA may be due to release of CMV from cells into plasma during storage. HSV DNA is stable in CSF specimens containing lymphocytes and monocytes for up to 30 days at temperatures ranging from 25 to −72°C (63). HIV-1 RNA is stable in dried whole blood or plasma stored at room temperature or at −70°C for up to 1 year (7). However, the integrity of HIV-1 RNA on dried blood or plasma spots is compromised at 37°C and high humidity (19). RNAlater, a RNA stabilization buffer (Qiagen), has been shown to stabilize hepatitis C virus and HIV RNA in plasma for up to 28 days at 37°C (39) as well as stabilizing the infectivity of enveloped and nonenveloped viruses stored at room temperature for up to 50 days (59). An RNA extraction reagent, buffer AVL (Qiagen), has also been shown to stabilize viral NA (6). Guidelines for collection, transport, preparation, and storage of specimens for molecular methods have been published by the CLSI (12).

Transport Medium

The ideal transport medium maintains viability of a broad range of cultivable viruses and is also compatible with the newer non-culture-based tests. VTM generally contains buffer to control pH, substances to maintain an appropriate osmotic environment, protein to stabilize the virus, and antibiotics to prevent growth of microbial contaminants. Many different transport media have been described and used successfully, including cell culture medium, bacteriological broth-based media, buffered salt solutions with added protein, sucrose-based solutions, bentonite-containing media, and swab-tube combinations. Although rarely used today, direct inoculation of cell monolayers and cell suspension at bedside has also been described (54). Some laboratories have reported that culturette swabs with Stuart's medium designed for collection and transport of bacteriology specimens are also acceptable for collection and transport of viral specimens (30). Historically, VTM was prepared in-house; however, many formulations are now commercially available (Table 5) and are sold as VTM alone or packaged with collection swabs.

Unfortunately, there have been no recent comprehensive comparisons of either commercially available or in-house-prepared VTM. The most comprehensive reviews of transport systems for viruses were published several years ago (32, 33), and many of these transport systems are no longer in use today. It is difficult to compare results of the few studies that have been performed because they were carried out in different laboratories under different conditions (with various viral inocula and detection methods). Ideally, direct comparisons of several different transport media that support growth of multiple viruses should be performed in a clinical setting. However, the cost and logistics of performing these types of comparative studies remain problematic.

Manufacturers of commercials assays for NA or Ag detection either supply transport media or make recommendations for transport systems that are compatible with their assays. The manufacturer's package insert should therefore be consulted for information on appropriate collection and transport systems. Thus far, VTM has not been shown to inhibit amplification assays such as PCR (34) and many Ag detection tests (21), although some media are not suitable for use with certain Ag detection tests. For example, M4RT interferes with and is not suitable for the 3M Rapid Detection Flu A+B Test.

Transportation Regulations

Few clinical virology laboratories can offer a complete battery of diagnostic tests for all human viruses. Therefore, shipment of samples to reference, specialty, state, or federal laboratories is common practice. A recent change in regulations has simplified the shipping process for most specimens (30a). Currently, the majority of diagnostic or clinical specimens can be shipped as biological substances, category B. Only specimens that have or may have a category A pathogen are classified as infectious substance. Strict attention must be paid to specimen packaging and labeling for the transport of infectious substances. Shipping specimens through the mail or by commercial courier is regulated by federal and international agencies. Regulations are published by the U.S. Public Health Service and are also available from the U.S. Department of Transportation on the Internet (http://www.dot.gov). Regulations stipulate that training must be provided within 90 days of assuming a job involving the transport of dangerous goods (30a). Retraining must take place every 24 months, and training records including time, place, instructor, and materials must be maintained. The 2010 document also defines infectious substances, containers, labels, and other packaging instructions required for shipping (30a).

TABLE 5 Commercial sources and formulations of VTM

Medium	Composition	Vol (ml)	Storage temp (°C)
BD Universal Viral Transport Medium[a] (BD Diagnostic Systems)	Basal constituents,[b] gelatin, vancomycin, colistin	1 or 3	2–25
Copan Universal Transport Medium (Copan Diagnostics Inc.)	Basal constituents, L-cysteine, gelatin, vancomycin, colistin	1 or 3	2–25
CVM Transport Media (Hardy Diagnostics)	Basal constituents, gelatin, vancomycin, colistin	2	2–8
Micro Test M4 (Remel)	Basal constituents, gelatin, vancomycin, colistin	3	−25–8
Micro Test M4RT (Remel)	Basal constituents, gelatin, gentamicin	3	2–30
Micro Test M5 (Remel)	Basal constituents, protein stabilizers, vancomycin, colistin	3	−25–8
Micro Test M6[a] (Remel)	Basal constituents, L-cysteine, gelatin, vancomycin, colistin	1.5	2–30
Multitrans Medium[a] (Starplex Scientific Inc.)	Basal constituents, gelatin, sodium bicarbonate, vancomycin, colistin	3	2–25
Virocult medium[a] (Medical Wire & Equipment Co.)	Balanced salt solution, disodium hydrogen orthophosphate, lactalbumin hydrolysate, chloramphenicol, amphotericin B	1.2	5–25
VCM[a] (Medical Wire & Equipment Co.)	Sucrose phosphate buffer, lactalbumin hydrolysate, amphotericin B, vancomycin, colistin	1 or 3	5–25

[a]Product available as swab-VTM tube combination.
[b]Basal constituents: Hanks balanced salt solution, bovine serum albumin, L-glutamic acid, sucrose, HEPES buffer (pH 7.3), phenol red, and amphotericin B.

SUMMARY

Diagnosis of virus infection is based on likely etiologies, assay performance (sensitivity, specificity, positive predictive value, and negative predictive value), time to result, and cost. Viruses in and of themselves put limitations on test options (viruses that are noncultivable must be identified directly in the specimen by electron microscopy, cytologic and histologic methods, Ag detection, or NA detection or indirectly by serology). Regardless of the test method, the proper selection, collection, transport, and processing of specimens will always be of the utmost importance. Many commercial assays have specific sample requirements that must be followed. If a sample is to be tested on diverse platforms, appropriate precautions in handling should be taken to ensure accurate results. For example, endocervical samples collected in liquid cytology medium should be handled in a manner appropriate for NA amplification given the growing menu of NA detection tests cleared for use with residual cytology samples. All aspects of user-defined assays, including specimen type, collection device, transport, and processing, as well as any changes to package insert specifications for commercial assays, must be verified in accordance with local, state, and federal regulations (9). Recommendations for NA test validation have been published by laboratory accreditation agencies (31). On the surface, the initial steps of viral detection appear simple and virtually static. However, as the field of diagnostic virology evolves, new collection devices, transport systems, and processing methods that enhance detection will continue to be developed.

REFERENCES

1. **Abu-Diab, A., M. Azzeh, R. Ghneim, M. Zoughbi, S. Turkuman, N. Rishmawi, A. E. Issa, I. Siriani, R. Dauodi, R. Kattan, and M. Y. Hindiyeh.** 2008. Comparison between pernasal flocked swabs and nasopharyngeal aspirates for detection of common respiratory viruses in samples from children. *J. Clin. Microbiol.* **46:**2414–2417.

2. **Ahluwalia, G., J. Embree, P. McNicol, B. Law, and G. W. Hammond.** 1987. Comparison of nasopharyngeal aspirate and nasopharyngeal swab specimens for respiratory syncytial virus diagnosis by cell culture, indirect immunofluorescence assay, and enzyme-linked immunosorbent assay. *J. Clin. Microbiol.* **25:**763–767.

3. **Baba, M., R. Pauwels, J. Balzarini, J. Arnout, J. Desmyter, and E. De Clercq.** 1988. Mechanism of inhibitory effect of dextran sulfate and heparin on replication of human immunodeficiency virus in vitro. *Proc. Natl. Acad. Sci. USA* **85:**6132–6136.

4. **Behzadbehbahani, A., P. E. Klapper, P. J. Vallely, and G. M. Cleator.** 1997. Detection of BK virus in urine by polymerase chain reaction: a comparison of DNA extraction methods. *J. Virol. Methods* **67:**161–166.

5. **Bennion, D. W., L. J. Wright, R. A. Watt, A. A. Whiting, and J. F. Carlquist.** 1998. Optimal recovery of cytomegalovirus from urine as a function of specimen preparation. *Diagn. Microbiol. Infect. Dis.* **31:**337–342.

6. **Blow, J. A., D. J. Dohm, D. L. Negley, and C. N. Mores.** 2004. Virus inactivation by nucleic acid extraction reagents. *J. Virol. Methods* **119:**195–198.

7. **Brambilla, D., C. Jennings, G. Aldrovandi, J. Bremer, A. M. Comeau, S. A. Cassol, R. Dickover, J. B. Jackson, J. Pitt, J. L. Sullivan, A. Butcher, L. Grosso, P. Reichelderfer, and S. A. Fiscus.** 2003. Multicenter evaluation of use of dried blood and plasma spot specimens in quantitative assays for human immunodeficiency virus RNA: measurement, precision, and RNA stability. *J. Clin. Microbiol.* **41:**1888–1893.

8. **Brenton, S.** 1997. RSV specimen collection methods: nasal vs. nasopharyngeal. *Pediatr. Nurs.* **23:**621–622, 629.

9. **Centers for Medicare and Medicaid Services, Department of Health and Human Services.** 2004. Clinical Laboratory Improvement Act, vol. 493.1253. Standard: establishment and verification of performance specifications. 42 CFR Ch. IV Subpart K Quality System for Nonwaived Testing, Analytical Systems. Centers for Medicare and Medicaid Services, Baltimore, MD. http://edocket.access.gpo.gov/cfr_2004/octqtr/pdf/42cfr493.1.pdf.

10. **Chan, K. H., J. S. Peiris, W. Lim, J. M. Nicholls, and S. S. Chiu.** 2008. Comparison of nasopharyngeal flocked swabs and aspirates for rapid diagnosis of respiratory viruses in children. *J. Clin. Virol.* **42:**65–69.

11. **Christensen, M. L.** 1989. Human viral gastroenteritis. *Clin. Microbiol. Rev.* **2:**51–89.

12. **CLSI.** 2005. *Collection, Transport, Preparation, and Storage of Specimens for Molecular Methods; Approved Guideline.* CLSI document MM13-A. CLSI, Wayne, PA.

13. **Daley, P., S. Castriciano, M. Chernesky, and M. Smieja.** 2006. Comparison of flocked and rayon swabs for collection of respiratory epithelial cells from uninfected volunteers and symptomatic patients. *J. Clin. Microbiol.* **44:**2265–2267.

14. **Dickover, R. E., S. A. Herman, K. Saddiq, D. Wafer, M. Dillon, and Y. J. Bryson.** 1998. Optimization of specimen-handling procedures for accurate quantitation of levels of human immunodeficiency virus RNA in plasma by reverse transcriptase PCR. *J. Clin. Microbiol.* **36:**1070–1073.

15. **Duan, S. M., X. S. Zhao, R. F. Wen, J. J. Huang, G. H. Pi, S. X. Zhang, J. Han, S. L. Bi, L. Ruan, and X. P. Dong.** 2003. Stability of SARS coronavirus in human specimens and environment and its sensitivity to heating and UV irradiation. *Biomed. Environ. Sci.* **16:**246–255.

16. **Esposito, S., C. G. Molteni, C. Daleno, A. Valzano, L. Cesati, L. Gualtieri, C. Tagliabue, S. Bosis, and N. Principi.** 2010. Comparison of nasopharyngeal nylon flocked swabs with universal transport medium and rayon-bud swabs with a sponge reservoir of viral transport medium in the diagnosis of paediatric influenza. *J. Med. Microbiol.* **59:**96–99.

17. **Fong, C. K. Y., and M. L. Landry.** 1994. Specimen collection, transport, and processing for virologic studies, p. 11–23. *In* G. D. Hsiung, C. K. Y. Fong, and M. L. Landry (ed.), *Diagnostic Virology.* Yale University Press, New Haven, CT.

18. **Forghani, B.** 2000. Laboratory diagnosis of infection, p. 351–353. *In* A. M. Arvin and A. A. Gerson (ed.), *Varicella-Zoster Virus, Virology and Clinical Management.* Cambridge University Press, Cambridge, United Kingdom.

19. **Garcia-Lerma, J. G., A. McNulty, C. Jennings, D. Huang, W. Heneine, and J. W. Bremer.** 2009. Rapid decline in the efficiency of HIV drug resistance genotyping from dried blood spots (DBS) and dried plasma spots (DPS) stored at 37 degrees C and high humidity. *J. Antimicrob. Chemother.* **64:**33–36.

20. **Ginocchio, C. C., X. P. Wang, M. H. Kaplan, G. Mulligan, D. Witt, J. W. Romano, M. Cronin, and R. Carroll.** 1997. Effects of specimen collection, processing, and storage conditions on stability of human immunodeficiency virus type 1 RNA levels in plasma. *J. Clin. Microbiol.* **35:**2886–2893.

21. **Gleaves, C. A., D. H. Rice, and C. F. Lee.** 1990. Evaluation of an enzyme immunoassay for the detection of herpes simplex virus (HSV) antigen from clinical specimens in viral transport media. *J. Virol. Methods* **28:**133–139.

22. **Grant, P. R., A. Kitchen, J. A. Barbara, P. Hewitt, C. M. Sims, J. A. Garson, and R. S. Tedder.** 2000. Effects of handling and storage of blood on the stability of hepatitis C virus RNA: implications for NAT testing in transfusion practice. *Vox Sang.* **78:**137–142.

23. **Greenfield, L., and T. J. White.** 1993. Sample preparation methods, p. 122–137. *In* D. H. Persing, T. F. Smith, F. C. Tenover, and T. J. White (ed.), *Diagnostic Molecular Biology: Principles and Applications.* ASM Press, Washington, DC.

24. **Griffith, B. P., and D. R. Mayo.** 2006. Increased levels of HIV RNA detected in samples with viral loads close to the detection limit collected in Plasma Preparation Tubes (PPT). *J. Clin. Virol.* **35:**197–200.

25. **Grys, T. E., and T. F. Smith.** 2009. Specimen requirements: selection, collection, transport, and processing, p. 18–35. *In* S. Specter, R. L. Hodinka, S. A. Young, and D. L. Wiedbrauk (ed.), *Clinical Virology Manual*, 4th ed. ASM Press, Washington, DC.

26. **Hambling, M. H.** 1964. Survival of the respiratory syncytial virus during storage under various conditions. *Br. J. Exp. Pathol.* **45:**647–655.

27. **Hoang, M. P., D. B. Dawson, Z. R. Rogers, R. H. Scheuermann, and B. B. Rogers.** 1998. Polymerase chain reaction amplification of archival material for Epstein-Barr virus, cytomegalovirus, human herpesvirus 6, and parvovirus B19 in children with bone marrow hemophagocytosis. *Hum. Pathol.* **29:**1074–1077.

28. **Hodinka, R. L., T. Nagashunmugam, and D. Malamud.** 1998. Detection of human immunodeficiency virus antibodies in oral fluids. *Clin. Diagn. Lab. Immunol.* **5:**419–426.

29. **Holodniy, M., S. Kim, D. Katzenstein, M. Konrad, E. Groves, and T. C. Merigan.** 1991. Inhibition of human immunodeficiency virus gene amplification by heparin. *J. Clin. Microbiol.* **29:**676–679.

30. **Huntoon, C. J., R. F. House, Jr., and T. F. Smith.** 1981. Recovery of viruses from three transport media incorporated into culturettes. *Arch. Pathol. Lab. Med.* **105:**436–437.

30a. **International Air Transport Association.** 2010. *IATA Dangerous Goods Regulations*, 51st ed. International Air Transport Association, Montreal, Quebec, Canada.

31. **Jennings, L., V. M. Van Deerlin, and M. L. Gulley.** 2009. Recommended principles and practices for validating clinical molecular pathology tests. *Arch. Pathol. Lab. Med.* **133:**743–755.

32. **Jensen, C., and F. B. Johnson.** 1994. Comparison of various transport media for viability maintenance of herpes simplex virus, respiratory syncytial virus, and adenovirus. *Diagn. Microbiol. Infect. Dis.* **19:**137–142.

33. **Johnson, F. B.** 1990. Transport of viral specimens. *Clin. Microbiol. Rev.* **3:**120–131.

34. **Josephson, S. L.** 1997. An update on the collection and transport of specimens for viral culture. *Clin. Microbiol. Newsl.* **19:**57–61.

35. **Khan, G., H. O. Kangro, P. J. Coates, and R. B. Heath.** 1991. Inhibitory effects of urine on the polymerase chain reaction for cytomegalovirus DNA. *J. Clin. Pathol.* **44:**360–365.

36. **Kran, A. M., T. O. Jonassen, M. Sannes, K. Jakobsen, A. Lind, A. Maeland, and M. Holberg-Petersen.** 2009. Overestimation of human immunodeficiency virus type 1 load caused by the presence of cells in plasma from plasma preparation tubes. *J. Clin. Microbiol.* **47:**2170–2174.

37. **Lambert, S. B., D. M. Whiley, N. T. O'Neill, E. C. Andrews, F. M. Canavan, C. Bletchly, D. J. Siebert, T. P. Sloots, and M. D. Nissen.** 2008. Comparing nose-throat swabs and nasopharyngeal aspirates collected from children with symptoms for respiratory virus identification using real-time polymerase chain reaction. *Pediatrics* **122:**e615–e620.

38. **Landry, M. L., S. Cohen, and D. Ferguson.** 2000. Impact of sample type on rapid detection of influenza virus A by cytospin-enhanced immunofluorescence and membrane enzyme-linked immunosorbent assay. *J. Clin. Microbiol.* **38:**429–430.

39. **Lee, D. H., L. Li, L. Andrus, and A. M. Prince.** 2002. Stabilized viral nucleic acids in plasma as an alternative shipping method for NAT. *Transfusion* **42:**409–413.

40. **Levin, M. J., S. Leventhal, and H. A. Masters.** 1984. Factors influencing quantitative isolation of varicella-zoster virus. *J. Clin. Microbiol.* **19:**880–883.

41. **Lipson, S. M., L. H. Falk, and S. H. Lee.** 1996. Effect of leukocyte concentration and inoculum volume on the laboratory identification of cytomegalovirus in peripheral blood by the centrifugation culture-antigen detection methodology. *Arch. Pathol. Lab. Med.* **120:**53–56.

42. **Navarro-Mari, J. M., S. Sanbonmatsu-Gamez, M. Perez-Ruiz, and M. De La Rosa-Fraile.** 1999. Rapid detection of respiratory viruses by shell vial assay using simultaneous culture of HEp-2, LLC-MK2, and MDCK cells in a single vial. *J. Clin. Microbiol.* **37:**2346–2347.

43. **Nesbitt, S. E., L. Cook, and K. R. Jerome.** 2004. Cytomegalovirus quantitation by real-time PCR is unaffected by delayed

44. **Nozawa, N., S. Koyano, Y. Yamamoto, Y. Inami, I. Kurane, and N. Inoue.** 2007. Real-time PCR assay using specimens on filter disks as a template for detection of cytomegalovirus in urine. *J. Clin. Microbiol.* **45:**1305–1307.

45. **Payne, C. M., C. G. Ray, V. Borduin, L. L. Minnich, and M. D. Lebowitz.** 1987. An eight-year study of the viral agents of acute gastroenteritis in humans: ultrastructural observations and seasonal distribution with a major emphasis on coronavirus-like particles. *Adv. Exp. Med. Biol.* **218:**579–580.

46. **Peyton, C. L., M. Schiffman, A. T. Lorincz, W. C. Hunt, I. Mielzynska, C. Bratti, S. Eaton, A. Hildesheim, L. A. Morera, A. C. Rodriguez, R. Herrero, M. E. Sherman, and C. M. Wheeler.** 1998. Comparison of PCR- and hybrid capture-based human papillomavirus detection systems using multiple cervical specimen collection strategies. *J. Clin. Microbiol.* **36:**3248–3254.

47. **Ratnamohan, V. M., A. L. Cunningham, and W. D. Rawlinson.** 1998. Removal of inhibitors of CSF-PCR to improve diagnosis of herpesviral encephalitis. *J. Virol. Methods* **72:**59–65.

48. **Rebeiro, P. F., A. Kheshti, S. S. Bebawy, S. E. Stinnette, H. Erdem, Y. W. Tang, T. R. Sterling, S. P. Raffanti, and R. T. D'Aquila.** 2008. Increased detectability of plasma HIV-1 RNA after introduction of a new assay and altered specimen-processing procedures. *Clin. Infect. Dis.* **47:**1354–1357.

49. **Roberts, T. C., R. S. Buller, M. Gaudreault-Keener, K. E. Sternhell, K. Garlock, G. G. Singer, D. C. Brennan, and G. A. Storch.** 1997. Effects of storage temperature and time on qualitative and quantitative detection of cytomegalovirus in blood specimens by shell vial culture and PCR. *J. Clin. Microbiol.* **35:**2224–2228.

50. **Romanowski, E. G., S. P. Bartels, R. Vogel, N. T. Wetherall, C. Hodges-Savola, R. P. Kowalski, K. A. Yates, P. R. Kinchington, and Y. J. Gordon.** 2004. Feasibility of an antiviral clinical trial requiring cross-country shipment of conjunctival adenovirus cultures and recovery of infectious virus. *Curr. Eye Res.* **29:**195–199.

51. **Salimnia, H., E. C. Moore, L. R. Crane, R. D. Macarthur, and M. R. Fairfax.** 2005. Discordance between viral loads determined by Roche COBAS AMPLICOR human immunodeficiency virus type 1 Monitor (version 1.5) standard and ultrasensitive assays caused by freezing patient plasma in centrifuged Becton-Dickinson Vacutainer brand plasma preparation tubes. *J. Clin. Microbiol.* **43:**4635–4639.

52. **Schafer, P., W. Tenschert, M. Schroter, K. Gutensohn, and R. Laufs.** 2000. False-positive results of plasma PCR for cytomegalovirus DNA due to delayed sample preparation. *J. Clin. Microbiol.* **38:**3249–3253.

53. **Shuster, E. A., J. S. Beneke, G. E. Tegtmeier, G. R. Pearson, C. A. Gleaves, A. D. Wold, and T. F. Smith.** 1985. Monoclonal antibody for rapid laboratory detection of cytomegalovirus infections: characterization and diagnostic application. *Mayo Clin. Proc.* **60:**577–585.

54. **Skinner, G. R., M. A. Billstrom, S. Randall, A. Ahmad, S. Patel, J. Davies, and A. Deane.** 1997. A system for isolation, transport and storage of herpes simplex viruses. *J. Virol. Methods* **65:**1–8.

55. **Smith, M. C., C. Creutz, and Y. T. Huang.** 1991. Detection of respiratory syncytial virus in nasopharyngeal secretions by shell vial technique. *J. Clin. Microbiol.* **29:**463–465.

56. **Smith, T. F.** 2000. Specimen requirements: selection, collection, transport, and processing, p. 11–26. *In* S. Specter, R. L. Hodinka, and S. A. Young (ed.), *Clinical Virology Manual*, 3rd ed. ASM Press, Washington, DC.

57. **St. George, K., M. J. Boyd, S. M. Lipson, D. Ferguson, G. F. Cartmell, L. H. Falk, C. R. Rinaldo, and M. L. Landry.** 2000. A multisite trial comparing two cytomegalovirus (CMV) pp65 antigenemia test kits, Biotest CMV Brite and Bartels/Argene CMV Antigenemia. *J. Clin. Microbiol.* **38:**1430–1433.

separation of plasma from whole blood. *J. Clin. Microbiol.* **42:**1296–1297.

58. **Tang, Y. W., S. E. Sefers, H. Li, D. J. Kohn, and G. W. Procop.** 2005. Comparative evaluation of three commercial systems for nucleic acid extraction from urine specimens. *J. Clin. Microbiol.* **43:**4830–4833.

59. **Uhlenhaut, C., and M. Kracht.** 2005. Viral infectivity is maintained by an RNA protection buffer. *J. Virol. Methods* **128:**189–191.

60. **Vizzi, E., D. Ferraro, A. Cascio, R. Di Stefano, and S. Arista.** 1996. Detection of enteric adenoviruses 40 and 41 in stool specimens by monoclonal antibody-based enzyme immunoassays. *Res. Virol.* **147:**333–339.

61. **Wadowsky, R. M., S. Laus, T. Libert, S. J. States, and G. D. Ehrlich.** 1994. Inhibition of PCR-based assay for *Bordetella pertussis* by using calcium alginate fiber and aluminum shaft components of a nasopharyngeal swab. *J. Clin. Microbiol.* **32:**1054–1057.

62. **Walsh, P., C. L. Overmyer, K. Pham, S. Michaelson, L. Gofman, L. DeSalvia, T. Tran, D. Gonzalez, J. Pusavat, M. Feola, K. T. Iacono, E. Mordechai, and M. E. Adelson.** 2008. Comparison of respiratory virus detection rates for infants and toddlers by use of flocked swabs, saline aspirates, and saline aspirates mixed in universal transport medium for room temperature storage and shipping. *J. Clin. Microbiol.* **46:**2374–2376.

63. **Wiedbrauk, D. L., and W. Cunningham.** 1996. Stability of herpes simplex virus DNA in cerebrospinal fluid specimens. *Diagn. Mol. Pathol.* **5:**249–252.

64. **Wiedbrauk, D. L., J. C. Werner, and A. M. Drevon.** 1995. Inhibition of PCR by aqueous and vitreous fluids. *J. Clin. Microbiol.* **33:**2643–2646.

65. **Wilson, M. L.** 1996. General principles of specimen collection and transport. *Clin. Infect. Dis.* **22:**766–777.

66. **World Health Organization.** 2000. *WHO Infection Control Guidelines for Transmissible Spongiform Encephalopathies.* World Health Organization, Geneva, Switzerland. http://www.who.int/csr/resources/publications/bse/WHO_CDS_CSR_APH_2000_3/en/.

67. **Young, N. S., and K. E. Brown.** 2004. Parvovirus B19. *N. Engl. J. Med.* **350:**586–597.

Reagents, Stains, Media, and Cell Cultures: Virology

CHRISTINE C. GINOCCHIO AND PATRICIA C. HARRIS

77

In 1915, vaccinia virus was first propagated in cell culture for the purpose of vaccine production (22). However, the potential role of cell culture for clinical diagnostics was not highlighted until 1949, when Enders et al. (5) first described the use of cultivated mammalian cells and the observation of cytopathic effect (CPE) for the detection of polioviruses. Today, living cells are used to support the growth of a number of cell-dependent organisms including viruses and certain bacteria such as *Chlamydia* spp. and, more rarely, *Mycoplasma* spp. In addition, cultured cells can be used to demonstrate the effects of bacterial toxins excreted from pathogens such as *Shigella* spp., toxigenic *Escherichia coli*, including O157:H7, and toxigenic *Clostridium difficile*, among others. Traditional tube cell culture and rapid cell culture methods (e.g., shell vial) are dependent on the interactions of viruses with a variety of animal, human, and/or insect cells and utilized within the laboratory setting as substrates for growth, identification, and enumeration of pathogenic viruses (13, 15).

In the era of molecular detection and quantification of viral pathogens, the applicability of viral isolation has been questioned. For many viruses it is well documented that molecular detection methods are preferred (i) for their greater sensitivity; (ii) for their faster potential for detection and reporting (hours versus overnight or days to weeks); (iii) for their ability to quantify more accurately the amount of virus present in the sample; and (iv) in instances where viral culture may place the laboratory at risk due to the highly pathogenic nature of the virus (e.g., variola virus, Ebola virus, avian influenza virus, etc.). However, cell culture methods have useful applications (i) when the potential viral agent is not known; (ii) when the cost of other methods of testing is greater than that of cell culture; (iii) for documentation of active infection; (iv) to perform antiviral susceptibility testing; (v) to assess response to antiviral treatment by the detection of viable virus; (vi) for serologic strain typing; (vii) for vaccine and therapeutic clinical trials; and (viii) for laboratories that do not have the ability to perform molecular detection methods. Some molecular assays, for practical reporting purposes, may take as long as overnight cell culture and may not lend themselves to single-specimen testing as well as cell culture does. For these reasons, cell cultures are still an indispensible research and clinical laboratory tool, particularly when combined with the use of highly specific monoclonal antibodies (MAbs)

for the detection of common viruses and *Chlamydia* spp. or when cell lines are engineered to produce virus-induced enzymes (19), such as beta-galactosidase for the detection of herpes simplex viruses (HSV) (21).

This chapter describes the cell lines, reagents, stains, and media used in association with traditional tube and rapid viral culture techniques. Sample collection, specimen processing, and culture requirements for individual or classes of viruses are discussed in the appropriate chapters. The reader is referred to a recent comprehensive review of cell culture (16) and reference document M41-A from the Clinical Laboratory Standards Institute, which provides guidance for viral culture methods, including the applicable biosafety measures required (3). The fourth edition of the *Clinical Virology Manual* lists the virology services offered by federal reference laboratories (17) and state public health laboratories (12). This chapter's appendix lists the manufacturers and suppliers of cell lines, media, and reagents referred to throughout the chapter.

REAGENTS

■ Balanced salt solutions (Hanks' and Earle's)
Hanks' balanced salt solution and Earle's balanced salt solution (EBSS) are the two most commonly used formulations. However, Hanks' balanced salt solution has a better buffering capacity with CO_2 and EBSS has a better buffering capacity with air.

■ Density gradient media
Density gradient media or cell preparation tubes (BD, Franklin Lakes, NJ) are used for the isolation of peripheral blood mononuclear and polymorphonuclear lymphocytes. Separated cells can be used for the direct detection of viruses, such as cytomegalovirus (CMV), using immunostaining methods. Detailed descriptions of the specific uses of the gradient media or tubes and commercial sources are listed in chapter 76.

■ Dulbecco's PBS
Dulbecco's phosphate-buffered saline (PBS) is a maintenance-type medium containing sodium pyruvate and glucose.

■ **HEPES**

HEPES is an organic chemical-buffering agent that maintains physiological pH despite changes in carbon dioxide concentration, in contrast to bicarbonate buffers. HEPES is used in culture media.

■ **Formalin for cell culture preservation**

Formalin can be used to preserve viral CPE in cell culture for both educational and research purposes.

Earle's minimal essential medium	81 ml
Formaldehyde (37 to 40% concentration)	30 ml

Fill CPE-positive culture tubes with the solution, seal, and store at room temperature.

■ **HAD test**

Hemadsorption (HAD) refers to the attachment of red blood cells (RBCs) to infected cell culture monolayers. Influenza A and B, parainfluenza 1, 2, 3, and 4, and mumps viruses possess a surface hemagglutinin protein that is expressed on the cell surface of infected cells (18). The hemagglutinin protein binds red blood cells and adsorbs them to the infected cell membrane. HAD is performed when there is no visual CPE in culture or as a rapid screen for the presence of an orthomyxovirus or paramyxovirus in cell culture with a suspicious CPE. HAD testing is usually performed at 3 to 7 days of incubation or at the end of the incubation period (generally 10 to 14 days).

Test procedure

Variations may occur from laboratory to laboratory. Positive- and negative-control tubes must be included when the test is performed.

1. Wash fresh guinea pig (GP) RBCs two or three times in PBS weekly, discarding the supernatant after each centrifugation. Prepare a final 4 to 10% GP-RBC stock suspension in PBS and store at 4°C. The GP-RBC suspension should be used within 7 days.

2. Using the 10% GP-RBC stock suspension, prepare a 0.4% suspension prior to testing (0.4 ml of the 10% suspension plus 9.6 ml of PBS).

3. Remove the cell culture tube media and replace with 1 ml cold PBS. Add 0.2 ml of the 0.4% GP-RBC suspension to the tube cultures and incubate at 4°C for 30 min.

4. Shake each tube and examine the tubes at 40× and 100× lens objectives for HAD to the monolayer or hemagglutination in the supernatant. Place HAD-positive tubes in the incubator at 37°C for 1 h to release the adsorbed RBCs.

5. To detect parainfluenza virus type 4, place HAD-negative tubes at room temperature for 30 min and reexamine for HAD.

■ **Saline**

Normal or physiological saline (0.85%) is commonly used as a diluent.

■ **10× Gentamicin-amphotericin B solution**

Several different combinations of antibiotics and amphotericin B are added to transport media, may be added to specimens such as stool prior to culture inoculation, or are used in refeed medium to reduce both bacterial and fungal contamination. Commercial media containing the appropriate strength of antibiotics and amphotericin B can be purchased. Alternatively, a 10× gentamicin-amphotericin B solution can be added by

the laboratory at a ratio of 1:10 (0.1 ml of 10× gentamicin-amphotericin B to every 1.0 ml of specimen). After centrifugation of transport medium, the specimen supernatant is inoculated onto the appropriate cell line(s).

Eagle's minimum essential medium (EMEM)	89 ml
Gentamicin (50 mg/ml)	1 ml
Amphotericin B (250 μg/ml)	10 ml

Combine all ingredients and store frozen at −20 to −70°C in working-size aliquots.

■ **Trypsin solutions**

In lieu of scraping cells from tubes or wells, trypsin solutions are used to disburse cells from the monolayer for repassage and for immunostaining of cell-associated viruses such as adenovirus, CMV, and varicella-zoster virus (VZV). Trypsin solutions made with 2.5% PBS or Versene EDTA solution are commercially available.

■ **Tween 20-PBS**

Tween 20-PBS is used to wash cell monolayers prior to staining with fluorescent MAbs. Store at room temperature and discard if solution is turbid or a precipitate develops.

VIROLOGY STAINS

Direct examination of clinical specimens using several methods, such as slide touch preps from unfixed tissue, cytologic examination of tissue scrapings (e.g., Tzanck assay for HSV), smears from mucous membrane scrapings (e.g., HSV or VZV), or sample concentration by cytospin or centrifugation (e.g., respiratory viruses), can provide relatively rapid results. Slides can be prepared at the bedside (e.g., skin scrapings for HSV or VZV) or in the laboratory (e.g., respiratory swabs in transport or respiratory washings, aspirates, and secretions) and fixed with either 80 to 100% reagent grade acetone, 95% alcohol, or a cytological fixative, depending on the method. Traditional staining with hematoxylin and eosin and Wright-Giemsa stains has largely been replaced with MAb staining, but these stains can demonstrate characteristic cell morphologies such as the "owl's eye" nuclear inclusions indicative of CMV or the "smudge cells" or large basophilic inclusions consistent with adenovirus. Definitive identification of certain viruses or *Chlamydia* spp. can be directly determined in clinical samples when using MAbs labeled with fluorescein isothiocyanate, methylrhodamine isothiocyanate, or phycoerythrin with an Evans blue and/or propidium iodide counterstain. Results are available within 15 to 60 min, depending on the application. Procedures require minimal equipment (incubator, fluorescent microscope, pipettes, and centrifuge) and basic technical expertise to perform and interpret the results (reviewed in reference 16). Commercial reagents, commonly provided at working strength and quality tested to ensure sensitive and specific reactions, cleared by the Food and Drug Administration (FDA) for in vitro diagnostic testing, are listed in Table 1.

CELL CULTURES

Good manufacturing practices-regulated commercial vendors (see the appendix) provide tissue culture cells that are sterile, stabilized at the proper pH, thoroughly tested for susceptibility to common pathogens, and carefully screened to be free of potentially harmful endogenous agents, such as foamy viruses

TABLE 1 Commercially available DFA and IFA reagents for the detection of chlamydiae and viruses[a]

Target[b]	Use as per manufacturer	Manufacturer and test name
Chlamydia spp.	DSD	Trinity Bartels Chlamydia DFA kit
Chlamydia spp.	CC	Trinity Bartels Chlamydia CC FA kit
C. trachomatis	CC	Trinity Biotech MicroTrak *C. trachomatis* Culture Confirmation
C. trachomatis	DSD	Trinity Biotech MicroTrak *C. trachomatis* Direct Specimen Kit
Chlamydia spp.	CC	BioRad Pathfinder Chlamydia
C. trachomatis	DSD	BioRad Pathfinder *C. trachomatis* Direct Specimen
Chlamydia spp.	CC	Quidel/Diagnostic Hybrids D³ DFA Chlamydia
Chlamydia spp.	CC	Meridian Merifluor Chlamydia
Chlamydia spp.	DSD and CC	Remel Imagen Chlamydia
CMV	DSD	Argene CMV CINA Antigenemia Kit
CMV	DSD	Millipore Light Diagnostics CMV pp65 Antigenemia IFA Kit
CMV	CC	Millipore Light Diagnostics CMV DFA Kit
CMV	CC	Millipore Light Diagnostics CMV IFA Kit
CMV	CC	Quidel/Diagnostic Hybrids D³ DFA CMV IE Kit
CMV	CC	Trinity Bartels CMV IEA Indirect Antibody Test
CMV	DSD and CC	Trinity Bartels CMV Fluorescent Monoclonal Antibody Test
CMV	CC	Trinity Biotech MicroTrak CMV Culture Identification Test
Enterovirus	CC	Millipore Light Diagnostics Pan-Enterovirus IFA
Enterovirus groups	CC	Millipore Light Diagnostics Enterovirus Blends IFA
Enterovirus	CC	Quidel/Diagnostic Hybrids D3 IFA Kit
Enterovirus	CC	Remel Imagen Enterovirus
HSV-1/2 detection	DSD and CC	Millipore Light Diagnostics SimulFluor HSV 1/2 Kit
HSV-1/2 and VZV	DSD and CC	Millipore Light Diagnostics SimulFluor HSV/VZV
VZV	DSD and CC	Millipore Light Diagnostics VZV DFA Kit
HSV species	CC	Quidel/Diagnostic Hybrids D³ HSV ID
HSV-1/2 typing	CC	Quidel/Diagnostic Hybrids D³ HSV Typing
HSV-1/2 species	CC	Quidel/Diagnostic Hybrids ELVIS HSV Identification
HSV-1/2 typing	CC	Quidel/Diagnostic Hybrids ELVIS HSV ID and Typing
HSV-1/2 detection and typing	CC	Remel Imagen Herpes Simplex Virus
HSV detection	CC	Trinity Bartels HSV Fluorescent Monoclonal Antibody Test
HSV-1/2 detection and typing	CC	Trinity Bartels HSV ID and Typing Kit
HSV detection	CC	Trinity Biotech MicroTrak HSV Culture ID Test
HSV-1/2 detection and typing	CC	Trinity Biotech MicroTrak HSV1/HSV2 Culture ID/typing Test
HSV-1/2 detection and typing	DSD	Trinity MicroTrak HSV1/HSV2 Direct Specimen ID/Typing
VZV	DSD	Meridian Merifluor VZV
Respiratory panel B pool	DSD and CC	Bartels Respiratory Viral Pool
Respiratory panel B/identification	CC	Bartels Viral Respiratory Screening and Identification Kit
RSV	DSD	Bartels RSV Direct Fluorescent Antibody Test
Respiratory panel B	CC	Millipore Light Diagnostics SimulFluor Respiratory Screen
Respiratory panel B	CC	Millipore Light Diagnostics Respiratory Screen DFA Kit
Respiratory panel B	CC	Millipore Light Diagnostics Respiratory Screen/ID DFA Kit
Influenza viruses A and B	DSD and CC	Millipore Light Diagnostics SimulFluor Flu A/B
Parainfluenza viruses 1, 2/3	CC	Millipore Light Diagnostics SimulFluor Para 1, 2/3
Parainfluenza viruses 1, 2, 3, adenovirus (dual)	CC	Millipore Light Diagnostics SimulFluor Para 1, 2, 3, /Adeno
RSV/influenza virus A (dual)	DSD and CC	Millipore Light Diagnostics SimulFluor RSV/Flu A
RSV/parainfluenza virus 3 (dual)	CC	Millipore Light Diagnostics SimulFluor RSV/Para 3
Respiratory panel A/identification	DSD and CC	Quidel/Diagnostic Hybrids D³ FastPoint L-DFA Respiratory Virus ID
Influenza viruses A and B	DSD and CC	Quidel/Diagnostic Hybrids D³ FastPoint L-DFA Influenza A/B ID
RSV and HMPV	DSD and CC	Quidel/Diagnostic Hybrids D³ FastPoint L-DFA RSV/MPV ID
Respiratory panel B/identification	DSD and CC	Quidel/Diagnostic Hybrids D³ Ultra Screening and Typing Kit
Respiratory panel C (dual)	DSD and CC	Quidel/Diagnostic Hybrids D³ FluA/respiratory Pool Kit
Respiratory panel D (dual)	DSD and CC	Quidel/Diagnostic Hybrids D³ RSV/respiratory Pool Kit
2009 FluA H1N1	DSD and CC	Quidel/Diagnostic Hybrids D³ Ultra 2009 H1N1
HMPV	DSD and CC	Quidel/Diagnostic Hybrids D³ MPV
Respiratory panel B pool	DSD and CC	Remel Imagen Respiratory Screen

(*Continued on next page*)

TABLE 1 Commercially available DFA and IFA reagents for the detection of chlamydiae and viruses (*Continued*)

Target[b]	Use as per manufacturer	Manufacturer and test name
Influenza viruses A and B	DSD and CC	Remel Imagen Influenza A and B
Parainfluenza virus group/typing	DSD and CC	Remel Imagen Parainfluenza Group and Typing
RSV	DSD	Remel Imagen RSV

[a]Refer to manufacturers' websites for FDA and in vitro diagnostic status of reagents. Although uses for the reagents may be suggested on manufacturers' websites, all suggested applications may not have been validated by the manufacturer. Abbreviations: adeno, adenovirus; CC, culture confirmation; DSD, direct specimen detection; dual, a 2-fluorophore stain; FluA, influenza virus A; ID, identification; IF, immunofluorescence; Para, parainfluenza virus; IFA, indirect fluorescent antibody; HSV-1/2, HSV type 1 or 2.
[b]Respiratory panel A: adenovirus, influenza viruses A and B, parainfluenza viruses 1, 2, and 3, RSV, HMPV; respiratory panel B: adenovirus, influenza viruses A and B, parainfluenza viruses 1, 2, and 3, RSV; respiratory panel C: adenovirus, influenza viruses A and B, parainfluenza viruses 1, 2, and 3, and differential identification of RSV; respiratory panel D: adenovirus, influenza virus B, parainfluenza viruses 1, 2, and 3, RSV, and differential detection of influenza virus A.

and mycoplasmas that will interfere with the detection of the intended pathogens. Monolayered, ready-to-use cells can be produced at the vendor facility within a day or two of order, allowing the laboratory flexibility in the quantity and delivery date. Culture cells are provided in a number of ready-to-use formats including traditional 16- by 125-mm glass round-bottom screw-cap tubes, 1-dram vials (shell vials), flasks, or cluster trays. Ready-to-use cell cultures have a shelf life that is defined by the manufacturer in days or weeks, depending on the cell line or intended pathogen to be recovered. Some cells are also supplied fresh in flasks or frozen in cryovials and other containers, and may be stored for months or years at −70°C or below. Cryovials of frozen cells, with a shelf life of up to 6 months frozen, are supplied in a stated density and require the laboratory to subculture them to obtain monolayers in a flask, multiwell plate, shell vial, or tube, depending on the end application (9). Frozen cells can be used as needed and for unexpected situations such as unanticipated increases in the volume of samples, sudden viral outbreaks, or delays in cell shipments.

For laboratories that require special cells not readily available from commercial sources, specific cell types can sometimes be obtained from research laboratories or the American Type Culture Collection (ATCC, Manassas, VA) and then propagated within the user laboratory, starting with stock cultures supplied in a frozen format or as a flask of living cells. Once the cells are received, the laboratory must confirm sterility, absence of mycoplasma, and the appropriate passage or cell duplication number necessary to ensure sensitivity for viral or chlamydial isolation and must maintain the cultures in an environment that allows appropriate cellular replication and proper utility for the tests desired (7). A number of references offer detailed procedures for growing cells from frozen or fresh flasks (3, 15); such procedures are not addressed in this chapter.

To ensure the safety of the technical staff and to prevent cell culture contamination, the laboratory must follow strict procedures for the handling of biohazardous materials (3, 7). These include (i) the use of class II or higher biological safety cabinets with HEPA filters and, if possible, external venting, certified at least annually; (ii) facilities and procedures that are appropriate to the biohazard level of the viruses tested as defined by the Centers for Disease Control and Prevention (CDC, Atlanta, GA); and (iii) training and annual competency assessment of the laboratory staff. Virology benches and safety cabinets should be disinfected at least daily with a high-level disinfectant, such as 10% sodium hypochlorite (bleach).

■ **Traditional cell culture**

The common culturable human viral pathogens causing significant infections are readily detected by using a variety of cell cultures, including the established cell lines listed in Table 2. Cell lines may be primary (e.g., rhesus monkey kidney), used for one or two passages; diploid (e.g., human embryonic lung), used for 20 to 50 passages; or heteroploid (e.g., human epidermoid lung carcinoma), which can be passaged indefinitely. The laboratory must maintain sufficient cell types and incubate cell cultures for an optimal length of time and under the appropriate conditions that permit the recovery of the potential range of detectable viruses for all specimen types processed by the laboratory (3, 4). Cell culture systems can be variable and are susceptible to conditions that can adversely affect results, including cell culture source and lineage, age and condition of the monolayer, number of passages, shipping conditions, and the presence of contaminating agents. Therefore, quality control procedures and specific testing guidelines must be followed (2, 3, 7). Shipments of cell culture material should be observed microscopically to confirm that the confluency of the monolayer is appropriate (75% to 90%), the cells are attached to the substratum, cell appearance is typical, and no evidence of contaminating viruses is present, usually signified by cytopathic appearance of the cells before use. Cell culture media should be free of contamination (clear) and near a neutral pH (salmon pink in color). If the laboratory introduces additives (e.g., L-glutamine or antibiotics) to commercial media, the final solution must be checked for sterility, pH, growth promotion, and the absence of toxicity to cells. The lot number and date of use for all media, buffers, reagents, and additives should also be recorded. Tubes of cell cultures should be stored in a slanted position with the cell monolayer covered by the medium. Tissue culture cells should ideally be inoculated within 7 days of receipt (8 to 10 days of seeding) for optimal propagation of cell-dependent organisms or demonstration of cytotoxicity. The laboratory should retain all documentation provided by the manufacturer, including cell culture records with cell types, source, passage number, and age of cells. Uninoculated lot-matched tubes, cluster plates, or shell vials that are incubated, maintained, and observed in the same manner as inoculated tissue cells serve as negative controls for CPE, toxicity, exogenous contamination, and procedures such as direct immunofluorescence (DFA), HAD, and hemagglutination. Daily inoculation of positive controls to monitor traditional tube culture performance is not routinely performed. However, commonly isolated viruses may be used to perform quality control on cell lines when new shipments are received in the laboratory, and they are a source of positive-control material for detection and confirmation methods such as HAD and DFA.

With the exception of a few viruses such as CMV, or when viruses are present at very low titers, the time to detection by traditional tube culture methods is generally between

TABLE 2 List of cell lines and virus susceptibility profiles

Cell line	Origin	Virus(es)[c]
A-549	Human lung carcinoma	Adenovirus, HSV, influenza virus, measles virus, mumps virus, parainfluenza virus, poliovirus, RSV, rotavirus, VZV
AGMK[a]	African green monkey kidney	Influenza virus, parainfluenza virus, enteroviruses
AP61	Mosquito	Arboviruses
B95 or B95a	EBV-transformed lymphoblastoid	Measles virus, mumps virus
BGMK	Buffalo green monkey kidney	*Chlamydia* spp., HSV, coxsackie B virus, poliovirus
C6/36	Mosquito	Arboviruses
Caco-2	Human epithelial colorectal adenocarcinoma	HCoV (NL63)
CV-1	African green monkey kidney	HSV, measles virus, mumps virus, rotavirus, SV40, VZV, some encephalitis viruses
Graham 293	Human embryonic kidney transformed with adenovirus type 5	Enteric adenoviruses
H292		Adenovirus, coxsackie B virus, echovirus, HSV, mumps virus, parainfluenza virus, poliovirus, RSV, rubella virus
HeLa	Human cervix adenocarcinoma	Adenovirus, coxsackie B virus, CMV, echovirus, HSV, poliovirus, rhinovirus, vesicular stomatitis virus (Indian strain), VZV
HeLa 229	Human cervix adenocarcinoma	Adenovirus, *Chlamydia* spp., CMV, echovirus, HSV, poliovirus, rhinovirus, vesicular stomatitis virus (Indian strain), VZV
HEL	Human embryonic lung	Adenovirus, CMV, echovirus, HSV, poliovirus, rhinovirus, vesicular stomatitis virus (Indian strain), VZV
HEK	Human embryonic kidney	Adenovirus, BK virus, enterovirus, HSV, measles virus, mumps virus, rhinovirus
HEK 293	Human embryonic kidney transformed with adenovirus Type 5	Enteric adenoviruses
HEp-2	Human epidermoid carcinoma	Adenovirus, *Chlamydia* spp., coxsackie B virus, HSV, measles virus, parainfluenza virus, poliovirus, RSV
HNK	Human neonatal kidney	Adenovirus, HSV, VZV
Hs27 (HFF)[b]	Human foreskin fibroblast	Adenovirus, CMV, echovirus, HSV, mumps virus, poliovirus, rhinovirus, VZV
HuH-7	Human hepatocyte	HCoVs (OC43, 229E)
LLC-MK2	Original, rhesus monkey kidney	Arboviruses (some), enteroviruses (including coxsackie virus groups A and B, echoviruses, polioviruses), HMPV (NL-63), influenza virus, mumps virus, parainfluenza virus, poxvirus groups, rhinovirus
Mv1Lu	Mink lung	CMV, HSV, influenza virus
McCoy[a]	Mouse fibroblast	*Chlamydia* spp., HSV
MDCK	Madin-Darby canine kidney	Adenovirus (some types), coxsackie virus, influenza virus, reovirus
MNA	Mouse neuroblastoma	Rabies virus
MRC-5	Human fetal lung	Adenovirus, coxsackie A virus, CMV, echovirus, HSV, influenza virus, mumps virus, poliovirus, rhinovirus, RSV, VZV, cytotoxicity for *C. difficile*
NCI-H292	Human pulmonary mucoepidermoid	Adenovirus, BK polyomavirus, enteroviruses (most), HSV, measles virus, reoviruses, rhinoviruses (most), RSV, vaccinia virus
RD	Human rhabdomyosarcoma	Adenovirus, coxsackie A virus, echovirus, HSV, poliovirus
RK[a]	Rabbit kidney	HSV, paramyxoviruses
RhMK[a]	Rhesus monkey kidney	Arboviruses, coxsackie A and B viruses, echoviruses, influenza virus, parainfluenza virus, measles virus, mumps virus, polioviruses
SF	Human foreskin	Adenovirus, coxsackie A virus, CMV, echovirus, HSV, poliovirus, VZV
Vero	African green monkey kidney	Adenovirus, arboviruses (some), *Chlamydia* spp., coxsackie B virus, HSV, HMPV, measles virus, mumps virus, poliovirus type 3, rotavirus, rubella virus
Vero E6	African green monkey kidney	Adenovirus, coxsackie B virus, HSV, measles virus, mumps virus, poliovirus type 3, rotavirus, rubella virus, SARS-CoV
Vero 76	African green monkey kidney	Adenovirus, coxsackie B virus, HSV, measles virus, mumps virus, poliovirus type 3, rotavirus, rubella virus, West Nile virus
WI-38	Human lung	Adenovirus, coxsackie A virus, CMV, echovirus, HSV, influenza virus, mumps virus, poliovirus, rhinovirus, RSV, VZV

[a]Primary cell cultures.
[b]Available as fresh and frozen ReadyCells (Quidel/Diagnostic Hybrids, Inc.).
[c]Abbreviations: HCoV, human coronavirus; EBV, Epstein-Barr virus; SARS-CoV, severe acute respiratory syndrome coronavirus.

1 and 7 days of inoculation (15). The standard approach for detecting viral proliferation is the microscopic examination of the unstained cell culture monolayer for the presence of CPE. The presence of a virus is indicated by degenerative changes in monolayer cells, including shrinking, swelling, rounding of cells, clustering, and formation of syncytia, or by complete destruction of the monolayer. Identification of the virus is then based on the CPE characteristics, the cell line involved, the time to detection, specimen type, and confirmation, generally by staining with virus-specific MAbs. Alternatively, for the identification of viruses for which MAbs may not be available, molecular methods or ancillary traditional testing (e.g., acid resistance for rhinoviruses) must be performed. In addition, for certain viruses (influenza, parainfluenza, and mumps viruses) that do not always demonstrate CPE, HAD testing may be done (18).

■ Centrifugation-enhanced rapid cell culture

Centrifugation-enhanced inoculation using cells grown on coverslips in 1-dram shell vials and pre-CPE detection of viral antigen in the monolayer cells by use of MAbs was first described for the detection of Chlamydia trachomatis. This technique was adapted for the routine detection of CMV using MRC-5 shell vials and staining with MAbs directed against early CMV proteins (8). This pioneering method has reduced the time for virus detection from as long as 10 to 30 days to 16 to 72 h. The important factor in reducing the time to detection is the stressing of the monolayer during centrifugation (11). This process has been shown to increase cell proliferation, decrease cell generation times, alter cell metabolism, increase cell longevity, and activate specific genes.

Rapid cell culture is now commonly used for the detection of Chlamydia spp. CMV, enteroviruses, VZV, HSV, mumps viruses, and the main respiratory viruses (adenovirus, human metapneumovirus [HMPV], influenza A and B viruses, parainfluenza viruses 1, 2, and 3, and respiratory syncytial virus [RSV]) (reviewed in reference 16). Centrifugation-enhanced rapid cell culture can be used with standard cell lines (Table 2) and has been adapted for use with cocultivated cells for the detection of respiratory viruses, HSV, and VZV (Table 3) (1, 6, 10) and with genetically

engineered cells for the detection of HSV and enteroviruses (Table 3) (14, 20). Identification of the viral pathogen when using centrifuge-enhanced rapid cell culture is not dependent on the visualization of CPE. Instead, the virus is detected either by "blind staining" with phycoerythrin, peroxidase, or fluorescein isothiocyanate-labeled virus-specific MAbs or by virus-specific induction of enzymes that are detected by using substrates such as beta-galactosidase (14, 20, 21). A significant benefit of using cocultivated cells is that they allow the identification of multiple viruses from a single shell vial or cluster tray well, rather than having to use multiple shell vials to cover the range of viruses that the laboratory may wish to detect in a particular sample type. One shell vial can be substituted for four different tube cell cultures that require much longer (10 to 14 days) to identify fewer subspecies of the group.

Since rapid detection formats are not based on the detection of CPE but use blind staining for either single viruses or multiple viruses, positive- and negative-control slides are required for each day of patient testing. When a single-culture system detects multiple viruses, the detection reagents must be validated for all targets (including any pooled MAb reagents) upon receipt in the laboratory (4, 7). Virus isolate controls can be tested daily and virus types rotated so that during the course of 1 week, the lots of cells and reagents have been tested against all the routinely isolated viruses.

■ ELVIS

ELVIS (enzyme-linked virus-inducible system) (Quidel/Diagnostic Hybrids) uses a genetically engineered cell line (BHKICP6LacZ) that was first described by Stabell and Olivo (21). The promoter sequence of the HSV UL97 gene and the Escherichia coli lacZ gene were used to stably transform a baby hamster kidney cell line. When the cell line is infected with HSV, the virion-associated transactivator protein VP16 and other transactivating factors such as ICP0 strongly transactivate the UL97 promoter, which in turn activates the lacZ gene, resulting in high levels of beta-galactosidase activity. Addition of 4-chloro-3-indol-β-D-galactopyranoside (X-Gal) turns a colorless substrate to blue, indicating the presence of HSV-infected cells. If

TABLE 3 List of cocultured cell lines and virus susceptibility profiles[a]

Cell mixture[b]	Cell types	Virus(es)
R-Mix[c]	Mv1Lu (mink lung)	CMV, HSV, influenza virus, SARS-CoV
	A549 (human lung carcinoma)	Adenovirus, HSV, influenza virus, measles virus, mumps virus, parainfluenza virus, poliovirus, rotavirus, RSV, VZV
R-Mix Too[c]	MDCK (Madin-Darby canine kidney)	Influenza virus
	A549 (human lung carcinoma)	Adenovirus, HSV, influenza virus, measles virus, mumps virus, parainfluenza virus, poliovirus, rotavirus, RSV, VZV
H&V-Mix	CV-1 (African green monkey kidney)	HSV, measles virus, mumps virus, rotavirus, SV40, VZV, some encephalitis viruses
	MRC-5 (human fetal lung)	Adenovirus, CMV, echovirus, HSV, influenza virus, mumps virus, poliovirus, rhinovirus, RSV, VZV
Super E-Mix[c]	sBGMK (buffalo green monkey kidney) (with degradation activating factor)	Chlamydia, HSV, coxsackie A and B viruses, echovirus, poliovirus
	A549 (human lung carcinoma)	Adenovirus, HSV, influenza virus, measles virus, mumps virus, parainfluenza virus, poliovirus, RSV, rotavirus, VZV
ELVIS	Transfected baby hamster kidney HSV UL97 promoter/E. coli lacZ gene	HSV-1, HSV-2

[a]Abbreviations: SARS-CoV, severe acute respiratory syndrome coronavirus.
[b]Available from Quidel/Diagnostic Hybrids, Inc.
[c]Available as both fresh and frozen cells which do not require propagation but are ready to use.

HSV typing is required, a fluorescence-labeled MAb that specifically detects HSV-2 and a nonlabeled MAb that specifically binds to HSV-1 are incorporated in the staining procedure. If the infected (blue) cells are not detected with the HSV-2 MAb, then the monolayers are stained with anti-mouse fluorescence-labeled Ab to detect the HSV-1 MAb. ELVIS is completed within 16 to 24 hours for both positive and negative results (14, 20).

■ Cell cytotoxicity assays

Tissue culture assays using cell types such as human foreskin fibroblasts (HFF), MRC-5 cells, and Vero epithelioid cells are commonly used for the detection of toxin-producing strains of *Clostridium difficile*. Cell culture testing for the presence of *C. difficile* cytotoxin has demonstrated improved sensitivity compared to *C. difficile* toxin A/B enzyme immunoassays. Enteroviruses can cause a CPE similar to that caused by *C. difficile* toxin; therefore, the procedure includes the use of a *C. difficile* antitoxin to *C. difficile* toxin, which creates a more specific assay. Fecal filtrate is diluted, bacteria are removed by membrane filtration, and the tissue culture cells are exposed to the patient material, with and without *C. difficile* antitoxin. Test wells without *C. difficile* antitoxin demonstrating CPE within 12 to 48 hours are presumed positive for *C. difficile* toxin if the control well with *C. difficile* antitoxin shows no evidence of CPE. As little as 1 picogram of toxin can cause a visible change in cells over a period of hours up to 1 to 2 days.

CELL CULTURE MEDIA

Transport Media and Collection Swabs

An important consideration in using cell culture is ensuring collection of cellular material and maintaining the viability of the organisms from the time of sample collection to inoculation in cell culture. Therefore, time to processing, transport temperature, and the use of transport media need to be evaluated for each sample type. Cell culture media with additives, such as antibiotics and fungicidal agents to inhibit microbial growth, are used to maintain the viability of viruses during sample transport. Transport media may be specific for virus isolation (viral transport media) or also allow the isolation of *Chlamydia*, *Mycoplasma*, and *Ureaplasma* (universal transport media). The types of transport media, uses and components, collection procedures, and swabs are detailed in chapter 76.

■ Growth medium with 10% fetal bovine serum

Cell culture media are an important part of the production and maintenance of cells. Cell culture stocks are generally grown in a richer medium than what is used for the maintenance of the cells. The higher level of serum or protein in growth medium rapidly enhances cell growth and is used for a day or more before it is replaced by maintenance medium. Standard growth medium consists of EMEM with EBSS and supplemented with 10% heat-inactivated fetal bovine serum (FBS), one or more antimicrobials (gentamicin, penicillin, streptomycin, vancomycin, and/or amphotericin B), and HEPES buffer. Since simian viruses are endogenous to primary monkey kidney cell cultures, media that contain simian virus 5 (SV5) and SV40 antisera are available (ViroMed, Minnetonka, MN, and Quidel/Diagnostic Hybrids, Inc.).

■ Maintenance medium

Maintenance medium contains nutrients and buffers that protect the cells during the stage when rapid growth is not desired but healthy monolayers must be controlled for inoculation of specimens and recovery of the etiologic agent. Seeded flasks, tubes, trays, or shell vials may be fed with medium multiple times prior to release from the vendor to ensure the cells are growing according to specifications and arrive at the user site ready to be used. At the user site, most cells remain stable for a period of a few days without needing changing of the medium with which they were shipped. However, before use, it is common to remove the shipping medium and add a maintenance medium such as 2% FBS EMEM or 0% FBS Hanks', MEM, or R-Mix refeed medium for those viruses that would be inhibited by serum proteins (myxoviruses and paramyxoviruses). Trypsin and antimicrobial agents can be added if indicated. Other refeeding media for viruses include E-Mix refeed medium and 5% or 10% FBS growth medium. Tube cell cultures may require refeeding on a weekly basis; however, the use of shell vial or cluster plate technology usually reduces refeeding to one time just prior to inoculation. Commercial media with and without enrichments are available, such as PBS, L-glutamine, trypsin, and bactericidal and fungicidal agents.

■ *Chlamydia* isolation medium

Some cell-dependent bacteria such as *C. trachomatis* require the cell host to restrict protein synthesis, thus allowing the infecting microbe to replicate more easily. For this reason, media used for propagation of *Chlamydia* spp. in cell culture commonly contain cycloheximide, a protein synthesis inhibitor. Isolation media for *Chlamydia* sp. detection using shell vials generally contain EMEM with EBSS, supplemented with 10% FBS, HEPES, glucose, nonessential amino acids, antibiotics (cycloheximide, gentamicin, or streptomycin), and amphotericin B.

■ EMEM pH 2–3

Rhinoviruses require a lower temperature of incubation than many other pathogenic human viruses, and their characteristic CPE can be confused with enterovirus CPE, which has a similar appearance. MAbs are not available to identify rhinoviruses, although such MAbs are being developed commercially. For this reason, the ability of acid solutions to neutralize rhinoviruses, thus reducing viral titers, can be used to differentiate rhinoviruses from enteroviruses, which are not sensitive to low pH. EMEM pH 2–3 (ViroMed) can be used to test for acid sensitivity testing.

■ RPMI 1640 medium

RPMI medium consists of glucose, essential amino acids, other amino acids, vitamins, HEPES buffer, antibiotics (such as penicillin and streptomycin), and phenol red as an indicator. This enriched medium is used for lymphocyte cell cultivation and culture of HIV.

Proprietary Media

■ CMV TurboTreat medium

CMV TurboTreat pretreatment medium (Quidel/Diagnostic Hybrids) consists of EMEM with EBSS without phenol red, 10% FBS, HEPES, and gentamicin. Pretreatment of Mv1Lu, R-Mix, and MRC-5 cultures overnight, prior to specimen addition, enhances the recovery of CMV (23).

■ **ELVIS replacement medium**

ELVIS replacement medium is used with the ELVIS test system (Quidel/Diagnostic Hybrids) and is comprised of EMEM, FBS, streptomycin, and amphotericin B.

■ **R-Mix refeed and rinse medium**

R-Mix refeed and rinse medium is used with R-Mix fresh and ReadyCell culture systems (Quidel/Diagnostic Hybrids) and is a defined serum-free medium with trypsin, penicillin, and streptomycin.

APPENDIX
Sources of Virology Reagents, Stains, Media, and Cell Lines

American Type Culture Collection
Manassas, VA 20110
http://www.atcc.org

BD Biosciences
Franklin Lakes, NJ 07417
http://www.bdbiosciences.com

BioRad Laboratories
Hercules, CA 94547
http://www.bio-rad.com

Cambrex Corporation (BioWhittaker Cell Products)
East Rutherford, NJ 07073
http://www.cambrex.com

Meridian Biosciences
Cincinnati, OH 45244
http://www.meridianbioscience.com

Lonza, Inc.
Allendale, NJ 07401
http://www.lonza.com

Millipore (Chemicon)
Billerica, MA 01821
http://www.millipore.com

Quidel Corporation/Diagnostic Hybrids
Athens, OH 45701
http://www.quidel.com

Remel
Lenexa, KS 66215
http://www.remelinc.com

Trinity Biotech (Bartels, MicroTrak)
Carlsbad, CA 92008
http://www.trinitybiotech.com

Trinity Biotech (Bartels)
Bray, County Wicklow, Ireland
http://www.trinitybiotech.com

ViroMed Laboratories
Minnetonka, MN 55343
http://www.viromed.com

REFERENCES

1. **Barenfanger, J., C. Drake, T. Mueller, T. Troutt, J. O'Brien, and K. Guttman.** 2001. R-Mix cells are faster, at least as sensitive and marginally more costly than conventional cell lines for the detection of respiratory viruses. *J. Clin. Virol.* **22:**101–110.
2. **Clinical and Laboratory Standards Institute.** 2006. *Quality Assurance for Commercially Prepared Microbiologic Culture Media. CLSI Document M22-A3.* Clinical and Laboratory Standards Institute, Wayne, PA.
3. **Clinical and Laboratory Standards Institute.** 2006. *Viral Culture. CLSI Document M41-A.* Clinical and Laboratory Standards Institute, Wayne, PA.
4. **College of American Pathologists.** 2010. *Laboratory Improvement: Laboratory Accreditation Program Checklists.* College of American Pathologists, Chicago, IL.
5. **Enders, J. F., T. H. Weller, and F. C. Robbins.** 1949. Cultivation of the Lansing strain of poliomyelitis virus in cultures of various human embryonic tissues. *Science* **109:**85–87.
6. **Fong, C. K. Y., M. K. Lee, and B. P. Griffith.** 2000. Evaluation of R-Mix FreshCells in shell vials for detection of respiratory viruses. *J. Clin. Microbiol.* **38:**4660–4662.
7. **Ginocchio, C. C.** 2009. Quality assurance in clinical virology, p. 3–17. *In* S. Spector, R. L. Hodinka, S. A. Young, and D. L. Wiedbrauk (ed.), *Clinical Virology Manual*, 4th ed. ASM Press, Washington, DC.
8. **Gleaves, C. A., T. F. Smith, E. A. Shuster, and G. R. Pearson.** 1984. Rapid detection of cytomegalovirus in MRC-5 cells inoculated with urine specimens by using low-speed centrifugation and monoclonal antibody to an early antigen. *J. Clin. Microbiol.* **19:**917–919.
9. **Huang, Y. T., H. Yan, Y. Sun, J. A. Jollick, Jr., and H. Baird.** 2002. Cryopreserved cell monolayers for rapid detection of herpes simplex virus and influenza virus. *J. Clin. Microbiol.* **40:**4301–4303.
10. **Huang, Y. T., S. Hite, V. Duane, and H. Yan.** 2002. CV-1 and MRC-5 mixed cells for simultaneous detection of herpes simplex viruses and varicella zoster virus in skin lesions. *J. Clin. Virol.* **24:**37–43.
11. **Hughes, J. D.** 1993. Physical and chemical methods for enhancing rapid detection of viruses and other agents. *Clin. Microbiol. Rev.* **6:**150–175.
12. **Humes, R.** 2009. State public health laboratory virology services, p. 663–671. *In* S. Spector, R. L. Hodinka, S. A. Young, and D. L. Wiedbrauk (ed.), *Clinical Virology Manual*, 4th ed. ASM Press, Washington, DC.
13. **Landry, M. L.** 2009. Primary isolation of viruses, p. 36–51. *In* S. Spector, R. L. Hodinka, S. A. Young, and D. L. Wiedbrauk (ed.), *Clinical Virology Manual*, 4th ed. ASM Press, Washington, DC.
14. **LaRocco, M. T.** 2000. Evaluation of an enzyme-linked viral inducible system for the rapid detection of herpes simplex virus. *Eur. J. Clin. Microbiol. Infect. Dis.* **19:**233–235.
15. **Leland, D. S.** 1996. *Clinical Virology.* W. B. Saunders, Philadelphia, PA.
16. **Leland, D. S., and C. C. Ginocchio.** 2007. Role of cell culture for virus detection in the age of technology. *Clin. Microbiol. Rev.* **20:**49–78.
17. **Mahy, B. W. J.** 2009. Virology services offered by the federal reference laboratories at the Centers for Disease Control and Prevention, p. 661–662. *In* S. Spector, R. L. Hodinka, S. A. Young, and D. L. Wiedbrauk (ed.), *Clinical Virology Manual*, 4th ed. ASM Press, Washington, DC.
18. **Minnich, L. L., and G. C. Ray.** 1987. Early testing of cell cultures for detection of hemadsorbing viruses. *J. Clin. Microbiol.* **25:**421–422.
19. **Olivo, P. D.** 1996. Transgenic cell lines for detection of animal viruses. *Clin. Microbiol. Rev.* **9:**321–334.
20. **Proffitt, M. R., and S. A. Schindler.** 1995. Rapid detection of HSV with an enzyme-linked virus inducible system™ (ELVIS™) employing a genetically modified cell line. *Clin. Diagn. Virol.* **4:**175–182.
21. **Stabell, E. C., and P. D. Olivo.** 1992. Isolation of a cell line for rapid and sensitive histochemical assay for the detection of herpes simplex virus. *J. Virol. Methods* **38:**195–204.
22. **Stinehardt, E., C. Israeli, and R. Lambert.** 1913. Studies on the cultivation of the virus of vaccinia. *J. Infect. Dis.* **13:**204–300.
23. **Yang, W., S. Hite, and Y. T. Huang.** 2005. Enhancement of cytomegalovirus detection in mink lung cells using CMV TurboTreat™. *J. Clin. Virol.* **34:**125–128.

Algorithms for Detection and Identification of Viruses

MARIE LOUISE LANDRY, ANGELA M. CALIENDO, CHRISTINE C. GINOCCHIO, YI-WEI TANG, AND ALEXANDRA VALSAMAKIS

78

Virology is a dynamic field that in recent decades has moved from the periphery to the mainstream of clinical laboratory practice. When the first edition of the *Manual of Clinical Microbiology* was published in 1970, diagnostic virology was practiced in a limited number of laboratories, primarily in public health, research, and academic settings. Methods focused on conventional cell cultures, classical serologic techniques, and light and electron microscopy. Time to result was slow, and it was often said the patient was dead or better by the time the result was received. Over the intervening years, diagnostic advances have transformed the field by allowing accurate results in a clinically useful time frame. These technology improvements include enzyme immunoassays for antigen and antibody detection, immunoglobulin M assays, monoclonal antibodies for rapid identification of culture isolates, and direct detection in clinical specimens by immunofluorescence, shell vial centrifugation cultures, and nucleic acid amplification techniques.

Since the last edition of this *Manual*, dramatic growth has occurred in the development and implementation of clinically useful molecular methods, which are both rapid and sensitive, can be largely automated, and can detect and quantify viruses not amenable to routine culture. The greater variety of instruments for nucleic acid extraction and real-time amplification and detection and the increasing availability of commercial reagents and FDA-cleared kits, including some requiring minimal molecular expertise, have facilitated this trend. Novel detection methods have permitted the diagnosis of multiple respiratory viruses in a single multiplex PCR test. Quantitative monitoring of viral load in blood has become more widely applied due to implementation of real-time PCR techniques. Increasingly, molecular assays are becoming the standard of care for the diagnosis of many viral infections, for predicting patient outcomes, and for monitoring response to antiviral therapies.

In addition to the advantages of molecular testing, some pitfalls are also becoming apparent as the tests are more widely used. For example, the sensitivities and specificities designed to detect the same virus can vary significantly among laboratories, especially for laboratory-developed tests. In addition, despite targeting conserved regions of the genome, strain variability and mutations can lead to under-quantification of viral load, or even falsely negative results. Furthermore, as tests become more sensitive, low levels of clinically irrelevant or nonviable viruses may be detected and can be misleading to clinicians. Similarly, interpreting the clinical relevance of multiple viral pathogens in the same sample when relative quantification is not available is problematic. Requirements for staff training, test validation, and quality control can also be challenging.

At the other end of the spectrum has been the proliferation of rapid tests requiring minimal or no equipment or reagent additions. These tests often employ immunochromatographic detection for viral antigen or antibody and can be used at the point of care for immediate impact on clinical decisions. However, the 2009 novel H1N1 influenza pandemic has revealed the need to improve the sensitivity of point-of-care rapid antigen tests.

Thus, with progress have come new challenges. Laboratories need to choose which tests to offer. Selecting the appropriate test will depend on the virus(es) sought, sample site, clinical presentation, clinical purpose (e.g., screening, confirmation, diagnosis, or monitoring), patient characteristics, and disease prevalence. Performance characteristics, staff expertise, and cost will also impact that choice. Laboratories must recognize the uses and also the limitations of each test in order to guide clinicians in interpreting the results. This *Manual* should serve as a key resource for accomplishing these tasks. The methods available for each virus differ and continue to evolve. Table 1 provides a concise overview for each virus group; however, the reader is referred to the specific chapters for more detailed discussions.

While it can be daunting for laboratories to acquire and maintain expertise in the variety of test methods now available, it is extremely gratifying to witness the impact of state-of-the-art testing on patient care. As we move forward, it is critical that laboratorians communicate with each other to address problems, including the optimization and standardization of methods, and, in addition, encourage input and feedback from clinicians. Due to the speed of methodological change and the continuing discovery of new viruses and new therapies, keeping abreast of the most recent literature is strongly recommended.

TABLE 1 Methods for detection and identification of viruses[a]

Virus(es)	Applicability[b] of:					Comments
	Virus isolation	Antigen detection	Nucleic acid detection	Electron microscopy	Antibody detection	
Adenoviruses	A	A	A	C	C	IFA, culture, and NAAT widely used for respiratory specimens. NAAT used to monitor viral load in compromised hosts. Rapid antigen assays used for ocular and enteric adenoviruses.
Arboviruses	C	D	B	C	A	Serology is primary diagnostic method. Most arboviruses are readily cultured; isolation of some agents may require BSL-3 or -4 facilities.
Bocaviruses	D	D	A	D	C	NAAT is the only test available for diagnosis. Clinical relevance awaits further investigation.
Coronaviruses	C	C	A	C	B	NAAT becoming more widely used for respiratory CoV as part of multiplex panels. Positive SARS-CoV NAAT and antibody results require confirmation by a reference laboratory.
Cytomegalovirus	A	A	A	C	B	Shell vial culture rapid and sensitive for nonblood specimens. Quantitative NAAT and pp65 antigenemia used to assess risk of disease and response to therapy. Serology primarily used to determine prior infection.
Enteroviruses and parechoviruses	A	D	A	D	D	Enterovirus NAAT preferred for CNS infection. Parechovirus NAAT required for optimal detection of infection.
Epstein-Barr virus	D	B	A	D	A	Serology is test of choice for routine diagnosis. NAAT useful for virus-related tumors. Quantitative NAAT useful for monitoring viral load in blood of transplant recipients. IHC or ISH can be used on tumor biopsy samples.
Filoviruses and arenaviruses	A	A	A	C	B	Testing confined to specialized laboratories. Antigen and NAAT key to rapid diagnosis. BSL-4 facility needed for culture, except for LCM. Patients with severe disease may die without developing antibody. LCM diagnosed primarily by serology.
Hantaviruses	C	B	A	C	A	Testing confined to specialized laboratories. Serology and NAAT equally useful for diagnosis. IHC used in fatal cases. BSL-4 facility needed for culture. Isolation difficult.
Hendra and Nipah viruses	B	B	A	C	A	Testing confined to specialized laboratories. Serology and NAAT equally useful for diagnosis. IHC used in fatal cases. BSL-4 facility needed for culture. Patients with severe disease may die without developing antibody.
Hepatitis A virus	D	C	C	D	A	Serology is standard diagnostic test. False-positive IgM problematic in low-prevalence areas.
Hepatitis B virus	D	A	A	C	A	Detection of specific viral antigens and antibodies allows diagnosis and monitoring of the course of infection. NAAT used to monitor therapy and determine genotype.

(Continued on next page)

TABLE 1 *(Continued)*

Virus(es)	Applicability[b] of:					Comments
	Virus isolation	Antigen detection	Nucleic acid detection	Electron microscopy	Antibody detection	
Hepatitis C virus	D	D	A	D	A	Serology is used for diagnosis. Qualitative NAAT used to confirm active infection. Quantitative NAAT used to monitor response to therapy. Genotyping helps determine duration of therapy.
Hepatitis D virus	D	B	B	D	A	Testing confined to reference laboratories. Diagnosis is relevant only in the presence of hepatitis B virus infection. IHC of biopsy tissue useful for diagnosis.
Hepatitis E virus	D	D	B	D	A	Serology is standard diagnostic test. False-positive IgM problematic in low-prevalence areas. NAAT specific for acute infection but lacks sensitivity.
HSV	A	A	A	C	B	IFA used for rapid detection in skin/mucous membrane lesions or tissue specimens. NAAT is test of choice for CNS infection and used for other sample types as well. Serology, including HSV-2-specific serology, used to determine prior infection.
Human herpesviruses 6 and 7	C	C	A	C	B	NAAT is test of choice for diagnosis. MAbs available to differentiate virus isolates and for IHC. Serology can document primary infection in children.
Human herpesvirus 8	D	B	B	C	A	Serology used to identify infected persons; sensitivity and specificity hampered by difficulty in setting cutoff values. NAAT of blood may be useful for monitoring KS risk. IHC more specific than NAAT for KS.
Human immunodeficiency virus	C	C	A	D	A	Serology is primary diagnostic method; rapid antibody testing becoming more widely available. Proviral DNA and plasma RNA tests used to diagnose neonatal infection. Quantitative RNA tests used to guide therapy and monitor response.
Human metapneumovirus	B	A	A	C	D	NAAT is test of choice for diagnosis. IFA and shell vial culture rapid and fairly sensitive. Conventional culture difficult.
HTLV	C	D	B	D	A	Serology is primary diagnostic method. NAAT useful for virus identification in HTLV Western blot-positive but untypeable specimens.
Influenza viruses	A	A	A	D	B	Rapid antigen tests widely used but suboptimal in sensitivity and specificity; IFA and rapid culture more sensitive. NAAT most sensitive, with increasing availability. Serology useful for epidemiological studies or retrospective diagnosis.
Measles viruses	B	B	C	C	A	Serology most useful for diagnosis and determination of immunity. Isolation useful only if attempted early (prodromal period to 4 days postrash).

(Continued on next page)

TABLE 1 Methods for detection and identification of viruses[a] *(Continued)*

Virus(es)	Applicability[b] of:					Comments
	Virus isolation	Antigen detection	Nucleic acid detection	Electron microscopy	Antibody detection	
Mumps virus	A	C	B	C	A	Serology used most commonly for diagnosis and determination of immunity. NAAT useful for diagnosing outbreaks among vaccinated individuals.
Noroviruses	D	C	B	B	D	NAAT challenging due to strain variability. Reagents for antigen detection not commercially available.
Parainfluenza viruses	A	A	A	D	C	IFA most common rapid detection method. NAAT more sensitive than isolation; usually performed as part of multiplex panel.
Papillomaviruses	D	D	A	C	D	NAAT is test of choice for detection and genotype differentiation. Cytopathology useful for diagnosis. Serologic diagnosis of past exposure not available.
Parvoviruses	D	C	A	C	A	Serology used to diagnose B19 infection in immunocompetent individuals. NAAT is the test of choice for exposed fetuses and immunocompromised hosts.
Polyomaviruses	C	B	A	B	C	NAAT is the test of choice, but genetic variability can lead to falsely low or negative results. JC virus DNA detection in CSF useful for presumptive diagnosis of PML. BK virus DNA quantification in plasma or urine used for preemptive diagnosis of PVAN. IHC and EM useful for biopsy tissues.
Poxviruses	A	C	A	A	A	EM is most useful routine test. NAAT allows virus inactivation and rapid detection. Smallpox virus isolation requires BSL-3 or -4 and should be attempted only in WHO Collaborating Centres. Vaccinia virus requires BSL-2 and grows readily in cell culture.
Rabies virus	B	A	B	C	B	IFA performed on fresh and frozen tissue at the CDC. Serology used to confirm immunization status and confirm exposure in absence of RIG. NAAT most useful for non-CNS samples when fresh CNS tissue not available.
Respiratory syncytial virus	A	A	A	C	C	Rapid antigen tests, especially IFA, more sensitive than culture. NAAT most sensitive but not yet widely used. Serology useful only for epidemiological studies.
Rhinoviruses	A	C	A	D	D	NAAT much more sensitive than culture; cross-reaction with enteroviruses can occur.
Rotaviruses	D	A	B	C	D	Antigen detection is test of choice for diagnosis. EM useful in suitably equipped laboratories. NAAT is promising.
Rubella virus	A	D	B	D	A	Serology most useful for diagnosis and determination of immunity. Isolation useful for postnatal rubella if attempted early (prodromal period to 4 days postrash). In CRS, virus can be isolated for weeks to months after birth.

(Continued on next page)

TABLE 1 *(Continued)*

Virus(es)	Applicability[b] of:					Comments
	Virus isolation	Antigen detection	Nucleic acid detection	Electron microscopy	Antibody detection	
Transmissible spongiform encephalopathy agents	D	C	B	C	D	Histology most useful diagnostic test. Surrogate markers popular but lack specificity. Western blot for PrP performed in specialized laboratories. Human genome sequencing useful for diagnosis of genetic disorders.
Varicella-zoster virus	A	A	A	C	B	IFA and NAAT are most commonly used tests. Culture less sensitive than IFA. Serology most useful for determination of immunity.

[a]Virus isolation includes conventional cell culture with detection of viral growth by cytopathic effects or hemadsorption, and shell vial centrifugation culture with detection of viral antigens by immunostaining. Viral antigens can be detected by a variety of immunoassays, such as enzyme-linked immunosorbent assays, agglutination assays, immunofluorescence or immunoperoxidase techniques, and immunochromatography. Viral nucleic acids (DNA or RNA) can be detected and quantified by direct hybridization or by the performance of amplification methods such as PCR. Electron microscopy involves the visualization of viral particles by negative staining or immunoelectron microscopy, or by thin-section techniques. Antibody detection involves measurement of total or class-specific immunoglobulins directed at specific viral antigens. Abbreviations: IFA, immunofluorescence assay; NAAT, nucleic acid amplification test; BSL, biosafety level; EM, electron microscopy; SARS, severe acute respiratory syndrome; CoV, coronavirus; CNS, central nervous system; LCM, lymphocytic choriomeningitis virus; IHC, immunohistochemistry; ISH, in situ hybridization; IgM, immunoglobulin M; HSV-2, herpes simplex virus type 2; MAb, monoclonal antibody; KS, Kaposi's sarcoma; HTLV, human T-cell lymphotropic virus; CSF, cerebrospinal fluid; PML, progressive multifocal leukoencephalopathy; PVAN, polyomavirus-associated nephropathy; RIG, rabies immune globulin; CRS, congenital rubella syndrome; PrP, prion protein.

[b]A, test is generally useful for the indicated diagnosis; B, test is useful under certain circumstances or for the diagnosis of specific forms of infection, as delineated in the right-hand column and in the text of the individual chapters; C, test is seldom useful for general diagnostic purposes but may be useful for epidemiological studies or for the diagnosis of unusual conditions; D, test is not available or not used for laboratory diagnosis of infection.

Human Immunodeficiency Viruses*

BRIGITTE P. GRIFFITH, SHELDON CAMPBELL, AND ANGELA M. CALIENDO

79

TAXONOMY

Origin and Historical Perspective

The human immunodeficiency virus (HIV) is the etiologic agent of AIDS. AIDS was first recognized clinically in 1981 (95), although the first known case of AIDS has been traced to 1959 (133, 156). HIV exists as two major viral species, HIV type 1 (HIV-1) and HIV-2. The more virulent of the two HIVs, HIV-1 is responsible for the worldwide AIDS pandemic, with more than 33.2 million people living with HIV/AIDS as of the end of 2007. HIV-2, on the other hand, is less pathogenic and has a more limited geographic distribution.

HIV-1 was initially discovered in 1983 (5) and was confirmed the following year to be the cause of AIDS (55, 84, 119). Clavel et al. first isolated HIV-2 in 1986 (25). Both HIV-1 and HIV-2 are related to simian immunodeficiency viruses (39, 70). Simian immunodeficiency virus strains have been found in more than 25 species of nonhuman African primates (70). Chimpanzees and a number of species of old-world monkeys are the natural hosts for these primate lentiviruses, and it has been suggested that both the HIV-1 and HIV-2 epidemics are the result of simian-to-human transmissions. The HIV-1 epidemic appears to be the result of zoonotic virus transmissions from chimpanzees to humans (56), while the sooty mangabey apparently is the source of HIV-2 infections in humans (133).

HIV Groups and Subgroups

Both types of HIV are members of the genus *Lentivirus* within the family *Retroviridae*. Because of the mutation and recombination capabilities of HIV, various genetic clades have evolved, and the genetic diversity of HIV-1 plays a significant role in the design and interpretation of HIV diagnostic assays (146). HIV-1 is subdivided into three genetic groups, designated M (for major), O (for outlier), and N (for non-M, non-O), based on sequence diversity within the HIV-1 *gag* and *env* genes. HIV-1 group M is divided into 9 subtypes (A through D, F through H, J, and K). Viruses belonging to different M subtypes have been isolated in distinct regions of the world. The initial epidemic in the early 1980s in North America and Europe was due to HIV-1 subtype B. Currently, subtype C dominates the global epidemic, although subtype B continues to be the major subtype in the United States, Europe, and Australia. Certain HIV-1 viral isolates appear to be recombinant, containing sequences from more than one subtype. These are referred to as circulating recombinant forms (CRFs). Group O viruses are only rarely isolated and mostly found in persons from Cameroon, Gabon, and Equatorial Guinea. Group N viruses have been recovered from Cameroon. Seven subtypes of HIV-2 (A through G) have been defined, although HIV-2 groups C through G have each only been recovered from a single individual.

DESCRIPTION OF THE AGENTS

Structure and Genomic Organization

HIVs are enveloped plus-stranded RNA viruses. The HIV genome is organized similarly to other retroviruses. It contains the *gag*, *pol*, and *env* genes which encode structural proteins, viral enzymes, and envelope glycoproteins, respectively. These are flanked by long terminal repeats. In addition, the genome comprises open reading frames for *trans*-acting transcriptional activator (Tat), the regulator of viral expression (Rev), and several other proteins such as Vif, Vpr, and Nef.

Mature viral particles measure 100 to 150 nm in diameter and have a conical core surrounded by a lipid envelope (Fig. 1). The core contains two identical copies of single-stranded RNA, approximately 10 kb in length, which are surrounded by structural proteins that form the nucleocapsid and the matrix shell as well as by-products of the *pol* gene. The lipid envelope is acquired as the virus buds from infected cells. The glycoprotein gp120/41 forms spikes protruding from this envelope. The glycoprotein, a product of the *env* gene, is synthesized as a precursor, gp160, which is cleaved into the heavily glycosylated gp120, forming the majority of the external portion and the transmembrane gp41 portion, which contains the membrane-spanning domain. The major structural proteins which are encoded by the *gag* gene include p17, p24, p7, and p9. Products of the *pol* gene include the protease, reverse transcriptase, RNase, and integrase.

HIV-2 is structurally analogous to HIV-1, but some of its protein components differ, most notably the outer envelope

*This chapter contains information presented by Brigitte P. Griffith, Sheldon Campbell, and Donald R. Mayo in chapter 83 of the ninth edition of this *Manual*.

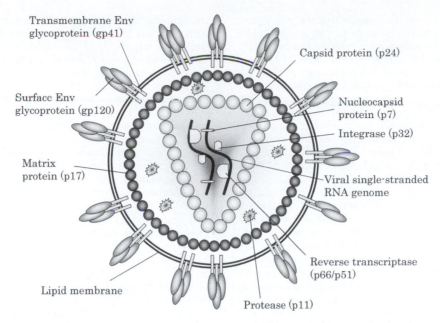

FIGURE 1 Schematic representation of a mature HIV virion showing the localization of viral proteins.

and transmembrane glycoproteins gp125 and gp36, as well as the core proteins p16 and p26. The major gene products that are of significance for the diagnosis of HIV-1 and HIV-2 are listed in Table 1.

Replication Cycle

The replication cycle of HIV-1 is accomplished in vivo in approximately 24 hours (115). Replication begins with the attachment of virus to the target cell via the interaction of gp120 and the cellular receptor CD4 (34). This binding results in gp120 conformational changes which allows the virus to interact with other cellular coreceptor sites, CXCR4 or CCR5. The interaction with CXCR4 occurs primarily with T-cell-tropic, syncytium-inducing viruses (51). In contrast, the β-chemokine receptor CCR5 is involved in macrophage-tropic non-syncytium-inducing HIVs (24).

Following fusion with the host cells, HIV enters the cell and RNA is released. HIV particles contain reverse

transcriptase (RT), an enzyme that plays a crucial role in the replication process. RT possesses three distinct functions: RNA-dependent DNA polymerase, which serves to synthesize cDNA; RNase H, which degrades RNA from the cDNA-RNA complex; and a DNA-dependent DNA polymerase, which duplicates the cDNA strand. The reverse-transcribed genome is associated with several viral proteins and transported into the nucleus. The DNA copy becomes integrated into the genome of the infected cell by the virally encoded integrase; this integrated retroviral DNA genome is called the provirus. The cDNA then serves as a template for viral RNA. Activation of HIV transcription and gene expression is modulated by cellular transcription factors and by viral regulatory proteins, including Tat, Rev, Nef, and Vrp. The regulatory genes *tat* and *rev* greatly influence the rate of viral replication. The Tat protein increases transcription from the long terminal repeat. The Rev protein facilitates export of unspliced or partially spliced RNAs encoding the viral structural proteins. At the end of the replication cycle, the virion assembles and buds through the plasma membrane.

EPIDEMIOLOGY AND TRANSMISSION

Epidemiology

The AIDS pandemic has had an enormous toll throughout the world, with over 6,800 persons becoming infected daily and HIV-1 reported in virtually every country on earth (149). In contrast, HIV-2 has remained limited primarily to West Africa and to European immigrants from West Africa. Two African countries which are not in West Africa, Angola and Mozambique, also have high HIV-2 seroprevalence rates, and additional spread of HIV-2 has been documented in Portugal, France, and India. Group M viruses are responsible for most HIV-1 infections, with a predominance of subtype C. Subtype B is most prevalent in the United States, Europe, and Australia but is rarely found in Africa. Subtypes A, C, and D predominate in Africa.

TABLE 1 Major HIV-1 and HIV-2 gene products

Gene	Description of gene products	Gene products of: HIV-1	Gene products of: HIV-2
Core (*gag*)	Precursor of Gag protein	p55	p53–55
	Capsid protein	p24	p26
	Matrix protein	p17	p16
Polymerase (*pol*)	RT component	p66	p68
	RT component	p51	
	Endonuclease component	p32	p33
Envelope (*env*)	Precursor of Env glycoprotein	gp160	gp125
	Outer Env glycoprotein	gp120	gp105
	Transmembrane Env glycoprotein	gp41	gp36

Epidemic updates from 2007 suggest that the global prevalence of HIV has reached a plateau in the past few years (149). In addition, there were reductions in both the number of HIV-associated deaths and the number of annual new infections. In 2007, an estimated 2.7 million people became newly infected with HIV. The AIDS epidemic killed 2.0 million people in 2007, with 76% of the deaths occurring in sub-Saharan Africa. South Africa is presently the country with the largest number of HIV-infected persons in the world. Globally, the overall proportion of HIV-positive women has remained stable; and women represented 50% of people living with HIV in 2007 (149). In sub-Saharan Africa and the Caribbean, 61% and 43% of adults living with HIV were women.

In the United States, the cumulative estimated number of AIDS cases diagnosed through 2007 was 1,051,875 and the cumulative estimated number of AIDS related deaths was 583,298 (20). In 2008, the CDC estimated that approximately 56,300 people acquired HIV-1 infection (20). The demographic characteristics of the epidemic have changed significantly since the 1980s. In the early days of the epidemic, the populations most affected in the United States included mostly homosexual and bisexual men. The epidemic now affects a large proportion of African-Americans and greater numbers of women (20), with approximately half of new infections reported among African-Americans. Most HIV-1 infections in men occur during injecting-drug use or sex between men. The main risk factor for women is heterosexual transmission from a male partner with undisclosed risk behaviors. AIDS-related deaths have steadily decreased since the introduction of antiretroviral therapy in 1995–1996. However, African-Americans have the poorest survival rates among individuals diagnosed with AIDS in the United States.

Transmission

Both HIV-1 and HIV-2 have the same modes of transmission. The most common mode of HIV infection is sexual transmission at the genital mucosa through direct contact with infected blood fluids, including blood, semen, and vaginal secretions (125). Infection may also occur through inoculation of infected blood, via transfusion of infected blood products, transplantation of infected tissues, or reuse of contaminated needles. The risk of HIV-1 infection following occupational percutaneous exposure to HIV-1-infected blood has been estimated to be 0.3% (58).

The vast majority of HIV transmission from mother to child occurs in resource-poor countries. Maternal HIV-1 RNA in blood and genital fluids has been documented to correlate strongly with mother-to-child transmission (101). HIV transmission can occur in utero, during labor and delivery, and during breast-feeding. In the absence of therapeutic intervention, the risk of mother-to-child transmission can range from 15 to 30% and is further increased in the setting of breast-feeding. However, the risk can be significantly reduced to below 2% if antiretroviral therapy is administered to women during pregnancy and labor (28). Antiretroviral treatment of the mother and infant after birth can also significantly decrease the risk of HIV-1 infection in the newborn.

CLINICAL SIGNIFICANCE

Virological Parameters during the Course of HIV Infection

The natural history of HIV-1 infection can be divided into three phases: a transient acute retroviral syndrome, a period of clinical latency, and finally, progression to AIDS. Each of these stages is associated with specific changes in virologic and immunologic parameters. Following HIV-1 infection, HIV-1-specific markers appear in the blood in the following chronological order: HIV-1 RNA, p24 antigen, and HIV-1 antibody (Fig. 2). The exact time when each of these 3 markers can be detected depends on a number of factors

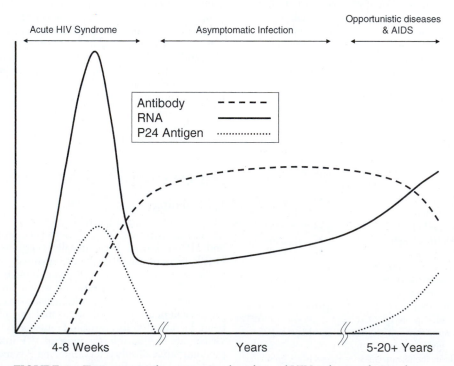

FIGURE 2 Time course of appearance of markers of HIV infection during the course of HIV infection.

including the type of test used, characteristics of the infecting virus, and host immune responses of the individual. During the first week after infection, HIV-1 RNA, antigen, and antibody are generally not detectable, although viral replication is occurring. Within 1 to 4 weeks after infection, HIV-1 RNA increases rapidly and viral antigen is detectable, but HIV antibody is usually not detectable. The time period when HIV antibody is not detectable is referred to as the window period. In most infected persons, HIV antibody is detected within 1 to 2 months, but in a small percentage of individuals, seroconversion may require up to 6 months. Following the initial HIV-1 RNA peak, viremia generally decreases to a lower comparatively stable level, which reflects ongoing viral replication and immune system damage. The HIV-1 RNA pattern in perinatally infected infants differs from that in infected adults, since high HIV-1 RNA levels may persist in HIV-infected children for prolonged time periods.

Acute Retroviral Syndrome

Acute HIV-1 infection is a transient symptomatic illness which is associated with high levels of HIV-1 replication and a developing virus-specific immune response. The diagnosis of acute HIV-1 infection is often missed because symptoms tend to be nonspecific and HIV-1-specific antibodies are not detectable. Symptoms present in 40 to 80% of the cases within 3 to 6 weeks after primary infection and usually last 7 to 14 days. The clinical symptoms of acute HIV-1 infection were first described as a mononucleosis-like syndrome in 1985 (32). Most commonly, fever, maculopapular rash, oral ulcers, lymphadenopathy, malaise, weight loss, arthralgia, pharyngitis and/or night sweats are seen (33, 72).

During acute HIV-1 infection, there is an initial rise in plasma viremia, reaching levels of up to 100 million copies of HIV-1 RNA per ml of plasma (79). In addition, destruction of HIV-1-specific $CD4^+$ T lymphocytes as well as widespread dissemination of the virus, with seeding of lymphoid organs and other tissue reservoirs, occurs. During resolution of primary infection, $CD4^+$ T-cell counts rebound and viremia declines before reaching a steady level, which has been shown to be an important predictor of disease progression (96, 97).

Clinical Latency

The asymptomatic period, which usually lasts several years, is the period between primary infection and the development of clinical immunodeficiency. During that period, the number of $CD4^+$ lymphocytes declines slowly and the virus continues to replicate, albeit at a relatively stable level. During this clinical latency period, high titers of virus can be found in lymphoid and other tissue compartments (112). The length of the clinical latency period can vary considerably but is 10 years on average. In rapid progressors, AIDS develops within 1 to 2 years, but the clinical latency period can be short, as in a well-publicized New York case, where the infection was reported to result in symptomatic AIDS in 4 to 20 months (93). In contrast, 5 to 10% of HIV-1-infected individuals are long-term nonprogressors and remain symptom-free for longer than 20 years (102). Several factors influence the steady-state level of viral replication and the rate of disease progression, including host immune responses, host genetic factors, and the fitness of the infecting virus. One of the most important host genetic factors reported to affect virus replication rates is the deletion of CCR5; most individuals homozygous for a 32-bp deletion in CCR5 are resistant to HIV-1 infection (127) and show slower HIV-1 replication (118). In addition to mutations in chemokine receptor genes, a number of HLA class I alleles have been found to be associated with lower steady-state viral levels and slow disease progression (1), and it has been suggested that rates of disease progression may also be influenced by other concurrent infections (138).

Disease Progression to AIDS

The continuous replication of HIV-1 in productively infected cells together with the elimination of host cells and chronic immune activation results over the years in deterioration of the immune system. Studies of HIV-1 replication dynamics have shown that, in productively infected lymphocytes, the interval between infection, virus production, and cell death is very short. The half-life of HIV-1 in plasma is thought to be 6 hours, the length of the replication cycle in $CD4^+$ lymphocytes has been estimated at 2.6 days, and 35 million $CD4^+$ cells are thought to be lost daily (76). As the ability of the host to eliminate productively infected cells declines, $CD4^+$ lymphocytes with integrated provirus accumulate. These resting memory $CD4^+$ lymphocytes serve as a long-lived reservoir for HIV-1. The mean half-life of this latent reservoir has been reported to be as long 40 months in many patients (53).

Clinical manifestations can affect nearly every organ system. In addition, destruction of the immune system is clinically manifested by the occurrence of opportunistic infections and tumors, and central nervous system involvement can be seen, most commonly the HIV-associated dementia complex (120). Opportunistic infections caused by viruses, bacteria, fungi, and protozoa, neoplastic disease, HIV encephalopathy, wasting syndrome, and progressive multifocal leukoencephalopathy can complicate the clinical course of HIV infections and are often the cause of death.

Several public health organizations, including the CDC and the WHO, have published HIV disease classification systems for both public health purposes and disease staging. All case definitions of HIV infection now require laboratory-confirmed evidence of HIV infection. The current CDC classification system for HIV-1-infected adolescents ($\geq$13 years) and adults is categorized by increasing severity as stage 1 ($CD4^+$ T lymphocyte count of $\geq$500 cells/μl), stage 2 ($CD4^+$ T lymphocyte count of 200 to 499 cells/μl), stage 3 (AIDS), or stage unknown (21).

The course of HIV-1 infection and the clinical characteristics of AIDS in children differ from those in adults, and the CDC has developed classification systems to describe the spectrum of HIV-1 disease in children less than 18 months of age and children 18 months to 13 years of age born to HIV-1-infected mothers (21). The disease progresses rapidly in infants with vertically acquired HIV-1 infection. The most common AIDS-defining conditions include *Pneumocystis jirovecii* pneumonia, lymphoid interstitial pneumonia/pulmonary lymphoid hyperplasia, and recurrent bacterial infections.

Therapy and Vaccination

Significant scientific advances in the development of effective antiretroviral therapy have occurred in the past 25 years. The first effective drug against HIV-1, zidovudine was approved by the FDA in March 1987. Currently, over 30 antiretroviral drugs or combinations of antiviral drugs have been approved by the FDA for the treatment of HIV infections (see www.aidsinfo.nih.gov for a list of FDA-approved drugs). Approved antiviral agents used to treat HIV-1 fall into 6 classes: nucleoside RT inhibitors, nonnucleoside

RT inhibitors, protease inhibitors, fusion inhibitors, integrase inhibitors, and CCR5 inhibitors. Guidelines for the use of antiretroviral agents in adults and in children evolve rapidly. These are updated on a regular basis, and the most recent guidelines can be obtained from the AIDSinfo website (http://aidsinfo.nih.gov).

Several obstacles have slowed down the progress toward the development of effective vaccines against HIV-1, including the inability of HIV-1 to produce neutralizing antibodies, the lack of understanding of correlates of protective immunity, the genetic diversity of the virus, and the limitation of animal models (4, 146).

COLLECTION, STORAGE, AND TRANSPORT OF SPECIMENS

Serum samples are used routinely for standard HIV antibody and antigen determinations, although plasma samples are also acceptable. The serum/plasma should be promptly separated from the clot/cellular elements and refrigerated at 2 to 8°C. If testing will not be performed within 7 days, the serum specimens should be frozen at −20°C or lower. Serum/plasma specimens can be transported either refrigerated (if transport takes places within 7 days of collection) or frozen in screw-cap plastic vials.

Dried blood spots, as well as noninvasive specimens such as urine or oral fluid, are approved for use in some of the HIV antibody kits. The OraSure HIV-1 specimen collection device (OraSure Technologies, Bethlehem, PA), which increases the flow of mucosal transudate across the mucosal surfaces onto an absorbent cotton pad, is available for collection of oral fluids. Rapid, point-of-care HIV assays usually require finger stick or venipuncture whole blood, although one of the assays is approved for use with oral fluid and some have been validated for use with serum samples.

HIV-1 RNA viral load assays are most commonly performed on plasma specimens. To ensure accurate HIV-1 RNA quantification in plasma, proper collection, processing, storage, and transport of plasma specimens are essential to avoid RNA degradation. The same collection system and procedures should be used to follow up patients over time because different collection systems may produce discrepant values. In addition, if a change in collection system or technology is planned, baseline HIV-1 viral load values should be determined. Each of the FDA-approved kits available for determination of HIV-1 viral load in plasma has specific volume and collection tube requirements (Table 2). For laboratories that test specimens from pediatric patients, flexibility of specimen volume should be investigated, as it may be difficult to obtain the 1 ml of plasma needed for several of the

TABLE 2 Comparison of FDA-approved HIV-1 viral load assay characteristics

Test	Amplification method and target	Anticoagulant(s)	Plasma vol[a]	Range (copies/ml)	Standards and controls
Amplicor HIV-1 Monitor version 1.5 (Roche Diagnostics, Indianapolis, IN)	RT-PCR, *gag* gene	EDTA, ACD			1 internal QS, 3 external controls
Standard			200 µl	400–750,000	
Ultrasensitive			500 µl	50–100,000	
Cobas Amplicor HIV-1 Monitor version 1.5					
Standard			200 µl	400–750,000	
Ultrasensitive			500 µl	50–100,000	
Cobas AmpliPrep/Cobas Amplicor HIV-1 Monitor version 1.5					
Standard			250 µl	500–1,000,000	
Ultrasensitive			750 µl	50–100,000	
Versant HIV-1 RNA 3.0 (bDNA) (Siemens Healthcare Diagnostics, Tarrytown, NY)	bDNA, *pol* gene	EDTA, ACD	1 ml	75–500,000	6 external standards, 3 external controls
NucliSens HIV-1 QT (BioMérieux, Inc., Durham, NC)	NASBA[b], *gag* gene	EDTA, ACD, heparin	1 ml	176–3,470,000	3 internal calibrators
Cobas AmpliPrep/Cobas TaqMan HIV-1 v1 (Roche Diagnostics, Indianapolis, IN)	Real-time RT-PCR, *gag* gene	EDTA	1 ml	48–10,000,000	1 internal QS, 3 external controls
Cobas AmpliPrep/Cobas TaqMan HIV-1 v2	Real-time RT-PCR, *gag* and LTR genes	EDTA	1 ml	20–10,000,000	1 internal QS, 3 external controls
RealTime TaqMan HIV-1 (Abbott Molecular, Des Plaines, IL)	Real-time RT-PCR, integrase gene	EDTA, ACD	1 ml	40–10,000,000	1 internal control, 3 external controls, calibration curve each new lot or 6 mo

[a]For tests that use an automated extraction instrument (AmpliPrep and RealTime), the specimen volume listed refers to the volume of sample that is loaded on the instrument, which is greater than the actual volume of specimen taken through the extraction.
[b]Nucleic acid sequence-based amplification.

assays. Some of the viral load assays have also been used to measure HIV-1 viral loads in specimens other than plasma, including dried blood spots, cerebrospinal fluid, cervical secretions, seminal plasma/semen, and serum. The RNA content in serum has been found to be lower than in the paired plasma sample (66). In addition, acid citrate dextrose (ACD) anticoagulated specimens have also been shown to yield results that are approximately 15% lower than results obtained with EDTA plasma (61, 85). For all assays, plasma must be separated from blood cells within 6 hours of collection because delays in the separation of plasma from cellular elements can result in RNA degradation. HIV-1 RNA is generally stable in cell-free plasma at refrigerated temperatures for several days and remains stable for at least three freeze-thaw cycles (66). For long-term storage, plasma samples should be stored at −70°C. Plasma preparation tubes (PPT) (BD Vacutainer PPT; Becton Dickinson, Franklin Lakes, NJ), which contain dried EDTA and a gel separator that after centrifugation forms a barrier between the plasma and cellular elements, have become available in recent years. PPT provide a closed collection system for the preparation and transport of plasma specimens. Plasma samples do not need to be poured off from PPT after centrifugation, and plasma transfer and relabeling steps are eliminated. This improves convenience, decreases risks of errors, and improves safety. Initial recommendations from the manufacturer allowed for either refrigerated or frozen transport of centrifuged PPT. However, discrepancies have been reported to occur in plasma samples that were frozen in situ (65, 126). The differences were noted only for samples with viral loads close to the limits of detection; a large proportion of samples with undetectable viral load in the standard EDTA aliquot were found to have detectable HIV-1 RNA in the corresponding PPT. As a result, the manufacturer has recommended that plasma in PPT be stored without freezing and that plasma from PPT should be transferred to a secondary tube if plasma samples need to be stored frozen.

For HIV-1 resistance assays, genotypic and phenotypic, plasma collected from EDTA, ACD, or PPT/EDTA tubes can be used. The plasma must be separated for the cellular elements within 6 hours of collection and frozen immediately. Plasma specimens should be transported frozen. Qualitative HIV-1 RNA testing is performed on plasma; samples can be collected in EDTA, sodium citrate, or PPT. For HIV-1 DNA and viral culture assays, whole blood is commonly used. It should be collected on either EDTA, ACD, or cell preparation tubes. HIV-1 can be cultured from plasma or from peripheral blood mononuclear cells (PBMCs), but HIV DNA assays require whole blood or PBMCs. For preparation of PBMCs, the blood specimen should not be refrigerated or frozen but instead should be kept at ambient temperature for no longer than 4 days.

DIRECT DETECTION

p24 Antigen Assays

In the early days of the AIDS epidemic, p24 antigen testing played an important role as a tool for the diagnosis, prognosis, and evaluation of antiretroviral activity and for monitoring of HIV-1-infected cultures. In 1996, the FDA approved the Coulter HIV-1 p24 Ag assay (Coulter Co., Miami, FL) for screening blood products. This test was used for screening blood and plasma donors in the United States for a few years until it was replaced with more sensitive nucleic acid tests in 1999. At present, use of antigen assays is very limited in the

United States. HIV-1 antigen assays are utilized more commonly in resource-limited areas for the detection of early HIV infection, for the diagnosis of HIV infection in the newborn, and for monitoring antiretroviral therapy because of its reduced cost and ease of performance.

The test is of diagnostic value during early infection. p24 antigen is usually not detectable during the first week after infection, but it is detectable thereafter during acute infection before HIV-1 antibody (Fig. 2). After HIV-1 antibody seroconversion, p24 antigen forms immune complexes with HIV-1 antibody and becomes undetectable. Therefore, p24 antigen is found in the blood either in a free form or in a complex with HIV-1 antibody. The presence of HIV p24 antigen can be detected in plasma or serum by antigen capture enzyme immunosorbent assay (EIA). Because p24 antigen tests can produce false-positive reactions due to interfering substances and immune complexes, positive samples need to be confirmed by a neutralization procedure.

Standard EIA procedures for HIV-1 antigen determination are insensitive, and modifications to the HIV-1 antigen test have been made to boost the sensitivity of the assay, including acid or heat treatment for dissociation of antigen-antibody complexes (104, 131); increased sensitivity has been achieved by the addition of signal amplification (103, 114, 121, 132, 134). These variants of HIV-1 antigen assays are of interest because they provide highly sensitive yet inexpensive and easy-to-use tools for use in resource-limited settings. The PerkinElmer ELAST (enzyme-linked immunosorbent assay [ELISA] amplification system tyramide) is designed to amplify the signal generated by horseradish peroxidase when applied to solid-phase EIA, and PerkinElmer has developed a kit, the ultrasensitive p24 antigen assay (Ultra p24), that combines heat denaturation and signal amplification-boosted detection of HIV-1 antigen (121, 132). Heat denaturation combined with tyramide signal amplification has been reported to increase the sensitivity of p24 antigen detection to levels comparable to detection of viral RNA by PCR and has been found to be effective for the monitoring of responses to antiretroviral therapy (10, 114, 121, 132) as well as for pediatric diagnosis (103, 134).

HIV RNA and DNA Qualitative Assays

The Aptima HIV-1 RNA qualitative assay (Gen-Probe, Inc., San Diego, CA) is the first FDA-approved nucleic acid test for the diagnosis of HIV-1 infection and has clinical utility for identification of acute and neonatal HIV-1 infection, resolution of indeterminate Western blots, and confirmation of a repeatedly positive antibody screen. With the APTIMA assay, HIV-1 RNA is detected 12 days earlier than antibody and 6 days earlier than p24 antigen. The test targets both the 5′ long terminal repeat and the *pol* gene of the HIV-1 genome, which allows detection of all HIV-1 group M, N, and O viruses. There are three general steps to the assay: target-specific capture of HIV-1 RNA from the clinical sample, transcription-mediated amplification, and detection using a hybridization protection assay. The dual kinetic nature of the test allows for detection of the HIV-1 RNA target and internal control in a single reaction. The assay has a limit of detection of 30 copies/ml of plasma with a specificity of 99.8%.

Detection of HIV-1 DNA can be used to supplement or substitute antibody testing for the diagnosis of HIV infection in special situations such as primary infection during the diagnostic window period or in newborns of infected mothers. HIV-1 DNA qualitative assays make use of PCR to amplify conserved regions of the HIV-1 genome to detect proviral HIV-1 DNA in blood mononuclear cells. Only one qualitative HIV-1 DNA PCR assay is commercially available (Roche Amplicor HIV DNA assay, version 1.5), but it is not approved by the FDA. Laboratory-developed tests based on nested as well as real-time PCR procedures are also used; the limit of detection and ability to detect non-B subtypes vary among these assays.

The sensitivity and specificity of standard HIV-1 DNA PCR assays for the diagnosis of neonatal HIV-1 infection have been reported to be 96% and 99% at 1 month of age for HIV-1 subtype B (45). The potential utility of qualitative DNA PCR assays in the diagnosis of vertical HIV-1 transmission has been greatly increased with the development of simple and sensitive procedures using dried blood spots. False-negative HIV-1 DNA results have been reported in infants with non-B subtypes (81), although the latest version 1.5 of the Amplicor assay appears to allow for the detection of most HIV-1 subtypes.

HIV RNA Viral Load Assays

Viral load assays, which measure the quantity of HIV-1 RNA present in plasma, are used as prognostic markers, to monitor response to therapy, and to determine infectiousness. HIV-1 plasma viral load is a strong predictor of the rate of disease progression (96, 108), but HIV-1 RNA load assays are most commonly used to guide HIV treatment decisions. In the United States, five commercial assays are FDA approved for the quantification of HIV-1 RNA in plasma, including two recently approved assays that utilize real-time RT-PCR technology. A comparison of the plasma specimen requirements and characteristics of the assays is shown in Table 2. The RealTime TaqMan HIV-1 assay (Abbott Molecular, Des Plaines, IL) is currently the only viral load test that detects group O virus. The other assays have not been optimized for group O virus and will likely underquantify HIV-1 RNA levels. None of the assays detect HIV-2.

The Amplicor HIV-1 Monitor assay (Roche Diagnostics, Indianapolis, IN) is based on reverse transcription of the target HIV-1 RNA and on PCR amplification of the resulting cDNA. The HIV-1 RNA copy number is calculated based on the input copy number of the quantitation standard (QS) RNA. The version of the assay currently in use (version 1.5) can adequately quantify all group M subtypes of HIV-1, in contrast to older versions of the assay. One advantage of the assay is that there is minimal risk of amplicon contamination because the kit includes UTP and uracil-N-glycosylase. One disadvantage of the Amplicor HIV-1 Monitor assay is that it has a limited dynamic range, requiring performance of both the standard and ultrasensitive assays for samples that fall outside the dynamic range. Three variations of these assays exist: the Amplicor HIV-1 Monitor assay, which is a manual test performed in microwell plates: the Cobas Amplicor HIV-1 Monitor assay in which amplicons are captured on magnetic beads, with the Cobas analyzer used to automate the amplification and detection steps; and the Cobas AmpliPrep/Cobas Amplicor assay, which provides automation of the nucleic acid extraction, followed by amplification and detection on the Cobas instrument.

The Versant HIV-1 RNA 3.0 assay (Siemens Healthcare Diagnostics, Tarrytown, NY) is a branched DNA (bDNA) method which quantifies HIV-1 RNA by signal amplification instead of target nucleic acid amplification (41). The quantity of HIV RNA is determined from an external standard curve run on the same plate; 6 kit standards of known viral concentration are used. When compared to other viral load assays, the reproducibility of the bDNA assay has been

reported to be superior, particularly at the low end of the dynamic range (86, 105). The Versant HIV-1 RNA 3.0 bDNA assay offers the advantages of high throughput; in the current version, 84 specimens can be run on one plate. In addition, the assay can reliably quantify all subtypes of HIV-1. Disadvantages of the bDNA assay include the requirement for a large volume of plasma, the absence of an internal QS for each sample tested, and lower specificity compared to target amplification methods. The Bayer System 340 bDNA analyzer provides semiautomation of the assay, while the System 440 provides even more extensive automation.

The NucliSens HIV-1 RNA QT assay (bioMérieux, Inc., Durham, NC) uses nucleic acid sequence-based amplification. The second-generation assay currently in use cannot reliably quantify subtypes A and G (59). Advantages of the Nuclisens HIV-1 QT assay include wide dynamic range (176 to 3,400,000 copies/ml) when a 1-ml input plasma volume is used. In addition, the assay can be used for measuring viral loads at other body sites because the RNA extraction procedure consistently generates RNA products that are free of interfering substances (54).

Three real-time RT-PCR tests have been FDA approved. These assays offer several advantages over the conventional viral load assays, including a very broad linear range, extensive automation, and decreased risk of carryover contamination. The RealTime TaqMan HIV-1 assay uses the automated m2000 system, which has two components: the m2000sp for nucleic acid extraction and loading of sample and master mix into the 96-well optical reaction plate and the m2000rt for amplification and detection. The assay contains an internal control, which is an unrelated RNA sequence that is added to the sample lysis buffer prior to extraction. RNA is captured by magnetic particles, washed to remove unbound material, and eluted. Once the master mix and sample are combined into the reaction plate, the reaction plate is covered and loaded into the m2000rt; these are the only manual steps of the assay. The amplification and detection utilize TaqMan technology, the HIV-1 oligonucleotide probe is a partially double-stranded complex, the long strand is complementary to the HIV-1 target (integrase region of the polymerase gene) and is labeled at the 5′ end with a fluorophore. The shorter strand is complementary to the 5′ end of the long strand and is labeled with a quencher moiety at its 3′ end. When HIV-1 target is present, the HIV-1-specific strand preferentially hybridizes to the target, allowing emission of fluorescence (143, 144). For calculation of viral load values, two assay calibrators are run in replicates of three to generate a calibration curve; the slope and intercept of the curve are stored on the instrument and used to calculate viral load values. The limit of detection of the assay is 40 copies/ml for a 1.0-ml sample volume, 75 copies/ml for a 0.5-ml sample volume, and 150 copies/ml for a 0.2-ml sample volume. The RealTime assay has been designed to quantify all group M and N viruses, CRFs, and group O virus (67, 144).

The Cobas AmpliPrep/Cobas TaqMan HIV-1 test (Roche Diagnostics) is also based on real-time TaqMan technology, and targets the HIV-1 *gag* gene. The extraction process is automated on the Cobas AmpliPrep instrument using a generic magnetic silica-based capture method and includes a QS that is added to each specimen at a known concentration along with the lysis buffer. The extracted sample and the reaction mix are added to amplification tubes on the AmpliPrep instrument, and the amplification and detection are completed on either the Cobas TaqMan analyzer or the Cobas TaqMan 48 analyzer. Docking the Cobas TaqMan analyzer to the AmpliPrep instrument creates a fully automated system;

alternatively, the amplification tubes can be manually loaded into the Cobas TaqMan 48 analyzer. For calculation of viral load values, the fluorescent readings for the QS and target are checked by the instrument software to ensure they are valid, crossing threshold values are determined, and the viral load value is calculated from lot-specific calibration constants provided by the manufacturer. The amount of QS added to each sample is constant, so if the critical threshold for the QS has been affected, the HIV-1 target concentration is adjusted accordingly. The Cobas AmpliPrep/Cobas Taq-Man HIV-1 test has been designed to quantify all group M viruses; the assay can also detect group N viruses and many CRFs (67, 130). Recently, version 2 of the Cobas Ampli-Prep/Cobas TaqMan HIV-1 test has been approved by the FDA. The version 2 test targets both the LTR and *gag* genes, and the limit of detection is 20 copies/ml. The most important improvements with the version 2 test are quantification of group O virus and more accurate quantification of CRFs than the version 1 test (113a).

The high cost and complex technical requirements of nucleic acid-based testing strategies have resulted in the development of other types of viral load assays for use in resource-limited settings. Two of these assays have received recent attention: the heat-denatured signal-boosted p24 antigen assays (Perkin Elmer, Wellesley, MA) and RT assay (Exa Vir Load assay; Cavidi AB, Uppsala, Sweden) (10, 139). Although both methods remain less sensitive and reproducible than the nucleic acid-based assays, they are affordable alternatives to HIV RNA quantification. Furthermore, an automated, low-cost real-time reverse transcription-PCR test is routinely used for diagnosis and monitoring of HIV-1 infection in a West African resource-limited setting (124).

ISOLATION PROCEDURES

Because HIV can be isolated from the blood of the majority of HIV-infected individuals, HIV culture was frequently utilized in the early years of the epidemic as a diagnostic or prognostic marker or for assessing the efficacy of antiviral therapy (77, 96). Although a positive culture provides direct evidence of HIV infection, HIV culture is no longer used for routine diagnosis but is utilized primarily in research laboratories. The procedure for HIV culture is elaborate and time-consuming (64, 77). To isolate HIV, the patient specimen is first cultured by mixing patient cells with cells from healthy donors stimulated with phytohemagglutinin and interleukin-2; fresh stimulated donor cells must be added weekly because HIV-1 produces cell death. In the second step, the presence of RT or p24 antigen released in the culture supernatants is assayed periodically.

Viral culture assays based on recombinant technology are now used in resistance assays and to determine the viral fitness of HIV-1 (48). The only commercially available fitness assay, also referred to as viral replication capacity (RC) assay, has been developed by Monogram BioSciences (South San Francisco, CA). It measures the ability of HIV-1 from a patient undergoing antiretroviral treatment to replicate in vitro compared to a wild-type reference virus. The patient RC value is expressed as a percentage of the RC of the wild-type reference standard. The assay uses a retroviral vector constructed from an infectious clone of HIV-1. The vector contains a luciferase expression cassette inserted within a deleted region of the envelope gene (117). HIV-1 protease and RT sequences are amplified from the patient plasma samples and inserted into the vector. The amount of luciferase produced by patient-derived viruses is then compared to the amount of luciferase produced

by well-characterized wild-type reference virus. RC has been suggested as an additional parameter for making decisions regarding antiretroviral therapy. Patients who do not experience increases in viral loads despite the accumulation of multiple resistance mutations have been shown to harbor virus with decreased RC (37). In addition, certain drug resistance mutations have been shown to reduce RC (40, 94), and low RC has been correlated with a lower rate of CD4 cell loss in individuals who have experienced viral rebound on treatment (142).

SEROLOGIC TESTS

Primary diagnosis of HIV infection is commonly accomplished via detection of HIV antibody using a screening test, followed by a subsequent confirmatory or supplementary test. Screening tests are highly sensitive and easy to perform; confirmatory tests are more specific (and generally, less sensitive) than screening tests and are more complex and difficult to perform and interpret (30). Because HIV infection typically lasts for years and the initial infection may be minimally symptomatic, most patients who are diagnosed with HIV are identified by antibody detection in the chronic phase of the illness.

Serological testing for HIV antibody is used for various purposes, including primary diagnosis, screening of blood products, management of untested persons in labor and delivery, evaluation of occupational exposures to blood/body fluid, and epidemiological surveillance. Screening of blood products for HIV and other viral transfusion-transmitted diseases has nearly eliminated a major source of HIV transmission in parts of the world where such screening has been implemented (140, 141). Rapid assays for detection of HIV antibody have played an increasingly important role in situations in which rapid provision of antiretroviral therapy may prevent HIV, including large-scale (154) and innovative outreach settings (128), labor and delivery (27), and in employee blood and body fluid exposures, where current guidelines call for postexposure prophylaxis within 2 hours of exposure (111). Rapid tests are also becoming widely used in parts of the world where laboratory infrastructure for HIV serodiagnosis is lacking (35, 98).

Tests for HIV antibody are the preferred method for diagnosis of HIV infection because they are rapid, economical, and highly sensitive and specific, but like all laboratory tests, they have limits. The most important limitation of HIV serodiagnostic tests is the window period: the time between initial infection and the production of detectable antibody (52). During the window period, active viral replication and often high levels of viremia occur; patients in the window period can be highly infectious (152). Different types of antibody tests have different window periods, but all tests based on detection of antibody miss patients early in infection.

Antibody Screening Tests

Standard and Automated EIAs

Great progress in the development of HIV antibody screening tests has been made since the discovery of the virus in 1983; current methods are summarized in Table 3. The first generation of HIV antibody assays relied on the detection of antibody to HIV viral protein lysates. Second-generation assays utilize HIV recombinant antigens as the source of antigen bound to the solid phase and include recombinant antigens for detection of HIV-2. Relative to first-generation tests, second-generation methods provided fewer false-positive results and the ability to detect HIV-2. Third-generation assays utilize solid phases coated with

TABLE 3 Major FDA-approved HIV-1/HIV-2 laboratory-based serodiagnostic tests[a]

Test	Analyte(s) used for detection	Reagent(s) detected	Generation
Conventional ELISA-type tests			
Abbott HIV AB HIV-1/HIV-2	Recombinant gp41, gp120, HIV-2 gp36	IgG and IgM	Third
Bio-Rad Genetic Systems HIV-1/HIV-2	Synthetic gp41, synthetic p32, HIV-2 gp36	IgG and IgM	Third
Bio-Rad Genetic Systems HIV-1/HIV-2 plus O	Recombinant p24, gp160, HIV-2 gp36, O	IgG	Second
bioMerieux Vironostika HIV-1	Viral lysate	IgG and IgM	Third
bioMerieux Vironostika HIV-1 plus O	Viral lysate, viral envelope, O	IgG and IgM	Third
Tests on random-access automated platforms			
Siemens Advia Centaur HIV 1/O/2	Recombinant gp41/120, p24, HIV-2 gp36, synthetic peptide for group O	IgG and IgM	Third
Ortho Vitros Anti-HIV 1+2	Recombinant gp41/120, 41, p24 HIV-2 gp36	IgG and IgM	Third
Architect HIV Ag/Ab Combo	Five recombinant proteins and two synthetic peptides derived from HIV-1 groups M and O and HIV-2; anti-HIV-1 p24 antibody to detect p24 antigen	IgG, IgM, and HIV-1 p24 antigen	Fourth

[a] Data from reference 155 and http://www.fda.gov/BiologicsBloodVaccines/BloodBloodProducts/ApprovedProducts/LicensedProductsBLAs/BloodDonorScreening/InfectiousDisease/ucm080466.htm.

recombinant antigens and peptides, and HIV antibody in the patient's sample is detected with labeled recombinant antigens. Relative to second-generation assays, third-generation methods provide earlier detection during seroconversion, since these antigen-antigen sandwich assays more efficiently detect immunoglobulin M (IgM) and other non-IgG antibodies. Some third-generation format assays use viral lysates instead of recombinant antigen. Fourth-generation assays combine antibody and antigen detection, further decreasing the time to detection during the window period (89, 90, 91). Because a reactive result from a fourth-generation assay may be produced by either antibody or antigen, confirmation of a reactive fourth-generation test should incorporate a nucleic acid test either as a primary confirmatory method or for samples which test negative with a Western blot, indirect fluorescent-antibody assay (IFA), or line probe method. Algorithms for confirmation of fourth-generation assays, as well as further algorithms for laboratory diagnosis of HIV, are found in CLSI document M-53-P (25a). At present, most of the commonly used assays provide for the simultaneous detection of antibodies to both HIV-1 and HIV-2 (Table 3).

The shortage of trained medical laboratory workers and increasing fiscal pressures on laboratories has driven increasing automation in clinical laboratories. Modern random-access immunochemistry platforms provide substantial labor savings over automated EIA screening tests. Tests performed on widely used random-access platforms have great potential to make laboratory-based HIV testing simpler, faster, and more widely available.

Rapid Assays

HIV prevalence continues to increase in the United States, and roughly a quarter of persons living with HIV are unaware that they are infected (20, 71). CDC goals for HIV prevention include making HIV testing a routine part of medical care, and recent publications suggest that expanded screening for HIV is a cost-effective health intervention (7, 9, 110, 123). Serving hard-to-reach populations has been limited by the logistics of conventional HIV testing, which require a follow-up visit before results of testing are available, even for seronegative patients. In addition, an immediate result is medically desirable in certain settings, for example, in assessment of the source patient in occupational blood and body fluid exposures and in labor and delivery settings with women of unknown HIV serostatus.

To address these problems, rapid HIV tests have been under development and in active use for over a decade (78, 137). Performed both in clinical laboratories and at the point of care, rapid HIV tests have a role when rapid results are necessary and when HIV testing is provided to previously inaccessible populations and situations. Rapid HIV tests fall mostly into two categories: membrane EIAs and immunochromatographic assays. Immunochromatographic or lateral flow assays require the addition of only one or no reagent and, thus, are extremely simple to perform. They are especially well suited for testing outside traditional laboratory settings. Six rapid HIV antibody tests were FDA approved in the United States as of July 2009 (Table 4).

Disadvantages of rapid assays include subjective interpretation, lack of automation, and possible errors if the reader has vision problems such as color blindness. Although these kits are easy to use, lack of attention to technique, weak positive tests, and often, less-skilled personnel can lead to errors (62, 63). Samples must be dispensed and tests read within specified time limits, control lines must be read, and instructions must be followed carefully. These formats are useful primarily for small-volume testing. Accurate timing of steps can be adversely affected when multiple samples are tested, and conventional EIAs and similar methods scale up to larger sample volumes more efficiently. Nevertheless, for clinical situations in which rapid results are essential and for outreach settings, rapid HIV tests have become valuable tools (14).

Published studies suggest that rapid tests perform similarly to laboratory-based standard EIA methods when performed by skilled staff. In the largest such study, the MIRIAD trial, HIV testing with OraQuick in point-of-care settings had equal sensitivity to a laboratory-based EIA and had fewer false positives (12). OraQuick was also found to perform as well as a laboratory-based EIA in a region with transmission of multiple HIV subtypes (122). While in most cases the rapid tests appear to have similar performance, one study addressed comparative sensitivity of two rapid tests in early HIV infection (88). A test using a sandwich-capture format and significantly more blood than other methods was more sensitive in early seroconversion.

TABLE 4 Rapid and point-of-care HIV tests approved for use in the United States[a]

Test	Manufacturer	Specimen types	CLIA category	Equipment required	Antigen(s) represented
OraQuick Advance Rapid HIV-1/2 antibody test	OraSure Technologies, Inc.	Whole blood, oral fluid, plasma	Waived; moderate complexity	Timer	gp41
Reveal G3, Rapid HIV-1 antibody test	MedMira, Inc.	Serum, plasma	Moderate complexity	Centrifuge, refrigerator	gp41 and gp120
Uni-Gold Recombigen HIV test	Trinity BioTech	Whole blood, serum, plasma	Waived; moderate complexity	Timer	gp41 and gp120
Multispot HIV-1/HIV-2 rapid test	Bio-Rad Laboratories	Serum, plasma	Moderate complexity	Centrifuge, refrigerator, lab equipment	gp41
Clearview HIV 1/2 Stat Pak	Chembio Diagnostic Systems, Inc.	Whole blood, serum, plasma	Waived; moderate complexity	Timer	gp41 and gp120
Clearview Complete HIV1/2	Chembio Diagnostic Systems, Inc.	Whole blood, serum, plasma	Moderate complexity	Timer	gp41 and gp120

[a]FDA-approved rapid HIV tests as of May 2009. Data derived from the CDC at http://www.cdc.gov/hiv/topics/testing/rapid/rt-purchasing.htm and http://www.cdc.gov/hiv/topics/testing/rapid/rt-comparison.htm and from manufacturers' package inserts and FDA data.

Alternative Samples for Antibody Screening

Alternative specimens to blood, serum, or plasma for HIV antibody testing include oral fluid and urine. Either may be useful in testing of patients who are reluctant to undergo phlebotomy or who have poor vascular access as well as in mass-screening settings and in locations in which phlebotomy is impossible. It is essential to employ only testing methods designed and validated for the specific sample in question.

Oral fluid is a complex mixture of secretions from several different sets of glands, as well as transudated plasma from the capillaries of the gum. Glandular secretions primarily contain secretory IgA, which may have a role in protection against infection but is not a reliable target for diagnostic testing. In contrast, the transudated gingival fluid contains primarily blood-derived IgG. Collection devices such as the OraSure specimen collection device are specifically targeted to enhance collection of gingival transudate. Oral-fluid-based HIV EIA, Western blot, and CLIA-waived rapid tests are FDA approved; indeterminate Western blots appear to be more common from oral fluid than from serum samples (30, 136, 145). Large-scale post-marketing studies found an elevated incidence of false-positive results in oral fluid testing at some sites using the OraSure rapid test (154); this has driven the use of blood-based supplemental testing for oral-fluid-positive patients, which promises to limit the impact of oral fluid false-positives in outreach settings (13, 44, 82).

IgG is found, usually in small quantities relative to serum, in the urine, and FDA-licensed ELISA and Western blots are available for urine (150).

Methods for Detecting Recent Seroconversion

Detuned EIAs are used to estimate the incidence of new infections by assessing the titer or affinity of HIV antibody by comparing the results of a standard, sensitive HIV antibody test with one whose sensitivity has been intentionally decreased—a detuned assay. Patients positive for both the standard and detuned tests are considered to have long-standing infections; patients positive on the standard but negative on the detuned test are considered to have recent infection. Approaches to detuning HIV tests include sample dilution, shortened incubation times, and chaotropic agents (42, 113). Protocols have also been described for using rapid tests in a detuned mode (83).

Serological Testing for Atypical HIV Infections

Most U.S. HIV infections are group M, subtype B HIV-1, but non-B infections are common in parts of Europe and group O and non-B infections are prevalent locally elsewhere, primarily in Africa. The ability to detect infections with these atypical viruses, as well as with HIV-2, varies between tests.

Early HIV tests were unreliable in the detection of HIV-2 (2, 38). Current screening tests include separate antigens for detection of HIV-2. When testing for HIV, the possibility of HIV-2 infection should be considered in persons with a direct or indirect epidemiologic link to West Africa and when discrepant HIV test results are obtained, such as:

- A repeatedly reactive HIV-1/HIV-2 immunoassay result but negative or indeterminate HIV-1 Western blot result
- Disease suggestive of AIDS but a nonreactive result with an HIV-1-specific test
- Confirmed HIV infection but undetectable HIV-1 RNA when patient is not on antiretroviral therapy

The Multispot HIV-1/HIV-2 rapid test (Bio-Rad, Redmond, WA) can distinguish between HIV-1 and HIV-2 infections; however, it is not labeled for use as a supplemental test.

Most group M non-B infections are reliably detected (122), but some have been missed by some immunoassays (57, 90). HIV-1 group O infections can be missed by immunoassays that do not contain specific reagents for the detection of antibodies to group O; 0 to 100% of group O infections were not detected (69, 129, 135, 157).

HIV Antibody Confirmation Assays

Both standard and rapid HIV screening tests require confirmation if the initial test result is positive (Fig. 3 and 4). Screening HIV tests are optimized to provide very high sensitivity at the expense of specificity. HIV testing algorithms therefore incorporate highly specific, but often less sensitive, confirmatory tests. The most commonly used confirmation test is the Western blot, but other confirmation methods and strategies are available, including IFA and line immunoassay. In addition to the traditional EIA screening confirmation algorithm, a number of alternative algorithms have been proposed which include the use of a second, different EIA, nucleic acid amplification test (NAAT), or rapid test as the

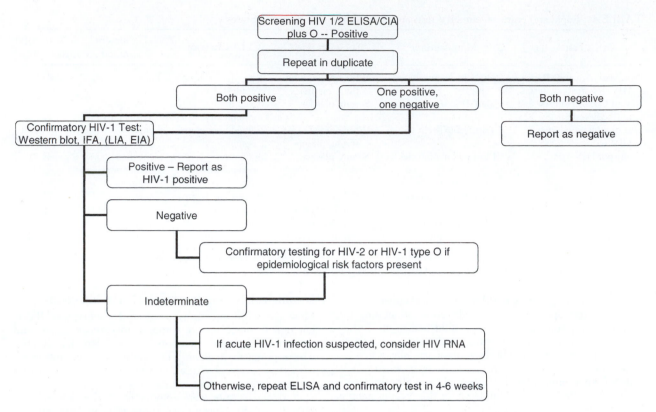

FIGURE 3 HIV antibody testing algorithm for samples initially reactive in a standard HIV-1/HIV-2 assay showing the sequence of suggested follow-up confirmatory testing. LIA, line immunoassay.

confirmatory method. Such schemes have been extensively examined and discussed by a joint CDC-Association of Public Health Laboratories task force (3, 8). Novel and alternative algorithms, incorporating nucleic acid supplementary tests and combinations of screening tests, may improve the availability or performance of testing for specific settings and populations, improve the sensitivity and specificity of screening, and reduce indeterminate Western blots if regulatory, scientific, and economic barriers can be overcome.

The Western blot is considered the gold standard for the confirmation of initially reactive HIV antibody samples. Western blots are supplied in kit form with HIV antigens separated by molecular weight by electrophoresis and blotted onto a membrane which is then cut into strips. The testing laboratory incubates the strips with patient serum and washes and then develops the reaction with an enzyme-labeled anti-human antibody, which detects patient antibodies bound to the specific viral proteins. Antibodies to the following HIV-1-associated antigens can be detected: gp160, gp120, p66, p55, p51, gp41, p31, p24, p17, and p15. Western blots are specific for HIV species and often subspecies. Therefore, it is necessary to use separate Western blots for HIV-1 and HIV-2, and results with subtypes other than M have been variable (22, 31). Western blots are prepared from HIV grown on cell culture; therefore, nonviral proteins may be present on the nitrocellulose strip and lead to nonspecific reactions.

The interpretation of Western blots predominantly follows CDC guidelines, which require detection of at least two of three antigens: p24, gp41, or gp120/160 (15, 16). The absence of all bands is a negative result. HIV-associated bands present but not meeting the criteria for positivity are read as indeterminate. Examples of HIV-1 Western blot results are shown in Fig. 5. Causes of indeterminate Western blots are

listed in Table 5. HIV-2-infected patients sometimes exhibit unusual indeterminate patterns on HIV-1 Western blots, consisting of reactivity to *gag* (p55, p24, or p17) and *pol* (p66, p51, or p32) gene products, in the absence of reactivity to envelope proteins. All indeterminate HIV-1 Western blots should be followed with a repeat screening test and Western blot after 2 weeks to 6 months, depending on the patient's risk factors. RNA or DNA PCR may be used to further assess cases in which the HIV-1 serological results are inconclusive; although except for the Aptima HIV-1 RNA qualitative assay (Gen-Probe, Inc., San Diego, CA), these tests are not approved for diagnosis of HIV infection.

An indirect fluorescence assay (Fluorognost) has also been used as both a screening and confirmatory test for HIV-1 infection. HIV-infected and uninfected lymphocytes are fixed on a slide. The slide is incubated first with patient serum and then with a fluorescent-labeled anti-human antibody. For interpretation, patterns of fluorescence in infected and uninfected cells are compared for each patient sample. Considerable skill is required, and indeterminate results can be produced in patients with autoantibodies and other conditions. In addition to their use as independent confirmatory tests, IFA can be used to resolve indeterminate Western blots. HIV-2-specific IFA has been described but is not FDA approved.

Line immunoassays employ a strategy similar to that of the Western blot. Recombinant or synthetic antigens are placed on a strip rather than transferred from an electrophoretic gel. This approach has the advantage of placing only viral antigens in the reaction, eliminating the background from cross-reactivity with nonspecific cell proteins. The manufacturer has control over the quantity and type of antigens represented and can include HIV-2 and type O antigens to confirm these infections in a single test (22, 23, 100). The

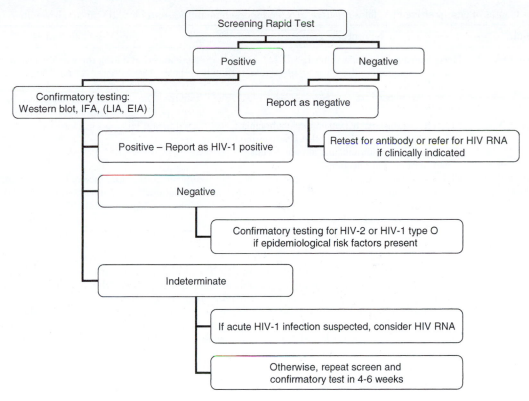

FIGURE 4 HIV antibody testing algorithm for samples tested with rapid HIV assays. LIA, line immunoassay.

Inno-LIA HIV1/11 Score test (Innogenetics, Zwijndrecht, Belgium) is widely available outside the United States.

ANTIVIRAL SUSCEPTIBILIES

Resistance testing has become a crucial element in the management of antiretroviral-experienced patients because it is useful for the selection of the antiretroviral treatment in patients who are failing their current regimen due to the development of antiviral resistance (http://aidsinfo.nih.gov). In addition, given the high rates of transmission of resistant

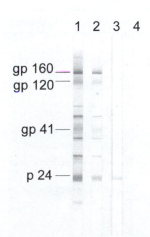

FIGURE 5 Examples of HIV-1 Western blot results. Samples with high and low positive results are shown in lanes 1 and 2, respectively. An indeterminate Western blot is illustrated in lane 3. A negative control is shown in lane 4.

viruses, resistance testing is also taking an increasingly important role in the choice of the initial antiretroviral therapy (87, 106). The clinical utility of HIV resistance testing has been evaluated in a number of prospective randomized clinical trials (6, 26, 46, 99, 148). Although not all of the trials demonstrated a clear benefit for using resistance testing (99), several of the studies showed that patients for whom the antiretroviral treatment was based on the results of resistance testing had greater decreases in viral load than patients in whom the antiretroviral regimen was based on prior antiretroviral usage (6, 26, 46, 148). One of these studies showed that expert advice further improved the benefit of using genotyping resistance testing (148). In addition, use of resistance testing to guide antiretroviral treatment has been reported to be cost-effective (153). Two types of methods are available to assay for HIV resistance. Genotyping tests examine the population of viral genomes in the patient sample for the presence of mutations known to confer decreased sensibility to antiretroviral drugs. Phenotypic assays measure viral replication of the patient's virus in the presence of antiretroviral drugs. Table 6 provides a list of the currently available HIV-1 resistance assays.

Genotyping Assays

Genotyping assays determine the sequence of nucleotides in the viral genome and compare the sequence to that of the wild-type virus. Mutations that appear during the course of antiretroviral therapy are considered to cause drug resistance if in vitro studies confirm that the presence of these mutations decreases the susceptibility of HIV-1 to a specific drug.

The initial steps of genotypic assays include extraction of viral RNA from plasma and RT-PCR to amplify viral RNA sequences which code for a portion of the patient RT

TABLE 5 Causes of false-positive EIA, false-negative EIA, and indeterminate Western blot HIV antibody results

Result	Nonspecific causes	HIV-specific causes
False-negative EIA	Hypogammaglobulinemia, other B-cell dysfunction, immunosuppressive therapies, archived sera, technical errors	Acute infection during the window period, fulminant primary disease, seroreversion,[a] advanced AIDS, HIV-2 (if EIA kit only detects HIV-1), HIV-1 subtype O (if EIA kit does not detect HIV-1 subtype O), other HIV strain variations
False-positive EIA	Multiple transfusions, hypergammaglobulinemia, hemodialysis, antibodies to HLAs, autoantibodies associated with autoimmune disease, recent vaccinations and infections	Experimental HIV vaccination
Indeterminate HIV-1 Western blot	Multiple transfusions, hypergammaglobulinemia, recent vaccinations, hemodialysis, antibodies to HLAs, autoantibodies associated with autoimmune disease, idiopathic	Early seroconversion, incomplete HIV-1 antibody evolution,[a] HIV-2 infection, HIV-1 subtype O infection, experimental HIV vaccination

[a] In acutely infected individuals treated with antiretroviral therapy.

and the entire protease gene, the targets of most available antiretroviral drugs. Next, the nucleotide sequence of amplified sequences is determined and examined for the presence of known resistance mutations. This can be accomplished most commonly in the clinical laboratory setting using automated sequencing technology. In this technology, the nucleotide sequence of the gene of interest is obtained and compared to the sequence of wild-type virus to identify resistance mutations. The process requires alignment and editing of the sequence, a comparison to the wild-type sequence, and final interpretation linking the mutations to specific antiretroviral drugs. Two FDA-approved kits, containing sequencing reagents as well as the software programs required for sequence alignment and interpretation, are commercially available. The databases used for interpretation of resistance mutations require regular updating as the number of new antiretroviral drugs continues to expand. Both of the assays, the Trugene HIV-1 genotyping kit and OpenGene DNA sequencing system (Siemens Healthcare Diagnostics), and the ViroSeq HIV-1 genotyping system (Abbott Molecular) have been found to perform in an equivalent manner (50). These tests detect mutations in the RT and protease genes but do not detect mutations associated with resistance to the fusion inhibitor, integrase inhibitors,

and CCR5 inhibitors. Laboratory-developed tests are available from referral laboratories that detect mutations associated with the other classes of drugs.

One limitation of genotypic assays is that they are only able to detect mutants comprising major fractions of the patient's virus; resistant variants must constitute at least 25 to 30% of the virus population (68). Although the clinical significance of resistant mutations present at low levels remains to be fully elucidated, there is evidence that minor mutations which are missed by standard genotyping assays can lead to failure of subsequent treatments. Because of the lack of sensitivity of standard genotyping assays for detection of low-frequency drug resistance mutations, efforts are under way to increase the sensitivity of detection of mutations through single-genome sequencing (109). Single-genome sequencing involves serially diluting the cDNA until there is a single copy present for amplification and sequencing. This is not presently a practical clinical tool as the process is expensive and labor-intensive.

Phenotyping Assays

In phenotyping assays, the ability of HIV-1 to grow in the presence of various concentrations of a given antiretroviral agent is measured. The amount of drug required to inhibit

TABLE 6 HIV-1 resistance assays

Assay (manufacturer)	Comment
Genotypic assays	
Trugene HIV-1 genotyping kit and Open Gene DNA sequencing system (Siemens Healthcare Diagnostics, Tarrytown, NY)	Detects only protease and RT mutations
Viroseq HIV-1 genotyping system (Abbott Molecular, Des Plaines, IL)	Detects only protease and RT mutations
Phenotypic assays	
Antivirogram (Virco Lab, Inc., Bridgewater, NJ)	
PhenoSense HIV for RT and protease inhibitors (Monogram Biosciences, South San Francisco, CA)	Measures susceptibility to RT and protease inhibitors
PhenoSense for entry inhibitor susceptibility (Monogram Biosciences, South San Francisco, CA)	Measures susceptibility to entry inhibitors (Fuzeon)
PhenoSense integrase (Monogram Biosciences, South San Francisco, CA)	Measures susceptibility to integrase inhibitors
Virco Type HIV-1 (virtual phenotype) (Virco Lab, Inc., Bridgewater, NJ)	
Tropism assays	
Trofile coreceptor tropism (Monogram Biosciences, South San Francisco, CA)	Used prior to initiating therapy with CCR5 inhibitors
SensiTrop II HIV coreceptor tropism (Pathway Diagnostics, Malibu, CA)	Used prior to initiating therapy with CCR5 inhibitors

virus replication by 50% or by 90% is determined and given as a 50% or 90% inhibitory concentration (IC_{50} or IC_{90}). The IC_{50} or IC_{90} obtained with the patient sample is compared to a control wild-type virus, and the result is reported as a relative difference. Early phenotypic resistance assays were labor-intensive because they necessitated the isolation and culture of HIV from the patient's specimen. Currently, commercially available methods use HIV-1 RNA amplified from plasma and are based on recombinant DNA technology. These phenotypic assays are automated but remain labor-intensive and technically complex. They have not been developed in a kit format and are only performed at two commercial laboratories: Virco Lab, Inc. (Bridgewater, NJ), and Monogram Biosciences (South San Francisco, CA). The first step involves extraction of HIV-1 RNA from plasma. Reverse transcription and PCR amplification of the protease and RT genes follow. The amplified genes from the patient's specimen are then inserted into vectors. The PhenoSense assay (Monogram BioSciences) uses an HIV-1 vector with a luciferase reporter gene replacing the viral envelope gene, allowing viral replication to be quantified by measuring luciferase activity (117). PhenoSense tests are also available to measure resistance to the entry inhibitor and integrase inhibitors. In the Antivirogram assay (Virco), patient and HIV-1 vector sequences are combined by recombination in vitro and viral replication is measured using a reporter gene system (73). As with genotypic testing, the phenotypic assays can only detect mutant variants that comprise at least 25% of the viral population.

The virtual phenotype, an approach developed by Virco, can be used as an alternative to phenotypic testing, although it is really a genotyping resistance interpreted with the aid of a large database of samples with paired genotypic and phenotypic data. The virtual phenotype is determined by entering the genotype into the database and finding the closest matching phenotyping results. The virtual phenotype has been shown to be at least as effective as conventional phenotypic testing for decisions regarding antiretroviral therapy (116). The virtual phenotype is a more rapid and less expensive approach to obtaining phenotypic data for the patient without directly performing phenotypic testing. Laboratories that perform genotyping can obtain virtual phenotype data electronically by accessing a Virco database. Alternatively, a plasma sample can be sent to Virco for both genotypic and virtual phenotypic testing. Although there is not always agreement between phenotype, virtual phenotype, and genotype, clinicians find the virtual phenotype to be a useful tool when resources for phenotypic resistance testing are limited and the patient is very antiretroviral experienced.

A new CCR5 inhibitor, maraviroc, has brought about a need for a tropism assay, as the drug is only effective against virus that uses CCR5 as a coreceptor for entry. The drug is not active against CXCR4-tropic virus or dual/mixed tropic virus. The tropism assay must be performed prior to initiating maraviroc, or any other CCR5 inhibitor, to determine whether the virus is CCR5 tropic. There are two commercially available tropism assays, the Trofile (Monogram Biosciences) and Sensitrop II HIV coreceptor tropism assay (Pathway Diagnostics, Malibu, CA). For the Trofile assay, env gene from the patient is amplified and used to construct pseudoviruses. Coreceptor tropism is then determined by measuring the ability of the pseudoviral population to infect $CD4^+/U87$ cells that express either CXCR4 or CCR5. Depending on which cells they infect, the viruses are then designated CXCR4 tropic, CCR5 tropic, or dual/mixed tropic (155). The Sensitrop assay utilizes a heteroduplex tracking assay combined with sequence analysis to identify minor viral populations that may be CXCR4 tropic. Only patients that are solely CCR5 tropic are candidates for a CCR5 inhibitor. Resistance to maraviroc has been reported and results from the development of mutations that allow the virus to use CXCR4 coreceptors or mutations that lead to structural changes in the envelope that prevent the drug from being effective (92, 147).

EVALUATION, INTERPRETATION, AND REPORTING OF RESULTS

Use and Interpretation of Antibody Assays

Currently available standard EIAs and other screening tests are exquisitely sensitive and specific. Causes of false-negative and false-positive screening tests are listed in Table 5. The currently approved rapid methods appear to have comparable sensitivity to conventional EIA methods, although occasional false-positive and false-negative results were seen in large panels but never in numbers sufficient to discriminate between different kits in a significant manner (151, 151a–151c).

The current standard algorithm for confirmation of rapid HIV tests is shown in Fig. 4. Given the overall good performance of rapid HIV tests, the CDC recommends that a screening EIA not be performed prior to confirmation of a positive rapid test. Requiring a second positive EIA could harm the sensitivity of the overall testing scheme, and a positive rapid or point-of-care EIA should be considered equivalent to a laboratory-based EIA as a screening test (18, 19).

The rapid HIV antibody tests have comparatively small antigen suites. In theory, this should limit sensitivity in some patients. The quality of testing is of concern at all times, but it is particularly of concern for rapid HIV assays when testing is performed outside standard laboratory settings and by personnel whose chief expertise is not performing laboratory tests. The CDC has issued extensive performance and quality assurance guidelines for use of rapid HIV tests (18). In addition, no laboratory test is 100% accurate, and results inconsistent with clinical findings should be repeated or assessed with different tests (29, 30).

Confirmatory tests also have limitations. The Western blot assay is less sensitive than either third- or fourth-generation screening tests during early infection. It can be up to 3 weeks following a positive result on a fourth-generation assay before the Western blot gives a positive result. At the other end of the disease spectrum, as the infection progresses to late AIDS, immune failure may lead to false-negative results.

Use and Interpretation of HIV RNA and DNA Qualitative Assays

In adults, HIV-1 RNA tests are primarily used to diagnose acute infection and for the resolution of indeterminate Western blot results. There is increasing interest in using this test to replace Western blot confirmation, but this is not the current standard of practice. The availability of an FDA-approved test (Aptima) may lead to changes in testing algorithms. Both HIV-1 RNA and DNA tests can be used for the diagnosis of neonatal HIV-1 infection, but DNA is often the preferred method used in the United States for determining an exposed infant's HIV-1 infection status. This is primarily due to the limited availability of a qualitative RNA test. Indeed, serological tests are not useful for the detection of HIV infection in infants, since maternal antibodies can be present in children until the age of 18 months. The DNA test can be performed on whole blood or on dried blood spots, but the specimen collected at birth must be a neonatal and not a cord blood sample; cord blood samples yield a high rate of false-positive results (80). Current recommendations are to test infants under the age of 18 months at 14 to 21 days, 1 to 2 months, and 4 to 6 months after birth, with some experts also recommending testing at birth. HIV-1 infection is diagnosed by two positive RNA or DNA tests performed on separate blood samples regardless of age. Infection is confirmed by a positive antibody test at $\geq$18 months of age (155a). The proviral DNA test has a sensitivity of 38% at 48 hours of life and 99% at 4 weeks of age (45). RNA and DNA tests have comparable sensitivities and specificities; to improve diagnostic accuracy, specimens with a low viral load (<10,000 copies/ml) should be repeated. The Aptima test may be more sensitive than HIV-1 DNA tests for the detection of non-B subtypes, CRFs, and group O virus. An advantage of proviral DNA tests is that they remain positive even in individuals receiving antiretroviral therapy. The impact of highly active antiretroviral therapy on the sensitivity of RNA tests is unknown.

Use and Interpretation of Viral Load Assays

The clinical utility of HIV-1 viral load testing has been well established (17) and can be found online at www.iasusa.org. Viral load assays are used widely to monitor changes in plasma viremia during antiretroviral therapy because they are useful for predicting time to progression to AIDS, determining when to initiate therapy, and monitoring responses to therapy. The magnitude of the decrease in viral load is dependent on the effectiveness of the antiretroviral therapy, and the optimum goal of therapy is to achieve viral loads below the detection limit of the assay. Baseline testing as well as repeated levels of HIV RNA should be obtained before initiating or changing antiretroviral therapy regimens. After initiation of therapy, patients should be tested within 2 to 8 weeks to assess drug efficacy and then every 3 to 4 months to assess durability of response.

Biological variation of HIV-1 RNA among clinically stable patients has been estimated to be approximately 0.3 $\log_{10}$ (36). In addition, commercial assays show reproducibility ranging from 0.1 to 0.3 $\log_{10}$ depending on the region of the assay's dynamic range. Generally, a change in viral load greater than 0.5 $\log_{10}$ copies/ml (threefold) is considered significant. Viral load changes for samples close to the 50-copies/ml low detection limit of assays should be interpreted with particular caution because at the low end of the dynamic range, assay variability has a greater impact on assay interpretation. For borderline viral load values in patients with no prior data, it may be indicated to verify patient status, scrutinize laboratory results, and consider repeat testing. Reporting viral load values as $\log_{10}$ copies/ml may help clinicians avoid overinterpreting small changes in viral load that are within the assay and biological variability.

Numerous studies comparing the performance of the conventional FDA-approved assays have been done (47, 49, 60, 74). Overall, high correlations between assays have been shown, and net changes in plasma RNA levels after antiretroviral therapy are similar. The current-generation assays have been standardized so that the differences in viral load are narrowing among assays. However, values do differ, and for a given sample, viral load obtained with the Bayer Versant 3.0 assay are consistently lower than the viral load values generated by the Amplicor and NucliSens assays. The few studies comparing viral load values between the two FDA-approved real-time RT-PCR assays have shown

good correlation and agreement between viral load values, with mean/median differences in viral load values ranging from 0.22 to 0.56 $\log_{10}$ copy/ml depending on the subtype of the samples, with the greatest differences seen with CRFs (11, 67, 113a). Overall, there is very good agreement between the different viral load tests, but it is optimal for patient care to monitor viral load values over time with a single assay.

HIV-1 RNA load testing is sometimes requested to resolve equivocal serologic findings or to facilitate the diagnosis of HIV-1 infection during the acute phase or in a pediatric setting. In these settings, it is important to keep in mind that these viral load tests are not approved by the FDA for the diagnosis of HIV-1 infection. In addition, false-positive results can be obtained because of contamination during specimen processing, carryover of amplified products, or incorrect thresholds. With the bDNA assay, nonspecific hybridization can also lead to false-positive results; overall, the specificity of the assay is 98%. In CDC proficiency surveys, false-positive results as high as 5,000 copies/ml have been reported. Furthermore, herpes simplex virus infections, acute respiratory infections, and vaccinations can cause transient increases in viral load; HIV-1 RNA viral loads usually return to baseline within 1 month (43, 107).

Use and Interpretation of Resistance Assays

Clinical guidelines for the use of HIV-1 resistance testing in adults are published and updated on a regular basis (75). In general, resistance testing is recommended for patients entering care regardless of whether the patient will be treated immediately, when initiating antiretroviral therapy, for patients failing therapy, for pregnant women, and for patients with acute infection. In contrast to phenotypic tests, genotypic assays are widely available, technically easier to perform, faster, and less expensive. In some cases, a resistance mutation may be detectable before a change in the phenotype has occurred, and therefore, genotypic and phenotypic results are not always correlated. One limitation of genotyping assays originates from the complexity of data generated by the genotyping assays. In the face of the rapid development in new drugs and new information of HIV-1 resistance, it remains a challenge to keep updated on which mutations are associated with each specific drug combination. A complete list of drug-resistant mutations for all classes of drug is available at the International AIDS Society—USA website (http://www.iasusa.org); this site is updated regularly.

The interpretation of HIV-1 genotyping results is complex. It requires knowledge of the identity of mutations associated with each specific drug, of the interactions of resistance mutations, and of the genetics of cross-resistance. Most systems use a rule-based approach; a group of experts establish interpretation algorithms based on the type of mutations or combination of mutations that are associated with resistance to specific drugs. In the Trugene and ViroSeq assays, these algorithms are used to generate automated HIV-1 genotyping reports. Depending on the mutations detected, the report will indicate, for each drug in each of the antiviral categories, whether virus contained in the sample shows no evidence of resistance, resistance, or possible resistance or if there is no sufficient evidence to place the virus in one of the three other categories. These rule-based systems provide easy-to-interpret information to clinicians, but the databases require regular updating. The manufacturer's database update may lag the published literature, so clinicians may refer to online databases (http://hivdb.stanford.edu/index.html). For this reason, it is very helpful to report the mutations as well as the interpretation so clinicians can easily use online databases.

Phenotyping assays offer the advantage that they provide results in a format that is more familiar to clinicians. Results are reported as a relative change in IC_{50} compared to wild-type virus. In addition, there appears to be less need for expert interpretation because susceptibility is measured directly. A problem with phenotypic resistance testing is that drugs are used in combination but are not tested in combination. The cutoffs for a significant change in IC_{50} can vary greatly depending on the drug. Initially, biological cutoffs were established based on the reproducibility of the assays; however, over time, clinical cutoffs correlated with outcome have been established for most drugs. The virtual phenotype provides an estimate of the probable phenotype, so the correlation between actual and virtual phenotype is likely to be lower in cases when there are few matches in the database as well as for newer drugs. One advantage of the virtual phenotype over phenotypic assays is the time to a result. Phenotypic testing can take 1 to 2 weeks for a result, while the virtual phenotype can be reported within an hour or so of completing the genotypic testing. In addition, the cost of the virtual phenotype is much lower than the cost of a phenotypic assay.

Both genotypic and phenotypic assays yield results only if the plasma used for testing contains at least 500 HIV-1 RNA copies per ml. Depending on the extraction method used, it may be possible to obtain results on specimens with a lower viral load. Concentration of the virions in plasma by high-speed centrifugation may allow sequencing of specimens with viral loads of <500 copies/ml, but the process may also concentrate inhibitors/interfering substances. Due to the labor and expenses of genotyping assays, laboratories should establish the lower viral load limit for obtaining reliable sequencing results. In addition, for both assays, the resistant viral mutant must constitute at least 20 to 30% of the viral quasispecies to be detected. Also, cross contamination can occur with both resistance assays because both procedures rely on an RT-PCR step to amplify the HIV-1 gene sequences. Both methods have clinical utility in managing patients and are widely used in clinical practice. However, given the wider availability, shorter turnaround time, and lower cost, most clinicians use genotyping for the initial evaluation of resistance. Phenotyping assays (or the virtual phenotype), on the other hand, can help in defining the significance of newly recognized resistance mutations, in elucidating the effects of complex mutation interactions, and may be very helpful in determining salvage regimens.

REFERENCES

1. Altfeld, M., M. Addo, E. S. Rosenberg, F. M. Hecht, P. K. Lee, M. Vogel, X. G. Yu, R. Draenert, M. N. Johnson, D. Strick, T. Allen, M. E. Feeney, J. O. Kahn, R. P. Sekaly, J. A. Levy, J. K. Rockstroh, K. Jurgen, P. J. Goulder, and B. D. Walker. 2003. Influence of HLA-B57 on clinical presentation and viral control during acute HIV-1 infection. *AIDS* **17:**2581–2591.
2. Andersson, S., Z. da Silva, H. Norrgren, F. Dias, and G. Biberfeld. 1997. Field evaluation of alternative testing strategies for diagnosis and differentiation of HIV-1 and HIV-2 infections in an HIV-1 and HIV-2 prevalent area. *AIDS* **11:**1815–1822.
3. Association of Public Health Laboratories and Centers for Disease Control and Prevention. 2007. *2007 HIV Diagnostics Conference Abstracts and Summary.* The Association of Public Health Laboratories, Silver Spring, MD. http://www.hivtestingconference.org.
4. Barouch, D. H. 2008. Challenges in the development of an HIV-1 vaccine. *Nature* **455:**613–617.
5. Barre-Sinoussi, F., J. C. Chermann, F. Rey, M. T. Nugeyre, S. Chamaret, J. Gruest, C. Dauguet, C. Axler-Blin, F. Brun-Vezinet, C. Rouzioux, W. Rosenbaum, and L. Montagnier. 1983. Isolation of a T-lymphotropic retrovirus from a patient at risk for acquired immune deficiency syndrome (AIDS). *Science* **220:**868–871.
6. Baxter, J. D., D. L. Mayers, D. N. Wentworth, J. D. Neaton, M. L. Hoover, M. A. Winters, S. B. Mannheimer, M. A. Thompson, D. I. Abrams, B. J. Brizz, J. P. Ioannidis, T. C. Merigan, and the CPCRA 046 Study team for the Terry Beirn Community Programs for Clinical Research on AIDS. 2000. A randomized study of antiretroviral management based on plasma genotypic antiretroviral resistance testing in patients failing therapy. *AIDS* **14:**F83–F93.
7. Beckwith, C. G., T. P. Flanigan, C. del Rio, E. Simmons, E. J. Wing, C. J. Carpenter, and J. G. Bartlett. 2005. It is time to implement routine, not risk-based, HIV testing. *Clin. Infect. Dis.* **40:**1037–1040.
8. Bennett, B., B. Branson, K. Delaney, M. Owen, M. Pentella, and B. Werner. 2009. *HIV Testing Algorithms: a Status Report.* The Association of Public Health Laboratories, Silver Spring, MD.
9. Branson, B. M., H. H. Handsfield, M. A. Lampe, R. S. Janssen, A. W. Taylor, S. B. Lyss, J. E. Clark, and Centers for Disease Control and Prevention. 2006. Revised recommendations for HIV testing of adults, adolescents, and pregnant women in health-care settings. *MMWR Recommend. Rep.* **55**(RR-14):1–17.
10. Braun, J., J. C. Plantier, M. F. Hellot, E. Tuaillon, M. Gueudin, F. Damond, A. Malmsten, G. E. Corrigan, and F. Simon. 2003. A new quantitative HIV load assay based on plasma virion reverse transcriptase activity for the different types, groups and subtypes. *AIDS* **17:**331–336.
11. Braun, P., R. Ehret, F. Wiesmann, F. Zabbai, M. Knickmann, R. Kuhn, S. Thamm, G. Warnat, and H. Knechten. 2007. Comparison of four commercial quantitative HIV-1 assays for viral load monitoring in clinical daily routine. *Clin. Chem. Lab. Med.* **45:**93–99.
12. Bulterys, M., D. J. Jamieson, M. J. O'Sullivan, M. H. Cohen, R. Maupin, S. Nesheim, M. P. Webber, R. Van Dyke, J. Wiener, B. M. Branson, et al. 2004. Rapid HIV-1 testing during labor: a multicenter study. *JAMA* **292:**219–223.
13. Cadoff, E. 2007. Retrospective application of the proposed CDC/APHL rapid testing algorithm in New Jersey 2004-2007, abstr. 15. *2007 HIV Diagn. Conf.* http://www.hivtestingconference.org/hivtesting2007/abstracts/abstract15.pdf.
14. Campbell, S. M., and Y. Fedoriw. 2009. Point-of-care immunodeficiency virus testing. *Point Care* **8:**32–35.
15. Centers for Disease Control. 1989. Interpretation and use of the Western blot assay for serodiagnosis of human immunodeficiency virus type 1 infections. *MMWR Morb. Mortal. Wkly. Rep.* **38**(Suppl. 7):1–7.
16. Centers for Disease Control. 1991. Interpretive criteria used to report Western blot results for HIV-1-antibody testing—United States. *MMWR Morb. Mortal. Wkly. Rep.* **40:**692–695.
17. Centers for Disease Control and Prevention. 2002. Guidelines for using antiretroviral agents among HIV-infected adults and adolescents. Recommendations of the panel on clinical practices for treatment of HIV. *MMWR Recommend. Rep.* **51**(RR-7):1–56.
18. Centers for Disease Control and Prevention. 2003. *Quality Assurance Guidelines for Testing Using the OraQuick Rapid HIV-1 Antibody Test.* U.S. Department of Health and Human Services, Washington, DC.
19. Centers for Disease Control and Prevention. 2004. Notice to readers: protocols for confirmation of reactive rapid HIV tests. *MMWR Morb. Mortal. Wkly. Rep.* **53:**221–222.

20. **Centers for Disease Control and Prevention.** 2007. *HIV/AIDS Surveillance Report. Cases of HIV Infection and AIDS in the United States and Dependent Areas.* Centers for Disease Control and Prevention, Atlanta, GA.

21. **Centers for Disease Control and Prevention.** 2008. Revised surveillance case definitions for HIV infection among adults, adolescents, and children aged <18 months and for HIV infection and AIDS among children aged 18 months to <13 years—United States, 2008. *MMWR Recommend. Rep.* **57**(RR-10):1–12.

22. **Chattopadhya, D., R. K. Aggarwal, and S. Kumari.** 1996. Profile of antigen-specific antibody response detectable by Western blot in relation to diagnostic criteria for human immunodeficiency virus type-1 (HIV-1) infection. *Clin. Diagn. Virol.* **7**:35–42.

23. **Chattopadhya, D., R. K. Aggarwal, U. K. Baveja, V. Doda, and S. Kumari.** 1998. Evaluation of epidemiological and serological predictors of human immunodeficiency virus type-1 (HIV-1) infection among high risk professional blood donors with Western blot indeterminate results. *J. Clin. Virol.* **11**:39–49.

24. **Choe, H., M Farzan, Y. Sun, N. Sullivan, B. Rollins, P. D. Ponath, L. Wu, C. R. Mackay, G. LaRosa, W. Neuman, N. Gerard, C. Gerard, and J. Sodroski.** 1996. The beta-chemokine receptors CCR3 and CCR5 facilitate infection by primary HIV-1 isolates. *Cell* **85**:1135–1148.

25. **Clavel, F., D. Guetard, F. Brun-Vezinet, S. Chamaret, M. A. Rey, M. O. Santos-Ferreira, A. G. Laurent, C. Dauguet, C. Katlama, and C. Rouzioux.** 1986. Isolation of a new human retrovirus from West African patients with AIDS. *Science* **233**:343–346.

25a. **Clinical and Laboratory Standards Institute.** 2010. *Criteria for Laboratory Testing and Diagnosis of HIV Infection, Proposed Guideline.* Document M-53-P. Clinical and Laboratory Standards Institute, Wayne, PA.

26. **Cohen, C. J., S. Hunt, M. Sension, C. Farthing, M. Conant, S. Jacobson, J. Nadler, W. Verbiest, K. Hertogs, M. Ames, A. R. Rinehart, N. M. Graham, and the VIRA3001 Study Team.** 2002. A randomized trial assessing the impact of phenotypic resistance testing on antiretroviral therapy. *AIDS* **16**:579–588.

27. **Cohn, S. E., and R. A. Clark.** 2005. Human immunodeficiency virus infections of women, p. 1617–1638. *In* G. L. Mandell, J. E. Bennett, and R. Dolin (ed.), *Principles and Practice of Infectious Diseases,* 6th ed. Elsevier, Philadelphia, PA.

28. **Connor, E. M., R. S. Sperling, R. D. Gelber, P. Kiselev, G. Scott, M. J. O'Sullivan, R. VanDyke, M. Bey, W. Shearer, R. L. Jacobson, E. Jimenez, E. O'Neill, B. Bazin, J. F. Delfraissy, M. Culnana, R. Coombs, M. Elkins, J. Moye, P. Stratton, and the Pediatric AIDS Clinical Trials Group Protocol 076 Study Group.** 1994. Reduction of maternal-infant transmission of human immunodeficiency virus type 1 with zidovudine treatment. *N. Engl. J. Med.* **331**:1173–1180.

29. **Constantine, N. T., and F. Ketema.** 2002. Rapid confirmation of HIV infection. *Int. J. Infect. Dis.* **6**:170–177.

30. **Constantine, N. T., and H. Zink.** 2005. HIV testing technologies after two decades of evolution. *Indian J. Med. Res.* **121**:519–538.

31. **Constantine, N. T., J. D. Callahan, and D. M. Watts.** 1992. *Retroviral Testing: Essentials for Quality Control and Laboratory Diagnosis.* CRC Publishers, Ann Arbor, MI.

32. **Cooper, D. A., J. Gold, P. Maclean, B. Donovan, R. Finlayson, T. G. Barnes, H. M. Michelmore, P. Brooke, and R. Penny for the Sydney AIDS Study Group.** 1985. Acute AIDS retrovirus infection. Definition of a clinical illness associated with seroconversion. *Lancet* **i**:537–540.

33. **Daar, E. S., S. Little, J. Pitt, J. Santangelo, P. Ho, N. Harawa, P. Kerndt, J. V. Glorgi, J. Bai, P. Gaut, D. D. Richman, S. Mandel, and S. Nichols.** 2001. Diagnosis of primary HIV-1 infection. *Ann. Intern. Med.* **134**:25–29.

34. **Dalgleish, A. G., P. C. L. Beverly, P. R. Clapham, D. H. Crawford, M. F. Greaves, and R. A. Weiss.** 1984. The CD4 (T4) antigen is an essential component of the receptor of the AIDS retrovirus. *Nature* **312**:763–767.

35. **De Cock, K. M., R. Bunnell, and J. Mermin.** 2006. Unfinished business—expanding HIV testing in developing countries. *N. Engl. J. Med.* **354**:440–442.

36. **Deeks, S. G., R. L. Coleman, R. White, C. Pachl, M. Schambelan, D. N. Chernoff, M. B. Feinberg.** 1997. Variance of plasma human immunodeficiency virus type 1 RNA levels measured by branched DNA within and between days. *J. Infect. Dis.* **176**:514–517.

37. **Deeks, S. G., T. Wrin, T. Liegler, R. Hoh, M. Hayden, J. D. Barbour, N. S. Hellmann, C. J. Petropoulos, J. M. McCune, M. K. Hellerstein, and R. M. Grant.** 2001. Virologic and immunologic consequences of discontinuing combination antiretroviral-drug therapy in HIV-1 infected patients with detectable viremia. *N. Engl. J. Med.* **344**:472–480.

38. **Denis, F., G. Leonard, and F. Barin.** 1988. Comparison of 10 enzyme immunoassays for detection of antibody to human immunodeficiency virus type 2 in West African sera. *J. Clin. Microbiol.* **26**:1000–1004.

39. **Desrosiers, R. C., M. D. Daniel, and Y. Li.** 1989. HIV-related lentiviruses of nonhuman primates. *AIDS Res. Hum. Retrovir.* **5**:465–473.

40. **Devereux, H. L., V. C. Emery, M. A. Johnson, and C. Loveday.** 2001. Replication fitness in vivo of HIV-1 variants with multiple drug resistance-associated mutations. *J. Med. Virol.* **65**:218–224.

41. **Dewar, R. L., H. C. Highbarger, M. D. Sarmiento, J. A. Todd, M. B. Vasudevachari, R. T. Davey, J. A. Kovacs, N. P. Salzman, H. C. Lane, and M. S. Urdea.** 1994. Application of branched DNA signal amplification to monitor human immunodeficiency virus type 1 burden in human plasma. *J. Infect. Dis.* **170**:1172–1179.

42. **Dobbs, T., S. Kennedy, C. P. Pau, J. S. McDougal, and B. S. Parekh.** 2004. Performance characteristics of the immunoglobulin G-capture BED-enzyme immunoassay, an assay to detect recent human immunodeficiency virus type 1 seroconversion. *J. Clin. Microbiol.* **42**:2623–2628.

43. **Donovan, R. M., C. E. Bush, N. P. Markowitz, D. M. Baxa, and L. D. Saravolatz.** 1996. Changes in viral load markers during AIDS associated opportunistic diseases in human immunodeficiency virus-infected persons. *J. Infect. Dis.* **174**:401–403.

44. **Dowling, T.** 2007. Training and quality assurance for a rapid test algorithm: lessons from implementation, San Francisco, CA 2007, abstr. 39. *2007 HIV Diagn. Conf.* http://www.hivtestingconference.org/hivtesting2007/abstracts/abstract39.pdf.

45. **Dunn, D. T., C. D. Brandt, A. Krivine, S. A. Cassol, P. Roques, V. Borkowsky, A. DeRossi, E. Denamur, A. Ehrnst, and C. Loveday.** 1995. The sensitivity of HIV-1 DNA polymerase chain reaction in the neonatal period and the relative contributions of intra-uterine and intra-partum transmission. *AIDS* **9**:F7–F11.

46. **Durant, J., P. Clevenbergh, P. Halfon, P. Delgiudice, S. Porsin, P. Simonet, N. Montagne, C. A. B. Boucher, J. M. Shapiro, and P. Dellamonica.** 1999. Drug-resistance genotyping in HIV-1 therapy: the VIRADAPT randomized controlled trial. *Lancet* **353**:2195–2199.

47. **Dyer, J. R., C. D. Pilcher, R. Shepard, J. Schock, J. J. Eron, and S. A. Fiscus.** 1999. Comparison of NucliSens and Roche monitor assays for quantitation of levels of human immunodeficiency virus type 1 RNA in plasma. *J. Clin. Microbiol.* **37**:447–449.

48. **Dykes, C., and L. M. Demeter.** 2007. Clinical significance of human immunodeficiency virus type 1 replication fitness. *Clin. Microbiol. Rev.* **20**:550–578.

49. **Elbeik, T. E., P. Charlebois, J. Nassos, J. Kahn, F. M. Hecht, D. Yajko, V. Ng, and K. Hadley.** 2000. Quantitative and cost comparison of ultrasensitive human immunodeficiency virus type 1 RNA viral load assays: Bayer bDNA quantiplex versions 3.0 and 2.0 and Roche PCR Amplicor Monitor version 1.5. *J. Clin. Microbiol.* **38**:1113–1120.

50. **Erali, M., S. Page, L. G. Reimer, and D. R. Hillyard.** 2001. Human immunodeficiency virus type 1 drug resistance testing: a comparison of three sequence-based methods. *J. Clin. Microbiol.* **39**:2157–2165.

51. **Feng, Y., C. C. Broder, P. E. Kennedy, and E. A. Berger.** 1996. HIV-1 entry cofactor: functional cDNA cloning of a seven-transmembrane, G-protein-coupled receptor. *Science* **272**:872–877.

52. Fiebig, E. W., D. J. Wright, B. D. Rawal, P. E. Garrett, R. T. Schumacher, L. Peddada, C. Heldebrant, R. Smith, A. Conrad, S. H. Kleinman, and M. P. Busch. 2003. Dynamics of HIV viremia and antibody seroconversion in plasma donors: implications for diagnosis and staging of primary HIV infection. *AIDS* **17:**1871–1879.

53. Finzi, D., J. Blankson, J. D. Siliciano, J. B. Margolick, K. Chadwick, T. Pierson, K. Smith, J. Lisziewicz, F. Lori, C. Flexner, T. C. Quinn, R. E. Chaisson, E. Rosenberg, B. Walker, S. Gange, J. Gallant, and R. F. Siliciano. 1999. Latent infection of CD4+ cells provides a mechanism for lifelong persistence of HIV-1, even in patients on effective combination therapy. *Nat. Med.* **5:**512–517.

54. Fiscus, S. A., D. Brambilla, R. W. Coombs, B. Yen-Lieberman, J. Bremer, A. Kovacs, S. Rasheed, M. Vahey, T. Schutzbank, and P. S. Reichelderfer. 2000. Multicenter evaluation of methods to quantitate human immunodeficiency virus type 1 RNA in seminal plasma. *J. Clin. Microbiol.* **38:**2348–2353.

55. Gallo, R. C., S. Z. Salahuddin, M. Popovic, G. M. Shearer, M. Kaplan, B. F. Haynes, T. J. Palker, R. Redfield, J. Oleske, and B. Safai. 1984. Frequent detection and isolation of cytopathic retroviruses (HTLV-III) from patients with AIDS and at risk for AIDS. *Science* **224:**500–503.

56. Gao, F., E. Bailes, D. L. Robertson, Y. L. Chen, C. M. Rodenburg, S. F. Michael, L. B. Cummins, L. O. Arthur, M. Peeters, G. M. Shaw, P. M. Sharp, and B. H. Hahn. 1999. Origin of HIV-1 in the chimpanzee *Pan troglodytes troglodytes*. *Nature* **397:**436–441.

57. Gaudy, C., A. Moreau, S. Brunet, J. M. Descamps, P. Deleplanque, D. Brand, and F. Barin. 2004. Subtype B human immunodeficiency virus (HIV) type 1 mutant that escapes detection in a fourth-generation immunoassay for HIV infection. *J. Clin. Microbiol.* **42:**2847–2849.

58. Gerberding, J. L., C. E. Bryant-LeBlanc, K. Nelson, A. R. Moss, D. Osmond, H. F. Chambers, J. R. Carlson, W. L. Drew, J. A. Levy, and M. A. Sande. 1987. Risk of transmitting the human immunodeficiency virus, cytomegalovirus, and hepatitis B virus to health care workers exposed to patients with AIDS and AIDS-related conditions. *J. Infect. Dis.* **156:**1–8.

59. Ginocchio, C., M. Kemper, K. Stellrecht, and D. J. Witt. 2003. Multicenter evaluation of the performance characteristics of the NucliSens HIV-1 QT assay used for the quantification of human immunodeficiency virus type 1 RNA. *J. Clin. Microbiol.* **41:**164–173.

60. Ginocchio, C. C., S. Tetali, D. Washburn, F. Zhang, and M. H. Kaplan. 1999. Comparison of levels of human immunodeficiency virus type 1 RNA in plasma as measured by the Nuclisens nucleic acid sequence-based amplification and Quantiplex branched-DNA assays. *J. Clin. Microbiol.* **37:**1210–1212.

61. Ginocchio, C. C., X. P. Wang, M. H. Kaplan, G. Mulligan, D. Witt, J. W. Romano, M. Cronin, and R. Carroll. 1997. Effects of specimen collection, processing, and storage conditions on stability of human immunodeficiency virus type 1 RNA levels in plasma. *J. Clin. Microbiol.* **35:**2886–2893.

62. Granade, T. C., B. S. Parekh, S. K. Phillips, and J. S. McDougal. 2004. Performance of the Oraquick and Hemastrip rapid HIV antibody detection assays by non-laboratorians. *J. Clin. Virol.* **30:**229–232.

63. Gray, R. H., F. Makumbi, D. Serwadda, T. Lutalo, F. Nalugoda, P. Opendi, G. Kigozi, S. J. Reynolds, N. K. Sewankambo, and M. J. Wawer. 2007. Limitations of rapid HIV-1 tests during screening for trials in Uganda: diagnostic test accuracy study. *BMJ* **335:**188–191.

64. Griffith, B. P. 1987. Principles of laboratory isolation and identification of the human immunodeficiency virus (HIV). *Yale J. Biol. Med.* **60:**575–587.

65. Griffith, B. P., and D. R. Mayo. 2006. Increased levels of HIV RNA detected in samples with viral loads close to the detection limit collected in Plasma Preparation Tubes (PPT). *J. Clin. Virol.* **35:**197–200.

66. Griffith, B. P., M. O. Rigsby, R. B. Garner, M. M. Gordon, and T. C. Chacko. 1997. Comparison of the Amplicor HIV-1 Monitor test and the nucleic acid sequence-based amplification assay for quantitation of human immunodeficiency virus RNA in plasma, serum, and plasma subjected to freeze-thaw cycles. *J. Clin. Microbiol.* **35:**3288–3291.

67. Gueudin, M., J. C. Plantier, V. Lemee, M. P. Schmitt, L. Chartier, T. Bourlet, A. Ruffault, F. Damond, M. Vray, and F. Simon. 2007. Evaluation of the Roche Cobas TaqMan and Abbott RealTime extraction-quantification systems for HIV-1 subtypes. *J. Acquir. Immune Defic. Syndr.* **44:**500–505.

68. Gunthard, H. F., J. K. Wong, C. C. Ignacio, D. V. Havlir, and D. D. Richman. 1998. Comparative performance of high-density oligonucleotide sequencing and dideoxynucleotide sequencing of HIV type 1 pol from clinical samples. *AIDS Res. Hum. Retrovir.* **14:**869–876.

69. Gürtler, L. G., L. Zekeng, F. Simon, J. Eberle, J. M. Tsague, L. Kaptue, S. Brust, and S. Knapp. 1995. Reactivity of five anti-HIV-1 subtype O specimens with six different anti-HIV screening ELISAs and three immunoblots. *J. Virol. Methods* **51:**177–184.

70. Hahn, B. H., G. M. Shaw, K. M. De Cock, and P. M. Sharp. 2000. AIDS as a zoonosis: scientific and public health implications. *Science* **287:**607–614.

71. Hall, H. I., R. Song, P. Rhodes, J. Prejean, Q. An, L. M. Lee, J. Karon, R. Brookmeyer, E. H. Kaplan, M. T. McKenna, and R. S. Janssen for the HIV Incidence Surveillance Group. 2008. Estimation of HIV incidence in the United States. *JAMA* **300:**520–529.

72. Hecht, F. M., M. P. Busch, B. Rawal, M. Webb, E. Rosenberg, M. Swanson, M. Chesney, J. Anderson, J. Levy, and J. O. Kahn. 2002. Use of laboratory tests and clinical symptoms for identification of primary infection. *AIDS* **16:**1119–1129.

73. Hertogs, K., M. P. de Bethune, V. Miller, T. Ivens, P. Schel, A. Van Cauwenberge, C. Van Den Eynde, V. Van Gerwen, H. Azijn, M. Van Houtte, F. Peeters, S. Staszewski, M. Conant, S. Bloor, S. Kemp, B. Larder, and R. Pauwels. 1998. A rapid method for simultaneous detection of phenotypic resistance to inhibitors of protease and reverse transcriptase in recombinant human immunodeficiency virus type 1 isolates from patients treated with antiretroviral drugs. *Antimicrob. Agents Chemother.* **42:**269–276.

74. Highbarger, H. C., W. G. Alvord, M. K. Jiang, A. S. Shah, J. A. Metcalf, H. C. Lane, and R. L. Dewar. 1999. Comparison of the Quantiplex version 3.0 assay and a sensitized Amplicor monitor assay for measurement of human immunodeficiency virus type 1 RNA levels in plasma samples. *J. Clin. Microbiol.* **37:**3612–3614.

75. Hirsch, M. S., H. F. Günthard, J. M. Schapiro, F. Brun-Vézinet, B. Clotet, S. M. Hammer, V. A. Johnson, D. R. Kuritzkes, J. W. Mellors, D. Pillay, P. G. Yeni, D. M. Jacobsen, and D. D. Richman. 2008. Antiretroviral drug resistance testing in adult HIV-1 infection: 2008 recommendations of an International AIDS Society-USA panel. *Clin. Infect. Dis.* **47:**266–285.

76. Ho, D. D., A. U. Neumann, A. S. Perelson, W. Chen, J. M. Leonard, and M. Markowitz. 1995. Rapid turnover of plasmas virions and CD4 lymphocytes in HIV-1 infection. *Nature* **373:**123–126.

77. Ho, D. D., T. Moudgil, and M. Alam. 1989. Quantitation of human immunodeficiency virus type 1 in the blood of infected persons. *N. Engl. J. Med.* **321:**1621–1625.

78. Irwin, K., N. Olivo, C. A. Schable, J. T. Weber, R. Janssen, J. Ernst, and the CDC-Bronx-Lebanon HIV Serosurvey Team. 1996. Performance characteristics of a rapid HIV antibody assay in a hospital with a high prevalence of HIV infection. *Ann. Intern. Med.* **125:**471–475.

79. Kahn, J. O., and B. D. Walker. 1998. Acute human immunodeficiency virus type 1 infection. *N. Engl. J. Med.* **339:**33–39.

80. King, S. M., for the Committee on Pediatric AIDS and Infectious Disease and Immunization Committee. 2004. Evaluation and treatment of the human immunodeficiency virus 1-exposed infant. *Pediatrics* **114:**497–505.

81. Kline, N. E., H. Schwarzwald, and M. W. Kline. 2002. False negative DNA polymerase chain reaction in an infant with subtype C human immunodeficiency virus type 1 infection. *Pediatr. Infect. Dis. J.* **21:**885–886.

82. Knoble, T. 2007. Implementing a multiple rapid HIV test algorithm to quickly identify false positive rapid tests and provide immediate referral to care for persons likely to be infected with HIV, San Francisco, CA 2007, abstr. 40. *2007 HIV Diagn. Conf.* http://www.hivtestingconference.org/hivtesting2007/abstracts/abstract40.pdf.

83. Kshatriya, R., A. A. Cachafeiro, R. J. S. Kerr, J. A. E. Nelson, and S. A. Fiscus. 2008. Comparison of two rapid human immunodeficiency virus (HIV) assays, Determine HIV-1/2 and OraQuick Advance Rapid HIV-1/2, for detection of recent HIV seroconversion. *J. Clin. Microbiol.* **46:**3482–3483.

84. Levy, J. A., A. D. Hoffman, S. M. Kramer, J. A. Landis, J. M. Shimabukuro, and L. S. Oshiro. 1984. Isolation of lymphocytopathic retroviruses from San Francisco patients with AIDS. *Science* **225:**840–842.

85. Lew, J., P. Reichelderfer, M. Fowler, J. Bremer, R. Carrol, S. Cassol, D. Chernoff, R. Coombs, M. Cronin, R. Dickover, S. Fiscus, S. Herman, B. Jackson, J. Kornegay, A. Kovacs, K. McIntosh, W. Meyer, N. Michael, L. Mofenson, J. Moye, T. Quinn, M. Robb, M. Vahey, B. Weiser, and T. Yeghiazarian. 1998. Determinations of levels of human immunodeficiency virus type 1 RNA in plasma: reassessment of parameters affecting assay outcome. *J. Clin. Microbiol.* **36:**1471–1479.

86. Lin, H. J., L. Pedneault, and F. B. Hollinger. 1998. Intra-assay performance characteristics of five assays for quantification of human immunodeficiency virus type 1 RNA in plasma. *J. Clin. Microbiol.* **36:**835–839.

87. Little, S. J., S. Holte, J. P. Routy, E. S. Daar, M. Markowitz, A. C. Collier, R. A. Koup, J. W. Mellors, E. Connick, B. Conway, M. Kilby, L. Wang, J. M. Whitcomb, N. S. Hellmann, and D. D. Richman. 2002. Antiretroviral-drug resistance among patients recently infected with HIV. *N. Engl. J. Med.* **347:**385–394.

88. Louie, B., E. Wong, J. D. Klausner, S. Liska, F. Hecht, T. Dowling, M. Obeso, S. S. Phillips, and M. W. Pandori. 2008. Assessment of rapid tests for detection of human immunodeficiency virus-specific antibodies in recently infected individuals. *J. Clin Microbiol.* **46:**1494–1497.

89. Ly, T. D., L. Martin, D. Daghfal, A. Sandridge, D. West, R. Bristow, L. Chalouas, X. Qiu, S. C. Lou, J. C. Hunt, G. Schochetman, and S. G. Devare. 2001. Seven human immunodeficiency virus (HIV) antigen-antibody combination assays: evaluation of HIV seroconversion sensitivity and subtype detection. *J. Clin. Microbiol.* **39:**3122–3128.

90. Ly, T. D., S. Laperche, C. Brennan, A. Vallari, A. Ebel, J. Hunt, L. Martin, D. Daghfal, G. Schochetman, and S. Devare. 2004. Evaluation of the sensitivity and specificity of six HIV combined p24 antigen and antibody assays. *J. Virol. Methods* **122:**185–194.

91. Ly, T. D., S. Laperche, and A. M. Courouce. 2001. Early detection of human immunodeficiency virus infection using third- and fourth-generation screening assays. *Eur. J. Clin. Microbiol. Infect. Dis.* **20:**104–110.

92. MacArthur, R. D., and R. M. Novak. 2008. Maraviroc: the first of a new class of antiretroviral agents. *Clin. Infect. Dis.* **47:**236–241.

93. Markowitz, M., H. Mohri, S. Mehandru, A. Shet, L. Berry, R. Kalyanaraman, A. Kim, C. Chung, P. Jean-Pierre, A. Horowitz, M. La Mar, T. Wrin, N. Parkin, M. Poles, C. Petropoulos, M. Mullen, D. Boden, and D. D. Ho. 2005. Infection with multidrug resistant, dual-tropic HIV-1 and rapid progression to AIDS: a case report. *Lancet* **365:**1031–1038.

94. Martinez-Picado, J., A. V. Savar, L. Sutton, and R. T. D'Aquila. 1999. Replication fitness of protease inhibitor-resistant mutants of human immunodeficiency virus type 1. *J. Virol.* **73:**3744–3752.

95. Masur, H., M. A. Michelis, J. B. Greene, I. Onorato, R. A. Stouwe, R. S. Holzman, G. Wormser, L. Breltman, M. Inage, H. W. Murray, and S. Cunningham-Rundles. 1981. An outbreak of community-acquired Pneumocystis carinii pneumonia: initial manifestation of cellular immune dysfunction. *N. Engl. J. Med.* **305:**1431–1438.

96. Mellors, J. W., C. R. Rinaldo, Jr., P. Gupta, R. M. White, J. A. Todd, and L. A. Kingsley. 1996. Prognosis in HIV-1 infection predicted by quantity of virus in plasma. *Science* **272:**1167–1170.

97. Mellors, J. W., L. A. Kingsley, C. R. Rinaldo, Jr., J. A. Todd, B. S. Hoo, R. P. Kokka, and P. Gupta. 1995. Quantitation of HIV-1 RNA in plasma predicts outcome after seroconversion. *Ann. Intern. Med.* **122:**573–579.

98. Menard, D., A. Mairo, M. J. Mandeng, P. Doyemet, T. A. Koyazegbe, C. Rochigneux, and A. Talarmin. 2005. Evaluation of rapid HIV testing strategies in under equipped laboratories in the Central African Republic. *J. Virol. Methods* **126:**75–80.

99. Meynard, J. L., M. Vray, L. Morand-Joubert, E. Race, D. Descamps, G. Peytavin, S. Matheron, C. Lamotte, S. Guiramand, D. Costagliola, F. Brun-Vezinet, F. Clavel, and P. M. Girard for the Narval Trial Group. 2002. Phenotyping or genotyping resistance testing for choosing antiretroviral therapy after treatment failure: a randomized trial. *AIDS* **16:**727–736.

100. Mingle, J. A. 1997. Differentiation of dual seropositivity to HIV 1 and HIV 2 in Ghanaian sera using line immunoassay (INNOLIA). *West Afr. J. Med.* **16:**71–74.

101. Montano, M., M. Russell, P. Gilbert, I. Thior, S. Lockman, R. Shapiro, S. Y. Chang, T. H. Lee, and M. Essex. 2003. Comparative prediction of perinatal human immunodeficiency virus type 1 transmission, using multiple virus load markers. *J. Infect. Dis.* **188:**406–413.

102. Munoz, A., A. J. Kirby, Y. D. He, J. B. Margolick, B. R. Visscher, C. R. Rinaldo, R. A. Kaslow, and J. P. Phair. 1995. Long-term survivors with HIV-1 infection: incubation period and longitudinal patterns of CD4+ lymphocytes. *J. Acquir. Immune Defic. Syndr. Hum. Retrovirol.* **8:**496–505.

103. Nadal, D., J. Boni, C. Kind, O. E. Varnier, F. Steiner, Z. Tomasik, and J. Schupbach. 1999. Prospective evaluation of amplification boosted ELISA for heat-denatured p24 antigen for diagnosis and monitoring of pediatric human immunodeficiency virus type 1 infection. *J. Infect. Dis.* **180:**1089–1095.

104. Nishanian, P., K. R. Huskins, S. Stehn, R. Detels, and J. L. Fahey. 1990. A simple method for improved assay demonstrates that HIV p24 antigen is present as immune complexes in most sera from HIV-infected individuals. *J. Infect. Dis.* **162:**21–28.

105. Nolte, F. S., J. Boysza, C. Thurmond, W. S. Clark, and J. L. Lennox. 1998. Clinical comparison of an enhanced sensitivity branched-DNA assay and reverse transcription PCR for quantitation of human immunodeficiency virus type 1 RNA in plasma. *J. Clin. Microbiol.* **36:**716–720.

106. Novak, R. M., L. Chen, R. D. MacArthur, J. D. Baxter, K. Huppler Hullsiek, G. Peng, Y. Xiang, C. Henely, B. Schmetter, J. Uy, M. van den Berg-Wolf, and M. Kozal. 2005. Prevalence of antiretroviral drug resistance mutations in chronically HIV-infected, treatment-naive patients: implications for routine resistance screening before initiation of antiretroviral therapy. *Clin. Infect. Dis.* **40:**468–474.

107. O'Brien, W. A., K. Grovit-Ferbas, A. Namazi, S. Ovcak-Derzic, H. J. Wang, J. Park, C. Yeramian, S. H. Mao, and J. A. Zack. 1995. Human immunodeficiency virus type 1 replication can be increased in peripheral blood of seropositive patients after influenza vaccination. *Blood* **86:**1082–1089.

108. O'Brien, W. A., P. M. Hartigan, D. Martin, J. Esinhart, A. Hill, M. Rubin, M. S. Simberkoff, J. D. Hamilton, et al. 1996. Changes in plasma HIV-1 RNA and CD4+ lymphocyte counts and the risk of progression to AIDS. *N. Engl. J. Med.* **334:**426–431.

109. **Palmer, S., M. Kearny, F. Maldarelli, E. K. Halvas, C. J. Bixby, H. Bazmi, D. Rock, J. Falloon, R. T. Davey, R. L. Dewar, J. A. Metcalf, S. Hammer, J. W. Mellors, and J. M. Coffin.** 2005. Multiple, linked human immunodeficiency virus type 1 drug resistance mutations in treatment-experienced patients are missed by standard genotype analysis. *J. Clin. Microbiol.* **43:**406–413

110. **Paltiel, A. D., M. C. Weinstein, A. D. Kimmel, G. R. Seage, E. Losina, S. M. Hong-Zang, K. A. Freedberg, and R. P. Wakensky.** 2005. Expanded screening for HIV in the United States–an analysis of cost-effectiveness. *N. Engl. J. Med.* **352:**586–595.

111. **Panlilio, A. L., D. M. Cardo, L. A. Grohskopf, W. Heneine, and C. S. Ross.** 2005. Updated U.S. Public Health Service guidelines for the management of occupational exposures to HIV and recommendations for postexposure prophylaxis. *MMWR Recommend. Rep.* **54**(RR-9)**:**1–17.

112. **Pantaleo, G., C. Graziosi, J. F. Desmarest, L. Butini, M. Montroni, C. H. Fox, J. M. Orenstein, D. P. Kotler, and A. S. Fauci.** 1993. HIV infection is active and progressive in lymphoid tissue during the clinically latent stage of disease. *Nature* **362:**355–358.

113. **Parekh, B. S., and J. S. McDougal.** 2005. Application of laboratory methods for estimation of HIV-1 incidence. *Indian J. Med. Res.* **121:**510–518.

113a. **Pas, S., J. W. A. Rossen, D. Schoener, D. Thamke, A. Pettersson, R. Babiel, and M. Schutten.** 2010. Performance evaluation of the new Roche Cobas AmpliPrep/Cobas Taqman HIV-1 Test version 2.0 for quantification of human immunodeficiency virus type 1 RNA. *J. Clin. Microbiol.* **48:**1195–1200.

114. **Pascual, A., A. Cachafeiro, M. L. Funk, and S. A. Fiscus.** 2002. Comparison of heat-dissociated "boosted" p24 antigen with the Roche monitor human immunodeficiency virus RNA assay. *J. Clin. Microbiol.* **40:**2472–2475.

115. **Perelson, A. S., A. U. Neuman, M. Markowitz, J. M. Leonard, and D. D. Ho.** 1996. HIV-1 dynamics in vivo: virion clearance rate, infected cells life span, and viral generation time. *Science* **271:**1582–1586.

116. **Perez-Elias, M. J., I. Garcia-Arota, V. Munoz, I. Santos, J. Sanz, V. Abraira, J. R. Arribas, J. Gonzalez, A. Moreno, F. Dronda, A. Antela, M. Pumares, P. Marti-Belda, J. L. Casado, P. Geijos, and S. Moreno.** 2003. Phenotype or virtual phenotype for choosing antiretroviral therapy after failure: a prospective, randomized study. *Antivir. Ther.* **8:**577–584.

117. **Petropoulos, C., N. Parkin, K. Limoli, Y. S. Lie, T. Wrin, W. Huang, H. Tian, D. Smith, G. A. Winslow, D. J. Capon, and J. M. Whitcomb.** 2000. A novel phenotyping drug susceptibility assay for human immunodeficiency virus type 1. *Antimicrob. Agents Chemother.* **44:**920–928.

118. **Picchio, G. R., R. J. Gulizia, and D. R. Mosier.** 1997. Chemokine receptor CCR5 genotype influences the kinetics of human immunodeficiency virus type 1 infection in human PBL-SCID mice. *J. Virol.* **71:**7124–7127.

119. **Popovic, M., M. G. Sarngadharan, E. Read, and R. C. Gallo.** 1984. Detection, isolation, and continuous production of cytopathic retrovirus (HTLV-III) from patients with AIDS and pre-AIDS. *Science* **224:**497–500.

120. **Price, R. W.** 1996. Neurological complications of HIV infection. *Lancet* **348:**445–452.

121. **Respess, R. A., A. Cachafeiro, D. Withum, S. A. Fiscus, D. Newman, B. Branson, O. E. Varnier, K. Lewis, and T. J. Dondero.** 2005. Evaluation of an ultrasensitive p24 antigen assay as a potential alternative to human immunodeficiency virus type 1 RNA viral load assay in resource-limited settings. *J. Clin. Microbiol.* **43:**506–508.

122. **Reynolds, S. J., L. M. Ndongala, C. C. Luo, K. Mwandagalirwa, A. J. Losoma, K. J. Mwamba, E. Bazepeyo, N. E. Nzilambi, T. C. Quinn, and R. C. Bollinger.** 2002. Evaluation of a rapid test for the detection of antibodies to human immunodeficiency virus type 1 and 2 in the setting of multiple transmitted viral subtypes. *Int. J. STD AIDS* **13:**171–173.

123. **Rothman, R. E., K. S. Ketlogetswe, T. Dolan, P. C. Wyer, and G. D. Kelen.** 2003. Preventive care in the emergency department: should emergency departments conduct routine HIV screening? A systematic review. *Acad. Emerg. Med.* **10:**278–285.

124. **Rouet, F., D. K. Ekouevi, M. L. Chaix, M. Burgard, A. Inwoley, T. D. Tony, C. Danel, X. Anglaret, V. Leroy, P. Msellati, F. Dabis, and C. Rouzioux.** 2005. Transfer and evaluation of an automated, low-cost real-time reverse transcriptase PCR test for diagnosis and monitoring of human immunodeficiency virus type 1 infection in a West African resource-limited setting. *J. Clin. Microbiol.* **43:**2709–2717.

125. **Royce, R. A., A. Sena, W. Cates, Jr., and M. S. Cohen.** 1997. Sexual transmission of HIV. *N. Engl. J. Med.* **336:**1072–1078.

126. **Salimnia, H., E. C. Moore, L. R. Crane, R. D. MacArthur, and M. R. Fairfax.** 2005. Discordance between viral loads determined by Roche COBAS AMPLICOR human immunodeficiency virus type 1 Monitor (version 1.5) standard and ultrasensitive assays caused by freezing patient plasma in centrifuged Becton-Dickinson vacutainer brand plasma preparation tubes. *J. Clin. Microbiol.* **43:**4635–4639.

127. **Samson, M., F. Libert, B. J. Doranz, J. Rucker, C. Liesnard, C. M. Farber, S. Saragosti, C. Lapoumeroulie, J. Cognaux, C. Forceille, G. Muyldermans, C. Verhofstede, G. Burtonboy, M. Georges, T. Imai, S. Rana, Y. Yi, R. J. Smyth, R. G. Collman, R. W. Doms, G. Vassart, and M. Parmentier.** 1996. Resistance to HIV-1 infection in Caucasian individuals bearing mutant alleles of the CCR-5 chemokine receptor gene. *Nature* **382:**722–725.

128. **Sanchez, T. H., and P. S. Sullivan.** 2008. Expanding the horizons: new approaches to providing HIV testing services in the United States. *Public Health Rep.* **123**(Suppl. 3)**:**1–4.

129. **Schable, C., C.-P. Pau, D. Hu, T. Dondero, G. Schochetman, H. Jaffe, J. R. George, L. Zekeng, L. Kaptue, J.-M. Tsague, and L. Gurtler.** 1994. Sensitivity of United States HIV antibody tests for detection of HIV-1 group O infections. *Lancet* **344:**1333–1334.

130. **Schumacher, W., E. Frick, M. Kauselmann, V. Maier-Hoyle, R. van der Vliet, and R. Babiel.** 2007. Fully automated quantification of human immunodeficiency virus (HIV) type 1 RNA in human plasma by the COBAS AmpliPrep/COBAS TaqMan system. *J. Clin. Virol.* **38:**304–312.

131. **Schupbach, J., and J. Boni.** 1993. Quantitative and sensitive detection of immune-complexed and free HIV antigen after boiling of serum. *J. Virol. Methods* **43:**247–256.

132. **Schupbach, J., M. Flepp, D. Pontelli, Z. Tomasik, R. Luthy, and J. Boni.** 1996. Heat-mediated immune complex dissociation and enzyme-linked immunosorbent assay signal amplification render p24 antigen detection in plasma as sensitive as HIV-1 RNA detection by polymerase chain reaction. *AIDS* **10:**1085–1090.

133. **Sharp, P. M., D. L. Robertson, D. L. Gao, and B. H. Hahn.** 1994. Origins and diversity of human immunodeficiency viruses. *AIDS* **8:**S27–S42.

134. **Sherman, G. G., G. Stevens, and W. S. Stevens.** 2004. Affordable diagnosis of human immunodeficiency virus infection in infants by p24 antigen detection. *Pediatr. Infect. Dis.* **23:**173–175.

135. **Simon, F., T. D. Ly, A. Baillou-Beaufils, V. Fauveau, J. De Saint-Martin, I. Loussert-Ajaka, M. L. Chaix, S. Saragosti, A. M. Courouce, D. Ingrand, C. Janot, and F. Brun-Vézinet.** 1994. Sensitivity of screening kits for anti-HIV-1 subtype O antibodies. *AIDS* **8:**1628–1629.

136. **Soto-Ramirez, L. E., L. Hernandez-Gomez, J. Sifuentes-Osornio, G. Barriga-Angulo, D. Duarte de Lima, M. Lopez-Portillo, and G. M. Ruiz-Palacios.** 1992. Detection of specific antibodies in gingival crevicular transudate by enzyme-linked immunosorbent assay for diagnosis of human immunodeficiency virus type 1 infection. *J. Clin. Microbiol.* **30:**2780–2783.

137. **Spielberg, F., and W. J. Kassler.** 1996. Rapid testing for HIV antibody: a technology whose time has come. *Ann. Intern. Med.* **125:**509–511.

138. **Stanley, S. K., M. A. Ostrowski, J. S. Justement, K. Gantt, S. Hedayati, M. Mannix, K. Roche, D. J. Schwartzentruber, C. H. Fox, and A. S. Fauci.** 1996. Effect of immunization with a common recall antigen on viral expression in patients infected with human immunodeficiency virus type 1. *N. Engl. J. Med.* **334:**1222–1230.

139. **Stevens, G., N. Rekhviashvili, L. E. Scott, R. Gonin, and W. Stevens.** 2005. Evaluation of two commercially available, inexpensive alternative assays used for assessing viral load in a cohort of human immunodeficiency virus type 1 subtype C-infected patients from South Africa. *J. Clin. Microbiol.* **43:**857–861.

140. **Stramer, S. L.** 2004. Viral diagnostics in the arena of blood donor screening. *Vox Sang.* **87**(Suppl. 2)**:**180–183.

141. **Stramer, S. L., S. A. Glynn, S. H. Kleinman, D. M. Strong, C. Sally, D. J. Wright, R. Y. Dodd, M. P. Busch, and the National Heart, Lung, and Blood Institute Nucleic Acid Test Study Group.** 2004. Detection of HIV-1 and HCV infections among antibody-negative blood donors by nucleic acid-amplification testing. *N. Engl. J. Med.* **351:**760–768.

142. **Sufka, S. A., G. Ferrari, V. E. Gryszowka, T. Wrin, S. A. Fiscus, G. D. Tomaras, H. F. Staats, D. P. Dhavalkumar, G. D. Sempowski, N. S. Hellmann, K. J. Wienhold, and C. B. Hicks.** 2003. Prolonged CD4+ cell/virus load discordance during treatment with protease inhibitor-based highly active antiretroviral therapy: immune response and viral control. *J. Infect. Dis.* **187:**1027–1037.

143. **Swanson, P., S. Huang, V. Holzmayer, P. Bodelle, J. Yamaguchi, C. Brennan, R. Badaro, C. Brites, K. Abravaya, S. G. Devare, and J. Hackett, Jr.** 2006. Performance of the automated Abbott RealTime HIV-1 assay on a genetically diverse panel of specimens from Brazil. *J. Virol. Methods* **134:**237–243.

144. **Swanson, P., V. Holzmayer, S. Huang, P. Hay, A. Adebiyi, P. Rice, K. Abravaya, S. Thamm, S. G. Devare, and J. Hackett, Jr.** 2006. Performance of the automated Abbott RealTime HIV-1 assay on a genetically diverse panel of specimens from London: comparison to VERSANT HIV-1 RNA 3.0, AMPLICOR HIV-1 Monitor v1.5, and LCx HIV RNA quantitative assays. *J. Virol. Methods* **137:**184–192.

145. **Tamashiro, H., and N. T. Constantine.** 1994. Serological diagnosis of HIV infection using oral fluid samples. *Bull. W. H. O.* **72:**135–143.

146. **Taylor, B. S., M. E. Sobieszczyk, F. E. McCutchan, and S. C. Hammer.** 2008. The challenge of HIV-1 subtype diversity. *N. Engl. J. Med.* **358:**1590–1602.

147. **Tsibris, A. M., M. Sagar, R. M. Gulick, Z. Su, M. Hughes, W. Greaves, M. Subramanian, C. Flexner, F. Giguel, K. E. Leopold, E. Coakley, and D. R. Kuritzkes.** 2008. In vivo emergence of vicriviroc resistance in an HIV-1 subtype C-infected subject. *J. Virol.* **82:**8210–8214.

148. **Tural, C., L. Ruiz, C. Holtzer, J. Schapiro, P. Viciana, J. Gonzalez, P. Domingo, C. Boucher, C. Rey-Joly, B. Clotet, and the Havana Study Group.** 2002. Clinical utility of HIV-1 genotyping and expert advice-the Havana trial. *AIDS* **16:**209–218.

149. **UNAIDS.** 2007. *2007 Report on the Global AIDS Epidemic.* UNAIDS, Geneva, Switzerland.

150. **Urnovitz, H. B., J. C. Sturge, and T. D. Gottfried.** 1997. Increased sensitivity of HIV-1 antibody detection. *Nat. Med.* **3:**1258.

151. **U.S. Food and Drug Administration.** 2002. Summary of safety and effectiveness. Oraquick Rapid HIV-1. http://www.fda.gov/downloads/BiologicsBloodVaccines/BloodBloodProducts/ApprovedProducts/PremarketApprovalsPMAs/UCM092003.pdf. Accessed 14 April 2005.

151a. **U.S. Food and Drug Administration.** 2003. Summary of safety and effectiveness. Unigold Recombigen HIV. http://www.fda.gov/downloads/BiologicsBloodVaccines/BloodBloodProducts/ApprovedProducts/PremarketApprovalsPMAs/ucm093447.pdf. Accessed 26 January 2011.

151b. **U.S. Food and Drug Administration.** 2009. Summary of safety and effectiveness. MedMira Reveal Rapid HIV-1 antibody test. http://www.fda.gov/BiologicsBloodVaccines/BloodBloodProducts/ApprovedProducts/PremarketApprovalsPMAs/ucm091872.htm. Accessed 26 January 2011.

151c. **U.S. Food and Drug Administration.** 2004. Summary of safety and effectiveness. Bio-Rad Multispot HIV-1/HIV-2 rapid test. http://www.fda.gov/downloads/BiologicsBloodVaccines/BloodBloodProducts/ApprovedProducts/PremarketApprovalsPMAs/ucm091383.pdf. Accessed 26 January 2011.

152. **Wawer, M. J., R. H. Gray, N. K. Sewankambo, D. Serwadda, X. Li, O. Laeyendecker, N. Kiwanuka, G. Kigozi, M. Kiddugavu, T. Lutalo, F. Nalugoda, F. Wabwire-Mangen, M. P. Meehan, and T. C. Quinn.** 2005. Rates of HIV-1 transmission per coital act, by stage of HIV-1 infection, in Rakai, Uganda. *J. Infect. Dis.* **191:**1403–1409.

153. **Weinstein, M. C., S. J. Goldie, E. Losina, C. J. Cohen, J. D. Baxter, H. Zhang, A. D. Kimmel, and K. A. Freedberg.** 2001. Use of genotyping testing to guide HIV therapy: clinical impact and cost-effectiveness. *Ann. Intern. Med.* **134:**440–450.

154. **Weslowski, L. G., D. A. Mackellar, S. F. Ethridge, J. H. Zhu, S. M. Owen, and P. S. Sullivan.** 2008. Repeat confirmatory testing for persons with discordant whole blood and oral fluid rapid HIV test results: findings from post marketing surveillance. *PLoS ONE* **3:**e1524.

155. **Whitcomb, J. M., W. Huang, S. Fransen, K. Limoli, J. Toma, T. Wrin, C. Chappey, L. D. Kiss, E. E. Paxinos, and C. J. Petropoulos.** 2007. Development and characterization of a novel single-cycle recombinant-virus assay to determine human immunodeficiency virus type 1 coreceptor tropism. *Antimicrob. Agents Chemother.* **51:**566–575.

155a. **Working Group on Antiretroviral Therapy and Medical Management of HIV-Infected Children.** 23 February 2009. *Guidelines for the Use of Antiretroviral Agents in Pediatric HIV Infection.* National Institutes of Health, Bethesda, MD. http://aidsinfo.nih.gov/ContentFiles/PediatricGuidelines.pdf. Accessed 29 January 2011.

156. **Zhu, T., B. T. Korber, A. J. Nahmias, E. Hooper, P. M. Sharp, and D. D. Ho.** 1998. An African HIV-1 sequence from 1959 and implications for the origin of the epidemic. *Nature* **391:**594–597.

157. **Zouhair, S., S. Roussin-Bretagne, A. Moreau, S. Brunet, S. Laperche, M. Maniez, F. Barin, and M. Harzic.** 2006. Group O human immunodeficiency virus type 1 infection that escaped detection in two immunoassays. *J. Clin. Microbiol.* **44:**662–665.

Human T-Cell Lymphotropic Virus Types 1 and 2

S. MICHELE OWEN, ANTOINE GESSAIN, CHARLENE S. DEZZUTTI,
ELLIOT P. COWAN, AND RENU B. LAL

80

TAXONOMY

Human T-cell lymphotropic virus types 1 and 2 (HTLV-1 and HTLV-2, respectively) are part of the *Retroviridae* family and members of the *Deltaretrovirus* genus. They are members of the primate T-lymphotropic virus (PTLV) group, along with their simian counterparts STLV-1, STLV-2, and STLV-3 and the recently identified human viruses HTLV-3 and HTLV-4 (11, 76). HTLVs are distinct from the *Lentivirus* genus, which includes human immunodeficiency virus types 1 and 2 (HIV-1 and HIV-2, respectively).

DESCRIPTION OF THE AGENT

HTLV is a complex retrovirus with regulatory genes in addition to the structural and enzymatic *gag*, *pol*, and *env* genes found in all classical retroviruses. Recent reports suggest that HTLV-1 and HTLV-2 use a receptor complex, including, minimally, GLUT-1, neuropilin, and heparan sulfate proteoglycan for cellular entry (22, 26, 34, 61). HTLV has made numerous cross-species jumps from nonhuman primates into humans and between nonhuman primate species (6, 11, 56, 76).

HTLV-1 and HTLV-2 are typical C-type retroviruses; they contain an electron-dense, centrally located nuclear core and bud from the cell surface. Within the core are two positive-sense single-stranded RNA genomes. Once a cell is infected, the RNA genome is converted by reverse transcriptase to DNA and integrates into the host genome. HTLV-1 and HTLV-2 have similar genomic organizations: *gag*, *pro/pol*, *env*, and *pX*, flanked by their long terminal repeats (LTRs) (Fig. 1). Further, they share approximately 60% of their nucleotide sequences. The *gag* gene encodes the structural proteins p19, p24, and p15. The *pro/pol* genes encode the protease and the reverse transcriptase, respectively. The *env* gene encodes the transmembrane and external envelope glycoproteins gp21 and gp46. HTLV-1 and HTLV-2 use alternative splicing and internal initiation codons to produce several regulatory and accessory proteins encoded by four open reading frames located in the pX region of the viral genome between *env* and the 3' *LTR*. The *pX* gene encodes the spliced regulatory proteins Tax and Rex and the products of several additional open reading frames (Fig. 1).

EPIDEMIOLOGY AND TRANSMISSION

HTLV-1 infects 15 to 20 million people worldwide, with foci of endemicity in southern Japan, the Caribbean, large parts of sub-Saharan Africa and Central and South America, and some areas (rare cases) in Melanesia and the Middle East (e.g., northern Iran) (18, 36, 46, 72). The seroprevalence rate in adults ranges from 1 to 5% in the Caribbean islands to approximately 5 to 25% in southern Japan (18). HTLV-2 is endemic in Amerindian tribes throughout the Americas, as well as in a few Pygmy tribes in Central Africa, with seroprevalence ranging from 1 to 30% in adults (18, 49). In all areas of endemicity, HTLV-1/2 seroprevalence increases with age, especially in women. In the United States and Europe, the seroprevalence for both HTLV-1 and HTLV-2 among low-risk populations is less than 1% (36, 62). However, high-risk populations, such as intravenous drug users (IDUs), in which HTLV-2 infection predominates over HTLV-1 infection, are reported to have a seroprevalence of up to 20% (18, 49).

HTLV-1 and HTLV-2 infections are transmitted sexually (mainly by males to females), vertically (from mother to child by prolonged breastfeeding), and parenterally (through drug use and blood transfusion) (18, 36, 62). IDU and sex with IDUs are the most important risk factors for HTLV-2 transmission (18, 49). Both cross-sectional and prospective studies support the spread by sexual transmission, and there was a strong concordance of seropositivity between spouses in an area where HTLV-2 is endemic (50). The mode of transmission may impact the rate of viral evolution (54). Lineages of the HTLV-2 virus evolve at a rate 150 to 350 times higher when the virus is transmitted between IDUs than when it is propagated by mother-to-infant transmission. Salemi et al. (54) postulated that the increase in the viral transmission rate between IDUs, which can be many transmissions per year, accounted for the increase in the HTLV-2 evolution rate, whereas vertical transmission is expected to occur just once every 14 to 30 years for a given viral lineage. This change in the mode of virus spread creates a possible risk for emergence of HTLV-2 strains with higher virulence.

Highly effective screening programs for volunteer blood donors have been implemented in Japan, Australia, the United States, Canada, and several Caribbean and European countries to reduce the risk of transfusion-related

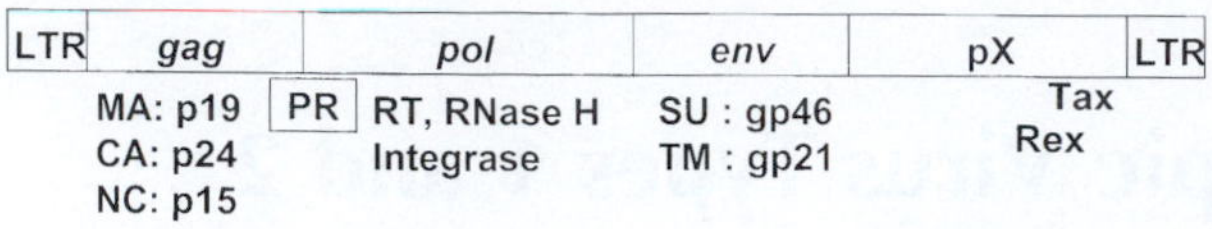

FIGURE 1 Organization of the HTLV-1 (9,046 bp) and -2 (8,952 bp) proviral genomes. MA, matrix; CA, capsid; NC, nucleocapsid; SU, surface; TM, transmembrane; RT, reverse transcriptase; PR, protease. The *gag* and *env* proteins are most immunogenic, and antibodies to these proteins are commonly detected by serological tests (EIA and WB). PCRs are designed to detect regions within the LTR region and the *gag*, *pol*, *env*, and/or *tax* gene.

HTLV-1 and HTLV-2 transmission (15, 23, 55, 62, 64). For example, in the United States between 1991 and 1996, the incidence rate of seroconversion associated with HTLV in blood donors was estimated to be 1.59 per 100,000 persons per year (23), and the residual risk of transmission of HTLV infection by transfusion of screened blood was estimated to be 1 in 641,000 (43). From 1998 to 2001, the estimated incidence of new infections among repeat blood donors to the American Red Cross was 0.239 per 100,000 person years, and the estimated risk of collecting blood during the infectious window period was 1:2,993,000 (17). A retrospective HTLV recipient-tracing study for the years 1999 to 2004, also carried out by the American Red Cross, found similar levels of HTLV incidence in U.S. blood donors. (59).

Both HTLV-1 and HTLV-2 are the result of zoonotic transmission of simian retrovirus from simian to human hosts. The phylogeny of PTLVs indicates that both HTLV-1 and HTLV-2 emerged from their respective primate lineages, PTLV-1 and PTLV-2, but that their subsequent evolution continued in different patterns (56). HTLV-1 includes at least four main subtypes, which evolved from PTLV-1 through several independent interspecies transmissions between simian and human hosts in different geographic locations (56, 70, 75). HTLV-2 includes three subtypes, which appear to originate from a common human ancestor virus that emerged possibly from only one simian-to-human transmission (6, 56). The possibility of additional zoonotic transfer of primate retroviruses from simian to human hosts and the impact that can result from such primate zoonotic transmission events remain a public health challenge (6, 56).

Molecular epidemiologic studies have shown HTLV proviruses to be remarkably stable genetically (44, 75). The different rates of evolution of HIV-1 and HTLV-1 are due to the clonal expansion of HTLV-infected cells versus the active replication of HIV-1 (73). While the overall genome of HTLV is highly conserved, nucleotide divergence in the LTR and the *gp21 env* gene has been exploited to genotypically subtype both HTLV-1 and HTLV-2 (56). The impact of diversity and emerging variants continues to challenge retroviral serology. An understanding of phylogenetic relationships is therefore useful (Fig. 2). There are at least four major geographic HTLV-1 subtypes: subtype A (cosmopolitan), subtype B (Central African), subtype C (Australo-Melanesian), and subtype D (Central African; mainly among Pygmy tribes) (56). Likewise, HTLV-2 has three subtypes: 2a, 2b, and 2d (6, 49, 56). Subtype 2a is commonly found among IDUs worldwide, whereas subtype 2b is found primarily among Amerindians and in some Pygmies from Cameroon. Subtype 2d has been found in only one Pygmy, from the Democratic Republic of the Congo. Earlier studies

had identified a molecular subtype, 2c; however, subsequent analysis confirmed this to be subtype 2b (68). This genetic heterogeneity within HTLV-1 and HTLV-2 has provided valuable information on geographic clustering, movement of ancient populations, and viral transmission (49, 56).

CLINICAL SIGNIFICANCE

HTLV-1 has been associated with two major diseases: adult T-cell leukemia (ATL) and HTLV-1-associated myelopathy/tropical spastic paraparesis (HAM/TSP) (18, 32, 46, 48, 60). ATL is a severe malignant lymphoproliferation of CD4-positive cells that is diagnosed biologically by seropositivity for HTLV-1, the presence of morphologically distinct $CD3^+$ $CD4^+$ $CD25^+$ lymphocytes with cleaved nuclei (flower cells), and clonal integration of HTLV-1 proviruses in tumor cells, as detected by Southern blotting or inverse PCR (32, 37, 48).

The clinical features of the chronic neuromyelopathy HAM/TSP are muscle weakness in the legs, hyperreflexia, clonus, extensor plantar responses, sensory disturbances, various urinary manifestations, impotence, and low-back pain (12, 60). Biological diagnosis includes the presence of high titers of HTLV-specific antibodies in the serum and cerebrospinal fluid. The estimated lifetime risk of developing HAM/TSP among HTLV-1-infected persons is less than 2% (18, 36) but can vary according to the geographic area. Other uncommon inflammatory disease associations include infective dermatitis, uveitis, myositis, and HTLV-associated arthropathy.

HTLV-2 has not been associated with malignancies; however, it has been associated rarely with a neurological disease resembling HAM/TSP (4, 49). The estimated lifetime risk of disease development for HTLV-2-infected persons is unknown but appears to be less than that estimated for persons with HTLV-1 infection. While the majority of HTLV-2-infected persons remain asymptomatic (>95%), recent studies report an increased incidence of infectious diseases (such as bronchitis and kidney and/or bladder infections) in HTLV-1- and HTLV-2-infected persons (4, 49).

HTLV coinfection with HIV can occur in high-risk groups, such as persons from areas of HTLV endemicity and IDUs. To date, a few studies evaluating the impact of HIV coinfection with HTLV have shown that there is an increased frequency of HTLV-associated clinical outcomes but that there is a delayed progression to AIDS (8). Moreover, HIV therapy that includes highly active antiretroviral therapy does not impact the HTLV proviral burden (9). These limited numbers of studies suggest that HIV coinfection may increase the morbidity of the HTLV-infected patients. However, additional studies are needed to determine if coinfection impacts the mortality of HTLV-infected patients.

There are limited treatment options for HTLV-associated diseases. Although zidovudine and alpha interferon (IFN-α) yield some responses and improve ATL prognosis, alternative therapies are needed. New drugs, such as arsenic trioxide, proteasome inhibitors, retinoids, and angiogenesis inhibitors, as well as cellular immunotherapy, are under investigation (7). Antiretroviral treatment, such as lamivudine and high-dose IFN-α and IFN-β have been evaluated with HAM/TSP patients and reductions in proviral loads (42, 53, 63). However, further follow-up of immunomodulatory therapies have been disappointing and antiretroviral therapies have been discouraging because of only partial or temporary success in reducing the proviral load. A recent study of HIV- and HTLV-2-coinfected individuals in which

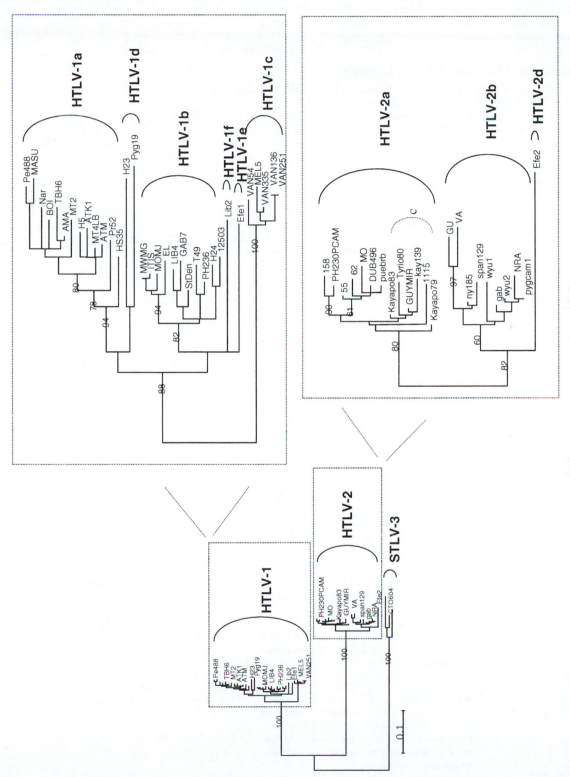

FIGURE 2 Unrooted phylogenetic tree generated by the neighbor-joining method using a fragment of the LTR region (622 bp) of representative sequences of the different subtypes of HTLV-1 and HTLV-2 strains. Bootstrap support (1,000 replicates) is noted on the branches of the tree. The branch lengths are drawn to scale, with the bar indicating 0.1 nucleotide replacement per site. The four main HTLV-1 subtypes (a, b, c, and d), as well as the three main subtypes of HTLV-2 (a, b, and d), are represented. HTLV-1e and HTLV-1f represent the two other rare HTLV-1 subtypes, which have so far been found in a few inhabitants of Central Africa.

highly active antiretroviral therapy was administered further illustrates the low efficacy of antiretrovirals for controlling HTLV infections (9). Symptomatic or targeted treatment is still the mainstay of therapy of HAM/TSP patients (5, 43). For uveitis, topical and systemic corticosteroids appear to improve sight, whereas infective dermatitis responds well to antibiotic treatment.

COLLECTION AND STORAGE OF SPECIMENS

Serum or plasma is suitable for use in serologic assays for HTLV-1 and HTLV-2 detection. These specimens can be drawn at the time of presentation. Seronegative patients who are suspected of having HTLV-1 or HTLV-2 or those with patterns that are seroindeterminate by Western blotting (WB) should be redrawn at 3 months and retested to capture potentially infected persons during the seroconversion window period (13). Serum and plasma specimens can be stored at 4°C or frozen for later use. Package inserts should be consulted for storage limitations and limitations on the number of freeze-thaw cycles permitted. Peripheral blood mononuclear cells (PBMCs) are appropriate specimens for nucleic acid detection and virus isolation

since HTLV-1 and HTLV-2 are cell-associated viruses. For nucleic acid amplification testing, whole blood is collected, and PBMCs are typically isolated on a Ficoll-Hypaque gradient (discussed in chapter 76 in this *Manual*). DNA is prepared using standard methods, and it can be stored at −20°C until needed. For virus culture, whole blood is collected in sodium citrate tubes and PBMCs are isolated on Ficoll-Hypaque gradient.

DIRECT DETECTION

Nucleic Acid Detection

Amplification of proviral DNA by PCR is the preferred method for determining infection status, testing the validity of serologic assays, distinguishing between HTLV-1 and HTLV-2, and studying tissue distribution in vivo. Two qualitative PCR procedures, utilizing primers in the *pol* or *tax* gene region, have been used to confirm and differentiate between HTLV-1 and HTLV-2 infections (Table 1) (24, 31). The first uses HTLV consensus primers that allow amplification of both viruses; typing is achieved either by hybridizing the product to an HTLV-1-specific or HTLV-2-specific

TABLE 1 Summary of serologic and supplemental confirmatory tests for HTLV-1 and HTLV-2 infections

Detection method	Description	Reference(s)	Availability in United States[a]
Serologic screening tests			
EIA	HTLV-1- and HTLV-2-infected cell lysates and/or recombinant antigens used to detect HTLV antibodies by colorimetric readout. Excellent sensitivity and specificity.	2, 31, 45	One FDA-licensed test
ChLIA	Similar to EIA but with chemiluminescent readout	47	One FDA-licensed test
Particle agglutination	Viral lysate coats gelatin or latex particles. Antigen-specific antibodies bind, which results in agglutination of particles. Visual readout by operator.		Not FDA licensed
Serologic supplementary tests			
WB	HTLV-1 viral lysates with or without recombinant antigens used to detect HTLV-1- and -2-specific antibodies. May contain recombinant antigens to differentiate antibodies to HTLV-1 and HTLV-2.	71	Not FDA licensed
LIA	Recombinant or peptide HTLV-1 and HTLV-2 antigens painted onto membrane. Antibodies to individual viral proteins are visualized.	52	Not FDA licensed, but CE marked for use outside the United States
IFA	Antibodies bind to HTLV-1- and HTLV-2-infected cells. Detected by secondary anti-human antibody with fluorescent label. Differentiates between antibodies to HTLV-1 and HTLV-2.	21	Not FDA licensed
Nucleic acid detection tests			
Qualitative PCR	Distinguishes between HTLV-1 and HTLV-2 either by using HTLV consensus primers, with typing done by HTLV-1- or HTLV-2-specific primers and probes in separate tests, or by differential patterns using restriction enzyme fragment length polymorphisms.	24, 31	Not FDA licensed
Quantitative PCR	Determines proviral DNA copy number by limiting dilution, quantitative competitive PCR, or real-time PCR using gene- and type-specific primers.	1, 25, 40, 66	Not FDA licensed

[a]FDA licensed, may be used for blood donor screening and as an aid in clinical diagnosis of HTLV-1 or HTLV-2 infection and related diseases. CE, Conformité Européenne.

probe or by specific restriction digestion pattern analysis (24, 31). A second approach employs type-specific primers and probes in separate amplifications. The PCR products can be detected with labeled internal probes by Southern blot hybridization (24). Most of these assays are performed for research use only.

Viral load assays are based on proviral DNA amplification; detection of RNA viral loads in plasma is not feasible for HTLV due to the cell-associated nature of these viruses (16). Quantitative nucleic acid amplification tests have been developed to determine HTLV-1 and HTLV-2 proviral DNA load using quantitative competitive PCR (1) or real-time PCR (25, 29, 40, 66). The real-time noncommercial PCR assay has excellent sensitivity and a broad dynamic range, from 10 to 10^6 copies/reaction (29), and has been used to study the relationship between proviral load and pathogenesis. Studies using these methods demonstrate that the proviral load is higher among HAM/TSP patients than among asymptomatic carriers (36, 60), suggesting that proviral load may be an indicator for future disease development (60). Follow-up of the proviral load or of the presence of a specific clone can also be done during ATL treatment (7, 48). Further, recent studies suggest that sexual transmission and mother-to-child transmission are associated with a higher HTLV proviral load in the index case (30, 41, 50). Thus, quantification of HTLV proviral load is providing a better understanding of correlates of transmission and disease progression (41, 50, 60).

VIRUS ISOLATION AND IDENTIFICATION

Viral isolation of HTLV-1 or HTLV-2 has been difficult due to the cell-associated nature of this virus (16). Nevertheless, cocultivation of HTLV-1- and HTLV-2-infected PBMCs with activated, allogeneic HTLV-negative PBMCs or cord blood cells is used to obtain viral isolates. The culture supernatants are collected weekly for up to 4 weeks, and the presence of p19 gag antigen in the supernatant is tested using a research use antigen capture assay (Zeptometrix Corp., Buffalo, NY). Because of the time required for and labor-intensive nature of this method, virus isolation and antigen detection are generally not done for diagnosis of HTLV infection but rather serve as a research tool.

GENOTYPING

PCR also has been used to genetically subtype HTLV-1 and HTLV-2 based on the LTR region. Earlier studies used restriction endonuclease digestion of PCR products; separation through an agarose gel with visualization of the bands by ethidium bromide allows for subtype determination (56). However, most recent studies now perform direct sequencing of the PCR products (56, 70). Likewise, sequence and phylogenetic analyses of the *env* and LTR regions have resulted in elucidation of the molecular epidemiology and the geographical distribution of virus-carrying populations (6, 56).

SEROLOGIC TESTS

Testing for antibodies to HTLV-1 and HTLV-2 should be performed for all blood donors and any patients presenting with relevant clinical signs and symptoms. In the United States, all blood donors have been screened for antibodies to both HTLV-1 and HTLV-2, using assays that include both HTLV-1 and HTLV-2 antigens (19) since 1997. Testing for HTLV-1 and HTLV-2 should also be offered

to persons who are from areas where HTLV is endemic, who engage in high-risk behaviors, such as needle sharing, and who have had sexual contact with persons from either group. Currently, HTLV-1 and HTLV-2 testing is not routinely performed for fertility or pregnancy testing in the United States. This is different in some European countries, including some islands in the West Indies, where recommendations have been made to test pregnant and breastfeeding women originating from areas of HTLV-1 endemicity (62, 64). In addition, in the United States, all donors of viable, leukocyte-rich cells or tissue (e.g., hematopoietic stem/progenitor cells and semen) are screened for HTLV-1 and HTLV-2 (20).

The most common screening assays detect antibodies in serum or plasma (15, 19, 65). The immunodominant regions of structural and regulatory proteins are well characterized (28) and are used in diagnostic assays that detect and differentiate HTLV-1 and HTLV-2. The major tests for HTLV-1 and HTLV-2 are described in Table 1. The serologic testing algorithm is comprised of a primary screening assay followed by testing for confirmation and identification of HTLV type (Fig. 3).

Primary screening assays include enzyme immunoassays (EIA), chemiluminescence immunoassays (ChLIA), particle agglutination (Fujirebio America, Fairfield, NJ), and immunofluorescence assays (IFAs) (Table 1). The EIA is a sensitive and simple colorimetric test that uses purified infected cell lysates and/or recombinant antigens or synthetic peptides (2, 15, 65). ChLIA is similar but uses chemiluminescence technology for the detection step. The addition of HTLV-2 antigens to screening test kits significantly improved the detection of antibodies to HTLV-2, compared with results using kits that contained only HTLV-1 antigens (2, 31, 45). The EIA and ChLIA can be automated and performed on a large scale (47). However, neither EIAs nor ChLIAs can differentiate between HTLV-1 and HTLV-2 infections because of the significant homology in structural proteins between the two viruses; therefore, these screening assays are referred to as tests for HTLV-1/2 (2, 15, 47, 65).

Comparative analysis of various commercial screening assays containing both HTLV-1 and HTLV-2 antigens indicates that sensitivity ranges from 98.9 to 100% for confirmed HTLV-1-positive specimens and 91.5 to 100% for confirmed HTLV-2-positive specimens. Specificity ranges from 90.2 to 100% (2, 15, 31, 45, 46, 65). Currently, one HTLV-1/2 EIA and one HTLV-1/2 ChLIA are licensed by the Food and Drug Administration (FDA) for use in the United States (Abbott HTLV-I/HTLV-II EIA and Abbott Prism HTLV-I/HTLV-II [Abbott Laboratories, Abbott Park, IL], respectively), with reports of overall sensitivity point estimates of 100% and specificities of 99.73 to 99.93%, according to data from clinical trials that supported the licensure of these tests. These licensed assays are used both for blood donor screening and as an aid in clinical diagnosis of HTLV-1 and HTLV-2 infection and related diseases. Further attempts have been made to develop a dual EIA algorithm to increase the predictive values of HTLV tests (58, 59). Pooling of samples for seroepidemiologic studies has been proposed; however, pooled testing is not recommended for blood donor testing (3).

While most screening assays are highly sensitive, specimens containing low titers of antibodies to HTLV-1 and HTLV-2 from certain areas of HTLV-2 endemicity or specimens from early seroconverters can be missed by current EIAs (35, 45). Nucleic acid assays can be used to detect infected individuals either with low antibody titers

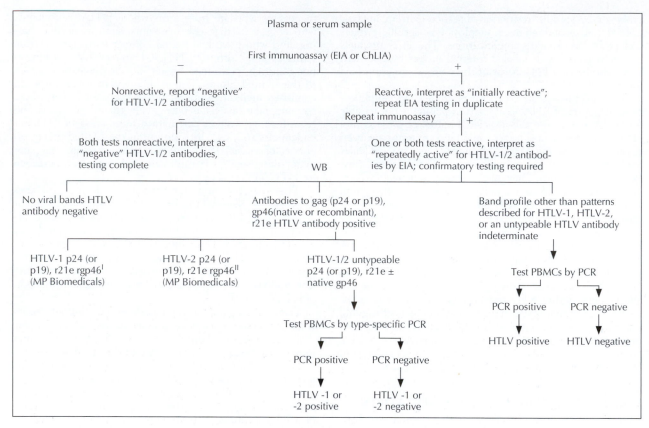

FIGURE 3 Serologic testing algorithm for the detection and confirmation of HTLV-1 and -2 infection. If the initial screening immunoassay (EIA or ChLIA) is reactive, a repeat assay with the same specimen is performed in duplicate. If one or both of the repeat tests are reactive, the specimen is classified as repeatedly reactive and supplemental testing is done for the purpose of confirmation. WB criteria shown are those used by the manufacturer and not the PHS working group. In some cases, further follow-up is done using PCR.

or within their window period prior to the development of an antibody response (median window period, 51 days; range, 36 to 72 days) (35). However, these assays are used mainly for research and are not in routine clinical use. It is important to note that a negative PCR result does not necessarily exclude infection since the period between infection and the consistent detection of HTLV proviral DNA is not well understood. Additional serologic and nucleic acid testing at a later date may therefore be indicated for an individual with potential risk factors.

Supplemental confirmatory or differentiation tests for HTLV-1 and HTLV-2 infection include the use of WBs containing the viral lysates supplemented with recombinant proteins (71), line immunoassays (LIAs) (Innogenetics, Ghent, Belgium) (52), and IFAs (21) (Table 1). Although WBs using purified viral lysates are highly sensitive for detecting p24 and p19 gag antibodies, they do not always detect antibodies to native envelope glycoproteins. An alternative approach used in a second-generation confirmatory assay is a modified WB assay (previously marketed as Genelabs W.B. 2.4) that contains type-specific gp46 env recombinant proteins from both viruses and a truncated form of recombinant 21e (r21e) that reduces nonspecific reactivity, improves performance (specificity and sensitivity), and allows differentiation between HTLV-1 and HTLV-2 (MP Diagnostics W.B. 2.4; MP Biomedicals, Science Park, Singapore) (Fig. 4) (31, 71).

Another supplementary test is the LIA, consisting of recombinant and synthetic HTLV-1 and HTLV-2 antigens painted onto strips (Innogenetics) (52). Some of these antigens are specific for HTLV-1 or HTLV-2; therefore, this assay can differentiate between HTLV-1 and HTLV-2 infections. IFAs that detect binding of antibodies from a specimen to HTLV-1- or HTLV-2-infected cells can be used to discriminate HTLV-1/2 infections and to determine antibody titer (21). No assay has been approved or licensed as a confirmatory test for clinical use by the U.S. FDA; however, WB and LIA have been certified for use in Europe and other areas of endemicity (Brazil, Argentina, West Indies, Iran, and Japan) to confirm any sample repeatedly reactive by EIA (62, 64).

EVALUATION, INTERPRETATION, AND REPORTING OF RESULTS

A typical algorithm for HTLV testing for diagnostic purposes is outlined in Fig. 3. If the initial screening immunoassay (EIA or ChLIA) is reactive, a repeat assay of the same specimen is performed in duplicate. If one or both of the repeat tests are reactive, the specimen is classified as repeatedly reactive. The repeatedly reactive specimens are subjected to confirmatory supplemental testing, which is typically done by WB, when available (Fig. 4 and Table 1). Based on the data available in 1992, the U.S. Public Health

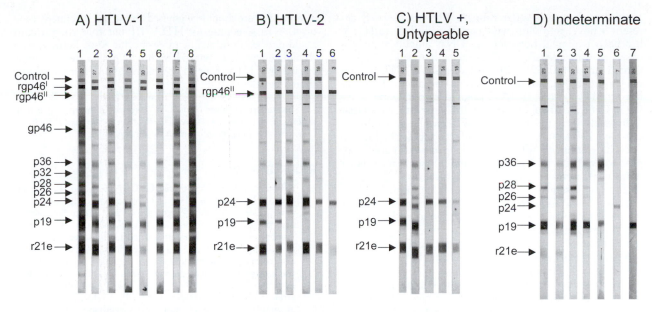

FIGURE 4 Western blot analysis of representative plasma or serum specimens from persons infected with HTLV-1 (A), HTLV-2 (B), and untypeable HTLV-1/2 (C). Representative seroreactivity patterns are shown for WBs from MP Biomedicals (previously Genelabs Diagnostics; HTLV-2.4 version), which contain HTLV-1 antigens spiked with r21e (common to HTLV-1 and HTLV-2) and two external recombinant envelope proteins specific for HTLV-1 (rgp46^I) and HTLV-2 (rgp46^{II}). (A) Typical patterns for HTLV-1 reactivity (lanes 1 to 5), atypical reactivity lacking a p24 response (lane 6), and specimens with high antibody titers showing reactivity to both rgp46 proteins (lanes 7 and 8) (titration of sera results in reactivity only to rgp46^I). (B) Typical patterns for HTLV-2 reactivity (lanes 1 to 6) (note that the p24 band is stronger than p19 reactivity, which is usually absent from HTLV-2-infected sera). (C) HTLV-1/2-positive but untypeable specimens, with reactivity to gag (p24, with or without p19) and r21e but not gp46^I or gp46^{II}. Lanes 1 and 2, characteristic patterns of specimens that are usually found to contain HTLV-1 after additional testing; lanes 3 to 5, characteristic patterns of specimens that are usually found to contain HTLV-2 after additional testing. (D) Typical patterns from HTLV-indeterminate specimens. Shown are typical HTLV gag-indeterminate profiles frequently found in plasma or sera from individuals originating from tropical regions (Central Africa and Papua New Guinea, etc.) (lanes 1 to 4) and those from low-risk populations (lanes 5 to 7). In the great majority of the cases, neither HTLV-1 nor HTLV-2 infection could be demonstrated in samples with such seroreactivity.

Service (PHS) recommended that the diagnostic criteria for confirmation of HTLV-1 or HTLV-2 seropositivity by supplemental tests include demonstration of antibodies to p24 gag and to native gp46 env and/or r21e (13). Subsequent data with more-sensitive assays suggest that alternative patterns of WB reactivity may be considered. The second-generation modified WB is the most commonly used WB worldwide (Genelabs W.B. 2.4). Specimens with reactivity to p19 gag (with or without p24 gag), r21e, and recombinant gp46^I (rgp46^I) are referred to as HTLV-1 (Fig. 4A). Sera with reactivity to p24 gag (with or without p19), r21e, and rgp46^{II} are referred to as HTLV-2 (Fig. 4B). Specimens with no immunoreactivity to any bands are considered negative for antibodies to HTLV-1 and HTLV-2 (false-positive EIA specimens). Specimens reacting with p24 gag (with or without p19 gag or native gp46) and r21e but with no reactivity to either rgp46^I or rgp46^{II} are referred to as untypeable and are considered to be HTLV positive since PCR analysis of these untypeable specimens has identified the presence of HTLV-specific sequences in some cases (Fig. 4C) (69). Individuals with this type of serologic reactivity who remain negative by type-specific PCR, after repeat testing, are most likely not infected with HTLV-1 or -2. Alternatively, this type of reactivity could indicate the presence of other, more divergent types of HTLV, such as HTLV-3 and HTLV-4, that have been recently identified (76). Similar interpretive criteria are used for LIA (see manufacturers' instructions).

Both the WB assays and LIA can give indeterminate results (immunoreactivity to a single HTLV gene product or multiple bands, conditions that do not meet the criteria for seropositivity [Fig. 4D]) (65, 71). Antibody only to gag proteins (p24, p19) is the most common indeterminate pattern that is observed in EIA-reactive specimens and is an area of intense investigation (10, 14, 27, 33, 38, 39, 51, 67, 69). In the case of both WB and LIAs, interpretation is often based on the intensity of bands observed. Specifically, with many commercial assays, bands are interpreted relative to their intensities observed on control strips on which highly and slightly reactive samples are included. However, interpretive criteria are kit or assay dependent, and results should be interpreted based on the manufacturer's recommendations.

Extensive PCR analyses using primers to detect multiple gene regions have failed to detect HTLV-1 or HTLV-2 proviral sequences in low-risk, seroindeterminate persons, thus indicating that these individuals are not likely to be infected with HTLV-1 or HTLV-2 (10, 14, 27, 39, 69). The possibility that such indeterminate WB results may represent a novel retrovirus with partial homology to HTLV has been explored; however, no DNA amplification was observed using generic PCR primers that detect HTLV-related viruses (10, 69), with the exception of HTLV-3 and HTLV-4 (11, 76), two novel human retroviruses closely related to HTLV-1 and HTLV-2 isolated from individuals living in Central Africa. Limited studies have established that individuals with indeterminate WB profiles generally do not have risk factors for HTLV infection (14, 38, 39, 51). Such indeterminate WB results among low-risk persons appear to represent antibodies to different viral and cellular antigens that cross-react with HTLV proteins (33).

In rare instances, specimens with confirmed HTLV infection have an indeterminate WB pattern of reactivity to p19 gag (in the absence of p24 gag) and r21e (14, 51). Likewise, in some instances, antibody to r21e may represent an early antibody response during seroconversion (36). Individuals with such reactivity should be retested in 3 months by EIA and/or PCR.

A very small number of patients with chronic progressive neurological disease from the United States with HTLV-indeterminate WB patterns may be infected with a defective HTLV or have HTLV-1 in low copy numbers (57, 74). Persons who have clinical neurological symptoms or are from high-prevalence areas (e.g., African, Asian, South American, and Caribbean countries) with HTLV-1/2-indeterminate reactivity should be further investigated for possible retroviral infection, including infection with the recently identified viruses HTLV-3 and HTLV-4. Further testing could include PCR in conjunction with serologic testing.

In the United States, decisions to accept or defer blood donations are currently based only on screening test (EIA or ChLIA) results because of the lack of FDA-licensed supplemental tests. Persons who are ultimately confirmed to be antibody positive to HTLV-1 or HTLV-2 (i.e., when licensed supplemental testing becomes available) are permanently barred from donating blood. Blood donors whose plasma specimens are repeatedly reactive upon screening but not confirmed as seropositive for HTLV-1 or HTLV-2 (including falsely EIA-reactive specimens and specimens for which supplemental testing was indeterminate or not performed) should be notified and required to defer donating if the same test result is obtained for two separate donations or if the same donation repeatedly tests reactive by screening tests from two different manufacturers (19). Screening tests are weighted toward better sensitivity than specificity because of the public health implications of false-negative results. Therefore, in the absence of known risk factors for a given blood donor, repeatedly reactive results from a single test kit or discrepant results between multiple test kits most likely represent false-positive reactions. Reactivity in a dual-screening test algorithm increases the probability of actual infection (58, 59).

Persons with HTLV-1- or HTLV-2-positive or -indeterminate test results are counseled according to the guidelines established by PHS Working Group (CDC) 13. These guidelines state that persons should be informed that HTLV is not the AIDS virus and that their risk of developing HTLV-related diseases is low. HTLV-1- or HTLV-2-infected persons are asked not to donate blood, semen, organs, or other tissues and not to share needles or syringes. To prevent transmission of HTLV, the infected person is counseled to use protective measures during sexual activity, and women are counseled to refrain from breastfeeding. Persons who have indeterminate results on two separate occasions at least 3 months apart should be advised that their specimens were reactive in screening for HTLV-1/2 but that these results could not be confirmed by more-specific tests. Further, they should be reassured that indeterminate results are very rarely caused by HTLV-1 or HTLV-2 infection. Repeat testing should be offered.

The authors employed by the U.S. government are writing as individual experts whose views should not be taken to represent those of the U.S. government agencies by which they are employed.

REFERENCES

1. **Albrecht, B., N. D. Collins, G. C. Newbound, L. Ratner, and M. D. Lairmore.** 1998. Quantification of human T-cell lymphotropic virus type 1 proviral load by quantitative competitive polymerase chain reaction. *J. Virol. Methods* **75:**123–140.
2. **Andersson, S., R. Thorstensson, K. G. Ramirez, A. Krook, M. von Sydow, F. Dias, and G. Biberfeld.** 1999. Comparative evaluation of 14 immunoassays for detection of antibodies to the human T-lymphotropic virus types I and II using panels of sera from Sweden and West Africa. *Transfusion* **39:**845–851.
3. **Andersson, S., A. Gessain, and G. P. Taylor.** 2001. Pooling of samples for seroepidemiological surveillance of human T-cell lymphotropic virus types I and II. *Virus Res.* **78:**101–106.
4. **Araujo, A., and W. W. Hall.** 2004. Human T-lymphotropic virus type II and neurological disease. *Ann. Neurol.* **56:**10–19.
5. **Araujo, A., and M. T. Silva.** 2006. The HTLV-1 neurological complex. *Lancet Neurol.* **5:**1068–1076.
6. **Azran, I., Y. Schavinsky-Khrapunsky, E. Priel, M. Huleihel, and M. Aboud.** 2004. Implications of the evolution pattern of human T-cell leukemia retroviruses on their pathogenic virulence. *Int. J. Mol. Med.* **14:**909–915.
7. **Bazarbachi, A., D. Ghez, Y. Lepelletier, R. Nasr, H. de The, M. E. El-Sabban, and O. Hermine.** 2004. New therapeutic approaches for adult T-cell leukaemia. *Lancet Oncol.* **5:**664–672.
8. **Beilke, M. A., K. P. Theall, M. O'Brien, J. L. Clayton, S. M. Benjamin, E. L. Winsor, and P. J. Kissinger.** 2004. Clinical outcomes and disease progression among patients coinfected with HIV and human T lymphotropic virus types 1 and 2. *Clin. Infect. Dis.* **39:**256–263.
9. **Beilke, M. A., V. L. Traina-Dorge, M. Sirois, A. Bhuiyan, E. L. Murphy, J. M. Walls, R. Fagan, E. L. Winsor, and P. J. Kissinger.** 2007. Relationship between human T lymphotropic virus (HTLV) type 1/2 viral burden and clinical and treatment parameters among patients with HIV type 1 and HTLV-1/2 coinfection. *Clin. Infect. Dis.* **44:**1229–1234.
10. **Busch, M. P., W. M. Switzer, E. L. Murphy, R. Thomson, and W. Heneine.** 2000. Absence of evidence of infection with divergent primate T-lymphotropic viruses in United States blood donors who have seroindeterminate HTLV test results. *Transfusion* **40:**443–449.
11. **Calattini, S., S. A. Chevalier, R. Duprez, S. Bassot, A. Froment, R. Mahieux, and A. Gessain.** 2005. Discovery of a new human T-cell lymphotropic virus (HTLV-3) in Central Africa. *Retrovirology* **2:**30.
12. **Castro, N. M., W. Rodrigues, D. M. Freitas, A. Muniz, P. Oliveira, and E. M. Carvalho.** 2007. Urinary symptoms associated with human T-cell lymphotropic virus I infection: evidence of urinary manifestations in large group of HTLV-I carriers. *Urology* **69:**813–818.
13. **Centers for Disease Control and Prevention and the U.S. Public Health Service Working Group.** 1993. Guidelines for counseling persons infected with human T-lymphotropic virus type I (HTLV-I) and type II (HTLV-II). *Ann. Intern. Med.* **118:**448–454.
14. **Cesaire, R., O. Bera, H. Maier, A. Lezin, J. Martial, M. Ouka, B. Kerob-Bauchet, A. K. Ould Amar, and J. C. Vernant.** 1999. Seroindeterminate patterns and seroconversions to human T-lymphotropic virus type I positivity in blood donors from Martinique, French West Indies. *Transfusion* **39:**1145–1149.

15. Courouce, A. M., J. Pillonel, and C. Saura. 1999. Screening of blood donations for HTLV-I/II. *Transfus. Med. Rev.* **13:**267–274.

16. Derse, D., G. Heidecker, M. Mitchell, S. Hill, P. Lloyd, and G. Princler. 2004. Infectious transmission and replication of human T-cell leukemia virus type 1. *Front. Biosci.* **9:**2495–2499.

17. Dodd, R. Y., E. P. Notari, and S. L. Stramer. 2002. Current prevalence and incidence of infectious disease markers and estimated window-period risk in the American Red Cross blood donor population. *Transfusion* **42:**975–979.

18. Ferreira, O. C., Jr., V. Planelles, and J. D. Rosenblatt. 1997. Human T-cell leukemia viruses: epidemiology, biology, and pathogenesis. *Blood Rev.* **11:**91–104.

19. Food and Drug Administration. 1997. *Guidance for Industry: Donor Screening for Antibodies to HTLV-II.* U.S. FDA, Washington, DC. [Online.] http://www.fda.gov/Biologics-BloodVaccines/GuidanceComplianceRegulatoryInformation/Guidances/Blood/ucm170786.htm.

20. Food and Drug Administration, Center for Biologics Evaluation and Research. 2007. *Guidance for Industry: Eligibility Determination for Donors of Human Cells, Tissues, and Cellular and Tissue-Based Products (HCT/Ps).* U.S. FDA, Washington, DC. [Online.] http://www.fda.gov/BiologicsBloodVaccines/GuidanceComplianceRegulatoryInformation/Guidances/CellularandGeneTherapy/ucm072929.htm.

21. Gallo, D., L. M. Penning, and C. V. Hanson. 1991. Detection and differentiation of antibodies to human T-cell lymphotropic virus types I and II by the immunofluorescence method. *J. Clin. Microbiol.* **29:**2345–2347.

22. Ghez, D., Y. Lepelletier, S. Lambert, J. M. Fourneau, V. Blot, S. Janvier, B. Arnulf, P. M. van Endert, N. Heveker, C. Pique, and O. Hermine. 2006. Neuropilin-1 is involved in human T-cell lymphotropic virus type 1 entry. *J. Virol.* **80:**6844–6854.

23. Glynn, S. A., S. H. Kleinman, G. B. Schreiber, M. P. Busch, D. J. Wright, J. W. Smith, C. C. Nass, A. E. Williams, and the Retrovirus Epidemiology Donor Study (REDS). 2000. Trends in incidence and prevalence of major transfusion-transmissible viral infections in US blood donors, 1991 to 1996. *JAMA* **284:**229–235.

24. Heneine, W., R. F. Khabbaz, R. B. Lal, and J. E. Kaplan. 1992. Sensitive and specific polymerase chain reaction assays for diagnosis of human T-cell lymphotropic virus type I (HTLV-I) and HTLV-II infections in HTLV-I/II-seropositive individuals. *J. Clin. Microbiol.* **30:**1605–1607.

25. Kamihira, S., N. Dateki, K. Sugahara, Y. Yamada, M. Tomonaga, T. Maeda, and M. Tahara. 2000. Real-time polymerase chain reaction for quantification of HTLV-1 proviral load: application for analyzing aberrant integration of the proviral DNA in adult T-cell leukemia. *Int. J. Hematol.* **72:**79–84.

26. Kinet, S., L. Swainson, M. Lavanya, C. Mongellaz, A. Montel-Hagen, M. Craveiro, N. Manel, J. L. Battini, M. Sitbon, and N. Taylor. 2007. Isolated receptor binding domains of HTLV-1 and HTLV-2 envelopes bind Glut-1 on activated CD4+ and CD8+ T cells. *Retrovirology* **4:**31.

27. Lal, R. B., D. L. Rudolph, J. E. Coligan, S. K. Brodine, and C. R. Roberts. 1992. Failure to detect evidence of human T-lymphotropic virus (HTLV) type I and type II in blood donors with isolated gag antibodies to HTLV-I/II. *Blood* **80:**544–550.

28. Lal, R. B. 1996. Delineation of immunodominant epitopes of human T-lymphotropic virus types I and II and their usefulness in developing serologic assays for detection of antibodies to HTLV-I and HTLV-II. *J. Acquir. Immune Defic. Syndr. Hum. Retrovirol.* **13**(Suppl. 1):S170–S178.

29. Lee, T. H., D. M. Chafets, M. P. Busch, and E. L. Murphy. 2004. Quantitation of HTLV-I and II proviral load using real-time quantitative PCR with SYBR Green chemistry. *J. Clin. Virol.* **31:**275–282.

30. Li, H. C., R. J. Biggar, W. J. Miley, E. M. Maloney, B. Cranston, B. Hanchard, and M. Hisada. 2004. Provirus load in breast milk and risk of mother-to-child transmission of human T lymphotropic virus type I. *J. Infect. Dis.* **190:**1275–1278.

31. Liu, H., M. Shah, S. L. Stramer, W. Chen, B. J. Weiblen, and E. L. Murphy. 1999. Sensitivity and specificity of human T-lymphotropic virus (HTLV) types I and II polymerase chain reaction and several serologic assays in screening a population with a high prevalence of HTLV-II. *Transfusion* **39:**1185–1193.

32. Mahieux, R., and A. Gessain. 2003. HTLV-1 and associated adult T-cell leukemia/lymphoma. *Rev. Clin. Exp. Hematol.* **7:**336–361.

33. Mahieux, R., P. Horal, P. Mauclere, O. Mercereau-Puijalon, M. Guillotte, L. Meertens, E. Murphey, and A. Gessain. 2000. Human T-cell lymphotropic virus type I gag indeterminate Western blot patterns in Central Africa: relationship to *Plasmodium falciparum* infection. *J. Clin. Microbiol.* **38:**4049–4057.

34. Manel, N., F. J. Kim, S. Kinet, N. Taylor, M. Sitbon, and J. L. Battini. 2003. The ubiquitous glucose transporter GLUT-1 is a receptor for HTLV. *Cell* **115:**449–459.

35. Manns, A., E. L. Murphy, R. Wilks, G. Haynes, J. P. Figueroa, B. Hanchard, M. Barnett, J. Drummond, D. Waters, and M. Cerney. 1991. Detection of early human T-cell lymphotropic virus type I antibody patterns during seroconversion among transfusion recipients. *Blood* **77:**896–905.

36. Manns, A., M. Hisada, and L. La Grenade. 1999. Human T-lymphotropic virus type I infection. *Lancet* **353:**1951–1958.

37. Matsuoka, M., and K. T. Jeang. 2007. Human T-cell leukemia virus type 1 (HTLV-1) infectivity and cellular transformation. *Nat. Rev. Cancer* **7:**270–280.

38. Mauclere, P., J. Y. Le Hesran, R. Mahieux, R. Salla, J. Mfoupouendoun, E. T. Abada, J. Millan, G. de The, and A. Gessain. 1997. Demographic, ethnic, and geographic differences between human T cell lymphotropic virus (HTLV) type I-seropositive carriers and persons with HTLV-I gag-indeterminate Western blots in Central Africa. *J. Infect. Dis.* **176:**505–509.

39. Medrano, F. J., V. Soriano, E. J. Calderon, C. Rey, M. Gutierrez, R. Bravo, M. Leal, J. Gonzalez-Lahoz, and E. Lissen. 1997. Significance of indeterminate reactivity to human T-cell lymphotropic virus in Western blot analysis of individuals at risk. *Eur. J. Clin. Microbiol. Infect. Dis.* **16:**249–252.

40. Miley, W. J., K. Suryanarayana, A. Manns, R. Kubota, S. Jacobson, J. D. Lifson, and D. Waters. 2000. Real-time polymerase chain reaction assay for cell-associated HTLV type I DNA viral load. *AIDS Res. Hum. Retrovir.* **16:**665–675.

41. Murphy, E. L., T. H. Lee, D. Chafets, C. C. Nass, B. Wang, K. Loughlin, D. Smith, and the HTLV Outcomes Study Investigators. 2004. Higher human T lymphotropic virus (HTLV) provirus load is associated with HTLV-I versus HTLV-II, with HTLV-II subtype A versus B, and with male sex and a history of blood transfusion. *J. Infect. Dis.* **190:**504–510.

42. Oh, U., Y. Yamano, C. A. Mora, J. Ohayon, F. Bagnato, J. A. Butman, J. Dambrosia, T. P. Leist, H. McFarland, and S. Jacobson. 2005. Interferon-beta1a therapy in human T-lymphotropic virus type I-associated neurologic disease. *Ann. Neurol.* **57:**526–534.

43. Oh, U., and S. Jacobson. 2008. Treatment of HTLV-I-associated myelopathy/tropical spastic paraparesis: toward rational targeted therapy. *Neurol. Clin.* **26:**781–797.

44. Overbaugh, J., and C. R. Bangham. 2001. Selection forces and constraints on retroviral sequence variation. *Science* **292:**1106–1109.

45. Poiesz, B. J., S. Dube, D. Choi, E. Esteban, J. Ferrer, M. Leon-Ponte, G. E. de Perez, J. Glaser, S. G. Devare, A. S. Vallari, and G. Schochetman. 2000. Comparative performances of an HTLV-I/II EIA and other serologic and PCR assays on samples from persons at risk for HTLV-II infection. *Transfusion* **40:**924–930.

46. Proietti, F. A., A. B. Carneiro-Proietti, B. C. Catalan-Soares, and E. L. Murphy. 2005. Global epidemiology of HTLV-I infection and associated diseases. *Oncogene* **24:**6058–6068.

47. Qiu, X., S. Hodges, T. Lukaszewska, S. Hino, H. Ara, J. Yamaguchi, P. Swanson, G. Schochetman, and S. Devare. 2008. Evaluation of a new fully automated immunoassay for the detection of HTLV-I and HTLV-II antibodies. *J. Med. Virol.* **80:**484–493.

48. Ratner, L. 2004. Adult T cell leukemia lymphoma. *Front. Biosci.* **9:**2852–2859.

49. Roucoux, D. F., and E. L. Murphy. 2004. The epidemiology and disease outcomes of human T-lymphotropic virus type II. *AIDS Rev.* **6:**144–154.

50. Roucoux, D. F., B. Wang, D. Smith, C. C. Nass, J. Smith, S. T. Hutching, B. Newman, T. H. Lee, D. M. Chafets, E. L. Murphy, and the HTLV Outcomes Study Investigators. 2005. A prospective study of sexual transmission of human T lymphotropic virus (HTLV)-I and HTLV-II. *J. Infect. Dis.* **191:**1490–1497.

51. Rouet, F., L. Meertens, G. Courouble, C. Herrmann-Storck, R. Pabingui, B. Chancerel, A. Abid, M. Strobel, P. Mauclere, and A. Gessain. 2001. Serological, epidemiological, and molecular differences between human T-cell lymphotropic virus type 1 (HTLV-1)-seropositive healthy carriers and persons with HTLV-I *gag* indeterminate Western blot patterns from the Caribbean. *J. Clin. Microbiol.* **39:**1247–1253.

52. Sabino, E. C., M. Zrein, C. P. Taborda, M. M. Otani, G. Ribeiro-Dos-Santos, and A. Saez-Alquezar. 1999. Evaluation of the INNO-LIA HTLV I/II assay for confirmation of human T-cell leukemia virus-reactive sera in blood bank donations. *J. Clin. Microbiol.* **37:**1324–1328.

53. Saito, M., M. Nakagawa, S. Kaseda, T. Matsuzaki, M. Jonosono, N. Eiraku, R. Kubota N. Takenouchi, M. Nagai, Y. Furukawa, K. Usuku, S. Izumo, and M. Osame. 2004. Decreased human T lymphotropic virus type I (HTLV-I) provirus load and alteration in T cell phenotype after interferon-alpha therapy for HTLV-I-associated myelopathy/tropical spastic paraparesis. *J. Infect. Dis.* **189:**29–40.

54. Salemi, M., M. Lewis, J. F. Egan, W. W. Hall, J. Desmyter, and A. M. Vandamme. 1999. Different population dynamics of human T cell lymphotropic virus type II in intravenous drug users compared with endemically infected tribes. *Proc. Natl. Acad. Sci. USA* **96:**13253–13258.

55. Schreiber, G. B., M. P. Busch, S. H. Kleinman, J. J. Korelitz, and the Retrovirus Epidemiology Donor Study Group. 1996. The risk of transfusion-transmitted viral infections. *N. Engl. J. Med.* **334:**1685–1690.

56. Slattery, J. P., G. Franchini, and A. Gessain. 1999. Genomic evolution, patterns of global dissemination, and interspecies transmission of human and simian T-cell leukemia/lymphotropic viruses. *Genome Res.* **9:**525–540.

57. Soldan, S. S., M. D. Graf, A. Waziri, A. N. Flerlage, S. M. Robinson, T. Kawanishi, T. P. Leist, T. J. Lehky, M. C. Levin, and S. Jacobson. 1999. HTLV-I/II seroindeterminate Western blot reactivity in a cohort of patients with neurological disease. *J. Infect. Dis.* **180:**685–694.

58. Stramer, S. L., J. P. Brodsky, J. Trenbeath, L. Taylor, B. Peoples, and R. Y. Dodd. 1999. Resolution testing of HTLV-I/II screening test repeatedly reactive donor samples by the use of a dual EIA algorithm. *Transfusion* **39:**106S.

59. Stramer, S. L., G. A. Foster, and R. Y. Dodd. 2006. Effectiveness of human T-lymphotropic virus (HTLV) recipient tracing (lookback) and the current HTLV-I and II confirmatory algorithm, 1999 to 2004. *Transfusion* **46:**703–707.

60. Takenouchi, N., K. Yao, and S. Jacobson. 2004. Immunopathogenesis of HTLV-I associated neurologic disease: molecular, histopathologic, and immunologic approaches. *Front. Biosci.* **9:**2527–2539.

61. Takenouchi, N., K. S. Jones, I. Lisinski, K. Fugo, K. Yao, S. W. Cushman, F. W. Ruscetti, and S. Jacobson. 2007 GLUT1 is not the primary binding receptor but is associated with cell-to-cell transmission of human T-cell leukemia virus type 1. *J. Virol.* **8:**1506–1510.

62. Taylor, G. P. 1996. The epidemiology of HTLV-I in Europe. *J. Acquir. Immune Defic. Syndr. Hum. Retrovirol.* **13**(Suppl. 1):S8–S14.

63. Taylor, G. P., S. E. Hall, S. Navarrete, C. A. Michie, R. Davis, A. D. Witkover, M. Rossor, M. A. Nowak, P. Rudge, E. Matutes, C. R. Bangham, and J. N. Weber. 1999. Effect of lamivudine on human T-cell leukemia virus type 1 (HTLV-1) DNA copy number, T-cell phenotype, and anti-tax cytotoxic T-cell frequency in patients with HTLV-1-associated myelopathy. *J. Virol.* **73:**10289–10295.

64. Taylor, G. P., M. Bodeus, F. Courtois, G. Pauli, A. Del Mistro, A. Machuca, E. Padua, S. Andersson, P. Goubau, L. Chieco-Bianchi, V. Soriano, J. Coste, A. E. Ades, and J. N. Weber. 2005. The seroepidemiology of human T-lymphotropic viruses: types I and II in Europe: a prospective study of pregnant women. *J. Acquir. Immune Defic. Syndr.* **38:**104–109.

65. Thorstensson, R., J. Albert, and S. Andersson. 2002. Strategies for diagnosis of HTLV-I and -II. *Transfusion* **42:**780–791.

66. Tosswill, J. H., G. P. Taylor, J. P. Clewley, and J. N. Weber. 1998. Quantification of proviral DNA load in human T-cell leukaemia virus type I infections. *J. Virol. Methods* **75:**21–26.

67. Tseliou, P. M., A. Spiliotakara, C. Politis, N. Spanakis, N. J. Legakis, and A. Tsakris. 2004. Prevalence of human T-cell lymphotropic virus-I/II-indeterminate reactivities in a Greek blood bank population. *Transfus. Med.* **14:**253–254.

68. Vallinoto, A. C., M. O. Ishak, V. N. Azevedo, A. C. Vicente, K. Otsuki, W. W. Hall, and R. Ishak. 2002. Molecular epidemiology of human T-lymphotropic virus type II infection in Amerindian and urban populations of the Amazon region of Brazil. *Hum. Biol.* **74:**633–644.

69. Vandamme, A. M., K. Van Laethem, H. F. Liu, M. Van Brussel, E. Delaporte, C. M. de Castro Costa, C. Fleischer, G. Taylor, U. Bertazzoni, J. Desmyter, and P. Goubau. 1997. Use of a generic polymerase chain reaction assay detecting human T-lymphotropic virus (HTLV) types I, II and divergent simian strains in the evaluation of individuals with indeterminate HTLV serology. *J. Med. Virol.* **52:**1–7.

70. Van Dooren, S., O. G. Pybus, M. Salemi, H. F. Liu, P. Goubau, C. Remondegui, A. Talarmin, E. Gotuzzo, L. C. Alcantara, B. Galvao-Castro, and A. M. Vandamme. 2004. The low evolutionary rate of human T-cell lymphotropic virus type-1 confirmed by analysis of vertical transmission chains. *Mol. Biol. Evol.* **21:**603–611.

71. Varma, M., D. L. Rudolph, M. Knuchel, W. M. Switzer, K. G. Hadlock, M. Velligan, L. Chan, S. K. Foung, and R. B. Lal. 1995. Enhanced specificity of truncated transmembrane protein for serologic confirmation of human T-cell lymphotropic virus type 1 (HTLV-1) and HTLV-2 infections by Western blot (immunoblot) assay containing recombinant envelope glycoproteins. *J. Clin. Microbiol.* **33:**3239–3244.

72. Verdonck, K., E. González, S. Van Dooren, A. M. Vandamme, G. Vanham, and E. Gotuzzo. 2007. Human T-lymphotropic virus 1: recent knowledge about an ancient infection. *Lancet Infect. Dis.* **7:**266–281.

73. Wattel, E., M. Cavrois, A. Gessain, and S. Wain-Hobson. 1996. Clonal expansion of infected cells: a way of life for HTLV-I. *J. Acquir. Immune Defic. Syndr. Hum. Retrovirol.* **13:**S92–S99.

74. Waziri, A., S. S. Soldan, M. D. Graf, J. Nagle, and S. Jacobson. 2000. Characterization and sequencing of prototypic human T-lymphotropic virus type 1 (HTLV-1) from an HTLV-1/2 seroindeterminate patient. *J. Virol.* **74:**2178–2185.

75. Wodarz, D., and C. R. Bangham. 2000. Evolutionary dynamics of HTLV-I. *J. Mol. Evol.* **50:**448.

76. Wolfe, N. D., W. Heneine, J. K. Carr, D. Albert, G. Herardo, V. Shanmugam, U. Tamoufe, J. N. Torimiro, A. T. Prosser, E. Mpoudi-Ngole, F. E. McCutchan, D. L. Birx, T. M. Folks, D. S. Burke, and W. M. Switzer. 2005. Emergence of unique primate T-lymphotropic viruses among central African bushmeat hunters. *Proc. Natl. Acad. Sci. USA* **102:**7994–7999.

Influenza Viruses

ROBERT L. ATMAR AND STEPHEN E. LINDSTROM

81

TAXONOMY

The influenza viruses are members of the family *Orthomyxoviridae*. Antigenic differences in two major structural proteins, the matrix protein (M) and the nucleoprotein (NP), are used to separate the influenza viruses into three genera within the family: *Influenzavirus A*, *Influenzavirus B*, and *Influenzavirus C*. Members of these three genera are also referred to as influenza type A, B, and C viruses, respectively. The influenza A viruses are further classified into subtypes based upon characteristics of the two major surface glycoproteins, hemagglutinin (HA) and neuraminidase (NA). Subtypes are recognized by the lack of cross-reactivity in double immunodiffusion assays with animal hyperimmune sera corresponding to each antigen (97). Sixteen HA subtypes and nine NA subtypes are now recognized (31). Within a subtype, strains may be further subclassified into lineages or clades based upon phylogenetic analysis of gene sequences. Criteria for classification of Eurasian-lineage highly pathogenic H5N1 strains into clades have been proposed (96).

The following information is used in the naming of individual virus strains: type, species of origin (if nonhuman), geographic location of isolation strain, laboratory identification number, year of isolation, and subtype (influenza A viruses only). Thus, an example of a human strain of influenza is A/California/7/2004 (H3N2), while A/quail/Vietnam/36/2004 (H5N1) is an example of an avian strain isolated in an epizootic in Asia.

DESCRIPTION OF THE AGENTS

Orthomyxoviruses are enveloped, single-stranded RNA viruses with segmented genomes of negative sense. Influenza A and B viruses have eight RNA segments, and influenza C viruses have only seven segments. Gene segments range from ~800 to ~2,500 nucleotides in length, and the entire genome ranges from 10 to 14.6 kb. The segmented genome of influenza viruses allows the exchange of one or more gene segments between two viruses when both infect a single cell. This exchange is called genetic reassortment and results in the generation of new strains containing a mix of genes from both parental viruses. Genetic reassortment between human and avian influenza virus strains led to the generation of the 1957 H2N2 and 1968 H3N2 pandemic strains, and it also played a role in the emergence of the novel 2009 H1N1 virus.

Influenza viruses are spherical and pleomorphic, with diameters of 80 to 120 nm after serial passage in culture. Filamentous forms also occur and may be up to several micrometers in size. The lipid envelope is derived from the host cell membrane through which maturing virus particles bud, and HA and NA form characteristic rod-like spikes (HA) and spikes with globular heads (NA) on the virus surface. As its name implies, the HA can agglutinate red blood cells from both mammalian (e.g., human [type O], guinea pig, and horse) and avian (e.g., chicken and turkey) species by binding to sialic acid residues. The HA protein is the major antigenic determinant and is used to identify viruses using immune sera. The lipid envelope surrounds the nucleocapsid, which has helical symmetry and consists of the genomic RNA segments, several copies of the polymerase proteins, and the NP. The matrix-1 (M1) protein is present between the nucleocapsid and the envelope, and the matrix-2 (M2) protein forms an ion channel across the envelope in influenza A viruses.

EPIDEMIOLOGY AND TRANSMISSION

Influenza viruses cause annual epidemics in areas with temperate climates, while in tropical climates seasonality is less apparent and influenza viruses can be isolated throughout the year. In the temperate regions of the Northern Hemisphere, epidemics generally occur between December and March, and in the Southern Hemisphere, the epidemic period is usually between May and August. Epidemics are characterized by a sudden increase in febrile respiratory illnesses and absenteeism from school and work, and within a community the epidemic period usually lasts from 3 to 8 weeks. A single subtype (A) or type (B) of influenza virus usually predominates, but epidemics have occurred in which both A and B viruses or two influenza A virus subtypes were isolated (16). Global epidemics, or pandemics, occur less frequently and are seen only with influenza A viruses. Pandemics occur following the emergence of an influenza A virus that carries a novel HA and that can be readily transmitted from person to person. The pandemic strain may develop due to genetic reassortment following coinfection of a susceptible host with human and avian influenza viruses or through gradual adaptation of an avian strain to mammalian hosts.

Influenza viruses are transmitted from person to person primarily via droplets generated by sneezing, coughing, and speaking. Direct or indirect (fomite) contact with contaminated secretions and small-particle aerosols are other potential routes of transmission that have been noted. The relative importance of these different routes has not been determined for influenza viruses (8). As for human infections caused by avian strains of influenza virus, direct contact with infected birds has been the most common factor of transmission, and direct inoculation into the pharynx or gastrointestinal tract may lead to infection (4).

There has been concern about the pandemic potential of avian strains of influenza A/H5N1 viruses since 1997, when several human cases occurred in Hong Kong in association with a large poultry outbreak. The outbreak was controlled by slaughtering all poultry in Hong Kong, but A/H5N1 viruses again caused outbreaks in poultry in China in 2003 and in several Southeast Asian countries in 2004 and 2005. By late 2005 and early 2006, the virus had spread to other parts of Asia, as well as to parts of Europe, Africa, and the Middle East (13). Human cases of A/H5N1 have been directly associated with outbreaks in poultry, and as of 2010, more than 500 human infections have been documented. Most cases have occurred in Southeast Asia, but several cases have also been documented in the Middle East and in northern Africa. Most human cases have been due to direct contact with infected birds, but limited human-to-human transmission has also occurred (4). A/H5N1 viruses continue to evolve and increase diversity, raising the possibility that they may acquire the ability to spread efficiently among humans (80).

In 2009, a novel swine-origin influenza A/H1N1 virus was identified as a cause of significant febrile respiratory illnesses in Mexico and the United States, demonstrating efficient human-to-human transmission (20). The virus rapidly spread to many countries around the world, prompting the World Health Organization (WHO) to declare an influenza pandemic. It appears that the pandemic strain emerged as a result of genetic reassortment involving North American and Eurasian swine influenza virus strains; this event likely occurred several years prior to recognition of the 2009 H1N1 virus as a cause of human illness (34, 82). The 2009 H1N1 hemagglutinin is antigenically distinct from seasonal human H1 strains, and children and young adults seem more susceptible to infection and less likely to have measurable levels of antibody than do older adults (14, 34).

CLINICAL SIGNIFICANCE

Influenza A and B virus infections typically cause a febrile respiratory illness characterized by fever, cough, upper respiratory tract symptoms (including sore throat, rhinorrhea, and nasal congestion), and systemic symptoms (including headache, myalgia, and malaise). This constellation of symptoms is called influenza, although other clinical presentations, ranging from asymptomatic infection to viral pneumonia, also occur. Illness begins abruptly after a 1- to 5-day incubation period (average, 2 days). Fever generally lasts for 3 to 5 days, but symptoms of dry cough and malaise may persist for several weeks. Complications include otitis media in children, sinusitis, viral pneumonia, secondary bacterial pneumonia, exacerbation of underlying cardiac or pulmonary disease, myositis (including rhabdomyolysis), neurologic problems (seizures, acute encephalitis, and postinfectious

encephalopathy), Reye's syndrome (associated with aspirin use), myopericarditis, and death (39, 85). In contrast, influenza C viruses cause mild respiratory illnesses that clinically are not distinguishable from common colds.

The 2009 H1N1 virus also causes a typical influenza-like illness, although up to 10% of infected persons may have an afebrile respiratory illness (20, 99). Gastrointestinal symptoms, such as nausea, vomiting, and diarrhea, have been seen in up to one-third of patients. Approximately half of the patients hospitalized in the United States have had high risk conditions other than age over 65 years (such as age under 5 years, chronic heart or lung disease, or pregnancy) that have been associated with severe seasonal influenza (20).

Influenza A/H5N1 virus also causes a febrile respiratory illness, although lower respiratory tract illness has been more prevalent. Upper respiratory tract symptoms may be absent, and gastrointestinal symptoms (watery diarrhea, vomiting, and abdominal pain) occur in some patients (4). Acute encephalitis may occur (21). Infection is associated with a high mortality (~60%), with most patients dying of progressive pneumonia. Viral replication is prolonged, and levels of several inflammatory mediators (e.g., interleukin-6, interleukin-8, and interleukin-1β) in plasma have been higher in fatal than in nonfatal cases. Surviving patients develop measurable serum antibody responses 10 to 14 days after symptom onset (4).

Influenza A and B virus infections spread rapidly through the community, with clinical attack rates having been documented to be as high as 70% following a common source exposure in an enclosed space (64). Epidemic disease is associated with an increase in hospitalization rates, especially in young children and in the elderly, and an increase in mortality rates in the elderly. Mortality rates have been higher in epidemics caused by influenza A/H3N2 viruses than in those caused by A/H1N1 or B viruses in the past 20 years. Additional information on the clinical presentation, manifestations, and complications of the diseases can be found in clinical textbooks (39, 85).

There are four licensed antiviral medications available for the treatment of influenza virus infection. Treatment with any of these medications must be initiated within 2 days of symptom onset to have demonstrable clinical benefit. Amantadine and rimantadine block the M2 ion channel and are active against only influenza A viruses. Zanamivir and oseltamivir are NA inhibitors and are active against both influenza A and B viruses. Clinically significant resistance has been seen following treatment of children or immunocompromised patients with amantadine and rimantadine, and the prevalence of resistance is high among influenza A/H3N2 and 2009 H1N1 virus isolates (37). Widespread resistance to oseltamivir among seasonal influenza A/H1N1 strains also limits the utility of this medication for these viruses (23). These drugs have also been used for prophylaxis, but annual immunization with a trivalent influenza vaccine is the primary means of prevention of influenza.

Both vaccines using inactivated virus and those using live attenuated virus are available (29). Influenza vaccines used in the United States are derived from viruses grown in embryonated chicken eggs, although vaccines derived from viruses grown in cell culture are in clinical development. For inactivated-virus vaccines, virus is harvested and then inactivated. Viral proteins are partially purified and standardized to contain 15 μg of HA per dose. The vaccine is trivalent, containing influenza A/H1N1, A/H3N2, and B virus strains. Due to constant virus evolution causing gradual antigenic changes in the HA protein, viruses included in the vaccine must be updated from time to time. The strains to be included in the vaccine are selected twice annually by the WHO. Vaccine strains for Northern Hemisphere countries are selected in January and February to make vaccine for use in September. Live attenuated influenza vaccines are also licensed for use in the United States. Live attenuated influenza vaccine is also trivalent and contains the same strains recommended for inactivated-virus vaccines. A reassortant vaccine virus for each strain to be included is derived to contain six internal genes from a parental attenuated influenza (A or B) virus and the HA and NA from the WHO-recommended vaccine strain. The vaccine is licensed in the United States for use in persons 2 to 49 years of age (29). It is given topically into the nose, and virus replicates in the upper respiratory tract. New vaccine alternatives, including those derived from viruses grown in mammalian cells and those containing larger amounts of HA or additional viral proteins, are currently under evaluation to improve on the efficacy of current influenza vaccines.

COLLECTION, TRANSPORT, AND STORAGE OF SPECIMENS

Influenza viruses infect the respiratory epithelium and can be found in respiratory secretions of all types. The level of virus shedding parallels the severity of clinical symptoms in uncomplicated influenza and is maximal in the first several days of illness. Samples should be collected during this time (first 2 to 3 days) to maximize the likelihood of virus detection. A variety of upper respiratory tract samples, including nasal aspirates, nasal wash fluids, nasal or nasopharyngeal

swabs, throat swabs, and throat wash fluids, alone or in combination, are routinely used for virus identification. Virus titers tend to be lower in samples collected from the throat, so assays of these samples alone tend to be less sensitive (17, 43). However, reports of human infection caused by H5N1 strains suggest that throat samples and lower respiratory tract samples may have better diagnostic yields than samples collected from the nose (4). Lower respiratory tract samples, including sputa, tracheal aspirates, and bronchoalveolar lavage fluids, may yield virus and can be assayed when indicated. Virus can occasionally be identified in nonrespiratory clinical samples (4, 56).

Once collected, the clinical samples should be placed in viral transport medium. A number of transport media are suitable for influenza viruses, including veal infusion broth, Hanks balanced salt solution, tryptose phosphate broth, sucrose phosphate buffer, and commercially available cell culture medium. All of these media are supplemented with 0.5% bovine serum albumin or 0.1% gelatin to stabilize the virus and antimicrobials (antibiotics and antifungals) to inhibit the growth of other respiratory flora. However, the use of transport medium may interfere with the test performance for certain commercially available virus detection assays; the package inserts of these assays should be consulted if they are to be used for diagnosis (Tables 1 and 2). Influenza virus infectivity is maintained for up to 5 days when samples are placed in transport media and maintained at 4°C (3). Clinical samples should be transported to the diagnostic laboratory as rapidly as possible after collection under these conditions. If a sample cannot be cultured during this time frame, it should be stored immediately at −70°C; storage at

TABLE 1 Commercially available kits for detection of influenza A or B viruses by FA staining[a]

Assay format	Kit name (manufacturer)	Acceptable clinical sample(s) for direct detection; cell culture confirmation	Comments	Influenza virus types detected	Assay sensitivity/specificity (%) per manufacturer brochure		Other virus(es) detected
					Direct detection	Isolate identification	
IFA	Bartels respiratory viral detection kit (Trinity Biotech)	NA, NPA, NPS, NW, TS; cell culture	Also available as individual influenza A or B components	A and B	A, 86/99; B, 65/98	A, 100/99.9; B, 100/100	Adenovirus, P1, P2, P3, RSV
DFA	D³ DFA respiratory virus screening and identification kit (Diagnostic Hybrids, Inc.)	NA, NPA, NW; cell culture	Also available as individual influenza A or B components	A and B	A, 96.6–100/100; B, 100/100	A, 100/99.5–100; B, 100/99.5–100	Adenovirus, P1, P2, P3, RSV
DFA	Imagen influenza virus A and B (Remel, Inc.)	NPA; cell culture		A and B	A, 96.2/100; B, 86.7/99.5	A, 100/100; B, 100/100	None
DFA	PathoDx respiratory virus panel (Oxoid)	Cell culture only	Not approved for direct use on clinical specimens	A and B	N/A	A, 100/100; B, 100/100	Adenovirus, P1, P2, P3, RSV
DFA	Light Diagnostics Simulfluor viral diagnostic screen (Millipore)	NPA, NPS, NW, TS; cell culture	Also available as Flu A/Flu B kit	A and B	A, 80/98.6; B, 50/100	A, 97.8/100; B, 100/100	Adenovirus, P1, P2, P3, RSV

[a]Abbreviations: IFA, indirect fluorescent antibody; DFA, direct fluorescent antibody; NA, nasal aspirate; NPA, nasopharyngeal aspirate; NPS, nasopharyngeal swab; NW, nasal wash fluid; TS, throat swab; N/A, not applicable; RSV, respiratory syncytial virus; P1, P2, and P3, parainfluenza virus types 1, 2, and 3, respectively.

TABLE 2 Commercially available kits for rapid (≤30-min) detection of influenza A or B viruses[a]

Assay format	Kit name (manufacturer)	Acceptable clinical sample(s)	Sample collection restriction(s)	Virus type(s) detected (differentiation of A and B)	Assay sensitivity/ specificity (%)[b]	Assay performance time (min)	Assay complexity[c]	Reference(s)
Dipstick chromatographic EIA	OSOM influenza A&B (Genzyme)	NS	Use only swabs supplied with the kit	A and B (yes)	No published studies	<15	CLIA moderate	No published studies
Dipstick chromatographic EIA	Tru Flu (Meridian Bioscience, Inc.)	NA, NPS, NS, NW	Do not use calcium alginate swabs	A and B (yes)	No published studies	<20	CLIA moderate	No published studies
Flowthrough EIA	Directigen Flu A (Becton-Dickinson)	NA, NPS, NW, TS	For swabs, use polyester- or rayon-tipped swabs with aluminum wire; do not use calcium alginate	A only	64–100/84–100	15	CLIA moderate	24, 55, 76, 91
Flowthrough EIA	Directigen Flu A+B (Becton-Dickinson)	BAL, NA, NPS, NS, NW, TS	For swabs, use polyester- or rayon-tipped swabs with aluminum wire; do not use calcium alginate	A and B (yes)	A, 41–87/98–100; B, 29–88/97–100	15	CLIA moderate	15, 73, 79, 94
Flowthrough EIA	Directigen Flu A+B/EZ (Becton-Dickinson)	NA, NPS, NW, TS	For swabs, use polyurethane foam swabs	A and B (yes)	A, 41–69/97–100; B, 30–33/100	15	CLIA moderate	42, 94
Lateral flow chromatographic EIA	BinaxNOW influenza A&B (Inverness Medical Professional Diagnostics)	NA, NPS, NW, NS	For swab samples, use cotton, rayon, foam, or polyester swabs; do not use calcium alginate	A and B (yes)	A, 52–78/96–100; B, 15–100/90–100	15	CLIA waived	18, 19, 49, 50, 94
Lateral flow chromatographic EIA	QuickVue influenza test (Quidel)	NA, NS, NW	Do not use any kind of transport medium to store or transport sample	A and B (no)	Combined, 37–95/76–99	10	CLIA waived	69, 70, 76
Lateral flow chromatographic EIA	QuickVue influenza A+B test (Quidel)	NA, NPS, NS, NW	Limited transport media supported	A and B (yes)	A, 26–93/92–100; B, 0–30/90–100	10	CLIA waived	42, 59, 89
Lateral flow chromatographic EIA	SAS FluAlert influenza A test (SA Scientific, Inc.)	NA, NW		A only	No published studies	<20	CLIA waived	No published studies
Lateral flow chromatographic EIA	SAS FluAlert influenza B test (SA Scientific, Inc.)	NA, NW		B only	No published studies	<20	CLIA waived	No published studies
Lateral flow chromatographic EIA	Xpect Flu A&B (Remel)	NS, NW, TS	For swab samples, use rayon- or dacron-tipped swabs with aluminum or plastic shafts; do not use calcium alginate	A and B (yes)	A, 48–92/99–100; B, 20–98/99–100	15	CLIA moderate	11, 18
Lateral flow chromatographic EIA	3M Rapid Detection Flu A+B	NA, NPS, NW	For swabs, use sterile foam, polyester, nylon, or rayon; do not use calcium alginate	A and B (yes)	A, 70–75/98–99.8; B, 31–87/99–100	<20	CLIA moderate	19, 35

[a]Abbreviations: EIA, enzyme immunoassay; BAL, bronchoalveolar lavage fluid; NA, nasal aspirate; NPS, nasopharyngeal swab; NS, nasal swab; NW, nasal wash fluid; TS, throat swab.

[b]Test characteristics were compiled from published literature.

[c]CLIA waived laboratory assays employ methodologies that are so simple and accurate as to render the likelihood of erroneous results negligible. CLIA moderate complexity assays require some knowledge, training, reagent preparation, processing, proficiency, ability to troubleshoot, or interpretation and judgment in the performance of the test.

1336

higher temperatures (e.g., −20°C) leads to the loss of virus viability. Immediate transport and processing of samples after collection are necessary for immunofluorescence detection of virus antigen in exfoliated epithelial cells.

DIRECT DETECTION

Microscopy

Influenza viruses have been detected in clinical specimens by direct and indirect visualization of their typical morphological appearance by electron microscopy (EM). Immune EM has been the most sensitive EM method and allows differentiation of virus type and subtype when specific hyperimmune sera are used in the assay (71). However, large numbers of viruses ($>10^5$ to 10^6 per ml) must be present in the clinical sample for successful detection using this diagnostic approach. Because of the need for an experienced microscopist and access to an electron microscope, the relatively high costs of assay performance, and the greater sensitivity of other diagnostic approaches, EM is not routinely used for the diagnosis of influenza virus infection.

Antigen Detection

Antigen detection assays are used in a variety of formats to rapidly detect influenza viruses in clinical specimens and to confirm the identity of isolates grown in culture. These assays are based upon detecting the interaction of viral proteins with specific antibodies. A variety of different formats are used, including direct and indirect fluorescent-antibody (FA) staining, radioimmunoassay, enzyme immunoassay, immunochromatographic assay, and fluoroimmunoassay.

FA assays identify viral antigens present on, or in, infected exfoliated epithelial cells present in respiratory secretions. Cells are collected on swabs or in aspirates or wash fluids and are washed in cold buffer to remove mucus before being applied and fixed to a microscope slide. Use of cytocentrifugation for application of the cells to slides can improve the number and morphology of cells for evaluation and enhance the accuracy of interpretation (48). Virus-specific antibodies are applied to the fixed cells; monoclonal antibodies directed against viral proteins that are conserved and expressed in large quantities (e.g., M and NP) are used because of their greater specificity compared to polyclonal sera and are available from a number of manufacturers. A fluorochrome is conjugated to the virus-specific antibody in direct FA (DFA) assays, and it is conjugated to a second antibody that reacts with the virus-specific antibody in indirect FA (IFA) assays. Antibody staining of cells is detected with a fluorescence microscope. Contaminating mucus can cause nonspecific fluorescence that can be reduced by treating the samples with N-acetylcysteine or dithiothreitol and by centrifuging cells through Percoll (60, 86). DFA and IFA assays take 2 to 4 h to perform, although some diagnostic laboratories batch samples and do not perform tests as soon as the sample is received, delaying the availability of results. In theory, IFA assays should be more sensitive and less specific than DFA assays, but there is significant overlap in the sensitivities (50 to 90%) and specificities (generally >90%) of these assays noted in published reports (87). An advantage of FA assays is that sample quality can be determined by observing whether an adequate number of epithelial cells are present. In addition, kits are available to screen for other respiratory viruses (e.g., respiratory syncytial virus, parainfluenza viruses, and adenovirus) as well as for influenza A and B viruses (Table 1). These multiplex assays allow for efficient screening for other viral causes of febrile respiratory disease. Disadvantages include the need for specialized equipment (a fluorescent microscope) and the impact of technician expertise on assay performance characteristics (i.e., sensitivity and specificity). Each laboratory should establish its own performance characteristics compared to those of cell culture.

A number of immunoassays that utilize different reporter formats (isotopic, colorimetric, fluorometric, and chromatographic) have been developed for the detection of influenza virus antigen in clinical specimens. Many of these assays take at least 2 h to perform and have 50 to 80% sensitivity compared to culture methods (57). A number of commercially available kits utilize the immunoassay format for rapid (≤30-min) detection of influenza A and B viruses in clinical specimens (Table 2). The kits utilize monoclonal antibodies to detect the presence of the influenza A or B nucleoprotein by enzyme immunoassay or chromatographic immunoassay. All of the kits provide results within 30 min, and some of them can be used as point-of-care tests (i.e., those classified by the Clinical Laboratory Improvement Amendments [CLIA] as waived). The types of specimens that are appropriate for testing vary among the kits, and specific instructions for sample collection and processing must be followed for optimal results. Assay performance characteristics in clinical settings are affected by the age of the patient (with generally lower sensitivity for adults) and by the type of specimen analyzed (36, 87). Recent studies suggest that the sensitivity of rapid antigen tests for identification of infection with influenza A virus strains containing novel hemagglutinins (e.g., H5 or 2009 H1) is lower than that for seasonal influenza A strains, so such tests should not be relied upon when such infections are suspected (35, 88, 89). The lower sensitivity of the rapid antigen tests for these viruses is not just due to using nucleic acid tests as a gold standard (35), and it varies depending upon the kit used (95).

A novel lateral flow immunochromatographic assay (AVantage; Arbor Vita, Sunnyvale, CA) has recently been approved by the FDA for the identification of some influenza A/H5N1 strains in nasal or throat swabs. The NS1 protein of clade 1 and 2 influenza A/H5N1 virus strains, but not clade 0 or seasonal influenza virus strains, contains a unique sequence that binds to PDZ domains (66). The test utilizes a recombinant protein containing a PDZ-binding domain and gold-labeled monoclonal antibody that recognizes a wide range of influenza A virus strains in a sandwich immunoassay. The performance of this assay with clinical samples has not yet been reported.

Nucleic Acid Analyses

Molecular methods are increasingly being used for both the detection and the characterization (see below) of influenza viruses. The most commonly used molecular method is reverse transcription-PCR (RT-PCR). Viral nucleic acids are first extracted from clinical samples. The use of guanidinium thiocyanate with silica particles or commercial kits based upon this approach reliably removes inhibitors of the enzymatic amplification that are often present in clinical specimens (7). Automated extraction instruments can be used in place of manual extraction, decreasing the amount of time personnel must spend in sample preparation while increasing the reproducibility of the procedure (28). Reverse transcriptase is used to synthesize cDNA from viral RNA by using random hexamers or a virus gene-specific oligonucleotide. The cDNA is then amplified by using virus gene-specific oligonucleotides as primers and a heat-stable

DNA polymerase. Resulting amplicons are identified as virus specific by using a variety of different methods (identification by size, hybridization, restriction enzyme mapping, and sequencing).

A large number of different RT-PCR assays have been developed since the initial description in 1991 of an RT-PCR method to detect and distinguish influenza A, B, and C viruses (103). Assays that identify and distinguish different influenza virus types have targeted conserved genes, such as the matrix gene, and subtype-specific assays have amplified a portion of the HA gene (2, 25). Nested PCR assays have been developed to improve assay sensitivity, but the inherent problem of carryover contamination associated with the use of this assay format limits its utility for most diagnostic laboratories. When a nested PCR format has been used, assay sensitivity has been better than that achieved with cell culture (102). Real-time RT-PCR assays, which are less vulnerable to cross-contamination, can directly and rapidly detect influenza viruses in clinical specimens with a sensitivity approaching or exceeding that of culture (90). Multiplexed assays able to identify both influenza viruses and other respiratory viruses have been developed and have performance characteristics that meet or exceed those of cell culture (52, 53, 65). Several of the multiplexed assays use bead arrays with virus-specific oligonucleotide probes individually linked to different bead types, and virus-specific amplification is identified by detection of fluorescently labeled amplicons hybridized to their respective beads using a process similar to flow cytometry (53, 65). The availability, and FDA clearance, of such assays (Table 3) may lead some diagnostic laboratories to use these assays for respiratory virus diagnosis in place of the more time-consuming cell culture methods. The currently available multiplexed respiratory virus panels may be less sensitive than monoplex molecular assays that target a single virus (53, 68, 74).

Another molecular method for direct detection of influenza viruses in clinical samples is nucleic acid sequence-based amplification (NASBA). NASBA is an isothermal method that amplifies a portion of the RNA genome by using avian myeloblastosis reverse transcriptase, T7 RNA polymerase, and RNase H. RNA amplicons complementary to the genomic RNA are generated and are detected by using a virus-specific probe, and when the probe is a molecular beacon, results can be obtained in real time. NASBA can be more sensitive than culture or immunofluorescent-antibody staining for the diagnosis of influenza virus infection, but additional experience with this method is needed (63).

ISOLATION PROCEDURES

Influenza virus isolation procedures should be performed under biosafety level 2 (BSL-2) conditions. When the clinical sample comes from a patient suspected to be infected with a highly pathogenic avian influenza (HPAI) virus strain, attempts at virus isolation should be performed under BSL-3 or higher conditions (12). Human clinical samples should be processed in separate laboratories and by staff members other than those handling clinical material from swine or birds (92).

Cell Culture

Influenza viruses can be grown in a number of different cell lines, including primary monkey kidney cells, Vero cells, human diploid lung fibroblasts, and Madin-Darby canine kidney (MDCK) cells (33, 75). Although some variability

can be seen from season to season, MDCK and primary monkey kidney cell lines have similar isolation frequencies (33), and MDCK cells are more sensitive than Vero or diploid lung fibroblast cells (75). Thus, MDCK cells (CCL 34; American Type Culture Collection, Manassas, VA), a continuous polarized cell line, are the most common cell line used for isolation of influenza viruses and support the growth of type A, B, and C strains. Continuous cell lines do not produce proteases that cleave the viral HA, a step necessary to produce infectious viral progeny, so exogenous protease must be added to the maintenance medium. L-(Tosylamido-2-phenyl) ethyl chloromethyl ketone (TPCK)-treated trypsin at a concentration of 1 to 2 μg/ml provides the necessary proteolytic activity and is the recommended protease for virus isolation. Chymotrypsin cleavage of the HA prevents the trypsin-mediated enhancement of viral infectivity, and TPCK treatment inactivates chymotrypsin activity which may contaminate pancreatic extracts of trypsin (47, 51).

MDCK cells are propagated in growth medium that contains 5 to 10% fetal calf serum (FCS). FCS contains inhibitors that prevent the production of infectious virus, so the FCS must be removed prior to inoculation of the clinical sample (26, 101). The inhibitory effects of FCS can be prevented by washing the cell sheet with Hanks buffer or serum-free medium sufficiently to remove the protein-containing growth medium and then adding serum-free medium to cover the cell sheet. The clinical sample is then inoculated into the medium. After a 2-h incubation, the inoculum-medium mixture is removed and replaced with serum-free medium supplemented with TPCK-treated trypsin. Alternatively, the sample can be inoculated directly onto cells with serum-free medium supplemented with TPCK-treated trypsin and incubated overnight prior to changing of the medium the next day. The cultures are maintained at 33 to 34°C and monitored for virus growth.

The replication of influenza viruses typically leads to cytopathic effects (CPE) and destruction of the cell sheet within a week following inoculation. CPE may be inapparent or absent in the presence of viral replication, but viral replication can be identified by the ability of the viral HA to bind to sialic residues on the erythrocytes of different animal species. Cultures should be screened every 2 to 3 days by hemadsorption (binding of erythrocytes to the viral HA of infected cells) or hemagglutination (cross-linking of erythrocytes by virus in the culture medium) for evidence of viral replication. To evaluate hemadsorption of cells grown in a tissue culture tube, CPE are first determined by microscopic examination (Fig. 1A), and then the medium is removed and stored. The cell sheet is rinsed three times with 1 ml of 0.05% guinea pig red blood cells. One milliliter of 0.05% guinea pig red blood cells is then added, and the tube is stored at 4°C for 20 min, with the red blood cell suspension covering the cells. The tube is then shaken, and adherence of red blood cells to the cell sheet is determined microscopically (Fig. 1B). If cytopathic changes are scored as less than 4+ (i.e., less than 75% of cell sheet with CPE), the tissue culture tubes are rinsed with phosphate-buffered saline and refed with culture medium. The media collected initially from tubes with 4+ cytopathic changes can be used for further characterization. All procedures are performed in a BSL-2 safety cabinet, and care must be taken to prevent cross-contamination between cultures. Guinea pig red blood cells are more sensitive for detection of influenza virus than are avian cells, but influenza C virus does not agglutinate guinea pig red blood cells. Chicken red blood cells

TABLE 3 Commercially available and selected other molecular detection assays for influenza viruses[a]

Assay format	Kit name (manufacturer)	Acceptable clinical sample(s)	Virus type(s) (subtypes) detected	FDA approval	Instrumentation	Other virus(es) detected	Reference(s)
Real-time RT-PCR	CDC human influenza virus real-time RT-PCR detection and characterization panel (CDC)[b]	NPS, NS	A (seasonal H1, H3, H5), B	Yes	ABI 7500 Fast DX real-time PCR instrument	None	No published studies
Real-time RT-PCR	CDC Influenza 2009 A(H1N1) pdm real-time RT-PCR panel (CDC)[b]	NPS, NS, NA, NW, NPS/TS, BAL, TA, BW	A (2009 H1)	Yes	ABI 7500 Fast DX Real-Time PCR instrument	None	No published studies
Multiplex RT-PCR, target-specific primer extension, Fluidic microbead microarray	MultiCode-PLx RVP panel (EraGen Biosciences)			No			65
Multiplex real-time RT-PCR	ProFlu+ Assay (Prodesse)	NPS	A, B	Yes	Cepheid SmartCycler II	RSV	52
Multiplex real-time RT-PCR	ProFAST+ Assay (Prodesse)	NPS	Seasonal H1, H3, 2009 H1	Yes	Cepheid SmartCycler II	None	No published studies
Multiplex real-time RT-PCR	Simplexa FluA/B & RSV (Focus Diagnostics)	NPS	A, B	Yes	3M Integrated Cycler	RSV	No published studies
Multiplex real-time RT-PCR	Simplexa Influenza A H1N1 (2009) (Focus Diagnostics)	NPS, NS, NPA	A, 2009 H1	Yes	3M Integrated Cycler	None	No published studies
Multiplex RT-PCR, target-specific primer extension, fluidic microbead microarray	ResPlex II assay (Qiagen)	NW, NPS	A, B	No	ABI 9700 SDS and Liquichip 200 or Luminex 100 or 200 system	RSV A, RSV B, P1, P2, P3, P4, hMPV, HRV, Ent, Ad, Boca	53
Multiplex RT-PCR, target-specific primer extension, fluidic microbead microarray	xTAG respiratory virus panel (Luminex Molecular Diagnostics)	NPS	A (seasonal H1, H3), B	Yes	Thermal cycler plus Luminex 100 or 200 system	RSV A, RSV B, P1, P2, P3, hMPV, HRV, Ad	54, 68
Multiplex RT-PCR, target-specific primer extension, microarray chip	Infiniti RVP Plus (AutoGenomics, Inc.)	NPA	A, B	No	Thermal cycler plus Infiniti Analyzer	RSV A, RSV B, P1, P2, P3, P4, hMPV, HRV, Ent, Ad, OC43, HKU1, 229E, NL63	74
Multiplex RT-PCR with auto-capillary electrophoresis	Seegene RV12 or RV15[b] ACE detection assay (Seegene, Inc.)	BAL, NPA, NPS	A, B	No	ScreenTape (Lab901), MCE-202 MultiNA	RSV A, RSV B, P1, P2, P3, P4,[c] hMPV, HRV, Ad, OC43, 229E/NL63, Boca,[c] Ent[c]	45
Multiplex RT-PCR	Verigene respiratory virus nucleic acid test (Nanosphere, Inc.)	NPS	A, B	Yes	Thermal cycler plus Verigene system	RSV	No published studies

[a] Not all available test kits may be listed here. Abbreviations: BAL, bronchoalveolar lavage fluid; BW, bronchial wash; NPA, nasopharyngeal aspirate; NPS, nasopharyngeal swab; NS, nasal swab; NW, nasal wash fluid; TA, tracheal aspirate; TS, throat swab; RSV, respiratory syncytial virus; P1, P2, P3, and P4, parainfluenza virus types 1, 2, 3, and 4, respectively; hMPV, human metapneumovirus; HRV, human rhinovirus; Ent, enterovirus; Ad, adenovirus; Boca, bocavirus; OC43, 229E, NL63, and HKU1, human coronavirus variants.
[b] Availability limited to U.S. public health laboratories.
[c] Additional virus strains identified in the RV15 panel.

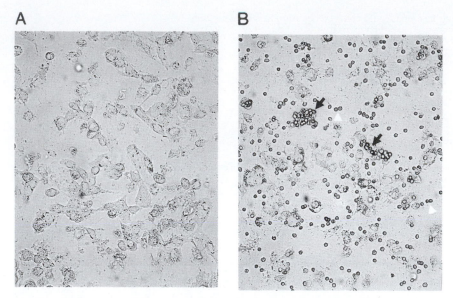

FIGURE 1 Influenza virus-infected MDCK cells. (A) Cytopathic changes. (B) Hemadsorption with guinea pig red blood cells. Red blood cells adsorb to both infected cells (black arrows) and the plastic surface, previously occupied by infected cells (white arrowheads).

can be used in agglutination assays to identify influenza C viruses. Although most isolates demonstrate growth within 1 week after inoculation, virus from samples with low infectious titers may require extended culture incubation for 10 to 14 days and additional blind passaging of negative cultures. Presumptive isolates are characterized further, as outlined below.

A disadvantage of traditional cell culture methods is the time needed to obtain a positive result (average, 4 to 5 days). More rapid methods have been developed by inoculating samples onto cell culture monolayers maintained in shell vials or multiwell plates. This approach can utilize either cell lines employed in traditional cell culture for identification of influenza virus (e.g., MDCK cells) or mixed cell cultures (e.g., A549 cells plus mink lung cells) to screen for multiple respiratory viruses (R-Mix FreshCells; Diagnostic Hybrids, Athens, OH) that are reported to detect seasonal influenza virus strains as well as strains with novel hemagglutinins (27, 30, 35, 61). The cells are fixed after 24 to 72 h, and type-specific monoclonal antibodies are used to detect viral antigen. Sensitivity can be lower than that achieved by using standard isolation methods, although R-Mix cells have been reported to have 82 to 100% sensitivity for detection of influenza A and B viruses (30, 35). Shell vial assays have the disadvantage of not producing virus for additional studies (e.g., antigenic characterization) (101). Screening for viral antigen by immunofluorescence can also be done at the end of the 10- to 14-day incubation period for standard culture prior to discarding of cells (93). This step is usually not necessary if screening by hemadsorption or hemagglutination is being performed, but it may detect virus in the absence of cytopathic changes if other strategies for virus detection are not utilized.

Isolation from Embryonated Chicken Eggs
The amniotic and allantoic cavities of 10- to 11-day-old embryonated chicken eggs are inoculated with the clinical sample for isolation of influenza A and B viruses. Seven- to eight-day-old eggs are used for isolation of influenza C

viruses, although these viruses are also isolated by using 10- to 11-day-old eggs. Embryonated eggs have endogenous proteases that are able to cleave the viral HA to yield infectious virus, so exogenous administration of proteases is not necessary. Inoculated eggs are incubated at 33 to 34°C for 2 to 3 days (5 days for influenza C viruses), and then both amniotic and allantoic fluids are collected and assayed for hemagglutination activity. Influenza A and B viruses can grow both in cells lining the allantoic cavities and in those lining the amniotic cavities, whereas influenza C virus grows only in cells lining the amniotic cavities of embryonated eggs. If no hemagglutination activity is detected, influenza viruses may still be recovered by performing one or two blind passages. A pool containing equal volumes of the amniotic and allantoic fluids is inoculated into eggs as described above (26).

IDENTIFICATION AND TYPING SYSTEMS
A variety of methods are used to identify and characterize influenza virus isolates. The most common are shown in Table 4 and are based upon immunologic or molecular approaches. The initial step is to identify the isolate as an influenza virus and to distinguish it from other respiratory viruses that have the ability to agglutinate or adsorb red blood cells (e.g., parainfluenza viruses and mumps virus). In many instances, it is sufficient to identify the virus by type, and this may be accomplished by using immunofluorescent or immunoperoxidase stains or an enzyme-linked immunosorbent assay (ELISA) using commercially available type-specific antibodies targeting the viral NP or M proteins. These assays are particularly useful for working with cell culture isolates. The rapid immunochromatographic assays described in Table 2 may be able to identify isolates and type them, but there are limited data on the use of these assays for this purpose, and these assays are not approved for this use. Importantly, the immunochromatographic assays may give false-negative results when the quantity of virus in a cell culture harvest is low.

TABLE 4 Methods to identify and characterize influenza virus isolates

Assay	Advantage(s)	Limitation(s)
Assays using type- or subtype-specific antisera		
ELISA	Standard assay with known performance characteristics; most labs experienced with assay format	For subtyping of influenza A strains, need to update sera periodically to detect circulating strain
Hemagglutination-inhibition	Standard assay with known performance characteristics; no special equipment needed	For subtyping of influenza A strains, need to update sera periodically to detect circulating strain; many clinical labs not experienced with this method
Immunofluorescence or immunoperoxidase staining of infected cells	Standard assay with known performance characteristics; most labs experienced with assay format	For subtyping of influenza A strains, need to update sera periodically to detect circulating strain
Molecular methods		
RT-PCR	Very sensitive assays	Potential for carryover contamination; need for stringent laboratory controls
Amplicon size	Ease of performance	Potential for false-positive results due to nonspecific amplification
Hybridization	Most commonly used approach for confirmation of PCR results	Depending on hybridization format used, may add time to performance of assay
Restriction analysis	Ease of performance	Need to know specific sequence; increased handling of post-PCR samples
Sequence	Obtain sequence data that may be used in other studies	Need for specialized equipment; increased cost
Microarray analysis	Potential to analyze multiple genetic sequences simultaneously	Investigational; limited experience

Hemagglutination inhibition (HAI) assays have been performed for more than 60 years and are still used for identification (40, 92). HAI assays can be type, subtype, or strain specific, and they are particularly useful for examining antigenic relationships among strains of the same subtype. HAI is the WHO gold standard for antigenic characterization of influenza virus isolates and vaccine strain selection. Immune sera are usually produced in ferrets, sheep, or chickens (101). The hemagglutination activity of the virus is quantitated, and a standard amount of viral HA (4 HA units) is mixed with serial twofold dilutions of the immune serum and turkey or guinea pig red blood cells. A fourfold or greater difference in HAI activities between the isolate and the reference strain is an indication that the isolate may be an antigenic variant. Because the HA undergoes antigenic change over time, subtype-specific antisera for interpandemic strains must be prepared and standardized periodically (2). Thus, subtype identification by HAI is usually performed only as part of surveillance activities or investigation of a case in which there is a strong epidemiologic suspicion of infection with a nonhuman strain.

Molecular assays are increasingly being used for virus identification and characterization. The same RT-PCR assays used for detection of viruses in clinical samples also can be used to identify clinical isolates. An advantage that molecular assays have over immunology-based assays is that the molecular assays can identify influenza A virus subtypes even after significant antigenic variation has occurred because there are well-conserved regions of the HA gene that serve as targets for the primers and probes used for identification (2). Multiplex assays can also be used to distinguish influenza A and B viruses or to identify HA and NA subtypes (54, 100). Results are determined by identification of amplicon size, by hybridization to type- or subtype-specific probes, and by direct sequencing of the amplicons. If the

sequences of different variants are known, it may be possible to identify unique differences by digesting amplified DNA with restriction endonucleases that generate restriction fragment length polymorphisms (RFLP) unique to each strain. For example, this method was used to distinguish two H3N2 variants that cocirculated during a single season (67). Influenza A/Wuhan/359/95 (H3N2) virus-like variants generated amplicons that could be digested with the BstF5I restriction enzyme, whereas amplicons from influenza A/Sydney/05/97 (H3N2) virus-like variants could be digested by HindIII. Given the difficulty of designing and performing RFLP analysis, together with the reduced cost and time required to perform DNA sequencing, direct sequencing of amplicons or of the entire HA gene has become a more common way to track and characterize specific strains.

DNA microarrays are increasingly being used in diagnostics for identification of specific pathogens. Oligonucleotide probes are arrayed on a chip or membrane, and hybridization of virus-specific sequences is then detected. The viral sequences can be generated by cDNA synthesis from viral genomic RNA or by amplification of fragments of genomic RNA by RT-PCR. Microarray analysis strategies that distinguish influenza virus types (A versus B) and subtypes (H1, H3, H5, N1, and N2) have been developed (41, 84) but at the present time are too costly for most individual laboratories to develop. Nevertheless, this technology has the promise of being able to more fully characterize strains in surveillance studies and to provide rapid and accurate identification of influenza virus strains.

SEROLOGIC TESTS

Influenza virus infections are also identified by using serologic methods. Most persons have been infected previously with influenza viruses, so detection of virus-specific immunoglobulin M or other immunoglobulin subclasses in a single serum sample has not been particularly useful (77). An exception may be detection of immunoglobulin M responses to novel HAs from avian strains (44). Instead, paired acute- and convalescent-phase serum samples collected at least 10 days apart are needed to detect a significant (fourfold or greater) increase in serum antibody levels. The requirement for paired sera to identify infection makes serology an impractical method for identification of influenza virus infection in the acutely ill individual. Instead, serology is used primarily in surveillance and in epidemiologic studies. The most widely used assay formats include complement fixation, HAI, neutralization, and enzyme immunoassay. Complement fixation identifies type-specific antibodies to the NP, but it is not as sensitive as the other commonly used serologic assays in detecting significant rises in antibody levels. HAI and neutralization antibodies in serum are functionally significant, in that higher serum antibody levels correlate with protection from infection and illness, and these antibody levels are used to measure responses to vaccination as well as to identify infection (16). HAI antibodies block the binding of the viral HA to sialic acid residues on red blood cells and thus inhibit hemagglutination. Each of the components in the HAI assay may affect the outcome of the test. Human and animal sera may contain nonspecific inhibitors of hemagglutination, but methods to remove these inhibitors have been developed (26). The source of the viral antigen can affect results, in that virus initially isolated in cell culture may detect a greater frequency of antibody rises than egg-grown virus (72). The species from which the red blood cells are derived can affect assay results. Chicken and turkey red blood cells are commonly used to measure HAI antibody to human strains of influenza viruses, but they may fail to detect HAI antibodies to avian strains (such as H5N1). Substitution of horse red blood cells can improve HAI assay sensitivity for detection of antibodies to avian influenza virus strains (83). Neutralizing antibodies block viral infectivity and provide a more sensitive assay for detection of antibodies to influenza A and B viruses (98). Although neutralization assays have been available for several decades, they are less standardized than are HAI antibody assays (78, 92). Nevertheless, neutralization assays are the preferred method for detection of antibody to HPAI virus strains (78). Because these assays require the use of live virus, their use with HPAI virus strains is restricted to those laboratories with BSL-3 or higher facilities (101). Enzyme immunoassays are also used for detection of antibody responses to whole-virus antigen or to specific viral proteins. The conjugate and the antigen used in the assay are factors that affect the performance characteristics (sensitivity and specificity) of these assays. Enzyme immunoassays are used to measure specific immunoglobulin responses in a variety of clinical specimens (serum samples and respiratory secretions) (10).

ANTIVIRAL SUSCEPTIBILITIES

Plaque inhibition assays are the gold standard for measuring susceptibility to amantadine and rimantadine, but the assays are cumbersome and time-consuming to perform (38). ELISA methods have also been used to measure decreases in the expression of viral antigens in the presence of these drugs. These assays can be used in combination with genotypic characterization of the M2 gene, since in vitro and in vivo resistance to these drugs is associated with specific M2 gene mutations (5). RT-PCR amplification followed by RFLP analysis or direct sequencing of amplicons is a genotypic method used to identify resistant viruses (9, 46). Amplification of the influenza A virus M2 gene followed by pyrosequencing is a rapid, high-throughput method that allows the rapid and reliable identification of adamantane (amantadine and rimantadine) resistance mutations (22, 46).

Cell culture assays do not reliably identify antiviral susceptibility to the NA inhibitors (NAIs) zanamivir and oseltamivir. Instead, NA enzyme inhibition assays with chemiluminescent or fluorescent substrates are used to identify resistance (58). A commercially available diagnostic assay (NA-Star, Applied Biosystems) is available for in vitro screening of influenza virus isolates (81). The results of these assays also correlate with mutations in the NA gene that can be identified by sequencing (1, 81). Molecular approaches can be used to identify known NA gene mutations associated with NAI resistance (e.g., E119V and R292K in A/H3N2, H274Y in A/H1N1, and R152K in influenza B) (30, 58). Both traditional terminal deoxynucleotide (Sanger) sequencing and pyrosequencing of the NA gene have been used successfully to identify these mutations (6, 23). Another strategy to quickly screen a large number of isolates is application of a real-time RT-PCR assay that utilizes a probe that recognizes wild-type (susceptible) NA sequence. This approach identified all A/H1N1 strains with an H274Y NA gene mutation (6).

Mutations in the HA gene may also lead to a resistance phenotype through decreased binding affinity of HA to cell surface receptors and decreased reliance on NA function to release budding viruses from infected cells. No reliable cell culture system currently exists for identifying HA resistance mutations, so identification relies upon sequencing of the receptor binding site of the HA gene.

EVALUATION, INTERPRETATION, AND REPORTING OF RESULTS

The results of a diagnostic test must be considered in the context of the overall setting in which the test is ordered. Clinicians play a critical role in assessing the plausibility of a test result, but the laboratory also can contribute to this appraisal. Seasonal, epidemiologic, and clinical factors are elements that must be evaluated in addition to the type of assay used. Unexpected laboratory results can be recognized by the laboratory as well as by the clinician. For example, a positive influenza test result when influenza is not recognized to be circulating in the community should prompt an assessment as to whether epidemiologic (e.g., travel history) or clinical (e.g., immunocompromised host) factors support the diagnosis of influenza virus infection. Close interactions between the laboratory and clinician are a vital component of a quality control program.

No diagnostic assay has 100% sensitivity and specificity, so false-negative and false-positive results can be expected to occur. Many factors that contribute to lowered sensitivity and specificity are known and can be addressed in ongoing quality control programs. False-negative results may be due to poor-quality or inappropriate clinical sample collection, delays in sample transportation or processing, inadequate sample storage (e.g., wrong temperature or transport medium), the time of sample collection during the clinical illness (e.g., later in the illness than recommended, when viral shedding has decreased), and the performance characteristics of the diagnostic assay (i.e., lower sensitivity). False-positive results may also be due to other characteristics of the diagnostic assay (i.e., nonspecific reactions), as well as to cross-contamination within the laboratory, mislabeling of specimens, and microbial contamination. Standard operating procedures in the collection, transportation, and processing of clinical samples should be established and followed to minimize the occurrence of inaccurate test results. Reagents should be standardized, and periodic assessments of assay performance should be performed with known positive and negative controls. The timing of these assessments will be based upon the type and number of tests being performed and the sources of reagents.

Each laboratory must decide upon the goals of its influenza virus diagnostic program in selecting the diagnostic assays to be performed. Rapid and sensitive assays can favorably impact patient management by allowing the prescription of targeted antiviral therapy and the institution of appropriate infection control isolation procedures. Positive test results may form the basis for offering prophylactic therapy to close contacts of infected patients, especially those contacts with high-risk medical conditions. Early and rapid laboratory diagnosis also can be important for evaluating influenza-like illnesses in the setting of a nosocomial outbreak, at the beginning of the influenza season (before influenza is recognized to be circulating in the community), and in persons with a history of contact with pigs or birds or travel to an area where influenza virus is circulating. The laboratory's expertise, staffing, and available equipment also influence test selection. For example, a fluorescence microscope and an experienced technician are necessary for the performance of immunofluorescence assays, and a thermal cycler along with other equipment is needed for RT-PCR assays. If the clinical specimen being tested comes from a patient who may be infected with an HPAI virus strain (e.g., H5N1), non-culture-based assays are currently recommended for laboratories that do not meet the BSL-3 or higher conditions recommended for growth of these strains (12). Commercially available antigen detection assays or the more sensitive H5-specific RT-PCR assays may be performed by using BSL-2 work practices. In the United States, influenza A virus-positive samples from patients meeting the clinical (febrile [>38°C] respiratory illness [cough, sore throat, or dyspnea]) and epidemiologic (contact with poultry or domestic birds or with a patient with known or suspected H5N1 virus infection in an H5N1-affected country) parameters for suspected A/H5N1 virus infection are referred to the CDC for further evaluation. Selected negative samples may also be sent to the CDC for analysis in consultation with the local public health department (12).

As new strains of influenza virus emerge, the sensitivities of established methods to detect these strains may change. For example, cell lines may have diminished sensitivity to new strains, or the ability to detect influenza virus antigen in infected tissue culture cells (e.g., by hemadsorption) may decrease (93). Thus, it is prudent to periodically reevaluate the performance characteristics of established methods, especially if results do not correlate with those expected based upon clinical and epidemiologic criteria.

Influenza diagnosis is also performed for reasons other than patient management. On the local level, knowledge that influenza is circulating in a community allows diagnosis of influenza based upon clinical symptoms (febrile respiratory illness with cough) with a sensitivity (60 to 80%) similar to that of many rapid antigen tests (62, 101). Influenza viruses isolated in national and global surveillance systems are characterized antigenically and genetically to identify variants. Information gained from these surveillance activities is used in the annual selection of strains for inclusion in updated trivalent influenza vaccines. Surveillance and characterization of isolates also allow the identification of infection with novel subtypes, as has occurred with influenza A/H5N1 viruses in Southeast Asia and A/H7N7 strains in The Netherlands (32).

REFERENCES

1. **Abed, Y., M. Baz, and G. Boivin.** 2006. Impact of neuraminidase mutations conferring influenza resistance to neuraminidase inhibitors in the N1 and N2 genetic backgrounds. *Antivir. Ther.* **11:**971–976.
2. **Atmar, R. L., and B. D. Baxter.** 1996. Typing and subtyping clinical isolates of influenza virus using reverse transcription-polymerase chain reaction. *Clin. Diagn. Virol.* **7:**77–84.
3. **Baxter, B. D., R. B. Couch, S. B. Greenberg, and J. A. Kasel.** 1977. Maintenance of viability and comparison of identification methods for influenza and other respiratory viruses of humans. *J. Clin. Microbiol.* **6:**19–22.
4. **Beigel, J. H., J. Farrar, A. M. Han, F. G. Hayden, R. Hyer, M. D. de Jong, S. Lochindarat, T. K. Nguyen, T. H. Nguyen, T. H. Tran, A. Nicoll, S. Touch, and K. Y. Yuen.** 2005. Avian influenza A (H5N1) infection in humans. *N. Engl. J. Med.* **353:**1374–1385.
5. **Belshe, R. B., M. H. Smith, C. B. Hall, R. Betts, and A. J. Hay.** 1988. Genetic basis of resistance to rimantadine emerging during treatment of influenza virus infection. *J. Virol.* **62:**1508–1512.
6. **Bolotin, S., A. V. Robertson, A. Eshaghi, C. De Lima, E. Lombos, E. Chong-King, L. Burton, T. Mazzulli, and S. J. Drews.** 2009. Development of a novel real-time reverse-transcriptase PCR method for the detection of H275Y positive influenza A H1N1 isolates. *J. Virol. Methods* **158:**190–194.
7. **Boom, R., C. J. Sol, M. M. Salimans, C. L. Jansen, P. M. Wertheim-van Dillen, and J. van der Noordaa.** 1990. Rapid and simple method for purification of nucleic acids. *J. Clin. Microbiol.* **28:**495–503.
8. **Bridges, C. B., M. J. Kuehnert, and C. B. Hall.** 2003. Transmission of influenza: implications for control in health care settings. *Clin. Infect. Dis.* **37:**1094–1101.
9. **Bright, R. A., D. K. Shay, B. Shu, N. J. Cox, and A. I. Klimov.** 2006. Adamantane resistance among influenza A viruses isolated early during the 2005–2006 influenza season in the United States. *JAMA* **295:**891–894.
10. **Burlington, D. B., M. L. Clements, G. Meiklejohn, M. Phelan, and B. R. Murphy.** 1983. Hemagglutinin-specific antibody responses in immunoglobulin G, A, and M isotypes as measured by enzyme-linked immunosorbent assay after primary or secondary infection of humans with influenza A virus. *Infect. Immun.* **41:**540–545.
11. **Cazacu, A. C., G. J. Demmler, M. A. Neuman, B. A. Forbes, S. Chung, J. Greer, A. E. Alvarez, R. Williams, and N. Y. Bartholoma.** 2004. Comparison of a new lateral-flow chromatographic membrane immunoassay to viral culture for rapid detection and differentiation of influenza A and B viruses in respiratory specimens. *J. Clin. Microbiol.* **42:**3661–3664.
12. **Centers for Disease Control and Prevention.** 2004. Outbreaks of avian influenza A (H5N1) in Asia and interim recommendations for evaluation and reporting of suspected cases—United States, 2004. *MMWR Morb. Mortal. Wkly. Rep.* **53:**97–100.
13. **Centers for Disease Control and Prevention.** 2006. New laboratory assay for diagnostic testing of avian influenza A/H5 (Asian lineage). *MMWR Morb. Mortal. Wkly. Rep.* **55:**127.
14. **Centers for Disease Control and Prevention.** 2009. Serum cross-reactive antibody response to a novel influenza A (H1N1) virus after vaccination with seasonal influenza vaccine. *MMWR Morb. Mortal. Wkly. Rep.* **58:**521–524.
15. **Chan, K. H., N. Maldeis, W. Pope, A. Yup, A. Ozinskas, J. Gill, W. H. Seto, K. F. Shortridge, and J. S. Peiris.** 2002. Evaluation of the Directigen FluA+B test for rapid diagnosis of influenza virus type A and B infections. *J. Clin. Microbiol.* **40:**1675–1680.

16. **Couch, R. B., J. A. Kasel, W. P. Glezen, T. R. Cate, H. R. Six, L. H. Taber, A. L. Frank, S. B. Greenberg, J. M. Zahradnik, and W. A. Keitel.** 1986. Influenza: its control in persons and populations. *J. Infect. Dis.* **153:**431–440.

17. **Covalciuc, K. A., K. H. Webb, and C. A. Carlson.** 1999. Comparison of four clinical specimen types for detection of influenza A and B viruses by optical immunoassay (FLU OIA test) and cell culture methods. *J. Clin. Microbiol.* **37:**3971–3974.

18. **Cruz, A. T., A. C. Cazacu, J. M. Greer, and G. J. Demmler.** 2008. Rapid assays for the diagnosis of influenza A and B viruses in patients evaluated at a large tertiary care children's hospital during two consecutive winter seasons. *J. Clin. Virol.* **41:**143–147.

19. **Dale, S. E., C. Mayer, M. C. Mayer, and M. A. Menegus.** 2008. Analytical and clinical sensitivity of the 3M rapid detection influenza A+B assay. *J. Clin. Microbiol.* **46:**3804–3807.

20. **Dawood, F. S., S. Jain, L. Finelli, M. W. Shaw, S. Lindstrom, R. J. Garten, L. V. Gubareva, X. Xu, C. B. Bridges, and T. M. Uyeki.** 2009. Emergence of a novel swine-origin influenza A (H1N1) virus in humans. *N. Engl. J. Med.* **360:**2605–2615.

21. **de Jong, M. D., V. C. Bach, T. Q. Phan, M. H. Vo, T. T. Tran, B. H. Nguyen, M. Beld, T. P. Le, H. K. Truong, V. V. Nguyen, T. H. Tran, Q. H. Do, and J. Farrar.** 2005. Fatal avian influenza A (H5N1) in a child presenting with diarrhea followed by coma. *N. Engl. J. Med.* **352:**686–691.

22. **Deyde, V. M., T. Nguyen, R. A. Bright, A. Balish, B. Shu, S. Lindstrom, A. I. Klimov, and L. V. Gubareva.** 2009. Detection of molecular markers of antiviral resistance in influenza A (H5N1) viruses using a pyrosequencing method. *Antimicrob. Agents Chemother.* **53:**1039–1047.

23. **Dharan, N. J., L. V. Gubareva, J. J. Meyer, M. Okomo-Adhiambo, R. C. McClinton, S. A. Marshall, K. St George, S. Epperson, L. Brammer, A. I. Klimov, J. S. Bresee, and A. M. Fry.** 2009. Infections with oseltamivir-resistant influenza A (H1N1) virus in the United States. *JAMA* **301:**1034–1041.

24. **Dominguez, E. A., L. H. Taber, and R. B. Couch.** 1993. Comparison of rapid diagnostic techniques for respiratory syncytial and influenza A virus respiratory infections in young children. *J. Clin. Microbiol.* **31:**2286–2290.

25. **Donofrio, J. C., J. D. Coonrod, and T. M. Chambers.** 1994. Diagnosis of equine influenza by the polymerase chain reaction. *J. Vet. Diagn. Investig.* **6:**39–43.

26. **Dowdle, W. R., A. P. Kendal, and G. R. Noble.** 1979. Influenza viruses, p. 585–609. *In* E. H. Lennette and N. J. Schmidt (ed.), *Diagnostic Procedures for Viral, Rickettsial, and Chlamydial Infections.* American Public Health Association, Washington, DC.

27. **Espy, M. J., T. F. Smith, M. W. Harmon, and A. P. Kendal.** 1986. Rapid detection of influenza virus by shell vial assay with monoclonal antibodies. *J. Clin. Microbiol.* **24:**677–679.

28. **Espy, M. J., J. R. Uhl, L. M. Sloan, S. P. Buckwalter, M. F. Jones, E. A. Vetter, J. D. Yao, N. L. Wengenack, J. E. Rosenblatt, F. R. Cockerill III, and T. F. Smith.** 2006. Real-time PCR in clinical microbiology: applications for routine laboratory testing. *Clin. Microbiol. Rev.* **19:**165–256.

29. **Fiore, A. E., D. K. Shay, K. Broder, J. K. Iskander, T. M. Uyeki, G. Mootrey, J. S. Bresee, and N. S. Cox.** 2008. Prevention and control of influenza: recommendations of the Advisory Committee on Immunization Practices (ACIP), 2008. *MMWR Recomm. Rep.* **57:**1–60.

30. **Fong, C. K., M. K. Lee, and B. P. Griffith.** 2000. Evaluation of R-Mix FreshCells in shell vials for detection of respiratory viruses. *J. Clin. Microbiol.* **38:**4660–4662.

31. **Fouchier, R. A., V. Munster, A. Wallensten, T. M. Bestebroer, S. Herfst, D. Smith, G. F. Rimmelzwaan, B. Olsen, and A. D. Osterhaus.** 2005. Characterization of a novel influenza A virus hemagglutinin subtype (H16) obtained from black-headed gulls. *J. Virol.* **79:**2814–2822.

32. **Fouchier, R. A., P. M. Schneeberger, F. W. Rozendaal, J. M. Broekman, S. A. Kemink, V. Munster, T. Kuiken, G. F. Rimmelzwaan, M. Schutten, G. J. Van Doornum, G. Koch, A. Bosman, M. Koopmans, and A. D. Osterhaus.** 2004. Avian influenza A virus (H7N7) associated with human conjunctivitis and a fatal case of acute respiratory distress syndrome. *Proc. Natl. Acad. Sci. USA* **101:**1356–1361.

33. **Frank, A. L., R. B. Couch, C. A. Griffis, and B. D. Baxter.** 1979. Comparison of different tissue cultures for isolation and quantitation of influenza and parainfluenza viruses. *J. Clin. Microbiol.* **10:**32–36.

34. **Garten, R. J., C. T. Davis, C. A. Russell, B. Shu, S. Lindstrom, A. Balish, W. M. Sessions, X. Xu, E. Skepner, V. Deyde, M. Okomo-Adhiambo, L. Gubareva, J. Barnes, C. B. Smith, S. L. Emery, M. J. Hillman, P. Rivailler, J. Smagala, M. de Graaf, D. F. Burke, R. A. Fouchier, C. Pappas, C. M. Alpuche-Aranda, H. Lopez-Gatell, H. Olivera, I. Lopez, C. A. Myers, D. Faix, P. J. Blair, C. Yu, K. M. Keene, P. D. Dotson, Jr., D. Boxrud, A. R. Sambol, S. H. Abid, K. St George, T. Bannerman, A. L. Moore, D. J. Stringer, P. Blevins, G. J. Demmler-Harrison, M. Ginsberg, P. Kriner, S. Waterman, S. Smole, H. F. Guevara, E. A. Belongia, P. A. Clark, S. T. Beatrice, R. Donis, J. Katz, L. Finelli, C. B. Bridges, M. Shaw, D. B. Jernigan, T. M. Uyeki, D. J. Smith, A. I. Klimov, and N. J. Cox.** 2009. Antigenic and genetic characteristics of swine-origin 2009 A (H1N1) influenza viruses circulating in humans. *Science* **325:**197–201.

35. **Ginocchio, C. C., F. Zhang, R. Manji, S. Arora, M. Bornfreund, L. Falk, M. Lotlikar, M. Kowerska, G. Becker, D. Korologos, M. de Geronimo, and J. M. Crawford.** 2009. Evaluation of multiple test methods for the detection of the novel 2009 influenza A (H1N1) during the New York City outbreak. *J. Clin. Virol.* **45:**191–195.

36. **Harper, S. A., J. S. Bradley, J. A. Englund, T. M. File, S. Gravenstein, F. G. Hayden, A. J. McGeer, K. M. Neuzil, A. T. Pavia, M. L. Tapper, T. M. Uyeki, and R. K. Zimmerman.** 2009. Seasonal influenza in adults and children—diagnosis, treatment, chemoprophylaxis, and institutional outbreak management: clinical practice guidelines of the Infectious Diseases Society of America. *Clin. Infect. Dis.* **48:**1003–1032.

37. **Hayden, F. G.** 2006. Antiviral resistance in influenza viruses—implications for management and pandemic response. *N. Engl. J. Med.* **354:**785–788.

38. **Hayden, F. G., K. M. Cote, and R. G. Douglas, Jr.** 1980. Plaque inhibition assay for drug susceptibility testing of influenza viruses. *Antimicrob. Agents Chemother.* **17:**865–870.

39. **Hayden, F. G., and P. Palese.** 2009. Influenza virus, p. 943–976. *In* D. D. Richman, R. J. Whitley, and F. G. Hayden (ed.), *Clinical Virology.* ASM Press, Washington, DC.

40. **Hirst, G. K.** 1942. The quantitative determination of influenza virus and antibodies by means of red cell agglutination. *J. Exp. Med.* **75:**47–64.

41. **Huang, Y., H. Tang, S. Duffy, Y. Hong, S. Norman, M. Ghosh, J. He, M. Bose, K. J. Henrickson, J. Fan, A. J. Kraft, W. G. Weisburg, and E. L. Mather.** 2009. Multiplex assay for simultaneously typing and subtyping influenza viruses by use of an electronic microarray. *J. Clin. Microbiol.* **47:**390–396.

42. **Hurt, A. C., R. Alexander, J. Hibbert, N. Deed, and I. G. Barr.** 2007. Performance of six influenza rapid tests in detecting human influenza in clinical specimens. *J. Clin. Virol.* **39:**132–135.

43. **Kaiser, L., M. S. Briones, and F. G. Hayden.** 1999. Performance of virus isolation and Directigen Flu A to detect influenza A virus in experimental human infection. *J. Clin. Virol.* **14:**191–197.

44. **Katz, J. M., W. Lim, C. B. Bridges, T. Rowe, J. Hu-Primmer, X. Lu, R. A. Abernathy, M. Clarke, L. Conn, H. Kwong, M. Lee, G. Au, Y. Y. Ho, K. H. Mak, N. J. Cox, and K. Fukuda.** 1999. Antibody response in individuals infected with avian influenza A (H5N1) viruses and detection of anti-H5 antibody among household and social contacts. *J. Infect. Dis.* **180:**1763–1770.

45. **Kim, S. R., C. S. Ki, and N. Y. Lee.** 2009. Rapid detection and identification of 12 respiratory viruses using a dual priming oligonucleotide system-based multiplex PCR assay. *J. Virol. Methods* **156:**111–116.

46. Klimov, A. I., E. Rocha, F. G. Hayden, P. A. Shult, L. F. Roumillat, and N. J. Cox. 1995. Prolonged shedding of amantadine-resistant influenzae A viruses by immunodeficient patients: detection by polymerase chain reaction-restriction analysis. *J. Infect. Dis.* **172:**1352–1355.

47. Kostka, V., and F. H. Carpenter. 1964. Inhibition of chymostrypsin activity in crystalline trypsin preparations. *J. Biol. Chem.* **239:**1799–1803.

48. Landry, M. L., S. Cohen, and D. Ferguson. 2000. Impact of sample type on rapid detection of influenza virus A by cytospin-enhanced immunofluorescence and membrane enzyme-linked immunosorbent assay. *J. Clin. Microbiol.* **38:**429–430.

49. Landry, M. L., S. Cohen, and D. Ferguson. 2004. Comparison of Binax NOW and Directigen for rapid detection of influenza A and B. *J. Clin. Virol.* **31:**113–115.

50. Landry, M. L., S. Cohen, and D. Ferguson. 2008. Real-time PCR compared to Binax NOW and cytospin-immunofluorescence for detection of influenza in hospitalized patients. *J. Clin. Virol.* **43:**148–151.

51. Lazarowitz, S. G., and P. W. Choppin. 1975. Enhancement of the infectivity of influenza A and B viruses by proteolytic cleavage of the hemagglutinin polypeptide. *Virology* **68:**440–454.

52. Legoff, J., R. Kara, F. Moulin, A. Si-Mohamed, A. Krivine, L. Belec, and P. Lebon. 2008. Evaluation of the one-step multiplex real-time reverse transcription-PCR ProFlu-1 assay for detection of influenza A and influenza B viruses and respiratory syncytial viruses in children. *J. Clin. Microbiol.* **46:**789–791.

53. Li, H., M. A. McCormac, R. W. Estes, S. E. Sefers, R. K. Dare, J. D. Chappell, D. D. Erdman, P. F. Wright, and Y. W. Tang. 2007. Simultaneous detection and high-throughput identification of a panel of RNA viruses causing respiratory tract infections. *J. Clin. Microbiol.* **45:**2105–2109.

54. Mahony, J., S. Chong, F. Merante, S. Yaghoubian, T. Sinha, C. Lisle, and R. Janeczko. 2007. Development of a respiratory virus panel test for detection of twenty human respiratory viruses by use of multiplex PCR and a fluid microbead-based assay. *J. Clin. Microbiol.* **45:**2965–2970.

55. Marcante, R., F. Chiumento, G. Palu, and G. Cavedon. 1996. Rapid diagnosis of influenza type A infection: comparison of shell-vial culture, Directigen flu-A and enzyme-linked immunosorbent assay. *New Microbiol.* **19:**141–147.

56. Maricich, S. M., J. L. Neul, T. E. Lotze, A. C. Cazacu, T. M. Uyeki, G. J. Demmler, and G. D. Clark. 2004. Neurologic complications associated with influenza A in children during the 2003–2004 influenza season in Houston, Texas. *Pediatrics* **114:**e626–e633.

57. McGeer, A. J. 2009. Diagnostic testing or empirical therapy for patients hospitalized with suspected influenza: what to do? *Clin. Infect. Dis.* **48**(Suppl. 1):S14–S19.

58. McKimm-Breschkin, J., T. Trivedi, A. Hampson, A. Hay, A. Klimov, M. Tashiro, F. Hayden, and M. Zambon. 2003. Neuraminidase sequence analysis and susceptibilities of influenza virus clinical isolates to zanamivir and oseltamivir. *Antimicrob. Agents Chemother.* **47:**2264–2272.

59. Mehlmann, M., A. B. Bonner, J. V. Williams, D. M. Dankbar, C. L. Moore, R. D. Kuchta, A. B. Podsiad, J. D. Tamerius, E. D. Dawson, and K. L. Rowlen. 2007. Comparison of the MChip to viral culture, reverse transcription-PCR, and the QuickVue influenza A+B test for rapid diagnosis of influenza. *J. Clin. Microbiol.* **45:**1234–1237.

60. Miller, H. R., P. H. Phipps, and E. Rossier. 1986. Reduction of nonspecific fluorescence in respiratory specimens by pretreatment with *N*-acetylcysteine. *J. Clin. Microbiol.* **24:**470–471.

61. Mills, R. D., K. J. Cain, and G. L. Woods. 1989. Detection of influenza virus by centrifugal inoculation of MDCK cells and staining with monoclonal antibodies. *J. Clin. Microbiol.* **27:**2505–2508.

62. Monto, A. S., S. Gravenstein, M. Elliott, M. Colopy, and J. Schweinle. 2000. Clinical signs and symptoms predicting influenza infection. *Arch. Intern. Med.* **160:**3243–3247.

63. Moore, C., S. Hibbitts, N. Owen, S. A. Corden, G. Harrison, J. Fox, C. Gelder, and D. Westmoreland. 2004. Development and evaluation of a real-time nucleic acid sequence based amplification assay for rapid detection of influenza A. *J. Med. Virol.* **74:**619–628.

64. Moser, M. R., T. R. Bender, H. S. Margolis, G. R. Noble, A. P. Kendal, and D. G. Ritter. 1979. An outbreak of influenza aboard a commercial airliner. *Am. J. Epidemiol.* **110:**1–6.

65. Nolte, F. S., D. J. Marshall, C. Rasberry, S. Schievelbein, G. G. Banks, G. A. Storch, M. Q. Arens, R. S. Buller, and J. R. Prudent. 2007. MultiCode-PLx system for multiplexed detection of seventeen respiratory viruses. *J. Clin. Microbiol.* **45:**2779–2786.

66. Obenauer, J. C., J. Denson, P. K. Mehta, X. Su, S. Mukatira, D. B. Finkelstein, X. Xu, J. Wang, J. Ma, Y. Fan, K. M. Rakestraw, R. G. Webster, E. Hoffmann, S. Krauss, J. Zheng, Z. Zhang, and C. W. Naeve. 2006. Large-scale sequence analysis of avian influenza isolates. *Science* **311:**1576–1580.

67. O'Donnell, F. T., F. M. Munoz, R. L. Atmar, L. Y. Hwang, G. J. Demmler, and W. P. Glezen. 2003. Epidemiology and molecular characterization of co-circulating influenza A/H3N2 virus variants in children: Houston, Texas, 1997–8. *Epidemiol. Infect.* **130:**521–531.

68. Pabbaraju, K., K. L. Tokaryk, S. Wong, and J. D. Fox. 2008. Comparison of the Luminex xTAG respiratory viral panel with in-house nucleic acid amplification tests for diagnosis of respiratory virus infections. *J. Clin. Microbiol.* **46:**3056–3062.

69. Poehling, K. A., Y. Zhu, Y. W. Tang, and K. Edwards. 2006. Accuracy and impact of a point-of-care rapid influenza test in young children with respiratory illnesses. *Arch. Pediatr. Adolesc. Med.* **160:**713–718.

70. Pregliasco, F., S. Puzelli, C. Mensi, G. Anselmi, R. Marinello, M. L. Tanzi, C. Affinito, M. C. Zambon, and I. Donatelli. 2004. Influenza virological surveillance in children: the use of the QuickVue rapid diagnostic test. *J. Med. Virol.* **73:**269–273.

71. Ptakova, M., and B. Tumova. 1985. Detection of type A and B influenza viruses in clinical materials by immunoelectron-microscopy. *Acta Virol.* **29:**19–24.

72. Pyhala, R., L. Pyhala, M. Valle, and K. Aho. 1987. Egg-grown and tissue-culture-grown variants of influenza A (H3N2) virus with special attention to their use as antigens in seroepidemiology. *Epidemiol. Infect.* **99:**745–753.

73. Rahman, M., B. A. Kieke, M. F. Vandermause, P. D. Mitchell, R. T. Greenlee, and E. A. Belongia. 2007. Performance of Directigen flu A+B enzyme immunoassay and direct fluorescent assay for detection of influenza infection during the 2004–2005 season. *Diagn. Microbiol. Infect. Dis.* **58:**413–418.

74. Raymond, F., J. Carbonneau, N. Boucher, L. Robitaille, S. Boisvert, W. K. Wu, G. De Serres, G. Boivin, and J. Corbeil. 2009. Comparison of automated microarray detection with real-time PCR assays for detection of respiratory viruses in specimens obtained from children. *J. Clin. Microbiol.* **47:**743–750.

75. Reina, J., V. Fernandez-Baca, I. Blanco, and M. Munar. 1997. Comparison of Madin-Darby canine kidney cells (MDCK) with a green monkey continuous cell line (Vero) and human lung embryonated cells (MRC-5) in the isolation of influenza A virus from nasopharyngeal aspirates by shell vial culture. *J. Clin. Microbiol.* **35:**1900–1901.

76. Rodriguez, W. J., R. H. Schwartz, and M. M. Thorne. 2002. Evaluation of diagnostic tests for influenza in a pediatric practice. *Pediatr. Infect. Dis. J.* **21:**193–196.

77. Rothbarth, P. H., J. Groen, A. M. Bohnen, R. de Groot, and A. D. Osterhaus. 1999. Influenza virus serology—a comparative study. *J. Virol. Methods* **78:**163–169.

78. Rowe, T., R. A. Abernathy, J. Hu-Primmer, W. W. Thompson, X. Lu, W. Lim, K. Fukuda, N. J. Cox, and J. M. Katz. 1999. Detection of antibody to avian influenza A (H5N1) virus in human serum by using a combination of serologic assays. *J. Clin. Microbiol.* **37:**937–943.

79. **Ruest, A., S. Michaud, S. Deslandes, and E. H. Frost.** 2003. Comparison of the Directigen flu A+B test, the QuickVue influenza test, and clinical case definition to viral culture and reverse transcription-PCR for rapid diagnosis of influenza virus infection. *J. Clin. Microbiol.* **41:**3487–3493.

80. **Russell, C. J., and R. G. Webster.** 2005. The genesis of a pandemic influenza virus. *Cell* **123:**368–371.

81. **Sheu, T. G., V. M. Deyde, M. Okomo-Adhiambo, R. J. Garten, X. Xu, R. A. Bright, E. N. Butler, T. R. Wallis, A. I. Klimov, and L. V. Gubareva.** 2008. Surveillance for neuraminidase inhibitor resistance among human influenza A and B viruses circulating worldwide from 2004 to 2008. *Antimicrob. Agents Chemother.* **52:**3284–3292.

82. **Smith, G. J., D. Vijaykrishna, J. Bahl, S. J. Lycett, M. Worobey, O. G. Pybus, S. K. Ma, C. L. Cheung, J. Raghwani, S. Bhatt, J. S. Peiris, Y. Guan, and A. Rambaut.** 2009. Origins and evolutionary genomics of the 2009 swine-origin H1N1 influenza A epidemic. *Nature* **459:**1122–1125.

83. **Stephenson, I., J. M. Wood, K. G. Nicholson, and M. C. Zambon.** 2003. Sialic acid receptor specificity on erythrocytes affects detection of antibody to avian influenza haemagglutinin. *J. Med. Virol.* **70:**391–398.

84. **Townsend, M. B., E. D. Dawson, M. Mehlmann, J. A. Smagala, D. M. Dankbar, C. L. Moore, C. B. Smith, N. J. Cox, R. D. Kuchta, and K. L. Rowlen.** 2006. Experimental evaluation of the FluChip diagnostic microarray for influenza virus surveillance. *J. Clin. Microbiol.* **44:**2863–2871.

85. **Treanor, J. J.** 2005. Influenza virus, p. 2060–2078. *In* G. L. Mandell, J. E. Bennett, and R. Dolin (ed.), *Principles and Practice of Infectious Diseases.* Churchill Livingstone, Inc., New York, NY.

86. **Ukkonen, P., and I. Julkunen.** 1987. Preparation of nasopharyngeal secretions for immunofluorescence by one-step centrifugation through Percoll. *J. Virol. Methods* **15:**291–301.

87. **Uyeki, T. M.** 2003. Influenza diagnosis and treatment in children: a review of studies on clinically useful tests and antiviral treatment for influenza. *Pediatr. Infect. Dis. J.* **22:**164–177.

88. **Uyeki, T. M.** 2009. Human infection with highly pathogenic avian influenza A (H5N1) virus: review of clinical issues. *Clin. Infect. Dis.* **49:**279–290.

89. **Uyeki, T. M., R. Prasad, C. Vukotich, S. Stebbins, C. R. Rinaldo, Y. H. Ferng, S. S. Morse, E. L. Larson, A. E. Aiello, B. Davis, and A. S. Monto.** 2009. Low sensitivity of rapid diagnostic test for influenza. *Clin. Infect. Dis.* **48:**e89–e92.

90. **van Elden, L. J., M. Nijhuis, P. Schipper, R. Schuurman, and A. M. van Loon.** 2001. Simultaneous detection of influenza viruses A and B using real-time quantitative PCR. *J. Clin. Microbiol.* **39:**196–200.

91. **Waner, J. L., S. J. Todd, H. Shalaby, P. Murphy, and L. V. Wall.** 1991. Comparison of Directigen FLU-A with viral isolation and direct immunofluorescence for the rapid detection and identification of influenza A virus. *J. Clin. Microbiol.* **29:**479–482.

92. **Webster, R., N. Cox, and K. Stohr.** 2004. *WHO Manual on Animal Influenza Diagnosis and Surveillance.* World Health Organization, Geneva, Switzerland. http://www.who.int/vaccine_research/diseases/influenza/WHO_manual_on_animal-diagnosis_and_surveillance_2002_5.pd.

93. **Weinberg, A., C. J. Mettenbrink, D. Ye, and C. F. Yang.** 2005. Sensitivity of diagnostic tests for influenza varies with the circulating strains. *J. Clin. Virol.* **33:**172–175.

94. **Weinberg, A., and M. L. Walker.** 2005. Evaluation of three immunoassay kits for rapid detection of influenza virus A and B. *Clin. Diagn. Lab. Immunol.* **12:**367–370.

95. **Welch, D. F., and C. C. Ginocchio.** 2010. Role of rapid immunochromatographic antigen testing in diagnosis of influenza A virus 2009 H1N1 infection. *J. Clin. Microbiol.* **48:**22–25.

96. **WHO/OIE/FAO H5N1 Evolution Working Group.** 2008. Toward a unified nomenclature system for highly pathogenic avian influenza virus (H5N1). *Emerg. Infect. Dis.* **14:**e1.

97. **World Health Organization.** 1980. A revision of the system of nomenclature for influenza viruses: a W.H.O. memorandum. *Bull. W. H. O.* **58:**585–591.

98. **World Health Organization.** 2003. Assays for neutralizing antibody to influenza viruses. Report of an informal scientific workshop, Dresden, 18–19 March 2003. *Wkly. Epidemiol. Rec.* **78:**290–293.

99. **World Health Organization.** 2009. Human infection with new influenza A (H1N1) virus: clinical observations from a school-associated outbreak in Kobe, Japan, May 2009. *Wkly. Epidemiol. Rec.* **84:**237–244.

100. **Wright, K. E., G. A. Wilson, D. Novosad, C. Dimock, D. Tan, and J. M. Weber.** 1995. Typing and subtyping of influenza viruses in clinical samples by PCR. *J. Clin. Microbiol.* **33:**1180–1184.

101. **Zambon, M.** 1998. Laboratory diagnosis of influenza, p. 291–313. *In* K. G. Nicholson, R. G. Webster, and A. J. Hay (ed.), *Textbook of Influenza.* Blackwell Science, London, England.

102. **Zambon, M., J. Hays, A. Webster, R. Newman, and O. Keene.** 2001. Diagnosis of influenza in the community: relationship of clinical diagnosis to confirmed virological, serologic, or molecular detection of influenza. *Arch. Intern. Med.* **161:**2116–2122.

103. **Zhang, W. D., and D. H. Evans.** 1991. Detection and identification of human influenza viruses by the polymerase chain reaction. *J. Virol. Methods* **33:**165–189.

Parainfluenza and Mumps Viruses

DIANE S. LELAND

82

TAXONOMY

The human parainfluenza viruses (HPIVs) and mumps virus are members of the *Paramyxoviridae* family. This family includes the *Paramyxovirinae* subfamily, to which both HPIV and mumps virus belong. However, within this subfamily, HPIV types 1, 2, 3, and 4 and mumps virus are classified into different genera. The *Respirovirus* genus is home for HPIV-1 and HPIV-3, and the *Rubulavirus* genus is home for HPIV-2, HPIV-4, and mumps virus. The *Paravirinae* subfamily includes two additional genera: *Morbillivirus*, to which measles virus belongs, and *Megamyxovirus*, to which Hendra and Nipah viruses belong. The *Pneumovirinae* subfamily completes the *Paramyxoviridae* family. Within this subfamily are the *Pneumovirus* genus, which includes respiratory syncytial virus (RSV), and the *Metapneumovirus* genus, which includes human metapneumovirus. The *Paramyxoviridae* family of viruses produces significant human and veterinary diseases, with its effects noted among virus families as "one of the most costly in terms of disease burden and economic impact to our planet" (21).

DESCRIPTION OF THE AGENTS

Although some of the HPIV types and mumps virus are classified into different genera, they are all pleomorphic, enveloped, medium-sized helical viruses, usually ranging from 150 to 250 nm in diameter. All have single-stranded, nonsegmented RNA with negative polarity. The genome encodes six common structural proteins. The largest, L, is a polymerase. L, along with the phosphoprotein P and the nucleocapsid protein N (or NP), is associated with the viral RNA to make up the viral nucleocapsid. The surface glycoproteins, hemagglutinin-neuraminidase (HN) and fusion protein (F), project from the viral envelope and can be seen with an electron microscope. The sixth structural protein is a membrane (M) protein. In viral replication, N protein binds to viral RNA, L and P function in transcription and replication, and the HN and F surface glycoproteins interact with the M protein, which attracts completed nucleocapsids to areas of infected membrane that will become the envelopes of the new virions during budding. The HN surface glycoproteins also function in virus-host cell attachment via sialic acid receptors, and the F proteins function in virus-host cell membrane fusion that allows the viral nucleocapsid to enter and infect a host cell.

Four serotypes of HPIV have been identified, namely, HPIV types 1, 2, 3, and 4. HPIV-4 can be subdivided further into HPIV-4A and HPIV-4B; because these are so closely related, they are considered HPIV-4 for the remainder of this discussion. Only one antigenic type of mumps virus has been identified, although strains show differences in expression of the SH gene; 12 genotypes have been identified and are designated A to L. HPIV and mumps virus are inactivated by temperatures above 50°C, organic solvents, UV irradiation, formalin treatment, low pH (3.0 to 3.4), drying, and desiccation. Preservation by freezing at −70°C or colder is effective, and the addition of 0.5% bovine serum albumin, skim milk, 5% dimethyl sulfoxide, or 2% chicken serum prior to freezing prolongs survival.

Although they are similar in structure and antigenic composition, HPIVs and mumps virus currently present very different pictures of disease production in the United States. The HPIVs are common agents of respiratory infections in children and adults in the United States, and virology laboratories routinely test for HPIV by direct antigen testing, virus isolation, and, often, molecular methods. In contrast, mumps virus, which was considered one of the common diseases of childhood prior to the introduction of an effective vaccine in 1968, is now relatively uncommon. Although sporadic mumps outbreaks occur, most virology laboratories no longer focus on the isolation and identification of mumps virus. Because of these differences, the HPIVs and mumps virus are discussed separately below.

PARAINFLUENZA VIRUSES

Epidemiology and Transmission

HPIVs are thought to be transmitted by large-droplet aerosols and by contact with contaminated surfaces. The viruses have been shown to survive for up to 10 h on porous surfaces; however, HPIV-3 experimentally placed on fingers was shown to lose more than 90% of its infectivity in the first 10 min (1). Currently, HPIV-1, -2, -3, and -4 represent approximately 5% of all viruses isolated in routine hospital diagnostic laboratories (29) and 13% of viruses isolated from respiratory specimens (6). HPIV-1 occurs most often in the fall of the year and biennially. The incidence of HPIV-2 is generally lower than that of HPIV-1 and HPIV-3. HPIV-2 may occur biennially with HPIV-1, in alternate years from

HPIV-1, or yearly. HPIV-3 occurs yearly, in spring and summer. HPIV-4 is seldom isolated, but diagnostic methods for this virus are admittedly suboptimal.

Clinical Significance

HPIV-1, -2, and -3 are associated with upper respiratory tract infections in infants, children, and adults. These are typically fairly mild and self-limited (33). Reinfection is common. HPIV accounts for the majority of cases of viral croup, which is the most common cause of upper airway obstruction in children of 6 months to 6 years of age. Croup is characterized by inspiratory stridor, barking cough, and hoarseness (31). As many as 7% of all hospitalizations for viral acute respiratory illness in children younger than 5 years of age have been shown to be due to HPIV infection (24). HPIV-1, -2, and -3 have also been found in as many as one-third of lower respiratory tract infections in children younger than 5 years of age in the United States and are second only to RSV as a cause of hospitalization for viral lower respiratory tract infections (19). Although associated with infections in children, HPIVs have the potential for serious pulmonary infections in adults, with HPIV-1 and HPIV-3 being among the four most common pathogens detected in adults requiring hospitalization for community-acquired pneumonia (34).

HPIVs also produce lower respiratory tract infections in the elderly and in those with chronic diseases, such as heart and lung disease or asthma. HPIV is increasingly recognized as a source of severe morbidity and mortality in immunocompromised patients, especially in those with congenital immunodeficiencies, and is capable of infecting tissues in the gastrointestinal and urinary systems in these individuals (33). In immunocompromised children, HPIV causes more than 50% of respiratory infections in bone marrow transplant recipients, 24% of those in patients with hematologic malignancies, and 19% of those in solid-organ transplant recipients (22). HPIVs are important causes of nosocomial respiratory infections (23).

HPIV-1 is associated with up to 50% of cases of croup reported in the United States, with the majority of cases occurring in children of 7 to 36 months of age. HPIV-2 causes typical lower respiratory tract syndromes in otherwise healthy children, with about 60% of infections occurring

in children younger than 5 years of age; peak incidence is in children between 1 and 2 years of age. HPIV-2 is associated with croup in immunocompromised or chronically ill children. HPIV-3 is more frequent in infants younger than 6 months of age, with 40% of infections occurring during the first year of life. Only RSV causes more lower respiratory tract infections in neonates and young infants than HPIV-3. Although HPIV-4 is rarely isolated, it can cause all of the different respiratory syndromes (19).

There are currently no U.S. Food and Drug Administration (FDA)-cleared antivirals for treatment of HPIV infection. Ribavirin has been used to treat HPIV infections in immunocompromised patients, but results have varied. Elizaga et al. (14) reported no efficacy for this therapy. In contrast, successful HPIV treatment has been reported for intravenous ribavirin therapy (23), oral ribavirin along with methylprednisolone (44), and high ribavirin doses used with early intervention (8). Management of symptoms through administration of corticosteroids has been recommended (31).

The diagnosis of HPIV infection may be based primarily on clinical signs and symptoms, and laboratory diagnostic studies may not be needed for all patients. However, laboratory assays to confirm HPIV infection, thus differentiating it from the many other viral infections that present with respiratory tract signs and symptoms, are widely available, and confirmation of infection may improve patient management and decrease costs (20, 21).

Collection, Transport, and Storage of Specimens

Testing to confirm HPIV infection may include virus isolation, antigen or nucleic acid detection, or antibody detection (Table 1). Viral specimen collection, transport, and storage guidelines are provided in chapter 76 in this *Manual*. Because detection of HPIV often involves immunofluorescence assays performed directly on the clinical material, care should be taken to include cellular material in samples collected from respiratory sites. The nasopharynx and oropharynx are primary locations of initial HPIV replication, and children shed virus from 3 to 4 days prior to the onset of clinical symptoms until approximately 10 days past onset. Virus recovery from adults is much more difficult than that from children, although immunocompromised patients and adults with chronic diseases,

TABLE 1 Diagnostic methods for parainfluenza and mumps virus detection

Virus	Virus isolation	Antigen detection[a]	Molecular methods	Antibody detection
HPIV-1, -2, and -3	Widely available; replicate in PMK cells in 4 to 8 days, little to no CPE; HAD positive	IF only; widely available as single tests or as part of respiratory virus panel; sensitivity, 70 to 83% compared to culture	Most sensitive method; available only at larger laboratories; one FDA-cleared RT-PCR method currently available	May be available at reference laboratories; cross-reactivity with other *Paramyxoviridae*
HPIV-4	Replicates in PMK cells in 4 to 8 days; HAD stronger at room temperature	IF only; testing not widely available	May be available at reference laboratories	Not available at most laboratories
Mumps virus	Widely available; replicates in PMK cells in 6 to 8 days, with little to no CPE; HAD positive	IF only; testing not widely available	May be available at reference laboratories	Immune status (IgG) testing widely available; seldom used to confirm acute infection due to cross reactivity with other *Paramyxoviridae*

[a]IF, immunofluorescence.

especially lung disease, have been shown to persistently shed HPIV for many months (19). Throat swabs, nasopharyngeal swabs, nasal washes, and nasal aspirates have all been used successfully to recover HPIV, but specimens from the nasopharynx—which is the primary location of initial HPIV replication—are best. Specimens should be collected, placed in viral transport medium, and kept at 4°C until cell culture inoculation. Inoculation within 24 h of collection is recommended (19).

Peripheral blood samples for use in HPIV antibody assays should be collected in tubes without anticoagulant, and serum should be separated from the clot as soon as possible to ensure sample integrity. Serum samples may be stored at 4°C if testing will be performed within 24 to 48 h but should be frozen at −20°C or lower if testing is delayed.

Direct Examination

Microscopy
Electron microscopy can easily demonstrate the presence of HPIV, but HPIV and the other paramyxoviruses appear the same. The lung, other bronchial tissues, pancreas, kidney, and bladder exhibit the typical appearance of giant-cell formation under a light microscope when they are infected with HPIV (33).

Antigen Detection
HPIV-1, -2, and -3 antigens are routinely detected in clinical specimens through the use of immunofluorescence techniques that employ monoclonal antibodies (MAbs). Cells from nasopharyngeal washes, aspirates, and swabs are fixed on the microscope slide, usually in several cell spots or dots or by cytocentrifugation (28). At least 20 columnar epithelial cells must be present if the assay is to be valid. Many laboratories use pooled MAbs containing antibodies against seven common respiratory pathogens; these are adenovirus, influenza A and B viruses, HPIV-1, -2, and -3, and RSV. These MAbs are applied in either a direct (DFA) or indirect (IFA) fluorescent-antibody staining protocol that detects antigens of all seven viruses. When a positive result is seen, further testing must be done to determine which virus is present. The sensitivity of HPIV antigen detection compared to virus isolation in cell culture varies from laboratory to laboratory and with the various DFA and IFA staining methods and reagents but has been reported to range from 70% (29) to 83% (28). Specificity is very high.

Pooled and individual MAbs for respiratory viruses, in DFA and IFA formats, are commercially marketed in the United States and are FDA cleared for use in direct specimen testing. Distributors of these reagents include but are not limited to the following: DakoCytomation USA, Carpinteria, CA; Diagnostic Hybrids, Inc., Athens, OH; Millipore Corporation Light Diagnostics, Temecula, CA; and Trinity Biotech, Carlsbad, CA. Brief overviews of the protocols used for one DFA and one IFA method for respiratory virus screening follow.

DFA (D³ Respiratory Virus Screening and ID Kit; Diagnostic Hybrids, Inc.)
The detailed instructions provided by the manufacturer should be followed. Briefly, smears from clinical specimens or of cells scraped from an infected cell culture monolayer are prepared on microscope slides. Shell vial monolayers may also be stained. All cells must be fixed in acetone (10 min) and dried prior to staining. Fixed smears may be stored for several days at 2 to 8°C or frozen at −20°C for up to a year when stored in an air-tight container. For smears

on microscope slides, 1 or 2 drops of fluorescein-labeled MAbs are added. For shell vial monolayers, 3 or 4 drops of MAbs are added. The preparations are incubated for 15 min at 37°C in a humidified environment. The smears are washed with diluted phosphate-buffered saline (PBS)–detergent solution (supplied in the kit) and then air dried. Mounting fluid and coverslips are added, and the smears are examined microscopically at a magnification of ×200 or higher, using a fluorescein isothiocyanate (FITC) filter system. HPIV-infected cells demonstrate bright apple-green fluorescence that is primarily cytoplasmic and often punctate, with irregular inclusions. Uninfected cells appear brick red due to Evans blue counterstaining and show no bright green fluorescence. The same protocol is followed both for the seven-virus screening assay and for subsequent staining of positive samples with the individual MAbs.

IFA (Bartels VRK Viral Respiratory Kit; Trinity Biotech)
Detailed instructions concerning all aspects of specimen handling, smear preparation, and staining/interpreting results are provided by the manufacturer and should be followed. The IFA test is appropriate for the same types of samples listed above for the DFA kit, with the same smear preparation and fixation guidelines. In IFA staining, briefly, sufficient unlabeled antiviral MAb reagent is added to each fixed preparation to cover the cells. The samples are incubated in a humidified environment at 35 to 37°C for 30 min. Smears are then washed in PBS for 5 to 10 min and air dried. Sufficient FITC-labeled anti-mouse antibodies are added to cover the cells, and the samples are again incubated at 35 to 37°C for 30 min. Following a 5-min wash in PBS and drying, buffered glycerol mounting medium and coverslips are added, and the smears are observed microscopically at a magnification of ×200 or higher, using an FITC filter system. Infected and uninfected cells appear as described above for the DFA procedure. The same protocol is followed for both the seven-virus screening assay and subsequent staining of positive samples with the individual MAbs. Cell culture confirmation is recommended for samples that produce a negative result.

MAb pools that screen for common respiratory viruses have also been marketed in a format that allows definitive identification of more than one virus simultaneously through the use of two different fluorescent dyes with overlapping spectra (Light Diagnostics SimulFluor reagents; Millipore Corp.). The reagents are cleared by the FDA for direct specimen testing and for culture confirmation. When stained preparations are examined with a fluorescence microscope with an FITC filter set, one antibody will produce apple-green fluorescence, and the second will appear gold or golden orange. SimulFluor reagents that are useful in HPIV antigen detection include a respiratory screen reagent by which RSV appears golden and the other six respiratory viruses, including HPIV-1, -2, and -3, appear green; an RSV/HPIV-3 reagent by which RSV appears green and HPIV-3 appears golden; an HPIV-1, -2, and -3/adenovirus reagent by which HPIV-1, -2, and -3 appear green and adenovirus appears golden; and an HPIV-1 and -2/HPIV-3 reagent by which HPIV-1 and HPIV-2 appear green and HPIV-3 appears golden. The SimulFluor reagents have shown excellent sensitivities and specificities, comparable to those of individual stains, for the respiratory viruses (28). Diagnostic Hybrids, Inc., also markets two MAb preparations with two different fluorescent labels; these are called Duet preparations. Staining with one of these preparations identifies influenza A virus with golden fluorescence while showing green fluorescence for the other six respiratory viruses, including HPIV-1, -2, and -3. The second Duet preparation identifies RSV with golden fluorescence while showing green fluorescence for the other six respiratory viruses.

A rapid format for staining cells in solution is also available (D^3 FastPoint; DHI, Inc.). This system features three dual-labeled (R-phycoerythrin versus FITC) Mab preparations also containing propidium iodide. One preparation stains influenza A virus yellow and influenza B virus green. Another stains RSV yellow and metapneumovirus green, and the third preparation stains HPIV-1, 2, and 3 yellow and adenovirus green. HPIV-1, -2, and -3 are not differentiated in this system. After a short incubation of specimen material with the three MAb preparations, the samples are placed on a microscope slide and examined in the wet state with a fluorescence microscope with an FITC filter set. Premarket trials by the manufacturer showed 85 to 100% sensitivity and 98% to 100% specificity for HPIV-1, -2, and -3 detection by the FastPoint method compared to other HPIV antigen detection methods.

HPIV-4 is the least frequently encountered of the HPIV types. It is not detected by most respiratory virus immunofluorescence screening reagent pools, which screen for only HPIV-1, -2, and -3. Although MAbs are available for immunofluorescence staining of HPIV-4 cell culture isolates, these are not FDA cleared for direct HPIV-4 antigen detection in clinical specimens.

Nucleic Acid Detection Techniques

Several different approaches for detecting HPIV RNAs have been described. These methods tend to be more sensitive than direct antigen tests or virus isolation for detecting HPIVs, with one method reported to detect double the number of HPIV-positive samples detected by cell culture (18).

A multiplexed nucleic acid amplification assay, the xTAG respiratory viral panel (Luminex Corp., Austin, TX), has received clearance from the FDA for testing nasopharyngeal swab samples for respiratory viruses. This is a bead microarray-based assay that targets adenovirus, influenza A and B viruses, HPIV-1, -2, and -3, metapneumovirus, rhinovirus, and RSV. In addition, it identifies the hemagglutinin (H) of influenza A virus as H1, H3, or "other" and differentiates RSV into types A and B. It has been cleared for use with two nucleic acid extraction platforms: the NucliSENS miniMAG extraction system (bioMerieux, Durham, NC) and the NucliSENS EasyMag extraction system (bioMerieux). The xTAG respiratory viral panel assay involves three main phases (36). Initially, a coupled multiplex reverse transcription-PCR (RT-PCR) produces amplicons for each of the viruses/subtypes present in the sample. Subsequently, shrimp alkaline phosphatase and exonuclease I are added to inactivate or degrade any unincorporated nucleotides and single-stranded primers. Next, the treated amplicons are hybridized to target-specific primers possessing unique DNA tags. A DNA polymerase extends perfectly formed complements, at the same time incorporating biotin-dCTP into the extension products. Finally, the extension products are added to microwells containing polystyrene microparticle beads, each of which contains an antitag sequence unique to a specific viral target and all of which are treated with colored dyes to distinguish each bead set. Each tagged primer hybridizes to its unique antitag complement; therefore, each bead detects a specific virus. Biotinylated extension products hybridizing to the bead surface are detected with a fluorescent reporter molecule, usually streptavidin-phycoerythrin. The Luminex

xMAP instrument sorts and analyzes the beads by interrogating with two lasers: one identifies the bead set by its unique color, and the other identifies the presence or absence of primer extension products through the phycoerythrin reporter. The xTAG system has been shown to be as sensitive as individual real-time PCR methods for detection of HPIV-1, -2, and -3 (36, 39). Because this is an end-point PCR rather than real-time PCR, testing requires at least 6 to 8 h to complete.

Gen-Probe Prodesse ProParaflu Plus (Gen-Probe Prodesse, Inc., Waukesha, WI) is a recently FDA-cleared multiplex RT-PCR test for detecting and differentiating HPIV-1, -2, and -3 in nasopharyngeal samples. Isolation and purification of nucleic acids are performed using the MagNA Pure LC system (Roche Applied Science, Germany) and a MagNa Pure total nucleic acid isolation kit (Roche) or the NucliSENS Easy MAG system (BioMerieux) and automated magnetic extraction reagents (bioMerieux). The system features *Taq* polymerase with dual-labeled probes and primers complementary to highly conserved regions of the hemagglutinin-neuraminidase genes of HPIV-1, -2, and -3. Amplification is performed in a Cepheid SmartCycler instrument (Cepheid, Sunnyvale, CA). Clinical trials by the manufacturer showed 88.9% to 97.3% sensitivity for HPIV-1, -2, and -3 detection compared to culture and DFA staining. The manufacturer noted that indications of dual or multiple HPIV infections reported with this system are likely artifacts due to signal bleed-over from the SmartCycler software. This system is new to the market, and peer-reviewed published evaluations are not yet available.

Reagents for other nucleic acid amplification assays are available commercially or can be prepared in-house for detection of the common respiratory viruses, including HPIVs (15, 16). Most have been shown to be more sensitive than cell culture for detection of HPIV and the other respiratory viruses (9, 15, 16, 26, 45). Extensive experimentation to establish analytical performance characteristics is required prior to implementation of assays using reagents that have not received regulatory clearance. Performance characteristics of cleared assays should also be investigated if sample types (e.g., nasopharyngeal aspirates or bronchoalveolar lavage fluid) and nucleic acid extraction platforms other than those specified in the manufacturer's package insert are used.

Isolation and Identification

Many commonly used cell lines support the growth of HPIV, but the best growth is seen in primary monkey kidney (PMK) cells, including rhesus, cynomolgus, and African green monkey cells (19). LLC-MK2 cells are also acceptable for primary isolation when 2 to 3 μg/ml of trypsin is added to the cell culture medium (19). Madin-Darby canine kidney (MDCK), HeLa, Vero, and HEp-2 cells may be used for transferring isolates but are not recommended for primary isolation (46). At this writing, commonly used cell lines are available commercially from two suppliers in the United States: Diagnostic Hybrids, Inc., Athens, OH; and Viromed Laboratories, Minnetonka, MN.

In preparing for cell culture inoculation of specimens collected on swabs and transported in a viral transport medium, the transport medium tube is mixed extensively on a vortex mixer, and excess fluid is expressed from the swab by pressing the swab against the side of the tube; the swab is then discarded. The transport medium is then centrifuged at $1,500 \times g$ for 10 min. The medium is decanted from cell culture tubes that are to be inoculated, and the supernatant from the centrifuged transport medium, usually 0.2 ml for each tube, is applied to each cell culture monolayer. The inoculated tubes are incubated in a horizontal position in a 35 to 37°C incubator for 1 h before excess inoculum is discarded and fresh cell culture medium is added. Inoculated cell culture tubes are incubated in rotating racks at 35 to 37°C and examined microscopically on alternate days for 14 days.

In PMK cells, some HPIVs produce a cytopathic effect (CPE) of rounded cells and syncytium formation in 4 to 8 days. However, many HPIVs will produce little, if any, CPE in traditional cell culture tubes. Fortunately, HPIVs produce hemagglutinin proteins that are inserted into the membranes of infected cells. These proteins have an affinity for erythrocytes, a phenomenon called hemadsorption (HAD), and this property can be used as another approach for detecting HPIVs in cell cultures. For HAD testing, culture medium is replaced with a dilute suspension of guinea pig erythrocytes, and the cell culture tubes are refrigerated at 4°C for 30 min; the tubes are then examined microscopically (29). When a hemadsorbing virus is present, erythrocytes adhere to the infected cell monolayer. If hemadsorbing virus is absent, erythrocytes will not adhere and will float free when the tube is tilted or tapped. Uninfected and infected control tubes should be included in HAD testing. HAD testing may be performed at the end of the typical incubation period of 14 days, or earlier, after 3 to 7 days of incubation (37). HPIV-4 hemadsorbs weakly compared to HPIV-1, -2, and -3 at 4°C and more strongly at room temperature. Other members of the *Paramyxoviridae* family, including mumps virus, and other viruses, such as influenza virus, also give positive HAD test results. Whether the presence of HPIV is suspected based on the appearance of typical CPE or by a positive HAD test result, confirmatory testing must be done to definitively identify the virus.

Confirmatory testing is routinely completed by immunofluorescence techniques involving the use of HPIV MAbs in DFA or IFA assays, as described for HPIV antigen detection in clinical samples. MAbs against HPIV-1, -2, and -3 are readily available in the various respiratory virus antibody testing kits. However, HPIV-4 antibodies are not included in most testing kits and must be purchased separately. Infected cells are scraped from the cell culture monolayer, applied to a microscope slide, fixed, and stained. The presence of apple-green fluorescence when the smear is viewed with a fluorescence microscope confirms the identification of HPIV. Confirmatory testing may also be accomplished by many other methods, including hemagglutination inhibition, complement fixation, and neutralization assays. These techniques are laborious and time-consuming compared to immunofluorescence methods and are seldom used.

Cell cultures grown on coverslips in shell vials or in microwell plates provide an alternative to traditional tube cell cultures for isolation of HPIVs. Centrifugation of the inoculated vials and plates, usually at 700 × g for 1 h, is an important feature of the inoculation process. Inoculated vials or plates are incubated for 24 to 48 h or as long as 5 days. Detection of viral proliferation depends on pre-CPE detection of viral antigens by application of HPIV MAbs to the monolayers in a typical DFA or IFA staining assay. Use of shell vial cultures with centrifugation-enhanced inoculation and pre-CPE detection by immunofluorescence staining has been shown to be very useful in HPIV detection.

Cocultivated mink lung (Mv1Lu) and A549 cells in shell vials, marketed as R-Mix (Diagnostic Hybrids, Inc.), are used with centrifugation-enhanced inoculation and pre-CPE detection by a DFA staining technique. Staining involves pooled MAbs to seven respiratory viruses (adenovirus, influenza A and B viruses, HPIV-1, -2, and -3, and RSV). In a recent comparison of respiratory virus detection in 3,800 clinical samples in R-Mix and in shell vials of PMK, A459, and MRC-5 cells, 33 of 38 (87%) HPIVs were detected after overnight incubation in the R-Mix cells (13). This included 26 of 30 HPIV-1 isolates, 2 of 2 HPIV-2 isolates, and 5 of 6 HPIV-3 isolates. Cocultivated MDCK cells and A549 cells comprise R-Mix Too (Diagnostic Hybrids, Inc.). This combination, which does not support the replication of severe acute respiratory syndrome coronavirus, was prepared as an alternative to R-Mix. The HPIVs proliferate very well in R-Mix Too (unpublished data) and are easily detected (Fig. 1).

An overview of the recommended protocol from the manufacturer of R-Mix and R-Mix Too (Diagnostic Hybrids, Inc.) is shown here; however, this may be adjusted to meet the needs of the laboratory. Briefly, the processed clinical specimen for respiratory virus detection is inoculated into three vials containing R-Mix or R-Mix Too cells, and the vials are spun in a centrifuge (700 × g for 1 h). At 16 to 24 h, one vial is stained with respiratory virus screening reagent (tests for seven respiratory viruses). If fluorescence is observed, the cells are scraped from one of the remaining shell vials, rinsed in PBS, and spotted onto an eight-well slide; seven of the wells are stained with individual MAbs against the seven respiratory viruses, and the eighth well is used as a control well. If no fluorescence is observed when the first vial is stained, the second vial is stained after an additional 16 to 24 h of incubation. If this vial is positive, the cells are scraped from the remaining vial and stained as described above. If the second vial is negative, the culture may be considered negative for the seven respiratory viruses (i.e., the remaining vial is discarded and the culture is terminated), or the third vial may be observed for CPE for up to 7 days.

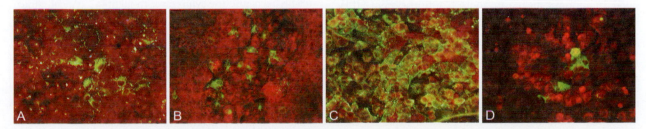

FIGURE 1 Immunofluorescence staining of HPIV-infected R-Mix Too and mumps virus-infected R-Mix cell cultures. R-Mix Too cells were infected with HPIV-1 (A), HPIV-2 (B), or HPIV-3 (C). (D) R-Mix cells infected with mumps virus. Magnification, ×200 (all). (A to C) Courtesy of Indiana Pathology Images; (D) courtesy of Diagnostic Hybrids, Inc., Athens, OH.

Serologic Tests

Most children are born with HPIV-neutralizing antibodies, but these diminish by 6 months of age, allowing more than two-thirds of children to be infected by HPIV during the first year of life. Most children have early serologic evidence of HPIV-3 infection, with HPIV-1 and -2 antibodies developing later, at 2 to 3 years of age. Antibodies to HPIV-4 peak in school-age children (19). Immunoglobulin M (IgM) is produced in most primary HPIV infections of children, so IgM detection in a single sample supports diagnosis of current infection. Likewise, measurement of a significant increase in the immunoglobulin G (IgG) antibody level, which is an increase of fourfold or more in assays that test serial twofold dilutions of serum samples collected 2 weeks apart, supports diagnosis of current infection. Cross-reactivity among the various HPIV types and other paramyxoviruses, such as mumps virus, makes serologic diagnosis more difficult. Serologic differentiation of the HPIV types is unreliable by all methods; this determination can be made only through virus isolation and antigen typing with MAbs or identification of the viral RNAs.

Antibodies to the HN protein may appear early, but both HN and F protein antibodies must be present for protection. Immune status determinations are not useful for HPIV. Serology in general is seldom used as a diagnostic approach for HPIV infection because of the wide availability of virus isolation and viral antigen and nucleic acid detection methods.

Principles of various serologic assays are described in detail in chapter 5 of this *Manual*. HPIV antibodies can be detected by many types of assays, including hemagglutination inhibition, complement fixation, and neutralization assays; all of these detect total antibody (IgG and IgM), and most laboratories do not offer these methods due to their cumbersome nature. A detailed procedure for hemagglutination inhibition testing for HPIV antibodies was published previously (46). HPIV antibody detection can be accomplished by enzyme immunoassay (EIA), but commercial kits are not available. Complement fixation is the least sensitive method for antibody detection, and EIA is the most sensitive.

Evaluation, Interpretation, and Reporting of Results

Isolation of HPIV-1, -2, -3, and -4 in traditional or shell vial/microwell cell cultures and detection of HPIV RNA in clinical samples are the best evidence for current or very recent infection because HPIV is seldom present in the absence of infection. These methods are the most sensitive and specific for HPIV. Rapid reporting of positive results is important (46). Although the sensitivity of HPIV antigen detection by immunofluorescence assay is lower than that of virus isolation in cell culture or molecular detection, the rapid availability of results makes such testing useful in patient management. Because these tests are widely available and have high specificities, they should be considered important diagnostic tools. Confirmation of HPIV infection via the serologic route and HPIV immune status determinations are seldom employed due to the difficulties with cross-reactions among the paramyxoviruses.

MUMPS VIRUS

Epidemiology and Transmission

More than 150,000 cases of mumps were expected each year in the United States before the aggressive vaccination programs implemented in the late 1960s. The mumps vaccine was combined with the measles and rubella vaccines to make a trivalent vaccine (MMR). In the United States,

the initial dose of MMR is administered to children between 12 and 15 months of age. Vaccination produced a dramatic decline in the incidence of mumps, resulting in fewer than 3,000 cases in the United States by 1985. There was a brief resurgence of mumps in 1986 and 1987 that peaked at 8,000 to 12,000 cases. Following the resurgence, a requirement for a second dose of the MMR vaccine was implemented. This dose is administered to children between ages 4 and 6 or 11 and 13 years (7) and has been expected to confer life-long immunity. The number of mumps cases continued to decline in the United States until the largest U.S. outbreak in 2 decades occurred in the midwestern states in 2006 (12). More than 6,500 cases were involved in this outbreak. The highest incidence of mumps was in persons aged 18 to 24 years; 83% of these were college students, and 84% of this group, as well as 63% of all those infected in the outbreak, had received two doses of mumps vaccine. The cause of this outbreak is unclear. Potential explanations include waning immunity and incomplete vaccine-induced immunity to circulating wild-type virus (12). At this writing, the incidence of mumps has returned to its pre-2006 outbreak levels, but it remains unclear whether a change in the vaccine itself or in vaccine administration schedules will be needed to prevent future outbreaks in the United States. Mumps remains common throughout much of the world, usually infecting 6- to 10-year old children in the spring in unvaccinated populations.

The virus is transmitted from person to person through respiratory droplets or contaminated fomites and is highly contagious, with approximately 85% of susceptible contacts becoming infected when first exposed. Humans are the only known host and reservoir for the virus. The virus replicates initially in epithelial cells in the upper respiratory tract and in regional lymph nodes. Initial replication is followed by viremia, which results in infection of the salivary glands and other sites. The period of communicability can be from 7 days before salivary gland involvement until 9 days after. The virus is excreted in the urine for as long as 14 days after the onset of illness.

Clinical Significance

The average incubation period for mumps is 16 to 18 days. Mumps virus infection is clinically inapparent in 25 to 30% of cases and is associated with nonspecific or respiratory symptoms in 50% of cases. Symptoms are typically mild and characterized by slightly elevated temperature and enlargement of one or both parotid glands in 30 to 40% of cases. Complications of mumps include meningoencephalitis (up to 15% of cases) and, in postpubertal individuals, orchitis in males (20 to 30%) and oophoritis in females (7%). Polyarthritis and pancreatitis have also been associated with mumps.

When mumps was a common disease of childhood, the diagnosis was made largely on clinical grounds alone. With the decrease in incidence of mumps, many physicians no longer readily recognize the symptoms. In addition, typical clinical signs and symptoms may be absent in underimmunized or immunocompromised individuals. Parotitis, the hallmark of clinical diagnosis, is now known to be present in other viral and nonviral diseases or conditions. Mumps-like symptoms in acutely ill children who previously received the MMR vaccine have been associated with Epstein-Barr virus, HPIV, adenovirus, and human herpesvirus type 6 (11). Therefore, laboratory confirmation of mumps virus infection is now more important in making the diagnosis.

Collection, Transport, and Storage of Specimens

The accepted laboratory criteria for the diagnosis of mumps virus infection are isolation of the virus from clinical specimens, detection of mumps virus RNA via molecular methods, a significant rise between acute- and convalescent-phase antibody titers in serum, or a positive IgM result for mumps. Guidelines for specimen collection, transport, and storage of specimens are presented in chapter 76 in this *Manual*. Most of the information that follows regarding specimen collection is applicable for diagnosing mumps virus infections in unvaccinated individuals. Specimen collection and expected test outcomes are different for vaccinated individuals who experience infection.

Specimens for mumps virus isolation in cell culture include the following: saliva, blood, urine, and cerebrospinal fluid (CSF). Virus can be isolated from saliva 9 days before and up to 8 days after the onset of parotitis, recovered from the urine for up to 2 weeks after onset of symptoms, isolated from CSF during meningitis, and detected rarely in peripheral blood. Throat swabs and urine samples have been shown to have similar efficacies as sources of mumps virus (43). It is always advisable to collect samples for virus isolation early in the course of the infection, when the viral titer is the highest. Recent studies have shown that samples collected from previously vaccinated individuals are unlikely to yield positive results by virus isolation or molecular methods unless they are collected within 3 days after the onset of parotitis (3).

The virus is stable for several days at 4°C, although inoculation of susceptible cell cultures within a few hours of specimen collection is recommended for optimal virus isolation. The virus may survive for months or longer when frozen at −70°C or lower.

Blood samples for use in mumps virus antibody testing should be collected and stored as described in "Parainfluenza Viruses" under "Collection, Transport, and Storage of Specimens." An alternative to serum collected by venipuncture is whole blood obtained by finger stick, heel prick, or venipuncture and then spotted on filter paper and dried. Following elution and dilution of the dried blood samples, commercial antibody assays may be used to test the sample for mumps virus antibody. Results of EIA in testing for mumps virus IgG and IgM by use of samples collected as blood spots have shown excellent correlation with those obtained in testing of fresh serum. The dried blood spots may be stored for 6 to 24 months without a significant change in antibody testing results (10).

In order to compare IgG or total antibody levels, two samples should be collected, the first (acute phase) as soon as possible after onset of symptoms and the second (convalescent phase) within 2 to 3 weeks following the acute-phase sample. A single serum sample collected within 4 to 10 days of onset is all that is required for IgM-specific antibody testing. If the purpose of the serologic testing is simply to determine the patient's mumps immune status, a single serum sample collected at random is sufficient. Neither comparison of IgG levels in sequential samples nor detection of IgM in a single sample collected early in the infection has been shown to be an effective diagnostic approach for confirming mumps virus infection in previously vaccinated individuals.

Direct Examination

Microscopy

Diagnosis of mumps does not typically involve examination of biopsy samples. However, microscopic examination of affected salivary glands reveals an edematous interstitium diffusely infiltrated by macrophages, lymphocytes, and plasma cells, which compress acini and ducts. Neutrophils and necrotic debris may fill the ductal lumen, causing focal damage to the ductal epithelium (35).

Antigen Detection

Mumps virus antigen detection by immunofluorescence in cells from CSF and salivary glands was described in the early 1970s (5, 32). More-recent studies of immunofluorescence staining of throat swab specimens for mumps virus antigen have shown sensitivities as high as 98 to 100% compared to mumps virus isolation in cell culture (43). Although mumps virus MAbs are available commercially, most are not FDA cleared for use in direct detection of mumps virus antigens in tissues and other clinical samples, and most virology laboratories do not offer direct antigen analysis for mumps virus.

Nucleic Acid Detection Techniques

Various molecular approaches have been developed to aid in mumps diagnosis. Mumps virus RNA has been detected by RT-PCR in oral fluid, CSF (40, 41), saliva or throat, and urine (41) specimens and in mumps virus isolates from cell culture (40). Recently, a multiplex real-time RT-PCR was developed for detection of mumps virus in clinical specimens (4). This assay uses oligonucleotide primers and a TaqMan probe that target an 86-bp fragment (nucleotide numbers 6249 to 6335) of the mumps virus SH gene. Also included are primers and a probe that target the human RNase P gene, which can signal the presence of PCR inhibitors as well as measure specimen quality. This assay, which reliably detects as few as 10 copies of mumps virus SH RNA, showed 100% correlation with mumps viral culture results and remained negative in the presence of closely related viruses such as HPIV-1 and -3 and RSV. Although molecular detection holds great promise in dealing with mumps virus detection and quantification, these methods are not well standardized, approved reagents are not commercially available at this writing, and testing is available only in specialized laboratories. In routine laboratories, virus isolation remains the standard method for diagnosing mumps virus infection.

Isolation and Identification

Mumps virus proliferates in traditional cell cultures of several cell lines commonly used in viral diagnostic laboratories. These include PMK, human neonatal kidney, HeLa, and Vero cells. Recently, a marmoset lymphoblastic cell line, B95a, was shown to be as sensitive for mumps virus isolation as PMK cells (27). A hybridized Vero cell line transfected with a plasmid carrying the gene for human CDw150—a signaling-lymphocytic activation molecule (SLAM)—and called Vero/SLAM, has been used for mumps virus isolation (38). Although used originally for isolation of measles virus, these cells have been shown to be effective for mumps virus isolation as well (3, 25). Directions for cell culture inoculation for swab samples in viral transport medium are the same as those described in "Parainfluenza Viruses" under "Isolation and Identification."

In cells infected with mumps virus, CPE characterized by rounded cells and multinucleated giant cells is typical, usually appearing after 6 to 8 days of incubation at 35 to 37°C. However, this characteristic CPE may be very subtle, may not appear at all, or may be confused with a similar CPE produced by endogenous contaminant viruses that sometimes infect PMK cells.

Mumps virus, like the HPIVs, inserts hemagglutinin proteins into the membranes of infected cells, so mumps virus-infected cells can be demonstrated through HAD testing. The HAD testing protocol is described in "Parainfluenza Viruses" under "Isolation and Identification." Whether mumps virus is detected by CPE production or by a positive HAD result, confirmatory testing must be performed. Confirmatory testing for mumps virus is routinely performed by IFA staining. The staining protocol for a typical IFA test is provided in "Parainfluenza Viruses" under "Direct Examination."

Many laboratories currently use centrifugation-enhanced inoculation and pre-CPE detection with MAbs to detect mumps virus within 24 to 48 h after inoculation. Various cell lines can be used in either shell vial or microwell plate formats for this purpose. The recommended centrifugation speeds and times may vary for inoculation, ranging from 700 × g for 45 min (43) to 3,000 × g for 20 min (13). Up to 66% of mumps virus-positive samples were identified within 2 days of inoculation in the shell vial system; after 5 days of incubation, the shell vial system was 96% sensitive compared to mumps virus isolation in traditional cell cultures (17). When various cell lines were compared for efficacy of mumps virus isolation in shell vials, Vero and LLC-MK2 cells were the most sensitive (100%), followed by MDCK (78%), MRC-5 (44%), and HEp-2 (22%) cells (42). Mumps virus can also be isolated in R-Mix cells (Fig. 1). An overview of the recommended protocol from the manufacturer of R-Mix (Diagnostic Hybrids, Inc.) is shown in "Parainfluenza Viruses" under "Isolation and Identification."

Because mumps virus infections in previously vaccinated individuals result in decreased levels of virus shedding into the buccal cavity, virus isolation may be difficult (2). Specimens collected and cultured within 3 days of onset of parotitis may aid in confirming the presence of mumps virus, but negative results do not rule out the infection (12).

Serologic Tests

In mumps virus infection, IgM is detectable initially within 3 to 4 days of appearance of clinical symptoms and persists for 8 to 12 weeks. IgG is detectable within 7 to 10 days of the onset of symptoms, is maintained at high levels for years, and remains detectable for life. Traditional serologic diagnosis of mumps is based on the detection of virus-specific IgM in a single sample or measurement of a significant increase in the titer of IgG or total antibody, i.e., fourfold or greater increase for methods that use serial twofold dilutions, between two specimens collected 2 weeks apart. Antibodies produced in mumps virus infection often cross-react with related viruses, which complicates the interpretation of results. Assays for mumps immune status indicate whether mumps virus IgG is present at detectable levels or is absent or undetectable. With the rarity of mumps cases in the United States at present, most laboratories focus mumps virus serology on immune status testing.

In previously vaccinated persons, serologic diagnosis has very limited use. IgM may be produced weakly or not at all in a secondary immune response. In a recent outbreak, mumps virus IgM antibodies were detected in fewer than 15% of mumps virus-infected persons who were previously immunized, and 95% of these patients were positive for mumps virus IgG (3).

Basic principles of serologic assays are described in chapter 5 in this *Manual*. Mumps virus antibodies can be detected by many types of assays, including hemagglutination inhibition, complement fixation, and neutralization assays; all of these detect total antibody (IgG and IgM). These methods are usually laborious and are available only at reference or specialty laboratories. A detailed procedure for mumps virus antibody hemagglutination inhibition testing was published previously (30). The complement fixation technique can be used with two different mumps virus antigens, V and S. Antibodies against the S antigen appear earlier and rise quickly, in contrast to the antibodies to the V antigen, which appear

later. The presence of both V and S antibodies is thought to signal a recent past infection, while V antibodies alone signal a long-past infection (46). An IgM-capture EIA was used recently for detection of mumps virus IgM (3).

Most diagnostic laboratories use commercially supplied mumps virus antibody EIA kits, in either manual or automated formats, or IFA testing systems for mumps virus antibody determinations. Most of these measure only mumps virus IgG. Antibodies are produced against various mumps virus proteins, but protection is most closely correlated with antibodies to the mumps virus HN protein. Most assays use whole virus or viral extract antigens that detect HN antibody effectively. Written protocols, along with the proper reagents and controls, are included with each commercial product, and each manufacturer's guidelines must be followed if assays are to yield high-quality results. The procedural steps for performance of antibody testing are not published here due to the need for strict adherence to manufacturers' guidelines. No specific recommendation on which specific mumps virus antibody test is most useful can be made at this time.

Evaluation, Interpretation, and Reporting of Results

Isolation of mumps virus in traditional or shell vial/microwell cell cultures is evidence of current or very recent infection. The same can be said for the detection of mumps virus RNA in clinical samples. Rapid antigen detection may also confirm the presence of mumps virus. However, neither molecular methods nor rapid antigen assays are routinely available in U.S. laboratories, so mumps virus isolation in culture remains the most sensitive approach. Confirmation of mumps virus infection via the serologic route is less straightforward. Mumps virus IgM may be detectable, along with significant increases in IgG, in patients infected with related viruses, including the other paramyxoviruses, such as HPIV-1, -2, -3, and -4. In general, cross-reactivity with related viruses can be ruled out by testing for antibodies to the related viruses in parallel with mumps virus antibody testing. The greatest increase in antibody level should identify the true infection. Given the potential lack of serologic test specificity, virus isolation and RNA detection in clinical samples (preferably buccal swabs) remain the most effective ways to confirm infection in unvaccinated individuals. Virus isolation and RNA detection have also been recommended for mumps diagnosis in individuals with a documented immunization history, in whom sporadic outbreaks are currently occurring (www.cdc.gov/mumps/lab/qa-lab-test-infect.html). Buccal swabs should be procured early (within 3 days of parotitis onset), as the duration of viral replication is likely to be shorter in these hosts. Despite these recommendations, it should be recognized that none of the traditional diagnostic approaches is highly effective for diagnosis of mumps in previously vaccinated individuals. IgM is not consistently observed and is therefore not a reliable indicator of recent infection. Virus detection can also be variable, presumably due to low viral loads. Conclusive mumps diagnosis in this setting can therefore be difficult (12).

REFERENCES

1. **Ansari, S. A., V. S. Springthorpe, S. A. Sattar, S. Rivard, and M. Rahman.** 1991. Potential role of hands in the spread of respiratory viral infections: studies with human parainfluenza virus 3 and rhinovirus. *J. Clin. Microbiol.* **29:**2115–2119.
2. **Bellini, W. J., J. P. Icenogle, and J. L. Sever.** 2009. Measles, mumps, and rubella, p. 562–577. *In* S. Specter, R. L. Hodinka, S. A. Young, and D. L. Wiedbrauk (ed.), *Clinical Virology Manual*, 4th ed. ASM Press, Washington, DC.

3. Bitsko, R. H., M. M. Cortese, G. H. Dayan, P.A. Rota, L. Lowe, S. C. Iversen, and W. J. Bellini. 2008. Detection of RNA of mumps virus during an outbreak in a population with a high level of measles, mumps, and rubella vaccine coverage. *J. Clin. Microbiol.* **46:**1101–1103.

4. Boddicker, J. D., P. A. Rota, T. Kreman, A. Wangeman, L. Lowe, K. B. Hummel, R. Thompson, W. J. Bellini, M. Pentella, and L. E. DesJardin. 2007. Real-time reverse transcription-PCR assay for detection of mumps virus RNA in clinical specimens. *J. Clin. Microbiol.* **45:**2902–2908.

5. Boyd, J. F., and V. Vince-Ribaric. 1973. The examination of cerebrospinal fluid cells by fluorescent antibody staining to detect mumps antigen. *Scand. J. Infect. Dis.* **5:**7–15.

6. Cazacu, A. C., S. E. Chung, J. Greer, and G. J. Demmler. 2004. Comparison of the Directigen Flu A+B membrane enzyme immunoassay with viral culture for rapid detection of influenza A and B viruses in respiratory specimens. *J. Clin. Microbiol.* **42:**3707–3710.

7. Centers for Disease Control and Prevention. 1998. Measles, mumps, and rubella-vaccine use and strategies for elimination of measles, rubella, and congenital rubella syndrome and control of mumps: recommendation of the Advisory Committee on Immunization Practices (ACIP). *Morb. Mortal. Wkly. Rep.* **47**(RR-8):6–16.

8. Chakrabarti, S., K. E. Collingham, K. Holder, S. Oyaide, D. Pillay, and D. W. Milligan. 2000. Parainfluenza virus type 3 infections in hematopoietic stem cell transplant recipients: response to ribavirin therapy. *Clin. Infect. Dis.* **31:**1516–1518.

9. Chonmaitree, T., and K. J. Henrickson. 2000. Detection of respiratory viruses in the middle ear fluids of children with acute otitis media by multiplex reverse transcription: polymerase chain reaction assay. *Pediatr. Infect. Dis. J.* **19:**258–260.

10. Condorelli, F., G. Scalia, A. Stivala, R. Gallo, A. Marino, C. M. Battaglini, and A. Castro. 1994. Detection of immunoglobulin G to measles virus, rubella virus, and mumps virus in serum samples and in microquantities of whole blood dried on filter paper. *J. Virol. Methods* **49:**25–36.

11. Davidkin, I., S. Jokinen, A. Paananen, P. Leinikki, and H. Peltola. 2005. Etiology of mumps-like illnesses in children and adolescents vaccinated for measles, mumps, and rubella. *J. Infect. Dis.* **1919:**719–723.

12. Dayan, G. H., M. P. Quinlisk, A. A. Parker, A. E. Barskey, M. L. Harris, J. M. Hill Schwartz, K. Hunt, C. G. Finley, D. P. Leschinsky, A. L. O'Keefe, J. Clayton, L. K. Kightlinger, E. G. Dietle, J. Berg, C. L. Kenyon, S. T. Goldstein, S. K. Stokley, S. B. Redd, P. A Rota, J. Rota, D. Bi, S. W. Roush, C. B. Bridges, T. A. Santibanez, U. Parashar, W. J. Bellini, and J. F. Seward. 2008. Recent resurgence of mumps in the United States. *N. Engl. J. Med.* **358:**1580–1589.

13. Dunn, J. J., R. D. Woolstenhulme, J. Langer, and K. C. Carroll. 2004. Sensitivity of respiratory virus culture when screening with R-Mix fresh cells. *J. Clin. Microbiol.* **42:**79–82.

14. Elizaga, J., E. Olavarria, J. Apperley, J. Goldman, and K. Ward. 2001. Parainfluenza virus 3 infection after stem cell transplant: relevance to outcome of rapid diagnosis and ribavirin treatment. *Clin. Infect. Dis.* **32:**413–418.

15. Fan, J., and K. J. Henrickson. 1996. Rapid diagnosis of human parainfluenza virus type 1 infection by quantitative reverse transcription-PCR-enzyme hybridization assay. *J. Clin. Microbiol.* **34:**1914–1917.

16. Fan, J., K. J. Henrickson, and L. L. Savatski. 1998. Rapid simultaneous diagnosis of infections with respiratory syncytial viruses A and B, influenza viruses A and B, and human parainfluenza virus types 1, 2, and 3 by multiplex quantitative reverse transcription-polymerase chain reaction-enzyme hybridization assay (Hexaplex). *Clin. Infect. Dis.* **26:**1397–1402.

17. Germann, D., M. Gorgievski, A. Strohle, and L. Matter. 1998. Detection of mumps virus in clinical specimens by rapid centrifugation culture and conventional tube cell culture. *J. Virol. Methods* **73:**59–64.

18. Griffin, M. R., F. J. Walker, M. K. Iwane, G. A. Weinberg, M. A. Staat, and D. D. Erdman. 2004. Epidemiology of respiratory infections in young children: insights from the new vaccine surveillance network. *Pediatr. Infect. Dis. J.* **23:**S188–S192.

19. Henrickson, K. J. 2003. Parainfluenza viruses. *Clin. Microbiol. Rev.* **16:**242–264.

20. Henrickson, K. J. 2004. Advances in the laboratory diagnosis of viral respiratory disease. *Pediatr. Infect. Dis. J.* **23:**S6–S10.

21. Henrickson, K. J. 2005. Cost-effective use of rapid diagnostic techniques in the treatment and prevention of viral respiratory infections. *Pediatr. Ann.* **34:**24–31.

22. Henrickson, K. J., S. Hoover, K. S. Kehl, and J. Weimin. 2004. National disease burden of respiratory viruses detected in children by polymerase chain reaction. *Pediatr. Infect. Dis. J.* **23:**S11–S18.

23. Hohenthal, U., J. Nikoskelainer, R. Vainionpaa, R. Peltonen, M. Routamaa, M. Itala, and P. Kotilainen. 2001. Parainfluenza virus type 3 infections in a hematology unit. *Bone Marrow Transplant.* **27:**295–300.

24. Iwane, M. K., K. M. Edwards, P. G. Szilagyi, F. J. Walker, M. R. Griffin, G. A. Weinberg, C. Coulen, K. A. Poehling, L. P. Shone, S. Balter, C. B. Hall, D. D. Erdman, J. Wooten, and B. Schwartz. 2004. Population-based surveillance for hospitalizations associated with respiratory syncytial virus, influenza virus, and parainfluenza viruses among young children. *Pediatrics* **113:**1758–1764.

25. Jin, L., Y. Feng, R. Parry, A. Cui, and Y. Lu. 2007. Real-time PCR and its application to mumps rapid diagnosis. *J. Med. Virol.* **79:**1761–1767.

26. Kehl, S. C., K. J. Henrickson, W. Hua, and J. Fan. 2001. Evaluation of the Hexaplex assay for detection of respiratory viruses in children. *J. Clin. Microbiol.* **39:**1696–1701.

27. Knowles, W. A., and B. J. Cohen. 2001. Efficient isolation of mumps virus from a community outbreak using the marmoset lymphoblastoid cell line B95a. *J. Virol. Methods* **96:**93–96.

28. Landry, M. L., and D. Ferguson. 2000. SimulFluor respiratory screen for rapid detection of multiple respiratory viruses in clinical specimens by immunofluorescence staining. *J. Clin. Microbiol.* **38:**708–711.

29. Leland, D. S. 1996. *Clinical Virology.* W. B. Saunders, Co., Philadelphia, PA.

30. Leland, D. S. 2002. Measles and mumps, p. 683–686. *In* N. R. Rose, R. G. Hamilton, and B. Detrick (ed.), *Manual of Clinical Laboratory Immunology*, 6th ed. ASM Press, Washington, DC.

31. Leung, A. K., J. D. Kellner, and D. W. Johnson. 2004. Viral croup: a current prospective. *J. Pediatr. Health Care* **18:**297–301.

32. Lindeman, J., W. K. Muller, J. Versteeg, G. T. A. M. Bots, and A. C. B. Peters. 1974. Rapid diagnosis of meningoencephalitis, encephalitis. Immunofluorescent examination of fresh and in vitro cultured cerebrospinal fluid cells. *Neurology* **24:**143–148.

33. Madden, J. F., J. L. Burchette, Jr., and L. P. Hale. 2004. Pathology of parainfluenza virus infection in patients with congenital immunodeficiency syndromes. *Hum. Pathol.* **35:**594–603.

34. Marx, A., H. E. Gary, Jr., B. J. Marston, D. D. Erdman, R. F. Breiman, T. J. Torok, J. F. Plouffe, T. M. File, Jr., and L. J. Anderson. 1999. Parainfluenza virus infection among adults hospitalized for lower respiratory tract infection. *Clin. Infect. Dis.* **29:**134–140.

35. McAdam, A. J., and A. H. Sharpe. 2005. Infectious diseases, p. 343–414. *In* V. Kumar, A. K. Abbas, and N. Fausto (ed.), *Robbins and Cotran Pathologic Basis of Disease*, 7th ed. Elsevier Saunders, Philadelphia, PA.

36. Merante, F., S. Yaghoubian, and R. Janeczko. 2007. Principles of the xTAG™ respiratory viral panel assay (RVP assay). *J. Clin. Virol.* **40**(Suppl. 1):S31–S35.

37. Minnich, L. L., and G. C. Ray. 1987. Early testing of cell cultures for detection of hemadsorbing viruses. *J. Clin. Microbiol.* **25:**421–422.

38. Ono, N., H. Tatsuo, Y. Hidaka, T. Aoki, H. Minagawa, and Y. Yanagi. 2001. Measles viruses on throat swabs from measles patients use signaling-lymphocytic activation molecule (CDw150) but not CD46 as a cellular receptor. *J. Virol.* **75:**4399–4401.

39. Pabbaraju, K., K. L. Tokaryk, S. Wong, and J. D. Fox. 2008. Comparison of the Luminex xTAG respiratory viral

panel with in-house nucleic acid amplification tests for diagnosis of respiratory virus infections. *J. Clin. Microbiol.* **46:**3056–3062.

40. Palacios, G., O. Jabado, D. Cisterna, F. DeOry, N. Renwick, J. E. Echevarria, A. Castellanos, M. Mosquera, M. C. Friere, R. H. Campos, and W. I. Lipkin. 2005. Molecular identification of mumps virus genotypes from clinical samples: standardized method of analysis. *J. Clin. Microbiol.* **43:**1869–1878.

41. Poggio, G. P., D. Rodriguez, D. Cisterna, M. C. Freire, and J. Cello. 2000. Nested PCR for rapid detection of mumps virus in cerebrospinal fluid from patients with neurological diseases. *J. Clin. Microbiol.* **38:**274–278.

42. Reina, J., F. Ballesteros, M. Mari, and M. Munar. 2001. Evaluation of different continuous cell lines in the isolation of mumps virus by the shell vial method from clinical samples. *J. Clin. Pathol.* **54:**924–926.

43. Reina, J., F. Ballesteros, E. Ruiz de Gopegui, M. Munar, and M. Mari. 2003. Comparison between indirect immunofluorescence assay and shell vial culture for detection of mumps virus from clinical samples. *J. Clin. Microbiol.* **41:**5186–5187.

44. Shima, T., G. Yoshimoto, A. Nonami, S. Yoshida, K. Kamezaki, H. Iwasaki, K. Takenaka, T. Miyamoto, N. Harada, T. Teshima, K. Akashi, and K. Nagafuji. 2008. Successful treatment of parainfluenza virus 3 pneumonia with oral ribavirin and methylprednisolone in a bone marrow transplant recipient. *Int. J. Hematol.* **88:**336–340.

45. Templeton, K. E., S. A. Scheltinga, M. F. C. Beersman, A. C. M. Kroes, and E. C. J. Claas. 2004. Rapid and sensitive method using multiplex real-time PCR for diagnosis of infections by influenza A and influenza B viruses, respiratory syncytial virus, and parainfluenza viruses 1, 2, 3, and 4. *J. Clin. Microbiol.* **42:**1564–1569.

46. Waner, J. L., and E. M. Swierkosz. 2003. Mumps and parainfluenza viruses, p. 1368–1377. *In* P. R. Murray, E. J. Baron, J. H. Jorgensen, M. A. Pfaller, and R. H. Yolken (ed.), *Manual of Clinical Microbiology*, 8th ed., vol. 2. ASM Press, Washington, DC.

Respiratory Syncytial Virus and Human Metapneumovirus

YI-WEI TANG AND JAMES E. CROWE, JR.

83

RESPIRATORY SYNCYTIAL VIRUS

Taxonomy

Respiratory syncytial virus (RSV), which was recovered from children with pulmonary disease in 1957 by cell culture, belongs to the *Pneumovirus* genus of the *Paramyxoviridae* family. Within this same genus are morphologically and biologically similar animal viruses, such as pneumonia virus of mice, bovine RSV, ovine RSV, and caprine RSV. Distinctive features of RSV include the number and order of genes and lack of hemagglutinin and neuraminidase activity. This virus derives its name from the characteristic formation of multinucleated giant cells (syncytia) in monolayer cell cultures of nonpolarized epithelial cells (22, 132).

Description of the Agent

The enveloped RSV virion consists of a single-stranded, negative-sense, nonsegmented RNA genome with 10 genes that are transcribed into 11 monocistronic polyadenylated mRNAs, each of which encodes a major polypeptide chain (Fig. 1). The N (nucleoprotein) protein serves as the major structural protein for the nucleocapsid, while P (phosphoprotein) and L (polymerase or large) are involved in transcription and replication (22, 132). The SH (short hydrophobic) protein accumulates within lipid-raft structures of the Golgi complex during RSV infection, the M (matrix) protein is present in detergent-solubilized cores, and M2-1 and M2-2 are expressed in infected cells. The two nonstructural proteins (NS1 and NS2) inhibit the induction of alpha/beta interferon in response to viral infection. The F (fusion) protein initiates viral penetration by fusing viral and cellular membranes and promotes viral spread by fusing the infected to adjacent uninfected cells. The G (glycosylated) protein mediates attachment of the virus to the host cells (22, 132). Two antigenic subgroups of RSV (designated A and B), which were initially identified on the basis of distinct reactivity patterns with postinfection sera or panels of monoclonal antibodies, are recognized and primarily based on variations in the structure of the G protein (22). Comparisons of the G ectodomains showed a 94% homology within subgroup A but revealed a 47% divergence between subgroup A and B RSVs. In contrast, the F protein is highly conserved, and antibodies against F cross-react with viruses from both subgroups A and B (22, 132).

RSV is one of the most vulnerable pathogens to environmental changes. Only 10% of RSVs remained infectious after exposure to 55°C for 5 min. At room temperature, 10% infectivity was present after 48 h, and at 4°C, 1% of the infectivity remained after 7 days. The RSV infectivity titer fell by approximately 90% after each freeze-thawing cycle (52, 132). The virus is inactivated quickly by ether, chloroform, and a variety of detergents, such as 0.1% sodium deoxycholate, sodium dodecyl sulfate, and Triton X-100. The survival of RSV in the environment depends in part on drying time as well as humidity (52). Long-term storage of RSV can be enhanced by flash freezing aliquots of virus in cryovials in an alcohol and dry ice bath and by adding stabilizing agents such as glycerin or sucrose.

Epidemiology and Transmission

RSV is the major cause of lower respiratory tract illnesses such as bronchiolitis, tracheobronchitis, and pneumonia among infants and young children worldwide. Early reports estimated that 100,000 hospitalizations and 4,500 deaths are related to RSV infection, with excess expenses from $300 million to $600 million for hospitalized infants with RSV in the United States (52). A recent study estimates that each year in the United States 2.1 million children under age 5 required medical attention for RSV, which is a far higher number than previously thought (53). RSV activity follows a seasonal pattern in temperate zones of the world, with annual outbreaks that occur from November through April. RSV neutralizing antibody levels in children in a community may play a role in the seasonal pattern (111). RSV is associated with 20% of hospitalizations, 18% of emergency department visits, and 15% of office visits during the peak season. The rates of hospitalization due to RSV were three times higher than those due to influenza (53) and have more than doubled in recent years for infants in Texas (48). The overall increased prevalence of RSV subgroup A over B viruses may be due to a more transient nature of subgroup A-specific immune protection (138). Virtually all children are infected by the time they reach 3 years of age, and repeated infections with RSV are common throughout life. No age group appears to be completely protected against reinfection due to prior exposure (48, 52). RSV infections are common but seldom severe in older children and immunocompetent adults, and they are usually manifested as upper respiratory infection or tracheobronchitis. Individuals

1357

RSV

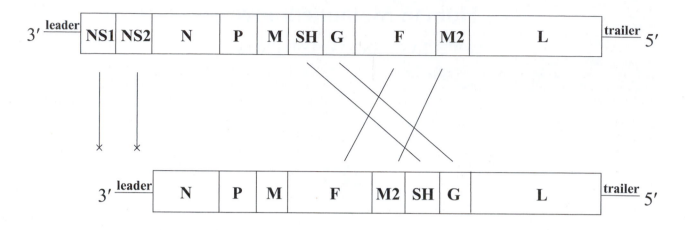

FIGURE 1 Schematic of RSV and hMPV genomic RNAs. The order of the genes from 3′ to 5′ is depicted. The virus-specific proteins encoded by these genes are shown.

at high risk for severe RSV infection include premature infants, young infants, asthmatics, immunocompromised individuals, and the elderly (39, 52, 85).

Crowding increases the attack rate of RSV. Schools and day care centers provide ideal settings for the spread of RSV to susceptible individuals. Population dynamics, with increased population density and urbanization, probably are responsible for the worsening of epidemics of the major respiratory viruses, including RSV (48). Infants who have not breast-fed appear to be at greater risk for developing severe RSV infections as determined by some studies, but a strong effect has not always been noted (77). Breast-feeding appears to have the strongest protective effect in female infants (76). RSV causes hazardous nosocomial infection and produces outbreaks each year with widespread infection in both children and adults, including medical personnel, who may have a mild enough illness so as to not cause absences from work (60, 116, 123). In a classic experiment, volunteers in close physical contact with RSV-infected infants were more readily infected than those who remained 6 ft away, suggesting that small-particle aerosol is less important in the spread of RSV than direct contact with infectious secretions via fomites or large-particle aerosols (52, 132). A targeted infection control intervention has been demonstrated to be cost-effective in reducing the rate of RSV nosocomial infections (77, 116). Contact isolation procedures are recommended for RSV-infected patients when they are hospitalized (52, 116).

Clinical Significance

Primary infections with RSV may be manifested as lower respiratory tract diseases, such as pneumonia, bronchiolitis, tracheobronchitis, or upper respiratory tract illness, often accompanied by a low-grade fever. The incubation period ranges from 2 to 8 days, with a median of 4.4 days based on a systematic review (73). Illness begins most frequently with rhinorrhea, sneezing, and cough. Most children diagnosed

with RSV infection were previously healthy and experience recovery from illness after 8 to 15 days (53). During their first RSV infection, 25 to 40% of infected infants and young children have signs or symptoms of bronchiolitis or pneumonia, and 0.5 to 2% require hospitalization (52). In contrast, hospitalization is required for up to 25% of high-risk children, such as those with a history of prematurity or chronic lung disease. In older persons or immunocompromised individuals, RSV infection typically begins as an upper respiratory tract infection and may evolve into lower respiratory tract disease in up to 50% of cases (39, 52). The clinical significance of differences of severity of infection with viruses of the two antigenic subgroups has been suggested to be important by some studies. Subgroup A RSV may be more virulent than subgroup B, and infection with subgroup A viruses may result in greater disease severity among hospitalized infants (126). Late bacterial superinfection of the airways that is confirmed by culture is unusual, although simultaneous bacterial-viral coinfection probably does occur (22, 52, 132).

For the majority of infants with mild disease, no specific treatment is necessary other than supportive care. In hospitalized and more severely infected infants, the quality of supportive care is of prime importance to reduce the RSV-associated morbidity (20, 52). Aerosolized ribavirin is now used infrequently and is restricted to immunocompromised patients or to those who are severely ill, because the efficacy of the medication in clinical practice has not been reproducible. Palivizumab (Synagis; MedImmune, Gaithersburg, MD) is a humanized murine monoclonal antibody that was licensed in the United States for prophylaxis against RSV disease in high-risk infants. Palivizumab prophylaxis reduces hospitalization due to RSV in young children with chronic lung disease, extremely premature birth, and significant congenital heart disease (41, 52). The antibody has not shown efficacy in clinical trials when given as a therapeutic intervention during severe disease. RSV604 (Arrow Therapeutics, London, United Kingdom), a novel benzodiazepine with submicromolar anti-RSV activity, has been proved to be equipotent against all clinical isolates tested from both A and B subgroups and has been tested in phase II clinical trials (17, 19). General use of high-dose inhaled corticosteroids should not be advocated, since such treatment has no major effect on duration of illness and may prolong virus shedding (36, 52). Antibiotics should not be administered routinely for therapy or to prevent secondary bacterial infection (52). Although there is a worldwide need for a preventative vaccine in the pediatric population, an effective and safe RSV vaccine is not yet licensed. Experimental live attenuated, vectored, and subunit vaccines are in development.

Collection, Transport, and Storage of Specimens

Appropriate respiratory specimens for RSV detection include aspirates and swabs, among which aspirates obtained by either wash or suction are optimal for culture or rapid antigen or nucleic acid detection (55, 110). The likelihood of identifying RSV as the etiology of a patient's infection is greatest when a specimen is obtained within the first several days of illness. Viral cultures or antigen tests usually become negative 1 week after onset of illness for about 50% of patients. However, excretion of live virus in immunocompromised infants has been documented up to 3 weeks after the onset of illness (21, 52, 65). The quantity of virus in the upper respiratory tract (nasal aspirates) is nearly equivalent to that found in the lower respiratory tract when tested by quantitative culture or real-time PCR methods (15, 96). Endotracheal tube aspirate or bronchoalveolar lavage fluid collection is preferred for immunocompromised adults who are being mechanically ventilated (35). The use of nasal or nasopharyngeal swabs is an alternative method for sample collection. Any synthetic cotton-tipped swabs without calcium alginate are acceptable (18), although flocked swabs collected significantly more epithelial cells than rayon swabs (1, 26). Throat swab and saliva specimens are inferior but might be acceptable when it is impractical to obtain nasal or nasopharyngeal specimens (103).

Most general viral specimen collection principles also apply to specimen collection for RSV detection and culture, such as collecting specimens during the acute phase of illness, maintaining recovered cells in intact form, delivering specimens promptly to the diagnostic laboratory, refrigerating specimens if stored temporarily, and sealing well in O-ring-sealed cryovials if stored on dry ice. Prompt collection and transportation of samples for diagnosis of RSV infection are especially critical for RSV, as the virus is extremely vulnerable to environmental changes (52, 132). Heating or freezing the specimen will result in a decreased number of infectious virions in the sample. To effectively isolate RSV, specimen containers should be transported to the laboratory on wet ice as quickly as possible. If specimens cannot be processed rapidly and inoculated into cell culture within 2 h of sample collection, they should be kept refrigerated. Samples should never be frozen without first consulting the virology laboratory.

Direct Detection

Microscopy
Although RSV can be visualized by electron microscopy, its application has been limited to research laboratories.

Antigen
Most clinical laboratories use rapid antigen detection assays to diagnose RSV infection. In contrast to cell culture, antigen tests do not require the presence of viable virus to detect an infection, and specimens obtained later in the course of the illness or those with suboptimal handling may yield a positive result. There are several rapid RSV antigen tests commercially available using platforms including immunofluorescent assay (IFA), enzyme immunoassay (EIA), dipstick immunoassay (DIA), and chromatographic immunoassay (CIA). Several novel direct antigen targeting techniques have been described and have potential diagnostic applications in RSV rapid antigen detection (6, 117). Key factors that influence choice include test accuracy, turnaround time, interference with commonly used medications, choice of specimen type, choice of transport products, and a reliable supply.

IFAs have widely been used for the rapid diagnosis of RSV infection. Reagents needed for performing the RSV IFA are commercially available from a number of companies (Table 1). Direct IFA (DFA) detection is comparable to that of cell culture (69, 98). Indirect IFA, on the other hand, consumes more test time but generally enhances test sensitivity. In general, when IFA is correctly performed, the sensitivity is higher than those of other rapid antigen tests (4, 69, 71, 98). The use of monoclonal antibodies in IFA has greatly improved the sensitivity and specificity, both of which range from 85 to 100% in various studies. Multiplex DFA reagents are available commercially to detect a panel of common respiratory viruses simultaneously (69). However, IFA testing requires an adequate number of respiratory epithelial cells and a skilled technologist for accurate interpretation. Test turnaround time is longer than for other rapid antigen tests.

In addition to IFA, several rapid antigen assays are commercially available (Table 2). These assays offer the advantages of ease of performance, objective reading of results, and very rapid results (15 to 30 min). The sensitivities and specificities of these kits are relatively poor (49, 88, 90), and a single negative rapid antigen test is not a reliable marker for RSV negativity (88). In comparison to a reverse transcriptase PCR (RT-PCR) assay, the BD Directigen RSV assay resulted in a 23% false-negativity rate (49). Another testing format, lateral flow CIA, has gained popularity due to its simplicity (Table 2). The sensitivity and specificity of these CIA kits were 83 and 93% when DFA and molecular assays were used as the "gold standard" (12, 67, 108). Two DIA assays, Respi-Strip from Coris BioConcept (Gembloux, Belgium) and QuickVue RSV from Quidel Corp. (San Diego, CA), have been reported that can generate RSV antigen test results within 15 min (51). All of these procedures possess extremely short hands-on time and fast test turnaround time, and they can be done at the point of care in emergency departments and clinician offices by personnel with no training in virology techniques (51, 79).

During the peak of the RSV season, a rapid antigen detection test may be helpful in diagnosing RSV as the cause of bronchiolitis and pneumonia among children. The positive predictive value of a positive test is low when prevalence is low; thus, the performance of these tests is much reduced during the RSV off-season (4, 56). In addition, the accuracy of these rapid tests can be influenced by the type of specimen obtained and the age of the patient. Rapid antigen detection tests for the diagnosis of RSV respiratory illness in adults are of limited value (39, 56). Several studies performed on RSV-infected older adults showed antigen detection in nasal specimens to be very insensitive (90). The extreme low sensitivity in adults is due to low magnitude and short duration of RSV shedding in adult respiratory secretions and the problems associated with obtaining nasal washes in frail older adults (13, 39, 132).

TABLE 1 Commercial RSV and hMPV DFA reagents and their performance[a]

Virus	Product (company)	Manufacturer's claimed performance[b]	Application	Remarks (references)
RSV	Bartels RSV DFA (Bartels, a Trinity Biotech Company, Carlsbad, CA)	Sensitivity, 88–100%; specificity, 100%	Direct specimen detection and culture confirmation	Single- or dual-reagent DFA available. Acquired recently by Trinity Biotech (4, 98).
	Light Diagnostics Respiratory DFA Viral Screening and Identification Kit (Millipore, Temecula, CA)	Sensitivity, 100%; specificity, 86%	Direct specimen detection and culture confirmation	In either single RSV or panel format. The panel covers RSV, influenza A and B viruses, adenovirus, and parainfluenza viruses 1–3.
	SimulFluor Respiratory Screen, RSV/flu A or RSV/Para 3 (Millipore)	Sensitivity, 83.3–100%; specificity, 83.8–100%	For screening in clinical specimens and culture	Three formats available. Covers RSV, influenza A and B viruses, adenovirus, and parainfluenza viruses 1–3 (51, 69).
	D³Ultra DFA Respiratory Kit (DHI)	Sensitivity, 93%; specificity, 99%	Direct specimen detection and culture confirmation	Covers influenza A and B viruses, RSV, parainfluenza viruses 1–3, and adenovirus
	Merifluor RSV (Meridian Bioscience Inc.)	NA	Culture confirmation	Subgroup differentiation available
	Imagen RSV (DakoCytomation, Glostrup, Denmark; Imagen, DAKO, Carpinteria, CA)	Sensitivity, 93%; specificity, 98%	Detection or identification in human clinical specimens	Mixture of three monoclonal antibodies covering RSV, and influenza A and B viruses (12, 71)
	PathoDx RSV and Respiratory Virus Panel (Remel Inc., Lenexa, KS)	Sensitivity, 77.6–100%; specificity, 98–100%	Clinical specimen detection and culture confirmation	The respiratory panel covers RSV, influenza A and B viruses, adenovirus, and parainfluenza viruses 1–3.
hMPV	D³Ultra DFA hMPV (DHI)	Sensitivity, 62.5%; specificity, 99.8%	Clinical specimen detection	Sensitivity and specificity were calculated by using culture and NAA assays as standards (4, 61).
	Imagen hMPV DFA test (Thermo Fisher Scientific, Ely, United Kingdom)	Sensitivity, 63.2%; specificity, 100.0%	Clinical specimen detection	Sensitivity and specificity were calculated by using culture and NAA assays as standards (4).
	Light Diagnostics Respiratory DFA Viral Screening and Identification Kit (Millipore)	ND	Direct specimen detection and culture confirmation	ASR kit carried by Millipore (68)

[a]NA, not applicable; ND, not done; ASR, analyte-specific reagent.
[b]Compared to cell culture unless specifically indicated. In many cases, the culture used for comparison and validation was suboptimal, making the rapid tests artificially look better. It should be recognized that performance in each laboratory may be different.

Nucleic Acid

Nucleic acid amplification (NAA) tests have been implemented increasingly in clinical laboratories for RSV detection and are superior to other methods in sensitivity and specificity (56, 134). The RSV N gene has been used as the principal target for developing NAA-based assays because (i) nucleotide sequences in the N gene are highly conserved and (ii) the N gene is preferentially transcribed because it is located nearer the 3' end of the genome, where transcription and replication initiate. Compared with conventional diagnostic tests, monoplex NAA assays have significantly enhanced diagnostic yields for RSV detection, with sensitivities ranging from 93.5 to 100% and specificities approaching 100% (49, 59, 93, 115). While cell culture remains the gold standard for RSV diagnosis, NAA assays have been considered the "platinum standard" to be used as the reference to validate new diagnostic kits in RSV detection (39, 56).

Different technical platforms have been described to detect RSV nucleic acids. PCR-based procedures incorporating one-step, nested, random, monoplex, or multiplex RT-PCR are the mainstay formats used in RSV NAA (13, 14, 40, 42, 49, 59, 64, 72, 75, 81, 88, 93, 99, 127). Other non-PCR amplification procedures have been described, including nucleic acid sequence-based amplification (NASBA) (30, 86), loop-mediated isothermal amplification (108, 118), and multiplex ligation-dependent probe amplification (101). Gel electrophoresis with or without restriction fragment length polymorphism (RFLP) or Southern blotting (42, 64, 93, 101), colorimetric EIAs (40, 115), sequence analysis (138), real-time probes (13, 30, 49, 59, 72, 86, 96), and microarrays (14, 75, 81, 84, 89, 99, 127) have been used for detection and identification of amplification products. Several diagnostic devices using different amplification and identification platforms are commercially available (Table 3).

Recently available multiplex RT-PCR-based devices have significantly improved the diagnostic yield of RSV testing and enhanced detection of coinfections of RSV and other viral pathogens (14, 75, 81). With more FDA-cleared devices becoming available, NAA-based assays will likely become the principal approach for the diagnosis of RSV infections, especially in adult patients, in whom viral shedding occurs for a short period and at a low titer, and during the RSV off-season (4, 46, 56), when false results are obtained frequently by rapid antigen tests. With implementation of the real-time format, rapid RSV viral load quantification by RT-PCR is possible, which is useful in some clinical settings (13, 45, 96). When test turnaround time improves and the test procedure becomes simplified, NAA assays may become the test of choice at the clinical point of care in the near future (74).

TABLE 2 Main commercially available RSV rapid antigen products and their performance characteristics[a]

Technique platform	Product (company)	Compatible specimens	Assay length (min)	Claimed sensitivity (%)[b]	Claimed specificity (%)[b]	Validated sensitivity (%)[b]	Validated specificity (%)[b]	Additional comments	Selected reference(s)
EIA, flow through	Directigen RSV (BD Diagnostic Systems, Sparks, MD)	NP washes, aspirates, and swabs and tracheal aspirates	15	93–97	90–97	61–86	69–95	Instant, clear-cut readings. Mucous specimen hard to pass through. Two antibodies utilized to detect two RSV antigens.	90
CIA, lateral flow	Directigen EZ RSV (BD Diagnostic Systems)	NP washes, aspirates, and swabs	15	89	93	59–86.5	92.3–98	Specific antibody used to avoid possible interference with immunoglobulin therapy	2, 49, 88, 90, 108
	BinaxNOW RSV (Inverness Medical, Princeton, NJ)	NWs or NP swabs	15	89–93	93–100	89–94.6	88.5–100	CLIA-waived test	2, 12, 90
	SAS RSV (SA Scientific, San Antonio, TX)	NP washes, aspirates, and swabs	15	95.6	94.1	57–97	73–100	The original equipment manufacturer for SAS, Sure-Vue, ImmunoCard, Xpect, and Clearview	67
	Sure-Vue RSV (Fisher Scientific)	NP washes, aspirates, and swabs	15	95.6	94.1	NA	NA	Has an 18-mo shelf life	
	ImmunoCard STAT! RSV Plus (Meridian Bioscience, Inc.)	NWs, NP, aspirates and swabs	15	Wash or aspirate, 77.8–84.2; swab, 89.5–94.4	Wash or aspirate, 78; swab, 94.4–100.0	NA	NA	Analytical sensitivity from 10 to 10,000 virions/ml for both subgroups A and B	
	Clearview RSV (Inverness Medical)	NP swabs or aspirates	15	93.7	97.7	NA	NA	CLIA-waived test. Formerly QuickLab RSV.	
	Xpect RSV (Remel Inc.)	NP specimens from neonatal and pediatric patients	15	95.6	94.1	67–78	96–98	Low rate of uninterpretable results. Even mildly mucoid specimens can fail to migrate.	12
DIA	RSV Respi-Strip (Coris BioConcept)	NP secretions and/ or culture supernatant	10	92	98	NA	NA	Two reagents (extraction buffer and the immunostrips), and results are available within 25 min	51
	QuickVue RSV (Quidel Corp.)	NP swabs and aspirates, NWs	15	83–99	90–92	NA	NA	Negative results do not preclude RSV infection and should be confirmed by culture or NAA tests.	

[a]Abbreviations: NA, not applicable or not available; NP, nasopharyngeal; NW, nasal wash; CLIA, Clinical Laboratory Improvement Amendments of 1988.
[b]Compared to cell culture unless specifically indicated.

TABLE 3 Commercial NAA kits and devices for detection and identification of RSV and hMPV[a]

Virus	Product (company)	Amplification	Detection and identification	Pathogen(s) covered	Published performance[b]	Comment (references)
RSV	NucliSENS EasyQ RSV (bioMérieux, Durham, NC)	Monoplex NASBA assay	Real time (molecular beacons)	RSV	Sensitivity, 99%; specificity, 87%	Basic ASR kit is available as well (30, 86)
	Cepheid RSV ASR (Cepheid, Sunnyvale, CA)	Monoplex RT-PCR	Real time (molecular beacons)	RSV and A and B subtyping	ND	Increases sensitivity by 23% in comparison to DFA (49)
	ProFlu+ Assay (GenProbe Inc., San Diego, CA)	Multiplex RT-PCR	Real time (TaqMan)	Flu-A, Flu-B, and RSV	Sensitivity, 95–100%; specificity, 97–99%	FDA cleared (72); has replaced the Hexaplex assay (40)
	Verigene Respiratory Virus Nucleic Acid Test (Nanosphere Inc., Northbrook, IL)	Multiplex RT-PCR	Fluidic cartridge (microarray)	Flu-A, Flu-B, RSV, and RSV subtyping	ND	FDA cleared but not currently available for commercial sale
	MGB Alert Influenza A&B/RSV Detection Reagent RUO (ELITech Group, Puteaux, France)	Multiplex RT-PCR	Real time (TaqMan MGB)	Flu-A, Flu-B, and RSV	ND	Not available in the United States (59)
hMPV	NucliSENS EasyQ hMPV (bioMérieux)	NASBA	Real time (molecular beacons)	hMPV	ND	Basic ASR kit is available as well (27, 47)
	MGB Alert hMPV Detection Reagent ASR (Nanogen, San Diego, CA); see above	RT-PCR	Real time (TaqMan MGB)	hMPV	ND	
	Pro hMPV Assay (GenProbe, Inc.)	RT-PCR	Real time (TaqMan)	hMPV	ND	FDA cleared (44)
RSV and hMPV	RespiFinder (PathoFinder BV, Maastricht, The Netherlands)	Multiplex ligation-dependent probe amplification	Gel electrophoresis and capillary electrophoresis	Flu-A (H5N1), Flu-B, PIV-1 to PIV-4, RSV-A, RSV-B, RhV, CoV-229E, CoV-VOC43, CoV-NL63, hMPV, and AdV	ND	Not available in the United States (101)
	ResPlex II assay (Qiagen, Valencia, CA)	Multiplex PCR and RT-PCR	Luminex xMAP suspension array (Luminex, Austin, TX)	Flu-A, Flu-B, PIV-1 to PIV-4, RSV, hMPV, RhV, EnV, and SARS-CoV	RSV: sensitivity, 95%; specificity, 100%. hMPV: sensitivity, 96%; specificity, 100%.	Unique TEM-PCR permits multitarget amplification without significant loss in sensitivity (14, 75)
	FilmArray Respiratory Pathogen Panel (Idaho Technology Inc., Salt Lake City, UT)	Nested multiplex RT-PCR	Solid array analyzer	AdV, bocavirus, four CoVs, Flu-A, Flu-B, hMPV, PIV-1, to PIV-4, RSV, RhV, and four bacterial pathogens	ND	Integrated and closed system
	Infiniti Respiratory Viral Panel (AutoGenomics, Inc., Carlsbad, CA)	Multiplex PCR and RT-PCR	Infiniti solid array analyzer	Flu-A, Flu-B, PIV-1, to PIV-4, RSV-A, RSV-B, hMPV-A, hMPV-B, RhV-A, RhV-B, EnV, CoV, and AdV	RSV: sensitivity, 100%; specificity, 100%. hMPV: sensitivity, 80–100%; specificity, 100%	Detection step by the Infiniti analyzer is completely automatic (99)
	MultiCode-PLx Respiratory Virus Panel (EraGen Biosciences, Madison, WI)[c]	Multiplex PCR and RT-PCR	BeadXpress Reader (Illumina Inc., San Diego, CA)	Flu-A, Flu-B, PIV-1, to, PIV-4, RSV, hMPV, RhV, AdV, and CoV	RSV: sensitivity, 92%; specificity, 99%. hMPV: ND.	Universal beads used for detection employ EraCode sequences (89)
	Seeplex Respiratory Virus Detection Assay (Seegene, Inc., Seoul, Korea)	Multiplex RT-PCR, two sets	Gel electrophoresis and capillary electrophoresis	AdV, hMPV, two CoVs, PIV-1, to PIV-3, Flu-A, Flu-B, RSV-A, RSV-B, and RhV	ND	Dual priming oligonucleotide system (64)
	xTAG Respiratory Viral Panel (Luminex Molecular Diagnostics, Toronto, Canada)	Multiplex PCR and RT-PCR	Luminex xMAP suspension array (Luminex)	Flu-A, Flu-B, PIV-1 to PIV-4, RSV-A, RSV-B, hMPV, AdV, EnV, CoV, and RhV	RSV: sensitivity, 97%. hMPV: sensitivity 100%; specificity, ND	FDA cleared; target-specific primer extension used in combination with universal detection beads (81)

[a] Abbreviations: ASR, analyte-specific reagent; Flu, influenza virus; ND, not determined; PIV, parainfluenza virus; RhV, rhinovirus; CoV, coronavirus; AdV, adenovirus; EnV, enterovirus; TEM, target-enriched multiplexing; SARS, severe acute respiratory syndrome.
[b] Performance varies significantly due to different standard references used for validation.
[c] Will be available as a research use only device.

1362

Isolation Procedures

Isolation of the virus from respiratory secretions by cell culture remains the gold standard method for RSV diagnosis due to its excellent specificity. Given the lability of the virus, diagnostic samples should be kept cold and should be inoculated as quickly as possible. Inadequate specimen collection or delays in processing may result in lower sensitivity by culture than by antigen tests. For primary isolation, human heteroploid cells, such as HEp-2, HeLa, and A549 cells, are usually preferred. Other cell lines that may be used but are usually less sensitive include human kidney, amnion, and diploid fibroblastic cells and monkey kidney cells (22, 52, 132). Cell line cultures show characteristic syncytial cytopathic effect (CPE) after 3 to 7 days of incubation (Fig. 2A). However, the degree of syncytium formation depends on the type of cell culture, the confluence of the cell monolayer, the medium, the strain of virus, the multiplicity of infection, and its laboratory adaptation. The reported sensitivities of conventional tube cell culture have ranged from 57 to 90% (56), in part due to compromise of virus viability, the technical expertise required, and the cell lines used in the laboratory for performing the viral isolation.

The shell vial assay has significantly shortened the length of time needed for detection of the virus, to about 16 h. This method combines centrifugation and immunofluorescence to detect expression of viral antigens on infected cells before development of CPE (56, 98). The use of R-Mix cultures (Diagnostic Hybrids, Inc. [DHI], Athens, OH), which contain a mixture of human lung carcinoma A549 and mink lung Mv1Lu cells, has been shown to be a rapid and sensitive method for the detection and identification of respiratory viruses (5, 33, 43, 112, 128). With significantly decreased costs compared to those of conventional culture, the use of R-Mix was slightly more sensitive than the use of RMK, HEp-2, and MRC-5 cell lines in conventional cultures, and it was several days faster (5). Screening of R-Mix cells after overnight incubation was more sensitive and produced more timely results for RSV and other respiratory viruses, and it was more reliable than direct antigen testing (71, 112). In addition, R-Mix cell cultures have the major advantage of identifying viruses not detected by direct staining (33). A cryopreserved R-Mix ReadyCells preparation can be stored frozen, thawed, and used as needed with minimal addition of refeeding media (63).

Identification

The appearance of characteristic syncytial CPE in cell culture, together with a negative hemadsorption test, may be adequate to establish the presence of RSV during the epidemic season. However, since other respiratory viruses, such as parainfluenza virus 3 and measles virus, can produce similar CPE in certain cell lines, clinical virology laboratories confirm RSV detection by performing subgroup-specific IFA on infected cells from cell culture vials as a standard practice (56, 98). Further subgroup identification can be performed by using RT-PCR followed by nucleotide sequence analysis and/or RFLP analysis (22, 42, 138).

Typing Systems

Infections with RSV subgroups A and B may result in differing clinical manifestations and outcomes; therefore, RSV subtype information can be useful in clinical patient management (52, 126). RSV subgroup information has been used widely to facilitate epidemiological investigations (138). DFA procedures have not been used routinely in the clinical laboratory for RSV subtyping.

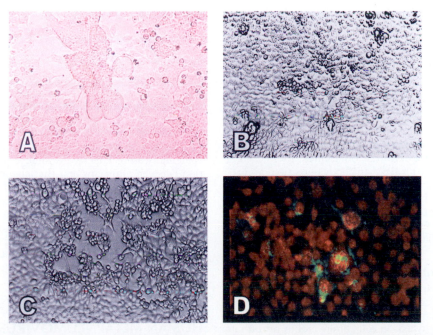

FIGURE 2   Microscopic detection of RSV and hMPV in cell cultures. (A) RSV-infected HEp-2 cells showing cells that have fused, forming large syncytia. (B and C) hMPV infection causes a focus of infection with rounding of LLC-MK2 cells and loss of monolayer integrity. (D) Indirect immunofluorescence of an hMPV-infected LLC-MK2 centrifugation culture stained with monoclonal antibody MAb-8 (70). Images courtesy of http://www.virology.org/hpphoto3.html (A), John Williams (B and C), and David Ferguson (D).

RT-PCR followed by subgroup-specific probe hybridization has been used for RSV subtyping directly from clinical specimens (40, 42, 75, 81, 99, 115). Further analysis on genomic differences among RSV isolates beyond subtyping has been used in epidemiological investigations (42, 138). There has been one study using heterogenous sequences in the RSV G gene to generate subgroups, and it demonstrated that different RSV subgroups were associated with the severity of clinical diseases (42). Another molecular epidemiology study confirmed that multiple subgroups cocirculate each year and that the predominant genotype may shift with the season. These highly discriminatory typing techniques have been useful in monitoring possible nosocomial RSV infections and facilitating the interruption of RSV outbreaks (138).

Serologic Tests

The diagnosis of RSV infections using serology has limited application for clinical use. Most children have serologic evidence of RSV infection by 2 years of age. A significant proportion (10 to 30%) of young patients with documented RSV infections remain serologically negative, probably due to the immaturity of the infant immune responses (48, 52, 56). Secretory antibodies to RSV in nasopharyngeal secretions may also be detected (28, 91, 100, 125), and low RSV-specific nasal immunoglobulin A (IgA) is an independent significant risk factor for RSV infection (125). Repeated infections with viruses of the same subgroup of RSV occur frequently; therefore, it is usually necessary to test acute- and convalescent-phase sera and observe an increase in titers to confirm the diagnosis. Furthermore, assays that detect IgM antibody to RSV show low sensitivity, particularly for infants less than 6 months of age, precluding a definitive diagnosis in a clinically relevant time frame (52, 82, 114).

Serologic diagnosis of RSV infection has been more useful for analysis of vaccine take, defined by a fourfold rise in titer, and for epidemiological monitoring of infections in the community (85, 97, 111). Current means of serologic diagnosis for RSV infections include IFA, EIA, complement fixation, and neutralization assays (52, 82, 91, 114). EIA is analytically more sensitive than complement fixation and has the feature of eliminating false IgM-positive results (82, 114). Oral-fluid samples have been used in the place of serum for RSV IgG and IgA antibody detection and surveillance by EIA (91). Virus neutralization tests have been developed as plaque reduction assays or in a microneutralization format. Indirect IFA has been used widely for RSV antibody detection, and reagents are commercially available from Bion Enterprises, Ltd. (Des Plaines, IL); BioWhittaker (Walkersville, MD); Diagnostic Products Corporation (Los Angeles, CA); Globalemed, LLC (Alexandria, VA); Hemagen Diagnostics, Inc. (Columbia, MD); and Meridian Bioscience Inc. (Cincinnati, OH).

Antiviral Susceptibilities

Resistance to ribavirin and palivizumab has not been recognized in the clinical setting. Several RSV escape mutants derived in the laboratory have been shown to be resistant to palivizumab prophylaxis in cell culture and in cotton rats (137). A total of 458 RSV isolates from treated subjects were recovered during the period from 1998 to 2002 and were tested for resistance. The evidence to date suggests that development of palivizumab-resistant mutants does not appear to play a significant role in hospitalizations for breakthrough RSV disease occurring in infants receiving palivizumab

prophylaxis. The nucleotide and amino acid sequences of the F protein epitope to which palivizumab binds appear to be highly conserved among clinical isolates, even in children receiving palivizumab prophylaxis (32). The RSV604 compound has a low rate of in vitro resistance, which is related to mutations that occur in the N gene (19).

Evaluation, Interpretation, and Reporting of Results

Test results should be interpreted with knowledge of the natural history of RSV infections in the context of the patient's clinical presentation and medical history. Serology is usually useless clinically, and rapid antigen and NAA-based molecular assays are the tests of choice for laboratory diagnostic needs. Culture remains the gold standard for RSV detection, but it is mainly used as a backup test, especially for those specimens yielding negative antigen results or when further characterization has been requested.

The availability of rapid antigen assays with a turnaround time as short as 15 min makes it possible for clinicians to receive results in a timely fashion. However, due to their relatively low sensitivity, false-negative results can be expected and should not be interpreted as excluding the possibility of RSV infection. To improve detection, culture or RT-PCR assays should be used as backup tests.

Cell culture is considered to have the highest specificity, followed by antigen tests and NAA assays. NAA assays, which have been demonstrated to be the most sensitive tests for RSV detection, are particularly useful to test respiratory specimens collected from adults and in the off-season. As more FDA-approved commercial kits become available, simultaneous detection and identification of common viral pathogens, including RSV, by multiplex NAA assays are expected to become the main tool for detection and subtyping of RSV. Special attention should be paid to potential carryover contamination and cross-reaction between tested viruses.

Whereas multiplex NAA assays are currently qualitative, real-time NAA assays can provide an estimate of viral load. Especially when more than one virus is detected, the viral load can be helpful in identifying the predominant pathogen. Nevertheless, the clinical relevance of quantitative respiratory virus PCR awaits further investigation and standardization.

The positive and negative predictive values of these tests vary according to the prevalence of the disease in a particular population during certain seasons. The diagnosis of RSV infection is often made with reasonable accuracy in combination with clinical and epidemiological findings in infants with lower respiratory tract disease during the epidemic season. Effective exchanges of relevant information between clinicians and the laboratory are essential to good patient care. RSV is extremely labile; due to improper specimen collection, transport, and processing, even when sensitive methods such as RT-PCR are used, false-negative results are possible. The importance of correct specimen collection and prompt specimen transport cannot be overemphasized. Prompt reporting of test results may assist clinicians in discontinuing unnecessary forms of therapy or in cohorting infected individuals, thereby preventing nosocomial spread of infection.

HUMAN METAPNEUMOVIRUS

Taxonomy

Human metapneumovirus (hMPV) is an RNA virus of the *Paramyxoviridae* family and is part of the *Pneumovirinae* subfamily along with RSV. The virus was discovered in 2001 (120). The *Paramyxoviridae* family is divided into two subfamilies, *Pneumovirinae* and *Paramyxovirinae*. The *Pneumovirinae* subfamily includes the two genera *Pneumovirus* and *Metapneumovirus*. The avian pneumoviruses (APV) are highly related to hMPV. APV and hMPV were separated by taxonomists into the separate genus *Metapneumovirus* because they can be distinguished from members of the *Pneumovirus* genus by their lack of genes encoding the non-structural proteins NS1 and NS2 and by a different gene order in the RNA genome. Sublineages of subgroup A2 also have been proposed (58).

Description of the Agent

hMPV is an enveloped respiratory virus with a single-stranded nonsegmented negative-sense RNA genome. Although APV and hMPV are related to the human and animal RSVs, they differ in that the gene order in the non-segmented genome is slightly altered and APV and hMPV lack the two nonstructural proteins NS1 and NS2, encoded at the 3' end of RSV genomes (Fig. 1). These RSV proteins are thought to counteract host type I interferons (109). Full-length sequences of a number of hMPV genomes have been reported (7, 57, 119). The genome is predicted to encode nine proteins in the order 3'-N-P-M-F-M2-SH-G-L-5' (the M2 gene is predicted to encode two proteins, M2-1 and M2-2, using overlapping open reading frames, as in RSV) (119). The genome also contains noncoding 3' leader, 5' trailer, and intergenic regions, consistent with the organization of most paramyxoviruses (57). The viral promoter is contained within the 3'-terminal 57 nucleotides of the genome (8). The F, G, and SH (short hydrophobic) proteins are integral membrane proteins on the surface of infected cells and virion particles. The F protein contains an Arg-Gly-Asp (RGD) sequence motif that facilitates interaction with the integrin $\alpha V\beta 1$, promoting attachment to epithelial cells (24). The predicted attachment (G) protein of hMPV exhibits the basic features of a glycosylated type II mucin-like protein. hMPV N and P interact and are recruited to cytoplasmic viral inclusion bodies in hMPV-infected cells that can be detected easily by immunofluorescent staining (31).

Epidemiology and Transmission

hMPV outbreaks occur in annual epidemics during late winter and early spring in temperate climates, often overlapping in part or in whole with the annual RSV epidemic. Nearly all children have evidence of prior infection by the age of 5 years, when they are tested by serology (120). A study of the association of the virus with respiratory disease was performed using prospectively collected data in a cohort of more than 2,000 subjects aged 0 to 5 years monitored during a 25-year period at Vanderbilt University Medical Center (131). This study showed that hMPV is associated with the common cold (complicated by otitis media in about one-third of cases) and with lower respiratory tract illnesses such as bronchiolitis, pneumonia, croup, and exacerbation of reactive airways disease. The signs and symptoms caused by hMPV are very similar to those caused by RSV; providers cannot distinguish the two infections based on clinical assessment alone. Approximately 12% of outpatient lower respiratory tract illness was associated with hMPV infection, which was second only to RSV in this regard. A prospective study of all infant hospitalizations for acute respiratory illness or fever without localizing symptoms in a multicenter study in the New Vaccine Surveillance Network organized by the Centers for Disease Control and Prevention (CDC) found that 3.9% of 668 such hospitalizations in children

were associated with hMPV (87). Children with RSV or hMPV infection required supplemental oxygen and medical intensive care at similar frequencies. Many other studies at referral hospitals, most performed as retrospective studies using samples referred to a diagnostic virology laboratory, suggested that approximately 5 to 10% of such patient specimens contain the hMPV genome. hMPV has been found in association with respiratory tract disease in every continent; dozens of country-specific case series have been reported.

Long-term studies have shown that sporadic infection does occur year-round (131). The incubation period is thought to be about 3 to 5 days. Humans are the only source of infection. The usual period of viral shedding has not been defined but is likely to be weeks following primary infection in infants. Formal transmission studies have not been reported, but experts believe that transmission occurs by close or direct contact with contaminated secretions involving large-particle aerosols, droplets, or contaminated surfaces. Nosocomial infections have been reported to occur in hospitalized children and adults, and contact isolation with excellent hand washing for health care providers is appropriate.

Clinical Significance

The virus causes upper and lower respiratory tract illnesses. About half of the cases of lower respiratory tract illness in children occur in the first 6 months of life, suggesting that young age is a major risk factor for severe disease (131). Both young adults and the elderly can suffer hMPV infection that leads to medically attended illnesses including hospitalization, but severe disease occurs at lower frequencies in adults than in young children (37, 38). Severe disease in older subjects is more common in immunocompromised patients (94, 121) and can be fatal in these subjects (16). A large proportion of respiratory tract secretion samples submitted to diagnostic virology laboratories are obtained from immunocompromised patients. hMPV infection is associated with wheezing more commonly in patients with underlying pulmonary disease, especially asthma (133). Although a significant number of patients with asthmatic exacerbation have hMPV infection, it is not yet clear whether there is a particular association of the virus with long-term wheezing. RSV and hMPV coinfections have been reported, which is not surprising given the overlapping seasons. Coinfection with bacteria is not common, except for the local complication of otitis media, which is frequent (106, 113, 131).

Collection, Transport, and Storage of Specimens

Reports in the literature suggest that the virus can be recovered or detected by RT-PCR from nasal aspirates, nasal washes, nasal or throat swabs, and bronchoalveolar lavage specimens. Typically, nasopharyngeal aspirates are collected from infants using a 10F catheter. Washing the catheter after dispensing, in addition to collecting material in the collection trap, may enhance yield over use of the trap material alone (107). Transport is generally performed using standard viral transport media, on ice. It is highly likely that optimal specimen collection and handling are very similar to those for RSV, which are discussed in detail above. Specimens should be processed as soon as possible after collection and stored at 4°C until processing. For long-term storage of specimens or laboratory stocks, a temperature of −70°C is preferred with specimens in O-ring-sealed cryovials.

Direct Detection

Microscopy

The virus can be seen by electron microscopy (10, 120). This method, however, is not sufficiently sensitive or reproducible for clinical detection.

Antigen Detection

Rapid antigen tests have been developed for use on nasopharyngeal aspirate samples using hMPV-specific monoclonal antibodies (34, 70, 104). A lateral flow CIA using two monoclonal antibodies against hMPV N proteins was described, and preliminary studies showed that the assay has good sensitivity and specificity for detecting hMPV from respiratory samples (62). An antigen detection EIA kit is commercially available from Biotrin (Dublin, Ireland). The assay had a sensitivity of 81%, a specificity of 100%, a positive predictive value of 100%, and a negative predictive value of 77% in comparison to viral culture and RT-PCR when frozen nasopharyngeal aspirate specimens from 93 individuals with acute respiratory illness were tested (66). A recent study reported an agreement of 94% between the Biotrin antigen test and RT-PCR results (44).

DFA staining has been gradually implemented for hMPV detection in the clinical setting. Mouse monoclonal antibodies specific for hMPV have been developed and used for DFA staining of nasopharyngeal samples. A number of DFA reagents have been developed, and several are commercially available (4, 61, 95) (Table 1). The sensitivity and specificity of these tests compared to RT-PCR have been reported as 62.5 and 99.8% for the DHI reagent (4) and 63.2 and 100% (4) or 73.9 and 94.1% (95) for the Imagen (Oxoid Ltd., Basingstoke, Hampshire, United Kingdom) reagent. The Light Diagnostics DFA reagent showed a sensitivity of 85% compared to the CDC real-time PCR (68). More recent testing of the DHI test showed a sensitivity of 95.2% compared to RT-PCR, and this test has been licensed (122). The DHI D^{3}Ultra DFA hMPV kit is the only FDA-cleared device that detects and identifies hMPV using antibodies (4). Human monoclonal antibodies for hMPV also have been isolated that function in experimental antigen detection formats, but they are more likely to be developed further for prophylactic therapy (130).

Nucleic Acid

The most sensitive test for identification of hMPV in clinical samples to date is RT-PCR. Many of the early clinical studies used an RT-PCR targeting the polymerase (L) gene (120, 131). Subsequently, real-time RT-PCRs have been developed, especially targeting the N and F genes, which offer enhanced sensitivity and specificity; these include an assay designed to detect viruses from the four known genetic lineages (4, 23, 29, 75, 78, 80, 105, 124, 129). Although the copy number of the N gene transcript should be higher than that of the F gene because of its more proximal position relative to the virus 3′ leader region, where transcription begins, both F and N primer sets have been shown to be sensitive in RT-PCRs. Two-stage testing targeting different genes has been evaluated (50). Quantitative RT-PCRs have been employed to define viral load in patient samples (105). A NASBA test also has been described; however, the sensitivity of this assay (lower limit of detection of 100 copies) appears to be lower than that of quantitative RT-PCR (27). At this time, the xTAG RVP assay is the only FDA-approved molecular test for hMPV (81, 83, 92). Several molecular devices are commercially available for detection of hMPV, and their performance characteristics are contrasted in Table 3.

Simultaneous testing for the presence of RNA from multiple respiratory viruses, including hMPV, reveals positive tests for more than one agent in a significant proportion of cases (14). Studies that identify coinfections solely on the basis of amplification of the viral genome by RT-PCR, however, should be interpreted with caution for several reasons. PCR is susceptible to false-positive results due to cross-contamination in some laboratories that perform frequent amplifications. Ideally, amplified PCR products should be confirmed by hybridization or, preferably, nucleotide sequence analysis to demonstrate diversity of isolates and lack of contamination by laboratory isolates. Second, the viral genome can be detected by RT-PCR in respiratory secretions for several weeks or more, even after live virus shedding has ceased. It is difficult to know in this situation if the presence of a positive RT-PCR signifies active infection or simply a recent acute infection. One potential future application of quantitative molecular tests is to differentiate acute infection from recent infection that has resolved (105). Because of the sensitivity of nucleic acid detection tests, viral RNA may be detected weeks after clinical resolution. If the kinetics of high and low viral RNA detection can be defined in future studies, quantitative RNA studies may be helpful to interpret a persistent RNA signal or the simultaneous presence of RNA signals from two viruses, one acute and one recent.

Isolation Procedures

hMPV replicates poorly in most conventional cell cultures used for respiratory virus diagnosis, such as HEK, HEp-2, and Madin-Darby canine kidney cells. Primary isolation is facilitated by the presence of a low concentration of trypsin, which is not used routinely in diagnostic virology cultures in many laboratories. The virus was first isolated in primary monkey kidney cells from a clean primate facility in The Netherlands that had been passaged twice (designated tertiary monkey kidney [tMK] cells). Monkey kidney cells in the United States generally cannot be used for this purpose because many of these commercial cell cultures contain simian foamy viruses that cause CPE during the prolonged culture necessary to grow hMPV. hMPV can be isolated and grown in LLC-MK2 cell or Vero cell monolayer cultures. Growth is slow in these cell lines and often requires several blind passages before CPE appears, especially following primary isolation. The CPE in tMK cells was reported to resemble that of RSV, although it usually appeared later than with RSV. The CPE in cell lines is not particularly striking, often appearing only as focal areas of rounding of cells and minor patches of cell-cell fusion in LLC-MK2 or Vero cell cultures (Fig. 2). Virus can be isolated in about half of cases in which nasopharyngeal samples are positive for hMPV by RT-PCR. Shell vial centrifugation cultures may enhance recovery and shorten the time to recovery. Investigators have used a monoclonal antibody (Chemicon MAB8510, prepared by the CDC) to detect hMPV in LLC-MK2, HEp-2, and A549 cells using shell vial culture, with equal success in the three lines on day 2 after inoculation (70). A shell vial culture method using R-Mix cells (DHI) and an hMPV-specific monoclonal antibody had a sensitivity of 100% compared with tube culture in one study (102).

Identification

The characteristics of the CPE are not distinct enough that the virus could be identified on this basis, even by trained observers. The virus can be suspected when a virus is isolated during the epidemic season in Vero or LLC-MK2 cells that is not identified by specific immunofluorescence tests for related viruses. Specific identification must be made using immunofluorescence with a commercial monoclonal antibody, or by a licensed RT-PCR on RNA extracted from cell lysates. Currently, the virus is best identified when a specific RT-PCR is found to be positive (optimally confirmed with sequence analysis of the cDNA copy of the RNA genome).

Typing Systems

The typing of strains of hMPV is principally of interest to epidemiologists at this time and does not currently provide guidance in clinical care or therapy. The nomenclature and classification of genotypes, subgroups, strains, variants, and isolates of hMPV are still being developed. Phylogenetic analyses of partial sequences of the viral genome have suggested in every case that there are at least two major genetic subgroups (designated A and B), and the phylogenetic groupings are consistent when analysis of any of five genes has been performed. Full-length sequences of hMPV genomes from viruses representing the two major subgroups have been obtained by two groups using isolates from The Netherlands (strains NL/1/00 and NL/1/99) or from Canada (strains CAN97-83 and CAN98-75). These studies show that the diversity between hMPV subgroup A and B sequences is greatest for the SH and G proteins. The G protein genes exhibit nucleotide and amino acid sequence identities ranging from 52 to 58% and 31 to 35%, respectively, between the two subgroups, while the hMPV F protein is highly conserved in hMPV strains even across subgroups (with amino acid identity of 93 to 96%). hMPV phylogeny studies also suggest that the virus sequences within subgroups A and B can be further divided into two clades per subgroup. Studies using experimental infection of animals and reciprocal cross-neutralization studies suggest for the most part that the viruses of various subgroups all fall within one serotype.

Serologic Tests

Serology is not used for clinical diagnosis of acute infections, because diagnosis requires a comparison of acute- and convalescent-phase titers. Most of the serologic tests for evidence of previous infection have used relatively crude methods to date. Most studies used microtiter plate-based enzyme-linked immunosorbent assays (ELISAs) with plates coated with virus-infected cell lysates or fixed and permeabilized infected cell monolayers as the viral antigen, which are susceptible to high-background reading and false-positive tests. Recombinant viral protein-based assays have been reported which hold promise as more reproducible assays (25, 54). Antibody detection by ELISA does not correlate well with RT-PCR results; thus, the usefulness of ELISA for diagnosing infections is very limited (37). Serum neutralizing antibody assays have been used to demonstrate the induction of functional antibodies in both humans and experimentally infected animals. Most of these tests have used reduction of virus plaques or CPE as the readout; however, a more objective microneutralization test using a recombinant hMPV expressing green fluorescent protein has been reported (9).

Antiviral Susceptibilities

There are no licensed therapies or prophylactic treatments for hMPV infection at this time. Ribavirin and intravenous immunoglobulin, which have activity against RSV, were tested in vitro and were found to have equivalent activities against hMPV and RSV (135). This combination has been used clinically, although its efficacy is uncertain (11).

Heparin and the sulfated sialyl lipid (NMSO$_3$) also have been shown to have activity against hMPV (136), and a low-molecular-weight benzimidazole derivative that inhibits hMPV has been reported (3). None of these inhibitory treatments has been tested clinically.

Evaluation, Interpretation, and Reporting of Results

FDA-approved tests are available for detection of hMPV. Therefore, the emphasis on clinical detection should be on the use of FDA-approved molecular tests to detect the genome or DFA to detect hMPV-infected cells in nasal secretions, washes, or aspirates. Currently, the diagnosis is best made when a specific RT-PCR is found to be positive. The virus can be suspected when a virus is isolated during the epidemic season in Vero or LLC-MK2 cells that is not identified by specific immunofluorescence tests for related viruses. Culture requires a very high level of technical experience, and even most research laboratories grow the virus with difficulty, especially from primary specimens. Diagnostic tests are helpful to distinguish the infection from RSV and other viral respiratory tract infections. Subgroup analysis is mostly of utility in studies of epidemiology at this time. Because the average duration of shedding during infection is not defined, and the role of coinfection in disease expression is not well understood, the clinical interpretation of a positive molecular test must be made with caution, especially when RNA from another virus is detected simultaneously in the same sample. In general, the diagnosis of hMPV infection is most likely when a positive nucleic acid test for hMPV infection is obtained when testing a respiratory secretion during late winter or early spring in temperate climates from a patient with acute respiratory illness and negative tests for other respiratory viruses.

REFERENCES

1. **Abu-Diab, A., M. Azzeh, R. Ghneim, R. Ghneim, M. Zoughbi, S. Turkuman, N. Rishmawi, A. E. Issa, I. Siriani, R. Dauodi, R. Kattan, and M. Y. Hindiyeh.** 2008. Comparison between pernasal flocked swabs and nasopharyngeal aspirates for detection of common respiratory viruses in samples from children. *J. Clin. Microbiol.* **46:**2414–2417.
2. **Aldous, W. K., K. Gerber, E. W. Taggart, J. Thomas, D. Tidwell, and J. A. Daly.** 2004. A comparison of Binax NOW to viral culture and direct fluorescent assay testing for respiratory syncytial virus. *Diagn. Microbiol. Infect. Dis.* **49:**265–268.
3. **Andries, K., M. Moeremans, T. Gevers, R. Willebrords, C. Sommen, J. Lacrampe, F. Janssens, and P. R. Wyde.** 2003. Substituted benzimidazoles with nanomolar activity against respiratory syncytial virus. *Antivir. Res.* **60:**209–219.
4. **Aslanzadeh, J., X. Zheng, H. Li, J. Tetreault, I. Ratkiewicz, S. Meng, P. Hamilton, and Y. W. Tang.** 2008. Prospective evaluation of rapid antigen tests for diagnosis of respiratory syncytial virus and human metapneumovirus infections. *J. Clin. Microbiol.* **46:**1682–1685.
5. **Barenfanger, J., C. Drake, T. Mueller, T. Troutt, J. O'Brien, and K. Guttman.** 2001. R-Mix cells are faster, at least as sensitive and marginally more costly than conventional cell lines for the detection of respiratory viruses. *J. Clin. Virol.* **22:**101–110.
6. **Bentzen, E. L., F. House, T. J. Utley, J. E. Crowe, Jr., and D. W. Wright.** 2005. Progression of respiratory syncytial virus infection monitored by fluorescent quantum dot probes. *Nano Lett.* **5:**591–595.
7. **Biacchesi, S., M. H. Skiadopoulos, G. Boivin, C. T. Hanson, B. R. Murphy, P. L. Collins, and U. J. Buchholz.** 2003. Genetic diversity between human metapneumovirus subgroups. *Virology* **315:**1–9.

8. Biacchesi, S., M. H. Skiadopoulos, K. C. Tran, B. R. Murphy, P. L. Collins, and U. J. Buchholz. 2004. Recovery of human metapneumovirus from cDNA: optimization of growth in vitro and expression of additional genes. *Virology* **321**:247–259.

9. Biacchesi, S., M. H. Skiadopoulos, L. Yang, B. R. Murphy, P. L. Collins, and U. J. Buchholz. 2005. Rapid human metapneumovirus microneutralization assay based on green fluorescent protein expression. *J. Virol. Methods* **128**:192–197.

10. Boivin, G., Y. Abed, G. Pelletier, L. Ruel, D. Moisan, S. Cote, T. C. Peret, D. D. Erdman, and L. J. Anderson. 2002. Virological features and clinical manifestations associated with human metapneumovirus: a new paramyxovirus responsible for acute respiratory-tract infections in all age groups. *J. Infect. Dis.* **186**:1330–1334.

11. Bonney, D., H. Razali, A. Turner, and A. Will. 2009. Successful treatment of human metapneumovirus pneumonia using combination therapy with intravenous ribavirin and immune globulin. *Br. J. Haematol.* **145**:667–669.

12. Borek, A. P., S. H. Clemens, V. K. Gaskins, D. Z. Aird, and A. Valsamakis. 2006. Respiratory syncytial virus detection by Remel Xpect, Binax Now RSV, direct immunofluorescent staining, and tissue culture. *J. Clin. Microbiol.* **44**:1105–1107.

13. Borg, I., G. Rohde, S. Loseke, J. Bittscheidt, G. Schultze-Werninghaus, V. Stephan, and A. Bufe. 2003. Evaluation of a quantitative real-time PCR for the detection of respiratory syncytial virus in pulmonary diseases. *Eur. Respir. J.* **21**:944–951.

14. Brunstein, J. D., C. L. Cline, S. McKinney, and E. Thomas. 2008. Evidence from multiplex molecular assays for complex multipathogen interactions in acute respiratory infections. *J. Clin. Microbiol.* **46**:97–102.

15. Buckingham, S. C., A. J. Bush, and J. P. Devincenzo. 2000. Nasal quantity of respiratory syncytial virus correlates with disease severity in hospitalized infants. *Pediatr. Infect. Dis. J.* **19**:113–117.

16. Cane, P. A., B. G. van den Hoogen, S. Chakrabarti, C. D. Fegan, and A. D. Osterhaus. 2003. Human metapneumovirus in a haematopoietic stem cell transplant recipient with fatal lower respiratory tract disease. *Bone Marrow Transplant.* **31**:309–310.

17. Carter, M. C., D. G. Alber, R. C. Baxter, S. K. Bithell, J. Budworth, A. Chubb, G. S. Cockerill, V. C. Dowdell, E. A. Henderson, S. J. Keegan, R. D. Kelsey, M. J. Lockyer, J. N. Stables, L. J. Wilson, and K. L. Powell. 2006. 1,4-Benzodiazepines as inhibitors of respiratory syncytial virus. *J. Med. Chem.* **49**:2311–2319.

18. Chan, K. H., J. S. Peiris, W. Lim, J. M. Nicholls, and S. S. Chiu. 2008. Comparison of nasopharyngeal flocked swabs and aspirates for rapid diagnosis of respiratory viruses in children. *J. Clin. Virol.* **42**:65–69.

19. Chapman, J., E. Abbott, D. G. Alber, R. C. Baxter, S. K. Bithell, E. A. Henderson, M. C. Carter, P. Chambers, A. Chubb, G. S. Cockerill, P. L. Collins, V. C. Dowdell, S. J. Keegan, R. D. Kelsey, M. J. Lockyer, C. Luongo, P. Najarro, R. J. Pickles, M. Simmonds, D. Taylor, S. Tyms, L. J. Wilson, and K. L. Powell. 2007. RSV604, a novel inhibitor of respiratory syncytial virus replication. *Antimicrob. Agents Chemother.* **51**:3346–3353.

20. Checchia, P. 2008. Identification and management of severe respiratory syncytial virus. *Am. J. Health Syst. Pharm.* **65**:S7–S12.

21. Cheng, F. W., V. Lee, M. M. Shing, and C. K. Li. 2008. Prolonged shedding of respiratory syncytial virus in immunocompromised children: implication for hospital infection control. *J. Hosp. Infect.* **70**:383–385.

22. Collins, P. L., and J. E. Crowe, Jr. 2007. Respiratory syncytial virus and metapneumovirus, p. 1601–1646. *In* D. M. Knipe, P. M. Howley, D. E. Griffin, R. A. Lamb, M. A. Martin, B. Roizman, and S. E. Straus (ed.), *Fields Virology*, 5th ed., vol. 2. Lippincott Williams & Wilkins, Philadelphia, PA.

23. Cote, S., Y. Abed, and G. Boivin. 2003. Comparative evaluation of real-time PCR assays for detection of the human metapneumovirus. *J. Clin. Microbiol.* **41**:3631–3635.

24. Cseke, G., M. S. Maginnis, R. G. Cox, S. J. Tollefson, A. B. Podsiad, D. W. Wright, T. S. Dermody, and J. V. Williams. 2009. Integrin $\alpha v\beta 1$ promotes infection by human metapneumovirus. *Proc. Natl. Acad. Sci. USA* **106**:1566–1571.

25. Cseke, G., D. W. Wright, S. J. Tollefson, J. E. Johnson, J. E. Crowe, Jr., and J. V. Williams. 2007. Human metapneumovirus fusion protein vaccines that are immunogenic and protective in cotton rats. *J. Virol.* **81**:698–707.

26. Daley, P., S. Castriciano, M. Chernesky, and M. Smieja. 2006. Comparison of flocked and rayon swabs for collection of respiratory epithelial cells from uninfected volunteers and symptomatic patients. *J. Clin. Microbiol.* **44**:2265–2267.

27. Dare, R., S. Sanghavi, A. Bullotta, M. C. Keightley, K. S. George, R. M. Wadowsky, D. L. Paterson, K. R. McCurry, T. A. Reinhart, S. Husain, and C. R. Rinaldo. 2007. Diagnosis of human metapneumovirus infection in immunosuppressed lung transplant recipients and children evaluated for pertussis. *J. Clin. Microbiol.* **45**:548–552.

28. De Alarcon, A., E. E. Walsh, H. T. Carper, J. B. La Russa, B. A. Evans, G. P. Rakes, T. A. Platts-Mills, and P. W. Heymann. 2001. Detection of IgA and IgG but not IgE antibody to respiratory syncytial virus in nasal washes and sera from infants with wheezing. *J. Pediatr.* **138**:311–317.

29. Deffrasnes, C., S. Cote, and G. Boivin. 2005. Analysis of replication kinetics of the human metapneumovirus in different cell lines by real-time PCR. *J. Clin. Microbiol.* **43**:488–490.

30. Deiman, B., C. Schrover, C. Moore, D. Westmoreland, and P. van de Wiel. 2007. Rapid and highly sensitive qualitative real-time assay for detection of respiratory syncytial virus A and B using NASBA and molecular beacon technology. *J. Virol. Methods* **146**:29–35.

31. Derdowski, A., T. R. Peters, N. Glover, R. Qian, T. J. Utley, A. Burnett, J. V. Williams, P. Spearman, and J. E. Crowe, Jr. 2008. Human metapneumovirus nucleoprotein and phosphoprotein interact and provide the minimal requirements for inclusion body formation. *J. Gen. Virol.* **89**:2698–2708.

32. DeVincenzo, J. P., C. B. Hall, D. W. Kimberlin, P. J. Sanchez, W. J. Rodriguez, B. A. Jantausch, L. Corey, J. S. Kahn, J. A. Englund, J. A. Suzich, F. J. Palmer-Hill, L. Branco, S. Johnson, N. K. Patel, and F. M. Piazza. 2004. Surveillance of clinical isolates of respiratory syncytial virus for palivizumab (Synagis)-resistant mutants. *J. Infect. Dis.* **190**:975–978.

33. Dunn, J. J., R. D. Woolstenhulme, J. Langer, and K. C. Carroll. 2004. Sensitivity of respiratory virus culture when screening with R-mix fresh cells. *J. Clin. Microbiol.* **42**:79–82.

34. Ebihara, T., R. Endo, X. Ma, N. Ishiguro, and H. Kikuta. 2005. Detection of human metapneumovirus antigens in nasopharyngeal secretions by an immunofluorescent-antibody test. *J. Clin. Microbiol.* **43**:1138–1141.

35. Englund, J. A., P. A. Piedra, A. Jewell, K. Patel, B. B. Baxter, and E. Whimbey. 1996. Rapid diagnosis of respiratory syncytial virus infections in immunocompromised adults. *J. Clin. Microbiol.* **34**:1649–1653.

36. Ermers, M. J., M. M. Rovers, J. B. van Woensel, J. L. Kimpen, and L. J. Bont. 2009. The effect of high dose inhaled corticosteroids on wheeze in infants after respiratory syncytial virus infection: randomised double blind placebo controlled trial. *BMJ* **338**:b897.

37. Falsey, A. R., M. C. Criddle, and E. E. Walsh. 2006. Detection of respiratory syncytial virus and human metapneumovirus by reverse transcription polymerase chain reaction in adults with and without respiratory illness. *J. Clin. Virol.* **35**:46–50.

38. Falsey, A. R., D. Erdman, L. J. Anderson, and E. E. Walsh. 2003. Human metapneumovirus infections in young and elderly adults. *J. Infect. Dis.* **187**:785–790.

39. Falsey, A. R., P. A. Hennessey, M. A. Formica, C. Cox, and E. E. Walsh. 2005. Respiratory syncytial virus infection in elderly and high-risk adults. *N. Engl. J. Med.* **352**:1749–1759.

40. **Fan, J., K. J. Henrickson, and L. L. Savatski.** 1998. Rapid simultaneous diagnosis of infections with respiratory syncytial viruses A and B, influenza viruses A and B, and human parainfluenza virus types 1, 2, and 3 by multiplex quantitative reverse transcription-polymerase chain reaction-enzyme hybridization assay (Hexaplex). *Clin. Infect. Dis.* **26:**1397–1402.

41. **Feltes, T. F., A. K. Cabalka, H. C. Meissner, F. M. Piazza, D. A. Carlin, F. H. Top, Jr., E. M. Connor, and H. M. Sondheimer.** 2003. Palivizumab prophylaxis reduces hospitalization due to respiratory syncytial virus in young children with hemodynamically significant congenital heart disease. *J. Pediatr.* **143:**532–540.

42. **Fletcher, J. N., R. L. Smyth, H. M. Thomas, D. Ashby, and C. A. Hart.** 1997. Respiratory syncytial virus genotypes and disease severity among children in hospital. *Arch. Dis. Child.* **77:**508–511.

43. **Fong, C. K. Y., M. K. Lee, and B. P. Griffith.** 2000. Evaluation of R-Mix FreshCells in shell vials for detection of respiratory viruses. *J. Clin. Microbiol.* **38:**4660–4662.

44. **Fuenzalida, L., J. Fabrega, S. Blanco, M. Del Mar Martinez, C. Prat, M. Perez, C. Ramil, J. Dominguez, V. Ausina, and C. Rodrigo.** 2010. Usefulness of two new methods for diagnosing metapneumovirus infections in children. *Clin. Microbiol. Infect.* **16:**1663–1668.

45. **Gerna, G., G. Campanini, V. Rognoni, A. Marchi, F. Rovida, A. Piralla, and E. Percivalle.** 2008. Correlation of viral load as determined by real-time RT-PCR and clinical characteristics of respiratory syncytial virus lower respiratory tract infections in early infancy. *J. Clin. Virol.* **41:**45–48.

46. **Ginocchio, C. C.** 2007. Detection of respiratory viruses using non-molecular based methods. *J. Clin. Virol.* **40**(Suppl. 1)**:**S11–S14.

47. **Ginocchio, C. C., R. Manji, M. Lotlikar, and F. Zhang.** 2008. Clinical evaluation of NucliSENS magnetic extraction and NucliSENS analyte-specific reagents for real-time detection of human metapneumovirus in pediatric respiratory specimens. *J. Clin. Microbiol.* **46:**1274–1280.

48. **Glezen, W. P.** 2004. The changing epidemiology of respiratory syncytial virus and influenza: impetus for new control measures. *Pediatr. Infect. Dis. J.* **23:**S202–S206.

49. **Goodrich, J. S., and M. B. Miller.** 2007. Comparison of Cepheid's analyte-specific reagents with BD Directigen for detection of respiratory syncytial virus. *J. Clin. Microbiol.* **45:**604–606.

50. **Greensill, J., P. S. McNamara, W. Dove, B. Flanagan, R. L. Smyth, and C. A. Hart.** 2003. Human metapneumovirus in severe respiratory syncytial virus bronchiolitis. *Emerg. Infect. Dis.* **9:**372–375.

51. **Gregson, D., T. Lloyd, S. Buchan, and D. Church.** 2005. Comparison of the RSV Respi-Strip with direct fluorescent-antigen detection for diagnosis of respiratory syncytial virus infection in pediatric patients. *J. Clin. Microbiol.* **43:**5782–5783.

52. **Hall, C. B., and C. A. McCarthy.** 2005. Respiratory syncytial virus, p. 2009–2021. *In* G. L. Mandell, J. E. Bennett, and R. Dolin (ed.), *Principles and Practice of Infectious Diseases*, 6th ed., vol. 3. Churchill Livingstone, Philadelphia, PA.

53. **Hall, C. B., G. A. Weinberg, M. K. Iwane, A. K. Blumkin, K. M. Edwards, M. A. Staat, P. Auinger, M. R. Griffin, K. A. Poehling, D. Erdman, C. G. Grijalva, Y. Zhu, and P. Szilagyi.** 2009. The burden of respiratory syncytial virus infection in young children. *N. Engl. J. Med.* **360:**588–598.

54. **Hamelin, M. E., and G. Boivin.** 2005. Development and validation of an enzyme-linked immunosorbent assay for human metapneumovirus serology based on a recombinant viral protein. *Clin. Diagn. Lab. Immunol.* **12:**249–253.

55. **Heikkinen, T., J. Marttila, A. A. Salmi, and O. Ruuskanen.** 2002. Nasal swab versus nasopharyngeal aspirate for isolation of respiratory viruses. *J. Clin. Microbiol.* **40:**4337–4339.

56. **Henrickson, K. J., and C. B. Hall.** 2007. Diagnostic assays for respiratory syncytial virus disease. *Pediatr. Infect. Dis. J.* **26:**S36–S40.

57. **Herfst, S., M. de Graaf, J. H. Schickli, R. S. Tang, J. Kaur, C. F. Yang, R. R. Spaete, A. A. Haller, B. G. van den Hoogen, A. D. Osterhaus, and R. A. Fouchier.** 2004. Recovery of human metapneumovirus genetic lineages A and B from cloned cDNA. *J. Virol.* **78:**8264–8270.

58. **Huck, B., G. Scharf, D. Neumann-Haefelin, W. Puppe, J. Weigl, and V. Falcone.** 2006. Novel human metapneumovirus sublineage. *Emerg. Infect. Dis.* **12:**147–150.

59. **Hymas, W. C., and D. R. Hillyard.** 2009. Evaluation of Nanogen MGB Alert Detection Reagents in a multiplex real-time PCR for influenza virus types A and B and respiratory syncytial virus. *J. Virol. Methods* **156:**124–128.

60. **Jalal, H., D. F. Bibby, J. Bennett, R. E. Sampson, N. S. Brink, S. MacKinnon, R. S. Tedder, and K. N. Ward.** 2007. Molecular investigations of an outbreak of parainfluenza virus type 3 and respiratory syncytial virus infections in a hematology unit. *J. Clin. Microbiol.* **45:**1690–1696.

61. **Kamboj, M., M. Gerbin, C. K. Huang, C. Brennan, J. Stiles, S. Balashov, S. Park, T. E. Kiehn, D. S. Perlin, E. G. Pamer, and K. A. Sepkowitz.** 2008. Clinical characterization of human metapneumovirus infection among patients with cancer. *J. Infect.* **57:**464–471.

62. **Kikuta, H., T. Ebihara, R. Endo, N. Ishiguro, C. Sakata, S. Ochiai, H. Ishiko, R. Gamo, and T. Sato.** 2007. Development of a rapid chromatographic immunoassay for detection of human metapneumovirus using monoclonal antibodies against nucleoprotein of hMPV. *Hybridoma* **26:**17–21.

63. **Kim, J. S., S. H. Kim, S. Y. Bae, C. S. Lim, Y. K. Kim, K. N. Lee, and C. K. Lee.** 2008. Enhanced detection of respiratory viruses using cryopreserved R-Mix ReadyCells. *J. Clin. Virol.* **42:**264–267.

64. **Kim, S. R., C. S. Ki, and N. Y. Lee.** 2009. Rapid detection and identification of 12 respiratory viruses using a dual priming oligonucleotide system-based multiplex PCR assay. *J. Virol. Methods* **156:**111–116.

65. **King, J. C., Jr., A. R. Burke, J. D. Clemens, P. Nair, J. J. Farley, P. E. Vink, S. R. Batlas, M. Rao, and J. P. Johnson.** 1993. Respiratory syncytial virus illnesses in human immunodeficiency virus- and noninfected children. *Pediatr. Infect. Dis. J.* **12:**733–739.

66. **Kukavica-Ibrulj, I., and G. Boivin.** 2009. Detection of human metapneumovirus antigens in nasopharyngeal aspirates using an enzyme immunoassay. *J. Clin. Virol.* **44:**88–90.

67. **Kuroiwa, Y., K. Nagai, L. Okita, S. Ukae, T. Mori, T. Hotsubo, and H. Tsutsumi.** 2004. Comparison of an immunochromatography test with multiplex reverse transcription-PCR for rapid diagnosis of respiratory syncytial virus infections. *J. Clin. Microbiol.* **42:**4812–4814.

68. **Landry, M. L., S. Cohen, and D. Ferguson.** 2008. Prospective study of human metapneumovirus detection in clinical samples by use of Light Diagnostics direct immunofluorescence reagent and real-time PCR. *J. Clin. Microbiol.* **46:**1098–1100.

69. **Landry, M. L., and D. Ferguson.** 2000. SimulFluor respiratory screen for rapid detection of multiple respiratory viruses in clinical specimens by immunofluorescence staining. *J. Clin. Microbiol.* **38:**708–711.

70. **Landry, M. L., D. Ferguson, S. Cohen, T. C. Peret, and D. D. Erdman.** 2005. Detection of human metapneumovirus in clinical samples by immunofluorescence staining of shell vial centrifugation cultures prepared from three different cell lines. *J. Clin. Microbiol.* **43:**1950–1952.

71. **LaSala, P. R., K. K. Bufton, N. Ismail, and M. B. Smith.** 2007. Prospective comparison of R-mix shell vial system with direct antigen tests and conventional cell culture for respiratory virus detection. *J. Clin. Virol.* **38:**210–216.

72. **Legoff, J., R. Kara, F. Moulin, A. Si-Mohamed, A. Krivine, L. Belec, and P. Lebon.** 2008. Evaluation of the one-step multiplex real-time reverse transcription-PCR ProFlu-1 assay for detection of influenza A and influenza B viruses and respiratory syncytial viruses in children. *J. Clin. Microbiol.* **46:**789–791.

73. **Lessler, J., N. G. Reich, R. Brookmeyer, T. M. Perl, K. E. Nelson, and D. A. Cummings.** 2009. Incubation periods of acute respiratory viral infections: a systematic review. *Lancet Infect. Dis.* **9:**291–300.

74. Letant, S. E., J. I. Ortiz, L. F. Bentley Tammero, J. M. Birch, R. W. Derlet, S. Cohen, D. Manning, and M. T. McBride. 2007. Multiplexed reverse transcriptase PCR assay for identification of viral respiratory pathogens at the point of care. *J. Clin. Microbiol.* **45:**3498–3505.

75. Li, H., M. A. McCormac, R. W. Estes, S. E. Sefers, R. K. Dare, J. D. Chappell, D. D. Erdman, P. F. Wright, and Y. W. Tang. 2007. Simultaneous detection and high-throughput identification of a panel of RNA viruses causing respiratory tract infections. *J. Clin. Microbiol.* **45:**2105–2109.

76. Libster, R., J. Bugna Hortoneda, F. R. Laham, J. M. Casellas, V. Israele, N. R. Polack, M. F. Delgado, M. I. Klein, and F. P. Polack. 2009. Breastfeeding prevents severe disease in full term female infants with acute respiratory infection. *Pediatr. Infect. Dis. J.* **28:**131–134.

77. Macartney, K. K., M. H. Gorelick, M. L. Manning, R. L. Hodinka, and L. M. Bell. 2000. Nosocomial respiratory syncytial virus infections: the cost-effectiveness and cost-benefit of infection control. *Pediatrics* **106:**520–526.

78. Mackay, I. M., S. Bialasiewicz, Z. Waliuzzaman, G. R. Chidlow, D. C. Fegredo, S. Laingam, P. Adamson, G. B. Harnett, W. Rawlinson, M. D. Nissen, and T. P. Sloots. 2004. Use of the P gene to genotype human metapneumovirus identifies 4 viral subtypes. *J. Infect. Dis.* **190:**1913–1918.

79. Mackie, P. L., E. M. McCormick, and C. Williams. 2004. Evaluation of Binax NOW RSV as an acute point-of-care screening test in a paediatric accident and emergency unit. *Commun. Dis. Public Health* **7:**328–330.

80. Maertzdorf, J., C. K. Wang, J. B. Brown, J. D. Quinto, M. Chu, M. de Graaf, B. G. van den Hoogen, R. Spaete, A. D. Osterhaus, and R. A. Fouchier. 2004. Real-time reverse transcriptase PCR assay for detection of human metapneumoviruses from all known genetic lineages. *J. Clin. Microbiol.* **42:**981–986.

81. Mahony, J., S. Chong, F. Merante, S. Yaghoubian, T. Sinha, C. Lisle, and R. Janeczko. 2007. Development of a respiratory virus panel test for detection of twenty human respiratory viruses by use of multiplex PCR and a fluid microbead-based assay. *J. Clin. Microbiol.* **45:**2965–2970.

82. Meddens, M. J., P. Herbrink, J. Lindeman, and W. C. van Dijk. 1990. Serodiagnosis of respiratory syncytial virus (RSV) infection in children as measured by detection of RSV-specific immunoglobulins G, M, and A with enzyme-linked immunosorbent assay. *J. Clin. Microbiol.* **28:**152–155.

83. Merante, F., S. Yaghoubian, and R. Janeczko. 2007. Principles of the xTAG respiratory viral panel assay (RVP Assay). *J. Clin. Virol.* **40**(Suppl. 1):S31–S35.

84. Miller, M. B., and Y. W. Tang. 2009. Basic concepts of microarrays and potential applications in clinical microbiology. *Clin. Microbiol. Rev.* **22:**611–633.

85. Mohapatra, S. S., and S. Boyapalle. 2008. Epidemiologic, experimental, and clinical links between respiratory syncytial virus infection and asthma. *Clin. Microbiol. Rev.* **21:**495–504.

86. Moore, C., M. Valappil, S. Corden, and D. Westmoreland. 2006. Enhanced clinical utility of the NucliSens EasyQ RSV A+B Assay for rapid detection of respiratory syncytial virus in clinical samples. *Eur. J. Clin. Microbiol. Infect. Dis.* **25:**167–174.

87. Mullins, J. A., D. D. Erdman, G. A. Weinberg, K. Edwards, C. B. Hall, F. J. Walker, M. Iwane, and L. J. Anderson. 2004. Human metapneumovirus infection among children hospitalized with acute respiratory illness. *Emerg. Infect. Dis.* **10:**700–705.

88. Myers, C., N. Wagner, L. Kaiser, K. Posfay-Barbe, and A. Gervaix. 2008. Use of the rapid antigenic test to determine the duration of isolation in infants hospitalized for respiratory syncytial virus infections. *Clin. Pediatr.* (Philadelphia) **47:**493–495.

89. Nolte, F. S., D. J. Marshall, C. Rasberry, S. Schievelbein, G. G. Banks, G. A. Storch, M. Q. Arens, R. S. Buller, and J. R. Prudent. 2007. MultiCode-PLx system for multiplexed detection of seventeen respiratory viruses. *J. Clin. Microbiol.* **45:**2779–2786.

90. Ohm-Smith, M. J., P. S. Nassos, and B. L. Haller. 2004. Evaluation of the Binax NOW, BD Directigen, and BD Directigen EZ assays for detection of respiratory syncytial virus. *J. Clin. Microbiol.* **42:**2996–2999.

91. Okiro, E. A., C. Sande, M. Mutunga, G. F. Medley, P. A. Cane, and D. J. Nokes. 2008. Identifying infections with respiratory syncytial virus by using specific immunoglobulin G (IgG) and IgA enzyme-linked immunosorbent assays with oral-fluid samples. *J. Clin. Microbiol.* **46:**1659–1662.

92. Pabbaraju, K., K. L. Tokaryk, S. Wong, and J. D. Fox. 2008. Comparison of the Luminex xTAG respiratory viral panel with in-house nucleic acid amplification tests for diagnosis of respiratory virus infections. *J. Clin. Microbiol.* **46:**3056–3062.

93. Paton, A. W., J. C. Paton, A. J. Lawrence, P. N. Goldwater, and R. J. Harris. 1992. Rapid detection of respiratory syncytial virus in nasopharyngeal aspirates by reverse transcription and polymerase chain reaction amplification. *J. Clin. Microbiol.* **30:**901–904.

94. Pelletier, G., P. Dery, Y. Abed, and G. Boivin. 2002. Respiratory tract reinfections by the new human Metapneumovirus in an immunocompromised child. *Emerg. Infect. Dis.* **8:**976–978.

95. Percivalle, E., A. Sarasini, L. Visai, M. G. Revello, and G. Gerna. 2005. Rapid detection of human metapneumovirus strains in nasopharyngeal aspirates and shell vial cultures by monoclonal antibodies. *J. Clin. Microbiol.* **43:**3443–3446.

96. Perkins, S. M., D. L. Webb, S. A. Torrance, C. El Saleeby, L. M. Harrison, J. A. Aitken, A. Patel, and J. P. DeVincenzo. 2005. Comparison of a real-time reverse transcriptase PCR assay and a culture technique for quantitative assessment of viral load in children naturally infected with respiratory syncytial virus. *J. Clin. Microbiol.* **43:**2356–2362.

97. Piedra, P. A., A. M. Jewell, S. G. Cron, R. L. Atmar, and W. P. Glezen. 2003. Correlates of immunity to respiratory syncytial virus (RSV) associated-hospitalization: establishment of minimum protective threshold levels of serum neutralizing antibodies. *Vaccine* **21:**3479–3482.

98. Rabalais, G. P., G. G. Stout, K. L. Ladd, and K. M. Cost. 1992. Rapid diagnosis of respiratory viral infections by using a shell vial assay and monoclonal antibody pool. *J. Clin. Microbiol.* **30:**1505–1508.

99. Raymond, F., J. Carbonneau, N. Boucher, L. Robitaille, S. Boisvert, W. K. Wu, G. De Serres, G. Boivin, and J. Corbeil. 2009. Comparison of automated microarray detection with real-time PCR assays for detection of respiratory viruses in specimens obtained from children. *J. Clin. Microbiol.* **47:**743–750.

100. Reed, J. L., T. P. Welliver, G. P. Sims, L. McKinney, L. Velozo, L. Avendano, K. Hintz, J. Luma, A. J. Coyle, and R. C. Welliver, Sr. 2009. Innate immune signals modulate antiviral and polyreactive antibody responses during severe respiratory syncytial virus infection. *J. Infect. Dis.* **199:**1128–1138.

101. Reijans, M., G. Dingemans, C. H. Klaassen, J. F. Meis, J. Keijdener, B. Mulders, K. Eadie, W. van Leeuwen, A. van Belkum, A. M. Horrevorts, and G. Simons. 2008. RespiFinder: a new multiparameter test to differentially identify fifteen respiratory viruses. *J. Clin. Microbiol.* **46:**1232–1240.

102. Reina, J., F. Ferres, E. Alcoceba, A. Mena, E. R. de Gopegui, and J. Figuerola. 2007. Comparison of different cell lines and incubation times in the isolation by the shell vial culture of human metapneumovirus from pediatric respiratory samples. *J. Clin. Virol.* **40:**46–49.

103. Robinson, J. L., B. E. Lee, S. Kothapalli, W. R. Craig, and J. D. Fox. 2008. Use of throat swab or saliva specimens for detection of respiratory viruses in children. *Clin. Infect. Dis.* **46:**e61–e64.

104. Rovida, F., E. Percivalle, M. Zavattoni, M. Torsellini, A. Sarasini, G. Campanini, S. Paolucci, F. Baldanti, M. G. Revello, and G. Gerna. 2005. Monoclonal antibodies versus reverse transcription-PCR for detection of respiratory viruses in a patient population with respiratory tract infections admitted to hospital. *J. Med. Virol.* **75:**336–347.

105. Scheltinga, S. A., K. E. Templeton, M. F. Beersma, and E. C. Claas. 2005. Diagnosis of human metapneumovirus and rhinovirus in patients with respiratory tract infections by an internally controlled multiplex real-time RNA PCR. *J. Clin. Virol.* **33:**306–311.

106. Schildgen, O., T. Geikowski, T. Glatzel, J. Schuster, and A. Simon. 2005. Frequency of human metapneumovirus in the upper respiratory tract of children with symptoms of an acute otitis media. *Eur. J. Pediatr.* **164:**400–401.

107. Semple, M. G., J. A. Booth, and B. Ebrahimi. 2007. Most human metapneumovirus and human respiratory syncytial virus in infant nasal secretions is cell free. *J. Clin. Virol.* **40:**241–244.

108. Shirato, K., H. Nishimura, M. Saijo, M. Okamoto, M. Noda, M. Tashiro, and F. Taguchi. 2007. Diagnosis of human respiratory syncytial virus infection using reverse transcription loop-mediated isothermal amplification. *J. Virol. Methods* **139:**78–84.

109. Spann, K. M., K. C. Tran, B. Chi, R. L. Rabin, and P. L. Collins. 2004. Suppression of the induction of alpha, beta, and lambda interferons by the NS1 and NS2 proteins of human respiratory syncytial virus in human epithelial cells and macrophages. *J. Virol.* **78:**4363–4369.

110. Spyridaki, I. S., I. Christodoulou, L. de Beer, V. Hovland, M. Kurowski, A. Olszewska-Ziaber, K. H. Carlsen, K. Lodrup-Carlsen, C. M. van Drunen, M. L. Kowalski, R. Molenkamp, and N. G. Papadopoulos. 2009. Comparison of four nasal sampling methods for the detection of viral pathogens by RT-PCR—a GA(2)LEN project. *J. Virol. Methods* **156:**102–106.

111. Stensballe, L. G., H. Ravn, K. Kristensen, T. Meakins, P. Aaby, and E. A. Simoes. 2009. Seasonal variation of maternally derived respiratory syncytial virus antibodies and association with infant hospitalizations for respiratory syncytial virus. *J. Pediatr.* **154:**296–298.

112. St. George, K., N. M. Patel, R. A. Hartwig, D. R. Scholl, J. A. Jollick, Jr., L. M. Kauffmann, M. R. Evans, and C. R. Rinaldo, Jr. 2002. Rapid and sensitive detection of respiratory virus infections for directed antiviral treatment using R-Mix cultures. *J. Clin. Virol.* **24:**107–115.

113. Suzuki, A., O. Watanabe, M. Okamoto, H. Endo, H. Yano, M. Suetake, and H. Nishimura. 2005. Detection of human metapneumovirus from children with acute otitis media. *Pediatr. Infect. Dis. J.* **24:**655–657.

114. Taggart, E. W., H. R. Hill, T. B. Martins, and C. M. Litwin. 2006. Comparison of complement fixation with two enzyme-linked immunosorbent assays for the detection of antibodies to respiratory viral antigens. *Am. J. Clin. Pathol.* **125:**460–466.

115. Tang, Y. W., P. J. Heimgartner, S. J. Tollefson, T. J. Berg, P. N. Rys, H. Li, T. F. Smith, D. H. Persing, and P. F. Wright. 1999. A colorimetric microtiter plate PCR system detects respiratory syncytial virus in nasal aspirates and discriminates subtypes A and B. *Diagn. Microbiol. Infect. Dis.* **34:**333–337.

116. Thorburn, K., S. Kerr, N. Taylor, and H. K. van Saene. 2004. RSV outbreak in a paediatric intensive care unit. *J. Hosp. Infect.* **57:**194–201.

117. Tripp, R. A., R. Alvarez, B. Anderson, L. Jones, C. Weeks, and W. Chen. 2007. Bioconjugated nanoparticle detection of respiratory syncytial virus infection. *Int. J. Nanomed.* **2:**117–124.

118. Ushio, M., I. Yui, N. Yoshida, M. Fujino, T. Yonekawa, Y. Ota, T. Notomi, and T. Nakayama. 2005. Detection of respiratory syncytial virus genome by subgroups—A, B specific reverse transcription loop-mediated isothermal amplification (RT-LAMP). *J. Med. Virol.* **77:**121–127.

119. van den Hoogen, B. G., T. M. Bestebroer, A. D. Osterhaus, and R. A. Fouchier. 2002. Analysis of the genomic sequence of a human metapneumovirus. *Virology* **295:**119–132.

120. van den Hoogen, B. G., J. C. de Jong, J. Groen, T. Kuiken, R. de Groot, R. A. Fouchier, and A. D. Osterhaus. 2001. A newly discovered human pneumovirus isolated from young children with respiratory tract disease. *Nat. Med.* **7:**719–724.

121. van den Hoogen, B. G., G. J. van Doornum, J. C. Fockens, J. J. Cornelissen, W. E. Beyer, R. de Groot, A. D. Osterhaus, and R. A. Fouchier. 2003. Prevalence and clinical symptoms of human metapneumovirus infection in hospitalized patients. *J. Infect. Dis.* **188:**1571–1577.

122. Vinh, D. C., D. Newby, H. Charest, and J. McDonald. 2008. Evaluation of a commercial direct fluorescent-antibody assay for human metapneumovirus in respiratory specimens. *J. Clin. Microbiol.* **46:**1840–1841.

123. Visser, A., S. Delport, and M. Venter. 2008. Molecular epidemiological analysis of a nosocomial outbreak of respiratory syncytial virus associated pneumonia in a kangaroo mother care unit in South Africa. *J. Med. Virol.* **80:**724–732.

124. von Linstow, M. L., H. H. Larsen, J. Eugen-Olsen, A. Koch, T. Nordmann Winther, A. M. Meyer, H. Westh, B. Lundgren, M. Melbye, and B. Høgh. 2004. Human metapneumovirus and respiratory syncytial virus in hospitalized Danish children with acute respiratory tract infection. *Scand. J. Infect. Dis.* **36:**578–584.

125. Walsh, E. E., and A. R. Falsey. 2004. Humoral and mucosal immunity in protection from natural respiratory syncytial virus infection in adults. *J. Infect. Dis.* **190:**373–378.

126. Walsh, E. E., K. M. McConnochie, C. E. Long, and C. B. Hall. 1997. Severity of respiratory syncytial virus infection is related to virus strain. *J. Infect. Dis.* **175:**814–820.

127. Wang, D., L. Coscoy, M. Zylberberg, P. C. Avila, H. A. Boushey, D. Ganem, and J. L. DeRisi. 2002. Microarray-based detection and genotyping of viral pathogens. *Proc. Natl. Acad. Sci. USA* **99:**15687–15692.

128. Weinberg, A., L. Brewster, J. Clark, and E. Simoes. 2004. Evaluation of R-Mix shell vials for the diagnosis of viral respiratory tract infections. *J. Clin. Virol.* **30:**100–105.

129. Whiley, D. M., M. W. Syrmis, I. M. Mackay, and T. P. Sloots. 2002. Detection of human respiratory syncytial virus in respiratory samples by LightCycler reverse transcriptase PCR. *J. Clin. Microbiol.* **40:**4418–4422.

130. Williams, J. V., Z. Chen, G. Cseke, D. W. Wright, C. J. Keefer, S. J. Tollefson, A. Hessell, A. Podsiad, B. E. Shepherd, P. P. Sanna, D. R. Burton, J. E. Crowe, Jr., and R. A. Williamson. 2007. A recombinant human monoclonal antibody to human metapneumovirus fusion protein that neutralizes virus in vitro and is effective therapeutically in vivo. *J. Virol.* **81:**8315–8324.

131. Williams, J. V., P. A. Harris, S. J. Tollefson, L. L. Halburnt-Rush, J. M. Pingsterhaus, K. M. Edwards, P. F. Wright, and J. E. Crowe, Jr. 2004. Human metapneumovirus and lower respiratory tract disease in otherwise healthy infants and children. *N. Engl. J. Med.* **350:**443–450.

132. Williams, J. V., P. A. Piedra, and J. A. Englund. 2009. Respiratory syncytial virus, human metapneumovirus, and parainfluenza viruses, p. 817–847. *In* D. D. Richman, R. J. Whitley, and F. G. Hayden (ed.), *Clinical Virology*, 3rd ed. ASM Press, Washington, DC.

133. Williams, J. V., S. J. Tollefson, P. W. Heymann, H. T. Carper, J. Patrie, and J. E. Crowe, Jr. 2005. Human metapneumovirus infection in children hospitalized for wheezing. *J. Allergy Clin. Immunol.* **115:**1311–1312.

134. Wu, W., and Y. W. Tang. 2009. Emerging molecular assays for detection and characterization of respiratory viruses. *Clin. Lab. Med.* **29:**673–693.

135. Wyde, P. R., S. N. Chetty, A. M. Jewell, G. Boivin, and P. A. Piedra. 2003. Comparison of the inhibition of human metapneumovirus and respiratory syncytial virus by ribavirin and immune serum globulin in vitro. *Antivir. Res.* **60:**51–59.

136. Wyde, P. R., E. H. Moylett, S. N. Chetty, A. Jewell, T. L. Bowlin, and P. A. Piedra. 2004. Comparison of the inhibition of human metapneumovirus and respiratory syncytial virus by NMSO3 in tissue culture assays. *Antivir. Res.* **63:**51–59.

137. Zhao, X., F. P. Chen, A. G. Megaw, and W. M. Sullender. 2004. Variable resistance to palivizumab in cotton rats by respiratory syncytial virus mutants. *J. Infect. Dis.* **190:**1941–1946.

138. Zlateva, K. T., L. Vijgen, N. Dekeersmaeker, C. Naranjo, and M. Van Ranst. 2007. Subgroup prevalence and genotype circulation patterns of human respiratory syncytial virus in Belgium during ten successive epidemic seasons. *J. Clin. Microbiol.* **45:**3022–3030.

Measles and Rubella Viruses

WILLIAM J. BELLINI AND JOSEPH P. ICENOGLE

84

Clinical differentiation of fever and rash illnesses caused by measles and rubella viruses has become increasingly difficult. The paucity of measles and rubella cases in the United States and other developed countries has led to a decline in clinical diagnostic acumen among physicians and health care workers (65, 105). Milder forms of measles have been reported to occur in previously vaccinated individuals (42), further obscuring diagnosis based on the clinical case definition. As global programs to control and eliminate measles expand, the medical and public health communities have become more dependent on laboratory confirmation of clinical diagnosis. Moreover, many countries where measles has been controlled by routine vaccination, coupled with mass vaccination and follow-up campaign strategies, are now implementing rubella control measures through the incorporation of rubella and measles combined vaccines in their programs. Laboratory diagnostic tests and laboratory surveillance activities for measles and rubella are performed in parallel in many clinical and public health laboratories worldwide (20). Consequently, this chapter combines the current laboratory diagnostic methods for measles and rubella for convenient review and reference. A summary of laboratory tests for confirmation of measles and rubella, including many of the tests described briefly here, has been published by the World Health Organization (131a).

MEASLES VIRUS

Taxonomy

Measles is the prototypic member of the genus *Morbillivirus* in the family *Paramyxoviridae*, and it is the only member of the genus that causes human disease (112). With rare exception, the members of this genus have restricted host ranges, indicative of long-term association with, and adaptation to, their respective zoonotic hosts. Other genus members include rinderpest virus, canine distemper virus, peste des petits ruminants virus, and cetacean and phocine distemper viruses.

Description of the Agent

Measles virus is an enveloped, nonsegmented, single-stranded, negative-sense RNA virus with a diameter of 120 to 250 nm. The measles virus genome is 15,894 nucleotides in length and contains six structural genes organized on the single strand of RNA in a gene order consistent with those of most of the paramyxoviruses, i.e., 3'-N, P, M, F, H, L-5'. The genome encodes at least eight proteins; three gene products are coded for by the phosphoprotein (P) cistron. The nucleoprotein (N) gene encodes the N protein, which encapsidates both full-length minus-strand (genome) and full-length plus-strand (antigenome) RNAs. The protein products of the P and the polymerase (L) genes interact with the full-length viral RNA and form the ribonucleoprotein complex. Viral nucleocapsid structures are surrounded by a membrane, derived from the plasma membrane, which includes the gene products from the M, F, and H genes (matrix, fusion, and hemagglutinin proteins, respectively). The F and H envelope proteins are N-linked transmembrane glycoproteins and are responsible for fusion of virus with host cell membranes (53, 112). The H glycoprotein is the major target for neutralizing antibody and interacts with the two formerly described cellular receptors for measles virus, CD46 (86) and hSLAM (119).

Although measles virus has only one serotype (monotypic), antigenic and genetic variability has been detected between and among wild-type viruses and vaccine viruses. The nucleotide sequence variability among wild-type viruses is most evident in the genes encoding the N and H proteins (7 to 10%), and the maximum sequence variability has been determined to reside in the last 450 nucleotides of the coding region of the N gene (~12%) (109). Based on this sequence region, a standard nomenclature has been established. For molecular epidemiological purposes, the genotype designations are considered the operational taxonomic unit, while related genotypes are grouped by clades. The World Health Organization (WHO) currently recognizes eight clades, designated A, B, C, D, E, F, G, and H. Within these clades, there are 23 recognized genotypes (109). A recent review by Rota et al. (109) provides an excellent overview of the current status of the molecular epidemiology of measles and the global distribution of the various genotypes.

Epidemiology and Transmission

Measles virus infections are transmitted via aerosols, droplets, or contaminated fomites. Measles is a highly contagious disease, and susceptible individuals who come into close contact with measles patients have a 99% probability of acquiring the disease. In the prevaccine era, more than 90% of individuals would acquire measles infections before 10 years of age.

In unvaccinated populations, measles causes periodic epidemics, with interepidemic periods of 2 to 5 years. These periods decrease as population size and density increase and are directly related to the availability of susceptible individuals for sustained disease transmission.

In vaccinated populations, the interval between measles outbreaks increases, and sufficiently high levels of vaccination can interrupt endemic transmission. With vaccination, the age distribution of cases is determined by which groups are likely to lack vaccine- or measles-induced immunity. In the United States, an extensive effort to achieve high levels of first-dose measles vaccination at 12 to 15 months of age and the addition of a recommended second dose of vaccine in school-age children have resulted in a decrease in reported measles cases from 400,000 to 500,000 per year in the 1960s to record lows of approximately 63 cases from 2000 to 2007, increasing somewhat due to importations in recent years (21, 22, 24). Endemic transmission of measles in the United States was interrupted in 1994, and subsequent cases have occurred through periodic introduction of measles from countries where measles is endemic, occasionally followed by only limited spread (108, 109). Given widespread international travel, measles will continue to occur even in highly vaccinated populations until global eradication is achieved.

Although measles remains a formidable disease of children in many areas of the world, tremendous strides have been made in global measles control and mortality rate reduction between 2000 and 2007. The global mortality rate decreased by 74% from an estimated 750,000 deaths in 2000 to 197,000 deaths in 2007 (25). The number of measles cases has fallen from 40 million to about 10 million cases accordingly over a similar period as estimated by the WHO. Effective use of available live attenuated measles vaccines and a variety of multidose vaccination strategies (second opportunities for vaccination) have combined to eliminate measles in many large geographic regions, including the Americas, Australia, the Scandinavian countries, and the United Kingdom.

Clinical Significance

Uncomplicated Clinical Course

Approximately 1 week to 10 days following exposure, the clinical presentation begins with cough, coryza, conjunctivitis, and fever. The prodromal stage then progresses over the next 3 to 4 days, with all symptoms intensifying and the associated fever reaching as high as 105°F.

Koplik's spots, pathognomonic for measles, appear on the buccal mucosa in 50 to 90% of cases 2 to 3 days before rash onset and may persist for 1 to 2 days following rash onset. These lesions are small, irregular red spots with a bluish white speck in the center. The erythematous rash appears approximately 2 weeks following exposure and is first evident on the forehead or behind the ears. The rash presents as red macules 1 to 2 mm in diameter, becoming maculopapules over the next 3 days. The exanthem is usually most confluent on the face and upper body and initially blanches on pressure. By the end of the second day the trunk and upper extremities are covered with rash, and by the third day the lower extremities are affected. The rash resolves in the same sequence, first disappearing from the face and neck. The lesions turn brown and persist for 7 to 10 days and then are followed by a fine desquamation. In most cases, recovery is rapid and complete.

Death resulting from respiratory and neurological causes (see below) occurs in 1 of every 1,000 measles cases, but estimates during the 1989 to 1991 outbreaks were three to four times higher (5). The risk of death is greater for infants and adults than for children and adolescents. However, rates of acute measles virus infections of infants and children in developing countries, particularly malnourished populations, can approach 10%, with rates of morbidity being much higher.

Complications

The most common complications associated with measles virus infection are otitis media (7 to 9%), pneumonia (1 to 6%), and diarrhea (6%). Pneumonia may occur as a primary viral pneumonia (Hecht pneumonia) or as a bacterial superinfection. Measles commonly involves the central nervous system (CNS), with as many as 50% of cases reported to have electroencephalogram abnormalities during the acute or convalescent phase of the illness (51).

Notable CNS complications include acute disseminated encephalomyelitis and subacute sclerosing panencephalitis (SSPE). Acute disseminated encephalomyelitis occurs approximately 1 week after rash onset in 1 per 1,000 cases and is manifested clinically by seizures, lethargy, irritability, and/or coma. It results in the death of 5 to 30% of patients and causes residual deficits in about 30% of survivors (16, 76). The disease is presently considered an autoimmune disease, since an immune response to myelin basic protein has been reported and measles virus has not been isolated from these patients (70).

SSPE is a progressive, inevitably fatal, late neurological complication caused by persistent measles virus infection of the CNS that occurs in approximately 1 per 100,000 measles cases (81), although recent studies estimate the rate to be 1 per 11,000 cases (8). Only wild-type measles virus nucleic acid sequences have been found in association with this disease. The average time from natural measles virus infection to manifestations of SSPE is 7 years. The disease characteristically involves personality changes, decreased motor and intellectual capabilities, involuntary movements, and muscular rigidity and ultimately leads to death of the patient. The virus is difficult to recover from brain specimens, requiring cocultivation or brain explant techniques, yet measles virus proteins and RNA can readily be detected in brain tissue (73, 115). Patients with SSPE usually have high titers of measles virus-specific antibodies in their sera and cerebrospinal fluid.

Infection during pregnancy is associated with an increased risk of miscarriage and prematurity, although there is no convincing evidence that maternal infection with measles virus is associated with congenital malformations. Clinical illness in the newborn after intrauterine exposure follows a shortened incubation period and may vary from mild to severe.

Atypical measles syndrome occurred in children who had been vaccinated with multiple doses of formalin-killed measles vaccine and subsequently exposed to wild-type measles virus. The syndrome was believed to occur as a result of immunopathological responses due to a combination of the Arthus reaction and delayed hypersensitivity (13). The syndrome has little relevance today, but the experience serves to emphasize the safety concerns that should be addressed by those wishing to develop alternative measles vaccines or to explore alternate routes of vaccine delivery.

The use of combined, live attenuated measles-mumps-rubella (MMR) vaccines has been the subject of controversy, particularly as their use might be associated with immune-mediated bowel disorders, ileal lymphonodular hyperplasia, and a regressive form of autism (125, 127). Reviews conducted by expert panels assembled by the Institute of Medicine, as well as numerous carefully controlled epidemiological and laboratory studies in many countries, including the United States and United Kingdom, have failed to confirm those reports (61, 120). Most recently, the Office of Special Masters of the U.S. Court of Federal Claims rejected test cases claiming compensation for injuries due, in part, to MMR vaccine playing a causal role in autism spectral disorders. A portion of the ruling was based on exhaustive review of the current literature regarding any causal relationship between MMR vaccine and autism spectral disorders. On 28 January 2010, a full retraction from the published record of the original paper by Wakefield and coworkers (127) was made by *The Lancet* (published online 2 February 2010).

Other described complications include thrombocytopenia, stomatitis, laryngotracheobronchitis, hepatitis, appendicitis and ileocolitis, pericarditis and myocarditis, glomerulonephritis, hypocalcemia, and Stevens-Johnson syndrome.

In immunocompromised patients, syndromes such as giant-cell pneumonia and measles inclusion body encephalitis (MIBE) have been observed (11, 84). Measles-induced giant-cell pneumonia is usually unrecognized due to the absence of rash. It usually occurs in patients with deficits in cell-mediated immunity, and several cases have been diagnosed following vaccination of children with severe combined immunodeficiency syndrome (82). MIBE is generally fatal and is best described as the unchecked replication of measles virus in the CNS in the face of an impaired or absent cell-mediated immune response. There are anecdotal reports of more severe and even fatal measles in patients with AIDS (3). However, vaccination is considered safe unless patients are severely immunocompromised.

Collection, Transport, and Storage of Specimens

In general, specimens for successful virus isolation should be collected early in the acute phase of the infection, when the virus is present in high concentrations, and transported to a laboratory under conditions that maintain the infectivity of labile viruses. Suitable samples for isolation of measles virus or for detection of viral antigen can be whole blood, serum, throat and nasopharyngeal secretions, urine, and, in special circumstances, brain and skin biopsy samples. Specimens should be processed as soon as possible after collection and are best kept at 4°C rather than frozen, since freezing causes significant loss of recoverable virus. Specimens should be frozen and shipped with dry ice only if the time between specimen collection and delivery to the laboratory is expected to exceed 48 h.

Transport medium should be used to maintain measles virus until isolation of virus from clinical specimens can be performed. Samples requiring viral transport medium and commercial sources of viral transport medium are reviewed in chapter 76. Measles virus is lymphotropic, and macrophages are a known source of infectious virus during natural infection (46). Thus, peripheral blood mononuclear cells are an excellent source for the isolation of measles virus. Peripheral blood mononuclear cells are obtained from heparinized blood (diluted 1:3 in saline) by sedimentation through density gradients.

Serum specimens from patients with suspected measles should be assayed in an immunoglobulin M (IgM) enzyme-linked immunoassay (EIA) within 7 to 10 days of rash onset, if possible. A single serum specimen is sufficient in most cases (123). To assess seroconversion following measles vaccination, serum specimens can be tested with IgG EIAs or plaque reduction neutralization (PRN) tests (see below). Ideally, paired specimens should be obtained: the first prior to vaccination and the second approximately 3 to 4 weeks later, so that a rise in measles virus-specific IgG can be measured. Serum samples should ideally be stored at −20°C, but antibody is stable for extended periods at 4°C. Samples for IgM determinations should not be frozen and thawed more than five times. Spinal fluid samples should also be obtained if neurological complications are present or suspected.

Respiratory specimens are appropriate for testing. Nasal aspirates or bronchial lavage samples yield virus more frequently than throat swabs, because of the greater likelihood of obtaining infected cells. For immunofluorescence assays (IFAs), slides of respiratory specimens should be fixed in cold acetone for 2 min and stored at 4°C.

For isolation of virus from urine, a large volume of midstream (clean-catch), preferably morning, urine should be collected into a sterile container. Measles virus is very cell associated; thus, the urine is centrifuged at 800 × g for 30 min. The pelleted cells and sediment are resuspended in 1 to 2 ml of Hanks' balanced salt solution in preparation for cell culture, PCR, or other diagnostic methods (107).

Two new approaches show promise in terms of alternatives to serum specimen collection for the diagnosis of measles: the use of oral mucosal transudates (OMT) (see chapter 76) and the use of blood spots on filter paper. OMT samples have been used both for detection of measles virus-specific IgM and IgG and for detection of hepatitis, rubella, mumps, and other viral infections (57, 91, 92, 94). This specimen collection method has been used successfully for many years for routine measles surveillance in the United Kingdom (14). The use of OMT samples has appeal because the collection method is noninvasive. The specimens can be used for rubella testing, do not require processing in the field, and offer the opportunity to detect measles virus-specific IgM for case confirmation and nucleic acids for molecular characterization (23, 69). Commercial serologic assays performed with OMT samples can result in heightened background reactivity and decreased sensitivity; cold chain issues remain a problem with OMT specimens in warmer climates. Devices (such as OraSure) containing compounds that stabilize IgM should be avoided if molecular testing is to be performed, as these additives inhibit nucleic acid amplification enzymes.

Like OMT samples, blood spots collected onto filter paper do not require processing in the field, but a cold chain does not appear to be necessary. They can be used to test for rubella as well as for measles (32, 33, 40, 58, 97, 111, 126), and they can be used for molecular characterization of the measles virus genome (41), although virus isolation would not be possible. In addition, the eluted serum from blood spots can likely be tested in commercially available measles virus EIAs without the loss of sensitivity and specificity (41, 58, 78), making this technology very attractive for widespread use. Although still considered an invasive technique, finger stick as a method for sample collection is often more acceptable to parents than phlebotomy (128).

In June 2007, the WHO convened a special meeting of the Laboratory Network collaborators to review the available data on use of OMT and dried blood spots (DBS). Among the recommendations that emerged, the committee endorsed the use of both methods as viable options for measles and rubella surveillance in all regions, especially where patients might resist venipuncture, or where special challenges exist with specimen storage or transportation (23).

Direct Examination

Cytologic Examination

Characteristic cytopathic effects (CPE) of measles virus infection include multinucleated cells and cellular inclusions (intracytoplasmic and intranuclear). Cytologic examination of various lymphoid tissue specimens and secretions frequently reveals the presence of giant cells with multiple overlapping nuclei, Warthin-Finkeldey giant cells. Slides can be stained with either Wright stain or hematoxylin and eosin. Tissue samples may be fixed in 10% formalin, embedded in paraffin, sectioned, and then stained with hematoxylin and eosin (50). Staining of tissue specimens with monoclonal antibodies (see below) to the measles virus N protein has been used for the diagnosis of giant-cell pneumonia and MIBE (132).

Immunofluorescence

Detection of measles virus can be achieved using an IFA to examine clinical specimens as well as cell cultures infected with clinical material. The standard assay uses a commercially available monoclonal antibody to the N protein of measles virus and fluorescein-conjugated goat anti-mouse antiserum (see "Confirmation of Measles Virus Isolation"). Nasal secretions are centrifuged at $800 \times g$ to pellet the cells. The cell pellets are then washed several times with sterile saline before being applied to a glass slide and fixed in cold 80% acetone for 10 min at $-20°C$ (79, 117).

Nucleic Acid Detection Techniques

Standard and real-time reverse transcriptase PCR (RT-PCR) assays have been used in research settings to detect measles virus RNA in a variety of clinical specimens and infected cells (49, 64, 85, 103, 107, 114). While measles virus IgM serology remains the recommended routine diagnostic test for acute measles virus infections, molecular detection methods can be more advantageous in certain circumstances. Therefore, RT-PCR should be considered for diagnostic use where IgM testing is compromised by the concurrent or recent use of measles virus-containing vaccine as part of an outbreak response or in settings of recent vaccine distribution, such as supplemental immunization activities (65). Likewise, molecular detection methods can be used when cell culture isolation is not a practical alternative, and/or when genetic characterization of the virus is required. RT-PCR amplification and nucleotide sequencing of the last 450 nucleotides of the coding region of the N protein gene permit genotype analysis of the sequence of the measles virus strain and delineation between vaccine and wild-type virus (see "Genotyping" below). Such techniques are still only performed in highly specialized laboratories such as the Global Specialized Laboratories and some regional reference laboratories or more advanced national laboratories of the WHO-LabNet and have been particularly useful in confirming MIBE, SSPE, and giant-cell pneumonia (8, 11, 82, 84).

Isolation and Identification of Measles Virus

Measles virus can be isolated from the conjunctiva, nasopharynx, and blood during the latter part of the prodromal period and during the early stages of rash development. Although virus has been isolated from the urine as late as 4 to 7 days after rash onset, viremia generally clears 2 to 3 days after rash onset, in parallel with the appearance of antibody. Thus, virus can be most readily isolated within a period from 2 to 4 days prior to rash onset to about 4 days after rash onset.

Though other cell cultures and lines, such as primary monkey kidney and Vero cells, have traditionally been used (53), an Epstein-Barr virus-transformed B lymphoblastoid cell line derived from marmoset lymphocytes until recently has been the preferred cell line for primary isolation of measles virus (75). These cells (B95a cells) were found to be as much as 10,000 times more sensitive for isolation of measles virus from clinical specimens than other cell lines. However, laboratorians should note that this cell line does produce Epstein-Barr virus and should be handled as infectious material at all times. B95a cells can no longer be obtained from commercial sources, thus dramatically restricting the widespread use of this cell line.

Recently, a Vero cell line transfected with a plasmid encoding the protein for the human signaling lymphocyte activation marker (hSLAM) molecule has been constructed (89). The hSLAM molecule has been shown to be a cell surface receptor for both wild-type and laboratory-adapted strains of measles virus. Testing conducted to date indicates that the sensitivity of Vero/hSLAM cells for isolation of measles virus is equivalent to that of B95a cells. Vero/hSLAM cells also express the simian CD46 molecule. The cell line has been recommended for use in the WHO Laboratory Network as a replacement for the B95a cell line. The CPE that results following measles virus infection is essentially that observed in measles virus-infected Vero cells (Fig. 1).

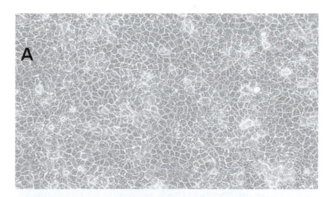
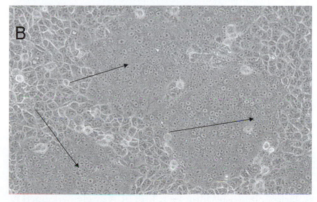

FIGURE 1 CPE of measles virus when propagated in Vero/hSLAM cells, a cell line that is transfected with a gene encoding the wild-type virus receptor (CDw150) for measles virus. The cell line naturally expresses the simian form of CD46 on the cell surface. (A) Uninfected monolayer of Vero/hSLAM cells; (B) measles virus-infected monolayer of Vero/hSLAM cells with apparent syncytium formation and multinucleated giant cells (arrows).

The advantage of Vero/hSLAM cells is that they are not persistently infected with Epstein-Barr virus, and therefore, they are not considered hazardous material like B95a cells. This provides a significant safety advantage for laboratorians and greatly facilitates international shipments. The disadvantage of Vero/hSLAM cells is that they must be cultured in medium containing Geneticin to retain hSLAM expression. This increases the cost of the cell culture medium. Laboratories (U.S. public health and WHO global laboratory network laboratories) should only accept Vero/hSLAM cells from a WHO-approved source (regional reference laboratory or global specialized laboratory). Upon receipt, the cells should be passaged in medium containing 400 μg of Geneticin/ml as described in the protocol distributed with the cell line. Laboratories should passage the cells two to four times in the presence of Geneticin to expand the number of cell culture vessels sufficient for preparation of 20 to 50 vials of seed stock for liquid nitrogen storage.

To prepare cells for virus isolation procedures, Vero/hSLAM cells can be recovered from liquid nitrogen and passaged up to 15 times in medium without the addition of Geneticin. These cells should be used for virus isolation attempts only and should be discarded after 15 passages. Even with addition of Geneticin to the medium, the cells should not be passaged forward beyond about 20 to 30 passages, as with the standard Vero cell line. Cells that have been passaged without Geneticin in the medium should never be used to prepare cell stocks for liquid nitrogen storage or shipped to another network laboratory for use in virus isolation.

Confirmation of Measles Virus Isolation

Confirmation of isolation is most often achieved by IFA and uses a monoclonal antibody to detect the N protein or another internal antigen of measles virus in infected cells. The infected cells are fixed onto a microscope slide. Binding of the measles virus-specific antibody is detected using a goat anti-mouse antibody that is conjugated to fluorescein isothiocyanate. Immunofluorescent-antibody test kits are available from Millipore Corporation, Billerica, MA (Light Diagnostics, catalog no. 3187). It is also possible to configure an indirect IFA without using a commercial kit. Most monoclonal antibodies to the N protein (Light Diagnostics, catalog no. 5030; available from Millipore Corporation) or other internal antigens (catalog no. 20-902-170205; GenWay BioTech, Inc., San Diego, CA) perform well in the IFA procedure described below. Monoclonal antibodies directed against other viral proteins, such as the H and F proteins, may recognize conformational epitopes that are not stable after acetone fixation. When configuring an in-house IFA, the appropriate working dilutions of monoclonal antibody and fluorescein isothiocyanate-labeled conjugate have to be determined by experimental titration. There are no commercial RT-PCR kits available for measles virus, and while the CDC does provide standard protocols, and validation standards to public health laboratories that wish to develop in-house assays, confirmation of cell culture isolation of measles virus by RT-PCR is rarely performed in the clinical laboratory.

Genotyping

Amplicon sequencing and phylogenetic analysis (genotyping) of the last 450 nucleotides of the measles N gene has proven useful in suggesting the possible source of virus involved in outbreaks, tracking transmission pathways during outbreaks, and differentiating between vaccine and wild-type strains of measles virus (106, 109). The latter application is the most pertinent to measles diagnostics but is rarely performed at the state or local public health laboratory level. In general, these laboratories are asked to collect appropriate viral specimens from suspected cases and send them to the CDC if the results of IgM serology are positive.

Molecular epidemiology in conjunction with conventional case investigation and epidemiology has permitted the linking of imported cases of measles from Japan (genotype D5) to a multistate outbreak associated with an international sporting event in 2007 (21), from Switzerland to clusters of measles cases in California and Arizona (genotype D5) in 2008 (22), and from India to a children's hospital in Pennsylvania in 2009 (genotype D8 [CDC, unpublished data]).

Genetic characterization of wild-type measles viruses provides a means to study the transmission pathways of the virus and is an essential component of laboratory-based surveillance. Laboratory-based surveillance for measles and rubella, including genetic characterization of wild-type viruses, is performed throughout the world by the WHO Measles and Rubella Laboratory Network, which serves 166 countries in all WHO regions. In particular, the genetic data can help confirm the sources of virus or suggest a source for unknown-source cases as well as to establish links, or lack thereof, between various cases and outbreaks. Virologic surveillance has helped to document the interruption of transmission of endemic measles in some regions. Thus, molecular characterization of measles viruses has provided a valuable tool for measuring the effectiveness of measles control programs, and virologic surveillance needs to be expanded in all areas of the world and conducted during all phases of measles control (20, 109). It must be emphasized, however, that conventional epidemiology and case investigation must be done hand in hand with the molecular studies to achieve the optimal outcome of this approach. Drawing conclusions from genotype determinations without proper epidemiological investigation can lead to false assumptions regarding geographic origin or source of infections.

Serologic Diagnosis

The recommended laboratory method for the confirmation of clinically diagnosed measles is a serum-based IgM EIA. Several serum-based IgM EIAs are commercially available and are used worldwide by public health, clinical, and commercial laboratories. These assays have been used as the primary confirmatory test by the laboratory network of the Pan American Health Organization-supported measles eradication effort throughout the Americas. The WHO Global Measles Laboratory Network has also recommended use of the IgM EIA for laboratory diagnosis of measles (20). The EIAs can be done using a single serum specimen, are relatively rapid (2 to 6 h), are simple to perform, and can be used to diagnose acute measles virus infection from the time of rash onset until at least 4 weeks after rash onset. Thus, the IgM EIAs fulfill all of the basic criteria for the accurate, effective, and efficient diagnosis of measles. Both indirect and IgM capture formats have been used (44, 63, 110). Though the IgM capture assay format is often regarded as more sensitive than the indirect format, comparative studies of some commercial indirect formatted EIA kits have demonstrated that the two formats have equivalent sensitivities and specificities (4, 100).

Traditional antibody tests such as hemagglutination inhibition (HI), PRN, and EIA have been used extensively in the serologic diagnosis of measles. However, because of the availability of sensitive and specific commercial kits, EIA has become the most widely used test format. Commercial EIAs also have the ability to measure measles virus-specific IgM as well as IgG responses and therefore have particular importance in diagnosis as well as measles control programs. Some of the available kits were found to have sensitivities and specificities that compared favorably with those of PRN (30, 38, 99). Most laboratories have trained personnel and are already equipped to run EIAs.

Standard EIAs

Several commercial assays now include measles virus antigens produced by recombinant DNA expression systems, such as baculovirus or a yeast, rather than antigen produced by infected cell cultures. EIAs using recombinant-expressed N protein in both capture and indirect formats have high sensitivity and specificity compared to those of other commercial EIAs (63, 110).

Though the configurations of the commercial measles virus IgM kits vary, the tests are simple and straightforward to perform by following the manufacturers' protocols. Indirect EIA has been successful in the detection of IgG (63). For this indirect test, either whole virus antigen diluted in 0.05 M bicarbonate buffer (pH 9.5) or recombinant antigen diluted in phosphate-buffered saline is distributed into polystyrene microtiter plates. Serum specimens are diluted in phosphate-buffered saline containing 4% normal goat serum (plus 4% Sf9 cell lysate for recombinant antigen) and 0.05% EDTA and then added to the washed plates. Bound antibody can be detected with standard commercial reagents such as goat anti-human IgG conjugated to either alkaline phosphatase or biotin. Assays are developed with the appropriate substrate, and the plates can be read either by eye or with the aid of a spectrophotometer.

PRN

The PRN assay, which measures neutralizing antibodies that are directed against the surface glycoproteins of measles virus, is more sensitive and specific than HI or EIA (2). Since functional antibodies are detected, the PRN provides the best serologic correlate for the assessment of immune protection (28, 31). However, the PRN test is not practical for routine serologic diagnosis because it is very labor-intensive, requires paired serum samples, and takes 5 to 7 days to complete. Recently, a fluorescence-based plaque reduction microneutralization assay for measles virus immunity (54) has been developed that permits higher-throughput processing of small quantities of serum specimens and is more amenable for use in large serosurveys for assessing immune status. This assay has been standardized against the conventional PRN assay (30) using the WHO 2nd International Standard for antimeasles serum and awaits further validation.

In the PRN assay, measles virus-specific antibody in serum combines with and neutralizes measles virus, preventing it from infecting a cell monolayer and forming a plaque under the overlay. The endpoint for the test is the highest dilution of serum which reduces the number of plaques by 50%. Serum dilutions are made in 96-well microtiter trays, making either two- or fourfold dilutions (depending on the expected titer of the serum). Once the dilutions of serum samples are made, an equal volume (120 µl) of a dilution of virus containing 25 to 35 PFU is added to each well and incubated for 2.5 h at 36°C. After incubation, 100 µl of the serum-virus

mixture is added to each of two 16-mm-diameter wells on a tissue culture plate(s) containing Vero cell monolayers. These plates are then incubated for 1 h at 36°C. Following incubation, the inoculum is removed by aspiration, and the monolayers are covered with overlay medium consisting of either 2% carboxymethyl cellulose in Leibovitz-15 medium or 1% agarose in Eagle's medium. The plates are then incubated for 4 days at 36°C, and the monolayers are stained with a solution of neutral red in cell culture medium. On day 5, the overlay is removed and the plaques are counted. The numbers of PFU in duplicate wells representing a given serum dilution are averaged.

New EIAs

A new and potentially promising development has been the use of EIAs to measure the avidity of IgG antibodies to measles virus (39, 124). As the immune response matures, low-avidity antibodies are replaced with high-avidity antibodies. These avidity differences can be detected by using protein denaturants, 6 to 8 M urea or diethylamine (S. Mercader, P. Garcia, and W. Bellini, CDC, unpublished data) in the washing step of the indirect EIA for measles virus IgG. An avidity index is then calculated by comparing the optical densities obtained with and without the denaturing agent in the wash buffer. These tests show promise in differentiating between primary and secondary responses to vaccination and to natural infection (93). However, the lack of appropriate guidelines for use of such assays coupled with the lack of performance standards and standard protocols for the assays places these assays in the realm of investigational tools for the time being.

Evaluation, Interpretation, and Reporting of Results

The interpretation of negative culture results should be made with caution, since many factors influence the outcome. Some of the most important considerations include the timing of sample collection, transportation to the laboratory, preparation for culture, and finally, and probably most importantly, the cell culture system used for virus isolation. In a recent survey of public health laboratories, of those that performed cell culture for measles virus, most were not using cell lines containing cell surface receptors that would optimize successful isolation of wild-type measles virus (http://www.aphl.org/aphlprograms/infectious/Documents/VPD_Report_2009.pdf). The same report indicated that very few (10 of 55) state and local public health laboratories responding to the survey performed measles virus real-time RT-PCR. Negative real-time RT-PCR results cannot be used to rule out a case of measles, since many of the same factors mentioned to influence culture also influence the outcome of this detection method. Moreover, genomic regions selected for amplification for measles virus RT-PCR assays do not distinguish between wild-type and vaccine viruses and thus would not be useful in many outbreak settings where vaccine is in use to control the outbreak.

The serum-based IgM assay is the recommended test for the confirmation of acute measles virus infection. False-negative results can occur when serum specimens taken too early with respect to rash onset are tested. For example, the CDC capture IgM assay, which has a sensitivity and specificity equivalent to those of commercial EIAs, has been shown to detect IgM in only 77% of true measles cases within the first day of rash onset (56). In the case of indirect IgM assays, false-negative values can be the result of insufficient removal of high levels of measles virus-specific IgG from a test specimen. The residual IgG competes with IgM

TABLE 1 Interpretation of measles virus EIA results[a]

IgM result	IgG result	Infection history	Current infection	Comment(s)
+	+ or −	Not previously vaccinated, no history of measles	Recent first MCV[b]	Seroconversion,[c] postvaccination, low-avidity IgG, if present
+	+ or −	Not vaccinated, no history of measles	Wild-type measles virus	Seroconversion,[c] classic measles, low-avidity IgG, if present
+	+ or −	Previously vaccinated, primary vaccine failure	Recent second MCV vaccination	Seroconversion,[c] postvaccination; low-avidity IgG confirms primary failure, if present
−	+	Previously vaccinated, IgG positive	Recent second MCV vaccination	IgG level may stay the same or increase; high-avidity IgG
+	+	Previously vaccinated, IgG positive	Wild-type measles virus	May have few or no symptoms[d]
+	+	Recently vaccinated	Exposed to wild-type measles virus	Cannot distinguish if vaccine or wild-type virus infection; evaluate on epidemiological grounds[e]
+ or −	+	Distant history of measles	Wild-type measles virus	May have few or no symptoms[d]; if clinically compatible, may have been misdiagnosed initially

[a]Modified from reference 7.
[b]MCV, measles virus-containing vaccine.
[c]IgG level depends on timing of specimen collection.
[d]Rare occurrence; do not consider contagious unless clinical presentation is consistent with measles.
[e]If result is IgM negative, it is helpful to rule out wild-type measles virus infection.

for viral antigen placed on the solid-phase support, thereby blocking IgM binding to the antigen and interfering with IgM detection. Present-day immune absorbent reagents are much improved over earlier reagents; thus, fewer problems of this nature occur.

False-positive tests due to the presence of rheumatoid factor (RF) appear to be more frequently encountered when using the indirect IgM assay. RF is an IgM class immunoglobulin that reacts with IgG and is produced as a result of some viral diseases and autoimmune diseases. Immune complexes may form that contain test antigen-specific IgG and RF IgM. By virtue of the IgG binding to the viral antigen, the IgM component of the RF immune complex is recognized by the detector system, thus rendering a false-positive result. Similar false-positive results can occur in capture assays but appear to be enhanced by the presence of high levels of both antigen-specific antibody and RF (44).

The inherent sensitivities and specificities of the EIAs in times of low disease prevalence become a factor in interpretation. This situation occurs in countries that have eliminated endemic measles but remain vigilant in performing case-based surveillance of rash illnesses. In these geographic regions, both measles virus IgM and IgG EIAs are performed on serum specimens from suspected cases due to high vaccine-induced seroprevalence. In this setting, if the IgG test is positive and the IgM test is negative, the case is discarded (depending upon the timing of serum collection).

Unfortunately, EIA specificity is not 100%. Serum specimens from patients with parvovirus B19 and rubella have inherent rates of false-positive reactions (overall rate of about 4%) when tested in measles virus IgM EIAs and vice versa (68, 121). The reason(s) for these false-positive reactions is not understood, and attempts to remove immune complexes using anti-RF have proven unsuccessful.

There is also evidence that case contacts that have a resident IgG response, due either to a history of natural infection or to vaccination, may develop a secondary IgG or an IgM response to currently circulating virus (45, 59). The IgM is generally fleeting and weakly positive and, except for

rare instances, should not pose a source of confusion to the diagnostic laboratory (66).

Table 1 summarizes the possible interpretations of EIA results. Despite the vagaries associated with the EIAs, they are the best assays available for laboratory confirmation of clinically diagnosed measles. It should be emphasized that the vast majority of serum specimens submitted for serology yield a test result that will be easily interpretable. However, laboratorians should be provided with as much information as possible about the clinical disease and epidemiological investigation to aid in the final interpretation of the test result.

RUBELLA VIRUS

Taxonomy

A number of small, enveloped viruses having the same overall genetic organization and replication strategy as rubella virus exist, and they are grouped into the *Togaviridae* family. The *Togaviridae* family consists of the *Rubivirus* genus, containing only rubella virus, and the *Alphavirus* genus, containing about 25 other viruses, all of which are transmitted by arthropods (e.g., western equine encephalitis virus). Rubella virus has a restricted host range and appears to infect only humans.

Description of the Agent

Rubella virus virions are particles about 70 nm in diameter that are comprised of a core surrounded by a lipid envelope. The core consists of the positive-strand genome ($\sim$9,760 nucleotides) and the virus protein C. The viral envelope contains two viral glycoproteins, E1 and E2. The viral RNA replicates in the cytoplasm of infected cells, with nonstructural proteins being translated from the 5′ two-thirds of the genomic RNA and the structural proteins being translated from a subgenomic RNA that is a copy of the 3′ one-third of the genomic RNA. New virions are produced when genomic RNA, the E1 glycoprotein, the E2 glycoprotein, and the C protein assemble at cellular membranes (26, 104).

Rubella viruses currently circulating in the world contain RNAs that differ sufficiently that two clades of rubella viruses, differing by about 10% in the nucleotide sequence, have so far been identified (48, 71). Groups of related viruses within the clades have been classified as genotypes. At present, nine genotypes and four provisional genotypes of rubella viruses have been recognized (131). Only minor immunologic differences exist among circulating viruses. Immunity to one rubella virus is sufficient to protect against clinical disease caused by other known rubella viruses.

Clinical Significance

Rubella (German measles or 3-day measles) was first described in the 18th century and was accepted as a disease independent of measles and scarlet fever in 1881 (34). Postnatal rubella is characterized by an acute onset and generalized maculopapular rash with mild fever (higher than 99°F) and may include arthritis or arthralgia (mostly in postpubertal females), lymphadenopathy (specifically postauricular and suboccipital nodes), and conjunctivitis. Because disease caused by rubella virus is mild, about 50% of postnatal rubella cases are not diagnosed. Although rubella had been largely ignored for 60 years, N. McAlister Gregg first recognized that cataracts in children followed maternal rubella during gestation (52). The association between congenital rubella and a spectrum of significant birth defects including sensorineural hearing loss, cardiovascular abnormalities, cataracts, congenital glaucoma, and meningoencephalitis is now accepted. Rubella virus is now recognized as the most potent infectious teratogenic agent yet identified (77, 113, 129).

When rubella occurs in a pregnant woman in the first 11 weeks of gestation, there is a high likelihood of defect(s) in the infant (about 90%). After 18 weeks, the likelihood of birth defect is much lower, although the infant may still be born infected with rubella virus. Congenital rubella virus infection (CRI) refers to infants born with rubella virus infection with or without birth defects. The pathogenesis of CRI leading to congenital rubella syndrome (CRS) is not well understood, but rubella virus infection early in gestation results in an altered immune response to the virus and altered organogenesis. The significant effect on the fetus of rubella virus infection during the first trimester is likely related to the facts that the fetus cannot synthesize IgM until about 20 weeks of gestation and cell-mediated immunity does not develop until late in gestation. Congenitally infected infants shed virus for long periods, have a slowly developing immune response to rubella virus, and respond to particular rubella virus proteins differently than individuals with postnatal rubella. These three characteristics of congenital infection are all consistent with selective immune tolerance to rubella virus proteins in such infants (26). Infection during the first 11 weeks of gestation often results in multiple organ involvement and necrosis in many tissues (77). Organogenesis is affected in CRS cases, since specific organs are abnormal and other apparently normal organs have a reduced number of cells. Reinfection with rubella virus can occur, but viremia is rare; reinfection of a pregnant woman poses low risk to the fetus (10, 77).

CRI results in both shedding of virus and IgM antibodies in the neonate. Diagnosis is based on detection of rubella virus or rubella virus-specific IgM in such patients. If congenital defects characteristic of CRS are not present, the infant is diagnosed as having CRI only. The clinical definition of CRS is standardized, but laboratory confirmation of rubella virus infection in the newborn by either serologic or culture techniques is critical, especially when only a single defect presents, since the defects characteristic of CRS can occur for other reasons (17).

Epidemiology and Transmission

Rubella virus was not isolated until 1962, largely because infected cells are difficult to identify in tissue culture (90, 130). Introduction of rubella vaccine (licensed in 1969) in the United States, mostly through childhood immunization, immediately broke the 6- to 9-year epidemic cycle of rubella. The last major U.S. rubella epidemic was in 1964 to 1965, when 20,000 CRS cases occurred (62). The combined MMR vaccine was recommended for the United States in 1972. The current incidence of CRS in the United States is very low (one case in 2005, one case in 2006, no cases in 2007 and 2008, and one provisional case in 2009). Most mothers of affected infants were born in countries without rubella immunization programs or with recently organized programs (102). Occasional outbreaks of rubella in some U.S. populations have not spread to the undervaccinated populations, suggesting that herd immunity has been protective (101). Indigenous rubella and CRS have been eliminated from the United States, and these diseases are targeted for elimination from the Americas and Europe by 2010 (15, 19) (http://www.euro.who.int/__data/assets/pdf.file/0008/79028/E87772.pdf). Despite the possibility of worldwide rubella eradication, rubella remains endemic in many countries and about 100,000 to 200,000 CRS cases occur annually in the world (6, 36, 96). Postnatal transmission of rubella virus is often by close contact with an infected individual, such as occurs in correctional institutions or day care centers.

The safety of live rubella virus vaccine strains is well documented (95). A recent summary indicated that only 1 of 833 infants born to rubella-susceptible mothers who were inadvertently vaccinated after conception were born with abnormalities consistent with CRS (10, 80). However, a small theoretical risk remains. Thus, the Advisory Committee on Immunization Practices recommends avoiding pregnancy after receipt of rubella-containing vaccine for 28 days (18).

Collection, Transport, and Storage of Specimens

Clinical specimens for culture of rubella virus are usually throat swabs or nasopharyngeal secretions diluted into transport medium (e.g., Culturette collection and transport devices). The virus can also be isolated from a number of other specimens, including cataract tissue and urine (provided that pH is controlled) (6). Urine is often a source of infectious virus from CRS patients. Specimens for virus detection should be stored at 4°C for short periods (days) or at −70°C for longer periods (weeks); virions lose infectivity at higher temperatures (e.g., 37°C). Virions are rapidly inactivated by mild heat (56°C), detergents, or lipid solvents. Rubella virus-specific IgG can be detected in urine (118). Specimens for serology or culture can be transported by standard methods (e.g., overnight carrier) at 4°C since virions are relatively stable at that temperature. Alternative specimens, such as DBS and OMT (see chapter 76), have been shown to be adequate for surveillance of rubella using IgM detection (DBS and OMT) and virus detection (OMT) (1, 23, 55, 58, 69, 88, 98). Two caveats should be considered if these alternative specimens are used. First, diagnostic kits are usually not approved by the FDA for use with DBS; second, low IgM levels in OMT necessitate the use of highly sensitive detection assays.

The timing of specimen collection is especially important in postnatal rubella. Rubella virus-specific IgM is the laboratory diagnostic criterion typically used for rubella, but about 50% of rubella cases are IgM negative on the day of rash (see Table 2 and related text below). Since postnatal rubella is a mild disease of short duration, special effort may be required to obtain a serum sample 5 to 7 days after rash, when most rubella patients are strongly IgM positive. Patients with CRS are IgM and virus positive for months; therefore, timing is less critical for these patients.

Direct Examination

Nucleic Acid Detection Techniques

Amplification of rubella virus RNA directly from a clinical specimen by RT-PCR can be used to determine if a patient is infected with rubella virus. Not all RT-PCR protocols are sufficiently sensitive to be used directly with clinical specimens. Assays that can reliably detect 3 to 10 copies of rubella virus RNA are sufficiently sensitive. Real-time and nested RT-PCR protocols, although difficult to maintain, usually meet this criterion (1, 12, 35).

Many postnatal rubella cases are IgM negative before 4 to 5 days postrash, and direct detection of viral RNA is the most sensitive test during this period (1). For example, on the day of rash onset, direct detection of rubella RNA by real-time assay will confirm about twice as many suspected rubella cases as commercial IgM enzyme-linked immunosorbent assays (ELISAs). No standard real-time or RT-PCR protocol for detection of viral RNA has been established, and there are currently a number of such tests being used. At present, real-time assays and RT-PCR are mostly used in national or reference laboratories.

Isolation and Identification of the Virus

Growth of rubella virus from clinical specimens can be used to diagnose postnatal rubella, CRS, and CRI (Table 2). Throat swabs taken on the day of rash, typically a convenient time for sample collection, are usually positive for rubella virus, even though a slightly higher percentage of cases are positive 2 days before rash onset. Virus shedding in the throat declines rapidly, and by 4 days after rash onset, only about 50% of cases are positive. In addition, viral culture is used to monitor virus in CRS and CRI patients for the purpose of determining when isolation of these patients from susceptible contacts can be stopped. The virus grows in a variety of cell types, including Vero, BHK21, AGMK, and RK-13 cells. The primary problem encountered with tissue culture is the lack of a cell type that produces CPE in a single passage of wild-type viruses. Historically, this problem was overcome by clever assays exploiting the fact that rubella virus growth interferes with the replication of lytic enteroviruses such as coxsackievirus A9. However, interference assays are quite difficult to maintain (29). Virus growth can now be identified in the absence of CPE using methods such as RT-PCR, IFA, and immunocolorimetric assays (ICA) to detect viral RNA or proteins (27, 133).

The sensitivity of the RT-PCR system used to detect viral RNA from infected tissue culture cells is not critical, since the amount of rubella viral RNA has been amplified by passage in tissue culture (about 10^6-fold) (48, 133). Detection of rubella virus-infected cell monolayers can also be accomplished by IFA or ICA. It is crucial that IFA and ICA reagents have low background, since rubella virus culture does not produce high levels of progeny virus (about 10^7 PFU/ml for laboratory strains such as f-Therien). Infected cells are easily identified when stained with high-quality reagents (Fig. 2). Dilution of specimens may be desirable since it is useful to have both infected and uninfected cells in the same field. Monoclonal antibodies to the E1, E2, and C proteins, which react with both reduced and nonreduced antigens on Western blots, often work well in IFA and ICA.

Utility of Sequences Derived from Viral RNA

Sequencing of the nucleic acid amplified directly from specimens or from tissue culture material can provide useful information. Vaccine virus can be differentiated from wild-type viruses (47). Useful information on the origin of imported cases of rubella and CRS can be obtained (74). Documentation of the elimination of rubella can be supported by analysis of sequences obtained over time (67).

Serologic Tests

ELISA

Detection of rubella virus-specific IgM by either IgM capture ELISA or indirect IgM ELISA is the fastest and most

TABLE 2 Timing of biological markers of rubella virus infection[a]

Diagnostic criterion	Convenient time when many cases are positive	Example of a time when >90% of cases are positive	Approx time for 50% decline[b]
Postnatal rubella			
Virus in throat by culture[c]	Day of rash (90%)	2 days *before* rash	4 days after rash
IgM in serum by ELISA[c]	Day of rash (50%)	5 days after rash	6 wk after rash
IgG in serum by ELISA	3 days after rash (50%)	8 days after rash	Lifetime
Virus in blood by culture[d]	Day of rash (50%)	5 days *before* rash	1 day after rash
CRS[e]			
Virus in throat by culture	At birth (almost all)	2 wk after birth	3 mo of age
IgM in serum by ELISA	At birth (80%)	1 mo of age	6 mo of age
IgG in serum by ELISA[f]			

[a]Times and percentages given are approximate and are meant to guide typical specimen collection. Percentages vary depending on the sensitivity of the assay used. Note that the times listed in the third column were chosen to help guide specimen collection and may not be the earliest time when >90% of cases are positive.
[b]After maximum number of cases are positive for a given criterion, the approximate time for 50% of cases to become negative.
[c]"Alternative" specimens, OMT and DBS, have been evaluated for detection of virus (OMT) and IgM (OMT and DBS). See references 1, 23, 55, 69, and 98.
[d]Data taken from reference 37.
[e]Information given is for fetal infection in the first trimester.
[f]Declining maternal IgG and developing IgG response in a CRS patient lead to high (steady) or increasing IgG levels in the CRS patient through the first year of life.

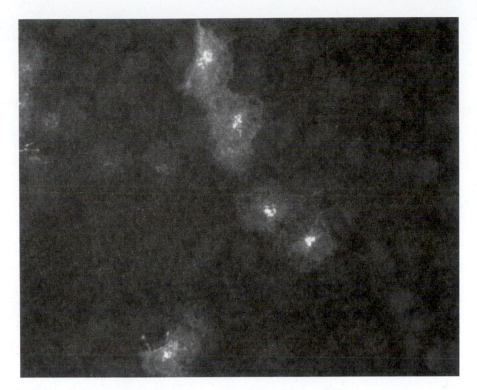

FIGURE 2   IFA of rubella virus-infected cells using monoclonal antibody to the E2 protein. Vero cells were infected with wild-type rubella virus and 3 days after infection were fixed with cold paraformaldehyde, followed by permeabilization with −20°C methanol. Reaction of infected cells with monoclonal antibody to the E2 protein (monoclonal antibody 24–26; Meridian Life Science, Saco, ME) was followed by detection of bound monoclonal antibody with Alexa Fluor 488-conjugated, highly cross-absorbed goat anti-mouse IgG (Molecular Probes Inc., Eugene, OR). Cell nuclei were visualized by staining with propidium iodide. About 25% of the cells which stained with propidium iodide were positive for E2 protein.

cost-effective diagnostic test for recent postnatal infection. Unfortunately, only about 50% of postnatal rubella cases are IgM positive on the day of symptom onset (Table 2) (1). Most postnatal rubella cases have virus-specific IgM detectable by capture ELISA from 5 until 40 days after symptom onset and IgG by indirect ELISA ≥8 days after symptom onset (Fig. 3) (43, 122). A negative IgM serologic result 4 to 5 days after onset should be followed with testing of a serum sample taken as soon as possible thereafter to avoid false-negative results (17). If acute- and convalescent-phase sera are available, a fourfold rise in rubella virus-specific IgG is diagnostic for postnatal rubella infection; such sera should be taken as early as possible after disease onset and about 2 to 3 weeks after disease onset. When IgG titers are used for diagnostic purposes, a dilution series of each serum sample should be made and ELISA results for each dilution series compared, since optical density values at a single dilution are an unreliable measure of the amount of IgG.

The same ELISAs may be used to confirm CRS. Most congenitally infected infants have IgM detectable from birth to 1 month of age (Table 2). The percentage of infants who are IgM positive declines over the first year of life. At 1 year, most infants are negative. In CRS patients, the IgG response increases gradually over the first 9 months, while maternal IgG declines. Thus, high or increasing IgG levels in the first year of life, in the absence of vaccination or significant risk of postnatal rubella, are consistent with CRS. Precise recommendations for the best times for collection

of samples from postnatal rubella and CRS cases have been published (17).

Latex Agglutination

Commercial rapid latex particle agglutination tests consist of latex spheres coated with rubella virus antigen. These particles aggregate in the presence of either rubella virus-specific IgG or IgM. Because high throughput is possible with these assays, they are often used in immunity screening programs (e.g., prenatal screening).

HI

The HI test was once the standard test for antibodies to rubella virus, and many current tests are calibrated using HI assays. However, indicator erythrocytes are not readily available, and the assay is difficult to perform as a diagnostic test since removal of nonspecific inhibitors and internal standardization are required.

IFA

IFA has been used for detection of IgG and IgM antibodies to rubella virus. Typically cells expressing rubella virus proteins and control cells are reacted with patient serum, and any rubella virus-specific antibodies are then detected with fluorescent dye-labeled goat anti-human IgG (or IgM) and fluorescence microscopy. Negative human sera and uninfected control cells are useful for detecting nonspecific signal. Fluorescence should be cell associated. Staining

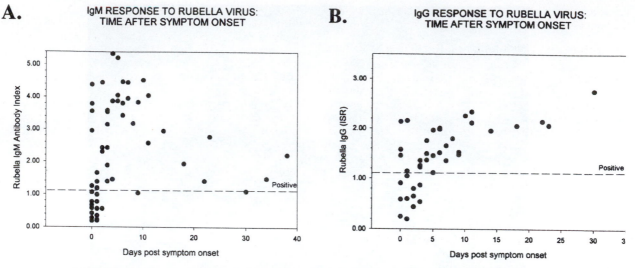

FIGURE 3 Time course of rubella virus-specific IgM and IgG detection by ELISA in sera of rubella patients. Commercial IgM capture ELISA (A) and IgG indirect ELISA (B) were used to detect rubella virus-specific antibodies at the indicated number of days after onset of symptoms (usually rash); antibody index and ISR are the commercial test designations for the ratio of the optical density obtained for the test serum to the optical density obtained for a standard (cutoff) serum. The minimum signal considered positive in each test is indicated by a dashed line. Only results from patients who tested positive for IgM to rubella virus at some time after the onset of symptoms are shown.

restricted to the periphery of the cell monolayer is artifactual and not indicative of a true-positive result.

PRN

PRN is performed when a quantitative assessment of the neutralizing capacity of an antiserum is necessary. A laboratory strain (e.g., f-Therien) should be used, since viruses from clinical specimens do not exhibit CPE. The assay follows a format common to many viruses. The initial step is incubation of 2- or 10-fold dilutions of antiserum and a standard amount of rubella virus (usually about 100 to 200 PFU) in medium or buffer containing protein to inhibit losses on surfaces (e.g., 0.1% bovine serum albumin) for 1 h at 35 to 37°C, followed by overnight in a refrigerator. A control consisting of virus alone must be included in the assay, since some reduction in the number of plaques is observed during the 1-h incubation. Virus-antiserum specimens are then allowed to attach to confluent Vero cell monolayers for 1 h at 35°C and then overlaid with DEAE dextran (100 μg/ml)-containing medium with 0.5% agar (e.g., Oxoid). Medium in the agar overlay is typically Dulbecco's modified Eagle's medium; 1% fetal calf serum may also be included to maintain the monolayer. After 6 days, agar is removed and plates are stained with neutral red. Crystal violet can also be used; however, a wash step to remove dead cells should be used prior to crystal violet staining. The ICA for rubella virus can also be used for virus detection (27). The neutralizing capacity of the antiserum is typically reported as the inverse of the antiserum dilution giving a standard reduction in plaques, typically 90% reduction. In both vaccination of nonimmune individuals and postnatal rubella cases the neutralizing capacity rises at least 100-fold, allowing the easy use of PRN data to confirm past exposure to rubella. However, information on the precise assay used is required to quantitatively compare neutralization capacities of antisera when assays are done in different

laboratories (e.g., rubella virus plaquing efficiency may vary among laboratories).

Other Serologic Tests

Avidity tests have been used when IgM detection does not reliably indicate recent infection (e.g., first serum sample was collected months after clinical symptoms). Low-avidity anti-rubella IgG suggests recent infection (60, 87, 121). This test compares the ability of detergents or chaotropic agents to dissociate case IgG and control IgGs from rubella virus proteins. Both high- and low-avidity control sera should be used in each assay. Avidity tests are not widely available and vary in performance (83).

Since the clinical symptoms of postnatal rubella and CRS are dramatically different, it is not surprising that there are significant differences in the immune responses of patients with these diseases. These differences can be observed on Western blots, in which antibodies in sera from CRS patients often demonstrate different reactivity to rubella glycoproteins than those from postnatal rubella patients (72). These tests are not widely used but have been developed in some diagnostic laboratories (10).

Prenatal Screening

The present description of laboratory testing for rubella emphasizes identification of postnatal and congenital rubella cases. However, in the United States much of the testing is for immunity to rubella, since health care providers should test for immunity by a serum IgG test in all pregnant women at the earliest prenatal visit. There are slightly different criteria for rubella immunity that are recommended by various groups (range is about 10 to 15 IU/ml) (95). Commonly used tests, e.g., ELISA, are standardized to give positive results for 10 IU/ml, the breakpoint defining immunity to rubella in the United States (116). Much of the screening for immunity to rubella virus in the United States is done by automated random-access systems using microparticle immunoassays.

Evaluation, Interpretation, and Reporting of Results

IgM and IgG testing should be done with most sera for both suspected postnatal rubella and CRS cases, since results from both immunoglobulin classes often provide additional information useful for diagnosis. For example, results from a serum sample taken at 8 days postrash which are positive for IgM but negative for IgG to rubella virus would be inconsistent with the immune response to rubella; usually the IgM result would be most suspect in this situation (e.g., cross-reaction with antibodies to parvovirus).

A positive result for rubella virus culture is obtained when a positive real-time assay or RT-PCR result is obtained from the culture or at least one cluster of cells is infected as determined by IFA or ICA. Control cultures must be negative. When an IFA or ICA is used, the expected distribution of viral proteins should be obtained (e.g., E1 glycoprotein distribution when using an E1 monoclonal antibody) (27).

Direct detection of rubella virus RNA by PCR-based protocols requires the laboratory to evaluate the significance of results from such tests. Multiple negative controls and amplified product in more than one specimen from a given patient will increase confidence of a positive diagnosis based on direct RT-PCR. The significance of negative results is usually difficult to determine, since false-negativity rates are usually not available. Sequence variation in wild-type viruses, which can lead to poor primer binding and poor amplification, must be considered when evaluating the significance of negative results. Nevertheless, when serum from a patient cannot be obtained, or when confirmation of serologic results is desired, direct detection of rubella virus RNA by RT-PCR may be necessary since it is more rapid than viral culture.

There is often a considerable burden on the laboratory in the diagnosis of rubella. For example, when primary rubella virus infection is suspected for a pregnant woman, false positives and false negatives may lead to incorrect clinical decisions (9). Thus, the laboratorian may be asked to go beyond just communicating false-positivity and false-negativity rates. Testing for recent infection with other viruses that cause clinically similar diseases (e.g., human parvovirus B19) is often prudent. Positive rubella results may be more believable if no other infection is found. Specimen retesting and testing of different specimen types with alternative methods (e.g., serology and viral culture [Table 2]) often yield consistent results and reduce the likelihood of false-positive results. False positives can occur even with IgM capture ELISA. For example, in one study, 1 of 87 sera testing positive for rubella virus-specific IgM by IgM capture ELISA was from a patient whose final diagnosis was primary human parvovirus B19 infection (121). False negatives can often be identified by testing multiple specimens from a patient (e.g., sera taken 1 week apart). If only a single specimen is available, it may be tested by multiple assays. For example, IgG avidity may resolve the diagnosis from a single serum sample that is IgM positive for both rubella virus and human parvovirus B19 (121).

Postnatal rubella can be clinically similar to other diseases, or it can be asymptomatic. Additionally, birth defects characteristic of CRS occur for other reasons. Thus, correct classification of suspected postnatal rubella and CRS is based on laboratory results rather than clinical presentation. Classification of a postnatal rubella case results in its categorization as suspected, probable, confirmed, or asymptomatic confirmed; for a case of congenital rubella, categories are suspected CRS, probable CRS, confirmed CRS, or infection only. Positive laboratory results are required to correctly classify asymptomatic confirmed or confirmed cases of postnatal rubella and CRS. Clinical, laboratory, and epidemiological information (e.g., international travel) all may enter into the final clinical decision(s). A full description of classification criteria and recommendations should be consulted (17). One specific diagnostic situation should be noted. A series of tests including a rubella virus IgM test should not be used to determine immunity in a pregnant woman because of the possibility of a false-positive result; immunity should be determined by IgG testing alone. Since standard TORCH (toxoplasmosis, other, rubella, cytomegalovirus, and herpes simplex virus) panels include testing for rubella virus IgM, they should not be used to determine immunity.

REFERENCES

1. **Abernathy, E., C. Cabezas, H. Sun, Q. Zheng, M.-H. Chen, C. Castillo-Solorzano, A. C. Ortiz, F. Osores, L. Oliveira, A. Whittembury, J. K. Andrus, R. F. Helfand, and J. Icenogle.** 2009. Confirmation of rubella within 4 days of rash onset: comparison of rubella virus RNA detection in oral fluid with immunoglobulin M detection in serum or oral fluid. *J. Clin. Microbiol.* **47:**182–188.
2. **Albrecht, P., K. Herrmann, and G. R. Burns.** 1981. Role of virus strain in conventional and enhanced measles plaque neutralization test. *J. Virol. Methods* **3:**251–260.
3. **Angel, J. B., P. Walpita, R. A. Lerch, M. S. Sidhu, M. Masurekar, R. A. DeLellis, J. T. Noble, D. R. Snydman, and S. A. Udem.** 1998. Vaccine-associated measles pneumonitis in an adult with AIDS. *Ann. Intern. Med.* **129:**104–106.
4. **Arista, S., D. Ferraro, A. Cascio, E. Vizzi, and R. di Stefano.** 1995. Detection of IgM antibodies specific for measles virus by capture and indirect enzyme immunoassays. *Res. Virol.* **146:**225–232.
5. **Atkinson, W. L., W. A. Orenstein, and S. Krugman.** 1992. The resurgence of measles in the United States, 1989–1990. *Annu. Rev. Med.* **43:**451–463.
6. **Banatvala, J. E., and D. W. G. Brown.** 2004. Rubella. *Lancet* **363:**1127–1137.
7. **Bellini, W. J., and P. A. Rota.** 1999. Measles (rubeola) virus, p. 603–621. *In* E. H. Lennette and T. F. Smith (ed.), *Laboratory Diagnosis of Viral Infections*, 3rd ed. Marcel Dekker, Inc., New York, NY.
8. **Bellini, W. J., J. S. Rota, L. E. Lowe, R. S. Katz, P. R. Dyken, S. R. Zaki, W.-J. Shieh, and P. A. Rota.** 2005. Subacute sclerosing panencephalitis: more cases of this fatal disease are prevented by measles immunization than previously recognized. *J. Infect. Dis.* **192:**1686–1693.
9. **Best, J. M., S. O'Shea, G. Tipples, N. Davies, S. M. Al-Khusaiby, A. Krause, L. M. Hesketh, L. Jin, and G. Enders.** 2002. Interpretation of rubella serology in pregnancy: pitfalls and problems. *Br. Med. J.* **325:**147–148.
10. **Best, J. M., J. P. Icenogle, and D. W. G. Brown.** 2009. Rubella, p. 561–592. *In* A. J. Zuckerman, J. E. Banatvala, B. D. Schoub, P. D. Griffiths, and P. Mortimer (ed.), *Principles and Practice of Clinical Virology*, 6th ed. Wiley-Blackwell, Singapore, Singapore.
11. **Bitnun, A., P. Shannon, A. Durward, P. A. Rota, W. J. Bellini, C. Graham, E. Wang, E. L. Ford-Jones, P. Cox, L. Becker, M. Fearon, M. Petric, and R. Tellier.** 1999. Measles inclusion body encephalitis caused by the vaccine strain of measles virus. *Clin. Infect. Dis.* **29:**855–861.
12. **Bosma, T. J., K. M. Corbett, S. O'Shea, J. E. Banatvala, and J. M. Best.** 1995. PCR for detection of rubella virus RNA in clinical samples. *J. Clin. Microbiol.* **33:**1075–1079.
13. **Brodsky, A. L.** 1972. Atypical measles: severe illness in recipients of killed measles virus vaccine upon exposure to natural infection. *JAMA* **222:**1415–1416.

14. Brown, D., M. Ramsey, A. Richards, and E. Miller. 1994. Salivary diagnosis of measles: a study of notified cases in the United Kingdom, 1991–3. *Br. Med. J.* **308:**1015–1017.

15. Castillo-Solórzano, C., and J. K. Andrus. 2004. Rubella elimination and improving health care for women. *Emerg. Infect. Dis.* **10:**2017–2021.

16. Centers for Disease Control. 1981. Measles encephalitis—United States, 1962–1979. *MMWR Morb. Mortal. Wkly. Rep.* **30:**362–364.

17. Centers for Disease Control and Prevention. 2001. Control and prevention of rubella: evaluation and management of suspected outbreaks, rubella in pregnant women, and surveillance for congenital rubella syndrome. *MMWR Morb. Mortal. Wkly. Rep.* **50**(RR-12):1–23.

18. Centers for Disease Control and Prevention. 2001. Notice to readers: revised ACIP recommendation for avoiding pregnancy after receiving a rubella-containing vaccine. *MMWR Morb. Mortal. Wkly. Rep.* **50:**1117.

19. Centers for Disease Control and Prevention. 2005. Achievements in public health: elimination of rubella and congenital rubella syndrome—United States, 1969–2004. *MMWR Morb. Mortal. Wkly. Rep.* **54:**279–282.

20. Centers for Disease Control and Prevention. 2005. Global Measles and Rubella Laboratory Network, January 2004–June 2005. *MMWR Morb. Mortal. Wkly. Rep.* **54:**1100–1104.

21. Centers for Disease Control and Prevention. 2008. Multistate measles outbreak associated with an international youth sporting event—Pennsylvania, Michigan, and Texas, August–September, 2007. *MMWR Morb. Mortal. Wkly. Rep.* **57:**169–173.

22. Centers for Disease Control and Prevention. 2008. Outbreak of measles—San Diego, California, January–February 2008. *MMWR Morb. Mortal. Wkly. Rep.* **57:**203–206.

23. Centers for Disease Control and Prevention. 2008. Recommendations from an ad hoc meeting of the WHO measles and rubella laboratory network (LabNet) on use of alternative diagnostic samples for measles and rubella surveillance. *MMWR Morb. Mortal. Wkly. Rep.* **57:**657–660.

24. Centers for Disease Control and Prevention. 2008. Update: measles—United States, January–July 2008. *MMWR Morb. Mortal. Wkly. Rep.* **57:**893–896.

25. Centers for Disease Control and Prevention. 2008. Progress in measles control and mortality reduction, 2000–2007. *MMWR Morb. Mortal. Wkly. Rep.* **57:**1303–1306.

26. Chantler, J., J. S. Wolinsky, and A. Tingle. 2001. Rubella virus, p. 963–990. *In* D. M. Knipe, P. M. Howley, D. E. Griffin, R. A. Lamb, M. A. Martin, B. Roizman, and S. E. Straus (ed.), *Fields Virology*, 4th ed. Lippincott Williams and Wilkins, Philadelphia, PA.

27. Chen, M.-H., Z. Zhen, Y. Zhang, S. Favors, W. Xu, D. A. Featherstone, and J. P. Icenogle. 2007. An indirect immunocolorimetric assay to detect rubella virus infected cells. *J. Virol. Methods* **146:**414–418.

28. Chen, R. T., L. E. Markowitz, P. Albrecht, J. A. Stewart, L. M. Mofenson, S. R. Preblud, and W. A. Orenstein. 1990. Measles antibody: reevaluation of protective titers. *J. Infect. Dis.* **162:**1036–1042.

29. Chernesky, M. A., and J. B. Mahony. 1999. Rubella virus, p. 964–969. *In* P. R. Murray, E. J. Baron, M. A. Pfaller, F. C. Tenover, and R. H. Yolken (ed.), *Manual of Clinical Microbiology*, 7th ed. ASM Press, Washington, DC.

30. Cohen, B. J., R. P. Parry, D. Doblas, D. Samuel, L. Warrener, N. Andrews, and D. Brown. 2006. Measles immunity testing: comparison of two measles IgG ELISAs with plaque reduction neutralisation assay. *J. Virol. Methods* **131:**209–212.

31. Cohen, B. J., S. Audet, N. Andrews, J. Beeler, and on Behalf of the WHO Working Group on Measles Plaque Reduction Neutralization Test. 2007. Plaque reduction neutralization test for measles antibodies: description of a standardised laboratory method for use in immunogenicity studies of aerosol vaccination. *Vaccine* **26:**59–66.

32. Condorelli, F., G. Scalia, A. Stivala, R. Gallo, A. Marino, C. M. Battaglini, and A. Castro. 1994. Detection of immunoglobulin G to measles virus, rubella virus, and mumps virus in serum samples and in microquantities of whole blood dried on filter paper. *J. Virol. Methods* **49:**25–36.

33. Condorelli, F., A. Stivala, R. Gallo, A. Marino, C. M. Battaglini, A. Messina, G. Russo, A. Castro, and G. Scalia. 1998. Use of a microquantity enzyme immunoassay in a large-scale study of measles, mumps, and rubella immunity in Italy. *Eur. J. Clin. Microbiol. Infect. Dis.* **17:**49–52.

34. Cooper, L. Z. 1985. The history and medical consequences of rubella. *Rev. Infect. Dis.* **7:**S2–S10.

35. Cooray, S., L. Warrener, and L. Jin. 2006. Improved RT-PCR for diagnosis and epidemiological surveillance of rubella. *J. Clin. Virol.* **35:**73–80.

36. Cutts, F. T., and E. Vynnycky. 1999. Modeling the incidence of congenital rubella syndrome in developing countries. *Int. J. Epidemiol.* **28:**1176–1184.

37. Davis, W. J., H. E. Larson, J. P. Simsarian, P. D. Parkman, and H. M. Meyer, Jr. 1971. A study of rubella immunity and resistance to infection. *JAMA* **215:**600–608.

38. de Sousa, V. A., C. S. Pannuti, L. M. Sumita, and P. Albrecht. 1991. Enzyme-linked immunosorbent assay (ELISA) for measles antibody. A comparison with hemagglutination inhibition, immunofluorescence and plaque neutralization tests. *Rev. Inst. Med. Trop. São Paulo* **33:**32–36.

39. de Souza, V. A., C. S. Pannuti, L. M. Sumita, and H. F. de Andrade. 1997. Enzyme-linked immunosorbent assay-IgG antibody avidity test for single sample serologic evaluation of measles vaccines. *J. Med. Virol.* **52:**275–279.

40. de Souza, V. A., L. M. Sumita, M. E. Otsubo, K. Trakei, and C. S. Pannuti. 1995. Enzyme linked immunosorbent assay for rubella antibodies: a simple method of antigen production. A preliminary report. *Rev. Inst. Med. Trop. São Paulo* **37:**357–359.

41. De Swart, R. L., Y. Nur, A. Abdallah, H. Kruining, H. S. Mubarak, S. A. Ibrahim, B. Van Den Hoogen, J. Groen, and A. D. Osterhaus. 2001. Combination of reverse transcriptase PCR analysis and immunoglobulin M detection on filter paper blood samples allows diagnostic and epidemiological studies of measles. *J. Clin. Microbiol.* **39:**270–273.

42. Edmonson, M. D. B., G. Addiss, J. T. McPherson, J. L. Berg, S. R. Circo, and J. P. Davis. 1990. Mild measles and secondary vaccine failure during a sustained outbreak in a highly vaccinated population. *JAMA* **263:**2467–2471.

43. Enders, G. 1985. Serologic test combinations for safe detection of rubella infections. *Rev. Infect. Dis.* **7:**S113–S122.

44. Erdman, D. D., L. J. Anderson, D. R. Adams, J. A. Stewart, L. E. Markowitz, and W. J. Bellini. 1991. Evaluation of monoclonal antibody-based capture enzyme immunoassays for detection of specific antibodies to measles virus. *J. Clin. Microbiol.* **29:**1466–1471.

45. Erdman, D. D., J. L. Heath, J. C. Watson, L. E. Markowitz, and W. J. Bellini. 1993. Immunoglobulin M antibody response to measles virus following primary and secondary vaccination and natural infection. *J. Med. Virol.* **41:**44–48.

46. Esolen, L. M., B. J. Ward, T. R. Moench, and D. E. Griffin. 1993. Infection of monocytes during measles. *J. Infect. Dis.* **168:**47–52.

47. Frey, T. K., and E. S. Abernathy. 1993. Identification of strain-specific nucleotide sequences in the RA27/3 rubella virus vaccine. *J. Infect. Dis.* **168:**854–864.

48. Frey, T. K., E. S. Abernathy, T. J. Bosma, W. G. Starkey, K. M. Corbett, J. M. Best, S. Katow, and S. C. Weaver. 1998. Molecular analysis of rubella virus epidemiology across three continents, North America, Europe, and Asia, 1961–1997. *J. Infect. Dis.* **178:**642–650.

49. Fujino, M., N. Yoshida, S. Yamaguchi, N. Hosaka, Y. Ota, T. Notomi, and T. Nakayama. 2005. A simple method for the detection of measles virus genome by loop-mediated isothermal amplification (LAMP). *J. Med. Virol.* **76:**406–413.

50. Gershon, A., and S. Krugman. 1979. Measles virus, p. 665–693. *In* E. H. Lennette and N. J. Schmidt (ed.), *Diagnostic Procedures for Viral, Rickettsial and Chlamydial Infections.* American Public Health Association, Washington, DC.

51. Gibbs, F. A., E. L. Gibbs, P. R. Carpenter, and H. W. Spies. 1959. Electroencephalographic abnormality to "uncomplicated" childhood diseases. *JAMA* **72:**1050–1055.

52. Gregg, N. M. 1941. Congenital cataract following German measles in the mother. *Trans. Ophthalmol. Soc. Aust.* **3:**35–46.

53. Griffin, D. E., and W. J. Bellini. 1996. Measles virus, p. 1267–1312. *In* B. N. Fields, D. M. Knipe, and P. M. Howley (ed.), *Fields Virology*, 3rd ed., vol. I. Lippincott-Raven Publishers, Philadelphia, PA.

54. Haralambieva, I. H., I. G. Ovsyannikova, R. A. Vierkant, and G. A. Poland. 2008. Development of a novel efficient fluorescent-based plaque reduction microneutralization assay for measles virus immunity. *Clin. Vaccine Immunol.* **15:**1054–1059.

55. Helfand, R. F., C. Cabezas, E. Abernathy, C. Castillo-Solorzano, A. C. Ortiz, H. Sun, F. Osores, L. Oliveira, A. Whittembury, M. Charles, J. Andrus, and J. Icenogle. 2007. Comparison of detection of rubella-specific IgM and IgG in dried blood spots and sera collected during a rubella outbreak in Peru. *Clin. Vaccine Immunol.* **14:**1522–1525.

56. Helfand, R. F., J. L. Heath, L. J. Anderson, E. F. Maes, D. Guris, and W. J. Bellini. 1997. Diagnosis of measles with an IgM capture EIA: the optimal timing of specimen collection after rash onset. *J. Infect. Dis.* **175:**195–199.

57. Helfand, R. F., S. Kebede, J. P. Alexander, W. Alemu, J. L. Heath, H. E. Gary, L. J. Anderson, H. Beyene, and W. J. Bellini. 1996. Comparative detection of measles-specific IgM in oral fluid and serum from children by an antibody-capture IgM EIA. *J. Infect. Dis.* **173:**1470–1474.

58. Helfand, R. F., H. L. Keyserling, I. Williams, A. Murray, J. Mei, C. Moscatiello, J. Icenogle, and W. J. Bellini. 2001. Comparative detection of measles and rubella IgM and IgG derived from filter paper blood and serum samples. *J. Med. Virol.* **65:**751–757.

59. Helfand, R. F., D. K. Kim, H. E. Gary, G. L. Edwards, G. P. Bisson, M. J. Papania, J. L. Heath, D. L. Schaff, W. J. Bellini, S. C. Redd, and L. J. Anderson. 1998. Nonclassic measles infections in an immune population exposed to measles during a college bus trip. *J. Med. Virol.* **56:**337–341.

60. Hofmann, J., M. Kortung, B. Pustowoit, R. Faber, U. Piskazeck, and U. G. Liebert. 2000. Persistent fetal rubella vaccine virus infection following inadvertent vaccination during early pregnancy. *J. Med. Virol.* **61:**155–158.

61. Hornig, M., T. Briese, T. Buie, M. L. Bauman, G. Lauwers, U.Siemetzki, K. Hummel, P. A. Rota, W. J. Bellini, J. J. O'Leary, O. Sheils, E. Alden, L. Pickering, and W. I. Lipkin. 2008. Lack of association between measles virus vaccine and autism with enteropathy: a case-control study. *PLoS One* **3:**e3140.

62. Horstmann, D. M. 1991. Rubella, p. 617–631. *In* A. S. Evens (ed.), *Viral Infections of Humans: Epidemiology and Control.* Plenum Medical Book Company, New York, NY.

63. Hummel, K. B., D. D. Erdman, J. L. Heath, and W. J. Bellini. 1992. Baculovirus expression of the nucleoprotein gene of measles virus and utility of the recombinant protein in diagnostic enzyme immunoassays. *J. Clin. Microbiol.* **30:**2874–2880.

64. Hummel, K. B., L. Lowe, W. J. Bellini, and P. A. Rota. 2006. Development of quantitative gene-specific real-time RT-PCR assays for the detection of measles virus in clinical specimens. *J. Virol. Methods* **132:**166–173.

65. Hutchins, S. S., L. E. Markowitz, P. Mead, D. Mixon, J. Sheline, N. Greenberg, S. R. Preblud, W. A. Orenstein, and H. F. Hull. 1990. A school-based measles outbreak: the effect of a selective revaccination policy and risk factors for vaccine failure. *Am. J. Epidemiol.* **132:**157–168.

66. Hyde, T. B., R. Nandy, C. J. Hickman, J. R. Langidrik, P. M. Strebel, M. J. Papania, J. F. Seward, and W. J. Bellini. 2009. Laboratory confirmation of measles in elimination settings: experience from the Republic of the Marshall Islands, 2003. *Bull. W. H. O.* **87:**93–98.

67. Icenogle, J. P., T. K. Frey, E. Abernathy, S. E. Reef, D. Schnurr, and J. A. Stewart. 2006. Genetic analysis of rubella viruses found in the United States between 1966 and 2004: evidence that indigenous rubella viruses have been eliminated. *Clin. Infect. Dis.* **43**(Suppl. 3):S127–S132.

68. Jenkerson, S. A., M. Beller, J. P. Middaugh, and D. D. Erdman. 1995. False positive rubeola IgM tests. *N. Engl. J. Med.* **332:**1103–1104.

69. Jin, L., A. Vyse, and D. W. Brown. 2002. The role of RT-PCR assay of oral fluid for diagnosis and surveillance of measles, mumps and rubella. *Bull. W. H. O.* **80:**76–77.

70. Johnson, R. T., D. E. Griffin, R. L. Hirsch, J. S. Wolinsky, S. Roedenbeck, I. Lindo de Soriano, and A. Vaisberg. 1984. Measles encephalomyelitis—clinical and immunologic studies. *N. Engl. J. Med.* **310:**137–141.

71. Katow, S. 1998. Rubella virus genome diagnosis during pregnancy and mechanism of congenital rubella. *Intervirology* **41:**163–169.

72. Katow, S., and A. Sugiura. 1985. Antibody response to individual rubella virus proteins in congenital and other rubella virus infections. *J. Clin. Microbiol.* **21:**449–451.

73. Katz, M., and H. Koprowski. 1973. The significance of failure to isolate infectious viruses in cases of subacute sclerosing panencephalitis. *Arch. Gesamte Virusforsch.* **41:**390–393.

74. Kellenberg, J., S. Buseman, K. Wright, J. F. Modlin, E. A. Talbot, J. T. Montero, S. Reef, E. Abernathy, J. Icenogle, and R. Plotinsky. 2005. Brief report: imported case of congenital rubella syndrome—New Hampshire, 2005. *MMWR Morb. Mortal. Wkly. Rep.* **54:**1160–1161.

75. Kobune, F., H. Sakata, and A. Sugiura. 1990. Marmoset lymphoblastoid cells as a sensitive host for isolation of measles virus. *J. Virol.* **64:**700–705.

76. LaBoccetta, A. C., and A. S. Tornay. 1964. Measles encephalitis. Report of 61 cases. *Am. J. Dis. Child.* **107:**247–255.

77. Lee, J.-Y., and D. S. Bowden. 2000. Rubella virus replication and links to teratogenicity. *Clin. Microbiol. Rev.* **13:**571–587.

78. Mercader, S., D. Featherstone, and W. J. Bellini. 2006. Comparison of available methods to elute serum from dried blood spot samples for measles serology. *J. Virol. Methods* **137:**140–149.

79. Minnich, L. L., F. Goodenough, and C. G. Ray. 1991. Use of immunofluorescence to identify measles virus infections. *J. Clin. Microbiol.* **29:**1148–1150.

80. Minussi, L., R. Mohrdieck, M. Bercini, T. Ranieri, M. T. V. Sanseverino, W. Momino, S. M. Callegari-Jacques, and L. Schuler-Faccini. 2008. Prospective evaluation of pregnant women vaccinated against rubella in southern Brazil. *Reprod. Toxicol.* **25:**120–123.

81. Modlin, J. F., J. T. Jabbour, J. J. Witte, and N. A. Halsey. 1977. Epidemiologic studies of measles, measles vaccine, and subacute sclerosing panencephalitis. *Pediatrics* **59:**505–512.

82. Monafo, W. J., D. B. Haslam, R. L. Roberts, S. Zaki, W. J. Bellini, and C. M. Coffin. 1994. Disseminated measles infection following vaccination in a child with a congenital immune deficiency. *J. Pediatr.* **124:**273–276.

83. Mubareka, S., H. Richards, M. Gray, and G. A.Tipples. 2007. Evaluation of commercial rubella immunoglobulin G avidity assays. *J. Clin. Microbiol.* **45:**231–233.

84. Mustafa, M. M., S. D. Weitman, N. J. Winick, W. J. Bellini, C. F. Timmons, and J. D. Siegel. 1993. Subacute measles encephalitis in the young immunocompromised host: report of two cases diagnosed by polymerase chain reaction and treated with ribavirin and review of the literature. *Clin. Infect. Dis.* **16:**654–660.

85. Nakayama, T., T. Mori, S. Yamaguchi, S. Sonoda, S. Asamura, R. Yamashita, Y. Takeuchi, and T. Urano. 1995. Detection of measles virus genome directly from clinical samples by reverse transcriptase-polymerase chain reaction and genetic variability. *Virus Res.* **35:**1–16.

86. Naniche, D., G. Varior-Krishnan, F. Cervoni, T. F. Wild, B. Rossi, C. Rabourdin-Combe, and D. Gerlier. 1993. Human membrane cofactor protein (CD46) acts as a cellular receptor for measles virus. *J. Virol.* **67:**6025–6032.

87. Nedeljkovic, J., T. Jovanovic, and C. Oker-Blom. 2001. Maturation of IgG avidity to individual rubella virus structural proteins. *J. Clin. Virol.* **22:**47–54.

88. Nokes, D. J., F. Enquselassie, W. Nigatu, A. J. Vyse, B. J. Cohen, D. W. Brown, and F. T. Cutts. 2001. Has oral fluid the potential to replace serum for the evaluation of population immunity levels? A study of measles, rubella and hepatitis B in rural Ethiopia. *Bull. W. H. O.* **79:**588–595.

89. **Ono, N., H. Tatsuo, Y. Hidaka, T. Aoki, H. Minagawa, and Y. Yanagi.** 2001. Measles viruses on throat swabs from measles patients use signaling-lymphocyte activation molecule (CDw150) but not CD46 as a cellular receptor. *J. Virol.* **75:**4399–4401.

90. **Parkman, P. D., and E. L. Buescher.** 1962. Recovery of rubella virus from army recruits. *Proc. Soc. Exp. Biol. Med.* **111:**225–230.

91. **Parry, J. V., K. R. Perry, and P. P. Mortimer.** 1987. Sensitive assays for viral antibodies in saliva: an alternative to tests on serum. *Lancet* ii:72–75.

92. **Parry, J. V., K. R. Perry, S. Panday, and P. P. Mortimer.** 1989. Diagnosis of hepatitis A and B by testing saliva. *J. Med. Virol.* **28:**255–260.

93. **Paunio, M., K. Hedman, I. Davidkin, and H. Peltola.** 2003. IgG avidity to distinguish secondary from primary vaccination failures: prospects for a more effective global measles elimination strategy. *Expert Opin. Pharmacother.* **4:**1215–1225.

94. **Perry, K., D. Brown, J. Parry, S. Panday, C. Pipkin, and A. Richards.** 1993. Detection of measles, mumps, and rubella antibodies in saliva using antibody capture radioimmunoassay. *J. Med. Virol.* **40:**235–240.

95. **Plotkin, S. A.** 1999. Rubella vaccine, p. 409–439. *In* S. A. Plotkin and W. A. Orenstein (ed.), *Vaccines*, 3rd ed. W. B. Saunders, Philadelphia, PA.

96. **Plotkin, S. A.** 2001. Rubella eradication. *Vaccine* **19:**3311–3319.

97. **Punnarugsa, V., and V. Mungmee.** 1991. Detection of rubella virus immunoglobulin G (IgG) and IgM antibodies in whole blood on Whatman paper: comparison with detection in sera. *J. Clin. Microbiol.* **29:**2209–2212.

98. **Ramsay, M. E., R. Brugha, D. W. Brown, B. J. Cohen, and E. Miller.** 1998. Salivary diagnosis of rubella: a study of notified cases in the United Kingdom, 1991–4. *Epidemiol. Infect.* **120:**315–319.

99. **Ratnam, S., V. Gadag, R. West, J. Burris, E. Oates, F. Stead, and N. Bouilianne.** 1995. Comparison of commercial enzyme immunoassay kits with plaque reduction neutralization test for detection of measles virus antibody. *J. Clin. Microbiol.* **33:**811–815.

100. **Ratnam, S., G. Tipples, C. Head, M. Fauvel, M. Fearon, and B. J. Ward.** 2000. Performance of indirect immunoglobulin M (IgM) serology tests and IgM capture assays for laboratory diagnosis of measles. *J. Clin. Microbiol.* **38:**99–104.

101. **Reef, S. E., T. K. Frey, K. Theall, E. Abernathy, C. L. Burnett, J. Icenogle, M. M. McCauley, and M. Wharton.** 2002. The changing epidemiology of rubella in the 1990s: on the verge of elimination and new challenges for control and prevention. *JAMA* **287:**464–472.

102. **Reef, S. E., S. Plotkin, J. F. Cordero, M. Katz, L. Cooper, B. Schwartz, L. Zimmerman-Swain, M. C. Danovaro-Holliday, and M. Wharton.** 2000. Preparing for elimination of congenital rubella syndrome (CRS): summary of a workshop on CRS elimination in the United States. *Clin. Infect. Dis.* **31:**85–95.

103. **Riddell, M. A., D. Chibo, H. A. Kelly, M. G. Catton, and C. G. Birch.** 2001. Investigation of optimal specimen type and sampling time for detection of measles virus RNA during a measles epidemic. *J. Clin. Microbiol.* **39:**375–376.

104. **Risco, C., J. L. Carrascosa, and T. K. Frey.** 2003. Structural maturation of rubella virus in the Golgi complex. *Virology* **312:**261–269.

105. **Robertson, S. E., L. E. Markowitz, D. A. Berry, E. F. Dini, and W. A. Orenstein.** 1992. A million dollar measles outbreak: epidemiology, risk factors, and a selective revaccination strategy. *Public Health Rep.* **107:**24–31.

106. **Rota, J. S., W. J. Bellini, and P. A. Rota.** 2000. Measles, p. 168–193. *In* R. C. A. Thompson (ed.), *Molecular Epidemiology of Infectious Diseases.* Kluwer Academic & Lippincott Raven Publishers, London, United Kingdom.

107. **Rota, P. A., A. L. Khan, E. Durigon, T. Yuran, Y. S. Villamarzo, and W. J. Bellini.** 1995. Detection of measles virus in RNA in urine specimens from vaccine recipients. *J. Clin. Microbiol.* **33:**2485–2488.

108. **Rota, P. A., J. S. Rota, S. Redd, M. Papania, and W. J. Bellini.** 2004. Genetic analysis of measles viruses isolated in the United States between 1989 and 2001: absence of an endemic genotype since 1994. *J. Infect. Dis.* **189**(Suppl. 1):160–164.

109. **Rota, P. A., D. A. Featherstone, and W. J. Bellini.** 2008. Molecular epidemiology of measles virus. *Curr. Top. Microbiol. Immunol.* **330:**129–150.

110. **Samuel, D., K, Sasnauskas, L. Jin, A. Gedvilaite, R. Slibinskas, S. Beard, A. Zvirbliene, S. A. Oliveira, J. Staniulis, B. Cohen, and D. Brown.** 2003. Development of a measles specific IgM ELISA for use with serum and oral fluid samples using recombinant measles nucleoprotein produced in Saccharomyces cerevisiae. *J. Clin. Virol.* **28:**121–129.

111. **Sanders, J., and C. Niehaus.** 1985. Screening for rubella IgG and IgM using an EIA test applied to dried blood on filter paper. *J. Pediatr.* **106:**457–461.

112. **Schneider-Schaulies, S., and W. J. Bellini.** 2005. Morbilliviruses: measles virus, p. 712–743. *In* B. M. J. Mahy and V. ter Meulen (ed.), *Topley and Wilson's Microbiology and Microbial Infections*, 10th ed., vol. 1 and 2. *Virology.* Hodder Arnold Publishers, London, United Kingdom.

113. **Shepard, T. H.** 1995. *Catalogue of Teratogenic Agents*, 8th ed. Johns Hopkins University Press, Baltimore, MD.

114. **Shimizu, H., C. A. McCarthy, M. F. Smaron, and J. C. Burns.** 1993. Polymerase chain reaction for detection of measles virus in clinical samples. *J. Clin. Microbiol.* **31:**1034–1039.

115. **Sidhu, M. S., J. Crowley, A. Lowenthal, D. Karcher, J. Menonna, S. Cook, S. Udem, and P. Dowling.** 1994. Defective measles virus in human subacute sclerosing panencephalitis brain. *Virology* **202:**631–641.

116. **Skendzel, L. P.** 1996. Rubella immunity. Defining the level of protective antibody. *Am. J. Clin. Pathol.* **106:**170–174.

117. **Smaron, M. F., E. Saxon, L. Wood, C. McCarthy, and J. A. Morello.** 1991. Diagnosis of measles by fluorescent antibody and culture of nasopharyngeal secretions. *J. Virol. Methods* **33:**223–229.

118. **Takahashi, S., F. Machikawa, A. Noda, T. Oda, and T. Tachikawa.** 1998. Detection of immunoglobulin G and A antibodies to rubella virus in urine and antibody responses to vaccine-induced infection. *Clin. Diagn. Lab. Immunol.* **5:**24–27.

119. **Tatsuo, H., N. Ono, K. Tanaka, and Y. Yanagi.** 2000. SLAM (CDw150) is a cellular receptor for measles virus. *Nature* **406:**893–897.

120. **Taylor, B., E. Miller, R. Lingam, N. Andrews, A. Simmons, and J. Stowe.** 2002. Measles, mumps and rubella vaccination and bowel problems or developmental regression in children with autism: population study. *Br. Med. J.* **324:**393–396.

121. **Thomas, H. I. J., E. Barrett, L. M. Hesketh, A. Wynne, and P. Morgan-Capner.** 1999. Simultaneous IgM reactivity by EIA against more than one virus in measles, parvovirus B19 and rubella infection. *J. Clin. Virol.* **14:**107–118.

122. **Tipples, G. A., R. Hamkar, T. Mohktari-Azad, M. Gray, J. Ball, C. Head, and S. Ratnam.** 2004. Evaluation of rubella IgM enzyme immunoassays. *J. Clin. Virol.* **30:**233–238.

123. **Tuokko, H.** 1984. Comparison of nonspecific reactivity in indirect and reverse immunoassays for measles and mumps immunoglobulin M antibodies. *J. Clin. Microbiol.* **20:**972–976.

124. **Tuokko, H.** 1995. Detection of acute measles infections by indirect and mu-capture enzyme immunoassays for immunoglobulin M antibodies and measles immunoglobulin G antibody avidity enzyme immunoassay. *J. Med. Virol.* **45:**306–311.

125. **Uhlmann, V., C. M. Martin, O. Sheils, L. Pilkington, I. Silva, A. Killalea, S. B. Murch, J. Walker-Smith, M. Thomson, A. J. Wakefield, and J. J. O'Leary.** 2002. Potential viral pathogenic mechanism for new variant inflammatory bowel disease. *J. Clin. Pathol. Mol. Pathol.* **55:**84–90.

126. **Veitorp, M., and J. Leerhoy.** 1981. Rubella IgG antibody detection by ELISA using capillary blood samples collected on filter paper and in microtainer tubes. *Acta Pathol. Microbiol. Scand. Sect. B* **89:**369–370.

127. **Wakefield, A. J., S. H. Murch, A. Anthony, J. Linnell, D. M.Casson, M. Malik, M. Berelowitz, A. P. Dhillon, M. A. Thomson, P. Harvey, A. Valentine, S. E. Davies, and J. A. Walker-Smith.** 1998. Ileal-lymphoid-nodular hyperplasia, non-specific colitis, and pervasive developmental disorder in children. *Lancet* **351:**637–641. (Retraction, **375:**445, 2010.)

128. **Wassilak, S. G., R. H. Bernier, H. L. Herrmann, W. A. Orenstein, K. J. Bart, and R. Amler.** 1984. Measles seroconfirmation using dried capillary blood specimens in filter paper. *Pediatr. Infect. Dis.* **3:**117–121.

129. **Webster, W. S.** 1998. Teratogen update: congenital rubella. *Teratology* **58:**13–23.

130. **Weller, T. H., and F. A. Neva.** 1962. Propagation in tissue culture of cytopathic agents from patients with rubella-like illness. *Proc. Soc. Exp. Biol. Med.* **111:**215–225.

131. **World Health Organization.** 2007. Update of standard nomenclature for wild-type rubella viruses, 2007. *Wkly. Epidemiol. Rec.* **82:**209–224.

131 a.**World Health Organization.** 2007. *Manual for the Laboratory Diagnosis of Measles and Rubella Virus Infection*, 2nd ed. World Health Organization, Geneva, Switzerland. http://www.who.int/immunization_monitoring/LabManualFinal.pdf.

132. **Zaki, S. R., and W. J. Bellini.** 1997. Measles, p. 233–244. *In* D. H. Connor, F. W. Chandler, D. A. Schwartz, H. J. Manz, and E. E. Lack (ed.), *Pathology of Infectious Diseases*. Appleton and Lange Publishers, Stamford, CT.

133. **Zhu, Z., W. Xu, E. A. Abernathy, M.-H. Chen, Q. Zheng, T. Wang, Z. Zhang, C. Li, C. Wang, W. He, S. Zhou, and J. Icenogle.** 2007. Comparison of four methods using throat swabs to confirm rubella virus infection. *J. Clin. Microbiol.* **45:**2847–2852.

Enteroviruses and Parechoviruses

KATHLEEN A. STELLRECHT, DARYL M. LAMSON,
AND JOSÉ R. ROMERO

85

TAXONOMY

Enteroviruses (EVs) are members of the *Picornaviridae* family, with "pico" meaning very small, "rna" indicating an RNA genome, and "viridae" signifying viruses. Traditional criteria for taxonomy and the identification of EVs to subgroups were based on patterns of replication in cell cultures, clinical syndromes or disease, and disease manifestations in suckling mice. The subgroups were poliovirus (PV), coxsackievirus A (CVA), coxsackievirus B (CVB), and echovirus (E). These criteria classified 67 distinct human EV (HEV) serotypes until this designation was dropped (78). All preceding serotypes were designated enterovirus followed by a number starting with enterovirus 68.

Due to the development of molecular sequencing and the limited availability of antisera for characterizing newly identified strains and variant stains, the traditional methods of taxonomy have become challenging. EV taxonomy was effectively redefined through phylogenetic analysis (97). EVs are now divided into four species: HEV A through D, with PV1, PV2, and PV3 as well as CVA1, CVA11, CVA13, CVA15, CVA17 to CVA22, and CVA24 classified in the HEV C group (Table 1) (97). The use of VP1 gene sequence analysis has led to a number of classification changes. Several EVs originally thought to be distinct serotypes are likely variants of the same strain (73), some strains have been reclassified into different groups, and new EVs have been identified from EV73 up to at least EV104 (15, 74, 103).

The genus *Parechovirus* (HPeV) is comprised of more than 14 different types (http://www.picornaviridae.com/parechovirus/hpev/hpev.htm). Originally identified in 1956 as members of the enterovirus genus, echoviruses 22 and 23 (renamed HPeV1 and HPeV2) are genetically distinct from other EVs (28, 45, 98). As with EVs, molecular techniques have led to the identification of 12 additional members of the HPeV genus, designated HPeV3 to 14, with more types soon to be reported.

DESCRIPTION OF THE AGENTS

Similar to other members of the family *Picornaviridae*, EVs are small (30-nm diameter in the hydrated state), nonenveloped viruses that possess a single-stranded positive (message)-sense RNA genome. Their buoyant density in cesium chloride is 1.30 to 1.34 g/cm^3 (46). The EVs are stable in acid, ether, and chloroform and are insensitive to nonionic detergent. They are inactivated by heat (>56°C), UV light, chlorination, and formaldehyde. The EVs replicate optimally at 36 to 37°C.

The EVs are quite stable in liquid environments and can survive for many weeks in water, body fluids, and sewage. This is due to a number of viral properties, including thermostability in the presence of divalent cations, acid stability, and the absence of a lipid envelope.

The EV RNA genome serves as a template for both viral protein translation and RNA replication (Fig. 1). The genome contains a 5′ nontranslated region (5′ NTR), which immediately precedes a single open reading frame (ORF) (Fig. 1). The ORF is translated into a single polyprotein that is posttranslationally cleaved into several functional intermediates and the final 11 proteins by virus-encoded proteases. Immediately downstream of the ORF is a short noncoding region of approximately 70 to 100 bases (3′ NTR) and a terminal polyadenylated tail.

The EV 5′ and 3′ NTRs play critical roles in the EV life cycle. The 5′ NTR contains multiple regions of predicted higher-order structure (i.e., stem-loops or domains). A domain located at the extreme 5′ terminus of the 5′ NTR is essential for viral RNA replication. Cap-independent translation of the EV genome is regulated by the internal ribosome entry site, which spans a discontinuous region within the 5′ NTR. For PV and several nonpolio enteroviruses (NPEVs), the 5′ NTR has been documented to be a determinant of virulence phenotype and cell type specificity (14, 63). Given the crucial nature of the functions controlled by the 5′ NTR, it is not surprising that nucleotide sequences with absolute (or near absolute) conservation among the EVs exist within this region. These regions of high nucleotide identity have been exploited for the design of primers and probes used for the detection of the EVs. The 3′ NTR has also been demonstrated to play a role in viral RNA replication.

The EV capsid is arranged in 60 repeating protomeric units that confer an icosahedral shape to the virion (Fig. 2). VP1, VP2, and VP3 comprise the surface of the virion and possess an eight-stranded "beta-barrel" core structure. The external loops that connect the beta strands are responsible for the differences in surface topography and antigenic diversity among the EVs. Neutralization sites, typically three or four per protomer, are most densely clustered on VP1. VP4 is located internally within the capsid and has no surface-exposed regions.

TABLE 1 HEVs and HPeVs

Virus	Serotypes[a]
Human enterovirus species	
HEV A (17 serotypes)	
Human coxsackieviruses	A2–8, A10, A12, A14, A16
Enteroviruses	71, 76, 89–92
HEV B (56 serotypes)	
Human coxsackieviruses	A9, B1–6
Human echoviruses	1–7, 9, 11–21, 24–27, 29–33
Enteroviruses	69, 73–75, 77–88, 93, 97, 98, 100, 101
HEV C (16 serotypes)	
Human coxsackieviruses	A1, A11, A13, A17, A19–22, A24
Human polioviruses	1–3
Enteroviruses	95, 96, 99, 102
HEV D (3 serotypes)	
Enteroviruses	68, 70, 94
Human rhinovirus A (75 serotypes)	1, 2, 7–13, 15, 16, 18–25, 28–34, 36, 38–41, 43–47, 49–51, 53–68, 71, 73–78, 80–82, 88–90, 94–96, 98, 100, Hanks
Human rhinovirus B (25 serotypes)	3–6, 14, 17, 26, 27, 35, 42, 48, 52, 69, 70, 72, 79, 83, 84, 86, 91–93, 97, 99
Human rhinovirus C	No serotypes yet defined[b]
Human parechovirus species	
Human parechovirus species (14 serotypes)	
Human parechovirus	1–14

[a]Classification adapted from the Picornavirus Study Group of the International Committee for the Taxonomy of Viruses (http://www.picornastudygroup.com) (97).
[b]As of February 2010 (http://www.picornaviridae.com/enterovirus/hrv-c/hrv-c_seqs.htm).

The resolution of the near-atomic structures of multiple human picornaviruses revealed that the EVs (and rhinoviruses) share a number of conserved structural motifs. Surrounding a conserved protrusion at the fivefold axis of each pentameric unit (i.e., five protomers) is a narrow deep cleft (25 Å) or canyon. It is into this site that the specific receptors for the EVs bind when the virus encounters a susceptible host cell.

The genomic organization of HPeVs is similar to that of EVs. However, unlike the EVs, HPeVs possess only three capsid proteins in VP0, VP3, and VP1. No crystallographic structural information exists for the HPeVs. Sequence similarities between HPeVs and the other picornaviruses suggest that the major capsid protein shares the typical beta-barrel core structure. Relative to the EVs, the HPeVs are predicted to have a flatter surface topography, with antigenic variants determined by the external loops, as with EVs.

EPIDEMIOLOGY AND TRANSMISSION

The EVs and HPeVs are ubiquitous agents found worldwide. In regions with temperate climates, the majority of EV infections (70 to 80%) occur in summer and fall. In tropical climates, EV infections occur year-round or with increased incidence during the rainy season. Seasonal differences in incidences have been seen among serotypes of HPeV. HPeV3 infections occur mainly during spring and summer, whereas HPeV1 circulates throughout the year, with a nadir in summer months (105, 114).

It is estimated that annually the EVs infect a billion or more individuals worldwide, with 30 to 50 million infections in the United States (19). EVs and HPeV are spread mainly by the fecal-oral or oral-oral routes, respiratory droplets, and fomites. Fecal-oral transmission may predominate in areas with poor sanitary conditions, whereas respiratory

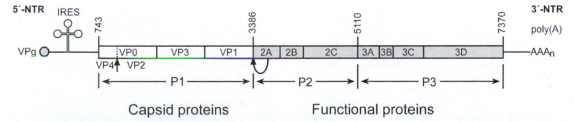

FIGURE 1 Genome organization of PV type 1. The PV genome is a single-stranded positive-sense RNA of approximately 7,500 nucleotides. Nucleotides 743 to 7370 encode in a single ORF the capsid proteins (white boxes in coding regions P1) and functional proteins (gray boxes in coding regions P2 and P3). The 5′ and 3′ NTRs are shown as lines. The internal ribosome entry site (IRES) is shown schematically with two-dimensional structure. The virus protein VPg is covalently linked to the terminal uracil of the 5′ NTR. Reprinted from reference 116 with permission of the publisher.

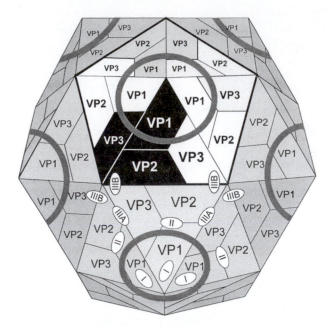

FIGURE 2 Schematic representation of the three-dimensional structure of a PV particle and the four neutralizing antigenetic (N-Ag) sites. The icosahedral capsid structure typical of EVs is composed of 60 protomers, each consisting of the capsid proteins VP1, VP2, and VP3 (black areas). Each of the 12 fivefold symmetry axes is surrounded by five protomers, forming a pentamer (surrounded by a bold black line). The attachment site for the virus-specific receptor is a depression around the fivefold symmetry axis, also called the canyon (dark gray circles). Each of the three surface-exposed capsid proteins contains immunodominant antigenic sites at which neutralizing antibodies bind. Four N-Ag sites (white ellipses) have been mapped to surface loop extensions. Reprinted from reference 116 with permission of the publisher.

transmission may be more important in more developed areas. These viruses may survive on environmental surfaces for periods long enough to allow transmission from fomites. Hospital nursery and other institutional outbreaks have occurred.

The highest incidence of EV infection is observed in young infants and children of 5 to 10 years of age, with children aged <1 year accounting for almost half of the reported cases in the United States (50). Generally, the incubation period is 3 to 6 days, except for acute hemorrhagic conjunctivitis, which is 24 to 72 hours (30), and secondary infections are observed in >50% of susceptible household members (64). The incidence of HPeV infection is highest in children <3 years of age, again with the majority of infections occurring in infants <1 year of age (13, 105).

Two major patterns of circulating enteroviruses between 1970 and 2005 have been observed: epidemic (e.g., E9, E13, E30, and CVB5) and endemic (e.g., CVA9, CVB2, CVB4, and EV71) (50). Epidemic serotypes were characterized by substantial fluctuations in numbers over time with occasional increased incidence. Endemic serotypes had stable and usually low levels of circulation with few changes in incidence. The five most commonly reported serotypes (E9, E11, E30, E6, and CVB5) accounted for 48.1% of cases. Interestingly, in 2007 three distinct clusters of CVB1, accounting for 25% of all EVs, were reported (21). In the 35 years prior, CVB1 accounted for a small proportion (2%) of all EVs in the United States (50).

Generally, mortality is not common with EV infections, with death being reported for 3.3% of cases with known outcomes. Infections with CVB4 and HPeV1 were associated with higher risk for death, and infections with E9 were associated with lower risk for death (50).

The Global Polio Eradication Initiative began in 1988; by 2006, indigenous transmission of wild poliovirus (WPV) type 2 infection had been interrupted globally, and indigenous transmission of type 1 and 3 (WPV1 and WPV3) infection had been interrupted in all but four countries worldwide (Afghanistan, India, Nigeria, and Pakistan) (22). Despite this success in controlling indigenous transmission, importations of WPV, with subsequent ongoing transmissions in some cases, have been occurring continuously into previously polio-free countries in Africa and Asia since 2002 (23). In particular, 18 countries which had previously controlled the disease were afflicted with outbreaks due to transmissions from Nigeria, and endemicity was reestablished in 6 of these countries (Fig. 3) (20). Still, the efforts of global polio eradication are to be commended, as the incidence of polio has decreased from an estimated 350,000 cases annually to 1,655 cases in 2008 (22).

CLINICAL SIGNIFICANCE

EVs and HPeVs cause a wide array of both localized and systemic infections, affecting many organ systems, in patients of all ages (Table 2). Generally, no disease is uniquely associated with any specific serotype, and no serotype is uniquely associated with any one disease. This is true even of paralytic poliomyelitis, which has been associated with numerous NPEV serotypes. However, different serotypes of EV have been associated with more severe disease and/or death in different age groups of children (49). Likewise, HPeV3 is associated with more severe disease (13, 40, 108).

The majority of EV and HPeV infections are asymptomatic. The most common symptomatic manifestation of infection is acute nonspecific febrile illness with or without an exanthem. This so-called viral syndrome is one of the most numerically important causes of fever among children. Although this illness in itself is benign, it is of great concern because it mimics other more serious illnesses in infants and young children. Distinguishing EV and HPeV infections from those due to common bacteria and other viruses on clinical grounds alone is often difficult, which leads to unnecessary treatment. During the summer and fall, the EVs are responsible for 50 to 60% of hospital admissions for the evaluation of acute febrile illness in children and infants (64).

By far the most vexing clinical EV/HPeV syndrome that the physician encounters is aseptic meningitis. The EVs are the most common cause of meningitis in the United States and account for over 80% of all viral meningitides (51, 101). More recently, HPeV3 has been recognized to cause a significant number of cases of neonatal sepsis and aseptic meningitis in children <5 years of age (12, 114). The onset of symptoms is usually sudden and generally includes a biphasic fever, headache, occasionally photophobia, vomiting, rash, and myalgias. In young children, symptoms include fever, lethargy, and anorexia (58), again mimicking bacterial infection. Currently, treatment is symptomatic, with illness generally resolving after a week with no long-term sequelae. An estimated 30,000 to 50,000 hospitalizations for NPEV meningitis occur each year. The echoviruses and CVB, particularly E4, E6, E9, E11, E16, E30, CVB2, and CVB5, constitute the principal EVs associated with this syndrome.

The term poliomyelitis refers to the inflammatory damage due to infection of the anterior horn cells of the spinal cord.

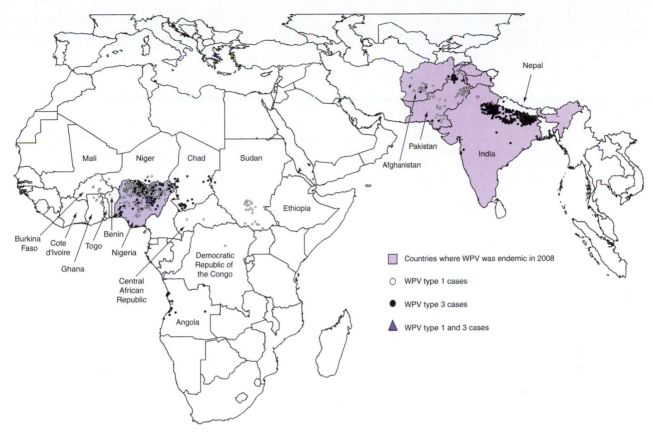

FIGURE 3 WPV cases worldwide, 2008. Data were reported for 2008 to the World Health Organization as of 3 March 2009 ($n = 1,655$). This excludes polioviruses detected by environmental surveillance and VDPV. Reprinted from reference 22.

Recognized clinically as acute-onset lower-motor-neuron paralysis of one or more muscles, the case fatality rate is 2 to 5%, and in epidemics, as high as 10% (78). Historically, this disease was most commonly associated with the PVs; however, in most countries, this is no longer the case. In regions of the world where the polioviruses have been eradicated, the NPEVs and circulating vaccine-derived PVs (VDPVs) are now the principal causes of acute flaccid paralysis (AFP). VDPVs are circulating strains derived from the vaccine (Sabin) strains of PV which have regained the capacity to cause paralytic poliomyelitis. Multiple NPEV serotypes are known to cause AFP, and at least six poliomyelitis outbreaks have been due to circulating VDPV (reviewed in reference 78). It is also important to point out that despite efforts towards polio eradication, this virus is still endemic in some

countries, where it has served as a reservoir for the reintroduction of polio to other areas.

Approximately 10 to 20% of viral encephalitides are due to EVs (65). CVAs are the predominant EV subgroup associated with this syndrome (64). HPeV has been shown to be a causative agent as well (108). A severe and often fatal form of brain stem encephalitis, rhombencephalitis, has been associated with EV71 infections in small children from several countries in Southeast Asia (24, 43, 44). Chronic EV meningoencephalitis in agammaglobulinemia occurs and is caused most frequently by the echoviruses, particularly E11.

Myocarditis was once an often fatal disease associated with EV; however, with current medical care mortality rates are low (~10%). Symptoms range from nonspecific (fever, myalgias, palpitations, or exertional dyspnea) to fulminant hemodynamic collapse and sudden death. Myocarditis has been implicated in 8.6 to 12% of cases of sudden cardiac death of young adults (34, 36). CVBs are responsible for one-third to one-half of all cases of acute myocarditis and pericarditis (7), with CVB2 and CVB5 being the most predominant serotypes identified in clinical studies. The echoviruses and PVs have also been associated with myopericarditis, but significantly less so than CVB.

Neonatal systemic enterovirus disease is associated with EV acquisition in utero, perinatally, or within the first 2 weeks of life. This syndrome is characterized by multiorgan involvement with symptoms including lethargy, feeding difficulty, vomiting, tachycardia, dyspnea, cyanosis, jaundice, and diarrhea, with or without fever. Typically, neonatal systemic enterovirus disease is associated with two severe clinical presentations: encephalomyocarditis, often with heart failure; and hemorrhage-hepatitis syndrome with hepatic failure

TABLE 2 Clinical syndromes associated with EV and HPeV infection

Organ system	Disease
Neurologic	Aseptic meningitis, encephalitis, poliomyelitis
Respiratory	Common cold, stomatitis, hand-foot-and-mouth disease, herpangina, lymphonodular pharyngitis, tonsillitis, rhinitis, pleurodynia (Bornholm disease), bronchiolitis, bronchitis, pneumonia
Cardiovascular	Myocarditis, pericarditis
Miscellaneous	AHC, febrile exanthematous illness, neonatal sepsis

and disseminated intravascular coagulation, although infants may present with combinations or organ system involvement (49, 112). The morbidity and mortality associated with this syndrome are significant, with death occurring rapidly. Recently, three distinct clusters of severe enterovirus illness due to CVB1, including six neonatal deaths, were reported in the United States in 2007 and 2008 (21, 112). However, other CVBs and echoviruses, particularly serotype 11, are also frequently associated with this syndrome.

Although originally described for agammaglobulinemic patients, persistent life-threatening EV infections can also occur in patients with combined variable immunodeficiency, severe combined immunodeficiency, hypogammaglobulinemia, or hyper-immunoglobulin M (hyper-IgM) syndrome and in those undergoing bone marrow and solid organ transplantation. Manifestations almost always include meningoencephalitis.

Other acute clinical EV syndromes of significance include acute hemorrhagic conjunctivitis (AHC; predominantly caused by EV70 and a variant, CVA24) and a wide variety of respiratory illnesses, such as the common cold, hand-foot-and-mouth syndrome (predominantly caused by CVA16), herpangina, Bornholm disease, pleurodynia (the major causes are CVB3 and CVB5), bronchitis, bronchiolitis, and pneumonia. Over the past several years, data suggesting a link between enterovirus infections and several chronic illnesses, including amyotrophic lateral sclerosis, chronic fatigue syndrome, polymyositis, congenital hydrocephalus, and attention-deficit/hyperactivity disorder, have been presented. However, definitive proof of causation is lacking (3). On the other hand, recent reports strengthen association between enteroviruses and type 1 insulin-dependent diabetes mellitus, although human genetic factors also play an important role (68, 81).

In general, the spectrum of diseases caused by HPeV is similar to that of EV. Symptomatic infections due to HPeVs are predominantly respiratory (i.e., colds or pneumonia) and gastrointestinal (gastroenteritis) in nature, particularly with HPeV1 (13, 41). However, as with the EV, cases of neonatal sepsis, AFP, aseptic meningitis, encephalitis, and myocarditis have been reported as a result of HPeV infection (particularly type 3). Interestingly, Ljungan virus, a parechovirus previously believed to infect exclusively rodents, has more recently been linked to human diseases, such as intrauterine fetal death in humans (69).

COLLECTION, TRANSPORT, AND STORAGE OF SPECIMENS

Specimen selection is important for making a diagnosis of EV infection, as asymptomatic shedding, especially in stool, is common. The specimen collected should correlate with the clinical syndrome (Table 3). Typically, EV infection begins with viral replication in the epithelial cells of the respiratory or gastrointestinal tract and the lymphoid follicles of the small intestine followed by viremia, leading to a secondary site of tissue infection. Hence, for patients with aseptic meningitis, cerebrospinal fluid (CSF) is generally the specimen of choice; however, if done early in the disease process, testing serum may yield better results. Likewise, if CSF is obtained >2 days after the onset of symptoms, the diagnostic yield may be lower. Prescreening of CSF for pleocytosis (lymphocytosis) is not recommended, as lack of pleocytosis, particularly in infants, is common (6, 67, 100). Furthermore, in the early stage of the disease, neutrophils may predominate for a few hours. On the other hand, patients with EV encephalitis often have negative CSF PCR results even when they have CSF pleocytosis; in these patients, throat and/or rectal swabs may be the specimen of choice. In cases of myocarditis and pericarditis, myocardial tissue is recommended over fluid (59). Analyses of blood samples by PCR have been almost uniformly negative (84). However, one report suggests that at least in pediatric patients, testing of tracheal aspirates may be an alternative to myocardial biopsy (5).

The EVs are quite stable in liquid environments and are able to survive many weeks in water, body fluids, and sewage; hence, rapid transport of specimens to the laboratory is generally not necessary. CSF and serum may be submitted to the laboratory in their original containers. Optimal specimens for virus isolation include stool, rectal swabs, throat swabs, and throat washings; swab specimens are best transported and stored in viral transport media. Viral infectivity for cell culture is preserved for long periods (years) at −70°C.

Specimen processing procedures for nucleic acid amplification methods should preserve viral capsid integrity so that the EV RNA genome is protected from ubiquitous nucleases in body fluids and the environment. Excessive freeze-thaw cycles should be avoided. Residual samples found in clinical laboratory refrigerators may be suitable for nucleic-acid-based detection of the EVs due to the inherent environmental stability of the EVs. Specimens that have been handled by automated chemistry or hematology analyzers should be considered compromised due to the potential for cross-contamination with other specimens.

Specimen storage at room temperature has been documented to negatively impact reverse transcription (RT)-PCR detection of EVs (107). No appreciable loss in PCR signal may be seen in specimens stored at 4°C to −20°C for up to a month. However, longer storage at these temperatures can result in a gradual decline of viral RNA copy number that could, in turn, potentially affect detection by nucleic acid amplification tests (NAATs). Thus, specimens are best stored at −70°C.

TABLE 3 EV and HPeV diseases and specimen selection

Disease	Acceptability of specimen[a]					
	Throat	Rectal/stool	Serum	CSF	Tissue	Conjunctival
Aseptic meningitis			±	+		
Encephalitis	+	+	±	±		
Poliomyelitis	+	+	±			
Respiratory disease	+					
Myocarditis					+	
AHC[b]						+
Febrile illness			+			
Neonatal sepsis			+			

[a]+, specimen is appropriate for testing; ±, specimen may be appropriate for testing.
[b]AHC, acute hemorrhagic conjunctivitis.

Certain clinical specimens require processing prior to inoculation of cell cultures. Feces (1 ml if liquid and approximately pea-sized samples if solid) are added to viral transport medium, vortexed, and centrifuged (1,000 × g, 30 min, 4°C). One milliliter of supernatant is removed and added to more viral transport media. Monolayers are inoculated with 0.2 to 0.3 ml of diluted supernatant. Nasopharyngeal aspirates and wash specimens are centrifuged (400 × g, 15 min, 4°C), and cell cultures are inoculated with 0.2 to 0.3 ml of supernatant. Serum, CSF, and urine need no pretreatment and may be inoculated directly onto the cell cultures. However, serum and urine can be toxic to monolayers. Cell death can often be prevented by replacing the culture medium within 24 hours of inoculation. Acid dissociation of antibodies bound to virus may improve detection when attempts are made to isolate EVs from serum and CSF (62).

Sera for antibody testing are best collected at both acute and convalescent stages, 2 to 4 weeks apart. The sera should be frozen at −20°C and tested simultaneously.

DIRECT DETECTION

Antigen

Historically, immunofluorescent techniques have not been used for the detection of respiratory infections due to EVs, since these viruses were believed to be associated with self-limited upper respiratory tract infection only. However, as the importance of these viruses in more severe respiratory diseases becomes more evident, the need for rapid antigen detection may emerge.

Nucleic Acid

There are numerous compelling reasons to use rapid diagnostic assays, such as NAAT, for the EVs. The time required for isolation and identification of EVs by traditional cell culture is too prolonged to be of clinical utility. Some serotypes, particularly within the CVA (i.e., CVA1, CVA19, and CVA22), fail to grow in cell culture, and some specimen types often have titers too low for detection by cell culture, i.e., 25 to 35% of CSF specimens (27). Furthermore, studies have demonstrated that the use of EV NAAT has a favorable impact on patient care. Correlations have been demonstrated between time to result and length of stay (100). Hence, when positive EV results are reported within 24 h, antibiotic usage is reduced, fewer ancillary tests are performed, and hospitalization is shortened and less costly (6, 80, 83).

EV RNA detection is best performed by nucleic acid amplification as opposed to direct hybridization techniques, which require considerably more viral nucleic acid than is typically found in CSF (113). The development of NAAT (RT-PCR or nucleic acid sequence-based amplification [NASBA]) has provided sensitive, specific, rapid, versatile, and clinically useful methods for the detection of EVs (38, 42, 85). NAAT of CSF is much more sensitive than cell culture, which has a sensitivity of 65 to 75% (85, 89, 109). Interestingly, the sensitivity of NAAT for the detection of EV in cases of aseptic meningitis ranges from 70 to 100% despite indications that EVs are the primary causative agent (77, 85, 87, 92, 99). One reason for this discrepancy is due in part to the fact that HPeV, which can account for a significant number of cases of neonatal sepsis and aseptic meningitis, is not detected by universal EV RT-PCR assays (28).

A limited number of studies have evaluated the sensitivity and specificity of RT-PCR with other sample types. For serum, the sensitivity and specificity of RT-PCR range from 81 to 92% and 98 to 100%, respectively (4, 89). In addition to the enhanced sensitivity of NAAT, this technology has the added benefit of rapid turnaround times, with results available in as little as 2.5 hours including extraction (54).

Prior to being tested by NAAT, EV RNA must be extracted from specimens to eliminate ubiquitous RNases and to remove potential amplification inhibitors. Only a small sample size, generally 100 to 200 μl of fluid or 1 mg of tissue, is required. The most common methods for RNA extraction are gel membrane or silica binding. Multiple automated extraction methods have been utilized, including the following: MagNA Pure LC and Compact (Roche Diagnostics System); easyMAG (bioMérieux); and M48, QIAcube, EZ One, and QIAsymphony (Qiagen). An EV RT-PCR assay on the GeneXpert system includes extraction, amplification, and detection all in one cartridge (54). All of the aspects of NAAT from the extraction to detection are discussed in more detail in chapter 4, of this *Manual*.

Currently, two Food and Drug Administration (FDA)-approved real-time assays are available for the detection of EV from CSF: Xpert EV and NucliSENS EasyQ Enterovirus (Table 4). Limited available data suggest that the sensitivities

TABLE 4 NAATs for EV and HPeV detection

Assay (manufacturer)	Method	Target	Regulatory status	Comment	Reference(s)
Xpert EV (Cepheid)	Real-time RT-PCR	5′ NTR	IVD[a]	Extraction, amplification, detection performed in single cartridge	54
NucliSENS EasyQ Enterovirus (bioMérieux)	NASBA[b]	5′ NTR	IVD	Separate extraction required; sensitivity comparable to Xpert EV	56, 60
MGB Alert Enterovirus (Nanogen)	Real-time RT-PCR	5′ NTR	ASR	Uses patented chemistry	
Multicode-RTx (Eragen Biosciences)	Real-time RT-PCR	5′ NTR	RUO	Uses labeled primer and proprietary chemistry	
Enterovirus Consensus kit (Argene)	Conventional RT-PCR	5′ NTR	RUO[c]	ELISA–based detection	56
Noncommercial EV reagents	Real-time and conventional RT-PCR	5′ NTR, VP2	LDA		25, 90, 96, 99
Noncommercial HPeV reagents	Real-time	5′ NTR,	LDA	Detects HPeV1–6	9, 70, 72

[a]IVD, in vitro diagnostic (FDA-approved test).
[b]NASBA, nucleic acid sequence-based amplification.
[c]RUO, research use only reagent.

of the two assays may be comparable (56, 60). However, a direct comparison of the two kits with clinical samples has yet to be performed.

Analyte-specific reagents (ASRs) and laboratory-developed assays (LDAs) for EV real-time RT-PCR are also widely used (Table 4). As with all ASRs and LDAs, laboratories must develop and validate the assays for themselves. One-step RT-PCR using a single reaction tube and higher RT temperatures has the advantage of decreased contamination risks, increased efficiency due to destabilization of secondary structures, and improved specificity. Most often, the LDAs target conserved sequences (81 to 100% homology) within the 5′ NTR or VP2 for nearly universal amplification of EVs (Table 4). The two 5′ NTR targets most frequently used are those reported by Rotbart (88) and Chapman et al. (25). While these primers do not detect HPeV (discussed below), they do amplify the genomes of several rhinoviruses (17, 47, 55).

Despite the increased availability and benefits of real-time PCR, conventional RT-PCR is still used, particularly for viral typing (18, 71). There is a wide array of detection systems for conventional PCR, ranging from agarose gel electrophoresis to dot or Southern blot to colorimetric assays using enzyme-linked immunosorbent assay (ELISA)-type formats (96, 99). Two commercial tests, Amplicor EV and the Enterovirus Consensus kit, have used this approach; the latter is still commercially available.

With regard to quality control, EV NAATs should include internal controls to detect amplification inhibitors and to assess nucleic acid recovery. Indeed, both of the FDA-approved EV detection kits include internal controls. EV RNA assay verification experiments and quality assurance performance demonstrate the need for a universal, nominal EV standard; however, none exists. Instead, most laboratories use either quantified EV isolates or transcripts from clones of target regions, both of which have to be lab generated. Multicenter proficiency testing programs for LDA EV NAATs indicate that properly designed tests can be equally effective in the detection of EV, regardless of the format used (66). However, other studies have reported marked center-to-center variation in testing proficiencies. In one survey, one-third of participating laboratories were nonproficient in the detection of EV by RT-PCR (107). In another report, 6.8% of participating laboratories recorded false positive results, pointing to the need for fastidious attention to methods for preventing cross-contamination (66). Overall, these findings underscore the importance of rigorous quality control and periodic proficiency reassessment to ensure uniformly high-quality testing.

Reports detailing the detection of HPeVs by RT-PCR have been published (13, 47, 57). Although the original methods were limited to the detection of HPeV1 and/or HPeV2 (48, 57, 75), some of the more recent reports detect at least types 1 to 6 (Table 4) (9, 70, 72).

ISOLATION AND IDENTIFICATION

A combination of human and primate cell lines is typically used for EV and HPeV isolation, since no single cell line supports the growth of all types. The general susceptibilities of commonly used cell lines are summarized in Table 5. Isolation times for EVs from CSF using traditional cell culture techniques range from 4 to 8 days but are shorter (1 to 3 days) from sites with higher viral titers. Recovery time for HPeV is variable and dependent upon type: for HPeV1 and HPeV2, 1 to 8 days; and for HPeV3, 14 to 17 days.

TABLE 5 Susceptibilities of cell lines commonly used for isolation of EV and HPeV

Cell line	Susceptibility to virus[a]						
	Poliovirus	Coxsackievirus		Echovirus	HPeV		
		Type A[b]	Type B		1	2	3
Monkey kidney							
Rhesus	+++	+	+++	+++	+	+	unk
Cynomolgus	++++	+	+++	+++	+	+	unk
Buffalo green (BGMK)	+++	+	++++	++	+	+	unk
African green (Vero)	+++	+	+++	++	+	+	+++[c]
LLCMK2	+++	+	+++	+++	++	++	+
Human							
HeLa	+++	+	+++	+	+	+	unk
Kidney (293)	+++	+	++	+++	++	++	−
WI-38	++	++	+	+++	+	+	unk
Embryonic lung (HELF)	+++	++	+	+++	+	+	unk
MRC-5	+++	+	+	+++	+	+	unk
Rhabdomyosarcoma (RD)	+++	+++[d]	+	+++	+	+	−
HEp-2	+++	+	+++	+	++	++	−
A549	+++	+	+++	+++	+	+	−
HuT-292	+++	+++	+++	+++	unk	unk	unk
HT-29	+++	+	+++	+++	+++	+++	−
Super E–mix (combination of BGMK-hDAF and CaCo[e])	++	unk	++++	++++	++	++	unk

[a]Relative susceptibilities: +, minimally susceptible; ++++, maximally susceptible; −, nonsusceptible; unk, unknown (no published reports). Some EVs are difficult to isolate even on minimally susceptible cell lines.
[b]Some type A coxsackieviruses (A1, A19, and A20) are not readily isolated.
[c]Improved yields after passage.
[d]Many types of type A coxsackie virus grow only in RD cells.
[e]BGMK-hDAF, BGMK cells expressing human decay-accelerating factor; CaCo, human colon adenocarcinoma cells.

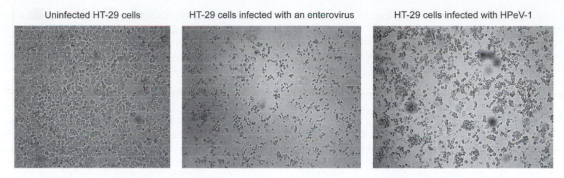

| Uninfected HT-29 cells | HT-29 cells infected with an enterovirus | HT-29 cells infected with HPeV-1 |

FIGURE 4 Cytopathic effects observed 3 days after infection of HT-29 cells with an EV or HPeV1 isolate after passage on this cell line. Reprinted from reference 2.

Infections of susceptible cell monolayers with EVs result in a characteristic cytopathic effect (CPE), consisting of shrinkage and rounding of individual cells within the monolayers. The nuclei of infected cells exhibit pyknosis. As infection progresses, the cells degenerate and separate from the surface of the plate. Often the CPE is so characteristic that a presumptive diagnosis of EV infection can be made (Fig. 4). However, experience is necessary, as toxic effects from primary specimens, such as *Clostridium difficile* toxin, can mimic CPE (37). CPE for HPeV appears as large, regularly shaped spheres compared to small irregular shapes caused by EVs (Fig. 4) (2).

The relatively low sensitivity of viral culture from CSF (65 to 75%; reviewed in reference 33) is likely due to the presence of neutralizing antibody, low viral load, and resistance of some serotypes to culture. Stool cultures have a much improved sensitivity (approaching 90% [104]) but lack specificity. These sensitivities can vary with fluctuations in the annual prevalence of different serotypes; improved sensitivity is observed when EV types that grow well in culture are circulating (91).

Shell vial culture (SVC), in which virus is detected with monoclonal antibodies in the absence of CPE, reduces the time to detection to 2 to 3 days. The sensitivity of SVC may or may not be higher than that of traditional cell culture (16, 53, 106) and is probably laboratory and cell line dependent (93). SVC using a mixture of cell lines in a single vial (Super E-Mix containing decay-accelerating factor-expressing BGMK cells and A549 cells; Diagnostic Hybrids Inc., Athens, OH) improves sensitivities (16, 93). The capacity of Super E-Mix to isolate HPeV has not been evaluated; however, it is presumed that at least HPeV1 and HPeV2 would grow in this cell mix, as A549 cells are susceptible to infection. The greatest limitation of SVC is the monoclonal antibodies used in the detection steps (discussed below).

Broadly reactive and serotype-specific EV monoclonal antibodies have been developed (62) and used for cell culture confirmation by immunofluorescence. While preliminary studies suggest that these reagents, used singly and in blends (DAKO-Enterovirus 5-D8/1 [Dako, Glostrup, Denmark] and Pan-Enterovirus blend [Chemicon International Inc.]), demonstrated an important role in serotype identifications, further studies have identified several limitations (53, 82, 106), most notably, cross-reactivity with the Chemicon blend (53) and the lack of EV71 detection with the Dako blend. More recently, Diagnostic Hybrids developed an EV blend (D3 IFA Enterovirus Identification) which reportedly has good sensitivity, including the detection of EV71 with little or no cross-reactivity; however, peer-reviewed publications using this antibody blend are lacking. The concordance of results for identification of clinical EV isolates to the species level using monoclonal blends versus the neutralization assay has demonstrated that the latter may be significantly superior for identification of the EVs (82). These studies appeared to indicate that monoclonal antibodies for EV identification should be used as a preliminary screen for species or serotype identification. With regard to HPeV, typing reagents are available only for types 1 and 2, and not all HPeV2 isolates are neutralized by specific antisera (1).

TYPING SYSTEMS

Determination of the specific serotypes of infecting EVs is often unnecessary for clinical purposes, because the diseases caused by the EVs are not serotype specific. Previously, the most common exception to this principle was in pediatrics, where distinguishing between VDPV and NPEVs was critical to the interpretation of viral culture results in areas where the Sabin PV strains were used for vaccination, as this live vaccine may be shed from the throat for 1 to 2 weeks and in the feces for several weeks to months (29). Identification of an NPEV-specific serotype is useful for epidemiological purposes and for the knowledge of the specific serotypes involved in unusual or novel clinical manifestations, such as flaccid paralysis due to NPEVs (reviewed in reference 78). Historically, EV serotype determinations involved neutralization with the Lim and Benyesh-Melnick (LBM) pools of antisera; however, several limitations exist for these methodologies. The pools identify only 40 of the 64 originally described EV serotypes, and genetic drift of the EVs over time has given rise to antigenic variants. Furthermore, the procedure is labor-intensive, and the supply of LBM pools available from the World Health Organization is limited (distribution is restricted to reference laboratories).

Sequencing of the VP1 gene is now the primary method used for typing. Specifically, a 340-bp region that encodes the serotype-specific neutralization epitopes of VP1 is amplified, sequenced, and analyzed against a sequence database for known EVs (71, 76). This method reduces the testing time by weeks (76). A pyrosequencing method has also been developed (95). These methods of "molecular serotyping" have been extremely useful in typing the isolates that could not be neutralized by traditional LBM pools and were therefore classified as "nontypeable" EVs and in identifying multiple new EV serotypes and novel HPeVs.

Various other molecular methods have been described for either species-specific typing (i.e., PV) or for the detection of multiple EV types. PV-specific typing includes PCR restriction fragment length polymorphism analysis (8), probe hybridization (32), and PV type-specific PCR assays (52). Rapid typing of multiple EV types has been demonstrated through the used line blot hybridization (117) and microwell oligonucleotide arrays (102).

SEROLOGIC TESTS

Classically, serologic diagnosis of EV infection involved comparing antibody titers in acute- and convalescent-phase serum in a neutralization assay, with a fourfold or greater rise in type-specific antibody titer considered diagnostic of recent infection. However, acute-phase sera are often not obtained due to nonspecific presentations early in EV disease.

Type-specific ELISAs for the detection of EV serotype-specific IgM antibodies (i.e., CVB-specific IgM and EV71-specific IgM), as well as a heterotypic assays for the detection of IgA, IgM, and IgG antibodies against EVs in general, have been developed (10, 11). Homotypic assays are more relevant to epidemiologic studies than to clinical diagnosis and have been successfully applied in such settings (78), as these assays appear to be less sensitive than PCR for the diagnosis of EV infection (31). Furthermore, the IgM response to EVs may be nonspecific and may lead to false-positive results (79, 110). Although cross-reactivity with non-EV pathogens has not been studied thoroughly, sera from patients infected with acute hepatitis A virus (a member of the *Picornaviridae* family) have been reported to produce a significant number of false-positive results in an ELISA for detection of enterovirus IgM antibodies (11). Recently, PCR-enhanced immunoassays for the detection of EV-specific IgM have been evaluated (35). Such systems improve the sensitivity and specificity of immunoassays, as the ligand is further amplified by PCR after immune capture (94). However, these methods are technically challenging to establish in the laboratory and are clearly investigational methods.

ANTIVIRAL SUSCEPTIBILITIES

There is no FDA-approved antiviral agent available for the treatment of EV or HPeV infections. However, several compounds targeting viral capsid proteins, proteases, polymerase, and other proteins are being developed, including some agents in phase III clinical trials (26). A promising investigational drug, the WIN compound pleconaril, has undergone extensive in vitro susceptibility testing against EVs and is undergoing clinical evaluation for the therapy of severe enteroviral infection in newborns (86, 111).

EVALUATION, INTERPRETATION, AND REPORTING OF RESULTS

An understanding of the sites where asymptomatic shedding and disease-induced replication occur is critical to the interpretation of EV test results. Detection of EV in the central nervous system, bloodstream, lower respiratory tract, and genitourinary tract implies a true invasive infection and a high-level likelihood of association with current illness. In contrast, EVs can be shed asymptomatically from the nasopharynx and the gastrointestinal tract for weeks to a month. Detection of EVs by virus isolation or NAAT at these sites must be interpreted cautiously, because their presence alone does not establish a diagnosis. EV in the feces or nasopharynx of a patient with

meningitis may represent residual shedding from an infection from weeks before and may have nothing to do with the current illness.

An additional factor potentially complicating the evaluation of results from these body sites in young children is the administration of live attenuated oral PV in the first years of life. While the vaccine is no longer used in the United States (29), the majority of countries worldwide, including some in Europe, still employ oral PV as part of their vaccination regimes. Reporting an EV isolate in a setting where oral PV is used without specifying if it is a PV or NPEV can lead the physician to wrongly discontinue antibiotic or antiherpes therapy in the belief that an EV ideology has been established. The distinction between PVs and NPEVs from the central nervous system, bloodstream, lower respiratory tract, and genitourinary tract is less important, since VDPVs have rarely been isolated from such specimens and, in those rare instances, may actually be causing the illness in question (39, 61).

A further cautionary note is warranted with regard to infections with dual agents. Rare reports of coinfection of the CSF by bacteria and EVs have appeared (115). In such cases, the bacterium-associated clinical sequelae dominated, i.e., the patients were clinically suspected of having bacterial meningitis and the virus was isolated incidentally. The patients were sick enough that identification of a virus before identification of the bacterium probably would not have dissuaded the clinician from continued use of the antibiotics. In the much more common situations where the clinical presentation is typical of viral meningitis, coinfection with a clinically "silent" bacterium would be extraordinarily unlikely. Hence, identification of an EV from a nonpermissive site in a patient with a clinically compatible illness is sufficient evidence for establishment of EV causality.

REFERENCES

1. **Abed, Y., and G. Boivin.** 2005. Molecular characterization of a Canadian human parechovirus (HPeV)-3 isolate and its relationship to other HPeVs. *J. Med. Virol.* **77:**566–570.
2. **Abed, Y., and G. Boivin.** 2006. Human parechovirus types 1, 2 and 3 infections in Canada. *Emerg. Infect. Dis.* **12:**969–975.
3. **Abzug, M. J.** 2008. The enteroviruses: an emerging infectious disease? The real, the speculative and the really speculative. *Adv. Exp. Med. Biol.* **609:**1–15. doi:10.1007/978-0-387-73960-1_1.
4. **Abzug, M. J., H. L. Keyserling, M. L. Lee, M. J. Levin, and H. A. Rotbart.** 1995. Neonatal enterovirus infection: virology, serology, and effects of intravenous immune globulin. *Clin. Infect. Dis.* **20:**1201–1206.
5. **Akhtar, N., J. Ni, D. Stromberg, G. L. Rosenthal, N. E. Bowles, and J. A. Towbin.** 1999. Tracheal aspirate as a substrate for polymerase chain reaction detection of viral genome in childhood pneumonia and myocarditis. *Circulation* **99:**2011–2018.
6. **Archimbaud, C., M. Chambon, J. L. Bailly, I. Petit, C. Henquell, A. Mirand, B. Aublet-Cuvelier, S. Ughetto, J. Beytout, P. Clavelou, A. Labbe, P. Philippe, J. Schmidt, C. Regagnon, O. Traore, and H. Peigue-Lafeuille.** 2009. Impact of rapid enterovirus molecular diagnosis on the management of infants, children, and adults with aseptic meningitis. *J. Med. Virol.* **81:**42–48.
7. **Baboonian, C., and T. Treasure.** 1997. Meta-analysis of the association of enteroviruses with human heart disease. *Heart* **78:**539–543.
8. **Balanant, J., S. Guillot, A. Candrea, F. Delpeyroux, and R. Crainic.** 1991. The natural genomic variability of poliovirus analyzed by a restriction fragment length polymorphism assay. *Virology* **184:**645–654.

9. Baumgarte, S., L. K. de Souza Luna, K. Gyrwna, M. Panning, J. F. Drexler, C. Karsten, H. I. Huppertz, and C. Drosten. 2008. Prevalence, types, and RNA concentrations of human parechoviruses, including a sixth parechovirus type, in stool samples from patients with acute enteritis. *J. Clin. Microbiol.* **46:**242–248.

10. Bell, E. J., R. A. McCartney, D. Basquill, and A. K. Chaudhuri. 1986. Mu-antibody capture ELISA for the rapid diagnosis of enterovirus infections in patients with aseptic meningitis. *J. Med. Virol.* **19:**213–217.

11. Bendig, J. W., and P. Molyneaux. 1996. Sensitivity and specificity of mu-capture ELISA for detection of enterovirus IgM. *J. Virol. Methods* **59:**23–32.

12. Benschop, K., X. Thomas, C. Serpenti, R. Molenkamp, and K. Wolthers. 2008. High prevalence of human parechovirus (HPeV) genotypes in the Amsterdam region and identification of specific HPeV variants by direct genotyping of stool samples. *J. Clin. Microbiol.* **46:**3965–3970.

13. Benschop, K. S., J. Schinkel, R. P. Minnaar, D. Pajkrt, L. Spanjerberg, H. C. Kraakman, B. Berkhout, H. L. Zaaijer, M. G. Beld, and K. C. Wolthers. 2006. Human parechovirus infections in Dutch children and the association between serotype and disease severity. *Clin. Infect. Dis.* **42:**204–210.

14. Bradrick, S. S., E. A. Lieben, B. M. Carden, and J. R. Romero. 2001. A predicted secondary structural domain within the internal ribosome entry site of echovirus 12 mediates a cell-type-specific block to viral replication. *J. Virol.* **75:**6472–6481.

15. Brown, B. A., K. Maher, M. R. Flemister, P. Naraghi-Arani, M. Uddin, M. S. Oberste, and M. A. Pallansch. 2009. Resolving ambiguities in genetic typing of human enterovirus species C clinical isolates and identification of enterovirus 96, 99 and 102. *J. Gen. Virol.* **90:**1713–1723. doi:10.1099/vir.0.008540-0.

16. Buck, G. E., M. Wiesemann, and L. Stewart. 2002. Comparison of mixed cell culture containing genetically engineered BGMK and CaCo-2 cells (Super E-Mix) with RT-PCR and conventional cell culture for the diagnosis of enterovirus meningitis. *J. Clin. Virol.* **25**(Suppl. 1):S13–S18.

17. Capaul, S. E., and M. Gorgievski-Hrisoho. 2005. Detection of enterovirus RNA in cerebrospinal fluid (CSF) using NucliSens EasyQ enterovirus assay. *J. Clin. Virol.* **32:**236–240.

18. Casas, I., G. F. Palacios, G. Trallero, D. Cisterna, M. C. Freire, and A. Tenorio. 2001. Molecular characterization of human enteroviruses in clinical samples: comparison between VP2, VP1, and RNA polymerase regions using RT nested PCR assays and direct sequencing of products. *J. Med. Virol.* **65:**138–148.

19. Centers for Disease Control and Prevention. 2000. Enterovirus surveillance—United States, 1997–1999. *MMWR Morb. Mortal. Wkly. Rep.* **49:**913–916.

20. Centers for Disease Control and Prevention. 2006. Resurgence of wild poliovirus type 1 transmission and consequences of importation—21 countries, 2002–2005. *MMWR Morb. Mortal. Wkly. Rep.* **55:**145–150.

21. Centers for Disease Control and Prevention. 2008. Increased detections and severe neonatal disease associated with coxsackievirus B1 infection—United States, 2007. *MMWR Morb. Mortal. Wkly. Rep.* **57:**553–556.

22. Centers for Disease Control and Prevention. 2009. Progress toward interruption of wild poliovirus transmission—worldwide, 2008. *MMWR Morb. Mortal. Wkly. Rep.* **58:**308–312.

23. Centers for Disease Control and Prevention. 2009. Wild poliovirus type 1 and type 3 importations—15 countries, Africa, 2008–2009. *MMWR Morb. Mortal. Wkly. Rep.* **58:**357–362.

24. Chan, L. G., U. D. Parashar, M. S. Lye, F. G. Ong, S. R. Zaki, J. P. Alexander, K. K. Ho, L. L. Han, M. A. Pallansch, A. B. Suleiman, M. Jegathesan, and L. J. Anderson for the Outbreak Study Group. 2000. Deaths of children during an outbreak of hand, foot, and mouth disease in Sarawak, Malaysia: clinical and pathological characteristics of the disease. *Clin. Infect. Dis.* **31:**678–683.

25. Chapman, N. M., S. Tracy, C. J. Gauntt, and U. Fortmueller. 1990. Molecular detection and identification of enteroviruses using enzymatic amplification and nucleic acid hybridization. *J. Clin. Microbiol.* **28:**843–850.

26. Chen, T.-C., K.-F. Weng, S.-C. Chang, J.-Y. Lin, P.-N. Huang, and S.-R. Shih. 2008. Development of antiviral agents for enteroviruses. *J. Antimicrob. Chemother.* **62:**1169–1173.

27. Chonmaitree, T., C. Ford, C. Sanders, and H. L. Lucia. 1988. Comparison of cell cultures for rapid isolation of enteroviruses. *J. Clin. Microbiol.* **26:**2576–2580.

28. Coller, B. A., N. M. Chapman, M. A. Beck, M. A. Pallansch, C. J. Gauntt, and S. M. Tracy. 1990. Echovirus 22 is an atypical enterovirus. *J. Virol.* **64:**2692–2701.

29. Committee on Infectious Diseases and American Academy of Pediatrics. 1999. Prevention of poliomyelitis: recommendations for use of only inactivated poliovirus vaccine for routine immunization. *Pediatrics* **104:**1404–1406.

30. Committee on Infectious Diseases and American Academy of Pediatrics. 2009. Enterovirus (nonpoliovirus) infections. In L. K. Pickering (ed.), *Red Book: 2009 Report*, 28th ed. American Academy of Pediatrics, Elk Grove Village, IL.

31. Craig, M. E., P. Robertson, N. J. Howard, M. Silink, and W. D. Rawlinson. 2003. Diagnosis of enterovirus infection by genus-specific PCR and enzyme-linked immunosorbent assays. *J. Clin. Microbiol.* **41:**841–844.

32. De, L., B. Nottay, C. F. Yang, B. P. Holloway, M. Pallansch, and O. Kew. 1995. Identification of vaccine-related polioviruses by hybridization with specific RNA probes. *J. Clin. Microbiol.* **33:**562–571.

33. Debiasi, R. L., and K. L. Tyler. 2004. Molecular methods for the diagnosis of viral enchephalitis. *Clin. Microbiol. Rev.* **17:**903–925.

34. Doolan, A., N. Langlois, and C. Semsarian. 2004. Causes of sudden cardiac death in young Australians. *Med. J. Aust.* **180:**110–112.

35. Elfaitouri, A., N. Mohamed, J. Fohlman, R. Aspholm, G. Frisk, G. Friman, L. Magnius, and J. Blomberg. 2005. Quantitative PCR-enhanced immunoassay for measurement of enteroviral immunoglobulin M antibody and diagnosis of aseptic meningitis. *Clin. Diagn. Lab. Immunol.* **12:**235–241.

36. Fabre, A., and M. N. Sheppard. 2006. Sudden adult death syndrome and other non-ischaemic causes of sudden cardiac death. *Heart* **92:**316–320. doi:10.1136/hrt.2004.045518.

37. Faden, H., P. H. Patel, and L. Campagna. 2006. Pitfalls in the diagnosis of enteroviral infection in young children. *Pediatr. Infect. Dis. J.* **25:**687–690. doi:10.1097/01.inf.0000226842.23106.a2.

38. Fox, J. D., S. Han, A. Samuelson, Y. Zhang, M. L. Neale, and D. Westmoreland. 2002. Development and evaluation of nucleic acid sequence based amplification (NASBA) for diagnosis of enterovirus infections using the NucliSens basic kit. *J. Clin. Virol.* **24:**117–130.

39. Gutierrez, K., and M. J. Abzug. 1990. Vaccine-associated poliovirus meningitis in children with ventriculoperitoneal shunts. *J. Pediatr.* **117:**424–427.

40. Harvala, H., I. Robertson, T. Chieochansin, E. C. McWilliam Leitch, K. Templeton, and P. Simmonds. 2009. Specific association of human parechovirus type 3 with sepsis and fever in young infants, as identified by direct typing of cerebrospinal fluid samples. *J. Infect. Dis.* **199:**1753–1760. doi:10.1086/599094.

41. Harvala, H., and P. Simmonds. 2009. Human parechoviruses: biology, epidemiology and clinical significance. *J. Clin. Virol.* **45:**1–9. doi:10.1016/j.jcv.2009.03.009.

42. Heim, A., and J. Schumann. 2002. Development and evaluation of a nucleic acid sequence based amplification (NASBA) protocol for the detection of enterovirus RNA in cerebrospinal fluid samples. *J. Virol. Methods* **103:**101–107.

43. Ho, M., E.-R. Chen, K.-H. Hsu, S.-J. Twu, K.-T. Chen, S.-F. Tsai, J.-R. Wang, and S.-R. Shih for the Taiwan Enterovirus Epidemic Working Group. 1999. An epidemic of enterovirus 71 infection in Taiwan. *N. Engl. J. Med.* **341:**929–935.

44. Huang, C. C., C. C. Liu, Y. C. Chang, C. Y. Chen, S. T. Wang, and T. F. Yeh. 1999. Neurologic complications in children with enterovirus 71 infection. *N. Engl. J. Med.* **341:**936–942.

45. Hyypia, T., C. Horsnell, M. Maaronen, M. Khan, N. Kalkkinen, P. Auvinen, L. Kinnunen, and G. Stanway. 1992. A distinct picornavirus group identified by sequence analysis. *Proc. Natl. Acad. Sci. USA* **89:**8847–8851.

46. **International Committee on Taxonomy.** 2000. Family Picornaviridae, p. 657–683. *In* M. H. V. van Regenmortel, C. M. Fauquet, D. H. L. Bishop, E. B. Carstens, M. K. Estes, S. M. Lemon, J. Maniloff, M. A. Mayo, D. J. McGeoch, C. R. Pringle, and R. B. Wickner (ed.), *Virus Taxonomy: Classification and Nomenclature of Viruses. Seventh Report of the International Committee on Taxonomy of Viruses.* Academic Press, San Diego, CA.

47. **Jokela, P., P. Joki-Korpela, M. Maaronen, V. Glumoff, and T. Hyypia.** 2005. Detection of human picornaviruses by multiplex reverse transcription-PCR and liquid hybridization. *J. Clin. Microbiol.* **43:**1239–1245.

48. **Joki-Korpela, P., and T. Hyypia.** 1998. Diagnosis and epidemiology of echovirus 22 infections. *Clin. Infect. Dis.* **27:**129–136.

49. **Khetsuriani, N., A. Lamonte, M. S. Oberste, and M. Pallansch.** 2006. Neonatal enterovirus infections reported to the national enterovirus surveillance system in the United States, 1983–2003. *Pediatr. Infect. Dis. J.* **25:**889–893. doi:10.1097/01.inf.0000237798.07462.32.

50. **Khetsuriani, N., A. Lamonte-Fowlkes, S. Oberst, and M. A. Pallansch.** 2006. Enterovirus surveillance—United States, 1970–2005. *MMWR Surveill. Summ.* **55:**1–20.

51. **Khetsuriani, N., E. S. Quiroz, R. C. Holman, and L. J. Anderson.** 2003. Viral meningitis-associated hospitalizations in the United States, 1988–1999. *Neuroepidemiology* **22:**345–352.

52. **Kilpatrick, D. R., K. Ching, J. Iber, R. Campagnoli, C. J. Freeman, N. Mishrik, H. M. Liu, M. A. Pallansch, and O. M. Kew.** 2004. Multiplex PCR method for identifying recombinant vaccine-related polioviruses. *J. Clin. Microbiol.* **42:**4313–4315.

53. **Klespies, S. L., D. E. Cebula, C. L. Kelley, D. Galehouse, and C. C. Maurer.** 1996. Detection of enteroviruses from clinical specimens by spin amplification shell vial culture and monoclonal antibody assay. *J. Clin. Microbiol.* **34:**1465–1467.

54. **Kost, C. B., B. Rogers, M. S. Oberste, C. Robinson, B. L. Eaves, K. Leos, S. Danielson, M. Satya, F. Weir, and F. S. Nolte.** 2007. Multicenter beta trial of the GeneXpert enterovirus assay. *J. Clin. Microbiol.* **45:**1081–1086.

55. **Lai, K. K., L. Cook, S. Wendt, L. Corey, and K. R. Jerome.** 2003. Evaluation of real-time PCR versus PCR with liquid-phase hybridization for detection of enterovirus RNA in cerebrospinal fluid. *J. Clin. Microbiol.* **41:**3133–3141.

56. **Landry, M. L., R. Garner, and D. Ferguson.** 2003. Comparison of the NucliSens Basic kit (nucleic acid sequence-based amplification) and the Argene Biosoft Enterovirus Consensus Reverse Transcription-PCR assays for rapid detection of enterovirus RNA in clinical specimens. *J. Clin. Microbiol.* **41:**5006–5010.

57. **Legay, V., J. J. Chomel, and B. Lina.** 2002. Specific RT-PCR procedure for the detection of human parechovirus type 1 genome in clinical samples. *J. Virol. Methods* **102:**157–160.

58. **Lepow, M. L., N. Coyne, L. B. Thompson, D. H. Carver, and F. C. Robbins.** 1962. A clinical, epidemiologic and laboratory investigation of aseptic meningitis during the four-year period, 1955–1958. II. The clinical disease and its sequelae. *N. Engl. J. Med.* **266:**1188–1193.

59. **Magnani, J. W., and G. W. Dec.** 2006. Myocarditis: current trends in diagnosis and treatment. *Circulation* **113:**876–890.

60. **Marlowe, E. M., S. M. Novak, J. J. Dunn, A. Smith, J. Cumpio, E. Makalintal, D. Barnes, and R. J. Burchette.** 2008. Performance of the GeneXpert enterovirus assay for detection of enteroviral RNA in cerebrospinal fluid. *J. Clin. Virol.* **43:**110–113.

61. **Melnick, J. L., R. O. Proctor, A. R. Ocampo, A. R. Diwan, and E. Ben Porath.** 1966. Free and bound virus in serum after administration of oral poliovirus vaccine. *Am. J. Epidemiol.* **84:**329–342.

62. **Melnick, J. L., H. A. Wenner, and C. A. Phillips.** 1979. Enteroviruses, p. 471–534. *In* E. H. Lennette and N. J. Schmidt (ed.), *Diagnostic Procedures for Viral, Rickettsial and Chlamydia Infections,* 5th ed. American Public Health Association, Washington, DC.

63. **Minor, P. D.** 1996. Poliovirus biology. *Structure* **4:**775–778.

64. **Modlin, J. F.** 1996. Update on enterovirus infections in infants and children. *Adv. Pediatr. Infect. Dis.* **12:**155–180.

65. **Modlin, J. F., R. Dagan, L. E. Berlin, D. M. Virshup, R. H. Yolken, and M. Menegus.** 1991. Focal encephalitis with enterovirus infections. *Pediatrics* **88:**841–845.

66. **Muir, P., A. Ras, P. E. Klapper, G. M. Cleator, K. Korn, C. Aepinus, A. Fomsgaard, P. Palmer, A. Samuelsson, A. Tenorio, B. Weissbrich, and A. M. van Loon.** 1999. Multicenter quality assessment of PCR methods for detection of enteroviruses. *J. Clin. Microbiol.* **37:**1409–1414.

67. **Mulford, W. S., R. S. Buller, M. Q. Arens, and G. A. Storch.** 2004. Correlation of cerebrospinal fluild (CSF) cell counts and elevated CSF protein levels with enterovirus reverse transcription-PCR results in pediatric and adult patients. *J. Clin. Microbiol.* **42:**4199–4203.

68. **Nejentsev, S., N. Walker, D. Riches, M. Egholm, and J. A. Todd.** 2009. Rare variants of IFIH1, a gene implicated in antiviral responses, protect against type 1 diabetes. *Science* **324:**387–389.

69. **Niklasson, B., A. Samsioe, N. Papadogiannakis, A. Kawecki, B. Hornfeldt, G. R. Saade, and W. Klitz.** 2007. Association of zoonotic Ljungan virus with intrauterine fetal deaths. *Birth Defects Res. A Clin. Mol. Teratol.* **79:**488–493. doi:10.1002/bdra.20359.

70. **Nix, W. A., K. Maher, E. S. Johansson, B. Niklasson, A. M. Lindberg, M. A. Pallansch, and M. S. Oberste.** 2008. Detection of all known parechoviruses by real-time PCR. *J. Clin. Microbiol.* **46:**2519–2524.

71. **Nix, W. A., M. S. Oberste, and M. A. Pallansch.** 2006. Sensitive, seminested PCR amplification of VP1 sequences for direct identification of all enterovirus serotypes from original clinical specimens. *J. Clin. Microbiol.* **44:**2698–2704. doi:10.1128/JCM.00542-06.

72. **Noordhoek, G. T., J. F. L. Weel, E. Poelstra, M. Hooghiemstra, and A. Brandenburge.** 2008. Clinical validation of a new real-time PCR assay for detection of enteroviruses and parechoviruses, and implications for diagnostic procedures. *J. Clin. Virol.* **41:**75–80.

73. **Oberste, M. S., K. Maher, D. R. Kilpatrick, and M. A. Pallansch.** 1999. Molecular evolution of the human enteroviruses: correlation of serotype with VP1 sequence and application to picornavirus classification. *J. Virol.* **73:**1941–1948.

74. **Oberste, M. S., K. Maher, S. M. Michele, G. Belliot, M. Uddin, and M. A. Pallansch.** 2005. Enteroviruses 76, 89, 90 and 91 represent a novel group within the species human enterovirus A. *J. Gen. Virol.* **86:**445–451.

75. **Oberste, M. S., K. Maher, and M. A. Pallansch.** 1999. Specific detection of echoviruses 22 and 23 in cell culture supernatants by RT-PCR. *J. Med. Virol.* **58:**178–181.

76. **Oberste, M. S., W. A. Nix, K. Maher, and M. A. Pallansch.** 2003. Improved molecular identification of enteroviruses by RT-PCR and amplicon sequencing. *J. Clin. Virol.* **26:**375–377.

77. **Olive, D. M., S. Al Mufti, W. Al Mulla, M. A. Khan, A. Pasca, G. Stanway, and W. Al Nakib.** 1990. Detection and differentiation of picornaviruses in clinical samples following genomic amplification. *J. Gen. Virol.* **71:**2141–2147.

78. **Pallansch, M. A., and M. S. Oberste.** 2009. Enteroviruses and parechoviruses, p. 249–282. *In* S. Specter, R. L. Hodinka, S. A. Young, and D. L. Wiedbrauk (ed.), *Clinical Virology Manual,* 4th ed. ASM Press, Washington, DC.

79. **Pozzetto, B., O. G. Gaudin, M. Aouni, and A. Ros.** 1989. Comparative evaluation of immunoglobulin M neutralizing antibody response in acute-phase sera and virus isolation for the routine diagnosis of enterovirus infection. *J. Clin. Microbiol.* **27:**705–708.

80. **Ramers, C., G. Billman, M. Hartin, S. Ho, and M. H. Sawyer.** 2000. Impact of a diagnostic cerebrospinal fluid enterovirus polymerase chain reaction test on patient management. *JAMA* **283:**2680–2685.

81. **Redondo, M. J., J. Jeffrey, P. R. Fain, G. S. Eisenbarth, and T. Orban.** 2008. Concordance for islet autoimmunity among monozygotic twins. *N. Engl. J. Med.* **359:**2849–2850.

82. **Rigonan, A. S., L. Mann, and T. Chonmaitree.** 1998. Use of monoclonal antibodies to identify serotypes of enterovirus isolates. *J. Clin. Microbiol.* **36:**1877–1881.

83. Robinson, C. C., M. Willis, A. Meagher, K. E. Gieseker, H. Rotbart, and M. P. Glode. 2002. Impact of rapid polymerase chain reaction results on management of pediatric patients with enteroviral meningitis. *Pediatr. Infect. Dis. J.* **21:** 283–286.

84. Rogers, B. B., L. C. Alpert, E. A. Hine, and G. J. Buffone. 1990. Analysis of DNA in fresh and fixed tissue by the polymerase chain reaction. *Am. J. Pathol.* **136:**541–548.

85. Romero, J. R. 1999. Reverse-transcription polymerase chain reaction detection of the enteroviruses. *Arch. Pathol. Lab. Med.* **123:**1161–1169.

86. Romero, J. R. 2001. Pleconaril: a novel antipicornaviral drug. *Expert Opin. Investig. Drugs* **10:**369–379.

87. Rotbart, H. A. 1990. Diagnosis of enteroviral meningitis with the polymerase chain reaction. *J. Pediatr.* **117:**85–89.

88. Rotbart, H. A. 1990. Enzymatic RNA amplification of the enteroviruses. *J. Clin. Microbiol.* **28:**438–442.

89. Rotbart, H. A., A. Ahmed, S. Hickey, R. Dagan, G. H. McCracken, Jr., R. J. Whitley, J. F. Modlin, M. Cascino, J. F. O'Connell, M. A. Menegus, and D. Blum. 1997. Diagnosis of enterovirus infection by polymerase chain reaction of multiple specimen types. *Pediatr. Infect. Dis. J.* **16:**409–411.

90. Rotbart, H. A., M. H. Sawyer, S. Fast, C. Lewinski, N. Murphy, E. F. Keyser, J. Spadoro, S. Y. Kao, and M. Loeffelholz. 1994. Diagnosis of enteroviral meningitis by using PCR with a colorimetric microwell detection assay. *J. Clin. Microbiol.* **32:**2590–2592.

91. Roth, B., M. Enders, A. Arents, A. Pfitzner, and E. Terletskaia-Ladwig. 2007. Epidemiologic aspects and laboratory features of enterovirus infections in Western Germany, 2000–2005. *J. Med. Virol.* **79:**956–962. doi:10.1002/jmv.20917.

92. Sawyer, M. H., D. Holland, N. Aintablian, J. D. Connor, E. F. Keyser, and N. J. Waecker, Jr. 1994. Diagnosis of enteroviral central nervous system infection by polymerase chain reaction during a large community outbreak. *Pediatr. Infect. Dis. J.* **13:**177–182.

93. She, R. C., G. Crist, E. Billetdeaux, J. Langer, and C. A. Petti. 2006. Comparison of multiple shell vial cell lines for isolation of enteroviruses: a national perspective. *J. Clin. Virol.* **37:**151–155. doi:10.1016/j.jcv.2006.06.009.

94. Shen, S., U. Desselberger, and T. A. McKee. 1997. The development of an antigen capture polymerase chain reaction assay to detect and type human enteroviruses. *J. Virol. Methods* **65:**139–144.

95. Silva, P. A., S. Diedrich, D. das Dores de Paula Cardoso, and E. Schreier. 2008. Identification of enterovirus serotypes by pyrosequencing using multiple sequencing primers. *J. Virol. Methods* **148:**260–264.

96. Smalling, T. W., S. E. Sefers, H. Li, and Y.-W. Tang. 2002. Molecular approaches to detecting herpes simplex virus and enteroviruses in the central nervous system. *J. Clin. Microbiol.* **40:**2317–2322.

97. Stanway, G., F. Brown, P. Christian, T. Hovi, T. Hyypiä, A. M. Q. King, N. J. Knowles, S. M. Lemon, P. D. Minor, et al. 2005. *Picornaviridae*, p. 757–788. In C. M. Fauquet, M. A. Mayo, J. Maniloff, U. Desselberger, and L. A. Ball (ed.), *Virus Taxonomy: Eighth Report of the International Committee on the Taxonomy of Viruses.* Elsevier Academic Press, Amsterdam, The Netherlands.

98. Stanway, G., N. Kalkkinen, M. Roivainen, F. Ghazi, M. Khan, M. Smyth, O. Meurman, and T. Hyypia. 1994. Molecular and biological characteristics of echovirus 22, a representative of a new picornavirus group. *J. Virol.* **68:**8232–8238.

99. Stellrecht, K. A., I. Harding, F. M. Hussain, N. G. Mishrik, R. T. Czap, M. L. Lepow, and R. A. Venezia. 2000. A one-step RT-PCR assay using an enzyme-linked detection system for the diagnosis of enterovirus meningitis. *J. Clin. Virol.* **17:**143–149.

100. Stellrecht, K. A., I. Harding, A. M. Woron, M. L. Lepow, and R. A. Venezia. 2002. The impact of an enteroviral RT-PCR assay on the diagnosis of aseptic meningitis and patient management. *J. Clin. Virol.* **25**(Suppl. 1):S19–S26.

101. Strikas, R. A., L. J. Anderson, and R. A. Parker. 1986. Temporal and geographic patterns of isolates of nonpolio enterovirus in the United States, 1970–1983. *J. Infect. Dis.* **153:**346–351.

102. Susi, P., L. Hattara, M. Waris, T. Luoma-aho, H. Siitari, T. Hyypia, and P. Saviranta. 2009. Typing of enteroviruses by use of microwell oligonucleotide arrays. *J. Clin. Microbiol.* **47:**1863–1870.

103. Tapparel, C., T. Junier, D. Gerlach, S. Van-Belle, L. Turin, S. Cordey, K. Muhlemann, N. Regamey, J. D. Aubert, P. M. Soccal, P. Eigenmann, E. Zdobnov, and L. Kaiser. 2009. New respiratory enterovirus and recombinant rhinoviruses among circulating picornaviruses. *Emerg. Infect. Dis.* **15:**719–726.

104. Terletskaia-Ladwig, E., S. Meier, R. Hahn, M. Leinmuller, F. Schneider, and M. Enders. 2008. A convenient rapid culture assay for the detection of enteroviruses in clinical samples: comparison with conventional cell culture and RT-PCR. *J. Med. Microbiol.* **57:**1000–1006. doi:10.1099/jmm.0.47799-0.

105. van der Sanden, S., E. de Bruin, H. Vennema, C. Swanink, M. Koopmans, and H. van der Avoort. 2008. Prevalence of human parechovirus in the Netherlands in 2000 to 2007. *J. Clin. Microbiol.* **46:**2884–2889. doi:10.1128/JCM.00168-08.

106. Van Doornum, G. J., and J. C. De Jong. 1998. Rapid shell vial culture technique for detection of enteroviruses and adenoviruses in fecal specimens: comparison with conventional virus isolation method. *J. Clin. Microbiol.* **36:**2865–2868.

107. Van Vliet, K. E., P. Muir, J. M. Echevarria, P. E. Klapper, G. M. Cleator, and A. M. van Loon. 2001. Multicenter proficiency testing of nucleic acid amplification methods for the detection of enteroviruses. *J. Clin. Microbiol.* **39:**3390–3392.

108. Verboon-Maciolek, M. A., F. Groenendaal, C. D. Hahn, J. Hellmann, A. M. van Loon, G. Boivin, and L. S. de Vries. 2008. Human parechovirus causes encephalitis with white matter injury in neonates. *Ann. Neurol.* **64:**266–273. doi:10.1002/ana.21445.

109. Vuorinen, T., R. Vainionpaa, and T. Hyypia. 2003. Five years' experience of reverse-transcriptase polymerase chain reaction in daily diagnosis of enterovirus and rhinovirus infections. *Clin. Infect. Dis.* **37:**452–455.

110. Wang, S. Y., T. L. Lin, H. Y. Chen, and T. S. Lin. 2004. Early and rapid detection of enterovirus 71 infection by an IgM-capture ELISA. *J. Virol. Methods* **119:**37–43.

111. Webster, A. D. B. 2005. Pleconaril—an advance in the treatment of enteroviral infection in immuno-compromised patients. *J. Clin. Virol.* **32:**1–6.

112. Wikswo, M. E., N. Khetsuriani, A. L. Fowlkes, X. Zheng, S. Penaranda, N. Verma, S. T. Shulman, K. Sircar, C. C. Robinson, T. Schmidt, D. Schnurr, and M. S. Oberste. 2009. Increased activity of coxsackievirus B1 strains associated with severe disease among young infants in the United States, 2007–2008. *Clin. Infect. Dis.* **49:**e44–e51. doi:10.1086/605090.

113. Wilfert, C. M., and J. Zeller. 1985. Enterovirus diagnosis, p. 85–107. In L. M. de la Maza and E. M. Peterson (ed.), *Medical Virology*, 4th ed. Lawrence Erlbaum Associates, Hillsdale, NJ.

114. Wolthers, K. C., K. S. Benschop, J. Schinkel, R. Molenkamp, R. M. Bergevoet, I. J. Spijkerman, H. C. Kraakman, and D. Pajkrt. 2008. Human parechoviruses as an important viral cause of sepsislike illness and meningitis in young children. *Clin. Infect. Dis.* **47:**358–363. doi:10.1086/589752.

115. Wright, H. T., Jr., R. M. Mcallister, and R. Ward. 1962. "Mixed" meningitis. Report of a case with isolation of Haemophilus influenzae type B and ECHO virus type 9 from the cerebrospinal fluid. *N. Engl. J. Med.* **267:**142–144.

116. Zeichhardt, H., and H.-P. Grunert. 2000. Enteroviruses, p. 252–269. In S. Specter, R. L. Hodinka, and S. A. Young (ed.), *Clinical Virology Manual*, 3rd ed. ASM Press, Washington, DC.

117. Zhou, F., F. Kong, K. McPhie, M. Ratnamohan, L. Donovan, F. Zeng, G. L. Gilbert, and D. E. Dwyer. 2009. Identification of 20 common human enterovirus serotypes by use of a reverse transcription-PCR-based reverse line blot hybridization assay. *J. Clin. Microbiol.* **47:**2737–2743.

Rhinoviruses

MARIE LOUISE LANDRY

86

TAXONOMY

Human rhinoviruses (HRV) are members of the family *Picornaviridae*. Previously a separate genus, rhinoviruses have recently been reclassified as species of the *Enterovirus* genus (http://www.ictvonline.org). Other genera in the *Picornaviridae* that are pathogenic for humans include *Parechovirus* and *Hepatovirus*. Recently, the *Cardiovirus* genus has been found to contain human pathogens as well (97).

The rhinovirus genus derives its name from the predominant site of its replication and symptomatology, the nose. On the basis of neutralization tests in cell culture, 100 rhinovirus serotypes have been designated: HRV1A, HRV1B, HRV2 to HRV86, and HRV88 to HRV100. HRV87 is now considered to be an acid-sensitive strain of enterovirus type 68 (7, 87). While some cross-neutralization occurs, there is no group antigen (52, 56). Based on receptor binding, rhinoviruses have been divided into two groups (87, 89). Intercellular adhesion molecule 1 (ICAM-1) is the cell receptor for the major group, comprising 88 known HRV serotypes. ICAM-1 is a member of the immunoglobulin supergene family and may be expressed on the surface of many different cells, including those that are active in respiratory immune responses (77). The minor group of serotypes binds to members of the low-density lipoprotein receptor family (40). Originally comprised of 10 serotypes, the minor group now includes two additional serotypes previously classified in the major group (89).

Based on antiviral susceptibility and sequencing of viral capsid protein genes VP4/VP2 and VP1, prototype rhinoviruses have been divided into two species, A (74 serotypes) and B (25 serotypes), which do not coincide with receptor groups (1, 56). Recently, a novel group of HRV has been detected by reverse transcription-PCR (RT-PCR) in patients with lower respiratory tract disease (53, 58, 66). Publications have variously referred to these novel strains as HRV-A2 (2), HRV-NY (53), HRV-QPM (66), HVR-X (48), and HRV-C (55). Comparisons have been difficult due to the different sequencing methods used and lack of full sequencing data. Since these viruses have not grown in cell culture, serotype information is not available. However, based on partial sequence data, these novel strains have been tentatively designated as a third rhinovirus species, group C (HRV-C) (8, 67). Molecular dating suggests that HRV-C strains have been circulating for at least 250 years (8). Recently, Palmenberg et al. completed the sequencing of all prototype HRV serotypes plus 10 field samples and postulated that many additional HRV-C strains are awaiting discovery (74). These authors also found divergence within HRV-A of a distinct clade, clade D, and evidence for recombination as a mechanism for HRV diversity. As more is learned about the molecular genetics of HRV, further revisions in classification and taxonomy are anticipated (74).

DESCRIPTION OF THE AGENT

The rhinovirus virion consists of a nonenveloped icosahedral nucleocapsid, 20 to 27 nm in diameter, with 60 protomeric units consisting of four protein subunits: VP1, VP2, VP3, and VP4. These structural polypeptides are obtained by posttranslational cleavage of a large polypeptide precursor. The 3C protease that participates in cleavage of this polypeptide is a target for antiviral drugs. VP1, VP2, and VP3 reside on the exterior of the virus and make up its protein coat. Located within VP1 is a hydrophobic pocket into which antiviral compounds such as pleconaril bind (96). VP4 resides inside the protein shell. X-ray crystallography and cryoelectron microscopy studies have identified large depressions or "canyons" on each of the 60 protomeric units, which appear to be sites for cell receptor binding and play a critical role in conformational changes that follow attachment (95). Conformational changes in the canyon floor can also be induced by certain antiviral agents, thus inhibiting virus attachment to cells or virus uncoating (96).

The HRV genome is single-stranded, plus-strand RNA, approximately 7,200 nucleotides in size, with a single open reading frame and coupled at the 5' noncoding region (5'NCR) with a short peptide (VPg). Rhinovirus replicates in the cytoplasm of infected cells, producing infectious virions that sediment at a buoyant density of 1.40 g/liter in cesium chloride. Empty capsids and particles lacking one or more structural polypeptides are also produced.

As they have no lipid envelope, rhinoviruses are fairly resistant to inactivation by organic solvents such as ether, chloroform, ethanol, and 5% phenol. Although rhinoviruses are relatively thermostable, heating at 50 to 56°C progressively decreases infectivity. Rhinoviruses are traditionally differentiated from enteroviruses by their loss of infectivity upon exposure to pH 3 for 3 h at room temperature, though this may not be the case with all serotypes and strains. Genetic variability is common, due to error-prone replication and, as only recently appreciated, recombination (74; X. Lu and D. D. Erdman, presented at the 25th Annual Clinical Virology Symposium, 19 to 22 April 2009, Daytona Beach, FL).

EPIDEMIOLOGY AND TRANSMISSION

In temperate zones, rhinovirus infections occur year-round, with a peak in September and a second peak in late spring (11). Seasonal fluctuations may relate in part to improved survival of rhinoviruses in conditions of high relative indoor humidity and herding together of children when school opens in the fall (70). Recent studies indicate, however, that circulation of newly recognized HRV-C strains may predominate in the fall, whereas HRV-A strains may predominate in the spring (69). As the disease burden and diversity of HRV infections have become evident, the interest in HRV discovery, genetic typing, and molecular epidemiology has intensified.

Studies with volunteers have shown that inoculation of virus into the nose or conjunctivae is the most efficient way to initiate infection (22). Rhinovirus is present in the highest titers in the nose of infected persons and commonly contaminates their hands. Consequently, investigators have found that rhinovirus can be transmitted via hand-to-hand contact (32) or by contaminated fomites, followed by self-inoculation of virus into the nose or conjunctivae (33). Furthermore, transmission can be interrupted by using tissues impregnated with virucidal agents for nose blowing, by treating surfaces with disinfectant, or by applying iodine to the fingers (39). Volunteer studies have also shown that with very prolonged exposure times, rhinovirus can also be transmitted by the aerosol route (21).

Rhinoviruses replicate primarily in ciliated epithelial cells in the nose, and the incubation period is 1 to 4 days. The peak of virus shedding coincides with the acute rhinitis. Symptoms last 7 days on average but can persist for 12 to 14 days or more (36, 63), and they typically include profuse watery discharge, nasal congestion, sneezing, headache, mild sore throat, cough, and little or no fever. By culture, virus may become undetectable at 4 to 5 days or may be present in low titers for up to 2 to 3 weeks (23). Using RT-PCR, however, rhinovirus RNA has been detected by some investigators for 4 to 5 weeks after the onset of symptoms, and even for 2 to 3 weeks prior to the onset of symptoms (43, 92). Though not proven, it is possible that prolonged detection represents a series of sequential rhinovirus infections, some asymptomatic. Indeed, asymptomatic infections are common, occurring in 20 to 30% of infected persons (11, 44, 92, 93).

Rhinovirus causes minimal pathology in the nasal epithelium, and the symptoms of rhinovirus infection parallel the rise and fall of chemical mediators of inflammation (33, 38). Psychological stress and inadequate sleep appear to increase susceptibility and the development of clinical symptoms (15, 16), whereas exposure to a cold environment does not (25). Early studies concluded that immunity is type specific and correlates best with local production of immunoglobulin A (IgA) (4, 12).

CLINICAL SIGNIFICANCE

Rhinoviruses cause approximately two-thirds of cases of the common cold and thus are responsible for more episodes of human illness than any other infectious agent (11, 38). Although a trivial illness, the common cold is acutely disabling and its cost, in days lost from work, cold remedies, and analgesics, is estimated at $40 billion annually in the United States (26). With the use of molecular methods in research studies, HRV has been increasingly implicated as the major viral cause of asthma exacerbations and decompensation of chronic lung disease (29, 65). Severe asthma exacerbations have been linked to prolonged shedding of rhinovirus RNA (49). Rhinoviruses can be the sole etiology of sinusitis and otitis media and can facilitate secondary bacterial infections (72, 78). Thus, the pathogenesis of rhinovirus infection is currently the subject of intense study.

Rhinovirus has been increasingly detected in lower respiratory tract infections (37, 76), especially in the very young (50), school-age children (84), the elderly (61, 71), and those with chronic illnesses, cancer, immunosuppressive illnesses or transplants (13, 31, 51, 88), or underlying pulmonary disease (54). The clinical manifestations of rhinovirus infection in hospitalized infants are similar to those caused by respiratory syncytial virus (RSV); however, the mean age of HRV-infected infants tends to be slightly older (50). Recently, investigators around the world have found that novel HRV-C strains appear to be the predominant HRV species linked to hospitalizations for fever, wheezing, and lower respiratory tract disease, especially in young infants and asthmatic children (46, 53, 58, 62, 66, 68, 69). Although rhinovirus viremia has rarely been found by culture, rhinovirus RNA has been detected using sensitive molecular methods in the blood of 11.4% of rhinovirus-infected young children, including 25% of those with rhinovirus-associated asthma exacerbations (94).

Since HRV have historically been difficult to culture and serotype, there is little information available on the relationships between serotype and clinical manifestations (47). With the development of genetic typing methods and increased awareness of the disease burden of HRV, this will likely change (11, 47).

Many antivirals show activity against rhinoviruses in the laboratory (20). However, inadequate drug delivery to the site of infection has reduced clinical benefit, and treatment remains experimental. Studies have included intranasal administration of soluble ICAM-1 in rhinovirus-infected volunteers, use of intranasal ipratropium bromide (an anticholinergic agent) or intranasal imiquimod, or administration of antivirals and antimediators in combination (14, 33, 35, 85). Efficacy studies in humans of echinacea, an herbal remedy, and zinc tablets have been mixed (86). Although the picornavirus capsid-binding agent pleconaril showed some benefit in clinical trials of natural colds (36), it was not approved for clinical use. A more recent phase II trial of a pleconaril nasal spray remains unpublished. Another capsid binding agent, BTA-798, is in clinical trials. Recently, inhibitors of rhinovirus 3C protease have shown potent antiviral activity, but trials of rupintrivir and compound 1 have been halted (20). Due to numerous HRV types, prospects for a vaccine have been considered negligible. However, it is hoped that full-genome sequencing will usher in a new era of antiviral and vaccine design (74).

COLLECTION, TRANSPORT, AND STORAGE OF SPECIMENS

In natural infections, rhinovirus can generally be isolated in culture from 1 day before to 6 days after onset of cold symptoms, but it is shed at the highest concentration on day 1 or 2 of illness. Since rhinovirus is excreted in the highest titers from the nose, nasal rather than throat or sputum specimens should be obtained for diagnosis. Earlier comparisons of nasal wash, nose swab, throat gargle, and throat swab specimens for the isolation of rhinovirus from clinical specimens revealed nasal wash to be the best (3, 12, 17). Nasal wash specimens are obtained as follows. Tilt the patient's head backwards and instill 1 ml of sterile phosphate-buffered saline (PBS) into one of the nostrils. Then ask the patient to lean forward and allow the washing to drip into a sterile petri dish or other collection container. Repeat with the other nostril until each nostril has been washed with 5 ml of PBS. Transfer the washings into a sterile container with an equal volume of viral transport medium (VTM) containing antibiotics. The inclusion of phenol red in the VTM allows the detection of acid pH, which would adversely affect the isolation of rhinovirus.

If a nasal wash cannot be obtained, a nasopharyngeal (NP) aspirate is preferred, or a deep nasal turbinate or NP swab (12, 38). Swabs are then immersed in a vial containing 2 ml of VTM. Well-collected NP swabs can provide results similar to those obtained with aspirates and are simpler to obtain (80). Endotracheal aspirate, bronchoalveolar lavage, or bronchial wash samples should be collected to diagnose lower respiratory tract disease.

Specimens should be transported promptly to the laboratory. For isolation, the best results are obtained with prompt inoculation of cell cultures; however, specimens can be held for up to 24 hours at 4°C in VTM with neutral pH. If longer delays are necessary, specimens should be frozen at −70°C and thawed just before inoculation. Freezing does not appear to be detrimental to virus recovery (3). In general, similar sample handling is acceptable for molecular analysis; however, the compatibility of various VTM with different extraction reagents must be confirmed in each laboratory.

DIRECT DETECTION

Antigen

Due to the large number of serotypes and the lack of a common group antigen, antigen detection assays are not used.

Nucleic Acid

Fortunately, picornavirus genomes have a high degree of nucleic acid sequence homology in the 5′NCR. Using primers or probes based on sequences in the 5′NCR, all rhinovirus serotypes can theoretically be detected in a single assay. RT-PCR and nucleic acid sequence-based amplification have been much more sensitive than culture methods, doubling or even tripling the number of HRV infections detected (6, 27, 41, 44, 60, 81, 88, 90). Nevertheless, culture can occasionally detect some rhinoviruses missed by RT-PCR due to variability in techniques and primer or probe mismatches (6, 41, 90). Although suboptimal culture conditions are often used in comparative studies (38), amplification methods are clearly superior and continue to improve in sensitivity and in time to result (63).

At present, molecular methods are not standardized, and published techniques have differed in types of samples tested, RNA extraction methods, primer selection, and amplification and detection protocols. Since primer pairs from the 5′NCR will commonly detect both enteroviruses and rhinoviruses, a universal problem is differentiating these two picornavirus groups from each other. Unfortunately, primers that are best able to distinguish rhinovirus from enterovirus may not be the most sensitive for detection of rhinovirus in clinical specimens (44). Thus, more broadly reactive primers are often used. Sequencing of amplicons to differentiate rhinovirus from enterovirus in clinical samples may be feasible in the future; however, the equipment and expertise are not currently available in the routine clinical laboratory (19). Earlier strategies to distinguish rhinovirus from enterovirus have included primer pair design to generate different-size amplicons for rhinovirus and enterovirus (34), restriction

enzyme digestion of a common-size amplicon (75), differential internal probe hybridization (6, 19, 34), and nested PCR with annealing and extension times optimized for rhinovirus detection (81). Most reported methods have failed to detect or accurately differentiate a few of the viruses tested, and none evaluated all rhinovirus and enterovirus serotypes.

More recently, real-time amplification using SYBR green, TaqMan hybridization probes, or molecular beacons (18, 19, 45, 60, 82, 88), as well as multiplex real-time PCR to detect multiple respiratory viruses (5, 9, 30, 79), has been developed. Real-time amplification methods have the advantages of simplicity, reduced risk of contamination, ability to estimate viral load, and a shortened time to result since detection occurs concurrently with amplification. Though SYBR green testing is less expensive than probe-based methods, results obtained by this method can be difficult to interpret (63).

Recently, Lu et al. obtained 5′NCR sequences of all 100 currently recognized HRV prototype strains and 85 recently circulating field isolates to develop and validate a real-time RT-PCR assay for comprehensive detection of HRV (63). The reverse primer and probe were highly conserved among all HRV/human enterovirus (HEV) sequences, but the forward primer was located in a variable region that distinguished all HRV from HEVs. Nevertheless, high-titer samples of HEV could give weakly positive reactions. It should be noted that protocol performance was optimized using a specific commercial one-step RT-PCR kit and platform and appeared to work with several different kits, but it failed completely with one RT-PCR kit. Thus, laboratories should be aware that deviations from the optimized protocol can have significant adverse effects on assay performance.

Two highly multiplexed commercial systems have been developed that detect 17 to 20 respiratory virus targets in a single tube. Both utilize multiplex PCR followed by amplicon identification using a fluid-microsphere-based array and a Luminex instrument (59, 64, 73). One of these, the Tm Bioscience respiratory virus panel, is currently the only FDA-approved molecular test that detects HRV. At present, few clinical laboratories are either interested or able to set up a homebrew HRV PCR, and even if available, HRV PCR may not be ordered unless it is included as part of a more comprehensive panel. These comprehensive multiplex assays have confirmed the frequent detection of rhinoviruses in culture-negative clinical samples and have revealed many mixed infections. Whereas real-time methods provide a cycle threshold value as an indicator of viral load that can be useful in assessing clinical relevance and potential contamination, highly multiplexed commercial assays are purely qualitative. They also do not incorporate uracil-N-glycosylase to prevent amplicon carryover.

Two highly multiplexed noncommercial methods that have been useful in research studies include MassTag PCR (53) and Virochip (48). MassTag PCR detects 22 respiratory virus and bacterial pathogens, and then amplification products are analyzed in a single-quadrupole mass spectrometer. When applied to samples from patients with influenza-like illness negative by other methods, MassTag PCR detected rhinoviruses in a large number of samples, including novel rhinovirus strains (53). The Virochip is a DNA microarray-based viral detection platform used to investigate virus infections in adults with and without asthma. In one study, Virochip detected over 20 serotypes of HRV, as well as 5 divergent viruses referred to as HRV-X but now thought to be HRV-C strains (48).

Although much effort has been devoted to distinguishing rhinovirus from enterovirus, in the clinical setting a single assay that detects both virus groups could ultimately prove to be an advantage, since some antivirals may be effective against both enterovirus and rhinovirus infections (36). Thus, some multiplexed assays have not attempted to separate the two genera but instead have targeted "picornaviruses" (53).

ISOLATION PROCEDURES

Cell Culture

Rhinoviruses grow only in cells of human or monkey origin. Although the original isolation of rhinoviruses was in primary monkey kidney cells, these cells have not been consistent in yielding a broad range of isolates. The most commonly used cells in clinical laboratories are the human embryonic lung fibroblast (HELF) lines WI-38 and MRC-5. WI-38 cells are significantly more sensitive than MRC-5 cells (3), but MRC-5 cells are more commonly available in clinical laboratories. Human embryonic kidney (HEK) cells can also support rhinovirus replication. Unfortunately, different lots of normally sensitive cell lines have been found to vary over 100-fold in sensitivity to rhinovirus (10); the reasons for this variation are not known. Therefore, for optimal results, simultaneous use of at least two sensitive systems is recommended.

In the research setting, several HeLa cell clones, such as HeLa M or Ohio HeLa cells, HeLa H, HeLa R-19, and HeLa I cells, have been shown to support the replication of rhinoviruses to high titers (3, 17). HeLa I cells were found to be more sensitive than WI-38, MRC-5, fetal tonsil, and HeLa H or M cells for recovery of rhinovirus from clinical specimens (3, 28). These specialized cell lines can be obtained only from research laboratories.

After inoculation, cultures are incubated in standard cell culture medium such as Eagle's minimum essential medium with 2% fetal calf serum and antibiotics at a neutral pH. To mimic conditions of the nose, cultures should be incubated at 33 to 35°C with continuous rotation in a roller drum to provide aeration of the monolayer. Rhinovirus cytopathic effects (CPE) can be observed as early as 24 to 48 hours after inoculation and are often detected by day 4. Passage of infected HeLa cell cultures may be necessary for some isolates before CPE is apparent. In fibroblasts, cellular changes are easier to read and are often detected earlier than in epithelial cell lines. Both large and small rounded, refractile cells with pyknotic nuclei are observed in foci that also contain cellular debris (Fig. 1). Rhinovirus CPE are similar to enterovirus CPE but may sometimes be confused with nonspecific changes. The CPE progresses over a 2- to 3-day period, with the degree of cellular change depending on the serotype and the inoculum dose. It should be noted that rhinovirus CPE can regress, or virus may inactivate if left too long. Therefore, cultures should be promptly passaged. Passage is also necessary to increase viral titers prior to the performance of identification tests.

HELF cell cultures should be observed for 14 days, with refeeding at 7 days to increase recovery of virus. HeLa cell cultures can be observed for only up to 7 to 8 days, when passage becomes necessary due to nonspecific cell degeneration and rounding.

Organ Culture

Organ cultures of human fetal nasal epithelium or trachea were used in the past to isolate rhinoviruses not grown in standard cell cultures, but they are no longer used for this purpose. Recently, however, cultures of nasal and tracheal mucosa obtained from biopsy material have been used for research studies of rhinovirus pathogenesis (42, 91).

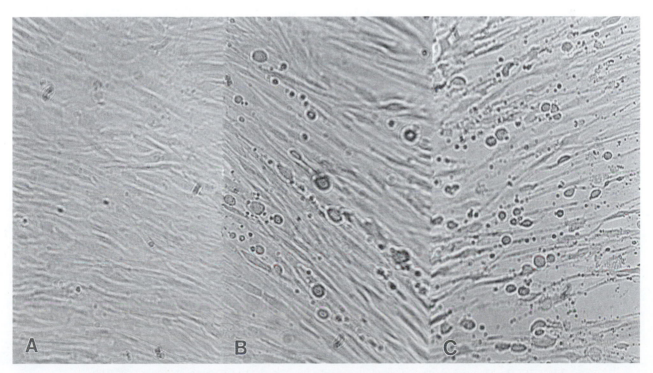

FIGURE 1 Rhinovirus CPE in HELF. (A) Uninfected cells; (B) early focus of rhinovirus CPE; (C) more advanced rhinovirus CPE. Magnification, ×100.

IDENTIFICATION OF VIRUS

A presumptive diagnosis of a rhinovirus isolate in cell culture is made by the appearance and progression of characteristic CPE in the appropriate clinical setting. In clinical laboratories, further identification of a presumed rhinovirus isolate is usually limited to differentiating it from enterovirus by determining sensitivity to acid pH (Fig. 2). Neutralization testing is time-consuming, costly, and not routinely available. In addition, the recently recognized HRV-C strains do not grow in culture, and no neutralizing sera are available.

Acid pH Stability

Rhinoviruses are sensitive to low pH, whereas enteroviruses are stable. Thus, a reduction in virus titer by 2 to 3 log_{10} tissue culture infective doses ($TCID_{50}$) can be expected upon exposure of rhinovirus to low pH. First, passage of the isolate will be necessary to obtain a minimum titer of 10^3 $TCID_{50}$/ml. Then, prepare two solutions of a buffer, such as HEPES, one at pH 3.0 and one at pH 7.0. Add 0.2 ml of unknown virus suspension to 1.8 ml of HEPES, pH 3.0, and 0.2 ml of virus to 1.8 ml of HEPES, pH 7.0. Keep the mixtures at room temperature for 3 hours, adjust the pH to 7.0, make serial dilutions of the mixtures, and inoculate into cell culture. If the unknown virus is a rhinovirus, a minimum 2-log_{10} reduction in viral titer should be evident in the acid-treated sample. A known rhinovirus and a known enterovirus should be treated in a similar fashion as controls.

Temperature Sensitivity

Since rhinoviruses often grow best at 33°C, they may be distinguished from enteroviruses by inoculation of serial dilutions of the unknown virus and incubation of one set of cultures at 33°C and a replicate set of cultures at 37°C.

The onset of CPE should be more rapid and the titer of virus obtained should be higher at the lower temperature. Some rhinovirus isolates may not show this temperature sensitivity, and this test is no longer used clinically (76).

Virus Identification by RT-PCR

Rhinovirus RT-PCR targeting highly conserved regions of the 5′NCR can be used for confirmation of rhinovirus isolates in cell culture. However, cross-reactions with enteroviruses can occur, especially with high-titer culture isolates (63, 83).

TYPING SYSTEMS

Serotyping of Virus Isolates by Neutralization

Rhinovirus serotyping is an expensive, labor-intensive research procedure that is rarely performed. Serotyping requires the neutralization of 30 to 100 $TCID_{50}$ of virus-induced CPE by 20 units of antiserum. Hyperimmune antisera for types 1A to 100 are available through the American Type Culture Collection. Intersecting serum pools similar to those used for enterovirus identification have been prepared, and culture isolates can be tested by microneutralization. Confirmation of serotype is then performed using monospecific antiserum. Detailed procedures are described elsewhere (17).

Genotyping by Sequencing

Molecular typing requires PCR amplification of a selected gene, usually 5′NCR, VP4/VP2, and/or VP1, followed by sequencing and phylogenetic analysis. The correlation of HRV serotype with genotype has not been thoroughly studied, but some discordance is known to occur.

The optimal genotyping strategy has not yet been established. The 5′NCR contains both highly conserved

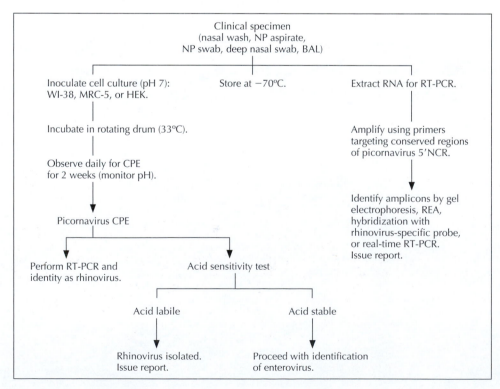

FIGURE 2 Flow scheme for the isolation or detection and identification of rhinovirus. REA, restriction enzyme analysis; BAL, bronchoalveolar lavage.

and variable sequences and has been reported by several groups as the most sensitive and reliable target for amplifying and typing clinical isolates, including directly from clinical specimens (47, 83). However, the 5′NCR cannot unequivocally determine HRV genotype. It is prone to recombination and should not be used for definitive typing of new strains (78; Lu and Erdman, 25th Annual Clinical Virology Symposium, 2009). Although VP1 sequence analysis requires multiple primer pairs and ongoing optimization as new HRV are recognized (56), it may correlate best with serotype and provide the most reliable results (52, 56; Lu and Erdman, 25th Annual Clinical Virology Symposium, 2009). It is likely that definitive genotyping results will need to be supported by data from multiple regions such as the 5′NCR, VP4/VP2, and VP1, and may require full genome sequencing (74).

SEROLOGIC TESTS

Determination of antibody response is impractical for the diagnosis of rhinoviruses in the clinical setting. The number of HRV serotypes and the lack of a common antigen make blind serologic testing impractical. Diagnosis by serology is also retrospective since antibody is usually not detectable until 1 to 3 weeks after onset of illness, with IgA predominant in nasal secretions and IgG predominant in serum (17). In research studies, antibody determination by neutralization test is the "gold standard" for serology (24). Enzyme-linked immunosorbent assay (ELISA) using specific-serotype antigens has been used to detect serum and nasal IgG and IgA in volunteers inoculated with known HRV serotypes, and ELISA was 100 to 10,000 times more sensitive than neutralization (4). Detailed procedures can be found elsewhere (17).

EVALUATION, INTERPRETATION, AND REPORTING OF RESULTS

A comparison of HRV diagnostic methods is shown in Table 1. The diagnosis of rhinovirus infection in most clinical laboratories is still based upon isolation of virus with characteristic CPE in commonly available conventional cell

TABLE 1 Comparison of diagnostic methods for rhinoviruses

Method	Advantages	Disadvantages and limitations	Clinical applicability	Key references
Virus isolation	Can recover in culture when rhinovirus not specifically requested Rhinovirus groups A and B replicate in conventional cell cultures used in clinical laboratories (e.g., WI-38, MRC-5, and HEK) These cultures may detect other viruses as well as rhinovirus (e.g., CMV, VZV, HSV, adenovirus, enterovirus, and RSV[a])	Optimal recovery of multiple rhinovirus serotypes requires use of additional sensitive cell cultures not routinely used in diagnostic laboratories (e.g., Ohio HeLa cells, HeLa I cells, or fetal tonsil) Normally sensitive cells can vary over 100-fold in sensitivity Differentiation of rhinovirus from enterovirus isolates is time-consuming (e.g., quantitative acid sensitivity test) Recently recognized novel HRV-C does not grow in culture	Most common means of detection in clinical laboratories	3, 10, 17, 28, 58
RT-PCR or other NAT[b]	Much more sensitive and rapid than culture methods for rhinoviruses Detects newly recognized HRV-C strains Broadly reactive primers that are most sensitive for detection of rhinoviruses in clinical specimens may also detect enteroviruses Real-time assays are more rapid, simpler to perform, and less prone to contamination than conventional or nested PCR assays Multiplex assays can detect multiple respiratory viruses Instrumentation can automate many steps	Most molecular assays must be established and validated in-house, which is time-consuming and expensive Differentiation of rhinovirus from enterovirus can be difficult Since the same clinical syndrome may be caused by other viruses, samples must be tested for additional viruses	Expected to increase	5, 9, 19, 27, 30, 45, 57, 59, 63, 65, 73, 79, 81, 88, 90, 93
Organ culture	May detect some infections not detected by virus isolation in cell culture Useful in studies of pathogenesis Biopsy or surgically removed tissues can be used	Fetal nasal or tracheal tissues are not readily available Supplanted by molecular assays for detection of rhinovirus in clinical specimens	Occasionally used in pathogenesis research	42, 91
Serology to detect antibody response	May detect some infections not detected by virus isolation Research tool used after infection of volunteers with a known HRV serotype or in epidemiologic studies	HRV antibody testing for clinical diagnosis is impractical due to the large number of HRV serotypes, the lack of a common antigen, and the need for acute- and convalescent-phase sera	Used only in research settings	4, 17, 24

[a]CMV, cytomegalovirus; VZV, varicella-zoster virus; HSV, herpes simplex virus.
[b]NAT, nucleic acid test.

systems, such as WI-38, MRC-5, or HEK. Incubation at 33 to 35°C and rotation of cultures provide optimal conditions for virus replication. Differentiation of rhinoviruses from enteroviruses, with which their CPE can be confused, is based primarily on acid stability testing of isolates. Specific identification of rhinovirus serotypes by neutralization test or sequence-based molecular methods is reserved for epidemiologic research studies. Serologic testing is not available.

Nucleic acid amplification assays have revolutionized rhinovirus detection. Yet in the clinical laboratory, rhinoviruses are rarely specifically requested. Rather, rhinoviruses are isolated in conventional culture when the suspected virus is influenza virus or RSV. Consequently, few clinical laboratories offer specific molecular testing for rhinoviruses, due to the expense and expertise required for in-house test development and the lack of clinical demand. The exceptions are multiplexed commercial (59, 64, 73) or real-time (5, 9, 30, 79) molecular assays, or respiratory virus PCR panels that include rhinovirus and thus allow HRV to be detected even when not specifically sought.

The interpretation of a positive rhinovirus PCR result in the individual case can be problematic. HRV are extremely common, occur in asymptomatic persons, exhibit prolonged shedding, and can occur as coinfections with other viruses or bacteria (11, 44, 68, 73, 93; Lu and Erdman, 25th Annual Clinical Virology Symposium, 2009). In these circumstances, reporting an assessment of viral load by real-time PCR may help determine its role in the acute illness. Quantitative results are not available, however, with commercial highly multiplexed assays.

Although molecular techniques applied in the research setting will continue to elucidate the important role of rhinoviruses as lower respiratory tract pathogens and as significant causes of asthma and chronic obstructive pulmonary disease exacerbation, the standard diagnostic approach may not change substantially until effective therapy becomes available, the impact of rapid and sensitive rhinovirus diagnosis on the management of hospitalized patients can be demonstrated, or highly multiplexed molecular assays incorporating rhinoviruses are more widely adopted.

REFERENCES

1. **Andries, K., B. Dewindt, J. Snoeks, L. Wouters, H. Moereels, P. J. Lewis, and P. A. Janssen.** 1990. Two groups of rhinoviruses revealed by a panel of antiviral compounds present sequence divergence and differential pathogenicity. *J. Virol.* **64:**1117–1123.
2. **Arden, K. E., P. McErlean, M. D. Nissen, T. P. Sloots, and I. M. Mackay.** 2006. Frequent detection of human rhinoviruses, paramyxoviruses, coronaviruses, and bocavirus during acute respiratory tract infections. *J. Med. Virol.* **78:**1232–1240.
3. **Arruda, E., C. E. Crump, B. S. Rollins, A. Ohlin, and F. G. Hayden.** 1996. Comparative susceptibilities of human embryonic fibroblasts and HeLa cells for isolation of human rhinoviruses. *J. Clin. Microbiol.* **34:**1277–1279.
4. **Barclay, W. S., and W. Al-Nakib.** 1987. An ELISA for the detection of rhinovirus specific antibody in serum and nasal secretion. *J. Virol. Methods* **15:**53–64.
5. **Bellau-Pujol, S., A. Vabret, L. Legrand, J. Dina, S. Gouarin, J. Petitjean-Lecherbonnier, B. Pozzetto, C. Ginevra, and F. Freymuth.** 2005. Development of three multiplex RT-PCR assays for the detection of 12 respiratory RNA viruses. *J. Virol. Methods* **126:**53–63.
6. **Blomqvist, S., A. Skytta, M. Roivainen, and T. Hovi.** 1999. Rapid detection of human rhinoviruses in nasopharyngeal aspirates by a microwell reverse transcription-PCR-hybridization assay. *J. Clin. Microbiol.* **37:**2813–2816.
7. **Blomqvist, S., C. Savolainen, L. Raman, M. Roivainen, and T. Hovi.** 2002. Human rhinovirus 87 and enterovirus 68 represent a unique serotype with rhinovirus and enterovirus features. *J. Clin. Microbiol.* **40:**4218–4223.
8. **Briese, T., N. Renwick, M. Venter, R. G. Jarman, D. Ghosh, S. Köndgen, S. K. Shrestha, A. M. Hoegh, I. Casas, E. V. Adjogoua, C. Akoua-Koffi, K. S. Myint, D. T. Williams, G. Chidlow, R. van den Berg, C. Calvo, O. Koch, G. Palacios, V. Kapoor, J. Villari, S. R. Dominguez, K. V. Holmes, G. Harnett, D. Smith, J. S. Mackenzie, H. Ellerbrok, B. Schweiger, K. Schønning, M. S. Chadha, F. H. Leendertz, A. C. Mishra, R. V. Gibbons, E. C. Holmes, and W. I. Lipkin.** 2008. Global distribution of novel rhinovirus genotype. *Emerg. Infect. Dis.* **14:**944–947.
9. **Brittain-Long, R., S. Nord, S. Olofsson, J. Westin, L. M. Anderson, and M. Lindh.** 2008. Multiplex real-time PCR for detection of respiratory tract infections. *J. Clin. Virol.* **41:**53–56.
10. **Brown, P. K., and D. A. J. Tyrrell.** 1964. Experiments on the sensitivity of strains of human fibroblasts to infection with rhinovirus. *Br. J. Exp. Pathol.* **45:**571–578.
11. **Brownlee, J. W., and R. B. Turner.** 2008. New developments in the epidemiology and clinical spectrum of rhinovirus infections. *Curr. Opin. Pediatr.* **20:**67–71.
12. **Cate, T. R., R. B. Couch, and K. M. Johnson.** 1964. Studies with rhinovirus in volunteers; production of illness, effect of naturally acquired antibody, and demonstration of a protective effect not associated with serum antibody. *J. Clin. Investig.* **43:**56–67.
13. **Christensen, M. S., L. P. Nielsen, and H. Hasle.** 2005. Few but severe viral infections in children with cancer: a prospective RT-PCR and PCR-based 12-month study. *Pediatr. Blood Cancer* **45:**945–951.
14. **Clejan, S., E. Mandrea, I. V. Pandrea, J. Dufour, S. Japa, and R. S. Veazey.** 2005. Immune responses induced by intranasal imiquimod and implications for therapeutics in rhinovirus infections. *J. Cell. Mol. Med.* **9:**457–461.
15. **Cohen, S., and D. A. J. Tyrrell.** 1991. Psychological stress and susceptibility to the common cold. *N. Engl. J. Med.* **325:**606–612.
16. **Cohen, S., W. J. Doyle, C. M. Alper, D. Janicki-Deverts, and R. B. Turner.** 2009. Sleep habits and susceptibility to the common cold. *Arch. Intern. Med.* **169:**62–67.
17. **Couch, R. B., and R. L. Atmar.** 1999. Rhinoviruses, p. 787–802. *In* E. H Lennette and T. F. Smith (ed.), *Laboratory Diagnosis of Viral Infections.* Marcel Dekker, Inc., New York, NY.
18. **Dagher, H., J. Donninger, P. Hutchinson, R. Ghildyal, and P. Bardin.** 2004. Rhinovirus detection: comparison of real-time and conventional PCR. *J. Virol. Methods* **117:**113–121.
19. **Deffernez, C., W. Wunderli, Y. Thomas, S. Yerly, L. Perrin, and L. Kaiser.** 2004. Amplicon sequencing and improved detection of human rhinovirus in respiratory samples. *J. Clin. Microbiol.* **42:**3212–3218.
20. **De Palma, A. M., I. Vliegen, E. De Clercq, and J. Neyts.** 2008. Selective inhibitors of picornavirus replication. *Med. Res. Rev.* **28:**823–884.
21. **Dick, E. C., L. C. Jennings, K. A. Mink, C. D. Wartgow, and S. L. Inhorn.** 1987. Aerosol transmission of rhinovirus colds. *J. Infect. Dis.* **156:**442–448.
22. **Douglas, R. G., Jr.** 1970. Pathogenesis of rhinovirus common colds in human volunteers. *Ann. Otol. Rhinol. Laryngol.* **79:**563–571.
23. **Douglas, R. G., Jr., T. R. Cate, P. J. Gerone, and R. B. Couch.** 1966. Quantitative rhinovirus shedding patterns in volunteers. *Am. Rev. Respir. Dis.* **94:**159–167.
24. **Douglas, R. G., Jr., W. F. Fleet, T. R. Cate, and R. B. Couch.** 1968. Antibody to rhinovirus in human sera. I. Standardization of a neutralization test. *Proc. Soc. Exp. Biol. Med.* **127:**497–502.
25. **Douglas, R. G., Jr., K. M. Lindgren, and R. B. Couch.** 1968. Exposure to cold environment and rhinovirus common cold. Failure to demonstrate effect. *N. Engl. J. Med.* **279:**742–747.
26. **Fendrick, A. M., A. S. Monto, B. Nightengale, and M. Sarnes.** 2003. The economic burden of non-influenza-related viral respiratory tract infection in the United States. *Arch. Intern. Med.* **163:**487–494.

27. Freymuth, F., A. Vabret, D. Cuvillon-Nimal, S. Simon, J. Dina, L. Legrand, S. Gouarin, J. Petitjean, P. Eckart, and J. Brouard. 2006. Comparison of multiplex PCR assays and conventional techniques for the diagnostic of respiratory virus infections in children admitted to hospital with an acute respiratory illness. *J. Med. Virol.* **78:**1498–1504.

28. Gcist, F. C., and F. G. Hayden. 1985. Comparative susceptibilities of strain MRC-5 human embryonic lung fibroblast cells and the Cooney strain of human fetal tonsil cells for isolation of rhinoviruses from clinical specimens. *J. Clin. Microbiol.* **22:**455–456.

29. Gern, J. E. 2009. Rhinovirus and the initiation of asthma. *Curr. Opin. Allergy Clin. Immunol.* **9:**73–78.

30. Gruteke, P., A. S. Glas, M. Dierdorp, W. B. Vreede, J. W. Pilon, and S. M. Bruisten. 2004. Practical implementation of a multiplex PCR for acute respiratory tract infections in children. *J. Clin. Microbiol.* **42:**5596–5603.

31. Gutman, J. A., A. J. Peck, J. Kuypers, and M. Boeckh. 2007. Rhinovirus as a cause of fatal lower respiratory tract infection in adult stem cell transplantation patients: a report of two cases. *Bone Marrow Transplant.* **40:**809–811.

32. Gwaltney, J. M., Jr., P. B. Moskalski, and J. O. Hendley. 1978. Hand-to-hand transmission of rhinovirus colds. *Ann. Intern. Med.* **88:**463–467.

33. Gwaltney, J. M., Jr. 1992. Combined antiviral and antimediator treatment of rhinovirus colds. *J. Infect. Dis.* **166:**776–782.

34. Halonen, P., E. Rocha, J. Hierholzer, B. Holloway, T. Hyypia, P. Hurskainen, and M. Pallansch. 1995. Detection of enteroviruses and rhinoviruses in clinical specimens by PCR and liquid-phase hybridization. *J. Clin. Microbiol.* **33:**648–653.

35. Hayden, F. G., L. Diamond, P. B. Wood, D. C. Korts, and M. T. Wecher. 1996. Effectiveness and safety of intranasal ipratropium bromide in common colds. *Ann. Intern. Med.* **125:**89–97.

36. Hayden, F. G., D. T. Herrington, T. L. Coats, K. Kim, E. C. Cooper, S. A. Villano, S. Liu, S. Hudson, D. C. Pevear, M. Collett, M. McKinlay, and the Pleconaril Respiratory Infection Study Group. 2003. Efficacy and safety of oral pleconaril for treatment of colds due to picornaviruses in adults: results of 2 double-blind, randomized, placebo-controlled trials. *Clin. Infect. Dis.* **36:**1523–1532.

37. Hayden, F. G. 2004. Rhinovirus and the lower respiratory tract. *Rev. Med. Virol.* **14:**17–31.

38. Hendley, J. O. 1999. Clinical virology of rhinoviruses. *Adv. Virus Res.* **54:**453–466.

39. Hendley, J. O., and J. M Gwaltney, Jr. 1988. Mechanisms of transmission of rhinovirus infections. *Epidemiol. Rev.* **10:**242–258.

40. Hofer, F., M. Gruenberger, H. Kowlaski, H. Machat, M. Huettinger, E. Kuechler, and D. Blaas. 1994. Members of the low density lipoprotein receptor family mediate cell entry of a minor-group common cold virus. *Proc. Natl. Acad. Sci. USA* **91:**1839–1842.

41. Hyypia, T., T. Puhakka, O. Ruuskanen, M. Makela, A. Arola, and P. Arstila. 1998. Molecular diagnosis of human rhinovirus infections: comparison with virus isolation. *J. Clin. Microbiol.* **36:**2081–2083.

42. Jang, Y. J., S. H. Lee, H. J. Kwon, Y. S. Chung, and B. J. Lee. 2005. Development of rhinovirus study model using organ culture of turbinate mucosa. *J. Virol. Methods* **125:**41–47.

43. Jartti, T., P. Lehtinen, T. Vuorinen, M. Koskenvuo, and O. Ruuskanen. 2004. Persistence of rhinovirus and enterovirus RNA after acute respiratory illness in children. *J. Med. Virol.* **72:**695–699.

44. Johnston, S. L., G. Sanderson, P. K. Pattemore, S. Smith, P. G. Vardin, C. B. Bruce, P. R. Lambden, D. A. J. Tyrrell, and S. T. Holgate. 1993. Use of polymerase chain reaction for diagnosis of picornavirus infection in subjects with and without respiratory symptoms. *J. Clin. Microbiol.* **31:**111–117.

45. Kares, S., M. Lonnrot, P. Vuorinen, S. Oikarinen, S. Taurianen, and H. Hyoty. 2004. Real-time PCR for rapid diagnosis of entero- and rhinovirus infections using LightCycler. *J. Clin. Virol.* **29:**99–104.

46. Khetsuriani, N., X. Lu, W. G. Teague, N. Kazerouni, L. J. Anderson, and D. D. Erdman. 2008. Novel human rhinoviruses and exacerbation of asthma in children. *Emerg. Infect. Dis.* **14:**1793–1796.

47. Kiang, D., I. Kalra, S. Yagi, J. K. Louie, H. Boushey, J. Boothby, and D. P. Schnurr. 2008. Assay for 5′ noncoding region analysis of all human rhinovirus prototype strains. *J. Clin. Microbiol.* **46:**3736–3745.

48. Kistler, A., P. C. Avila, S. Rouskin, D. Wang, T. Ward, S. Yagi, D. Schnurr, D. Ganem, J. L. DeRisi, and H. A. Boushey. 2007. Pan-viral screening of respiratory tract infections in adults with and without asthma reveals unexpected human coronavirus and human rhinovirus diversity. *J. Infect. Dis.* **196:**817–825.

49. Kling, S., H. Donninger, Z. Williams, J. Vermeulen, E. Weinberg, K. Latiff, R. Ghildyal, and P. Bardin. 2005. Persistence of rhinovirus RNA after asthma exacerbation in children. *Clin. Exp. Allergy* **35:**672–678.

50. Korppi, M., A. Kotaniemi-Syrjanen, M. Waris, R. Vainionpaa, and T. M. Reijonen. 2004. Rhinovirus-associated wheezing in infancy. Comparison with respiratory syncytial virus bronchiolitis. *Pediatr. Infect. Dis. J.* **23:**995–999.

51. Kumar, D., D. Erdman, S. Keshavjee, T. Peret, R. Tellier, D. Hadjiliadis, G. Johnson, M. Ayers, D. Siegal, and A. Humar. 2005. Clinical impact of community-acquired respiratory viruses on bronchiolitis obliterans after lung transplant. *Am. J. Transplant.* **5:**2031–2036.

52. Laine, P., C. Savolainen, S. Blomqvist, and T. Hovi. 2005. Phylogenetic analysis of human rhinovirus capsid protein VP1 and 2A protease coding sequences confirms shared genus-like relationships with human enteroviruses. *J. Gen. Virol.* **86:**697–706.

53. Lamson, D., N. Renwick, V. Kapoor, Z. Liu, G. Palacios, J. Ju, A. Dean, K. St. George, T. Briese, and W. I. Lipkin. 2006. MassTag polymerase-chain-reaction detection of respiratory pathogens, including a new rhinovirus genotype, that caused influenza-like illness in New York State during 2004–2005. *J. Infect. Dis.* **194:**1398–1402.

54. Las Heras, J., and V. L. Swanson. 1983. Sudden death of an infant with rhinovirus infection complicating bronchial asthma: case report. *Pediatr. Pathol.* **1:**319–323.

55. Lau, S. K., C. C. Yip, H. W. Tsoi, R. A. Lee, L. Y. So, Y. L. Lau, K. H. Chan, P. C. Woo, and K. Y. Yuen. 2007. Clinical features and complete genome characterization of a distinct human rhinovirus (HRV) genetic cluster, probably representing a previously undetected HRV species, HRV-C, associated with acute respiratory illness in children. *J. Clin. Microbiol.* **45:**3655–3664.

56. Ledford, R. M., N. R. Patel, T. M. Demenczuk, A. Watanyar, T. Herbertz, M. S. Collet, and D. C. Pevear. 2004. VP1 sequencing of all human rhinovirus serotypes: insights into genus phylogeny and susceptibility to antiviral capsid-binding compounds. *J. Virol.* **78:**3663–3674.

57. Lee, B. E., J. L. Robinson, V. Khurana, X. L. Pang, J. K. Preiksaitis, and J. D. Fox. 2006. Enhanced identification of viral and atypical bacterial pathogens in lower respiratory tract samples with nucleic acid amplification tests. *J. Med. Virol.* **78:**702–710.

58. Lee, W. M., C. Kiesner, T. Pappas, I. Lee, K. Grindle, T. Jartti, B. Jakiela, R. F. Lemanske, Jr., P. A. Shult, and J. E. Gern. 2007. A diverse group of previously unrecognized human rhinoviruses are common causes of respiratory illnesses in infants. *PLoS ONE* **2:**e966.

59. Lee, W. M., K. Grindle, T. Pappas, D. J. Marshall, M. J. Moser, E. L. Beaty, P. A. Shult, J. R. Prudent, and J. E. Gern. 2007. High-throughput, sensitive, and accurate multiplex PCR-microsphere flow cytometry system for large-scale comprehensive detection of respiratory viruses. *J. Clin. Microbiol.* **45:**2626–2634.

60. Loens, K., H. Goossens, C. de Laat, H. Foolen, P. Oudshoorn, S. Pattyn, P. Sillekens, and M. Ieven. 2006. Detection of rhinoviruses by tissue culture and two independent amplification techniques, nucleic acid sequence-based amplification and reverse transcription-PCR, in children with acute respiratory infections during a winter season. *J. Clin. Microbiol.* **44:**166–171.

61. Louie, J. K., S. Yagi, F. A. Nelson, D. Kiang, C. A. Glaser, J. Rosenberg, C. K. Cahill, and D. P. Schnurr. 2005. Rhinovirus outbreak in a long term care facility for elderly persons associated with unusually high mortality. *Clin. Infect. Dis.* **41:**262–265.

62. Louie, J. K., A. Roy-Burman, L. Guardia-Labar, E. J. Boston, D. Kiang, T. Padilla, S. Yagi, S. Messenger, A. M. Petru, C. A. Glaser, and D. P. Schnurr. 2009. Rhinovirus associated with severe lower respiratory tract infections in children. *Pediatr. Infect. Dis. J.* **28:**337–339.

63. Lu, X., B. Holloway, R. K. Dare, J. Kuypers, S. Yagi, J. V. Williams, C. B. Hall, and D. D. Erdman. 2008. Real-time reverse transcription-PCR assay for comprehensive detection of human rhinoviruses. *J. Clin. Microbiol.* **46:**533–539.

64. Mahony, J., S. Chong, F. Merante, S. Yaghoubian, T. Sinha, C. Lisle, and R. Janeczko. 2007. Development of a respiratory virus panel test for detection of twenty human respiratory viruses by use of multiplex PCR and a fluid microbead-based assay. *J. Clin. Microbiol.* **45:**2965–2970.

65. Mallia, P., and S. L. Johnston. 2006. How viral infections cause exacerbation of airway diseases. *Chest* **130:**1203–1210.

66. McErlean, P., L. A. Shackelton, S. B. Lambert, M. D. Nissen, T. P. Sloots, and I. M. Mackay. 2007. Characterisation of a newly identified human rhinovirus, HRV-QPM, discovered in infants with bronchiolitis. *J. Clin. Virol.* **39:**67–75.

67. McErlean, P., L. A. Shackelton, E. Andrews, D. R. Webster, S. B. Lambert, M. D. Nissen, T. P. Sloots, and I. M. Mackay. 2008. Distinguishing molecular features and clinical characteristics of a putative new rhinovirus species, human rhinovirus C (HRV C). *PLoS ONE* **3:**e1847.

68. Miller, E. K., X. Lu, D. D. Erdman, K. A. Poehling, Y. Zhu, M. R. Griffin, T. V. Hartert, L. J. Anderson, G. A. Weinberg, C. B. Hall, M. K. Iwane, and K. M. Edwards for the New Vaccine Surveillance Network. 2007. Rhinovirus-associated hospitalizations in young children. *J. Infect. Dis.* **195:**773–781.

69. Miller, E. K., K. M. Edwards, G. A. Weinberg, M. K. Iwane, M. R. Griffin, C. B. Hall, Y. Zhu, P. G. Szilagyi, L. L. Morin, L. H. Heil, X. Lu, and J. V. Williams for the New Vaccine Surveillance Network. 2009. A novel group of rhinoviruses is associated with asthma hospitalizations. *J. Allergy Clin. Immunol.* **123:**98–104.

70. Monto, A. S. 2002. The seasonality of rhinovirus infections and its implications for clinical recognition. *Clin. Ther.* **24:**1987–1997.

71. Nicholson, K. G., J. Kent, V. Hammersley, and E. Cancio. 1996. Risk factors for lower respiratory complications of rhinovirus infections in elderly people living in the community: prospective cohort study. *BMJ* **313:**1119–1123.

72. Nokso-Koivisto, J., R. Raty, S. Blomqvist, M. Kleemola, R. Syrjanen, A. Pitkaranta, T. Kilpi, and T. Hovi. 2004. Presence of specific viruses in the middle ear fluids and respiratory secretions of young children with acute otitis media. *J. Med. Virol.* **72:**241–248.

73. Nolte, F. S., D. J. Marshall, C. Rasberry, S. Schievelbein, G. G. Banks, G. A. Storch, M.Q. Arens, R. S. Buller, and J. R. Prudent. 2007. MultiCode-PLx system for multiplexed detection of seventeen respiratory viruses. *J. Clin. Microbiol.* **45:**2779–2786.

74. Palmenberg, A. C., D. Spiro, R. Kuzmickas, S. Wang, A. Djikeng, J. A. Rathe, C. M. Fraser-Liggett, and S. B. Liggett. 2009. Sequencing and analyses of all known human rhinovirus genomes reveal structure and evolution. *Science* **324:**55–59.

75. Papadopoulos, N. G., J. Hunter, G. Sanderson, J. Meyer, and S. L. Johnston. 1999. Rhinovirus identification by BglI digestion of picornavirus RT-PCR amplicons. *J. Virol. Methods* **80:**179–185.

76. Papadopoulos, N. G., P. J. Bates, P. G. Bardin, A. Papi, S. H. Leir, D. J. Fraenkel, J. Meyer, P. M. Lackie, G. Sanderson, S. T. Holgate, and S. L. Johnston. 2000. Rhinoviruses infect the lower airways. *J. Infect. Dis.* **181:**1875–1884.

77. Rossmann, M. G., J. Bella, P. R. Kolatkar, Y. He, E. Wimmer, R. J. Kuhn, and T. S. Baker. 2000. Cell recognition and entry by rhino- and enteroviruses. *Virology* **269:**239–247.

78. Savolainen-Kopra, C., S. Blomqvist, T. Kilpi, M. Roivainen, and T. Hovi. 2009. Novel species of human rhinoviruses in acute otitis media. *Pediatr. Infect. Dis. J.* **28:**59–61.

79. Scheltinga, S. A., K. E. Templeton, M. F. C. Beersma, and E. C. J. Claas. 2005. Diagnosis of human metapneumovirus and rhinovirus in patients with respiratory tract infections by an internally controlled multiplex real-time RNA PCR. *J. Clin. Virol.* **33:**306–311.

80. Spyridaki, I. S., I. Christodoulou, L. de Beer, V. Hovland, M. Kurowski, A. Olszewska-Ziaber, K. H. Carlsen, K. Lødrup-Carlsen, C. M. van Drunen, M. L. Kowalski, R. Molenkamp, and N. G. Papadopoulos. 2009. Comparison of four nasal sampling methods for the detection of viral pathogens by RT-PCR—a GA(2)LEN project. *J. Virol. Methods* **156:**102–106.

81. Steininger, C., S. W. Aberle, and T. Popow-Kraupp. 2001. Early detection of acute rhinovirus infections by a rapid reverse transcription-PCR assay. *J. Clin. Microbiol.* **39:**129–133.

82. Templeton, K. E., C. B. Forde, A. M. Loon, E. C. Claas, H. G. Niesters, P. Wallace, and W. F. Carman. 2006. A multicentre pilot proficiency programme to assess the quality of molecular detection of respiratory viruses. *J. Clin. Virol.* **35:**51–58.

83. Torgersen, H., T. Skern, and D. Blaas. 1989. Typing of human rhinoviruses based on sequence variations in the 5′ non-coding region. *J. Gen. Virol.* **70:**3111–3116.

84. Tsolia, M. N., S. Psarras, A. Bossios, H. Audi, M. Paldanius, D. Gourgiotis, K. Kallergi, D. A. Kafetzis, A. Constantopoulos, and N. G. Papadopoulos. 2004. Etiology of community-acquired pneumonia in hospitalized school-age children: evidence for high prevalence of viral infections. *Clin. Infect. Dis.* **39:**681–686.

85. Turner, R. B., M. T. Wecker, G. Pohl, T. J. Witek, E. McNally, R. St. George, B. Winther, and F. G. Hayden. 1999. Efficacy of tremacamra, a soluble intercellular adhesion molecule 1 alpha, for experimental rhinovirus infection. *JAMA* **281:**1797–1804.

86. Turner, R. B., R. Bauer, K. Woelkart, T. C. Hulsey, and J. D. Gangemi. 2005. An evaluation of Echinacea angustifolia in experimental rhinovirus infections. *N. Engl. J. Med.* **353:**341–348.

87. Uncapher, C. R., C. M. DeWitt, and R. J. Colonno. 1991. The major and minor group receptor families contain all but one human rhinovirus serotype. *Virology* **180:**814–817.

88. Van Kraaij, M. G. J., L. J. R. van Elden, A. M. van Loon, K. A. W. Hendriksen, L. Laterveer, A. W. Dekker, and M. Nijhuis. 2005. Frequent detection of respiratory viruses in adult recipients of stem cell transplants with the use of real-time polymerase chain reaction, compared with viral culture. *Clin. Infect. Dis.* **40:**662–669.

89. Vlasak, M., M. Roivainen, M. Reithmayer, I. Goesler, P. Laine, L. Snyers, T. Hovi, and D. Blaas. 2005. The minor receptor group of human rhinovirus (HRV) includes HRV23 and HRV25, but the presence of a lysine in the VP1 HI loop is not sufficient for receptor binding. *J. Virol.* **79:**7389–7395.

90. Vuorinen, T., R. Vainionpaa, and T. Hyypia. 2003. Five years' experience of reverse-transcriptase polymerase chain reaction in daily diagnosis of enterovirus and rhinovirus infections. *Clin. Infect. Dis.* **37:**452–455.

91. Wang, J. H., H. J. Kwon, Y. S. Chung, B. J. Lee, and Y. J. Jang. 2008. Infection rate and virus-induced cytokine secretion in experimental rhinovirus infection in mucosal organ culture: comparison between specimens from patients with chronic rhinosinusitis with nasal polyps and those from normal subjects. *Arch. Otolaryngol. Head Neck Surg.* **134:**424–427.

92. Winther, B., F. G. Hayden, and J. O. Hendley. 2006. Picornavirus infections in children diagnosed by RT-PCR during longitudinal surveillance with weekly sampling: association with symptomatic illness and effect of season. *J. Med. Virol.* **78:**644–650.

93. Wright, P. F., A. M. Deatly, R. A. Karron, R. B. Belshe, J. R. Shi, W. C. Gruber, Y. Zhu, and V. B. Randolph. 2007. Comparison of results of detection of rhinovirus by PCR and viral culture in human nasal wash specimens from subjects

with and without clinical symptoms of respiratory illness. *J. Clin. Microbiol.* **45:**2126–2129.

94. **Xatzipsalti, M., S. Kyrana, M. Tsolia, S. Psarras, A. Bossios, V. Laza-Stanca, S. L. Johnston, and N. G. Papadopoulos.** 2005. Rhinovirus viremia in children with respiratory infections. *Am. J. Respir. Crit. Care Med.* **172:**1037–1040.

95. **Xing, l., J. M. Casasnovvas, and R. H. Cheng.** 2003. Structural analysis of human rhinovirus complexed with ICAM-1 reveals the dynamics of receptor-mediated virus uncoating. *J. Virol.* **77:**6101–6107.

96. **Zhang, Y., A. A. Simpson, R. M. Ledford, C. M. Bator, S. Chakravarty, G. A. Skochko, T. M. Demenczuk, A. Watanyar, D. C. Pevear, and M. G. Rossmann.** 2004. Structural and virological studies of the stages of virus replication that are affected by antirhinovirus compounds. *J. Virol.* **78:**11061–11069.

97. **Zoll, J., S. Erkens Hulshof, K. Lanke, F. Verduyn Lunel, W. J. Melchers, E. Schoondermark-van de Ven, M. Roivainen, J. M. Galama, and F. J. van Kuppeveld.** 2009. Saffold virus, a human Theiler's-like cardiovirus, is ubiquitous and causes infection early in life. *PLoS Pathog.* **5:**e1000416.

Coronaviruses*

KANTI PABBARAJU AND JULIE D. FOX

87

TAXONOMY

The family *Coronaviridae* includes the genera *Torovirus* and *Coronavirus* in the order *Nidovirales*. Coronaviruses (CoVs) were first identified by electron microscopy (EM) of cultured samples and were named for the distinct crown-like morphology of the long surface spikes, as illustrated in Fig. 1.

CoVs were separated initially into serologically distinct groups, and there is thought to be no (or very limited) serological cross-reactivity between the groups. Antigenic criteria and neutralization are still used for grouping viruses, but increasingly, CoVs are also identified and differentiated based on sequence. Representative CoVs and the phylogenetic relationships among them are illustrated in Fig. 2. The same groupings emerge regardless of the structural protein compared for this type of analysis. In the future, the CoV family may be reorganized based on full genome analysis of representative CoVs (84).

The group 1 human CoVs (HCoVs), HCoV-229E and HCoV-NL63, are more closely related to each other than to any other HCoV (63), yet they share only 65% sequence identity and use different cell receptors (17). This group also contains multiple examples of nonhuman CoVs.

The group 2 virus HCoV-OC43 clusters tightly with bovine, porcine, and equine CoVs, and they likely share a recent common ancestor (76, 78). Although clearly a group 2 virus, HCoV-HKU1 is not part of the same cluster as HCoV-OC43 (Fig. 2). The causative agent of severe acute respiratory syndrome (SARS-CoV) was identified in 2003 and is of animal origin, with recent molecular phylogeny studies confirming that the civet cat SARS-CoV and bat SARS-CoV are very close relatives within group 2. However, SARS-CoV appears to be quite divergent from other group 2 viruses (Fig. 2), and in some analyses, SARS-CoV has been split into a putative group 4 (75).

Group 3 CoVs, to date, have been found exclusively in domestic poultry and are highly divergent from the other CoV groups. One hypothesis is that these viruses originated in bats and evolved via raptors (75).

DESCRIPTION OF THE AGENTS

HCoVs have the largest genomes of RNA viruses (27 to 32 kb). Purified genomic RNA is infectious and associates with the N phosphoprotein to form a long flexible helical nucleocapsid (N). This virus core is enclosed by a lipoprotein envelope containing the transmembrane (M) glycoprotein and envelope (E) protein. Two types of spikes line the outside of the CoV virion. The long spikes (20 nm) consist of the spike (S) glycoprotein, and the short spikes consist of the hemagglutinin-esterase (HE) glycoprotein (the latter is present only in a subset of CoVs). The functions of CoV genes and proteins were reviewed recently (51).

HCoV-229E and HCoV-OC43 were first identified by virus isolation and propagation procedures in the mid-1960s. However, isolation is often inefficient without the use of primary organ cultures. The SARS outbreak occurred in Southeast Asia in 2003, and based on serological studies, SARS-CoV was confirmed as a virus newly introduced into the human population (12, 19, 56). Since 2003, two further CoVs, HCoV-NL63 and HCoV-HKU1, have been discovered and reported to be circulating in the human population (20, 22, 37, 73, 81). These two most recently identified HCoVs are not new introductions into the human population but were not identified before nucleic acid-based discovery methods were available. HCoV-NL63 and related viruses were found to replicate relatively efficiently in culture (20, 22, 73). An example of the HCoV-NL63 cytopathic effect (CPE) in LLC-MK2 cells is provided in Fig. 3. To date, HCoV-HKU1 has not been propagated in vitro (81, 84).

EPIDEMIOLOGY AND TRANSMISSION

HCoV-229E and HCoV-OC43 were first isolated from patients with upper respiratory tract infections, and these viruses seem to be spread mainly by the respiratory route. CoVs identified subsequently were also isolated from respiratory samples, although other, nonrespiratory routes of transmission may occur, as shown for animal CoVs. CoVs first replicate in epithelial cells. In very young or immunocompromised individuals, widespread distribution of HCoVs has been reported. In animals, group 2 CoVs are associated with gastrointestinal symptoms. Some CoVs isolated from fecal samples of patients with diarrhea

---

*This chapter contains figures presented in chapter 91 by James B. Mahony in the ninth edition of this *Manual*.

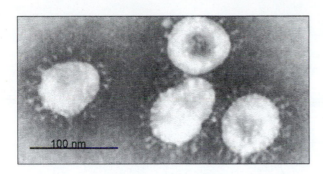

FIGURE 1 Electron micrograph of HCoV-OC43 showing pleomorphic shape and characteristic coronas made up of surrounding peplomers.

seem to be more closely related to bovine CoV than to the prototype human group 2 CoV, HCoV-OC43.

Serological studies have shown that HCoV infections are common and that reinfection with the same HCoV is possible even in the presence of neutralizing antibody. Infection with the group 1 viruses HCoV-229E and HCoV-NL63 likely occurs very early in life, with up to 75% of children having detectable antibodies against these viruses after 3.5 years of age (16, 67). Studies using nucleic acid amplification tests (NAATs) for screening of respiratory samples showed that the group 1 HCoVs are generally the most commonly found CoVs (21). However, the relative prevalence of different HCoVs seems to vary from season to season (72). There is evidence from some studies that group 1 viruses may circulate in different seasons (with, for example, HCoV-229E and HCoV-NL63 being dominant in alternate years) (28). HCoV-NL63 has been detected in 1.7% to 9.3% of respiratory samples tested, with a worldwide distribution. Seasonal peaks have been reported for January to March in temperate climates, and coinfections are common (2, 3, 5, 13, 21, 26). (Figure 4 shows example results for the currently circulating HCoVs. Samples from individuals with a range of respiratory symptoms were tested over a 1-year period by use of a sensitive nucleic acid amplification procedure. Over this period, the peaks for detection of HCoV-229E and HCoV-NL63 occurred at different times (December to February versus April-May, respectively). HCoV-OC43 was identified mainly in the winter, and detection of HCoV-HKU1 was rare, as reported previously (21), although other studies have reported a predominance of HCoV-HKU1 in pediatric patients (40). Analysis by age demonstrated some enhanced detection of HCoVs in the very young and in older adults compared with that for children and young adults.

HCoV-HKU1 was first detected in 2005 in Hong Kong and has since been shown to have a global distribution. Seroepidemiological studies have shown that >10% of the studied population aged 21 to 70 years has evidence of HCoV-HKU1 infection, suggesting that the virus is endemic, at least in Hong Kong (6). Infections with HCoV-HKU1 are detected more commonly in the winter season; adults are infected frequently worldwide, with prevalences ranging from 1.0% to 3.1% of respiratory samples tested (5, 40), although the majority of studies report lower detection rates for HCoV-HKU1 than for the other circulating group 1 and 2 viruses (excluding SARS-CoV, which has not been reported in the last 3 to 4 years). One study reported this virus as a significant cause of community-acquired pneumonia in adults (82).

Serological studies reported the absence of antibodies to SARS-CoV prior to the SARS outbreak in 2003 (8). Although SARS-CoV was originally introduced into the human population by zoonotic transmission, global spread was by human-to-human transmission, and studies of the adaptation of this virus to the human host are critical to our understanding and management of possible future zoonotic events.

The epidemiological data from surveillance of wild animals suggest that horseshoe bats are the natural reservoir for SARS-CoV (12). The virus was transmitted from bats to animals such as palm civets, raccoons, and dogs in food markets and then spread to humans from these secondary animals, which were amplification hosts. The majority of SARS-CoV isolates identified worldwide are genetically closely linked. However, phylogenetically distinct SARS-CoV isolates were identified, suggesting that several introductions of the virus had occurred but that only one was associated with the outbreak in Hong Kong, which subsequently spread globally (12, 30). At least initially, human-to-human transmission of SARS-CoV was likely inefficient, but analysis of the virus throughout the SARS outbreak showed the development of mutations reflecting adaptation to a new host. Nosocomial transmission of SARS-CoV was reported frequently. Health care workers were recognized as being at increased risk of acquiring the virus if they undertook activities related to intubation (45), with the use of a mask (especially an N95 mask) offering protection. Virus shedding studies have shown that the peaks of SARS-CoV shedding tend to occur relatively late in the course of infection, when those severely affected are hospitalized (9). A deletion mutation identified late in the outbreak likely contributed to viral fitness and human-to-human transmission (31). Some patients with SARS also had gastrointestinal symptoms, with high viral titers in stool samples (12), making a fecal-oral route of transmission likely (in addition to respiratory transmission). Several animal CoVs can replicate in the respiratory and enteric tracts, suggesting that both modes of transmission are possible. SARS-CoV is the most recent example of animal-to-human transmission of a CoV, but this is likely a fairly common event.

CLINICAL SIGNIFICANCE AND MANAGEMENT

Before the SARS epidemic, HCoVs were associated mainly with upper respiratory tract infections and occasionally were linked to severe pulmonary disease in the elderly, newborn, and immunocompromised. The group 1 virus HCoV-229E has long been known to cause a significant number of upper respiratory tract infections with symptoms of the "common cold," characterized by a relatively long incubation period, short duration of symptoms, and prominent nasal discharge compared with rhinovirus infections (17). Outbreaks of HCoV-229E are thought to occur every few years. The impact of HCoV-229E as a cause of nosocomial infections in high-risk infants, such as those in pediatric and neonatal intensive care units, was recently investigated (25), and this virus may be associated with pneumonia more commonly in such vulnerable individuals. For hospitalized patients, coinfection with HCoV-229E and other respiratory viruses is reported frequently (17).

HCoV-OC43 infection has been associated mainly with upper respiratory tract symptoms and, in early volunteer studies, was indistinguishable in presentation from infections caused by rhinoviruses (70). The most common symptoms

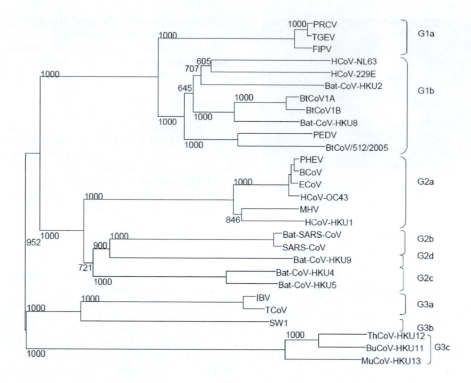

FIGURE 2 Phylogenetic analysis of the RNA-dependent RNA polymerase gene showing the grouping of CoVs. Analysis was undertaken by use of complete genome sequences available by the end of 2008. The tree was constructed by the neighbor-joining method, using Kimura's two-parameter correction and bootstrap values calculated from 1,000 trees. Nine hundred fifty-eight amino acid positions were included in the analysis. The scale bar indicates the estimated number of substitutions per 50 amino acids. The following viral sequences (GenBank accession number) were used: HCoV-229E, human coronavirus 229E (GenBank accession no. NC_002645); PEDV, porcine epidemic diarrhea virus (NC_003436); TGEV, porcine transmissible gastroenteritis virus (NC_002306); FCoV, feline coronavirus (AY994055); PRCV, porcine respiratory coronavirus (DQ811787); HCoV-NL63, human coronavirus NL63 (NC_005831); bat-CoV-HKU2 (EF203064), -HKU4 (NC_009019), -HKU5 (NC_009020), -HKU8 (NC_010438), -HKU9 (NC_009021), -1A (NC_010437), -1B (NC_010436), and -512/2005 (NC_009657); HCoV-HKU1, human coronavirus HKU1 (NC_006577), HCoV-OC43, human coronavirus OC43 (NC_005147); MHV, mouse hepatitis virus (NC_006852); BCoV, bovine coronavirus (NC_003045); PHEV, porcine hemagglutinating encephalomyelitis virus (NC_007732); ECoV, equine coronavirus (NC_010327); SARS-CoV, SARS coronavirus (NC_004718); bat-SARS-CoV-HKU3, bat SARS coronavirus HKU3 (NC_009694); IBV, infectious bronchitis virus (NC_001451); TCoV, turkey coronavirus (NC_010800); SW1, beluga whale coronavirus (NC_010646); BuCoV-HKU11, bulbul coronavirus HKU11 (NC_011548); ThCoV-HKU12, thrush coronavirus HKU12 (NC_011549); and MuCoV-HKU13, munia coronavirus HKU13 (NC_011550). (Reproduced from reference 84.)

are cough and rhinitis, but HCoV-OC43 has been associated with exacerbation of asthma and pneumonia in some groups and institutional settings (13). Outbreaks of HCoV-OC43 have been reported, but there is some evidence that they occur only when circulating levels of HCoV-229E (and perhaps other HCoVs) are low, with year-to-year variation in clinical impact (14). In one study, HCoV-OC43 was the most commonly identified HCoV in bronchoalveolar lavage (BAL) samples from hospitalized adults (26).

Patients with HCoV-NL63 infection show symptoms ranging from fever, cough, sore throat, and rhinitis to severe lower respiratory tract infections, which may require hospitalization (2, 5). HCoV-NL63 was first identified from a patient with bronchiolitis (17, 72, 73) and has also been

linked with laryngotracheitis (croup), asthma exacerbation, and febrile seizures (13).

HCoV-HKU1 was first described for an elderly patient with underlying respiratory and cardiovascular problems (81). Several reports have described HCoV-HKU1 infections in children with underlying conditions, suggesting that it may aggravate problems in these patients. Respiratory symptoms of HCoV-HKU1 infections include rhinorrhea, fever, cough, and wheezing; disease conditions may include bronchiolitis and pneumonia. Involvement in gastrointestinal disease has also been suggested (5).

SARS-CoV causes severe respiratory disease with a high mortality rate (10%) (56). The clinical disease consists of a prodrome with a respiratory stage beginning 3 to 7 days later,

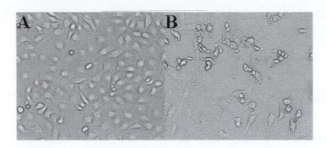

FIGURE 3 HCoV CPE at 5 days postinfection. (A) Uninfected LLC-MK2 cells. (B) HCoV-NL63-infected LLC-MK2 cells.

with rapid clinical deterioration. Respiratory failure and the need for mechanical ventilation were common in adult patients during the outbreak in 2003. Disease in children younger than 12 years of age was milder than that in adults, but a case fatality rate of 10% has been reported (5, 12).

In general, CoV infections are not treated specifically, with management being supportive for those with severe symptoms. However, diagnosis of CoV infections enhances our understanding of viral epidemiology, prompts the rapid initiation of appropriate infection control procedures, and avoids inappropriate treatment for bacterial or other viral infections which may present in a similar way. SARS-CoV

infections have a high mortality rate. Some theoretical and experimental work has been undertaken to identify therapeutic targets for SARS-CoV which may prove useful should the virus reemerge. Studies with animal models have demonstrated the efficacy of SARS-CoV-specific monoclonal antibodies, pegylated alpha interferon, and small interfering RNAs against the virus (reviewed in reference 69).

COLLECTION, TRANSPORT, AND HANDLING OF SPECIMENS

A comparison of diagnostic procedures for detection of HCoVs is provided in Table 1. The presence of HCoVs has been reported for nasopharyngeal swabs/aspirates, throat swabs, and lower respiratory samples such as BAL fluid, although other samples (such as blood and stool) may also be useful (1, 11, 55). For the most complete diagnostic investigation, it may be necessary to collect a range of samples, as was recommended for identification of SARS cases during the outbreak in 2003. However, although the positive rate was highest for lower respiratory tract specimens such as BAL fluid and lung biopsy specimens from patients with SARS, collection risks related to the generation of infectious aerosols must be considered. Samples for cases with a nontypical presentation or where SARS is suspected should not be manipulated in laboratories lacking the ability to undertake such handling under enhanced level 2 conditions (biosafety level 2 facilities

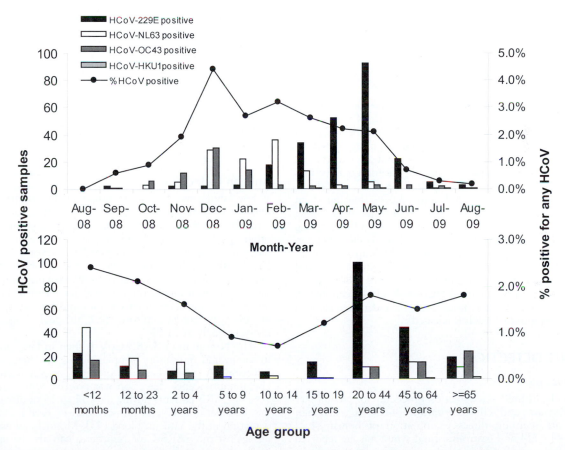

FIGURE 4 Circulating HCoVs in respiratory samples. Samples received from community and hospitalized patients with respiratory symptoms were tested for HCoVs by use of a multiplex panel test as described previously (54). The total number of samples tested was 25,799, with 437 HCoV-positive samples (overall, 1.7% of samples were positive for any HCoV).

TABLE 1 Comparison of diagnostic procedures for detection of HCoVs

Method	Advantages	Disadvantages	Example diagnostic applications (references)
EM	Rapid. Does not require virus-specific reagents.	Insensitive. Viral load can be low in respiratory specimens.	Confirmation of novel CoV isolation in vitro. Analysis of tissue samples in index cases. Visualization of HCoVs directly in stool samples (22, 56).
Antigen detection	Rapid. Has high specificity.	Antibodies not widely available. Requires a good cellular sample. Insensitive compared with NAAT.	Application to respiratory samples and blood (24, 28, 43, 44)
NAATs	Most sensitive method. Can identify all HCoVs or be virus specific.	Requires prior knowledge of circulating HCoV sequences, which may be subject to variation	Virus-specific and HCoV-generic formats available. Wide range of formats and platforms are used. Commercial assays including HCoVs in respiratory virus panels are becoming available (1, 4, 8–11, 13–15, 18, 21, 26–28, 34, 38–40, 46, 48, 49, 52–60, 62, 73, 74, 79, 81, 82, 85, 86).
Virus isolation	Excellent specificity. Confirms presence of infectious virus.	Many CoVs do not grow in routine cell cultures. SARS-CoV is a biosafety level 3 pathogen; there are safety concerns if virus is isolated inadvertently. Too slow for routine diagnosis.	Initial identification of HCoVs. Modified cell culture (with antigen, nucleic acid, or other confirmation) has been reported. Some procedures prescreen samples by NAAT and then culture the positive samples (8, 9, 19, 28, 29, 33, 41, 53, 62, 65, 68, 73).
Antibody detection	Fast and inexpensive for population screening	Diagnosis is usually retrospective. SARS-CoV IgM is not detectable early and persists. Only IgG assays are available for most HCoVs, and most adults have evidence of past infection.	Useful in SARS-CoV case confirmation. Useful for studying epidemiologic impact of CoVs (6, 8, 16, 42, 50, 55, 66, 67, 83).

with biosafety level 3 practices). In the case of a potential novel virus infection or suspected reemergence of SARS-CoV in humans, updated safety guidelines will likely be developed for classification of "high-risk" samples, and protocols will be suggested for manipulation of samples and for undertaking any procedure that might result in amplification of infectious virus. Nucleic acid extraction procedures have the advantage of inactivating viruses before analysis, making them the most likely front-line test in such circumstances. Public health guidelines for investigation of cases and monitoring the outbreak need to be followed so that sample collection and testing are focused on individuals for whom a test result will alter management or provide critical infection control information. The likelihood of a false-positive result because of cross-reaction with related HCoVs should be considered, and detailed confirmatory tests should be undertaken before a SARS-CoV-positive result is released.

DIRECT DETECTION

Microscopy
EM can be utilized as a detection procedure for preliminary identification and characterization of CoVs. Although CoVs are seen on direct examination of human stool samples by EM and gastrointestinal symptoms are reported for HCoV infection (5, 21), the sensitivity of such direct examination is not likely good enough for routine diagnostics. Also, such an approach would not be suitable for the majority of analyses, which are undertaken on dilute respiratory samples. EM has proved most useful in the identification of novel HCoVs that replicate in vitro. This includes early identification of the first HCoVs in the 1960s and then later identifications for preliminary investigation of the novel SARS-CoV and HCoV-NL63 strains after their isolation in vitro.

Antigen Detection
A few laboratories use noncommercial laboratory-developed and validated reagents for direct antigen detection. Antigen assays for detection of CoVs in respiratory and other specimens can provide rapid results, especially in laboratories that are not equipped to perform NAATs. HCoV antigen detection using a range of labels and formats (e.g., immunofluorescence assay, enzyme immunoassay, and time-resolved fluorimetry) has been utilized for direct detection in cellular samples and for confirmation of viruses isolated in culture (68), although reagents are not yet widely available.

The N protein of SARS-CoV is shed in large amounts in serum and respiratory samples during the first week of infection. A SARS-CoV N protein antigen assay with chemiluminescence detection was positive with sera from 90% of SARS patients during days 11 to 15 of disease and may be superior to reverse transcription-PCR (RT-PCR) for detection of the virus in blood (43). Monoclonal antibodies against the SARS-CoV N protein can also be used for direct detection of the virus in nasopharyngeal aspirates (24). One study reported that 65% of patients with SARS had N antigen in throat washings that was detectable by immunofluorescence, with a trend toward positive results being related to higher viral loads (44).

Nucleic Acid Detection

The most common diagnostic approach for identification of HCoVs is now amplification and detection of virus-specific RNA. Assays utilizing one-step or two-step RT-PCR procedures for the amplification stage have dominated most diagnostic formats. The first-generation NAATs utilized gel-based detection, with nested reactions performed to enhance assay sensitivity and specificity. In recent years, real-time RT-PCR assays have been shown to provide additional sensitivity and specificity and shorter turnaround times and to avoid problems relating to cross-contamination because of the absence of postamplification steps. Alternatives to PCR amplification include isothermal amplification methods, such as nucleic acid sequence-based amplification (NASBA) (bioMérieux, Boxtel, The Netherlands) and loop-mediated amplification (LAMP) assays, some of which have also been combined with real-time detection of products (34, 38, 61). Other probe-based detection systems for detection of amplified products include amplification followed by hybridization with a low-density DNA microarray which can be read manually (15). The preferred format for HCoV RNA amplification and detection will depend on the need for automation and availability of resources in the diagnostic laboratory.

The majority of NAATs for detection of HCoV-229E, HCoV-OC43, and HCoV-NL63 have targeted the N, M, and *pol* genes. Primer pairs for amplification of the N genes of HCoV-OC43 and HCoV-229E in a nested PCR format were designed by Myint and colleagues and combined with gel-based detection (53). Several other authors also reported direct amplification of individual HCoVs by use of single-round or nested amplification assays targeting the N gene, with detection of products by gel analysis and/or sequencing (2, 3, 28, 71, 73). The other commonly used gene target for detection of HCoVs is the *pol* gene. One- and two-step RT-PCR assays targeting the 1a and 1b regions of the *pol* gene of HCoVs have been reported (2, 73, 82). A summary of gel-based detection assays for HCoV-HKU1 targeting both the *pol* and N genes has been published (84).

Generic detection of HCoVs may be useful as a screening step for viral diagnosis and can help in identification of potentially novel viruses (as was seen for SARS-CoV). The 1b region of the *pol* gene is the most conserved region of the genome and has been used for the design of consensus PCRs ("pan-corona" assays) for amplification of all HCoVs (1, 13, 52, 62). However, for diagnostic purposes, the sensitivity of such assays tends to be lower than that of virus-specific assays, presumably because of genetic variability (13, 28). For detection of a range of circulating CoVs by use of pan-corona primers, amplification using virus-specific primers or sequencing of the amplified product must be undertaken for confirmation and epidemiological purposes.

Multiplexing assays for the detection of individual HCoVs may be useful in reducing technical time and costs for diagnosis, especially as in many cases it would be difficult to differentiate among infections caused by HCoV-229E, HCoV-OC43, HCoV-NL63, and HCoV-HKU1 based on clinical criteria. In some studies where a direct comparison has been made, such multiplex assays have been shown to be as sensitive as the individual virus assays for diagnosis (71).

Real-time NAATs were described recently for detection of the currently circulating HCoVs, targeting the M, N, and *pol* genes. Some methodological details and key references are provided in Table 2 for those assays which have undergone extensive evaluation in a diagnostic setting. The "real-time" approach combines the amplification and detection phases of PCR (or another amplification method) with detection of the product, generally using a target-specific probe. The most common HCoV target in such assays is the N gene, with some primers and amplification regions adapted from previously reported single-round and nested PCR assays. In some studies, enhanced clinical sensitivity was confirmed when the individual HCoV real-time assay was compared with gel detection (74).

Multiplex approaches with real-time detection have been evaluated, with some reporting no apparent loss in clinical sensitivity (32). Kuypers et al. (40) used eight primers and three probes for detection of all four currently circulating HCoVs, with positive results confirmed by individual HCoV-specific assays. Similar sensitivity was obtained using the virus-specific and consensus assays. Real-time PCR assays may be adapted to provide quantitative data for HCoVs by use of hydrolysis probe chemistry or intercalating dyes (35, 55, 77, 81, 85). Although quantification of target RNA is not necessary for diagnostics, such assays may prove useful in epidemiological studies and when responses to interventions are measured.

SARS-CoV has been detected by NAATs in specimens obtained from the respiratory tract, cerebrospinal fluid, feces, and urine, but most reported studies have utilized respiratory specimens. Soon after SARS-CoV was identified, primers reported by Drosten and colleagues (19) were developed by a collaboration of laboratories participating in the World Health Organization SARS Laboratory Consortium. These primers, which target the *pol* 1b region, have been used by different groups in nested and nonnested formats for one-step and two-step RT-PCRs for gel-based detection and to develop real-time assays. Peiris et al. (56) performed RT-PCR with random primers for initial identification of SARS-CoV, and based on this sequence, they developed a gel-based two-step RT-PCR targeting the *pol* 1b region. They have published detailed methodologies for conventional and real-time PCR-based amplification and detection of SARS-CoV (57). Other authors have also described and evaluated RT-PCR assays targeting the *pol* 1b region (55, 60, 62, 79). Several modifications to the RNA extraction and RT steps reported by others were made to enhance detection sensitivity (59, 79). The N gene target has also been used in SARS-CoV NAATs (4, 48). In one study, a real-time assay targeting the N gene was found to be more sensitive than commercially available assays (18). Houng et al. used the 3'-noncoding region (NCR) of the SARS-CoV genome to develop a quantitative hydrolysis probe-based assay, using a recombinant plasmid as a quantitation standard (35).

Early in the SARS epidemic, commercial NAATs became available and were compared with "in-house" procedures. In one study, the first-generation LightCycler SARS-CoV quantification assay (Roche, Penzberg, Germany) and the RealArt HPA coronavirus LC assay (Artus, Hamburg, Germany [now Qiagen Molecular Diagnostics, Valencia, CA]) were found to be more sensitive than a two-step gel-based RT-PCR for a range of clinical sample types (86). The specimen type and timing of specimen collection affect the detection of SARS-CoV RNA (as is likely the case for other HCoVs). In a large evaluation of assays for detection of SARS-CoV by NAATs, assay sensitivities ranged from 83.3% to 100%, and specificities ranged from 94% to 100% (48). The authors reported a good overall performance for all assays, with the commercial approaches being more expensive than the in-house assays. A comparison of three commercial kits (from Artus, Roche, and EraGen Biosciences [Madison, WI]) showed various degrees of sensitivity and specificity for detection of SARS-CoV for a range of positive and negative samples (49).

A

TABLE 2 Real-time RT-PCR methods for detection of currently-circulating HCoVs

Virus (target gene)	Primer or probe designation: sequence (5'-3')	PCR format	Assay performance and diagnostic evaluation [reference(s)]
HCoV-OC43 (M)	Forward: ATGTTAGGCCGATAATTGAGGACTAT Reverse: AATGTAAAGATGGCCGCGTATT Probe: CATACTCTGACGGTCACAAT	One-step virus-specific real-time RT-PCR assays using hydrolysis probe chemistry. Performed with ABI 7700 platform.	Set up as separate quantitative assays using standard curves. Evaluation on 100 clinical samples. Sensitivity reported as 20 copies of cDNA (77).
HCoV-229E (M)	Forward: TTCCGACGTGCTCGAACTTT Reverse: CCAACACGGTTGTGACAGTGA Probe: TCCTGAGGTCAATGCA		
HCoV-NL63 (N)	Forward: GACCAAAGCACTGAATAACATTTTCC Reverse: ACCTAATAAGCCTCTTTCTCAACCC Probe: AACACGCT"T"CCAAGGAGGTTTCTTCAACTGAG	One-step virus-specific real-time RT-PCR assays using hydrolysis probe chemistry. Performed with iCycler iQ real-time detection system and regents (Bio-Rad).	Evaluation on 1,890 samples. Sensitivity reported as 5 copies of synthetic RNA/reaction (14).
HCoV-HKU1 (pol 1b)	Forward: CCTTGCGAATGAATGTGCT Reverse: TTGCATCACCACTGCTAGTACCAC Probe: TGTGTGGCGGTTGCTATTATGTTAAGCCTG		
HCoV-OC43 (N)	Primer 1: CGATGAGGCTATTCCGACTAGGT Primer 2: CCTTCCTGAGCCTTCAATATAGTAACC Probe: TCCGCCTGGCACGGTACTCCCT	Two-step virus-specific RT-PCR. Real-time cDNA amplification undertaken under universal amplification conditions with hydrolysis probe chemistry, using ABI Prism 7700 platform.	Evaluation on 504 clinical samples. Sensitivity equal to or better than that of nested PCR (74).
HCoV-229E (N)	Primer 1: CAGTCAAAATGGGCTGATGCA Primer 2: AAAGGGCTATAAAGAGAATAAGGTATTCT Probe: CCCTGACGACCACGTTGTGGTTCA		
HCoV-NL63 (N)	Forward: CTAGTTCTTCTGGTACTTCCACTCC Reverse: TCTGGTAGGAACACGCTTCCAA Probe: TAAGCCTCTTTTCTCAACCCAGGGC	Real-time amplification undertaken with LightCycler platform (Roche)	Evaluation on 539 clinical samples. Assay sensitivity not quoted (85).
HCoV-229E (N)	Sense primer: CGCAAGAATTCAGAACCAGAG Antisense primer: GGGAGTCAGGTTCTTCAACAA Probe: CCACACTTCAATCAAAAGCTCCCAAATG	Individual, single-tube, two-step virus-specific real-time RT-PCRs with hydrolysis probe chemistry, using ABI 7700 or ABI 7500 platform	Sensitivity quoted as <500 to 1,000 copies/ml for each assay. Assays evaluated on 2,060 clinical samples (21).
HCoV-OC43 (N)	Sense primer: GCTCAGGAAGGTCTGCTCC Antisense primer: TCCTGCACTAGAGGCTCTGC Probe: TTCCAGATCTACTTCGCGCACATCC		
HCoV-NL63 (N)	Sense primer: AGGACCTTAAATTCAGACAACGTTCT Antisense primer: GATTACGTTTGCGATTACCAAGACT Probe: TAACAGTTTTAGCACCTTCCTTAGCAACCCAAACA		
HCoV-HKU1 (N)	Sense primer: AGTTCCCATTGCTTTCGGAGTA Antisense primer: CCGGCTGTGTCTATACCAATATCC Probe: CCCCTTCTGAAGCAA		

Target	Primer/Probe sequences	Description
HCoV-229E, HCoV-OC43, HCoV-NL63, and HCoV-HKU1 (pol 1b)	F1: TGGTGGCTGGGACGATATGT F2: TTTATGTGGTTGGAATAATATGTTG F3: TGGCGGGTGGGATAATATGT F-OC: CCTTATTAAAGATGTTGACAATCCTGTAC R1: GGCATAGCACGATCACACTTAGG R2: GGCAAAGCTCTATCACATTTGG R3: GAGGGCATAGCTCTATCACACTTAGG R-OC: AATACGTAGTAGGTTTGGCATAGCAC P1: ATAATCCCAACCCATRAG P2: ATAGTCCCATCCCATCAA P-OC: CACACTTAGGATAGTCCCA	One-step real-time RT-PCR with hydrolysis probe chemistry, using RNA UltraSense One-Step quantitative RT-PCR system (Invitrogen Life Technologies). Assay multiplexed to provide a consensus HCoV screen or individual primers and probes selected for each specific HCoV. Consensus PCR used as a screen with primers F1, F2, F3, R1, R2, and R3, with sensitivity quoted as 10 viral copies/reaction. Assay setup evaluated on 1,061 clinical samples (40).
HCoV-HKU1 (pol)	Forward: GAA TTT TGT TGT TCA CAT GGT GAT AGA Reverse: GCA ACC GCC ACA CAT AAC TAT TT Probe: TTT ATC GCC TTG CGA ATG AAT GTG CTC	Two-step RT-PCR. Real-time cDNA amplification undertaken under universal amplification conditions with hydrolysis probe chemistry, using ABI 7900 platform. HCoV-HKU1 assay evaluated on 540 samples (26). Other HCoV assays evaluated in two separate studies, with 540 and 148 clinical samples. Assay sensitivities reported as 1 to 18 copies/μl of RNA (26, 27).
HCoV-OC43 (pol)	Forward: CGC CGC CTT ATT AAA GAT GTT G Reverse: GGC ATA GCA CGA TCA CAC TTA GG Probe: AAT CCT GTA CTT ATG GGT TGG GAT T	
HCoV-229E (pol)	Forward: TGG AGC GAG GAT CGT GTT C Reverse: TAG GCT GTG ACA GCT TTT GCA Probe: TGT TCT CAC GCT GCT GTT GAT TCG CT	
HCoV-NL63 (replicase)	Forward: TGT TGT AGT AGG TGG TTG TGT AAC ATCT Reverse: AAT TTT TGT GCA CCA GTA TCA AGT TT Probe: ATG TTT CAC CAA TTG TTA GTG AGA AAA TTT CTG TTA TGG	

Isothermal NAATs were also developed for amplification and detection of SARS-CoV. A NASBA assay (bioMérieux) targeted the *pol* and N genes, with the N gene being more sensitive (38). Real-time NASBA demonstrated equal or enhanced sensitivity compared with those of other real-time RT-PCR assays (10). A real-time LAMP assay was shown to be more sensitive than a comparator conventional RT-PCR assay in one study (34), although in another investigation, the LAMP approach, while easy to perform, was found to be less sensitive than quantitative RT-PCR (61). Juang et al. combined multiplex PCR and hybridization of amplified products to specific probes immobilized on a chip to increase the sensitivity and specificity of SARS-CoV detection (36). Their study confirmed the strategy to be equally sensitive to real-time nested PCR.

The data from all studies to date indicate that the sensitivity of NAATs for detection of SARS-CoV cannot be improved further by altering the target or extraction protocol. The only way to improve clinical sensitivity for identification of SARS cases might be to test multiple samples per patient (18, 56, 58, 86).

Consensus PCR assays may allow simultaneous detection of SARS-CoV and other HCoVs (1, 13, 52, 62). These assays have been shown to be sensitive, but it would be prudent to use specific assays for confirmation of SARS-CoV infections should this virus reemerge in the human population.

Infections with the currently circulating HCoVs present with symptoms similar to those for other respiratory virus infections. Several commercial assays based on NAATs are available for broad detection of respiratory viruses, including HCoVs, in respiratory samples. These are based mainly on multiplexed amplification reactions with separate probe-specific detection of amplified products in different formats. Kits using end-point detection which identify some HCoV targets include the Seeplex range of assays (Seegene, Seoul, Korea) (39). Kits using nucleic acid amplification with suspension microarray detection of a broad range of respiratory viruses (including HCoVs) have been developed and evaluated. Such assays include the xTAG respiratory viral panel from Luminex Molecular Diagnostics (Austin, TX) (46). The xTAG respiratory viral panel assay has been evaluated extensively, and its results have been compared with those of individual NAATs for HCoVs (example results are provided in Fig. 4 and in previously published reports [46, 54]). Broad detection of respiratory viruses is particularly important in analyses of outbreaks, and recent studies have shown the added value of broad respiratory virus detection in such diagnostic situations (80). The cost-effective nature of such a multiplex approach compared with individual culture, antigen detection, and NAATs has also been confirmed (47). Other broad respiratory virus detection assays geared toward diagnostics and epidemiological studies are at various stages of regulatory approval. These include the Respiratory MultiCode-PLx assay (EraGen), the Infiniti Respiratory Viral Panel Plus assay (Autogenomics Inc., Vista, CA), and the ResPlex assay (Qiagen Molecular Diagnostics), as reviewed recently (23).

ISOLATION PROCEDURES

HCoVs are fastidious in their in vitro requirements for isolation and propagation, and thus culture-based methods are not routinely used for diagnosis. Virus isolation procedures are used more often for analysis of novel CoVs or for antigenic studies. HCoVs tend to induce subtle CPE, and many cell types are not susceptible. For diagnostic purposes, culture may be used for initial amplification of virus, with detection of HCoV antigens by antigen detection or PCR-based

methods. Both nucleic acid and antigen detection methods were found to be useful for detection of HCoV-229E and -OC43 after culture, with PCR being the most sensitive (68). Although initially isolated in organ cultures, HCoV-OC43- and HCoV-229E-like viruses can be cultured in Huh-7 cell lines, with syncytium formation appearing 24 to 48 h after inoculation (17, 28). Modified antigen detection can be utilized for titration of HCoV-229E and HCoV-OC43 stocks grown in culture or, potentially, for quantification of virus levels in clinical samples (41), although reagents for such an approach are not yet available commercially.

HCoV-NL63 can replicate to some degree in tertiary monkey kidney cells and hepatocytes (17), and the LLC-MK2 (73) and Caco-2 (33) cell lines have been used to support its growth. Figure 3 shows the CPE for LLC-MK2 cells. A plaque assay has been reported for quantification of infectious virus (33). However, growth of HCoV-NL63 is often slow (22), with low viral titers resulting in a diffuse CPE (65). Thus a cell culture system suitable for long-term propagation of HCoV-NL63-like strains remains to be identified (28). HCoV-HKU1 has still not been cultured successfully (84).

For initial identification of SARS-CoV, patient specimens were inoculated into a variety of continuous cell lines (reviewed in reference 64). Culture detection of SARS-CoV is relatively insensitive (compared with detection by NAATs) and requires biosafety level 3 facilities and expertise, which limits the number of laboratories where it can be performed. Since most laboratories do not stain their cultures with antibodies to HCoVs, they are not likely to identify SARS-CoV (or other novel CoVs) during routine procedures. One study showed that R-Mix cells (Diagnostic Hybrids Inc. [DHI]), which contain a fresh mixture of Mv1Lu (mink lung cells) and A549 cells, could support growth of SARS-CoV (29). This means that laboratories using this cell mix for routine analysis of respiratory samples should be particularly careful when handling samples from patients with an atypical presentation of symptoms or where SARS-CoV or another novel virus may emerge. DHI has developed a cell line (R-Mix Too) which uses MDCK and A549 cells and does not support growth of SARS or other CoVs. DHI has also developed a medium for feeding RhMK cells which avoids the risk of CoV isolation. If a laboratory were to inadvertently isolate a novel virus (including CoVs), it should cease manipulation of the sample/culture and notify the local public health laboratory for follow-up.

SEROLOGIC TESTS

Studies have shown that a large proportion of the population was exposed to the currently circulating HCoVs early in life (6, 7, 16, 50, 66, 84), with reinfection being common. Thus, serological approaches are difficult to use for primary diagnosis, and detection of HCoV-specific antibody has been used largely for seroepidemiological studies or retrospective diagnosis and confirmation of cases. Blood may be used for serum storage and possible follow-up for unusual presentations or in outbreak situations.

The S and N proteins of HCoVs are expressed most abundantly during virus infection, and these proteins have been used in both native and recombinant forms to develop antibody detection assays for HCoVs, using a range of detection systems and labels. Enzyme-linked immunosorbent assays (ELISAs) developed for detection of N-specific antibodies to HCoV-NL63 and HCoV-229E were shown to be species specific, with no detectable cross-reactivity between these closely related viruses (16). Line immunoassays using recombinant N proteins as antigens could be used to detect HCoV antibodies (42). The use of recombinant N and S proteins for detection of HCoV-HKU1 immunoglobulin G (IgG) and IgM in patient sera by use of Western blotting and ELISA has been reported (6, 84). Recent serological studies of adults, using recombinant N protein enzyme immunoassays, reported a seroprevalence of >90% for HCoV-229E, HCoV-NL63, and HCoV-OC43 and of 59.2% for HCoV-HKU1 (66).

Antibody detection by an ELISA for the N protein is considered a useful and economic method for diagnosis of SARS-CoV, with the main neutralizing antibody response targeting the S protein (reviewed in reference 69). The IgM response to SARS-CoV infection is delayed and is detectable for longer periods (up to 180 days) than those for other viral infections (83). Although profiling of IgM, IgG, and IgA antibodies against SARS-CoV has been undertaken, it is difficult to make an acute diagnosis by use of serological methods alone, and this approach is inevitably retrospective for case identification (12, 64). Ruling out SARS-CoV infection by use of serological methods would require a negative result at least 28 days after the onset of illness.

EVALUATION, INTERPRETATION, AND REPORTING OF RESULTS

CoVs are a unique group of viruses with the potential for widespread recombination and the ability to cross between species, resulting in diseases in unrelated hosts, as seen for SARS. HCoV infection does not present in a way that is clinically distinguishable from other causes of respiratory virus infection. Laboratory diagnosis is helpful for appropriate management, even though specific treatment is not available. Thus, direct detection of HCoVs in respiratory specimens by use of NAATs is increasing, particularly for acute diagnosis in university-based hospital settings.

Nucleotide changes and mutations are common in HCoVs because of error-prone replication. While NAATs are dominant among the main diagnostic approaches for detection of HCoVs, the published assays must be evaluated continually to ensure that they do not miss circulating viruses and variants. Many different NAATs have been reported for generic detection of HCoVs and for specific detection of the individual viruses. In evaluating the validation data available, it is important to consider the number and range of clinical samples tested, sensitivity, specificity, reproducibility, dynamic range, positive predictive value, and negative predictive value. If pan-corona assays are used, special attention must be paid to the fact that sequence conservation among HCoVs is low, and relatively conserved regions of the genome with functions that are not prone to change must be selected. Confirmation tests should be performed by using a specific assay targeting a different gene. Pan-corona assays may be used in adjunct testing alongside virus-specific assays, providing a "catch-all" approach to identifying novel CoVs that might have crossed over into the human population or may be insertion or deletion mutants with altered pathogenicity. As is the case for all NAATs, extraction of RNA is critical for downstream assay sensitivity and performance, and internal controls which copurify with the HCoV nucleic acid should be incorporated wherever possible to identify problems. The specificities of NAATs are generally very good, but as shown for SARS-CoV, sensitivities may vary greatly depending on the type of sample and the collection time relative to the course of infection. For diagnosis of SARS or identification of other potential new CoV infec-

tions of humans, a combination of serological assays and NAATs is recommended. A diagnostic laboratory should not report a positive SARS result (preliminary or confirmed) without first notifying the local public health laboratory, because confirmation of cases will involve a public health response with global implications.

REFERENCES

1. **Adachi, D., G. Johnson, R. Draker, M. Ayers, T. Mazzulli, P. J. Talbot, and R. Tellier.** 2004. Comprehensive detection and identification of human coronaviruses, including the SARS-associated coronavirus, with a single RT-PCR assay. *J. Virol. Methods* **122:**29–36.
2. **Arden, K. E., M. D. Nissen, T. P. Sloots, and I. M. Mackay.** 2005. New human coronavirus, HCoV-NL63, associated with severe lower respiratory tract disease in Australia. *J. Med. Virol.* **75:**455–462.
3. **Bastien, N., J. L. Robinson, A. Tse, B. E. Lee, L. Hart, and Y. Li.** 2005. Human coronavirus NL-63 infections in children: a 1-year study. *J. Clin. Microbiol.* **43:**4567–4573.
4. **Bressler, A. M., and F. S. Nolte.** 2004. Preclinical evaluation of two real-time, reverse transcription-PCR assays for detection of the severe acute respiratory syndrome coronavirus. *J. Clin. Microbiol.* **42:**987–991.
5. **Brodzinski, H., and R. M. Ruddy.** 2009. Review of new and newly discovered respiratory tract viruses in children. *Pediatr. Emerg. Care* **25:**352–360.
6. **Chan, C. M., H. Tse, S. S. Wong, P. C. Woo, S. K. Lau, L. Chen, B. J. Zheng, J. D. Huang, and K. Y. Yuen.** 2009. Examination of seroprevalence of coronavirus HKU1 infection with S protein-based ELISA and neutralization assay against viral spike pseudotyped virus. *J. Clin. Virol.* **45:**54–60.
7. **Chan, K. H., V. C. C. Cheng, P. C. Woo, S. K. Lau, L. L. Poon, Y. Guan, W. H. Seto, K. Y. Yuen, and J. S. Peiris.** 2005. Serological responses in patients with severe acute respiratory syndrome coronavirus infection and cross-reactivity with human coronaviruses 229E, OC43, and NL63. *Clin. Diagn. Lab. Immunol.* **12:**1317–1321.
8. **Chan, K. H., L. L. M. Poon, V. C. C. Cheng, Y. Guan, I. F. N. Hung, J. Kong, L. Y. C. Yam, W. H. Seto, K. Y. Yuen, and J. S. M. Peiris.** 2004. Detection of SARS coronavirus in patients with suspected SARS. *Emerg. Infect. Dis.* **10:**294–299.
9. **Chan, P. K., W. K. To, K. C. Ng, R. K. Lam, T. K. Ng, R. C. Chan, A. Wu, W. C. Yu, N. Lee, D. S. Hui, S. T. Lai, E. K. Hon, C. K. Li, J. J. Sung, and J. S. Tam.** 2004. Laboratory diagnosis of SARS. *Emerg. Infect. Dis.* **10:**825–831.
10. **Chantratita, W., W. Pongtanapisit, W. Piroj, C. Srichunrasmi, and S. Seesuai.** 2004. Development and comparison of the real-time amplification based methods—NASBA-Beacon, RT-PCR Taqman and RT-PCR hybridization probe assays—for the qualitative detection of SARS coronavirus. *Southeast Asian J. Trop. Med. Public Health* **35:**623–629.
11. **Cheng, P. K., D. A. Wong, L. K. Tong, S. M. Ip, A. C. Lo, C. S. Lau, E. Y. Yeung, and W. W. Lim.** 2004. Viral shedding patterns of coronavirus in patients with probable severe acute respiratory syndrome. *Lancet* **363:**1699–1700.
12. **Cheng, V. C., S. K. Lau, P. C. Woo, and K. Y. Yuen.** 2007. Severe acute respiratory syndrome coronavirus as an agent of emerging and reemerging infection. *Clin. Microbiol. Rev.* **20:**660–694.
13. **Chiu, S. S., K. H. Chan, K. W. Chu, S. W. Kwan, Y. Guan, L. L. Poon, and J. S. Peiris.** 2005. Human coronavirus NL63 infection and other coronavirus infections in children hospitalized with acute respiratory disease in Hong Kong, China. *Clin. Infect. Dis.* **40:**1721–1729.
14. **Dare, R. K., A. M. Fry, M. Chittaganpitch, P. Sawanpanyalert, S. J. Olsen, and D. D. Erdman.** 2007. Human coronavirus infections in rural Thailand: a comprehensive study using real-time reverse-transcription polymerase chain reaction assays. *J. Infect. Dis.* **196:**1321–1328.

15. de Souza Luna, L. K., V. Heiser, N. Regamey, M. Panning, J. F. Drexler, S. Mulangu, L. Poon, S. Baumgarte, B. J. Haijema, L. Kaiser, and C. Drosten. 2007. Generic detection of coronaviruses and differentiation at the prototype strain level by reverse transcription-PCR and nonfluorescent low-density microarray. *J. Clin. Microbiol.* **45**:1049–1052.

16. Dijkman, R., M. F. Jebbink, N. B. El Idrissi, K. Pyrc, M. A. Muller, T. W. Kuijpers, H. L. Zaaijer, and L. van der Hoek. 2008. Human coronavirus NL63 and 229E seroconversion in children. *J. Clin. Microbiol.* **46**:2368–2373.

17. Dijkman, R., and L. van der Hoek. 2009. Human coronaviruses 229E and NL63: close yet still so far. *J. Formos. Med. Assoc.* **108**:270–279.

18. Drosten, C., L. L. Chiu, M. Panning, H. N. Leong, W. Preiser, J. S. Tam, S. Gunther, S. Kramme, P. Emmerich, W. L. Ng, H. Schmitz, and E. S. Koay. 2004. Evaluation of advanced reverse transcription-PCR assays and an alternative PCR target region for detection of severe acute respiratory syndrome-associated coronavirus. *J. Clin. Microbiol.* **42**:2043–2047.

19. Drosten, C., S. Gunther, W. Preiser, S. van der Werf, H. R. Brodt, S. Becker, H. Rabenau, M. Panning, L. Kolesnikova, R. A. Fouchier, A. Berger, A. M. Burguiere, J. Cinatl, M. Eickmann, N. Escriou, K. Grywna, S. Kramme, J. C. Manuguerra, S. Muller, V. Rickerts, M. Sturmer, S. Vieth, H. D. Klenk, A. D. Osterhaus, H. Schmitz, and H. W. Doerr. 2003. Identification of a novel coronavirus in patients with severe acute respiratory syndrome. *N. Engl. J. Med.* **348**:1967–1976.

20. Esper, F., C. Weibel, D. Ferguson, M. L. Landry, and J. S. Kahn. 2005. Evidence of a novel human coronavirus that is associated with respiratory tract disease in infants and young children. *J. Infect. Dis.* **191**:492–498.

21. Esposito, S., S. Bosis, H. G. Niesters, E. Tremolati, E. Begliatti, A. Rognoni, C. Tagliabue, N. Principi, and A. D. Osterhaus. 2006. Impact of human coronavirus infections in otherwise healthy children who attended an emergency department. *J. Med. Virol.* **78**:1609–1615.

22. Fouchier, R. A., N. G. Hartwig, T. M. Bestebroer, B. Niemeyer, J. C. de Jong, J. H. Simon, and A. D. Osterhaus. 2004. A previously undescribed coronavirus associated with respiratory disease in humans. *Proc. Natl. Acad. Sci. USA* **101**:6212–6216.

23. Fox, J. D. 2007. Nucleic acid amplification tests for the detection and analysis of respiratory viruses: the future for diagnostics? *Future Microbiol.* **2**:199–211.

24. Fujimoto, K., K. H. Chan, K. Takeda, K. F. Lo, R. H. Leung, and T. Okamoto. 2008. Sensitive and specific enzyme-linked immunosorbent assay using chemiluminescence for detection of severe acute respiratory syndrome viral infection. *J. Clin. Microbiol.* **46**:302–310.

25. Gagneur, A., S. Vallet, P. J. Talbot, M. C. Legrand-Quillien, B. Picard, C. Payan, and J. Sizun. 2008. Outbreaks of human coronavirus in a pediatric and neonatal intensive care unit. *Eur. J. Pediatr.* **167**:1427–1434.

26. Garbino, J., S. Crespo, J. D. Aubert, T. Rochat, B. Ninet, C. Deffernez, W. Wunderli, J. C. Pache, P. M. Soccal, and L. Kaiser. 2006. A prospective hospital-based study of the clinical impact of non-severe acute respiratory syndrome (non-SARS)-related human coronavirus infection. *Clin. Infect. Dis.* **43**:1009–1015.

27. Garbino, J., M. W. Gerbase, W. Wunderli, C. Deffernez, Y. Thomas, T. Rochat, B. Ninet, J. Schrenzel, S. Yerly, L. Perrin, P. M. Soccal, L. Nicod, and L. Kaiser. 2004. Lower respiratory viral illnesses: improved diagnosis by molecular methods and clinical impact. *Am. J. Respir. Crit. Care Med.* **170**:1197–1203.

28. Gerna, G., G. Campanini, F. Rovida, E. Percivalle, A. Sarasini, A. Marchi, and F. Baldanti. 2006. Genetic variability of human coronavirus OC43-, 229E-, and NL63-like strains and their association with lower respiratory tract infections of hospitalized infants and immunocompromised patients. *J. Med. Virol.* **78**:938–949.

29. Gillim-Ross, L., J. Taylor, D. R. Scholl, J. Ridenour, P. S. Masters, and D. E. Wentworth. 2004. Discovery of novel human and animal cells infected by the severe acute respiratory syndrome coronavirus by replication-specific multiplex reverse transcription-PCR. *J. Clin. Microbiol.* **42**:3196–3206.

30. Guan, Y., J. S. Peiris, B. Zheng, L. L. Poon, K. H. Chan, F. Y. Zeng, C. W. Chan, M. N. Chan, J. D. Chen, K. Y. Chow, C. C. Hon, K. H. Hui, J. Li, V. Y. Li, Y. Wang, S. W. Leung, K. Y. Yuen, and F. C. Leung. 2004. Molecular epidemiology of the novel coronavirus that causes acute respiratory syndrome. *Lancet* **363**:99–104.

31. Guan, Y., B. J. Zheng, Y. Q. He, X. L. Liu, Z. X. Zhuang, C. L. Cheung, S. W. Luo, P. H. Li, L. J. Zhang, Y. J. Guan, K. M. Butt, K. L. Wong, K. W. Chan, W. Lim, K. F. Shortridge, K. Y. Yuen, J. S. Peiris, and L. L. Poon. 2003. Isolation and characterization of viruses related to the SARS coronavirus from animals in southern China. *Science* **302**:276–278.

32. Gunson, R. N., T. C. Collins, and W. F. Carman. 2005. Real-time RT-PCR detection of 12 respiratory viral infections in four triplex reactions. *J. Clin. Virol.* **33**:341–344.

33. Herzog, P., C. Drosten, and M. A. Muller. 2008. Plaque assay for human coronavirus NL63 using human colon carcinoma cells. *Virol. J.* **5**:138.

34. Hong, T. C., Q. L. Mai, D. V. Cuong, M. Parida, H. Minekawa, T. Notomi, F. Hasebe, and K. Morita. 2004. Development and evaluation of a novel loop-mediated isothermal amplification method for rapid detection of severe acute respiratory syndrome coronavirus. *J. Clin. Microbiol.* **42**:1956–1961.

35. Houng, H. S., D. Norwood, G. V. Ludwig, W. Sun, M. Lin, and D. W. Vaughn. 2004. Development and evaluation of an efficient 3′-noncoding region based SARS coronavirus (SARS-CoV) RT-PCR assay for detection of SARS-CoV infections. *J. Virol. Methods* **120**:33–40.

36. Juang, J. L., T. C. Chen, S. S. Jiang, C. A. Hsiung, W. C. Chen, G. W. Chen, S. M. Lin, J. H. Lin, S. C. Chiu, and Y. K. Lai. 2004. Coupling multiplex RT-PCR to a gene chip assay for sensitive and semiquantitative detection of severe acute respiratory syndrome-coronavirus. *Lab. Invest.* **84**:1085–1091.

37. Kahn, J. S., and K. McIntosh. 2005. History and recent advances in coronavirus discovery. *Pediatr. Infect. Dis. J.* **24**:S223–S227.

38. Keightley, M. C., P. Sillekens, W. Schippers, C. Rinaldo, and K. S. George. 2005. Real-time NASBA detection of SARS-associated coronavirus and comparison with real-time reverse transcription-PCR. *J. Med. Virol.* **77**:602–608.

39. Kim, S. R., C. S. Ki, and N. Y. Lee. 2009. Rapid detection and identification of 12 respiratory viruses using a dual priming oligonucleotide system-based multiplex PCR assay. *J. Virol. Methods* **156**:111–116.

40. Kuypers, J., E. T. Martin, J. Heugel, N. Wright, R. Morrow, and J. A. Englund. 2007. Clinical disease in children associated with newly described coronavirus subtypes. *Pediatrics* **119**:e70–e76.

41. Lambert, F., H. Jacomy, G. Marceau, and P. J. Talbot. 2008. Titration of human coronaviruses, HcoV-229E and HCoV-OC43, by an indirect immunoperoxidase assay. *Methods Mol. Biol.* **454**:93–102.

42. Lehmann, C., H. Wolf, J. Xu, Q. Zhao, Y. Shao, M. Motz, and P. Lindner. 2008. A line immunoassay utilizing recombinant nucleocapsid proteins for detection of antibodies to human coronaviruses. *Diagn. Microbiol. Infect. Dis.* **61**:40–48.

43. Li, Y. H., J. Li, X. E. Liu, L. Wang, T. Li, Y. H. Zhou, and H. Zhuang. 2005. Detection of the nucleocapsid protein of severe acute respiratory syndrome coronavirus in serum: comparison with results of other viral markers. *J. Virol. Methods* **130**:45–50.

44. Liu, I. J., P. J. Chen, S. H. Yeh, Y. P. Chiang, L. M. Huang, M. F. Chang, S. Y. Chen, P. C. Yang, S. C. Chang, and W. K. Wang. 2005. Immunofluorescence assay for detection of the nucleocapsid antigen of the severe acute respiratory syndrome (SARS)-associated coronavirus in cells derived from throat wash samples of patients with SARS. *J. Clin. Microbiol.* **43**:2444–2448.

45. Loeb, M., A. McGeer, B. Henry, M. Ofner, D. Rose, T. Hlywka, J. Levie, J. McQueen, S. Smith, L. Moss, A. Smith, K. Green, and S. D. Walter. 2004. SARS among critical care nurses, Toronto. *Emerg. Infect. Dis.* **10:**251–255.

46. Mahony, J., S. Chong, F. Merante, S. Yaghoubian, T. Sinha, C. Lisle, and R. Janeczko. 2007. Development of a respiratory virus panel test for detection of twenty human respiratory viruses by use of multiplex PCR and a fluid microbead-based assay. *J. Clin. Microbiol.* **45:**2965–2970.

47. Mahony, J. B., G. Blackhouse, J. Babwah, M. Smieja, S. Buracond, S. Chong, W. Ciccotelli, T. O'Shea, D. Alnakhli, M. Griffiths-Turner, and R. Goeree. 2009. Cost analysis of multiplex PCR testing for diagnosing respiratory virus infections. *J. Clin. Microbiol.* **47:**2812–2817.

48. Mahony, J. B., A. Petrich, L. Louie, X. Song, S. Chong, M. Smieja, M. Chernesky, M. Loeb, and S. Richardson. 2004. Performance and cost evaluation of one commercial and six in-house conventional and real-time reverse transcription-PCR assays for detection of severe acute respiratory syndrome coronavirus. *J. Clin. Microbiol.* **42:**1471–1476.

49. Mahony, J. B., and S. Richardson. 2005. Molecular diagnosis of severe acute respiratory syndrome: the state of the art. *J. Mol. Diagn.* **7:**551–559.

50. Manopo, I., L. Lu, Q. He, L. L. Chee, S. W. Chan, and J. Kwang. 2005. Evaluation of a safe and sensitive spike protein-based immunofluorescence assay for the detection of antibody responses to SARS-CoV. *J. Immunol. Methods* **296:**37–44.

51. Masters, P. S. 2006. The molecular biology of coronaviruses. *Adv. Virus Res.* **66:**193–292.

52. Moës, E., L. Vijgen, E. Keyaerts, K. Zlateva, S. Li, P. Maes, K. Pyrc, B. Berkhout, L. van der Hoek, and M. Van Ranst. 2005. A novel pancoronavirus RT-PCR assay: frequent detection of human coronavirus NL63 in children hospitalized with respiratory tract infections in Belgium. *BMC Infect. Dis.* **5:**6.

53. Myint, S., S. Johnston, G. Sanderson, and H. Simpson. 1994. Evaluation of nested polymerase chain methods for the detection of human coronaviruses 229E and OC43. *Mol. Cell. Probes* **8:**357–364.

54. Pabbaraju, K., K. L. Tokaryk, S. Wong, and J. D. Fox. 2008. Comparison of the Luminex xTAG respiratory viral panel with in-house nucleic acid amplification tests for diagnosis of respiratory virus infections. *J. Clin. Microbiol.* **46:**3056–3062.

55. Peiris, J. S., C. M. Chu, V. C. Cheng, K. S. Chan, I. F. Hung, L. L. Poon, K. I. Law, B. S. Tang, T. Y. Hon, C. S. Chan, K. H. Chan, J. S. Ng, B. J. Zheng, W. L. Ng, R. W. Lai, Y. Guan, and K. Y. Yuen. 2003. Clinical progression and viral load in a community outbreak of coronavirus-associated SARS pneumonia: a prospective study. *Lancet* **361:**1767–1772.

56. Peiris, J. S., S. T. Lai, L. L. Poon, Y. Guan, L. Y. Yam, W. Lim, J. Nicholls, W. K. Yee, W. W. Yan, M. T. Cheung, V. C. Cheng, K. H. Chan, D. N. Tsang, R. W. Yung, T. K. Ng, and K. Y. Yuen. 2003. Coronavirus as a possible cause of severe acute respiratory syndrome. *Lancet* **361:**1319–1325.

57. Peiris, J. S., and L. L. Poon. 2008. Detection of SARS coronavirus in humans and animals by conventional and quantitative (real time) reverse transcription polymerase chain reactions. *Methods Mol. Biol.* **454:**61–72.

58. Poon, L. L., K. H. Chan, O. K. Wong, T. K. Cheung, I. Ng, B. Zheng, W. H. Seto, K. Y. Yuen, Y. Guan, and J. S. Peiris. 2004. Detection of SARS coronavirus in patients with severe acute respiratory syndrome by conventional and real-time quantitative reverse transcription-PCR assays. *Clin. Chem.* **50:**67–72.

59. Poon, L. L., K. H. Chan, O. K. Wong, W. C. Yam, K. Y. Yuen, Y. Guan, Y. M. Lo, and J. S. Peiris. 2003. Early diagnosis of SARS coronavirus infection by real time RT-PCR. *J. Clin. Virol.* **28:**233–238.

60. Poon, L. L., B. W. Wong, K. H. Chan, C. S. Leung, K. Y. Yuen, Y. Guan, and J. S. Peiris. 2004. A one step quantitative RT-PCR for detection of SARS coronavirus with an internal control for PCR inhibitors. *J. Clin. Virol.* **30:**214–217.

61. Poon, L. L., B. W. Wong, K. H. Chan, S. S. Ng, K. Y. Yuen, Y. Guan, and J. S. Peiris. 2005. Evaluation of real-time reverse transcriptase PCR and real-time loop-mediated amplification assays for severe acute respiratory syndrome coronavirus detection. *J. Clin. Microbiol.* **43:**3457–3459.

62. Poutanen, S. M., D. E. Low, B. Henry, S. Finkelstein, D. Rose, K. Green, R. Tellier, R. Draker, D. Adachi, M. Ayers, A. K. Chan, D. M. Skowronski, I. Salit, A. E. Simor, A. S. Slutsky, P. W. Doyle, M. Krajden, M. Petric, R. C. Brunham, and A. J. McGeer. 2003. Identification of severe acute respiratory syndrome in Canada. *N. Engl. J. Med.* **348:**1995–2005.

63. Pyrc, K., R. Dijkman, L. Deng, M. F. Jebbink, H. A. Ross, B. Berkhout, and L. van der Hoek. 2006. Mosaic structure of human coronavirus NL63, one thousand years of evolution. *J. Mol. Biol.* **364:**964–973.

64. Richardson, S. E., R. Tellier, and J. Mahony. 2004. The laboratory diagnosis of severe acute respiratory syndrome: emerging laboratory tests for an emerging pathogen. *Clin. Biochem. Rev.* **25:**133–142.

65. Schildgen, O., M. F. Jebbink, M. de Vries, K. Pyrc, R. Dijkman, A. Simon, A. Muller, B. Kupfer, and L. van der Hoek. 2006. Identification of cell lines permissive for human coronavirus NL63. *J. Virol. Methods* **138:**207–210.

66. Severance, E. G., I. Bossis, F. B. Dickerson, C. R. Stallings, A. E. Origoni, A. Sullens, R. H. Yolken, and R. P. Viscidi. 2008. Development of a nucleocapsid-based human coronavirus immunoassay and estimates of individuals exposed to coronavirus in a U.S. metropolitan population. *Clin. Vaccine Immunol.* **15:**1805–1810.

67. Shao, X., X. Guo, F. Esper, C. Weibel, and J. S. Kahn. 2007. Seroepidemiology of group 1 human coronaviruses in children. *J. Clin. Virol.* **40:**207–213.

68. Sizun, J., N. Arbour, and P. J. Talbot. 1998. Comparison of immunofluorescence with monoclonal antibodies and RT-PCR for the detection of human coronaviruses 229E and OC43 in cell culture. *J. Virol. Methods* **72:**145–152.

69. Suresh, M. R., P. K. Bhatnagar, and D. Das. 2008. Molecular targets for diagnostics and therapeutics of severe acute respiratory syndrome (SARS-CoV). *J. Pharm. Pharm. Sci.* **11:**1s–13s.

70. Tyrrell, D. A., S. Cohen, and J. E. Schlarb. 1993. Signs and symptoms in common colds. *Epidemiol. Infect.* **111:**143–156.

71. Vabret, A., T. Mourez, J. Dina, L. van der Hoek, S. Gouarin, J. Petitjean, J. Brouard, and F. Freymuth. 2005. Human coronavirus NL63, France. *Emerg. Infect. Dis.* **11:**1225–1229.

72. van der Hoek, L., K. Pyrc, and B. Berkhout. 2006. Human coronavirus NL63, a new respiratory virus. *FEMS Microbiol. Rev.* **30:**760–773.

73. van der Hoek, L., K. Pyrc, M. F. Jebbink, W. Vermeulen-Oost, R. J. Berkhout, K. C. Wolthers, P. M. Wertheim-van Dillen, J. Kaandorp, J. Spaargaren, and B. Berkhout. 2004. Identification of a new human coronavirus. *Nat. Med.* **10:**368–373.

74. van Elden, L. J., A. M. van Loon, F. van Alphen, K. A. Hendriksen, A. I. Hoepelman, M. G. van Kraaij, J. J. Oosterheert, P. Schipper, R. Schuurman, and M. Nijhuis. 2004. Frequent detection of human coronaviruses in clinical specimens from patients with respiratory tract infection by use of a novel real-time reverse-transcriptase polymerase chain reaction. *J. Infect. Dis.* **189:**652–657.

75. Vijaykrishna, D., G. J. Smith, J. X. Zhang, J. S. Peiris, H. Chen, and Y. Guan. 2007. Evolutionary insights into the ecology of coronaviruses. *J. Virol.* **81:**4012–4020.

76. Vijgen, L., E. Keyaerts, P. Lemey, P. Maes, K. Van Reeth, H. Nauwynck, M. Pensaert, and M. Van Ranst. 2006. Evolutionary history of the closely related group 2 coronaviruses: porcine hemagglutinating encephalomyelitis virus, bovine coronavirus, and human coronavirus OC43. *J. Virol.* **80:**7270–7274.

77. Vijgen, L., E. Keyaerts, E. Moes, P. Maes, G. Duson, and M. Van Ranst. 2005. Development of one-step, real-time,

quantitative reverse transcriptase PCR assays for absolute quantitation of human coronaviruses OC43 and 229E. *J. Clin. Microbiol.* **43:**5452–5456.

78. **Vijgen, L., E. Keyaerts, E. Moes, I. Thoelen, E. Wollants, P. Lemey, A. M. Vandamme, and M. Van Ranst.** 2005. Complete genomic sequence of human coronavirus OC43: molecular clock analysis suggests a relatively recent zoonotic coronavirus transmission event. *J. Virol.* **79:**1595–1604.

79. **Wang, H., Y. Mao, L. Ju, J. Zhang, Z. Liu, X. Zhou, Q. Li, Y. Wang, S. Kim, and L. Zhang.** 2004. Detection and monitoring of SARS coronavirus in the plasma and peripheral blood lymphocytes of patients with severe acute respiratory syndrome. *Clin. Chem.* **50:**1237–1240.

80. **Wong, S., K. Pabbaraju, B. E. Lee, and J. D. Fox.** 2009. Enhanced viral etiological diagnosis of respiratory system infection by use of a multitarget nucleic acid amplification assay. *J. Clin. Microbiol.* **47:**3839–3845.

81. **Woo, P. C., S. K. Lau, C. M. Chu, K. H. Chan, H. W. Tsoi, Y. Huang, B. H. Wong, R. W. Poon, J. J. Cai, W. K. Luk, L. L. Poon, S. S. Wong, Y. Guan, J. S. Peiris, and K. Y. Yuen.** 2005. Characterization and complete genome sequence of a novel coronavirus, coronavirus HKU1, from patients with pneumonia. *J. Virol.* **79:**884–895.

82. **Woo, P. C., S. K. Lau, H. W. Tsoi, Y. Huang, R. W. Poon, C. M. Chu, R. A. Lee, W. K. Luk, G. K. Wong, B. H.** Wong, V. C. Cheng, B. S. Tang, A. K. Wu, R. W. Yung, H. Chen, Y. Guan, K. H. Chan, and K. Y. Yuen. 2005. Clinical and molecular epidemiological features of coronavirus HKU1-associated community-acquired pneumonia. *J. Infect. Dis.* **192:**1898–1907.

83. **Woo, P. C., S. K. Lau, B. H. Wong, K. H. Chan, C. M. Chu, H. W. Tsoi, Y. Huang, J. S. Peiris, and K. Y. Yuen.** 2004. Longitudinal profile of immunoglobulin G (IgG), IgM, and IgA antibodies against the severe acute respiratory syndrome (SARS) coronavirus nucleocapsid protein in patients with pneumonia due to the SARS coronavirus. *Clin. Diagn. Lab. Immunol.* **11:**665–668.

84. **Woo, P. C., S. K. Lau, C. C. Yip, Y. Huang, and K. Y. Yuen.** 2009. More and more coronaviruses: human coronavirus HKU1. *Viruses* **1:**57–71.

85. **Wu, P. S., L. Y. Chang, B. Berkhout, L. van der Hoek, C. Y. Lu, C. L. Kao, P. I. Lee, P. L. Shao, C. Y. Lee, F. Y. Huang, and L. M. Huang.** 2008. Clinical manifestations of human coronavirus NL63 infection in children in Taiwan. *Eur. J. Pediatr.* **167:**75–80.

86. **Yam, W. C., K. H. Chan, K. H. Chow, L. L. Poon, H. Y. Lam, K. Y. Yuen, W. H. Seto, and J. S. Peiris.** 2005. Clinical evaluation of real-time PCR assays for rapid diagnosis of SARS coronavirus during outbreak and post-epidemic periods. *J. Clin. Virol.* **33:**19–24.

Hepatitis A and E Viruses*

DAVID A. ANDERSON AND NATALIE A. COUNIHAN

88

Viral hepatitis is the general term for inflammatory diseases of the liver caused by at least five different viruses, with hepatitis A, B, C, D, and E viruses having a definite association with acute viral hepatitis. Of these, only hepatitis A virus (HAV) and hepatitis E virus (HEV) are enterically transmitted, and both cause acute and generally self-limiting infections without significant long-term carrier status. While there are no serious long-term sequelae in patients who recover from hepatitis A or hepatitis E, both viruses are associated with significant risks of acute, fulminant hepatitis and liver failure, and chronic hepatitis E has been reported to occur in immunosuppressed patients. Severe outcomes are most commonly seen in patients with acute hepatitis A on a background of chronic hepatitis C or hepatitis B virus infection, and for patients with acute hepatitis E during pregnancy, especially during the third trimester. In the absence of these cofactors, the diseases show a general trend towards greater severity with increasing age, with the majority of infections being subclinical in children; however, severe and fulminant HAV and HEV infections can occur at any age.

TAXONOMY

Hepatitis A Virus

HAV is the type species of the *Hepatovirus* genus within the family *Picornaviridae*. HAV is distinguished from other picornaviruses (such as poliovirus) by its tropism for the liver, high thermal stability, and a unique assembly process (Fig. 1). There are two major genotype groups found in humans and a third genotype considered to be a true simian strain (AGM-27) (35). Although there is significant genetic diversity among HAV strains, all strains of HAV represent a single serotype and this diversity does not affect the performance of serologic assays. Genotyping of HAV is based on sequence analysis around the VP1-2A region and is useful as a research tool for outbreak investigations (84).

Hepatitis E Virus

HEV is the type species of the *Hepevirus* genus within the family *Hepeviridae* (38). Four genotypes of HEV have been described to occur in humans, at least two of which appear to represent zoonotic infections originating from viruses endemic in swine and other mammals (see below) (54, 89, 115). An avian genotype of HEV was first recognized as causing "big liver and spleen disease"/hepatosplenomegaly (50, 81). Due to the rather low sequence homology between avian HEV and human and swine strains (around 50% at the nucleotide level, compared to a minimum of 75% between mammalian strains), avian HEV is tentatively considered a second species of the *Hepevirus* genus, but it may eventually be considered a member of a separate genus within the *Hepeviridae* family. This would be analogous to the taxonomy for mammalian and avian hepatitis B viruses (*Orthohepadnavirus* genus and *Avihepadnavirus* genus, respectively, within the family *Hepadnaviridae*).

DESCRIPTION OF THE AGENTS

Hepatitis A Virus

HAV is a small virus with a nonenveloped, icosohedral capsid approximately 27 nm in diameter. The viral genome is composed of linear, positive-sense RNA and is about 7,500 nucleotides (nt) in length (Fig. 1A). Its structure is characteristic of all picornaviral genomes, being organized into an uncapped 5′ untranslated region (UTR), then a single open reading frame (ORF) encoding all known viral proteins, and a short 3′ UTR (86). Viral particles have a sedimentation coefficient of around 156S and a buoyant density of 1.325 g/cm^3 in cesium chloride (67). HAV is resistant to low pH (<3.0) and shows remarkable thermal stability, especially in the presence of magnesium salts (3). Thorough cooking is necessary to inactivate HAV in contaminated foods.

An outline of the viral replication mechanism is shown in Fig. 1A (see reference 86 for a comprehensive review of picornaviral replication). The positive-strand RNA genome contains a single ORF, which is translated to yield the sole polyprotein. The virus-encoded 3C protease liberates eight individual proteins, including the three capsid proteins: VP0, VP1-2A (also known as PX), and VP3 (6). Five copies of each of the three proteins associate to form pentamers, and 12 pentamers are then assembled into empty capsids or combined with RNA to form virions.

Following assembly, HAV is exported from infected hepatocytes, although the precise mechanism by which

*This chapter contains information presented in chapter 95 by Edwin A. Brown and Jack T. Stapleton and chapter 98 by George G. Schlauder and George J. Dawson in the eighth edition of this *Manual*.

A HAV

B HEV

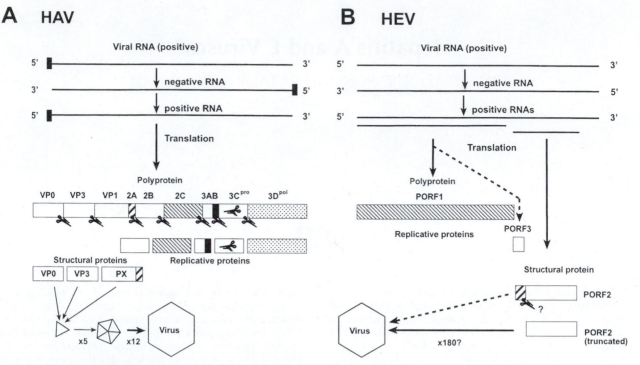

FIGURE 1 Genome replication and proteins of HAV and HEV. Both viruses have positive-strand RNA genomes of around 7,200 to 7,500 nt. (A) HAV replication proceeds via transcription from the genome to give full-length negative-strand RNA and then positive-strand RNA, which can either be assembled into the virus particle or used to translate further copies of a single, giant polyprotein which is processed by viral protease to yield the replicative proteins and capsid proteins. Assembly of five copies of each of the three capsid proteins (VP0, VP3, and PX) into pentamers and then 12 pentamers into capsids is required to form the antigenic sites of the virus. (B) Details of HEV replication are unknown, but it most likely produces a full-length negative-strand RNA and then full-length positive-strand RNA (new viral genomes) as well as subgenomic mRNAs which are used to translate the ORF2 (capsid) and ORF3 proteins, as well as the ORF1 polyprotein, which is cleaved at unknown sites to yield the replicative proteins. Cleavage of full-length PORF2 results in assembly of virus-like particles from the truncated product, but the size of the authentic viral capsid protein is unknown. Modified from reference 4, with permission.

this occurs is unknown. In vivo, hepatocytes are organized into a complex three-dimensional structure with surfaces facing both the bile (apical surface) and blood (basolateral surface [Fig. 2]). Any substrates exported from the apical membrane, including bile, can travel to the small intestine via bile canaliculi. As HAV is an enterically transmitted virus, it must enter the gastrointestinal tract for excretion in feces. Export of virus directly from hepatocytes via the apical surface would facilitate this transport; however, recent studies have shown that secretion is towards the hepatic blood supply from the basolateral surface (97). Presumably HAV must then traverse the hepatocyte for delivery to the gastrointestinal tract via bile, possibly via transcytosis (Fig. 2, inset). This type of indirect transport for apical-surface-destined cargo is a common mechanism in hepatocytes. Export mechanisms of HEV have not been examined.

Diagnosis and immunization for hepatitis A are not complicated by strain differences, despite significant levels of amino acid variation in the capsid proteins, because HAV exists as a single serotype worldwide. This is especially notable in the case of the highly divergent AGM-27, which is considered a true simian strain of HAV causing disease in African green monkeys and other lower primates (35).

The antigenic sites of HAV are formed through the complex interactions of the proteins within and between pentamers (100), which has hampered the production of HAV antigenic material through recombinant DNA techniques. As a result, cell culture remains the only reliable source of HAV antigens for serologic diagnostic tests and for vaccines. The replication of HAV in cell culture is rather inefficient compared to that of most picornaviruses, which necessitates very-large-scale cell culture production, but the virus is highly immunogenic. A number of highly effective, licensed vaccines are available against HAV: Havrix (GlaxoSmithKline) and Vaqta (Merck) within the United States, together with Avaxim (Sanofi Pasteur) and Epaxal (Berna Biotech) worldwide. A combination hepatitis A and hepatitis B vaccine, Twinrix (GlaxoSmithKline), is also widely available.

Hepatitis E Virus

Virions of HEV are nonenveloped, icosahedral particles approximately 32 to 34 nm in diameter, most likely comprising a single viral protein which encapsidates the single-stranded, positive-sense RNA genome of approximately 7,200 nt. Virions of HEV are much less stable than those of HAV, being sensitive to conditions (such as CsCl and

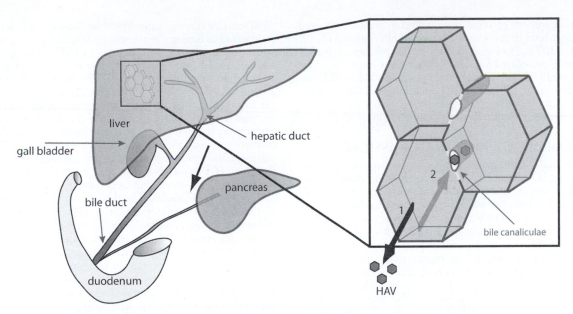

FIGURE 2 Export of HAV from hepatocytes. Polarized hepatocytes are organized in complex structures within the liver, with bile canaliculi representing grooves formed from the apical domains of adjacent hepatocytes (inset). Bile is secreted into the canaliculi via the apical membranes and then flows into the small intestine via a network of ducts. The basolateral surfaces of hepatocytes are in contact with the hepatic blood supply and underlying tissue. Following replication in hepatocytes, HAV is exported via basolateral membranes towards the blood supply (step 1, arrow). The virus is then transported back through the cell (step 2, arrow), possibly by transcytosis, to the apical surface and secreted into bile canaliculi.

freeze-thawing) that have no effect on HAV, and showing much greater sensitivity to heat than those of HAV (31). This lower stability is likely to be a major factor in the low secondary attack rate for HEV. Virions have a sedimentation coefficient of 183S and a buoyant density of 1.29 g/cm³ (16). The single capsid protein is encoded by ORF2, expected to yield a protein of 660 amino acids; however, the capsid protein of authentic viral particles has not been characterized.

Extensive progress has been made in the development of HEV diagnostics and experimental vaccines based on heterologous expression systems for viral proteins, but modestly robust, continuous cell culture systems for HEV have only recently been reported. The first of these uses a subclone of hepatocyte-derived HepG2 cells, and while virus yields remain low, it has allowed some key questions of virus replication to be addressed (33, 34, 44, 45), as well as providing a system for the study of virus neutralization (32). Recent reports have described relatively efficient cell culture systems for PLC/PRF/5 and A549 cells with HEV isolates of genotypes 3 and 4 from patients with fulminant hepatitis (102, 103). These initial reports show great promise, including the preliminary characterization of progeny viral particles and the potential incorporation of PORF3 (see below) in viral particles (102). Infectious cDNA clones of HEV were first described by Emerson and colleagues in 2001 (36), and studies using these systems have revealed many aspects of HEV replication. An infectious cDNA clone of one of the cell culture-adapted HEV strains has recently been reported (117).

A schematic of the HEV genome and encoded proteins is shown in Fig. 1B. The 7,204-nt infectious cDNA clone of the SAR-55 strain of HEV described by Emerson and colleagues (36) can be assumed to be full-length. Most isolates of HEV are close to this length, while avian HEV is substantially smaller, at 6,654 nt, due to deletions in both ORF1 and ORF2 (56).

The 5′ end of the genome has a 7-methylguanosine cap, while both the 5′ and 3′ ends of the viral RNA have short, highly conserved UTRs. Three ORFs, organized as 5′-ORF1-ORF3-ORF2-3′, encode the viral proteins (described here as PORFs): PORF1 (replicative polyprotein), PORF3 (unknown functions, possibly including virus export), and PORF2 (capsid protein) (Fig. 1B).

HEV shows a much greater degree of genetic diversity than HAV (see reference 56 for a detailed review of HEV genotypes). HEV can be classified into four putative "genotypes" (as defined by Wang and colleagues) (115); the Burmese and related strains (including most Chinese strains) are classified as genotype 1, the Mexican strain is classified as genotype 2, the swine HEV strain discovered in the United States (73) and closely related strains isolated from patients infected in the United States (88) are classified as genotype 3, and distinct isolates from patients in the People's Republic of China (T1 strain) (115) and both patients and swine in Taiwan (53, 54) are classified as genotype 4. Some strains isolated in Nigeria appear to be genotype 2 (17), whereas most other African strains have been identified as genotype 1 (111).

In contrast to HAV, the genotypic differences among HEV strains are associated with significant antigenic differences, with corresponding effects on the sensitivities of many serologic assays (see below). However, these antigenic differences appear to lie outside the principal neutralizing antibody domains, since HEV appears to exist as a single serotype, with experimental vaccines providing strong cross-genotype protection (108, 123). Similarly, the identification of conserved, immunodominant epitopes has resulted in greatly improved diagnostic tests that appear to detect all HEV strains (5, 19, 39, 43, 52, 72, 78, 119, 121). Extensive preclinical studies have been completed for a candidate HEV vaccine based on a truncated HEV ORF2 protein (amino acids 112 to 607) expressed in insect cells (108, 125), and it showed very positive results in a phase III trial conducted in Nepal during 2003 (95); however, no vaccine is yet commercially available.

EPIDEMIOLOGY AND TRANSMISSION

Despite sharing the primary mode of transmission via human feces, HAV and HEV have very different distributions of both disease and infection worldwide. These differences appear to be linked at least partly to the efficiency of virus transmission, with HAV being excreted in very high titers allowing waterborne as well as person-to-person spread, whereas HEV is more commonly seen in waterborne outbreaks. However, unresolved questions remain regarding the prevalence of HEV infection in areas of high endemicity such as Nepal, where infection with HAV is almost universal and yet less than 50% of the population show evidence of exposure to HEV (5, 22). Notably, the precise source of presumed zoonotic infections with HEV in developed countries remains obscure since most cases have no evidence of contact with swine, the species most clearly recognized to be a reservoir of HEV.

Hepatitis A Virus

Transmission

The generalized course of infection and serologic responses for both HAV and HEV is shown in Fig. 3. Due to its en-

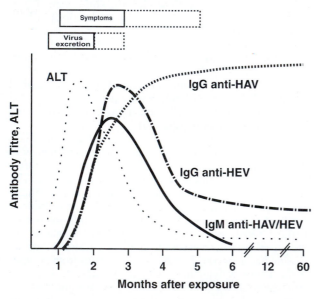

FIGURE 3 Serologic and virologic courses of infection with HAV or HEV. For HAV, the serologic responses shown are typical of those detected with numerous commercially available assays. For HEV, the serologic responses shown are those that probably occur in most patients, but the detection of these responses will vary widely depending on the assays used. High levels of HAV-specific IgG provide lifelong protection from reinfection, but HEV-specific IgG declines rapidly during the first 6 months and might not persist at protective levels for life. Modified from reference 4 with permission.

teric route of transmission, HAV has been widely assumed to infect cells lining the alimentary tract. However, studies with Caco-2 cells suggest that progeny HAV from intestinal epithelial cells is released back into the lumen of the gut rather than into the circulation (15) and that the virus is around 10,000-fold more infectious when administered by the intravenous route rather than the oral route (82). This is consistent with early studies that suggested the liver as the primary site of replication, with amplification in the alimentary tract making little or no contribution (63). During the incubation period of 4 to 6 weeks after first exposure to the virus, HAV spreads throughout the liver without causing any cytolytic effects, but liver damage eventually results and is most likely mediated by the cellular immune response to the virus, with infections in young children generally following a benign course. Virus is excreted through bile to the gut, and very high titers of infectious HAV are present in most patients at the onset of illness. Virus is generally cleared within several weeks, although prolonged excretion of HAV has been reported to occur in a significant proportion of cases. In general, titers of excreted virus are highest before the onset of obvious symptoms.

Although the vast majority of progeny virus is excreted in the feces, HAV patients display a viremia that may last for some weeks around the time of clinical presentation, consistent with the initial release of progeny virus into the hepatic blood supply from the basolateral surface of infected hepatocytes (97). Transmission of HAV via blood products has been demonstrated (77), and inactivation procedures to eliminate HAV are clearly required in the manufacture of blood products (66). Fortunately, such processes have now been validated for HAV, and further transmission is unlikely (1, 59, 65).

Epidemiology: High, Low, and Intermediate Rates of Infection

HAV is found worldwide, but with widely varying epidemiological patterns that largely reflect sanitation standards (13). In countries or areas with poor sanitation, high levels of HAV exposure result in most individuals becoming infected at an early age, but in these circumstances HAV is not a major public health problem because the symptoms tend to be mild or absent in children and very few members of the adult population are susceptible. However, HAV can certainly cause clinical disease in children, most obviously in foodborne outbreaks in schools of developed countries (57, 83) but also in endemic populations in countries such as Nepal (I. L. Shrestha, personal communication) and Turkey, where HAV was the most commonly identified cause of fulminant hepatic failure in children from 1 month to 17 years of age (11).

Conversely, in countries or populations with high standards of personal and public sanitation, relatively few individuals are exposed at an early age. In many countries of Western Europe, uniformly high standards of sanitation result in very low rates of HAV disease even though the vast majority of the population is susceptible. Prior to the widespread use of vaccines, sporadic HAV infection continued at a significant level in the United States, Australia, and other countries with generally high sanitation levels but a wide diversity of socioeconomic circumstances, especially in the very young and in disadvantaged communities where standards of personal hygiene are low. Acute infection rates have been reduced considerably since 1996 due to the progressive introduction of vaccination to at-risk groups, communities, and states and to the general pediatric population

(25). Focal circulation of this highly transmissible virus in some populations and geographic areas provides an ongoing source of virus for sustained transmission throughout the broader community, and the most profound reductions in overall attack rates followed the introduction of nationwide pediatric immunization.

In the United States in 2007, international travel was the most frequently identified risk factor for HAV infection (17.5%), while household or sexual contact with an infected person was next at 7.8%, but risk factor data were not available for 67.7% of reported cases (25). Children in day care centers were identified as a risk factor in 4.6% of cases, but children are likely to be a factor in a large proportion of the cases where no risk factor is identified (25, 99). An important aspect in the epidemiology and transmission of HAV is the high titer of virus produced, combined with the very great physical stability of the viral particle, which is relatively insensitive to extremes of heat: infectious virus is readily recovered after heating for 10 min at 60°C, and at as much as 78°C when in the presence of 1 M $MgCl_2$ (3).

HAV disease burden in the United States was estimated at more than 140,000 cases and 80 deaths annually in 1990 (48) but has declined rapidly since then (see reference 14 for a comprehensive review), and the lowest ever incidence rate was recorded in 2007 (25). This decline has been most pronounced in children, from a peak incidence of 39 cases/100,000 in 1990 to around 2 cases/100,000 in 2002, coincident with the introduction of targeted immunization of children from high-risk ethnic and racial groups and geographic areas, but the rate in adults (>18 years) also fell from around 17 cases/100,000 to 2 cases/100,000 during the same period (14). During the period from 2001 to 2007, the lowest rates were among children under 5 years of age (25). However, the figure may be underestimated, as asymptomatic infection is common among children of this age. The public health problem of HAV in the United States and other low-endemicity countries is compounded by the potential for large outbreaks of HAV spread by contaminated foods. Food- and waterborne infection with HAV was identified as a factor in 6.5% of cases in 2007 (25), but this proportion is likely to increase because such cases will not be prevented by targeted immunization strategies.

In the past, such foodborne outbreaks were largely confined to shellfish, which concentrate viruses such as HAV from large volumes of water and which are generally eaten raw or only lightly cooked. Examples are provided by outbreaks seen in Shanghai, People's Republic of China, in 1988 (49), the United States in 1991 (30), and Australia in 1997 (23). However, the increased trade in foodstuffs among countries now creates additional sources of infection. A number of outbreaks within the United States have been traced to fresh and frozen foods imported from Mexico (57, 83, 94, 116), where they had presumably been exposed to contaminated water during production or processing.

Intravenous and other illicit drug use is also positively associated with a higher risk of HAV infection and may play a major role in the epidemiology of HAV in some societies (92). Men who have sex with men are at increased risk, and outbreaks in this population in different countries have been described in recent years (14).

Residents from developed countries who travel to regions of endemicity, especially those visiting friends and relatives in regions of endemicity, are at greatly increased risk of HAV infection (8). The relative contribution of travel to the HAV disease burden may be underestimated, because travel history is often overlooked in diagnosis.

The greatest disease burden for HAV worldwide falls on countries that have previously had high rates of HAV infection but are now undergoing rapid economic growth and improvements in public sanitation and infrastructure, resulting in intermediate rates of HAV infection. Improved sanitation has the effect of sparing many young children from infection, but this results in a much larger pool of susceptible older children and young adults, in whom disease is more pronounced. HAV may continue to circulate widely within households and other close contacts, resulting in high rates of clinical disease. Routine infant immunization is likely to have the most impact on disease burden by interrupting transmission cycles as seen in other countries, but the cost of universal immunization programs is a major barrier to control of HAV in many countries.

Hepatitis E Virus

Transmission

Hepatitis E is primarily transmitted via the fecal-oral route. HEV RNA is detectable in the feces of 50% of patients 2 weeks after onset (21), and in one uncomplicated case was detected at 52 days after onset (79). Chronic HEV infection appears to be limited to patients on immunosuppressive therapy (60) and is unlikely to contribute significantly to transmission. Consumption of contaminated water is by far the most common route of transmission for clinical cases of HEV in countries where HEV is endemic, with household contact being much less important than for HAV.

Travel to areas where HEV is endemic is the most common source of HEV infections in areas of nonendemicity such as the United States and Western Europe, but locally acquired HEV infections also occur, representing zoonotic infections from pigs or other, unidentified hosts (50, 53, 73, 88). Genotyping has demonstrated close relationships between viruses from human cases of HEV and local swine HEV strains in many developed countries (for examples, see reference 53), and cross-species infection has been experimentally established for swine and human HEV (75), although other strains are unable to cross species (74). The route of transmission for these HEV cases is unknown, as clinical cases generally have no evidence of contact with swine. In Japan, a number of reports have demonstrated HEV infection following the consumption of raw or partially cooked liver or meat from swine or deer harboring corresponding strains of HEV (76, 98, 101, 120), but this is unlikely to be a significant source of infection in other countries.

HEV exhibits a significant viremia, with the majority of patients being positive by reverse transcriptase PCR (RT-PCR) at the time of disease onset, and there have been several reported cases of hepatitis E associated with transfusion both in countries where HEV is endemic and in countries where it is not endemic (10, 71).

Epidemiology: Countries Where the Virus Is Endemic and Where It Is Nonendemic

In countries where HEV is endemic, sporadic HEV infection is often the most common form of viral hepatitis on an annual basis, accounting for around 70% of cases in Kathmandu, Nepal (7), but above this background major epidemics also occur with a periodicity of around 7 to 10 years. For example, HEV was shown retrospectively to be responsible for 16 of 17 epidemics of enterically transmitted hepatitis in India (9), but HEV is also responsible for at least 25% of sporadic hepatitis between epidemics (61). Epidemics are most often associated with the wet season; however, one study has shown an increased rate of infection associated with a period of unusually low rainfall, presumably by concentrating human wastes in a riverine ecology (24).

Clinical HEV infection in countries where HEV is endemic is most common in adolescents and young adults, but it occurs to a lesser extent in childhood (58) and in late ages. There appear to be considerable differences in exposure rates among countries where HEV is considered endemic: in Egypt around 60% of children were exposed to HEV by the age of 10, and this rate did not increase further with age (26), whereas in Nepal only 16% of 12-year-olds had evidence of exposure to HEV, and the rate peaked at 31% later in life (22).

It is likely that the risk of clinical disease increases with age, as for hepatitis A, but while clinical HAV infection is uncommon in many developing countries because of high exposure rates in children, HEV exposure rates are never as high as for HAV and a large proportion of the population remains susceptible throughout adulthood.

In developing countries, exposure to water contaminated with human waste is a clear risk factor for disease, and close contact with domestic animals may also be a risk factor. Importantly, boiling of drinking water appears to be protective (51), but while this will not be practical for all residents in many developing countries, it is advisable for pregnant women because of the high risk of fulminant hepatitis E in this population (see below). The low rate of person-to-person spread of HEV is likely to be due to a combination of lower particle stability (31) and lower virus titers in excreta compared to those for HAV.

Reported seroprevalence rates for anti-HEV immunoglobulin G (IgG) in countries where HEV is presumed to be nonendemic vary widely, at least partly due to the different assays used which show very poor concordance (70). Observed rates of antibody between 1 and 5% are most common, at least some of which can be considered to represent true anti-HEV reactivity on the basis of neutralization tests (126). Experimental infections of macaques have demonstrated a strong dose-response for the development of clinical HEV disease (110), and the unexpectedly high rate of HEV seroprevalence in countries where clinical HEV is very rare may represent subclinical infection with low doses of zoonotic strains of HEV. There is some evidence for increased exposure to HEV in groups with occupational exposure to swine (62).

Travel to countries where HEV is endemic remains the greatest risk factor for clinical HEV infection in residents of countries where HEV is nonendemic (developed countries) (90). This risk can be assumed to be especially great for travelers visiting friends and relatives, as for HAV (8). However, with the very clear evidence for low rates of presumably zoonotic HEV infection from a large number of studies across many different developed countries, HEV infection must be considered in cases of unexplained hepatitis.

CLINICAL SIGNIFICANCE

Acute infections with any of the hepatitis viruses cannot be distinguished on clinical characteristics or pathological examinations, and the diseases caused by HAV and HEV are considered together here. However, HEV infection is unique among the hepatitis viruses in being associated with a high mortality rate during pregnancy due to fulminant hepatitis with a very rapid onset, approaching 30% in the third trimester, and the rate of fulminant hepatitis

for HEV outside of pregnancy is probably around 10-fold higher than for HAV (1% versus 0.1%) (12). The reasons for such severe outcomes for HEV infection are not known, but it is clear that women should take all possible precautions to avoid exposure to HEV during pregnancy. A major risk factor in this regard is travel from countries where it is nonendemic to areas where it is endemic, such as India and Pakistan.

Infection with HAV or HEV can result in a broad range of clinical outcomes, from subclinical infections (especially in children, or with low doses of HEV) to fulminant hepatitis. Disease severity shows a general increase with age; however, clinical and even fulminant hepatitis A and E do occur in children, and there is no reason to exclude the enterically transmitted hepatitis viruses from diagnostic consideration on the basis of patient age. A retrospective study in Turkey has shown HAV to be the most common identifiable cause of fulminant hepatitis in children (11).

Clinical presentation of acute viral hepatitis commonly begins with nonspecific, "flu-like" symptoms such as fever, headache, anorexia, nausea, and abdominal discomfort. Physical examination usually reveals an enlarged, tender liver. The first distinctive sign of hepatitis is usually dark urine (excretion of conjugated bilirubin), followed by pale feces and jaundice (yellow discoloration of the skin and sclera), but many patients do not show visible signs of jaundice despite severe symptoms, even when raised levels of serum bilirubin are present. However, it must be stressed that these nonspecific symptoms alone are not sufficient to infer acute viral hepatitis in a patient without jaundice, and liver function tests are an important adjunct to diagnosis (18), with raised levels of aspartate aminotransferase (AST) and alanine aminotransferase (ALT) detectable at the time of onset. Unless there are strong epidemiological grounds for suspicion, hepatitis A or E should not be considered in the absence of one of these biochemical markers or jaundice.

In most developed countries, hepatitis A is much more likely than hepatitis E unless there are specific indications to suggest HEV, such as past HAV infection or recent travel to areas where HEV is endemic combined with a history of receiving inactivated HAV vaccine. Patients with proven evidence of past HAV infection will not have HAV, other than those very rare cases that represent relapses after recent HAV infection (96). In developing countries with poor sanitation, clinical cases of HEV are often more common than HAV due to almost universal childhood exposure to that virus, although HEV appears to be relatively infrequent in many parts of South America. Coinfection with HAV and HEV has also been reported, with 14 of 33 outbreaks investigated in Cuba during the period from 1998 to 2003 showing strong serologic evidence of exposure to both viruses; however, a larger proportion of individual patients were infected exclusively with HAV (85), consistent with its more efficient secondary transmission.

Serum aminotransferase levels usually resolve after a period of 3 to 4 weeks. Normalization of liver enzymes usually marks complete recovery; however, many patients report an intolerance to fatty foods which may last for years. Relapses are rare for hepatitis A, occurring in around 7 to 12% of patients beyond 1 month (96). Protracted hepatitis A has been associated with a particular HLA allele (37). Prolonged disease with hepatitis E has also been observed in some areas where HEV is endemic and is frequently characterized by cholestasis with jaundice and itching. Cholestasis can occur with both hepatitis A and hepatitis E.

While both HAV and HEV (outside pregnancy) have low overall rates of fulminant hepatitis, the onset of encephalopathy can be quite rapid (around 7 days from onset of dark urine for hepatitis A). HEV has been found to be responsible for around 62% of fulminant hepatitis cases in studies from India (80) and Bangladesh (93), where the virus is highly endemic. Acute HAV infection on a background of chronic hepatitis C or hepatitis B is associated with more severe outcomes (113).

While chronic HEV infection has rarely been reported to occur in healthy individuals, a significant number of cases have been reported among patients receiving immunosuppressive therapy after solid-organ transplantation (42, 47, 60). There is no suggestion that transplantation was the source of infection in these cases, with cases occurring many months or years after transplantation. Rather, these represent sporadic cases of HEV infection that have progressed to chronicity due to ongoing immunosuppression. In the largest study, of 217 French patients with elevated liver enzymes and with no evidence of drug toxicities or other viral causes, 14 patients (6.5%) tested positive for serum HEV RNA, and 8 of these progressed to chronic infection (60).

HAV and HEV differ markedly in the relationship between infecting dose and the course of infection and disease. For HAV, studies with tamarins have shown a very clear correlation between higher infectious doses and reduced incubation period to develop disease, but no correlation with disease severity (82). This is consistent with the high secondary clinical attack rates seen for HAV. Low-dose infections of cynomolgus macaques with HEV have also demonstrated an increased time to seroconversion, but HEV disease severity showed a positive correlation with high infectious doses (2, 110). This attenuation of low-dose infections may help to explain the low secondary attack rates of HEV, and the rarity of clinical HEV disease in countries where it is considered nonendemic despite seroprevalence rates of around 2%.

Vaccines and Antiviral Agents

Passive immunization with human gamma globulin has been used for many years to provide short-term protection against hepatitis A, and it is still used for postexposure prophylaxis (<2 weeks postexposure) and for infants less than 1 year of age. As noted above, there are now a number of highly efficacious, inactivated vaccines available against hepatitis A (Havrix and Vaqta in the United States, plus Avaxim and Epaxal worldwide) or hepatitis A and B (Twinrix), and these have replaced the use of gamma globulin for protection of individuals with future risk of HAV infection. In the United States, progressively expanded programs of active immunization against hepatitis A have been implemented, beginning in 1996 with children (>2 years of age) living in communities with elevated rates of hepatitis A, travelers to countries where standards of hygiene and sanitation are low, men who have sex with men, recipients of clotting factors, injecting drug users, and patients with chronic hepatitis (where disease severity is exacerbated) (18). Extension of this program in 1999 to include children in all states or counties reporting more than 10 cases/100,000 population contributed to the rapid decline in HAV disease rates over the subsequent 7 years, and since 2006 the inclusion of children nationwide from 12 to 24 months of age (following the licensure of vaccines for use beginning at 12 months age) has led to further-reduced disease rates, reaching historical lows of 1 per 100,000 in 2007 (25).

No vaccines are yet commercially available for protection against hepatitis E. Studies by Purcell, Emerson, and colleagues at the NIH have demonstrated that antibody to PORF2 is sufficient to protect against hepatitis E (109), and active immunization of macaques with 53-kDa subunit antigen (amino acids 112 to 607) expressed in the baculovirus system has conferred protection against viral challenge with both homologous and heterologous HEV strains (108, 109, 125).

This candidate vaccine completed a phase III clinical trial in Army recruits in Nepal in 2003, with results published in 2007 (95). A total of 1,794 healthy HEV-seronegative adults received three doses of either the 53-kDa vaccine or placebo at months 0, 1, and 6 and were monitored for a median of 804 days. Hepatitis E developed in 66 of 896 placebo recipients, versus 3 of 898 vaccine recipients, yielding an efficacy of 95.5% (95). If and when it is commercially produced, it is likely that this vaccine would be most useful for travelers (including the military, Peace Corps, etc.) and for residents of countries where HEV is endemic, although further studies are required to determine the duration of protection in these populations.

No antivirals are available for treatment of hepatitis A or E, and it is unlikely that antivirals would be useful because the acute disease is largely immunopathogenic in mechanism. Experimental inhibitors have been developed that are active against the 3C protease of HAV, but clinical development of these is unlikely.

No specific symptomatic or anti-inflammatory treatments can be advised for hepatitis A or E. Bed rest and attention to diet (avoiding fatty foods) are commonly recommended to minimize symptoms and speed recovery; alcohol intake should be minimized. Pruritus is a feature of cholestatic hepatitis that may justify the cautious use of corticosteroids.

Intensive supportive medical care, as for acute liver failure due to other causes, is required in cases of fulminant hepatitis A or E. Fulminant hepatitis A has a better prognosis for spontaneous recovery than hepatitis B (69% versus 19% [87]). Liver transplantation is less frequently performed, and there is some risk of graft reinfection (41).

COLLECTION, TRANSPORT, AND STORAGE OF SPECIMENS

Standard methods for collection, transport, and storage of sera or plasma are adequate for the detection of both IgG and IgM antibodies to HAV and HEV, which are the only standard diagnostic tests performed. Sera or plasma can be stored at 4°C for weeks but should be frozen under other circumstances (−20 or −70°C for storage and dry ice for shipping). Shipping is most often an issue with HEV testing, which is not available in many routine diagnostic laboratories. IgM is more sensitive to freezing and thawing than is IgG, and repetitive cycles should be avoided. Feces may be collected for epidemiological studies of HAV (genotyping of strains) and are stable as a solid mass or slurries in phosphate-buffered saline or water for years at −70°C. HEV is difficult to detect in feces, and serum is preferred for RT-PCR and genotyping. Because HEV is more labile than HAV, sera for HEV RT-PCR studies must be tested within 24 h or frozen and shipped at −70°C.

Rapid, point-of-care (RPOC) tests for HEV-specific IgM are now available outside the United States (19, 78), which can overcome the need for collection and shipping of venous blood. These tests can be used for either fresh whole blood, or for serum and plasma as for laboratory assays.

DIRECT DETECTION

Electron Microscopy

Electron microscopy and, especially, immunoelectron microscopy are of historical importance for their roles in identifying HAV (40) and HEV particles (16) before the characterization and molecular cloning of the viruses and development of specific diagnostic tests, but they are insensitive and technically difficult and have no diagnostic value.

Antigen Detection

HAV

HAV antigen (HAAg) is very stable and is readily detected in the acute-phase fecal samples collected from many patients. Viral antigen is detected by enzyme-linked immunosorbent assay (ELISA) using monoclonal antibodies and may be present in very high titers in some patients, but antigen detection is less sensitive than RT-PCR or follow-up serology for detecting the uncommon cases in which IgM has not yet developed at initial presentation. There are no commercially available tests for HAAg.

HEV

HEV antigen is less stable than HAAg, and no reliable tests are available (either commercially or on a research-only basis) for the detection of antigen in clinical samples. It is unlikely that antigen detection would have any clinical value relative to serology or RT-PCR performed on sera (see below).

Nucleic Acid Detection

HAV

HAV patients are viremic in the prodromal phase, and one study from Brazil has reported around 12% of children during a common-source outbreak to have been RT-PCR positive but IgM negative ("window period") at the time of testing (29). The high proportion of window period cases found in this study contrasts with the high sensitivity of HAV IgM detection in other studies and may be related to high-dose infections with short incubation periods, and/or early case detection due to active surveillance of the outbreak. The authors also reported the detection of HAV RNA in 26% of patients initially classified as having acute, sporadic non-A, non-C hepatitis (29). All patients available for follow-up seroconverted, highlighting the utility of follow-up IgM serology or RT-PCR in the uncommon cases of acute hepatitis with unknown etiology, especially in a country where HAV is endemic. Serum is the preferred specimen for nucleic acid detection, but plasma is acceptable provided that anticoagulants do not interfere in the reactions; feces are least suitable, with variable levels of virus and high levels of inhibitors. While RT-PCR is useful for detection of very early (window period) infections and the confirmation of questionable IgM results, accredited assays are not commercially available for routine diagnostic testing of possible acute hepatitis A. In the absence of a mandate for screening of the blood supply for HAV RNA, there may be insufficient test numbers for such assays to be made commercially available; conversely, many manufacturers now routinely conduct HAV RT-PCR screens on pools of source plasma for blood products, although virus inactivation methods provide the most important protection for such products. HAV RNA can also be used for genotyping

of virus for research purposes using RT-PCR primers in the region of VP1-2A (Fig. 1) (20).

HEV

RT-PCR remains the "gold standard" for specificity in the diagnosis of acute HEV infection. However, levels of HEV RNA are generally low and the sensitivity of RT-PCR for diagnosis is very dependent on (i) patient presentation early in disease, (ii) rapid and careful processing of serum or plasma samples and appropriate transport at −70°C, and (iii) reference laboratories for testing and quality control. Serologic tests are preferable for routine diagnosis (see below). RT-PCR has provided the vast majority of information on zoonotic infections with HEV around the world (54, 64, 71, 89, 115, 120, 122) and will remain useful for confirmatory testing in areas of low endemicity such as the United States and Western Europe.

VIRAL ISOLATION

Many primary isolates of HAV have been adapted to cell culture, but virus isolation is insensitive and generally requires multiple passages over a period of many months and is not useful in diagnosis or epidemiological studies. Individual strains of HEV appear to replicate well in cell lines (103, 104), but in general the virus has proven refractory to propagation in standard cell cultures and virus isolation is not useful for diagnosis.

VIRAL IDENTIFICATION AND TYPING SYSTEMS

As described above, the direct detection of HAV and HEV RNA by RT-PCR and sequence-based genotyping has been used for the identification of potential sources of sporadic cases of HEV in countries where it is nonendemic, and for the investigation of common-source outbreaks of HAV. HEV genotyping is usually based on the ORF1 region and, to a lesser extent, on the ORF2 region (54, 64, 89, 115), while HAV strains and genotypes are determined by sequencing in the VP1-2A region of the genome (20).

SEROLOGIC TESTS

Despite the very good specificity of most serologic tests for HAV and HEV, their appropriate use and interpretation are dependent on patients meeting the clinical criteria for acute hepatitis, particularly in areas where the viruses have low incidence, such as the United States and other developed countries. The clinical criteria for the HAV surveillance case definition in the United States are "an acute illness with discrete onset of symptoms (e.g. fatigue, abdominal pain, loss of appetite, intermittent nausea, and vomiting) and jaundice or elevated serum aminotransferase levels" (18). Serologic testing should be limited to persons who meet the clinical criteria or to persons likely to have been exposed to HAV (18), and in light of the nonspecific nature of the symptoms, the importance of jaundice or elevated ALT or AST in meeting the case definition must be stressed. The same criteria are clearly relevant to HEV. In the absence of these clinical criteria for patients in regions of nonendemicity, the positive predictive value of the tests will be severely compromised. This is especially relevant given the very low rates of clinical HAV disease in countries with successful immunization programs, and of HEV disease in most developed countries.

Hepatitis A Virus

Tests for HAV-specific IgM are commercially available from numerous sources in a variety of formats (ELISA, enzyme immunoassay, and AxSym). The technology for detection of HAV-specific IgM is sufficiently well established that there are no significant differences in the diagnostic performance (sensitivity and specificity) among the laboratory-based testing platforms. Choices of diagnostic assays for HAV may reasonably be made on the basis of convenience for the testing laboratory, with a range from single-strip ELISAs for small numbers of specimens to completely automated systems for high-volume laboratories.

Test principles are either IgM class capture or indirect ELISA. In the IgM class capture assays, plates coated with anti-human IgM are used to capture IgM from patient samples, with HAV-specific IgM being detected by binding of labeled HAAg (inactivated HAV derived from cell culture). Indirect ELISAs use plates coated with HAAg, to which HAV-specific IgM will bind, and bound IgM is then detected using anti-human IgM conjugates. In both cases, assay reactivity and cutoffs are determined from internal controls supplied with the kits. Because HAAg binding to plates is generally inefficient, monoclonal antibodies are sometimes used to facilitate the binding of antigen to plates. All commercially available HAV serologic assays use inactivated, whole HAV derived from cell culture and thus detect the same antibody specificities.

Total or IgG anti-HAV does not have diagnostic value because antibody persists for life, although a rising titer of IgG (greater than fourfold in specimens taken 2 weeks apart) is indicative of acute HAV. Total HAV-specific antibody is a marker of immunity and can be used for prevaccination screening to identify those who require immunization, but the cost-effectiveness of screening depends on many factors (112). Postvaccination tests are not required due to the very high efficacy of available HAV vaccines. Tests for the measurement of total anti-HAV use a competitive ELISA format, in which HAAg is used to coat plates and specific antibody in patient serum binds to the antigen, resulting in a proportionately reduced assay signal from the binding of labeled monoclonal antibodies to HAAg.

In addition to serum or plasma, saliva can be used for detection of anti-HAV IgM or total antibody (107, 114), but the use of saliva or other samples, such as urine, falls outside the manufacturers' recommendations for current tests. These samples can be useful for research and investigational purposes but require internal validation.

RPOC tests for HAV-specific IgM have been developed (4) but are not yet commercially available. In common with the RPOC test for HEV-specific IgM (19, 78) (see below), such tests could prove especially useful in outbreak investigations.

Hepatitis E Virus

A number of research and commercial immunoassays for HEV-specific IgG and IgM are available in various countries, but with major differences in their sensitivities and specificities (see below). Only IgG ELISAs are currently approved for routine diagnostic use in the United States; in-house IgM ELISAs are available in reference laboratories. The appropriate use and interpretation of current serologic assays for HEV infection must take into account differences in assay sensitivity and specificity, the pattern of serologic responses (IgG and IgM and, in some cases, IgA) to various antigens, and the widely varying prevalence of clinical HEV infection worldwide.

Laboratory-Based HEV Serologic Tests

Many recombinant and synthetic peptide antigens have been used in diagnostics for HEV. Antigens included in early HEV diagnostic tests were notable for the transient IgG response observed in most patients (27, 28), which provided some specificity for acute infection but at the cost of sensitivity (7). This variability in detected IgG responses also contributes to the uncertainty regarding seroprevalence rates around the world, as studies using different antigens cannot be compared. Using more advanced antigens (such as the truncated forms of PORF2 expressed in insect cells, and ORF2.1 expressed in *Escherichia coli*), IgG levels appear to persist for many years (Fig. 3). High titers of IgG in patients are suggestive of acute infection, but this correlation is imperfect (5, 43) and the detection of IgG antibody is thus of little use for diagnosis of acute infection, especially in those developing countries where HEV is endemic and large numbers of patients will have antibody from past infections.

HEV-specific IgM is therefore preferable for diagnosis. As in the case of IgG, antigens vary significantly in their rates of reactivity with HEV-specific IgM. Second-generation commercial tests used a cocktail of three antigens (119), each of which has IgM reactivity with a proportion of HEV patient sera; however, positive sera show widely variable reactivities, presumably related to the number of individual antigens recognized by each patient, and the total reactivity rate is still low, at around 60% (118). An artificial recombinant mosaic protein, incorporating numerous linear peptide epitopes, has also been used in research settings (39) but suffers from a similar variability in patient reactivity, which decreases assay performance.

Improved IgM ELISAs have now been developed, based on highly conserved and immunodominant antigens derived from the capsid protein, PORF2. The ORF2.1 antigen, representing amino acids 394 to 660 of PORF2 expressed in *E. coli*, was originally shown to be highly conserved and immunodominant in the IgG response to HEV infection (68, 69), and it forms the basis of the MP Biomedicals (Singapore) HEV IgM ELISA 3.0 (19). This test has an overall sensitivity of 98.7% (149 positive of 151 confirmed HEV patients) and a specificity of 97.6% (203 negative of 208 patients with other forms of viral hepatitis or other diseases) (19), and it is commercially available outside the United States. The ORF2.1 antigen is also used in a double-antigen sandwich assay for total HEV-specific immunoglobulin (HEV ELISA 4.0), which is notable in being useful for detection of antibody in potential zoonotic hosts such as pigs, as well as in humans (55).

Sensitive and specific tests for HEV-specific IgM have also been developed using the truncated r55k antigen, representing amino acids 112 to 607 of PORF2 expressed in insect cells, in both indirect ELISA and IgM class capture ELISA formats (91, 121), but these are not commercially available. ELISA-based HEV IgM kits manufactured by Adaltis (Rome, Italy) and Biokit (Lliçà d'Amunt, Spain) are commercially available in many developing countries, but to date there have been no published evaluations of assay performance for these tests, and no details are available on the antigens used. HEV-specific IgA has also been reported to have utility in HEV diagnosis (106, 124), but these tests are not commercially available and require further evaluation.

RPOC HEV Serologic Tests

The major disease burden of HEV falls on developing countries and is especially severe among displaced populations such as refugees, with major epidemics observed

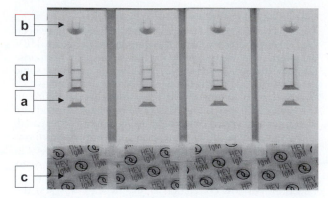

FIGURE 4 RPOC tests for HEV-specific IgM. Undiluted serum (25 μl) was added to the specimen window (a) and allowed to migrate through part of the membrane. Approximately 30 s later, 3 drops of buffer were added to the buffer window (b), the separator was removed by pulling the protruding end (c), and 1 drop of wash buffer was added to the specimen window. Results were visible through the viewing window (d) after 8 min. Samples are considered positive for IgM anti-HEV if two colored lines appear in the viewing window, and negative for IgM anti-HEV if a colored line appears only at the control line. Test kits are as described previously (19, 78), kindly provided by MP Biomedicals. Data are from our laboratory.

during 2004–2005 in the Greater Darfur region of Sudan (46). Timely access to sophisticated laboratory facilities is not available in these situations, highlighting the need for rapid diagnostic assays that can provide reliable diagnosis at the point of care, with minimal training or infrastructure. RPOC tests for HEV-specific IgM have now been developed using the ORF2.1 antigen and corresponding monoclonal antibodies in a novel format of immunochromatographic test (Fig. 4) (19, 78); these tests are commercially available in many countries outside the United States.

The HEV IgM RPOC test has been evaluated in two separate studies. In the first study (19), the RPOC test showed a sensitivity of 96.7% (146 of 151) and an overall specificity between 98.6% (205 of 208) and 96.9% (220 of 227), depending on exclusion or inclusion of sera having high levels of rheumatoid factor (RF), a common source of false-positive reactivity in rapid assays. In the second study (78), the RPOC test showed the slightly lower sensitivity of 93% (186 of 200) but a specificity of 99.7% (320 of 321) against a panel including RF-positive sera and sera from patients with acute Epstein-Barr virus infection, a further source of problems in many RPOC tests. The positive predictive value (PPV) and negative predictive value of the test were estimated at 98.0 to 99.5% and 97.6 to 95.0%, respectively (19, 78). These results suggest that the RPOC tests will certainly prove useful for the diagnosis of HEV in field situations of regions of endemicity and may also be considered as an alternative to ELISAs for laboratory use in both regions where HEV is nonendemic and regions where it is endemic.

These RPOC tests offer the further benefit of reduced collection of venous blood, which is difficult in small children and not well tolerated in some cultural settings.

Serologic Diagnosis of HEV Infection in Areas of Low Prevalence

In areas with a low incidence of clinical HEV infection, such as the United States and Western Europe, assay specificity will have a very large impact on the predictive value of HEV serologic tests. In order to be useful, HEV diagnostic assays will need to demonstrate very high specificity, high sensitivity, and the ability to detect infections caused by the diverse range of HEV strains (including potentially zoonotic strains) that are present worldwide. Commercially available assays for the detection of HEV-specific IgG have considerable value for the diagnosis of acute hepatitis in travelers returned from areas where HEV is endemic, among whom the incidence may be much higher than the approximate 2% prevalence detected in the healthy population. However, with the recognition that HEV should be considered in the diagnosis of sporadic acute hepatitis *without* a travel history, the need for more specific tests becomes evident. For example, if the incidence of HEV infection among acute hepatitis patients in the United States was 0.2%, then only 1 in 10 patients reactive in a test for HEV-specific IgG would be a true positive, leading to an unacceptable PPV. Notably, some research assays detect much higher HEV IgG prevalence rates among healthy populations in the United States (105); the reasons for this are not clear, but IgG detected in such assays would have an even lower PPV for acute HEV infection.

The detection of HEV-specific IgM should therefore become the method of choice for diagnosis of acute HEV infection in areas of low prevalence. Early assays for HEV-specific IgM showed false-positive reactivity in 3% of U.S. blood donors (technical bulletin; Genelabs Diagnostics, Singapore, 1998), roughly equivalent to the rate of IgG reactivity, which limited their usefulness in areas where HEV is nonendemic. A prototype IgM ELISA based on the ORF2.1 antigen was positive for only 1 of 500 Australian blood donors (specificity of 99.8% [2a]). A modified version of this test demonstrated a higher level of false-positive reactivity (2.4%) in studies to evaluate the RPOC test (19), which suggests that caution should also be used with this test pending further evaluation of false-positivity rates. The quantitative indirect IgM ELISA (91) and the IgM class capture assay (121) using r55k antigen have reported specificities of around 100%. Notably, the RPOC assay is also IgM class capture and has a specificity between 98.6 and 99.7% in different studies (19, 78). Many of these new tests should be suitable for use in regions of nonendemicity.

Serologic Diagnosis of HEV Infection in Areas of High Prevalence

Although the titer of HEV-specific IgG tends to decline markedly in the first year after infection (Fig. 3), this relationship is not reliable enough to form the basis of differential diagnosis (5, 43). The detection of HEV-specific IgG is therefore of little use for diagnosis of acute infection in developing countries where HEV is endemic and large numbers of patients will have antibody from past infections. Detection of HEV-specific IgM must therefore be the method of choice in areas where HEV is endemic.

As HEV accounts for as much as 70% of the acute sporadic hepatitis cases in countries where HEV is endemic, the specificity of assays is less critical in these settings, and assay sensitivity is of primary concern. The HEV IgM assays based on recombinant antigens expressed using the baculovirus system (91, 121), or the ORF2.1 antigen expressed in *E. coli* (5, 19), all appear to have sufficient sensitivity to allow their use in settings of endemicity. The robustness of assays should also be considered. For example, assays will sometimes be processed and interpreted manually where equipment such as ELISA washers and readers is not available. The ORF2.1 IgM ELISA has been evaluated in routine clinical laboratories based in regions of endemicity, allowing the identification of acute sporadic hepatitis E in a large proportion of patients in Nepal (7).

EVALUATION, INTERPRETATION, AND REPORTING OF RESULTS

In many developed countries, including the United States, the rarity of HEV infection and rapid decline in rates of HAV infection, coupled with increasing rates and recognition of hepatitis C and hepatitis B virus infections, provide a challenge in the correct diagnostic test selection for individual patients. In particular, testing for HAV IgM in the absence of clinical or epidemiological features consistent with acute hepatitis A is likely to result in false-positive results (18), and the same is true of HEV. Close attention should be paid to the clinical characteristics and patient history, including overseas travel, in interpretation of test results.

Hepatitis A is a reportable disease in the United States, Australia, and many other developed countries, where patient contacts are generally managed by active or passive immunoprophylaxis. In routine laboratories, interpretation of HAV and HEV IgM serologic tests is based on reference to internal test controls according to manufacturers' specifications. Many laboratories test for total HAV immunoglobulin and, if this is positive, retest for HAV IgM, which may be more convenient for sample throughput in areas of low endemicity. There are no standard confirmatory tests for HAV and HEV, again highlighting the need for test requests to be justified on clinical and/or epidemiological grounds in order to reduce false-positive results. False-negative results are uncommon for HAV and should be uncommon with the more recently developed HEV tests, because patients almost always have IgM present by the time of clinical presentation and the window period for seroconversion is very narrow. When false negatives are strongly suspected, for example, a negative HAV IgM test for a patient with raised ALTs and contact with a confirmed case of HAV, it may be appropriate to request a second specimen for retesting.

REFERENCES

1. **Adcock, W. L., A. MacGregor, J. R. Davies, M. Hattarki, D. A. Anderson, and N. H. Goss.** 1998. Chromatographic removal and heat inactivation of hepatitis A virus during manufacture of human albumin. *Biotechnol. Appl. Biochem.* **28:**85–94.
2. **Aggarwal, R., S. Kamili, J. Spelbring, and K. Krawczynski.** 2001. Experimental studies on subclinical hepatitis E virus infection in cynomolgus macaques. *J. Infect. Dis.* **184:**1380–1385.
2a. **Anderson, D., M. Riddell, F. Li, I. Shrestha, T. Howard, G. Perry, and G. Mearns.** 2000. *Abstr. 10th Int. Symp. Viral Hepatitis Liver Dis.*, abstr. E001.
3. **Anderson, D. A.** 1987. Cytopathology, plaque assay, and heat inactivation of hepatitis A virus strain HM175. *J. Med. Virol.* **22:**35–44.
4. **Anderson, D. A.** 2000. Waterborne hepatitis, p. 295–305. *In* S. C. Specter, R. L. Hodinka, and S. A. Young (ed.), *Clinical Virology Manual*, 3rd ed. ASM Press, Washington, DC.
5. **Anderson, D. A., F. Li, M. A. Riddell, T. Howard, H.-F. Seow, J. Torresi, G. Perry, D. Sumarsidi, S. M. Shrestha, and I. L. Shrestha.** 1999. ELISA for IgG-class antibody to hepatitis E virus based on a highly conserved, conformational epitope expressed in *Escherichia coli. J. Virol. Methods* **81:**131–142.
6. **Anderson, D. A., and B. C. Ross.** 1990. Morphogenesis of hepatitis A virus: isolation and characterization of subviral particles. *J. Virol.* **64:**5284–5289.
7. **Anderson, D. A., and I. L. Shrestha.** 2002. Hepatitis E virus, p. 1061–1074. *In* D. D. Richman, R. J. Whitley, and F. G. Hayden (ed.), *Clinical Virology.* ASM Press, Washington, DC.
8. **Angell, S. Y., and R. H. Behrens.** 2005. Risk assessment and disease prevention in travelers visiting friends and relatives. *Infect. Dis. Clin. N. Am.* **19:**49–65.
9. **Arankalle, V. A., M. S. Chadha, S. A. Tsarev, S. U. Emerson, A. R. Risbud, K. Banerjee, and R. H. Purcell.** 1994. Seroepidemiology of water-borne hepatitis in India and evidence for a third enterically-transmitted hepatitis agent. *Proc. Natl. Acad. Sci. USA* **91:**3428–3432.
10. **Arankalle, V. A., and L. P. Chobe.** 2000. Retrospective analysis of blood transfusion recipients: evidence for post-transfusion hepatitis E. *Vox Sang.* **79:**72–74.
11. **Aydogdu, S., F. Ozgenc, S. Yurtsever, S. A. Akman, Y. Tokat, and R. V. Yagci.** 2003. Our experience with fulminant hepatic failure in Turkish children: etiology and outcome. *J. Trop. Pediatr.* **49:**367–370.
12. **Balayan, M. S.** 1997. Epidemiology of hepatitis E virus infection. *J. Viral Hepat.* **4:**155–165.
13. **Bell, B. P.** 2002. Global epidemiology of hepatitis A: implications for control strategies, p. 359–365. *In* H. S. Margolis, M. J. Alter, and T. J. Liang (ed.), *Viral Hepatitis and Liver Disease.* International Medical Press, London, United Kingdom.
14. **Bell, B. P., D. A. Anderson, and S. M. Feinstone.** 2005. Hepatitis A virus, p. 2162–2185. *In* G. L. Mandell, J. E. Bennett, and R. Dolin (ed.), *Principles and Practice of Infectious Diseases*, 6th ed. Elsevier, Philadelphia, PA.
15. **Blank, C. A., D. A. Anderson, M. Beard, and S. M. Lemon.** 2000. Infection of polarized cultures of human intestinal epithelial cells with hepatitis A virus: vectorial release of progeny virions through apical cellular membranes. *J. Virol.* **74:**6476–6484.
16. **Bradley, D., A. Andjaparidze, E. H. Cook, Jr., K. McCaustland, M. Balayan, H. Stetler, O. Velazquez, B. Robertson, C. Humphrey, M. Kane, and I. Weisfuse.** 1988. Aetiological agent of enterically transmitted non-A, non-B hepatitis. *J. Gen. Virol.* **69:**731–738.
17. **Buisson, Y., M. Grandadam, E. Nicand, P. Cheval, H. van Cuyck-Gandre, B. Innis, P. Rehel, P. Coursaget, R. Teyssou, and S. Tsarev.** 2000. Identification of a novel hepatitis E virus in Nigeria. *J. Gen. Virol.* **81:**903–909.
18. **Centers for Disease Control and Prevention.** 2005. Positive test results for acute hepatitis A virus infection among persons with no recent history of acute hepatitis—United States, 2002–2004. *MMWR Morb. Mortal. Wkly. Rep.* **54:**453–456.
19. **Chen, H. Y., Y. Lu, T. Howard, D. Anderson, P. Y. Fong, W. P. Hu, C. P. Chia, and M. Guan.** 2005. Comparison of a new immunochromatographic test to enzyme-linked immunosorbent assay for rapid detection of immunoglobulin M antibodies to hepatitis E virus in human sera. *Clin. Diagn. Lab. Immunol.* **12:**593–598.
20. **Chen, Y., J. Mao, Y. Hong, L. Yang, Z. Ling, and W. Yu.** 2001. Genetic analysis of wild-type hepatitis A virus strains. *Chin. Med. J. (Engl.)* **114:**422–423.
21. **Clayson, E. T., K. S. Myint, R. Snitbhan, D. W. Vaughn, B. L. Innis, L. Chan, P. Cheung, and M. P. Shrestha.** 1995. Viremia, fecal shedding, and IgM and IgG responses in patients with hepatitis E. *J. Infect. Dis.* **172:**927–933.
22. **Clayson, E. T., M. P. Shrestha, D. W. Vaughn, R. Snitbhan, K. B. Shrestha, C. F. Longer, and B. L. Innis.** 1997. Rates of hepatitis E virus infection and disease among adolescents and adults in Kathmandu, Nepal. *J. Infect. Dis.* **176:**763–766.
23. **Conaty, S., P. Bird, G. Bell, E. Kraa, G. Grohmann, and J. M. McAnulty.** 2000. Hepatitis A in New South Wales, Australia from consumption of oysters: the first reported outbreak. *Epidemiol. Infect.* **124:**121–130.
24. **Corwin, A., K. Jarot, I. Lubis, K. Nasution, S. Suparmawo, A. Sumardiati, S. Widodo, S. Nazir, G. Orndorff, Y. Choi, R. Tan, A. Sie, S. Wignall, R. Graham, and K. Hyams.** 1995. Two years' investigation of epidemic hepatitis E virus transmission in West Kalimantan (Borneo), Indonesia. *Trans. R. Soc. Trop. Med. Hyg.* **89:**262–265.

25. **Daniels, D., S. Grytdal, and A. Wasley.** 2009. Surveillance for acute viral hepatitis—United States, 2007. *MMWR Morb. Mortal. Wkly. Rep.* **58:**1–27.

26. **Darwish, M. A., R. Faris, J. D. Clemens, M. R. Rao, and R. Edelman.** 1996. High seroprevalence of hepatitis A, B, C, and E viruses in residents in an Egyptian village in the Nile Delta: a pilot study. *Am. J. Trop. Med. Hyg.* **54:**554–558.

27. **Dawson, G. J., K. H. Chau, C. M. Cabal, P. O. Yarbough, G. R. Reyes, and I. K. Mushahwar.** 1992. Solid-phase enzyme-linked immunosorbent assay for hepatitis E virus IgG and IgM antibodies utilizing recombinant antigens and synthetic peptides. *J. Virol. Methods* **38:**175–186.

28. **Dawson, G. J., I. K. Mushahwar, K. H. Chau, and G. L. Gitnick.** 1992. Detection of long-lasting antibody to hepatitis E virus in a US traveller to Pakistan. *Lancet* **340:**426–427.

29. **de Paula, V. S., L. M. Villar, L. M. Morais, L. L. Lewis-Ximenez, C. Niel, and A. M. Gaspar.** 2004. Detection of hepatitis A virus RNA in serum during the window period of infection. *J. Clin. Virol.* **29:**254–259.

30. **Desenclos, J. C., K. C. Klontz, M. H. Wilder, O. V. Nainan, H. S. Margolis, and R. A. Gunn.** 1991. A multistate outbreak of hepatitis A caused by the consumption of raw oysters. *Am. J. Public Health* **81:**1268–1272.

31. **Emerson, S. U., V. A. Arankalle, and R. H. Purcell.** 2005. Thermal stability of hepatitis E virus. *J. Infect. Dis.* **192:**930–933.

32. **Emerson, S. U., P. Clemente-Casares, N. Moiduddin, V. A. Arankalle, U. Torian, and R. H. Purcell.** 2006. Putative neutralization epitopes and broad cross-genotype neutralization of hepatitis E virus confirmed by a quantitative cell-culture assay. *J. Gen. Virol.* **87:**697–704.

33. **Emerson, S. U., H. Nguyen, J. Graff, D. A. Stephany, A. Brockington, and R. H. Purcell.** 2004. In vitro replication of hepatitis E virus (HEV) genomes and of an HEV replicon expressing green fluorescent protein. *J. Virol.* **78:**4838–4846.

34. **Emerson, S. U., H. Nguyen, U. Torian, and R. H. Purcell.** 2006. ORF3 protein of hepatitis E virus is not required for replication, virion assembly, or infection of hepatoma cells in vitro. *J. Virol.* **80:**10457–10464.

35. **Emerson, S. U., S. A. Tsarev, and R. H. Purcell.** 1991. Biological and molecular comparisons of human (HM-175) and simian (AGM-27) hepatitis A viruses. *J. Hepatol.* **13**(Suppl. 4):S144–S145.

36. **Emerson, S. U., M. Zhang, X. J. Meng, H. Nguyen, M. St. Claire, S. Govindarajan, Y. K. Huang, and R. H. Purcell.** 2001. Recombinant hepatitis E virus genomes infectious for primates: importance of capping and discovery of a cis-reactive element. *Proc. Natl. Acad. Sci. USA* **98:**15270–15275.

37. **Fainboim, L., M. C. Canero Velasco, C. Y. Marcos, M. Ciocca, A. Roy, G. Theiler, M. Capucchio, S. Nuncifora, L. Sala, and M. Zelazko.** 2001. Protracted, but not acute, hepatitis A virus infection is strongly associated with HLA-DRB*1301, a marker for pediatric autoimmune hepatitis. *Hepatology* **33:**1512–1517.

38. **Fauquet, C. M., M. A. Mayo, J. Maniloff, U. Desselberger, and L. A. Ball (ed.).** 2005. *Virus Taxonomy. Eighth Report of the International Committee on Taxonomy of Viruses.* Elsevier Academic Press, San Diego, CA.

39. **Favorov, M. O., Y. E. Khudyakov, E. E. Mast, T. L. Yashina, C. N. Shapiro, N. S. Khudyakova, D. L. Jue, G. G. Onischenko, H. S. Margolis, and H. A. Fields.** 1996. IgM and IgG antibodies to hepatitis E virus (HEV) detected by an enzyme immunoassay based on an HEV-specific artificial recombinant mosaic protein. *J. Med. Virol.* **50:**50–58.

40. **Feinstone, S. M., A. Z. Kapikian, and R. H. Purcell.** 1973. Hepatitis A: detection by immune electron microscopy of a viruslike antigen associated with acute illness. *Science* **182:**1026–1028.

41. **Gane, E., R. Sallie, M. Saleh, B. Portmann, and R. Williams.** 1995. Clinical recurrence of hepatitis A following liver transplantation for acute liver failure. *J. Med. Virol.* **45:**35–39.

42. **Gerolami, R., V. Moal, and P. Colson.** 2008. Chronic hepatitis E with cirrhosis in a kidney-transplant recipient. *N. Engl. J. Med.* **358:**859–860.

43. **Ghabrah, T. M., S. Tsarev, P. O. Yarbough, S. U. Emerson, G. T. Strickland, and R. H. Purcell.** 1998. Comparison of tests for antibody to hepatitis E virus. *J. Med. Virol.* **55:**134–137.

44. **Graff, J., H. Nguyen, C. Kasorndorkbua, P. G. Halbur, M. St. Claire, R. H. Purcell, and S. U. Emerson.** 2005. In vitro and in vivo mutational analysis of the 3′-terminal regions of hepatitis E virus genomes and replicons. *J. Virol.* **79:**1017–1026.

45. **Graff, J., U. Torian, H. Nguyen, and S. U. Emerson.** 2006. A bicistronic subgenomic mRNA encodes both the ORF2 and ORF3 proteins of hepatitis E virus. *J. Virol.* **80:**5919–5926.

46. **Guthmann, J. P., H. Klovstad, D. Boccia, N. Hamid, L. Pinoges, J. Y. Nizou, M. Tatay, F. Diaz, A. Moren, R. F. Grais, I. Ciglenecki, E. Nicand, and P. J. Guerin.** 2006. A large outbreak of hepatitis E among a displaced population in Darfur, Sudan, 2004: the role of water treatment methods. *Clin. Infect. Dis.* **42:**1685–1691.

47. **Haagsma, E. B., A. P. van den Berg, R. J. Porte, C. A. Benne, H. Vennema, J. H. Reimerink, and M. P. Koopmans.** 2008. Chronic hepatitis E virus infection in liver transplant recipients. *Liver Transpl.* **14:**547–553.

48. **Hadler, S. C.** 1991. Global impact of hepatitis A virus infection: changing patterns, p. 14–20. *In* F. B. Hollinger, S. M. Lemon, and H. S. Margolis (ed.), *Viral Hepatitis and Liver Disease.* Williams & Wilkins, Baltimore, MD.

49. **Halliday, M. L., L. Y. Kang, T. K. Zhou, M. D. Hu, Q. C. Pan, T. Y. Fu, Y. S. Huang, and S. L. Hu.** 1991. An epidemic of hepatitis A attributable to the ingestion of raw clams in Shanghai, China. *J. Infect. Dis.* **164:**852–859.

50. **Haqshenas, G., H. L. Shivaprasad, P. R. Woolcock, D. H. Read, and X. J. Meng.** 2001. Genetic identification and characterization of a novel virus related to human hepatitis E virus from chickens with hepatitis-splenomegaly syndrome in the United States. *J. Gen. Virol.* **82:**2449–2462.

51. **Hau, C. H., T. T. Hien, N. T. Tien, H. B. Khiem, P. K. Sac, V. T. Nhung, R. P. Larasati, K. Laras, M. P. Putri, R. Doss, K. C. Hyams, and A. L. Corwin.** 1999. Prevalence of enteric hepatitis A and E viruses in the Mekong River delta region of Vietnam. *Am. J. Trop. Med. Hyg.* **60:**277–280.

52. **He, J., A. W. Tam, P. O. Yarbough, G. R. Reyes, and M. Carl.** 1993. Expression and diagnostic utility of hepatitis E virus putative structural proteins expressed in insect cells. *J. Clin. Microbiol.* **31:**2167–2173.

53. **Hsieh, S. Y., X. J. Meng, Y. H. Wu, S. T. Liu, A. W. Tam, D. Y. Lin, and Y. F. Liaw.** 1999. Identity of a novel swine hepatitis E virus in Taiwan forming a monophyletic group with Taiwan isolates of human hepatitis E virus. *J. Clin. Microbiol.* **37:**3828–3834.

54. **Hsieh, S. Y., P. Y. Yang, Y. P. Ho, C. M. Chu, and Y. F. Liaw.** 1998. Identification of a novel strain of hepatitis E virus responsible for sporadic acute hepatitis in Taiwan. *J. Med. Virol.* **55:**300–304.

55. **Hu, W. P., Y. Lu, N. A. Precioso, H. Y. Chen, T. Howard, D. Anderson, and M. Guan.** 2008. Double-antigen enzyme-linked immunosorbent assay for detection of hepatitis E virus-specific antibodies in human or swine sera. *Clin. Vaccine Immunol.* **15:**1151–1157.

56. **Huang, F. F., Z. F. Sun, S. U. Emerson, R. H. Purcell, H. L. Shivaprasad, F. W. Pierson, T. E. Toth, and X. J. Meng.** 2004. Determination and analysis of the complete genomic sequence of avian hepatitis E virus (avian HEV) and attempts to infect rhesus monkeys with avian HEV. *J. Gen. Virol.* **85:**1609–1618.

57. **Hutin, Y. J., V. Pool, E. H. Cramer, O. V. Nainan, J. Weth, I. T. Williams, S. T. Goldstein, K. F. Gensheimer, B. P. Bell, C. N. Shapiro, M. J. Alter, and H. S. Margolis for the National Hepatitis A Investigation Team.** 1999. A multistate, foodborne outbreak of hepatitis A. *N. Engl. J. Med.* **340:**595–602.

58. **Hyams, K. C., M. C. McCarthy, M. Kaur, M. A. Purdy, D. W. Bradley, M. M. Mansour, S. Gray, D. M. Watts, and M. Carl.** 1992. Acute sporadic hepatitis E in children living in Cairo, Egypt. *J. Med. Virol.* **37:**274–277.

59. **Johnston, A., A. Macgregor, S. Borovec, M. Hattarki, K. Stuckly, D. Anderson, N. H. Goss, A. Oates, and E. Uren.**

2000. Inactivation and clearance of viruses during the manufacture of high purity factor IX. *Biologicals* **28:**129–136.

60. **Kamar, N., J. Selves, J. M. Mansuy, L. Ouezzani, J. M. Peron, J. Guitard, O. Cointault, L. Esposito, F. Abravanel, M. Danjoux, D. Durand, J. P. Vinel, J. Izopet, and L. Rostaing.** 2008. Hepatitis E virus and chronic hepatitis in organ-transplant recipients. *N. Engl. J. Med.* **358:**811–817.

61. **Kar, P., S. Budhiraja, A. Narang, and A. Chakravarthy.** 1997. Etiology of sporadic acute and fulminant non-A, non-B viral hepatitis in north India. *Indian J. Gastroenterol.* **16:**43–45.

62. **Karetnyi, Y. V., M. J. Gilchrist, and S. J. Naides.** 1999. Hepatitis E virus infection prevalence among selected populations in Iowa. *J. Clin. Virol.* **14:**51–55.

63. **Krawczynski, K. K., D. W. Bradley, B. L. Murphy, J. W. Ebert, T. E. Anderson, I. L. Doto, A. Nowoslawski, W. Duermeyer, and J. E. Maynard.** 1981. Pathogenetic aspects of hepatitis A virus infection in enterally inoculated marmosets. *Am. J. Clin. Pathol.* **76:**698–706.

64. **Kwo, P. Y., G. G. Schlauder, H. A. Carpenter, P. J. Murphy, J. E. Rosenblatt, G. J. Dawson, E. E. Mast, K. Krawczynski, and V. Balan.** 1997. Acute hepatitis E by a new isolate acquired in the United States. *Mayo Clin. Proc.* **72:**1133–1136.

65. **Lemon, S. M.** 1995. Hepatitis A virus and blood products: virus validation studies. *Blood Coagul. Fibrinolysis* **6**(Suppl. 2):S20–S22.

66. **Lemon, S. M.** 1994. The natural history of hepatitis A: the potential for transmission by transfusion of blood or blood products. *Vox Sang.* **4:**19–23.

67. **Lemon, S. M., R. W. Jansen, and J. E. Newbold.** 1985. Infectious hepatitis A virus particles produced in cell culture consist of three distinct types with different buoyant densities in CsCl. *J. Virol.* **54:**78–85.

68. **Li, F., J. Torresi, S. A. Locarnini, H. Zhuang, W. Zhu, X. Guo, and D. A. Anderson.** 1997. Amino-terminal epitopes are exposed when full-length open reading frame 2 of hepatitis E virus is expressed in *Escherichia coli*, but carboxy-terminal epitopes are masked. *J. Med. Virol.* **52:**289–300.

69. **Li, F., H. Zhuang, S. Kolivas, S. Locarnini, and D. Anderson.** 1994. Persistent and transient antibody responses to hepatitis E virus detected by Western immunoblot using open reading frame 2 and 3 and glutathione S-transferase fusion proteins. *J. Clin. Microbiol.* **32:**2060–2066.

70. **Mast, E. E., M. J. Alter, P. V. Holland, and R. H. Purcell for the Hepatitis E Virus Antibody Serum Panel Evaluation Group.** 1998. Evaluation of assays for antibody to hepatitis E virus by a serum panel. *Hepatology* **27:**857–861.

71. **Matsubayashi, K., Y. Nagaoka, H. Sakata, S. Sato, K. Fukai, T. Kato, K. Takahashi, S. Mishiro, M. Imai, N. Takeda, and H. Ikeda.** 2004. Transfusion-transmitted hepatitis E caused by apparently indigenous hepatitis E virus strain in Hokkaido, Japan. *Transfusion* **44:**934–940.

72. **McAtee, C. P., Y. Zhang, P. O. Yarbough, T. Bird, and T. R. Fuerst.** 1996. Purification of a soluble hepatitis E open reading frame 2-derived protein with unique antigenic properties. *Protein Expr. Purif.* **8:**262–270.

73. **Meng, X.-J., R. H. Purcell, P. G. Halbur, J. R. Lehman, D. M. Webb, T. S. Tsareva, J. S. Haynes, B. J. Thacker, and S. U. Emerson.** 1997. A novel virus in swine is closely related to the human hepatitis E virus. *Proc. Natl. Acad. Sci. USA* **94:**9860–9865.

74. **Meng, X. J., P. G. Halbur, J. S. Haynes, T. S. Tsareva, J. D. Bruna, R. L. Royer, R. H. Purcell, and S. U. Emerson.** 1998. Experimental infection of pigs with the newly identified swine hepatitis E virus (swine HEV), but not with human strains of HEV. *Arch. Virol.* **143:**1405–1415.

75. **Meng, X. J., P. G. Halbur, M. S. Shapiro, S. Govindarajan, J. D. Bruna, I. K. Mushahwar, R. H. Purcell, and S. U. Emerson.** 1998. Genetic and experimental evidence for cross-species infection by swine hepatitis E virus. *J. Virol.* **72:**9714–9721.

76. **Mizuo, H., Y. Yazaki, K. Sugawara, F. Tsuda, M. Takahashi, T. Nishizawa, and H. Okamoto.** 2005. Possible risk factors

for the transmission of hepatitis E virus and for the severe form of hepatitis E acquired locally in Hokkaido, Japan. *J. Med. Virol.* **76:**341–349.

77. **Mosley, J. W., M. J. Nowicki, C. K. Kasper, E. A. Operskalski, E. Donegan, L. M. Aledort, M. W. Hilgartner, and The Transfusion Safety Study Group.** 1994. Hepatitis A virus transmission by blood products in the United States. *Vox Sang.* **67**(Suppl. 1):24–28.

78. **Myint, K. S., M. Guan, H. Y. Chen, Y. Lu, D. Anderson, T. Howard, H. Noedl, and M. P. Mammen, Jr.** 2005. Evaluation of a new rapid immunochromatographic assay for serodiagnosis of acute hepatitis E infection. *Am. J. Trop. Med. Hyg.* **73:**942–946.

79. **Nanda, S. K., I. H. Ansari, S. K. Acharya, S. Jameel, and S. K. Panda.** 1995. Protracted viremia during acute sporadic hepatitis E virus infection. *Gastroenterology* **108:**225–230.

80. **Nanda, S. K., K. Yalcinkaya, A. K. Panigrahi, S. K. Acharya, S. Jameel, and S. K. Panda.** 1994. Etiological role of hepatitis E virus in sporadic fulminant hepatitis. *J. Med. Virol.* **42:**133–137.

81. **Payne, C. J., T. M. Ellis, S. L. Plant, A. R. Gregory, and G. E. Wilcox.** 1999. Sequence data suggests big liver and spleen disease virus (BLSV) is genetically related to hepatitis E virus. *Vet. Microbiol.* **68:**119–125.

82. **Purcell, R. H., D. C. Wong, and M. Shapiro.** 2002. Relative infectivity of hepatitis A virus by the oral and intravenous routes in 2 species of nonhuman primates. *J. Infect. Dis.* **185:**1668–1671.

83. **Reid, T. M. S., and H. G. Robinson.** 1987. Frozen raspberries and hepatitis A. *Epidemiol. Infect.* **98:**109–112.

84. **Robertson, B. H., M. J. Alter, B. P. Bell, B. Evatt, K. A. McCaustland, C. N. Shapiro, S. D. Sinha, and J. M. Souci.** 1998. Hepatitis A virus sequence detected in clotting factor concentrates associated with disease transmission. *Biologicals* **26:**95–99.

85. **Rodriguez Lay, L. D. L. A., A. Quintana, M. C. M. Villalba, G. Lemos, M. B. Corredor, A. G. Moreno, P. A. Prieto, M. G. Guzman, and D. Anderson.** 2008. Dual infection with hepatitis A and E viruses in outbreaks and in sporadic clinical cases: Cuba 1998–2003. *J. Med. Virol.* **80:**798–802.

86. **Rueckert, R. R.** 1990. Picornaviridae and their replication, p. 507–548. *In* B. N. Fields, D. M. Knipe, R. M. Chanock, M. S. Hirsch, J. L. Melnick, T. P. Morath, and B. Roizman (ed.), *Virology*, 2nd ed. Raven Press, New York, NY.

87. **Schiodt, F. V., and W. M. Lee.** 2003. Fulminant liver disease. *Clin. Liver Dis.* **7:**331–349, vi.

88. **Schlauder, G. G., G. J. Dawson, J. C. Erker, P. Y. Kwo, M. F. Knigge, D. L. Smalley, J. E. Rosenblatt, S. M. Desai, and I. K. Mushahwar.** 1998. The sequence and phylogenetic analysis of a novel hepatitis E virus isolated from a patient with acute hepatitis reported in the United States. *J. Gen. Virol.* **79:**447–456.

89. **Schlauder, G. G., S. M. Desai, A. R. Zanetti, N. C. Tassopoulos, and I. K. Mushahwar.** 1999. Novel hepatitis E virus (HEV) isolates from Europe: evidence for additional genotypes of HEV. *J. Med. Virol.* **57:**243–251.

90. **Schwartz, E., N. P. Jenks, P. Van Damme, and E. Galun.** 1999. Hepatitis E virus infection in travelers. *Clin. Infect. Dis.* **29:**1312–1314.

91. **Seriwatana, J., M. P. Shrestha, R. M. Scott, S. A. Tsarev, D. W. Vaughn, K. S. Myint, and B. L. Innis.** 2002. Clinical and epidemiological relevance of quantitating hepatitis E virus-specific immunoglobulin M. *Clin. Diagn. Lab. Immunol.* **9:**1072–1078.

92. **Shaw, D. D., D. C. Whiteman, A. D. Merritt, D. M. El-Saadi, R. J. Stafford, K. Heel, and G. A. Smith.** 1999. Hepatitis A outbreaks among illicit drug users and their contacts in Queensland, 1997. *Med. J. Aust.* **170:**584–587.

93. **Sheikh, A., M. Sugitani, N. Kinukawa, M. Moriyama, Y. Arakawa, K. Komiyama, T. C. Li, N. Takeda, S. M. Ishaque, M. Hasan, and K. Suzuki.** 2002. Hepatitis E virus infection in fulminant hepatitis patients and an apparently healthy population in Bangladesh. *Am. J. Trop. Med. Hyg.* **66:**721–724.

94. Shieh, Y., Y. Khudyakov, G. Xia, L. Ganova-Raeva, F. Khambaty, J. Woods, M. Motes, M. Glatzer, S. Bialek, and A. Fiore. 2007. Molecular confirmation of oysters as the vector for hepatitis A virus in a 2005 multistate outbreak. *J. Food Prot.* **70:**145–150.

95. Shrestha, M. P., R. M. Scott, D. M. Joshi, M. P. Mammen, Jr., G. B. Thapa, N. Thapa, K. S. Myint, M. Fourneau, R. A. Kuschner, S. K. Shrestha, M. P. David, J. Seriwatana, D. W. Vaughn, A. Safary, T. P. Endy, and B. L. Innis. 2007. Safety and efficacy of a recombinant hepatitis E vaccine. *N. Engl. J. Med.* **356:**895–903.

96. Sjogren, M. H., H. Tanno, O. Fay, S. Sileoni, B. D. Cohen, D. S. Burke, and R. J. Feighny. 1987. Hepatitis A virus in stool during clinical relapse. *Ann. Intern. Med.* **106:**221–226.

97. Snooks, M. J., P. Bhat, J. Mackenzie, N. A. Counihan, N. Vaughan, and D. A. Anderson. 2008. Vectorial entry and release of hepatitis A virus in polarized human hepatocytes. *J. Virol.* **82:**8733–8742.

98. Sonoda, H., M. Abe, T. Sugimoto, Y. Sato, M. Bando, E. Fukui, H. Mizuo, M. Takahashi, T. Nishizawa, and H. Okamoto. 2004. Prevalence of hepatitis E virus (HEV) infection in wild boars and deer and genetic identification of a genotype 3 HEV from a boar in Japan. *J. Clin. Microbiol.* **42:**5371–5374.

99. Staes, C. J., T. L. Schlenker, I. Risk, K. G. Cannon, H. Harris, A. T. Pavia, C. N. Shapiro, and B. P. Bell. 2000. Sources of infection among persons with acute hepatitis A and no identified risk factors during a sustained community-wide outbreak. *Pediatrics* **106:**E54.

100. Stapleton, J. T., V. Raina, P. L. Winokur, K. Walters, D. Klinzman, E. Rosen, and J. H. McLinden. 1993. Antigenic and immunogenic properties of recombinant hepatitis A virus 14S and 70S subviral particles. *J. Virol.* **67:**1080–1085.

101. Takahashi, M., T. Nishizawa, H. Miyajima, Y. Gotanda, T. Iita, F. Tsuda, and H. Okamoto. 2003. Swine hepatitis E virus strains in Japan form four phylogenetic clusters comparable with those of Japanese isolates of human hepatitis E virus. *J. Gen. Virol.* **84:**851–862.

102. Takahashi, M., K. Yamada, Y. Hoshino, H. Takahashi, K. Ichiyama, T. Tanaka, and H. Okamoto. 2008. Monoclonal antibodies raised against the ORF3 protein of hepatitis E virus (HEV) can capture HEV particles in culture supernatant and serum but not those in feces. *Arch. Virol.* **153:**1703–1713.

103. Tanaka, T., M. Takahashi, E. Kusano, and H. Okamoto. 2007. Development and evaluation of an efficient cell-culture system for hepatitis E virus. *J. Gen. Virol.* **88:**903–911.

104. Tanaka, T., M. Takahashi, H. Takahashi, K. Ichiyama, Y. Hoshino, S. Nagashima, H. Mizuo, and H. Okamoto. 2009. Development and characterization of a genotype 4 hepatitis E virus cell culture system using a HE-JF5/15F strain recovered from a fulminant hepatitis patient. *J. Clin. Microbiol.* **47:**1906–1910.

105. Thomas, D. L., P. O. Yarbough, D. Vlahov, S. A. Tsarev, K. E. Nelson, A. J. Saah, and R. H. Purcell. 1997. Seroreactivity to hepatitis E virus in areas where the disease is not endemic. *J. Clin. Microbiol.* **35:**1244–1247.

106. Tian, D. Y., Y. Chen, and N. S. Xia. 2006. Significance of serum IgA in patients with acute hepatitis E virus infection. *World J. Gastroenterol.* **12:**3919–3923.

107. Tilzey, A. J., S. J. Palmer, S. Barrow, K. R. Perry, H. Tyrell, A. Safary, and J. E. Banatvala. 1992. Effect of hepatitis A vaccination schedules on immune response. *Vaccine* **10(Suppl. 1):**S121–S123.

108. Tsarev, S. A., T. S. Tsareva, S. U. Emerson, S. Govindarajan, M. Shapiro, J. L. Gerin, and R. H. Purcell. 1997. Recombinant vaccine against hepatitis E: dose response and protection against heterologous challenge. *Vaccine* **15:**1834–1838.

109. Tsarev, S. A., T. S. Tsareva, S. U. Emerson, S. Govindarajan, M. Shapiro, J. L. Gerin, and R. H. Purcell. 1994. Successful passive and active immunization of cynomolgus monkeys against hepatitis E. *Proc. Natl. Acad. Sci. USA* **91:**10198–10202.

110. Tsarev, S. A., T. S. Tsareva, S. U. Emerson, P. O. Yarbough, L. J. Legters, T. Moskal, and R. H. Purcell. 1994. Infectivity titration of a prototype strain of hepatitis E virus in cynomolgus monkeys. *J. Med. Virol.* **43:**135–142.

111. van Cuyck, H., F. Juge, and P. Roques. 2003. Phylogenetic analysis of the first complete hepatitis E virus (HEV) genome from Africa. *FEMS Immunol. Med. Microbiol.* **39:**133–139.

112. Van Doorslaer, E., G. Tormans, and P. Van Damme. 1994. Cost-effectiveness analysis of vaccination against hepatitis A in travellers. *J. Med. Virol.* **44:**463–469.

113. Vento, S., T. Garofano, C. Renzini, F. Cainelli, F. Casali, G. Ghironzi, T. Ferraro, and E. Concia. 1998. Fulminant hepatitis associated with hepatitis A virus superinfection in patients with chronic hepatitis C. *N. Engl. J. Med.* **338:**286–290.

114. Wang, Y. 1992. Study on diagnosis of hepatitis A by testing salivary IgM anti-HAV. *Zhonghua Liu Xing Bing Xue Za Zhi* **13:**9–11.

115. Wang, Y., R. Ling, J. C. Erker, H. Zhang, H. Li, S. Desai, I. K. Mushahwar, and T. J. Harrison. 1999. A divergent genotype of hepatitis E virus in Chinese patients with acute hepatitis. *J. Gen. Virol.* **80:**169–177.

116. Wheeler, C., T. M. Vogt, G. L. Armstrong, G. Vaughan, A. Weltman, O. V. Nainan, V. Dato, G. Xia, K. Waller, J. Amon, T. M. Lee, A. Highbaugh-Battle, C. Hembree, S. Evenson, M. A. Ruta, I. T. Williams, A. E. Fiore, and B. P. Bell. 2005. An outbreak of hepatitis A associated with green onions. *N. Engl. J. Med.* **353:**890–897.

117. Yamada, K., M. Takahashi, Y. Hoshino, H. Takahashi, K. Ichiyama, T. Tanaka, and H. Okamoto. 2009. Construction of an infectious cDNA clone of hepatitis E virus strain JE03-1760F that can propagate efficiently in cultured cells. *J. Gen. Virol.* **90:**457–462.

118. Yarbough, P. O., E. Garza, A. W. Tam, Y. Zhang, P. McAtee, and T. R. Fuerst. 1996. Assay development of diagnostic tests for IgM and IgG antibody to hepatitis E virus, p. 294–296. *In* Y. Buisson, P. Coursaget, and M. Kane (ed.), *Enterically-Transmitted Hepatitis Viruses.* La Simarre, Joue-les-Tours, France.

119. Yarbough, P. O., A. W. Tam, K. Gabor, E. Garza, R. A. Moeckli, I. Palings, C. Simonsen, and G. R. Reyes. 1994. Assay development of diagnostic tests for hepatitis E, p. 367–370. *In* K. Nishioka, H. Suzuki, S. Mishiro, and T. Oda (ed.), *Viral Hepatitis and Liver Disease.* Springer-Verlag, Tokyo, Japan.

120. Yazaki, Y., H. Mizuo, M. Takahashi, T. Nishizawa, N. Sasaki, Y. Gotanda, and H. Okamoto. 2003. Sporadic acute or fulminant hepatitis E in Hokkaido, Japan, may be food-borne, as suggested by the presence of hepatitis E virus in pig liver as food. *J. Gen. Virol.* **84:**2351–2357.

121. Yu, C., R. E. Engle, J. P. Bryan, S. U. Emerson, and R. H. Purcell. 2003. Detection of immunoglobulin M antibodies to hepatitis E virus by class capture enzyme immunoassay. *Clin. Diagn. Lab. Immunol.* **10:**579–586.

122. Zanetti, A. R., G. G. Schlauder, L. Romano, E. Tanzi, P. Fabris, G. J. Dawson, and I. K. Mushahwar. 1999. Identification of a novel variant of hepatitis E virus in Italy. *J. Med. Virol.* **57:**356–360.

123. Zhang, M., S. U. Emerson, H. Nguyen, R. E. Engle, S. Govindarajan, J. L. Gerin, and R. H. Purcell. 2001. Immunogenicity and protective efficacy of a vaccine prepared from 53 kDa truncated hepatitis E virus capsid protein expressed in insect cells. *Vaccine* **20:**853–857.

124. Zhang, S., D. Tian, Z. Zhang, J. Xiong, Q. Yuan, S. Ge, J. Zhang, and N. Xia. 2009. Clinical significance of anti-HEV IgA in diagnosis of acute genotype 4 hepatitis E virus infection negative for anti-HEV IgM. *Dig. Dis. Sci.* **54:**2512–2518.

125. Zhou, Y. H., R. H. Purcell, and S. U. Emerson. 2005. A truncated ORF2 protein contains the most immunogenic site on ORF2: antibody responses to non-vaccine sequences following challenge of vaccinated and non-vaccinated macaques with hepatitis E virus. *Vaccine* **23:**3157–3165.

126. Zhou, Y. H., R. H. Purcell, and S. U. Emerson. 2004. An ELISA for putative neutralizing antibodies to hepatitis E virus detects antibodies to genotypes 1, 2, 3, and 4. *Vaccine* **22:**2578–2585.

Hepatitis C Virus

MICHAEL S. FORMAN AND ALEXANDRA VALSAMAKIS

89

TAXONOMY

Hepatitis C virus (HCV) is classified within the family *Flaviviridae* in its own genus, *Hepacivirus*. Phylogenetic analysis of helicase sequences has been used to probe its relatedness to other viruses in the family (110). The data suggest that HCV is most closely related to the nonpathogenic human virus GBV-C. The next closest relatives appear to be the pestiviruses, viruses that infect nonhuman hosts (bovine viral diarrhea virus and hog cholera virus). HCV is more distantly related to arthropod-borne viruses in the *Flavivirus* genus that infect humans (yellow fever virus, dengue virus, and West Nile virus).

DESCRIPTION OF THE AGENT

HCV has an ~9.6-kb positive-sense RNA genome composed of a long open reading frame flanked by terminal 5′ and 3′ untranslated regions (UTRs) (Fig. 1). The 5′ UTR is highly conserved, and the 3′ UTR has a short variable sequence, a poly(U) tract, and a highly conserved element. Core, p7, E1, and E2 are structural protein genes that encode nucleocapsid, transmembrane, gp33, and gp72 proteins, respectively.

During replication, the HCV open reading frame is translated into a single polyprotein (approximately 3,000 amino acids) that is subsequently cleaved by host and viral proteases encoded by NS2, NS3, and NS4A genes. The NS3 gene also encodes a helicase. The p7 region encodes a protein that is essential for replication of infectious virus (66); however, its specific function is unknown. The RNA-dependent RNA polymerase NS5B lacks efficient proofreading activity, resulting in extensive genome mutation during replication and quasispecies generation within an infected individual.

Currently, there are six major genotypes of HCV and more than 50 known subtypes based on genomic sequence heterogeneity. Genotypes and subtypes differ by 30 to 35% and 20 to 25% of nucleotides, respectively. Genotypes 1 to 3 (Gt1 to Gt3) have a worldwide distribution and account for most HCV infections in Europe and North America. In the United States, the majority of HCV infections in all age groups are caused by Gt1 (75%), followed by Gt2 (13.5%) and Gt3 (5.5%). Gt4 is most prevalent in the Middle East and North and Central Africa; Gt5 is found primarily in South Africa; Gt6 occurs throughout Asia.

EPIDEMIOLOGY AND TRANSMISSION

HCV is a globally significant pathogen, infecting over 150 million individuals. In the United States, it is the most common blood-borne infection, causing an estimated 3 million chronic infections (8). Acute hepatitis C occurs in the United States at a rate of approximately 0.3 per 100,000, with estimates of 19,000 new infections per year after adjusting for underreporting and asymptomatic infection (164). In the blood-screening era, most transmission occurs after exposure to a low viral inoculum through intravenous drug use, multiple sexual partners, sex with a chronically infected partner, iatrogenic exposure, and occupational exposure to blood such as needlestick (163).

CLINICAL SIGNIFICANCE

The clinical features of acute infection are depicted in Fig. 2. The majority of individuals are thought to be asymptomatic. Spontaneous clearance is observed in approximately 25% of acute infections; the remaining individuals become chronically infected. Signs of hepatitis during acute infection are actually positive indicators as they represent early, vigorous T-cell responses associated with spontaneous virus clearance; these responses are minimal or absent in individuals who progress to chronicity (123). Disease progression occurs in a relatively small proportion of patients. Over decades, progressive liver damage produces cirrhosis in 10 to 20% of chronic infections and liver failure or hepatocellular carcinoma in approximately 5% of chronic infections (141). However, the overall disease burden is significant due to the number of infected individuals. In fact, liver failure due to chronic hepatitis C infection is the leading cause of liver transplantation in the United States (113). Risk factors for disease progression include diseases or behaviors that induce additional hepatic injury (such as concomitant hepatitis B virus infection and alcohol consumption) or impair antiviral immunity (such as HIV infection). Epidemiologic descriptors such as male gender and age at infection are also associated with higher risk and faster rate of disease progression.

Unlike other chronic viral infections such as HIV and hepatitis B virus, virologic parameters including viral load and genotype do not predict disease progression or indicate disease severity in chronic hepatitis C (2, 168). Viral load

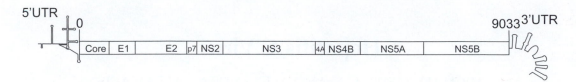

Protein	Role	nuc pos$_{H77}$	aa pos	aa length	size
Core	Encapsidation	342	1	191	p21
E1	Receptor binding, entry?	915	192	192	gp31
E2	Receptor binding, entry?	1491	384	363	gp70
p7	viroporin?	2580	747	63	p7
NS2	NS2/3 Zn-dependent protease	2769	810	217	p21
NS3	NS2/3 Zn-dependent protease, NS3/4A protease, helicase-NTPase	3420	1027	631	p70
NS4A	cofactor for NS3-4A protease	5313	1658	54	p8
NS4B	membranous web organization	5475	1712	261	p27
NS5A	phosphoprotein	6258	1973	448	p58
NS5B	RNA-dependent RNA polymerase	7602	2421	591	p68

FIGURE 1 HCV genome and protein coding scheme. E, envelope; NS, nonstructural gene; nuc, nucleotide; pos, position; aa, amino acid; gp, glycoprotein. Numbering is according to references 21 and 85.

remains fairly constant once chronic hepatitis C infection is established (168), and rates of progression have been found to correlate more with disease severity in the liver, as manifested by the extent of fibrosis on initial liver biopsy (167), than on the level of HCV replication represented by viremia (44).

Treatment for HCV infection has undergone significant evolution in regard to available agents, duration, and dosing strategy. A 15% response rate to alpha interferon (IFN-α) in non-A, non-B hepatitis was demonstrated early, even before the identification of the causative agent (62). All current (and likely future) treatment regimens contain IFN as a backbone. The addition of ribavirin resulted in improved

overall (~45%) and genotype-specific (Gt1, 35%; Gt2 and Gt3, 70%) responses. Further gains in overall (~55%) and genotype-specific (Gt1, 45%; Gt2 and Gt3, 80%) were achieved by the addition of a polyethylene glycol (peg) moiety to IFN-α, which prolongs drug half-life and allows for decreased dosing frequency (from three times per week to once weekly). The increased efficacy of combination therapy with pegylated interferon (peg-IFN) and ribavirin is likely due to greater sustained IFN-α levels and improved adherence resulting from decreased severity of IFN-associated side effects afforded by less frequent dosing.

Response definitions and treatment milestones are synopsized in Table 1. The goal of treatment is sustained

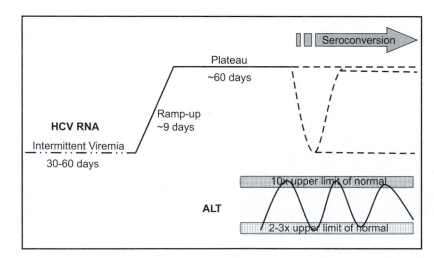

FIGURE 2 Clinical features of acute hepatitis C following exposure to low viral inoculum such as occupational needlestick exposure or community-based exposure (56, 84, 143). Characteristics following higher-dose exposure (transfusion with contaminated blood products) may be different. The intermittent viremia phase was estimated from needlestick exposure (143). Kinetics of other characteristics were derived from seroconversion panels (56). ALT, alanine aminotransferase. Dashed lines indicate potential viremia patterns as defined by HCV RNA levels in peripheral blood. Adapted from reference 56.

TABLE 1 Response and milestone definitions in chronic hepatitis C treatment

Treatment response or milestone (abbreviation)	Definition
Rapid virologic response (RVR)	No detectable HCV RNA in plasma at treatment wk 4[a]
Early virologic response (EVR)	$\geq 2 \log_{10}$ decline in HCV RNA in plasma at treatment wk 12
End of treatment (EOT)	End of drug treatment, as appropriate for genotype, viremia clearance kinetics, and baseline viral load
Virologic response (VR)	No detectable HCV RNA in plasma at EOT[a]
End of follow-up (EFU)	Last time point for HCV RNA testing in individuals with virologic response (VR); typically 6 months (24 wks) after EOT
Sustained virologic response (SVR)	No detectable HCV RNA at EFU[a]

[a]As detected by assay with limit of detection of ≤ 50 IU/ml.

virologic response (SVR), defined as the absence of detectable viremia by highly sensitive nucleic acid amplification tests at the end of follow-up (EFU), 6 months after the end of treatment (EOT). A 5-year follow-up study of 150 patients who achieved SVR demonstrated no evidence of virologic relapse, demonstrating the validity of this end point (51). Genotype is an important SVR predictor. Gt1 infections are generally associated with lower SVR rates and generally require longer treatment to attain SVR than Gt2 and Gt3 infections. Although Gt2 and Gt3 infections are more responsive to treatment than those caused by Gt1, SVR rates are greater in Gt2 infections than in Gt3 infections (75% to 92% versus 66% to 73%, depending upon the study), suggesting that there are important differences between the two (87, 137, 161).

Viremia clearance kinetics are also important predictors of virologic response (VR), relapse rate, and SVR (36, 41). Individuals with a rapid virologic response (RVR), defined as no detectable HCV RNA after 4 weeks of treatment and no subsequent detectable viremia, have the highest SVR rates. EOT response rates are uniformly high if a decline or disappearance of viremia occurs at any time before 12 weeks. Longer durations of detectable virus result in increased relapse rates and diminished SVR rates.

Therapy to attain SVR has evolved from a "one size fits all" paradigm in which all patients were treated for 48 weeks to one of tailored treatment based on an individual's genotype and viremia clearance kinetics (Fig. 3). The key concepts underlying the current treatment regimens are treatment of responders for a period that is sufficient to achieve SVR and early identification of nonresponders through viral load testing at defined time points to avoid unnecessary therapy. In infections with Gt1, Gt2, and Gt3, a low baseline viral load (<400,000 IU/ml) is predictive of RVR and associated with high SVR rates (≥80%) after shortened treatment (24 weeks for Gt1 and 12 to 16 weeks for Gt2 and Gt3 [86, 102, 137, 161, 169]). A shortened treatment course may therefore be an option for these individuals. One drawback to shortened treatment is a two- to threefold increase in relapse rates (27, 75); however, many of these patients can be treated successfully with an additional course of therapy (87). Three points are worth mentioning in regard to shortened treatment in patients with low baseline viral load and RVR. First, the cutoff of 400,000 IU/ml is the viral load that optimally differentiates high from low probability of SVR in Gt1-infected individuals as shown by receiver operator characteristic (ROC) analysis of data from the two phase III trials of peg-IFN/ribavirin

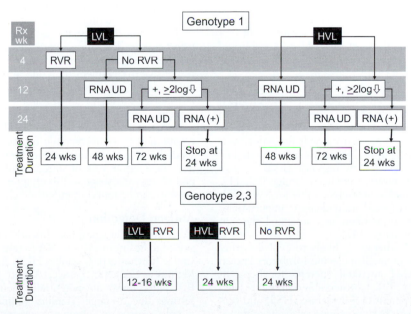

FIGURE 3 Individualized chronic hepatitis C therapy algorithms based on genotype, baseline viral load, and response kinetics. Rx wk, treatment week; LVL, low baseline viral load (<400,000 IU/ml); HVL, high baseline viral load (≥400,000 IU/ml); UD, undetectable; +, detectable HCV RNA. Adapted from reference 120.

that used the Cobas Monitor assay for HCV quantification (170). The applicability of this cutoff to the probability of SVR in rapid virologic responders has been inferred and appears to be useful given that viremia of <400,000 IU/ml is predictive of RVR and identifies individuals most likely to achieve SVR with a shortened treatment course. However, its utility has not been formally proven through receiver operating characteristic (ROC) analysis of clinical trial data. Secondly, this cutoff certainly does not represent a consensus value based on quantification with different assays; whether it would vary in an assay-dependent manner is unknown. Lastly, shortened treatment courses with peg-IFN/ribavirin have been approved by the European Medical Association (Europe's version of the U.S. Food and Drug Administration [FDA]), but not by the FDA.

In Gt1 infections, early stopping rules are advocated by current guidelines (55) to avoid further treatment of individuals with a low likelihood of treatment success. Failure to achieve EVR (Table 1), indicated by a reduction in viral load of 2.0 $\log_{10}$ IU/ml at 12 weeks compared to baseline, is associated with a negative predictive value of 97% for SVR (47). In addition, low SVR rates (1%) were found when EVR was achieved but viremia was still detectable at 24 weeks (31). Treatment is therefore usually stopped after 12 weeks if EVR is not achieved or after 24 weeks if viremia is still detectable due to the limited benefit of further therapy. Early identification of nonresponders is more critical in Gt1 infections than Gt2 or Gt3 infections because Gt1-infected patients are more refractory to combination therapy and generally require longer treatment courses to attain SVR (59) while most individuals with Gt2 or Gt3 infections respond to 24 weeks of therapy.

Gt1-infected individuals with delayed clearance require progressively longer treatment courses. Forty-eight weeks of treatment appears optimal if viremia is cleared by 12 weeks. Even longer courses (72 weeks) are required to obtain maximum SVR rates if viremia is cleared between 12 and 24 weeks (86, 131).

For patients infected with genotypes other than Gt1 through Gt3, treatment data are available only for Gt4. Overall responsiveness, positive predictive value of RVR, and negative predictive value of EVR in treatment of Gt4 infections are similar to those of Gt1 (42, 68). Published guidelines have therefore recommended that Gt4 infections be treated similarly to Gt1 infections (141).

Other than lower response rates (40% overall, approximately 30% for Gt1 and 60% for Gt2 and Gt3 [14, 152]) necessitating longer treatment, therapy of HCV- and HIV-1-coinfected individuals closely parallels monoinfection therapy. As in monoinfected individuals, genotype is predictive of SVR (34, 136) and therapy can be tailored by assessing RVR and early virologic response (EVR), which respectively have high positive predictive value (92, 117, 136) and excellent negative predictive value for SVR (76). Treatment of HIV-coinfected individuals is important as disease progression is more rapid in coinfected than in HCV-monoinfected patients (147).

Chronic hepatitis C therapy is likely to evolve further with the introduction of small-molecule inhibitors known as "specifically targeted antiviral therapy for hepatitis C" (STAT-C) drugs (139). Considerable effort has been devoted to the development of polymerase (NS5) and protease (NS3/4) inhibitors, but none have yet been approved for use. The majority of compounds have failed due to lack of efficacy or unsatisfactory side effect profile. Telaprevir, an orally bioavailable inhibitor of the viral NS3/4A protease, is the most promising STAT-C agent for use in the treatment of Gt1 infections. Although not yet approved by the FDA, initial published phase I and phase II trials of Gt1 treatment using telaprevir in combination with peg-IFN-α/ribavirin demonstrate improved RVR and SVR (~60%) compared to standard peg-IFN-α/ribavirin therapy for 48 weeks (61, 96). These therapeutic gains were observed with as little as 24 total weeks of therapy (12 weeks of triple drug, followed by 12 weeks of peg-IFN-α/ribavirin). A drug-induced maculopapular rash appeared to be the major side effect, which approximately doubled the rate of treatment discontinuation compared to standard therapy.

COLLECTION, TRANSPORT, AND STORAGE OF SPECIMENS

Serum or plasma is acceptable for HCV nucleic acid tests (NATs). Plasma collected in heparin-containing tubes is not acceptable for PCR-based assays, since *Taq* polymerase is inhibited by this anticoagulant. Serum and plasma should be obtained from whole blood as per standard technique, described in chapter 76. Serum is used conventionally for serologic assays, but plasma is acceptable. Information on assay-specific specimen requirements, recommended intervals between collection and processing, storage conditions, and freeze-thaw cycles can be found in Table 4 in chapter 76. Whole-blood specimens can be transported at 25°C prior to processing. Liver tissue is not typically tested, except for histologic assessment of fibrosis in Gt1-infected individuals.

DIRECT DETECTION

Microscopy

By electron microscopy, HCV virions are 55- to 65-nm spheres with 6-nm surface projections. HCV antigens and nucleic acids are detectable in liver sections by immunohistochemistry and in situ hybridization, respectively. However, these methods are insensitive and nonspecific; therefore, HCV detection by microscopy has minimal clinical utility.

Liver fibrosis is usually assessed histologically in Gt1 infections to determine liver disease status and the need for therapeutic intervention. Since Gt1 infections are less responsive to treatment than Gt2 and Gt3 infections, treatment of Gt1 infections is usually reserved for patients with advanced fibrosis, in an attempt to prevent cirrhosis. In response to the disadvantages of liver biopsy (its invasive nature, potential complications, and sampling error), surrogate markers of fibrosis that can be assessed in peripheral blood have been developed. The literature on liver biopsies and the relative role of surrogate fibrosis markers is large and beyond the scope of this chapter. An encapsulated discussion can be found in published clinical guidelines (55).

Antigen Detection

Core antigen detection/quantification assays that were envisioned to be alternatives to NATs tests have been developed (*trak-c* [Ortho/J&J]; Monolisa HCV Ag-Ab Ultra [Bio-Rad, Marnes-la-Coquette, France; Abbott Murex, Abbott Park, IL). These assays are potentially useful in resource-limited settings due to target stability (eliminating the need for sample storage at ultralow temperatures), simplified instrumentation, and easier technical protocols that reduce labor/training pressures. Good quantitative correlation was observed between these tests and end point PCR assays;

however, the antigen-based assays had a limit of detection (LOD) of ~4.0 log$_{10}$ IU/ml (149, 156), were ~98% sensitive in samples from high-risk populations compared to end point PCR tests (6, 39, 49), and were 70% sensitive compared to minipool NA blood screening tests (78). The utility of these tests was limited due to their insensitivity compared to NAT, and they are no longer widely available. A new-generation test (Architect HCV Ag Test, Abbott, Wiesbaden-Delkenheim, Germany) with sensitivity comparable to that of end point PCR (~1,000 IU/ml) but less than that of real-time PCR in clinical samples has been reported (97, 104).

Nucleic Acid Tests

Clinical Utility

NAT Usage in the Diagnosis of Acute Hepatitis C
HCV NATs are useful in establishing the diagnosis of acute HCV infection in seronegative individuals because HCV RNA can be detected as early as 1 week after exposure via needlestick or transfusion (40, 105, 146) and at least 4 to 6 weeks prior to seroconversion in a number of transmission settings (56). Available guidelines do not make recommendations on the specific NAT type for the diagnosis of acute hepatitis C. However, early after a known exposure, when viral loads are known to be low and HCV RNA in peripheral blood is intermittently detected (56), it would be reasonable to use the most sensitive assays (Tables 2 and 3). Establishing this diagnosis is useful due to the availability and efficacy of therapy. Without therapy, approximately 75% of infected individuals develop chronic infection and may require future therapy. Large prospective trials have not been performed, but two meta-analyses report sustained clearance rates of 60 to 70% of patients treated with IFN-α monotherapy compared to 12 to 35% of untreated patients (3, 80). Treatment initiation is usually considered after 12 weeks of documented acute infection to allow for spontaneous clearance.

NAT Usage in the Diagnosis of Chronic Hepatitis C
Given the asymptomatic nature of most acute HCV infections, the majority of patients present symptomatically, in the chronic phase. The diagnosis of chronic HCV infection is established with antibody screening tests to document infection and HCV RNA NAT to document replication. Universal screening for HCV has been recommended in HIV-1-infected patients due to common virus transmission routes and the high prevalence of coinfection (141). NAT is particularly advisable for those patients with potential impaired humoral immunity before excluding the diagnosis of chronic HCV infection. Approximately 5% of

HIV-1-infected individuals have HCV viremia but no HCV antibodies as detected by second- and third-generation serologic assays; low CD4 cell counts (<200 cells/microliter) have been found to be a risk factor (18, 58).

NAT Usage in the Management of Chronic Hepatitis C Therapy
NATs are the cornerstones of chronic HCV treatment since therapeutic tailoring is based on genotype and viral load determinations. Genotype and viral load should be determined at baseline. These parameters are used to counsel patients on the likelihood of SVR and the potential duration of treatment (Fig. 3). Viral load assessment at baseline is also critical for determining response kinetics during therapy.

During treatment, viremia should be assessed at specific times and with certain assay types. Gt1-infected individuals should be tested with a quantitative assay after 12 weeks of treatment to assess EVR, and all patients should be tested for the absence of viremia at week 4 (to determine RVR), at EOT, and at EFU. Assays with sensitivity of ≤50 IU/ml should be used at EOT and EFU to avoid misidentification of nonresponders (13) (see "Evaluation, Reporting, and Interpretation of Results" below for further discussion).

Real-time PCR-based tests have greatly simplified the task of therapeutic monitoring since they are quantitative and highly sensitive. A single test can therefore be used to evaluate EVR in Gt1 infections and to determine all other responses. Laboratories performing quantification with other, less sensitive test methods will additionally need to offer qualitative testing to accurately determine RVR, EOT response, and SVR.

Nucleic Acid Preparation for HCV NAT
Any discussion of HCV NATs must first address nucleic acid extraction due to its contribution to assay performance characteristics. Some extraction methodologies are HCV specific, while others target total RNA or total nucleic acids in clinical samples. HCV RNA can be extracted manually with chaotropic salts or silica-based columns (as reviewed in chapter 4). More recently, automated extraction platforms with different sizes, throughput capacities, and chemistries have been introduced. The performances of different HCV NATs after extraction with ABI PRISM 6100 Nucleic Acid PrepStation (Applied Biosystems), AmpliPrep (Roche), BioRobot M48 (Qiagen), BioRobot 9604 (Qiagen), m1000 (Abbott), MagNAPure LC (Roche), and NucliSens Extractor (bioMérieux) have been reported (9, 22, 45, 46, 67, 72, 138). Unfortunately there have been no comprehensive comparisons of these automated extraction platforms using a single HCV NAT to determine extraction efficiencies and overall performance.

Qualitative Tests
Qualitative NATs have historically been considered the most sensitive methods for HCV RNA detection in serum or plasma. A variety of tests are available in commercial and laboratory-developed formats. Currently there are four FDA-approved commercial qualitative assays for HCV detection, including two tests that employ conventional reverse transcription-PCR (RT-PCR) in either manual microwell plate or semiautomated formats (Table 2) (this method is reviewed in chapter 4). Two FDA-approved tests employ transcription-mediated amplification (TMA) (Table 2; see also chapter 4 for a description). TMA is more sensitive than conventional RT-PCR and can detect HCV in 33% of RT-PCR-negative EOT samples from patients

TABLE 2 HCV RNA qualitative tests[a]

Test (manufacturer)	Chemistry	LOD (IU/ml)
Amplicor HCV v2.0 (Roche)	Manual RT-PCR	50
Cobas Amplicor HCV v2.0 (Roche)	Semiautomated RT-PCR	50
Aptima HCV (Gen-Probe)	TMA	10
Versant HCV RNA (Siemens)	TMA	10

[a]All tests are FDA approved and Conformité Européenne (CE) marked according to European In Vitro Diagnostic Directive 98/79/EC.

who relapse (33). TMA test formats have been reported to have faster time-to-result and greater throughput than conventional PCR-based tests (73).

Quantitative Tests

Before 1997, the interpretation of quantitative HCV RNA data was hampered by the use of individual reporting units that were specific to individual assays. In response to this, The World Health Organization (WHO) established a preparation of HCV to be used as a globally recognized standard for characterization of qualitative assay sensitivity and calibration of quantitative assays. The First International Standard for HCV RNA is a Gt1 virus preparation that was established in 1997 (130). The Second International Standard for HCV RNA was established in 2004 and is currently in use (129). A Third Standard for HCV RNA has been evaluated for future use. These standards have been the basis for converting reportable results from copies/ml to IU/ ml. Due to differences in assay chemistries, the conversion factor varies from one assay to another (Table 2).

Commercial (Table 3) and laboratory-developed NATs are used for quantification of HCV RNA. Results are reported in IU/ml. The Versant HCV RNA 3.0 is a branched-DNA (bDNA)-based microwell plate assay that does not require nucleic acid extraction. HCV virions are lysed, and viral genomes are captured with probes. Genomes are quantified by hybridization using a series of probes that contain iso-C and iso-G oligonucleotides to reduce nonspecific hybridization and increase assay sensitivity. Luminescent signal emission is enhanced through preamplifier and amplifier probe hybridization. Quantification is performed using external calibrators that are included on each plate. The advantages of this assay are its simple genomic isolation procedure, high upper limit of quantification, and reproducibility. The greatest drawback is its lower limit of quantification, which is greater than that of real-time RT-PCR assays.

Quantitative testing by PCR can be performed with commercially available analyte-specific reagents (ASRs), research use only (RUO) kits (Table 3), and FDA-approved in vitro diagnostic tests. Tests utilizing ASRs or RUO products must be completely verified by individual laboratories, as manufacturers are prohibited from making claims regarding performance characteristics of these products.

Commercial conventional PCR HCV quantification products include manual Amplicor Monitor HCV v2.0 and semiautomated Cobas Amplicor Monitor HCV v2.0 RUO tests (Table 3). These tests require viral RNA extraction. The 5′ UTR is amplified; quantification is performed through internal calibration. The limitations of these methods are their narrow measurable range (4 orders of magnitude) and high LOD (615 IU/ml).

HCV RNA quantification can be performed by real-time PCR with commercially available reagents (Table 3) that amplify 5′ UTR sequences but employ slightly different amplicon detection chemistry. The probe in the Abbott RealTime HCV ASR assay is labeled with a 5′ fluorophore and a 3′ quencher. Unhybridized probe is randomly coiled and fails to fluoresce due to fluorophore and quencher proximity. Major fluorescence occurs upon probe hybridization; a minor amount of fluorescence is produced due to cleavage of the 5′ labeled nucleotide by *Taq* polymerase. Reduced genotype bias is achieved through low-temperature hybridization that permits binding of probes despite probe-target mismatches. Quantification is performed via an internal calibrator. Assays based on these reagents have a low LOD and a broad measurable range.

In the Cobas AmpliPrep/Cobas TaqMan HCV real-time PCR test, total nucleic acid extraction and reaction setup are performed by the AmpliPrep. Amplification occurs on the TaqMan instrument. The assay is calibrated externally by the manufacturer; lot-specific calibration coefficients are used by the system software to calculate HCV RNA concentrations. An internal quantitative standard is added prior to extraction to quantitatively correct for potential inhibitors within individual samples. The inability of this assay to detect HCV RNA in two Gt4 samples found to have viral loads in excess of 5.0 $\log_{10}$ IU/ml has been reported, and two single-nucleotide polymorphisms (a G-to-A substitution at nucleotide 145 and an A-to-T substitution at nucleotide 165) were implicated (20). Follow-up studies with a large number of Gt4 samples could not replicate this detection failure; however, underquantification by approximately 1.0 $\log_{10}$ IU/ml was observed; the implicated sequence polymorphisms were found to be rare but did not abrogate virus detection (52, 60).

Real-time PCR-based quantitative assays have a broader measurable range than conventional RT-PCR and bDNA-based assays (12, 46, 72) and LODs that are comparable to those of conventional PCR-based qualitative tests. Diagnostic testing and therapeutic monitoring can therefore be performed with a single assay, greatly simplifying HCV

TABLE 3 Commercial HCV RNA quantification tests

Test or reagent (manufacturer)	Method	Measurable range (IU/ml)[a]	IU/ml-to-copies/ml conversion[b]	U.S. regulatory status[c]	Reference(s)
Versant HCV RNA 3.0 (Siemens)	bDNA	615–7.7 × 10⁶	5.2	FDA approved	37
Amplicor HCV Monitor v2.0 (Roche)	Manual RT-PCR	600–5 × 10⁵	0.9	RUO	
Cobas Amplicor Monitor HCV v2.0 (Roche)	Semiautomated RT-PCR	600–5 × 10⁵	2.7	RUO	
RealTime HCV (Abbott)	RT-real-time PCR	10–1 × 10⁷ᵈ	3.8	ASR	12, 128
Cobas AmpliPrep/Cobas TaqMan (Roche)	RT-real-time PCR	43–6. 9 × 10⁷ᵉ	ND[f]	FDA approved	Package insert
High Pure/Cobas TaqMan (Roche)	RT-real-time PCR	25–3.9 × 10⁸ᵍ	ND	RUO	25, 128

[a]Lower limit of quantification to upper limit of quantification of undiluted specimens.
[b]1 IU/ml = x copies/ml..
[c]All products are Conformité Européenne (CE) marked and approved according to European In Vitro Diagnostic Directive 98/79/EC. U.S. regulatory status is shown.
[d]LOD, 10 IU/ml.
[e]Analytical measuring range. Expanded clinical reportable range (43–6.9 × 10⁹ IU/ml) can be obtained by maximum dilution of 1:100. LOD, 18 IU/ml.
[f]ND, not determined. The test was developed after universal institution of IU.
[g]LOD reported as genotype dependent, from 6 IU/ml for Gt4 to 18 IU/ml for Gt5.

nucleic acid testing. In comparison, conventional RT-PCR and bDNA assays require a combination of qualitative and quantitative testing for these clinical uses.

Several user-defined HCV RNA quantification assays have been reported in the literature. A laboratory-developed, conventional RT-PCR assay, HCV SuperQuant (National Genetics Institute), was used in a number of clinical trials for early anti-HCV therapies. This assay used multicycle amplification of HCV and internal control cDNA, followed by Southern blot hybridization and densitometry to quantify HCV RNA. It was performed at a single site with proprietary reagents and technology. Its performance characteristics were never independently verified. A plethora of user-defined real-time PCR assays employing TaqMan chemistry and noncommercial oligonucleotide reagents have been described to quantify the six major genotypes of HCV. In general these assays have high upper limits of quantification and good precision (15, 38). However, their lower limits of quantification are higher than those of assays using commercial real-time PCR reagents, limiting their utility for EOT and SVR assessment. One reported assay has a low LOD (50 IU/ml), but a lower limit of quantification was not reported (29).

ISOLATION PROCEDURES AND IDENTIFICATION

Until recently there have been no known in vitro cell culture systems for HCV recovery. The chimpanzee animal model was the only means to study infection, life cycle, and pathobiology of HCV. Systems for recovery of infectious virus after transfecting permissive cells with HCV molecular clones have been reported (81, 162, 171). Although this advance is a powerful tool, it has not been adopted for diagnostic use.

GENOTYPING

HCV genotyping is useful for counseling patients on the likelihood of response to treatment and is used to determine therapy duration in conjunction with baseline viremia and viral load kinetics during treatment (Fig. 3). Subtype is often reported with genotype, although it is currently not clinically useful. It may become more important as protease inhibitors such as telaprevir are incorporated into therapeutic regimens (see "Antiviral Susceptibility" below).

HCV genotypes and subtypes can be determined with numerous commercial and user-developed NATs based on a variety of biochemical methods (summarized in Tables 4 and 5).

TABLE 4 Commercial HCV RNA genotyping tests[a]

Test (manufacturer)	Method	Target(s)	Subtyping	Comments	Reference(s)
Trugene HCV[b] (Siemens)	Direct bidirectional sequencing using forward/reverse primers labeled with unique fluorophores	5′ UTR	No	Suitable for use with Roche Amplicor HCV or Amplicor HCV Monitor test amplicons. Subtyping unreliable due to 5′ UTR conservation. Resolution of mixed genotypes (9:1 ratio) reported.	108
Versant HCV Genotype (LiPA) 2.0 (Siemens)[c,d]	Reverse hybridization with detection on strips (line probe); automated blot processor and band interpretation instrumentation available.	5′ UTR and core gene	Yes	In contrast to direct sequencing, mixed genotype infections are readily detected. Compared to version 1.0 (5′ UTR analysis only) version 2.0 demonstrates improved genotype and subtype accuracy (particularly Gt1 and Gt6). Some difficulty in reliably distinguishing Gt2 and Gt4 subtypes reported. Ghost bands that complicate result interpretation occur less commonly than in version 1.0 (A. Caliendo, personal communication).	10, 140, 157
Gen-Eti-K DEIA (Sorin Biomedica)	Reverse hybridization with detection on multiwell plate	Core gene		Performance reported as similar to LiPA 2.0.	126, 159
HCV DNA Chip v2.0 (Bio-Core)	Amplicon hybridization to chip	5′ UTR	Yes	Agreement with direct sequencing reported as 100% and 95% for genotype and subtype.	114
Invader (Hologic)[e]	RT-PCR plus Invader detection	5′ UTR	No	Two genotypes detected in single well by distinct genotype-specific probes, Invader oligonucleotides and FRET probes with different fluorophores. HCV genotype determination therefore requires three wells per sample.	53
RealTime HCV Genotype II[c,e] (Abbott)	Real-time RT-PCR	NS5b (Gt1a, 1b), 5′ UTR (Gt2a, 2b, 3, 4, 5, 6)	Yes	96% genotype agreement with LiPA 2.0 and NS5b-based direct sequencing.	95

[a]Genotypes 1 through 6 can be determined with all assays.
[b]Available globally as RUO product.
[c]CE marked and approved according to European In Vitro Diagnostic Directive 98/79/EC.
[d]U.S. regulatory status, RUO.
[e]Available for sale outside the United States only.

TABLE 5 User-defined HCV RNA genotyping tests[a]

Test	Method	Target(s)	Genotyping	Subtyping	References
Direct sequencing	Sanger and CLIP biochemistries	NS5b, core, core-E1	1–6	Yes	91, 106, 127, 155
Reverse hybridization	Amplicon detection on multiwell plates (enzyme-linked oligosorbent nucleotide assay) or microarrays	5′ UTR	1–6	Yes	64, 89
RFLP	RT-PCR with restriction enzyme digestion of amplicons; more sensitive than subtype-specific PCR	5′ UTR	1–6	Yes	30, 107
Heteroduplex mobility analysis	Differential electrophoretic mobility of matched versus mismatched duplexes	5′ UTR, NS5b	1–4, 6	Yes	90, 166
PSEA or PSMEA	Fluorescent PCR products of different lengths detected on DNA sequencer; highly sensitive detection of mixed genotypes (level of minority genotypes detected by PSEA, ~3%; by PSMEA, ~1%).	5′ UTR	PSEA: Gt1a and b, 2a/c, 2b, 3, 4; PSMEA: Gt1a and b, 2a and b, 3a and b, 4, 6a	Partial	7, 63
Subtype-specific PCR	PCR with subtype-specific primers; amplicons of different size detected by gel electrophoresis	Core, NS5b	Gt1a and b, 2a and b, 3a and b, 4, 5a, 6a	Yes	111, 112
Real-time PCR	TaqMan or FRET chemistries with specific robes or melt curve analysis	5′ UTR	1–4	Yes	4, 82, 101, 125, 135

[a]Abbreviations: RFLP, restriction fragment length polymorphism; PSEA, primer-specific extension analysis; PSMEA, primer-specific mispair extension analysis; FRET, fluorescent resonance energy transfer.

Assays based on 5′ UTR sequences are generally acceptable for genotype determination but must be carefully designed for subtyping due to the degree of sequence conservation among different viruses. More accurate subtype determination can be achieved through analysis of NS5b, core, and core-E1 genes.

Direct sequencing is considered the gold standard in accuracy for HCV genotype and subtype determination. Sequences generated from samples are compared to reference genotype and subtype sequence libraries. Mixed genotype infections can be difficult to detect when the proportion of one genotype greatly exceeds the other. Although it is too laborious for use in clinical laboratories, amplicon cloning may help to detect minority genotype populations (below 10%); however, analysis of large numbers of clones may be required. Sequencing methods require specialized instrumentation and analysis software. These methods are generally labor-intensive, and time to result is usually longer than in other methods.

Methods other than direct sequencing do not usually require highly sophisticated technical expertise and specialized instrumentation. Reverse hybridization is probably the most common method adopted by clinical laboratories. It is more reliable than direct sequencing for the detection of mixed infections. Low-throughput formats use paper strips; higher-throughput microwell plate and microarray formats have been developed (Table 4).

As of this writing, there are no FDA-approved HCV genotyping products available in the United States. Therefore, the task of determining assay performance prior to implementation falls to the individual laboratory. Defining genotyping accuracy for the more common viruses (Gt1 through Gt3) is fairly straightforward, as these samples are readily accessible. Gt4 through Gt6 are more problematic as they are found less commonly. Samples containing HCV are available commercially (Gt1 through Gt3 from ProMedDx, Norton, MA; Gt1 through Gt4 from Acrometrix, Benicia, CA; Gt1 through Gt6 from BocaBiolistics, Coconut Creek,

FL, and SeraCare, Milford, MA) for use in preimplementation accuracy studies. One strategy for samples found to putatively contain these less common genotypes is to refer them to a reference laboratory for genotype confirmation.

SEROLOGIC TESTS

The diagnosis of chronic HCV infection is usually established with serology assays. Given the asymptomatic nature of most acute and chronic infections, recommendations have been made regarding screening individuals at risk of chronic infection by using serology followed by NAT for seropositive individuals (55) (synopsized in Table 6). The first serologic assay was comprised of a single NS4 peptide (c-100-3) and was introduced in 1990 shortly after HCV was identified as a major cause of non-A, non-B hepatitis. This assay represented a significant advance, particularly in identifying contaminated blood products and preventing transfusion-transmitted hepatitis C; however, its flaws of low sensitivity and specificity were soon apparent

TABLE 6 Recommendations for chronic hepatitis C screening[a]

Serology should be performed in individuals with the following risk factors:

Injection drug use (recent or remote; single or multiple episodes)
Conditions associated with hepatitis C prevalence
  HIV
  Hemophilia with receipt of clotting factors prior to 1987
  Hemodialysis
  Unexplained aminotransferase elevations
Blood transfusion or organ transplant prior to 1992
Children born to HCV-infected mothers
Needlestick injury or mucosal exposure to HCV-positive blood
Current sexual partners of HCV-infected persons

[a]Synopsized from reference 55.

(sensitivity, ~70%; positive predictive values in low- and high-prevalence populations, 30 to 50% and 70 to 85%, respectively [57]). Increased sensitivity and specificity were achieved in second-generation blood screening tests. These tests (one of which is still marketed) were better able to detect acute infections due to the incorporation of NS3 and core antigens (Table 7 and Fig. 4), two targets of early antibody responses. The reasons for improved performance of third-generation blood screening assays that incorporate NS5 and contain reconfigured NS3 antigen (Fig. 4) are unclear. Improved antigenicity of the alternate NS3 antigen leading to increased detection during early seroconversion has been argued (154). However, the finding of HCV RNA-positive donors who were consistently reactive by enzyme immunoassay (EIA) 3.0 but remained unreactive by EIA 2.0 for over 6 months suggests that more complex immunologic factors may be responsible (151).

Using seroconversion panels in which infection has been documented by serology only, the seroconversion window has been documented to decrease from approximately 16 to 10 to 8 weeks with the introduction of first-, second-, and third-generation serology tests, respectively. It is important to note that when infection is documented with NAT, the seroconversion window using second- and third-generation serology screening tests is much longer (Fig. 2) (56, 143). Table 7 contains information on HCV serology screening, diagnostic, and supplemental tests available in the United States; numerous other assays are also available globally (134).

Despite improvements in performance characteristics, spurious serology results can still be observed. Second-generation assays are still available (Abbott HCV EIA 2.0 [Table 7]) and can yield false-negative results due to low sensitivity compared to third-generation assays. Therefore, in the appropriate clinical setting (for example, an individual with sudden-onset hepatitis, or an occupational exposure such as needlestick from an HCV-infected individual), alternative testing (third-generation EIA or NAT) should be considered for a patient with a negative EIA 2.0 result. Alternative testing should also be considered

for any negative serology test result if acute hepatitis C is suspected (see "Interpretation of Results in Acute Hepatitis C" in "Evaluation, Interpretation, and Reporting of Results" below for additional discussion). False-negative results have also been observed in immunocompromised patients (HIV-infected patients with CD4 counts of <100 or chemotherapy-treated oncology patients); therefore, NAT should be performed to definitively exclude infection in these patients (58, 83).

For most antibody screening assays, a positive result is considered initially reactive and repeat testing in duplicate is required. Results are reported as reactive if two or more replicates are positive. One advantage of certain chemiluminescent and microparticle immunoassays (AxSYM Anti-HCV [Abbott]; Architect anti-HCV [Abbott]; Vitros Anti-HCV [Ortho], and Advia Centaur HCV [Siemens] [Table 7]) is that initial positive results can be reported as reactive; repeat testing is not required due to the high sensitivities and specificities of these tests.

HCV serologic tests were originally developed as screening assays, with an emphasis on sensitivity and consequent potential for false-positive results. Early recommendations (16) therefore advised confirming all positive results by recombinant immunoblot (RIBA) before proceeding to NAT to avoid erroneous diagnoses. These tests are based on Western blot technology: HCV antigens (recombinant antigens and peptides) and control human immunoglobulin G (IgG) (at low and high concentrations) are attached to membranes; then, membrane strips are incubated sequentially with specimen (serum or plasma), peroxidase-labeled anti-human IgG antibody, and colorimetric detector (hydrogen peroxide and 4-chloro-1-naphthol). HCV antibodies are detected by the presence of bands at expected locations for each HCV antigen that meets intensity requirements (Fig. 5). Some recombinant HCV antigens are chimeras of HCV proteins and human superoxide dismutase (hSOD); therefore, hSOD is also placed on each strip, allowing distinction between reactivity to HCV antigens from false-positive reactivity to hSOD. Band intensity is scored relative to level I and level II (low- and

TABLE 7 Serologic assays for the detection of anti-HCV antibodies[a]

Test (manufacturer)	Assay type	S/CO threshold[b]	Sensitivity (%)	Specificity (%)	Approved for donor screening	Reference(s)
Abbott HCV EIA 2.0 (Abbott)	Enzyme immunoassay	≥3.8	85.6	98.4	Yes	1
AxSYM Anti-HCV (Abbott)	Microparticle immunoassay	≥10.0	100[c]	94[d]	No	Package insert
Architect Anti-HCV (Abbott)	Chemiluminescent microparticle	≥5.0	99.7[c]	97.7[d]	No	Package insert
Abbott Prism HCV (Abbott)	Chemiluminescent immunoassay	NA[e]	100	100	Yes	Package insert
Ortho HCV version 3.0 EIA (Ortho)	Enzyme immunoassay	≥3.8	96.9–100	100	Yes	23
VITROS Anti-HCV (Ortho)	Chemiluminescent immunoassay	≥8.0	100	96.5–98.1	No	65, 70
Advia Centaur HCV (Siemens)	Chemiluminescent immunoassay	≥11.0	100	99.9	No	32

[a]All assays approved for diagnostic use by U.S. Food and Drug Administration.
[b]>95% of samples with S/CO ratios above indicated threshold predicted to be confirmed positive.
[c]Expressed in package insert as percent positive agreement.
[d]Expressed in package insert as percent negative agreement.
[e]NA, not available.

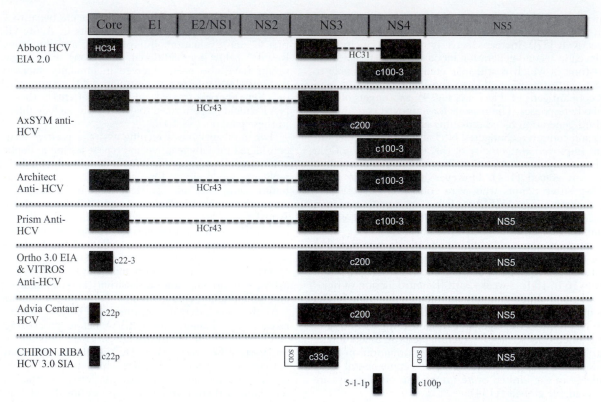

FIGURE 4 Antigens in serology tests and supplemental RIBA currently available commercially in the United States. Abbott HCV EIA 2.0 is the only second-generation screening test currently available. AxSYM, Architect, Ortho 3.0 EIA, Ortho Vitros, and Advia Centaur are third-generation HCV antibody screening tests. HC34, recombinant antigen containing HCV core protein (amino acids [aa] 1 to 150); HC31, recombinant antigen containing NS3 (aa 1192 to 1457) and NS4 (aa 1676 to 1931) separated by an 8-aa linker. c100-3, recombinant antigen containing NS3-4 (aa 1569 to 1931). HCr43, fusion protein of two noncontiguous antigens, c33c and core protein (aa 1 to 150). c200, recombinant antigen containing NS3-4 (aa 1192 to 1931). NS5, recombinant antigen (aa 2054 to 2995). c22-3, recombinant antigen containing core protein (aa 2 to 120). c22p, peptide containing core protein major epitope (aa 10 to 53). 5-1-1p and c100p, NS4 peptides (aa 1694 to 1735 and aa 1920 to 1935, respectively). SOD, superoxide dismutase. First-generation RIBA contained c100-3 and 5-1-1p expressed as a recombinant antigen. Second-generation RIBA contained these two antigens plus c33c and c22-3. Compared to RIBA 2.0, RIBA 3.0 contains an additional antigen (NS5) and peptides have replaced recombinant core and NS4 antigens.

high-concentration) human IgG controls as follows: (−), absent; +/−, <level I; 1+, level I; 2+, >level I but < level II; 3+, level II; 4+, >level II. Although band intensity is an indicator of serologic reactivity and putatively reflects the strength of antibody response, the primary interpretive criterion is the intensity of the level I control. In addition, no interpretive significance is ascribed to the number of reactive bands other than the criterion of ≥2, although the presence of ≥3 positive HCV bands has been found to correlate with the presence of viremia (28, 35).

Negative RIBA results indicate either a false-positive serology screening test result or a false-negative RIBA result, as can occur in acute infection (Fig. 6). Assessment of risk factors and additional follow-up testing (serology and NAT, particularly for the diagnosis of acute infection; see "Interpretation of Results in Acute Hepatitis C" below for additional discussion) should be considered. Positive RIBA results confirm HCV infection; additional testing should be performed as indicated in Fig. 6. Indeterminate results are problematic as infection cannot be excluded. These samples can be han-

dled in the same way as specimens yielding negative RIBA results (Fig. 6). Indeterminate results occur at varying frequencies depending on the test generation and population. Refinements in antigen composition (addition of NS5 and conversion of recombinant 5-1-1, c100-3, and c22-3 antigens to corresponding peptides) in the latest-generation assay (Chiron RIBA HCV 3.0 SIA) (Fig. 4 and 5) have resulted in lower rates of indeterminate results and improved detection of positives compared to RIBA 2.0 as demonstrated by an 85% reduction in specimens reactive for c22-3 alone and a concomitant increase in specimens reactive to c22-3 plus an additional antigen (c100p or c33c) (116). Despite this improvement, indeterminate results continue to be problematic, with rates of ~20% among screening-test-positive blood donations (71, 118) and ~10% among patients who are being tested for diagnostic purposes (115).

The most noteworthy indeterminate band patterns are reactivity to hSOD plus multiple HCV antigens/peptides, reactivity to c33p (major antibody epitope of core protein) or c22p (N3 peptide) alone, and reactivity to c100p/5-1-1p

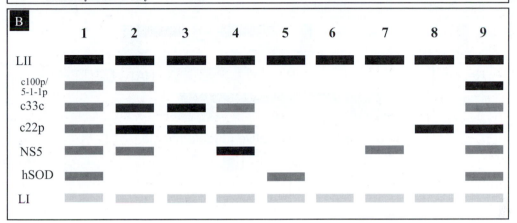

FIGURE 5 RIBA interpretation. (A) Interpretive criteria; (B) illustrations of sample results. Lane 1, illustration of band locations for human IgG (LI, level one, low-concentration IgG control; LII, level two, high-concentration IgG control), hSOD, and HCV recombinant antigens and peptides. Lanes 2 to 9, sample results. Lanes 2 to 4, RIBA positive. Lanes 5 to 7, RIBA negative. Lanes 8 and 9, RIBA indeterminate. See Fig. 4 for location of HCV antigens/peptides.

(NS4) or NS5 alone. Reactivity to hSOD and multiple HCV antigens/peptides is uncommon (frequencies between 1 in 120,000 and 1 in 1,000,000 blood donations have been described; there are no published data on diagnostic populations) and most likely represents true infection, as the majority of these individuals have detectable HCV RNA (71, 150). Isolated reactivity to c33p (core) or c22p (N3) can indicate acute infection. Studies demonstrating the utility of NAT in narrowing the time to detection of acute HCV infection have shown that this reactivity pattern occurs early during seroconversion (48, 142). Isolated c33p or c22p has also been found rarely in chronic infection (79). In contrast to these patterns, isolated reactivity to NS4 or NS5 is likely not associated with HCV infection, as individuals with these results have no evidence of infection (79, 99).

Confirmation of all reactive screening test results was never widely adopted by clinicians or laboratorians outside the blood screening arena, largely due to the availability of more definitive NATs and the conviction that RIBA did not represent an adequate confirmatory test as it employed the same antigens as antibody screening tests. Subsequent recommendations have outlined a more reasonable, circumscribed approach, advising the confirmation of screening results with low signal/cutoff (S/CO) ratios, since false positives were most likely to occur in these samples (5). A high rate of false-positive results in low S/CO ranges has been confirmed in a number of clinical studies (26, 109, 165). The most efficient way to incorporate confirmatory testing may be as a reflex test after a low positive screening result (outlined in Fig. 6). S/CO ratios that can serve as thresholds for confirmatory testing have now been determined for a number of commercially available antibody screening assays (see Table 7 for assays available in the United States and Europe; S/CO ratios for other assays are described in reference 124).

ANTIVIRAL SUSCEPTIBILITY

Virologic breakthrough and relapse (Fig. 3) can occur during combination therapy; however, the viral genetic determinants associated with these suboptimal responses are poorly understood and are not directly determined. Testing for viral determinants of resistance could become more important diagnostically if small-molecule inhibitors such as telaprevir are approved for use. Virologic breakthrough occurred commonly (in 30 to 50% of cases [69, 133]) and rapidly, within 14 days of telaprevir monotherapy (69), demonstrating that a single-drug regimen was not viable. Trials of triple-drug (telaprevir/peg-IFN-α/ribavirin) therapy demonstrated a lower rate of breakthrough (less than 7%) that occurred primarily by week 4 but was also observed up to week 12.

Telaprevir resistance mutations likely lie near the protease active site and decrease enzyme affinity for drug, as determined by modeling based on protease crystallographic structure (133). Distinct protease variants have been found in Gt1a and Gt1b, likely due to the fact that a single nucleotide change can produce a mutant protein in one subtype, whereas two nucleotide changes are required for codon change in the other (69).

The exact mechanisms governing the emergence of protease-resistant viruses are not completely understood. They could arise de novo during treatment or they may be minor components of the pretreatment quasispecies that emerge as

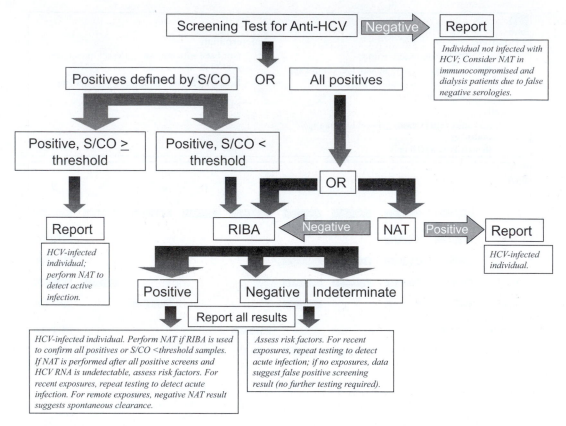

FIGURE 6 Algorithms for HCV antibody screening and confirmation. Interpretations and suggested follow-up are indicated by boxed, italicized text. Derived from www.cdc.gov/hepatitis/HCV/LabTesting.htm.

a result of selective advantage during treatment. The rapid occurrence of breakthrough suggests that the emergence of a minor population during protease inhibitor treatment may explain resistance in certain individuals. In addition, resistant viruses have been demonstrated to occur sporadically in the quasispecies of treatment-naïve individuals (74).

Measurement of recombinant mutant protease activity in vitro and assessment of mutant virus replication in a genome replication system have been used to classify mutations biologically as producers of high- and low-level resistance. The clinical significance of these in vitro characteristics is unclear. Both types have been observed in individuals with virologic breakthrough after mono- and triple therapy. Interestingly, high- and low-level resistance mutations have also been noted in individuals with virologic relapse, suggesting that salvage therapy regimens containing similar protease inhibitors may have minimal efficacy in these patients.

Given the accumulating protease inhibitor data, a number of potential changes in diagnostic testing could occur as a result of approval for use. For instance, Gt1 subtyping may become important to identify patients at risk of treatment failure due to subtype-dependent resistance mutations. Baseline protease gene sequence determination may become useful to identify treatment-naïve individuals at risk of treatment failure due to preexisting protease-inhibitor mutants. This will likely require novel sequence determination methods as current protocols are too insensitive to detect low-prevalence quasispecies constituents. Finally identification of specific protease gene mutations may become important after protease-inhibitor treatment failure if drugs with nonoverlapping genetic determinants of resistance become available.

Although virus-associated parameters of antiviral resistance are the conventional focus of diagnostic testing, host genetics may become important in hepatitis C treatment paradigms. Recent genome-wide association studies have identified single nucleotide polymorphisms in the host interleukin 28B gene that are associated with treatment response (50, 122, 144, 145) and spontaneous HCV clearance during acute infection (148). In the future, host genotype determination may therefore be implemented to identify who should be treated for acute and chronic HCV infections.

EVALUATION, INTERPRETATION, AND REPORTING OF RESULTS

Interpretation of Results in Acute Hepatitis C

Establishing the diagnosis of acute hepatitis C can be challenging. Most cases of acute hepatitis C are asymptomatic; therefore, serum aminotransferase elevations can be helpful if present but should not be relied upon as the sole indicator of infection. Additionally, seroconversion can be delayed and viremia can be sporadic. Serology and RNA assessment should therefore both be performed to optimally detect infection. Diagnostic accuracy also requires testing at multiple time points. Single HCV NAT results do not reliably predict exposure outcome. Transient HCV RNA negativity has been documented early postinfection in individuals who become chronically infected and later, at the time of seroconversion (Fig. 2) (11). Transient positive results have been found in those who spontaneously clear virus (56, 160).

Antibody screening has been recommended 4 to 6 months after a known exposure, since the majority of individuals seroconvert by this time (17). These public health guidelines have not been updated since the accumulation of evidence regarding early treatment efficacy and the increasing adoption of acute HCV treatment into clinical practice. More recent practitioner recommendations advocate serologic testing (and NAT) at multiple time points prior to 6 months since it may provide complementary and confirmatory information that is helpful in shaping the decision to start treatment.

Interpretation of Results in Chronic Hepatitis C

Issues in regard to NAT interpretation in chronic hepatitis C include reporting of quantitative data, interassay variability in quantification, the impact of test selection on the interpretation of EOT and EFU status, and subtype reporting by genotyping assays.

Reporting Quantitative Data

Linearity is one of the important parameters used to define the measurable range of a quantitative assay. With currently available quantitative tests, linearity can only be achieved using logarithmically transformed (base 10) data. HCV RNA levels should therefore be reported and interpreted in $\log_{10}$ format. This requirement is fairly unique to viral load measurement and is difficult to grasp by care providers since most quantitative interpretations are performed with arithmetic data. Laboratorians should nonetheless strive to educate care providers regarding the need for logarithmic interpretation, to facilitate proper patient management. Quantitative data and assay precision can be reported in logarithmic and arithmetic formats to assist with this educational effort.

Sources of Variability in HCV RNA Quantification

Despite the implementation of an international standard for calibration of quantitative assays, HCV RNA measurement is not equivalent between different assays (77, 100, 121). Patients should therefore be tested with a single viral load assay to avoid inconsistent results that could potentially be interpreted erroneously and lead to management errors.

The factors that contribute to interassay quantification variability are complex. The WHO international standard and the properties of individual assays, such as inherent genotype bias, are likely contributors. The development of a WHO standard that functions as a common calibrator has been extremely useful in improving the comparability of different assays. However, it is an imperfect calibrator from the perspective of physical standardization since it is a single genotype (Gt1) and its value represents a consensus concentration obtained by diverse assays in numerous laboratories rather than a concentration that is traceable to a physically quantifiable substance such as phosphorus content.

Sequence diversity between HCV genotypes can also affect HCV RNA quantification resulting in genotype-dependent quantitative bias. For example, assays based on primers and probes that have varying, genotype-dependent degrees of complementarity may favor the quantification of one genotype over another or extraction methods may favor the amplification of certain genotypes. Evidence of such genotypic bias in quantification has been reported and has been serious enough to require assay reformulation as in the cases of Amplicor Monitor

HCV v. 1.0, which underquantified Gt2 through Gt6 (94); of the first-generation HCV bDNA assay, which had lower sensitivities for Gt2 and Gt3 (98); and of High Pure/COBAS TaqMan, which underquantified Gt2a/c and Gt3 through Gt5 (132). Genotype-dependent quantification variability has been reported in multiple studies comparing the performances of different quantitative tests (19, 24, 93, 119, 153, 158). These findings underscore the importance of monitoring treatment efficacy with a single assay.

Parameters such as interlaboratory variability, specimen type, and tube type do not seem to play a major role in quantification variability, although the available data are not exhaustive. In a study of four different quantitative assays (Versant HCV RNA 3.0, Cobas Amplicor Monitor, Cobas TaqMan, and RealTime HCV), reasonable quantitative agreement was observed among four labs that performed testing on a standardized panel (12). No significant differences in quantification have been reported between serum and plasma specimens for Versant HCV RNA 3.0 and Cobas AmpliPrep/Cobas TaqMan tests (37, 138), and quantification by Versant HCV RNA 3.0 has been reported to be equivalent across a broad range of tube types (SST, K_2-EDTA, K_2-PPT, and ACD). Laboratories that are planning to offer testing from a sample or tube type that has not been approved for use with a given platform should establish the assay performance (including quantitative equivalence) in any alternative sample source to prevent the introduction of unanticipated quantification variability.

Interpreting Changes in Viremia

Changes in viremia must be interpreted in the context of assay precision and variability in viremia over time in untreated chronic infection. Using a quantitative assay with excellent precision, viral load was observed to vary up to 10-fold in most individuals with stable, untreated chronic hepatitis C (168). During treatment, a viral load change of at least this magnitude must therefore occur in order to be biologically significant.

Impact of Test Selection on EOT and EFU Response

Correct interpretation of EOT results and accurate prediction of virologic response at EOT are highly dependent upon utilization of the proper test at EOT. Undetectable results obtained by quantitative tests with high LODs and high lower limits of quantification could lead to the erroneous conclusion that an EOT response had been achieved. EOT response should therefore be assessed with highly sensitive assays that have an LOD of ≤50 IU/ml. Use of less sensitive tests such as quantitative tests with conventional PCR or bDNA-based formats at these time points can lead to the misidentification of responders (13).

Whether sensitive (LOD, 50 IU/ml) or ultrasensitive (LOD, ≤10 IU/ml) NATs are preferable at EOT is not clear, as there are advantages and disadvantages to both. Relapse rates of approximately 15% have been observed with sensitive assays (47, 88). Higher accuracy may be achieved with ultrasensitive formats such as TMA, since these tests can detect residual RNA in a proportion of samples with no detectable HCV RNA by sensitive PCR tests (43, 54, 103). However, sensitive tests may be more accurate for predicting final therapeutic outcome, since 5% of patients with SVR and no evidence of recurrent disease after prolonged follow-up have been found to have residual viremia at EFU by TMA (103). The lack of detectable

HCV RNA at EOT should therefore be interpreted in the context of the NAT used, and patients should be counseled appropriately regarding the likelihood of SVR.

REFERENCES

1. **Abdel-Hamid, M., M. El-Daly, S. El-Kafrawy, N. Mikhail, G. T. Strickland, and A. D. Fix.** 2002. Comparison of second- and third-generation enzyme immunoassays for detecting antibodies to hepatitis C virus. *J. Clin. Microbiol.* **40:**1656–1659.

2. **Adinolfi, L. E., R. Utili, A. Andreana, M. F. Tripodi, P. Rosario, G. Mormone, E. Ragone, G. Pasquale, and G. Ruggiero.** 2000. Relationship between genotypes of hepatitis C virus and histopathological manifestations in chronic hepatitis C patients. *Eur. J. Gastroenterol. Hepatol.* **12:**299–304.

3. **Alberti, A., S. Boccato, A. Vario, and L. Benvegnu.** 2002. Therapy of acute hepatitis C. *Hepatology* **36:**S195–S200.

4. **Alfaresi, M. S., and A. A. Elkoush.** 2007. Determination of hepatitis C virus genotypes by melting-curve analysis of quantitative polymerase chain reaction products. *Indian J. Med. Microbiol.* **25:**249–252.

5. **Alter, M. J., W. L. Kuhnert, and L. Finelli.** 2003. Guidelines for laboratory testing and result reporting of antibody to hepatitis C virus. *MMWR Recommend. Rep.* **52:**1–13, 15; quiz CE11-14.

6. **Alzahrani, A. J.** 2008. Simultaneous detection of hepatitis C virus core antigen and antibodies in Saudi drug users using a novel assay. *J. Med. Virol.* **80:**603–606.

7. **Antonishyn, N. A., V. M. Ast, R. R. McDonald, R. K. Chaudhary, L. Lin, A. P. Andonov, and G. B. Horsman.** 2005. Rapid genotyping of hepatitis C virus by primer-specific extension analysis. *J. Clin. Microbiol.* **43:**5158–5163.

8. **Armstrong, G. L., A. Wasley, E. P. Simard, G. M. McQuillan, W. L. Kuhnert, and M. J. Alter.** 2006. The prevalence of hepatitis C virus infection in the United States, 1999 through 2002. *Ann. Intern. Med.* **144:**705–714.

9. **Beuselinck, K., M. van Ranst, and J. van Eldere.** 2005. Automated extraction of viral-pathogen RNA and DNA for high-throughput quantitative real-time PCR. *J. Clin. Microbiol.* **43:**5541–5546.

10. **Bouchardeau, F., J. F. Cantaloube, S. Chevaliez, C. Portal, A. Razer, J. J. Lefrere, J. M. Pawlotsky, P. De Micco, and S. Laperche.** 2007. Improvement of hepatitis C virus (HCV) genotype determination with the new version of the INNO-LiPA HCV assay. *J. Clin. Microbiol.* **45:**1140–1145.

11. **Busch, M. P.** 2001. Insights into the epidemiology, natural history and pathogenesis of hepatitis C virus infection from studies of infected donors and blood product recipients. *Transfus. Clin. Biol.* **8:**200–206.

12. **Caliendo, A. M., A. Valsamakis, Y. Zhou, B. Yen-Lieberman, J. Andersen, S. Young, A. Ferreira-Gonzalez, G. J. Tsongalis, R. Pyles, J. W. Bremer, and N. S. Lurain.** 2006. Multilaboratory comparison of hepatitis C virus viral load assays. *J. Clin. Microbiol.* **44:**1726–1732.

13. **Carlsson, T., A. Quist, and O. Weiland.** 2008. Rapid viral response and treatment outcome in genotype 2 and 3 chronic hepatitis C: comparison between two HCV RNA quantitation methods. *J. Med. Virol.* **80:**803–807.

14. **Carrat, F., F. Bani-Sadr, S. Pol, E. Rosenthal, F. Lunel-Fabiani, A. Benzekri, P. Morand, C. Goujard, G. Pialoux, L. Piroth, D. Salmon-Ceron, C. Degott, P. Cacoub, and C. Perronne.** 2004. Pegylated interferon alfa-2b vs standard interferon alfa-2b, plus ribavirin, for chronic hepatitis C in HIV-infected patients: a randomized controlled trial. *JAMA* **292:**2839–2848.

15. **Castelain, S., V. Descamps, V. Thibault, C. Francois, D. Bonte, V. Morel, J. Izopet, D. Capron, P. Zawadzki, and G. Duverlie.** 2004. TaqMan amplification system with an internal positive control for HCV RNA quantitation. *J. Clin. Virol.* **31:**227–234.

16. **Centers for Disease Control and Prevention.** 1998. Recommendations for prevention and control of hepatitis C virus (HCV) infection and HCV-related chronic disease. *MMWR Recommend. Rep.* **47:**1–39.

17. **Centers for Disease Control and Prevention.** 2001. Updated U.S. Public Health Service guidelines for the management of occupational exposures to HBV, HCV, and HIV and recommendations for postexposure prophylaxis. *MMWR Recommend. Rep.* **50:**1–52.

18. **Chamie, G., M. Bonacini, D. R. Bangsberg, J. T. Stapleton, C. Hall, E. T. Overton, R. Scherzer, and P. C. Tien.** 2007. Factors associated with seronegative chronic hepatitis C virus infection in HIV infection. *Clin. Infect. Dis.* **44:**577–583.

19. **Chevaliez, S., M. Bouvier-Alias, R. Brillet, and J. M. Pawlotsky.** 2007. Overestimation and underestimation of hepatitis C virus RNA levels in a widely used real-time polymerase chain reaction-based method. *Hepatology* **46:**22–31.

20. **Chevaliez, S., M. Bouvier-Alias, L. Castera, and J. M. Pawlotsky.** 2009. The Cobas AmpliPrep-Cobas TaqMan real-time polymerase chain reaction assay fails to detect hepatitis C virus RNA in highly viremic genotype 4 clinical samples. *Hepatology* **49:**1397–1398.

21. **Choo, Q. L., K. H. Richman, J. H. Han, K. Berger, C. Lee, C. Dong, C. Gallegos, D. Coit, R. Medina-Selby, P. J. Barr, et al.** 1991. Genetic organization and diversity of the hepatitis C virus. *Proc. Natl. Acad. Sci. USA* **88:**2451–2455.

22. **Clancy, A., B. Crowley, H. Niesters, and C. Herra.** 2008. The development of a qualitative real-time RT-PCR assay for the detection of hepatitis C virus. *Eur. J. Clin. Microbiol. Infect. Dis.* **27:**1177–1182.

23. **Colin, C., D. Lanoir, S. Touzet, L. Meyaud-Kraemer, F. Bailly, and C. Trepo.** 2001. Sensitivity and specificity of third-generation hepatitis C virus antibody detection assays: an analysis of the literature. *J. Viral Hepat.* **8:**87–95.

24. **Colson, P., A. Motte, and C. Tamalet.** 2006. Broad differences between the COBAS Ampliprep total nucleic acid isolation-COBAS TaqMan 48 hepatitis C virus (HCV) and COBAS HCV monitor v2.0 assays for quantification of serum HCV RNA of non-1 genotypes. *J. Clin. Microbiol.* **44:**1602–1603.

25. **Colucci, G., J. Ferguson, C. Harkleroad, S. Lee, D. Romo, S. Soviero, J. Thompson, M. Velez, A. Wang, Y. Miyahara, S. Young, and C. Sarrazin.** 2007. Improved COBAS TaqMan hepatitis C virus test (Version 2.0) for use with the High Pure system: enhanced genotype inclusivity and performance characteristics in a multisite study. *J. Clin. Microbiol.* **45:**3595–3600.

26. **Contreras, A. M., C. M. Tornero-Romo, J. G. Toribio, A. Celis, A. Orozco-Hernandez, P. K. Rivera, C. Mendez, M. I. Hernandez-Lugo, L. Olivares, and M. A. Alvarado.** 2008. Very low hepatitis C antibody levels predict false-positive results and avoid supplemental testing. *Transfusion* **48:**2540–2548.

27. **Dalgard, O., K. Bjoro, H. Ring-Larsen, E. Bjornsson, M. Holberg-Petersen, E. Skovlund, O. Reichard, B. Myrvang, B. Sundelof, S. Ritland, K. Hellum, A. Fryden, J. Florholmen, and H. Verbaan.** 2008. Pegylated interferon alfa and ribavirin for 14 versus 24 weeks in patients with hepatitis C virus genotype 2 or 3 and rapid virological response. *Hepatology* **47:**35–42.

28. **Damen, M., H. L. Zaaijer, H. T. Cuypers, H. Vrielink, C. L. van der Poel, H. W. Reesink, and P. N. Lelie.** 1995. Reliability of the third-generation recombinant immunoblot assay for hepatitis C virus. *Transfusion* **35:**745–749.

29. **Daniel, H. D., G. M. Chandy, and P. Abraham.** 2008. Quantitation of hepatitis C virus using an in-house real-time reverse transcriptase polymerase chain reaction in plasma samples. *Diagn. Microbiol. Infect. Dis.* **61:**415–420.

30. **Davidson, F., P. Simmonds, J. C. Ferguson, L. M. Jarvis, B. C. Dow, E. A. Follett, C. R. Seed, T. Krusius, C. Lin, G. A. Medgyesi, et al.** 1995. Survey of major genotypes and subtypes of hepatitis C virus using RFLP of sequences amplified from the 5' non-coding region. *J. Gen. Virol.* **76:**1197–1204.

31. **Davis, G. L., J. B. Wong, J. G. McHutchison, M. P. Manns, J. Harvey, and J. Albrecht.** 2003. Early virologic response to treatment with peginterferon alfa-2b plus ribavirin in patients with chronic hepatitis C. *Hepatology* **38:**645–652.

32. **Denoyel, G., J. van Helden, R. Bauer, and B. Preisel-Simmons.** 2004. Performance of a new hepatitis C assay on the Bayer ADVIA Centaur Immunoassay System. *Clin. Lab.* **50:**75–82.

33. **Desombere, I., H. Van Vlierberghe, S. Couvent, F. Clinckspoor, and G. Leroux-Roels.** 2005. Comparison of qualitative

(COBAS AMPLICOR HCV 2.0 versus VERSANT HCV RNA) and quantitative (COBAS AMPLICOR HCV monitor 2.0 versus VERSANT HCV RNA 3.0) assays for hepatitis C virus (HCV) RNA detection and quantification: impact on diagnosis and treatment of HCV infections. *J. Clin. Microbiol.* **43:**2590–2597.

34. Dore, G. J., F. J. Torriani, M. Rodriguez-Torres, N. Brau, M. Sulkowski, R. S. Lamoglia, C. Tural, N. Clumeck, M. R. Nelson, M. C. Mendes-Correa, E. W. Godofsky, D. T. Dieterich, E. Yetzer, E. Lissen, and D. A. Cooper. 2007. Baseline factors prognostic of sustained virological response in patients with HIV-hepatitis C virus co-infection. *AIDS* **21:**1555–1559.

35. Dow, B. C., I. Buchanan, H. Munro, E. A. Follett, F. Davidson, L. E. Prescott, P. L. Yap, and P. Simmonds. 1996. Relevance of RIBA-3 supplementary test to HCV PCR positivity and genotypes for HCV confirmation of blood donors. *J. Med. Virol.* **49:**132–136.

36. Drusano, G. L., and S. L. Preston. 2004. A 48-week duration of therapy with pegylated interferon alpha 2b plus ribavirin may be too short to maximize long-term response among patients infected with genotype-1 hepatitis C virus. *J. Infect. Dis.* **189:**964–970.

37. Elbeik, T., J. Surtihadi, M. Destree, J. Gorlin, M. Holodniy, S. A. Jortani, M. Kuramoto, V. Ng, R. Valdes, Jr., A. Valsamakis, and N. A. Terrault. 2004. Multicenter evaluation of the performance characteristics of the Bayer VERSANT HCV RNA 3.0 assay (bDNA). *J. Clin. Microbiol.* **42:**563–569.

38. Engle, R. E., R. S. Russell, R. H. Purcell, and J. Bukh. 2008. Development of a TaqMan assay for the six major genotypes of hepatitis C virus: comparison with commercial assays. *J. Med. Virol.* **80:**72–79.

39. Fabrizi, F., G. Lunghi, F. Aucella, S. Mangano, F. Barbisoni, S. Bisegna, D. Vigilante, A. Limido, and P. Martin. 2005. Novel assay using total hepatitis C virus (HCV) core antigen quantification for diagnosis of HCV infection in dialysis patients. *J. Clin. Microbiol.* **43:**414–420.

40. Farci, P., H. J. Alter, D. Wong, R. H. Miller, J. W. Shih, B. Jett, and R. H. Purcell. 1991. A long-term study of hepatitis C virus replication in non-A, non-B hepatitis. *N. Engl. J. Med.* **325:**98–104.

41. Ferenci, P., M. W. Fried, M. L. Shiffman, C. I. Smith, G. Marinos, F. L. Goncales, Jr., D. Haussinger, M. Diago, G. Carosi, D. Dhumeaux, A. Craxi, M. Chaneac, and K. R. Reddy. 2005. Predicting sustained virological responses in chronic hepatitis C patients treated with peginterferon alfa-2a (40 KD)/ribavirin. *J. Hepatol.* **43:**425–433.

42. Ferenci, P., H. Laferl, T. M. Scherzer, M. Gschwantler, A. Maieron, H. Brunner, R. Stauber, M. Bischof, B. Bauer, C. Datz, K. Loschenberger, E. Formann, K. Staufer, and P. Steindl-Munda. 2008. Peginterferon alfa-2a and ribavirin for 24 weeks in hepatitis C type 1 and 4 patients with rapid virological response. *Gastroenterology* **135:**451–458.

43. Ferraro, D., M. Giglio, C. Bonura, V. Di Marco, M. U. Mondelli, A. Craxi, and R. Di Stefano. 2008. Assessment of hepatitis C virus-RNA clearance under combination therapy for hepatitis C virus genotype 1: performance of the transcription-mediated amplification assay. *J. Viral. Hepat.* **15:**66–70.

44. Ferreira-Gonzalez, A., and M. L. Shiffman. 2004. Use of diagnostic testing for managing hepatitis C virus infection. *Semin. Liver Dis.* **24**(Suppl. 2):9–18.

45. Fiebelkorn, K. R., B. G. Lee, C. E. Hill, A. M. Caliendo, and F. S. Nolte. 2002. Clinical evaluation of an automated nucleic acid isolation system. *Clin. Chem.* **48:**1613–1615.

46. Forman, M. S., and A. Valsamakis. 2004. Verification of an assay for quantification of hepatitis C virus RNA by use of an analyte-specific reagent and two different extraction methods. *J. Clin. Microbiol.* **42:**3581–3588.

47. Fried, M. W., M. L. Shiffman, K. R. Reddy, C. Smith, G. Marinos, F. L. Goncales, Jr., D. Haussinger, M. Diago, G. Carosi, D. Dhumeaux, A. Craxi, A. Lin, J. Hoffman, and J. Yu. 2002. Peginterferon alfa-2a plus ribavirin for chronic hepatitis C virus infection. *N. Engl. J. Med.* **347:**975–982.

48. Galel, S. A., D. M. Strong, G. E. Tegtmeier, P. V. Holland, I. K. Kuramoto, M. Kemper, L. Pietrelli, and J. Gallarda.

2002. Comparative yield of HCV RNA testing in blood donors screened by 2.0 versus 3.0 antibody assays. *Transfusion* **42:**1507–1513.

49. Gaudy, C., C. Thevenas, J. Tichet, N. Mariotte, A. Goudeau, and F. Dubois. 2005. Usefulness of the hepatitis C virus core antigen assay for screening of a population undergoing routine medical checkup. *J. Clin. Microbiol.* **43:**1722–1726.

50. Ge, D., J. Fellay, A. J. Thompson, J. S. Simon, K. V. Shianna, T. J. Urban, E. L. Heinzen, P. Qiu, A. H. Bertelsen, A. J. Muir, M. Sulkowski, J. G. McHutchison, and D. B. Goldstein. 2009. Genetic variation in IL28B predicts hepatitis C treatment-induced viral clearance. *Nature* **461:**399–401.

51. George, S. L., B. R. Bacon, E. M. Brunt, K. L. Mihindukulasuriya, J. Hoffmann, and A. M. Di Bisceglie. 2009. Clinical, virologic, histologic, and biochemical outcomes after successful HCV therapy: a 5-year follow-up of 150 patients. *Hepatology* **49:**729–738.

52. Germer, J. J., C. E. Bommersbach, D. M. Schmidt, J. L. Bendel, and J. D. Yao. 2009. Quantification of genotype 4 hepatitis C virus RNA by the COBAS AmpliPrep/COBAS TaqMan hepatitis C virus test. *Hepatology* **50:**1679–1680.

53. Germer, J. J., D. W. Majewski, B. Yung, P. S. Mitchell, and J. D. Yao. 2006. Evaluation of the invader assay for genotyping hepatitis C virus. *J. Clin. Microbiol.* **44:**318–323.

54. Gerotto, M., F. Dal Pero, G. Bortoletto, A. Ferrari, R. Pistis, G. Sebastiani, S. Fagiuoli, S. Realdon, and A. Alberti. 2006. Hepatitis C minimal residual viremia (MRV) detected by TMA at the end of Peg-IFN plus ribavirin therapy predicts post-treatment relapse. *J. Hepatol.* **44:**83–87.

55. Ghany, M. G., D. B. Strader, D. L. Thomas, and L. B. Seeff. 2009. Diagnosis, management, and treatment of hepatitis C: an update. *Hepatology* **49:**1335–1374.

56. Glynn, S. A., D. J. Wright, S. H. Kleinman, D. Hirschkorn, Y. Tu, C. Heldebrant, R. Smith, C. Giachetti, J. Gallarda, and M. P. Busch. 2005. Dynamics of viremia in early hepatitis C virus infection. *Transfusion* **45:**994–1002.

57. Gretch, D. R. 1997. Diagnostic tests for hepatitis C. *Hepatology* **26:**43S–47S.

58. Hadlich, E., M. R. Alvares-Da-Silva, R. K. Dal Molin, R. Zenker, and L. Z. Goldani. 2007. Hepatitis C virus (HCV) viremia in HIV-infected patients without HCV antibodies detectable by third-generation enzyme immunoassay. *J. Gastroenterol. Hepatol.* **22:**1506–1509.

59. Hadziyannis, S. J., H. Sette, Jr., T. R. Morgan, V. Balan, M. Diago, P. Marcellin, G. Ramadori, H. Bodenheimer, Jr., D. Bernstein, M. Rizzetto, S. Zeuzem, P. J. Pockros, A. Lin, and A. M. Ackrill. 2004. Peginterferon-alpha2a and ribavirin combination therapy in chronic hepatitis C: a randomized study of treatment duration and ribavirin dose. *Ann. Intern. Med.* **140:**346–355.

60. Halfon, P., M. Martinot-Peignoux, H. Khiri, and P. Marcellin. 2010. Quantification of genotype 4 serum samples: impact of hepatitis C virus genetic variability. *Hepatology* **52:**401.

61. Hezode, C., N. Forestier, G. Dusheiko, P. Ferenci, S. Pol, T. Goeser, J. P. Bronowicki, M. Bourliere, S. Gharakhanian, L. Bengtsson, L. McNair, S. George, T. Kieffer, A. Kwong, R. S. Kauffman, J. Alam, J. M. Pawlotsky, and S. Zeuzem. 2009. Telaprevir and peginterferon with or without ribavirin for chronic HCV infection. *N. Engl. J. Med.* **360:**1839–1850.

62. Hoofnagle, J. H., K. D. Mullen, D. B. Jones, V. Rustgi, A. Di Bisceglie, M. Peters, J. G. Waggoner, Y. Park, and E. A. Jones. 1986. Treatment of chronic non-A, non-B hepatitis with recombinant human alpha interferon. A preliminary report. *N. Engl. J. Med.* **315:**1575–1578.

63. Hu, Y. W., E. Balaskas, M. Furione, P. H. Yen, G. Kessler, V. Scalia, L. Chui, and G. Sher. 2000. Comparison and application of a novel genotyping method, semiautomated primer-specific and mispair extension analysis, and four other genotyping assays for detection of hepatitis C virus mixed-genotype infections. *J. Clin. Microbiol.* **38:**2807–2813.

64. Huang, R. Y., H. T. Chang, C. Y. Lan, T. W. Pai, C. N. Wu, C. M. Ling, and M. D. Chang. 2008. Development

and evaluation of a sensitive enzyme-linked oligonucleotide-sorbent assay for detection of polymerase chain reaction-amplified hepatitis C virus of genotypes 1-6. *J. Virol. Methods* **151:**211–216.

65. Ismail, N., G. E. Fish, and M. B. Smith. 2004. Laboratory evaluation of a fully automated chemiluminescence immunoassay for rapid detection of HBsAg, antibodies to HBsAg, and antibodies to hepatitis C virus. *J. Clin. Microbiol.* **42:**610–617.

66. Jones, C. T., C. L. Murray, D. K. Eastman, J. Tassello, and C. M. Rice. 2007. Hepatitis C virus p7 and NS2 proteins are essential for production of infectious virus. *J. Virol.* **81:**8374–8383.

67. Jongerius, J. M., M. Bovenhorst, C. L. van der Poel, J. A. van Hilten, A. C. Kroes, J. A. van der Does, E. F. van Leeuwen, and R. Schuurman. 2000. Evaluation of automated nucleic acid extraction devices for application in HCV NAT. *Transfusion* **40:**871–874.

68. Kamal, S. M., S. S. El Kamary, M. D. Shardell, M. Hashem, I. N. Ahmed, M. Muhammadi, K. Sayed, A. Moustafa, S. A. Hakem, A. Ibrahiem, M. Moniem, H. Mansour, and M. Abdelaziz. 2007. Pegylated interferon alpha-2b plus ribavirin in patients with genotype 4 chronic hepatitis C: the role of rapid and early virologic response. *Hepatology* **46:**1732–1740.

69. Kieffer, T. L., C. Sarrazin, J. S. Miller, M. W. Welker, N. Forestier, H. W. Reesink, A. D. Kwong, and S. Zeuzem. 2007. Telaprevir and pegylated interferon-alpha-2a inhibit wild-type and resistant genotype 1 hepatitis C virus replication in patients. *Hepatology* **46:**631–639.

70. Kim, S., J. H. Kim, S. Yoon, Y. H. Park, and H. S. Kim. 2008. Clinical performance evaluation of four automated chemiluminescence immunoassays for hepatitis C virus antibody detection. *J. Clin. Microbiol.* **46:**3919–3923.

71. Kleinman, S. H., S. L. Stramer, J. P. Brodsky, S. Caglioti, and M. P. Busch. 2006. Integration of nucleic acid amplification test results into hepatitis C virus supplemental serologic testing algorithms: implications for donor counseling and revision of existing algorithms. *Transfusion* **46:**695–702.

72. Konnick, E. Q., S. M. Williams, E. R. Ashwood, and D. R. Hillyard. 2005. Evaluation of the COBAS Hepatitis C Virus (HCV) TaqMan analyte-specific reagent assay and comparison to the COBAS Amplicor HCV Monitor V2.0 and Versant HCV bDNA 3.0 assays. *J. Clin. Microbiol.* **43:**2133–2140.

73. Krajden, M., R. Ziermann, A. Khan, A. Mak, K. Leung, D. Hendricks, and L. Comanor. 2002. Qualitative detection of hepatitis C virus RNA: comparison of analytical sensitivity, clinical performance, and workflow of the Cobas Amplicor HCV test version 2.0 and the HCV RNA transcription-mediated amplification qualitative assay. *J. Clin. Microbiol.* **40:**2903–2907.

74. Kuntzen, T., J. Timm, A. Berical, N. Lennon, A. M. Berlin, S. K. Young, B. Lee, D. Heckerman, J. Carlson, L. L. Reyor, M. Kleyman, C. M. McMahon, C. Birch, J. Schulze Zur Wiesch, T. Ledlie, M. Koehrsen, C. Kodira, A. D. Roberts, G. M. Lauer, H. R. Rosen, F. Bihl, A. Cerny, U. Spengler, Z. Liu, A. Y. Kim, Y. Xing, A. Schneidewind, M. A. Madey, J. F. Fleckenstein, V. M. Park, J. E. Galagan, C. Nusbaum, B. D. Walker, G. V. Lake-Bakaar, E. S. Daar, I. M. Jacobson, E. D. Gomperts, B. R. Edlin, S. M. Donfield, R. T. Chung, A. H. Talal, T. Marion, B. W. Birren, M. R. Henn, and T. M. Allen. 2008. Naturally occurring dominant resistance mutations to hepatitis C virus protease and polymerase inhibitors in treatment-naive patients. *Hepatology* **48:**1769–1778.

75. Lagging, M., N. Langeland, C. Pedersen, M. Farkkila, M. R. Buhl, K. Morch, A. P. Dhillon, A. Alsio, K. Hellstrand, J. Westin, and G. Norkrans. 2008. Randomized comparison of 12 or 24 weeks of peginterferon alpha-2a and ribavirin in chronic hepatitis C virus genotype 2/3 infection. *Hepatology* **47:**1837–1845.

76. Laguno, M., M. Larrousse, J. Murillas, J. L. Blanco, A. Leon, A. Milinkovic, M. Lonca, E. Martinez, J. M. Sanchez-Tapias, E. de Lazzari, J. M. Gatell, J. Costa, and J. Mallolas. 2007. Predictive value of early virologic response in HIV/hepatitis C virus-coinfected patients treated with an interferon-based regimen plus ribavirin. *J. Acquir. Immune Defic. Syndr.* **44:**174–178.

77. Laperche, S., F. Bouchardeau, V. Thibault, B. Pozzetto, S. Vallet, A. R. Rosenberg, A. M. Roque-Afonso, M. Gassin, F. Stoll-Keller, P. Trimoulet, E. Gault, B. Chanzy, B. Mercier, M. Branger, J. M. Pawlotsky, C. Henquell, F. Lunel, C. Gaudy-Graffin, S. Alain, M. L. Chaix, G. Duverlie, J. Izopet, and J. J. Lefrere. 2007. Multicenter trials need to use the same assay for hepatitis C virus viral load determination. *J. Clin. Microbiol.* **45:**3788–3790.

78. Laperche, S., M. H. Elghouzzi, P. Morel, M. Asso-Bonnet, N. Le Marrec, A. Girault, A. Servant-Delmas, F. Bouchardeau, M. Deschaseaux, and Y. Piquet. 2005. Is an assay for simultaneous detection of hepatitis C virus core antigen and antibody a valuable alternative to nucleic acid testing? *Transfusion* **45:**1965–1972.

79. Lemaire, J. M., A. M. Courouce, C. Defer, F. Bouchardeau, J. Coste, O. Agulles, J. F. Cantaloube, V. Barlet, and F. Barin. 2000. HCV RNA in blood donors with isolated reactivities by third-generation RIBA. *Transfusion* **40:**867–870.

80. Licata, A., D. Di Bona, F. Schepis, L. Shahied, A. Craxi, and C. Camma. 2003. When and how to treat acute hepatitis C? *J. Hepatol.* **39:**1056–1062.

81. Lindenbach, B. D., M. J. Evans, A. J. Syder, B. Wolk, T. L. Tellinghuisen, C. C. Liu, T. Maruyama, R. O. Hynes, D. R. Burton, J. A. McKeating, and C. M. Rice. 2005. Complete replication of hepatitis C virus in cell culture. *Science* **309:**623–626.

82. Lindh, M., and C. Hannoun. 2005. Genotyping of hepatitis C virus by Taqman real-time PCR. *J. Clin. Virol.* **34:**108–114.

83. Macedo de Oliveira, A., K. L. White, B. D. Beecham, D. P. Leschinsky, B. P. Foley, J. Dockter, C. Giachetti, and T. J. Safranek. 2006. Sensitivity of second-generation enzyme immunoassay for detection of hepatitis C virus infection among oncology patients. *J. Clin. Virol.* **35:**21–25.

84. Maheshwari, A., S. Ray, and P. J. Thuluvath. 2008. Acute hepatitis C. *Lancet* **372:**321–332.

85. Major, M. E., and S. M. Feinstone. 1997. The molecular virology of hepatitis C. *Hepatology* **25:**1527–1538.

86. Mangia, A., N. Minerva, D. Bacca, R. Cozzolongo, G. L. Ricci, V. Carretta, F. Vinelli, G. Scotto, G. Montalto, M. Romano, G. Cristofaro, L. Mottola, F. Spirito, and A. Andriulli. 2008. Individualized treatment duration for hepatitis C genotype 1 patients: a randomized controlled trial. *Hepatology* **47:**43–50.

87. Mangia, A., R. Santoro, N. Minerva, G. L. Ricci, V. Carretta, M. Persico, F. Vinelli, G. Scotto, D. Bacca, M. Annese, M. Romano, F. Zechini, F. Sogari, F. Spirito, and A. Andriulli. 2005. Peginterferon alfa-2b and ribavirin for 12 vs. 24 weeks in HCV genotype 2 or 3. *N. Engl. J. Med.* **352:**2609–2617.

88. Manns, M. P., J. G. McHutchison, S. C. Gordon, V. K. Rustgi, M. Shiffman, R. Reindollar, Z. D. Goodman, K. Koury, M. Ling, and J. K. Albrecht. 2001. Peginterferon alfa-2b plus ribavirin compared with interferon alfa-2b plus ribavirin for initial treatment of chronic hepatitis C: a randomised trial. *Lancet* **358:**958–965.

89. Mao, H., Z. Lu, H. Zhang, K. Liu, J. Zhao, G. Jin, S. Gu, and M. Yang. 2008. Colorimetric oligonucleotide array for genotyping of hepatitis C virus based on the 5' non-coding region. *Clin. Chim. Acta* **388:**22–27.

90. Margraf, R. L., M. Erali, M. Liew, and C. T. Wittwer. 2004. Genotyping hepatitis C virus by heteroduplex mobility analysis using temperature gradient capillary electrophoresis. *J. Clin. Microbiol.* **42:**4545–4551.

91. Margraf, R. L., S. Page, M. Erali, and C. T. Wittwer. 2004. Single-tube method for nucleic acid extraction, amplification, purification, and sequencing. *Clin. Chem.* **50:**1755–1761.

92. Martin-Carbonero, L., M. Nunez, A. Marino, F. Alcocer, L. Bonet, J. Garcia-Samaniego, P. Lopez-Serrano, M. Cordero, J. Portu, and V. Soriano. 2008. Undetectable hepatitis C virus RNA at week 4 as predictor of sustained virological response in HIV patients with chronic hepatitis C. *AIDS* **22:**15–21.

93. **Martinot-Peignoux, M., H. Khiri, L. Leclere, S. Maylin, P. Marcellin, and P. Halfon.** 2009. Clinical performances of two real-time PCR assays and bDNA/TMA to early monitor treatment outcome in patients with chronic hepatitis C. *J. Clin. Virol.* **46:**216–221.

94. **Martinot-Peignoux, M., V. Le Breton, S. Fritsch, G. Le Guludec, N. Labouret, F. Keller, and P. Marcellin.** 2000. Assessment of viral loads in patients with chronic hepatitis C with AMPLICOR HCV MONITOR version 1.0, COBAS HCV MONITOR version 2.0, and QUANTIPLEX HCV RNA version 2.0 assays. *J. Clin. Microbiol.* **38:**2722–2725.

95. **Martro, E., V. Gonzalez, A. J. Buckton, V. Saludes, G. Fernandez, L. Matas, R. Planas, and V. Ausina.** 2008. Evaluation of a new assay in comparison with reverse hybridization and sequencing methods for hepatitis C virus genotyping targeting both 5′ noncoding and nonstructural 5b genomic regions. *J. Clin. Microbiol.* **46:**192–197.

96. **McHutchison, J. G., G. T. Everson, S. C. Gordon, I. M. Jacobson, M. Sulkowski, R. Kauffman, L. McNair, J. Alam, and A. J. Muir.** 2009. Telaprevir with peginterferon and ribavirin for chronic HCV genotype 1 infection. *N. Engl. J. Med.* **360:**1827–1838.

97. **Mederacke, I., H. Wedemeyer, S. Ciesek, E. Steinmann, R. Raupach, K. Wursthorn, M. P. Manns, and H. L. Tillmann.** 2009. Performance and clinical utility of a novel fully automated quantitative HCV-core antigen assay. *J. Clin. Virol.* **46:**210–215.

98. **Mellor, J., A. Hawkins, and P. Simmonds.** 1999. Genotype dependence of hepatitis C virus load measurement in commercially available quantitative assays. *J. Clin. Microbiol.* **37:**2525–2532.

99. **Melve, G. K., H. Myrmel, G. E. Eide, and T. Hervig.** 2009. Evaluation of the persistence and characteristics of indeterminate reactivity against hepatitis C virus in blood donors. *Transfusion* **49:**2359–2365.

100. **Michelin, B. D., Z. Muller, E. Stelzl, E. Marth, and H. H. Kessler.** 2007. Evaluation of the Abbott RealTime HCV assay for quantitative detection of hepatitis C virus RNA. *J. Clin. Virol.* **38:**96–100.

101. **Moghaddam, A., N. Reinton, and O. Dalgard.** 2006. A rapid real-time PCR assay for determination of hepatitis C virus genotypes 1, 2 and 3a. *J. Viral Hepat.* **13:**222–229.

102. **Moreno, C., P. Deltenre, J. M. Pawlotsky, J. Henrion, M. Adler, and P. Mathurin.** 2010. Shortened treatment duration in treatment-naive genotype 1 HCV patients with rapid virologic response: a meta-analysis. *J. Hepatol.* **52:**25–31.

103. **Morishima, C., T. R. Morgan, J. E. Everhart, E. C. Wright, M. C. Apodaca, D. R. Gretch, M. L. Shiffman, G. T. Everson, K. L. Lindsay, W. M. Lee, A. S. Lok, J. L. Dienstag, M. G. Ghany, and T. M. Curto.** 2008. Interpretation of positive transcription-mediated amplification test results from polymerase chain reaction-negative samples obtained after treatment of chronic hepatitis C. *Hepatology* **48:**1412–1419.

104. **Morota, K., R. Fujinami, H. Kinukawa, T. Machida, K. Ohno, H. Saegusa, and K. Takeda.** 2009. A new sensitive and automated chemiluminescent microparticle immunoassay for quantitative determination of hepatitis C virus core antigen. *J. Virol. Methods* **157:**8–14.

105. **Mosley, J. W., E. A. Operskalski, L. H. Tobler, Z. J. Buskell, W. W. Andrews, B. Phelps, J. Dockter, C. Giachetti, L. B. Seeff, and M. P. Busch.** 2008. The course of hepatitis C viraemia in transfusion recipients prior to availability of antiviral therapy. *J. Viral Hepat.* **15:**120–128.

106. **Murphy, D. G., B. Willems, M. Deschenes, N. Hilzenrat, R. Mousseau, and S. Sabbah.** 2007. Use of sequence analysis of the NS5B region for routine genotyping of hepatitis C virus with reference to C/E1 and 5′ untranslated region sequences. *J. Clin. Microbiol.* **45:**1102–1112.

107. **Nakao, T., N. Enomoto, N. Takada, A. Takada, and T. Date.** 1991. Typing of hepatitis C virus genomes by restriction fragment length polymorphism. *J. Gen. Virol.* **72:**2105–2112.

108. **Nolte, F. S., A. M. Green, K. R. Fiebelkorn, A. M. Caliendo, C. Sturchio, A. Grunwald, and M. Healy.** 2003. Clinical evaluation of two methods for genotyping hepatitis C virus based on analysis of the 5′ noncoding region. *J. Clin. Microbiol.* **41:**1558–1564.

109. **Oethinger, M., D. R. Mayo, J. Falcone, P. K. Barua, and B. P. Griffith.** 2005. Efficiency of the ortho VITROS assay for detection of hepatitis C virus-specific antibodies increased by elimination of supplemental testing of samples with very low sample-to-cutoff ratios. *J. Clin. Microbiol.* **43:**2477–2480.

110. **Ohba, K., M. Mizokami, J. Y. Lau, E. Orito, K. Ikeo, and T. Gojobori.** 1996. Evolutionary relationship of hepatitis C, pesti-, flavi-, plantviruses, and newly discovered GB hepatitis agents. *FEBS Lett.* **378:**232–234.

111. **Ohno, O., M. Mizokami, R. R. Wu, M. G. Saleh, K. Ohba, E. Orito, M. Mukaide, R. Williams, and J. Y. Lau.** 1997. New hepatitis C virus (HCV) genotyping system that allows for identification of HCV genotypes 1a, 1b, 2a, 2b, 3a, 3b, 4, 5a, and 6a. *J. Clin. Microbiol.* **35:**201–207.

112. **Okamoto, H., S. Kobata, H. Tokita, T. Inoue, G. D. Woodfield, P. V. Holland, B. A. Al-Knawy, O. Uzunalimoglu, Y. Miyakawa, and M. Mayumi.** 1996. A second-generation method of genotyping hepatitis C virus by the polymerase chain reaction with sense and antisense primers deduced from the core gene. *J. Virol. Methods* **57:**31–45.

113. **O'Leary, J. G., R. Lepe, and G. L. Davis.** 2008. Indications for liver transplantation. *Gastroenterology* **134:**1764–1776.

114. **Park, J. C., J. M. Kim, O. J. Kwon, K. R. Lee, Y. G. Chai, and H. B. Oh.** 2010. Development and clinical evaluation of a microarray for hepatitis C virus genotyping. *J. Virol. Methods* **163:**269–275.

115. **Pawlotsky, J. M., A. Bastie, C. Pellet, J. Remire, F. Darthuy, L. Wolfe, C. Sayada, J. Duval, and D. Dhumeaux.** 1996. Significance of indeterminate third-generation hepatitis C virus recombinant immunoblot assay. *J. Clin. Microbiol.* **34:**80–83.

116. **Pawlotsky, J. M., A. Fleury, V. Choukroun, L. Deforges, F. Roudot-Thoraval, P. Aumont, J. Duval, and D. Dhumeaux.** 1994. Significance of highly positive c22-3 "indeterminate" second-generation hepatitis C virus (HCV) recombinant immunoblot assay (RIBA) and resolution by third-generation HCV RIBA. *J. Clin. Microbiol.* **32:**1357–1359.

117. **Payan, C., A. Pivert, P. Morand, S. Fafi-Kremer, F. Carrat, S. Pol, P. Cacoub, C. Perronne, and F. Lunel.** 2007. Rapid and early virological response to chronic hepatitis C treatment with IFN alpha2b or PEG-IFN alpha2b plus ribavirin in HIV/HCV co-infected patients. *Gut* **56:**1111–1116.

118. **Piro, L., S. Solinas, M. Luciani, A. Casale, T. Bighiani, D. Santonocito, and G. Girelli.** 2008. Prospective study of the meaning of indeterminate results of the recombinant immunoblot assay for hepatitis C virus in blood donors. *Blood Transfus.* **6:**107–111.

119. **Pisani, G., K. Cristiano, F. Marino, F. Luciani, G. M. Bisso, C. Mele, D. Adriani, G. Gentili, and M. Wirz.** 2009. Quantification of hepatitis C virus (HCV) RNA in a multicenter study: implications for management of HCV genotype 1-infected patients. *J. Clin. Microbiol.* **47:**2931–2936.

120. **Poordad, F., K. R. Reddy, and P. Martin.** 2008. Rapid virologic response: a new milestone in the management of chronic hepatitis C. *Clin. Infect. Dis.* **46:**78–84.

121. **Pyne, M. T., E. Q. Konnick, A. Phansalkar, and D. R. Hillyard.** 2009. Evaluation of the Abbott investigational use only RealTime hepatitis C virus (HCV) assay and comparison to the Roche TaqMan HCV analyte-specific reagent assay. *J. Clin. Microbiol.* **47:**2872–2878.

122. **Rauch, A., Z. Kutalik, P. Descombes, T. Cai, J. di Iulio, T. Mueller, M. Bochud, M. Battegay, E. Bernasconi, J. Borovicka, S. Colombo, A. Cerny, J. F. Dufour, H. Furrer, H. F. Gunthard, M. Heim, B. Hirschel, R. Malinverni, D. Moradpour, B. Mullhaupt, A. Witteck, J. S. Beckmann, T. Berg, S. Bergmann, F. Negro, A. Telenti, and P. Y. Bochud.** 2010. Genetic variation in IL28B is associated with chronic hepatitis C and treatment failure—a genome-wide association study. *Gastroenterology* **138:**1338–1345.

123. **Rehermann, B.** 2009. Hepatitis C virus versus innate and adaptive immune responses: a tale of coevolution and coexistence. *J. Clin. Investig.* **119:**1745–1754.

124. **Ren, F. R., Q. S. Lv, H. Zhuang, J. J. Li, X. Y. Gong, G. J. Gao, C. L. Liu, J. X. Wang, F. Z. Yao, Y. R. Zheng, F. M. Zhu, M. H. Tiemuer, X. H. Bai, and H. Shan.** 2005. Significance of the signal-to-cutoff ratios of anti-hepatitis C virus enzyme immunoassays in screening of Chinese blood donors. *Transfusion* **45:**1816–1822.

125. **Rolfe, K. J., G. J. Alexander, T. G. Wreghitt, S. Parmar, H. Jalal, and M. D. Curran.** 2005. A real-time Taqman method for hepatitis C virus genotyping. *J. Clin. Virol.* **34:**115–121.

126. **Ross, R. S., S. Viazov, and M. Roggendorf.** 2007. Genotyping of hepatitis C virus isolates by a new line probe assay using sequence information from both the 5′ untranslated and the core regions. *J. Virol. Methods* **143:**153–160.

127. **Ross, R. S., S. Viazov, B. Wolters, and M. Roggendorf.** 2008. Towards a better resolution of hepatitis C virus variants: CLIP sequencing of an HCV core fragment and automated assignment of genotypes and subtypes. *J. Virol. Methods* **148:**25–33.

128. **Sabato, M. F., M. L. Shiffman, M. R. Langley, D. S. Wilkinson, and A. Ferreira-Gonzalez.** 2007. Comparison of performance characteristics of three real-time reverse transcription-PCR test systems for detection and quantification of hepatitis C virus. *J. Clin. Microbiol.* **45:**2529–2536.

129. **Saldanha, J., A. Heath, C. Aberham, J. Albrecht, G. Gentili, M. Gessner, and G. Pisani.** 2005. World Health Organization collaborative study to establish a replacement WHO international standard for hepatitis C virus RNA nucleic acid amplification technology assays. *Vox Sang.* **88:**202–204.

130. **Saldanha, J., N. Lelie, A. Heath, et al.** 1999. Establishment of the first international standard for nucleic acid amplification technology (NAT) assays for HCV RNA. *Vox Sang.* **76:**149–158.

131. **Sanchez-Tapias, J. M., M. Diago, P. Escartin, J. Enriquez, M. Romero-Gomez, R. Barcena, J. Crespo, R. Andrade, E. Martinez-Bauer, R. Perez, M. Testillano, R. Planas, R. Sola, M. Garcia-Bengoechea, J. Garcia-Samaniego, M. Munoz-Sanchez, and R. Moreno-Otero.** 2006. Peginterferon-alfa2a plus ribavirin for 48 versus 72 weeks in patients with detectable hepatitis C virus RNA at week 4 of treatment. *Gastroenterology* **131:**451–460.

132. **Sarrazin, C., B. C. Gartner, D. Sizmann, R. Babiel, U. Mihm, W. P. Hofmann, M. von Wagner, and S. Zeuzem.** 2006. Comparison of conventional PCR with real-time PCR and branched DNA-based assays for hepatitis C virus RNA quantification and clinical significance for genotypes 1 to 5. *J. Clin. Microbiol.* **44:**729–737.

133. **Sarrazin, C., T. L. Kieffer, D. Bartels, B. Hanzelka, U. Muh, M. Welker, D. Wincheringer, Y. Zhou, H. M. Chu, C. Lin, C. Weegink, H. Reesink, S. Zeuzem, and A. D. Kwong.** 2007. Dynamic hepatitis C virus genotypic and phenotypic changes in patients treated with the protease inhibitor telaprevir. *Gastroenterology* **132:**1767–1777.

134. **Scheiblauer, H., M. El-Nageh, S. Nick, H. Fields, A. Prince, and S. Diaz.** 2006. Evaluation of the performance of 44 assays used in countries with limited resources for the detection of antibodies to hepatitis C virus. *Transfusion* **46:**708–718.

135. **Schroter, M., B. Zollner, P. Schafer, O. Landt, U. Lass, R. Laufs, and H. H. Feucht.** 2002. Genotyping of hepatitis C virus types 1, 2, and 4 by a one-step LightCycler method using three different pairs of hybridization probes. *J. Clin. Microbiol.* **40:**2046–2050.

136. **Shea, D. O., H. Tuite, G. Farrell, M. Codd, F. Mulcahy, S. Norris, and C. Bergin.** 2008. Role of rapid virological response in prediction of sustained virological response to Peg-IFN plus ribavirin in HCV/HIV co-infected individuals. *J. Viral Hepat.* **15:**482–489.

137. **Shiffman, M. L., F. Suter, B. R. Bacon, D. Nelson, H. Harley, R. Sola, S. D. Shafran, K. Barange, A. Lin, A. Soman, and S. Zeuzem.** 2007. Peginterferon alfa-2a and ribavirin for 16 or 24 weeks in HCV genotype 2 or 3. *N. Engl. J. Med.* **357:**124–134.

138. **Sizmann, D., C. Boeck, J. Boelter, D. Fischer, M. Miethke, S. Nicolaus, M. Zadak, and R. Babiel.** 2007. Fully automated quantification of hepatitis C virus (HCV) RNA in human plasma and human serum by the COBAS AmpliPrep/COBAS TaqMan system. *J. Clin. Virol.* **38:**326–333.

139. **Soriano, V., M. G. Peters, and S. Zeuzem.** 2009. New therapies for hepatitis C virus infection. *Clin. Infect. Dis.* **48:**313–320.

140. **Stelzl, E., C. van der Meer, R. Gouw, M. Beld, M. Grahovac, E. Marth, and H. H. Kessler.** 2007. Determination of the hepatitis C virus subtype: comparison of sequencing and reverse hybridization assays. *Clin. Chem. Lab. Med.* **45:**167–170.

141. **Strader, D. B., T. Wright, D. L. Thomas, and L. B. Seeff.** 2004. Diagnosis, management, and treatment of hepatitis C. *Hepatology* **39:**1147–1171.

142. **Stramer, S. L., S. A. Glynn, S. H. Kleinman, D. M. Strong, S. Caglioti, D. J. Wright, R. Y. Dodd, and M. P. Busch.** 2004. Detection of HIV-1 and HCV infections among antibody-negative blood donors by nucleic acid-amplification testing. *N. Engl. J. Med.* **351:**760–768.

143. **Sulkowski, M. S., S. C. Ray, and D. L. Thomas.** 2002. Needlestick transmission of hepatitis C. *JAMA* **287:**2406–2413.

144. **Suppiah, V., M. Moldovan, G. Ahlenstiel, T. Berg, M. Weltman, M. L. Abate, M. Bassendine, U. Spengler, G. J. Dore, E. Powell, S. Riordan, D. Sheridan, A. Smedile, V. Fragomeli, T. Muller, M. Bahlo, G. J. Stewart, D. R. Booth, and J. George.** 2009. IL28B is associated with response to chronic hepatitis C interferon-alpha and ribavirin therapy. *Nat. Genet.* **41:**1100–1104.

145. **Tanaka, Y., N. Nishida, M. Sugiyama, M. Kurosaki, K. Matsuura, N. Sakamoto, M. Nakagawa, M. Korenaga, K. Hino, S. Hige, Y. Ito, E. Mita, E. Tanaka, S. Mochida, Y. Murawaki, M. Honda, A. Sakai, Y. Hiasa, S. Nishiguchi, A. Koike, I. Sakaida, M. Imamura, K. Ito, K. Yano, N. Masaki, F. Sugauchi, N. Izumi, K. Tokunaga, and M. Mizokami.** 2009. Genome-wide association of IL28B with response to pegylated interferon-alpha and ribavirin therapy for chronic hepatitis C. *Nat. Genet.* **41:**1105–1109.

146. **Thimme, R., D. Oldach, K. M. Chang, C. Steiger, S. C. Ray, and F. V. Chisari.** 2001. Determinants of viral clearance and persistence during acute hepatitis C virus infection. *J. Exp. Med.* **194:**1395–1406.

147. **Thomas, D. L.** 2008. The challenge of hepatitis C in the HIV-infected person. *Annu. Rev. Med.* **59:**473–485.

148. **Thomas, D. L., C. L. Thio, M. P. Martin, Y. Qi, D. Ge, C. O'Huigin, J. Kidd, K. Kidd, S. I. Khakoo, G. Alexander, J. J. Goedert, G. D. Kirk, S. M. Donfield, H. R. Rosen, L. H. Tobler, M. P. Busch, J. G. McHutchison, D. B. Goldstein, and M. Carrington.** 2009. Genetic variation in IL28B and spontaneous clearance of hepatitis C virus. *Nature* **461:**798–801.

149. **Tillmann, H. L., J. Wiegand, I. Glomb, A. Jelineck, G. Picchio, H. Wedemeyer, and M. P. Manns.** 2005. Diagnostic algorithm for chronic hepatitis C virus infection: role of the new HCV-core antigen assay. *Z. Gastroenterol.* **43:**11–16.

150. **Tobler, L. H., S. L. Stramer, S. H. Kleinman, J. P. Brodsky, D. S. Todd, and M. P. Busch.** 2001. Misclassification of HCV-viremic blood donors as indeterminate by RIBA 3.0 because of human superoxide dismutase reactivity. *Transfusion* **41:**1625–1626.

151. **Tobler, L. H., S. L. Stramer, S. R. Lee, B. L. Masecar, J. E. Peterson, E. A. Davis, W. E. Andrews, J. P. Brodsky, S. H. Kleinman, B. H. Phelps, and M. P. Busch.** 2003. Impact of HCV 3.0 EIA relative to HCV 2.0 EIA on blood-donor screening. *Transfusion* **43:**1452–1459.

152. **Torriani, F. J., M. Rodriguez-Torres, J. K. Rockstroh, E. Lissen, J. Gonzalez-Garcia, A. Lazzarin, G. Carosi, J. Sasadeusz, C. Katlama, J. Montaner, H. Sette, Jr., S.

Passe, J. De Pamphilis, F. Duff, U. M. Schrenk, and D. T. Dieterich. 2004. Peginterferon Alfa-2a plus ribavirin for chronic hepatitis C virus infection in HIV-infected patients. *N. Engl. J. Med.* **351:**438–450.

153. Tuaillon, E., A. M. Mondain, L. Ottomani, L. Roudiere, P. Perney, M. C. Picot, F. Seguret, F. Blanc, D. Larrey, P. Van de Perre, and J. Ducos. 2007. Impact of hepatitis C virus (HCV) genotypes on quantification of HCV RNA in serum by COBAS AmpliPrep/COBAS TaqMan HCV test, Abbott HCV realtime assay [corrected] and VERSANT HCV RNA assay. *J. Clin. Microbiol.* **45:**3077–3081.

154. Uyttendaele, S., H. Claeys, W. Mertens, H. Verhaert, and C. Vermylen. 1994. Evaluation of third-generation screening and confirmatory assays for HCV antibodies. *Vox Sang.* **66:**122–129.

155. van Doorn, L. J., B. Kleter, I. Pike, and W. Quint. 1996. Analysis of hepatitis C virus isolates by serotyping and genotyping. *J. Clin. Microbiol.* **34:**1784–1787.

156. Veillon, P., C. Payan, G. Picchio, M. Maniez-Montreuil, P. Guntz, and F. Lunel. 2003. Comparative evaluation of the total hepatitis C virus core antigen, branched-DNA, and Amplicor monitor assays in determining viremia for patients with chronic hepatitis C during interferon plus ribavirin combination therapy. *J. Clin. Microbiol.* **41:**3212–3220.

157. Verbeeck, J., M. J. Stanley, J. Shieh, L. Celis, E. Huyck, E. Wollants, J. Morimoto, A. Farrior, E. Sablon, M. Jankowski-Hennig, C. Schaper, P. Johnson, M. Van Ranst, and M. Van Brussel. 2008. Evaluation of Versant hepatitis C virus genotype assay (LiPA) 2.0. *J. Clin. Microbiol.* **46:**1901–1906.

158. Vermehren, J., A. Kau, B. C. Gartner, R. Gobel, S. Zeuzem, and C. Sarrazin. 2008. Differences between two real-time PCR-based hepatitis C virus (HCV) assays (RealTime HCV and Cobas AmpliPrep/Cobas TaqMan) and one signal amplification assay (Versant HCV RNA 3.0) for RNA detection and quantification. *J. Clin. Microbiol.* **46:**3880–3891.

159. Viazov, S., A. Zibert, K. Ramakrishnan, A. Widell, A. Cavicchini, E. Schreier, and M. Roggendorf. 1994. Typing of hepatitis C virus isolates by DNA enzyme immunoassay. *J. Virol. Methods* **48:**81–91.

160. Villano, S. A., D. Vlahov, K. E. Nelson, S. Cohn, and D. L. Thomas. 1999. Persistence of viremia and the importance of long-term follow-up after acute hepatitis C infection. *Hepatology* **29:**908–914.

161. von Wagner, M., M. Huber, T. Berg, H. Hinrichsen, J. Rasenack, T. Heintges, A. Bergk, C. Bernsmeier, D. Haussinger, E. Herrmann, and S. Zeuzem. 2005. Peginterferon-alpha-2a (40KD) and ribavirin for 16 or 24 weeks in patients with genotype 2 or 3 chronic hepatitis C. *Gastroenterology* **129:**522–527.

162. Wakita, T., T. Pietschmann, T. Kato, T. Date, M. Miyamoto, Z. Zhao, K. Murthy, A. Habermann, H. G. Krausslich, M. Mizokami, R. Bartenschlager, and T. J. Liang. 2005. Production of infectious hepatitis C virus in tissue culture from a cloned viral genome. *Nat. Med.* **11:**791–796.

163. Wang, C. C., E. Krantz, J. Klarquist, M. Krows, L. McBride, E. P. Scott, T. Shaw-Stiffel, S. J. Weston, H. Thiede, A. Wald, and H. R. Rosen. 2007. Acute hepatitis C in a contemporary US cohort: modes of acquisition and factors influencing viral clearance. *J. Infect. Dis.* **196:**1474–1482.

164. Wasley, A., S. Grytdal, and K. Gallagher. 2008. Surveillance for acute viral hepatitis—United States, 2006. *MMWR Surveill. Summ.* **57:**1–24.

165. Watterson, J. M., P. Stallcup, D. Escamilla, P. Chernay, A. Reyes, and S. C. Trevino. 2007. Evaluation of the Ortho-Clinical Diagnostics Vitros ECi Anti-HCV test: comparison with three other methods. *J. Clin. Lab. Anal.* **21:**162–166.

166. White, P. A., X. Zhai, I. Carter, Y. Zhao, and W. D. Rawlinson. 2000. Simplified hepatitis C virus genotyping by heteroduplex mobility analysis. *J. Clin. Microbiol.* **38:**477–482.

167. Yano, M., H. Kumada, M. Kage, K. Ikeda, K. Shimamatsu, O. Inoue, E. Hashimoto, J. H. Lefkowitch, J. Ludwig, and K. Okuda. 1996. The long-term pathological evolution of chronic hepatitis C. *Hepatology* **23:**1334–1340.

168. Yeo, A. E., M. Ghany, C. Conry-Cantilena, J. C. Melpolder, D. E. Kleiner, J. W. Shih, J. H. Hoofnagle, and H. J. Alter. 2001. Stability of HCV-RNA level and its lack of correlation with disease severity in asymptomatic chronic hepatitis C virus carriers. *J. Viral Hepat.* **8:**256–263.

169. Yu, M. L., C. Y. Dai, J. F. Huang, C. F. Chiu, Y. H. Yang, N. J. Hou, L. P. Lee, M. Y. Hsieh, Z. Y. Lin, S. C. Chen, L. Y. Wang, W. Y. Chang, and W. L. Chuang. 2008. Rapid virological response and treatment duration for chronic hepatitis C genotype 1 patients: a randomized trial. *Hepatology* **47:**1884–1893.

170. Zeuzem, S., M. W. Fried, K. R. Reddy, P. Marcellin, M. Diago, A. Craxi, P. Pockros, M. Rizzetto, D. Berstein, M. L. Shiffman, A. Lin, and S. Hadziyannis. 2006. Improving the clinical relevance of pre-treatment viral load as a predictor of sustained virologic response (SVR) in patients infected with hepatitis C genotype 1 treated with peginterferon alfa-2A (40KD) (Pegasys) plus ribavirin (Copegus). *Hepatology* **44S1:**267A.

171. Zhong, J., P. Gastaminza, G. Cheng, S. Kapadia, T. Kato, D. R. Burton, S. F. Wieland, S. L. Uprichard, T. Wakita, and F. V. Chisari. 2005. Robust hepatitis C virus infection in vitro. *Proc. Natl. Acad. Sci. USA* **102:**9294–9299.

Gastroenteritis Viruses*

XIAOLI PANG AND XI JIANG

90

Common causes of viral gastroenteritis include rotavirus, calicivirus (norovirus and sapovirus), astrovirus, and enteric adenovirus (EAdV). Rotaviruses are the most important cause of severe acute gastroenteritis in young children. Noroviruses have been recognized as the most important cause of nonbacterial epidemics of gastroenteritis. Sapoviruses, astroviruses, and EAdVs are important causes of pediatric gastroenteritis. Other viruses, such as coronavirus, torovirus, Aichi virus, picobirnavirus, and bocavirus, have been implicated in human gastroenteritis, but their etiologic role is not well established.

TAXONOMY

Rotaviruses

Rotaviruses are classified as members of the *Rotavirus* genus within the *Reoviridae*, which contains 10 other distinct genera (Table 1). Based on group-specific antigens of the major viral structural protein VP6, rotaviruses are divided into seven groups (A to G) (21). Group-specific epitopes are also found on other structural proteins as well as on some nonstructural proteins. Group A to C rotaviruses infect both humans and animals, with the group A rotaviruses infecting humans most frequently and causing disease mainly in young children. Group D to G rotaviruses are mainly animal pathogens. Within each group, rotaviruses are further classified into serotypes based on neutralization assays using antibodies against two major outer capsid proteins, VP4 and VP7. VP4 is a spike protein on the capsid surface which is sensitive to protease cleavage; therefore, the types based on the VP4 protein are also called P types (protease sensitive). VP7 is a glycoprotein, and the types based on this protein are also called G types. Both P and G types are also classified based on the sequences of the VP4 and VP7 genes (genotypes). In 2008, a new classification system was recommended (68, 69) and a Rotavirus Classification Working Group including specialists in molecular virology, infectious diseases,

epidemiology, and public health was formed to assist in the delineation of new genotypes. Scientists discovering a potentially new rotavirus genotype for any of the 11 gene segments are invited to send the novel sequence to the Rotavirus Classification Working Group; the sequence will be analyzed, and a new nomenclature will be advised as appropriate.

Caliciviruses

Caliciviruses belong to the family *Caliciviridae*, which includes six genera, *Norovirus*, *Sapovirus*, *Lagovirus*, *Vesivirus*, and the newly proposed *Becovirus* and *Recovirus* (25, 32, 78). *Norovirus* and *Sapovirus* genera cause mainly gastroenteritis in humans. They were also called "Norwalk-like viruses" and "Sapporo-like viruses" after their prototype strains, the Norwalk and Sapporo viruses, respectively. Within each genus, strains are further grouped into genogroups (G) and genotypes or clusters. Noroviruses can be classified into five genogroups; GI, GII, and GIV are found mainly among human isolates, whereas GIII has been isolated from cattle and GV has been isolated from mice (100). A single genotype of norovirus (genogroup II, genotype 4 [GII.4]) has been found to be predominant in the past decade, causing up to 80% of all norovirus gastroenteritis outbreaks (10, 86) in many countries. Genetic analysis also showed that the GII.4 viruses may undergo an epochal evolution selected by herd immunity (62, 87). Similar to noroviruses, sapoviruses are grouped into 14 genotypes within 5 genogroups (26, 38). Genogroups GI, GII, GIV, and GV contain human isolates, and genogroup GIII contains the porcine strains (26).

Enteric Adenoviruses

Until recently, there were 51 serotypes of human AdV (HAdV) grouped into six subgroups (A to F) based on their antigenic and genetic properties. This number has now been increased to 54, with a new type (HAdV-52) potentially causing gastroenteritis (50) and two more types (HAdV-53 and HAdV-54) causing keratoconjunctivitis (44, 95). HAdV-52 has also been proposed to represent a new species (HAdV-G) based on genetic analysis, although classification of this strain into a new type and a new species remains debatable due to a lack of antigenic characterization (17).

Many AdVs are readily isolated from human stool specimens, but their role in acute gastroenteritis is unclear.

---

*This chapter contains information presented in chapter 94 by Martin Petric and Raymond Tellier in the eighth edition and by Tibor Farkas and Xi Jiang in the ninth edition of this *Manual*.

TABLE 1 Taxonomy and virologic properties of gastroenteritis viruses[a]

Virus	Family	Size (nm)	Appearance under EM	Viral genome	Genetic or antigenic types
Rotavirus	*Reoviridae*	70	Wheel-shaped, triple-layered capsid	dsRNA	7 antigenic groups (A–F) and 14 G and 23 P types
Norovirus	*Caliciviridae*	30–38	SRSV	ss(+)RNA	5 genogroups and >20 genetic types (clusters)
Sapovirus	*Caliciviridae*	30–38	SRSV, with Star of David appearance	ss(+)RNA	5 genogroups and >9 genetic types (clusters)
Adenovirus	*Adenoviridae*	70–100	Icosahedral capsid	dsDNA	Ad40 and Ad41, linked to gastroenteritis
Astrovirus	*Astroviridae*	28–30	SRSV, star shaped	ss(+)RNA	8 serotypes
Coronavirus	*Coronaviridae*	60–200	Pleomorphic, with club-shaped projections	ss(+)RNA	Unknown
Torovirus	*Coronaviridae*	100–150	Pleomorphic, with torus-shaped core	ss(+)RNA	Unknown
Aichi virus	*Picornaviridae*	30	Small round virus	ss(+)RNA	Unknown
Picobirnavirus	*Picobirnaviridae*	35	Small round virus	dsRNA	Unknown, genetic variation found
Bocavirus	*Parvoviridae*	18–26	Isometric capsid	ssDNA	Unknown

[a]dsRNA, double-stranded RNA; ss(+)RNA, single-stranded positive-sense RNA; dsDNA, double-stranded DNA; SRSV, small, round, structured virus.

However, there are two serotypes, Ad40 and Ad41 in subgroup F, that have been evidently associated with infantile diarrhea and are referred as EAdVs (29). These EAdVs are also known as "fastidious," as they are difficult to grow in cell culture. Recently, a plaque assay was developed to detect EAdV types 40 and 41 (15).

Astroviruses

Astroviruses, which belong to the *Astroviridae* family, were named for their characteristic star-like (*astron* = star in Greek) surface structure. Two genera of astroviruses, *Mamastrovirus* and *Avastrovirus*, have been described according to their host species (96). Human astroviruses have been divided into eight types based on antigenic and genetic typing (7, 43, 59).

Other Viruses Causing Gastroenteritis

Other enteric viruses that are implicated in acute gastroenteritis of humans include coronaviruses and toroviruses, two genera in the *Coronaviridae* family (40), Aichi virus in the genus *Kobuvirus* of the *Picornaviridae* family (94), picobirnaviruses in the *Picobirnaviridae* family (28), and human bocavirus in the genus *Bocavirus* within the *Parvoviridae* family (63) (Table 1).

DESCRIPTION OF THE AGENTS

Rotaviruses

Viral particles of around 70 nm with a wheel-like appearance from a number of animal species had been described during the 1960s. Similar human viruses were first identified in 1973 by thin-section electron microscopy (EM) of the duodenal mucosa from children with acute gastroenteritis. Later these viruses were designated rotaviruses (*rota* = wheel in Latin). Mature rotavirus particles are about 70 nm in diameter and nonenveloped, and they possess a triple-layered icosahedral protein capsid composed of an outer layer, an intermediate layer, and an inner core (Fig. 1). The rotavirus genome contains 11 segments of double-stranded RNA ranging from ~660 (segment 11) to ~3,300 (segment 1) bp. The gene coding assignments of the 11 genome segments have been determined; these segments code for six major structural proteins (VP1, VP2, VP3, VP4, VP6,

and VP7) that appear on the mature viral particles and six nonstructural proteins (NSP1 to NSP6) that are expressed in infected cells and play important roles in viral genome replication, protein synthesis, capsid assembly, and maturation. One of the nonstructural proteins, NSP4, has been found to be a viral enterotoxin (4, 22).

Caliciviruses

Caliciviruses are small (30 to 38 nm), round, nonenveloped viruses. Sapoviruses have the typical calicivirus morphology, with the "star of David" appearance (Fig. 1). Noroviruses reveal a smoother surface structure and therefore are also called small, round, structured viruses (31). Cryo-EM and X-ray crystallography analysis of recombinant virus-like particles (VLPs) revealed that noroviruses possess a T = 3 icosahedral capsid composed of 180 capsid monomers that form 90 dimeric capsomers. Each capsid protein possesses two major domains, the shell (S) and the protrusion (P) domains. An expression of the P domain in *Escherichia coli* has resulted in self-formation of a subviral particle, the P particle, which maintains the VLPs' properties of receptor binding and antigenic recognition (88). This P particle is highly stable and easy to make and has been proposed as a subunit vaccine for noroviruses.

Noroviruses contain a single-stranded, positive-sense, poly(A)-tailed RNA genome of ~7.5 kb (47, 48). It is organized into three open reading frames (ORFs), with ORF1 encoding the nonstructural proteins, ORF2 the capsid protein, and ORF3 a minor structural protein. The sapovirus genome is slightly different in that sequences encoding the nonstructural and capsid proteins are fused into one large ORF.

Enteric Adenoviruses

AdVs were named from the Greek word *aden*, meaning "gland," after their original isolation from adenoid tissue and were also called "adenoid-associated viruses." HAdVs have been linked to a number of diseases, including respiratory illness, conjunctivitis, and diarrhea (41). AdVs are nonenveloped, icosahedral particles that are 70 to 100 nm in diameter (Fig. 1). Mature virions consist of a DNA-containing core surrounded by a protein shell. The genome is a linear double-stranded DNA of 30 to 38 kb (size varies from group to group). The protein shell (capsid) is composed of 252 capsomeres, of which 240 are hexons and 12

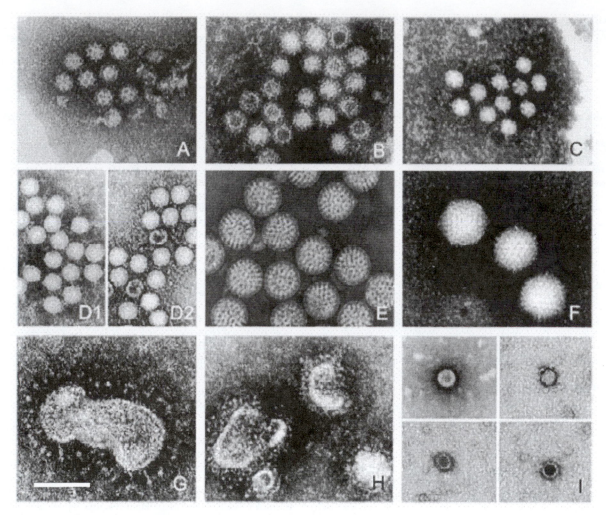

FIGURE 1 Electron micrographs of gastroenteritis viruses. (A) Sapoviruses; (B) noroviruses; (C) astroviruses; (D1) Aichi virus; (D2) picornaviruses; (E) rotaviruses; (F) AdVs; (G) coronaviruses; (H) torovirus-like particles; (I) picobirnaviruses. Bar = 100 nm. Modified from Fig. 2 of reference 81a. Panel D1 was provided by Teruo Yamashita, and panels E and I were provided by Charles Humphrey.

are pentons. There are a total of 11 viral structural proteins, and three of them (hexon, penton base, and fiber) are of important clinical relevance. These proteins are involved in viral entry (fiber) and intracellular transportation. The hexon and fiber contain the major neutralization epitopes.

Astroviruses

Astroviruses are small (28 to 30 nm in diameter), round, and nonenveloped viruses with a typical star-like appearance (Fig. 1). The virions contain a single-stranded, positive-sense RNA genome of about 6.8 kb. The viral genome contains three ORFs. ORF-1a and ORF-1b encode the nonstructural proteins. ORF-1a has a protease motif, transmembrane helices, nuclear localization signals, and a ribosomal frame-shifting signal, whereas ORF-1b has an RNA polymerase motif. ORF-2 encodes the capsid precursor protein (~87 kDa), which is further cleaved to smaller peptides of 25 to 34 kDa to form mature virions.

EPIDEMIOLOGY AND TRANSMISSION

Gastroenteritis viruses are transmitted by the fecal-oral pathway and through person-to-person and environmental surface contact (Table 2). These viruses can also be transmitted by contaminated water and food, which usually results in large outbreaks. Most viral diarrhea diseases are endemic, with significant disease burden, in both developing and developed countries. Caliciviruses, particularly the noroviruses, also cause epidemics of acute gastroenteritis, which is an important public health concern. In temperate countries, viral gastroenteritis does not have the typical summer peak of most bacterium- and parasite-caused gastroenteritis. Instead, viral gastroenteritis is more common in colder seasons, with a typical winter-spring peak.

Rotaviruses

Rotaviruses usually cause severe dehydration in infants and children less than 2 years of age, which makes rotaviruses a major cause of childhood deaths in developing countries. Rotavirus mortality is much lower in developed countries, but the disease burden remains high, representing approximately 2.7 million diarrheal episodes each year in the United States, with significant numbers of physician visits and hospitalizations and high medical and societal costs. Infants usually acquire the disease from their siblings or from their parents, who may have subclinical infection.

TABLE 2 Epidemiology, transmission, and clinical significance of gastroenteritis viruses

Virus	Mode of transmission	Target population	Clinical significance	Disease control and prevention
Rotavirus	Fecal-oral	Children <5 yr old	Acute severe gastroenteritis, mostly sporadic, nosocomial infection can occur	Rehydration for severely affected patients, vaccines are developed
Norovirus	Fecal-oral, close contact, water and food	All age groups	Moderate to severe gastroenteritis, commonly causes outbreaks in a variety of settings	Good personal hygiene, hand washing, avoid crowding, control food handling
Sapovirus	Fecal-oral, close contact	Mainly children	Mild to moderate gastroenteritis, subclinical infection occurs, sporadic, but outbreaks occur	Good personal hygiene, hand washing
Adenovirus	Fecal-oral	Mainly children <5 yr old	Moderate to severe gastroenteritis, sporadic, nosocomial infection, persists in immunocompromised patients	Good personal hygiene, hand washing
Astrovirus	Fecal-oral	Mainly children	Mild to moderate gastroenteritis, subclinical infection occurs, sporadic, but outbreaks occur	Good personal hygiene, hand washing
Coronavirus	Unknown, possibly fecal-oral	Possibly all age groups	Possibly sporadic, mild to moderate gastroenteritis	Good personal hygiene, hand washing
Torovirus	Unknown, possibly fecal-oral	Possibly all age groups	Possibly sporadic, mild to moderate gastroenteritis	Good personal hygiene, hand washing
Aichi virus	Unknown, possibly fecal-oral	Children and adults	Possibly sporadic, mild to moderate gastroenteritis	Good personal hygiene, hand washing
Picobirnavirus	Unknown, possibly fecal-oral	Children and adults	Possibly sporadic, mild to moderate gastroenteritis	Good personal hygiene, hand washing
Bocavirus	Unknown, possibly aerosol, fecal-oral	Mainly children but also adults	Uncertain	Good personal hygiene, hand washing

Shedding of rotavirus in stools can occur prior to onset of disease and continue following cessation of diarrhea. Rotaviruses are able to survive on environmental surfaces at ambient temperature and are resistant to physical inactivation, both of which may contribute to their efficient transmission (1). Cross-species transmission of rotaviruses has been demonstrated, indicating a zoonotic potential for rotavirus disease (5). In temperate countries, rotavirus diarrhea usually exhibits a typical winter-spring peak, during which time over one-third of the diarrhea cases seen in emergency rooms and outpatient clinics are caused by rotaviruses. This seasonal pattern of rotavirus infection observed in temperate climates does not occur uniformly in tropical countries.

Caliciviruses

Noroviruses are highly contagious and have been recognized as the most important causes of nonbacterial acute gastroenteritis in both developing and developed countries (23). The disease is endemic in children, but all ages can be infected due to potential incomplete immunity following a childhood infection or reinfection with antigenically different strains. Noroviruses commonly cause large outbreaks in closed communities and in a variety of settings, such as hospitals, child care centers, schools, restaurants, nursing homes for the elderly, cruise ships, and military communities or camps. Particular attention has been paid to foodborne outbreaks occurring in nursing homes for the elderly and onboard cruise ships in the United States and European countries. Recently, noroviruses have been found to recognize the ABH (secretor) and Lewis histo-blood

group antigens as receptors (42), and significant progress has been made in the elucidation of the diversity and structure/function relationship of the receptor binding interfaces of these viruses. Direct evidence of zoonotic transmission of noroviruses remains lacking, although noroviruses closely related to human noroviruses have been detected in domestic and wild animals.

Sapoviruses cause disease mainly in children, although outbreaks have been reported to occur in adults.

Enteric Adenoviruses

While the role of EAdVs in acute gastroenteritis is widely accepted, the incidences of AdV-related gastroenteritis differ considerably in various studies and locations, with an average of ~5% of cases of pediatric diarrhea being caused by EAdVs. Outbreaks of EAdV-related diarrhea have been reported in hospitals and child day care centers. Human EAdV infection does not have the typical winter seasonality of the rotaviruses and caliciviruses, and sporadic cases are reported year-round. Like other enteric pathogens, human EAdVs are frequently detected in stools of children without gastroenteritis. Many children acquire EAdV infection (as many as 41% of children) during hospitalization for other diseases (11). EAdVs also cause prolonged or chronic diarrhea in immunocompromised patients, which is an increasing concern in the clinical care of these patients (84, 91).

Astroviruses

Human astroviruses cause mainly pediatric gastroenteritis. Cases in care givers of sick children, immunocompromised adults (34), military troops (8), and nursing homes (61, 71) have been reported. Astrovirus infection can be linked to 2 to 10% of cases of pediatric gastroenteritis worldwide, depending on settings and diagnostic tests used. Asymptomatic infections are common in all ages. Among school-aged children, there is a 70 to 90% seroprevalence of astroviruses, indicating frequent infections during childhood.

CLINICAL SIGNIFICANCE

Clinical symptoms of viral gastroenteritis include watery diarrhea, vomiting, anorexia, abdominal pain, and fever, with rotavirus gastroenteritis being the most severe. The disease lasts for 2 to 3 days in most cases; however, viral shedding in some cases can continue for several weeks. There are no effective antivirals against gastroenteritis viruses. Rehydration therapy is the most important procedure for severe cases and for reducing mortality in developing countries. A prompt diagnosis of viral gastroenteritis is important to avoid unnecessary use of antibiotics and to help with institutional measures to control transmission.

Rotaviruses

The major symptoms of rotavirus gastroenteritis include watery diarrhea, vomiting, abdominal pain, and fever. Symptoms can be mild and last for a few days, but prolonged illness with severe dehydration can occur if the children are not treated with rehydration procedures. Severe dehydration can be lethal and remains an important cause of infant mortality in developing countries. Rotaviruses can cause chronic infection in immunocompromised individuals, such as patients who have undergone organ transplantation and those infected with human immunodeficiency virus (HIV), and in rare cases, the viruses can disseminate systemically and cause hepatic infection. Like other enteric viruses, rotaviruses may also cause subclinical infection in children. Subclinical infections can be due to maternal antibody or previous exposure to antigenically related strains. Immunity to rotaviruses is believed to be long-lasting following natural infection.

The lack of antiviral drugs against rotaviruses and the significant disease burden of rotavirus gastroenteritis encouraged development of a vaccine. After decades of efforts by many scientists and the failure of some earlier vaccine products, two live attenuated-rotavirus vaccines—Rotarix (RV1) and RotaTeq (RV5)—were licensed worldwide in 2004 and 2006, respectively. Rotarix is a monovalent vaccine containing one attenuated human rotavirus, and RotaTeq is a pentavalent human-bovine (WC3) reassortant vaccine. Both vaccines are safe and effective, providing 80 to 100% protection against severe disease and 70 to 80% protection against rotavirus gastroenteritis of any severity in high- and middle-income countries. The Advisory Committee on Immunization Practices (ACIP) recently updated its rotavirus vaccine recommendations to include the use of RV1 and RV5 for prevention of rotavirus gastroenteritis (14).

Caliciviruses

The clinical symptoms of norovirus gastroenteritis have been reported to be milder than that of rotaviruses. However, increasing data show that noroviruses are frequently detected in children hospitalized with acute gastroenteritis, indicating that noroviruses may also cause severe gastroenteritis. The major symptoms of norovirus gastroenteritis include watery diarrhea, vomiting, anorexia, abdominal pain, and fever. Diarrhea and vomiting are serious symptoms

and vary in different populations. Norovirus has also been reported to cause chronic diarrhea, with prolonged viral shedding in the stools of recipients of transplanted tissue and solid organs (58, 97), and to cause necrotizing enterocolitis in children (66, 93). At present, preventive strategies for norovirus infection are aimed at eliminating the source of infection by increasing personal hygiene, disinfecting environmental surfaces, identifying sick food handlers, and adequately disposing of contaminated food and water. Diagnosis of norovirus infection in transplant recipients and other immunocompromised patients also may be important. The clinical symptoms of sapovirus gastroenteritis are, in general, milder than those of norovirus gastroenteritis.

Since noroviruses cause the great majority of epidemics of viral gastroenteritis, development of a vaccine and antivirals against noroviruses is needed. Approaches to develop a norovirus vaccine include transgenic plant-, baculovirus-, or *E. coli*-expressed recombinant VLPs or P particles as a subunit vaccine. Challenges in developing these vaccines include our lack of understanding of immunity, particularly the mechanism of the short duration of protective immunity following a natural infection, and the lack of a cell culture and suitable animal model for efficacy studies. The high genetic and antigenic diversity of noroviruses also makes it difficult to select vaccine targets for broad protection.

Enteric Adenoviruses

AdV-associated acute gastroenteritis is usually milder but lasts longer (5 to 12 days) than other viral gastroenteritis viruses. AdV infection in immunodeficient individuals, such as hematopoietic stem cell and solid organ transplant recipients, HIV patients, and other immunosuppressed individuals, has a growing clinical importance (27). AdV infection in these individuals can be mild gastroenteritis, asymptomatic infection, or severe disease, including gastroenteritis, pneumonitis, hemorrhagic cystitis, hepatitis, and disseminated infection associated with high mortality. Patients can excrete AdVs in stool for weeks to months after infection. Potential treatment of AdV infection in such clinical settings includes reduction of immunosuppressive drugs, intravenous immunoglobulin, and intravenous antiviral therapy (cidofovir).

Astroviruses

The major symptoms of astrovirus gastroenteritis include diarrhea, vomiting, anorexia, abdominal pain, and fever, which symptoms are generally milder than those of rota- and norovirus gastroenteritis. Astroviruses are frequently detected in stools of children without acute gastroenteritis.

COLLECTION, TRANSPORT, AND STORAGE OF SPECIMENS

Gastroenteritis viruses replicate and cause disease mainly in the intestine, and stool is the major specimen for laboratory diagnosis. Specimens are preferably collected within the first 48 hours of illness. Specimens collected in later stages have a lower detection rate, although prolonged shedding of some gastroenteritis viruses have been reported after the onset of illness. Stool specimens of a few grams are sufficient for detection by EM and antigen or nucleic acid detection methods. The samples can be collected with a bed pan and then transferred into smaller containers or test tubes. Specimens can be recovered from a diaper with a wooden tongue depressor. Rectal swabs may be easy to obtain, but they are poor specimens for viral diagnosis and not recommended.

In general, the best results are obtained by testing fresh stool samples, particularly for good viral morphology by EM. Stool samples can be stored at 4°C for weeks if they are not tested immediately after collection or after transport to a diagnostic laboratory. For prolonged storage, specimens should be kept frozen, preferably at −70°C. If multiple tests are planned for multiple pathogens or for confirmation of results, aliquots of the samples are usually prepared to avoid repeated freezing and thawing of the bulk samples, which usually destroys the viral structures and results in decreased detection rates. Stool samples can be shipped on ice or dry ice, depending on their storage conditions (e.g., short- or long-term storage). Unnecessary freezing and thawing between shipment and storage should be avoided.

Serum samples are used for detection of antibodies against gastroenteritis viruses. Documenting seroconversion between acute- and convalescent-phase serum samples has been particularly useful for diagnosis of viral infection in outbreak investigations; however, it is used mainly in research laboratories and is not suitable for clinical diagnosis because collection of the convalescent-phase samples is required within 2 to 3 weeks after the onset of illness. Blood and serum samples should be handled with precautions for transmission of blood-borne pathogens. For long-term storage, it is preferred that samples are processed to separate serum from cell components and kept at −20°C or −70°C in aliquots.

Drinking water, food, or other environmental specimens are used in research on viral (mainly noroviral) gastroenteritis outbreaks. If a food item or water is suspected as the source of an outbreak, a sample should be obtained as early as possible and stored at 4°C. Since testing of these items for the presence of viruses is not routinely done in most of the diagnostic laboratories and often requires special methodology (e.g., filter concentration of 5 to 100 liters of water and processing of food to remove food debris), a laboratory with the capacity to test these specimens should be contacted (e.g., local health departments or the Centers for Disease Control and Protection).

DIRECT DETECTION

Direct EM

Direct EM is used to visualize the negatively stained viral particles on a grid without additional steps of grid preparation (81). It is fast, does not require specific reagents, and can be used for any viruses, but it is relatively less sensitive (minimum of ~10^6 viral particles/ml) than other techniques and requires expensive equipment and maintenance. Liquid stool samples can be applied to the grid following a low-speed centrifugation (5,000 rpm for 10 min) to remove large debris. For solid stool samples, a 10 to 20% stool suspension in either distilled water or a 1% ammonium acetate solution is made. One drop (5 to 10 μl) of the sample is then applied to a copper EM grid (300- to 400-mesh size), which is coated with Formvar (polyvinyl formal) and reinforced by carbon shadowing (commercially available). The sample drop can also be placed on a piece of Parafilm, and then the grid is floated on the top of the drop. After incubation for approximately 1 min, excess specimen is removed from the grid with filter paper. Longer incubation may be used, but drying of the samples should be avoided. If the resulting grid is too thick, the sample may be diluted or the grid washed with a drop of distilled water. The grid is then stained with a drop of 2% phosphotungstic acid (pH 7) for

10 to 30 s and then blotted with filter paper. The dried grid is ready for EM examination.

For specimens containing a low concentration of viruses, a concentration step by ultracentrifugation may be used. The Beckman Airfuge with an EM-90 rotor is useful for depositing the specimens on the EM grid for small-volume samples. Centrifugation at 100,000 × g for 1 h is used to pellet most of the viral particles. Following the centrifugation, the pellet is resuspended in distilled water and processed for making the grids as outlined above. The samples may be further diluted if the sample layer on the grid is too thick. A step of low-speed centrifugation to remove large aggregates may also help to avoid overloading.

The stool suspension can also be subjected to agar diffusion to concentrate the virus particles. Briefly, the stool specimen is placed on a small block of 1% agar made up in distilled water, and the grid is floated on the surface of the drop. After incubation at room temperature until the drop is absorbed into the agar, the grid is removed and processed for EM as described above. This procedure not only concentrates the viruses but also removes excessive quantities of salts, which may precipitate on the grid, obscuring the viruses.

Under EM, negatively stained virus particles appear as lighter structures surrounded by a dark background (Fig. 1) (81). The most definitive of the spherical structures are the AdVs and rotaviruses, whose icosahedral capsids are readily discerned. Each of the smaller round viruses, including the norovirus, sapovirus, astrovirus, and Aichi virus, has a unique surface appearance: sapovirus reveals a rigid surface structure with the cup-like depressions of a typical Star of David, norovirus has a less rigid surface appearance and does not have the Star of David structure, astrovirus has a distinct five-point star appearance, and Aichi virus reveals a smooth surface indistinguishable from those of other picornaviruses (Fig. 1). However, viral particles lacking well-defined features, which can pose diagnostic dilemmas, particularly when they are seen as individual particles, are commonly seen. Thus, a confident diagnosis relies on a repeated observation of identical particles in more than one EM field, with some particles revealing typical morphology.

Among the nonspherical particles, the coronavirus forms pleomorphic structures with well-delineated dumbbell-shaped peplomers, or spikes. Generally, the peplomers form a dark halo around the enveloped capsid. Torovirus-like particles have a less well defined peplomer fringe. A proportion of them are kidney shaped, while others have well-established darker-staining regions in the center of the particle (Fig. 1). The bacteriophages in stool specimens may pose problems since they may be confused with small gastroenteritis viruses, especially if their tails are absent. Membrane blebs can be confused with toroviruses.

Immune EM

The immune EM (IEM) technique has played an important role in the discovery of a number of gastroenteritis viruses, including the prototype Norwalk virus (55, 81). The principle of the technique is to allow virions to form aggregates with specific antibodies by incubation of stool samples with specific antibodies; these aggregates are much easier to identify than the virions alone by EM. A solid-phase IEM is also used to reduce the background of the grid by capture of viruses on an EM grid precoated with specific antibodies (60). IEM is also used to measure antibody responses by comparison of the numbers and sizes of virus-antibody aggregates at different concentrations of serum samples.

Antigen Detection Assays

Antigen detection assays can be highly sensitive and specific if hyperimmune or high-titer monoclonal antibodies are used. Common formats of antigen detection assays include enzyme-linked immunosorbent assay (ELISA) or enzyme immunoassay (EIA), latex agglutination, and rapid membrane-based assays. These assays are simple, fast, and suitable for clinical diagnosis. Due to the difficulty of propagating many gastroenteritis viruses, reliable antigen detection assays remain unavailable for many viral families because of the lack of specific antibodies. In addition, due to the high degrees of genetic and antigenic variations, even existing assays need to be improved for better sensitivity and specificity.

Monoclonal or hyperimmune antibodies against specific viral capsid proteins, such as the VP6 protein of rotaviruses and the capsid protein or the P domain of the capsid protein of noroviruses, have been used in the development of antigen detection assays for diagnosis of gastroenteritis viruses. Due to the lack of a cell culture for human noroviruses, recombinant viral capsid proteins expressed in an in vitro system have been used as the source of reagents for development of the assays. The 96-well plates or the break-away strips are common formats of commercial ELISA kits. Stool suspensions (10 to 20%) are prepared in phosphate-buffered saline (pH 7.4) or sodium carbonate buffer (pH 9.5) for the assays. The assay is usually completed within 2 hours and has a sensitivity equal to or greater than that of EM.

Rapid membrane-based EIAs (immunochromatography) are valuable for small laboratories with demand for diagnosis of sporadic viral gastroenteritis (18). Immunochromatographic kits usually include negative and built-in positive controls to ensure that the reaction has been performed appropriately. The test requires minimal equipment (such as a centrifuge), and the results can be visualized rapidly. Because of their speed, simplicity, and low cost, immunochromatographic kits are amenable for point-of-care testing. In general, immunochromatographic assays have a slightly lower sensitivity and specificity than the ELISA-based kits.

The latex agglutination tests are based on the agglutination of latex beads, coated with virus-specific immunoglobulins, by the virus particles or viral antigens present in the specimens. Since some fecal specimens can cause nonspecific agglutination, negative-control latex beads coated with nonspecific immunoglobulins are also included in the test. Large particles are usually removed from a 10% stool suspension by low-speed centrifugation, and the supernatant is mixed with the latex reagent. A positive reaction is indicated by visible clumping (agglutination) occurring within minutes. The assays are generally less sensitive than ELISAs but are useful in small diagnostic laboratories.

While commercial antigenic detection assays are available for different gastroenteritis viruses, only assays for rotaviruses and EAdVs are recommended for clinical diagnosis (Table 3). The conventional ELISAs for rotaviruses have been on the market for years and are still widely used due to their high sensitivity and specificity and consistent test results. The immunochromatographic tests were introduced at later stages and are useful for rapid diagnosis. In a comparison of seven commercially available immunochromatographic assays with an EIA for the detection of group A rotaviruses in fecal samples, six immunochromatographic assays revealed results comparable with those of the EIA, and only one immunochromatographic assay had a significantly lower detection rate (9). Immunochromatographic tests for the detection of multiple pathogens, such as both rotaviruses and AdVs (bioMérieux and Operon), have also been developed. Direct-comparison studies have shown that these assays have a sensitivity and specificity comparable to those of the EIAs and are useful for rapid diagnosis in ambulatory practice (19, 90).

Not all antigen detection tests for noroviruses and astroviruses are available in the United States. Due to their limited sensitivity and specificity, currently available norovirus antigen assays are used mainly in research laboratories and are not recommended for clinical diagnosis (16). A comparison of two commercial ELISAs, the IDEIA norovirus kit (Dakocytomation Ltd., Ely, United Kingdom) and the Ridascreen norovirus kit (R-Biopharm AG, Darmstadt, Germany), using a panel of 158 fecal samples from 23 outbreaks revealed sensitivities of 38% and 36% and specificities of 96% and 88%, respectively, compared with those of

TABLE 3 Commercial antigen detection tests available for diagnosis of viral gastroenteritis

Manufacturer (URL)	Virus(es) (test[s])
Inverness Medical Professional Diagnostics (www.invernessmedicalpd.com)	Rotavirus (Virogen Rotatest)
Bio-Rad Laboratories (www.bio-rad.com)	Rotavirus (Pastorex Rotavirus, Pathfinder Rotavirus)
Meridian Bioscience (www.meridianbioscience.com)	Rotavirus, AdV (ImmunoCard STAT! Rotavirus ImmunoCard STAT! Adenovirus, Premier Rotaclone, Premier Adenoclone, type 40/41, Rapid Strip Rota-Adeno)
bioMérieux (www.biomerieux.com)	Rotavirus, AdV (Slidex Rota-Kit 2, Slidex Rota-Adeno kit, VIKIA Rota-Adeno)
Orion Diagnostica (www.oriondiagnostica.fi)	Rotavirus, AdV (Rotalex, Adenolex, Diarlex, Diarlex MB)
ANI Biotech (www.anibiotech.fi)	Rotavirus, AdV (Biocard Rota, Biocard Adeno, ANI Rotatest, Biocard Rota Stick, Biocard Adeno Stick)
Dako (www.dako.com)	Rotavirus, AdV, astrovirus, norovirus (IDEIA Rotavirus, IDEIA Adenovirus, IDEIA Astrovirus, IDEIA Norovirus)
R Biopharm AG (www.r-biopharm.com)	Rotavirus, AdV, astrovirus, norovirus (Ridascreen Rotavirus, Ridascreen Adenovirus, Ridascreen Astrovirus, Ridascreen Norovirus)
SA Scientific, San Antonio, TX (http://www.sascientific.com)	Rotavirus, AdV (SAS Rotavirus and SAS)
Denka Seiken Co. Ltd., Tokyo, Japan (http://www.denka-seiken.co.jp)	Norovirus (NV-AD)

reverse transcription-PCR (RT-PCR). Significant numbers of GI and GII viruses were not detected by either ELISA or both ELISAs (16).

In another study, statistical analysis was performed to determine the minimal number of positive samples and the probability of detecting the number of positive samples required to assign norovirus as the causative agent of an outbreak of acute gastroenteritis. The results showed that the probability of detecting a required minimum number of positive samples is low for ELISA compared to that for RT-PCR when small numbers of samples are tested (57% when two samples are tested and 72% when three samples are tested). Thus, using ELISA instead of RT-PCR for the detection of norovirus in stool samples will result in considerable numbers of false-negative results unless a minimum of six samples are tested per outbreak (20).

NAT Assays

Diagnosis based on the detection of viral genomes includes detecting viral DNA or RNA by electrophoresis, hybridization, amplification of the viral DNA or RNA by PCR or RT-PCR, and DNA sequencing. Due to continual improvement of technology, including automation and computerization of methods, nucleic acid detection (NAT) methods are more commonly used in diagnostic laboratories than in the past.

Direct Staining following Electrophoresis

The segmented, double-stranded RNA genome of rotaviruses has traditionally been the target for detection and genotyping (73). The viral RNA is extracted from stool specimens and then subjected to electrophoresis followed by silver staining for detection. This method is as sensitive as EM. It is also applied in the classification of rotaviruses, in which the appearance of an unusual electropherotype may denote a novel strain or group of rotaviruses. Schematic diagrams of electropherotypes of group A to G rotaviruses have been compiled as a reference. Similar methods of electrophoresis have been used for the detection of picobirnaviruses. Direct detection and genotyping of viral DNA has also been used for diagnosis of human EAdVs following treatment of adenoviral genomic DNA with a restriction enzyme.

PCR and RT-PCR

Extraction of Nucleic Acid for PCR or RT-PCR

One of the major challenges of viral detection in stool specimens by PCR or RT-PCR is the presence of inhibitors in the samples, which could lead to a false-negative result. Such inhibitors can be monitored by adding an internal control to the sample during the nucleic acid extraction or purification process. Approaches to reduce inhibition include dilution of extracted nucleic acids; treatment of samples with chelating agents (Chelex 100; Bio-Rad Laboratories), detergents, or denaturing chemicals during RNA extraction (83); and inclusion of amplification facilitators such as bovine serum albumin and betain during the PCR (3). Most commercial nucleic acid extraction protocols use a spin column or magnetic beads, the use of which is simple and efficient, to improve the recovery and purity of nucleic acids from stool specimens.

Nucleic acids extracted from stool specimens usually contain large amounts of nonviral nucleic acids from different microorganisms and host cells that may be nonspecifically amplified by virus-specific primers. These nonspecific PCR products cannot be completely eliminated even under the high-stringency conditions of the reactions. In this case, hybridization with virus-specific probes usually is required to confirm the results (85).

cPCR

Conventional PCR (cPCR or cRT-PCR) refers to the PCR procedures used before the introduction of real-time PCR. cPCR relies on the detection of PCR products by size fractionation, such as by electrophoresis, which is straightforward. By using type-specific primers, cPCR has been widely used to determine the molecular epidemiology of viral gastroenteritis. For example, cRT-PCR is used for genotyping of group A rotaviruses by using primers specific to individual serotypes determined by the two major viral surface neutralization proteins VP7 (G types) and VP4 (P types) (30, 74). cPCR followed by sequencing of the PCR products was also commonly used for determining the molecular epidemiology of gastroenteritis for assessment of genetic variation and for outbreak investigations because most gastroenteritis viruses are genetically diverse (100). Disadvantages of cPCR include the requirement of multiple labor-intensive steps, the risk of contamination due to the open-tube system, and at times the requirement for confirmation by hybridization or sequencing. Thus, while cPCR remains commonly used in research laboratories, real-time PCR has been increasingly used in diagnostic laboratories.

Real-Time PCR

Real-time PCR detects the fluorescent signals from the target sequences of the viral genome in each cycle of amplification, which is rapid and quantitative. The results are analyzed automatically by user-friendly software. Real-time PCR is a closed-tube system which reduces the risk of carryover contamination of amplified DNA. In addition, many of the steps in the primer and probe design and thermal cycling conditions are computerized. Furthermore, many of the reagents used in the assays are commercially available, which further simplifies the procedures and allows reproducible results by reducing variation in the assays. Finally, multiplex real-time PCR has also been developed for the detection of several viruses in a single PCR, which is valuable for broad detection.

Although the real-time PCR technology has been around for a decade, there was no diagnostic kit commercially available for gastroenteritis viruses until recently. Most of the kits were first announced through the Internet (Table 4); examples are kits for norovirus (AnDiaTec, Kornwestheim, Germany), AdV (PrimerDesign Ltd.), and both rotavirus and norovirus (Zj Bio-Tech Co., Ltd., Shanghai, China). Some kits (from Zj Bio-Tech) are flexible and can be applied to different instruments, while others (from AnDiaTec) are specific for the LightCycler (Roche). Due to the lack of information on the designs of these assays, such as the primer sequences that they use, and their performance, such as their specificity, their sensitivity, and the reproducibility of their results for diagnosis in clinical laboratories, the value of these kits for clinical application remains unknown at this point.

In addition to commercial assays, a number of laboratory-developed assays for diagnosis of gastroenteritis viruses have been reported (Table 4). These assays are highly specific and sensitive, with detection limits of 1.5 to 3.6 viral particles per PCR for rotavirus (52) and less than 10 RNA copies per PCR for norovirus (92). The primers of these assays have been selected according to highly conserved regions of the viral genomes, such as those in the VP6,

TABLE 4 Summary of commercial and laboratory development assays using real-time PCR and RT-PCR for detection of enteric viruses associated with gastroenteritis in stool specimens

Virus	Assay[a]	Primers[b]	Probe	Target gene	Length(s) (bp)	Platform(s)	Reference(s) or supplier
Rotavirus	LD	NSP3F/R, NSP3F2[c]	TaqMan	NSP3	87	ABI 7700/7000/7300/7500	79, 79a
	LD	RotaAF1.2/RotaA R1.2	MGB[c]	VP6	145	ABI 7000	65
	LD	VP2F1-5/VP2R1.2	MGB	VP2	79	ABI 7900HT	37
	LD	JVKF/JVKR	TaqMan	NSP3	131	Bio-Rad iCycler	52
	CM	ASR	TaqMan	Not available	Not available	ABI 7000/7300/7500/7900, Smart Cycler-II, iCycler iQ 4/iQ 5, Rotor Gene 2000/3000, Mx3000P/3005P, MJOption2/Chromo4	Zj Bio-Tech
Norovirus	LD	COG1F/G1R, COG2F/G2R (multiplex PCR)	TaqMan	ORF1-ORF2 junction region	85 for G1, 98 for G2	ABI 7700/7000/7300/7500	54, 80
	LD	NV192/193-G1, NV107a,c/ NV119-GII (multiplex RT-PCR)	MGB	ORF1-ORF2 junction region	98 for G1, 94 for G2	ABI PRISM 7700	39
	LD	JJV1F/R-GI, JJV2F/ COG2R-GII	TaqMan	ORF1-ORF2 junction region	96 for G1, 98 for G2	Bio-Rad iCycler, Cepheid SmartCycler, ABI 5700	53
	LD	COG1F/G1R-GI, COG2F/ G2R-GII, Mon4F/R-GIV	TaqMan	ORF1-ORF2 junction region	85 for G1, 98 for G2, 98 for G4	Roche LightCycler	92
	LD	GIF/GIR-GI, GIIF, GIVF/GII&IVR	MGB	ORF1-ORF2 junction region	85 for G1, 97 for G2 and G4	ABI 7000	64
	CM	ASR	TaqMan	Not available	Not available	ABI 7000/7300 /7500/7900, Smart Cycler-II, iCycler iQ 4/iQ 5, Rotor Gene 2000/3000, Mx3000P/3005P, MJOption2/Chromo4	Zj Bio-Tech
	CM	ASR	TaqMan	Not available	Not available	Roche LightCycler	AnDiaTec
Sapovirus	LD	sapoFa&Fb/sapoR SaV124F, SaV1F, SaV5F/SaV1245R	MGB	Polymerase	104	ABI 7000	64
			MGB	Polymerase-capsid junction	104	ABI 7500 Fast	77
		SapoF/R	TaqMan	Polymerase	Not Available	ABI 7500	36
		CU-SVF1, CU-SVF2/ Cu-SVR	TaqMan	Polymerase-capsid junction	104	Bio-Rad iCycler	12
EAdV	LD	AdenoF/AdenoR	MGB	Hexon	130	ABI 7000	65
	LD	EAdVF/R	TaqMan	Hexon	135	ABI 7500	56
	CM	ASR	TaqMan	Hexon	Not available	Real-time PCR instruments (not specific)	PrimerDesign Ltd.
Astrovirus	LD	AV1/AV2	TaqMan	Capsid	90	ABI 7700/7000	57
	LD	AstU1-4/AstL1-2	TaqMan	Capsid	218	ABI 7000	33
	LD	HastF/HastR	MGB	Capsid	67	ABI 7000	64
Bocavirus	LD	Fwd/Rev	TaqMan	NS1/NP-1	88/81	Bio-Rad iCycler	67

[a]LD, laboratory development assay; CM, commercial assay.
[b]ASR, analyte-specific reagents.
[c]MGB, minor groove buffer.

VP2, and NP3 genes of rotaviruses. The primers targeting the NP3 gene are particularly useful for broad detection and have been demonstrated to be able to detect most of the common genotypes (G1 to G4 and G9) as well as some rare genotypes, such as G10 and G12 of rotaviruses (52).

Primers targeting the highly conserved junction regions between ORF1 and ORF2 of the norovirus genome have been used for the detection of human noroviruses by real-time PCR, and the assays are highly sensitive for broad detection of many genotypes of noroviruses (54). With primers specific to individual genogroups (GI and GII), a multiplex real-time PCR (using the ABI Prism PCR system) which is highly sensitive and useful for typing noroviruses has been developed (80). It also increases testing efficiency by reducing test time (50%) and test reagent costs compared with those of other real-time PCR methods. A LightCycler real-time RT-PCR assay with additional primers and a probe targeting the GIV norovirus has also been developed (92). Currently, this and the multiplex assays are widely used in clinical as well as research laboratories worldwide, especially in North America.

There are only a few laboratory-developed real-time PCR assays for the detection of EAdV. A real-time PCR assay targeting the conserved hexon gene was reported using two minor groove binder/nonfluorescent quencher probes in an ABI Prism 7000 (65). This assay showed a high sensitivity and specificity and an increased detection rate (175%) in comparison with those of EM.

DNA Oligonucleotide Microarray

The DNA oligonucleotide microarray is another NAT-based detection technique that has been explored for the detection of norovirus and rotavirus (13, 46). Microarray methods require a small volume of sample and can detect multiple pathogens simultaneously, which is useful for disease surveillance, such as in identifying the source of outbreaks and monitoring epidemic patterns for disease control and prevention. The method is basically qualitative and may require a step to clean up the clinical samples for best hybridization results. However, this method has not been used for clinical diagnosis.

ISOLATION PROCEDURES

Cell Culture

While growth in cell culture has a major impact on the detection of some viruses from clinical specimens, it is generally time-consuming and not considered sufficiently rapid to contribute to meaningful management of a disease like acute gastroenteritis. In addition, most of the enteric viruses causing human gastroenteritis are fastidious in cell culture and require multiple passages before they can readily grow in cell culture from their primary isolation. Therefore, cell culture is not routinely used in clinical diagnosis of viral gastroenteritis. Propagation of human caliciviruses, human coronaviruses, toroviruses, picobirnaviruses, and bocaviruses in cell culture has not yet been achieved.

Rotaviruses

Cell lines for isolation of rotaviruses include MDBK, PK-15, BSC-1, LLC-MK2, MA104, CaCo-2, and HRT-29. To grow the viruses in cell culture, the medium must be supplemented with proteases such as trypsin or pancreatin. This approach was adapted for titration of viruses by plaque assay and serotyping by virus neutralization.

Human Caliciviruses

Propagation of human caliciviruses in cell culture has not yet been achieved. A method of using a three-dimensional organoid model of human small intestinal epithelium for cultivation of human noroviruses was reported but has not been reproduced by other laboratories. The porcine enteric calicivirus, a sapovirus, has been successfully adapted in porcine kidney cell lines but only in the presence of intestinal contents of pigs as a supplement in the culture medium. The murine norovirus has been reported to replicate in primary dendritic cells and macrophages (98).

Enteric Adenoviruses

EAdV types 40 and 41 grow best in the Graham 293 human embryonic kidney cell line, which has been transformed by AdV type 5 DNA. A plaque assay has been developed recently for the detection of EAdVs types 40 and 41 (15).

Astroviruses

Isolation of astroviruses from clinical samples is difficult, although most of the astrovirus serotypes have been adapted in HEK or LLC-MK2 cell culture (89). Propagation of astroviruses in cell culture requires the presence of trypsin in the culture medium.

IDENTIFICATION

Typing Systems

Both antigenic and genetic typing methods are important in understanding the classification and epidemiology of many gastroenteritis viruses and for developing preventive strategies against the diseases caused by these pathogens. Typing does not affect clinical treatment. Therefore, typing of gastroenteritis viruses is used mainly in research laboratories.

Rotaviruses

According to antigenic and genetic variations in the two major surface proteins of rotaviruses, VP7 and VP4, a dual system of antigenic (serotyping) and genetic typing has been used for the classification of human group A rotaviruses. The antigenic typing is accomplished by characterizing the specific interaction of a rotavirus with a panel of monoclonal antibodies representing individual G (VP7) and P (VP4) types of rotaviruses. The genetic typing is performed by RT-PCR using type-specific primers targeting unique regions of the VP7 and VP4 genes. Using this classification system, each strain of rotaviruses is dually assigned to a G and [P] type by either the antigenic or the genetic typing method. The antigenic typing results are highly correlated with the genetic typing for the G types, while the correlation between antigenic and genetic typing for the P types is low. Due to a limited supply of type-specific antibodies, P genotyping is commonly used. Frequent genetic and antigenic drifting of rotaviruses may result in newly emerging variants which are no longer detectable by the current typing assays (45, 82). It becomes necessary to update the methods and reagents continuously, such as with type-specific monoclonal antibodies for the antigenic typing and primers for the genotyping.

Rotaviruses are also typeable based on the genetic variations in the major structure protein VP6 and the putative viral enterotoxin NSP4 genes. The recently recommended new classification system based on sequence information for all 11 genomic RNA segments is an extension of the previous classification systems (69). While this new system is challenging due to the requirement of sequencing all 11 genomic segments, it will eventually impact our understanding of the genetic variation, host-pathogen interaction, evolution, and potentially zoonotic nature of human rotaviruses.

Caliciviruses

Genetic typing has been used mainly for human norovirus identification and classification due to the lack of an efficient cell culture or animal model for a neutralization assay. The wide genetic diversity of human noroviruses also restricts the methods used for the G and P typing of human rotaviruses based on type-specific primers, although genogroup-specific RT-PCR using the GI and GII group-specific primers has been developed (70). Thus, genetic typing of human noroviruses is based mainly on sequencing of the amplified DNA products following RT-PCR detection. Primers from the highly conserved RNA-dependent RNA polymerase genes have been commonly used. However, primers targeting the viral capsid proteins are recommended because the viral capsids are directly involved in host-receptor interaction and immune responses. Sequence alignment followed by phylogenetic analysis has been commonly applied for the classification of human noroviruses, and there are ~30 genotypes associated with acute human gastroenteritis in two major genogroups (GI and GII) of noroviruses.

Enteric Adenoviruses

Genomic DNA restriction enzyme analysis was commonly used before monoclonal antibody-based EIA typing was developed for the detection and typing of EAdVs (72). In addition, typing PCR or PCR in combination with restriction enzyme analysis has also been developed for the detection and typing of AdVs (2, 99). Recently, a quantitative real-time PCR assay was described for detecting HAdVs and identifying AdVs of types 40 and 41 (51). Field surveillance using various methods suggests that the choice of diagnostic method may influence the epidemiologic picture and disease burden attributed to EAdV infections (6).

Astroviruses

For typing of astroviruses, immunologic assays, such as IEM and typing ELISA, have been described but are not commercially available (75, 76). The most commonly used RT-PCR typing methods for astroviruses are summarized in a recent review by Guix et al. (35).

SEROLOGIC TESTS

Antibody neutralization tests based on plaque reduction or epitope-blocking assays using type-specific monoclonal antibodies have been described for rotaviruses. There is no neutralization-based serologic test for most other gastroenteritis viruses. However, ELISAs for antibody detection using specific viral proteins as the capture antigens have been used in epidemiology studies of gastroenteritis viruses. Recombinant viral capsid proteins of caliciviruses and astroviruses generated in the baculovirus and other systems are an excellent source of viral antigens for these studies (49). Application of these assays in sero-surveillance against gastroenteritis viruses has played an important role in understanding the importance of these viruses in different populations. Monitoring seroconversion based on a collection of paired acute- and convalescent-phase sera has been used in outbreak investigations.

ANTIVIRAL SUSCEPTIBILITIES

There are no effective antiviral agents available for the prevention or treatment of viral gastroenteritis. Candidate antivirals have been tested in animal models or in vitro but are not used for human treatment.

EVALUATION, INTERPRETATION, AND REPORTING OF RESULTS

Although a laboratory diagnosis may not help for treating the disease, a prompt diagnosis of viral gastroenteritis is important to avoid unnecessary use of antibiotics. Increasing data have shown that the major gastroenteritis viruses, such as EAdVs, rotaviruses, and noroviruses, can cause chronic gastroenteritis with prolonged shedding of viruses in the stools of recipients of transplanted organs, HIV patients, and other immunocompromised individuals. Prompt diagnosis in these clinical settings is important to adjust immunosuppressive therapy, to assess prognosis, and to stop the transmission of the disease. Rapid identification and monitoring of the source of infection in outbreaks of acute gastroenteritis, such as water, food, and environmental surfaces, is also important for disease control and prevention in the community. Early identification of food handlers with subclinical infection or chronic shedding of viruses is believed to be important for the prevention of food-borne outbreaks.

EM remains a simple and rapid method for clinical diagnosis of viral gastroenteritis, although it is less sensitive than most molecular diagnostic methods. It also requires experienced individuals who are familiar with the morphologies of different gastroenteritis viruses and who are able to differentiate atypical viral particles from unrelated cellular and microbial debris and structures commonly seen in stool specimens. The use of reference grids (81) with typical viral morphologies of gastroenteritis viruses is helpful for a person who is new to the field to gain such experience. IEM is useful for identifying unknown viral pathogens that may be an etiology of acute gastroenteritis, but this method is not widely used in diagnostic laboratories.

The antigen detection methods are highly sensitive and specific and therefore the best choice for clinical diagnosis if available. Commercial antigen detection assays for rotaviruses, EAdVs, and astroviruses are useful for clinical diagnosis (Table 3). Antigenic tests based on type-specific monoclonal antibodies against the G and P types of rotaviruses and various types of astroviruses are widely used in research laboratories. Commercial antigen detection assays for human noroviruses suffer from a lack of sensitivity and specificity and are not recommended for clinical diagnosis, although they may be useful for outbreak investigations.

Nucleic acid-based assays, such as PCR and RT-PCR, are highly sensitive and specific and increasingly used for clinical diagnosis; real-time PCR methods have the added benefit of being rapid and potentially providing quantitative results. While less useful in clinical diagnosis, cPCR with type-specific primers and sequencing of the amplified product is useful for determining the molecular epidemiology of viral gastroenteritis.

Most gastroenteritis viral families are genetically diverse, which makes clinical diagnosis using PCR and RT-PCR difficult. Human noroviruses have over 30 recognized genetic clusters within three genogroups (32). Using primers targeting highly conserved regions of the genomes, the majority of known human noroviruses are detected, but there is probably no single primer pair that can detect all strains.

In this case, multiple primer sets targeting different regions of the genome can be used to enhance the detection rates. In addition, degenerate primers based on sequence variations of known viral family members have also been used (23, 24, 26).

Diagnosis of viral gastroenteritis remains difficult because of the lack of readily available commercial kits for many viral families. The fact that a variety of microbial pathogens, including bacterial and parasitic agents, in addition to viruses, as well as noninfectious agents, cause acute gastroenteritis in humans further complicates the situation. Furthermore, many viral pathogens are known to cause subclinical infection. Others, such as AdV, can be shed for prolonged periods in stools. In some cases, more than one pathogen is detected in the same clinical sample or during the same episode of clinical illness, complicating efforts to determine the true etiology. Thus, care needs to be taken in the interpretation of laboratory results for gastroenteritis viruses. Proper epidemiologic case-control studies are necessary to address these issues.

REFERENCES

1. **Abad, F. X., R. M. Pinto, and A. Bosch.** 1994. Survival of enteric viruses on environmental fomites. *Appl. Environ. Microbiol.* **60:**3704–3710.
2. **Allard, A., B. Albinsson, and G. Wadell.** 2001. Rapid typing of human adenoviruses by a general PCR combined with restriction endonuclease analysis. *J. Clin. Microbiol.* **39:**498–505.
3. **Al-Soud, W. A., and P. Radstrom.** 2001. Purification and characterization of PCR-inhibitory components in blood cells. *J. Clin. Microbiol.* **39:**485–493.
4. **Ball, J. M., P. Tian, C. Q. Zeng, A. P. Morris, and M. K. Estes.** 1996. Age-dependent diarrhea induced by a rotaviral nonstructural glycoprotein. *Science* **272:**101–104.
5. **Banyai, K., A. Bogdan, G. Domonkos, P. Kisfali, P. Molnar, A. Toth, B. Melegh, V. Martella, J. R. Gentsch, and G. Szucs.** 2009. Genetic diversity and zoonotic potential of human rotavirus strains, 2003–2006, Hungary. *J. Med. Virol.* **81:**362–370.
6. **Banyai, K., P. Kisfali, A. Bogdan, V. Martella, B. Melegh, D. Erdman, and G. Szucs.** 2009. Adenovirus gastroenteritis in Hungary, 2003–2006. *Eur. J. Clin. Microbiol. Infect. Dis.* **28:**997–999.
7. **Belliot, G., H. Laveran, and S. S. Monroe.** 1997. Detection and genetic differentiation of human astroviruses: phylogenetic grouping varies by coding region. *Arch. Virol.* **142:**1323–1334.
8. **Belliot, G., H. Laveran, and S. S. Monroe.** 1997. Outbreak of gastroenteritis in military recruits associated with serotype 3 astrovirus infection. *J. Med. Virol.* **51:**101–106.
9. **Bon, F., J. Kaplon, M. H. Metzger, and P. Pothier.** 2007. Evaluation of seven immunochromatographic assays for the rapid detection of human rotaviruses in fecal specimens. *Pathol. Biol.* (Paris) **55:**149–153. (In French.)
10. **Buesa, J., R. Montava, R. Abu-Mallouh, M. Fos, J. M. Ribes, R. Bartolome, H. Vanaclocha, N. Torner, and A. Dominguez.** 2008. Sequential evolution of genotype GII.4 norovirus variants causing gastroenteritis outbreaks from 2001 to 2006 in eastern Spain. *J. Med. Virol.* **80:**1288–1295.
11. **Carraturo, A., V. Catalani, and L. Tega.** 2008. Microbiological and epidemiological aspects of rotavirus and enteric adenovirus infections in hospitalized children in Italy. *New Microbiol.* **31:**329–336.
12. **Chan, M. C., J. J. Sung, R. K. Lam, P. K. Chan, R. W. Lai, and W. K. Leung.** 2006. Sapovirus detection by quantitative real-time RT-PCR in clinical stool specimens. *J. Virol. Methods* **134:**146–153.
13. **Chizhikov, V., M. Wagner, A. Ivshina, Y. Hoshino, A. Z. Kapikian, and K. Chumakov.** 2002. Detection and genotyping of human group A rotaviruses by oligonucleotide microarray hybridization. *J. Clin. Microbiol.* **40:**2398–2407.
14. **Cortese, M. M., and U. D. Parashar.** 2009. Prevention of rotavirus gastroenteritis among infants and children: recommendations of the Advisory Committee on Immunization Practices (ACIP). *MMWR Recomm. Rep.* **58:**1–25.
15. **Cromeans, T. L., X. Lu, D. D. Erdman, C. D. Humphrey, and V. R. Hill.** 2008. Development of plaque assays for adenoviruses 40 and 41. *J. Virol. Methods* **151:**140–145.
16. **de Bruin, E., E. Duizer, H. Vennema, and M. P. Koopmans.** 2006. Diagnosis of norovirus outbreaks by commercial ELISA or RT-PCR. *J. Virol. Methods* **137:**259–264.
17. **de Jong, J. C., A. D. Osterhaus, M. S. Jones, and B. Harrach.** 2008. Human adenovirus type 52: a type 41 in disguise? *J. Virol.* **82:**3809–3810. (Letter.)
18. **Dennehy, P. H., M. Hartin, S. M. Nelson, and S. F. Reising.** 1999. Evaluation of the ImmunoCardSTAT! rotavirus assay for detection of group A rotavirus in fecal specimens. *J. Clin. Microbiol.* **37:**1977–1979.
19. **de Rougemont, A., J. Kaplon, G. Billaud, B. Lina, S. Pinchinat, T. Derrough, E. Caulin, P. Pothier, and D. Floret.** 2008. Sensitivity and specificity of the VIKIA® Rota-Adeno immuno-chromatographic test (bioMérieux) and the ELISA IDEIA™ rotavirus kit (Dako) compared to genotyping. *Pathol. Biol.* (Paris) **57:**86–89. (In French.)
20. **Duizer, E., A. Pielaat, H. Vennema, A. Kroneman, and M. Koopmans.** 2007. Probabilities in norovirus outbreak diagnosis. *J. Clin. Virol.* **40:**38–42.
21. **Estes, M.** 2001. Rotaviruses and their replication, p. 1747–1785. D. M. Knipe, P. M. Howley, D. E. Griffin, R. A. Lamb, M. A. Martin, B. Roizman, and S. E. Straus (ed.), *Fields Virology*, 4th ed. Lippincott Williams & Wilkins, Philadelphia, PA.
22. **Estes, M. K., and A. P. Morris.** 1999. A viral enterotoxin. A new mechanism of virus-induced pathogenesis. *Adv. Exp. Med. Biol.* **473:**73–82.
23. **Fankhauser, R. L., S. S. Monroe, J. S. Noel, C. D. Humphrey, J. S. Bresee, U. D. Parashar, T. Ando, and R. I. Glass.** 2002. Epidemiologic and molecular trends of "Norwalk-like viruses" associated with outbreaks of gastroenteritis in the United States. *J. Infect. Dis.* **186:**1–7.
24. **Farkas, T., T. Berke, G. Reuter, G. Szucs, D. O. Matson, and X. Jiang.** 2002. Molecular detection and sequence analysis of human caliciviruses from acute gastroenteritis outbreaks in Hungary. *J. Med. Virol.* **67:**567–573.
25. **Farkas, T., K. Sestak, C. Wei, and X. Jiang.** 2008. Characterization of a rhesus monkey calicivirus representing a new genus of *Caliciviridae*. *J. Virol.* **82:**5408–5416.
26. **Farkas, T., W. M. Zhong, Y. Jing, P. W. Huang, S. M. Espinosa, N. Martinez, A. L. Morrow, G. M. Ruiz-Palacios, L. K. Pickering, and X. Jiang.** 2004. Genetic diversity among sapoviruses. *Arch. Virol.* **149:**1309–1323.
27. **Fischer, S. A.** 2008. Emerging viruses in transplantation: there is more to infection after transplant than CMV and EBV. *Transplantation* **86:**1327–1339.
28. **Fregolente, M. C., E. de Castro-Dias, S. S. Martins, F. R. Spilki, S. M. Allegretti, and M. S. Gatti.** 2009. Molecular characterization of picobirnaviruses from new hosts. *Virus Res.* **143:**134–136.
29. **Gary, G. W., Jr., J. C. Hierholzer, and R. E. Black.** 1979. Characteristics of noncultivable adenoviruses associated with diarrhea in infants: a new subgroup of human adenoviruses. *J. Clin. Microbiol.* **10:**96–103.
30. **Gouvea, V., R. I. Glass, P. Woods, K. Taniguchi, H. F. Clark, B. Forrester, and Z. Y. Fang.** 1990. Polymerase chain reaction amplification and typing of rotavirus nucleic acid from stool specimens. *J. Clin. Microbiol.* **28:**276–282.
31. **Green, K., R. Chanock, and A. Kapikian.** 2001. Human calicivirus, p. 841–874. *In* D. M. Knipe, P. M. Howley, D. E. Griffin, R. A. Lamb, M. A. Martin, B. Roizman, and S. E. Straus (ed.), *Fields Virology*, 4th ed., vol. 2. Lippincott Williams & Wilkins, Philadelphia, PA.
32. **Green, K. Y., T. Ando, M. S. Balayan, T. Berke, I. N. Clarke, M. K. Estes, D. O. Matson, S. Nakata, J. D. Neill, M. J. Studdert, and H. J. Thiel.** 2000. Taxonomy of the caliciviruses. *J. Infect. Dis.* **181**(Suppl. 2):S322–S330.

33. **Grimm, A. C., J. L. Cashdollar, F. P. Williams, and G. S. Fout.** 2004. Development of an astrovirus RT-PCR detection assay for use with conventional, real-time, and integrated cell culture/RT-PCR. *Can. J. Microbiol.* **50:**269–278.

34. **Grohmann, G. S., R. I. Glass, H. G. Pereira, S. S. Monroe, A. W. Hightower, R. Weber, and R. T. Bryan, for the Enteric Opportunistic Infections Working Group.** 1993. Enteric viruses and diarrhea in HIV-infected patients. *N. Engl. J. Med.* **329:**14–20.

35. **Guix, S., A. Bosch, and R. M. Pinto.** 2005. Human astrovirus diagnosis and typing: current and future prospects. *Lett. Appl. Microbiol.* **41:**103–105.

36. **Gunson, R. N., T. C. Collins, and W. F. Carman.** 2006. The real-time detection of sapovirus. *J. Clin. Virol.* **35:**321–322.

37. **Gutierrez-Aguirre, I., M. Banjac, A. Steyer, M. Poljsak-Prijatelj, M. Peterka, A. Strancar, and M. Ravnikar.** 2008. Concentrating rotaviruses from water samples using monolithic chromatographic supports. *J. Chromatogr. A* **1216:**2700–2704.

38. **Hansman, G. S., T. Oka, K. Katayama, and N. Takeda.** 2007. Human sapoviruses: genetic diversity, recombination, and classification. *Rev. Med. Virol.* **17:**133–141.

39. **Hoehne, M., and E. Schreier.** 2006. Detection of norovirus genogroup I and II by multiplex real-time RT-PCR using a 3'-minor groove binder-DNA probe. *BMC Infect. Dis.* **6:**69.

40. **Holmes, K.** 2001. Coronaviruses, p. 1187–1203. *In* D. M. Knipe, P. M. Howley, D. E. Griffin, R. A. Lamb, M. A. Martin, B. Roizman, and S. E. Straus (ed.), *Fields Virology,* 4th ed., vol. 2. Lippincott Williams & Wilkins, Philadelphia, PA.

41. **Horowitz, M.** 2001. Adenoviruses, p. 2301–2326. *In* D. M. Knipe, P. M. Howley, D. E. Griffin, R. A. Lamb, M. A. Martin, B. Roizman, and S. E. Straus (ed.), *Fields Virology,* 4th ed. Lippincott Williams & Wilkins, Philadelphia, PA.

42. **Huang, P., T. Farkas, W. Zhong, M. Tan, S. Thornton, A. L. Morrow, and X. Jiang.** 2005. Norovirus and histo-blood group antigens: demonstration of a wide spectrum of strain specificities and classification of two major binding groups among multiple binding patterns. *J. Virol.* **79:**6714–6722.

43. **Hudson, R. W., J. E. Herrmann, and N. R. Blacklow.** 1989. Plaque quantitation and virus neutralization assays for human astroviruses. *Arch. Virol.* **108:**33–38.

44. **Ishiko, H., and K. Aoki.** 2009. Spread of epidemic keratoconjunctivitis due to a novel serotype of human adenovirus in Japan. *J. Clin. Microbiol.* **47:**2678–2679.

45. **Iturriza-Gomara, M., G. Kang, and J. Gray.** 2004. Rotavirus genotyping: keeping up with an evolving population of human rotaviruses. *J. Clin. Virol.* **31:**259–265.

46. **Jaaskelainen, A. J., and L. Maunula.** 2006. Applicability of microarray technique for the detection of noro- and astroviruses. *J. Virol. Methods* **136:**210–216.

47. **Jiang, X., D. Y. Graham, K. N. Wang, and M. K. Estes.** 1990. Norwalk virus genome cloning and characterization. *Science* **250:**1580–1583.

48. **Jiang, X., M. Wang, K. Wang, and M. K. Estes.** 1993. Sequence and genomic organization of Norwalk virus. *Virology* **195:**51–61.

49. **Jiang, X., N. Wilton, W. M. Zhong, T. Farkas, P. W. Huang, E. Barrett, M. Guerrero, G. Ruiz-Palacios, K. Y. Green, J. Green, A. D. Hale, M. K. Estes, L. K. Pickering, and D. O. Matson.** 2000. Diagnosis of human caliciviruses by use of enzyme immunoassays. *J. Infect. Dis.* **181**(Suppl. 2)**:**S349–S359.

50. **Jones, M. S., II, B. Harrach, R. D. Ganac, M. M. Gozum, W. P. Dela Cruz, B. Riedel, C. Pan, E. L. Delwart, and D. P. Schnurr.** 2007. New adenovirus species found in a patient presenting with gastroenteritis. *J. Virol.* **81:**5978–5984.

51. **Jothikumar, N., T. L. Cromeans, V. R. Hill, X. Lu, M. D. Sobsey, and D. D. Erdman.** 2005. Quantitative real-time PCR assays for detection of human adenoviruses and identification of serotypes 40 and 41. *Appl. Environ. Microbiol.* **71:**3131–3136.

52. **Jothikumar, N., G. Kang, and V. R. Hill.** 2009. Broadly reactive TaqMan assay for real-time RT-PCR detection of rotavirus in clinical and environmental samples. *J. Virol. Methods* **155:**126–131.

53. **Jothikumar, N., J. A. Lowther, K. Henshilwood, D. N. Lees, V. R. Hill, and J. Vinje.** 2005. Rapid and sensitive detection of noroviruses by using TaqMan-based one-step reverse transcription-PCR assays and application to naturally contaminated shellfish samples. *Appl. Environ. Microbiol.* **71:**1870–1875.

54. **Kageyama, T., S. Kojima, M. Shinohara, K. Uchida, S. Fukushi, F. B. Hoshino, N. Takeda, and K. Katayama.** 2003. Broadly reactive and highly sensitive assay for Norwalk-like viruses based on real-time quantitative reverse transcription-PCR. *J. Clin. Microbiol.* **41:**1548–1557.

55. **Kapikian, A. Z., R. G. Wyatt, R. Dolin, T. S. Thornhill, A. R. Kalica, and R. M. Chanock.** 1972. Visualization by immune electron microscopy of a 27-nm particle associated with acute infectious nonbacterial gastroenteritis. *J. Virol.* **10:**1075–1081.

56. **Ko, G., N. Jothikumar, V. R. Hill, and M. D. Sobsey.** 2005. Rapid detection of infectious adenoviruses by mRNA real-time RT-PCR. *J. Virol. Methods* **127:**148–153.

57. **Le Cann, P., S. Ranarijaona, S. Monpoeho, F. Le Guyader, and V. Ferre.** 2004. Quantification of human astroviruses in sewage using real-time RT-PCR. *Res. Microbiol.* **155:**11–15.

58. **Lee, B. E., X. L. Pang, J. L. Robinson, D. Bigam, S. S. Monroe, and J. K. Preiksaitis.** 2008. Chronic norovirus and adenovirus infection in a solid organ transplant recipient. *Pediatr. Infect. Dis. J.* **27:**360–362.

59. **Lee, T. W., and J. B. Kurtz.** 1994. Prevalence of human astrovirus serotypes in the Oxford region 1976–92, with evidence for two new serotypes. *Epidemiol. Infect.* **112:**187–193.

60. **Lewis, D., T. Ando, C. D. Humphrey, S. S. Monroe, and R. I. Glass.** 1995. Use of solid-phase immune electron microscopy for classification of Norwalk-like viruses into six antigenic groups from 10 outbreaks of gastroenteritis in the United States. *J. Clin. Microbiol.* **33:**501–504.

61. **Lewis, D. C., N. F. Lightfoot, W. D. Cubitt, and S. A. Wilson.** 1989. Outbreaks of astrovirus type 1 and rotavirus gastroenteritis in a geriatric in-patient population. *J. Hosp. Infect.* **14:**9–14.

62. **Lindesmith, L. C., E. F. Donaldson, A. D. Lobue, J. L. Cannon, D. P. Zheng, J. Vinje, and R. S. Baric.** 2008. Mechanisms of GII.4 norovirus persistence in human populations. *PLoS Med.* **5:**e31.

63. **Lindner, J., and S. Modrow.** 2008. Human bocavirus—a novel parvovirus to infect humans. *Intervirology* **51:**116–122.

64. **Logan, C., J. O'Leary, and N. O'Sullivan.** 2007. Real-time reverse transcription PCR detection of norovirus, sapovirus and astrovirus as causative agents of acute viral gastroenteritis. *J. Virol. Methods* **146:**36–44.

65. **Logan, C., J. J. O'Leary, and N. O'Sullivan.** 2006. Real-time reverse transcription-PCR for detection of rotavirus and adenovirus as causative agents of acute viral gastroenteritis in children. *J. Clin. Microbiol.* **44:**3189–3195.

66. **Long, S. S.** 2008. Evidence of norovirus causing necrotizing enterocolitis (NEC) in a NICU. *J. Pediatr.* **153:**A2.

67. **Lu, X., M. Chittaganpitch, S. J. Olsen, I. M. Mackay, T. P. Sloots, A. M. Fry, and D. D. Erdman.** 2006. Real-time PCR assays for detection of bocavirus in human specimens. *J. Clin. Microbiol.* **44:**3231–3235.

68. **Matthijnssens, J., M. Ciarlet, E. Heiman, I. Arijs, T. Delbeke, S. M. McDonald, E. A. Palombo, M. Iturriza-Gomara, P. Maes, J. T. Patton, M. Rahman, and M. Van Ranst.** 2008. Full genome-based classification of rotaviruses reveals a common origin between human Wa-like and porcine rotavirus strains and human DS-1-like and bovine rotavirus strains. *J. Virol.* **82:**3204–3219.

69. **Matthijnssens, J., M. Ciarlet, M. Rahman, H. Attoui, K. Banyai, M. K. Estes, J. R. Gentsch, M. Iturriza-Gomara, C. D. Kirkwood, V. Martella, P. P. Mertens, O. Nakagomi, J. T. Patton, F. M. Ruggeri, L. J. Saif, N. Santos, A. Steyer, K. Taniguchi, U. Desselberger, and M. Van Ranst.** 2008. Recommendations for the classification of group A rotaviruses using all 11 genomic RNA segments. *Arch. Virol.* **153:**1621–1629.

70. **Mattison, K., E. Grudeski, B. Auk, H. Charest, S. J. Drews, A. Fritzinger, N. Gregoricus, S. Hayward, A. Houde, B. E. Lee, X. L. Pang, J. Wong, T. F. Booth, and J. Vinje.** 2009. Multicenter comparison of two norovirus ORF2-based genotyping protocols. *J. Clin. Microbiol.* **47:**3927–3932.

71. **Midthun, K., H. B. Greenberg, J. B. Kurtz, G. W. Gary, F. Y. Lin, and A. Z. Kapikian.** 1993. Characterization and seroepidemiology of a type 5 astrovirus associated with an outbreak of gastroenteritis in Marin County, California. *J. Clin. Microbiol.* **31:**955–962.

72. **Moore, P. L., A. D. Steele, and J. J. Alexander.** 2000. Relevance of commercial diagnostic tests to detection of enteric adenovirus infections in South Africa. *J. Clin. Microbiol.* **38:**1661–1663.

73. **Moosai, R. B., M. J. Carter, and C. R. Madeley.** 1984. Rapid detection of enteric adenovirus and rotavirus: a simple method using polyacrylamide gel electrophoresis. *J. Clin. Pathol.* **37:**1404–1408.

74. **Nakagomi, O., H. Oyamada, and T. Nakagomi.** 1991. Experience with serotyping rotavirus strains by reverse transcription and two-step polymerase chain reaction with generic and type-specific primers. *Mol. Cell. Probes* **5:**285–289.

75. **Noel, J., and D. Cubitt.** 1994. Identification of astrovirus serotypes from children treated at the Hospitals for Sick Children, London 1981–93. *Epidemiol. Infect.* **113:**153–159.

76. **Noel, J. S., T. W. Lee, J. B. Kurtz, R. I. Glass, and S. S. Monroe.** 1995. Typing of human astroviruses from clinical isolates by enzyme immunoassay and nucleotide sequencing. *J. Clin. Microbiol.* **33:**797–801.

77. **Oka, T., K. Katayama, G. S. Hansman, T. Kageyama, S. Ogawa, F. T. Wu, P. A. White, and N. Takeda.** 2006. Detection of human sapovirus by real-time reverse transcription-polymerase chain reaction. *J. Med. Virol.* **78:**1347–1353.

78. **Oliver, S. L., E. Asobayire, A. M. Dastjerdi, and J. C. Bridger.** 2006. Genomic characterization of the unclassified bovine enteric virus Newbury agent-1 (Newbury1) endorses a new genus in the family Caliciviridae. *Virology* **350:**240–250.

79. **Pang, X., B. Lee, L. Chui, J. K. Preiksaitis, and S. S. Monroe.** 2004. Evaluation and validation of real-time reverse transcription-PCR assay using the LightCycler system for detection and quantitation of norovirus. *J. Clin. Microbiol.* **42:**4679–4685.

79a. **Pang, X., M. Cao, M. Zhang, and B. Lee.** 2011. Increased sensitivity for various rotavirus genotypes in stool specimens by amending three mismatched nucleotides in the forward primer of a real-time RT-PCR assay. *J. Virol. Methods* **172:**85–87.

80. **Pang, X. L., J. K. Preiksaitis, and B. Lee.** 2005. Multiplex real time RT-PCR for the detection and quantitation of norovirus genogroups I and II in patients with acute gastroenteritis. *J. Clin. Virol.* **33:**168–171.

81. **Petric, M., and M. T. Szymanski.** 2000. Electron microscopy and immunoelectron microscopy, p. 54–65. *In* S. Specter, R. L. Hodinka, and S. A. Young (ed.), *Clinical Virology Manual*, 3rd ed. ASM Press, Washington, DC.

81a. **Petric, M., and R. Tellier.** 2003. Rotaviruses, caliciviruses, astroviruses, and other diarrheic viruses, p. 1439–1451. *In* P. R. Murray, E. J. Baron, J. H. Jorgensen, M. A. Pfaller, and R. H. Yolken (ed.), *Manual of Clinical Microbiology*, 8th ed. ASM Press, Washington, DC.

82. **Rahman, M., R. Sultana, G. Podder, A. S. Faruque, J. Matthijnssens, K. Zaman, R. F. Breiman, D. A. Sack, M. Van Ranst, and T. Azim.** 2005. Typing of human rotaviruses: nucleotide mismatches between VP7 gene and primer are associated with genotyping failure. *Virol. J.* **2:**24.

83. **Rasool, N. B., S. S. Monroe, and R. I. Glass.** 2002. Determination of a universal nucleic acid extraction procedure for PCR detection of gastroenteritis viruses in faecal specimens. *J. Virol. Methods* **100:**1–16.

84. **Schofield, K. P., D. J. Morris, A. S. Bailey, J. C. de Jong, and G. Corbitt.** 1994. Gastroenteritis due to adenovirus type 41 in an adult with chronic lymphocytic leukemia. *Clin. Infect. Dis.* **19:**311–312.

85. **Schwab, K. J., M. K. Estes, F. H. Neill, and R. L. Atmar.** 1997. Use of heat release and an internal RNA standard control in reverse transcription-PCR detection of Norwalk virus from stool samples. *J. Clin. Microbiol.* **35:**511–514.

86. **Siebenga, J. J., H. Vennema, E. Duizer, and M. P. Koopmans.** 2007. Gastroenteritis caused by norovirus GGII.4, The Netherlands, 1994–2005. *Emerg. Infect. Dis.* **13:**144–146.

87. **Siebenga, J. J., H. Vennema, B. Renckens, E. de Bruin, B. van der Veer, R. J. Siezen, and M. Koopmans.** 2007. Epochal evolution of GGII.4 norovirus capsid proteins from 1995 to 2006. *J. Virol.* **81:**9932–9941.

88. **Tan, M., and X. Jiang.** 2005. The P domain of norovirus capsid protein forms a subviral particle that binds to histo-blood group antigen receptors. *J. Virol.* **79:**14017–14030.

89. **Taylor, M. B., W. O. Grabow, and W. D. Cubitt.** 1997. Propagation of human astrovirus in the PLC/PRF/5 hepatoma cell line. *J. Virol. Methods* **67:**13–18.

90. **Tellez, C. J., R. Montava, J. M. Ribes, M. D. Tirado, and J. Buesa.** 2008. Evaluation of two immunochromatography kits for rapid diagnosis of rotavirus infections. *Rev. Argent. Microbiol.* **40:**167–170. (In Spanish.)

91. **Trevino, M., E. Prieto, D. Penalver, A. Aguilera, A. Garcia-Zabarte, C. Garcia-Riestra, and B. J. Regueiro.** 2001. Diarrhea caused by adenovirus and astrovirus in hospitalized immunodeficient patients. *Enferm. Infecc. Microbiol. Clin.* **19:**7–10. (In Spanish.)

92. **Trujillo, A. A., K. A. McCaustland, D. P. Zheng, L. A. Hadley, G. Vaughn, S. M. Adams, T. Ando, R. I. Glass, and S. S. Monroe.** 2006. Use of TaqMan real-time reverse transcription-PCR for rapid detection, quantification, and typing of norovirus. *J. Clin. Microbiol.* **44:**1405–1412.

93. **Turcios-Ruiz, R. M., P. Axelrod, K. St. John, E. Bullitt, J. Donahue, N. Robinson, and H. E. Friss.** 2008. Outbreak of necrotizing enterocolitis caused by norovirus in a neonatal intensive care unit. *J. Pediatr.* **153:**339–344.

94. **Van Regenmortel, M., C. M. Fauquet, D. H. L. Bishop, E. Carstens, M. K. Estes, S. Lemon, J. Maniloff, M. A. Mayo, D. J. McGeoch, C. R. Pringle, and R. Wickner.** 1999. *Virus Taxonomy: Classification and Nomenclature of Viruses. Seventh Report of the International Committee on Taxonomy of Viruses.* Academic Press, New York, NY.

95. **Walsh, M. P., A. Chintakuntlawar, C. M. Robinson, I. Madisch, B. Harrach, N. R. Hudson, D. Schnurr, A. Heim, J. Chodosh, D. Seto, and M. S. Jones.** 2009. Evidence of molecular evolution driven by recombination events influencing tropism in a novel human adenovirus that causes epidemic keratoconjunctivitis. *PLoS One* **4:**e5635.

96. **Walter, J. E., and D. K. Mitchell.** 2003. Astrovirus infection in children. *Curr. Opin. Infect. Dis.* **16:**247–253.

97. **Westhoff, T. H., M. Vergoulidou, C. Loddenkemper, S. Schwartz, J. Hofmann, T. Schneider, W. Zidek, and M. van der Giet.** 2009. Chronic norovirus infection in renal transplant recipients. *Nephrol. Dial. Transplant.* **24:**1051–1053.

98. **Wobus, C. E., S. M. Karst, L. B. Thackray, K. O. Chang, S. V. Sosnovtsev, G. Belliot, A. Krug, J. M. Mackenzie, K. Y. Green, and H. W. Virgin.** 2004. Replication of norovirus in cell culture reveals a tropism for dendritic cells and macrophages. *PLoS Biol.* **2:**e432.

99. **Xu, W., M. C. McDonough, and D. D. Erdman.** 2000. Species-specific identification of human adenoviruses by a multiplex PCR assay. *J. Clin. Microbiol.* **38:**4114–4120.

100. **Zheng, D. P., T. Ando, R. L. Fankhauser, R. S. Beard, R. I. Glass, and S. S. Monroe.** 2006. Norovirus classification and proposed strain nomenclature. *Virology* **346:**312–323.

Rabies Virus

LILLIAN A. ORCIARI AND CHARLES E. RUPPRECHT

91

TAXONOMY

The etiologic agents responsible for the acute, progressive viral encephalomyelitis known as rabies belong to the genus *Lyssavirus*. These are single-stranded RNA viruses of the order *Mononegavirales* and family *Rhabdoviridae*, bullet-shaped RNA viruses. The genus includes the prototype species, *Rabies virus*; the less commonly known species of nonrabies lyssaviruses, *Lagos bat virus*, *Mokola virus*, *Duvenhage virus*, *European bat lyssavirus 1*, *European bat lyssavirus 2*, *Australian bat lyssavirus*, *Aravan virus*, *Khujand virus*, *Irkut virus*, and *West Caucasian bat virus*; and the proposed species *Shimoni bat virus* (9, 13). Differences among lyssaviruses were first noticed by serologic cross neutralization studies, which were used to divide them into serogroups (28). More recently differences were based on nucleotide sequence analysis, and lyssaviruses were grouped as different genotypes or species. Current commercial human and animal vaccines are based upon rabies virus and provide adequate cross-protection against most other lyssaviruses, with the exception of *Lagos bat virus*, *Mokola virus*, and *West Caucasian bat virus*.

DESCRIPTION OF THE AGENT

The virions are rod shaped, approximately 180 by 75 nm, consisting of five structural proteins: the glycoprotein (G), matrix protein (M), nucleoprotein (N), phosphoprotein (P), and large polymerase (L). The virus is contained in an envelope bilayer derived from the host cell cytoplasmic membrane during budding (Fig. 1). Peplomers, G protein trimeric spike inserts of approximately 10 nm, are found within the surface of the virus envelope. The rabies virus G protein binds with host cell surface receptors (adsorption), thus initiating a cascade in the infectious cycle and replication. Virus-neutralizing antibodies (VNAs) produced against the G protein after vaccination or natural infection may inhibit this process. The inner surface lining of the envelope is formed by the M protein, which binds with the G protein and envelope and the ribonucleoprotein (RNP) core.

The RNP is composed of tightly wound RNA, encapsidated by the phosphorylated N protein, and associated with the P and L proteins. All lyssaviruses contain nonsegmented genomes (RNA) of approximately 12 kb. The RNA-nucleoprotein complex is responsible for transcription of genomic RNA to five polyadenylated mRNAs which are translated into the structural proteins, and viral replication by providing a template to synthesize complementary full-length (negative-sense) genomic RNA. During assembly the coiling of RNP-M protein binds with the G protein as the completed virus buds from the plasma membrane (30). From a diagnostic viewpoint, the N and G proteins have been the focus of most laboratory research evaluations. Rabies diagnosis is based on the ability to detect intracellular viral inclusions, which are collections of RNP. Since the rabies virus G protein and host cell receptor interactions initiate the infection cycle, the G protein is directly involved in pathogenesis and virulence, induction of immune responses, and binding of neutralizing antibodies. Vaccines prepared from whole virions or purified rabies virus G proteins or recombinant viral vaccines encoding rabies virus G proteins have been used to successfully immunize and protect animals from rabies virus infections (18, 26). Additionally, detection of antibody to the G protein has been used as a method to evaluate vaccine potency. More detailed reviews of virus replication and virus pathogenesis have been published (8). Descriptions of the rabies virus epidemiology, transmission, clinical signs, and diagnosis are generalizable to the other lyssaviruses.

EPIDEMIOLOGY AND TRANSMISSION

Rabies is a zoonotic disease (primarily an animal disease which may be transmitted to humans). All mammals are susceptible. Although rabies viruses are endemic on five of the seven continents, the geographical distributions of the other lyssaviruses are more localized: Lagos bat, Shimoni bat, Mokola, and Duvenhage viruses were detected only in Africa; European bat lyssaviruses, only in Europe; Australian bat virus, exclusively in Australia; Aravan, Khujand, Irkut, and West Caucasian bat viruses, restricted to Eurasia (13). Approximately 7,000 rabies cases occur in animals annually in the United States. In the United States, the predominant terrestrial host species are skunks in California and the north-central and south-central states, gray foxes in Texas and Arizona, Arctic and red foxes in Alaska, mongooses in the U.S. territory of Puerto Rico, and raccoons in the eastern states. Bats are ubiquitous. Although dogs represent a major reservoir species in most developing nations, enzootic canine rabies transmission has been eliminated in

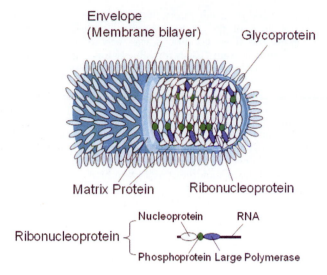

Envelope
(Membrane bilayer)

Glycoprotein

Matrix Protein

Ribonucleoprotein

Ribonucleoprotein { Nucleoprotein RNA Phosphoprotein Large Polymerase

FIGURE 1 Diagram of lyssavirus morphology and structural proteins.

the United States and other developed countries primarily due to canine vaccination programs (1).

Human rabies cases are rare in developed countries, which have controlled canine rabies. Fewer than eight cases are reported annually in the United States. The disease has a significant impact on global health, accounting for an estimated 55,000 human deaths annually. Methods to reduce viral exposures include avoiding contact with stray domestic animals and avoiding contact with wild animals.

Rabies viruses are usually transmitted in infected saliva via the bite of a rabid animal. Human rabies cases due to nonbite exposures are extremely rare. Nonbite exposures include contamination of scratches, open wounds, and mucous membranes with a source of rabies virus, such as infected saliva or central nervous system (CNS) tissues from a rabid animal. Nosocomial infection (inhalation of an aerosolized highly infectious dose of rabies virus) and subsequent mucous membrane contact is a potential source of nonbite exposure. Infection by this route is rare but has been documented (4, 29). No human rabies cases from fomite (surface contamination) exposures have been substantiated, most likely because the virus is inactivated by drying and by the UV rays of sunlight. Immediate wound cleansing with soap and water should be performed if an exposure is suspected, and medical care should be obtained.

Lyssaviruses are susceptible to a number of common laboratory disinfectants, such as 1:256 quaternary ammonium compound, 0.5% sodium hypochlorite (10% bleach), 70% isopropanol, or 70% ethanol. Chemical disinfectants are less effective when used on items contaminated with brain tissues or heavy suspensions of brain tissue. Decontamination of instruments, laboratory glassware, and disposable waste is best achieved by autoclaving at a minimum of 121°C, 15 lb, for 60 min.

CLINICAL SIGNIFICANCE

In the early stages of the clinical course, human rabies may be misdiagnosed because of the nonspecific symptoms, such as flu-like symptoms, associated with the prodromal period.

The usual incubation period is approximately 30 to 90 days after exposure. Following the prodromal period, an acute neurological phase occurs. The majority of rabies cases manifest as an encephalitic form, and less than 20% are observed as a paralytic presentation. Among patients exhibiting classical encephalitic symptoms, generalized arousal or hyperexcitability with intermittent lucid periods may appear, including periods of confusion, hallucinations, agitation or aggressive behavior, autonomic dysfunction, difficulty swallowing, hypersalivation, lacrimation, sweating, and dilated pupils. Cranial nerve deficits include anisocoria and facial or tongue paralysis. Hydrophobic and aerophobic spasms can be dramatic. In the end stage, disease presentation includes cardiopulmonary problems and instability leading to coma, cardiac arrest, and death.

The paralytic form of presentation includes flaccid muscle weakness, frequently spreading in an ascending pattern to the other extremities. In some cases laryngeal and facial muscle weakness or bilateral deafness occurs. These cases may resemble Guillain-Barré syndrome. Other symptoms include urinary incontinence and priapism. Hydrophobia is less common with the paralytic form, but mild inspiratory spasms may be present. Cardiopulmonary complications and instability usually result in cardiac arrest and death (12).

There is no definitive treatment for rabies after clinical signs are apparent. Management of a patient with rabies may be palliative or aggressive. Aggressive treatment of laboratory-confirmed human rabies cases was once considered futile, but the successful treatment of a high school student from Wisconsin in 2004 has broadened treatment options. Experimental treatment of rabies cases is a dynamic process. The latest information on the Wisconsin treatment protocol may be found at the rabies registry website of the Medical College of Wisconsin (http://www.mcw .edu/display/router.asp?DocID=11655). Administration of vaccine and rabies immunoglobulin (RIG) to patients with laboratory-confirmed rabies has no proven efficacy, complicates antemortem testing, and may accelerate the disease process and patient demise.

All potential rabies virus exposures need to be evaluated on a case-by-case basis. True exposures (bite or mucous membrane) to suspect animals or animals proven rabid should receive prompt medical intervention and postexposure prophylaxis as outlined in the Advisory Committee on Immunization Practices guidelines.

Unvaccinated individuals exposed to a rabid animal should receive human RIG at dosage of 20 IU/kg of body weight. The RIG should be infiltrated around the wound and any remaining given at a site distant from where the vaccine was administered. In addition, four doses of a human rabies vaccine licensed for use in the United States should be administered on days 0, 3, 7, and 14 postexposure. Individuals who have received preexposure vaccinations require only two doses of vaccine on days 0 and 3, regardless of the preexposure VNA titer (5).

Individuals who are at high risk for a rabies virus exposure (laboratorians, field biologists, and veterinarians) are recommended to receive preexposure rabies prophylaxis. According to the current Advisory Committee on Immunization Practices guidelines for prevention of rabies in humans, 1.0 ml of cell culture-derived rabies vaccine (licensed for use in the United States) should be administered intramuscularly to the deltoid on days 0, 7, and 14. For all individuals working in a routine rabies diagnostic laboratory, determination of rabies VNA titer every 2 years is recommended. Individuals working in high-volume rabies research facilities should check VNA levels more frequently, every 6 months. Preexposure vaccination and maintenance of detectable neutralizing antibodies do not equate with protection or eliminate the need for postexposure prophylaxis if a rabies virus exposure should occur.

COLLECTION, TRANSPORT, AND STORAGE OF SPECIMENS

A summary of tests, required samples, and shipping and storage conditions may be found in Table 1. Diagnosis of rabies in animals requires postmortem examination of brain tissues. Full cross section of the brain stem (either pons, medulla, or midbrain area) and cerebellum (vermis and right and left lateral lobes inclusive) are required to test the maximum ascending and descending nerve tracts (Fig. 2). Removal of CNS tissues should be performed by trained vaccinated personnel wearing personal protective equipment (gown or lab coat with sleeves, double latex or heavy rubber gloves, and face shield). Information on sample collection for postmortem rabies diagnosis in animals is found at http://www.cdc.gov/ncidod/dvrd/rabies/Professional/publications/DFA_diagnosis/DFA_protocol-b.htm#IV.

Information regarding samples for diagnosis of rabies in humans is available at http://www.cdc.gov/RABIES/healthcare.html. Four antemortem clinical samples (collected with limited invasiveness) are required: saliva for nested reverse transcription-PCR (RT-PCR) and/or virus isolation, nuchal skin biopsy for antigen detection and nested RT-PCR, and serum and cerebrospinal fluid (CSF) for immunoglobulin M (IgM) and IgG antibody determination. Other samples such as brain biopsy and corneal impressions may be useful in diagnosis of rabies but are discouraged because of the invasiveness of collection procedures and potential harmful sequelae. No single antemortem sample or test has been able to diagnose all cases. Patient submission forms may be obtained on the CDC website (http://www.cdc.gov/RABIES/docs/ror_form.pdf). The CDC should be consulted before sample submission for primary diagnosis or confirmation[(404) 639-1050].

The recommended samples for postmortem diagnosis of rabies in humans are brain tissues (cross section brain stem and cerebellum, vermis, and right and left lobes). Tests for antigen detection, antigenic typing, and genetic typing can be performed on these samples. Formalin-fixed tissues may be used for histopathology and antigen detection; however, these samples are not recommended for primary diagnosis unless fresh brain tissues are unavailable because of the increased preparation required for processing, embedding in paraffin, and sectioning prior to test initiation. Other samples (serum and CSF) may be tested for detection of rabies virus antibodies.

The shipment of samples to a testing laboratory for rabies diagnosis should follow the U.S. Department of Transportation's *Transporting Infectious Substances Safely* (23a). Packaging of clinical samples for rabies diagnosis should fulfill the International Air Transport Association (IATA) regulations for shipment of biological substances, category B, UN 3373. Packaging of cell culture isolates and stock virus suspensions constitutes a higher infectious risk and should fulfill the IATA regulations for category A, UN 2814, infectious substances affecting humans, and UN 2900, infectious substances affecting animals. Samples for rabies testing should be shipped on dry ice (or ice packs for same-day delivery) to the diagnostic laboratory by the most expedient method.

The validity of laboratory diagnostic tests depends on maintenance of the optimal storage conditions for the samples, and these conditions vary according to sample type. Unfixed brain tissues for rabies virus antigen detection, virus isolation, and RT-PCR require long-term storage at $-80°C$. Samples for antigen detection only may be stored for short periods (≤48 h) at $4°C$ or for 4 weeks at $-20°C$. Tissues placed in 10% buffered formalin should remain in the fixative for a minimum of 24 to 48 h at ambient temperature. Formalin-fixed brain tissues should be stored in 70% ethanol at room temperature for long-term storage and never frozen. Paraffin-blocked tissues and tissue sections (slides) should be stored at ambient temperatures and never frozen.

Saliva samples for RT-PCR and virus isolation should be stored at $-80°C$ or below. Nuchal biopsy samples for RT-PCR and antigen detection should be stored at $-80°C$. Samples for antigen detection may be stored for short periods at $-20°C$ prior to testing. Serum and CSF samples for rabies serologic testing should be stored at $-20°C$ or below. Samples may be stored for short periods prior to testing at $4°C$. Whole-blood samples should be centrifuged and serum removed before freezing. Whole blood should never be shipped in the same container as samples on dry ice, since there is a risk of freezing and hemolysis regardless of packing insulation. Hemolyzed and chylous serum samples are unsatisfactory for testing. Other biological fluids (vitreous fluids, tracheal washings, tears, and others) for RT-PCR or virus isolation require storage at $-80°C$ or below.

DIRECT DETECTION METHODS

Direct methods may be used to detect histopathological changes or viral antigen and to observe virion morphology. These methods provide rapid diagnosis (within minutes to hours) without the need for amplification (e.g., isolation in cell cultures or RT-PCR).

Microscopic Methods

Microscopic examination methods may utilize routine stains (e.g., hematoxylin and eosin) to examine abnormal histopathology consistent with encephalomyelitis or more specialized stains (e.g., Sellers, Mann's, or Giemsa stain) to observe typical viral eosinophilic intracytoplasmic inclusions, such as classical Negri bodies within neurons (15, 23). Sellers stain (methylene blue and basic fuchsin, 2:1), is most frequently used for Negri body detection. In contrast to antigen detection methods, this staining procedure is most successfully performed on brain tissues infected in the later stages of disease (hippocampus, cerebral cortex pyramidal cells, cerebellum, and Purkinje cells). Brain impression slides are stained for 2 to 10 min in Sellers stain (the time varies depending on the thickness of the impression) and then rinsed with tap water. Typically, rabies virus infection demonstrates magenta intracytoplasmic inclusions that are oval or round, with dark blue basophilic granules inside. Although of historical importance, these methods lack both the specificity and sensitivity of modern methods to detect specific rabies virus antigen. Properly performed, the Sellers staining technique may identify Negri bodies in 50 to 80% of rabid animals. Observation of virions by electron microscopy allows for examination of the ultrastructure, shape, and size. The technique provides supportive evidence of a rhabdovirus infection but is less sensitive and costly for routine diagnosis (11).

TABLE 1 Routine tests for rabies diagnosis[a]

Analysis	Test method	Detection	Sample	Source	Requirements	Provider	Results
Microscopic examination	Specialized stains, e.g., H&E and Sellers	Eosinophilic intracytoplasmic inclusions	Postmortem CNS	Human or animal	Brain stem, cerebellum, hippocampus	Pathology laboratories (hospital, veterinary)	Detects eosinophilic intracytoplasmic inclusions, low sensitivity (60–80%)
Antigen detection by immunofluorescence	DFA	Rabies virus antigen	Postmortem CNS	Human or animal	Full cross-section of brain stem and cerebellum	State PH laboratories, veterinary laboratories, CDC	Detects rabies virus specific antigen, very high sensitivity (100%)
Antigen detection by immunofluorescence	DFA (cryostat)	Rabies virus antigen	Antemortem nuchal biopsy sample	Human	Full thickness of skin (5- to 6-μm cryosections)	CDC, some regional or national laboratories	Detects rabies virus specific antigen
Antigen detection by immunofluorescence	FFDFA	Rabies virus antigen	Formalin-fixed postmortem CNS	Human or animal	Full cross-section of brain stem and cerebellum	CDC, some regional or national laboratories	Detects rabies virus specific antigen, very high sensitivity (~100%)
Antigen detection by immunohistochemistry	Immunohistochemistry	Rabies virus antigen	Formalin-fixed postmortem CNS	Human or animal	Full cross section of brain stem and cerebellum	CDC, some regional or national laboratories	Detects rabies virus specific antigen, very high sensitivity (~100%)
Antigen detection by immunohistochemistry	DRIT	Rabies virus antigen	Postmortem CNS	Human or animal	Full cross section of brain stem and cerebellum	CDC, USDA, some regional or national laboratories	Detects rabies virus specific antigen, very high sensitivity (~100%)
Nucleic acid	RT-PCR	Rabies virus RNA	Postmortem CNS	Human or animal	50 mg of brain stem and cerebellum	CDC, some regional or national laboratories	Produces specific RT-PCR amplicons. Very high sensitivity. (detects ~1 infectious unit), but related to primer specificity.
Nucleic acid	Nested RT-PCR	Rabies virus RNA	Antemortem saliva, throat, skin, other	Human	100 μl of fluid samples or ≤50 mg of tissue	CDC, some regional or national laboratories	Produces specific RT-PCR amplicons. Very high sensitivity (detects less than 1 infectious unit), but related to primer specificity.
Virus isolation	Cell culture (e.g., MNA) and animal inoculation (e.g., MI)	Infectious rabies virus	Postmortem CNS	Human or animal	20% brain homogenate (brain stem and cerebellum)	State PH laboratories, veterinary laboratories, CDC	Detects infectious rabies virus
Serology (virus neutralization)	RFFIT, FAVN, MNT	Rabies VNA	Antemortem or postmortem serum or CSF	Human or animal	Serum or CSF	CDC, some commercial, regional, or national laboratories	Detects neutralizing antibodies. Neutralization tests are useful in determining immunization status.
Serology by indirect immunofluorescence	IFA	Rabies virus IgG or IgM antibodies	Antemortem or postmortem	Human or animal	Serum or CSF	CDC, some regional or national laboratories	Detects specific rabies virus IgM and IgG antibodies from serum or CSF. Very sensitive as a diagnostic technique.

[a]H&E, hematoxylin and eosin; PH, public health; USDA, U.S. Department of Agriculture; MI, mouse inoculation; MNI, mouse neutralization.

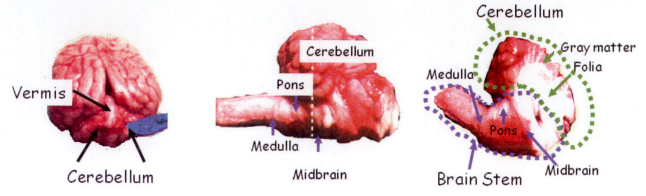

FIGURE 2 (Left) Dorsal view of a dog brain with the cerebellum (vermis and right and left lobes) labeled. (Middle) Lateral view of the cerebellum and brain stem. A cross section of the tissues demonstrated by the dotted line includes the tissues required by the standard DFA for rabies diagnosis (cross section of brain stem and right, left, and vermis of the cerebellum). (Right) View of cross section of brain stem and cerebellum. Tissue characteristics are demonstrated for orientation during dissection.

Antigen Detection

DFA Test

The standard test for rabies virus antigen detection in CNS tissues is the direct fluorescent-antibody (DFA) test. This test is easy to perform, is highly specific, approximates 100% sensitivity, and can be completed within 3 to 4 h. A copy of the standard DFA may be obtained at http://www.cdc.gov/ncidod/dvrd/rabies/Professional/publications/DFA_diagnosis/DFA_protocol-b.htm. In contrast to the nonspecific staining of viral inclusions observed with histologic stains, the rabies virus diagnostic conjugates consist of antibodies to the whole virion or to the RNP, labeled with fluorescein isothiocyanate (FITC). Within infected brain cells there are abundant collections of rabies virus proteins (antigen), especially RNP. The conjugates may be hyperimmune polyclonal or monoclonal antibodies directed against highly conserved rabies virus epitopes.

Impression slides are prepared from a cross section of brain stem and cerebellum (right, left, and vermis) or hippocampus (right and left) (Fig. 2) and are fixed in acetone for a minimum of 1 h at −20°C. The brain impression slides are tested with two different anti-rabies virus conjugates to ensure antigen detection. When the conjugates are added to rabies virus-infected brain impressions and incubated for 30 min at 37°C, the labeled antibodies bind with the rabies virus proteins (antigens) and form specific antigen-antibody-FITC complexes. After the impression slides are washed in phosphate-buffered saline (PBS) (twice for 3 to 5 min each time), only specific antigen-antibody complexes remain. These complexes fluoresce an intense sparkling apple green color when observed with a fluorescence microscope equipped with a FITC filter combination. Morphologically, rabies virus antigen may be fluorescent large or small (oval or round) inclusions, dust-like particles, or strands (Fig. 3).

DRIT

The direct rapid immunohistochemistry (IHC) test (DRIT) is an alternate procedure for rabies virus antigen detection (14). The DRIT uses a cocktail of purified biotinylated antirabies virus nucleocapsid monoclonal antibodies to detect rabies virus antigen. The test has demonstrated preliminary

sensitivity and specificity equal to those of the DFA test in detecting rabies virus antigen. Suggested uses include application to confirmatory DFA testing and enhanced surveillance. The test is currently used in the field in samples without human exposures. Advantages of this procedure include rapidity of the test protocol (1 h to completion), fixation of brain touch impression slides in formalin (inactivates rabies virus), and minimal equipment requirements (ambient incubation temperatures and standard light microscope). The sample requirements for DRIT are the same as for the DFA and other antigen detection methods. (Refer to "Collection, Transport, and Storage of Specimens" above for detailed information.) The DRIT is performed on brain touch impressions as with the DFA. Slides are fixed in 10% buffered formalin for 10 min, rinsed in PBS with 1% Tween 20 (TPBS), and then pretreated with hydrogen peroxide for 10 min before primary antibodies are applied. The test is a multistep process (biotin–streptavidin–peroxidase–3-amino-9-ethylcarbazole [AEC]): first an incubation with a biotinylated cocktail of rabies virus monoclonal antibodies for 10 min, followed by rinsing in 1% TPBS and then incubation with streptavidin-peroxidase for 10 min, followed by rinsing with TPBS and incubation with peroxidase substrate for 10 min (AEC) to initiate (red) color development and rinsing with distilled water. Slides are counterstained with Gill's hematoxylin for 2 min and rinsed with water; a coverslip is added with water-soluble mounting medium, and then the slides are observed with a standard light microscope. Rabies virus antigen appears as bright red large or small (oval or round) inclusions, dust-like particles, or strands against a contrasting blue background (Fig. 3) (14). Additional information and training for the DRIT may be obtained by contacting the CDC Rabies Program.

Formalin-Fixed Tissues

Routine formalin-fixed CNS tissue samples cannot be tested by the standard DFA test. The fixation process causes chemical cross-linking of proteins. Formalin-fixed tissue samples which have been processed, embedded in paraffin, and sectioned may be tested by a formalin-fixed DFA (FFDFA). All tests for rabies virus antigen require the same thorough tissue sampling (complete cross section of brain stem and cerebellum) as the standard DFA test. The FFDFA includes modifications of the standard DFA, such

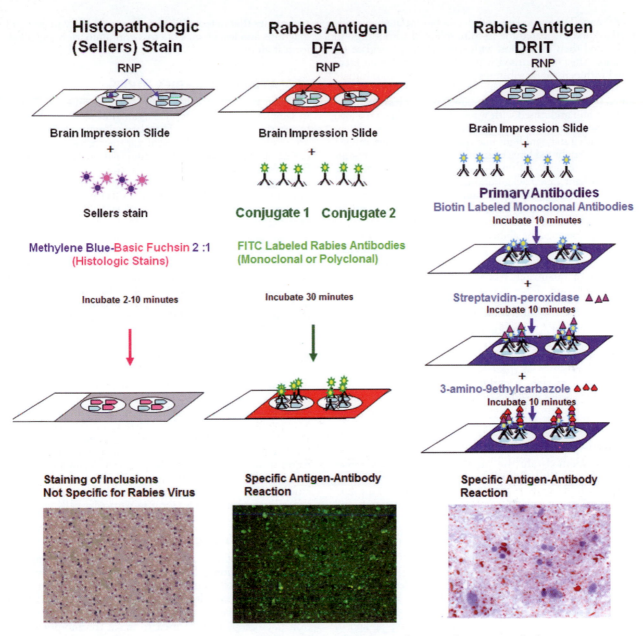

FIGURE 3   Comparison of nonspecific histologic staining and antigen detection methods.

as heating the slides to 55 to 60°C to melt the paraffin, deparaffinization in xylene, and rehydration of tissue sections in graded alcohols. In addition, the FFDFA requires proteinase K digestion for 30 min at 37°C to disassociate chemical bonds and to expose rabies virus epitopes. The incubation with anti-rabies virus FITC conjugate is increased to 1 h instead of 30 min to maximize reaction efficiency, and the wash times in PBS (twice for 15 min each time) are increased to clear unbound conjugate from tissue sections (27). The reliability of the FFDFA is dependent upon the availability of a high-affinity, high-titer commercial source of polyclonal anti-rabies virus conjugate, since the FFDFA test may require 5 to 10 times more concentrated working dilutions of rabies virus conjugate to detect 100% of the antigen in formalin-fixed tissues.

An immunohistochemistry test for rabies virus antigen detection is an alternative protocol for formalin-fixed tissue samples which have been processed, embedded in paraffin, and sectioned (10). The sample requirements are the same as for the FFDFA. Like the FFDFA, the immunohistochemistry protocol requires enzyme digestion (pronase instead of proteinase K) to disassociate cross-linking of protein bonds. The immunohistochemistry test is similar to the DRIT but is done with paraffin-embedded tissues. It is a multistep process: first digestion with pronase, followed by a rinse in TPBS and then 3% hydrogen peroxide for 20 min to remove endogenous peroxidase activity; normal goat serum is added and slides incubated for 20 min to block nonspecific binding of the primary antibody. The primary anti-rabies virus monoclonal or polyclonal antibodies are added, and the slides are incubated for 60 min. The secondary antispecies biotinylated antibody is added and incubated for 15 min, followed with a rinse in TPBS and then incubation with streptavidin-peroxidase for 15 min. After being rinsed with TPBS, the slides are incubated with peroxidase substrate (AEC) for 15 min to initiate (red) color development, followed by a rinse with distilled water. Finally, slides are counterstained with Gill's hematoxylin for 2 min and rinsed with water, and coverslips are added with water-soluble mounting medium. The slides are observed with a standard light microscope. Rabies virus antigen appears as bright red large or small (oval or round) inclusions or dust-like particles within the cytoplasm of infected neurons against a light blue background of the hematoxylin-stained tissue. Advantages of the immunohistochemistry test over the FFDFA include the ability to test for rabies virus antigen and other etiologies simultaneously by including antibodies to the other agents, the ability to examine the histopathology of tissues, and the ability to observe slides with a standard light microscope. Disadvantages are the time required for the procedure, approximately 6 h, and the number of test components to optimize.

DFA Test of Nuchal (Neck) Biopsy Specimens

Antemortem DFA tests for rabies virus antigen are performed on serial 5- to 6-μm tissue cryosections of neck skin biopsy samples and provide a rapid method for viral antigen detection in nerves at the base of hair follicles. The DFA test on tissue sections is performed exactly the same as the standard DFA test on CNS tissues. This is an alternate and less invasive method than brain biopsies to diagnose rabies in antemortem samples.

Nucleic Acid Detection

RT-PCR methods are the most sensitive tests for rabies virus diagnosis if all conditions are optimal. The reliability of RT-PCR depends in part upon the sample (type and condition), the particular method of RNA extraction and RT-PCR, the primers selected for amplification, the quality of reagents, individual technical expertise, avoidance of contamination, interpretation of the results, and confirmatory methods. The usefulness of RT-PCR as a routine diagnostic test on postmortem (fresh and fixed) CNS tissues is limited. Highly sensitive, broadly reactive, less expensive, and less time-consuming procedures for antigen detection by DFA are more efficient routine tests for rabies diagnosis. RT-PCR may be a useful tool for molecular typing and in some cases for confirming a positive diagnosis in CNS tissues, but the maximum utility is the detection of nucleic acid in non-CNS samples (e.g., antemortem saliva, skin, cornea impressions, tears, eye swabs, and throat swabs or postmortem vitreous fluid) when fresh CNS tissues are unavailable (19). When all conditions are optimal, RT-PCR detects RNA in 1 infectious unit of rabies virus and nested RT-PCR increases the sensitivity (10- to 100-fold) to below an infectious unit of virus (20). RNA may be limited or degraded when examining non-CNS samples, and nested (or heminested) RT-PCR is usually required. The diversity among rabies virus variants and lack of specific nondegenerate universal primers have discouraged use of real-time PCR until recently for detection of rabies virus RNA in non-CNS samples when the rabies virus variant is unknown. A real-time RT-PCR for human antemortem diagnosis has been developed with degenerate primers and probes with reported sensitivity to detect all major rabies virus variants (genotype 1), including Aravan virus and Khujand virus. The future incorporation of real-time

techniques that detect all lyssaviruses will allow more rapid diagnosis and less chance of cross-contamination and allow for test automation (16).

ISOLATION OF RABIES VIRUS

Isolation methods are useful in detecting infectious virus in samples and may be applied as an alternate confirmatory test to the standard DFA. The classical methods include in vivo isolation in animals (usually intracerebral inoculation of suckling mice) and in vitro virus isolation in cell cultures. For most routine diagnostic needs, the inoculation of cell cultures, such as mouse neuroblastoma (MNA; obtained from Diagnostic Hybrids, Athens, OH) or an alternative similar cell culture line, CCL 131 (ATCC, Rockville, MD), provides the same sensitivity as animal inoculation, but with quicker results and without the maintenance required for the use of laboratory animals. For these purposes, 0.4 ml of supernatant from a 20% brain suspension prepared in the tissue culture medium with 10% fetal calf serum (MEM10) is inoculated into suspension of 4×10^6 MNA cells/2 ml and incubated for 1 h at 37°C. To maximize infection of the cells, gentle mixing of the suspension is performed every 15 min. The cell suspension is diluted to a volume of 10 ml with MEM10; 6 ml is transferred to a 25-ml cell culture flask and the remaining suspension (4 ml) to 12 Teflon-coated 6-mm slides (or other cell culture slides). At least one slide should be acetone fixed daily and examined by the DFA test for rabies virus antigen. At least one additional passage of the cell culture (performed in 3 to 5 days) is required to rule out rabies. Ideally, in vivo testing use should be reserved for purposes of efficacy and safety studies for biologics or for virulence and pathogenesis studies. Cell cultures may be useful in the propagation, amplification, and quantification of virus and antibodies, to produce vaccines, to determine the safety of vaccine lots, and to study the pathogenesis of rabies virus in particular cells (24, 25).

IDENTIFICATION

Identification of a lyssavirus infection is made typically by direct examination of brain impressions and demonstration of specific viral inclusions (antigen) by the DFA test or DRIT. Isolates are also identified in brains of inoculated mice and cell cultures by the DFA test or DRIT. Electron microscopy may be used to make the morphological identification of lyssaviruses by examination of the virion ultrastructure in cell cultures or CNS tissues.

Lyssavirus identification and variant determination can be made by antigenic typing with monoclonal antibodies, genetic typing with sequence analysis, and studies of patterns of cross neutralization.

TYPING SYSTEMS

Rabies viruses are separated into carnivore and bat variants using antigenic and molecular methods. In the United States, there are at least five major reservoirs detectable among carnivores, as identified by antigenic typing. Genetic typing adds resolution and identifies seven distinct virus lineages among the current variants. Antigenic typing is less useful in certain cases involving rabid bats. Nucleotide sequence analysis adds resolution when studying these samples. Typing methods are useful in a variety of circumstances, such as determining the rabies virus variants in human cases with unclear or unknown virus exposure histories, discovering the emergence of new viruses, monitoring the epidemiological spread or reemergence of virus in defined geographical areas, detecting spillover or host switching of variants from the predominant host species to another species, and monitoring the success of rabies vaccination programs through typing of surveillance samples.

Antigenic Typing

Antigenic typing with monoclonal antibodies is done by an indirect fluorescent-antibody test (IFA) that can be performed on acetone-fixed brain impression slides and rabies virus-infected cell culture slides. If direct brain impressions are used, the best results are obtained if 75 to 100% of the microscope fields contain viral antigen. If there is insufficient antigen present, it is necessary to amplify virus by inoculating cell cultures or animals. Murine anti-rabies virus N protein monoclonal antibodies (panel of seven commercially available) are used to distinguish rabies virus variants by the different reaction patterns. Antigenic typing is an inexpensive, rapid, and easily performed method to determine rabies virus variants in a few hours. Limitations include the necessity for amplification when antigen amounts are inadequate and a lack of resolution for certain terrestrial and bat rabies virus variants. If antigenic typing results are inconclusive, additional testing can be performed at reference laboratories, such as of the CDC, which have a more extensive panel of monoclonal antibodies and resources for sequence analysis (21).

Nucleotide Sequence Analysis

Genetic typing methods for molecular epidemiological studies have become routine since more laboratories are able to extract RNA, perform RT-PCR tests, and sequence viruses. The N protein gene has been the one most frequently utilized in molecular epidemiology studies. Studies have focused the analyses on short sequences, less than 400 nucleotides; however, current technologies have expanded focus from single gene sequences to whole viral genomes (13). At present, there are thousands of N gene sequences (complete and partial) in GenBank for comparisons. Lyssavirus researchers now focus on the G, P, and L genes (2, 17). These data may assist in understanding specific gene functions in host species, viral pathogenesis, replication, and virion formation.

SEROLOGIC TESTS

The serologic tests for rabies virus antibody include neutralization and IFA tests. Each varies in sensitivity, specificity, type of antibody detected, and the viral antigen (protein) recognized. Neutralization and IFA tests are routinely used to diagnose rabies in humans (7, 22, 24). Enzyme-linked immunosorbent assay methods to confirm or rule out human rabies diagnosis have had inconsistent results.

Neutralization Tests

Neutralization tests are the standard tests for detection of antibodies to the rabies virus G protein. The rapid fluorescent focus inhibition test (RFFIT), fluorescent-antibody virus neutralization test (FAVN), and mouse neutralization are highly specific tests which measure the ability of rabies virus antibodies in serum or CSF samples to neutralize a known standard challenge virus dose. The RFFIT and FAVN, a modification of the RFFIT microneutralization test performed in microtiter plates instead of chamber slides, are most frequently used to determine the immunization status of vaccinated humans and animals, respectively. These tests exhibit the same sensitivity

and specificity in determining rabies VNAs, and tests results are comparable and are equivalent when converted to international units per milliliter (3, 7, 22).

IFA Test

IFA tests are sensitive methods for detection of specific rabies virus IgM and IgG antibodies in human serum and CSF for antemortem diagnosis (19). Unlike the neutralization tests, the IFA detects antibodies to rabies virus proteins other than G protein and predominantly to the RNP. Serum or CSF samples are titrated and added to acetone-fixed cell culture slides infected with rabies virus (CVS-11). The endpoint antibody titer is the last dilution demonstrating specific fluorescence. The IFA titers cannot be interpreted as neutralizing antibody levels since the test is not G-protein specific.

ANTIVIRAL SUSCEPTIBILITIES

No biologics are licensed for rabies antiviral activity. Human antiviral treatment recommendations and treatment protocols are dynamic. For the most current information, consult the rabies registry at the Medical College of Wisconsin website (http://www.mcw.edu/display/router.asp?DocID=11655). Antiviral drugs previously used in human treatment regimens include ribavirin, ketamine, amantadine, and alpha interferon. Although effective against RNA virus infections, ribavirin is contraindicated for rabies treatment due to depression of the immune responses. However, ketamine (anesthetic and antiviral) and amantadine (neuroprotectant and antiviral) are included in current human rabies treatment. Alpha interferon has demonstrated toxicity and is now contraindicated. Please refer to the above website for detailed information on antiviral treatments.

EVALUATION, INTERPRETATION, AND REPORTING OF RESULTS

Written protocols, which include quality assurance and quality control measures, are essential for all diagnostic tests. All reagents should be optimized before use with known positive samples from two or more rabies virus variants endemic to the geographical region and known negative control samples. The accuracy and limitations of each diagnostic test should be understood before interpretation of the test results (Table 1). The national standard protocol in the United States for rabies diagnosis in postmortem brain tissues is the DFA test. Procedural requirements of the standard DFA, DRIT, RT-PCR, and isolation methods maximize sensitivity by testing the CNS tissues most likely to be positive in rabid animals (brain stem and cerebellum). Problems of cross-contamination in direct detection and amplification methods can be avoided by processing necropsy samples separately, using separate containers for acetone fixation and washing of DFA tests, and using different areas for processing RNA and cDNA samples for RT-PCR. Multiple readers are required to evaluate each of the diagnostic tests and provide quality assurance. Since there are no universal primers for all lyssaviruses, multiple broadly reactive or degenerate primers are needed to rule out rabies by RT-PCR. Confirmatory testing is required for all rabies diagnostic tests with weak reactions or unusual results (atypical morphology, atypical reaction patterns, and epidemiological inconsistencies). Samples with nonspecific reactions and inconclusive results should be sent to a reference laboratory for confirmation and alternative testing methods. The timeliness of reporting results directly affects medical intervention; ideally rabies diagnosis from CNS tissues should be made within 24 to 48 h.

We thank Pamela Yager for her assistance in the preparation of this chapter and acknowledge the contributions of the CDC DVRD Rabies Program members.

Use of trade names and commercial sources is for identification only and does not imply endorsement by the U.S. Department of Health and Human Services. The findings and conclusions in this chapter are those of the authors and do not necessarily represent the views of the funding agency.

REFERENCES

1. **Blanton, J. D., K. Robertson, D. Palmer, and C. E. Rupprecht.** 2009. Rabies surveillance in the United States in 2008. *J. Am. Vet. Med. Assoc.* **235:**676–689.

2. **Bourhy, H., J. A. Cowley, F. Larrous, E. C. Holmes, and P. J. Walker.** 2005. Phylogenetic relationships among rhabdoviruses inferred using the L polymerase gene. *J. Gen. Virol.* **86:**2849–2858.

3. **Briggs, D. J., J. S. Smith, F. L. Mueller, J. Schwenke, R. D. Davis, C. R. Gordon, K. Schweitzer, L. A. Orciari, P. A. Yager, and C. E. Rupprecht.** 1998. A comparison of two serological methods for detecting the immune response after rabies vaccination in dogs and cats being exported to rabies-free areas. *Biologicals* **26:**347–355.

4. **Center for Disease Control.** 1977. Follow-up on rabies—New York. *MMWR Morb. Mortal. Wkly. Rep.* **26:**249–250.

5. **Centers for Disease Control and Prevention.** 2010. Use of (4-dose) reduced vaccine schedule for post-exposure prophylaxis to prevent human rabies. Recommendations of the Advisory Committee on Immunization Practices. *MMWR Recommend. Rep.* **59**(RR-2):1–8.

6. **Centers for Disease Control and Prevention and National Institutes of Health.** 1999. Agent Summary Statements—rabies virus, p. 170–171. *In* J. Y. Richmond and R. W. McKinney (ed.), *Biosafety in Microbiological and Biomedical Laboratories,* 4th ed. U.S. Government Printing Office, Washington, DC.

7. **Cliquet, F., M. Aubert, and L. Sagne.** 1998. Development of a fluorescent antibody virus neutralisation test (FAVN test) for the quantitation of rabies-neutralising antibody. *J. Immunol. Methods* **212:**79–87.

8. **Dietzschold, B., J. Li, M. Faber, and M. Schnell.** 2008. Concepts in the pathogenesis of rabies. *Future Virol.* **3:**481–490.

9. **Fauquet, C. M., M. A. Mayo, J. Maniloff, U. Desselberger, and L. A. Ball (ed.).** 2005. *Virus Taxonomy. Eighth Report of the International Committee on Nomenclature of Viruses.* Elsevier Academic Press, Inc., San Diego, CA.

10. **Hamir, A. N., G. Moser, Z. F. Fu, B. Dietzschold, and C. E. Rupprecht.** 1995. Immunohistochemical test for rabies: identification of a diagnostically superior monoclonal antibody. *Vet. Rec.* **136:**295–296.

11. **Hummeler, K., and P. Atanasiu.** 1973. Electron microscopy, p. 158–164. *In* M. M. Kaplan and H. Koprowski (ed.), *Laboratory Techniques in Rabies,* 3rd ed. World Health Organization, Geneva, Switzerland.

12. **Jackson, A. C.** 2007. Human disease, p. 309–340. *In* A. C. Jackson and W. H. Wunner (ed.), *Rabies,* 2nd ed. Academic Press, San Diego, CA.

13. **Kuzmin, I. V., A. E. Mayer, M. Niezgoda, W. Markotter, B. Agwanda, R. F. Breiman, and C. E. Rupprecht.** 2010. Shimoni bat virus, a new representative of the *Lyssavirus* genus. *Virus Res.* **149:**197–210.

14. **Lembo, T., M. Niezgoda, A. Velasco-Villa, S. Cleaveland, E. Ernest, and C. E. Rupprecht.** 2005. Evaluation of a direct immunohistochemical test for rabies diagnosis. *Emerg. Infect. Dis.* **12:**310–313.

15. **Lepine, P., and P. Atanasiu.** 1996. Histopathological diagnosis, p. 66–79. *In* F. X. Meslin, M. M. Kaplan, and H. Koprowski (ed.), *Laboratory Techniques in Rabies,* 4th ed. World Health Organization, Geneva, Switzerland.

16. **Nadin-Davis, S. A., M. Sheen, and A. I. Wandeler.** 2009. Development of real-time reverse transcriptase polymerase chain reaction methods for human rabies diagnosis. *J. Med. Virol.* **81:**1484–1497.

17. **Nadin-Davis, S. A., F. Muldoon, and A. I. Wandeler.** 2006. A molecular epidemiological analysis of the incursion of the raccoon strain of rabies virus into Canada. *Epidemiol. Infect.* **134:**534–547.

18. **National Association of State Public Health Veterinarians Committee.** 2008. Compendium of animal rabies vaccines, 2008. *J. Am. Vet. Med. Assoc.* **232:**1478–1486.

19. **Noah, D. L., C. L. Drenzek, J. S. Smith, J. W. Krebs, L. Orciari, J. Shaddock, D. Sanderlin, S. Whitfield, M. Fekadu, J. G. Olson, C. E. Rupprecht, and J. E. Childs.** 1998. Epidemiology of human rabies in the United States, 1980 to 1996. *Ann. Intern. Med.* **128:**922–930.

20. **Orciari, L. A., M. Niezgoda, C. A. Hanlon, J. H. Shaddock, D. W. Sanderlin, P. A. Yager, and C. E. Rupprecht.** 2001. Rapid clearance of SAG-2 from dogs after oral rabies vaccination. *Vaccine* **19:**4511–4518.

21. **Smith, J. S.** 1989. Rabies virus epitopic variation: use in ecologic studies. *Adv. Virus Res.* **36:**215–253.

22. **Smith, J. S., P. A. Yager, and G. M. Baer.** 1996. A rapid fluorescent focus inhibition test (RFFIT) for determining rabies virus neutralizing antibody, p. 181–192. *In* F. X. Meslin, M. M. Kaplan, and H. Koprowski (ed.), *Laboratory Techniques in Rabies,* 4th ed. World Health Organization, Geneva, Switzerland.

23. **Tierkel, E. S., and P. Atanasiu.** 1996. Rapid microscopic examination for Negri bodies and preparation of specimens for biological tests, p. 55–65. *In* F. X. Meslin, M. M. Kaplan, and H. Koprowski (ed.), *Laboratory Techniques in Rabies,* 4th ed. World Health Organization, Geneva, Switzerland.

23a. **U.S. Department of Transportation.** 2006. *Transporting Infectious Substances Safely.* U.S. Department of Transportation, Washington, DC. https://hazmatonline.phmsa.dot.gov/services/publication_documents/Transporting%20Infectious%20Substances%20Safely.pdf.

24. **Webster, L. T., and J. R. Dawson.** 1935. Early diagnosis of rabies by mouse inoculation. Measurement of humoral immunity to rabies by mouse protection test. *Proc. Soc. Exp. Biol. Med.* **32:**570–573.

25. **Webster, W. A., and G. A. Casey.** 1996. Virus isolation in neuroblastoma cell culture, p. 96–104. *In* F. X. Meslin, M. M. Kaplan, and H. Koprowski (ed.), *Laboratory Techniques in Rabies,* 4th ed. World Health Organization, Geneva, Switzerland.

26. **Weyer, J., C. E. Rupprecht, and L. H. Nel.** 2009. Pox-vectored vaccines for rabies—a review. *Vaccine* **27:**7198–7201.

27. **Whitfield, S. G., M. Fekadu, J. H. Shaddock, M. Niezgoda, C. K. Warner, S. L. Messenger, and Rabies Working Group.** 2001. A comparative study of the fluorescent antibody test for rabies diagnosis in fresh and formalin-fixed brain tissue specimens. *J. Virol. Methods* **95:**145–151.

28. **Wiktor, T. J., A. Flamand, and H. Koprowski.** 1980. Use of monoclonal antibodies in diagnosis of rabies virus infection and differentiation of rabies and rabies-related viruses. *J. Virol. Methods* **1:**33–46.

29. **Winkler, W. G., T. R. Fashinell, L. Leffingwell, P. Howard, and P. Conomy.** 1973. Airborne rabies transmission in a laboratory worker. *JAMA* **226:**1219–1221.

30. **Wunner, W. H.** 2007. Rabies virus, p. 23–56. *In* A. C. Jackson and W. H. Wunner (ed.), *Rabies,* 2nd ed. Academic Press, San Diego, CA.

Hendra and Nipah Viruses

PIERRE E. ROLLIN, PAUL A. ROTA, SHERIF ZAKI, AND THOMAS G. KSIAZEK

92

In September 1994, a respiratory disease was responsible for the sickness and death of several thoroughbred horses in Hendra, near Brisbane, Queensland, Australia (45, 46, 53). Two persons involved in the care and training of the horses developed a severe flu-like sickness within days after exposure. Both were hospitalized, and one died. The causal virus, previously undescribed, was initially named equine morbillivirus but was subsequently renamed Hendra virus. In October 1995, a second outbreak near Mackay, central Queensland, was retrospectively recognized when a horse owner died of a relapsing encephalitic disease. His probable infection occurred in August 1994, when two horses died after exhibiting severe respiratory distress and neurological symptoms. Since no known link could be traced between the two outbreaks, extensive surveys of domestic and wildlife animals were initiated around the two foci. In April 1996, anti-Hendra virus antibodies were detected in flying foxes (frugivorous bats, genus *Pteropus*) in Queensland. In September 1996, a virus identical to that found in the infected horses and humans was isolated from the reproductive tract of a grey-headed flying fox (*Pteropus poliocephalus*). Extensive serologic surveillance among flying foxes in Queensland as well as other areas within geographic range of these bats demonstrated a very high prevalence of antibodies against Hendra virus. Since then, several outbreaks occurred, mostly in the western fringe of Queensland (19, 65) (Table 1). On several occasions, fatal cases occurred in veterinary personnel after unprotected exposure to infected horses (19, 48, 53).

In September 1998, a highly contagious respiratory disease in pigs, with a low mortality, emerged in the northern part of peninsular Malaysia. In the early months of 1999, an outbreak of severe febrile encephalitis in humans with a high mortality rate was recognized, and Nipah virus, a previously unrecognized virus, was identified as the agent (9). The majority of affected humans had a history of contact with pigs, most of them being pig farmers. The outbreak subsequently spread to various states of the country and Singapore due to the movement of infected pigs. A total of 265 clinical cases were identified, and 105 of these patients died. The associated outbreak among pig abattoir workers in Singapore during March 1999 led to 22 cases, with one death. These workers had been handling pigs that had been imported from the outbreak areas in Malaysia. Antibodies were found in flying foxes in Malaysia (34). Nipah and Hendra viruses share ultrastructural, antigenic, and molecular characteristics.

Successive outbreaks of Nipah virus encephalitis have occurred in Bangladesh since 2001 (1, 41) (Table 1). In India, human encephalitis cases in Siliguri in 2001 and in Nadia in 2007 were retrospectively diagnosed as Nipah virus infections (5, 30, 37).

TAXONOMY AND DESCRIPTION OF THE AGENTS

Members of the family *Paramyxoviridae* are nonsegmented, negative-stranded RNA viruses composed of helical nucleocapsids enclosed within an envelope to form roughly spherical, pleomorphic virus particles (39). Within the family *Paramyxoviridae*, there are two subfamilies, the *Paramyxovirinae* and *Pneumovirinae*. The subfamily *Paramyxovirinae* has been divided into five genera: four of these are *Rubulavirus* (prototype, mumps virus), *Respirovirus* (prototype, human parainfluenza virus 1), *Avulavirus* (prototype, Newcastle disease virus), and *Morbillivirus* (prototype, measles virus). The fifth genus, *Henipavirus*, has been added recently, with Hendra virus as the prototype virus and Nipah virus as the second member. The complete sequences of Hendra and Nipah viruses are available on GenBank. The structure of the genome is consistent with the other members of the subfamily. The six transcription units encode six structural proteins: nucleocapsid protein (N), phosphoprotein (P), matrix protein (M), fusion protein (F), glycoprotein (G), and large protein (L) or RNA polymerase, in the order 3'-N-P-M-F-G-L-5' (39). The Nipah virus genome is 18,246 nucleotides in length, while the Hendra virus genome is 18,234 nucleotides.

EPIDEMIOLOGY AND TRANSMISSION

The geographic distribution of Hendra and Nipah viruses should overlap with the distribution of the bat reservoirs, the flying foxes (genus *Pteropus*). About 60 species of bats, which inhabit an area extending from Madagascar and Mauritius to Australia and into the western Pacific islands, are described in that genus (http://www.bucknell.edu/msw3/browse.asp?s=y&id=13800239). Many species are restricted to islands, but others are widespread in Australia and South and Southeast Asia. At this time, antibodies

TABLE 1 Hendra and Nipah virus outbreaks in Australia, Bangladesh, and India, 1994 to January 2010

Month and year	Virus	Location	No. of human cases (deaths)	Other cases
August 1994	Hendra	Mackay, Queensland, Australia	1 (fatal)	2 horses
September 1994	Hendra	Hendra, Queensland, Australia	2 (1 death in 1995)	20 horses
September 1998–December 1999	Nipah	Malaysia	265 (105 deaths)	More than 1 million pigs culled
January 1999	Hendra	Cairns, Queensland, Australia		1 horse
March 1999	Nipah	Singapore	22 (1 death)	
February 2001	Nipah	Siliguri, India	66 (45 deaths)	
April 2001	Nipah	Meherpur, Bangladesh	13 (9 deaths)	
January 2003	Nipah	Naogaon, Bangladesh	12 (8 deaths)	
January 2004	Nipah	Rajbari, Bangladesh	31 (10 deaths)	
April 2004	Nipah	Faridpur, Bangladesh	36 (18 deaths)	
October 2004	Hendra	Cairns, Queensland, Australia	1	1 horse
January 2005	Nipah	Tangail, Bangladesh	11 (1 death)	
June 2005	Hendra	Peachester, Queensland, Australia		1 horse
October 2006	Hendra	Murwillumbah, New South Wales, Australia		1 horse
February 2007	Nipah	Thakurgeon, Bangladesh	7 (3 deaths)	
March 2007	Nipah	Kushtia, Bangladesh	8 (5 deaths)	
April 2007	Nipah	Nadia, India	5 (5 deaths)	
June 2007	Hendra	Peachester, Queensland, Australia		1 horse
July 2007	Hendra	Clifton Beach, Queensland, Australia		1 horse
February 2008	Nipah	Manikgonj, Bangladesh	4	
February 2008	Nipah	Rajbari, Bangladesh	6 (3 deaths)	
July 2008	Hendra	Thornlands, Queensland, Australia	2 (1 death)	5 horses
July 2008	Hendra	Proserpine, Queensland, Australia		3 horses
August 2009	Hendra	Cawarral, Queensland, Australia	1 (fatal)	4 horses
September 2009	Hendra	Bowen, Queensland, Australia		2 horses
January 2010	Nipah	Faridpur, Bangladesh	8 (7 deaths)	
May 2010	Hendra	Tewantin, Queensland, Australia		1 horse

have been found in only a few species. In Australia, Hendra virus antibodies were identified in black flying foxes (*Pteropus alecto*), grey-headed flying foxes (*P. poliocephalus*), little red flying foxes (*Pteropus scapulatus*), and spectacled flying foxes (*Pteropus conspicillatus*). Hendra virus has been isolated from grey-headed flying foxes (*P. poliocephalus*) and from one black flying fox (*P. alecto*) (28). Hendra virus antibodies have been detected in *Pteropus* bats in Papua New Guinea. Serological evidence of Nipah virus infection has been found in *Pteropus hypomelanus* and *Pteropus vampyrus* in Malaysia (34); *Pteropus lylei* in Cambodia (47); *P. hypomelanus*, *P. lylei*, *P. vampyrus*, and *Hipposideros larvatus* in Thailand (62); *P. vampyrus* in Indonesia (54); and *Pteropus giganteus* in Bangladesh and India (14). Nipah virus has been isolated from *P. lylei* urine specimen in Cambodia (52) and more recently from a wild-caught *P. vampyrus* bat in Malaysia (55). Antibodies and viral sequences suggestive of henipaviral infections have been detected in *Eidolon helvum* in West Africa (13, 31).

Several aspects of the epidemiological features of both viruses are not fully understood. The densities of bats and the prevalence of Hendra virus antibody positives among them can be very high in certain areas, but the frequency of transmission to human or susceptible intermediate animal hosts (horses or other mammals) fortunately seems to be rare. The virus has been circulating in bats since at least 1982 (18). Only a few bat isolates of Hendra virus are available despite numerous attempts at isolation. In bats, urine is the most likely route of excretion and source of infection of susceptible animals, such as pigs or horses.

Nipah and Hendra viruses are capable of infecting a wide range of mammalian species in nature and under experimental conditions. But under laboratory conditions, the transmissibility of Hendra virus was very low. There was no transmission from bats to horses, horses to horses, or horses to cats, and only one case of transmission from infected cats to one horse was observed (66). Transmission and maintenance of Nipah virus among pigs, mostly via the respiratory route, were very efficient in Malaysia, as demonstrated by the epidemic spread within farms; farmers were mostly responsible for the transmission between farms by moving infected animals within states in Malaysia and to Singapore. Only a very severe culling strategy was effective in stopping the epidemic (20, 38). No nosocomial cases were described during the large Nipah virus outbreak in Malaysia; human-to-human transmission among community care givers, but not among health care workers (27), has been observed several times in Bangladesh (40) and India (5). Like Hendra virus in Australia, Nipah virus was present earlier in Malaysia (retrospective diagnosis of pig disease in 1996). For both viruses, the amplification through a secondary host (horse or pig) was necessary for the infection of humans. In Bangladesh, no secondary host has been described, and direct transmission from Nipah virus-contaminated palm sap, contaminated fruit trees, or contaminated fruits to human is strongly suspected. Ecological investigations have incriminated *Pteropus* bats in the contamination of the sap and sap-collecting devices (40).

CLINICAL SIGNIFICANCE

Only seven persons are known to have been infected by Hendra virus, and four of them died (18, 45, 49, 50). In all cases, the disease started with a nonspecific flu-like syndrome including fever, myalgia, headache, lethargy, sore throat, nausea, and vomiting. Two patients recovered without sequelae, and one had a slow and still-incomplete neurological recovery. Despite supportive treatment, some patients developed progressive encephalitis associated with multiorgan (respiratory and renal) failure and died. One patient recovered fully from this initial stage, but a year later the patient developed neurological signs with seizure and loss of consciousness and died 25 days after hospital admission. The pathogenesis of this patient's illness could be similar to that of a persistent measles virus infection, subacute sclerosing panencephalitis.

During the Malaysian epidemic, Nipah virus was identified as the cause of the encephalitis outbreak among pig farmers in Malaysia (7, 9, 23, 56). The incubation period ranged from 2 days to 1 month but in most of the cases was between 1 and 2 weeks. Prodromal signs and symptoms are nonspecific, with fever, headache, myalgia, and sore throat followed by drowsiness, confusion, and reduced level of consciousness after a few days (Table 2). Neurological symptoms usually appeared within a week postonset. The most common neurological signs were coma, hyporeflexia or areflexia, segmental myoclonus, gaze palsy, and limb weakness. Notable laboratory findings include thrombocytopenia, elevated alanine aminotransferase and aspartate aminotransferase, and abnormal cerebrospinal fluid (CSF; elevated protein and white-cell count). Systolic hypertension, tachycardia, high fever, and severe brain stem involvement were associated with poor outcome. Mortality occurred in 30 to 40% of the patients and was more frequent in patients with rapidly developing severe neurological signs (56). Residual neurological signs were common among the survivors.

Treatment is supportive, including mechanical ventilatory support in patients with deep coma. Ribavirin was used in humans during the Nipah virus outbreak in Malaysia with equivocal results: one study suggests that ribavirin was able to reduce the mortality of acute Nipah virus encephalitis (8); another saw no significant difference in outcome (23). Ribavirin showed no efficacy in in vitro tests and in a guinea pig or hamster model of Nipah virus disease (21, 22; P. E. Rollin, unpublished data). Ribavirin delayed but did not prevent death in a Hendra virus guinea pig model; it was

used to treat a Hendra virus-infected patient with equivocal results. Human monoclonal antibody showed very promising results in pre- and even postexposure therapy in a ferret model of Hendra virus disease (3).

There are no vaccines currently available for either Hendra virus or Nipah virus. Recombinant expressed soluble versions of the G glycoprotein from Nipah virus were used to vaccinate cats and produced high antibody titers along with complete protection from Nipah virus challenge. Canarypox virus-based vaccine vectors expressing Nipah virus G or F (or both) protected pigs against challenge and prevented viral shedding (42, 44, 63).

In horses, Hendra virus is responsible for a severe pulmonary syndrome with encephalitis in some animals (25, 64, 66). Experimentally infected cats develop an acute febrile disease with respiratory signs similar to those observed in horses (66). Hamster, guinea pig, and ferret models of Hendra virus infection have been described (1, 3, 67). In experimental infections, grey-headed flying foxes (*P. poliocephalus*) seroconverted without clinical disease (66, 67).

Nipah virus is pathogenic for several animals. In pigs, during the Malaysian outbreak and in experimental infections, the virus induces a respiratory and less commonly a neurological syndrome. Some animals remain asymptomatic, but in these animals, as in those showing clinical signs, virus can be found in the respiratory secretions. Nipah virus is easily transmitted to contact animals (43). Respiratory and neurological disease was also produced in cats. Nipah virus can be recovered from urine and oropharyngeal secretions of human patients (45). During the Malaysian outbreak, fatal infections in dogs were described, and a Nipah serological survey found that several dogs had antibody in areas adjacent to infected pig farms (2). Models of Nipah virus disease have been described for hamsters (21, 68) and guinea pigs (61).

COLLECTION, TRANSPORT, AND STORAGE OF SPECIMENS

Hendra and Nipah viruses are classified as biosafety level 4 (BSL-4) agents in the United States and Australia, as there is a risk of infection of laboratory personnel and appropriate precautions must be taken (4). The guidelines

TABLE 2 Signs and symptoms of patients with confirmed Nipah or Hendra virus infection

Parameter	Nipah virus infection			Hendra virus infection	
Reference no.	23	56	7	48	53
No. of patients in the series	94	18	103	1	2
No. of patients exhibiting:					
Fever	91 (97%)	17 (94%)	100 (97%)	1	2
Headache	61 (65%)	12 (67%)	90 (88%)	1	2
Dizziness	34 (3%)	8 (44%)	40 (39%)	1	2
Vomiting	25 (27%)	7 (39%)	37 (36%)	1	1
Reduced consciousness or loss of consciousness	20 (21%)			1	
Sore throat			21 (21%)	1	
Diarrhea		1 (5%)	21 (21%)		
Nonproductive cough	13 (14%)	3 (17%)			
Myalgia	11 (12%)	4 (22%)	48 (47%)		
Neurological signs	10 (11%)	(1–89%)	5 (5%)	1	
Mortality	30 (32%)	11 (61%)	42 (41%)	1	1
Residual neurologic deficits	14 (15%)	6 (33%)	19 (19%)		0

for veterinarians handling potential Hendra virus infection in horses have been recently updated and are available at http://www.dpi.qld.gov.au/documents/Biosecurity_General AnimalHealthPestsAndDiseases/Hendra-GuidelinesFor Vets.pdf. In the United States, the viruses are also classified as select agents by both the U.S. Department of Agriculture and HHS and should be handled as such (http://www .selectagents.gov/Select%20Agents%20and%20Toxins%20 List.html; see also chapters 10, 11, and 12 in this *Manual*).

For virus isolation, CSF, urine, or oropharyngeal secretions should be collected during the acute, febrile stages of illness and frozen on dry ice or in liquid nitrogen. Nasal or oral swabs, bronchial wash, and urine specimens can also be collected and mixed with an equal volume of buffered diluents containing serum proteins to stabilize viral infectivity prior to freezing. In fatal infections, Nipah virus could easily be isolated from different parts of the central nervous system (CNS). Specimens collected for viral isolation are also suitable for testing by reverse transcriptase PCR (RT-PCR) and TaqMan; formalin-fixed tissues and paraffin-embedded blocks are also suitable for immunohistochemical identification of viral antigens and should be conserved and shipped at room temperature. Maintenance of samples at −20°C or below is sufficient to preserve antibody, but lower temperatures are required to preserve infectivity.

Manipulation of these specimens and tissues, including sera obtained from convalescent patients, may pose a serious biohazard and should be minimized. Although no nosocomial transmissions were described in Malaysia, proper barrier nursing procedures should be implemented, and personnel caring for the patient and handling diagnostic specimens should wear disposable caps, gowns, shoe covers, surgical gloves, and face masks (N99 or N100 [HEPA] filters). Procedures generating aerosols (e.g., centrifugation) should be minimized and performed only if additional protective equipment, such as a flexible plastic film isolator capable of maintaining negative pressure and HEPA-filtered exhaust, is available. For specialized procedures, the infectivity of samples may be greatly reduced, if not totally inactivated, by the addition of Triton X-100 and heating, and the samples may be safely tested by serologic or antigen capture assays in the field. Heating to 60°C for 1 h renders diagnostic specimens noninfectious and is acceptable for measurement of heat-stable substances, such as electrolytes, blood urea nitrogen, and creatinine. When the equipment is available, sterilization by ^{60}Co γ-irradiation is the preferred method. Extraction of RNA from infectious samples by using the guanidinium acid-phenol method should be conducted in a laminar-flow safety cabinet, but the extracted RNA is no longer infectious and can be manipulated at BSL-2.

For all testing of infectious material, samples should be packaged in accordance with current recommendations (from the International Airline Transportation Association [http://www.iata.org/index.htm]) and forwarded, after consultation, to one of the following laboratories that maintain BSL-4 facilities and a diagnostic capability for these agents:

> Special Pathogens Branch, MS G-14, Division of Viral and Rickettsial Diseases, National Center for Zoonotic, Vector-Borne, and Enteric Diseases, Centers for Disease Control and Prevention, Atlanta, GA 30333. Phone: (404) 639-1115. Fax: (404) 639-1118.

> AAHL Geelong, Chief, Diagnostic Sciences, 5 Portarlington Road, East Geelong, Private Bag 24 Geelong, Victoria 3220, Australia. Phone: 61 (3) 5227 5115. Fax: 61 (3) 5227 5555.

DIRECT DETECTION

Electron Microscopy

Electron microscopy (EM) examination (thin-section and negative-stain preparations) shows extracellular virions as tangled collections of filamentous, helical nucleocapsids surrounded by the viral envelope. Particles are pleomorphic and vary greatly in size, averaging about 500 nm in diameter (range, 180 to 1,900 nm). Negative-stain EM reveals nucleocapsids with the typical herringbone appearance that is characteristic for paramyxoviruses. These measure an average of 21 nm in diameter, with a 5-nm periodicity, and up to 1.67 μm in length. In thin-section preparations, nucleocapsids average 18 nm in diameter, and spikes along the viral envelope, when seen, measure 12 nm in length (24) (Fig. 1).

EM examination of CNS specimens collected from fatal cases of Nipah virus infection showed typical *Paramyxoviridae* inclusions consisting of smooth, filamentous nucleocapsids associated with dense amorphous material. These inclusions were seen mostly in neurons and occasionally within endothelial cells. In addition, unusual cytoplasmic inclusions composed of aggregates of smooth curvilinear membranes were found in neurons (69).

Pathology and Immunohistopathology

During the Malaysian Nipah virus outbreak, tissues were collected in several fatal human cases. Histopathologic findings included a systemic vasculitis with extensive

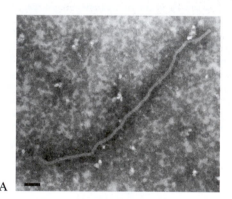

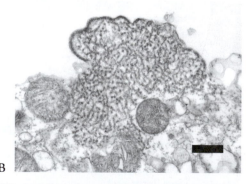

FIGURE 1 Ultrastructural characteristics of Nipah virus isolate in cell culture as seen by negative-stain (A) and thin-section (B) EM (courtesy of C. S. Goldsmith). (A) A single nucleocapsid shows the typical herringbone appearance characteristic of the family *Paramyxoviridae*. (B) Nipah virus nucleocapsids become tightly aligned along the plasma membrane as particle prepares to bud. Scale bar, 100 nm.

thrombosis and adjacent parenchymal necrosis, particularly in the CNS. Endothelial cell damage, necrosis, and syncytial giant cell formation could be observed in affected vessels. Intracytoplasmic eosinophilic inclusions can be seen on hematoxylin and eosin staining in neurons and other cell types (Fig. 2). Widespread presence of Nipah virus antigens could be seen by immunohistochemistry (IHC) in endothelial and smooth muscle cells of blood vessels and in various parenchymal cells, particularly in neurons (Fig. 3). Plaques with various degrees of necrosis were found in both the gray and white matter. In non-CNS organs, multinucleated giant cells with intranuclear inclusions were occasionally noted in lung, spleen, lymph nodes, and kidneys. Infection of endothelial cells and neurons as well as vasculitis and thrombosis appear to be critical to the pathogenesis of this disease (33, 69).

The IHC technique is adapted from previously published hantavirus or filovirus antigen detection techniques (71). Briefly, 4-μm sections were predigested by proteinase K (Boehringer-Mannheim Corporation, Indianapolis, IN) for 15 minutes at room temperature and blocked with normal serum. Primary antibodies were applied for 1 hour at room temperature. For anti-Hendra virus and anti-Nipah virus antibodies, the dilutions of the hyperimmune mouse ascitic fluids were 1:4,000 and 1:2,000, respectively. This step was followed by sequential application of biotinylated link antibody, alkaline phosphatase-conjugated streptavidin, and naphthol fast red according to the manufacturer's protocol (LSAB2 Universal Alkaline Phosphatase kit; Dako Corporation, Carpinteria, CA). Sections were then counterstained in Meyer's hematoxylin (Fisher Scientific, Pittsburgh, PA).

Molecular Detection

During outbreaks, RT-PCR assays have been used successfully to detect RNA from Nipah and Hendra viruses in a variety of clinical samples, including CSF, throat swabs, and urine samples (5, 9, 29). RNA can be extracted from samples by using the guanidinium acid-phenol method or by using a standard commercial RNA extraction kit. RT-PCR is performed using standard conditions, with one-step

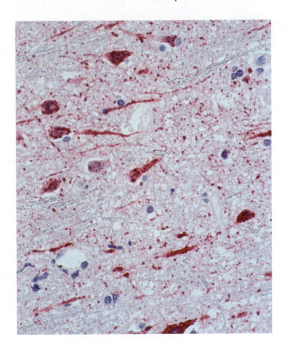

FIGURE 3 Nipah virus encephalitis: viral antigen present among numerous neurons. Note the abundance of extracellular antigen (immunoalkaline phosphatase with naphthol fast red substrate and light hematoxylin counterstain; magnification, ×120).

RT-PCRs being preferred. PCR products are detected by agarose gel electrophoresis. The primers targeting 159- to 320-nucleotide regions of the N and M genes have given the best results with diagnostic specimens thus far (5, 29). Primer sequences can be designed to detect both Hendra and Nipah viruses or to detect each virus separately. For recent outbreak investigations, two primer pairs consisting of NVNF-4 (5′GGAGTTATCAATCTAAGTTAG3′) and NVNBR4 (5′CATAGAGATGAGTGTAAAAGC3′), which amplify a 159-nucleotide region of the N gene, and NVBMFC1 (5′CAATGGAGCCAGACATCAAGAG3′) and NVBMFR2 (5′CGGAGAGTAGGAGTTCTA-GAAG3′), which amplify a 320-nucleotide region of the M gene, were used. Sequence analysis of the PCR products should be used to confirm the positive reactions, and sequence analysis allows differentiation between Hendra and Nipah viruses. In addition, phylogenetic analysis of the sequences can be used to study the evolution and transmission pathways of the viruses (5, 29).

Compared to standard RT-PCR techniques, real-time RT-PCR assays have greater sensitivity and higher throughput and are less labor-intensive and faster to perform. In addition, the TaqMan format provides increased specificity, because the identity of the amplified product is confirmed by hybridization to a target-specific, fluorogenic probe. Real-time RT-PCR assays have been developed to detect RNA from Hendra and Nipah viruses by targeting sequences in the N and P genes (26, 57). The lower limit of detection of Nipah virus RNA ranged from 10 to 1,000 copies of RNA (26), with excellent specificity. In addition to their critical role in diagnosis, real-time RT-PCR assays will facilitate research into the pathogenesis of Hendra and Nipah viruses. For example, a real-time assay was used to determine viral loads in serum samples from experimentally infected hamsters (25).

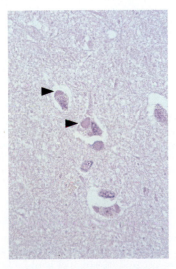

FIGURE 2 Typical eosinophilic viral inclusions (black arrowheads) in the cytoplasm of neurons (hematoxylin and eosin stain; original magnification, ×250).

ISOLATION PROCEDURES

Hendra and Nipah viruses are classified as BSL-4 agents in the United States and Australia, as there is a risk of infection of laboratory personnel and appropriate precautions must be taken (4). Virus isolation should be attempted only when the required laboratory containment is available.

African green monkey kidney (Vero) cells inoculated with high-titer samples contain antigen within a few days of inoculation. Cytopathic effect (CPE) is usually seen within 3 to 5 days. The CPE is noticeable by the formation of syncytia containing several nuclei. If no CPE is detected by 5 to 7 days, the sample is considered negative, but supernatant fluids should be blind-passaged to confirm the absence of virus. CPE is usually observed faster with Nipah virus than with Hendra virus. To confirm the presence and identity of the virus, fixed cells are tested by immunofluorescence assay (see below), or supernatant fluids can be tested for evidence of viral replication by RT-PCR techniques (see above). Hendra and Nipah viruses can be reliably distinguished from each other only by neutralization tests. Other cells, such as rabbit kidney cells (RK-13), are susceptible to Hendra and Nipah viruses. Suckling mice are susceptible by intracerebral or intraperitoneal inoculations and die, while adult mice survive (64).

SEROLOGIC TESTS

Immunofluorescence Assay

Detection of antibodies by immunofluorescence is possible but is not in routine use. Preparation of spot slides with infected Vero cells would be identical to the procedure described for other viruses (35) and requires a BSL-4 facility for production.

Enzyme-Linked Immunosorbent Assay

Enzyme-linked immunosorbent assay (ELISA) procedures for Hendra and Nipah virus-specific immunoglobulin G (IgG) and immunoglobulin M (IgM) have been successfully used. The viruses are closely related antigenically, so Hendra or Nipah virus antigens could be used interchangeably in the ELISAs. Antigens irradiated with 50 kGy before use can be used under BSL-2 conditions.

IgM Detection

A Nipah or Hendra virus-Vero E6 cell slurry antigen is prepared in a BSL-4 laboratory and γ-irradiated with 5×10^6 rads (50,000 Gy). A mock-infected Vero E6 control antigen is similarly prepared. Microtiter plates are coated with goat anti-Mu chain antibody (Biosource International, Camarillo, CA) in coating buffer at a dilution of 1:500, held overnight at 4°C, and then washed. Fourfold serial dilutions of test sera (1:100 to 1:6,400) or CSF (1:20 to 1:1,280) in diluent and of a sample of negative and positive controls (to validate the cutoff values for the assays) are added, and the plates are incubated and washed. The Hendra or Nipah virus-Vero E6 cell slurry and mock-infected control are added to the top and bottom halves of the plate, respectively, at a dilution of 1:20. After incubation and washing, Nipah or Hendra virus hyperimmune mouse ascitic fluid is added at a dilution of 1:2,000, and the plates are again incubated and washed. Horseradish peroxidase-labeled anti-mouse IgG antibody (Biosource International, Camarillo, CA) is added at a dilution of 1:2,000 before incubating and washing once more. The addition of substrate and the final incubation and wash steps are identical to those described

above. A specimen is considered positive for the IgM assay if the sum of the adjusted optical densities from all of the dilutions (infected antigen less the mock-infected antigen) is >0.75 through the entire dilution series and the titer is ≥1:400 (≥1:80 for CSF).

IgG Detection

A Hendra or Nipah virus-Vero E6 and a mock-infected Vero E6 control antigen cell lysate are prepared in the BSL-4 and then γ-irradiated as described above. Microtiter plates are again divided into positive and negative halves and coated with the respective antigens, both at a dilution of 1:1,000 as determined by checkerboard titration. Plates are kept overnight at 4°C and washed to remove unbound antigen, and fourfold serial dilutions of test sera (1:100 to 1:6,400) or CSF (1:20 to 1:1,280) are added. A sample of negative and positive controls is used to validate the cutoff values for the assays. After incubation and washing, horseradish peroxidase-labeled mouse gamma-chain-specific anti-human IgG antibody (Accurate Chemical, Grand Island, NY) is added at a dilution of 1:10,000. The addition of substrate, final incubation, and wash steps are performed as described above. A specimen is considered positive in the IgG assay if the sum for the adjusted optical densities from all of the dilutions (infected antigen less the mock-infected antigen) is >0.90 through the entire dilution series and if the titer is ≥1:400 (≥1:80 for CSF).

Nipah virus antigens have been expressed by recombinant DNA technology. These antigens, which are produced at BSL-2, have the potential to be used to configure serological diagnostic tests. So far, the extracellular domain of the G protein and the N protein virus have been expressed from recombinant baculoviruses and *Escherichia coli* (6, 15–17, 60, 70) and have produced promising results in initial tests.

Virus Neutralization

Virus neutralization assays are the reference standard for confirmation of results obtained from ELISAs. Because of antigenic differences in the G and F proteins of the viruses, neutralization is the only serologic test that can distinguish between infections with Hendra or Nipah virus. The procedure involves handling infectious Nipah or Hendra virus in a BSL-4 laboratory. Several techniques are available.

In the 50% tissue culture infective dose (TCID$_{50}$) assay, a constant challenge dose (between 30 and 300 TCID$_{50}$ of Nipah or Hendra virus) is incubated for 60 minutes at 37°C with various dilutions of heat-inactivated serum to be tested, as well as negative and positive controls. Each virus-serum mixture is then inoculated onto susceptible Vero cells and incubated at 37°C in 5% CO$_2$ for 6 days. The cells are then observed for signs of CPE. The CPE in the wells can be scored by microscopic observation or after staining the monolayer with crystal violet. For the latter, 10% buffered Formalin is added to the well, and then crystal violet stain is added, allowed to absorb, and rinsed with distilled water. If the staining is done outside of BSL-4, the plates are fixed with formalin, double bagged for removal from BSL-4, and irradiated with 2×10^6 rads before staining.

The virus control (back titration) of the test dose should confirm that the input dose of virus was between 30 and 300 TCID$_{50}$. Neutralization titers of test samples are reported as the highest dilution in which cells are protected from CPE (the last well in which at least half of the monolayer was protected and that also stains purple).

A rapid immune plaque assay is also available (11), and more recently, a neutralization assay using vesicular stomatitis virus pseudotype particles expressing the F and G proteins of Nipah virus as target antigens has been described previously (36, 59). These assays are rapid and offer the advantage of being performed at BSL-2.

Western Blotting and Immunoprecipitation

In some cases, Western blot assays and immunoprecipitation assays have been used to confirm serologic results from ELISAs. Both Western blotting and immunoprecipitation can confirm the presence of IgG antibodies to individual structural proteins of Nipah or Hendra virus. Western blot assays are conducted using standard sodium dodecyl sulfate-polyacrylamide gel electrophoresis (10%) and blotting techniques. No infectious Nipah or Hendra virus is required for the assays. Baculovirus-expressed Nipah or Hendra virus nucleoprotein or inactivated native proteins are available for use as the test antigen, and lysates of uninfected insect cells are used for the control antigen. The nucleoprotein antigens can be detected with a monoclonal antibody in the positive control reactions (P. A. Rota and B. H. Harcourt, unpublished data).

To prepare radiolabeled antigen for immunoprecipitation experiments, cells are infected with recombinant vaccinia viruses expressing the G, F, and N of Nipah or Hendra virus. Radiolabeling and immunoprecipitation are performed using standard conditions, as previously described (58). Hyperimmune mouse ascites fluid, which recognizes all of the structural proteins of Nipah or Hendra viruses, is used as the positive control. Though this immunoprecipitation assay has been used to detect antibodies to Nipah virus in human serum samples, some samples may contain a high background of reactivity with vaccinia antigens if the patient has received smallpox vaccination.

EVALUATION, INTERPRETATION, AND REPORTING OF RESULTS

As for any infectious disease, the diagnosis should be based on a combination of clinical, epidemiological, and laboratory data. Several reviews have been published on the laboratory diagnosis of Nipah and Hendra virus infections in humans and animals (12, 20). The proper timing and the type of the specimens collected are essential. Virus can be isolated from throat or nasal swabs, tracheal secretions, CSF, and urine at the early stage of the disease, and the excretion rate decreases in the late phase, when anti-Nipah virus antibodies are present (10, 23). Isolation could also be attempted from brain tissues collected at autopsy. Ideally, any virus isolation attempt should be performed in a BSL-4. In the absence of BSL-4, primary virus isolation from suspect samples could be conducted under strict BSL-3 conditions. Cell culture and the manipulation of potentially infectious specimens should be stopped with the appearance of a CPE with syncytia. Fixed cells should be stained with proper reagents to confirm the diagnosis; in the case of positive results, the specimen should be transferred to an appropriate laboratory.

Molecular diagnosis using standard or real-time RT-PCR techniques can be used on oropharyngeal swabs or secretions, CSF, CNS or other tissues, or viral isolates in cell culture. The specimens are inactivated by adding the lysis buffer used for the first step of the RNA extraction (usually containing 4 M guanidinium isothiocyanate), and the remainder of the RNA extraction and PCRs can be performed in any BSL-2 laboratory that is equipped for these techniques. Molecular techniques can be used to confirm Nipah or Hendra virus infection in a patient or to confirm isolation in cell culture. Positive PCRs should always be confirmed by amplification of more than one target sequence and by sequencing the PCR products. This sequence information will clearly identify the virus as being either Hendra or Nipah virus and may allow use of molecular epidemiologic techniques to study viral transmission pathways between and during outbreaks. However, the sensitivity of RT-PCR for identifying cases of Hendra or Nipah virus infection will, most likely, be lower than the sensitivity of serologic testing; the timing and the type of specimen obtained and the condition and handling of the specimen will all have effects on the quantity and quality of detectable RNA in the sample. In addition to molecular detection and identification assays, efforts should be made to obtain virus isolates to allow comparative pathogenesis studies and therapeutic or vaccination studies.

The ELISA IgM test has been the most important technique for serological confirmation in acute patients. The rate of serum IgM positivity increased from 50% on the first day of illness to nearly 100% a week after onset. In Nipah virus-infected patients, 88% of the first samples tested were positive for IgM (51). Fewer patients have CSF IgM at onset, but nearly all are positive by days 10 to 15. In contrast, very few patients have IgG detectable by ELISA either in the serum or in the CSF at onset. All have IgG in the serum by day 17 to 18. There was no difference in the prevalence of IgM and IgG antibodies between encephalitic and nonencephalitic Nipah virus infection. As mentioned before, neutralization tests should be used to determine the specificity (between Nipah virus and Hendra virus) of the antibodies detected by ELISA, particularly if no virus or viral RNA is available to facilitate molecular typing. Neutralizing antibody titers in bats are usually very low and may be not the best way to detect and monitor the immune response in wild-caught bats.

In some patients, rapid neurological deterioration and death may occur, and the only specimens available for testing are tissues collected at autopsy; or patients may die before antibodies appear. In these patients, histopathological findings and IHC staining are essential to confirm the diagnosis and to understand the pathogenesis of the disease (32).

The findings and conclusions in this chapter are those of the authors and do not necessarily represent the views of the funding agency.

REFERENCES

1. **Anonymous.** 2003. Outbreaks of encephalitis due to Nipah/Hendra-like viruses, Western Bangladesh. *Health Sci. Bull.* (English) 1:1–6.
2. **Asiah, N. M., J. N. Mills, B. L. Ong, and T. G. Ksiazek.** 2001. Epidemiological investigation of Nipah virus infection in peridomestic animals in peninsular Malaysia and future plans, p. 47–50. *In* Office International des Epizooties and Department of Veterinary Services, Malaysia, *Report of the Regional Seminar on Nipah Virus Infection; Kuala Lumpur, Malaysia.* OIE Representation for Asia and the Pacific, Tokyo, Japan.
3. **Bossart, K. N., Z. Zhu, D. Middleton, J. Klippel, G. Crameri, J. Bingham, J. A. McEachern, D. Green, T. J. Hancock, E. P. Chan, A. C. Hickey, D. S. Dimitrov, L. F. Wang, and C. C. Broder.** 2009. A neutralizing human monoclonal antibody protects against lethal disease in a new ferret model of acute Nipah virus infection. *PLoS Path.* 5:e1000642.
4. **Centers for Disease Control and Prevention and the National Institutes of Health.** 2009. *Biosafety in Microbiological and Biomedical Laboratories,* 5th ed. U.S. Department

of Health and Human Services, Washington, DC. http://www.cdc.gov/od/ohs/biosfty/bmbl5/BMBL_5th_Edition.pdf.

5. Chadha, M. S., A. C. Mishra, N. K. Ganguly, T. G. Ksiazek, P. E. Rollin, J. A. Comer, P. A. Rota, W. J. Bellini, and L. Lowe. 2006. Nipah virus associated with an encephalitis outbreak, Siliguri, India, 2001. *Emerg. Infect. Dis.* **12:**235–240.

6. Chong, F. C., W. S. Tan, D. R. Biak, T. C. Ling, and B. T. Tey. 2009. Purification of histidine-tagged nucleocapsid protein of Nipah virus using immobilized metal affinity chromatography. *J. Chromatogr. B* **877:**1561–1567.

7. Chong, H. T., S. R. Kunjapan, T. Thayaparan, J. M. G. Tong, V. Patharunam, M. R. Jusoh, and C. T. Tan. 2000. Nipah encephalitis outbreak in Malaysia, clinical features in patients from Seremban. *Neurol. J. Southeast Asia* **5:**61–67.

8. Chong, H. T., A. Kamarulzaman, C. T. Tan, K. J. Goh, T. Thayaparan, S. R. Kunjapan, N. K. Chew, K. B. Chua, and S. K. Lam. 2001. Treatment of acute Nipah encephalitis with ribavirin. *Ann. Neurol.* **49:**810–813.

9. Chua, K. B., W. J. Bellini, P. A. Rota, B. H. Harcourt, A. Tamin, S. K. Lam, T. G. Ksiazek, P. E. Rollin, S. R. Zaki, W. Shieh, C. S. Goldsmith, D. J. Gubler, J. T. Roehrig, B. Eaton, A. R. Gould, J. Olson, H. Field, P. Daniels, A. E. Ling, C. J. Peters, L. J. Anderson, and B. W. Mahy. 2000. Nipah virus: a recently emergent deadly paramyxovirus. *Science* **288:**1432–1435.

10. Chua, K. B., S. K. Lam, K. J. Goh, P. S. Hooi, T. G. Ksiazek, A. Kamarulzaman, J. Olson, and C. T. Tan. 2001. The presence of Nipah virus in respiratory secretions and urine of patients during an outbreak of Nipah virus encephalitis in Malaysia. *J. Infect.* **42:**40–43.

11. Crameri, G., L. F. Wang, C. Morrissy, J. White, and B. T. Eaton. 2002. A rapid immune plaque assay for the detection of Hendra and Nipah viruses and anti-virus antibodies. *J. Virol. Methods* **99:**41–51.

12. Daniels, P., T. Ksiazek, and B. T. Eaton. 2001. Laboratory diagnosis of Nipah and Hendra virus infections. *Microbes Infect.* **3:**289–295.

13. Drexler, J. F., V. M. Corman, F. Gloza-Rausch, A. Seebens, A. Annan, A. Ipsen, T. Kruppa, M. A. Muller, E. K. Kalko, Y. Adu-Sarkodie, S. Oppong, and C. Drosten. 2009. Henipavirus RNA in African bats. *PLoS One* **4:**e6367.

14. Epstein, J. H., V. Prakash, C. S. Smith, P. Daszak, A. B. McLaughlin, G. Meehan, H. E. Field, and A. A. Cunningham. 2008. Henipavirus infection in fruit bats (*Pteropus giganteus*), India. *Emerg. Infect. Dis.* **14:**1309–1311.

15. Eshaghi, M., W. S. Tan, T. B. Mohidin, and K. Yusoff. 2004. Nipah virus glycoprotein: production in baculovirus and application in diagnosis. *Virus Res.* **106:**71–76.

16. Eshaghi, M., W. S. Tan, W. K. Chin, and K. Yusoff. 2005. Purification of the extra-cellular domain of Nipah virus glycoprotein produced in *Escherichia coli* and possible application in diagnosis. *J. Biotechnol.* **116:**221–226.

17. Eshaghi, M., W. S. Tan, S. T. Ong, and K. Yusoff. 2005. Purification and characterization of Nipah virus nucleocapsid protein produced in insect cells. *J. Clin. Microbiol.* **43:**3172–3177.

18. Field, H., P. Young, J. M. Yob, J. N. Mill, L. Hall, and J. Mackenzie. 2001. The natural history of Hendra and Nipah viruses. *Microbes Infect.* **3:**307–314.

19. Field, H. 2009. Hendra virus infection risks. *Neurol. Asia* **14:**77–78.

20. Food and Agriculture Organization. 2002. *Manual on the Diagnosis of Nipah Virus Infection in Animals.* RAP publication no. 2002/01. FAO, Regional Office for Asia and the Pacific, Bangkok, Thailand.

21. Freiberg, A. N., M. N. Worthy, B. Lee, and M. R. Holbrook. 2010. Combinatorial chloroquine and ribavirin treatment does not prevent death in a hamster model of Nipah and Hendra virus infection. *J. Gen. Virol.* **91:**765–772.

22. Georges-Courbot, M. C., H. Contamin, C. Faure, P. Loth, S. Baize, P. Leyssen, J. Neyts, and V. Deubel. 2006. Poly(I)-poly(C$_{12}$U) but not ribavirin prevents death in a hamster model of Nipah virus infection. *Antimicrob. Agents Chemother.* **50:**1768–1772.

23. Goh, K. J., C. T. Tan, N. K. Chew, P. S. Tan, A. Kamarulzaman, S. A. Sarji, K. T. Wong, B. J. J. Abdullah, K. B. Chua, and S. K. Lam. 2000. Clinical features of Nipah virus encephalitis among pig farmers in Malaysia. *N. Engl. J. Med.* **342:**1229–1235.

24. Goldsmith, C. S., T. Whistler, P. E. Rollin, T. G. Ksiazek, P. Rota, W. J. Bellini, P. Daszak, K. T. Wong, W.-J. Shieh, T. G. Ksiazek, and S. R. Zaki. 2003. Elucidation of Nipah virus morphogenesis and replication using ultrastructural and molecular approaches. *Virus Res.* **92:**89–98.

25. Guillaume, V., H. Contamin, P. Loth, M.-C. Georges-Courbot, A. Lefeuvre, P. Marianneau, K. B. Chua, S. K. Lam, R. Buckland, V. Deubel, and T. F. Wild. 2004. Nipah virus: vaccination and passive protection studies in a hamster model. *J. Virol.* **78:**834–840.

26. Guillaume, V., A. Lefeuvre, C. Faure, P. Marianneau, R. Buckland, S. K. Lam, T. F. Wild, and V. Deubel. 2004. Specific detection of Nipah virus using real-time RT-PCR (TaqMan). *J. Virol. Methods* **120:**229–237.

27. Gurley, E. S., J. M. Montgomery, M. J. Hossain, M. Jahangir, M. R. Islam, M. A. R. Molla, S. M. Shamsuzzaman, K. Akram, K. Zaman, N. Asgari, J. A. Comer, A. K. Azad, P. E. Rollin, T. G. Ksiazek, and R. F. Breiman. 2007. Risk of nosocomial transmission of Nipah virus in a Bangladesh hospital. *Infect. Control Hosp. Epidemiol.* **28:**740–742.

28. Halpin, K., P. L. Young, H. E. Field, and J. S. Mackenzie. 2000. Isolation of Hendra virus from pteropid bats: a natural reservoir of Hendra virus. *J. Gen. Virol.* **81:**1927–1932.

29. Harcourt, B. H., L. Lowe, A. Tamin, X. Liu, B. Bankamp, N. Bowden, P. E. Rollin, J. A. Comer, T. G. Ksiazek, J. H. Mohammed, E. S. Gurley, R. Breiman, W. J. Bellini, and P. A. Rota. 2005. Genetic characterization of Nipah virus, Bangladesh, 2004. *Emerg. Infect. Dis.* **11:**1594–1597.

30. Harit, A. K., R. L. Ichhpujani, S. Gupta, K. S. Gill, S. Lal, N. K. Ganguly, and S. P. Agarwal. 2006. Nipah/Hendra virus outbreak in Siliguri, West Bengal, India in 2001. *Indian J. Med. Res.* **23:**553–560.

31. Hayman, D. T., R. Suu-Ire, A. C. Breed, J. A. McEachern, L. Wang, J. L. Wood, and A. A. Cunningham. 2008. Evidence of henipavirus infection in West African fruit bats. *PLoS One* **3:**e2739.

32. Hooper, P., S. Zaki, P. Daniels, and D. Middleton. 2001. Comparative pathology of the diseases caused by Hendra and Nipah viruses. *Microbes Infect.* **3:**315–322.

33. Hyatt, A. D., S. R. Zaki, C. S. Goldsmith, T. G. Wise, and S. G. Hengstberger. 2001. Ultrastructure of Hendra virus and Nipah virus within cultured cells and host animals. *Microbes Infect.* **3:**297–306.

34. Johara, M. Y., H. Field, R. A. Mohd, C. Morrissy, B. van der Heide, P. Rota, A. bin Adzhar, J. White, P. Daniels, A. Jamaluddin, and T. G. Ksiazek. 2001. Nipah virus infection in bats (order Chiroptera) in peninsular Malaysia. *Emerg. Infect. Dis.* **7:**439–441.

35. Johnson, K. M., L. H. Elliott, and D. L. Heymann. 1981. Preparation of polyvalent viral immunofluorescent intracellular antigens and use in human serosurveys. *J. Clin. Microbiol.* **14:**527–529.

36. Kaku, Y., A. Noguchi, G. A. Marsh, J. A. McEachern, A. Okutani, K. Hotta, B. Bazartseren, S. Fukushi, C. C. Broder, A. Yamada, S. Inoue, and L. F. Wang. 2009. A neutralization test for specific detection of Nipah virus antibodies using pseudotyped vesicular stomatitis virus expressing green fluorescent protein. *J. Virol. Methods* **160:**7–13.

37. Krishanan, S., and K. Biswas. 2007. Nipah outbreak in India and Bangladesh. *Commun. Dis. Dep. Newsl.* **4:**3.

38. Lam, S. K., and K. B. Chua. 2002. Nipah virus encephalitis outbreak in Malaysia. *Clin. Infect. Dis.* **34:**S48–S51.

39. Lamb, R. A., and D. Kolakofsky. 2001. *Paramyxoviridae:* the viruses and their replication, p. 1305–1340. *In* D. M. Knipe, P. M. Howley, D. E. Griffin, R. A. Lamb, M. A. Martin, B. Roizman, and S. E. Straus (ed.), *Fields Virology*, 4th ed., vol. 1. Lippincott Williams & Wilkins, Philadelphia, PA.

40. Luby, S. P., E. S. Gurley, and M. J. Hossain. 2009. Transmission of human infection with Nipah virus. *Clin. Infect. Dis.* **49:**1743–1748.

41. Luby, S. P., M. J. Hossain, E. Gurley, B. N. Ahmed, S. Banu, S. U. Khan, N. Homaira, P. Rota, P. E. Rollin, J. A. Comer, K. Eben, T. G. Ksiazek, and M. Rahman. 2009. Recurrent zoonotic transmission of Nipah virus into humans, Bangladesh, 2001–2007. *Emerg. Infect. Dis.* **15:**1229–1235.

42. McEachern, J. A., J. Bingham, G. Crameri, D. J. Green, T. J. Hancock, D. Middleton, Y. R. Feng, C. C. Broder, L. F. Wang, and K. N. Bossart. 2008. A recombinant subunit vaccine formulation protects against lethal Nipah virus challenge in cats. *Vaccine* **26:**3842–3952.

43. Middleton, D. J., H. A. Westbury, C. J. Morrissy, B. M. van der Heide, G. M. Russell, M. A. Braun, and A. D. Hyatt. 2002. Experimental Nipah virus infection in pigs and cats. *J. Comp. Pathol.* **126:**124–136.

44. Mungall, B. A., D. Middleton, G. Crameri, J. Bingham, K. Halpin, G. Russell, D. Green, J. McEachern, L. I. Pritchard, B. T. Eaton, L. F. Wang, K. N. Bossart, and C. C. Broder. 2006. Feline model of acute Nipah virus infection and protection with a soluble glycoprotein-based subunit vaccine. *J. Virol.* **80:**12293–12302.

45. Murray, K., R. Rogers, L. Selvey, P. Selleck, A. Hyatt, A. Gould, L. Gleeson, P. Hooper, and H. Westbury. 1995. A novel morbillivirus pneumonia of horses and its transmission to humans. *Emerg. Infect. Dis.* **1:**31–33.

46. Murray, K., P. Selleck, P. Hooper, A. Hyatt, A. Gould, L. Gleeson, H. Westbury, L. Hiley, L. Selvey, and B. Rodwell. 1995. A morbillivirus that caused fatal disease in horses and humans. *Science* **268:**94–97.

47. Olson, J. G., C. Rupprecht, P. E. Rollin, U. S. An, M. Niezgoda, T. Clemins, J. Walston, and T. G. Ksiazek. 2002. Antibodies to Nipah-like virus in bats (*Pteropus lylei*), Cambodia. *Emerg. Infect. Dis.* **8:**987–988.

48. O'Sullivan, J. D., A. M. Allworth, D. L. Paterson, T. M. Snow, R. Boots, L. J. Gleeson, A. R. Gould, A. D. Hyatt, and J. Bradfield. 1997. Fatal encephalitis due to novel paramyxovirus transmitted from horses. *Lancet* **349:**93–95.

49. Paterson, D. L., P. K. Murray, and J. G. McCormack. 1998. Zoonotic disease in Australia caused by a new member of the paramyxoviridae. *Clin. Infect. Dis.* **27:**112–118.

50. Playford, E. G., B. McCall, G. Smith, V. Slinko, G. Allen, I. Smith, F. Moore, C. Taylor, Y. H. Kung, and H. Field. 2010. Human Hendra virus encephalitis associated with equine outbreak, Australia, 2008. *Emerg. Infect. Dis.* **16:**219–223.

51. Ramasundrum, V., C. T. Tan, K. B. Chua, H. T. Chong, K. J. Goh, N. K. Chew, K. S. Tan, T. Thayaparan, S. R. Kunjapan, V. Petharunam, V. L. Loh, T. G. Ksiazek, and S. K. Lam. 2000. Kinetics of IgM and IgG seroconversion in Nipah virus infection. *Neurol. J. Southeast Asia* **5:**23–28.

52. Reynes, J.-M., D. Counor, S. Ong, C. Faure, V. Seng, S. Molia, J. Walston, M. C. Georges-Courbot, V. Deubel, and J.-L. Sarthou. 2005. Nipah virus in Lyle's flying foxes, Cambodia. *Emerg. Infect. Dis.* **11:**1042–1047.

53. Selvey, L. A., R. M. Wells, J. G. McCormack, A. J. Ansford, K. Murray, R. J. Rogers, P. S. Lavercombe, P. Selleck, and J. W. Sheridan. 1995. Infection of humans and horses by a newly described morbillivirus. *Med. J. Aust.* **162:**642–645.

54. Sendow, I., H. E. Field, J. Curran, Darminto, C. Morrissy, G. Meehan, T. Buick, and P. Daniels. 2006. Henipavirus in *Pteropus vampyrus* bats, Indonesia. *Emerg. Infect. Dis.* **12:**711–712.

55. Sharifah, S. H., A. R. Sohayati, M. Maizan, L. Y. Chang, M. Sharina, K. Latiffah, S. S. Arshad, C. M. Zaini, F. Humes, P. Daszak, and J. Epstein. 2009. Genetic characterization of a Nipah virus isolated from a *Pteropus vampyrus* in Malaysia. *Neurol. Asia* **14:**67–69.

56. Sim, B. F., R. Jusoh, C. C. Chang, and R. Khalid. 2002. Nipah encephalitis: a report of 18 patients from Kuala Lumpur Hospital. *Neurol. J. Southeast Asia* **7:**13–18.

57. Smith, I. L., K. Halpin, D. Warrilow, and G. A. Smith. 2001. Development of a fluorogenic RT-PCR assay (TaqMan) for the detection of Hendra virus. *J. Virol. Methods* **98:**33–40.

58. Tamin, A., B. H. Harcourt, T. G. Ksiazek, P. E. Rollin, W. J. Bellini, and P. A. Rota. 2002. Functional properties of the fusion and attachment glycoproteins of Nipah virus. *Virology* **296:**190–200.

59. Tamin, A., B. H. Harcourt, M. K. Lo, J. A. Roth, M. C. Wolf, B. Lee, H. Weingartl, J. C. Audonnet, W. J. Bellini, and P. A. Rota. 2009. Development of a neutralization assay for Nipah virus using pseudotype particles. *J. Virol. Methods* **160:**1–6.

60. Tan, W. S., S. T. Ong, M. Eshaghi, S. S. Foo, and K. Yusoff. 2004. Solubility, immunogenicity and physical properties of the nucleocapsid protein of Nipah virus produced in *Escherichia coli*. *J. Med. Virol.* **73:**105–112.

61. Torres-Velez, F. J., W. J. Shieh, P. E. Rollin, T. Morken, C. Brown, T. G. Ksiazek, and S. R. Zaki. 2008. Histopathologic and immunohistochemical characterization of Nipah virus infection in the guinea pig. *Vet. Pathol.* **45:**576–585.

62. Wacharapluesadee, S., B. Lumlertdacha, K. Boongird, S. Wanghongsa, L. Chanhome, P. E. Rollin, P. Stockton, C. E. Rupprecht, T. G. Ksiazek, and T. Hemachudha. 2005. Bat Nipah virus, Thailand. *Emerg. Infect. Dis.* **11:**1949–1951.

63. Weingartl, H. M., Y. Berhane, J. L. Caswell, S. Loosmore, J. C. Audonnet, J. A. Roth, and M. Czub. 2006. Recombinant Nipah virus vaccines protect pigs against challenge. *J. Virol.* **80:**7929–7938.

64. Westbury, H. A., P. T. Hooper, P. W. Selleck, and P. K. Murray. 1995. Equine morbillivirus pneumonia: susceptibility of laboratory animals to the virus. *Aust. Vet. J.* **72:**278–279.

65. Westbury, H. A. 2000. Hendra virus disease in horses. *Rev. Sci. Tech. Off. Int. Epizoot.* **19:**151–159.

66. Williamson, M. M., P. T. Hooper, P. W. Selleck, L. J. Gleeson, P. W. Daniels, H. A. Westbury, and P. K. Murray. 1998. Transmission studies of Hendra virus (equine morbillivirus) in fruit bats, horses and cats. *Aust. Vet. J.* **76:**813–818.

67. Williamson, M. M., P. T. Hooper, P. W. Selleck, H. A. Westbury, and R. F. Slocombe. 1999. Experimental Hendra virus infection in pregnant guinea-pigs and fruit bats (*Pteropus poliocephalus*). *J. Comp. Pathol.* **122:**201–207.

68. Wong, K. T., I. Grosjean, C. Brisson, B. Blanquier, M. Fevre-Montange, A. Bernard, P. Loth, M. C. Georges-Courbot, M. Chevallier, H. Akaoka, P. Marianneau, S. K. Lam, T. F. Wild, and V. Deubel. 2003. A golden hamster model for human acute Nipah virus infection. *Am. J. Pathol.* **163:**2127–2137.

69. Wong, K. T., W. J. Shieh, S. Kumar, K. Norain, W. Abdullah, J. Guarner, C. S. Goldsmith, K. B. Chua, S. K. Lam, C. T. Tan, K. J. Goh, H. T. Chong, R. Jusoh, P. E. Rollin, T. G. Ksiazek, S. R. Zaki, and the Nipah Virus Pathology Working Group. 2002. Nipah virus infection. Pathology and pathogenesis of an emerging paramyxoviral zoonosis. *Am. J. Pathol.* **161:**2153–2167.

70. Yu, F., N. S. Khairullah, S. Inoue, V. Balasubramaniam, S. J. Berendam, L. K. Teh, N. S. W. Ibrahim, S. Abdul Rahman, S. S. Hassan, F. Hasebe, M. Sinniah, and K. Morita. 2006. Serodiagnosis using recombinant Nipah virus nucleocapsid protein expressed in *Escherichia coli*. *J. Clin. Microbiol.* **44:**3134–3138.

71. Zaki, S., P. W. Greer, L. M. Coffield, C. S. Goldsmith, K. B. Nolte, K. Foucar, R. M. Feddersen, R. Zumwalt, G. L. Miller, A. S. Khan, P. E. Rollin, T. G. Ksiazek, S. T. Nichol, B. W. J. Mahy, and C. J. Peters. 1995. Hantavirus pulmonary syndrome: pathogenesis of an emerging infectious disease. *Am. J. Pathol.* **146:**552–579.

Arboviruses*

ROBERT S. LANCIOTTI AND THEODORE F. TSAI

93

TAXONOMY

The term "arbovirus," a shortened form of "arthropod-borne virus," is used to describe a taxonomically diverse group of viruses that share the common feature of being transmitted biologically to vertebrate hosts by the bite of arthropod vectors (mosquitoes, sand flies, ticks, midges, etc.). This ecological grouping includes more than 500 viruses belonging to at least seven families, including the *Togaviridae, Flaviviridae, Bunyaviridae, Reoviridae, Rhabdoviridae, Orthomyxoviridae,* and *Asfarviridae* (17, 30). Over 100 of these agents have been associated with naturally acquired disease in humans and/or domestic animals. The *International Catalogue of Arboviruses* (30) also includes a number of other zoonotic viruses (i.e., hantaviruses, arenaviruses, and filoviruses) that are transmitted from animals to humans without the agency of a vector; these agents are not true arboviruses and are not included in this chapter.

DESCRIPTION OF THE AGENTS

All of the arboviruses affecting humans are RNA viruses (Table 1). Complete or partial genome nucleotide sequences have been determined for many of the medically important arboviruses, facilitating the use of nucleic acid detection techniques and the production of synthetic antigens for use in diagnosis and as candidate vaccines. Important antigenic determinants have been elucidated for the most important arboviruses, and virus- and group-specific monoclonal antibodies are available for taxonomic and diagnostic purposes.

Most arboviruses elaborate hemagglutinins that aggregate goose, chick, and/or human group O erythrocytes. Hemagglutination (HA) occurs optimally within a narrow and specific pH range, a property that may aid in viral identification. In general, serologic cross-relationships are most evident in hemagglutination inhibition (HI) and binding assays, e.g., enzyme-linked immunosorbent assays (ELISAs) and immunofluorescent antibody (IFA) tests, and occur to a lesser extent in complement fixation (CF) tests. These broad antigenic relationships can be refined in virus neutralization tests that differentiate individual viruses and even more specific subtype relationships through ratios of homologous and heterologous neutralization antibody titers. Genomic sequence divergence among strains of a single virus in separate geographic locations differentiates viral topotypes, which apparently result from the isolation and evolutionary divergence of these strains in distinct ecologic niches. Topotypic differences among populations of Japanese encephalitis (JE), tick-borne encephalitis (TBE), yellow fever (YF), dengue (DEN), West Nile (WN), eastern equine encephalitis (EEE), Venezuelan equine encephalitis (VEE), snowshoe hare, and LaCrosse (LAC; a serotype of California encephalitis virus) viruses, among others, have been described. Such genetic changes have been linked to differences in clinical expression of EEE, Sindbis (SIN), VEE, and St. Louis encephalitis (SLE) virus infections.

EPIDEMIOLOGY AND TRANSMISSION

The epidemiologic and clinical characteristics of the medically important arboviruses are summarized in Table 2. More comprehensive descriptions can be found elsewhere (18, 47, 59, 72). Current information on arboviral outbreaks and transmission patterns can be obtained from state health departments, from the World Health Organization (WHO) (http://www.who.org), and from the Centers for Disease Control and Prevention (CDC) (http://www.cdc.gov).

CLINICAL SIGNIFICANCE

The majority of arboviral infections in humans result in simple febrile illnesses that usually cannot be distinguished clinically from other common viral or bacterial infections. Clinical features that characterize acute arboviral fevers usually include a sudden onset of debilitating symptoms, such as malaise, extreme headache, myalgia, lumbar pain, and sometimes nausea, vomiting, and dizziness. In general, these illnesses are of relatively short duration (1 to 6 days) and resolve without sequelae, except for weakness and lethargy, which can persist for a week or more. In a few arboviral illnesses (e.g., Colorado tick fever [CTF] and Oropouche [ORO] fever), a recrudescent course of fever and systemic symptoms can occur 10 to 14 days after the initial symptoms occur. In cases of Kyasanur Forest disease and Rift Valley fever (RVF), delayed syndromes of encephalitis or retinitis may follow weeks after the initial illness. Some important arboviruses, such as DEN, Ross River (RR), and WN viruses, may also produce a rash, but these exanthems are not

*This chapter contains information presented in chapter 103 by Theodore F. Tsai and Laura J. Chandler in the eighth edition of this *Manual*.

TABLE 1 Charactertistics of arboviruses

Family	Representative arboviruses affecting humans	Genome (no. of segments)	Vector(s)
Togaviridae	EEE, WEE, and VEE viruses	Positive, single-stranded RNA (1)	Mosquitoes, ticks
Flaviviridae	WN, SLE, DEN, YF, POW, and JE viruses	Positive, single-stranded RNA (1)	Mosquitoes, ticks
Bunyaviridae	LAC, Crimean-Congo hemorrhagic fever, and sandfly fever viruses	Negative- and ambisense single-stranded RNA (3)	Mosquitoes, ticks
Reoviridae	CTF virus	Double-stranded RNA (10)	Mosquitoes, ticks
Rhabdoviridae	Vesicular stomatitis virus	Negative, single-stranded RNA (1)	Sand flies
Orthomyxoviridae	Thogoto virus	Negative, single-stranded RNA (6 or 7)	Ticks
Asfarviridae	None	Double-stranded DNA	Ticks

distinctive; in fact, even when outbreaks occur in epidemic proportions, diseases such as DEN fever are sometimes incorrectly diagnosed as rubella or measles. Likewise, diseases such as influenza, leptospirosis, and some rickettsial infections are sometimes misdiagnosed as DEN fever. Several alphaviruses, such as the chikungunya (CHIK), O'nyong-nyong, Mayaro (MAY), RR, SIN, and Barmah Forest viruses, produce an acute febrile illness with polyarthritis and exanthem that must be differentiated clinically from rubella or cytomegalovirus, parvovirus, or mycoplasma infection (70). Arboviruses can also cause congenital infections, especially when introduced into immunologically naïve populations (75).

Neurotropic arboviruses such as JE, WN, SLE, TBE, Murray Valley encephalitis (MVE), and LAC viruses cause aseptic meningitis, encephalitis, or even flaccid paralysis in only a small percentage of infected persons; most infections are asymptomatic or lead to a mild illness, sometimes with headache. Pathologically, global involvement of cortical, subcortical, and brain stem structures and spinal cord myelitis are typical in more-severe forms. Consequently, various neurologic presentations are possible, with combinations of coma, weakness, cerebellar and extrapyramidal movement disorders, cranial palsies, and other manifestations of bulbar dysfunction and myelitis.

Viscerotropic disease can occur with YF, DEN, RVF, and certain other arboviral infections, resulting in hepatitis and jaundice. Generalized hemorrhage and multisystem organ failure are sometimes the end results of fulminant YF, RVF, and DEN hemorrhagic fever, mimicking malaria, leptospirosis, and the viral hemorrhagic fevers produced by Lassa virus and other arenaviruses, the Ebola and Marburg filoviruses, and Crimean-Congo hemorrhagic fever virus. Although YF, RVF, and DEN viruses pose a low risk for person-to-person nosocomial transmission (e.g., through needlestick exposures), the other viruses are proven hazards to hospital and laboratory workers (45, 76).

Although more than 100 of the recognized arboviruses can cause illness in humans, the laboratory diagnosis of these infections can be simplified by first considering the patient's history of travel or exposure. Some arboviruses, such as the DEN viruses, are transmitted virtually everywhere in the tropics and subtropics, but others are much more limited in their geographic distribution. By considering the known incubation periods of the principal arboviral infections in the context of the itinerary of places and circumstances under which infection may have been acquired, the differential diagnosis can be narrowed considerably. However, microbiologists and clinicians should be mindful that arboviruses can occasionally appear unexpectedly in new geographic regions, as illustrated by the 1999 introduction of WN virus into North America

and by cases of chikungunya arthritis imported into Europe in 2006 from an Indian Ocean island outbreak.

Currently, there is no specific therapy available for arboviral infections; supportive care (e.g., fluid replacement, analgesics, control of convulsions, and use of blood products in the case of severe hemorrhage) is all that is available. The rationale for promptly establishing the laboratory diagnosis of an arboviral infection is to hasten the confirmation of other treatable conditions, to avoid unnecessary treatment, and to assist public health officials in identifying arboviral infections with epidemic potential so that appropriate control measures (e.g., vector control or vaccination) can be implemented.

COLLECTION AND STORAGE OF SPECIMENS

Other than perhaps serologic testing for WN virus infection, few primary diagnostic laboratories can justify routine arboviral diagnosis as a service; instead, most laboratories should focus on the collection of appropriate specimens for submission to a reference laboratory. Assistance with diagnosis of arboviral infections can be obtained from some commercial reference laboratories, selected university research groups, the Division of Vector-Borne Infectious Diseases of the CDC [phone: (970) 221-6400], some state public health laboratories in the United States, and the WHO Collaborating Centers for Arbovirus Reference and Research. A listing of the WHO Collaborating Centers may be found at http://www.bireme.br/whocc.

Most arboviruses produce a brief, low level of viremia in humans, and it is only by chance that a viral isolate can be recovered from blood in these instances. However, other arboviruses, notably DEN and YF viruses, produce higher levels of viremia ($>10^{3.5}$ PFU/ml) of sufficient duration (ca. 5 to 6 days after the onset of fever) that humans serve as hosts for epidemic transmission. From the perspective of the clinical laboratory, these infections can be diagnosed by isolating virus from blood obtained during the acute phase of illness or by detecting genomic sequences by use of nucleic acid amplification techniques (NAAT) such as reverse transcriptase PCR (RT-PCR). Viruses causing encephalitis usually can be recovered from blood only during the preneuroinvasive phase of illness, and then usually by chance. When donors are in the viremic phase of infection, both WN virus and DEN virus can be transmitted via blood transfusion or organ transplantation (8, 29, 51, 58). Retrospective testing of the donors' blood in such instances has confirmed viremia (67). CTF virus is exceptional among human arboviruses in that it infects bone marrow erythrocytic

(Text continues on page 1494)

TABLE 2 Arboviruses associated with human illness by geographic region, mode of transmission, and clinical syndrome[a]

Location, mode of transmission, and virus	Febrile illness			Meningoencephalitis	Hemorrhagic fever	Other
	Nondescript	With rash	With arthritis			
North America						
Mosquito borne						
Cache Valley	○			○		
California encephalitis				○		
DEN viruses 1–4 (DEN 1–4)	●	●			●	Hepatitis[b]
EEE				●		
Everglades (VEE type II)				○		
Jamestown Canyon				○		Respiratory symptoms
Keystone				○		
LAC				●		
SLE				●		
Snowshoe hare				○		
Tensaw				○		
Trivittatus				○		Respiratory symptoms
VEE (sylvatic subtypes 1D and 1E)	○			○		
WEE[b]				●		Pneumonitis
WN[b]	●	●	●	●		Flaccid paralysis, hepatitis, pancreatitis, myocarditis, chorioretinitis
Sand fly borne						
Vesicular stomatitis (New Jersey and Indiana)	○			○		
Tick borne						
CTF	●			○	○	
POW/deer tick				○		
Salmon River	○					
Central and South America						
Mosquito borne						
Bussuquara	○					
Cache Valley	○					
Catu	○					
Cotia	○					
DEN 1–4	●	●		○	●	Hepatitis[b]
EEE						
Fort Sherman	○					
Group C viruses (Apeu, Caraparu, Itaqui, Madrid, Marituba, Murutucu, Nepuyo, Oriboca, Ossa, Restan)	○					
Guama	○			?		
Guaroa	○			○		Hepatitis
Ilheus	○					
Maguari	○					
MAY	●	●	●			
Mucambo (VEE type IIIA)	○			○		

(Continued on next page)

TABLE 2 *(Continued)*

Location, mode of transmission, and virus	Febrile illness			Meningoencephalitis	Hemorrhagic fever	Other
	Nondescript	With rash	With arthritis			
ORO	•			°		
Piry	°					
Rocio				•		
SLE	°			°		
Tacaiuma						Two cases with concurrent malaria were fatal
Tonate (VEE type IIIB)	°			°		
Tucunduba				°		
VEE (epizootic subtypes IABC)	•			•		Abortion, CNS malformation after first-trimester infection
VEE (sylvatic subtypes 1D, 1E, and 1F)	°			°		Pneumonitis
WEE					•	
WN[b]	•	•	•	•		Flaccid paralysis, hepatitis, pancreatitis, myocarditis
Wyeomyia	°					
Xingu	°					Hepatitis?
YF	•				•	Hepatitis
Sand fly and/or midge borne						
Alenquer	°					
Candiru	°					
Chagres	°					
Changuinola	°					
Morumbi	°					
ORO	•	°		°		
Punta Toro	°					
Serra Norte	°					
Vesicular stomatitis (New Jersey, Indiana, and Alagoas)	°			°		
Europe						
Mosquito borne						
Batai	°					
CHIK[b]		•	•	°	°	Exanthems, retinitis, Guillain-Barré syndrome, acute disseminated encephalomyelitis, acute flaccid paralysis
Inkoo	°			°		Respiratory illness
SIN (Ockelbo)	•	•	•			
Snowshoe hare				°		
Tahyna	•			°		Respiratory illness
WN[b]	°	°	°	•		Flaccid paralysis, hepatitis, pancreatitis, myocarditis, chorioretinitis
Sand fly borne						
Sandfly fever (Naples)	•					
Sandfly fever (Sicilian)	•					
Toscana	•	°		•		Hepatosplenomegaly, DIC, cerebral vasculitis

(Continued on next page)

TABLE 2 Arboviruses associated with human illness by geographic region, mode of transmission, and clinical syndrome (*Continued*)

Location, mode of transmission, and virus	Febrile illness			Meningoencephalitis	Hemorrhagic fever	Other
	Nondescript	With rash	With arthritis			
Tick borne						
Bhanja	○			○		
Central European encephalitis[c,d]	●			●		Hepatitis, thrombocytopenia
Crimean-Congo hemorrhagic fever[d]						
Dhori	○			○[e]		
Kemerovo				○		
Lipovnik				○		
Louping ill[d]				○		
Thogoto	○			○		Hepatitis, optic neuritis
Tribec					○	
Asia						
Mosquito borne						
Batai	○			○		
Chandipura	●			●		
CHIK[b]		●	●	○	○	Exanthems, retinitis, Guillain-Barré syndrome, acute disseminated encephalomyelitis, acute flaccid paralysis
DEN 1–4	●	●		○	●	Hepatitis[b]
JE						Abortion after congenital first- and second-trimester infection
Kunjin (WN)		○	○	○		
Semliki Forest (Metri)				○		
SIN	●	●	●	○	○	
Snowshoe hare				○		
Tahyna	●			○		Respiratory illness
WN[b]	●	●	●	○		Flaccid paralysis, hepatitis, pancreatitis, myocarditis, chorioretinitis
Yunnan	○					
Zika		●				Conjunctivitis
Sand fly borne						
Chandipura	●			●		
Sandfly fever (Naples)	●					
Sandfly fever (Sicilian)	●					
Tick borne						
Alma-Arasan	○					
Banna				●		
Crimean-Congo hemorrhagic fever[d]					●	
Dhori			○[e]			
Ganjam	○					
Issyk-kul	○					
Karshi	○					
Kemerovo				○		
Kyasanur Forest (Alkhurma)[d]				●	●	Pneumonia, retinitis
Negishi				○		

(Continued on next page)

TABLE 2 *(Continued)*

Location, mode of transmission, and virus	Febrile illness			Meningoencephalitis	Hemorrhagic fever	Other
	Nondescript	With rash	With arthritis			
Omsk hemorrhagic fever				●	●	Pneumonia
POW				○		
Russian spring-summer encephalitis[c]				●		
Syr-Darya Valley		○				
Tamdy	○					
Wanowrie				○	○	
Africa						
Mosquito borne						
Babanki	●	●	●			
Bangui		○				
Banzi	○					
Bhanja	○			○		
Bunyamwera		●		○		
Bwamba		●		○		
CHIK[b]		●	●	○	○	Exanthems, retinitis, Guillain-Barré syndrome, acute disseminated encephalomyelitis, acute flaccid paralysis
DEN 1–4		●		○	●	Hepatitis[b]
Garissa (Ngari)		○		○	●	Reassortant of Bunyamwera virus
Germiston		○		○		
Ilesha		●		○	○	
Koutango		○				
Lebombo	○					
Ngari				○		
Nyando	○					
O'nyong-nyong		●	●			
Orungo	●					
Pongola			○			
RVF[b,d]	●			●	●	Hepatitis, retinitis
Semliki Forest	○			○		
Shokwe	○					
Shuni	○					
SIN		●	●		○	
Spondweni		○				
Tahyna	●			○		Respiratory illness
Tataguine		●				
Usutu		○				
Wesselsbron	○					Hepatitis
WN[b]	●	●	●	●		Flaccid paralysis, hepatitis, pancreatitis, myocarditis, chorioretinitis
YF	●				●	Hepatitis
Zika		○				Conjunctivitis
Sand fly borne						
Chandipura	●			●		
Sandfly fever (Naples)	●					
Sandfly fever (Sicilian)	●					
Tick borne						
Abadina	○					
Bhanja	○			○		

(Continued on next page)

TABLE 2 Arboviruses associated with human illness by geographic region, mode of transmission, and clinical syndrome (*Continued*)

Location, mode of transmission, and virus	Febrile illness			Meningoencephalitis	Hemorrhagic fever	Other
	Nondescript	With rash	With arthritis			
Crimean-Congo hemorrhagic fever[d]					•	
Dugbe	o			o		
Nairobi sheep disease	o					
Quaranfil	o			o		
Thogoto	o			o		Hepatitis, optic neuritis
Australia and Oceania						
Mosquito borne						
Barmah Forest			•	o		Glomerulonephritis
DEN 1–4	•	•				Hepatitis[b]
Edge Hill			o			
GanGan			o			
JE				o		
Kokobera			o			
Kunjin (WN)	o		o	o		
MVE				•		
RR		•	•	o		Glomerulonephritis
Sepik	o					
SIN	o	o	o			
Trubanaman	o					
Zika		•				Conjunctivitis

[a]Key: o, rare or sporadic; •, frequent, epidemic. Only arboviruses causing illness after natural infection are listed; viruses causing illness after laboratory exposure only are excluded.
[b]Perinatal illness following third-trimester infection has also been described.
[c]Transmissible by ingestion of infected milk products.
[d]Transmissible through meat of infected animals.
[e]Syndrome reported only after laboratory-acquired infection.

precursors, leading to infection of the erythrocyte for its lifetime; consequently, the virus can be recovered from blood obtained for several weeks after clinical recovery and can be transmitted through transfusion (41, 80). TBE virus has also been transmitted by transfusion (41).

Viral isolates can sometimes be recovered by biopsy or at autopsy from the viscera of patients with acute YF, DEN hemorrhagic fever, or other viscerotropic arboviral infections and from brain tissue or cerebrospinal fluid (CSF) of patients with central nervous system (CNS) infections. Brain samples should be taken from several areas, including the cortex, brain nuclei, cerebellum, and brain stem. Neurotropic arboviruses can occasionally be isolated from CSF obtained by lumbar puncture during the acute stages of encephalitis or aseptic meningitis. RT-PCR has often proved to be more sensitive in detecting specific arboviral genomic sequences in brain tissue or CSF. Alphaviruses have rarely been isolated from vesicular skin lesions, the joint fluids of patients with acute polyarthritis, or the upper respiratory tracts of patients with acute febrile illnesses. Under certain circumstances, arboviruses or their antigens have been detected in urine, milk, semen, and vitreous fluid (5, 73). Clinical laboratories sometimes also receive arthropods for viral isolation. These samples can be referred to a reference laboratory in the same manner as tissues, where they can be processed for virus isolation or nucleic acid or antigen detection procedures.

A plan for dividing available tissues or fluids for viral isolation, electron microscopy, and direct detection assays of antigen and genomic sequences should be devised. Tissues should be collected aseptically and rapidly transported to the laboratory in a viral transport medium or on a moist sponge. If the aliquot for viral isolation cannot be processed within 24 h, it can be maintained at 4°C; otherwise, the sample should be frozen immediately at −70°C or stored on dry ice. Samples for virus isolation and nucleic acid detection should be kept frozen continuously, avoiding freeze-thaw cycles, which may inactivate virus or disrupt nucleic acids. The aliquot for electron microscopy should be minced and placed directly in glutaraldehyde or another fixative. Autolytic changes occur rapidly, and tissues should be fixed as quickly as possible. To prepare sections for immunohistochemical (IHC) examination, a portion of the sample should either be fixed in 10% buffered formalin or, preferably, added to freezing medium and frozen. Touch preparations are less reliable. Aliquots for antigen detection by other means and for PCR should be frozen at −70°C. Samples should be shipped by express mail in double-sealed containers according to local transport regulations. Frozen samples should be shipped separately on dry ice and labeled appropriately. International shipments usually require import and/or customs permits and clearances.

Serologic studies are best done by comparing antibody titers in paired serum samples drawn during the first week of illness and 2 to 3 weeks later. A single serum specimen may be sufficient for diagnosis of certain arboviral infections for which immunoglobulin M (IgM) assays are available. Detection of virus-specific IgM in CSF is a sensitive and highly specific approach to diagnosing CNS infection, but both CSF and serum samples should be tested. IgM capture ELISAs for arboviral CNS infections transmitted in the

United States are offered by several reference and some state public health laboratories. Serum and CSF samples should be collected aseptically, stored either refrigerated or frozen, and transported according to current shipping regulations. Freeze-thaw cycles may reduce antibody titers and should be avoided. Blood or serum blotted and dried on filter paper may be suitable for some serologic assays.

No specific procedures for patient preparation are required. The isolation of certain arboviruses from host systems could be inhibited in patients treated with antiviral agents, such as ribavirin, or immunomodulators, such as alpha or gamma interferon. Some preparations of gamma globulin, including preparations for intravenous use, may contain arboviral antibodies and could interfere with the isolation of arboviruses from patient specimens or with arboviral serologic tests.

DIRECT EXAMINATION

Clinical application and experience with direct arbovirus detection methods generally have been limited, and specimens should be evaluated in parallel with conventional viral isolation, molecular testing, and serologic procedures.

Electron Microscopy

When tissue is available, direct examination by electron microscopy can sometimes provide rapid evidence of an arboviral infection. Experienced observers can identify virions morphologically, often to the level of a viral family, in thin tissue sections. Visualization of togaviruses in brain tissue has helped to establish a diagnosis of EEE in some reported cases. Newer techniques using confocal microscopy combined with transmission electron microscopy have been used to diagnose human flavivirus infections (12). Virions may be absent, however, from autopsy tissues of patients who died after a prolonged course of illness and from whom infection had previously been cleared.

Detection of Viral Antigens by Use of IHC Staining or Immunofluorescence

IHC staining of peripheral blood mononuclear cells or tissue sections has been successful in detecting arboviral antigens in CSF and brain specimens from encephalitis patients; in the viscera of patients with YF, DEN fever, and other viscerotropic infections; and in joint fluids of patients with acute arthritis (15, 22). CTF virus-infected erythrocytes occasionally can be identified directly by staining a simple smear of peripheral or clotted blood. Postmortem diagnosis of arboviral infections can be made from formalin-fixed sections by using IHC staining. Formalin-fixed tissue or paraffin-embedded tissue block samples can be used. The advantage of IHC staining is that samples can be examined months after collection and storage. For best results, formalin-fixed specimens should be transferred to 70% ethanol after 48 h for storage. Monoclonal antibodies specific for many medically important arboviruses are available; for more obscure arboviruses, hyperimmune mouse antibodies can be employed. Antibodies and information on their working dilutions can be obtained from the CDC and other reference laboratories. Although trypsinized, formalin-fixed tissues are suitable for IFA examination, frozen sections are generally preferred because trypsinization procedures have not been standardized for all arboviruses and because success varies with the duration of formalin fixation.

Formalin-fixed tissue or paraffin-embedded tissue block samples can also be sent to the CDC or to some academic pathology groups (e.g., University of Texas Medical Branch) for detection of specific arboviruses, such as WN virus. Arrangements can be made with the CDC pathology staff [phone: (404) 639-3133] before shipping any specimen.

Antigen Capture ELISA

Antigen capture ELISAs have been developed to detect several arboviruses in mosquitoes and DEN virus in acute-phase blood samples. The detection thresholds of antigen capture ELISAs for SLE, WN, and JE viruses (ca. $10^{3.5}$ PFU/ml) are sufficiently sensitive for their application in the epidemiologic surveillance of infected arthropod vectors (28, 74). Several commercial antigen assay kits are available for detection of WN, SLE, and EEE viral antigens in mosquitoes (VecTest; Medical Analysis Systems).

Commercially available ELISA (Platelia Dengue NS1 AG; Bio-Rad) and lateral-flow rapid tests (Dengue NS1 Ag strip; Bio-Rad) that detect soluble DEN viral NS1 circulating in the blood are highly specific (99 to 100%) in differentiating DEN from JE virus and other viruses causing acute infections (23, 83). The assays are more sensitive in the early phase of primary DEN virus infection (92 to 96%) than IgM capture ELISA and RT-PCR, but their sensitivity is reduced in the presence of IgM and IgG antibodies that complex the antigen. Consequently, the assays' sensitivities for detecting secondary DEN virus infection range from 66 to 78%. A serotype-specific DEN virus 1 (DEN 1) NS1 antigen detection assay using specific monoclonal antibodies has been reported.

Nucleic Acid Detection Techniques

A number of nucleic acid amplification strategies have been developed for the detection and identification of medically important arboviruses, including standard RT-PCR (with agarose gel analysis), real-time RT-PCR using fluorescent probes, nucleic acid sequence-based amplification (NASBA), and the recently developed reverse transcription–loop-mediated isothermal amplification (LAMP) method. A review of the current literature reveals that in nearly all cases, the analytical sensitivity of any of the amplification assays is equal to or exceeds that of the most sensitive antigen detection assays or viral isolation procedures performed with either cultured cells or neonatal mice. In addition, amplification assays can provide results in a much shorter time than isolation methods, while allowing for the processing of larger numbers of samples. However, the clinical sensitivity of amplification assays is highly dependent upon the dynamics of in vivo viral replication and the tissue tropism of the virus. For example, WN virus infection produces a relatively short viremia which is often low or absent at the time of clinical presentation of CNS symptoms; in one study, WN viral RNA was detected in the CSF of patients with serologically confirmed cases only 57% of the time with a real-time RT-PCR assay, with an analytical sensitivity of 0.1 PFU (38). However, in another study, RT-PCR and/or NASBA testing of acute specimens obtained early during the febrile phase provided very useful diagnostic data which complemented serologic testing to confirm infection in 94.2% of the patients. Interestingly, in that study, in which 82.6% of patients had WN fever, not neuroinvasive disease, 36.1% of acute specimens were RT-PCR positive and IgM negative (72a). A real-time assay for detection of DEN virus with a similar analytical sensitivity can detect and correctly serotype DEN viruses from nearly all clinical cases, since the DEN viruses typically achieve a much higher level of viremia, with a longer duration (82). In general, amplification assays have been successful in detecting arboviruses in tissues obtained from fatal human cases when the appropriate tissue target is known and assayed (i.e., brain tissue in cases of WN fever, LAC fever, or EEE, liver tissue in cases of YF, etc.). A commercially available WN viral RNA detection system is approved by the U.S. Food and Drug Administration (FDA) for screening of donor blood, organs, cells, and tissues (Procleix WNV assay; Gen-Probe Inc.).

The use of amplification assays for the detection of arboviruses in surveillance protocols, particularly in mosquitoes collected in the field, has become the method of choice because large numbers of samples can be tested with minimum labor and the sensitivity often exceeds that of virus isolation or antigen detection assays. With the addition of automation, amplification approaches have been used to test hundreds of mosquito specimens in a single day (64). Amplification assays have also been utilized successfully in environmental surveillance by detecting arboviruses in tissues obtained from vertebrate hosts collected in the field. WN virus detection in dead birds collected in the field and EEE virus detection in fatal equine cases are typical applications of this technology.

Careful consideration and planning must be undertaken in the formulation of a molecular testing algorithm for arboviruses due to the potential for cross-contamination inherent with all amplification assays. In general, a good testing algorithm for an amplification assay would include independent confirmation of all positive results by another virus detection assay, such as an alternate amplification strategy, virus isolation, antigen capture ELISA, or direct IFA. In addition, the inclusion of an internal positive control (see below) is desired to ensure that all reagents and amplification parameters are optimal for target amplification. At minimum, all positive amplification results should be confirmed by retesting with the same technology (e.g., RT-PCR) with a different primer set. Testing algorithms must also incorporate appropriate controls to ensure against false-positive or false-negative results. Negative controls should include reaction mixes with no RNA added (reagent controls) to ensure that amplification reagents are not contaminated with target RNA or DNA, as well as RNA extracted from negative specimens (extraction controls) to monitor contamination during sample processing. Positive controls included in each assay should contain various levels of target RNA (high, medium, low, etc.) to ensure that the sensitivity of the current assay is similar to those of previous tests. The use of an exogenously added RNA target along with a corresponding amplification primer set allows for the monitoring of every amplification reaction and can detect false-negative results. This strategy is particularly useful for testing specimens that may contain inhibitors of RT-PCR (e.g., blood, mosquito lysates, etc.). For all amplification-based technologies, it is essential that proper laboratory procedures be followed to prevent cross-contamination of clinical samples with amplified DNA or RNA, which would result in the generation of false-positive results. In general, there should be a complete physical separation of pre- and postamplification laboratory space and equipment. Finally, clinical samples should be tested in duplicate wells, at minimum, and ideally two primer sets should be utilized in independent reactions.

RNA Extraction and Purification

The majority of arboviruses of medical importance are enveloped single-stranded RNA viruses, and therefore the sensitivity and specificity of any amplification strategy are highly dependent on the efficient extraction and purification of the target RNA template. Highly efficient RNA extraction and purification protocols are now commercially available from a number of sources. Many of these commercial RNA extraction kits—both manual and automated—have been evaluated and compared to one another in several multicenter studies, and all performed well, with minimal differences in RNA extraction sensitivity (10, 56). Most of these utilize a chaotropic lysis buffer which allows for both efficient solubilization of the sample and stabilization of the RNA, followed by binding to silica, subsequent washing, and then elution in a low-salt solution. Some purification protocols have also been automated, and hundreds of samples can be processed within a single day. The use of a chaotropic lysis buffer has also enabled the efficient extraction of intact RNA from sources that were problematic in the past due to RNase activity, including serum/plasma, whole blood, CSF, tissues, and homogenized ticks or mosquitoes. Ticks and mosquitoes are particularly useful for environmental surveillance of arboviruses.

RT-PCR

Standard RT-PCR-based assays (as opposed to real-time assays [described below]) to detect arbovirus genomic sequences have been developed for a number of the medically important arboviruses (31). Most of the assays use virus-specific primers designed to amplify a single virus species or, in a few cases, serologically related viruses (i.e., the DEN viruses). The assays typically involve RT-PCR amplification followed by agarose gel electrophoresis, with DNA visualization by staining with ethidium bromide to characterize the amplified DNA by molecular weight. Visualization of a DNA fragment of the predicted size is considered diagnostic in some cases. Because nontarget amplification in some instances can generate DNA products with similar mobilities in agarose gels to that of the predicted fragment, generating false-positive results, additional characterization of the amplified DNA is often utilized. A variety of sequence-specific technologies for detecting and confirming the identity of the amplified DNA include hybridization with virus-specific probes (e.g., Southern blot, dot blot, or microtiter plate hybridization and simultaneous detection of multiple target sequences by capture oligonucleotide microarrays), PCR amplification with primers internal to the original primers (nested or seminested PCR), restriction endonuclease digestion of the DNA product, or nucleic acid sequence analysis (19). With the advent of automated DNA sequencing instrumentation, this approach is becoming the method of choice in many diagnostic laboratories due to the unambiguous identification achievable in a short time frame. Virus-specific RT-PCR assays are available to detect, among others, DEN, YF, JE, western equine encephalitis (WEE), EEE, SLE, VEE, MVE, Powassan (POW), TBE, and WN viruses; the California serogroup viruses; and the RR, Ockelbo, and CTF viruses. In contrast to virus-specific RT-PCR assays, there are also RT-PCR amplification strategies which utilize primers designed to amplify most or all viruses within a genus. Consensus RT-PCR assays have been described for alphaviruses, flaviviruses, orthobunyaviruses, phleboviruses, and nairoviruses (34, 53, 62). When consensus primers are utilized, a sequence-specific detection method (as described above) must be employed to specifically identify the resulting DNA, since by the design of the assay, all related viruses would generate DNA amplicons of identical size.

Real-Time 5′-Exonuclease Fluorogenic Assays

Real-time RT-PCR assays with exonuclease digestion of target-specific probes (commonly referred to as TaqMan assays) combine RT-PCR amplification with concurrent sequence-based detection of amplified DNA, using fluorescently labeled, virus-specific DNA probes. The assays offer many advantages over standard RT-PCR, namely, increased sensitivity, increased specificity, quantification, high throughput, a decreased likelihood of cross-contamination, and rapid results. These advantages are due to the use of a fluorescently labeled internal probe, which rapidly and specifically detects amplified DNA via hybridization. Subsequent *Taq* polymerase digestion of the probe releases the 5′-labeled nucleotide and results in a measurable increase in fluorescence. This sequence-specific detection obviates the need for any postamplification characterization of the amplified DNA, resulting in a much more rapid result. In addition, the likelihood of contamination is reduced because amplified DNA is not manipulated in the laboratory, as occurs with gel electrophoresis and standard RT-PCR. Real-time fluorogenic assays also offer the added advantage of multiplexing, the ability to detect multiple targets at the same time in the same amplification reaction mix by including additional primers and probes containing unique fluorescent dyes. Several TaqMan assays for the detection of arboviruses have been described, including assays for WN, SLE, TBE, DEN, EEE, WEE, LAC, VEE, CTF, RVF, YF, CHIK, and Zika viruses (33, 35–39, 50, 79).

NASBA

Another nucleic acid amplification technology that has been used for the detection and identification of arboviruses is NASBA. The initial stage of NASBA is similar to RT-PCR in that single-stranded target RNA is copied into double-stranded DNA via virus-specific primers in an RT reaction. However, NASBA subsequently differs significantly from RT-PCR in a number of ways: the amplification reaction is isothermic (41°C), different enzymes are used (RT, RNase H, and T7 RNA polymerase), and the final amplification product is single-stranded RNA. In NASBA, the oligonucleotide used to prime cDNA synthesis contains the T7 promoter sequence. The resultant reverse-transcribed DNA serves as a template for transcription by T7 RNA polymerase. Amplification is generally more rapid because it is not dependent on thermal cycling. Amplified RNA can be detected by hybridization to a virus-specific oligonucleotide probe either by utilizing an electrochemiluminescence detection format or by using (in real time) a fluorescently labeled molecular beacon probe. Both detection approaches have been employed successfully to detect a number of arboviruses, including WN, SLE, EEE, WEE, LAC, CHIK, and DEN viruses (36, 37, 68, 82).

LAMP

A number of reports describing the detection of arboviruses by LAMP have recently been described in the literature (49). The amplification is based upon strand displacement DNA polymerization utilizing six target-specific oligonucleotide primers. After reverse transcription, isothermal (63°C) DNA amplification proceeds by use of a DNA polymerase with high displacement activity (Bst DNA polymerase). The LAMP strategy generates double-stranded DNA stem-loop molecules of various stem lengths based upon primer design, specifically the incorporation of complementary target sequences into the 5′ region of some of the primers. The final DNA products can be visualized as a DNA ladder on an agarose gel. Alternatively, amplification can be detected in real time by measuring the turbidity (using a photometer/turbidimeter) of the reaction mixture, which increases with the amount of DNA synthesized due to the accumulation of magnesium pyrophosphate. The specificity in LAMP is due to the binding of the six oligonucleotide primers, and specific identification of the amplified DNA is not considered necessary, so the final detection is completely nonspecific turbidity. LAMP reagent kits and detection equipment are available commercially, and the overall reaction costs are similar to those of real-time PCR. LAMP assays have been described for the detection of WN, RVF, CHIK, JE, and DEN viruses (42, 49).

VIRUS ISOLATION

Novel arboviruses continue to be discovered, usually as orphan viruses first identified in vector surveys but, remarkably, also from human clinical specimens. For this reason, despite the availability of rapid analytical assays, attempts to recover viruses from diagnostic specimens should not be regarded as an anachronism in the contemporary viral diagnostic laboratory.

Many of the medically important arboviruses have caused infections in laboratory workers. The pathogenesis of infections acquired from aerosols created by pipetting tissue, homogenization, centrifugation, and other procedures may differ from that of natural infection, with the possibility of direct CNS invasion through the olfactory epithelium (52). On the basis of this experience, the joint CDC-National Institutes of Health guidelines for biosafety in microbiological and biomedical laboratories recommend biosafety level 2 to 4 containment facilities for laboratory work with arboviruses (76). The essential elements of the various biosafety levels for activities with arboviruses and laboratory animals infected with them are detailed in these guidelines (76). Some arboviruses are also designated select agents and require additional levels of security. Laboratory staff should be immunized with available arboviral vaccines. Laboratories that process CNS specimens from patients with encephalitis should consider immunizing staff with rabies vaccine as well.

Most arboviruses can be cultivated in a variety of primary and continuous cell lines, including primary duck and chicken embryo cells, primary monkey and hamster kidney cells, C6/36 *Aedes albopictus* and AP61 *Aedes pseudoscutellaris* mosquito cell lines, and Vero, LLC-MK2, BHK-21, CER, SW13, and PK cell lines. The time to develop cytopathic effects (CPE) as well as the pattern of CPE varies in each virus-cell system, e.g., primary duck and BHK-21 cells are rapidly destroyed by most arboviruses, while the development of CPE in monkey kidney cell lines is generally slower. AP61 and C6/36 cells exhibit nearly universal susceptibility to the mosquito-associated arboviruses, including the DEN viruses, which grow poorly in continuous monkey kidney cell lines. The mosquito cell lines, which are generally incubated at 28°C, exhibit little evidence of viral CPE, and replication must be identified by an IFA test or other means. Many alphaviruses and some flavivirus strains produce CPE or form cell syncytia in these lines, but most arboviruses do not. The majority of arboviruses are lethal to suckling (2- to 3-day-old) mice, which exhibit signs of illness, paralysis, and death within days to 2 weeks after intracerebral inoculation. Some field isolates (e.g., DEN and sandfly fever group viruses) exhibit virulence for mice only after adaptation through blind passages. Infected suckling mouse brain is still the preferred antigen for many serologic tests and for the preparation of clean, high-titer immune reagents.

Since no single isolation system detects all arboviruses, tissues, fluids, and sera collected in the acute (febrile) phase of illness should be inoculated into cultures of several cell lines, including C6/36 or AP61 mosquito cells, Vero, LLC-MK2, or BHK-21 cells, or primary embryonic cells, and into

2- to 4-day-old suckling mice (33, 57, 72). Direct inoculation of live colony-reared mosquitoes can also be used (61). Ideally, serum specimens should be inoculated undiluted and in 10^{-1} and 10^{-2} dilutions to avoid prozone effects due to viral autointerference and antiviral antibodies present in the specimen. Tissues should be homogenized and diluted similarly, on a weight-to-volume basis (10 to 20%), with a protein- and antibiotic-containing medium, e.g., phosphate-buffered saline with 0.75% bovine serum albumin and 1% gentamicin. After adsorption to the drained cell monolayer, cell cultures are fed with medium and observed daily or more often for signs of CPE. Small flasks (12.5 or 25 cm^2), tubes, or coverslips in shell vials may be used. Viral growth in C6/36 and AP61 cells does not reliably produce CPE, and these cells must be examined for viral antigen and replication by an IFA test or other means (69). When medium from infected cultures is harvested for passage or storage, fetal calf serum should be added to a final concentration of 20 to 40% before the medium is frozen at −70°C.

Intracerebrally inoculated mice (one litter of 6 to 10 mice for each dilution) should be observed twice daily for up to 2 weeks for signs of illness and death (40). Ill and dead mice should be frozen at −70°C until infected organs can be harvested and passaged in cell culture. When a bunyaviral or orthomyxoviral etiology is suspected, it is prudent to harvest livers in addition to brains, since certain orthobunyaviruses and thogotoviruses replicate to higher titers in the mouse liver than in the brain.

Although NAAT have the advantages of speed and sensitivity, virus isolation remains the "gold standard" against which other methods are compared. Virus isolation can detect new or unsuspected agents, as well as those agents for which NAAT have not yet been developed. Furthermore, genetic variants and mutations can lead to false-negative NAAT results, yet the virus may be detected in culture.

VIRAL IDENTIFICATION

While identification of arboviral isolates previously depended upon their antigenic characterization, PCR and other molecular tests are now available for many of the medically important arboviruses. Provided that sufficient sequence information is available, sequence analysis of the PCR product can provide more-specific identification of the isolates than ELISA, IFA, or other rapid serologic assays. PCR-based assays that amplify sequences conserved among medically important alphaviruses, bunyaviruses, or flaviviruses permit the assignment of an unknown virus within a broad taxon, and sequence analysis of the amplified products can give their precise identification. Such omnibus primers have been reported for alphaviruses and flaviviruses and for certain groups of bunyaviruses and reoviruses (11, 16, 32, 34). Sequence information can also be used for molecular epidemiology, including identification of source strains during outbreaks and investigation of strain relationships that may have epidemiologic or clinical importance.

The identity of a suspected arbovirus can often be narrowed down from information on the circumstance, source, location, or other aspects of collection (Table 2). If no particular agent is suspected, polyclonal or monoclonal antibodies against selected prototype virus strains can be used to provide a provisional identification of the agent. Antibody panels prepared against representative serogroups of viruses, such as those prepared against the suspected etiologic agents of a specific clinical syndrome (i.e., encephalitis) or against viruses present in the area where the sample was collected or the patient was infected, are particularly useful. Once the virus is provisionally identified, PCR or specific antibodies can be used to type the virus.

Any of several standard serologic tests (ELISA, IFA, HI, and CF tests) can be used in this preliminary phase of identification. Complete identification requires partial sequencing or serologic comparison between reactivity levels of antisera prepared against the new isolate and a prototype strain. The neutralization test is the preferred and accepted method for such antigenic comparisons.

When screening with broadly reactive antibodies fails to place an unknown virus within a group of arboviruses, morphologic examination of the unknown by negative-stain electron microscopy can categorize the virus within a taxon (12). Virions generally can be found in cell culture medium or directly in clinical specimens that have infectivity titers of ≥10^6 PFU/ml. Although most pathology laboratories do not routinely prepare negatively stained grids, examination of thin sections of infected cell cultures can often be arranged.

SEROLOGIC TESTS

In most laboratories, diagnosis of arboviral infections relies mainly on serology. The classical serologic tests, HI and CF, have been abandoned by many diagnostic laboratories in favor of IgM capture ELISA or IFA. The HI and CF tests are now used mainly in research laboratories. A number of serologic assay kits are now available commercially for specific pathogens (Table 3). In the United States, indirect

TABLE 3 Serologic assays commercially available in the United States for diagnosis of arbovirus infections

Assay type	Virus(es)	Manufacturer	FDA status[a]
IFA for IgG or IgM	WEE, EEE, LAC, SLE	Focus Diagnostics	IVD
	WEE, EEE, LAC, SLE, WN, POW	PanBio	ASR
	WN	PanBio	ASR
ELISA for IgG and IgM	WN	Focus Diagnostics	IVD
	WN	PanBio	IVD
	DEN 1–4	Focus Diagnostics	RUO
	DEN 1–4	PanBio	ASR
ELISA for IgM	WN	InBios	IVD
ELISA for IgG	WN	InBios	RUO
Immunochromatographic test	WN	Spectral	

[a]IVD, for in vitro diagnostics; ASR, analyte-specific reagent; RUO, for research use only. Additional products available for sale outside the United States include IFAs for WN, VEE, JE, YF, and DEN viruses; rapid lateral-flow and strip immunochromatographic tests for DEN virus, and IgM and IgG ELISAs for JE virus.

IFA and ELISA reagents and kits are confined to those for arboviruses most likely to be encountered by U.S. residents. The FDA status varies for each product. In some cases, a kit may be approved for diagnostic use for serum samples but not for CSF (55). Additional products, including rapid lateral-flow and strip immunochromatographic tests, are available for a number of arboviruses important outside the United States.

ELISA

The antibody capture format for detection of IgM in serum or CSF is more sensitive and specific than indirect methods of IgM detection (2, 7, 77). Virus-specific IgM can be detected in the sera of 90 to 95% of patients with primary DEN virus infections by the sixth day after the onset of illness, but earlier and more sensitive diagnosis can be achieved with detection of the NS1 antigen in blood (23, 77). IgM to WN virus is usually detected in CSF 3 to 5 days into clinical illness, although up to 8 days may be required (24, 55, 72). IgM in serum appears 3 days after IgM in CSF. Four commercial kits are available in the United States for rapid presumptive diagnosis (PanBio WNV IgM capture and IgG ELISA [Inverness Medical Innovations Australia Pty. Ltd.], West Nile detect IgM capture ELISA [Bios International, Inc.], DxSelect West Nile virus IgM capture [Focus Diagnostics, Inc.], and Spectral RapidWN West Nile virus IgM test [Spectral Diagnostics, Inc.]); however, positive results should be confirmed in reference laboratories. WN virus can be detected earlier in infection by PCR or culture, but once clinical illness develops, PCR is generally less sensitive than antibody-based methods. The presence of virus-specific IgM in CSF reflects intrathecal antibody production and is considered diagnostic of recent CNS infection. In serum, a declining level of virus-specific IgM can usually be detected for several months after infection and for up to a year after infection in some cases. In WN virus infection, specific IgM antibodies have been reported for some patients for up to 2 years or more (60); therefore, a positive IgM result for a single serum sample is considered only presumptive evidence of recent infection. An analogous IgA capture ELISA for RR polyarthritis was shown to be better suited for diagnosis of recent infection because the level of virus-specific IgA declined more rapidly than that of IgM (9). In addition, IgG avidity tests on acute-phase sera have been used to discriminate between primary and secondary infections (43, 46). Low-avidity antibodies are characteristic of recent infections, whereas high-avidity IgG antibodies are seen 6 months or more after the onset of symptoms. Arboviral IgG antibodies are usually detected by an indirect sandwich method.

Heterologous reactions among antibodies to antigenically related viruses are a vexing problem in areas where several related viruses cocirculate. Cross-reactions between DEN viruses and JE virus, between YF virus and the numerous flaviviruses that circulate in West Africa, and between SLE, WN, and POW viruses in the United States frequently produce overlapping values that may be uninterpretable. Serologic cross-reactions of WN virus with other flaviviruses, and less frequently with bunyaviruses, enteroviruses, and cytomegalovirus, can occur, especially with IgG in serum (55). Because of cross-reactivity, a positive IgM assay should be followed by a neutralization test to determine the etiology of illness.

Numerous schemes have been devised to define the threshold of a positive or significant ELISA absorbance value. Some laboratories define a positive reaction in multiples (units) of the absorbance of a weak positive specimen, an approach that controls plate-to-plate variations in specimen reactivity. An alternative approach is to define the threshold

absorbance as a multiple (e.g., 5 standard deviations) above the mean absorbance for samples from a population of uninfected persons. A simple multiple of 2 times the absorbance of a negative control generally produces a conservative interpretation, exceeding 5 standard deviations above the mean value for negative samples.

Indirect IFA

Some laboratories use IFA for differentiation of IgG and IgM responses. Infected cells fixed on microscope slides with multiple wells are the usual antigen substrate. Kits for detection of antibodies to the most common arboviruses in the United States are commercially available (Table 3). The kits provide multivalent slides with four (EEE, WEE, LAC, and SLE viruses) or six (WN and POW viruses, in addition to the other four) infected cell spots and uninfected control cells. WN viral antigen is also available as a single analyte (45). Positive and negative sera are supplied with the kits, and all reagents are ready to use and do not have to be titrated. As with other assays, sera from persons previously infected with WN, DEN, JE, POW, or other flaviviruses may cross-react with the SLE antigen in these tests and vice versa; thus, confirmation of the diagnosis should be obtained with a neutralization test.

IgM antibodies detected by immunofluorescence become detectable within a few days after the onset of illness, and IgG antibodies appear shortly thereafter. IgG antibodies detected by IFA are long-lived, paralleling the longevity of HI and neutralizing antibodies. Fourfold changes are diagnostic of recent infection, and in some circumstances, single or stable elevated titers (>1:128) may indicate recent infection. The sensitivities and specificities of the IFA and HI tests are similar. Thus, cross-reactions among related flaviviruses, e.g., among SLE, WN, and DEN viruses, sometimes present a problem in interpretation.

HI Test

For the arboviruses that hemagglutinate erythrocytes, i.e., members of the families *Flaviviridae*, *Bunyaviridae*, and *Togaviridae* and certain members of the *Rhabdoviridae* and *Orthomyxoviridae*, the HI test is a convenient screening serologic procedure (2, 25). HI antibodies rise rapidly, within the first week after the onset of illness, and are long-lived, persisting at low levels for decades in some instances. These kinetics are consistent with the mixed IgM and IgG isotype distribution of HI antibodies. Gander erythrocytes are preferred, although chick and trypsinized human O erythrocytes have also been used. Inactivated sucrose-acetone extracts of infected mouse brains provide a high-titer source of antigen; for viruses such as ORO and group C viruses that do not propagate to high titers in mouse brain, livers, antigens from infected cell culture, or twice-acetone-extracted sera from infected mice or hamsters can be used. For each virus, HA is optimal within a narrow pH range of less than one-half a pH unit. Before the HI test is performed, a preliminary HA test is done to determine the specific pH optimum and the antigen titer.

Serum samples are conventionally tested at a 1:10 dilution and at further twofold dilutions to the end point. A fourfold change between acute- and convalescent-phase samples is diagnostic of recent infection, a titer of >1:80 may be interpreted as presumptive evidence of recent infection, and a titer of >1:2,560 is evidence of a recent secondary antibody response to flaviviral infection.

The HI test is highly sensitive in confirming an infection when adequately timed serum pairs are available, but it is considerably less useful when applied to a single serum sample. Furthermore, HI antibodies tend to be broadly reactive, recognizing common epitopes within antigenic groups or complexes. For this reason, the HI test is useful for screening unknown samples and for demonstrating group relationships among arboviruses. But as noted before, while a primary infection may lead to a specific antibody response, repeated infections with related viruses produce increasing levels of heterologous antibodies to the related viruses, often rendering the HI test results uninterpretable.

The HI test is useful in epidemiologic surveys because of its broad reactivity and the longevity of HI antibodies and because the procedure is robust. Blood samples collected on filter paper and dried can be stored for short periods without refrigeration, mailed, and tested by the HI test after reconstitution. Another advantage of the HI test is that the procedure does not require species-specific reagents and can be used for wildlife and animal surveys involving sera from a variety of birds, mammals, and reptiles.

CF Test

The CF test is moderately specific and is often used to narrow the definition of a heterologous HI antibody response (66). The half-lives of CF antibodies vary, but the antibodies may persist for several years. CF antibodies to some flaviviruses (DEN, WN, JE, MAY, and YF viruses) persist for many years. Thus, some laboratories use the HI test to screen samples and the CF test to define the specificities of reactive samples. Some arboviruses, such as CTF virus, certain rhabdoviruses, and the orbiviruses, do not hemagglutinate erythrocytes, so the HI test cannot be used and the CF test is then used for primary diagnosis. Because the test is relatively insensitive, it should be used in combination with some other procedure. A fourfold change is diagnostic of recent infection, and in some circumstances, a single or stable elevated titer of 1:32 may be accepted as presumptive evidence of recent infection.

CF antibodies generally rise slowly after infection, often peaking as late as 6 weeks after the onset of illness. Convalescent-phase serum samples should be obtained 2 to 3 months after onset to ensure against missing a late-rising CF antibody response. Some individuals fail to produce detectable CF antibodies, and advanced age may be associated with a blunted, delayed, or undetectable response.

Neutralization

The neutralization test is the most specific of the common serologic procedures and is used principally to sort out heterologous reactions observed in other assays (2, 26). The presence of virus-neutralizing antibodies is also considered the best indication of protective immunity, and the response to immunization is usually monitored by following neutralizing antibody levels. Neutralizing antibodies generally become detectable within the first or second week after the onset of illness, peak in the following 2 weeks, and decay slowly, persisting for years and often over a lifetime. Reexposures and infections with related viruses (i.e., sequential DEN virus infections) may stimulate an accelerated secondary response. Although the neutralizing antibody response is relatively specific, repeated infections with related viruses produce a progressively broader heterologous immune response, with the possible extension of cross-protection in some instances. Sometimes, as in the case of repeated flavivirus infections, these extensive heterologous reactions cannot be resolved with cross-neutralization tests.

Infectious virus is used in the neutralization test; consequently, the procedure should be performed only in laboratories capable of working safely at the appropriate biosafety level. Neutralizing antibodies are best quantitated with a plaque reduction assay, in which dilutions of heat-inactivated serum are mixed with a fixed dose of virus and incubated for 1 h at 37°C or overnight at 5°C. The longer incubation time usually gives slightly higher antibody titers (greater sensitivity). Sometimes, exogenous complement is also added to the mixture. The highest serum dilution inhibiting 80 to 90% of the infectious virus dose observed in virus control wells is the end point. In a typical test using 100 PFU as the viral input dose, the 90% end point is the last well showing 10 or fewer plaques. Serum samples are generally diluted 1:5, and with the addition of an equal volume of virus, the initial test dilution is 1:10. A fourfold change in titer is considered diagnostic of recent infection.

The neutralizing capacity of a serum sample can also be measured by testing a single dilution of the serum against a series of virus dilutions. The result is expressed as the serum's log neutralization index. For viruses that do not form readable plaques, neutralization tests can also be done by inoculation of laboratory animals (i.e., newborn or weanling mice) or by a fluorescent focus technique.

Other Procedures

Rapid procedures such as dipstick, dot blot, microsphere immunoassay, and immunochromatographic tests are commercially available outside the United States for several arboviruses (Table 3). These tests have shown good sensitivity and specificity for some arboviruses, including DEN and JE viruses (3, 13, 14, 21, 27, 78, 81), although their diagnostic accuracy may be well below manufacturers' claims (3). The assay format is usually simple and robust enough for use in primary care hospitals or outpatient facilities and in field situations where the capacity for more complex testing, such as ELISA, is not available. Further clinical evaluations are needed, but such kits may bring the capacity for serologic diagnosis within the reach of a wider range of laboratories and medical care facilities in developed and developing countries.

As stated above, heterologous serologic reactions in patients who have had repeated arboviral infections are difficult to sort out, even after all available conventional tests have been exhausted. In an attempt to improve specificity, the narrow reactivity provided by viral monoclonal antibodies has been utilized in the development of serologic tests that combine a serum sample with a virus-specific monoclonal antibody in a competitive ELISA (4, 6). Virus-specific antibodies present in the test sample block binding of the monoclonal conjugate to viral antigen, thus reducing the absorbance. Synthetic antigens, expressed as polyproteins including areas of the envelope glycoprotein or produced by proteolytic cleavage, have allowed some differentiation of flaviviral antibody responses by ELISA, by IHC staining of expressed antigens on cell surfaces, or by Western blotting (immunoblotting). Although these techniques may be applicable to population surveys, they are still largely research techniques, and their discriminatory power for routine clinical diagnostic purposes requires further confirmation.

Recently, discrimination between primary and secondary infections was performed by using IgG avidity tests on acute-phase serum samples (43, 46). This type of determination is especially helpful for hospitalized patients with DEN fever (46).

EVALUATION AND INTERPRETATION OF TEST RESULTS

Unlike herpesviruses, adenoviruses, and other viruses that produce persistent or latent infections, nearly all human arboviral infections are acute and are terminated by viral clearance. Thus, the isolation of an arbovirus from an ill patient or detection of viral nucleic acid in blood or tissues is virtually diagnostic. However, rare subacute, progressive, and recrudescent infections and experimental models of persistent infection have been reported for TBE, WN, SLE, JE, and ORO viruses (20, 54, 57, 60, 63, 71).

Due to the possibility of cross-reactivity, serologic results should always be interpreted in view of the patient's prior residence history, exposure, and immunization record. For example, recent immigrants may have resided in regions where DEN, YF, or JE is endemic and may have antibodies to the agents of these diseases that may produce positive results in commercial WN virus serologic assays. Vaccines for YF, JE, and TBE are commercially available in the United States and abroad and are widely used in some countries or for high-risk groups (e.g., military personnel). A vaccination history should be sought from the patient because evidence of prior immunization might militate against certain diagnoses and because vaccine-induced antibodies can interfere with the interpretation of serologic test results. The influence of immunosuppression on antibody responses to arbovirus infections is not well characterized, but results should be interpreted with caution, and in this instance, nonserologic methods should be employed. It is known, for example, that the antibody responses of human immunodeficiency virus-infected children to live YF virus vaccine, essentially an attenuated infection, are poorer than those of healthy control children (65).

Finally, laboratory detection of a recent arboviral infection does not necessarily secure the clinical diagnosis, because concurrent infections are possible. Arboviral infections may occur coincidentally with or may predispose patients to more serious secondary infections. In a review of ~2,800 pediatric DEN fever cases in Thailand, concurrent bacteremia and other infections complicated the illness in 14 cases (48). Furthermore, acute DEN fever has also been associated with reactivation of latent human herpesvirus 6 infection (1). Dual infection with an arbovirus and a protozoan or bacterium may also occur because certain vector species participate simultaneously in several transmission cycles. *Ixodes ricinus* ticks in Europe, for example, are vectors for TBE virus, anaplasmosis, and *Borrelia* sp., and *Ixodes scapularis* ticks in the United States can transmit POW virus, *Babesia microti*, and *Borrelia burgdorferi*. Dual human infections have been reported, possibly occurring from a single, dually infected tick or after simultaneous exposure to more than one tick, each infected with a different agent (44). Similarly, because some vectors participate in the transmission of multiple arboviruses in the same locale (e.g., DEN viruses of all serotypes and CHIK virus by *Aedes aegypti* or, in the United States, WN virus by mosquito species that also function as vectors of neurotropic SLE and WEE viruses), the targeted identification of an agent or an antibody rise could be misleading, as dual infections may have occurred.

REFERENCES

1. **Balachandra, K., K. Chimabutra, P. Supromajakr, C. Wasi, T. Yamamoto, T. Mukai, T. Okuno, and K. Yamanishi.** 1994. High rate of reactivation of human herpesvirus 6 in children with dengue hemorrhagic fever. *J. Infect. Dis.* **170:**746–748.

2. **Beaty, B. J., C. H. Calisher, and R. E. Shope.** 1995. Arboviruses, p. 189–212. *In* E. H. Lennette, P. A. Lennette, and E. T. Lennette (ed.), *Diagnostic Procedures for Viral, Rickettsial, and Chlamydial Infections*, 7th ed. American Public Health Association, Washington, DC.

3. **Blacksell, S. D., P. N. Newton, D. Bell, J. Kelley, M. P. Mammen, Jr., D. W. Vaughn, V. Wuthiekanun, A. Sungkakum, A. Nisalak, and N. P. J. Day.** 2006. The comparative accuracy of 8 commercial rapid immunochromatographic assays for the diagnosis of acute dengue infection. *Clin. Infect. Dis.* **42:**1127–1134.

4. **Blitvich, B. J., R. A. Bowen, N. L. Marlenee, R. A. Hall, M. L. Bunning, and B. J. Beaty.** 2003. Epitope-blocking enzyme-linked immunosorbent assays for detection of West Nile virus antibodies in domestic mammals. *J. Clin. Microbiol.* **41:**2676–2679.

5. **Burke, D. S., and T. P. Monath.** 2001. Flaviviruses, p. 1043–1125. *In* D. M. Knipe, P. M. Howley, D. E. Griffin, R. A. Lamb, M. A. Martin, B. Roizman, and S. E. Straus (ed.), *Fields Virology*, 4th ed., vol. 1. Lippincott Williams & Wilkins, Philadelphia, PA.

6. **Burke, D. S., A. Nisalak, and M. K. Gentry.** 1987. Detection of flavivirus antibodies in human serum by epitope blocking immunoassay. *J. Med. Virol.* **23:**165–173.

7. **Burke, D. S., A. Nisalak, M. A. Ussery, T. Laorakpongse, and S. Chantavibul.** 1985. Kinetics of IgM and IgG responses to Japanese encephalitis virus in human serum and cerebrospinal fluid. *J. Infect. Dis.* **151:**1093–1099.

8. **Busch, M. P., S. Caglioti, E. F. Robertson, J. D. McAuley, L. H. Tobler, H. Kamel, J. M. Linnen, V. Shyamala, P. Tomasulo, and S. H. Kleinman.** 2005. Screening the blood supply for West Nile virus RNA by nucleic acid amplification testing. *N. Engl. J. Med.* **353:**460–467.

9. **Carter, I. W. J., J. R. E. Fraser, and M. J. Cloonan.** 1987. Specific IgA antibody response in Ross River virus infection. *Immunol. Cell Biol.* **65:**511–513.

10. **Chan, K. H., W. C. Yam, C. M. Pang, K. M. Chan, S. Y. Lam, K. F. Lo, L. L. Poon, and J. S. Peiris.** 2008. Comparison of the NucliSens easyMAG and Qiagen BioRobot 9604 nucleic acid extraction systems for detection of RNA and DNA respiratory viruses in nasopharyngeal aspirate samples. *J. Clin. Microbiol.* **46:**2195–2199.

11. **Chang, G. J., D. W. Trent, A. V. Vorndam, E. Vergene, R. M. Kinney, and C. J. Mitchell.** 1994. An integrated target sequence and signal amplification assay, reverse transcriptase-PCR-enzyme-linked immunosorbent assay, to detect and characterize flaviviruses. *J. Clin. Microbiol.* **32:**477–483.

12. **Chu, C. T., D. N. Howell, J. C. Morgenleander, C. M. Hulette, R. E. McLendon, and S. E. Miller.** 1999. Electron microscopic diagnosis of human flavivirus encephalitis: use of confocal microscopy as an aid. *Am. J. Surg. Pathol.* **23:**1217–1226.

13. **Cuzzubbo, A. J., T. P. Endy, D. W. Vaughn, T. Solomon, A. Nisalak, S. Kalayanarooj, N. M. Dung, D. Warrilow, J. Aaskov, and P. L. Devine.** 1999. Evaluation of a new commercially available immunoglobulin M capture enzyme-linked immunosorbent assay for diagnosis of Japanese encephalitis infections. *J. Clin. Microbiol.* **37:**3738–3741.

14. **Cuzzubbo, A. J., D. W. Vaughn, A. Nisalak, T. Solomon, S. Kalayanarooj, J. Aaskov, N. M. Dung, and P. L. Devine.** 2000. Comparison of PanBio Dengue Duo IgM and IgG capture ELISA and Venture Technologies dengue IgM and IgG dot blot. *J. Clin. Virol.* **16:**135–144.

15. **De Brito, T., S. A. C. Siqueira, R. T. M. Santos, E. S. Nassar, T. L. M. Coimbra, and V. A. F. Alves.** 1992. Human fatal yellow fever. Immunohistochemical detection of viral antigens in the liver, kidney and heart. *Pathol. Res. Pract.* **188:**177–181.

16. **Fang, M. Y., H. S. Chen, C. H. Chen, X. D. Tian, and H. Jiang.** 1997. Detection of flaviviruses by reverse transcriptase-polymerase chain reaction with the universal primer set. *Microbiol. Immunol.* **41:**209–213.

17. **Fauquet, C. M., M. A. Mayo, J. Maniloff, U. Desselberger, and L. A. Ball.** 2005. *Virus Taxonomy: Classification and Nomenclature of Viruses*, 8th ed. Elsevier, Academic Press, San Diego, CA.

18. Feigin, R. D., J. D. Cherry, G. J. Demmier, and S. L. Kaplan (ed.). 2004. *Textbook of Pediatric Infectious Diseases*, 5th ed., vol. 2. Saunders, Philadelphia, PA.

19. Fitzgibbon, J. E., and J. L. Sagripanti. 2006. Simultaneous identification of orthopoxviruses and alphaviruses by oligonucleotide macroarray with special emphasis on detection of variola and Venezuelan equine encephalitis viruses. *J. Virol. Methods* **131:**160–167.

20. Gritsun, T. S., T. V. Frolova, A. I. Zhankov, M. Armesto, S. L. Turner, M. P. Frolova, V. V. Pogodina, V. A. Lashkevich, and E. A. Gould. 2003. Characterization of a Siberian virus isolated from a patient with progressive chronic tick-borne encephalitis. *J. Virol.* **77:**25–36.

21. Groen, J., P. Koraka, J. Velzing, C. Copra, and A. D. Osterhaus. 2000. Evaluations of six immunoassays for detection of dengue virus-specific immunoglobulin M and G antibodies. *Clin. Diagn. Lab. Immunol.* **7:**867–871.

22. Hall, W. C., T. P. Crowell, D. M. Watts, V. L. R. Barros, H. Kruger, F. Pinheiro, and C. L. Peters. 1991. Demonstration of yellow fever and dengue antigens in formalin-fixed paraffin-embedded human liver by immunohistochemical analysis. *Am. J. Trop. Med. Hyg.* **45:**408–417.

23. Hang, V. T., N. M. Nguyet, D. T. Trung, V. Tricou, S. Yoksan, N. M. Dung, T. Van Ngoc, T. T. Hien, J. Farrar, B. Wills, and C. P. Simmons. 2009. Diagnostic accuracy of NS1 ELISA and lateral flow rapid tests for dengue sensitivity, specificity and relationship to viraemia and antibody responses. *PLoS Negl. Trop. Dis.* **3:**e360.

24. Hayes, E. B., J. J. Sejvar, S. Zaki, R. S. Lanciotti, A. V. Bode, and G. L. Campbell. 2005. Virology, pathology and clinical manifestations of West Nile virus disease. *Emerg. Infect. Dis.* **11:**1174–1179.

25. Hsiung, G. D. 1994. Hemagglutination and hemagglutination-inhibition test, p. 69–75. *In* G. D. Hsiung, C. K. Y. Fong, and M. L. Landry (ed.), *Hsiung's Diagnostic Virology*, 4th ed. Yale University Press, New Haven, CT.

26. Hsiung, G. D. 1994. Virus assay, neutralization test and antiviral assay, p. 46–55. *In* G. D. Hsiung, C. K. Y. Fong, and M. L. Landry (ed.), *Hsiung's Diagnostic Virology*, 4th ed. Yale University Press, New Haven, CT.

27. Hunsperger, E. A., S. Yoksan, P. Buchy, V. C. Nguyen, S. D. Sekaran, D. A. Enria, J. L. Pelegrino, S. Vázquez, H. Artsob, M. Drebot, D. J. Gubler, S. B. Halstead, M. G. Guzmán, H. S. Margolis, C. M. Nathanson, N. R. Rizzo Lic, K. E. Bessoff, S. Kliks, and R. W. Peeling. 2009. Evaluation of commercially available anti-dengue virus immunoglobulin M tests. *Emerg. Infect. Dis.* **15:**436–440.

28. Hunt, A. R., R. A. Hall, A. J. Kerst, R. S. Nasci, H. M. Savage, N. A. Panella, K. L. Gottfried, K. L. Burkhalter, and J. T. Roehrig. 2002. Detection of West Nile virus antigen in mosquitoes and avian tissues by a monoclonal antibody-based capture enzyme immunoassay. *J. Clin. Microbiol.* **40:**2023–2030.

29. Iwamoto, M., D. B. Jernigan, A. Guasch, M. J. Trepka, C. G. Blackmore, W. C. Hellinger, S. M. Pham, S. Zaki, R. S. Lanciotti, S. E. Lance-Parker, C. A. Diaz-Granados, A. G. Winquist, C. A. Perlino, S. Wiersma, K. L. Hillyer, J. L. Goodman, A. A. Marfin, M. E. Chamberland, L. R. Petersen, and the West Nile Virus in Transplant Recipients Investigation Team. 2003. Transmission of West Nile virus from an organ donor to four transplant recipients. *N. Engl. J. Med.* **348:**2196–2203.

30. Karabatsos, N. 1985. *International Catalogue of Arboviruses 1985, Including Certain Other Viruses of Vertebrates*, 3rd ed. American Society of Tropical Medicine and Hygiene, San Antonio, TX.

31. Kuno, G. 1998. Universal diagnostic RT-PCR protocol for arboviruses. *J. Virol. Methods* **72:**27–41.

32. Kuno, G., C. J. Mitchell, G. J. Chang, and G. C. Smith. 1996. Detecting bunyaviruses of the Bunyamwera and California serogroups by a PCR technique. *J. Clin. Microbiol.* **34:**1184–1188.

33. Lambert, A. J., O. Kosoy, J. O. Velez, B. J. Russell, and R. S. Lanciotti. 2007. Detection of Colorado tick fever viral RNA in acute human serum samples by a quantitative real-time RT-PCR assay. *J. Virol. Methods* **140:**43–48.

34. Lambert, A. J., and R. S. Lanciotti. 2009. Consensus amplification and novel multiplex sequencing method for S segment species identification of 47 viruses of the *Orthobunyavirus*, *Phlebovirus*, and *Nairovirus* genera of the family *Bunyaviridae*. *J. Clin. Microbiol.* **47:**2398–2404.

35. Lambert, A. J., D. A. Martin, and R. S. Lanciotti. 2003. Detection of North American Eastern and Western equine encephalitis viruses by nucleic acid amplification assays. *J. Clin. Microbiol.* **41:**379–385.

36. Lambert, A. J., R. S. Nasci, B. C. Cropp, D. A. Martin, B. C. Rose, B. J. Russell, and R. S. Lanciotti. 2005. Nucleic acid amplification assays for detection of La Crosse virus RNA. *J. Clin. Microbiol.* **43:**1885–1889.

37. Lanciotti, R. S., and A. J. Kerst. 2001. Nucleic acid sequence-based amplification assays for the rapid detection of West Nile and St. Louis encephalitis viruses. *J. Clin. Microbiol.* **39:**4506–4513.

38. Lanciotti, R. S., A. J. Kerst, R. S. Nasci, M. S. Godsey, C. J. Mitchell, H. M. Savage, N. Komar, N. A. Panella, B. C. Allen, K. E. Volpe, B. S. Davis, and J. T. Roehrig. 2000. Rapid detection of West Nile virus from human clinical specimens, field-collected mosquitoes, and avian samples by a TaqMan reverse transcriptase PCR assay. *J. Clin. Microbiol.* **38:**4066–4071.

39. Lanciotti, R. S., O. L. Kosoy, J. J. Laven, J. O. Velez, A. J. Lambert, A. J. Johnson, S. M. Stanfield, and M. R. Duffy. 2008. Genetic and serologic properties of Zika virus associated with an epidemic, Yap State, Micronesia, 2007. *Emerg. Infect. Dis.* **14:**1232–1239.

40. Landry, M. L., and G. D. Hsiung. 2000. Primary isolation of viruses, p. 27–42. *In* S. Specter, R. L. Hodinka, and S. A. Young (ed.), *Clinical Virology Manual*, 3rd ed. ASM Press, Washington, DC.

41. Leiby, D. A., and J. E. Gill. 2004. Transfusion-transmitted tick-borne infections: a cornucopia of threats. *Transfus. Med. Rev.* **18:**293–306.

42. Le Roux, C. A., T. Kubo, A. A. Grobbelaar, P. J. van Vuren, J. Weyer, L. H. Nel, R. Swanepoel, K. Morita, and J. T. Paweska. 2009. Development and evaluation of a real-time reverse transcription-loop-mediated isothermal amplification assay for rapid detection of Rift Valley fever virus in clinical specimens. *J. Clin. Microbiol.* **47:**645–651.

43. Levett, P. N., K. Sonnenberg, F. Sidaway, S. Shead, M. Niedrig, K. Steinhagen, G. B. Horsman, and M. A. Drebot. 2005. Use of immunoglobulin G avidity assays for differentiation of primary from previous infections with West Nile virus. *J. Clin. Microbiol.* **43:**5873–5875.

44. Lotric-Furlan, S., M. Petrovec, T. Avsic-Zupanc, and F. Srle. 2005. Concomitant tickborne encephalitis and human granulocytic ehrlichiosis. *Emerg. Infect. Dis.* **11:**485–488.

45. Malan, A. K., P. J. Stipanovich, T. B. Martins, H. R. Hill, and C. M. Litwin. 2003. Detection of IgG and IgM to West Nile virus. Development of an immunofluorescence assay. *Am. J. Clin. Pathol.* **119:**508–515.

46. Matheus, S., X. Deparis, B. Labeau, J. Lelarge, J. Morvan, and P. Dussart. 2005. Discrimination between primary and secondary dengue virus infection by an immunoglobulin G avidity test using a single acute-phase serum sample. *J. Clin. Microbiol.* **43:**2793–2797.

47. Monath, T. P. (ed.). 1988. *The Arboviruses: Epidemiology and Ecology*, vol. I to V. CRC Press, Inc., Boca Raton, FL.

48. Pancharoen, C., and U. Thisyakorn. 1998. Coinfections in dengue patients. *Pediatr. Infect. Dis. J.* **17:**81–82.

49. Parida, M., S. Sannarangaiah, P. K. Dash, P. V. Rao, and K. Morita. 2008. Loop mediated isothermal amplification (LAMP): a new generation of innovative gene amplification technique; perspectives in clinical diagnosis of infectious diseases. *Rev. Med. Virol.* **18:**407–421.

50. Pastorino, B., M. Bessaud, M. Grandadam, S. Murri, H. J. Tolou, and C. N. Peyrefitte. 2005. Development of a TaqMan RT-PCR assay without RNA extraction step for the detection and quantification of African Chikungunya viruses. *J. Virol. Methods* **124:**65–71.

51. Pealer, L. N., A. A. Marfin, R. S. Petersen, L. R. Lanciotti, P. L. Page, S. L. Stramer, M. G. Stobierski, K. Signs, B. Newman, H. Kapoor, J. L. Goodman, M. E. Chamberland, and the West Nile Virus Transmission Investigation Team. 2003. Transmission of West Nile virus through blood transfusion in the United States in 2002. N. Engl. J. Med. **349:**1236–1245.

52. Peters, C. J., P. B. Jahrling, and A. S. Khan. 1996. Patients infected with high-hazard viruses: scientific basis for infection control. Arch. Virol. **11**(Suppl. 1):141–158.

53. Pfeffer, M., B. Proebster, R. M. Kinney, and O. R. Kaaden. 1997. Genus-specific detection of alphaviruses by a semi-nested reverse transcription-polymerase chain reaction. Am. J. Trop. Med. Hyg. **57:**709–718.

54. Pogodina, V. V., M. P. Frolova, G. V. Malenko, G. I. Fokina, L. S. Levina, L. L. Mamonenko, G. V. Koreshkova, and N. M. Ralf. 1981. Persistence of tick-borne encephalitis virus in monkeys. 1. Features of experimental infection. Acta Virol. **25:**337–343.

55. Prince, H. E., M. Lape-Nixon, R. J. Moore, and W. R. Hogrefe. 2004. Utility of the Focus Technologies West Nile virus immunoglobulin M capture enzyme-linked immunosorbent assay for testing cerebrospinal fluid. J. Clin. Microbiol. **42:**12–15.

56. Rasmussen, T. B., A. Uttenthal, M. Hakhverdyan, S. Belák, P. R. Wakeley, S. M. Reid, K. Ebert, and D. P. King. 2009. Evaluation of automated nucleic acid extraction methods for virus detection in a multicenter comparative trial. J. Virol. Methods **155:**87–90.

57. Ravi, V., A. S. Desai, P. K. Shenoy, P. Satishchandra, A. Chandramuki, and M. Gourie-Devi. 1993. Persistence of Japanese encephalitis virus in the human nervous system. J. Med. Virol. **40:**326–329.

58. Ravindra, K. V., A. G. Freifeld, A. C. Kalil, D. F. Mercer, W. J. Grant, J. F. Botha, L. E. Wrenshall, and R. B. Stevens. 2004. West Nile virus-associated encephalitis in recipients of renal and pancreas transplants: case series and literature review. Clin. Infect. Dis. **38:**1257–1260.

59. Richman, D. D., R. J. Whitley, and F. G. Hayden (ed.). 2002. Clinical Virology, 2nd ed. ASM Press, Washington, DC.

60. Roehrig, J. T., D. Nash, B. Maldin, A. Laborvitz, D. A. Martin, R. S. Lanciotti, and G. L. Campbell. 2003. Persistence of virus-reactive serum immunoglobulin M antibody in confirmed West Nile encephalitis cases. Emerg. Infect. Dis. **9:**376–379.

61. Rosen, L. 1984. Use of mosquitoes to detect and propagate viruses. Methods Virol. **8:**281–292.

62. Scaramozzino, N., J. M. Crance, A. Jouan, D. A. DeBriel, F. Stoll, and D. Garin. 2001. Comparison of flavivirus universal primer pairs and development of a rapid, highly sensitive heminested reverse transcription-PCR assay for detection of flaviviruses targeted to a conserved region of the NS5 gene sequences. J. Clin. Microbiol. **39:**1922–1927.

63. Sharma, S., A. Mathur, R. Prakash, R. Kulshreshtha, R. Kumar, and U. C. Chaturvedi. 1991. Japanese encephalitis virus latency in peripheral blood lymphocytes and recurrence of infection in children. Clin. Exp. Immunol. **85:**85–89.

64. Shi, P. Y., E. B. Kauffman, P. Ren, A. Felton, J. H. Tai, A. P. Dupuis II, S. A. Jones, A. Ngo, D. C. Nicholas, J. Maffei, G. D. Ebel, K. A. Bernard, and L. D. Kramer. 2001. High-throughput detection of West Nile virus RNA. J. Clin. Microbiol. **39:**1264–1271.

65. Sibailly, T. S., S. Z. Wiktor, T. F. Tsai, B. C. Cropp, E. R. Ekpini, G. Adjorlolo-Johnson, E. Gnaore, K. M. DeCock, and A. E. Greenberg. 1997. Poor antibody response to yellow fever vaccination in children infected with human immunodeficiency virus type 1. Pediatr. Infect. Dis. J. **16:**1177–1179.

66. Stark, L. M., and A. L. Lewis. 2000. Complement fixation test, p. 112–126. In S. Spector, R. L. Hodinka, and S. A. Young (ed.), Clinical Virology Manual, 3rd ed. ASM Press, Washington, DC.

67. Stramer, S. L., C. T. Fang, G. A. Foster, A. G. Wagner, J. P. Brodsky, and R. Y. Dodd. 2005. West Nile virus among blood donors in the United States, 2003 and 2004. N. Engl. J. Med. **353:**451–459.

68. Telles, J. N., K. Leroux, P. Grivard, G. Vernet, and A. Michault. 2009. Evaluation of real-time nucleic acid sequence-based amplification for detection of Chikungunya virus in clinical samples. J. Med. Microbiol. **58:**1168–1172.

69. Tesh, R. B. 1979. A method for the isolation of dengue viruses, using mosquito cell cultures. Am. J. Trop. Med. Hyg. **28:**1053–1059.

70. Tesh, R. B. 1982. Arthrites caused by mosquito-borne viruses. Annu. Rev. Med. **33:**31–40.

71. Tesh, R. B., M. Siirin, H. Guzman, A. P. A. Travassos da Rosa, X. Wu, T. Duan, H. Lei, M. R. Nunes, and S. Y. Xiao. 2005. Persistent West Nile virus infection in the golden hamster: studies on its mechanism and possible implications for other flavivirus infections. J. Infect. Dis. **192:**287–295.

72. Tilley, P. A. G., R. Walle, A. Chow, G. C. Jayuaraman, K. Fonseca, M. A. Drebot, J. Preiksaitis, and J. Fox. 2005. Clinical utility of commercial enzyme immunoassays during the inaugural season of West Nile virus activity, Alberta, Canada. J. Clin. Microbiol. **43:**4691–4695.

72a. Tilley, P. A., J. D. Fox, G. C. Jayaraman, and J. K. Preiksaitis. 2006. Nucleic acid testing for West Nile virus RNA in plasma enhances rapid diagnosis of acute infection in symptomatic patients. J. Infect. Dis. **193:**1361–1364.

73. Tonry, J. H., C. B. Brown, C. B. Cropp, J. K. G. Co, S. N. Bennett, V. R. Nerurkar, T. Kuberski, and D. J. Gubler. 2005. West Nile virus detection in urine. Emerg. Infect. Dis. **11:**1294–1296.

74. Tsai, T. F., R. A. Bolin, M. Montoya, R. E. Bailey, D. B. Francy, M. Jozan, and J. T. Roehrig. 1987. Detection of St. Louis encephalitis virus antigen in mosquitoes by capture enzyme immunoassay. J. Clin. Microbiol. **25:**370–376.

75. Tsai, T. F. 2006. Congenital arboviral infections: something new, something old. Pediatrics **117:**936–939.

76. U.S. Department of Health and Human Services. 2007. Biosafety in Microbiological and Biomedical Laboratories, 5th ed. U.S. Government Printing Office, Washington, DC.

77. Vaughn, D. W., S. Greens, S. Kalayanarooj, B. L. Innis, S. Nimmannitya, S. Suntayakom, A. L. Rothman, F. A. Ennis, and A. Nisalak. 1997. Dengue in the early febrile phase: viremia and antibody response. J. Infect. Dis. **176:**322–330.

78. Vaughn, D. W., A. Nisalak, S. Kalayanarooj, T. Solomon, N. M. Dung, A. Cuzzubboo, and P. L. Devine. 1998. Evaluation of a rapid immunochromatographic test for diagnosis of dengue virus infection. J. Clin. Microbiol. **36:**234–238.

79. Wicki, R., P. Sauter, C. Mettler, A. Natsch, T. Enzler, N. Pusterla, P. Kuhnert, G. Egli, M. Bernasconi, R. Lienhard, H. Lutz, and C. M. Leutenegger. 2000. Swiss Army survey in Switzerland to determine the prevalence of Francisella tularensis, members of the Ehrlichia phagocytophila genogroup, Borrelia burgdorferi sensu lato, and tick-borne encephalitis virus in ticks. Eur. J. Clin. Microbiol. Infect. Dis. **19:**427–432.

80. Wong, J. K. 2002. Colorado tick fever virus and other arthropod-borne Reoviridae, p. 731–741. In D. O. Richman, R. J. Whitley, and F. G. Hayden (ed.), Clinical Virology, 2nd ed. ASM Press, Washington, DC.

81. Wong, S. J., V. L. Demarest, R. H. Doyle, T. Wang, M. Ledizet, K. Kar, L. D. Kramer, E. Fikrig, and R. A. Koski. 2004. Detection of human anti-flavivirus antibodies with a West Nile virus recombinant antigen microsphere immunoassay. J. Clin. Microbiol. **42:**65–72.

82. Wu, S. J., E. M. Lee, R. Putvatana, R. N. Shurtliff, K. R. Porter, W. Suharyono, D. M. Watts, C. C. King, G. S. Murphy, C. G. Hayes, and J. W. Romano. 2001. Detection of dengue viral RNA using a nucleic acid sequence-based amplification assay. J. Clin. Microbiol. **39:**2794–2798.

83. Zainah, S., A. H. Wahab, M. Mariam, M. K. Fauziah, A. H. Khairul, I. Roslina, A. Sairulakhma, S. S. Kadimon, M. S. Jais, and K. B. Chua. 2009. Performance of a commercial rapid dengue NS1 antigen immunochromatography test with reference to dengue NS1 antigen-capture ELISA. J. Virol. Methods **155:**157–160.

Hantaviruses

CHARLES F. FULHORST AND MICHAEL D. BOWEN

94

TAXONOMY

Hemorrhagic fever with renal syndrome (HFRS) and hantavirus pulmonary syndrome (HPS; also referred to as hantavirus cardiopulmonary syndrome) are rodent-borne zoonoses caused by certain members of the virus family *Bunyaviridae*, genus *Hantavirus*. The International Committee on Taxonomy of Viruses currently recognizes 23 species in the genus *Hantavirus* (http://ictvonline.org/virusTaxonomy.asp?version=2009) (79), 11 of which have been causally associated with either HFRS or HPS. (The terms species, strain, and hantavirus have been used synonymously in the literature.)

Specific rodents (i.e., one or two closely related members of the order Rodentia) are the principal hosts of the hantaviruses known to cause human disease. Other natural hosts of hantaviruses include shrews and moles (order Soricomorpha) (48, 94, 109).

The rodent-borne hantaviruses are divided into three groups based upon the taxonomic assignment of their principal host(s): family Muridae, subfamily Murinae (Old World rats and mice); family Cricetidae, subfamily Arvicolinae (voles and lemmings); and family Cricetidae, subfamilies Sigmodontinae and Neotominae (New World rats and mice). Murine rodents are the principal hosts of the hantaviruses associated with severe HFRS (Table 1). Voles are the principal hosts of Puumala virus, which is the cause of a relatively mild form of HFRS named nephropathia epidemica. Sigmodontine and neotomine rodents are the principal hosts of hantaviruses known to cause HPS (Table 1). Many rodent-borne hantaviruses, particularly those associated with rodents of the subfamily Arvicolinae, have not been associated with human disease.

The degree of genetic and antigenic relatedness among rodent-borne hantaviruses typically correlates with the degree of (phylo)genetic relatedness among their respective rodent hosts. This observation has been attributed to virus-host coevolution and codivergence or, alternatively, preferential host switching and local adaptation (77, 78, 94).

DESCRIPTION OF THE AGENTS

Hantavirus virions are pleomorphic, average 100 nm in diameter, and possess a lipid-bilayer envelope (79). The envelope displays a grid-like pattern that is apparent when negatively stained virions are viewed by electron microscopy

(Fig. 1) (74). Protruding from the lipid envelope are spikes, approximately 6 nm in length, which are formed from the virus glycoproteins Gn and Gc (formerly G1 and G2, respectively) (79). The virion interior contains ribonucleocapsids—segments of single-stranded genomic RNA complexed with nucleocapsid protein and L protein (an RNA-dependent RNA polymerase).

The genomes of hantaviruses consist of three unique negative-sense, single-stranded RNA molecules, designated L (large, approximately 6.5 kb long), M (medium, 3.6 to 3.7 kb), and S (small, 1.6 to 2.0 kb) (92). These RNA molecules encode the L protein, the glycoprotein precursor (which is cotranslationally cleaved to yield the envelope glycoproteins, Gn and Gc), and the nucleocapsid protein, respectively (79). In some hantaviruses the S segment also encodes a functional nonstructural (NSs) protein (43). The ribonucleocapsids display helical symmetry and form circular structures as a result of base pairing by conserved, inverse complementary sequences at the termini of each genomic RNA (79).

EPIDEMIOLOGY AND TRANSMISSION

Hantaan virus, the prototypical member of the genus *Hantavirus*, is the cause of a severe form of HFRS that is endemic in Korea, China, and eastern Russia. Dobrava-Belgrade virus is an agent of a severe form of HFRS in the Balkans, Greece, and Russia; Seoul virus is an agent of a relatively mild form of HFRS in Asia, Europe, and the Americas (59); and as indicated above, Puumala virus is the agent of nephropathia epidemica, which is endemic in Europe and western Russia. Other hantaviruses known to cause HFRS include Saaremaa virus in Europe and Amur virus in eastern Russia (115, 124). The case fatality rate of HFRS ranges from 0.2% (Puumala virus) to 15% (Hantaan virus). Approximately 150,000 HFRS cases occur each year worldwide (14). The majority (>100,000) of these cases are caused by Hantaan or Seoul virus and occur in China.

The hantaviruses causally associated with HPS include Sin Nombre virus, Bayou virus, Black Creek Canal virus, New York virus, and Choclo virus in North America and Andes virus and Laguna Negra virus in South America (Table 1) (54, 93). From May 1993 through March 2007, 465 HPS cases were reported in the United States (http://www.cdc.gov/ncidod/diseases/hanta/hps/noframes/caseinfo.htm). In addition, HPS

TABLE 1 Hantaviral species associated with human disease[a]

Virus species or strain	Natural rodent host(s)	Known geographical distribution	Human disease
Principally associated with family Muridae, subfamily Murinae[b]			
Dobrava-Belgrade virus	Apodemus flavicollis (yellow-necked field mouse) and other Apodemus spp.	Balkans, Greece, Russia	HFRS
Hantaan virus	Apodemus agrarius (striped field mouse)	China, Korea, Russia	HFRS
Saaremaa virus	Apodemus agrarius	Europe	HFRS
Seoul virus	Rattus norvegicus (Norway rat) and Rattus rattus (black rat)	Worldwide	HFRS
Principally associated with family Cricetidae, subfamily Arvicolinae[b]			
Puumala virus	Myodes glareolus (red bank vole) and other Myodes spp.	Scandinavia, Western Europe	HFRS
Principally associated with family Cricetidae, subfamily Sigmodontinae or Neotominae[b]			
Andes virus	Oligoryzomys longicaudatus (long-tailed pygmy rice rat)	Argentina, Chile	HPS
Bayou virus	Oryzomys palustris (marsh rice rat)	United States	HPS
Black Creek Canal virus	Sigmodon hispidus (hispid cotton rat)	United States	HPS
Laguna Negra virus	Calomys laucha and Calomys callosus (vesper mouse)	Argentina, Bolivia, Brazil, Paraguay	HPS
New York virus	Peromyscus leucopus (white-footed mouse)	United States	HPS
Sin Nombre virus	Peromyscus maniculatus (deer mouse)	United States, Canada	HPS

[a]Adapted from references 54, 79, 91, 93, and 124. Amur virus has been associated with HFRS in eastern Russia; Apodemus peninsulae is the natural host. Additional hantaviruses associated with HPS include Monongahela virus in the United States; Central Plata virus in Uruguay; Choclo virus in Panama; Bermejo, Lechiguanas, and Oran viruses in Argentina; and Anajatuba, Araraquara, Castelo dos Sonhos, and Juquitiba viruses in Brazil. Monongahela virus is a strain of Sin Nombre virus, and Bermejo, Lechiguanas, and Oran viruses are considered strains of Andes virus. Sigmodontine rodents are the natural hosts of Anajatuba, Araraquara, Bermejo, Central Plata, Choclo, Juquitiba, Lechiguanas, and Oran viruses. The natural host of Castelo dos Sonhos virus is not known.

[b]Murinae, Old World rats and mice; Arvicolinae, voles and lemmings; Sigmodontinae and Neotominae, New World rats and mice.

has been reported in Canada, Panama, Argentina, Bolivia, Brazil, Chile, Paraguay, and Uruguay (http://www.paho.org/english/ad/dpc/cd/hantavirus-1993-2004.htm). Undoubtedly, Sin Nombre virus and Andes virus are the major causes of HPS in North America and South America, respectively. Although there are far fewer HPS cases than HFRS cases each year,

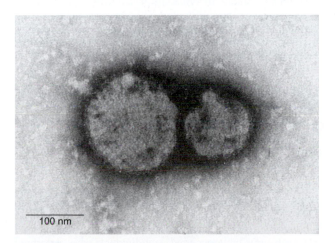

FIGURE 1 Electron micrograph of negatively stained Sin Nombre virus (2% phosphotungstic acid stain, pH 6.5). Courtesy of Charles Humphrey, Centers for Disease Control and Prevention.

outbreaks of HPS usually are highly lethal, with case fatality rates of 40 to 60%.

Humans usually become infected with hantaviruses by inhalation of aerosolized droplets of urine, saliva, or respiratory secretions from infected rodents or inhalation of aerosolized particles of feces, dust, or other organic matter contaminated with secretions or excretions from infected rodents. The aerosol transmission of hantaviruses from rodents to humans has been well documented (49, 110). Other means of infection include contamination of cutaneous injuries with infectious virus, contact of infectious materials with mucous membranes, ingestion of food contaminated with infectious rodent secretions or excretions, laboratory-acquired infections (7, 49, 58, 63, 118), and—only in the case of Andes virus—contact with an HPS patient during the acute phase of illness (84). Note that person-to-person hantavirus transmission has never been documented in Europe, Asia, or North America.

In nature, the risk of infection in humans depends upon occupational or recreational activities, ecological factors which affect the abundance of infectious rodents, and other variables that affect the frequency and intensity of human exposure to infected rodents and their excreta. The cleaning of closed quarters occupied by infected rodents has been repeatedly associated with an increased risk of infection (2, 15, 75, 76, 113, 119).

CLINICAL SIGNIFICANCE

The clinical features of HFRS, including nephropathia epidemica, and the clinical features of HPS were reviewed recently (54, 62). Both syndromes are associated with acute thrombocytopenia and a reversible increase in microvascular (capillary) permeability. A major difference between the two syndromes is that the retroperitoneum is the major site of the vascular leak in HFRS, whereas the lungs and thoracic cavity are the major sites of the vascular leak in HPS.

The length of the incubation period in HFRS and HPS usually is 2 to 4 weeks but can range from a few days to 2 months. The clinical course of HFRS can be divided into five phases: prodrome, hypotensive, oliguric, diuretic, and convalescent. Similarly, the clinical course of HPS can be divided into four phases: prodrome, pulmonary edema and shock, diuretic, and convalescent. Death in HFRS usually is due to shock in the hypotensive or diuretic phase. Death in HPS usually is attributed to hypoxia or shock in the cardiopulmonary phase.

Nephropathia epidemica and other forms of HFRS usually include renal and hemostatic disturbances. In severe HFRS caused by Hantaan virus or Dobrava-Belgrade virus, the prodrome usually lasts 3 to 7 days; it begins with an abrupt onset of high fever, chills, headache, blurred vision, malaise, and anorexia and then includes severe abdominal or lumbar pain, gastrointestinal symptoms, facial flushing, petechiae, and an erythematous rash or conjunctival hemorrhage. The hypotensive phase lasts from several hours to 3 days, begins with a characteristic drop in platelet number, and is followed by defervescence and abrupt onset of hypotension, which may progress to shock and more apparent hemorrhagic manifestations. In the oliguric phase, which typically lasts 3 to 7 days, blood pressure returns to normal or becomes high, urinary output falls dramatically, concentrations of serum creatinine and blood urea nitrogen increase, and severe hemorrhage may occur. Spontaneous diuresis, with polyuria greater than 3 liters per day, heralds the onset of recovery. Distinct clinical phases are less obvious in HFRS caused by Seoul virus and nephropathia epidemica (Puumala virus), and visible superficial hemorrhages usually do not occur in nephropathia epidemica (59). Pathological findings in HFRS at autopsy include effusions in body cavities, retroperitoneal edema, and enlarged, congested, hemorrhagic kidneys (66).

HPS was first recognized in 1993 as a highly fatal disease in the southwestern United States (80). The original description of HPS (17) subsequently was modified to include mild infections that do not result in radiographic evidence of pulmonary disease (52). It is now recognized that HPS sometimes may include renal impairment and, at least in South America, bleeding manifestations (6, 96). The prodrome in HPS typically lasts 3 to 5 days (range, 1 to 12 days) and is characterized by fever, myalgia, and malaise. Symptoms that may occur during the prodrome include headache, dizziness, anorexia, abdominal pain, nausea, vomiting, and diarrhea. Nonproductive cough and tachypnea usually mark the onset of pulmonary edema. Fully developed HPS is characterized by rapidly progressive (time span, 4 to 24 h) noncardiogenic pulmonary edema, hypoxemia, large volumes of pleural effusion, and cardiogenic shock. Hypotension and oliguria are the result of shock; myocardial depression may occur and contribute to shock (54). The diuretic phase is characterized by rapid clearance of pulmonary edema and resolution of fever and shock. Hematologic abnormalities in HPS at hospitalization include thrombocytopenia, hemoconcentration, and the presence of large, reactive (immunoblastic) lymphocytes (53, 83). Other laboratory abnormalities may include elevated levels of hepatic enzymes, hypoalbuminemia,

metabolic acidosis, and, in severe cases, lactic acidosis. The gross features of HPS at autopsy have been reported previously (126) and include copious amounts of frothy fluid in bronchi and other airways; heavy, edematous lungs; and large volumes of pleural fluid.

Therapy

Successful management of HFRS and HPS begins with prompt recognition of the disease and hospitalization of the patient. Shock in HFRS usually can be effectively managed by judicious administration of vasopressors and intravenous fluids. Intravenous ribavirin given within the first few days of the onset of clinical disease has been shown to significantly decrease morbidity and the mortality rate in HFRS (37). The oxygen status of an HPS patient should be closely monitored so that oxygen supplementation and mechanical ventilation can be provided if required. Transfer to a state-of-the-art critical care facility with the capacity for extracorporeal membrane oxygenation should be an early consideration because life-threatening pulmonary disease and cardiogenic shock can develop rapidly in HPS (22, 54). Hyperimmune (neutralizing) serum may prove beneficial in the treatment of HPS because (i) survival has been positively correlated with neutralizing antibody titers at admission (125) and (ii) postexposure passive antibody therapy can protect hamsters against lethal HPS-like disease caused by Andes virus (16). The effect of ribavirin on the course and outcome of HPS has not yet been rigorously investigated (see "Antiviral Agents" below).

Vaccines

There are no WHO-approved hantavirus vaccines available; however, inactivated vaccines have been developed in Asia and used locally in Korea and China for protection of humans against HFRS (70). These vaccines were prepared from the brains of suckling rats or mice or from cell cultures infected with Hantaan virus or Seoul virus (10, 65, 108, 123). Hantavax (GreenCross Vaccine Corp., Seoul, Korea) and other inactivated vaccines that have been tested in humans yielded only low levels of neutralizing antibodies at 1 year after the last vaccine dose, raising concern about the duration of protection afforded by these vaccines (9, 87, 107). Optimization of vaccination schedules and advances in adjuvant technology may increase the duration of immunity elicited by inactivated vaccines. Strategies for the development of new hantavirus vaccines include recombinant viruses, virus-like particles, alphavirus replicons, and naked DNA (70, 100).

COLLECTION, TRANSPORT, AND STORAGE OF SPECIMENS

Hantavirus RNA can be detected in HFRS and HPS clinical samples, and virus has been isolated from blood, serum, urine, and cerebrospinal fluid samples collected soon after the onset of clinical disease (7). Thus, blood, serum, urine, respiratory secretions, and other biological materials from HFRS and HPS patients, especially specimens collected during the acute phase of illness, should be considered potentially infectious to humans. Laboratorians should note that laboratory-acquired infections with cell culture-adapted Hantaan virus have occurred in individuals who performed centrifugation of concentrated virus (95) and that dried, cell culture-grown virus maintained at room temperature has been infectious for up to 2 days (7). The U.S. Department of Health and Human Services has recommended the following precautions for the handling of hantavirus clinical specimens: (i) sera from potential HFRS or HPS patients should be handled at biosafety level 2 (BSL-2), (ii) potentially infectious tissue specimens should be handled at BSL-2 using BSL-3 practices, (iii) all procedures that could result in splatter or aerosolization of human body fluids should be done inside a certified biological safety cabinet, and (iv) propagation of virus in cell culture and virus purification should be carried out in a BSL-3 facility using BSL-3 practices and procedures (16a). Hantaviruses are thermolabile (99) and can be inactivated by acids, alcohols, bleach, paraformaldehyde, detergents which disrupt lipid membranes, many commercial disinfectants, and UV irradiation (7, 55, 73, 115).

Blood, serum, or plasma samples for serology may be stored at 4°C and shipped to the diagnostic laboratory on cold packs if there is no significant delay between collection and testing. Otherwise, these specimens should be stored at −20°C or colder and shipped on dry ice. Blood, blood clots, solid tissues, and other samples intended for RNA isolation and subsequent testing by reverse transcription-PCR (RT-PCR) or virus isolation should be stored continuously at −70°C or colder and shipped on dry ice in order to preserve the integrity of the viral RNA and infectivity of the virus. Samples should be subjected to a minimum number of freeze-thaw cycles. Samples shipped by air should be packaged, documented, and shipped in accordance with International Air Transport Association Dangerous Goods Regulations (http://www.iata.org). In the United States, ground shipments must comply with regulations issued by the U.S. Department of Transportation (22a, 22b).

DIRECT DETECTION

Laboratory assays that have been used for diagnosis of hantaviral infections in humans have not been standardized. Consequently, no hantavirus diagnostic assays have received approval from the U.S. Food and Drug Administration (32). Diagnostic test kits that are commercially produced in Europe are sold "for research use only" in the United States.

Microscopy

Direct electron microscopic examination of tissues is of limited diagnostic value but has been used to detect virions and viral replicative structures in postmortem samples. Electron microscopic examination of autopsy tissues from HFRS and HPS patients found that mature virions are infrequent in tissues and can be difficult to identify due to considerable polymorphism in size and shape (40, 83, 126). Structures determined to be hantaviral inclusion bodies were seen more often than intact virions (40, 126).

Antigen Detection

Immunohistochemistry has been used to detect hantaviral antigens in formalin-fixed tissues from patients with fatal HPS (Fig. 2) (126, 127). Polyclonal antibodies (e.g., immune sera from humans, experimentally infected rabbits or rodents, or naturally infected rodents) and murine monoclonal antibodies have been used as primary antibodies in immunohistochemistry assays. Fatal HPS is associated with the widespread distribution of hantaviral antigen in lung, liver, spleen, kidney, and heart tissues, with antigen primarily localized within endothelial cells of capillaries and other small blood vessels (126). Immunohistochemistry assays for diagnosis of hantaviral infections in humans are limited to the few institutions that have access to the appropriate primary antibodies and control (comparison) tissues.

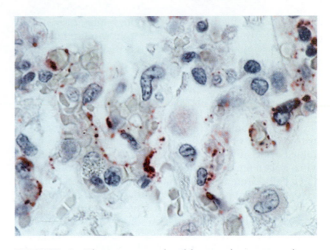

FIGURE 2 Photomicrograph of human lung tissue showing hantaviral antigens in pulmonary microvasculature by using immunohistochemistry. Viral antigens are stained in red. Courtesy of Sherif Zaki, Centers for Disease Control and Prevention.

Nucleic Acid Detection

Since the 1993 outbreak of HPS in the southwestern United States (80), RT-PCR assays have been employed extensively to detect hantaviral RNA in clinical samples from HPS and HFRS patients and to obtain amplified products for viral characterization by DNA sequencing. Sets of oligonucleotide primers have been designed that anneal to regions of the S and M genomic segments that are highly conserved among the hantaviruses (45, 80, 121). RNA can be isolated from tissues, blood, and serum and protected from ribonuclease degradation by using methods employing chaotropic salts such as guanidinium isothiocyanate. RT of hantaviral RNA and subsequent PCR amplification of the resulting cDNA usually can be accomplished by using a "one-step" single-tube format in which a single set of oligonucleotide primers is used for both enzymatic reactions. Clinical specimens rarely yield a RT-PCR product that can be visualized by UV translumination of agarose gels stained with ethidium bromide or other DNA-binding dyes; consequently, a second "nested" PCR amplification must be performed to obtain amplicons that can be detected on gels and purified for sequencing (80). The lower limit of detection for nested RT-PCR assays for hantaviruses has been reported to be less than one viral fluorescent focus unit, or (approximately) 316 median cell culture infectious doses of virus per 1.0 ml (25, 36). RT-PCR assays have been used to detect hantavirus RNA in fixed, paraffin-embedded tissues (102). Real-time RT-PCR assays have been developed for some hantaviruses and are being used increasingly for routine diagnosis (1, 18, 21, 25, 86, 98, 111, 116, 120). These assays match or exceed the sensitivity of nested RT-PCR assays, with less manipulation of reaction components and shorter times to detection, and can provide precise estimates of viral load in clinical samples.

ISOLATION PROCEDURES

Isolation of infectious hantaviruses from blood, serum, urine, or tissues using cultured cells or live laboratory animals is significantly less sensitive and requires considerably more time than for established RT-PCR assays for hantavirus-specific RNA. In addition, hantaviruses usually are extremely difficult to isolate from clinical materials. Thus, virus isolation is not commonly used for the diagnosis of hantaviral infections in humans.

The Vero E6 cell line (ATCC CRL-1586) has been used to isolate infectious hantaviruses from blood, solid tissue, and/or urine samples from HFRS patients and from serum and urine of patients with Andes virus HPS (24, 27). Typically, monolayer cultures of Vero E6 cells are inoculated with a crude or clarified tissue homogenate and then maintained under a fluid overlay for 10 to 14 days. Successful virus isolation may require repeated blind passages of inoculated cell culture material. Hantaviruses usually are neither cytopathic in cultured cells nor pathogenic in laboratory rodents. Consequently, detection of infection in cultured cells and in tissues of laboratory rodents often requires an indirect method, e.g., a fluorescent-antibody test for viral antigen or RT-PCR assay for hantavirus-specific RNA.

IDENTIFICATION

Serologic Methods

Historically, serologic methods were used to define taxonomic relationships among the hantaviruses. Neutralization of infectivity in vitro, immunofluorescent-antibody assays (IFAs), enzyme-linked immunosorbent assays (ELISAs), and a host of other serologic methods have been used to characterize hantaviruses isolated from clinical samples and rodents. The antibodies used in these assays have included sera from HFRS or HPS patients (11, 60), sera from experimentally infected animals and naturally infected rodents, and immune mouse ascitic fluids. Overall, serologic cross-reactivity within the genus *Hantavirus* is greatest between hantaviruses principally associated with phylogenetically closely related rodent species and usually is higher in antigen-binding assays such as IFA and ELISA than in neutralization assays. Neutralization of infectivity has been measured by plaque reduction in monolayer cultures of Vero E6 cells maintained under an overlay containing agarose and by focus reduction in monolayer cultures of Vero E6 cells maintained under an overlay containing agarose (114) or methylcellulose (3). The focus reduction neutralization test is used more widely than the plaque reduction neutralization test because some hantaviral strains do not consistently produce readily discernible plaques in monolayer cultures of cells stained with neutral red (81). Foci of infected cells (viral antigen) in the focus reduction neutralization test can be revealed by immunochemical staining (26) or chemiluminescence (30).

Genetic Methods

The use of genetic sequence data to define taxonomic relationships within the genus *Hantavirus* has become increasingly important, in part because some hantaviruses have never been adapted to growth in cultured cells and because our knowledge of the serologic relationships among some of the hantaviral species is based on one strain per species. Since a RT-PCR or nested PCR product can be amplified directly from RNA isolated from clinical materials and then sequenced, analysis of sequence data (particularly from the nucleocapsid protein gene or Gc region of the glycoprotein precursor gene) may provide the most rapid and specific means for determination of the species identity of a hantavirus. Sequence data can also be used for subtyping of viruses (see next section).

TYPING SYSTEMS

Analysis of hantaviral sequence data provides the fastest and most discriminating method for hantavirus typing. An advantage of sequence data is that they are not affected by variation between different sources (e.g., hosts or tissues) or variation between different lots of antibodies and antigens used in serologic typing of hantaviruses (88). Additionally, sequence analysis may enable the detection of hantaviral strains that have arisen by genetic reassortment of genomic RNA segments or homologous recombination, two processes for which there is evidence in hantavirus evolution (31, 61, 104, 105). The *Eighth Report of the International Committee on Taxonomy of Viruses* differentiates hantaviral species by a minimum 7% difference in amino acid sequence identity in comparisons of complete nucleocapsid protein amino acid sequences and comparisons of complete glycoprotein precursor amino acid sequences (79); however, more recently proposed criteria are minimum 10% and 12% differences in pairwise comparisons of amino acid identity for complete nucleocapsid protein and glycoprotein precursor sequences, respectively (72). Analysis of sequence data also enables subtyping of hantaviruses, which often can identify geographic variants and variants associated with particular rodent host subspecies or populations (69, 89, 90, 104, 116). Phylogenetic analysis of sequence data permits reconstruction of virus evolutionary trees, which have been invaluable in the establishment of virus-host relationships, virus evolutionary processes, and molecular epidemiology (34, 80, 114, 122).

SEROLOGIC TESTS

Virtually all HFRS and HPS patients have high levels of hantavirus-specific immunoglobulin M (IgM) in serum or plasma at or soon after the onset of clinical disease (13, 44, 56, 82). Many of these patients also have measurable levels of hantavirus-specific IgG during the acute phase of their illnesses (5, 19, 20, 44, 85). The IgM and IgG responses are directed first against the nucleocapsid protein and then against the glycoproteins (23, 29, 33, 44, 67). Hantavirus-specific IgM may persist as long as 6 months after the end of the acute phase of illness in nephropathia epidemica (20) and longer than 2 months after the end of the acute phase of illness in HPS (5). The level of hantavirus-specific IgG increases through the end of the acute phase of illness, remains high for months or years, and then declines gradually (67). Hantavirus-specific IgG may persist as long as 10 years in HFRS cases (67) and for more than 3 years in HPS cases (125).

Neutralizing antibodies may appear during the acute phase of HFRS and HPS and are reactive against the glycoproteins, Gn and Gc. A strong neutralizing antibody response early in the course of infection has been positively associated with successful recovery from HPS caused by Sin Nombre virus (3). High titers of neutralizing antibodies have been found in nephropathia epidemica patients 10 to 20 years after infection (35) and as long as 11 years after infection in HPS patients (112).

Antibodies (IgM and IgG) from patients infected with one hantavirus may cross-react with the nucleocapsid proteins or glycoproteins of other hantaviruses (19, 23, 39, 106), but IgG against Gn usually is more specific than anti-nucleocapsid protein IgG (12, 44). Neutralizing antibody, even in acute- or early convalescent-phase sera, can efficiently neutralize strains of several different hantaviral species and thus may not yield a species-specific diagnosis (68).

A variety of methods have been used to detect antibodies against hantaviruses in serum or plasma. These methods include high-density particle agglutination, indirect IFA, immunoprecipitation, radioimmunoassay, hemagglutination inhibition, plaque and focus reduction neutralization, Western (immuno)blotting, μ capture (IgM capture) ELISA, and IgG ELISA. The most widely accessible and perhaps the best serologic method for diagnosis of HFRS and HPS is the IgM capture ELISA, which is done by many national, regional, and state public health laboratories and by some commercial reference laboratories.

The IgM capture ELISA typically uses a lysate of hantavirus-infected cells for the test antigen and should include an uninfected cell lysate for the control (comparison) antigen and appropriate positive and negative control sera (41, 56, 57, 82). The IgM capture ELISA can be highly sensitive for detection of antihantavirus IgM but may not be specific for the virus that was used to prepare the test antigen. For example, an IgM capture assay for detection of antibody to a Sin Nombre virus antigen has detected IgM to all known agents of HPS in the Americas (23, 42, 50, 51, 56, 64, 117).

The antigens used in serologic assays for antihantavirus antibodies traditionally were prepared from cultures of virus-infected cells, concentrated virus, or tissues of naturally or experimentally infected rodents. Antigens must be rendered noninfectious prior to use. Inactivation of hantavirus usually is accomplished by gamma irradiation (Co^{60} source). Heat treatment is an alternative method for making hantavirus antigens noninfectious prior to use in serologic assays (99).

Recombinant nucleocapsid proteins or glycoproteins expressed in bacteria, yeasts, insect cells, or mammalian cells, as well as synthetic peptides, have been used as antigens in IFAs and ELISAs for the detection of antihantavirus antibodies (23, 28, 46, 47, 71, 101). The recombinant protein and synthetic peptide antigens can be more specific than native viral proteins in distinguishing between possible etiological agents of HFRS or HPS.

ANTIVIRAL AGENTS

Currently, there are no antiviral compounds approved by the U.S. Food and Drug Administration for the prevention or treatment of HFRS or HPS. However, ribavirin (1-β-D-ribo-furanosyl-1,2,4-triazole-3-carboxamide) has been shown to have activity against Hantaan virus in vitro (103), in laboratory mice (38), and in clinical studies (37, 97). In a double-blind, placebo-controlled study done in the People's Republic of China, intravenous ribavirin therapy significantly reduced the morbidity and lethality of HFRS (37). In contrast, an open-label study done in the United States failed to demonstrate an appreciable effect of intravenous ribavirin therapy on the lethality of HPS (8).

EVALUATION, INTERPRETATION, AND REPORTING OF RESULTS

Early diagnosis is critical to the successful management of HFRS and HPS and, at least in the case of HPS caused by Andes virus, implementation of appropriate isolation procedures to prevent virus transmission to health care providers and other people. Diagnosis early in the course of disease is difficult because the hantaviral prodrome is similar to the prodrome of many other diseases. Fever and severe myalgia are prominent during the prodrome phase. These symptoms, especially in patients who develop thrombocytopenia,

should lead health care providers in regions of endemicity to suspect hantaviral disease.

The laboratory criteria for diagnosis of HPS established by the Centers for Disease Control and Prevention (see http://www.cdc.gov/ncidod/diseases/hanta/hps/noframes/phys/casedefn.htm) are as follows:

- Presence of hantavirus-specific IgM in persons who meet the case definition for HPS (see http://www.cdc.gov/ncphi/disss/nndss/casedef/hantaviruscurrent.htm) or a fourfold or greater increase in titers of hantavirus-specific IgG in paired acute- and convalescent-phase serum samples
- Positive RT-PCR assay for hantavirus-specific RNA
- Positive assay for hantaviral antigens in lung, spleen, kidney, or other tissues

These criteria could be used for laboratory diagnosis of HFRS as well. Note that the extreme sensitivity of RT-PCR assays, especially those employing nested PCR or real-time PCR, predisposes these tests to generating false-positive results as a consequence of template contamination. Nucleic acid detection assays should include the proper negative controls and be supported by the results of tests for hantavirus-specific antibodies or antigen in clinical or autopsy specimens. Also note that proper controls for μ capture and IgG ELISAs (e.g., sera from laboratory-confirmed HPS cases) and immunohistochemical assays are essential for correct interpretation of the results of these assays. Most local laboratories do not have direct access to these materials. Thus, diagnostic testing is often limited to federal laboratories and research institutions that have a specific interest in HFRS or HPS and a small number of commercial laboratories.

As noted previously (32), testing procedures for detection of hantaviral infections in humans have not been standardized. Thus, confidence in the results reported from individual laboratories varies substantially according to the tests used and the rigor of the standards for diagnosis. In an external quality control study for serological diagnosis of hantavirus infections involving 18 laboratories in Europe and Canada, only 53 and 76% of IgM- and IgG-positive samples, respectively, were diagnosed correctly (4).

The requirement for reporting HFRS and HPS varies among local health agencies and from country to country. In the United States, reporting of HPS cases is mandated at the state level. HPS is listed as a notifiable disease in the National Notifiable Diseases Surveillance System maintained by the Centers for Disease Control and Prevention, although reporting is not compulsory.

REFERENCES

1. **Aitichou, M., S. S. Saleh, A. K. McElroy, C. Schmaljohn, and M. S. Ibrahim.** 2005. Identification of Dobrava, Hantaan, Seoul, and Puumala viruses by one-step real-time RT-PCR. *J. Virol. Methods* **124:**21–26.
2. **Armstrong, L. R., S. R. Zaki, M. J. Goldoft, R. L. Todd, A. S. Khan, R. F. Khabbaz, T. G. Ksiazek, and C. J. Peters.** 1995. Hantavirus pulmonary syndrome associated with entering or cleaning rarely used, rodent-infested structures. *J. Infect. Dis.* **172:**1166.
3. **Bharadwaj, M., R. Nofchissey, D. Goade, F. Koster, and B. Hjelle.** 2000. Humoral immune responses in the hantavirus cardiopulmonary syndrome. *J. Infect. Dis.* **182:**43–48.
4. **Biel, S. S., O. Donoso Mantke, K. Lemmer, A. Vaheri, A. Lundkvist, P. Emmerich, M. Hukic, and M. Niedrig.** 2003. Quality control measures for the serological diagnosis of hantavirus infections. *J. Clin. Virol.* **28:**248–256.

5. **Bostik, P., J. Winter, T. G. Ksiazek, P. E. Rollin, F. Villinger, S. R. Zaki, C. J. Peters, and A. A. Ansari.** 2000. *Sin Nombre* virus (SNV) Ig isotype antibody response during acute and convalescent phases of hantavirus pulmonary syndrome. *Emerg. Infect. Dis.* **6:**184–187.

6. **Castillo, C., J. Naranjo, A. Sepulveda, G. Ossa, and H. Levy.** 2001. Hantavirus pulmonary syndrome due to Andes virus in Temuco, Chile: clinical experience with 16 adults. *Chest* **120:**548–554.

7. **Centers for Disease Control and Prevention.** 1994. Laboratory management of agents associated with hantavirus pulmonary syndrome: interim biosafety guidelines. *MMWR Recommend. Rep.* **43:**1–7.

8. **Chapman, L. E., G. J. Mertz, C. J. Peters, H. M. Jolson, A. S. Khan, T. G. Ksiazek, F. T. Koster, K. F. Baum, P. E. Rollin, A. T. Pavia, R. C. Holman, J. C. Christenson, P. J. Rubin, R. E. Behrman, L. J. Bell, G. L. Simpson, R. F. Sadek, and the Ribavirin Study Group.** 1999. Intravenous ribavirin for hantavirus pulmonary syndrome: safety and tolerance during 1 year of open-label experience. *Antivir. Ther.* **4:**211–219.

9. **Cho, H. W., C. R. Howard, and H. W. Lee.** 2002. Review of an inactivated vaccine against hantaviruses. *Intervirology* **45:**328–333.

10. **Choi, Y., C. J. Ahn, K. M. Seong, M. Y. Jung, and B. Y. Ahn.** 2003. Inactivated Hantaan virus vaccine derived from suspension culture of Vero cells. *Vaccine* **21:**1867–1873.

11. **Chu, Y. K., G. Jennings, A. Schmaljohn, F. Elgh, B. Hjelle, H. W. Lee, S. Jenison, T. Ksiazek, C. J. Peters, P. Rollin, and C. S. Schmaljohn.** 1995. Cross-neutralization of hantaviruses with immune sera from experimentally infected animals and from hemorrhagic fever with renal syndrome and hantavirus pulmonary syndrome patients. *J. Infect. Dis.* **172:**1581–1584.

12. **Chu, Y. K., C. Rossi, J. W. Leduc, H. W. Lee, C. S. Schmaljohn, and J. M. Dalrymple.** 1994. Serological relationships among viruses in the Hantavirus genus, family Bunyaviridae. *Virology* **198:**196–204.

13. **Clement, J., P. McKenna, J. Groen, A. Osterhaus, P. Colson, T. Vervoort, G. van der Groen, and H. W. Lee.** 1995. Epidemiology and laboratory diagnosis of hantavirus (HTV) infections. *Acta Clin. Belg.* **50:**9–19.

14. **Clement, J., and P. McKenna.** 1998. Hantaviruses, p. 331–351. *In* S. R. Palmer, E. J. L. Soulsby, and D. I. H. Simpson (ed.), *Zoonoses, Biology, Clinical Practice and Public Health Control.* Oxford University Press, New York, NY.

15. **Crowcroft, N. S., A. Infuso, D. Ilef, B. Le Guenno, J. C. Desenclos, F. Van Loock, and J. Clement.** 1999. Risk factors for human hantavirus infection: Franco-Belgian collaborative case-control study during 1995-6 epidemic. *Br. Med. J.* **318:**1737–1738.

16. **Custer, D. M., E. Thompson, C. S. Schmaljohn, T. G. Ksiazek, and J. W. Hooper.** 2003. Active and passive vaccination against hantavirus pulmonary syndrome with Andes virus M genome segment-based DNA vaccine. *J. Virol.* **77:**9894–9905.

16a. **Department of Health and Human Services.** 2009. *Biosafety in Microbiological and Biomedical Laboratories,* 5th ed. U.S. Government Printing Office, Washington, DC. http://www.cdc.gov/biosafety/publications/bmbl5/BMBL.pdf.

17. **Duchin, J. S., F. T. Koster, C. J. Peters, G. L. Simpson, B. Tempest, S. R. Zaki, T. G. Ksiazek, P. E. Rollin, S. Nichol, E. T. Umland, R. L. Moolenaar, S. E. Reef, K. B. Nolte, M. M. Gallaher, J. C. Butler, R. F. Breiman, and The Hantavirus Study Group.** 1994. Hantavirus pulmonary syndrome: a clinical description of 17 patients with a newly recognized disease. *N. Engl. J. Med.* **330:**949–955.

18. **Dzagurova, T. K., B. Klempa, E. A. Tkachenko, G. P. Slyusareva, V. G. Morozov, B. Auste, and D. H. Kruger.** 2009. Molecular diagnostics of hemorrhagic fever with renal syndrome during a Dobrava virus infection outbreak in the European part of Russia. *J. Clin. Microbiol.* **47:**4029–4036.

19. **Elgh, F., M. Linderholm, G. Wadell, A. Tarnvik, and P. Juto.** 1998. Development of humoral cross-reactivity to the nucleocapsid protein of heterologous hantaviruses in nephropathia epidemica. *FEMS Immunol. Med. Microbiol.* **22:**309–315.

20. **Elgh, F., G. Wadell, and P. Juto.** 1995. Comparison of the kinetics of Puumala virus specific IgM and IgG antibody responses in nephropathia epidemica as measured by a recombinant antigen-based enzyme-linked immunosorbent assay and an immunofluorescence test. *J. Med.Virol.* **45:**146–150.

21. **Evander, M., I. Eriksson, L. Pettersson, P. Juto, C. Ahlm, G. E. Olsson, G. Bucht, and A. Allard.** 2007. Puumala hantavirus viremia diagnosed by real-time reverse transcriptase PCR using samples from patients with hemorrhagic fever and renal syndrome. *J. Clin. Microbiol.* **45:**2491–2497.

22. **Fabbri, M., and M. J. Maslow.** 2001. Hantavirus pulmonary syndrome in the United States. *Curr. Infect. Dis. Rep.* **3:**258–265.

22a. **Federal Register.** 2002. Hazardous materials: revision to standards for infectious substances, final rule. *Fed. Regist.* **67:**53118–53144.

22b. **Federal Register.** 2006. Hazardous materials: infectious substances; harmonization with the United Nations Recommendations, final rule. *Fed. Regist.* **71:**32244–32263.

23. **Feldmann, H., A. Sanchez, S. Morzunov, C. F. Spiropoulou, P. E. Rollin, T. G. Ksiazek, C. J. Peters, and S. T. Nichol.** 1993. Utilization of autopsy RNA for the synthesis of the nucleocapsid antigen of a newly recognized virus associated with hantavirus pulmonary syndrome. *Virus Res.* **30:**351–367.

24. **Galeno, H., J. Mora, E. Villagra, J. Fernandez, J. Hernandez, G. J. Mertz, and E. Ramirez.** 2002. First human isolate of Hantavirus (Andes virus) in the Americas. *Emerg. Infect. Dis.* **8:**657–661.

25. **Garin, D., C. Peyrefitte, J. M. Crance, A. Le Faou, A. Jouan, and M. Bouloy.** 2001. Highly sensitive Taqman PCR detection of Puumala hantavirus. *Microbes Infect.* **3:**739–745.

26. **Gavrilovskaya, I. N., M. Shepley, R. Shaw, M. H. Ginsberg, and E. R. Mackow.** 1998. β3 Integrins mediate the cellular entry of hantaviruses that cause respiratory failure. *Proc. Natl. Acad. Sci. USA* **95:**7074–7079.

27. **Godoy, P., D. Marsac, E. Stefas, P. Ferrer, N. D. Tischler, K. Pino, P. Ramdohr, P. Vial, P. D. Valenzuela, M. Ferres, F. Veas, and M. Lopez-Lastra.** 2009. Andes virus antigens are shed in urine of patients with acute hantavirus cardiopulmonary syndrome. *J. Virol.* **83:**5046–5055.

28. **Gott, P., R. Stohwasser, P. Schnitzler, G. Darai, and E. K. Bautz.** 1993. RNA binding of recombinant nucleocapsid proteins of hantaviruses. *Virology* **194:**332–337.

29. **Groen, J., J. Dalrymple, S. Fisher-Hoch, J. G. Jordans, J. P. Clement, and A. D. Osterhaus.** 1992. Serum antibodies to structural proteins of Hantavirus arise at different times after infection. *J. Med. Virol.* **37:**283–287.

30. **Heider, H., B. Ziaja, C. Priemer, A. Lundkvist, J. Neyts, D. H. Kruger, and R. Ulrich.** 2001. A chemiluminescence detection method of hantaviral antigens in neutralisation assays and inhibitor studies. *J. Virol. Methods* **96:**17–23.

31. **Henderson, W. W., M. C. Monroe, S. C. St. Jeor, W. P. Thayer, J. E. Rowe, C. J. Peters, and S. T. Nichol.** 1995. Naturally occurring Sin Nombre virus genetic reassortants. *Virology* **214:**602–610.

32. **Hjelle, B.** 2002. Vaccines against hantaviruses. *Expert Rev. Vaccines* **1:**373–384.

33. **Hjelle, B., F. Chavez-Giles, N. Torrez-Martinez, T. Yamada, J. Sarisky, M. Ascher, and S. Jenison.** 1994. Dominant glycoprotein epitope of Four Corners hantavirus is conserved across a wide geographical area. *J. Gen. Virol.* **75:**2881–2888.

34. **Hjelle, B., S. Jenison, N. Torrez-Martinez, T. Yamada, K. Nolte, R. Zumwalt, K. MacInnes, and G. Myers.** 1994. A novel hantavirus associated with an outbreak of fatal respiratory disease in the southwestern United States: evolutionary relationships to known hantaviruses. *J. Virol.* **68:**592–596.

35. **Horling, J., A. Lundkvist, J. W. Huggins, and B. Niklasson.** 1992. Antibodies to Puumala virus in humans determined by neutralization test. *J. Virol. Methods* **39:**139–147.

36. **Horling, J., A. Lundkvist, K. Persson, M. Mullaart, T. Dzagurova, A. Dekonenko, E. Tkachenko, and B. Niklasson.** 1995. Detection and subsequent sequencing of Puumala virus from human specimens by PCR. *J. Clin. Microbiol.* **33:**277–282.

37. Huggins, J. W., C. M. Hsiang, T. M. Cosgriff, M. Y. Guang, J. I. Smith, Z. O. Wu, J. W. LeDuc, Z. M. Zheng, J. M. Meegan, Q. N. Wang, D. D. Oland, X. E. Gui, P. H. Gibbs, G. H. Yuan, and T. M. Zhang. 1991. Prospective, double-blind, concurrent, placebo-controlled clinical trial of intravenous ribavirin therapy of hemorrhagic fever with renal syndrome. J. Infect. Dis. 164:1119–1127.

38. Huggins, J. W., G. R. Kim, O. M. Brand, and K. T. McKee, Jr. 1986. Ribavirin therapy for Hantaan virus infection in suckling mice. J. Infect. Dis. 153:489–497.

39. Hujakka, H., V. Koistinen, I. Kuronen, P. Eerikainen, M. Parviainen, A. Lundkvist, A. Vaheri, O. Vapalahti, and A. Narvanen. 2003. Diagnostic rapid tests for acute hantavirus infections: specific tests for Hantaan, Dobrava and Puumala viruses versus a hantavirus combination test. J. Virol. Methods 108:117–122.

40. Hung, T., J. Y. Zhou, Y. M. Tang, T. X. Zhao, L. J. Baek, and H. W. Lee. 1992. Identification of Hantaan virus-related structures in kidneys of cadavers with haemorrhagic fever with renal syndrome. Arch. Virol. 122:187–199.

41. Ivanov, A., O. Vapalahti, H. Lankinen, E. Tkachenko, A. Vaheri, B. Niklasson, and A. Lundkvist. 1996. Biotin-labeled antigen: a novel approach for detection of Puumala virus-specific IgM. J. Virol. Methods 62:87–92.

42. Iversson, L. B., A. P. da Rosa, M. D. Rosa, A. V. Lomar, G. Sasaki Mda, and J. W. LeDuc. 1994. Human infection by Hantavirus in southern and southeastern Brazil. Rev. Assoc. Med. Bras. 40:85–92. (In Portuguese.)

43. Jaaskelainen, K. M., P. Kaukinen, E. S. Minskaya, A. Plyusnina, O. Vapalahti, R. M. Elliott, F. Weber, A. Vaheri, and A. Plyusnin. 2007. Tula and Puumala hantavirus NSs ORFs are functional and the products inhibit activation of the interferon-beta promoter. J. Med. Virol. 79:1527–1536.

44. Jenison, S., T. Yamada, C. Morris, B. Anderson, N. Torrez-Martinez, N. Keller, and B. Hjelle. 1994. Characterization of human antibody responses to Four Corners hantavirus infections among patients with hantavirus pulmonary syndrome. J. Virol. 68:3000–3006.

45. Johnson, A. M., M. D. Bowen, T. G. Ksiazek, R. J. Williams, R. T. Bryan, J. N. Mills, C. J. Peters, and S. T. Nichol. 1997. Laguna Negra virus associated with HPS in western Paraguay and Bolivia. Virology 238:115–127.

46. Kallio-Kokko, H., R. Leveelahti, M. Brummer-Korvenkontio, A. Lundkvist, A. Vaheri, and O. Vapalahti. 2001. Human immune response to Puumala virus glycoproteins and nucleocapsid protein expressed in mammalian cells. J. Med. Virol. 65:605–613.

47. Kallio-Kokko, H., A. Lundkvist, A. Plyusnin, T. Avsic-Zupanc, A. Vaheri, and O. Vapalahti. 2000. Antigenic properties and diagnostic potential of recombinant Dobrava virus nucleocapsid protein. J. Med. Virol. 61:266–274.

48. Kang, H. J., S. N. Bennett, L. Sumibcay, S. Arai, A. G. Hope, G. Mocz, J. W. Song, J. A. Cook, and R. Yanagihara. 2009. Evolutionary insights from a genetically divergent hantavirus harbored by the European common mole (Talpa europaea). PLoS One 4:e6149.

49. Kawamata, J., T. Yamanouchi, K. Dohmae, H. Miyamoto, M. Takahaski, K. Yamanishi, T. Kurata, and H. W. Lee. 1987. Control of laboratory acquired hemorrhagic fever with renal syndrome (HFRS) in Japan. Lab. Anim. Sci. 37:431–436.

50. Khan, A. S., M. Gaviria, P. E. Rollin, W. G. Hlady, T. G. Ksiazek, L. R. Armstrong, R. Greenman, E. Ravkov, M. Kolber, H. Anapol, E. D. Sfakianaki, S. T. Nichol, C. J. Peters, and R. F. Khabbaz. 1996. Hantavirus pulmonary syndrome in Florida: association with the newly identified Black Creek Canal virus. Am. J. Med. 100:46–48.

51. Khan, A. S., C. F. Spiropoulou, S. Morzunov, S. R. Zaki, M. A. Kohn, S. R. Nawas, L. McFarland, and S. T. Nichol. 1995. Fatal illness associated with a new hantavirus in Louisiana. J. Med. Virol. 46:281–286.

52. Kitsutani, P. T., R. W. Denton, C. L. Fritz, R. A. Murray, R. L. Todd, W. J. Pape, J. Wyatt Frampton, J. C. Young, A. S. Khan, C. J. Peters, and T. G. Ksiazek. 1999. Acute Sin Nombre hantavirus infection without pulmonary syndrome, United States. Emerg. Infect. Dis. 5:701–705.

53. Koster, F., K. Foucar, B. Hjelle, A. Scott, Y. Y. Chong, R. Larson, and M. McCabe. 2001. Rapid presumptive diagnosis of hantavirus cardiopulmonary syndrome by peripheral blood smear review. Am. J. Clin. Pathol. 116:665–672.

54. Koster, F. T., and H. Levy. 2007. Hantavirus Cardiopulmonary Syndrome: a New Twist to an Established Pathogen. Springer, New York, NY.

55. Kraus, A. A., C. Priemer, H. Heider, D. H. Kruger, and R. Ulrich. 2005. Inactivation of Hantaan virus-containing samples for subsequent investigations outside biosafety level 3 facilities. Intervirology 48:255–261.

56. Ksiazek, T. G., C. J. Peters, P. E. Rollin, S. Zaki, S. Nichol, C. Spiropoulou, S. Morzunov, H. Feldmann, A. Sanchez, A. S. Khan, B. W. J. Mahy, K. Wachsmuth, and J. C. Butler. 1995. Identification of a new North American hantavirus that causes acute pulmonary insufficiency. Am. J. Trop. Med. Hyg. 52:117–123.

57. LeDuc, J. W., T. G. Ksiazek, C. A. Rossi, and J. M. Dalrymple. 1990. A retrospective analysis of sera collected by the Hemorrhagic Fever Commission during the Korean Conflict. J. Infect. Dis. 162:1182–1184.

58. Lee, H. W., and K. M. Johnson. 1982. Laboratory-acquired infections with Hantaan virus, the etiologic agent of Korean hemorrhagic fever. J. Infect. Dis. 146:645–651.

59. Lee, H. W., and G. van der Groen. 1989. Hemorrhagic fever with renal syndrome. Prog. Med. Virol. 36:62–102.

60. Lee, P. W., C. J. Gibbs, Jr., D. C. Gajdusek, and R. Yanagihara. 1985. Serotypic classification of hantaviruses by indirect immunofluorescent antibody and plaque reduction neutralization tests. J. Clin. Microbiol. 22:940–944.

61. Li, D., A. L. Schmaljohn, K. Anderson, and C. S. Schmaljohn. 1995. Complete nucleotide sequences of the M and S segments of two hantavirus isolates from California: evidence for reassortment in nature among viruses related to hantavirus pulmonary syndrome. Virology 206:973–983.

62. Linderholm, M., and F. Elgh. 2001. Clinical characteristics of hantavirus infections on the Eurasian continent. Curr. Top. Microbiol. Immunol. 256:135–151.

63. Lloyd, G., and N. Jones. 1986. Infection of laboratory workers with hantavirus acquired from immunocytomas propagated in laboratory rats. J. Infect. 12:117–125.

64. Lopez, N., P. Padula, C. Rossi, M. E. Lazaro, and M. T. Franze-Fernandez. 1996. Genetic identification of a new hantavirus causing severe pulmonary syndrome in Argentina. Virology 220:223–226.

65. Lu, Q., Z. Zhu, and J. Weng. 1996. Immune responses to inactivated vaccine in people naturally infected with hantaviruses. J. Med. Virol. 49:333–335.

66. Lukes, R. 1954. The pathology of thirty-nine fatal cases of epidemic hemorrhagic fever. Am. J. Med. 16:639–650.

67. Lundkvist, A., S. Bjorsten, and B. Niklasson. 1993. Immunoglobulin G subclass responses against the structural components of Puumala virus. J. Clin. Microbiol. 31:368–372.

68. Lundkvist, A., M. Hukic, J. Horling, M. Gilljam, S. Nichol, and B. Niklasson. 1997. Puumala and Dobrava viruses cause hemorrhagic fever with renal syndrome in Bosnia-Herzegovina: evidence of highly cross-neutralizing antibody responses in early patient sera. J. Med. Virol. 53:51–59.

69. Lundkvist, A., D. Wiger, J. Horling, K. B. Sjolander, A. Plyusnina, R. Mehl, A. Vaheri, and A. Plyusnin. 1998. Isolation and characterization of Puumala hantavirus from Norway: evidence for a distinct phylogenetic sublineage. J. Gen. Virol. 79(Pt. 11):2603–2614.

70. Maes, P., J. Clement, and M. Van Ranst. 2009. Recent approaches in hantavirus vaccine development. Expert Rev. Vaccines 8:67–76.

71. Maes, P., E. Keyaerts, J. Clement, V. Bonnet, A. Robert, and M. Van Ranst. 2004. Detection of Puumala hantavirus antibody with ELISA using a recombinant truncated nucleocapsid protein expressed in Escherichia coli. Viral Immunol. 17:315–321.

72. **Maes, P., B. Klempa, J. Clement, J. Matthijnssens, D. C. Gajdusek, D. H. Kruger, and M. Van Ranst.** 2009. A proposal for new criteria for the classification of hantaviruses, based on S and M segment protein sequences. *Infect. Genet. Evol.* **9:**813–820.

73. **Maes, P., S. Li, J. Verbeeck, E. Keyaerts, J. Clement, and M. Van Ranst.** 2007. Evaluation of the efficacy of disinfectants against Puumala hantavirus by real-time RT-PCR. *J. Virol. Methods* **141:**111–115.

74. **Martin, M. L., H. Lindsey-Regnery, D. R. Sasso, J. B. McCormick, and E. Palmer.** 1985. Distinction between Bunyaviridae genera by surface structure and comparison with Hantaan virus using negative stain electron microscopy. *Arch. Virol.* **86:**17–28.

75. **Mills, J. N., B. R. Amman, and G. E. Glass.** 2010. Ecology of hantaviruses and their hosts in North America. *Vector Borne Zoonotic Dis.* **10:**563–574.

76. **Mills, J. N., A. Corneli, J. C. Young, L. E. Garrison, A. S. Khan, and T. G. Ksiazek.** 2002. Hantavirus pulmonary syndrome—United States: updated recommendations for risk reduction. *MMWR Recommend. Rep.* **51:**1–12.

77. **Monroe, M. C., S. P. Morzunov, A. M. Johnson, M. D. Bowen, H. Artsob, T. Yates, C. J. Peters, P. E. Rollin, T. G. Ksiazek, and S. T. Nichol.** 1999. Genetic diversity and distribution of *Peromyscus*-borne hantaviruses in North America. *Emerg. Infect. Dis.* **5:**75–86.

78. **Morzunov, S. P., J. E. Rowe, T. G. Ksiazek, C. J. Peters, S. C. St. Jeor, and S. T. Nichol.** 1998. Genetic analysis of the diversity and origin of hantaviruses in *Peromyscus leucopus* mice in North America. *J. Virol.* **72:**57–64.

79. **Nichol, S. T., B. J. Beaty, R. M. Elliott, R. Goldbach, A. Plyusnin, C. S. Schmaljohn, and R. B. Tesh.** 2005. Family *Bunyaviridae*, p. 695–716. *In* C. M. Fauquet, M. A. Mayo, J. Maniloff, U. Desselberger, and L. A. Ball (ed.), *Virus Taxonomy: Eighth Report of the International Committee on Taxonomy of Viruses.* Elsevier Academic Press, San Diego, CA.

80. **Nichol, S. T., C. F. Spiropoulou, S. Morzunov, P. E. Rollin, T. G. Ksiazek, H. Feldmann, A. Sanchez, J. Childs, S. Zaki, and C. J. Peters.** 1993. Genetic identification of a hantavirus associated with an outbreak of acute respiratory illness. *Science* **262:**914–917.

81. **Niklasson, B., M. Jonsson, A. Lundkvist, J. Horling, and E. Tkachenko.** 1991. Comparison of European isolates of viruses causing hemorrhagic fever with renal syndrome by a neutralization test. *Am. J. Trop. Med. Hyg.* **45:**660–665.

82. **Niklasson, B., and T. Kjelsson.** 1988. Detection of nephropathia epidemica (Puumala virus)-specific immunoglobulin M by enzyme-linked immunosorbent assay. *J. Clin. Microbiol.* **26:**1519–1523.

83. **Nolte, K. B., R. M. Feddersen, K. Foucar, S. R. Zaki, F. T. Koster, D. Madar, T. L. Merlin, P. J. McFeeley, E. T. Umland, and R. E. Zumwalt.** 1995. Hantavirus pulmonary syndrome in the United States: a pathological description of a disease caused by a new agent. *Hum. Pathol.* **26:**110–120.

84. **Padula, P. J., A. Edelstein, S. D. Miguel, N. M. Lopez, C. M. Rossi, and R. D. Rabinovich.** 1998. Hantavirus pulmonary syndrome outbreak in Argentina: molecular evidence for person-to-person transmission of Andes virus. *Virology* **241:**323–330.

85. **Padula, P. J., C. M. Rossi, M. O. Della Valle, P. V. Martinez, S. B. Colavecchia, A. Edelstein, S. D. Miguel, R. D. Rabinovich, and E. L. Segura.** 2000. Development and evaluation of a solid-phase enzyme immunoassay based on Andes hantavirus recombinant nucleoprotein. *J. Med. Microbiol.* **49:**149–155.

86. **Papa, A., H. Zelena, D. Barnetova, and L. Petrousova.** 2010. Genetic detection of Dobrava/Belgrade virus in a Czech patient with haemorrhagic fever with renal syndrome. *Clin. Microbiol. Infect.* **16:**1187–1190.

87. **Park, K., C. S. Kim, and K. T. Moon.** 2004. Protective effectiveness of hantavirus vaccine. *Emerg. Infect. Dis.* **10:**2218–2220.

88. **Plyusnin, A.** 2002. Genetics of hantaviruses: implications to taxonomy. *Arch. Virol.* **147:**665–682.

89. **Plyusnin, A., Y. Cheng, O. Vapalahti, M. Pejcoch, J. Unar, Z. Jelinkova, H. Lehvaslaiho, A. Lundkvist, and A. Vaheri.** 1995. Genetic variation in Tula hantaviruses: sequence analysis of the S and M segments of strains from Central Europe. *Virus Res.* **39:**237–250.

90. **Plyusnin, A., and S. P. Morzunov.** 2001. Virus evolution and genetic diversity of hantaviruses and their rodent hosts. *Curr. Top. Microbiol. Immunol.* **256:**47–75.

91. **Plyusnin, A., A. Vaheri, and A. Lundkvist.** 2006. Saaremaa hantavirus should not be confused with its dangerous relative, Dobrava virus. *J. Clin. Microbiol.* **44:**1608–1609. (Author's reply, **44:**1609–1611.)

92. **Plyusnin, A., O. Vapalahti, and A. Vaheri.** 1996. Hantaviruses: genome structure, expression and evolution. *J. Gen. Virol.* **77:**2677–2687.

93. **Puerta, H., C. Cantillo, J. Mills, B. Hjelle, J. Salazar-Bravo, and S. Mattar.** 2006. The new-world hantaviruses. Ecology and epidemiology of an emerging virus in Latin America. *Medicina* (Buenos Aires) **66:**343–356. (In Spanish.)

94. **Ramsden, C., E. C. Holmes, and M. A. Charleston.** 2009. Hantavirus evolution in relation to its rodent and insectivore hosts: no evidence for codivergence. *Mol. Biol. Evol.* **26:**143–153.

95. **Richmond, J. Y., and R. W. McKinney (ed.).** 1999. *Biosafety in Microbiological and Biomedical Laboratories,* 4th ed. U.S. Government Printing Office, Washington, DC.

96. **Riquelme, R., M. Riquelme, A. Torres, M. L. Rioseco, J. A. Vergara, L. Scholz, and A. Carriel.** 2003. Hantavirus pulmonary syndrome, southern Chile. *Emerg. Infect. Dis.* **9:**1438–1443.

97. **Rusnak, J. M., W. R. Byrne, K. N. Chung, P. H. Gibbs, T. T. Kim, E. F. Boudreau, T. Cosgriff, P. Pittman, K. Y. Kim, M. S. Erlichman, D. F. Rezvani, and J. W. Huggins.** 2009. Experience with intravenous ribavirin in the treatment of hemorrhagic fever with renal syndrome in Korea. *Antivir. Res.* **81:**68–76.

98. **Saksida, A., D. Duh, M. Korva, and T. Avsic-Zupanc.** 2008. Dobrava virus RNA load in patients who have hemorrhagic fever with renal syndrome. *J. Infect. Dis.* **197:**681–685.

99. **Saluzzo, J. F., B. Leguenno, and G. Van der Groen.** 1988. Use of heat inactivated viral haemorrhagic fever antigens in serological assays. *J. Virol. Methods* **22:**165–172.

100. **Schmaljohn, C.** 2009. Vaccines for hantaviruses. *Vaccine* **27**(Suppl. 4):D61–D64.

101. **Schmidt, J., B. Jandrig, B. Klempa, K. Yoshimatsu, J. Arikawa, H. Meisel, M. Niedrig, C. Pitra, D. H. Kruger, and R. Ulrich.** 2005. Nucleocapsid protein of cell culture-adapted Seoul virus strain 80-39: analysis of its encoding sequence, expression in yeast and immuno-reactivity. *Virus Genes* **30:**37–48.

102. **Schwarz, T. F., S. R. Zaki, S. Morzunov, C. J. Peters, and S. T. Nichol.** 1995. Detection and sequence confirmation of Sin Nombre virus RNA in paraffin-embedded human tissues using one-step RT-PCR. *J. Virol. Methods* **51:**349–356.

103. **Severson, W. E., C. S. Schmaljohn, A. Javadian, and C. B. Jonsson.** 2003. Ribavirin causes error catastrophe during Hantaan virus replication. *J. Virol.* **77:**481–488.

104. **Sibold, C., H. Meisel, D. H. Kruger, M. Labuda, J. Lysy, O. Kozuch, M. Pejcoch, A. Vaheri, and A. Plyusnin.** 1999. Recombination in Tula hantavirus evolution: analysis of genetic lineages from Slovakia. *J. Virol.* **73:**667–675.

105. **Sironen, T., A. Vaheri, and A. Plyusnin.** 2001. Molecular evolution of Puumala hantavirus. *J. Virol.* **75:**11803–11810.

106. **Sjolander, K. B., and A. Lundkvist.** 1999. Dobrava virus infection: serological diagnosis and cross-reactions to other hantaviruses. *J. Virol. Methods* **80:**137–143.

107. **Sohn, Y. M., H. O. Rho, M. S. Park, J. S. Kim, and P. L. Summers.** 2001. Primary humoral immune responses to formalin inactivated hemorrhagic fever with renal syndrome vaccine (Hantavax): consideration of active immunization in South Korea. *Yonsei Med. J.* **42:**278–284.

108. **Song, G., Y. C. Huang, C. S. Hang, F. Y. Hao, D. X. Li, X. L. Zheng, W. M. Liu, S. L. Li, Z. W. Huo, L. J. Huei, and Q. F. Zhang.** 1992. Preliminary human trial of inactivated golden

hamster kidney cell (GHKC) vaccine against haemorrhagic fever with renal syndrome (HFRS). *Vaccine* **10:**214–216.

109. **Song, J. W., L. J. Baek, C. S. Schmaljohn, and R. Yanagihara.** 2007. Thottapalayam virus, a prototype shrew-borne hantavirus. *Emerg. Infect. Dis.* **13:**980–985.

110. **Tsai, T. F.** 1987. Hemorrhagic fever with renal syndrome: mode of transmission to humans. *Lab. Anim. Sci.* **37:**428–430.

111. **Vaheri, A., O. Vapalahti, and A. Plyusnin.** 2008. How to diagnose hantavirus infections and detect them in rodents and insectivores. *Rev. Med. Virol.* **18:**277–288.

112. **Valdivieso, F., P. Vial, M. Ferres, C. Ye, D. Goade, A. Cuiza, and B. Hjelle.** 2006. Neutralizing antibodies in survivors of Sin Nombre and Andes hantavirus infection. *Emerg. Infect. Dis.* **12:**166–168.

113. **Van Loock, F., I. Thomas, J. Clement, S. Ghoos, and P. Colson.** 1999. A case-control study after a hantavirus infection outbreak in the south of Belgium: who is at risk? *Clin. Infect. Dis.* **28:**834–839.

114. **Vapalahti, O., A. Lundkvist, V. Fedorov, C. J. Conroy, S. Hirvonen, A. Plyusnina, K. Nemirov, K. Fredga, J. A. Cook, J. Niemimaa, A. Kaikusalo, H. Henttonen, A. Vaheri, and A. Plyusnin.** 1999. Isolation and characterization of a hantavirus from *Lemmus sibiricus:* evidence for host switch during hantavirus evolution. *J. Virol.* **73:**5586–5592.

115. **Vapalahti, O., J. Mustonen, A. Lundkvist, H. Henttonen, A. Plyusnin, and A. Vaheri.** 2003. Hantavirus infections in Europe. *Lancet Infect. Dis.* **3:**653–661.

116. **Weidmann, M., P. Schmidt, M. Vackova, K. Krivanec, P. Munclinger, and F. T. Hufert.** 2005. Identification of genetic evidence for Dobrava virus spillover in rodents by nested reverse transcription (RT)-PCR and TaqMan RT-PCR. *J. Clin. Microbiol.* **43:**808–812.

117. **Wells, R. M., S. Sosa Estani, Z. E. Yadon, D. Enria, P. Padula, N. Pini, J. N. Mills, C. J. Peters, E. L. Segura, and the Hantavirus Pulmonary Syndrome Study Group for Patagonia.** 1997. An unusual hantavirus outbreak in southern Argentina: person-to-person transmission? *Emerg. Infect. Dis.* **3:**171–174.

118. **Wong, T. W., Y. C. Chan, E. H. Yap, Y. G. Joo, H. W. Lee, P. W. Lee, R. Yanagihara, C. J. Gibbs, Jr., and D. C. Gajdusek.** 1988. Serological evidence of hantavirus infection in laboratory rats and personnel. *Int. J. Epidemiol.* **17:**887–890.

119. **Woods, C., R. Palekar, P. Kim, D. Blythe, O. de Senarclens, K. Feldman, E. C. Farnon, P. E. Rollin, C. G. Albarino, S. T. Nichol, and M. Smith.** 2009. Domestically acquired Seoul virus causing hemorrhagic fever with renal syndrome—Maryland, 2008. *Clin. Infect. Dis.* **49:**e109–e112.

120. **Xiao, R., S. Yang, F. Koster, C. Ye, C. Stidley, and B. Hjelle.** 2006. Sin Nombre viral RNA load in patients with hantavirus cardiopulmonary syndrome. *J. Infect. Dis.* **194:**1403–1409.

121. **Xiao, S. Y., Y. K. Chu, F. K. Knauert, R. Lofts, J. M. Dalrymple, and J. W. LeDuc.** 1992. Comparison of hantavirus isolates using a genus-reactive primer pair polymerase chain reaction. *J. Gen. Virol.* **73:**567–573.

122. **Xiao, S. Y., J. W. Leduc, Y. K. Chu, and C. S. Schmaljohn.** 1994. Phylogenetic analyses of virus isolates in the genus *Hantavirus*, family *Bunyaviridae*. *Virology* **198:**205–217.

123. **Yamanishi, K., O. Tanishita, M. Tamura, H. Asada, K. Kondo, M. Takagi, I. Yoshida, T. Konobe, and K. Fukai.** 1988. Development of inactivated vaccine against virus causing haemorrhagic fever with renal syndrome. *Vaccine* **6:**278–282.

124. **Yashina, L. N., N. A. Patrushev, L. I. Ivanov, R. A. Slonova, V. P. Mishin, G. G. Kompanez, N. I. Zdanovskaya, I. I. Kuzina, P. F. Safronov, V. E. Chizhikov, C. Schmaljohn, and S. V. Netesov.** 2000. Genetic diversity of hantaviruses associated with hemorrhagic fever with renal syndrome in the far east of Russia. *Virus Res.* **70:**31–44.

125. **Ye, C., J. Prescott, R. Nofchissey, D. Goade, and B. Hjelle.** 2004. Neutralizing antibodies and Sin Nombre virus RNA after recovery from hantavirus cardiopulmonary syndrome. *Emerg. Infect. Dis.* **10:**478–482.

126. **Zaki, S. R., P. W. Greer, L. M. Coffield, C. S. Goldsmith, K. B. Nolte, K. Foucar, R. M. Feddersen, R. E. Zumwalt, G. L. Miller, A. S. Khan, P. E. Rollin, T. G. Ksiazek, S. T. Nichol, B. W. J. Mahy, and C. J. Peters.** 1995. Hantavirus pulmonary syndrome. Pathogenesis of an emerging infectious disease. *Am. J. Pathol.* **146:**552–579.

127. **Zaki, S. R., A. S. Khan, R. A. Goodman, L. R. Armstrong, P. W. Greer, L. M. Coffield, T. G. Ksiazek, P. E. Rollin, C. J. Peters, and R. F. Khabbaz.** 1996. Retrospective diagnosis of hantavirus pulmonary syndrome, 1978–1993: implications for emerging infectious diseases. *Arch. Pathol. Lab. Med.* **120:**134–139.

Arenaviruses and Filoviruses

PIERRE E. ROLLIN, STUART T. NICHOL, SHERIF ZAKI, AND THOMAS G. KSIAZEK

95

This chapter focuses on the viral hemorrhagic fever (VHF) viruses from two taxa, the families *Arenaviridae* (10) and *Filoviridae* (82). Some, but not all, members of these virus families cause severe, frequently fatal VHF in localized areas of the world. Although exotic in North America, these viruses are important public health problems in Africa and South America and have the potential of being introduced into the United States by travelers returning from these areas. The arenavirus and particularly the filovirus pathogens have been associated with serious nosocomial outbreaks involving health care workers and laboratory personnel. A document, *Interim Guidance for Managing Patients with Suspected Viral Hemorrhagic Fever in U.S. Hospitals*, has been recently published (15a). Continuing isolation of new arenavirus and filovirus species from new geographic locations categorizes these agents as the causes of emerging infections, whose potential importance to public health is only recently becoming recognized (53). The similarity of initial isolation, clinical management, and viral diagnostic procedures for patients with suspected arenavirus or filovirus infections is the rationale for grouping these taxonomically distinct viruses in this chapter. Viruses from other taxonomic groups, including *Bunyaviridae* and *Flaviviridae* (chapter 93), have also been associated with VHF (75).

TAXONOMY AND DESCRIPTION OF THE AGENTS

Arenaviridae

The family *Arenaviridae* comprises 29 named viruses, which have unique morphologic and physiochemical characteristics. Antigenic relationships are established mainly on the basis of broadly reactive antibody binding assays: historically, the complement fixation test (13) and the indirect fluorescent-antibody (IFA) test (103), and more recently, the enzyme-linked immunosorbent assay (ELISA). Both serologic and phylogenetic analyses of the viruses divide the arenaviruses into two complexes. The LCM or Old World complex contains lymphocytic choriomeningitis (LCM) virus and the Lassa viruses, including a number of apparently benign Lassa-like but unique viruses, Mopeia from Mozambique and Zimbabwe, and Mobala and Ippy from the Central African Republic. All have been isolated from rodents of the family Muridae. More recently, new arenaviruses have been isolated either from rodents, such as Kodoko virus (52) and Morogoro virus (34), or from human fatal hemorrhagic fever patients (Lujo virus) (7, 74). The Tacaribe or New World complex includes Tacaribe, Junin, Machupo, Amapari, Cupixi, Parana, Latino, Pichinde, Tamiami, Flexal, Guanarito, Sabia, Oliveros, Whitewater Arroyo, Pirital, Bear Canyon (26), Allpahuayo (65), Catarina (11), Pampa (59), Skinner Tank (12), and Chapare (21) viruses. All the rodent isolates of New World complex viruses have been from rodents of the family Muridae, subfamily Sigmodontinae, and Tacaribe virus has been isolated from bats. The Old and New World Arenavirus complexes are distantly related; only when very-high-titer antisera are used can cross-reactions be observed. Monoclonal antibodies with specificities for structural proteins of arenaviruses suggest that the N protein is the group-reactive determinant whereas the envelope glycoproteins (G1 and G2) are responsible for type specificity (9, 10).

The morphology of arenaviruses is distinctive in thin-section electron microscopy (66, 67) and was the basis for first associating LCM virus with Machupo virus and ultimately associating these viruses with all the viruses in the present family. Three major virion structural proteins are usually found (9). Two are glycosylated, G1 (50,000 to 72,000 Da) and G2 (31,000 to 41,000 Da), which constitute the virion envelope and spikes and which both serve as highly type-specific neutralization targets. The third, the N protein (63,000 to 72,000 Da), is clearly associated with the virion RNA and is considered the nucleocapsid protein. Four RNA species can be isolated from intact arenavirus virions. Two are virus specific and are ambisense in coding strategy: the small (S) RNA (22S) encodes the N protein and GPC, the precursor of G1 and G2, and the large (L) RNA (31S) codes for the viral polymerase and the Z protein, a regulatory element (10). The 28S and 18S species, isolated in different proportions depending on external conditions, are ribosomal.

Arenaviruses mature by budding at the cytoplasmic membrane, and host proteins are incorporated into the virion envelope. Vero cells infected with each of the viruses contain distinctive intracytoplasmic inclusion bodies, immunoreactive with anti-N but not anti-G1 or anti-G2 antibody. All arenaviruses are readily inactivated by ethyl ether, chloroform, sodium deoxycholate, and acidic media (pH, <5). β-Propiolactone (95) and gamma irradiation (24) are both reported to inactivate arenavirus infectivity while preserving reactivity in standard serologic tests.

Filoviridae

The filoviruses, Marburg and Ebola viruses, have a common morphology and similar genomic organization and complement of structural proteins (46). Marburg and Ebola virion RNAs are nonsegmented, negative, and single-stranded RNAs, 19.1 kb long, and with molecular masses of 4.0×10^6 to 4.5×10^6 Da. The viral genomes are linearly arranged in a manner consistent with other nonsegmented, negative, and single-stranded RNA viruses. Some sequence similarity to the paramyxoviruses, especially in the nucleocapsid and polymerase proteins, was noted. However, comparison with other filovirus protein sequences confirms that filoviruses are distinct. Furthermore, filoviruses are sufficiently distinct by ultrastructural and serologic criteria to warrant separate taxonomic status as members of the family Filoviridae (47, 82).

Marburg and Ebola viruses have at least seven virus-specific structural proteins, expressed from seven genes (82). For Ebola virus, the ribonucleoprotein complex contains L (180 kDa), N (104 kDa), VP30 (30 kDa), and VP35 (35 kDa) in loose association. L is an RNA-dependent RNA polymerase, and VP35 may play a role similar to that of the P protein of paramyxoviruses and rhabdoviruses. GP (125 kDa) is the major spike protein; VP40 (a matrix protein) and VP24 make up the remaining protein content of the multilayered envelope (47, 83). The GP of Ebola virus and that of Marburg virus can be differentiated by the presence or absence of N- and O-linked glycans and by the lack, in Marburg virus, of the second open reading frame coding for the small/soluble glycoprotein expressed during Ebola infection in vitro and in vivo. When grown in Vero (or Vero E6) or MA-104 cells, the GP of Marburg virus is totally devoid of terminal sialic acid, whereas that of Ebola virus has abundant (2-3)-linked sialic acid. Phylogenetic analysis of GP genes from filoviruses clearly separates Marburg and Ebola viruses into two genera, Ebolavirus and Marburgvirus, and furthermore, defines one species for Marburg virus (86) and five for Ebola virus: Zaire ebolavirus, Sudan ebolavirus, Reston ebolavirus, Cote d'Ivoire ebolavirus (formerly known as Ivory Coast ebolavirus), and Bundibugyo ebolavirus (92).

Despite their unusual long-rod-like morphologic properties, Marburg and Ebola viruses resemble the other lipid-enveloped viruses, including the arenaviruses, in being susceptible to heat, lipid solvents, β-propiolactone (95), formaldehyde, UV light, and gamma radiation (24). These viruses are stable at room temperature for several hours but are inactivated by incubation at 60°C for 1 h.

EPIDEMIOLOGY AND TRANSMISSION

Arenaviridae

Arenaviruses are maintained in nature by association with specific rodent hosts (Table 1), in which they produce chronic viremia and/or viruria. The viruses are routinely isolated from blood and urine samples of their specific rodent host. Naturally occurring human disease can usually be traced to direct or indirect contact with infected rodents. Aerosol infectivity is thought to be an important natural route of infection as well. Attempts to implicate arthropod vectors have been unsuccessful, but ectoparasites taken from viremic mammalian

hosts have occasionally yielded arenavirus isolates. Of the 29 named members of the family Arenaviridae (10), 9 are known to be human pathogens. Nosocomial transmission is well described for Lassa and Machupo viruses. Lujo virus was identified recently during a nosocomial outbreak involving five persons, four of whom died (74). Because of the high level of virus circulation in West Africa, Lassa fever is the most frequently exported viral hemorrhagic fever to areas where the disease is not endemic.

Filoviridae

Marburg and Ebola hemorrhagic fevers are caused by taxonomically distinct viruses, which form two genera, Ebolavirus and Marburgvirus, within the family Filoviridae (82). Marburg virus was first recognized in 1967, when 31 persons in Germany and Yugoslavia became infected following contact with monkey kidneys, primary tissue cultures derived from monkeys imported from Uganda, or sick patients (62). Ebola virus first emerged in two major disease outbreaks, which occurred almost simultaneously in Zaire and Sudan in 1976. Over 500 cases were reported, with case-fatality rates of 88% in Zaire and 53% in Sudan. Despite the simultaneous emergence of Ebola virus species from Zaire (Zaire ebolavirus ZEBO) and Sudan (Sudan ebolavirus SEBO) in 1976, these isolates are distinct species by serologic and sequence analysis criteria (87). In 1989 and 1990, a new species of Ebola virus (Reston ebolavirus REBO) was isolated from cynomolgus monkeys being held in quarantine in Reston, VA, and Perkasie, PA, following their importation from the Philippines (40). REBO reappeared in monkeys exported from the Philippines to Siena, Italy, in 1992 and to Alice, TX, in 1996 (77). In 1994, another genetically distinct species of Ebola virus (Cote d'Ivoire CEBO) was associated with disease in a human and deaths among chimpanzees in the Ivory Coast (Cote d'Ivoire) (54). In 1995, ZEBO reappeared in Zaire, and subsequently (in 1996 and 2001 to 2005) a number of outbreaks have occurred in Gabon and adjacent areas of the Republic of Congo among apes and humans. Some human cases were associated with exposure to infected nonhuman primates (31, 79, 98). In 2000, SEBO was responsible for a large outbreak in Gulu, in the northwest of Uganda. Approximatively 425 persons were infected, and 53% of them died (70, 90). In Yambio (south Sudan) in 2004, 17 persons were infected by SEBO-S, and 7 of them died (71). An outbreak due to Marburg virus, involving gold miners and secondary contacts, started in 1999 and continued into 2000 in eastern Democratic Republic of Congo (98). Several bats collected in the mine were found positive for Marburg virus by reverse transcriptase (RT) PCR (88). In the spring of 2005, a large outbreak of Marburg hemorrhagic fever occurred in Uige, northern Angola. A total of 252 cases and 227 deaths from Marburg hemorrhagic fever were reported as of 24 August 2005 (91, 99, 100).

In 2005, Ebola RT-PCR-positive fruit bats were found (56). In 2007 and 2008 ZEBO was responsible for two small outbreaks in the same area of Kasai-Occidental (Democratic Republic of Congo) (57; WHO, 2009 [http://www.who.int/csr/don/2009_02_17/en/index.html]). A new species of Ebola (Bundibugyo ebolavirus BEBO) was isolated during an outbreak, centered around Bundibugyo in western Uganda (92). One hundred thirty-one cases of suspected, probable, or confirmed cases were reported from August to December 2007. In 2008, REBO was isolated from swine tissues during the laboratory investigation of samples from a 2007 outbreak with high mortality in

TABLE 1 Currently recognized arenaviruses and filoviruses and associated human diseases

Virus	Yr isolated	Natural host	Geographic distribution	Naturally occurring human disease	Human laboratory infections
Old World arenaviruses					
LCM virus	1933	Mus musculus (house mouse)	Americas, Europe	Undifferentiated febrile illness, aseptic meningitis; rarely serious	Common; usually mild, but 5 were fatal
Lassa virus	1969	Mastomys sp. (multimammate rat)	West Africa, imported cases in Europe, Japan, United States	Lassa fever; mild to severe and fatal disease	Common; often severe
Mopeia virus	1977	Mastomys natalensis	Mozambique, Zimbabwe	Unknown	None; little experience
Mobala virus	1983	Praomys sp.	Central African Republic	Unknown	None; little experience
Ippy virus	1984	Arvicanthus sp.	Central African Republic	Unknown	None
Kodoko virus	2007	Mus (Nannomys) minutoides	Guinea	Unknown	None
Lujo virus	2008	Unknown	Zambia, South Africa	Fatal hemorrhagic fever	None
Morogoro virus	2009	Mastomys natalensis	Tanzania	Unknown	None
New World arenaviruses					
Tacaribe virus	1956	Artibeus sp. bats	Trinidad, West Indies	Unknown	One suspected; moderately symptomatic
Junin virus	1958	Calomys musculinus	Argentina	Argentinian hemorrhagic fever	Common; often severe
Machupo virus	1963	Calomys callosus	Bolivia	Bolivian hemorrhagic fever	Common; often severe
Cupixi virus	1965	Oryzomys gaeldi	Brazil	Unknown	None detected
Amapari virus	1965	Neacomys guianae	Brazil	Unknown	None detected
Parana virus	1970	Oryzomys buccinatus	Paraguay	Unknown	None detected
Tamiami virus	1970	Sigmodon hispidus	Florida	Antibodies detected	None detected
Pichinde virus	1971	Oryzomys albigularis	Columbia	Unknown	Occasional; mild to asymptomatic
Latino virus	1973	Calomys callosus	Bolivia	Unknown	None detected
Flexal virus	1977	Oryzomys spp.	Brazil	None detected	One recognized (severe)
Guanarito virus	1989	Zygodontomys brevicauda	Venezuela	Venezuelan hemorrhagic fever	None detected
Sabia virus	1993	Unknown	Brazil	Viral hemorrhagic fever	Two recognized (both severe)
Oliveros virus	1996	Bolomys obscuris	Argentina	Unknown	None detected
Whitewater Arroyo virus	1997	Neotoma spp.	New Mexico, Oklahoma, Utah, California	Unknown	None detected
Pirital virus	1997	Sigmodon alstoni	Venezuela	Unknown	None detected
Pampa virus	1997	Bolomys sp.	Argentina	Unknown	None detected
Allpahuayo virus	2001	Aecomys bicolor, Aecomys paricola	Peru	Unknown	None detected
Bear Canyon virus	2002	Peromyscus californicus	California	Unknown	None detected
Catarina virus	2007	Neotoma micropus	Texas	Unknown	None detected
Skinner Tank virus	2008	Neotoma mexicana	Arizona	Unknown	None detected
Chapare virus	2008	Unknown	Venezuela	Single fatal hemorrhagic fever case	None detected

(Continued on next page)

TABLE 1 *(Continued)*

Virus	Yr isolated	Natural host	Geographic distribution	Naturally occurring human disease	Human laboratory infections
Filoviruses					
Marburg virus	1967	Bats?, *Rousettus aegyptiacus*	Imported in Germany and Yugoslavia; Kenya, Zimbabwe, Democratic Republic of Congo, Angola, Uganda, imported single cases in The Netherlands and the United States	Fatal hemorrhagic fever (mortality, 30 to 80%)	Severe hemorrhagic fever
Zaire Ebola virus	1976	Bats?	Democratic Republic of Congo, Gabon, Republic of Congo, imported case in South Africa	Fatal hemorrhagic fever (mortality, up to 90%)	Severe hemorrhagic fever
Sudan Ebola virus	1976	Bats?	Sudan, Uganda	Fatal hemorrhagic fever (mortality, around 55%)	None detected
Reston Ebola virus	1989	Bats?	Philippines, imported infected primates in United States and Italy	Asymptomatic cases	Seroconversion in nonhuman primates handlers, pig farmers, and slaughterhouse workers
Côte d'Ivoire Ebola virus	1994	Bats?	Ivory Coast	One febrile illness, survived	None detected
Bundibugyo Ebola virus	2007	Bats?	Uganda	Fatal hemorrhagic fever case (mortality, 30–35%)	None detected

swine in farms in the Philippines, which was thought to be atypical porcine reproductive and respiratory syndrome (2). Porcine reproductive and respiratory syndrome and Circo 2 viruses were also isolated from the swine, leaving unclear the extent to which REBO was contributing to the disease symptoms. The exact role of REBO in the clinical process is still under investigation through field surveillance and experimental infections in the laboratory. This virus species may be less virulent for humans than are other filovirus species, since four workers at the U.S. quarantine facility in 1990 seroconverted to REBO without experiencing disease and several slaughterhouse and pig farm workers were also found to have the antibody without associated clinical disease (WHO report, http://www.who.int/csr/resources/publications/HSE_EPR_2009_2.pdf). In 2007, four workers from a lead ore mine near Ibanda, Uganda, were infected with Marburg viruses. Two patients died, and the subsequent investigations led to the detection of Marburg virus RT-PCR-positive *Rousettus aegyptiacus* fruit bats and to the first isolation of Marburg viruses from this potential reservoir (93). In 2008, Marburg disease was diagnosed in two tourists who independently visited the same bat-inhabited cave (Python Cave) in western Uganda. The first case was a Dutch woman, who subsequently died of Marburg hemorrhagic fever in The Netherlands (89). The second patient was an American woman from Colorado, who recovered and was diagnosed retrospectively (18).

CLINICAL SIGNIFICANCE

Patients with VHF frequently present with similar, nonspecific clinical signs resembling malaria, typhoid fever, and pharyngitis. A detailed travel history, coupled with a high index of suspicion and availability of definitive virologic tools, should facilitate rapid diagnosis and the timely implementation of appropriate patient isolation, clinical management procedures, and public health measures. Therapy for various VHFs follows the same general principles: symptomatic treatment with careful maintenance of fluid balances and management of bleeding diasthesis. The antiviral drug ribavirin, if used early in the course of the disease, is effective in reducing the mortality and duration of arenavirus diseases. The side effects are limited, but the drug is teratogenic. No antiviral drugs against filovirus are available.

Arenaviridae

Among the known arenavirus human pathogens, LCM virus produces the least severe infection (55). A modest proportion of LCM infections are subclinical. A "typical" LCM case is usually heralded by fever, myalgia, retro-orbital headache, weakness, and anorexia. Especially during the first week, prominent symptoms include sore throat, chills, vomiting, cough, retrosternal pain, and arthralgia. Rash occurs but is infrequent. In about one-third of the patients, fever recurs, coinciding with the onset of frank neurologic involvement, usually aseptic meningitis, but less frequently meningoencephalitis.

Complete recovery is almost always the rule. Thus, LCM virus infections are temporarily debilitating but rarely fatal, even when neurologic complications arise. Although recognized only recently, in utero infections with LCM virus are a cause of significant birth defects of the central nervous and ocular systems (64, 101). Fatal forms of LCM virus infections were reported recently in several clusters following transplantation of organs from LCM virus-infected donors to immunosuppressed recipients (17, 25).

Lassa, Junin, and Machupo virus infections are much more severe. Lassa fever patients usually present at the hospital within 5 to 7 days of onset and complain of sore throat, severe lower back pain, and conjunctivitis. Despite the usual antimalaria treatment, these symptoms usually increase in severity during the following week and are accompanied by nausea, vomiting, diarrhea, chest and abdominal pain, headache, cough, dizziness, and tinnitus. Later, pneumonitis and pleural and pericardial effusions with friction rub frequently occur. A maculopapular rash may develop, but frank hemorrhage is seen in only a proportion of the more severe cases. Bleeding from puncture sites and mucous membranes and melena are more common. Approximately 15 to 20% of hospitalized patients die. Death occurs as a result of sudden cardiovascular collapse resulting from hepatic, pulmonary, and myocardial damage. Few Lassa fever patients develop central nervous system signs, although tinnitus or deafness may develop as recovery begins. Lassa fever is a particularly severe disease among pregnant women, for whom mortality rates are somewhat higher. The disease course in children is similar to that in adults, but in infants a condition described as swollen-baby syndrome, characterized by anasarca, abdominal distension, and bleeding, is typical. Clinical laboratory studies are not usually helpful for Lassa fever; specific virologic testing is required, especially in a setting where Lassa fever is less common or where mild, atypical cases are occurring.

The clinical pictures for Argentinian hemorrhagic fever, due to Junin virus, and Bolivian hemorrhagic fever, due to Machupo virus, are well characterized; for Venezuelan hemorrhagic fever (due to Guanarito virus), Sabia virus infection in Brazil, or more recently, Chapare virus infection in Bolivia, less information is available (75). However, all these infections are sufficiently similar to each other to be discussed as a single entity, termed South American or New World arenavirus hemorrhagic fevers. Incubation periods range from 7 to 14 days, and very few subclinical cases are thought to occur. Following gradual onset of fever, anorexia, and malaise over several days, constitutional signs involving the gastrointestinal, cardiovascular, and central nervous systems become apparent by the time patients present to the hospital. On initial examination, Argentinian hemorrhagic fever and Bolivian hemorrhagic fever patients are febrile, acutely ill, and mildly hypotensive. They frequently complain of back pain, epigastric pain, headache, retro-orbital pain, photophobia, dizziness, constipation or diarrhea, and coughing. Flushing of the face, neck, and chest and bleeding from the gums are common. Enanthem is almost invariably present; petechiae or tiny vesicles spread over the erythematous palate and fauces. Neurologic involvement, ranging from mild irritability and lethargy to abnormalities in gait, tremors of the upper extremities, and in severely ill patients, coma, delirium, and convulsions, occurs in more than one-half of the patients. During the second week of illness, clinical improvement may begin or complications may develop. Complications include extensive petechial hemorrhages, blood oozing from puncture wounds, melena, and hematemesis. These manifestations of capillary damage and thrombocytopenia do not result in life-threatening blood loss. However, hypotension and shock may develop, often in combination with serious

neurologic signs, among the 15% of patients who die. Survivors begin to show improvement by the third week. Recovery is slow; weakness, fatigue, and mental difficulties may last for weeks, and a significant proportion of patients relapse with a "late neurologic syndrome," which includes headache, cerebellar tremor, and cranial nerve palsies. In contrast to Lassa fever, clinical laboratory studies are frequently useful. Total leukocyte counts usually fall to 1,000 to 2,000 cells/mm^3, although the differential remains normal. Platelet counts fall precipitously, usually to between 25,000 and 100,000/mm^3. Routine clotting parameters are usually normal or slightly abnormal; however, patients with severe cases may show evidence of disseminated intravascular coagulation.

All the Lujo virus patients presented with nonspecific febrile illness with headache and myalgia, following an incubation ranging from 7 to 13 days (74). A morbilliform rash was evident in three Caucasian patients on days 6 to 8 of illness, but not in two African patients. In the four fatal cases, the disease course was biphasic. The second phase, starting around 1 week after disease onset, was characterized by a rapid deterioration with respiratory distress, neurological signs, and circulatory collapse. All patients had thrombocytopenia on admission to the hospital (platelet count range, 20×10^9 to 104×10^9/liter). Three patients had normal white cell counts and two had leukopenia on admission, while four developed leukocytosis during the illness. The last patient (the only one surviving) was treated with the antiviral drug ribavirin.

Filoviridae

Marburg and Ebola virus infections are clinically similar, although the frequencies of reported signs and symptoms vary among individuals. Following incubation periods of 4 to 16 days, onset is sudden and is marked by fever, chills, headache, anorexia, and myalgia. These signs are soon followed by nausea, vomiting, sore throat, abdominal pain, and diarrhea. When first examined, patients are usually overtly ill, dehydrated, apathetic, and disoriented. Pharyngeal and conjunctival injection is usual. Within several days, a characteristic maculopapular rash over the trunk, petechiae, and mucous membrane hemorrhages appear. Gastrointestinal bleeding, accompanied by intense epigastric pain, is common, as are petechiae and bleeding from puncture wounds and mucous membranes. Shock develops shortly before death, often 6 to 16 days after the onset of illness. Abnormalities in coagulation parameters include fibrin split products and prolonged prothrombin and partial thromboplastin times, suggesting that disseminated intravascular coagulation is a terminal event and is usually associated with multiorgan failure (78). Clinical laboratory studies usually reveal profound leukopenia early, sometimes moderately elevated at a later stage. Platelet counts decline to 50,000 to 100,000/mm^3 during the hemorrhagic phase.

COLLECTION, TRANSPORT, AND STORAGE OF SPECIMENS

Safety and Security

Some arenaviruses (Lassa, Junin, Machupo, Sabia, Guanarito, Chapare, and Lujo viruses) and all the filoviruses are classified as biosafety level 4 (BSL-4) agents, as there is a high risk of infection of laboratory personnel and appropriate precautions must be taken (16). In the United States, most are also classified as select agents by the U.S. Department of Health and Human Services and should be handled as such (http://www.selectagents.gov/Select%20Agents%20and%20Toxins%20List.html). See also chapter 12 in this *Manual*. At a minimum, barrier nursing procedures should be implemented and personnel caring for the patient and handling diagnostic specimens should wear disposable caps, gowns, shoe covers, surgical gloves, and face masks (preferably full-face respirators equipped with HEPA filters) (14, 15). Gloves should be disinfected immediately if they come in direct contact with infected blood or secretions. Manipulation of these specimens and tissues, including sera obtained from convalescent patients, may pose a serious biohazard and should be minimized outside a BSL-4 laboratory (15, 16). Use of Vacutainer tubes is considered safer than use of syringes and needles, which must be disassembled before their contents are transferred to another tube. Procedures that generate aerosols (e.g., centrifugation) should be minimized and performed only if additional protective measures, such as keeping the equipment in a class I or II laminar flow hood, are taken. For specialized procedures, the infectivity of samples may be greatly reduced, if not totally inactivated, by the addition of Triton X-100 and heating. Heating to 60°C for 1 h renders diagnostic specimens noninfectious and is acceptable for measurement of heat-stable substances such as electrolytes, blood urea nitrogen, and creatinine. When the equipment is available, sterilization by ^{60}Co γ-irradiation is the preferred method of inactivation. Extraction of RNA from infectious samples by using guanidinium thiocyanate (with a proper ratio, at least 1 to 5 or 1 to 10 of lysis reagents) should be conducted in a laminar flow hood, but after extraction, the extracted RNA is no longer infectious.

Specimen Collection

For virus isolation, antigen detection, and RT-PCR, serum, heparinized plasma, or whole blood should be collected during the acute, febrile stages of illness and frozen on dry ice or in liquid nitrogen vapor. Storage at higher temperatures (above 240°C) leads to rapid losses in infectivity. Blood obtained in early convalescence for serodiagnosis may be infectious despite the presence of antibodies, and it should be handled accordingly (14–16). In addition to blood samples, throat wash specimens have also been used for virus isolation during infections with arenaviruses (Lassa, Junin, and Machupo viruses). LCM virus may be recovered from acute-phase serum samples obtained during the first week after onset but more likely from cerebrospinal fluid during the period of meningeal involvement, and from the brain at autopsy but is rarely, if ever, recovered from throat washings or urine specimens. LCM virus is easily isolated from the blood of the immunocompromised organ transplant recipients. Chapare and Lujo viruses were isolated from blood during the acute phase of the disease. Marburg and Ebola viruses are usually recovered from acute-phase serum samples; various specimens including throat washings, saliva, urine, soft tissue effusions, semen, and anterior eye fluid have yielded filovirus isolates, even when the specimens were obtained late in convalescence.

Postmortem Specimens

Lassa, Machupo, Junin, Marburg, and Ebola viruses are all readily isolated from specimens of spleen, lymph nodes, liver, and kidney obtained at autopsy but rarely, if ever, from brain or other central nervous system tissues. Notably, Lassa virus is usually isolated from the placentas of infected pregnant women. In the recent severe and fatal clinical forms observed after organ transplant, LCM virus was isolated from several organs at autopsy. Lujo virus was isolated from liver at autopsy. Formaldehyde-fixed tissues and paraffin-embedded blocks are also suitable for histopathology and immunohistochemical identification of viral antigens and should be conserved and shipped at room temperature.

Shipping

For all testing of infectious material, samples should be packaged in accordance with current recommendations (International Airline Transportation Association, http://www.iata.org/index.htm) and forwarded, after consultation, to one of the following laboratories that maintain BSL-4 facilities and a diagnostic capability for these agents:

1. Centers for Disease Control and Prevention, Special Pathogens Branch, Division of Viral and Rickettsial Diseases, Center for Infectious Diseases, Atlanta, GA 30333. Phone: (404) 639-1115. Fax: (404) 639-1118.
2. U.S. Army Medical Research Institute of Infectious Diseases, Headquarters, Fort Detrick, Frederick, MD 21702-5011. Phone: (301) 619-2833. Fax: (301) 610-4625.
3. Center for Applied Microbiology and Research, Special Pathogens Unit, Salisbury, Porton Down, Wiltshire SP4 0JG, England. Phone: 44 980-612224. Fax: 44 980-611310.
4. National Institute for Communicable Diseases, Private Bag X4, Sandringham, Johannesburg, South Africa. Phone: 27 (11) 386 6336. Fax: 27 (11) 882 3741.

Several BSL-4 laboratories are available in Europe (http://www.enivd.de/index.htm), and in the United States other BSL-4 facilities may be available in the near future.

DIRECT EXAMINATION

Electron Microscopy

Individual arenavirus virions are pleomorphic and range in size from 60 to 280 nm (mean, 110 to 130 nm) (Fig. 1A).

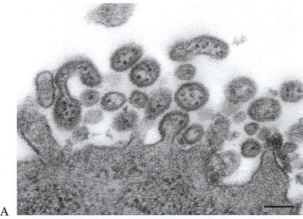

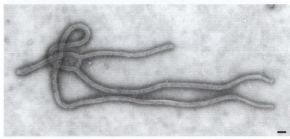

FIGURE 1 Ultrastructural characteristics of LCMV and Ebola virus as seen in tissue culture cells. (A) LCM virus, an arenavirus, showing pleomorphic enveloped particles with internal ribosome-like granules; scale bar, 100 nm. (Courtesy of C. S. Goldsmith.) (B) Ebola virus isolate, a filovirus, showing enveloped filamentous particles around 80 nm wide. Some filaments can occasionally measure up to 15,000 nm in length; scale bar, 100 nm. (Courtesy of C. S. Goldsmith.)

A unit membrane envelops the structure and is covered with club-shaped, 10-nm projections. No symmetry has been discerned. The most prominent and distinctive feature of these virions is the presence of different numbers of electron-dense particles (usually 2 to 10), which may be connected by fine filaments. These particles, 20 to 25 nm in diameter, are identical to host cell ribosomes by biochemical and oligonucleotide analysis (67). Immunoelectron microscopy techniques also work well for diagnosis of arenavirus infections, although the morphology of the virions is less striking for arenaviruses than filoviruses.

Marburg and Ebola viruses have been successfully visualized directly by electron microscopy of both heparinized blood and urine obtained during the febrile period as well as in tissue culture supernatant fluids. The combination of the size and shape of the virions is sufficiently characteristic to allow a morphologic diagnosis of filovirus (27, 40, 66). The virus particles are very large, typically 790 to 970 nm long and consistently 80 nm in diameter. Bizarre structures of widely different lengths are frequently found in negatively stained preparations, sometimes exceeding 14,000 nm, as well as branching, circular, or "6" shapes, probably resulting from coenvelopment of multiple nucleocapsids during budding (Fig. 1B) (27, 28, 66).

Several Ebola viral inclusions are seen in thin-section electron micrograph of liver. The inclusions consist of viral nucleocapsids mostly seen in longitudinal section. Numerous viral particles are also seen in sinusoidal spaces (Fig. 2B). These virions can be differentiated and identified as Marburg or Ebola virus by immunoelectron microscopy techniques (28–30).

Antigen Detection

Immunohistochemistry

IFA staining of impression smears or air-dried suspensions of the liver, spleen, or kidney has been used successfully to detect cytoplasmic inclusion bodies associated with Marburg virus infection; clumps of Marburg virus antigen have also been observed by IFA examination of infected, dried, citrated blood smears. This approach was successfully adapted to the diagnosis of REBO infection in impression smears from blood, tissues, and nasal turbinates, as it was to the detection of Junin virus-infected cells in peripheral blood and urinary sediment. Hematoxylin and eosin staining of the liver reveals hepatocellular necrosis, numerous intracytoplasmic, eosinophilic Ebola viral inclusions, as well as sinusoidal dilatation and congestion (Fig. 2A). The development of immunohistochemical techniques for detection of filovirus and arenavirus antigens in formalin-fixed tissues has recently advanced to the point that their results are far more satisfactory than those of IFA examination of frozen, acetone-fixed sections (19, 20, 39, 72, 104). Obtaining frozen sections for diagnosis is rarely worth the biohazard incurred, especially since the threshold sensitivity for detection exceeds 6 $\log_{10}$ PFU per g. For filoviruses, paraffin blocks of tissues are sectioned. Sections are deparaffinized, hydrated, digested with protease, and stained for the presence of viral antigens with immune rabbit serum or cocktails of murine monoclonal antibodies (39, 40, 104). Biotinylated antiserum is then allowed to react, and the product is developed with a streptavidin-alkaline phosphatase system. Substitution of other chromogens can further increase sensitivity while

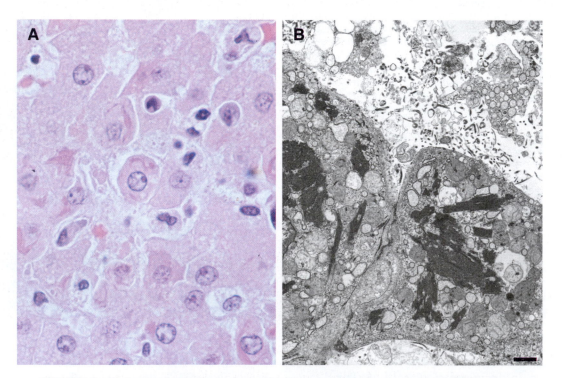

FIGURE 2 Ebola virus hemorrhagic fever. (A) Section of liver showing hepatocellular necrosis and numerous intracytoplasmic, eosinophilic Ebola virus inclusions, as well as sinusoidal dilatation and congestion. Hematoxylin and eosin stain; original magnification, ×250. (B) Several Ebola virus inclusions are seen in this thin-section electron micrograph of liver. The inclusions consist of viral nucleocapsids mostly seen in longitudinal section. Numerous viral particles are also seen in sinusoidal spaces. Scale bar, 100 nm. (Courtesy of C. S. Goldsmith.)

reducing background (19). In the recent epizootic of Ebola Reston virus in swine in the Philippines (2), Ebola virus antigens were detected in different tissues including lymph nodes (Fig. 3A). Remarkable success was reported in the application of immunohistochemistry to the demonstration of Ebola virus antigens in formalin-fixed skin biopsy specimens obtained from deceased Ebola virus patients in Zaire in 1995 (76, 104) (Fig. 3B). Immunohistochemistry

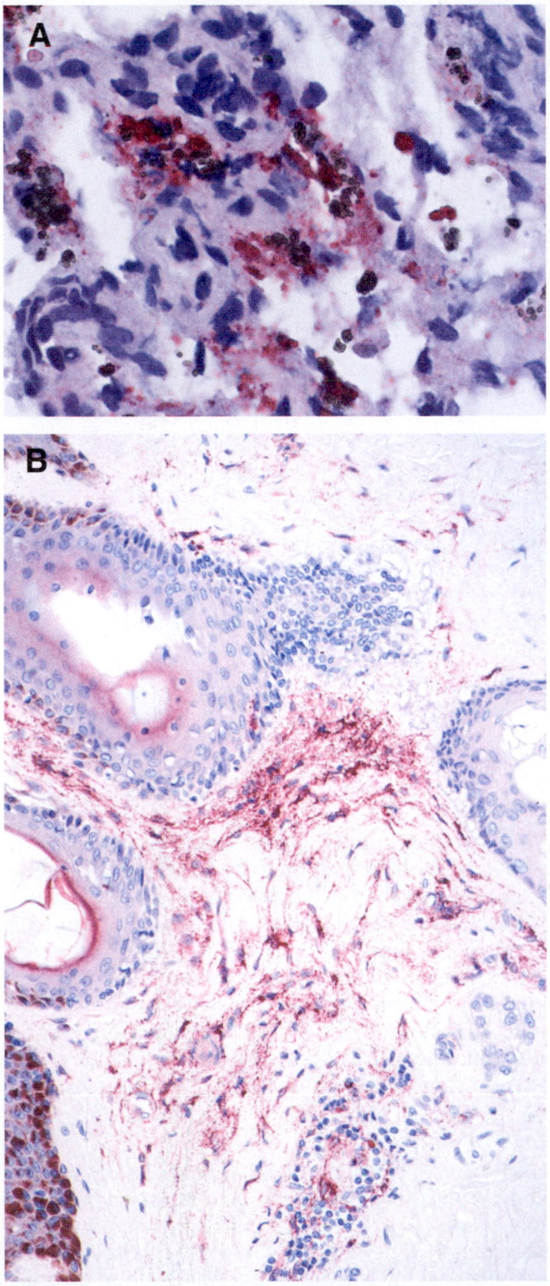

FIGURE 3 (A) By use of immunohistochemistry, abundant Ebola virus antigens (in red) are seen in the lymph node of a pig infected by Ebola Reston virus. Original magnification, ×158. (B) Skin showing massive viral burden as seen in this section immunostained for Ebola virus antigens; original magnification, ×50. (Immunoalkaline phosphatase staining, naphthol fast red substrate with light hematoxylin counterstain.)

was used to confirm the diagnosis of a fatal Lassa fever in a New Jersey patient returning from West Africa (Fig. 4A). More recently, it was the immunohistochemistry assays on a liver biopsy (Fig. 4B) that first indicated the arenavirus etiology of a disease observed in South Africa, leading to the description of Lujo virus (74). In the cluster of LCM cases occurring through organ transplants (17, 25), very abundant LCM virus antigen was found in different organs (Fig. 4C).

Antigen Capture ELISA

Development of an antigen capture ELISA for quantitative detection of arenavirus and filovirus antigens in viremic sera and tissue culture supernatants has facilitated the early detection and identification of these agents (3, 48, 49, 69). These tests reliably detect antigens in samples inactivated by either β-propiolactone or irradiation; therefore, they can be conducted safely without elaborate containment facilities. The threshold sensitivities for these assays are approximately 2.1 to 2.5 $\log_{10}$ PFU per ml, and so they are sufficiently sensitive to detect antigen in most acute-phase VHF viremias and to detect viruses at the concentrations present in throat wash and urine samples. Substitution of one or several monoclonal antibodies of high avidity and appropriate specificities for polyclonal sera (mostly against nucleoprotein and VP40) generally increases the sensitivities and specificities of these antigen capture ELISAs (37, 60, 61, 68, 69, 81).

Based on the same capture principles, a rapid, colorimetric, column immunofiltration assay for the direct detection of Ebola virus antigen has been used in field conditions for the first time, during an Ebola virus outbreak in the Republic of Congo (60, 61).

Nucleic Acid Detection

RT-PCR followed by genome analysis is rapidly replacing identification methods based on antigen-antibody methods criteria and has the advantage of complete inactivation of the samples in the first extraction step. However, as RT-PCR is more prone to cross-contamination problems, we would still encourage its use in combination with traditional methods (virus isolation and/or serology). Real-time PCR combined with classical cell culture could also be used for testing antivirals against Lassa and Ebola viruses (33).

Arenaviridae

RT-PCR has also been evaluated in a small series of serum samples from Lassa fever patients in West Africa (22, 94). The sensitivity of PCR relative to that of conventional virus isolation was 82%, and the specificity was 68%. PCR was positive throughout more of the disease course than was isolation, perhaps because of its greater sensitivity in the presence of the early antibodies associated with acute Lassa fever. Although systematic comparison with other techniques has not been made, improvement in the technique has occurred and suggests that considerable genetic variation among Lassa viruses requires the need for caution in primer design if diagnosis of infections in more than one geographic area is being considered (4–6). Real-time PCR assays are available for Lassa fever diagnosis but still lack field validation (96). Likewise, various strategies for RT-PCR have been devised to detect Junin virus RNA in clinical materials (4, 5, 58, 59). Some of these are reputed to be far more sensitive than conventional isolation procedures, especially in the presence of antibody. Any method that

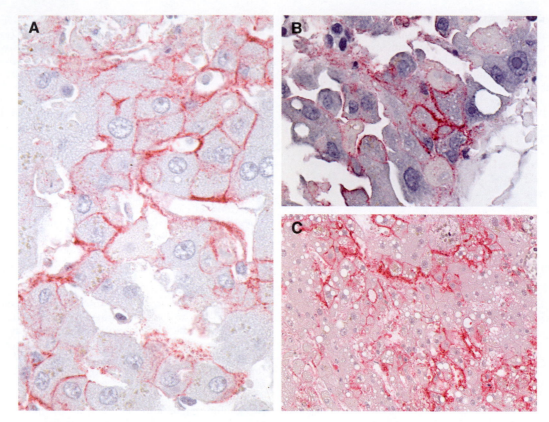

FIGURE 4 By use of immunohistochemistry, abundant virus antigens are seen within the cytoplasm of hepatocytes and sinusoidal lining cells in the liver of patients infected by Lassa virus (original magnification, ×158) (A); by Lujo virus (original magnification, ×158) (B); and by LCM virus (transplant patient) (original magnification, ×50) (C). (Immunoalkaline phosphatase staining, naphthol fast red substrate with light hematoxylin counterstain.)

promises to be a reliable substitute for procedures that entail the manipulation of infectious BSL-4 virus deserves attention. However, the ability to isolate and retain the virus has obvious advantages and should not be abandoned. The shipment of clinical material to an appropriate reference laboratory should be encouraged.

Filoviridae

Protocols that maximize detection are usually based on conserved sequences within the N, VP35, or L genes, while fine discrimination and phylogeny are based on the more variable GP region (82, 84, 86, 97). The sensitivity of RT-PCR for various Ebola virus species is similar to that of conventional isolation. During the SEBO virus outbreak in Gulu, RT-PCR-based assay was very valuable because of its ability to identify patients early, prior to identification by any other available tests, and for early convalescents, after clearing of detectable antigen. Using NP-based real-time quantitative RT-PCR, the viral load was found to correlate with disease outcome (90, 91). During the recent outbreak in Angola, Marburg virus real-time PCR assays were developed and effectively applied in the laboratory in Luanda and in the field in Uige, respectively (32, 91). Other platforms are available (73, 97), and recently reverse-transcription-loop-mediated-isothermal amplification has been proposed but has not yet been field tested (51).

ISOLATION PROCEDURES

Cell Culture

Clinical specimens and clarified tissue homogenates (usually 10% [wt/vol]) are diluted in a suitable maintenance medium and adsorbed in small volumes to cell monolayers grown in suitable vessels, such as T-25 tissue culture flasks. If no antigen is detected by IFA by 14 days, the sample is considered negative, but supernatant fluids should be blind-passaged to confirm the absence of virus. To confirm the presence and identity of the virus, scraped cells are tested by immunofluorescence assay and supernatant fluids are tested by antigen capture ELISA or RT-PCR techniques.

Arenaviridae

Cocultivation of Hypaque-Ficoll-separated peripheral blood leukocytes with susceptible cells has increased the isolation frequency of Junin virus. Cocultivation of lymphocytes from spleens of experimentally infected animals has yielded Lassa virus late in convalescence, even after neutralizing antibody has appeared. The technique merits systematic development for the remaining arenavirus and filovirus pathogens.

Although historically Machupo and Junin viruses were isolated by inoculation of newborn hamsters and mice, respectively, Vero cells are approximately as sensitive and are far less cumbersome to manage in BSL-4 containment.

Furthermore, Vero cells usually permit isolation and identification within 1 to 5 days, a significant advantage over the use of animals, since 7 to 20 days of incubation is required for illness to develop in the animals.

Filoviridae

The best general method currently available for isolation of filoviruses is the inoculation of appropriate cell cultures (usually Vero cells) followed by IFA or other immunologically specific testing of the inoculated cells for the presence of viral antigens at intervals. Other cell lines, including human diploid lung (MRC-5) and BHK-21 cells, also work; MA-104 cells (a fetal rhesus monkey kidney cell line) may be more sensitive than Vero cells for some strains.

Animal Inoculation

Arenaviridae

Intracranial (i.c.) inoculation of weanling mice is still regarded by some as the most sensitive established indicator of LCM virus (35), although adequate cell culture systems exist for the isolation of LCM virus. Care must be taken to use mice from a colony known to be free of LCM virus. Many LCM virus isolates produce a characteristic convulsive disease within 5 to 7 days, which is nearly pathognomonic. Brains from dead mice may be used to prepare ELISA antigens or may be subjected to IFA or immunohistochemical staining to obtain presumptive identification. Clarified mouse brain may also be used as the antigen for confirmatory testing by neutralization or RT-PCR.

Most LCM virus strains are also lethal for guinea pigs. The pathogenicity of virulent Lassa virus strains for outbred Swiss albino mice inoculated i.c. seems to vary with different sources; mice should not be seriously considered for Lassa virus isolations.

For the New World arenaviruses, particularly Junin virus, young adult guinea pigs inoculated either i.c. or peripherally have been used. Guinea pigs die 7 to 18 days after Junin virus inoculation. Strain 13 guinea pigs are exquisitely sensitive to most Lassa virus strains and uniformly die 12 to 18 days after inoculation; outbred Hartley strain guinea pigs are somewhat less susceptible. Newborn mice (1 to 3 days old) are highly susceptible to Junin virus inoculated i.c.; newborn hamsters are believed to be more sensitive to Machupo virus.

Filoviridae

Marburg virus and the ZEBO and SEBO species of Ebola virus produce febrile responses in guinea pigs 4 to 10 days after inoculation; however, none of these viruses kills guinea pigs consistently on primary inoculation, and only ZEBO and Marburg virus have been adapted to uniform lethality by sequential guinea pig passages. ZEBO is usually pathogenic for newborn mice inoculated i.c., but SEBO, REBO, and Marburg virus are not.

IDENTIFICATION OF VIRUSES

Typing Antisera

Detection of viral antigens in infected tissue culture cells (usually Vero or MA-104) permits a presumptive diagnosis, provided that the serologic reagents have been tested against all the reference arenaviruses and filoviruses expected in a given laboratory, thus permitting an interpretation of virus cross-reactions. Virus isolates in cell culture supernatant fluids or tissue homogenates are presumptively or specifically identified by their reactivity with diagnostic antisera in various serologic tests (see below). Specific polyclonal antisera are prepared in adult guinea pigs, hamsters, rabbits, rats, or mice inoculated intraperitoneally with infectious virus. Rhesus and cynomolgus monkeys that are convalescent from experimental infections are also reasonable sources for larger quantities of immune sera. Polyvalent polyclonal "typing" sera or ascitic fluids made by immunization with a number of viruses within the families have also been useful in early identification of virus isolates and in immunohistochemistry on unknown patient materials. Diagnostic antisera produced by single injection of infectious virus are less cross-reactive and usually have higher titers than those produced by multiple injections of inactivated antigens. To further reduce the induction of extraneous antibodies, input virus should be derived from tissues or cells homologous to the species being immunized; likewise, the virus suspension should be stabilized with homologous serum or serum proteins. Sera produced for use in the IFA tests and ELISA should be collected 30 to 60 days after inoculation; sera for neutralization tests should be collected later. All sera must be inactivated and rigorously tested for the presence of live virus before being removed from a BSL-4 environment.

Production and use of specific murine monoclonal antibodies with fine specificities for N and GP epitopes of LCM virus, Lassa virus, Junin virus (8, 85), and other arenaviruses have been reported, as well as monoclonal antibodies against the different proteins of the filoviruses. Reference reagents for all of these viruses are not generally available outside the appropriately equipped specialized laboratories.

Immunofluorescence

To process infected cells for IFA examination and presumptive identification, inoculated cell monolayers are dispersed by using glass beads or a rubber policeman or trypsinization, washed, and placed onto circular areas of specially prepared Teflon-coated slides. These "spot slides" are air dried, fixed in acetone at room temperature for 10 min, and either stained quickly or stored frozen at −70°C. Although acetone fixation greatly reduces the number of infectious intracellular viruses, spot slides prepared in this manner should still be considered infectious and handled accordingly. Gamma irradiation has been used to render spot slides noninfectious (24), with no diminution in fluorescent-antigen intensity. Alternatively, infected cells may be biologically inactivated with β-propiolactone (95). Gamma irradiation is recommended if the appropriate equipment is available.

For direct FA tests, specific immunoglobulins conjugated to fluorescein are used with Evans blue counterstain. Specific viral fluorescence is characterized as intense, punctate to granular aggregates confined to the cytoplasm of infected cells. Specific Marburg virus and Ebola virus fluorescence may include large, bizarrely shaped aggregates up to 10 μm across. Nonspecific fluorescence is rarely a problem in IFA procedures for these viruses. Detection of Marburg, Ebola, Lassa, and LCM virus antigens by the IFA test is usually considered sufficient for a definitive diagnosis, although Lassa and LCM viruses cross-react at low levels in this test (103). Detection of Junin or Machupo virus antigens by the IFA test constitutes a presumptive diagnosis, since these viruses can be reliably distinguished from each other only by neutralization tests. IFA formats for viral detection are more cumbersome and cross-reactive but can be used if direct conjugates are unavailable. Immunohistochemical techniques for detecting arenaviruses (19) and filoviruses (20, 39) with a variety of chromogens can also be applied.

SEROLOGIC DIAGNOSIS

IFA Test

Until recently, the IFA test was widely regarded as the most practical single method for documenting recent infections with Marburg and Ebola viruses or large prevalence studies (1). Preparation of spot slides with infected Vero cells is identical to the procedure described above. Some refinements to enhance reproducibility and quality between spot slide lots have been suggested (23). Although monovalent spot slides are usually desired and are prepared with cells optimally infected with a single virus, polyvalent spot slides can also be prepared by mixing cells infected with different viruses selected from these or other taxonomic groups that have similar geographic distributions (44). The BSL-4 facility requirement to produce the spot slides could be avoided by using recombinant antigen-expressing cells (36). Discrepancies in titers determined by different laboratories, or even different investigators, are common. In addition, in most of the severe and fatal forms of these diseases, the patients never develop a humoral response and die without antibodies. This technique is not recommended for acute diagnosis of hemorrhagic fevers.

ELISA for Detection of IgG and IgM Antibodies

For all intents and purposes, the immunoglobulin G (IgG) and IgM ELISAs have replaced the more subjective IFA tests as the serologic tests of choice (48, 102). ELISA procedures for Lassa virus-specific IgG and IgM have been developed and successfully used on field-collected human sera (3, 69). When this ELISA is used in combination with the Lassa antigen capture ELISA described above, virtually all Lassa fever patients can be specifically diagnosed within hours of hospital admission. A simplification of this procedure, which entails the use of infected Vero cell detergent lysate as the antigen, diluted in phosphate-buffered saline and adsorbed directly to the microtiter plate wells, has been developed for Ebola virus (48–50). Test sera are serially diluted, initially 1:100, and incubated with antigen in a format analogous to that used in the antigen capture ELISA described above. Following incubation, washing, and addition of horseradish peroxidase-conjugated anti-human serum, ABTS [2,2′-azinobis(3-ethylbenzthiazoinesulfonic acid)] substrate is added for color development. Species-specific conjugates allow testing of other animal species during epidemiological studies. To avoid the use of several conjugates during epidemiological studies, protein A-protein G conjugate can be used. More recently a competition assay using antibody-phage indicator has been proposed, but it has never been used in the field (63). Samples are considered positive if the optical density at 410 nm exceeds the mean plus 3 standard deviations for the normal-serum controls. This procedure can be further modified to detect virus-specific IgM by coating the plates with anti-human IgM followed by test serum dilutions and cell slurry antigens and then using the antigen capture protocol. These IgG and IgM ELISA procedures have worked well with specimens obtained from humans during natural infection and

from animals experimentally infected with Lassa, Machupo, Junin, Marburg, and Ebola viruses. A simplification of the ELISA plate procedure, substituting filter paper disks, has been reported for REBO virus (45); it appears to sacrifice some sensitivity and precision in comparison with the more established procedures but may find application in a field setting. All of these developmental assays are sufficiently robust to warrant field testing. Recombinant full or truncated proteins have also been proposed and used as antigen for ELISAs (38, 80).

Neutralization Tests

For the arenaviruses, plaque reduction tests with Vero cells are generally used. For measuring the levels of neutralizing antibody to Lassa and LCM viruses, which are both difficult to neutralize and poor inducers of this antibody, test sera are diluted, usually 1:10, in medium containing 10% guinea pig serum as a complement source and mixed with serial dilutions of challenge virus. Titers are expressed as a $\log_{10}$ neutralization index, defined as ($\log_{10}$ PFU in control) − ($\log_{10}$ PFU in test serum). For Junin and Machupo viruses, the more conventional serum dilution-constant virus format is normally used, although the constant serum-virus dilution format is equally useful for distinguishing among virus strains. Neutralizing-antibody responses require weeks to months to evolve but persist for years (43). Performance of these tests is restricted to laboratories equipped to handle the infectious viruses.

In survivors, neutralizing antibodies to Lassa virus first appear very late in convalescence (6 weeks or later), long after the viremia has disappeared. This pattern of early IFA and delayed neutralizing-antibody response is similar for LCM virus infections. Neutralizing antibodies against Junin and Machupo viruses become detectable 3 to 4 weeks after onset, soon after the termination of viremia. While these antibodies are thought to be important in protection against reinfection, their role in the resolution of acute infections is less firmly established (41, 42).

As described above, reliable tests for measuring the levels of neutralizing antibody to Marburg and Ebola viruses are not currently available.

Western Blotting

Western blotting is feasible for demonstrating antibodies to arenaviruses and filoviruses. However, it has never been applied systematically or routinely to diagnosis, although it was proposed as a confirmatory test to supplement the IFA test for filovirus antibodies (23). Detection of the nucleocapsid (N) band plus either VP30 or VP24 was taken as diagnostic. The Western blotting procedure was further refined by miniaturization, using the Phast system sodium dodecyl sulfate-polyacrylamide gel electrophoresis and transblot apparatus (Phast Western blot system). This test is not used anymore for antibody detection.

Other Serologic Tests

Other serologic tests have been applied to diagnosis but are now abandoned: gel diffusion for arenaviruses, complement fixation tests, reverse passive-hemagglutination (and inhibition) test involving Lassa virus antibody-coated erythrocytes, and a radioimmunoassay using ^{125}I-labeled staphylococcal protein A for Ebola. Western blotting and radioimmunoassay procedures are used in specialized laboratories to determine the fine specificities of monoclonal antibodies and occasionally to confirm the results of serosurveys based on ELISA.

EVALUATION AND INTERPRETATION OF RESULTS

Early diagnosis of arenavirus and filovirus infection is desirable, since specific immune plasma and appropriately selected antiviral drugs are in certain cases effective when treatment is initiated soon after disease onset. Early recognition of these infections should also trigger strict isolation procedures to prevent the spread of disease to patient contacts. In areas where specific viruses are endemic, the index of suspicion is often high and experienced clinicians may be remarkably accurate in rendering an accurate diagnosis of fully developed cases on clinical grounds alone. However, even in these areas, specific virologic and serologic tests are required to confirm clinical impressions, since many other diseases, including malaria, typhoid, rickettsial infections, idiopathic thrombocytopenia, and viral hepatitis, may masquerade as an arenavirus or filovirus infection.

Since patients with most of the severe and fatal forms of these diseases can die without developing detectable levels of antibody, timely diagnosis requires a means of detecting infectious virus or antigen in the field. The antigen capture ELISA holds promise for use in detecting clinically relevant concentrations of virus in infectious or gamma-irradiation-inactivated or β-propiolactone-inactivated sera, body fluids, and tissues, and in blood and tissues of humans and nonhuman primates infected with Machupo, Lassa, Ebola, and Marburg viruses (3, 40, 48, 49, 77).

RT-PCR assays may eventually eliminate almost all need to isolate infectious virus to establish a definitive diagnosis, but virus isolation remains important for subsequent genetic and pathogenesis studies. The ability to amplify viral genomes from infected tissues and even from formalin-fixed tissues and to sequence the reaction products has eclipsed serologic methods of identification and classification of arenaviruses (4–6) and filoviruses (90, 92). With the exception of LCM virus, which may be handled at a lower containment level, attempts to isolate these viruses should not be done outside a BSL-4 laboratory (16). A combination of several laboratory techniques should be used to confirm any clinical suspicion of hemorrhagic fever.

Among arenavirus infections, Lassa virus is usually recovered (by isolation, antigen detection, or RT-PCR) from acute-phase sera of hospitalized patients soon after admission, frequently in the presence of specific IgM antibody, and a detectable antibody response does not necessarily signal imminent recovery; viremia frequently persists, and some patients die despite an antibody response. Junin, Machupo, and LCM viruses are recovered less frequently, and diagnosis is usually based on seroconversion. The presence of specific IgM ELISA titers in the cerebrospinal fluid of LCM patients constitutes a definitive diagnosis, and for all arenavirus infections, the presence of specific IgM antibodies is indicative of recent infection. The extent to which heterologous arenavirus infection and/or reinfection broadens antibody specificity has not been systematically evaluated for any of the available serologic tests. Neutralizing antibodies against arenaviruses persist for long periods, perhaps for life, and thus provide the most reliable basis for determining the minimum resistance of a population to reinfection. The role of neutralizing antibody in acute recovery is less clear. The protective efficacy of passively administered immune plasma is believed to be a function of neutralizing-antibody titers, and plasma should be selected on this basis, especially for Junin and Lassa fevers (41, 42).

For filoviruses, the combination of antigen detection, RT-PCR, and IgM titer is the most valuable for acute-case diagnosis. Because of the time required for culture and the biohazard, virus isolation data for these viruses are usually available only retrospectively. Marburg virus and Ebola viruses are usually isolated from acute-phase serum samples. A rising IgM or IgG ELISA titer constitutes a strong presumptive diagnosis. Since IgM titers do not persist for long, a decreasing titer suggests a recent infection that occurred perhaps several months previously. The IFA test has yielded misleading results when applied to diagnostic and population-based serosurveys and should be abandoned. For unknown reasons, the filoviruses are notoriously poor inducers of neutralizing antibody. The role of neutralizing antibodies for Ebola virus protective immunity is unclear, although passively administered IgG with very high neutralizing-antibody titers conferred only partial protection to experimentally infected primates (42).

The highest priority for future development is refinement of the available diagnostic tools to permit definitive virus identification in the field. PCR-based assays add another dimension to the capability of field laboratories to diagnose acute disease almost in real time. Proper tailoring of primers should permit the design of tests with the proper degree of specificity. The emergence of new arenaviruses, as well as BEBO, in the past decade, serves as a reminder that broadly reactive, grouping reagents are still required to augment the newly evolving tools of conventional and real-time PCR and capture ELISAs based on extremely specific monoclonal antibodies and gene sequences.

An investment in rapid diagnosis should result in more timely intervention with effective treatment regimens and, through implementation of appropriate public health measures, contribute to reduce the dissemination of these highly virulent viral pathogens.

REFERENCES

1. **Ambrosio, A. M., M. R. Feuillade, G. S. Gamboa, and J. I. Maiztegui.** 1994. Prevalence of lymphocytic choriomeningitis virus infection in a human population in Argentina. *Am. J. Trop. Med. Hyg.* **50:**381–386.
2. **Barrette, R. W., S. A. Metwally, J. M. Rowland, L. Xu, S. R. Zaki, S. T. Nichol, P. E. Rollin, J. S. Towner, W. J. Shieh, B. Batten, T. K. Sealy, C. Carrillo, K. E. Moran, A. J. Bracht, G. A. Mayr, M. Sirios-Cruz, D. P. Catbagan, E. A. Lautner, T. G. Ksiazek, W. R. White, and M. T. McIntosh.** 2009. Discovery of swine as a host for the Reston ebolavirus. *Science* **325:**204–206.
3. **Bausch, D. G., P. E. Rollin, A. H. Demby, M. Coulibaly, J. Kanu, A. S. Conteh, K. D. Wagoner, L. K. McMullan, M. D. Bowen, C. J. Peters, and T. G. Ksiazek.** 2000. Diagnosis and clinical virology of Lassa fever as evaluated by enzyme-linked immunosorbent assay, indirect fluorescent-antibody tests, and virus isolation. *J. Clin. Microbiol.* **38:**2670–2677.
4. **Bowen, M. D., C. J. Peters, and S. T. Nichol.** 1996. The phylogeny of new world (Tacaribe complex) arenaviruses. *Virology* **219:**285–290.
5. **Bowen, M. D., C. J. Peters, and S. T. Nichol.** 1997. Phylogenetic analysis of the *Arenaviridae:* patterns of virus evolution and evidence for cospeciation between arenaviruses and their rodent hosts. *Mol. Phylogenet. Evol.* **8:**301–316.
6. **Bowen, M. D., P. E. Rollin, T. G. Ksiazek, H. L. Hustad, D. G. Bausch, A. H. Demby, M. D. Bajani, C. J. Peters, and S. T. Nichol.** 2000. Genetic diversity among Lassa virus strains. *J. Virol.* **74:**6992–7004.
7. **Briese, T., J. T. Paweska, L. K. McMullan, S. K. Hutchison, C. Streer, G. Palacios, M. L. Khristova, J. Weyer, R. Swanepoel, M. Egholm, S. T. Nichol, and I. W. Lipkin.** 2009. Genetic detection and characterization of Lujo virus, a new hemorrhagic fever–associated arenavirus from Southern Africa. *PLoS Pathog.* **4**(5):e1000455.

8. **Buchmeier, M. J., H. A. Lewicki, O. Tomori, and M. B. A. Oldstone.** 1981. Monoclonal antibodies to lymphocytic choriomeningitis and Pichinde viruses: generation, characterization, and cross-reactivity with other arenaviruses. *Virology* **113:**73–85.

9. **Buchmeier, M. J., and B. S. Parekh.** 1987. Protein structure and expression among arenaviruses. *Curr. Top. Microbiol. Immunol.* **133:**41–58.

10. **Buchmeier, M. J., J. C. de la Torre, and C. J. Peters.** 2007. Arenaviridae: the viruses and their replication, p. 1791–1827. *In* D. M. Knipe and P. M. Howley (ed.), *Fields Virology*, 5th ed. Lippincott Williams & Wilkins, Philadelphia, PA.

11. **Cajimat, M. N. B., M. L. Milazzo, R. D. Bradley, and C. F. Fulhorst.** 2007. Catarina virus, an arenaviral species principally associated with *Neotoma micropus* (southern plains woodrat) in Texas. *Am. J. Trop. Med. Hyg.* **77:**732–736.

12. **Cajimat, M. N. B., M. L. Milazzo, J. N. Borchert, K. D. Abbott, R. D. Bradley, and C. F. Fulhorst.** 2008. Diversity among Tacaribe serocomplex viruses (family Arenaviridae) naturally associated with the Mexican woodrat (*Neotoma mexicana*). *Virus Res.* **133:**211–217.

13. **Casals, J.** 1977. Serologic reactions with arenaviruses. *Medicina* (Buenos Aires) **37**(Suppl. 3):59–68.

14. **Centers for Disease Control.** 1988. Management of patients with suspected viral hemorrhagic fever. *MMWR Morb. Mortal. Wkly. Rep.* **37**(Suppl. 3):1–16.

15. **Centers for Disease Control and Prevention.** 1995. Update. Management of patients with suspected viral hemorrhagic fever—United States. *MMWR Morb. Mortal. Wkly. Rep.* **44:**475–479.

15a. **Centers for Disease Control and Prevention.** 19 May 2005. *Interim Guidance for Managing Patients with Suspected Viral Hemorrhagic Fever in U.S. Hospitals.* Centers for Disease Control and Prevention, Atlanta, GA. http://www.cdc.gov/ncidod/dhqp/pdf/bbp/VHFinterimGuidance05_19_05.pdf.

16. **Centers for Disease Control and Prevention—National Institutes of Health.** 2007. *Biosafety in Microbiological and Biomedical Laboratories,* 5th ed. U.S. Department of Health and Human Services, Washington, DC. http://www.cdc.gov/od/ohs/biosfty/bmbl5/BMBL_5th_Edition.pdf.

17. **Centers for Disease Control and Prevention.** 2008. Lymphocytic choriomeningitis virus transmitted through solid organ transplantation—Massachusetts, 2008. *MMWR Morb. Mortal. Wkly. Rep.* **57:**799–801.

18. **Centers for Disease Control and Prevention.** 2009. Imported case of Marburg hemorrhagic fever—Colorado, 2008. *MMWR Morb. Mortal. Wkly. Rep.* **58:**1377–1381.

19. **Connolly, B. M., A. B. Jenson, C. J. Peters, S. J. Geyer, J. F. Barth, and R. A. McPherson.** 1993. Pathogenesis of Pichinde virus infection in strain 13 guinea pigs: an immunocytochemical, virologic, and clinical chemistry study. *Am. J. Trop. Med. Hyg.* **49:**10–23.

20. **Connolly, B. M., K. E. Steele, K. J. Davis, T. W. Geisbert, W. M. Kell, N. K. Jaax, and P. B. Jahrling.** 1999. Pathogenesis of experimental Ebola virus infection in guinea pigs. *J. Infect. Dis.* **179**(Suppl.):S203–S217.

21. **Delgado, S., B. R. Erickson, R. Agudo, P. J. Blair, E. Vallejo, C. G. Albarino, J. Vargas, J. A. Comer, P. E. Rollin, T. G. Ksiazek, J. G. Olson, and S. T. Nichol.** 2008. Chapare Virus, a newly discovered arenavirus isolated from a fatal hemorrhagic fever case in Bolivia. *PLoS Pathog.* **4**(4):e1000047.

22. **Drosten, C., S. Gottig, S. Schilling, M. Asper, M. Panning, H. Schmitz, and S. Gunther.** 2002. Rapid detection and quantification of RNA of Ebola and Marburg viruses, Lassa virus, Crimean-Congo hemorrhagic fever virus, Rift Valley fever virus, Dengue virus, and Yellow fever virus by real-time reverse transcription-PCR. *J. Clin. Microbiol.* **40:**2323–2330.

23. **Elliott, L. H., S. P. Bauer, G. Perez-Oronoz, and E. S. Lloyd.** 1993. Improved specificity of testing methods for filovirus antibodies. *J. Virol. Methods* **43:**85–100.

24. **Elliott, L. H., J. B. McCormick, and K. M. Johnson.** 1982. Inactivation of Lassa, Marburg, and Ebola viruses by gamma irradiation. *J. Clin. Microbiol.* **16:**704–708.

25. **Fischer, S. A., M. B. Graham, M. J. Kuehnert, C. N. Kotton, A. Srinivasan, F. M. Marty, J. A. Comer, J. Guarner, C. D. Paddock, D. L. DeMeo, W. J. Shieh, B. R. Erickson, U. Bandy, A. DeMaria, J. P. Davis, F. L. Delmonico, B. Pavlin, A. Likos, M. J. Vincent, T. K. Sealy, C. S. Goldsmith, D. B. Jernigan, P. E. Rollin, M. M. Packard, M. Patel, C. Rowland, R. F. Helfand, S. T. Nichol, J. A. Fishman, T. G. Ksiazek, S. R. Zaki, R. Sherif, and the LCMV in Transplant Recipients Investigation team.** 2006. Transmission of lymphocytic choriomeningitis virus by organ transplantation. *N. Engl. J. Med.* **354:**2235–2249.

26. **Fulhorst, C. F., S. G. Bennet, M. L. Malazza, H. L. Murray, Jr., J. P. Webb, M. J. Cajima, and R. D. Bradley.** 2002. Bear Canyon virus: an arenavirus naturally associated with the California mouse (*Peromyscus californicus*). *Emerg. Infect. Dis.* **8:**717–721.

27. **Geisbert, T. W., and P. B. Jahrling.** 1995. Differentiation of filoviruses by electron microscopy. *Virus Res.* **39:**129–150.

28. **Geisbert, T. W., and N. K. Jaax.** 1997. Marburg hemorrhagic fever: report of a case studied by immunohistochemistry and electron microscopy. *Ultrastruct. Pathol.* **22:**3–17.

29. **Geisbert, T. W., and P. B. Jahrling.** 1990. Use of immunoelectron microscopy to show Ebola virus during the 1989 United States epizootic. *J. Clin. Pathol.* **43:**813–816.

30. **Geisbert, T. W., P. B. Jahrling, M. A. Hanes, and P. M. Zack.** 1992. Association of Ebola-related Reston virus particles and antigen with tissue lesions of monkeys imported to the United States. *J. Comp. Pathol.* **106:**137–152.

31. **Georges-Courbot, M. C., A. Sanchez, C. Y. Lu, S. Baize, E. Leroy, J. Lansoud-Soukate, C. Tevi-Benissan, A. J. Georges, S. G. Trappier, S. R. Zaki, R. Swanepoel, P. A. Leman, P. E. Rollin, C. J. Peters, S. T. Nichol, and T. G. Ksiazek.** 1997. Isolation and phylogenetic characterization of Ebola viruses causing different outbreaks in Gabon. *Emerg. Infect. Dis.* **3:**59–62.

32. **Grolla, A., A. Lucht, D. Dick, J. E. Strong, and H. Feldmann.** 2005. Laboratory diagnosis of Ebola and Marburg hemorrhagic fever. *Bull. Soc. Path. Exot.* **98:**205–209.

33. **Gunther, S., M. Asper, C. Roser, L. K. S. Luna, C. Drosten, B. Becker-Ziaja, P. Borowski, H.-M. Chen, and R. S. Hosmane.** 2004. Application of real-time PCR for testing antiviral compounds against Lassa virus, SARS Coronavirus and Ebola virus in vitro. *Antivir. Res.* **63:**209–215.

34. **Gunther, S., G. Hoofd, R. Charrel, C. Roser, B. Becker-Ziaja, G. Lloyd, C. Sabuni, R. Verhagen, G. van der Groen, J. Kennis, A. Katakweba, R. Machang'u, R. Makundi, and H. Leirs.** 2009. Mopeia virus-related arenavirus in natal multimammate mice, Morogoro, Tanzania. *Emerg. Infect. Dis.* **15:**2008–2012.

35. **Hotchin, J., and E. Sikora.** 1975. Laboratory diagnosis of lymphocytic choriomeningitis. *Bull. W. H. O.* **52:**555–558.

36. **Ikegami, T., M. Saijo, M. Niikura, M. E. G. Miranda, A. B. Calaor, M. Hernandez, D. L. Manalo, I. Kurane, Y. Yoshikawa, and S. Morikawa.** 2002. Development of an immunofluorescence method for the detection of antibodies to Ebola virus subtype Reston by the use of recombinant nucleoprotein-expressing HeLa cells. *Microbiol. Immunol.* **46:**633–638.

37. **Ikegami, T., M. Niikura, M. Saijo, M. E. Miranda, A. B. Calaor, M. Hernandez, L. P. Acosta, D. L. Manalo, I. Kurane, Y. Yoshikawa, and S. Morikawa.** 2003. Antigen capture enzyme-linked immunosorbent assay for specific detection of Reston Ebola virus nucleoprotein. *Clin. Diagn. Lab. Immunol.* **10:**552–557.

38. **Ikegami, T., M. Saijo, M. Niikura, M. E. Miranda, A. B. Calaor, M. Hernandez, D. L. Manalo, I. Kurane, Y. Yoshikawa, and S. Morikawa.** 2003. Immunoglobulin G enzyme-linked immunosorbent assay using truncated nucleoproteins of Reston Ebola virus. *Epidemiol. Infect.* **130:**533–539.

39. **Jaax, N. K., K. J. Davis, T. W. Geisbert, A. P. Vogel, G. P. Jaax, M. Topper, and P. B. Jahrling.** 1996. Lethal experimental infection of rhesus monkeys with Ebola-Zaire (Mayinga) virus by the oral and conjunctival route of exposure. *Arch. Pathol. Lab. Med.* **120:**140–155.

40. **Jahrling, P. B., T. W. Geisbert, D. W. Dalgard, E. D. Johnson, T. G. Ksiazek, W. C. Hall, and C. J. Peters.** 1990. Preliminary report: isolation of Ebola virus from monkeys imported to USA. *Lancet* **335:**502–505.

41. **Jahrling, P. B., and C. J. Peters.** 1984. Passive antibody therapy of Lassa fever in cynomolgus monkeys. *Infect. Immun.* **44:**528–533.

42. **Jahrling, P. B., T. W. Geisbert, J. B. Geisbert, J. R. Swearengen, M. Bray, N. K. Jaax, J. W. Huggins, J. W. LeDuc, and C. J. Peters.** 1999. Evaluation of immune globulin and recombinant interferon α-2b for treatment of experimental Ebola virus infections. *J. Infect. Dis.* **179**(Suppl.): S224–S234.

43. **Jahrling, P. B., T. W. Geisbert, N. K. Jaax, M. A. Hanes, T. G. Ksiazek, and C. J. Peters.** 1996. Experimental infection of cynomolgus macaques with Ebola-Reston filoviruses from the 1989–1990 U.S. epizootic. *Arch. Virol. Suppl.* **11:** 115–134.

44. **Johnson, K. M., L. H. Elliott, and D. L. Heymann.** 1981. Preparation of polyvalent viral immunofluorescent intracellular antigens and use in human serosurveys. *J. Clin. Microbiol.* **14:**527–529.

45. **Kalter, S. S., R. L. Heberling, J. D. Barry, and P. Y. Tian.** 1995. Detection of Ebola-Reston (filoviridae) virus antibody by dot-immunobinding assay. *Lab. Anim. Sci.* **45:**523–525.

46. **Kiley, M. P., E. T. W. Bowen, G. A. Eddy, M. Isaacson, K. M. Johnson, J. B. McCormick, F. A. Murphy, S. R. Pattyn, D. Peters, O. W. Prozesky, R. L. Regnery, D. I. H. Simpson, W. Slenczka, P. Sureau, G. Van der Groen, P. A. Webb, and H. Wulff.** 1982. Filoviridae: taxonomic home for Marburg and Ebola viruses? *Intervirology* **18:**24–32.

47. **Kiley, M. P., N. J. Cox, L. H. Elliott, A. Sanchez, R. Defries, M. J. Buchmeier, D. D. Richman, and J. B. McCormick.** 1988. Physiochemical properties of Marburg virus: evidence for three distinct virus strains and their relationship to Ebola virus. *J. Gen. Virol.* **69:**1957–1967.

48. **Ksiazek, T. G., P. E. Rollin, A. J. Williams, D. S. Bressler, M. L. Martin, R. Swanepoel, F. J. Burt, P. A. Leman, A. K. Rowe, R. Mukunu, A. Sanchez, and C. J. Peters.** 1999. Clinical virology of Ebola hemorrhagic fever (EHF) virus: virus, virus antigen, and IgG and IgM findings among EHF patients in Kikwit, Democratic Republic of Congo, 1995. *J. Infect. Dis.* **179**(Suppl.):S177–S187.

49. **Ksiazek, T. G., P. E. Rollin, P. B. Jahrling, E. Johnson, D. W. Dalgard, and C. J. Peters.** 1992. Enzyme immunosorbent assay for Ebola virus antigens in tissues of infected primates. *J. Clin. Microbiol.* **30:**947–950.

50. **Ksiazek, T. G., C. P. West, P. E. Rollin, P. B. Jahrling, and C. J. Peters.** 1999. ELISA for the detection of antibodies to Ebola viruses. *J. Infect. Dis.* **179**(Suppl. 1):S191–S198.

51. **Kurosaki, Y., A. Takada, H. Ebihara, A. Grolla, N. Kamo, H. Feldmann, Y. Kawacka, and J. Yasuda.** 2007. Rapid and simple detection of Ebola virus by reverse transcription-loop-mediated isothermal amplification. *J. Virol. Methods* **141:**78–83.

52. **Lecompte, E., J. ter Meulen, S. Emonet, S. Daffis, and R. N. Charrel.** 2007. Genetic identification of Kodoko virus, a novel arenavirus of the African pigmy mouse (*Mus Nannomys minutoides*) in West Africa. *Virology* **364:**178–183.

53. **Lederberg, J., R. E. Shope, and S. C. Oals, Jr. (ed.).** 1992. *Emerging Infections. Microbial Threats to Health in the United States.* National Academy Press, Washington, DC.

54. **Le Guenno, B., P. Formenty, M. Wyers, P. Gounon, F. Walker, and C. Boesch.** 1995. Isolation and partial characterisation of a new strain of Ebola virus. *Lancet* **345:** 1271–1274.

55. **Lehmann-Grube, F.** 1971. Lymphocytic choriomeningitis virus. *Virol. Monogr.* **10:**1–173.

56. **Leroy, E. M., B. Kumulungui, X. Pourrut, P. Rouquet, A. Hassanin, P. Yaba, A. Delicat, J. T. Paweska, J. P. Gonzalez, and R. Swanepoel.** 2005. Fruit bats as reservoirs of Ebola virus. *Nature* **438:**575–576.

57. **Leroy, E. M., A. Epelboin, V. Mondonge, X. Pourrut, J. P. Gonzalez, J. J. Muyembe-Tamfum, and P. Formenty.** 2009. Human Ebola outbreak resulting from direct exposure to fruit bats in Luebo, Democratic Republic of Congo, 2007. *Vector Borne Zoon. Dis.* **9:**723–728.

58. **Lozano, M. E., D. Enria, J. I. Maiztegui, O. Grau, and V. Romanowski.** 1995. Rapid diagnosis of Argentine hemorrhagic fever by reverse transcriptase PCR-based assay. *J. Clin. Microbiol.* **33:**1327–1332.

59. **Lozano, M. E., D. M. Posik, C. G. Albarino, G. Schujman, P. D. Ghiringhelli, G. Calderon, M. Sabattini, and V. Romanowski.** 1997. Characterization of arenaviruses using a family-specific primer set for RT-PCR amplification and RFLP analysis. Its potential use for detection of uncharacterized arenaviruses. *Virus Res.* **49:**79–89.

60. **Lucht, A., R. Grunow, C. Otterbein, P. Möller, H. Feldmann, and S. Becker.** 2004. Production of monoclonal antibodies and development of an antigen capture ELISA directed against the envelope glycoprotein GP of Ebola virus. *Med. Microbiol. Immunol.* **193:**181–187.

61. **Lucht, A., P. Formenty, H. Feldmann, M. Gotz, E. Leroy, P. Bataboukila, A. Grolla, F. Feldmann, T. Wittmann, P. Campbell, C. Atsangandoko, P. Boumandoki, E. J. Finke, P. Miethe, S. Becker, and R. Grunow.** 2007. Development of an immunofiltration-based antigen-detection assay for rapid diagnosis of Ebola virus infection. *J. Infect. Dis.* **196**(Suppl. 2):S184–S192.

62. **Martini, G. A.** 1971. Marburg virus disease. Clinical syndrome, p. 1–9. *In* G. A. Martini and R. Siegert (ed.), *Marburg Virus Disease.* Springer-Verlag, New York, NY.

63. **Meissner, F., T. Maruyama, M. Frentsch, A. Hessell, L. Rodriguez, T. Geisbert, P. Jahrling, D. Burton, and P. Parren.** 2002. Detection of antibodies against the four subtypes of Ebola virus in sera from any species using a novel antibody-phage indicator assay. *Virology* **300:**236–243.

64. **Mets, M. B., L. J. Barton, A. S. Khan, and T. G. Ksiazek.** 2000. Lymphocytic choriomeningitis virus: an underdiagnosed cause of congenital chorioretinitis. *Am. J. Ophthalmol.* **130:**209–215.

65. **Moncayo, A., C. L. Hice, D. M. Watts, A. P. A. Travassos da Rosa, H. Guzman, K. L. Russell, C. Calampa, A. Gozalo, V. L. Popov, S. C. Weaver, and R. B. Tesh.** 2001. Allpahuayo virus, a newly recognized arenavirus (*Arenaviridae*) from arboreal rice rats (*Oecomys bicolor* and *Oecomys paricola*) in Northeastern Peru. *Virology* **284:**277–286.

66. **Murphy, F. A., G. Van der Groen, S. G. Whitfield, and J. V. Lange.** 1978. Ebola and Marburg virus morphology and taxonomy, p. 61–84. *In* S. R. Pattyn (ed.), *Ebola Virus Haemorrhagic Fever.* Elsevier/North Holland Biomedical Press, Amsterdam, The Netherlands.

67. **Murphy, F. A., and S. G. Whitfield.** 1975. Morphology and morphogenesis of arenaviruses. *Bull. W. H. O.* **52:**409–419.

68. **Niikura, M., T. Ikegami, M. Saijo, I. Kurane, M. E. Miranda, and S. Morikawa.** 2001. Detection of Ebola viral antigen by enzyme-linked immunosorbent assay using a novel monoclonal antibody to nucleoprotein. *J. Clin. Microbiol.* **39:**3267–3271.

69. **Niklasson, B. S., P. B. Jahrling, and C. J. Peters.** 1984. Detection of Lassa virus antigens and Lassa-specific IgG and IgM by enzyme-linked immunosorbent assay. *J. Clin. Microbiol.* **20:**239–244.

70. **Okware, S. I., F. G. Omaswa, S. Zaramba, A. Opio, J. J. Lutwama, J. Kamugisha, E. B. Rwaguma, P. Kagwa, and M. Lamunu.** 2002. An outbreak of Ebola in Uganda. *Trop. Med. Intern. Health* **7:**1068–1075.

71. **Onyango, C. O., M. L. Opoka, T. G. Ksiazek, P. Formenty, A. Ahmed, P. M. Tukei, R. C. Sang, V. O. Ofula, S. L. Konongoi, R. L. Coldren, T. G. Grein, D. Legros, M. Bell, K. M. De Cock, W. J. Bellini, J. S. Towner, S. T. Nichol, and P. E. Rollin.** 2007. Laboratory diagnosis of Ebola hemorrhagic fever during an outbreak in Yambio, Sudan, 2004. *J. Infect. Dis.* **196**(Suppl. 2):S193–S198.

72. **Paddock, C., T. Ksiazek, J. A. Comer, P. Rollin, S. Nichol, W. J. Shieh, J. Guarner, C. Goldsmith, P. Greer, A. Srinivasan, D. Jernigan, S. Kehl, M. Graham, and S. Zaki.** 2005. Pathology of fatal lymphocytic choriomeningitis virus

infection in multiple organ transplant recipients from a common donor. *Mod. Pathol.* **18**(Suppl.):263A–264A.

73. **Panning, M., T. Laue, S. Olschlager, M. Eickmann, S. Becker, S. Raith, M. C. Georges-Courbot, M. Nilsson, R. Gopal, A. Lundkvist, A. di Caro, D. Brown, H. Meyer, G. Lloyd, B. M. Kummerer, S. Gunther, and C. Drosten.** 2007. Diagnostic reverse-transcription polymerase chain reaction kit for filoviruses based on the strain collections of all European biosafety level 4 laboratories. *J. Infect. Dis.* **196**(Suppl. 2): S199–S204.

74. **Paweska, J. T., N. H. Sewlall, T. G. Ksiazek, L. H. Blumberg, M. J. Hale, I. Lipkin, J. Weyer, S. T. Nichol, P. E. Rollin, L. K. McMullan, C. D. Paddock, T. Briese, J. Mnyaluza, T. H. Dinh, V. Mukonka, P. Ching, A. Duse, G. Richards, G. de Jong, C. Cohen, B. Ikalafeng, C. Mugero, C. Asomugha, M. M. Molotle, D. M. Nteo, E. Misiani, R. Swanepoel, S. R. Zaki, and members of the Outbreak Control and Investigation Teams.** 2009. Nosocomial outbreak of novel arenavirus infection, Southern Africa. *Emerg. Infect. Dis.* **15**:1598–1602.

75. **Peters, C. J.** 1997. Viral hemorrhagic fevers, p. 779–799. *In* N. Nathanson (ed.), *Viral Pathogenesis.* Lippincott-Raven Publishers, Philadelphia, PA.

76. **Rodriguez, L., A. De Roo, Y. Guimard, S. Trappier, A. Sanchez, D. Bressler, A. J. Williams, T. G. Ksiazek, C. J. Peters, and S. T. Nichol.** 1999. Persistence and genetic stability of Ebola virus during the outbreak in Kikwit, Zaire 1995. *J. Infect. Dis.* **179**(Suppl. 1):S170–S176.

77. **Rollin, P. E., R. J. Williams, D. S. Bressler, S. Pearson, M. Cottingham, G. Pucak, A. Sanchez, S. G. Trappier, R. L. Peters, P. W. Greer, S. Zaki, T. Demarcus, K. Hendricks, M. Kelley, D. Simpson, T. W. Geisbert, P. B. Jahrling, C. J. Peters, and T. G. Ksiazek.** 1999. Ebola-Reston virus among quarantine nonhuman primates recently imported from the Philippines to the United States. *J. Infect. Dis.* **179**(Suppl.):S108–S114.

78. **Rollin, P. E., D. G. Bausch, and A. Sanchez.** 2007. Blood chemistry measurements and D-dimer levels associated with fatal and nonfatal outcomes in humans infected with Sudan Ebola virus. *J. Infect. Dis.* **196**(Suppl. 2):S364–S371.

79. **Rouquet, P., J.-M. Froment, M. Bermejo, A. Kilbourn, W. Karesh, P. Reed, B. Kumulungui, P. Yaba, A. Délicat, P. E. Rollin, and E. M. Leroy.** 2005. Wild animal mortality monitoring and human Ebola outbreaks, Gabon and Republic of Congo, 2001–2003. *Emerg. Infect. Dis.* **11**:283–290.

80. **Saijo, M., M. Niikura, S. Morikawa, T. G. Ksiazek, R. F. Meyer, C. J. Peters, and I. Kurane.** 2001. Enzyme-linked immunosorbent assays for detection of antibodies to Ebola and Marburg viruses using recombinant nucleoproteins. *J. Clin. Microbiol.* **39**:1–7.

81. **Saijo, M., M. C. Georges-Courbot, S. Fukushi, T. Mizutani, P. Marianneau, A. J. Georges, I. Kurane, and S. Morikawa.** 2006. Marburgvirus nucleoprotein-capture enzyme-linked immunosorbent assay using monoclonal antibodies to recombinant nucleoprotein: detection of authentic marburgvirus. *Jpn. J. Infect. Dis.* **59**:323–325.

82. **Sanchez, A., T. W. Geisbert, and H. Feldmann.** 2007. Filoviridae: Marburg and Ebola viruses, p. 1409–1448. *In* D. M. Knipe and P. M. Howley (ed.), *Fields Virology,* 5th ed. Lippincott Williams & Wilkins, Philadelphia, PA.

83. **Sanchez, A., M. P. Kiley, B. P. Holloway, and D. D. Auperin.** 1993. Sequence analysis of the Ebola virus genome: organization, genetic elements, and comparison with the genome of Marburg virus. *Virus Res.* **29**:215–240.

84. **Sanchez, A., T. G. Ksiazek, P. E. Rollin, M. E. G. Miranda, S. G. Trappier, A. S. Khan, C. J. Peters, and S. T. Nichol.** 1999. Detection and molecular characterization of Ebola viruses causing disease in humans and nonhuman primates. *J. Infect. Dis.* **179**(Suppl. 1):S164–S169.

85. **Sanchez, A., D. Y. Pifat, R. H. Kenyon, C. J. Peters, J. B. McCormick, and M. P. Kiley.** 1989. Junin virus monoclonal antibodies: characterization and cross-reactivity with other arenaviruses. *J. Gen. Virol.* **70**:1125–1132.

86. **Sanchez, A., S. G. Trappier, U. Stroher, S. T. Nichol, M. D. Bowen, and H. Feldmann.** 1998. Variation in the glycoprotein and VP35 genes of Marburg virus strains. *Virology* **240**:138–146.

87. **Sanchez, A., S. G. Trappier, B. W. Mahy, C. J. Peters, and S. T. Nichol.** 1996. The virion glycoproteins of Ebola virus are encoded in two reading frames and are expressed through transcriptional editing. *Proc. Natl. Acad. Sci. USA* **93**:3602–3607.

88. **Swanepoel, R., S. B. Smit, P. E. Rollin, P. Formenty, P. A. Leman, A. Kemp, F. J. Burt, A. A. Grobbelaar, J. Croft, D. G. Bausch, H. Zeller, H. Leirs, L. E. O. Braack, M. L. Libande, S. Zaki, S. T. Nichol, T. G. Ksiazek, and J. T. Paweska.** 2007. Studies of reservoir hosts for Marburg virus. *Emerg. Infect. Dis.* **13**:1847–1851.

89. **Timen, A., M. P. Koopmans, A. C. Vossen, G. J. van Doornum, S. Gunther, F. van den Berkmortel, K. M. Verduin, S. Dittrich, P. Emmerich, A. D. Osterhaus, J. T. van Dissel, and R. A. Coutinho.** 2009. Response to imported case of Marburg hemorrhagic fever, the Netherland. *Emerg. Infect. Dis.* **15**:1171–1175.

90. **Towner, J. S., P. E. Rollin, D.G. Bausch, A. Sanchez, S. M. Crary, M. Vincent, W. F. Lee, C. F. Spiropoulou, T. G. Ksiazek, M. Lukwiya, F. Kaducu, R. Downing, and S.T. Nichol.** 2004. Rapid diagnosis of Ebola hemorrhagic fever by reverse transcription-PCR in an outbreak setting and assessment of patient viral load as a predictor of outcome. *J. Virol.* **78**:4330–4341.

91. **Towner, J. S., M. L. Khristova, T. K. Sealy, M. J. Vincent, B. R. Erickson, D. A. Bawiec, A. L. Hartman, J. A. Comer, S. R. Zaki, U. Stroher, F. Gomes da Silva, F. del Castillo, P. E. Rollin, T. G. Ksiazek, and S. T. Stuart.** 2006. Marburgvirus genomics and association with a large hemorrhagic fever outbreak in Angola. *J. Virol.* **80**:6497–6516.

92. **Towner, J. S., T. K. Sealy, M. L. Khristova, C. G. Albarino, S. Conlan, S. A. Reeder, P. L. Quan, W. I. Lipkin, R. Downing, J. W. Tappero, S. Okware, J. Lutwama, B. Bakamutumaho, J. Kayiwa, J. A. Comer, P. E. Rollin, T. G. Ksiazek, and S. T. Nichol.** 2008. Newly discovered Ebola virus associated with hemorrhagic fever outbreak in Uganda. *PLoS Pathog.* **4**(11):e1000212.

93. **Towner, J. S., B. R. Amman, T. K. Sealy, S. A. Reeder, J. A. Comer, A. Kemp, R. Swanepoel, C. D. Paddock, S. Balinandi, M. L. Khristova, P. B. H. Formenty, C. G. Albarino, D. M. Miller, Z. D. Reed, J. T. Kayiwa, J. N. Mills, D. L. Cannon, P. W. Greer, E. Byaruhanga, E. C. Farnon, P. Atimnedi, S. Okware, E. Katongole-Mbidde, R. Downing, J. W. Tappero, S. R. Zaki, T. G. Ksiazek, S. T. Nichol, and P. E. Rollin.** 2009. Isolation of genetically diverse Marburg viruses from Egyptian fruit bats. *PLoS Pathog.* **5**(7):e1000536.

94. **Trappier, S. G., A. L. Conaty, B. B. Farrar, D. D. Auperin, J. B. McCormick, and S. P. Fisher-Hoch.** 1993. Evaluation of the polymerase chain reaction for diagnosis of Lassa virus infection. *Am. J. Trop. Med. Hyg.* **49**:214–221.

95. **Van der Groen, G., and L. H. Elliott.** 1982. Use of betapropiolactone-inactivated Ebola, Marburg, and Lassa intracellular antigens in immunofluorescent antibody assay. *Ann. Soc. Belg. Med. Trop.* **62**:49–54.

96. **Vieth, S., C. Drosten, O. Lenz, M. Vincent, S. Omilabu, M. Hass, B. Becker-Ziaja, J. ter Meulen, S. T. Nichol, H. Schmitz, and S. Gunther.** 2007. RT-PCR assay for detection of Lassa virus and related Old World arenaviruses targeting the L gene. *Trans. R. Soc. Trop. Med. Hyg.* **101**: 1253–1264.

97. **Weidmann, M., E. Muhlberger, and F. T. Hufert.** 2004. Rapid detection protocol for filoviruses. *J. Clin. Virol.* **30**:94–99.

98. **World Health Organization.** 1999. Viral haemorrhagic fever/Marburg. Democratic Republic of the Congo. *Wkly. Epidemiol. Rec.* **50**(5):73–77.

99. **World Health Organization.** 2005. Ebola haemorrhagic fever, Angola, Congo. 2005. *Wkly Epidemiol. Rec.* **80**:178. (Erratum, Marburg instead of Ebola.)

100. **World Health Organization.** 24 August 2005. Marburg haemorrhagic fever in Angola—update 25. World Health Organization, Geneva, Switzerland. http://www.who.int/csr/don/2005_08_24/en/index.html.

101. **Wright, R., D. Johnson, M. Neumann, T. G. Ksiazek, P. Rollin, R. V. Keech, D. J. Bonthius, P. Hitchon, C. F. Grose, W. E. Bell, and J. F. Bale.** 1997. Congenital lymphocytic choriomeningitis virus syndrome: a disease that mimics congenital toxoplasmosis or cytomegalovirus infection. *Pediatrics* **100:**E91–E96.

102. **Wulff, H., and K. M. Johnson.** 1979. Immunoglobulin M and G responses measured by immunofluorescence in patients with Lassa or Marburg virus infections. *Bull. W. H. O.* **57:**631–635.

103. **Wulff, H., J. V. Lange, and P. A. Webb.** 1978. Interrelationships among arenaviruses measured by indirect immunofluorescence. *Intervirology* **9:**344–350.

104. **Zaki, S. R., W.-J. Shieh, P. W. Greer, C. J. Goldsmith, T. Ferebee, J. Katshitshi, K. Tchioko, M. A. Bwaki, R. Swanepoel, P. Calain, A. S. Khan, E. Lloyd, P. E. Rollin, T. G. Ksiazek, C. J. Peters, and the EHF Study Group.** 1999. A novel immunohistochemical assay for detection of Ebola virus in skin: implications for diagnosis, spread, and surveillance of Ebola hemorrhagic fever. *J. Infect. Dis.* **177**(Suppl. 1)**:**S36–S47.

Herpes Simplex Viruses and Herpes B Virus

KEITH R. JEROME AND RHODA ASHLEY MORROW

96

HERPES SIMPLEX VIRUSES

Taxonomy

Herpes simplex virus types 1 and 2 (HSV-1 and HSV-2), formally designated human herpesvirus 1 and human herpesvirus 2, respectively, are members of the family *Herpesviridae*. Along with varicella-zoster virus (human herpesvirus 3) and a number of viruses primarily affecting nonhuman hosts, they comprise the subfamily *Alphaherpesvirinae*.

Description of the Agents

Historical Aspects

The herpesviruses are thought to have coevolved with their hosts (61, 62), and thus the earliest documentation of presumptive HSV infection appeared shortly after the development of writing and clinical observation. The infectious nature of HSV was demonstrated in 1919 (101). The concepts of seropositivity and recurrence developed in the 1930s (17, 23). In the 1960s, antigenically distinct strains (HSV-1 and HSV-2) were identified. HSV-1 and HSV-2 are two of eight known human herpesviruses (135). In addition, herpes B virus (also called herpesvirus simiae), a cercopithecine herpesvirus, is an important zoonotic pathogen in humans.

Genetic Structure

The linear, double-stranded genome is 152 kbp for HSV-1 and 155 kbp for HSV-2. HSV-1 and HSV-2 share 83% nucleotide identity within their protein coding regions. The genome is organized into unique long (UL) and unique short (US) regions, each of which is flanked by inverted-repeat regions. Although significant stretches of sequence are conserved between unrelated clinical isolates, identification of isolates can be achieved by restriction endonuclease digestion (136), PCR (103), or sequencing (106, 119).

Virion Structure

The HSV virion is 120 to 300 nm in diameter, with a central electron-dense core containing the DNA, an icosahedral capsid consisting of 162 capsomeres surrounding the core, and a tegument layer surrounded by a spiked envelope containing viral glycoproteins that aid in attachment, penetration, and immune evasion (135). The envelope is a trilaminar, lipid-rich layer derived largely from the nuclear membrane of the infected cell. Because the viral envelope is lipid rich, the virus is readily inactivated. Lipid solvents such as 70% ethanol or isopropanol (but not alcohol at >95%), Lysol, bleach, exposure to pHs of <5 or >11, and temperatures of >56°C for 30 min will all eliminate infectivity (40, 159).

Life Cycle

Viral replication begins with attachment to the target cell via cell-type-dependent host receptors (66, 150). After attachment, the viral envelope and cell membrane fuse, releasing the capsid into the cell. The capsid is translocated to the nuclear pores (12, 158), and DNA is released into the nucleus. The tegument protein VP16 induces expression of the immediate-early, or alpha, proteins, which in turn transactivate the expression of the early, or beta, genes. The early genes are maximally expressed 5 to 7 h after infection and are involved in the synthesis of progeny viral DNA. DNA replication is required for optimal synthesis of the late, or gamma, genes, which are mainly structural proteins. Progeny DNA is processed and assembled into preformed capsids within the cell nucleus. The DNA-containing capsids attach to patches of the nuclear membrane that contain viral tegument proteins and viral glycoproteins. In neurons, nucleocapsids are transported anterograde to the axon terminus, where the final assembly of enveloped virus occurs (48). The replication cycle is complete within about 20 h in epithelial cells.

Immunobiology

Innate immune mechanisms such as activation of macrophages and NK cells and interferon production play a predominant role in the control of primary infection, while both innate and adaptive immune responses are important in the control of recurrences. Although both cellular and humoral forms of immunity are thought to be important, persons with defective cellular immunity often show severe HSV infections, while those with agammaglobulinemia do not (6). CD4$^+$ T cells infiltrate mucocutaneous lesions early in lesion development (41), followed by cytotoxic T lymphocytes (87). HSV-specific T cells can be detected early in lesion development, and they persist at the lesion site after healing (182). T cells also play an important role in controlling viral reactivation from the dorsal root ganglia, via noncytotoxic mechanisms that do not result in neuronal death (86).

Functional antibody responses include complement-independent and complement-dependent virus neutralization (49). Immunoglobulin G (IgG), IgM, and IgA responses to individual viral proteins arise within the first weeks after infection (6). IgM wanes after 2 to 3 months, appearing sporadically thereafter and in about one-third of patients after recurrent genital herpes episodes. Antibody titer may or may not rise after recurrences (132). However, IgG titers are maintained for years after primary infection.

Most epitopes are shared between HSV-1 and HSV-2. As a result, it is difficult to distinguish antibodies to HSV-1 from those to HSV-2 (5). In particular, in HSV-1-seropositive patients, seroconversion to HSV-2 is accompanied by brisk anamnestic responses to HSV-1, resulting in the predominant antibody response being directed toward HSV-1 rather than to HSV-2 for prolonged periods (5). While type-specific epitopes have been demonstrated on the major viral proteins, only glycoprotein G (gG) elicits predominantly type-specific responses.

Epidemiology and Transmission

HSV infections occur worldwide, with no seasonal distribution. The virus is spread by direct contact with virus in secretions. Incubation periods range from 1 to 26 days. The prevalence of HSV-1 infection increases gradually from childhood, reaching 80% or more in later years (117). In contrast, the seroprevalence of HSV-2 remains low until adolescence and the onset of sexual activity. The incidence of antibodies to HSV-2 in the United States reached 21% in the period from 1988 to 1994 (56); however, in recent years, seropositivity rates have apparently declined, to 17% for the period from 1999 to 2004 (179). Rates of seropositivity vary widely, reaching more than 50% in some demographic groups (76, 179). In general, the seroprevalence of HSV-2 is higher in the United States than in other developed countries (104, 149).

Importantly, a large percentage of individuals seropositive for HSV-1 and/or HSV-2 are unaware of the infection (56, 179). Such persons comprise an important reservoir of infection. The risk of genital HSV transmission can be reduced approximately 50% by disclosure of HSV infection status to sexual partners (164), 30 to 50% through the use of condoms (107, 165), and approximately 50% with suppressive antiviral therapy in the source partner (37). It is likely that combining these approaches further reduces risk.

Clinical Significance

Primary Infection

Most HSV-1 infections are acquired early in childhood as subclinical or unrecognized infections (152). Young children may present with classic primary HSV-1 infection, characterized by gingivostomatitis, fever, and marked submandibular lymphadenopathy. Oral lesions progress to ulceration and heal without scarring over 2 to 3 weeks. Adolescents may present with pharyngitis and mononucleosis.

Primary infection with HSV-2 classically presents as herpes genitalis, with extensive, bilateral vesicles, fever, inguinal lymphadenopathy, and dysuria (32). Lesions ulcerate and heal without scarring within 3 weeks. Secondary lesions may develop in the second to third week. Subclinical or unrecognized primary infection with HSV-2 is common.

The proportion of primary genital infections due to HSV-1 is increasing (22), from about 10% in 1983 to 32% in 1995 (32, 166); in fact, HSV-1 may now represent the cause of the majority of first-episode anogenital infections in certain populations (134, 137). This trend is thought to result from changing sexual practices, including increased oral-genital exposure (134). The clinical presentation of primary genital HSV-1 infection cannot be distinguished from that of HSV-2 infection. However, recurrent disease (see below) is less common with genital HSV-1 than HSV-2 infection (32, 53), and thus determining the infecting virus type is useful for prognostic purposes.

Latency and Recurrent Disease

Primary infection with HSV-1 or HSV-2 is followed by the establishment of latency in the dorsal root ganglia, typically the trigeminal ganglia for orolabial disease and the lumbosacral ganglia for genital disease. Periodically, the virus reactivates and travels via the nerve axon to oral or genital sites, resulting in release of infectious virus and, in some cases, lesion formation. Recurrent disease has milder symptoms and a shorter time to lesion healing than do primary episodes (32, 152). The frequencies of HSV-2 genital recurrences vary widely among individuals, ranging from none to 12 or more per year (13), with a mean rate of 0.33 recurrence/month. Orolabial HSV-1 recurrence rates are lower, with a mean of 0.12 episode/month, while genital HSV-1 infection occurs even less frequently (mean of 0.02 episode/month) (94). While HSV-2 may be isolated from the pharynx during primary genital herpes episodes, orolabial HSV-2 recurrences are extremely infrequent (94).

Asymptomatic or Subclinical Infection

Approximately 70 to 90% of individuals with HSV-2 antibodies have not been diagnosed with genital herpes (56, 179). Over one-half of such persons recognize and present with symptoms after education regarding manifestations of HSV disease (58, 98). In addition, about 20% of patients presenting with first episodes of genital herpes have serologic evidence of having been infected for some time (47). These episodes most closely resemble recurrent disease, with mild symptoms. The risks of recurrence are similar between patients presenting with true primary and first recognized recurrent episodes (132). Most patients with genital herpes have episodes of subclinical virus excretion from anogenital sites; these constitute an important source of transmission. The copy number of HSV DNA can sometimes be as high during subclinical episodes as when symptoms occur (163). In general, oral shedding of HSV-1 occurs somewhat less frequently than genital shedding of HSV-2 (100). Oral shedding of HSV-2 or genital shedding of HSV-1 is comparatively rare, particularly outside the setting of newly acquired disease (94, 100, 162).

Neonatal Herpes

The most serious consequence of genital HSV infection is neonatal herpes (36). Infection usually occurs during vaginal delivery, when the infant is exposed to HSV in maternal secretions. The risk of mother-to-infant transmission is 10-fold higher in mothers experiencing unrecognized primary infection during the time of labor than in those shedding HSV as a result of recurrent, subclinical reactivation. This conclusion was drawn in part from the finding that the neonatal infection rate is 54 per 100,000 among HSV-seronegative mothers, 26 per 100,000 among mothers with only HSV-1 antibody, and 22 per 100,000 among all mothers with HSV-2 antibody (21, 129). Transmission of HSV-1 occurs at a significantly higher rate than that of HSV-2 (21, 90). The high rate of transmission during primary disease means that 50 to 80% of all cases of neonatal herpes occur in children of women who acquire genital

HSV infection near term (20, 155). Pregnant women who present with HSV infection should undergo both a type-specific serologic assay and viral typing to identify those infants at highest risk for infection (2).

Infected neonates can present with HSV disease localized to the skin, eyes, and mucosa or with more-serious central nervous system (CNS) or disseminated disease but often have a nonspecific presentation (36, 88). The mortality rate for untreated neonates with disseminated disease exceeds 70%. Early diagnosis and antiviral therapy while disease is localized to the skin can substantially reduce the morbidity and mortality associated with neonatal infections (173, 175). PCR should be used to test samples from skin lesions, cerebrospinal fluid (CSF), plasma, and peripheral blood mononuclear cells (36, 46).

Herpes CNS Disease in the Immunocompetent Host

HSV is the most common cause of fatal sporadic encephalitis in the United States (121). HSV encephalitis presents as fever, behavioral changes, and altered consciousness, resulting from localized temporal lobe involvement. Without treatment, mortality exceeds 70%, and few survivors recover normal neurologic function. Early treatment with acyclovir reduces morbidity and mortality; however, residual neurologic impairment is common (63). HSV PCR of CSF is the test of choice, being far more sensitive than culture (27, 51).

Genital HSV may be followed by sporadic meningitis or recurrent meningitis (Mollaret's syndrome), characterized by headache, fever, photophobia, and lymphocytic pleocytosis (144, 180). The condition is self-limiting and typically resolves within 1 week (180). HSV also can be associated with myelitis, radiculitis, ascending paralysis, autonomic nerve dysfunction, and possibly Bell's palsy.

Ocular Herpes Infections

HSV is the most common viral cause of corneal infection in the United States, affecting 400,000 to 500,000 people (43, 126). Most corneal HSV infections are limited to the epithelial layer, causing characteristic branching ulcerations, pain, photophobia, and blurred vision. HSV epithelial keratitis responds well to oral or topical therapy (see below). Such superficial infections heal without loss of vision. HSV infection may extend to the corneal stroma, leading to scarring and opacification of the cornea. Stromal HSV infections respond favorably to a combination of corticosteroids and topical or oral antivirals (79, 85).

Herpes in the Immunocompromised Host

Immunosuppressed individuals with defective cell-mediated immunity frequently develop symptomatic HSV disease. HSV infections in such individuals can be severe, with extensive mucocutaneous necrosis and involvement of contiguous tissues leading to esophagitis or proctitis. Disseminated HSV, which can lead to meningoencephalitis, pneumonitis, hepatitis, and coagulopathy, may be more common in immunocompromised and hospitalized patients than is generally recognized (14). Disseminated infections require intravenous antiviral therapy and monitoring for development of antiviral resistance.

Antiviral Therapy

Several antiviral drugs, including acyclovir, valacyclovir, penciclovir, and famciclovir, are now widely used to treat mucocutaneous and genital herpes (24a, 156) and for long-term suppression of recurrent episodes. These drugs are selectively activated by the viral thymidine kinase and have minimal side effects. Suppressive therapy reduces the risk of viral transmission between HSV-discordant partners (37). N-Docosanol, a nonprescription topical medication, and topical acyclovir are used for the treatment of herpes labialis. HSV conjunctivitis, blepharitis, and dendritic keratitis are treated either topically with trifluridine, idoxuridine, or vidarabine or orally with acyclovir, valacyclovir, or famciclovir (79). In cases with stromal involvement, the addition of topical corticosteroids reduces the persistence of inflammation (79). Neonatal herpes, herpes encephalitis, and severe infections in immunocompromised patients require prompt intravenous antiviral therapy (45). The alternative agents foscarnet, cidofovir, and vidarabine are generally reserved for acyclovir-resistant herpesvirus infections (80, 156).

Collection, Transport, and Storage of Specimens

Specimens from lesions or mucocutaneous sites should be placed in a viral transport medium (VTM) and kept at a controlled temperature to retain optimal infectivity for culture. VTMs are made of balanced salt solutions, such as Hanks balanced salt solution, Stuart's medium, Leibovitz-Emory medium, veal infusion broth, or tryptose phosphate broth buffered to maintain a neutral pH. Protein stabilizing agents, such as gelatin or bovine serum albumin, are added in addition to antibiotics to prevent bacterial overgrowth (151). Most VTMs are inappropriate for bacterial or chlamydial transport. However, Multi-Microbe M4 medium from Remel (Lenexa, KS) can be used for bacterial, chlamydial, or viral specimens, and Universal Transport Medium (UTM) from Copan is suitable for viruses, *Chlamydia*, *Mycoplasma*, and *Ureaplasma*. It is important that laboratories validate the suitability of the selected media for their particular applications, as performances can vary. For example, in one recent study, M4 or the CVM system from Copan (Corona, CA) supported detection of low-titer HSV better than other media did (52).

Necrotic debris or exudate should be removed from mucosal sites (endocervix, anogenital areas, conjunctiva, and throat) or lesions with a cotton swab prior to sampling. The area must be rubbed vigorously with Dacron, rayon, or cotton swabs on aluminum shafts to ensure that infected cells at the base of the lesion are collected. Calcium alginate swabs and swabs with wooden shafts inhibit infectivity (39, 151). Swabs are then placed into VTM for transport. Several manufacturers offer combined swab/medium packaging, such as the Copan UTM system and the Remel Multi-Microbe M4 system.

Samples should be shipped cold (on ample ice packs) but not frozen. Prolonged (>48 h) storage should be at −70°C. HSV stability is reduced significantly at 22°C compared with that at 4°C; in one study, median half-lives of virus in Copan CVM were 6.8 days (HSV-1) and 4.9 days (HSV-2) at 4°C but only 1.9 (HSV-1) and 3.8 (HSV-2) days at 22°C (52). With other transport media, reported half-lives of HSV-1 have ranged from 0.5 to 4 days at 22°C and from 1 to 180 days at 4°C (74).

A single transport vial may provide specimen for both viral culture and direct antigen detection tests. Alternatively, slides for direct fluorescent-antibody (DFA) detection can be prepared immediately after collection by gently spreading the material on a swab in a thin layer over a clean microscope slide. The slide is air dried and fixed in cold acetone before transport.

Samples for DNA amplification (PCR) require careful collection and handling to ensure an adequate amount of specimen and to avoid contamination of the sample with exogenous viral DNA. For lesions or mucocutaneous sites, a dedicated specimen should be collected with a Dacron swab in VTM or digestion buffer (138). Serum, plasma, and CSF do not require special handling. Blood from neonates is collected in lavender-topped tubes (EDTA) for PCR of peripheral blood mononuclear cells and plasma (46). Heparin can inhibit PCR and therefore is not an acceptable anticoagulant. Specimens for PCR can be maintained at 4°C for up to 72 h, but longer storage should be at −20°C (75, 168).

Fluids such as tracheal aspirates should be collected aseptically and transported without VTM. Urine should be collected by the clean-catch method and refrigerated before transport. Once in the laboratory, urine is diluted 1:1 with culture medium. Corneal samples are obtained with a scalpel blade, and cells are suspended in VTM. Tissue is placed in VTM in a sterile container. Prolonged storage of tissue requires immersion in sterile 50% neutral glycerol in saline or, alternatively, in culture medium with 5% fetal bovine serum. Fresh tissue samples can also be frozen, sectioned, applied to slides, and fixed in acetone.

Direct Detection

Detection of virus in patient samples without an intervening culture amplification step provides the most rapid diagnosis. Immunostaining methods to detect antigen require less expertise than cytopathic effect (CPE)-based culture methods and are usually less expensive than culture. PCR provides the best sensitivity of the direct detection approaches.

Microscopy

Changes that are characteristic of HSV are sometimes visible in fixed, stained cells from lesions (Tzanck preparations) or cervical scrapings (Papanicalou stains) or in hematoxylin and eosin stains of fixed tissue (116). Enlarged or degenerating cells, syncytium formation, chromatin margination, a "ground glass" appearance of the cytoplasm, and nuclear inclusions are typical of HSV-infected cells. These methods are widely available but lack sensitivity and specificity (35). Virus-specific methods are preferred.

Antigen

Slides are prepared with cells from the patient's fixed specimen and coated with antibody preparations against HSV-1 and HSV-2 or against type-common epitopes. If the antibodies are linked to a fluorophore such as fluorescein isothiocyanate, the test is a DFA assay. If bound anti-HSV antibodies are detected with secondary antibodies conjugated to a fluorophore, the test is an indirect fluorescent-antibody (IFA) assay. Same-well testing can be performed by using antibody conjugates with different fluorophores for

HSV-1 and HSV-2 (25). DFA is 10 to 87% as sensitive as culture, with a higher sensitivity for vesicular lesions and poor sensitivity for healing lesions (94). DFA is far less sensitive than PCR (38), and validated commercial kits for DFA are not readily available.

An effective modification of DFA testing employs a cell centrifugation (cytospin) step to apply cells from the sample to slides for subsequent DFA testing. The cytospin step results in better adherence of cells to the slides and fewer inadequate specimens than those obtained with drip application methods (97), while allowing a turnaround time of <2 h. The reported sensitivities of cytospin DFA assays have varied; in one study, the sensitivity was higher than that of culture for detecting HSV from swab specimens (97), while another study, using different DFA and cell culture systems, reported a sensitivity of 31% versus culture (140). The Light Diagnostics Simulfluor assay (Millipore, Billerica, MA) has been reported to have a sensitivity of 80.0% and a specificity of 98.8% compared to culture (25).

Antibodies give their own distinct patterns, depending on the viral antigens recognized (Table 1). Staining patterns require skill to interpret; nonspecific staining can be distinguished from staining of viral antigen by a trained reader. It is important to ensure that antibody reagents are validated for use directly on clinical samples, as some antibodies intended for culture confirmation can give spurious results in other settings.

Enzyme immunoassay (EIA) is rapid and amenable to automation. Sensitivity can be as high as that of culture for diagnosis from lesions (31) or as low as 35% for asymptomatic patients (18, 160). EIA for direct detection of virus has largely been supplanted by other methods.

Nucleic Acid

In situ hybridization or solution hybridization methods are not as widely used as IFA or DFA assay. These tests use DNA or RNA probes, some of which are type specific. The sensitivity of direct hybridization methods is limited (approximately 1×10^5 copies/ml), and thus these approaches have largely been replaced by PCR.

PCR is the most sensitive method for direct detection of HSV (147). Precautions to prevent contamination of the sample and the inclusion of frequent negative controls within the assay are critical (92, 96). Some laboratories include isopsoralens or uracil N-glycosylase in their PCR amplification mixtures, preventing the amplification of PCR products in subsequent reactions.

The likelihood of laboratory contamination by amplicons is reduced by using real-time PCR detection systems that eliminate the need for postamplification manipulation of

TABLE 1 Monoclonal antibodies for HSV-1 and HSV-2 detection, confirmation, and typing by immunofluorescence

Test	Source	Intended Use	Comments
Light Diagnostics SimulFluor HSV 1/2	Millipore, Billerica, MA	Confirmation of CPE in cell culture, antigen detection in cells from patient specimens	HSV-1: whole cell stain (apple green); HSV-2: cytoplasmic or membrane stain (yellow); simultaneous testing for HSV-1 and HSV-2
D³ DFA idenfication and typing kit	Diagnostic Hybrids Inc., Athens, OH	Confirmation of CPE and typing in cell culture	HSV-1, strong focal nuclear staining; HSV-2: strong nuclear and perinuclear staining
MicroTrak HSV 1 & 2 culture identification/ typing test	Trinity Biotech, Jamestown, NY	Confirmation of CPE and typing in cell culture, antigen detection prior to CPE by shell vial culture	HSV-1: nuclear staining; HSV-2: strong nuclear stain, with speckled cytoplasmic staining

the PCR product. There is currently only one FDA-approved PCR assay for HSV-1 and/or HSV-2, the MultiCode-RTx HSV 1&2 Kit from EraGen BioSciences, Madison, WI (146a). Note that this assay is approved only for vaginal lesion swabs, not for other specimen types. Laboratories performing PCR testing should participate in a regular proficiency testing program, such as those provided by the College of American Pathologists (www.cap.org) and Quality Control for Molecular Diagnostics (www.qcmd.org).

Depending on the primers and detection methods, PCR can be set up to detect both HSV-1 and HSV-2 (91, 138) or to allow distinction of HSV-1 from HSV-2 (84, 138). PCR primers have been described to amplify portions of HSV genes encoding thymidine kinase (U_L23), DNA polymerase (U_L30), DNA binding protein (U_L42), glycoproteins B, C, D, and G (U_L27, U_L44, U_S6, and U_S4, respectively), and many others (157). The choice of target gene is probably not a critical factor for HSV PCR, and efficient and sensitive assays have been developed using a variety of target genes. Instead, laboratories should ensure that the primers and probes in any contemplated assay follow the principles of efficient PCR assay design (89). Distinction of HSV-1 and HSV-2 can be achieved by using type-specific primers and/or probes, melting curve analysis, restriction enzyme analysis, or direct sequencing. At our institution, we detect both HSV-1 and HSV-2 by PCR in a real-time detection system (see below), using the type-common gB forward primer CCG TCA GCA CCT TCA TCG A, reverse primer CGC TGG ACC TCC GTG TAG TC, and probe CCA CGA GAT CAA GGA CAG CGG CC (75). To differentiate HSV-1 from HSV-2, we use a multiplex PCR assay containing the type-common gB forward primer CGC ATC AAG ACC ACC TCC TC and reverse primer GCT CGC ACC ACG CGA, which amplify both viruses with equal efficiencies. Differentiation is achieved by using an HSV-1 probe (TGG CAA CGC GGC CCA AC) labeled at the 5′ end with VIC and at the 3′ end with 6-carboxytetramethylrhodamine (TAMRA) and an HSV-2 probe (CGG CGA TGC GCC CCA G) labeled at the 5′ end with 6-carboxyfluorescein and at the 3′ end with TAMRA (34). Test results are available on the same day as receipt of specimen.

Methods to detect PCR products include intercalating agents such as ethidium bromide, Southern blot hybridization, and liquid hybridization (30, 69, 70, 138). A recent improvement has been the development of HSV assays using real-time detection of PCR products (55, 78, 118, 138, 141). Real-time systems allow constant monitoring of the amount of PCR product by detection of a fluorescent signal generated as the PCR product accumulates. These systems decrease the likelihood of laboratory contamination and allow more accurate quantification than is possible with older quantitative-competitive assays (138). Laboratory contamination is of particular concern for CSF specimens, where reliable detection of low viral loads is of major clinical significance, and can occur when such specimens are processed together with lesion or other specimens with high viral loads. Careful, systematic monitoring of negative controls is essential. Quantitation of virus may be useful in monitoring responses to antiviral therapy, particularly in HSV encephalitis or neonatal herpesvirus infections (1).

As stated above, there are currently no FDA-approved PCR assays for HSV-1 or HSV-2. Note that a CE-marked HSV-1/2 PCR kit is available from Qiagen (Hilden, Germany) to non-U.S. customers, as is a CE-marked nucleic acid sequence-based amplification assay from bioMérieux (Marcy l'Etoile, France). In the United States, analyte specific reagents for HSV-1 and HSV-2 are available from Cepheid (Sunnyvale, CA), Nanogen (San Diego, CA), and Roche (Indianapolis, IN). Other manufacturers offer primer and probe sets on a research-use-only basis, including Abbott (Abbott Park, IL). Using these or other primer-probe sets, a large number of labs offer in-house validated assays with real-time detection and quantitation. Despite the paucity of FDA-approved tests, PCR is the gold standard for detection of HSV in CSF, neonatal, and ocular specimens and is increasingly used for other sample types as well. Substantial differences in performance have been reported in interlaboratory comparisons, particularly in sensitivity for detection of low-level positive specimens (143). Thus, it is important to carefully consider the laboratory's reputation, performance data, and test turnaround times before selecting a provider of DNA amplification testing.

Isolation Procedures

Virus detection methods, including culture and modified culture, are used to diagnose mucocutaneous, genital, and ocular lesions (Table 2). Conventional culture uses cells that are permissive for HSV-1 and HSV-2 as well as other

TABLE 2 Selected diagnostic tests for HSV

Syndrome	Sample	Lab tests	Comment
Oral or genital lesion	Swab in VTM	Culture, shell vial	Viability must be preserved
		FA, cytospin FA	Cell architecture must be maintained
		PCR	Better stability than culture
Recurrent genital symptoms; culture-negative	Serum	Western blot	Limited availability; good confirmatory test
	Serum	gG-specific ELISA	FDA approved
	Capillary blood	gG-based point-of-care tests	FDA approved
	Swab in VTM	PCR	Better sensitivity than culture
Neonatal herpes	CSF, blood in EDTA	PCR	Collect separate CSF for PCR; use blood in EDTA (purple top)
	Eye, mouth, nasal and rectal swabs	Culture, FA, PCR	
Ocular herpes	Swab in VTM	Culture, FA, PCR	Clinical presentation may be sufficient for diagnosis
Conjunctivitis, dendritic corneal ulcers	Corneal scraping	Culture, FA, PCR	
Encephalitis	CSF	PCR	Culture is far less sensitive than PCR and is not recommended
Recurrent lymphocytic meningitis	CSF	PCR	

viruses that may be of diagnostic importance. Inoculated cells are examined frequently for CPE (see below). In our laboratory, 95% of HSV isolates produce CPE by day 5; only 5% require 5 to 14 days. Mink lung cells, rhabdomyosarcoma cells, human diploid fibroblasts such as MRC-5 and WI-38, and human epidermoid carcinoma lines such as Hep-2 and A549 are commercially available. Direct comparisons suggest that test sensitivity can be affected markedly by the type of cells used, particularly with a low-titer HSV inoculum. Mink lung cells are reportedly more sensitive than MRC-5 cells, while Vero cells have had low sensitivity reported even with high-titer isolates (181).

Infected cells develop cytoplasmic granulation and then become large, round, and refractile. Clusters or "foci" of infected cells appear early after inoculation in diploid fibroblast or epidermoid carcinoma lines (Fig. 1). CPE in A549

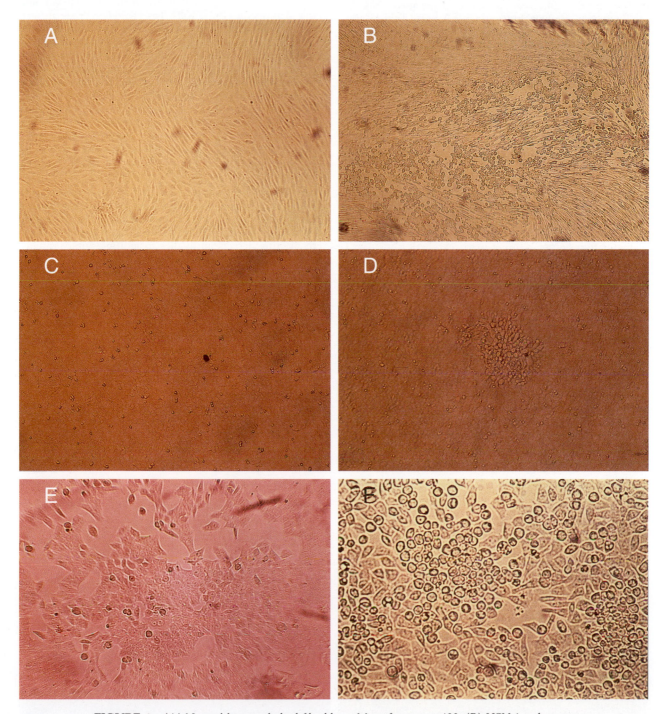

FIGURE 1 (A) Normal human diploid fibroblasts. Magnification, ×400. (B) HSV-1 in human diploid fibroblasts. Magnification, ×400. (C) Normal mink lung cells. Magnification, ×100. (D) HSV-2 in mink lung cells. Magnification, ×100. (E) Normal HEp-2 cells. Magnification, ×400. (F) HSV-2 in HEp-2 cells. Magnification, ×400.

cells is characterized by syncytium formation, particularly with HSV-2 (72). Cells then lyse and detach from the substrate, with eventual destruction of the monolayer.

Identification and Typing

Other viruses as well as toxic factors in specimens can mimic the CPE of HSV (Fig. 2A). Confirmation of putative HSV CPE is accomplished by use of commercially available polyclonal or monoclonal antibodies against type-common or type-specific epitopes. The most widely used reagents are fluorescein conjugated for use in FA tests (Table 1 and Fig. 2B). Trinity Biotech (Bray, Ireland) and Diagnostic Hybrids Inc. (Athens, OH) both supply these reagents. The SimulFluor HSV1/2 test (Millipore, Billerica, MA) can detect and type HSV from a single sample. Peroxidase-conjugated antibodies against HSV-1 and HSV-2 are also used for in situ EIA formats (181).

Spin amplification methods reduce the time required to detect HSV in culture by detecting viral proteins before CPE develops (181). The most widely used technique involves centrifuging the sample onto monolayers of cells on coverslips that are placed in the bottom of small vials (shell vials) or in the wells of flat-bottomed plates. After 16 to 48 h of incubation, the coverslips or plates are subjected to antigen detection tests for HSV (25). Compared to standard culture, reported sensitivities range from 71% to 97% (54, 127, 178). Sensitivity is affected by the time of incubation before staining, with incubation for 48 to 72 h yielding more positive results than incubation for 16 to 24 h. The cell line also affects sensitivity, with mink lung or A549 cells having greater sensitivity than MRC-5 cells (127).

The ReadyCells HSV system (Diagnostic Hybrids Inc., Athens, OH) is a mixture of cryopreserved CV-1 and MRC-5 cells (73) in a shell vial format supporting growth of HSV-1 and HSV-2. Combined with immunodetection, this approach allows rapid definitive diagnosis and differentiation of HSV-1 and HSV-2 from lesions.

The enzyme-linked virus-inducible system (ELVIS) is based on BHK cells with a reporter gene for β-galactosidase that is driven by the promoter from the HSV-1 UL39 gene (153). Other viruses do not transactivate this promoter. Infected cells express the reporter gene, resulting in a color change visualized by light microscopy. The ELVIS HSV

test system (Diagnostic Hybrids) allows HSV-positive cells to be tested further to distinguish HSV-1 from HSV-2. ELVIS-based systems can have comparable sensitivities to those of standard culture (125) and spin-amplified cell culture (99).

Serologic Tests

Because nearly all HSV structural proteins have extensive antigenic cross-reactivity, only IgG tests based on the type-specific HSV gG accurately distinguish HSV-1 and HSV-2 antibodies (5, 7, 108). Tests based on crude antigen mixtures are still marketed, but they have unacceptably low sensitivity and specificity, especially for detecting new HSV-2 infections in those with prior HSV-1 infection (5, 108, 112, 113). Type-specific IgM tests are not available. FDA-approved IgM tests decrease the time to detecting seroconversion in new infections but cannot accurately distinguish new from established infections (111). Tests for HSV-2 antibody avidity can discriminate accurately between first episodes (low avidity) and recurrent episodes (high avidity) in most cases (114). However, these tests are not commercially available.

Western blotting

The HSV Western blot assay used by the University of Washington laboratory uses nitrocellulose blots prepared with human diploid fibroblast-infected cell proteins. Western blotting detects antibodies to multiple viral proteins, including those to the type-specific glycoproteins gG-1 and gG-2 (9). About 20% of sera must be preabsorbed against Sepharose beads coated with HSV-1 or HSV-2 proteins and retested to give definitive results. This combination of tests gives a very accurate determination of HSV-1 versus HSV-2 antibody status (9).

Commercial Type-Specific gG-Based Assays

A number of manufacturers now offer FDA-approved assays using gG as the target antigen. As noted above, gG-based assays are preferred over those based on crude antigen mixtures due to their ability to distinguish antibodies to HSV-1 from those to HSV-2. Microplate EIAs include the Herpe-Select enzyme-linked immunosorbent assay (ELISA) from Focus Diagnostics (Cypress, CA), the Captia HSV 1 and HSV 2 IgG type-specific ELISA test kits (Trinity Biotech,

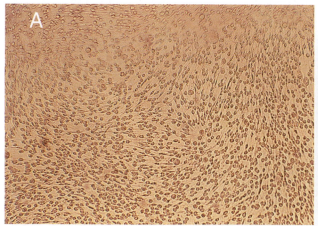
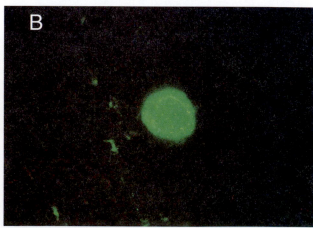

FIGURE 2   (A) Toxicity in human diploid fibroblasts. Magnification, ×100. (B) HSV-2 DFA confirmatory test.

Bray, Ireland), and the Anti-HSV-1 and Anti-HSV-2 ELISA IgG kits from Euroimmun (Lubeck, Germany). Some newer assays utilize microparticle-based detection technology, which provides the possibility of multiplexing and offers potential advantages in assay throughput and reproducibility. The BioPlex 2200 HSV 1 and 2 test (Bio Rad) and the AtheNA Multi-Lyte HSV1&2 test (Zeus Scientific, Raritan, NJ) utilize Luminex detection technology (Luminex, Austin, TX). The Liaison HSV-1 and HSV-2 type-specific IgG tests are bead-based chemiluminescence immunoassays requiring the use of a Liaison analyzer (Diasorin, Saluggia, Italy). Finally, simple gG-based lateral-flow assays are available that are designed for point-of-care testing. These include the HerpeSelect Express IgG test (Focus Diagnostics), which distinguishes antibodies to HSV-1 and HSV-2, and the Biokit HSV-2 Rapid test (Biokit, Barcelona, Spain).

The commercial gG-based tests perform well in clinical use in North America. Compared with the University of Washington Western blot assay, HerpeSelect ELISA for HSV-1 had 91 to 96% sensitivity and 92 to 95% specificity (7). The HerpeSelect immunoblot assay had 99 to 100% sensitivity and 93 to 96% specificity. For HSV-2, HerpeSelect ELISA had 96 to 100% sensitivity and 96 to 97% specificity, while the HerpeSelect immunoblot assay for HSV-2 had 97 to 100% sensitivity and 94 to 98% specificity. The BioPlex assay had a sensitivity and specificity for HSV-1 of 85% and 98%, respectively, and for HSV-2 of 100% and 95%, respectively, compared to Western blotting (111). For point-of-care tests, the POCkit-HSV-2 test (now called the Biokit HSV-2 Rapid test) had 93 to 96% sensitivity and 95 to 98% specificity in comparison tests (7). While performance characteristics against Western blotting are not available, the HerpeSelect Express IgG assay had 100% sensitivity and 97.3% specificity compared to HerpeSelect ELISA (93).

The median time to seroconversion is approximately 3 weeks for HerpeSelect HSV ELISA and about 2 weeks for the Biokit HSV-2 Rapid test, the only FDA-approved tests for which extensive data are available (8, 11).

Antiviral Susceptibilities
Acyclovir-resistant strains of HSV typically result from mutation of the gene encoding the viral thymidine kinase and, more rarely, from mutations in the HSV polymerase. Prolonged use of antivirals can lead to selection of resistant strains, especially in immunocompromised individuals and neonates (172). Strains with detectable in vitro resistance can also be isolated from patients who have never received acyclovir (124). Such isolates are rarely of clinical significance in immunocompetent individuals, and these persons generally respond well to acyclovir (110). However, in infants or immunocompromised individuals, acyclovir-resistant HSV can lead to treatment failure (110), and thus laboratory confirmation of resistance can inform patient management decisions (26). Some patients with suspected acyclovir-resistant virus will respond to an increased dosage of drug. For most patients, second-line therapy requires the use of less-desirable drugs, such as foscarnet or cidofovir. However, since some mutations in the HSV polymerase cause acyclovir resistance but do not affect sensitivity to penciclovir, testing for susceptibility to individual antivirals may be warranted in certain circumstances (172). as it may allow use of a less toxic drug.

Susceptibility testing is best performed by phenotypic assays. A major drawback of genotypic assays is that frameshift or nonsense mutations are possible throughout the thymidine kinase gene, requiring complete sequencing of the gene for definitive results (172). Among phenotypic assays, plaque reduction assay is considered the gold standard (110, 172). Alternative phenotypic assays include antigen reduction assay by EIA and genome reduction assay by DNA hybridization (172). In general, a 50% inhibitory concentration of <2 μg/ml is used as the threshold for susceptibility and correlates relatively well with clinical response (139). However, false determinations of resistance are common in the various phenotypic assays, and interlaboratory variability is significant (172). Thus, clinical correlation of testing results is essential.

Evaluation, Interpretation, and Reporting of Results
Laboratory results are best interpreted in the context of the patient's presentation and history and with the knowledge of the natural history of HSV infection.

Interpretation of Virus Detection Tests
Interpretation of positive test results depends upon the specificity of the test. The specificity of culture is virtually 100% if confirmatory tests are performed. In situ techniques for antigen detection (FA or immunoperoxidase staining of infected cells) have higher specificities than those of other antigen detection methods because the staining pattern allows the technologist to confirm that the signal is specific (Table 1). Given its extreme sensitivity, PCR is most reliable when closed-system methods are used and lab practices are strictly met to avoid contamination of specimens with exogenous HSV DNA. Given these caveats, in practice positive culture or PCR results are highly diagnostic for patients with lesions due to gingivostomatitis, genital herpes, or ocular infections. Positive FA tests for lesions or ocular swabs are considered reliable. HSV found in the CNS, tissues, blood, or eye by culture or PCR is diagnostic. Positive cultures or positive PCR tests for symptomatic infants at 1 to 3 weeks of life are highly diagnostic (81).

For other patients, interpretation of a positive viral detection test requires caution. One potential confounding issue is the simultaneous presence of multiple potential pathogens. For example, respiratory secretions from immunocompromised patients may contain HSV in addition to the presumably causative agent, such as respiratory syncytial virus, influenza virus, parainfluenza virus, or adenovirus (42, 44). HSV may also be shed concurrently with other pathogens from oral or anogenital sites or may not be the cause of the episodic syndrome that triggered testing. Syphilis and chancroid are the most likely alternative causes of genital ulcers in the United States. In a series of patients with genital ulcers other than those typical of herpes (vesiculopustular lesions), 65% had only herpes detected, while 20% had both syphilis and herpes detected (109). HSV results for such patients need to be interpreted in the context of laboratory testing for other pathogens in the differential diagnosis. Symptoms of HSV gingivostomatitis or genital infection can be mimicked by noninfectious causes, such as Stephens-Johnson syndrome, or by infectious agents. Because of the sporadic nature of asymptomatic HSV shedding (105), swabs of oral or anogenital sites may yield positive HSV culture, PCR, or antigen tests when the underlying cause of disease is not herpesvirus.

Positive cultures or PCR results from skin, conjunctival, mouth, or nasal swabs from neonates of <24 h old may reflect maternal virus rather than neonatal infection. Neonates born to mothers shedding HSV from the genital tract at labor and delivery may be tested 24 to 72 h after birth, the likely time frame for receiving maternal culture or PCR results. Most babies developing neonatal herpes present at between 9 and 14 days of life (176), well beyond the time frame where maternal viral contamination would be a problem. However, early initiation of therapy is strongly associated with a favorable outcome (82), and thus current opinion favors aggressive monitoring and treatment (36).

False-negative culture, DFA, or PCR tests may occur because of poor technique in sampling resulting in the failure to obtain infected cells. For culture, false-negative results can occur because of prolonged transport time or exposure of samples to high ambient temperature or because the specimen has low levels of virus; these are less problematic for PCR testing. Recurrent episodes yield lower titers of virus for shorter periods (32). In many cases, a combination of tests or repeat testing is the most sensitive approach. Performing both culture and FA testing can increase sensitivity by 20% or more for genital lesions; repeating testing at a later recurrence nearly doubles the sensitivity (95). PCR is the most sensitive test available and is the test of choice for herpes encephalitis, disseminated neonatal herpes, and, increasingly, diagnosis of anogenital herpes (154, 163). However, in areas without local PCR testing, DFA or IFA methods and culture may yield more timely results. Antiviral therapy should be started empirically if disseminated herpes, neonatal herpes, or encephalitis is suspected.

Interpretation of PCR Results

PCR has adequate sensitivity to detect shedding of HSV in individuals with asymptomatic infection or negative cultures (15, 161, 167) and also to detect HSV in CSF, a specimen with a low yield of HSV by culture. The sensitivity of HSV PCR for HSV encephalitis has been reported to be about 96%, and the specificity is 99% (16). Since the viral load in CSF can be quite low in HSV encephalitis, it is critical that PCR assays be optimized to provide the lowest possible limit of detection. Similarly, PCR has much greater sensitivity than culture for detection of genital HSV-2 both from lesions and during periods of subclinical shedding (163). PCR can detect virus early in lesion development, before culture positivity, and can remain positive for several days after HSV lesions become negative by culture (15, 131). PCR positivity in such cases probably represents infectious virus below the limit of detection by culture, and PCR positivity is quickly lost in the absence of active shedding (161). False-negative results can occur with PCR, due to reaction failure or the presence of inhibitors in clinical specimens (24, 65, 133). It is therefore critical that only negative reactions accompanied by positive internal controls be accepted as true negative results (29). Importantly, a negative PCR result for HSV does not rule out HSV disease, since specimens taken very early or late in the course of disease may not have viral DNA (130). This is especially true in pediatric populations; for example, in one series, nearly 25% of infants with CNS HSV infections had negative CSF PCR results (81). The specificity of PCR for detection of HSV encephalitis has been reported to be >98% (174); thus, all HSV-positive PCR results demand immediate attention. In patients with CNS HSV infections, HSV PCR may become negative after about 7 days of antiviral therapy (16). The persistence or reemergence of virus after antiviral therapy has been associated with a poor clinical outcome (83).

Quantitative PCR may be useful in monitoring the response to antiviral therapy. Successful therapy is associated with a decline in viral load in the CSF (1, 50, 133, 177), and a long duration of viral detectability is associated with poor outcome (142). Quantitation of HSV may also have prognostic value; patients with >100 copies/μl of CSF (100,000 copies/ml) were reported to have worse outcomes than those of patients with lower levels (50). However, other groups have reported no association between CSF viral load and clinical outcome (68, 133, 142, 177).

Interpretation of Type-Specific Serology

Type-specific serology is useful when culture or other virus detection methods are not available or when specimen collection or transport is inadequate. Serology based on gG-1 and gG-2 is vital for diagnosing subclinical and unrecognized HSV infections. In fact, many experts believe that better recognition of genital HSV-2 infections by increased use of accurate gG-based serologic tests could help to slow the spread of genital herpes (19, 33, 64).

As with other herpes laboratory tests, serology tests based on gG must be ordered and interpreted with care. First, due to the low specificity of non-gG-based commercial tests, it is important to ensure that a gG-based test is used. If so, a positive test for HSV-2 antibodies in a patient with genital lesions is highly likely to be a true positive result. A positive HSV-2 antibody test for a patient without a history compatible with genital herpes may be a false-positive result and should be confirmed by testing with a different type-specific test (115). Negative HSV-2 test results for a patient with symptomatic genital disease may indicate genital HSV-1 infection; no test can distinguish between antibodies elicited by oral versus genital HSV-1, and definitive diagnosis rests on direct detection of virus. False-negative tests may also occur during seroconversion; sera drawn 4 to 6 weeks later should be tested. While "index values" in HSV-2 EIAs have been shown to rise during seroconversion, index values alone are not reliable indicators of early versus established infection (10). IgM tests based on gG-1 and gG-2 are not available commercially. The available IgM tests cannot distinguish new from established symptomatic episodes with sufficient accuracy and are not recommended (111).

As noted above, type-specific serology is critical for identifying pregnant women with new HSV infections, who are at high risk for transmitting virus to their neonates (19, 36). Determining HSV-2 serostatus early in pregnancy has been recommended so that treatment options can be considered (19). If a herpesvirus culture from the anogenital region is positive at labor or delivery, a negative maternal type-specific serology indicates a high risk (30 to 50%) for neonatal herpes. A positive maternal serology result by Western blotting or an equivalent test indicates a lower risk of transmission (1 to 3%).

HERPES B VIRUS

Description of the Agent

Herpes B virus, also known as cercopithecine herpesvirus 1 or monkey B virus, is similar to HSV in terms of genome size and structure and in terms of virion morphology. Herpes B virus DNA has 161 ± 12 kbp (102) and is extremely (approximately 75%) G+C rich.

The replication cycle of herpes B virus is very similar to that of HSV. Herpes B virus is detectable as soon as 6 h postinfection, and titers of virus stabilize by 24 to 36 h (67). At least nine herpes B virus glycoproteins have been identified, and at least two of these share antigenic determinants with glycoproteins B and D of HSV (120). As an enveloped virus, herpes B virus can be inactivated by lipid solvents, UV light, or heat, and thus cell-free virus is inactivated rapidly in the environment.

Clinical Significance

Herpes B virus is the simian counterpart of HSV in Old World monkeys of the genus *Macaca*, including the rhesus, cynomolgus, Japanese, Taiwan, and stumptail macaques. The virus can affect the oropharynx or genital area and is spread between animals via biting, sexual activity, or other close contact (169, 171). The seroprevalence of herpes B virus among adult macaques in the wild is nearly 75% (122). Among animals housed in outdoor breeding corrals, the seroprevalence is approximately 22% before 2.5 years of age, rising to >97% among animals 2.5 years or older (170). Primary infection in the macaque is often asymptomatic, but the virus establishes latency and can reactivate. Reactivation can be triggered by stress, such as the transition of animals from freedom to captivity or crowded conditions. Recurrent disease in macaques is typically characterized by vesicular lesions of the tongue and buccal mucosa, progressing to ulceration. Encephalitis is rare but can occur. Asymptomatic shedding of virus can occur.

In 1932, a researcher was bitten by a macaque and developed ascending myelitis and encephalitis culminating in death. Herpes B virus was subsequently described (60). Sporadic cases of herpes B virus infection in humans have subsequently been described in the literature. Humans can be infected via animal bites, mucosal or eye exposure (4), inoculation of broken skin, needle sticks, or potentially aerosols. The possibility of herpes B virus transmission makes macaques unsuitable as pets (123). Safety precautions for workers with close contact with macaques and recommendations for postexposure management have been published (28). Primary cell cultures from macaques also represent a potential source of virus (28).

Herpes B virus disease is severe in humans, with a mortality rate of 70% or higher without treatment. The first symptoms usually appear 3 to 5 days after exposure (although they can appear up to several weeks later) and include a localized vesicular lesion at the site of inoculation, erythema, and edema. Lymphangitis and lymphadenopathy follow, with fever, myalgia, vomiting, and cramping. Neurologic signs develop quickly, starting with meningeal irritation, diplopia, and altered sensation and progressing to paralysis, altered mentation, respiratory depression, seizures, and death within 10 days to 6 weeks. Human-to-human transmission appears to be extremely rare (3). Asymptomatic infection in humans also appears to be rare. In one study of over 300 primate handlers (among whom more than 150 had a history of exposures), none had antibody to herpes B virus (57).

Acyclovir is effective against herpes B virus, although the 50% effective dose is 10-fold higher than that for HSV. Ganciclovir is somewhat more effective than acyclovir (183), although clinical experience with ganciclovir is limited. Foscarnet has also been used in some cases (4). Postexposure therapy can often prevent the development of acute disease (71). The preferred drug for postexposure prophylaxis is oral valacyclovir (28), due to its improved bioavailability (28). Clinical disease necessitates intravenous antiviral therapy. Intravenous therapy should be continued until symptoms resolve and two or more viral cultures are negative after having been held for 10 to 14 days, at which time therapy can be switched to oral antivirals (28). Reactivation and relapse have occurred in some patients upon cessation of antiviral therapy. Many clinicians therefore recommend continuing oral antiviral therapy indefinitely.

Collection, Transport, and Storage of Specimens

Because herpes B virus should be propagated only under biosafety level 4 conditions, diagnostic specimens are best handled by specialized reference laboratories (see below). Precautions should be taken by other laboratories to ensure that herpes B virus specimens are not confused with HSV specimens and thus cultured under lower biosafety conditions, since amplification of virus in culture increases the risk to laboratory personnel. Lesion swabs should be taken from each collection site by use of a separate, sterile Dacron or cotton swab with a wooden or plastic shaft. Swabs or biopsy tissue should be placed into separate tubes containing 1 to 2 ml of VTM. Specimens can be stored in the refrigerator for up to 1 week or at < −60°C indefinitely.

Reference Laboratory for Herpes B Virus

Advice regarding proper specimen collection and submission of specimens for herpes B diagnosis can be obtained from the National B Virus Resource Laboratory, Atlanta, GA [phone, (404) 413-6550; website, http://www.gsu.edu/bvirus].

Identification of Virus and Serodiagnosis

Herpes B virus can be cultured in monkey kidney and chick embryo cells. A characteristic CPE similar to that of HSV is seen, with polykaryon formation and intranuclear Cowdry type A inclusion bodies. Confirmation of herpes B virus in culture can be done using monoclonal antibodies or molecular techniques. PCR for herpes B virus (145, 146, 148) is generally preferred over culture for diagnostic purposes, since it is comparatively rapid, is highly sensitive and specific, and avoids the need to amplify infectious virus to high titers.

Serodiagnosis of herpes B virus infections has been complicated by extensive cross-reactivity with HSV-1 and HSV-2. However, careful ELISA tests have been developed that allow discrimination of antibodies to herpes B virus, HSV-1, and HSV-2 (59, 77). Serologic testing can be useful for evaluation of potentially infected animals involved in human exposures and for screening of research animals. Serial determinations of serostatus for potentially exposed individuals are also useful adjuncts for diagnosis (4, 28).

REFERENCES

1. **Ando, Y., H. Kimura, H. Miwata, T. Kudo, M. Shibata, and T. Morishima.** 1993. Quantitative analysis of herpes simplex virus DNA in cerebrospinal fluid of children with herpes simplex encephalitis. *J. Med. Virol.* **41:**170–173.
2. **Anonymous.** June 2007. Clinical management guidelines for obstetrician-gynecologists. Management of herpes in pregnancy. *Obstet. Gynecol.* **109:**1489–1498.
3. **Anonymous.** 1987. B virus infection in humans—Pensacola, Florida. *MMWR Morb. Mortal. Wkly. Rep.* **36:**289–290.
4. **Anonymous.** 1998. Fatal cercopithecine herpesvirus 1 (B virus) infection following mucocutaneous exposure and interim recommendations for worker protection. *MMWR Morb. Mortal. Wkly. Rep.* **47:**1073–1076.
5. **Ashley, R., A. Cent, V. Maggs, A. Nahmias, and L. Corey.** 1991. Inability of enzyme immunoassays to discriminate between infections with herpes simplex virus types 1 and 2. *Ann. Intern. Med.* **115:**520–526.
6. **Ashley, R., and D. M. Koelle.** 1992. Immune responses to genital herpes infection, p. 201–238. *In* T. C. Quinn (ed.), *Advances in Host Defense Mechanisms: Sexually Transmitted Diseases*, vol. 8. Raven Press, New York, NY.

7. **Ashley, R. L.** 2001. Sorting out the new HSV type specific antibody tests. *Sex. Transm. Infect.* **77:**232–237.

8. **Ashley, R. L., M. Eagleton, and N. Pfeiffer.** 1999. Ability of a rapid serology test to detect seroconversion to herpes simplex virus type 2 glycoprotein G soon after infection. *J. Clin. Microbiol.* **37:**1632–1633.

9. **Ashley, R. L., J. Militoni, F. Lee, A. Nahmias, and L. Corey.** 1988. Comparison of Western blot (immunoblot) and glycoprotein G-specific immunodot enzyme assay for detecting antibodies to herpes simplex virus types 1 and 2 in human sera. *J. Clin. Microbiol.* **26:**662–667.

10. **Ashley Morrow, R., E. Krantz, D. Friedrich, and A. Wald.** 2006. Clinical correlates of index values in the focus HerpeSelect ELISA for antibodies to herpes simplex virus type 2 (HSV-2). *J. Clin. Virol.* **36:**141–145.

11. **Ashley-Morrow, R., E. Krantz, and A. Wald.** 2003. Time course of seroconversion by HerpeSelect ELISA after acquisition of genital herpes simplex virus type 1 (HSV-1) or HSV-2. *Sex. Transm. Dis.* **30:**310–314.

12. **Batterson, W., D. Furlong, and B. Roizman.** 1983. Molecular genetics of herpes simplex virus. VIII. Further characterization of a *ts* mutant defective in release of viral DNA and in other stages of viral reproductive cycle. *J. Virol.* **45:**397–407.

13. **Benedetti, J., L. Corey, and R. Ashley.** 1994. Recurrence rates in genital herpes after symptomatic first-episode infection. *Ann. Intern. Med.* **121:**847–854.

14. **Berrington, W. R., K. R. Jerome, L. Cook, A. Wald, L. Corey, and C. Casper.** 2009. Clinical correlates of herpes simplex virus viremia among hospitalized adults. *Clin. Infect. Dis.* **49:**1295–1301.

15. **Boggess, K. A., D. H. Watts, A. C. Hobson, R. L. Ashley, Z. A. Brown, and L. Corey.** 1997. Herpes simplex virus type 2 detection by culture and polymerase chain reaction and relationship to genital symptoms and cervical antibody status during the third trimester of pregnancy. *Am. J. Obstet. Gynecol.* **176:**443–451.

16. **Boivin, G.** 2004. Diagnosis of herpesvirus infections of the central nervous system. *Herpes* **11**(Suppl. 2):48A–56A.

17. **Brain, R. T.** 1932. The demonstration of herpetic antibody in human sera by complement fixation, and the correlation between its presence and infection with herpes virus. *Br. J. Exp. Pathol.* **13:**166–167.

18. **Brinker, J. P., and J. E. Herrmann.** 1995. Comparison of three monoclonal antibody-based enzyme immunoassays for detection of herpes simplex virus in clinical specimens. *Eur. J. Clin. Microbiol. Infect. Dis.* **14:**314–317.

19. **Brown, Z. A.** 2000. HSV-2 specific serology should be offered routinely to antenatal patients. *Rev. Med. Virol.* **10:**141–144.

20. **Brown, Z. A., S. Selke, J. Zeh, J. Kopelman, A. Maslow, R. L. Ashley, D. H. Watts, S. Berry, M. Herd, and L. Corey.** 1997. The acquisition of herpes simplex virus during pregnancy. *N. Engl. J. Med.* **337:**509–515.

21. **Brown, Z. A., A. Wald, R. A. Morrow, S. Selke, J. Zeh, and L. Corey.** 2003. Effect of serologic status and cesarean delivery on transmission rates of herpes simplex virus from mother to infant. *JAMA* **289:**203–209.

22. **Brugha, R., K. Keersmaekers, A. Renton, and A. Meheus.** 1997. Genital herpes infection: a review. *Int. J. Epidemiol.* **26:**698–709.

23. **Burnet, F. M., and S. W. Williams.** 1939. Herpes simplex: a new point of view. *Med. J. Aust.* **1:**637–642.

24. **Cassinotti, P., H. Mietz, and G. Siegl.** 1996. Suitability and clinical application of a multiplex nested PCR assay for the diagnosis of herpes simplex virus infections. *J. Med. Virol.* **50:**75–81.

24a. **Centers for Disease Control and Prevention.** 2002. Guidelines for treatment of sexually transmitted diseases. *MMWR Morb. Mortal. Wkly. Rep.* **51:**12–17.

25. **Chan, E. L., K. Brandt, and G. B. Horsman.** 2001. Comparison of Chemicon SimulFluor direct fluorescent antibody staining with cell culture and shell vial direct immunoperoxidase staining for detection of herpes simplex virus and with cytospin direct immunofluorescence staining for detection of varicella-zoster virus. *Clin. Diagn. Lab. Immunol.* **8:**909–912.

26. **Chilukuri, S., and T. Rosen.** 2003. Management of acyclovir-resistant herpes simplex virus. *Dermatol. Clin.* **21:**311–320.

27. **Cinque, P., G. M. Cleator, T. Weber, P. Monteyne, C. J. Sindic, and A. M. van Loon.** 1996. The role of laboratory investigation in the diagnosis and management of patients with suspected herpes simplex encephalitis: a consensus report. The EU concerted action on virus meningitis and encephalitis. *J. Neurol. Neurosurg. Psychiatry* **61:**339–345.

28. **Cohen, J. I., D. S. Davenport, J. A. Stewart, S. Deitchman, J. K. Hilliard, and L. E. Chapman.** 2002. Recommendations for prevention of and therapy for exposure to B virus (cercopithecine herpesvirus 1). *Clin. Infect. Dis.* **35:**1191–1203.

29. **Cone, R. W., A. C. Hobson, and M. L. Huang.** 1992. Coamplified positive control detects inhibition of polymerase chain reactions. *J. Clin. Microbiol.* **30:**3185–3189.

30. **Cone, R. W., A. C. Hobson, J. Palmer, M. Remington, and L. Corey.** 1991. Extended duration of herpes simplex virus DNA in genital lesions detected by the polymerase chain reaction. *J. Infect. Dis.* **164:**757–760.

31. **Cone, R. W., P. D. Swenson, A. C. Hobson, M. Remington, and L. Corey.** 1993. Herpes simplex virus detection from genital lesions: a comparative study using antigen detection (HerpChek) and culture. *J. Clin. Microbiol.* **31:**1774–1776.

32. **Corey, L., H. G. Adams, Z. A. Brown, and K. K. Holmes.** 1983. Genital herpes simplex virus infections: clinical manifestations, course, and complications. *Ann. Intern. Med.* **98:**958–972.

33. **Corey, L., and H. H. Handsfield.** 2000. Genital herpes and public health: addressing a global problem. *JAMA* **283:**791–794.

34. **Corey, L., M. L. Huang, S. Selke, and A. Wald.** 2005. Differentiation of herpes simplex virus types 1 and 2 in clinical samples by a real-time Taqman PCR assay. *J. Med. Virol.* **76:**350–355.

35. **Corey, L., and P. G. Spear.** 1986. Infections with herpes simplex viruses. *N. Engl. J. Med.* **314:**686–691.

36. **Corey, L., and A. Wald.** 2009. Maternal and neonatal herpes simplex virus infections. *N. Engl. J. Med.* **361:**1376–1385.

37. **Corey, L., A. Wald, R. Patel, S. L. Sacks, S. K. Tyring, T. Warren, J. M. Douglas, Jr., J. Paavonen, R. A. Morrow, K. R. Beutner, L. S. Stratchounsky, G. Mertz, O. N. Keene, H. A. Watson, D. Tait, and M. Vargas-Cortes.** 2004. Once-daily valacyclovir to reduce the risk of transmission of genital herpes. *N. Engl. J. Med.* **350:**11–20.

38. **Coyle, P. V., A. Desai, D. Wyatt, C. McCaughey, and H. J. O'Neill.** 1999. A comparison of virus isolation, indirect immunofluorescence and nested multiplex polymerase chain reaction for the diagnosis of primary and recurrent herpes simplex virus type 1 and type 2 infections. *J. Virol. Methods* **83:**75–82.

39. **Crane, L. R., P. A. Gutterman, T. Chapel, and A. M. Lerner.** 1980. Incubation of swab materials with herpes simplex virus. *J. Infect. Dis.* **141:**531.

40. **Croughan, W. S., and A. M. Behbehani.** 1988. Comparative study of inactivation of herpes simplex virus types 1 and 2 by commonly used antiseptic agents. *J. Clin. Microbiol.* **26:**213–215.

41. **Cunningham, A. L., R. R. Turner, A. C. Miller, M. F. Para, and T. C. Merigan.** 1985. Evolution of recurrent herpes simplex lesions. An immunohistologic study. *J. Clin. Investig.* **75:**226–233.

42. **Daubin, C., S. Vincent, A. Vabret, D. du Cheyron, J. J. Parienti, M. Ramakers, F. Freymuth, and P. Charbonneau.** 2005. Nosocomial viral ventilator-associated pneumonia in the intensive care unit: a prospective cohort study. *Intensive Care Med.* **31:**1116–1122.

43. **Dawson, C.** 1995. Management of herpes simplex eye diseases, p. 127–136. *In* P. D. Griffiths (ed.), *Clinical Management of Herpes Viruses.* IOS Press, Washington, DC.

44. **De Vos, N., L. Van Hoovels, A. Vankeerberghen, K. Van Vaerenbergh, A. Boel, I. Demeyer, L. Creemers, and H. De Beenhouwer.** 2009. Monitoring of herpes simplex virus in the lower respiratory tract of critically ill patients using real-time PCR: a prospective study. *Clin. Microbiol. Infect.* **15:**358–363.

45. **Diamond, C., and L. Corey.** 1999. Antiviral drugs and therapy, p. 349–364. *In* R. K. Root, W. Stamm, F. Waldvogel, and L. Corey (ed.), *Clinical Infectious Diseases: a Practical Approach.* University Press, Oxford, United Kingdom.

46. **Diamond, C., K. Mohan, A. Hobson, L. Frenkel, and L. Corey.** 1999. Viremia in neonatal herpes simplex virus infections. *Pediatr. Infect. Dis. J.* **18:**487–489.

47. **Diamond, C., S. Selke, R. Ashley, J. Benedetti, and L. Corey.** 1999. Clinical course of patients with serologic evidence of recurrent genital herpes presenting with signs and symptoms of first episode disease. *Sex. Transm. Dis.* **26:**221–225.

48. **Diefenbach, R. J., M. Miranda-Saksena, M. W. Douglas, and A. L. Cunningham.** 2008. Transport and egress of herpes simplex virus in neurons. *Rev. Med. Virol.* **18:**35–51.

49. **Dix, R. D., L. Pereira, and J. R. Baringer.** 1981. Use of monoclonal antibody directed against herpes simplex virus glycoproteins to protect mice against acute virus-induced neurological disease. *Infect. Immun.* **34:**192–199.

50. **Domingues, R. B., F. D. Lakeman, M. S. Mayo, and R. J. Whitley.** 1998. Application of competitive PCR to cerebrospinal fluid samples from patients with herpes simplex encephalitis. *J. Clin. Microbiol.* **36:**2229–2234.

51. **Domingues, R. B., A. M. Tsanaclis, C. S. Pannuti, M. S. Mayo, and F. D. Lakeman.** 1997. Evaluation of the range of clinical presentations of herpes simplex encephalitis by using polymerase chain reaction assay of cerebrospinal fluid samples. *Clin. Infect. Dis.* **25:**86–91.

52. **Dunn, J. J., E. Billetdeaux, L. Skodack-Jones, and K. C. Carroll.** 2003. Evaluation of three Copan viral transport systems for the recovery of cultivatable, clinical virus isolates. *Diagn. Microbiol. Infect. Dis.* **45:**191–197.

53. **Engelberg, R., D. Carrell, E. Krantz, L. Corey, and A. Wald.** 2003. Natural history of genital herpes simplex virus type 1 infection. *Sex. Transm. Dis.* **30:**174–177.

54. **Espy, M. J., and T. F. Smith.** 1988. Detection of herpes simplex virus in conventional tube cell cultures and in shell vials with a DNA probe kit and monoclonal antibodies. *J. Clin. Microbiol.* **26:**22–24.

55. **Espy, M. J., J. R. Uhl, P. S. Mitchell, J. N. Thorvilson, K. A. Svien, A. D. Wold, and T. F. Smith.** 2000. Diagnosis of herpes simplex virus infections in the clinical laboratory by LightCycler PCR. *J. Clin. Microbiol.* **38:**795–799.

56. **Fleming, D. T., G. M. McQuillan, R. E. Johnson, A. J. Nahmias, S. O. Aral, F. K. Lee, and M. E. St. Louis.** 1997. Herpes simplex virus type 2 in the United States, 1976 to 1994. *N. Engl. J. Med.* **337:**1105–1111.

57. **Freifeld, A. G., J. Hilliard, J. Southers, M. Murray, B. Savarese, J. M. Schmitt, and S. E. Straus.** 1995. A controlled seroprevalence study of primate handlers for evidence of asymptomatic herpes B virus infection. *J. Infect. Dis.* **171:**1031–1034.

58. **Frenkel, L. M., E. M. Garratty, J. P. Shen, N. Wheeler, O. Clark, and Y. J. Bryson.** 1993. Clinical reactivation of herpes simplex virus type 2 infection in seropositive pregnant women with no history of genital herpes. *Ann. Intern. Med.* **118:**414–418.

59. **Fujima, A., Y. Ochiai, A. Saito, Y. Omori, A. Noda, Y. Kazuyama, H. Shoji, K. Tanabayashi, F. Ueda, Y. Yoshikawa, and R. Hondo.** 2008. Discrimination of antibody to herpes B virus from antibody to herpes simplex virus types 1 and 2 in human and macaque sera. *J. Clin. Microbiol.* **46:**56–61.

60. **Gay, F. P., and M. Holden.** 1933. The herpes encephalitis problem. *J. Infect. Dis.* **53:**287–303.

61. **Gentry, G. A., M. Lowe, G. Alford, and R. Nevins.** 1988. Sequence analyses of herpesviral enzymes suggest an ancient origin for human sexual behavior. *Proc. Natl. Acad. Sci. USA* **85:**2658–2661.

62. **Gentry, G. A., S. Rana, M. Hutchinson, and P. Starr.** 1988. Evolution of herpes and pox viruses and their hosts: a problem with the molecular clock. *Intervirology* **29:**277–280.

63. **Gordon, B., O. A. Selnes, J. J. Hart, D. F. Hanley, and R. J. Whitley.** 1990. Long-term cognitive sequelae of acyclovir-treated herpes simplex encephalitis. *Arch. Neurol.* **47:**646–647.

64. **Handsfield, H. H.** 2000. Public health strategies to prevent genital herpes: where do we stand? *Curr. Infect. Dis. Rep.* **2:**25–30.

65. **Hardy, D. A., A. M. Arvin, L. L. Yasukawa, R. N. Bronzan, D. M. Lewinsohn, P. A. Hensleigh, and C. G. Prober.** 1990. Use of polymerase chain reaction for successful identification of asymptomatic genital infection with herpes simplex virus in pregnant women at delivery. *J. Infect. Dis.* **162:**1031–1035.

66. **Heldwein, E. E., and C. Krummenacher.** 2008. Entry of herpesviruses into mammalian cells. *Cell. Mol. Life Sci.* **65:**1653–1668.

67. **Hilliard, J. K., R. Eberle, S. L. Lipper, R. M. Munoz, and S. A. Weiss.** 1987. Herpesvirus simiae (B virus): replication of the virus and identification of viral polypeptides in infected cells. *Arch. Virol.* **93:**185–198.

68. **Hjalmarsson, A., F. Granath, M. Forsgren, M. Brytting, P. Blomqvist, and B. Skoldenberg.** 2009. Prognostic value of intrathecal antibody production and DNA viral load in cerebrospinal fluid of patients with herpes simplex encephalitis. *J. Neurol.* **256:**1243–1251.

69. **Hobson, A., A. Wald, N. Wright, and L. Corey.** 1997. Evaluation of a quantitative competitive PCR assay for measuring herpes simplex virus DNA content in genital tract secretions. *J. Clin. Microbiol.* **35:**548–552.

70. **Hofgartner, W. T., A. F. Huhmer, J. P. Landers, and J. A. Kant.** 1999. Rapid diagnosis of herpes simplex encephalitis using microchip electrophoresis of PCR products. *Clin. Chem.* **45:**2120–2128.

71. **Holmes, G. P., L. E. Chapman, J. A. Stewart, S. E. Straus, J. K. Hilliard, and D. S. Davenport.** 1995. Guidelines for the prevention and treatment of B-virus infections in exposed persons. *Clin. Infect. Dis.* **20:**421–439.

72. **Hsiung, G. D.** 1994. Diagnostic virology, p. 241–248. *In* G. D. Hsiung, C. K. Y. Fong, and M. L. Landry (ed.), *Hsiung's Diagnostic Virology.* Yale University Press, London, United Kingdom.

73. **Huang, Y. T., S. Hite, V. Duane, and H. Yan.** 2002. CV-1 and MRC-5 mixed cells for simultaneous detection of herpes simplex viruses and varicella zoster virus in skin lesions. *J. Clin. Virol.* **24:**37–43.

74. **Jensen, C., and F. B. Johnson.** 1994. Comparison of various transport media for viability maintenance of herpes simplex virus, respiratory syncytial virus, and adenovirus. *Diagn. Microbiol. Infect. Dis.* **19:**137–142.

75. **Jerome, K. R., M. L. Huang, A. Wald, S. Selke, and L. Corey.** 2002. Quantitative stability of DNA after extended storage of clinical specimens as determined by real-time PCR. *J. Clin. Microbiol.* **40:**2609–2611.

76. **Johnson, R. E., A. J. Nahmias, L. S. Magder, F. K. Lee, C. A. Brooks, and C. B. Snowden.** 1989. A seroepidemiologic survey of the prevalence of herpes simplex virus type 2 infection in the United States. *N. Engl. J. Med.* **321:**7–12.

77. **Katz, D., J. K. Hilliard, R. Eberle, and S. L. Lipper.** 1986. ELISA for the detection of group-specific and virus-specific antibodies in human and simian sera induced by herpes simplex and related simian viruses. *J. Virol. Methods* **14:**99–109.

78. **Kessler, H. H., G. Muhlbauer, B. Rinner, E. Stelzl, A. Berger, H. W. Dorr, B. Santner, E. Marth, and H. Rabenau.** 2000. Detection of herpes simplex virus DNA by real-time PCR. *J. Clin. Microbiol.* **38:**2638–2642.

79. **Khan, B. F., and D. Pavan-Langston.** 2004. Clinical manifestations and treatment modalities in herpes simplex virus of the ocular anterior segment. *Int. Ophthalmol. Clin.* **44:**103–133.

80. **Kimberlin, D. W., D. M. Coen, K. K. Biron, J. I. Cohen, R. A. Lamb, M. McKinlay, E. A. Emini, and R. J. Whitley.** 1995. Molecular mechanisms of antiviral resistance. *Antivir. Res.* **26:**369–401.

81. **Kimberlin, D. W., F. D. Lakeman, A. M. Arvin, C. G. Prober, L. Corey, D. A. Powell, S. K. Burchett, R. F. Jacobs, S. E. Starr, R. J. Whitley, et al.** 1996. Application of the polymerase chain reaction to the diagnosis and management of neonatal herpes simplex virus disease. *J. Infect. Dis.* **174:**1162–1167.

82. Kimberlin, D. W., C. Y. Lin, R. F. Jacobs, D. A. Powell, L. Corey, W. C. Gruber, M. Rathore, J. S. Bradley, P. S. Diaz, M. Kumar, A. M. Arvin, K. Gutierrez, M. Shelton, L. B. Weiner, J. W. Sleasman, T. M. de Sierra, S. Weller, S. J. Soong, J. Kiell, F. D. Lakeman, and R. J. Whitley. 2001. Safety and efficacy of high-dose intravenous acyclovir in the management of neonatal herpes simplex virus infections. *Pediatrics* **108:**230–238.

83. Kimura, H., K. Aso, K. Kuzushima, N. Hanada, M. Shibata, and T. Morishima. 1992. Relapse of herpes simplex encephalitis in children. *Pediatrics* **89:**891–894.

84. Kimura, H., M. Shibata, K. Kuzushima, K. Nishikawa, Y. Nishiyama, and T. Morishima. 1990. Detection and direct typing of herpes simplex virus by polymerase chain reaction. *Med. Microbiol. Immunol.* **179:**177–184.

85. Knickelbein, J. E., R. L. Hendricks, and P. Charukamnoetkanok. 2009. Management of herpes simplex virus stromal keratitis: an evidence-based review. *Surv. Ophthalmol.* **54:**226–234.

86. Knickelbein, J. E., K. M. Khanna, M. B. Yee, C. J. Baty, P. R. Kinchington, and R. L. Hendricks. 2008. Noncytotoxic lytic granule-mediated CD8+ T cell inhibition of HSV-1 reactivation from neuronal latency. *Science* **322:**268–271.

87. Koelle, D. M., C. M. Posavad, G. R. Barnum, M. L. Johnson, J. M. Frank, and L. Corey. 1998. Clearance of HSV-2 from recurrent genital lesions correlates with infiltration of HSV-specific cytotoxic T lymphocytes. *J. Clin. Investig.* **101:**1500–1508.

88. Kohl, S. 2002. The diagnosis and treatment of neonatal herpes simplex virus infection. *Pediatr. Ann.* **31:**726–732.

89. Kramer, M. F., and D. M. Coen. 2001. Enzymatic amplification of DNA by PCR: standard procedures and optimization. *Curr. Protoc. Immunol.* **Chapter 10:**Unit 10.20.

90. Kropp, R. Y., T. Wong, L. Cormier, A. Ringrose, S. Burton, J. E. Embree, and M. Steben. 2006. Neonatal herpes simplex virus infections in Canada: results of a 3-year national prospective study. *Pediatrics* **117:**1955–1962.

91. Kudelova, M., M. Muranyiova, O. Kudela, J. Rajcani, M. Lehtinen, J. Stankovic, M. Arvaja, and O. Balint. 1995. Detection of herpes simplex virus DNA by polymerase chain reaction in the cerebrospinal fluid of patients with viral meningoencephalitis using primers for the glycoprotein D gene. *Acta Virol.* **39:**11–17.

92. Kwok, S., and R. Higuchi. 1989. Avoiding false positives with PCR. *Nature* **339:**237–238.

93. Laderman, E. I., E. Whitworth, E. Dumaual, M. Jones, A. Hudak, W. Hogrefe, J. Carney, and J. Groen. 2008. Rapid, sensitive, and specific lateral-flow immunochromatographic point-of-care device for detection of herpes simplex virus type 2-specific immunoglobulin G antibodies in serum and whole blood. *Clin. Vaccine Immunol.* **15:**159–163.

94. Lafferty, W. E., R. W. Coombs, J. Benedetti, C. Critchlow, and L. Corey. 1987. Recurrences after oral and genital herpes simplex virus infection: influence of anatomic site and viral type. *N. Engl. J. Med.* **316:**1444–1449.

95. Lafferty, W. E., S. Krofft, M. Remington, R. Giddings, C. Winter, A. Cent, and L. Corey. 1987. Diagnosis of herpes simplex virus by direct immunofluorescence and viral isolation from samples of external genital lesions in a high-prevalence population. *J. Clin. Microbiol.* **25:**323–326.

96. Landry, M. L. 1995. False-positive polymerase chain reaction results in the diagnosis of herpes simplex encephalitis. *J. Infect. Dis.* **172:**1641–1643.

97. Landry, M. L., D. Ferguson, and J. Wlochowski. 1997. Detection of herpes simplex virus in clinical specimens by cytospin-enhanced direct immunofluorescence. *J. Clin. Microbiol.* **35:**302–304.

98. Langenberg, A., J. Benedetti, J. Jenkins, R. Ashley, C. Winter, and L. Corey. 1989. Development of clinically recognizable genital lesions among women previously identified as having "asymptomatic" herpes simplex virus type 2 infection. *Ann. Intern. Med.* **110:**882–887.

99. LaRocco, M. T. 2000. Evaluation of an enzyme-linked viral inducible system for the rapid detection of herpes simplex virus. *Eur. J. Clin. Microbiol. Infect. Dis.* **19:**233–235.

100. Leone, P., T. Warren, K. Hamed, K. Fife, and A. Wald. 2007. Famciclovir reduces viral mucosal shedding in HSV-seropositive persons. *Sex. Transm. Dis.* **34:**900–907.

101. Lowenstein, A. 1919. Aetiologische untersuchungen über den fieberhaften, Herpes. *Meunch. Med. Wochenschr.* **66:**769–770.

102. Ludwig, H. 1972. Untersuchen am genetischn Material von Herpesvirus I. Biophysikalisch-chemische. Charakterisierung von Herpesvirus-Desoxyribonukleinsauren. *Med. Microbiol. Immunol.* **157:**186–211.

103. Maertzdorf, J., L. Remeijer, A. Van Der Lelij, J. Buitenwerf, H. G. Niesters, A. D. Osterhaus, and G. M. Verjans. 1999. Amplification of reiterated sequences of herpes simplex virus type 1 (HSV-1) genome to discriminate between clinical HSV-1 isolates. *J. Clin. Microbiol.* **37:**3518–3523.

104. Malkin, J. E. 2004. Epidemiology of genital herpes simplex virus infection in developed countries. *Herpes* **11**(Suppl. 1):2A–23A.

105. Mark, K. E., A. Wald, A. S. Magaret, S. Selke, L. Olin, M. L. Huang, and L. Corey. 2008. Rapidly cleared episodes of herpes simplex virus reactivation in immunocompetent adults. *J. Infect. Dis.* **198:**1141–1149.

106. Martin, E. T., D. M. Koelle, B. Byrd, M. L. Huang, J. Vieira, L. Corey, and A. Wald. 2006. Sequence-based methods for identifying epidemiologically linked herpes simplex virus type 2 strains. *J. Clin. Microbiol.* **44:**2541–2546.

107. Martin, E. T., E. Krantz, S. L. Gottlieb, A. S. Magaret, A. Langenberg, L. Stanberry, M. Kamb, and A. Wald. 2009. A pooled analysis of the effect of condoms in preventing HSV-2 acquisition. *Arch. Intern. Med.* **169:**1233–1240.

108. Martins, T. B., R. D. Woolstenhulme, T. D. Jaskowski, H. R. Hill, and C. M. Litwin. 2001. Comparison of four enzyme immunoassays with a Western blot assay for the determination of type-specific antibodies to herpes simplex virus. *Am. J. Clin. Pathol.* **115:**272–277.

109. Mertz, K. J., D. Trees, W. C. Levine, J. S. Lewis, B. Litchfield, K. S. Pettus, S. A. Morse, M. E. St. Louis, J. B. Weiss, J. Schwebke, J. Dickes, R. Kee, J. Reynolds, D. Hutcheson, D. Green, I. Dyer, G. A. Richwald, J. Novotny, I. Weisfuse, M. Goldberg, J. A. O'Donnell, R. Knaup, et al. 1998. Etiology of genital ulcers and prevalence of human immunodeficiency virus coinfection in 10 US cities. *J. Infect. Dis.* **178:**1795–1798.

110. Moellering, R. C., Jr., J. R. Graybill, J. E. McGowan, Jr., and L. Corey. 2007. Antimicrobial resistance prevention initiative—an update: proceedings of an expert panel on resistance. *Am. J. Infect. Control* **35:**S1–S23.

111. Morrow, R., and D. Friedrich. 2006. Performance of a novel test for IgM and IgG antibodies in subjects with culture-documented genital herpes simplex virus-1 or -2 infection. *Clin. Microbiol. Infect.* **12:**463–469.

112. Morrow, R. A., and Z. A. Brown. 2005. Common use of inaccurate antibody assays to identify infection status with herpes simplex virus type 2. *Am. J. Obstet. Gynecol.* **193:**361–362.

113. Morrow, R. A., and D. Friedrich. 2003. Inaccuracy of certain commercial enzyme immunoassays in diagnosing genital infections with herpes simplex virus types 1 or 2. *Am. J. Clin. Pathol.* **120:**839–844.

114. Morrow, R. A., D. Friedrich, E. Krantz, and A. Wald. 2004. Development and use of a type-specific antibody avidity test based on herpes simplex virus type 2 glycoprotein G. *Sex. Transm. Dis.* **31:**508–515.

115. Morrow, R. A., D. Friedrich, A. Meier, and L. Corey. 2005. Use of "Biokit HSV-2 Rapid Assay" to improve the positive predictive value of Focus HerpeSelect HSV-2 ELISA. *BMC Infect. Dis.* **5:**84.

116. Nahass, G. T., B. A. Goldstein, W. Y. Zhu, U. Serfling, N. S. Penneys, and C. L. Leonardi. 1992. Comparison of Tzanck smear, viral culture, and DNA diagnostic methods in detection of herpes simplex and varicella-zoster infection. *JAMA* **268:**2541–2544.

117. Nahmias, A. J., F. K. Lee, and S. Beckman-Nahmias. 1990. Sero-epidemiological and -sociological patterns of herpes

simplex virus infection in the world. *Scand. J. Infect. Dis.* **69**(Suppl.):19–36.

118. **Nicoll, S., A. Brass, and H. A. Cubie.** 2001. Detection of herpes viruses in clinical samples using real-time PCR. *J. Virol. Methods* **96**:25–31.

119. **Norberg, P., T. Bergstrom, E. Rekabdar, M. Lindh, and J. A. Liljeqvist.** 2004. Phylogenetic analysis of clinical herpes simplex virus type 1 isolates identified three genetic groups and recombinant viruses. *J. Virol.* **78**:10755–10764.

120. **Norrild, B., H. Ludwig, and R. Rott.** 1978. Identification of a common antigen of herpes simplex virus, bovine herpes mammilitis virus, and B virus. *J. Virol.* **26**:712–717.

121. **Olson, L. C., E. L. Buescher, and M. S. Artenstein.** 1967. Herpesvirus infections of the human central nervous system. *N. Engl. J. Med.* **277**:1271–1276.

122. **Orcutt, R. P., G. J. Pucak, H. L. Foster, J. T. Kilcourse, and T. Ferrell.** 1976. Multiple testing for the detection of B virus antibody in specially handled rhesus monkeys after capture from virgin trapping grounds. *Lab. Anim. Sci.* **26**:70–74.

123. **Ostrowski, S. R., M. J. Leslie, T. Parrott, S. Abelt, and P. E. Piercy.** 1998. B-virus from pet macaque monkeys: an emerging threat in the United States? *Emerg. Infect. Dis.* **4**:117–121.

124. **Parris, D. S., and J. E. Harrington.** 1982. Herpes simplex virus variants resistant to high concentrations of acyclovir exist in clinical isolates. *Antimicrob. Agents Chemother.* **22**:71–77.

125. **Patel, N., L. Kauffmann, G. Baniewicz, M. Forman, M. Evans, and D. Scholl.** 1999. Confirmation of low-titer, herpes simplex virus-positive specimen results by the enzyme-linked virus-inducible system (ELVIS) using PCR and repeat testing. *J. Clin. Microbiol.* **37**:3986–3989.

126. **Pepose, J. D.** 1996. Herpes simplex virus diseases: anterior segment of the eye, p. 905–932. *In* J. D. Pepose, G. N. Holland, and K. R. Wilhelmus (ed.), *Ocular Infection and Immunity*. Mosby, St. Louis, MO.

127. **Peterson, E. M., B. L. Hughes, S. L. Aarnaes, and L. M. de la Maza.** 1988. Comparison of primary rabbit kidney and MRC-5 cells and two stain procedures for herpes simplex virus detection by a shell vial centrifugation method. *J. Clin. Microbiol.* **26**:222–224.

128. Reference deleted.

129. **Prober, C. G., W. M. Sullender, L. L. Yasukawa, D. S. Au, A. S. Yeager, and A. M. Arvin.** 1987. Low risk of herpes simplex virus infections in neonates exposed to the virus at the time of vaginal delivery to mothers with recurrent herpes simplex virus infections. *N. Engl. J. Med.* **316**:240–244.

130. **Puchhammer-Stockl, E., E. Presterl, C. Croy, S. Aberle, T. Popow-Kraupp, M. Kundi, H. Hofmann, U. Wenninger, and I. Godl.** 2001. Screening for possible failure of herpes simplex PCR in cerebrospinal fluid for the diagnosis of herpes simplex encephalitis. *J. Med. Virol.* **64**:531–536.

131. **Ramaswamy, M., C. McDonald, M. Smith, D. Thomas, S. Maxwell, M. Tenant-Flowers, and A. M. Geretti.** 2004. Diagnosis of genital herpes by real time PCR in routine clinical practice. *Sex. Transm. Infect.* **80**:406–410.

132. **Reeves, W. C., L. Corey, H. G. Adams, L. A. Vontver, and K. K. Holmes.** 1981. Risk of recurrence after first episodes of genital herpes. Relation to HSV type and antibody response. *N. Engl. J. Med.* **305**:315–319.

133. **Revello, M. G., F. Baldanti, A. Sarasini, D. Zella, M. Zavattoni, and G. Gerna.** 1997. Quantitation of herpes simplex virus DNA in cerebrospinal fluid of patients with herpes simplex encephalitis by the polymerase chain reaction. *Clin. Diagn. Virol.* **7**:183–191.

134. **Roberts, C.** 2005. Genital herpes in young adults: changing sexual behaviours, epidemiology and management. *Herpes* **12**:10–14.

135. **Roizman, B., and D. M. Knipe.** 2001. Herpes simplex viruses and their replication, p. 2399–2459. *In* D. M. Knipe et al. (ed.), *Fields Virology*, 4th ed., vol. 2. Lippincott Williams and Wilkins, Philadelphia, PA.

136. **Roizman, B., and M. Tognon.** 1983. Restriction endonuclease patterns of herpes simplex virus DNA: application to diagnosis and molecular epidemiology. *Curr. Top. Microbiol. Immunol.* **104**:275–286.

137. **Ryder, N., F. Jin, A. M. McNulty, A. E. Grulich, and B. Donovan.** 2009. Increasing role of herpes simplex virus type 1 in first-episode anogenital herpes in heterosexual women and younger men who have sex with men, 1992–2006. *Sex. Transm. Infect.* **85**:416–419.

138. **Ryncarz, A. J., J. Goddard, A. Wald, M.-L. Huang, B. Roizman, and L. Corey.** 1999. Development of a high-throughput quantitative assay for detecting herpes simplex virus DNA in clinical samples. *J. Clin. Microbiol.* **37**:1941–1947.

139. **Safrin, S., T. Elbeik, L. Phan, D. Robinson, J. Rush, A. Elbaggari, and J. Mills.** 1994. Correlation between response to acyclovir and foscarnet therapy and in vitro susceptibility result for isolates of herpes simplex virus from human immunodeficiency virus-infected patients. *Antimicrob. Agents Chemother.* **38**:1246–1250.

140. **Sanders, C., C. Nelson, M. Hove, and G. L. Woods.** 1998. Cytospin-enhanced direct immunofluorescence assay versus cell culture for detection of herpes simplex virus in clinical specimens. *Diagn. Microbiol. Infect. Dis.* **32**:111–113.

141. **Schalasta, G., A. Arents, M. Schmid, R. W. Braun, and G. Enders.** 2000. Fast and type-specific analysis of herpes simplex virus types 1 and 2 by rapid PCR and fluorescence melting-curve-analysis. *Infection* **28**:85–91.

142. **Schloss, L., K. I. Falk, E. Skoog, M. Brytting, A. Linde, and E. Aurelius.** 2009. Monitoring of herpes simplex virus DNA types 1 and 2 viral load in cerebrospinal fluid by real-time PCR in patients with herpes simplex encephalitis. *J. Med. Virol.* **81**:1432–1437.

143. **Schloss, L., A. M. van Loon, P. Cinque, G. Cleator, J. M. Echevarria, K. I. Falk, P. Klapper, J. Schirm, B. F. Vestergaard, H. Niesters, T. Popow-Kraupp, W. Quint, and A. Linde.** 2003. An international external quality assessment of nucleic acid amplification of herpes simplex virus. *J. Clin. Virol.* **28**:175–185.

144. **Schmutzhard, E.** 2001. Viral infections of the CNS with special emphasis on herpes simplex infections. *J. Neurol.* **248**:469–477.

145. **Scinicariello, F., R. Eberle, and J. K. Hilliard.** 1993. Rapid detection of B virus (herpesvirus simiae) DNA by polymerase chain reaction. *J. Infect. Dis.* **168**:747–750.

146. **Scinicariello, F., W. J. English, and J. Hilliard.** 1993. Identification by PCR of meningitis caused by herpes B virus. *Lancet* **341**:1660–1661.

146a. **Selvaraju, S. B., M. Wurst, R. T. Horvat, and R. Selvarangan.** 2009. Evaluation of three analyte-specific reagents for detection and typing of herpes simplex virus in cerebrospinal fluid. *Diagn. Microbiol. Infect. Dis.* **63**:286–291.

147. **Slomka, M. J.** 2000. Current diagnostic techniques in genital herpes: their role in controlling the epidemic. *Clin. Lab.* **46**:591–607.

148. **Slomka, M. J., D. W. Brown, J. P. Clewley, A. M. Bennett, L. Harrington, and D. C. Kelly.** 1993. Polymerase chain reaction for detection of herpevirus simiae (B virus) in clinical specimens. *Arch. Virol.* **131**:89.

149. **Smith, J. S., and N. J. Robinson.** 2002. Age-specific prevalence of infection with herpes simplex virus types 2 and 1: a global review. *J. Infect. Dis.* **186**(Suppl. 1):S3–S28.

150. **Spear, P. G.** 2004. Herpes simplex virus: receptors and ligands for cell entry. *Cell. Microbiol.* **6**:401–410.

151. **Specter, S., and D. Jeffries.** 1996. Detection of virus and viral antigens, p. 309–322. *In* B. W. Mahy and H. L. Kangro (ed.), *Virology Methods Manual*. Harcourt, New York, NY.

152. **Spruance, S. L.** 1992. The natural history of recurrent oral-facial herpes simplex virus infection. *Semin. Dermatol.* **11**:200–206.

153. **Stabell, E. C., S. R. O'Rourke, G. A. Storch, and P. D. Olivo.** 1993. Evaluation of a genetically engineered cell line and a histochemical beta-galactosidase assay to detect herpes simplex virus in clinical specimens. *J. Clin. Microbiol.* **31**:2796–2798.

154. Strick, L. B., and A. Wald. 2006. Diagnostics for herpes simplex virus: is PCR the new gold standard? *Mol. Diagn. Ther.* **10:**17–28.

155. Sullender, W. M., L. L. Yasukawa, M. Schwartz, L. Pereira, P. A. Hensleigh, C. G. Prober, and A. M. Arvin. 1988. Type-specific antibodies to herpes simplex virus type 2 (HSV-2) glycoprotein G in pregnant women, infants exposed to maternal HSV-2 infection at delivery, and infants with neonatal herpes. *J. Infect. Dis.* **157:**164–171.

156. Superti, F., M. G. Ammendolia, and M. Marchetti. 2008. New advances in anti-HSV chemotherapy. *Curr. Med. Chem.* **15:**900–911.

157. Tang, Y. W., P. S. Mitchell, M. J. Espy, T. F. Smith, and D. H. Persing. 1999. Molecular diagnosis of herpes simplex virus infections in the central nervous system. *J. Clin. Microbiol.* **37:**2127–2136.

158. Tognon, M., D. Furlong, A. J. Conley, and B. Roizman. 1981. Molecular genetics of herpes simplex virus. V. Characterization of a mutant defective in ability to form plaques at low temperatures and in a viral function which prevents accumulation of coreless capsids at nuclear pores late in infection. *J. Virol.* **40:**870–880.

159. Tyler, R., and G. A. Ayliffe. 1987. A surface test for virucidal activity of disinfectants: preliminary study with herpes virus. *J. Hosp. Infect.* **9:**22–29.

160. Verano, L., and F. J. Michalski. 1995. Comparison of a direct antigen enzyme immunoassay, Herpchek, with cell culture for detection of herpes simplex virus from clinical specimens. *J. Clin. Microbiol.* **33:**1378–1379.

161. Wald, A., L. Corey, R. Cone, A. Hobson, G. Davis, and J. Zeh. 1997. Frequent genital herpes simplex virus 2 shedding in immunocompetent women. Effect of acyclovir treatment. *J. Clin. Investig.* **99:**1092–1097.

162. Wald, A., M. Ericsson, E. Krantz, S. Selke, and L. Corey. 2004. Oral shedding of herpes simplex virus type 2. *Sex. Transm. Infect.* **80:**272–276.

163. Wald, A., M. L. Huang, D. Carrell, S. Selke, and L. Corey. 2003. Polymerase chain reaction for detection of herpes simplex virus (HSV) DNA on mucosal surfaces: comparison with HSV isolation in cell culture. *J. Infect. Dis.* **188:**1345–1351.

164. Wald, A., E. Krantz, S. Selke, E. Lairson, R. A. Morrow, and J. Zeh. 2006. Knowledge of partners' genital herpes protects against herpes simplex virus type 2 acquisition. *J. Infect. Dis.* **194:**42–52.

165. Wald, A., A. G. Langenberg, E. Krantz, J. M. Douglas, Jr., H. H. Handsfield, R. P. DiCarlo, A. A. Adimora, A. E. Izu, R. A. Morrow, and L. Corey. 2005. The relationship between condom use and herpes simplex virus acquisition. *Ann. Intern. Med.* **143:**707–713.

166. Wald, A., J. Zeh, S. Selke, R. L. Ashley, and L. Corey. 1995. Virologic characteristics of subclinical and symptomatic genital herpes infections. *N. Engl. J. Med.* **333:**770–775.

167. Wald, A., J. Zeh, S. Selke, T. Warren, A. J. Ryncarz, R. Ashley, J. N. Krieger, and L. Corey. 2000. Reactivation of genital herpes simplex virus type 2 infection in asymptomatic seropositive persons. *N. Engl. J. Med.* **342:**844–850.

168. Waldhuber, M. G., I. Denham, C. Wadey, W. Leong-Shaw, and G. F. Cross. 1999. Detection of herpes simplex virus in genital specimens by type-specific polymerase chain reaction. *Int. J. STD AIDS* **10:**89–92.

169. Weigler, B. J., D. W. Hird, J. K. Hilliard, N. W. Lerche, J. A. Roberts, and L. M. Scott. 1993. Epidemiology of cercopithecine herpesvirus 1 (B virus) infection and shedding in a large breeding cohort of rhesus macaques. *J. Infect. Dis.* **167:**256–263.

170. Weigler, B. J., J. A. Roberts, D. W. Hird, N. W. Lerche, and J. K. Hilliard. 1990. A cross sectional survey for B virus antibody in a colony of group housed rhesus macaques. *Lab. Anim. Sci.* **40:**257–261.

171. Weigler, B. J., F. Scinicariello, and J. K. Hilliard. 1995. Risk of venereal B virus (cercopithecine herpesvirus 1) transmission in rhesus monkeys using molecular epidemiology. *J. Infect. Dis.* **171:**1139–1143.

172. Weinberg, A., J. J. Leary, R. T. Sarisky, and M. J. Levin. 2007. Factors that affect in vitro measurement of the susceptibility of herpes simplex virus to nucleoside analogues. *J. Clin. Virol.* **38:**139–145.

173. Whitley, R., A. Arvin, C. Prober, S. Burchett, L. Corey, D. Powell, S. Plotkin, S. Starr, C. Alford, J. Connor, et al. 1991. A controlled trial comparing vidarabine with acyclovir in neonatal herpes simplex virus infection. *N. Engl. J. Med.* **324:**444–449.

174. Whitley, R. J. 2006. Herpes simplex encephalitis: adolescents and adults. *Antivir. Res.* **71:**141–148.

175. Whitley, R. J., and A. M. Arvin. 1995. Herpes simplex virus infection, p. 354–378. *In* J. Remingon and J. Klein (ed.), *Infectious Diseases of the Fetus and Newborn*, 4th ed. The W. B. Saunders Co., Philadelphia, PA.

176. Whitley, R. J., and D. W. Kimberlin. 1997. Treatment of viral infections during pregnancy and the neonatal period. *Clin. Perinatol.* **24:**267–283.

177. Wildemann, B., K. Ehrhart, B. Storch-Hagenlocher, U. Meyding-Lamade, S. Steinvorth, W. Hacke, and J. Haas. 1997. Quantitation of herpes simplex virus type 1 DNA in cells of cerebrospinal fluid of patients with herpes simplex virus encephalitis. *Neurology* **48:**1341–1346.

178. Woods, G. L., and R. D. Mills. 1988. Effect of dexamethasone on detection of herpes simplex virus in clinical specimens by conventional cell culture and rapid 24-well plate centrifugation. *J. Clin. Microbiol.* **26:**1233–1235.

179. Xu, F., M. R. Sternberg, B. J. Kottiri, G. M. McQuillan, F. K. Lee, A. J. Nahmias, S. M. Berman, and L. E. Markowitz. 2006. Trends in herpes simplex virus type 1 and type 2 seroprevalence in the United States. *JAMA* **296:**964–973.

180. Yamamoto, L. J., D. G. Tedder, R. Ashley, and M. J. Levin. 1991. Herpes simplex virus type 1 DNA in cerebrospinal fluid of a patient with Mollaret's meningitis. *N. Engl. J. Med.* **325:**1082–1085.

181. Zhao, L. S., M. L. Landry, E. S. Balkovic, and G. D. Hsiung. 1987. Impact of cell culture sensitivity and virus concentration on rapid detection of herpes simplex virus by cytopathic effects and immunoperoxidase staining. *J. Clin. Microbiol.* **25:**1401–1405.

182. Zhu, J., D. M. Koelle, J. Cao, J. Vazquez, M. L. Huang, F. Hladik, A. Wald, and L. Corey. 2007. Virus-specific CD8+ T cells accumulate near sensory nerve endings in genital skin during subclinical HSV-2 reactivation. *J. Exp. Med.* **204:**595–603.

183. Zwartouw, H. T., C. R. Humphreys, and P. Collins. 1989. Oral chemotherapy of fatal B virus (herpesvirus simiae) infection. *Antivir. Res.* **11:**275–283.

Varicella-Zoster Virus*

ELISABETH PUCHHAMMER-STÖCKL AND STEPHAN W. ABERLE

97

TAXONOMY

Varicella-zoster virus (VZV) belongs to the family *Herpesviridae*, based on morphological criteria, and is one of the eight human-pathogenic herpesviruses identified so far. On the basis of its biological properties, it is classified, together with herpes simplex virus, as a member of the subfamily *Alphaherpesvirinae* (genus *Varicellovirus*, species *Human herpesvirus 3* [HHV-3]).

DESCRIPTION OF THE AGENT

VZV is an enveloped virus with a diameter of about 180 to 200 nm (Fig. 1). It contains an icosahedral nucleocapsid surrounded by a tegument structure, a lipid envelope that allows the virus to be degraded by lipid solvents, and a linear double-stranded DNA genome (21). The viral genome has an approximate length of 125,000 bp, making it the smallest of the human herpesviruses (24), and it encodes at least 70 viral genes. The VZV genome consists of a unique long region, a unique short region, and flanking internal and terminating repeat regions, and it can exist in four isomeric forms (Fig. 2).

VZV may infect susceptible cells either by fusion at the cell surface or by endocytosis. Virus replication takes place in the nucleus of the infected cell, and similar to what is observed in other herpesviruses, the progression of viral gene expression is highly regulated. Not all VZV gene functions are yet known. The especially well characterized ones include some transcription regulator proteins (IE 61 through IE 63), viral enzymes such as thymidine kinase (TK; open reading frame 36 [ORF 36]) and the DNA polymerase (ORF 28), and various VZV glycoproteins (gp), such as gB (ORF 31), gE (ORF 68), and gH (ORF 37), which are required for virus attachment and for inducing a host immune response.

VZV exhibits low genomic diversity among isolates in comparison to other herpesviruses (81). Currently, complete sequences are available for at least 18 VZV isolates (70), and so far, five major VZV genomic groups have been established (63). There is no evidence that naturally circulating VZV strains differ significantly in virulence.

EPIDEMIOLOGY AND TRANSMISSION

VZV is ubiquitous and highly contagious, and primary infection with VZV therefore usually already occurs in early childhood. Prevaccination seroepidemiological studies in 11 European countries have shown that in most areas, more than 90% of 10- to 15-year-olds were already seropositive for VZV (73). In the United States, the incidence of varicella has declined significantly since 1995, when the VZV vaccine was generally introduced (15).

Primary infection with VZV is most likely acquired by virus transmission through aerosols. Cell-free virus is also produced at high levels in the skin vesicles, and thus the fluid from these vesicles is also highly infectious. Infection occurs by inoculation of the respiratory tract mucosa and replication in tonsillar lymphoid tissue, from which the virus is then disseminated, most likely by T cells (21). The incubation period is 10 to 21 days. During this incubation time, the virus is spread by viremia, may also replicate in reticuloendothelial organs, and finally infects cutaneous epithelial cells, which are the major sites of virus replication (21). Eventually, the infected host begins to shed virus by the respiratory route. New vesicles containing infectious fluid may appear for several days after rash onset. Individuals are no longer infectious once the last set of vesicles have dried and crusted.

After primary VZV infection, the virus remains latent in ganglia. Upon reactivation, herpes zoster may develop. Herpes zoster rash vesicles are filled with virus-containing fluid and may be also a source of primary infection for susceptible, VZV-seronegative individuals. The virus can also be transmitted from mother to child during pregnancy (30).

CLINICAL SIGNIFICANCE

Varicella (chicken pox) is the manifestation of primary infection with VZV. The clinical appearance of chicken pox is usually dominated by a generalized vesicular rash. Sometimes, symptoms such as fever, malaise, or abdominal pain are seen as prodromal symptoms 24 to 48 hours before and during the first days after the onset of the rash. New vesicles develop during the first 3 to 6 days of varicella. Due to its characteristic clinical appearance, the diagnosis of varicella is often a clinical one and does not require laboratory confirmation. Clinical reinfection with VZV has been described for immunocompetent and

---

*This chapter contains figures presented in chapter 101 by Anne A. Gershon, Jingxian Chen, Philip LaRussa, and Sharon P. Steinberg in the ninth edition of this *Manual*.

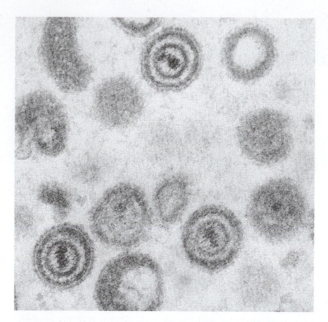

FIGURE 1 Electron micrograph of VZV in skin vesicle fluid from a patient with varicella (magnification, ×100,000). Reprinted from reference 16.

immunosuppressed individuals (42) and might occur more frequently than usually supposed (47).

Complications associated with chicken pox can occur, and before vaccination was introduced, up to 4 of 1,000 cases of chicken pox in the United States required hospitalization each year (39). Older age, immunosuppression, and pregnancy are considered to be generally associated with a higher complication rate with varicella. The most frequent complications seen with chicken pox are secondary bacterial infections of the skin lesions, which can lead to abscesses, lymphadenitis, and, rarely, also to bacteremia and sepsis. In healthy adults especially, varicella may be complicated by VZV pneumonia, which is 25 times more frequent in these patients than in children and has been described to be especially severe in pregnant women (52). The hospitalization rate among adults with varicella is about 32 per 1,000 reported cases, which is more than six times higher than in children (68).

VZV encephalitis can occur during chicken pox, due to primary infection or to postinfectious processes, and often presents with symptoms of acute cerebellar ataxia (108). Other varicella complications include hepatitis, nephritis, and acute thrombocytopenia. In immunosuppressed patients, extensive general dissemination can occur, leading to multiorgan infection and death if not treated early.

Primary infection with VZV during the first 21 weeks of gestation may lead to congenital varicella syndrome in the fetus, characterized by cutaneous scarifications, atrophy of the extremities, and in rare cases, seizures, microcephaly, and other sequelae. The association between the clinical syndrome and VZV has been confirmed by detection of viral DNA by PCR in fetal tissue (79). The incidence is low, <1% in the first two trimesters (96). Neonatal varicella can result in severe disseminated infection in babies born within 4 days before to 2 days after the maternal varicella rash appears.

After primary infection, VZV persists in the host in a latent state in sensory trigeminal and dorsal root ganglia. VZV reaches the sensory ganglia, most likely by retrograde axonal transport from skin lesions, and eventually also by hematogenous spread (21). Variable amounts of virus, ranging from 10 to about 55,000 viral genome copies per 100,000 ganglion cells, have been detected in latently infected hosts (22, 64, 77). During VZV latency, transcription and translation of different genes are observed (53). The virus is kept under control mostly by the host's VZV-specific T-cell immunity. When this immunity decreases due to immunosuppression or older age, reactivation of the virus may occur.

Reactivation of VZV can lead to limited subclinical local infection, or the virus may spread via neurons to the skin, resulting in the clinical syndrome herpes zoster. Herpes zoster is mostly characterized as a vesicular rash, typically limited in immunocompetent hosts to the dermatome innervated by a single sensory nerve (21). It is often preceded and accompanied by intense neuropathic pain due to sensory neuron involvement. The eye may be affected, resulting in zoster ophthalmicus. An increase in the VZV-specific T-cell response limits viral spread. The most frequent complication of herpes zoster is postherpetic neuralgia, which presents as severe pain and may last for up to several months after herpes zoster.

In immunocompetent hosts, the most severe complications of herpes zoster are associated with VZV infections of the central nervous system (CNS). Viral meningitis, myelitis, or encephalitis may be observed, with encephalitis probably occurring due to neuronal spread. Cases of facial

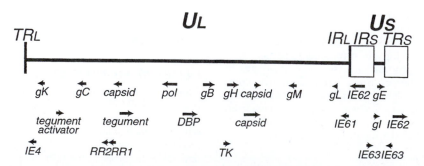

FIGURE 2 Schematic of the VZV linear double-stranded DNA genome. UL, long unique segment (100 kbp); US, short unique segment (5.4 kbp); TRS and TRL, terminal repeats; IRS and IRL, internal repeats. The arrows indicate the direction of the transcription of the viral genes indicated. RR, ribonucleotide reductase; DBP, DNA binding protein. Reprinted from reference 40

palsy syndrome are also seen. In most cases, the diagnosis of herpes zoster is a clinical one, based on its characteristic appearance and the distribution of vesicles. In some cases, however, reactivation may also result in "zoster sine herpete," a syndrome of undefined local pain that is sometimes also associated with CNS infection that occurs in the absence of a vesicular rash. The diagnosis of "zoster sine herpete" can be provided only by virological investigation. It may occur more commonly than previously thought. Approximately 25% of cases with CNS complications due to virologically confirmed VZV reactivation occurred in the context of zoster sine herpete (1).

In the immunosuppressed host, primary infection and reactivation can lead to severe and possibly life-threatening generalized infection. In the prevaccine era, severe disseminated primary infection associated with high mortality was a particular concern in immunosuppressed children. This remains an important entity in undervaccinated populations. After bone marrow or solid-organ transplantation, patients frequently exhibit episodes of VZV reactivation, which sometimes proceed to severe disseminated infection and to the development of visceral zoster, a clinical picture characterized by severe abdominal pain and associated with the involvement of internal organs, such as the liver, colon, or lung (for reviews, see references 45 and 71). Among solid-organ transplant recipients, lung transplant patients especially have an increased risk for VZV complications (14), but VZV can also cause substantial problems in patients with hematological malignancies or after hematopoietic stem cell transplantation (for a review, see reference 101). HIV-infected individuals may also undergo severe episodes of VZV reactivation and dissemination, especially during AIDS, and they may exhibit an unusual clinical presentation (34, 44, 107). VZV can also play a role in the development of immune reconstitution inflammatory syndrome, and mucocutaneous zoster may occur within 4 weeks after the initiation of highly active antiretroviral therapy (HAART) (32).

Disease caused by VZV can be prevented by vaccination. A live attenuated varicella vaccine derived from the Japanese Oka strain was developed in the early 1970s. It was approved in the United States in 1995 for persons who are susceptible to chicken pox and is currently also recommended in various European countries (94). The childhood vaccination policy in the United States has led to a substantial decrease in varicella incidence (95), disease severity, and associated complications (110). An Oka-derived vaccine has also been developed to boost T-cell immunity against VZV in older patients in order to prevent zoster reactivation (48).

Varicella-zoster immunoglobulin may prevent severe varicella and is thus given to high-risk patient populations to avoid the development of disease. Seronegative women during the first 21 weeks of pregnancy receive the commercially available VZV immunoglobulin up to 72 hours after VZV exposure, to avoid the development of congenital varicella syndrome in the fetus (30). In immunosuppressed VZV-seronegative patients, such as hematopoietic cell transplant patients, application of VZV immunoglobulin has been recommended up to 96 hours postexposure to inhibit the development of severe generalized infections (115).

Early and rapid diagnosis of VZV infection is important. Different detection methods are available (summarized in Table 1). Due to its sensitivity, PCR has largely supplanted culture and become the preferred method in many instances. Antigen detection is still useful, as it can be

TABLE 1 Diagnostic tests for VZV-induced disease

Method	Target	Suitable specimen(s) (disease or clinical procedure)	Comments
PCR	ORF 17, 29, 31, 62, 69	Fluid, cells, or crust from lesions (varicella, herpes zoster) Blood (disseminated infection, zoster sine herpete) CSF (encephalitis, meningitis, myelitis, facial palsy, zoster sine herpete) Tissue (autopsy)	Most sensitive method. Shorter time to result than with culture. Quantification possible.
Direct fluorescent-antibody assay	gE	Cells from lesions (varicella, herpes zoster) Tissue (autopsy)	More sensitive than culture. Rapid time to results (<2 h); random access.
Culture	Infectious virus	Lesion fluid or cells (varicella, herpes zoster) Blood (disseminated infection, zoster sine herpete) Tissue (autopsy)	Positive early in disease (<2 days after rash onset). Recovery can be difficult as virus is very labile. Traditional diagnostic standard now largely replaced by PCR due to lack of sensitivity and long time to result (7–10 days for CPE).
Serology	Anti-VZV IgM, IgG	Serum (primarily to assess immunity)	Not recommended for use in disease diagnosis; false-positive and false-negative IgM results may arise. To test IgG levels, 7–10 days required between acute- and convalescent-phase samples.

performed rapidly and in a random-access format. Serology is most useful to ascertain immunity.

Specific antiviral treatment of VZV infection and reactivation is possible. If treatment is necessary, it is usually performed with nucleoside analogues such as acyclovir or penciclovir, or with the better orally bioavailable prodrugs valacyclovir and famciclovir (10, 97). Brivudine is another nucleoside analogue that has proven effective against VZV (25). Anti-VZV treatment is applied in immunosuppressed hosts and in immunocompetent patients when clinical complications arise. In addition, herpes zoster reactivation is also treated to limit the development of postherpetic neuralgia and to prevent ocular involvement.

COLLECTION, TRANSPORT, AND STORAGE OF SPECIMENS

Various specimens can be used for diagnosis (Table 1), depending on the clinical presentation and test method. Vesicular fluid contains cell-free virus, mostly at high concentration. Since nearly all patients with varicella and many patients with herpes zoster show a vesicular rash, and because collection of vesicular fluid is very convenient, laboratory diagnosis from vesicular fluid is a major diagnostic tool for detection or confirmation of VZV infection or reactivation. The vesicular fluid can be collected by use of capillary pipettes or syringes. For PCR analysis, vesicular fluid can also be collected on swabs and submitted to the laboratory in physiological saline or in viral transport medium. If further virus culture is planned, it should be kept in mind that virus collected on swabs is less stable and is also further diluted in the medium, which may decrease the efficiency of virus culture.

VZV DNA is detectable by PCR in plasma, serum, whole blood, and peripheral blood mononuclear cells (PBMCs). Plasma or serum is conventionally used due to ease of preparation. Whole-blood specimens should be submitted in anticoagulants other than heparin if PCR testing is to be performed, as heparin can inhibit *Taq* polymerases. Virus can be recovered from PBMCs early in disease; however, this is primarily a method used in research. Cerebrospinal fluid (CSF) should be submitted in a sterile container. Usually, uncentrifuged CSF is used for detection of VZV DNA, but virus can also be detected in the cellular fraction or in the supernatant.

Tissue is tested primarily at autopsy. In disseminated disease, tissue testing has now largely been replaced by PCR of blood specimens due to test sensitivity and ease of specimen procurement. Cells from tissue can be stained by immunofluorescence. Touch preparations of cells are prepared by pressing tissue (typically 10 to 15 mm) against the clean surface of a glass slide multiple times, over a length of 30 to 40 mm. Slides are air dried, fixed in cold acetone, and stained with reagents used in antigen detection (see below). Tissue homogenates can be prepared as described in chapter 76 and tested by culture or PCR.

Generally, VZV DNA, which is ultimately amplified by PCR methods, is quite stable during collection, transport, and storage. VZV virions, however, are quite labile; therefore, specimens should be placed into culture as quickly as possible after collection if isolation is required. Samples for PCR can be stored at −20°C. Virus isolation from frozen samples is largely ineffective unless cellular fractions are stored in cryoprotectant medium at −80°C.

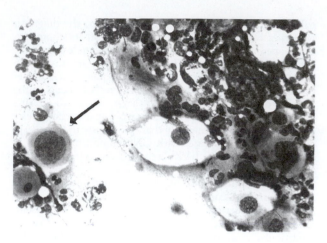

FIGURE 3 Giemsa-stained preparation of material from the base of a vesicular lesion. Magnification, ×102. The arrow indicates a giant cell with a folded nucleus characteristic of VZV or HSV.

DIRECT DETECTION

Microscopy

One of the oldest and simplest direct detection methods is the Tzanck test. In this assay, cellular material is scraped from the base of vesicular lesion and put onto glass slides. These smears are then stained, examined under a microscope, and screened for multinucleated giant cells, which contain multiple eosinophilic intranuclear inclusions representing viral capsids (Fig. 3). However, since the presence of these cells is characteristic of both HSV and VZV infections, a specific diagnosis of VZV cannot be made with this test. VZV can be visualized by electron microscopy, but this method also does not allow a clear differentiation between the different herpesviruses (Fig. 1).

Antigen Detection

VZV antigen detection is still used in different hospitals as a first front-line diagnostic test for rapid detection of VZV infection in hospitalized patients. For antigen detection, cell-containing material is required. Cell suspensions obtained by skin scrapings from the base of the vesicle are applied onto glass slides, fixed with cold acetone, and dried. Then, cells are stained with fluorescently labeled monoclonal antibodies (MAbs) for 30 min at 37°C in a humidified chamber. After a washing step cells are covered with a coverslip, and staining is visualized by fluorescence microscopy (20). VZV-specific MAbs are commercially available (Merifluor; Meridian Diagnostics, Meridian Bioscience Inc., Cincinnati, OH; and Light Diagnostics; Chemicon/Millipore, Billerica, MA); mixtures of HSV- and VZV-specific MAbs labeled with different fluorophores are also available (Light Diagnostics Simulfluor HSV/VZV kit; Millipore/Chemicon). These products allow the detection of either virus from a single slide. While superior to culture in regard to sensitivity and time to result, antigen detection is clearly less sensitive than PCR-based methods for direct detection of virus from clinical material.

Nucleic Acid Detection

Over the last decade, nucleic acid amplification-based techniques, especially PCR assays, have become standard tools for the diagnosis of VZV disease. These techniques have revolutionized the diagnosis of VZV disease of the CNS and of disseminated VZV infection in immunocompromised patients and the identification of herpes zoster in patients who do not develop the typical rash. The advantages of these molecular techniques are that they require only small volumes of input material and are highly sensitive and rapid.

Since the description of the first detection of VZV DNA in CSF by conventional PCR (80), the PCR techniques used have changed substantially. Real-time PCR methods (reviewed in chapter 4) that are more sensitive and can be quantitative have replaced older PCR techniques and are now routinely performed in many diagnostic laboratories. Numerous in-house PCR tests have been published for amplifying various gene segments of the VZV genome (Table 1), and in addition, an increasing number of commercially available VZV PCR kits are being developed, as for instance VZV tracer (affigene; Cepheid), VZV PCR kit (Abbott Laboratories),

and LightCycler VZV Qual kit (Roche Diagnostics). Protocols have also been designed for simultaneous amplification of VZV together with various other viruses causing similar clinical pictures. Commercially available tests include artus Herpes Virus LC-PCR kits (Qiagen; CE marked for in vitro diagnostic use in Europe, available for research use only in Canada, and not available in the United States) or HSV1 HSV2 VZV R-gene (Argene Inc.; CE marked for in vitro diagnostic use in Europe and available for research use only in the United States). These multiplex PCRs are able to identify a variety of diagnostically important viruses simultaneously, either within one tube or by parallel detection in a single PCR run (99, 112). VZV detection and quantification by PCR can be performed in various clinical materials (for an overview, see Table 2). Quantified VZV DNA for use as nucleic acid

TABLE 2 Quantitative VZV DNA results with different clinical materials from patients with different VZV-associated diseases[a]

Material	Clinical syndrome	No. investigated	PCR positive (%)	Viral load (median, mean, geometric mean)	Viral load range	Reference
Vesicle	Varicella	3		1.0×10^8 co/ml		55
	Zoster	3		7.4×10^8 co/ml		55
CSF	Varicella	1		10^2 co/ml		2
	Varicella	1		91 co/ml		87
	Zoster	30		1.4×10^4 co/ml	$50–2.6 \times 10^8$ co/ml	1
	Zoster	16		3.1×10^3 co/ml	$1.1 \times 10^2–4 \times 10^4$ co/ml	87
Saliva	Ramsay Hunt syndrome	25	52		$30–1.4 \times 10^6$ co/50 μl	38
	Facial palsy without rash	31	55		$10–1 \times 10^5$ co/50 μl	38
Whole blood	Varicella in adults	34	100	5×10^2 co/ml	$20–10^5$ co/ml	66
	Varicella	8	87.5	1.6×10^3 co/ml	$2 \times 10^2–1.1 \times 10^4$ co/ml	26
	Zoster, dermatomal	9	90	2×10^2 co/ml	$10^2–9 \times 10^2$ co/ml	26
	Zoster, multi-dermatomal	5	100	2.7×10^3 co/ml	$9 \times 10^2–3 \times 10^5$ co/ml	26
	Healthy control	20	0			26
	Blood donors	100	0			49
PBMCs	Varicella	9	100	12 co/10^5 cells		50
	Varicella	19	73	4.9×10^2 co/10^5 cells	$5–5 \times 10^3$ co/10^5 cells	55
	Varicella	21	48		$1.4 \times 10^2–3.4 \times 10^3$ co/10^5 cells	65
	Zoster	10	20	10 co/10^5 cells		55
	Zoster	71	16		$10–10^2$ co/10^5 cells	65
	Zoster	130	78	9×10^2 co/10^5 cells	$40–2.9 \times 10^4$ co/10^5 cells	84
	Healthy controls	28	0			55
	Healthy controls (50 ml blood)	53	5	1.3×10^3 co/10^5 cells	$6 \times 10^2–5 \times 10^3$ co/10^5 cells	84
Serum, plasma	Varicella	18	88.9	2.0×10^3 co/ml	$100–2 \times 10^5$ co/ml	26
	Varicella	5	100	10^4 co/ml		50
	Disseminated varicella	1		1.2×10^7 co/ml		6
	Zoster, dermatomal	9	66.7	100 co/ml		26
	Zoster, multidermatomal	6	100	2.7×10^3 co/ml		26
	Zoster	9	100	1.7×10^3 co/ml	$1.8 \times 10^2–10^4$ co/ml	57
	Zoster	12		7×10^3 co/ml	$4 \times 10^2–2 \times 10^5$ co/ml	51
	Zoster, disseminated	4	100	2.1×10^5 co/ml	$2.5 \times 10^3–7.4 \times 10^5$ co/ml	57
	Zoster, visceral disseminated	1		2×10^5 co/ml		85
	Healthy control	10	0			26
Aqueous humor	Acute retinal necrosis	2			9×10^2 and 5.5×10^6 co/ml	5
	Anterior uveitis	8		2.5×10^5 co/ml	$3.8 \times 10^2–1.2 \times 10^7$ co/ml	54
Tissue	Postmortem	32	68		$6–28$ co/10^5 GC	64
	Postmortem	14	79	2.6×10^2 co/10^5 GC		77
	Postmortem	17	100	9×10^3 co/10^5 GC	$5.8 \times 10^2–5.5 \times 10^4$ co/10^5 GC	22

[a]Abbreviations: co, copies; GC, ganglion cells.

detection and quantification test controls is provided by various manufacturers such as Advances Biotechnologies, Inc. (Columbia, MD) and Zeptometrix Corp. (Buffalo, NY) or by the National Institute for Biological Standards and Control (Potters Bar, Hertfordshire, United Kingdom).

VZV DNA from vesicular fluid and skin scrapings can be detected easily by PCR. This helps to discriminate quickly between vesicular lesions caused by VZV and those due to various other causes, especially HSV type 1 or type 2 infection. PCR is more sensitive than virus isolation or direct immunofluorescence for the detection of VZV in vesicular lesions (9, 109). VZV DNA can be detected by PCR in crusting lesions and in skin scrapings in VZV-associated facial palsy in the absence of visible vesicular lesions (114). The easy access and the high virus detection rates make dermal lesions an ideal material to be used not only for diagnosis but also for further genotyping of vaccine and wild-type strains, using genotype-specific PCR strategies (75, 90).

Analysis of CSF by nucleic acid amplification has become the method of choice for diagnosis of neurological disease associated with VZV, such as cerebellitis, aseptic meningitis, and encephalitis. Using PCR, it was found that neurological disease is an important and not infrequent complication in immunocompetent as well as immunosuppressed patients. VZV DNA was detected in CSF of up to 10% of patients presenting with clinical symptoms of aseptic meningitis and (meningo-) encephalitis (58, 69). PCR analysis is also useful for the diagnosis of VZV-induced neurological symptoms in cases where the characteristic CNS vesicular rash appears only after the start of CNS infection, or even in cases of zoster sine herpete (1, 7, 29, 56, 76). No rash was observed in about a quarter of all cases of patients suffering from VZV-associated neurological symptoms (1, 56, 76). Higher mean VZV DNA loads were found in CSF of patients with herpes-zoster-associated encephalitis than with meningitis (Fig. 4A) and in patients requiring intensive-care treatment than in those who did not, although overlap was observed among individual patients in each of the compared groups (Fig. 4B) (1). Virus is predominantly detected within 1 week after the onset of clinical symptoms, but in cases of VZV-induced neurological symptoms without rash, virus can be detected in the second week of disease (1, 56). VZV may be occasionally detected in CSF from individuals with uncomplicated zoster, but viral loads are lower than in patients with

neurological complications. In cases of varicella-induced cerebellar ataxia the amount of viral DNA was shown to be generally low (2, 80, 87), supporting the theory that these symptoms might be mediated by the antiviral immune response. After initiation of antiviral therapy, CSF usually becomes negative for VZV DNA in the follow-up in uncomplicated cases (80). In contrast, the continuous presence of viral DNA has been found in individual HIV-infected patients in spite of therapy, and this was associated with the death of these patients (18).

PCR testing plays an important role in the diagnosis of acute VZV-associated peripheral facial palsy occurring as a neurological complication in the course of VZV reactivation. In cases of Ramsay Hunt syndrome, virus can be detected not only in vesicles of the auricles and the oral cavity but also in the facialis nerve sheath, middle ear mucosa, and CSF (72). As the rash is mostly hidden in the ear or mouth and may be faint or delayed, only sensitive testing for the presence of VZV by PCR has shown that a considerable number of "idiopathic" peripheral facial palsy or Bell's palsy cases are due to VZV reactivation. By use of PCR methods, VZV was detected in saliva samples of 58% of patients with VZV-induced facial palsy, with 64% of those cases presenting without the characteristic rash (37). Virus was shown to be present in oropharyngeal swabs until day 12 in patients with acute peripheral facial palsy (36). VZV DNA levels in saliva were about 10^4 copies higher and recovery of facial function was worse in patients with facial palsy and oropharyngeal lesions than in those with facial palsy alone (35a). VZV can be detected rarely in CSF samples of patients with facial palsy (72, 98), indicating that in some cases of facial palsy VZV may lead to an accompanying VZV meningitis. But overall, lower amounts of virus are found in these patients than in those presenting with meningitis and encephalitis (Fig. 4C) (1, 76).

VZV DNA is also detectable in PBMCs (43, 50, 55, 65) and in whole blood (8, 26, 66, 84), and although the viremia is assumed to be cell associated, viral DNA can also be detected in serum or plasma (26, 28, 50, 51, 57). Viremia is detected by PCR in up to 100% of cases of acute varicella, but virus can also be detected in the blood compartment in cases of herpes zoster. VZV DNA was detected in 47% of serum samples obtained within the first 8 days after the start of herpes zoster from otherwise healthy patients (28). In a small cohort of nine immunocompetent patients with herpes zoster, all were found to be VZV DNA positive when the amount

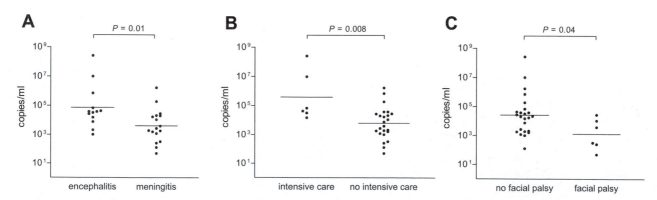

FIGURE 4 Comparison of the amount of VZV DNA in CSF according to the neurological diagnosis (A), the severity of disease (B), and the presence of acute peripheral facial palsy (C). The geometric mean value is shown by a horizontal line. The P value was calculated using the Mann-Whitney U test. (Modified from reference 1, with permission.)

of plasma analyzed was increased to 1 ml (57). Quantitative analysis showed that viral loads may range from 5 to 5×10^3 copies/10^5 cells in PBMCs, from 20 to 10^5 copies/ml in whole blood, and from 100 to 2×10^5 copies/ml in plasma or serum. The virus load is higher in patients with acute varicella than in those with herpes zoster (26). A higher viral load correlates with a larger number of skin lesions and more severe disease (66) as well as with the presence of multidermatomal zoster (26). The viral load was lower in samples taken only a few days after the start of varicella symptoms (55) and was found to be negative in convalescent-phase sera of patients with shingles (28). When applying a highly sensitive nested-PCR assay, VZV DNA was also detected in PBMCs of patients with facial palsy without dermal lesions (105).

Virus detection in blood is important for the diagnosis of complicated or clinically unclear courses of varicella or herpes zoster, especially in cases in which the appearance of a rash is delayed or completely lacking, and also in cases of visceral dissemination (6, 57, 85, 86). In immunocompromised patients, quantitative PCR analysis proved to be an important tool for monitoring the clinical course of disease and assessing therapeutic success (6, 51, 57, 85).

VZV is not detectable in the blood in the majority of healthy control patients, even with sensitive PCR methods (49), unless a very large volume of blood (50 ml) is used (84). In other studies, VZV was detectable in 2 to 3% of PBMC samples taken from immunocompetent individuals without clinical signs of VZV illness (65, 93). These findings support the assumption that asymptomatic reactivation of latent virus may occur and may be important for boosting host immunity to the virus (3).

VZV PCR can be performed from aqueous humor and has been found to be helpful in confirming VZV-associated ocular disease. The viral load in the aqueous humor of patients with anterior uveitis corresponds to the extent of iris atrophy (54).

Identification of VZV by PCR in bronchoalveolar lavage specimens has been reported and seems to be useful for the successful early diagnosis of severe VZV pneumonitis (23). The detection of VZV DNA in tissue samples by PCR is also possible and has been used to confirm the association between VZV and congenital varicella syndrome (74, 79). Generally, the use of highly sensitive PCR techniques may be especially important for confirming the diagnosis of VZV-related disease in cases of less disseminated or milder disease associated with lower viral loads (65, 114) or for samples obtained later in the course of disease after the initiation of antiviral therapy.

ISOLATION AND IDENTIFICATION

Cell Culture Methods

Virus isolation provides the basis for phenotypic characterization of individual VZV strains, for generating VZV-infected cells for serologic tests such as the fluorescent antibody to membrane antigen (FAMA) test, and for the phenotypic analysis of VZV drug resistance. Many laboratories use human foreskin fibroblasts for isolation of VZV from clinical samples. Other sensitive host cells include diploid human cell lines, preferably derived from fetal kidney, fetal lung, human lung carcinoma (A549), or human melanoma cell lines, and nonhuman cell lines such as primary monkey kidney cells (20, 46). A cell mixture (CV-1 and MRC-5) is commercially available for the recovery of herpesviruses including VZV (H&V

Mix; Diagnostic Hybrids, Inc., Athens, OH). In contrast to other herpesviruses, VZV maintains a high level of genetic stability during the culturing procedure. Cell cultures are performed at 37°C under sterile conditions, and the medium used is usually Eagle's minimal essential medium, prepared in Hanks' or Earle's balanced salt solution containing neomycin and glutamine and supplemented with 10% fetal bovine serum for the growth medium and 1 to 2% fetal bovine serum for maintenance. The medium is heat inactivated at 56°C for 30 min. The need for a medium change is indicated by a drop in pH, and this is required at least once weekly. When virus culture is done for diagnostic purposes, the clinical material is adsorbed onto the cell monolayer or inoculated directly into the medium, and the cells are then incubated at 37°C and evaluated daily by microscopy. The development of a cytopathic effect (CPE) is variable but is usually visible from 4 days up to maximally 2 weeks. The CPE consists of small foci of rounded and swollen cells (Fig. 5). Confirmation of VZV infection is done by PCR or by staining monolayer cells with VZV-specific MAbs (described below). Shell vial centrifugation cultures can provide results in 2 to 5 days and are more sensitive than conventional cultures for VZV but less sensitive than PCR (31).

Virus Identification from Cell Culture

Specific identification of VZV from clinical material in cell culture after the emergence of a CPE is necessary because it may be difficult to distinguish VZV from other herpesviruses. VZV-specific PCR analysis may be performed for identification. For this purpose, supernatant is taken from the culture, and DNA is extracted and subjected to PCR. Monolayers can also be stained with VZV-specific MAbs when approximately 50% of the monolayer demonstrates CPE suggestive of VZV. For this purpose, cell monolayers are washed with phosphate-buffered saline (PBS). Then, monolayer cells are scraped into 0.5 ml of PBS. Slides are prepared by directly applying the suspension to a glass slide by using a cytocentrifuge. Slides are air dried and then fixed in cold acetone for 10 minutes. Following wash with PBS, cells are stained with VZV-specific MAbs. Commercial reagents approved for use in culture confirmation include D^3 DFA VZV Detection kit (DHI) as well as the MAbs listed in "Antigen Detection" above. After a 30-min incubation at 37°C, monolayers are washed in PBS and rinsed in distilled water.

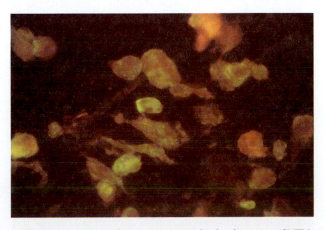

FIGURE 5 Immunofluorescence assay for the detection of VZV-positive cells from a patient with zoster. A smear of a skin vesicle was fixed and stained with MAb to VZV gE. Magnification, ×200.

Excess moisture is removed by blotting around wells. Stained cells should not be allowed to dry as this produces artifactual fluorescence. Mounting medium and a coverslip are applied, and the staining is visualized by fluorescence microscopy.

Genetic Identification of VZV Strains

Genetic identification of VZV is performed by different molecular methods, directly from clinical specimens, but primarily on a research basis rather than as a routine clinical test. Characterization of VZV strains is usually done by PCR assays followed by restriction fragment length polymorphism analysis or by sequencing of characteristic fragments and determination of single nucleotide polymorphisms (for a review, see reference 81). Genetic analysis of virus strains has proven that the VZV strains identified during varicella are identical within an outbreak and are also identical to those present in subsequent herpes zoster (100). It has been shown that VZV strains vary between geographic areas (81).

Characterization of VZV strains may be especially important for differentiating between wild-type (WT) strains and Oka vaccine strains after vaccination, for determining the etiology of a postvaccination rash, for analyzing the association between vaccination and the development of herpes zoster, and also for assessing whether transmission of vaccine virus to susceptible persons has occurred. Different methods for discrimination between WT and vaccine strains have been published, and in this regard, much attention has been focused on the VZV ORF 62 because most nonsynonymous VZV vaccine mutations occur in this ORF. In particular, SmaI and NaeI sites in ORF 62 have been shown to allow the discrimination of vaccine strains from WT strains and also from the Oka parental strain (83). Restriction fragment length polymorphism analysis has also been described for other ORFs, for example, ORF 6 (103), with differences in the AluI sites, and ORFs 38 and 54 in combination, with differences in the PstI and BglI sites (59).

Real-time PCR assays based on sequence polymorphisms, especially in ORF 62 or ORF 38, have also been established (13, 62, 75, 106). In addition, a considerable amount of sequence data for various ORFs in the VZV genome have been obtained so far in the search for single nucleotide polymorphisms that would allow further VZV strain discrimination (for an overview, see reference 81).

The analysis of the Oka vaccine itself has shown that it contains a mixture of different strains that also differ in the R2 repeat region (92). The development of rash after vaccination seems to be associated with the emergence of certain strains that are closely related to the Oka parental strain (82).

SEROLOGIC TESTS

Antibodies (Abs) against VZV develop in the course of primary infection, are directed against various proteins of the virus, and can be detected in most cases within 3 days after the appearance of the rash. Serologic testing can be used for confirmation of primary infections, where it is applied especially in clinically atypical cases. Detection of VZV-specific Abs is also routinely used for determining immune status. This may be required for patients who cannot remember their varicella history and is especially important in pretransplantation evaluations as well as after virus exposure to guide prophylaxis with varicella immunoglobulin in high-risk individuals such as solid-organ or bone marrow transplant patients, pregnant women, and health care workers. In addition, it may be used for monitoring a patient's immune status after vaccination, although assessment of vaccine efficacy is not routinely performed. A variety of serologic methods that differ in specificity and sensitivity are available for detecting VZV-specific Abs. The method considered to be the "gold standard" for serologic testing is the FAMA test (reviewed in reference 12), which correlates best with protection against varicella (113). The FAMA titer, however, is not predictive of long-term protection after vaccination. Although high seroconversion rates have been described after vaccination, a loss of FAMA-detectable Abs is generally observed over time (89).

The serology test most frequently used by laboratories is the enzyme-linked immunosorbent assay (ELISA) (see below). Other methods include the anticomplement immunofluorescence test, the indirect immunofluorescence antibody test, and the latex agglutination (LA) test. Neutralizing Abs against varicella can also be detected in plaque-reduction assays, but these are not used for routine testing.

Enzyme-Linked Immunosorbent Assays

ELISAs are used most commonly by clinical laboratories, and numerous commercial tests are available. These assays have the advantage of being less laborious than the FAMA test, do not require any additional VZV cell culture procedures, are in an automated format, and can be judged objectively. The different tests use either whole VZV-infected cell lysate as the specific antigen or, in some cases, purified gp, and the test procedure is done according to the manufacturer's protocol provided. In various routine diagnostic laboratories, noncommercial, in-house ELISAs have also been established for routine detection of VZV-specific Abs, mostly with whole viral lysates as test antigen (17, 27, 67, 91). Validation of the commercial ELISAs is usually done by comparison to FAMA, and the results obtained show that ELISAs are generally less sensitive. Commercial ELISAs have been shown to detect Abs in 43% to 92% of naturally infected individuals identified as seropositive by FAMA or an adapted FAMA protocol (60). In their specificity, the ELISAs are more similar to the FAMA test (27). Considering that one aim of an Ab test is usually to determine if a person is susceptible to infection and thus a candidate for vaccination, the lower sensitivity of the ELISAs leads to more unnecessary vaccinations. The risks associated with this, however, are low compared to the risk of infection of a person who has been falsely declared immune. A noncommercial and apparently very sensitive ELISA developed by Merck, based on the detection of VZV gp preparations, has been used for extended postvaccination serostudies. ELISA titer levels of 5 gp ELISA units/ml or more at 6 weeks after vaccination have been associated with a high degree of protection against breakthrough for the following 7 years (61). However, the fact that breakthroughs have also been observed after this Ab level has been achieved suggests that gp ELISA levels correlating with long-term protection have not been adequately defined. The ELISA is usually used to determine VZV-specific Abs in blood, but it may also serve to detect Abs in CSF.

Other Serologic Tests

The LA method is a commercially available test system (41) in which VZV antigen-coated latex particles are used. Serial twofold dilutions are prepared from patient serum, and each dilution is spread on a wax-coated card. A latex emulsion is then added, and agglutination can then be observed. The test is simple and rapid to perform, and false-positive reactions are rare. However, prozone reactions may be observed, leading to false-negative results at high antibody titers. In the United States, testing at 1:2 and 1:40 (to detect prozone artifact) is recommended by the manufacturer. However, antibody levels corresponding to 1:2 dilutions do not correlate well with immunity. Therefore, results at 1:4 are preferred. Other disadvantages of this assay are the facts that the results are interpreted individually and that the test cannot be automated. LA results correlate well with those obtained by FAMA. The anticomplement immunofluorescence test is also similar in sensitivity to FAMA and LA and shows a high specificity (78), but it is not simple to perform and cannot distinguish between immunoglobulin G (IgG) and IgM.

Cellular Immunity

It has been shown that VZV-specific cellular immunity is the key factor in keeping VZV in a latent state. A decrease in cellular immunity, which is observed with increasing age or during immunosuppression, facilitates VZV reactivation and development of herpes zoster (4). Cellular immunity against VZV can be measured with a gamma-interferon enzyme-linked immunospot assay and intracellular cytokine staining followed by fluorescence-activated cell sorter analysis (35, 88, 111); however, these methods are purely investigational.

ANTIVIRAL THERAPY AND SUSCEPTIBILITY

Most VZV strains are fully susceptible to antiviral drugs. Resistance against acyclovir or penciclovir has been observed primarily in HIV-infected individuals in the pre-HAART era or in transplant recipients. Development of resistance may lead to uncontrolled viral dissemination, visceral complication, and death of the patient (11). Data from in vitro studies and investigation of resistant WT isolates have shown that acyclovir resistance is mostly associated with mutations in the VZV TK gene and only rarely due to mutations in the VZV DNA polymerase (19). Foscarnet and cidofovir can be used for treatment of acyclovir-resistant strains.

Screening for drug-resistant virus strains is only rarely performed. Antiviral susceptibility of VZV strains can be determined. Changes in virus replication in the presence of different concentrations of various drugs are measured in most cases by plaque reduction assay. Using plaque reduction in human diploid lung cells, 50% effective doses of acyclovir have been shown to range from 2.06 μM to 6.28 μM (10). Individual differences between VZV strains are observed. Other methods that have been described include the late-antigen synthesis reduction assay (33) and phenotypic characterization of the TK gene without the need for virus isolation (102).

Genotypic resistance testing can also be performed and is usually done by sequencing the VZV TK gene. Defined mutations identified in certain regions of the VZV TK gene are associated with a TK-negative function and are clearly associated with resistance to acyclovir (104). Single mutations in the VZV polymerase region are associated with foscarnet resistance.

EVALUATION, INTERPRETATION, AND REPORTING OF RESULTS

For appropriate evaluation and interpretation of test results, knowledge about the clinical background of the individual patient is of utmost importance. The interpretation of the results is dependent on whether a primary infection with VZV is suspected or whether the patient has already had

chicken pox. In addition, it is important to know whether a patient is immunosuppressed or not.

Primary infection is usually diagnosed based on clinical presentation. Virus detection, particularly from vesicles, can be performed if necessary. The results of serologic tests can be suggestive but are not definitively diagnostic of primary infection. For example, IgM (alone or in the presence of low IgG) or a fourfold increase in IgG in convalescent-phase serum can be observed during primary infection; however, these antibody responses can also be detected during reactivation.

Herpes zoster can also be diagnosed clinically, but confirmation may be necessary if vesicles are limited or otherwise indistinct in appearance from other types of infection. Detection of virus in vesicle fluid is preferred.

The presence of VZV in blood can be observed by PCR assays during chicken pox and sometimes during VZV reactivation. In most immunocompromised hosts, detection of VZV in blood by PCR is generally indicative of severe disease, although VZV DNA can also be detected in the blood of HIV patients with localized zoster. Detection of VZV DNA in CSF is also generally considered a pathological finding. Both clinical situations usually require immediate antiviral treatment.

However, highly sensitive detection of virus DNA does not always prove the causality of disease. VZV DNA may also be found due to secondary and/or subclinical reactivation but will then be observed mostly at clearly lower levels than during VZV disease. In this context the quantitative evaluation and reporting of VZV DNA levels is gaining significance. Within the immunocompromised patients, so far no defined VZV DNA thresholds in blood exist for distinguishing subclinical reactivation from clinically relevant and potentially fatal disease. However, severe visceral infections are clearly associated with higher virus load levels in blood (Table 2). Studies have also shown that high VZV DNA levels in CSF may be associated with the expression and severity of CNS disease (Fig. 4). It may therefore be useful to assess and report quantitative results in the setting of VZV CNS disease. In the pre-PCR era, Ab detection in CSF and quantitation in comparison to blood Ab levels was used for diagnosis of VZV infections of the CNS. The detection of IgM Abs is considered a proof for intrathecal Ab production, as is a significantly higher Ab level in CSF than that in blood when it is associated with an intact blood-brain barrier. The clinical significance of these tests, however, is limited because positive results are obtained too late in the course of disease to be of value for therapeutic decisions.

The major importance of Ab assays, of which ELISAs are currently the most commonly used, lies in their ability to identify previously infected individuals, as indicated by anti-VZV IgG Abs in the absence of IgM. This information can be used to guide further vaccination decisions. However, this may result in the vaccination of seropositive individuals since ELISA tests are not as sensitive as other gold standard formats.

REFERENCES

1. Aberle, S. W., J. H. Aberle, C. Steininger, and E. Puchhammer-Stöckl. 2005. Quantitative real time PCR detection of Varicella-zoster virus DNA in cerebrospinal fluid in patients with neurological disease. Med. Microbiol. Immunol. 194:7–12.
2. Aberle, S. W., and E. Puchhammer-Stöckl. 2002. Diagnosis of herpesvirus infections of the central nervous system. J. Clin. Virol. 25(Suppl. 1):S79–S85.

3. **Arvin, A.** 2005. Aging, immunity, and the varicella-zoster virus. *N. Engl. J. Med.* **352**:2266–2267.

4. **Arvin, A. M.** 2008. Humoral and cellular immunity to varicella-zoster virus: an overview. *J. Infect. Dis.* **197**(Suppl. 2):S58–S60.

5. **Asano, S., T. Yoshikawa, H. Kimura, Y. Enomoto, M. Ohashi, H. Terasaki, and Y. Nishiyama.** 2004. Monitoring herpesvirus DNA in three cases of acute retinal necrosis by real-time PCR. *J. Clin. Virol.* **29**:206–209.

6. **Beby-Defaux, A., S. Brabant, D. Chatellier, A. Bourgoin, R. Robert, T. Ruckes, and G. Agius.** 2009. Disseminated varicella with multiorgan failure in an immunocompetent adult. *J. Med. Virol.* **81**:747–749.

7. **Bergstrom, T.** 1996. Polymerase chain reaction for diagnosis of varicella zoster virus central nervous system infections without skin manifestations. *Scand. J. Infect. Dis. Suppl.* **100**:41–45.

8. **Bezold, G., M. Lange, H. Pillekamp, and R. U. Peter.** 2002. Varicella zoster viraemia during herpes zoster is not associated with neoplasia. *J. Eur. Acad. Dermatol. Venereol.* **16**:357–360.

9. **Bezold, G. D., M. E. Lange, H. Gall, and R. U. Peter.** 2001. Detection of cutaneous varicella zoster virus infections by immunofluorescence versus PCR. *Eur. J. Dermatol.* **11**:108–111.

10. **Biron, K. K., and G. B. Elion.** 1980. In vitro susceptibility of varicella-zoster virus to acyclovir. *Antimicrob. Agents Chemother.* **18**:443–447.

11. **Breton, G., A. M. Fillet, C. Katlama, F. Bricaire, and E. Caumes.** 1998. Acyclovir-resistant herpes zoster in human immunodeficiency virus-infected patients: results of foscarnet therapy. *Clin. Infect. Dis.* **27**:1525–1527.

12. **Breuer, J., D. S. Schmid, and A. A. Gershon.** 2008. Use and limitations of varicella-zoster virus-specific serological testing to evaluate breakthrough disease in vaccinees and to screen for susceptibility to varicella. *J. Infect. Dis.* **197**(Suppl. 2):S147–S151.

13. **Campsall, P. A., N. H. Au, J. S. Prendiville, D. P. Speert, R. Tan, and E. E. Thomas.** 2004. Detection and genotyping of varicella-zoster virus by TaqMan allelic discrimination real-time PCR. *J. Clin. Microbiol.* **42**:1409–1413.

14. **Carby, M., A. Jones, M. Burke, A. Hall, and N. Banner.** 2007. Varicella infection after heart and lung transplantation: a single-center experience. *J. Heart Lung Transplant.* **26**:399–402.

15. **Centers for Disease Control and Prevention.** 2003. Decline in annual incidence of varicella—selected states, 1990–2001. *MMWR Morb. Mortal. Wkly. Rep.* **52**:884–885.

16. **Chen, J. J., Z. Zhu, A. A. Gershon, and M. D. Gershon.** 2004. Mannose 6-phosphate receptor dependence of varicella zoster virus infection in vitro and in the epidermis during varicella and zoster. *Cell* **119**:915–926.

17. **Chris Maple, P. A., A. Gunn, J. Sellwood, D. W. Brown, and J. J. Gray.** 2009. Comparison of fifteen commercial assays for detecting Varicella Zoster virus IgG with reference to a time resolved fluorescence immunoassay (TRFIA) and the performance of two commercial assays for screening sera from immunocompromised individuals. *J. Virol. Methods* **155**:143–149.

18. **Cinque, P., S. Bossolasco, L. Vago, C. Fornara, S. Lipari, S. Racca, A. Lazzarin, and A. Linde.** 1997. Varicella-zoster virus (VZV) DNA in cerebrospinal fluid of patients infected with human immunodeficiency virus: VZV disease of the central nervous system or subclinical reactivation of VZV infection? *Clin. Infect. Dis.* **25**:634–639.

19. **Coen, D. M., and D. D. Richman.** 2007. Antiviral agents, p. 447–486. *In* D. M. Knipe, P. M. Howley, D. E. Griffin, R. A. Lamb, M. A. Martin, B. Roizman, and S. E. Straus (ed.), *Fields Virology*, 5th ed. Lippincott Williams and Wilkins, Philadelphia, PA.

20. **Coffin, S. E., and R. L. Hodinka.** 1995. Utility of direct immunofluorescence and virus culture for detection of varicella-zoster virus in skin lesions. *J. Clin. Microbiol.* **33**:2792–2795.

21. **Cohen, J., S. E. Straus, and A. M. Arvin.** 2007. Varicella zoster virus, replication, pathogenesis and management, p. 2773–2818. *In* D. M. Knipe, P. M. Howley, D. E. Griffin, R. A. Lamb, M. A. Martin, B. Roizman, and S. E. Straus (ed.), *Fields Virology*, 5th ed. Lippincott Williams and Wilkins, Philadelphia, PA.

22. **Cohrs, R. J., J. Randall, J. Smith, D. H. Gilden, C. Dabrowski, H. van Der Keyl, and R. Tal-Singer.** 2000. Analysis of individual human trigeminal ganglia for latent herpes simplex virus type 1 and varicella-zoster virus nucleic acids using real-time PCR. *J. Virol.* **74**:11464–11471.

23. **Cowl, C. T., U. B. S. Prakash, P. S. Mitchell, and M. R. Migden.** 2000. Varicella-zoster virus detection by polymerase chain reaction using bronchoalveolar lavage specimens. *Am. J. Respir. Crit. Care Med.* **162**:753–754.

24. **Davison, A. J., and J. E. Scott.** 1986. The complete DNA sequence of varicella-zoster virus. *J. Gen. Virol.* **67**(Pt. 9): 1759–1816.

25. **de Clercq, E., H. Degreef, J. Wildiers, G. de Jonge, A. Drochmans, J. Descamps, and P. de Somer.** 1980. Oral (E)-5-(2-bromovinyl)-2'-deoxyuridine in severe herpes zoster. *Br. Med. J.* **281**:1178.

26. **de Jong, M. D., J. F. Weel, T. Schuurman, P. M. Wertheim-van Dillen, and R. Boom.** 2000. Quantitation of varicella-zoster virus DNA in whole blood, plasma, and serum by PCR and electrochemiluminescence. *J. Clin. Microbiol.* **38**:2568–2573.

27. **de Ory, F., J. M. Echevarria, G. Kafatos, C. Anastassopoulou, N. Andrews, J. Backhouse, G. Berbers, B. Bruckova, D. I. Cohen, H. de Melker, I. Davidkin, G. Gabutti, L. M. Hesketh, K. Johansen, S. Jokinen, L. Jones, A. Linde, E. Miller, J. Mossong, A. Nardone, M. C. Rota, A. Sauerbrei, F. Schneider, Z. Smetana, A. Tischer, A. Tsakris, and R. Vranckx.** 2006. European seroepidemiology network 2: standardisation of assays for seroepidemiology of varicella zoster virus. *J. Clin. Virol.* **36**:111–118.

28. **Dobec, M., W. Bossart, F. Kaeppeli, and J. Mueller-Schoop.** 2008. Serology and serum DNA detection in shingles. *Swiss Med. Wkly.* **138**:47–51.

29. **Echevarria, J. M., I. Casas, A. Tenorio, F. de Ory, and P. Martinez-Martin.** 1994. Detection of varicella-zoster virus-specific DNA sequences in cerebrospinal fluid from patients with acute aseptic meningitis and no cutaneous lesions. *J. Med. Virol.* **43**:331–335.

30. **Enders, G., E. Miller, J. Cradock-Watson, I. Bolley, and M. Ridehalgh.** 1994. Consequences of varicella and herpes zoster in pregnancy: prospective study of 1739 cases. *Lancet* **343**:1548–1551.

31. **Espy, M. J., R. Teo, T. K. Ross, K. A. Svien, A. D. Wold, J. R. Uhl, and T. F. Smith.** 2000. Diagnosis of varicella-zoster virus infections in the clinical laboratory by LightCycler PCR. *J. Clin. Microbiol.* **38**:3187–3189.

32. **Feller, L., N. H. Wood, and J. Lemmer.** 2007. Herpes zoster infection as an immune reconstitution inflammatory syndrome in HIV-seropositive subjects: a review. *Oral. Surg. Oral. Med. Oral. Pathol. Oral. Radiol. Endod.* **104**:455–460.

33. **Fillet, A. M., B. Dumont, E. Caumes, B. Visse, H. Agut, F. Bricaire, and J. M. Huraux.** 1998. Acyclovir-resistant varicella-zoster virus: phenotypic and genetic characterization. *J. Med. Virol.* **55**:250–254.

34. **Franco-Paredes, C., T. Bellehemeur, A. Merchant, P. Sanghi, C. DiazGranados, and D. Rimland.** 2002. Aseptic meningitis and optic neuritis preceding varicella-zoster progressive outer retinal necrosis in a patient with AIDS. *AIDS* **16**:1045–1049.

35. **Frey, C. R., M. A. Sharp, A. S. Min, D. S. Schmid, V. Loparev, and A. M. Arvin.** 2003. Identification of CD8+ T cell epitopes in the immediate early 62 protein (IE62) of varicella-zoster virus, and evaluation of frequency of CD8+ T cell response to IE62, by use of IE62 peptides after varicella vaccination. *J. Infect. Dis.* **188**:40–52.

35a. **Furuta, Y., H. Aizawa, F. Ohtani, H. Sawa, and S. Fukuda.** 2004. Varicella-zoster virus DNA level and facial paralysis in Ramsay Hunt syndrome. *Ann. Otol. Rhinol. Laryngol.* **113**:700–705.

36. Furuta, Y., S. Fukuda, S. Suzuki, T. Takasu, Y. Inuyama, and K. Nagashima. 1997. Detection of varicella-zoster virus DNA in patients with acute peripheral facial palsy by the polymerase chain reaction, and its use for early diagnosis of zoster sine herpete. *J. Med. Virol.* **52**:316–319.

37. Furuta, Y., F. Ohtani, H. Kawabata, S. Fukuda, and T. Bergstrom. 2000. High prevalence of varicella-zoster virus reactivation in herpes simplex virus-seronegative patients with acute peripheral facial palsy. *Clin. Infect. Dis.* **30**:529–533.

38. Furuta, Y., F. Ohtani, H. Sawa, S. Fukuda, and Y. Inuyama. 2001. Quantitation of varicella-zoster virus DNA in patients with Ramsay Hunt syndrome and zoster sine herpete. *J. Clin. Microbiol.* **39**:2856–2859.

39. Galil, K., C. Brown, F. Lin, and J. Seward. 2002. Hospitalizations for varicella in the United States, 1988 to 1999. *Pediatr. Infect. Dis. J.* **21**:931–935.

40. Gershon, A., and S. Silverstein. 2002. Varicella-zoster virus, p. 413–432. *In* D. Richman, R. Whitley, and F. Hayden (ed.), *Clinical Virology*, 2nd ed. ASM Press, Washington, DC.

41. Gershon, A. A., P. Larussa, and S. Steinberg. 1994. Detection of antibodies to varicella-zoster virus using a latex agglutination assay. *Clin. Diagn. Virol.* **2**:271–277.

42. Gershon, A. A., S. P. Steinberg, and L. Gelb. 1984. Clinical reinfection with varicella-zoster virus. *J. Infect. Dis.* **149**:137–142.

43. Gilden, D. H., M. Devlin, M. Wellish, R. Mahalingham, C. Huff, A. Hayward, and A. Vafai. 1989. Persistence of varicella-zoster virus DNA in blood mononuclear cells of patients with varicella or zoster. *Virus Genes* **2**:299–305.

44. Gnann, J. W., Jr. 2002. Varicella-zoster virus: atypical presentations and unusual complications. *J. Infect. Dis.* **186**(Suppl. 1):S91–S98.

45. Gourishankar, S., J. C. McDermid, G. S. Jhangri, and J. K. Preiksaitis. 2004. Herpes zoster infection following solid organ transplantation: incidence, risk factors and outcomes in the current immunosuppressive era. *Am. J. Transplant.* **4**:108–115.

46. Grose, C., and P. A. Brunel. 1978. Varicella-zoster virus: isolation and propagation in human melanoma cells at 36 and 32 degrees C. *Infect. Immun.* **19**:199–203.

47. Hall, S., T. Maupin, J. Seward, A. O. Jumaan, C. Peterson, G. Goldman, L. Mascola, and M. Wharton. 2002. Second varicella infections: are they more common than previously thought? *Pediatrics* **109**:1068–1073.

48. Harpaz, R., I. R. Ortega-Sanchez, and J. F. Seward. 2008. Prevention of herpes zoster: recommendations of the Advisory Committee on Immunization Practices (ACIP). *MMWR Recommend. Rep.* **57**:1–30; quiz CE2–CE4.

49. Hudnall, S. D., T. Chen, P. Allison, S. K. Tyring, and A. Heath. 2008. Herpesvirus prevalence and viral load in healthy blood donors by quantitative real-time polymerase chain reaction. *Transfusion* **48**:1180–1187.

50. Ito, Y., H. Kimura, S. Hara, S. Kido, T. Ozaki, Y. Nishiyama, and T. Morishima. 2001. Investigation of varicella-zoster virus DNA in lymphocyte subpopulations by quantitative PCR assay. *Microbiol. Immunol.* **45**:267–269.

51. Kalpoe, J. S., A. C. Kroes, S. Verkerk, E. C. Claas, R. M. Barge, and M. F. Beersma. 2006. Clinical relevance of quantitative varicella-zoster virus (VZV) DNA detection in plasma after stem cell transplantation. *Bone Marrow Transplant.* **38**:41–46.

52. Kaneko, T., and Y. Ishigatsubo. 2004. Varicella pneumonia in adults. *Intern. Med.* **43**:1105–1106.

53. Kennedy, P. G., E. Grinfeld, and J. E. Bell. 2000. Varicella-zoster virus gene expression in latently infected and explanted human ganglia. *J. Virol.* **74**:11893–11898.

54. Kido, S., S. Sugita, S. Horie, M. Miyanaga, K. Miyata, N. Shimizu, T. Morio, and M. Mochizuki. 2008. Association of varicella zoster virus load in the aqueous humor with clinical manifestations of anterior uveitis in herpes zoster ophthalmicus and zoster sine herpete. *Br. J. Ophthalmol.* **92**:505–508.

55. Kimura, H., S. Kido, T. Ozaki, N. Tanaka, Y. Ito, R. K. Williams, and T. Morishima. 2000. Comparison of quantitations of viral load in varicella and zoster. *J. Clin. Microbiol.* **38**:2447–2449.

56. Koskiniemi, M., H. Piiparinen, T. Rantalaiho, P. Eranko, M. Farkkila, K. Raiha, E. M. Salonen, P. Ukkonen, and A. Vaheri. 2002. Acute central nervous system complications in varicella zoster virus infections. *J. Clin. Virol.* **25**:293–301.

57. Kronenberg, A., W. Bossart, R. P. Wuthrich, C. Cao, S. Lautenschlager, N. D. Wiegand, B. Mullhaupt, G. Noll, N. J. Mueller, and R. F. Speck. 2005. Retrospective analysis of varicella zoster virus (VZV) copy DNA numbers in plasma of immunocompetent patients with herpes zoster, of immunocompromised patients with disseminated VZV disease, and of asymptomatic solid organ transplant recipients. *Transpl. Infect. Dis.* **7**:116–121.

58. Kupila, L., T. Vuorinen, R. Vainionpaa, V. Hukkanen, R. J. Marttila, and P. Kotilainen. 2006. Etiology of aseptic meningitis and encephalitis in an adult population. *Neurology* **66**:75–80.

59. LaRussa, P., O. Lungu, I. Hardy, A. Gershon, S. P. Steinberg, and S. Silverstein. 1992. Restriction fragment length polymorphism of polymerase chain reaction products from vaccine and wild-type varicella-zoster virus isolates. *J. Virol.* **66**:1016–1020.

60. Larussa, P., S. Steinberg, E. Waithe, B. Hanna, and R. Holzman. 1987. Comparison of five assays for antibody to varicella-zoster virus and the fluorescent-antibody-to-membrane-antigen test. *J. Clin. Microbiol.* **25**:2059–2062.

61. Li, S., I. S. Chan, H. Matthews, J. F. Heyse, C. Y. Chan, B. J. Kuter, K. M. Kaplan, S. J. Vessey, and J. C. Sadoff. 2002. Inverse relationship between six week postvaccination varicella antibody response to vaccine and likelihood of long term breakthrough infection. *Pediatr. Infect. Dis. J.* **21**:337–342.

62. Loparev, V. N., K. McCaustland, B. P. Holloway, P. R. Krause, M. Takayama, and D. S. Schmid. 2000. Rapid genotyping of varicella-zoster virus vaccine and wild-type strains with fluorophore-labeled hybridization probes. *J. Clin. Microbiol.* **38**:4315–4319.

63. Loparev, V. N., E. N. Rubtcova, V. Bostik, D. Govil, C. J. Birch, J. D. Druce, D. S. Schmid, and M. C. Croxson. 2007. Identification of five major and two minor genotypes of varicella-zoster virus strains: a practical two-amplicon approach used to genotype clinical isolates in Australia and New Zealand. *J. Virol.* **81**:12758–12765.

64. Mahalingam, R., M. Wellish, W. Wolf, A. N. Dueland, R. Cohrs, A. Vafai, and D. Gilden. 1990. Latent varicella-zoster viral DNA in human trigeminal and thoracic ganglia. *N. Engl. J. Med.* **323**:627–631.

65. Mainka, C., B. Fuss, H. Geiger, H. Hofelmayr, and M. H. Wolff. 1998. Characterization of viremia at different stages of varicella-zoster virus infection. *J. Med. Virol.* **56**:91–98.

66. Malavige, G. N., L. Jones, S. D. Kamaladasa, A. Wijewickrama, S. L. Seneviratne, A. P. Black, and G. S. Ogg. 2008. Viral load, clinical disease severity and cellular immune responses in primary varicella zoster virus infection in Sri Lanka. *PLoS One* **3**:e3789.

67. Maple, P. A., J. Gray, J. Breuer, G. Kafatos, S. Parker, and D. Brown. 2006. Performance of a time-resolved fluorescence immunoassay for measuring varicella-zoster virus immunoglobulin G levels in adults and comparison with commercial enzyme immunoassays and Merck glycoprotein enzyme immunoassay. *Clin. Vaccine Immunol.* **13**:214–218.

68. Marin, M., T. L. Watson, S. S. Chaves, R. Civen, B. M. Watson, J. X. Zhang, D. Perella, L. Mascola, and J. F. Seward. 2008. Varicella among adults: data from an active surveillance project, 1995–2005. *J. Infect. Dis.* **197**(Suppl. 2):S94–S100.

69. Markoulatos, P., A. Georgopoulou, N. Siafakas, E. Plakokefalos, G. Tzanakaki, and J. Kourea-Kremastinou. 2001. Laboratory diagnosis of common herpesvirus infections of the central nervous system by a multiplex PCR assay. *J. Clin. Microbiol.* **39**:4426–4432.

70. McGeoch, D. J. 2009. Lineages of varicella-zoster virus. *J. Gen. Virol.* **90**:963–969.

71. Miller, G. G., and J. S. Dummer. 2007. Herpes simplex and varicella zoster viruses: forgotten but not gone. *Am. J. Transplant.* **7**:741–747.

72. **Murakami, S., Y. Nakashiro, M. Mizobuchi, N. Hato, N. Honda, and K. Gyo.** 1998. Varicella-zoster virus distribution in Ramsay Hunt syndrome revealed by polymerase chain reaction. *Acta Otolaryngol.* **118:**145–149.

73. **Nardone, A., F. de Ory, M. Carton, D. Cohen, P. van Damme, I. Davidkin, M. C. Rota, H. de Melker, J. Mossong, M. Slacikova, A. Tischer, N. Andrews, G. Berbers, G. Gabutti, N. Gay, L. Jones, S. Jokinen, G. Kafatos, M. V. de Aragon, F. Schneider, Z. Smetana, B. Vargova, R. Vranckx, and E. Miller.** 2007. The comparative seroepidemiology of varicella zoster virus in 11 countries in the European region. *Vaccine* **25:**7866–7872.

74. **Nikkels, A. F., K. Delbecque, G. E. Pierard, B. Wienkotter, G. Schalasta, and M. Enders.** 2005. Distribution of varicella-zoster virus DNA and gene products in tissues of a first-trimester varicella-infected fetus. *J. Infect. Dis.* **191:**540–545.

75. **Parker, S. P., M. Quinlivan, Y. Taha, and J. Breuer.** 2006. Genotyping of varicella-zoster virus and the discrimination of Oka vaccine strains by TaqMan real-time PCR. *J. Clin. Microbiol.* **44:**3911–3914.

76. **Persson, A., T. Bergstrom, M. Lindh, L. Namvar, and M. Studahl.** 2009. Varicella-zoster virus CNS disease—viral load, clinical manifestations and sequel. *J. Clin. Virol.* **46:**249–253.

77. **Pevenstein, S. R., R. K. Williams, D. McChesney, E. K. Mont, J. E. Smialek, and S. E. Straus.** 1999. Quantitation of latent varicella-zoster virus and herpes simplex virus genomes in human trigeminal ganglia. *J. Virol.* **73:**10514–10518.

78. **Preissner, C. M., S. P. Steinberg, A. A. Gershon, and T. F. Smith.** 1982. Evaluation of the anticomplement immunofluorescence test for detection of antibody to varicella-zoster virus. *J. Clin. Microbiol.* **16:**373–376.

79. **Puchhammer-Stöckl, E., C. Kunz, G. Wagner, and G. Enders.** 1994. Detection of varicella zoster virus (VZV) DNA in fetal tissue by polymerase chain reaction. *J. Perinat. Med.* **22:**65–69.

80. **Puchhammer-Stöckl, E., T. Popow-Kraupp, F. X. Heinz, C. W. Mandl, and C. Kunz.** 1991. Detection of varicella-zoster virus DNA by polymerase chain reaction in the cerebrospinal fluid of patients suffering from neurological complications associated with chicken pox or herpes zoster. *J. Clin. Microbiol.* **29:**1513–1516.

81. **Quinlivan, M., and J. Breuer.** 2006. Molecular studies of Varicella zoster virus. *Rev. Med. Virol.* **16:**225–250.

82. **Quinlivan, M., A. A. Gershon, S. P. Steinberg, and J. Breuer.** 2005. An evaluation of single nucleotide polymorphisms used to differentiate vaccine and wild type strains of varicella-zoster virus. *J. Med. Virol.* **75:**174–180.

83. **Quinlivan, M., K. Hawrami, W. Barrett-Muir, P. Aaby, A. Arvin, V. T. Chow, T. J. John, P. Matondo, M. Peiris, A. Poulsen, M. Siqueira, M. Takahashi, Y. Talukder, K. Yamanishi, M. Leedham-Green, F. T. Scott, S. L. Thomas, and J. Breuer.** 2002. The molecular epidemiology of varicella-zoster virus: evidence for geographic segregation. *J. Infect. Dis.* **186:**888–894.

84. **Quinlivan, M. L., K. Ayres, H. Ran, S. McElwaine, M. Leedham-Green, F. T. Scott, R. W. Johnson, and J. Breuer.** 2007. Effect of viral load on the outcome of herpes zoster. *J. Clin. Microbiol.* **45:**3909–3914.

85. **Rau, R., C. D. Fitzhugh, K. Baird, K. J. Cortez, L. Li, S. H. Fischer, E. W. Cowen, J. E. Balow, T. J. Walsh, J. I. Cohen, and A. S. Wayne.** 2008. Triad of severe abdominal pain, inappropriate antidiuretic hormone secretion, and disseminated varicella-zoster virus infection preceding cutaneous manifestations after hematopoietic stem cell transplantation: utility of PCR for early recognition and therapy. *Pediatr. Infect. Dis. J.* **27:**265–268.

86. **Roque-Afonso, A. M., M. P. Bralet, P. Ichai, D. Desbois, P. Vaghefi, D. Castaing, D. Samuel, and E. Dussaix.** 2008. Chickenpox-associated fulminant hepatitis that led to liver transplantation in a 63-year-old woman. *Liver Transplant.* **14:**1309–1312.

87. **Ruzek, D., N. Piskunova, and E. Zampachova.** 2007. High variability in viral load in cerebrospinal fluid from patients with herpes simplex and varicella-zoster infections of the central nervous system. *Clin. Microbiol. Infect.* **13:**1217–1219.

88. **Sadaoka, K., S. Okamoto, Y. Gomi, T. Tanimoto, T. Ishikawa, T. Yoshikawa, Y. Asano, K. Yamanishi, and Y. Mori.** 2008. Measurement of varicella-zoster virus (VZV)-specific cell-mediated immunity: comparison between VZV skin test and interferon-gamma enzyme-linked immunospot assay. *J. Infect. Dis.* **198:**1327–1333.

89. **Saiman, L., P. LaRussa, S. P. Steinberg, J. Zhou, K. Baron, S. Whittier, P. Della-Latta, and A. A. Gershon.** 2001. Persistence of immunity to varicella-zoster virus after vaccination of healthcare workers. *Infect. Control Hosp. Epidemiol.* **22:**279–283.

90. **Sauerbrei, A., U. Eichhorn, S. Gawellek, R. Egerer, M. Schacke, and P. Wutzler.** 2003. Molecular characterisation of varicella-zoster virus strains in Germany and differentiation from the Oka vaccine strain. *J. Med. Virol.* **71:**313–319.

91. **Sauerbrei, A., and P. Wutzler.** 2006. Serological detection of varicella-zoster virus-specific immunoglobulin G by an enzyme-linked immunosorbent assay using glycoprotein antigen. *J. Clin. Microbiol.* **44:**3094–3097.

92. **Sauerbrei, A., R. Zell, and P. Wutzler.** 2007. Analysis of repeat units in the R2 region among different Oka varicella-zoster virus vaccine strains and wild-type strains in Germany. *Intervirology* **50:**40–44.

93. **Schunemann, S., C. Mainka, and M. H. Wolff.** 1998. Subclinical reactivation of varicella-zoster virus in immunocompromised and immunocompetent individuals. *Intervirology* **41:**98–102.

94. **Sengupta, N., R. Booy, H. J. Schmitt, H. Peltola, P. Van-Damme, R. F. Schumacher, M. Campins, C. Rodrigo, T. Heikkinen, J. Seward, A. Jumaan, A. Finn, P. Olcen, N. Thiry, C. Weil-Olivier, and J. Breuer.** 2008. Varicella vaccination in Europe: are we ready for a universal childhood programme? *Eur. J. Pediatr.* **167:**47–55.

95. **Seward, J. F., B. M. Watson, C. L. Peterson, L. Mascola, J. W. Pelosi, J. X. Zhang, T. J. Maupin, G. S. Goldman, L. J. Tabony, K. G. Brodovicz, A. O. Jumaan, and M. Wharton.** 2002. Varicella disease after introduction of varicella vaccine in the United States, 1995–2000. *JAMA* **287:**606–611.

96. **Smith, C. K., and A. M. Arvin.** 2009. Varicella in the fetus and newborn. *Semin. Fetal Neonatal Med.* **14:**209–217.

97. **Snoeck, R., G. Andrei, and E. De Clercq.** 1994. Chemotherapy of varicella zoster virus infections. *Int. J. Antimicrob. Agents* **4:**211–226.

98. **Stjernquist-Desatnik, A., E. Skoog, and E. Aurelius.** 2006. Detection of herpes simplex and varicella-zoster viruses in patients with Bell's palsy by the polymerase chain reaction technique. *Ann. Otol. Rhinol. Laryngol.* **115:**306–311.

99. **Stöcher, M., V. Leb, M. Bozic, H. H. Kessler, G. Halwachs-Baumann, O. Landt, H. Stekel, and J. Berg.** 2003. Parallel detection of five human herpes virus DNAs by a set of real-time polymerase chain reactions in a single run. *J. Clin. Virol.* **26:**85–93.

100. **Straus, S. E., J. Hay, H. Smith, and J. Owens.** 1983. Genome differences among varicella-zoster virus isolates. *J. Gen. Virol.* **64:**1031–1041.

101. **Styczynski, J., P. Reusser, H. Einsele, R. de la Camara, C. Cordonnier, K. N. Ward, P. Ljungman, and D. Engelhard.** 2009. Management of HSV, VZV and EBV infections in patients with hematological malignancies and after SCT: guidelines from the Second European Conference on Infections in Leukemia. *Bone Marrow Transplant.* **43:**757–770.

102. **Suzutani, T., M. Saijo, M. Nagamine, M. Ogasawara, and M. Azuma.** 2000. Rapid phenotypic characterization method for herpes simplex virus and varicella-zoster virus thymidine kinases to screen for acyclovir-resistant viral infection. *J. Clin. Microbiol.* **38:**1839–1844.

103. **Takayama, M., and N. Takayama.** 2004. New method of differentiating wild-type varicella-zoster virus (VZV) strains from Oka varicella vaccine strain by VZV ORF 6-based PCR and restriction fragment length polymorphism analysis. *J. Clin. Virol.* **29:**113–119.

104. **Talarico, C. L., W. C. Phelps, and K. K. Biron.** 1993. Analysis of the thymidine kinase genes from acyclovir-resistant mutants of varicella-zoster virus isolated from patients with AIDS. *J. Virol.* **67:**1024–1033.

105. **Terada, K., T. Niizuma, S. Kawano, N. Kataoka, T. Akisada, and Y. Orita.** 1998. Detection of varicella-zoster virus DNA in peripheral mononuclear cells from patients with Ramsay Hunt syndrome or zoster sine herpete. *J. Med. Virol.* **56:**359–363.

106. **Tipples, G. A., D. Safronetz, and M. Gray.** 2003. A real-time PCR assay for the detection of varicella-zoster virus DNA and differentiation of vaccine, wild-type and control strains. *J. Virol. Methods* **113:**113–116.

107. **Vafai, A., and M. Berger.** 2001. Zoster in patients infected with HIV: a review. *Am. J. Med. Sci.* **321:**372–380.

108. **van der Maas, N. A., P. E. Bondt, H. de Melker, and J. M. Kemmeren.** 2009. Acute cerebellar ataxia in the Netherlands: a study on the association with vaccinations and varicella zoster infection. *Vaccine* **27:**1970–1973.

109. **van Doornum, G. J., J. Guldemeester, A. D. Osterhaus, and H. G. Niesters.** 2003. Diagnosing herpesvirus infections by real-time amplification and rapid culture. *J. Clin. Microbiol.* **41:**576–580.

110. **Vazquez, M., P. S. LaRussa, A. A. Gershon, S. P. Steinberg, K. Freudigman, and E. D. Shapiro.** 2001. The effectiveness of the varicella vaccine in clinical practice. *N. Engl. J. Med.* **344:**955–960.

111. **Vossen, M. T., M. R. Gent, J. F. Weel, M. D. de Jong, R. A. van Lier, and T. W. Kuijpers.** 2004. Development of virus-specific CD4+ T cells on reexposure to Varicella-Zoster virus. *J. Infect. Dis.* **190:**72–82.

112. **Weidmann, M., K. Armbruster, and F. T. Hufert.** 2008. Challenges in designing a Taqman-based multiplex assay for the simultaneous detection of Herpes simplex virus types 1 and 2 and Varicella-zoster virus. *J. Clin. Virol.* **42:**326–334.

113. **Williams, V., A. Gershon, and P. A. Brunell.** 1974. Serologic response to varicella-zoster membrane antigens measured by direct immunofluorescence. *J. Infect. Dis.* **130:**669–672.

114. **Yamakawa, K., M. Hamada, and T. Takeda.** 2007. Different real-time PCR assays could lead to a different result of detection of varicella-zoster virus in facial palsy. *J. Virol. Methods* **139:**227–229.

115. **Zaia, J., L. Baden, M. J. Boeckh, S. Chakrabarti, H. Einsele, P. Ljungman, G. B. McDonald, and H. Hirsch.** 2009. Viral disease prevention after hematopoietic cell transplantation. *Bone Marrow Transplant.* **44:**471–482.

Human Cytomegalovirus

RICHARD L. HODINKA

98

TAXONOMY

Human cytomegalovirus (CMV), formally designated human herpesvirus 5 (HHV-5) by the International Committee on Taxonomy of Viruses, is a member of the family *Herpesviridae*, which includes herpes simplex virus types 1 (HHV-1) and 2 (HHV-2), varicella-zoster virus (HHV-3), Epstein-Barr virus (HHV-4), and human herpesviruses 6, 7, and 8. It is classified in the subfamily *Betaherpesvirinae* with cytomegaloviruses of other animal species based on its tropism for salivary glands, slow growth in cell culture, and strict species specificity. Human CMV is the type species of the genus *Cytomegalovirus*, and its name is derived from the enlargement of cells (cyto = cell, mega = large) infected by the virus. Regions of genome sequence homology between CMV and herpesviruses 6 and 7 have been identified, and HHV-6 and HHV-7 are now classified with CMV among the betaherpesviruses.

DESCRIPTION OF THE AGENT

Complete CMV particles have a diameter of 120 to 200 nm and consist of a core containing a 220- to 240-kb linear double-stranded DNA genome, an icosahedral capsid with 162 capsomeres, an amorphous tegument or matrix, and a surrounding phospholipid-rich envelope. The CMV genome consists of more than 200 open reading frames that encode structural and regulatory proteins and proteins that function to modulate the immune system of the host. Electron microscopic features of CMV include virions morphologically indistinguishable from those of other herpesviruses, a high ratio of defective viral particles, and the presence of spherical particles called dense bodies. Viral replication occurs in the nucleus of the host cell and involves the expression of immediate-early (α), early (β), and late (γ) classes of genes. The viral envelope is formed as assembled nucleocapsids bud from the inner surface of the nuclear membrane.

Molecular and immunologic techniques have been used to study variation among CMV strains. Although it has been shown that different strains of CMV are 95% homologous to the standard laboratory reference strains AD-169 and Towne, genetically distinct CMV genotypes that display polymorphisms in multiple coding and noncoding regions of the virus genome have been identified. Strain diversity has been associated with specific differences in geographic distribution, transmission, tissue tropism, immunopathogenesis, and clinical manifestations of disease, but the exact role and importance of CMV genotypes in infection and disease are largely unknown (for a review, see reference 96).

CMV is inactivated by a number of physical and chemical treatments, including heat (56°C for 30 min), low pH, lipid solvents, UV light, and cycles of freezing and thawing.

EPIDEMIOLOGY AND TRANSMISSION

CMV has a worldwide distribution and infects humans of all ages, with no seasonal or epidemic patterns of transmission. The seroprevalence of CMV increases with age in all populations and ranges from 40 to 100%; the virus is acquired earlier in life, and the prevalence is highest among lower socioeconomic groups in crowded living conditions. CMV can be transmitted vertically and horizontally, and infections are classified as being acquired before birth (congenital), at the time of delivery (perinatal), or later in life (postnatal).

Most infections are acquired by direct close personal contact with individuals who are shedding virus. Since CMV has been detected in many body fluids, including saliva, urine, breast milk, tears, stool, vaginal and cervical secretions, blood, and semen, it is clear that transmission can occur in a variety of ways. Prolonged shedding of virus after congenital or acquired CMV infection contributes to the ease of virus spread; virus may be excreted for weeks, months, or even years following a primary infection.

Transplacental infection of the fetus can occur following primary or recurrent infection of a pregnant woman, but the risk of CMV transmission to the fetus and the rate of symptomatic fetal infection are much higher with primary maternal infection. The incidence of fetal damage is highest if infection occurs during the first 12 to 16 weeks of pregnancy. Newborns can also acquire infection at the time of delivery by contact with virus in the birth canal. Nearly 10% of women shed CMV in the genital tract at or near the time of delivery, and virus is transmitted to approximately 50% of the newborns. Such infants begin to excrete virus at 3 to 12 weeks of age but usually remain asymptomatic. Mother-to-infant transmission of CMV through breast milk is very common; low-birth-weight premature infants are at greatest risk for developing disease. Of children who attend day care centers and enter as toddlers, 20 to 70% experience

CMV infection over a 1- to 2-year period. Infection is usually asymptomatic, but the children may transmit CMV to their parents and other caregivers, posing a risk to an unborn fetus if a woman is pregnant at the time. In adolescents and adults, sexual transmission of CMV may occur and is an important route of CMV spread.

Similar to infections with other herpesviruses, primary infection with CMV results in the establishment of a persistent or latent infection. The sites of latent infection are thought to include various tissues, endothelial cells, and leukocytes. Therefore, CMV can be transmitted by blood transfusion and organ transplantation. Reactivation of the virus can occur in response to different stimuli, particularly immunosuppression.

CLINICAL SIGNIFICANCE

CMV infections are common and usually asymptomatic in otherwise healthy children and adults; however, the incidence and spectrum of disease in newborns and in immunocompromised hosts establish this virus as an important human pathogen.

CMV infection has been detected in 0.2 to 2.5% of newborn infants and is the most common identified cause of congenital infection. Approximately 10 to 15% of congenitally infected infants develop symptoms during the newborn period; possible manifestations range from severe disease with any combination of intrauterine growth retardation, jaundice, hepatosplenomegaly, petechiae, thrombocytopenic purpura, myocarditis, pneumonitis, central nervous system abnormalities, deafness, and chorioretinitis to more limited involvement. Symptomatic infants may die of complications within the first months of life; more commonly, they survive but are neurologically damaged. It is now recognized that even congenitally infected infants who are asymptomatic at birth may develop sensorineural hearing loss, visual impairment, or psychomotor and/or intellectual disabilities later in life. Thus far, it appears that perinatally infected infants do not develop late neurologic sequelae of infection.

The vast majority of immunocompetent children and adults who acquire CMV infection postnatally remain asymptomatic. In high-risk premature newborns infected as a result of blood transfusions, morbidity and mortality can be significant and hepatosplenomegaly, thrombocytopenia, atypical lymphocytosis, and hemolytic anemia have been described. Symptoms in young adults can mimic the infectious mononucleosis syndrome caused by Epstein-Barr virus and include prolonged fever (persisting for 2 to 3 weeks), malaise, an atypical lymphocytosis, and mild hepatitis without the production of heterophile antibody. A link between CMV infection in the immunocompetent host and atherosclerosis has been suggested, and there is growing evidence that CMV is a contributing factor to vascular disease in certain individuals (for a review, see reference 86). More recently, there has been an increase in the number of reports of severe CMV infection associated with poor outcomes in hospitalized immunocompetent patients (89, 98).

CMV infections are frequent and occasionally severe in children or adults with congenital or acquired defects of cellular immunity, such as patients with AIDS, cancer patients (particularly those with leukemia and lymphoma receiving chemotherapy), and recipients of solid-organ and hematopoietic stem cell transplants. Infections in these patients may be due to reactivation of latent virus or primary infection or reinfection with exogenous virus, which may be introduced by blood transfusions or by the grafted organ. Symptoms tend to be most severe after primary infection; however, reactivation infection or reinfection in a severely immunocompromised host may also cause serious illness. Active infection usually occurs between 1 and 4 months after transplantation, when patients are at the height of their immunosuppression, or when CD4$^+$ lymphocyte counts drop below 50 to 100 cells/μl for individuals infected with HIV. The widespread use of antiviral drugs for prophylaxis or preemptive therapy following transplantation has resulted in the emergence of late-onset (>90 days posttransplant) CMV disease (for a review, see reference 60). The frequency and severity of CMV infection in organ transplant recipients are variable and depend on the type of transplant, the source of the donated organ, the immune status of the recipient, and the duration of the immunosuppressive therapy. The major symptoms in these patients usually include fever, malaise, lethargy, myalgia or arthralgia, leukopenia, thrombocytopenia, and hepatitis. Specific organ damage may lead to pneumonitis in recipients of lung or heart-lung transplants; the development of myocarditis, retinitis, or accelerated vascular damage and atherosclerosis after cardiac transplantation; hepatitis and pancreatitis in liver and pancreas transplant recipients, respectively; and gastrointestinal disease. CMV infection in transplant recipients has also been associated with delayed or failed bone marrow engraftment, an increased incidence or severity of graft-versus-host disease, and an increased risk of graft rejection in solid-organ transplants. Death may occur as a result of various complications, including bacterial and fungal superinfections. CMV infection, particularly when associated with pneumonitis, is an important cause of morbidity and mortality after hematopoietic stem cell transplantation. In patients infected with HIV, CMV is an important cause of fever, sight-threatening retinitis, encephalitis, polyradiculomyelopathy, and gastrointestinal infections including esophagitis, gastritis, and ulcerative colitis. However, there has been a significant decline in severe CMV disease in AIDS patients with the introduction of highly active antiretroviral therapy.

Antiviral drugs, including ganciclovir, valganciclovir, foscarnet, cidofovir, and fomivirsen, have been licensed by the U.S. Food and Drug Administration (FDA) for treatment of CMV retinitis in immunocompromised hosts, particularly in patients with AIDS. Ganciclovir, valganciclovir, valacyclovir, cidofovir, and foscarnet have been used with or without immunoglobulin products containing CMV-specific antibodies in various strategies as universal prophylaxis, preemptive therapy, and treatment for CMV disease in transplant recipients (for a review, see reference 102). Experience in using these antiviral drugs in the settings of congenital and perinatal CMV infection is limited. There are currently no licensed vaccines available for prevention of CMV disease. A number of candidate vaccines have been developed and are in various stages of preclinical and clinical evaluation (for a review, see reference 109).

COLLECTION, TRANSPORT, AND STORAGE OF SPECIMENS

At present, a variety of methods are available for use in the diagnosis and management of patients infected with CMV. These include isolation of the virus in cell culture, histologic and cytologic techniques, assays for the direct detection and/or quantification of viral proteins or nucleic acids, serologic tests, and phenotypic and genotypic tests to screen for antiviral drug resistance. The selection of assays to perform and the choice of specimen(s) to be tested depend on the patient population and clinical situation and the intended use of the individual tests.

Specimens for Direct Detection

Tissue specimens, respiratory secretions, urine sediment, cerebrospinal fluid (CSF), umbilical cord blood, amniotic fluid, aqueous humor and vitreous fluid, and peripheral blood leukocytes have been used for the direct detection of CMV antigens or nucleic acids from various patient populations. Blood specimens have proven most useful for identification and monitoring of CMV disease in immunocompromised hosts. Purified blood leukocytes are used when performing the CMV antigenemia assay, while whole blood, plasma obtained from anticoagulated whole blood, serum obtained from clotted blood, or purified peripheral blood leukocytes have all been used to quantify CMV DNA in molecular amplification assays (26, 81, 101, 115). EDTA is currently the preferred anticoagulant for molecular testing since it is considered to be the most effective stabilizer of nucleic acids in blood. The optimal frequency of blood collection remains to be established for surveillance of different patient groups, although it is common practice to submit blood specimens once or twice a week to monitor viral loads during preemptive antiviral therapy (102). There is considerable debate about which blood compartment is best suited for the detection of CMV DNA (35, 62). The most experience to date is with peripheral blood leukocytes and plasma. More recently, whole blood has been shown to yield the highest levels of CMV DNA of all blood compartments examined (101) and may represent the most practical specimen for laboratories to process for use in the diagnosis and monitoring of CMV disease since it requires little processing prior to extraction of the DNA. Also, delays in sample preparation can result in lysis of leukocytes after blood collection, which may result in inaccurate quantification of CMV DNA if either purified leukocytes or plasma is used as a specimen source (106). A potential limitation for the use of whole blood is the possibility of variation in leukocyte counts from patient to patient; this may lead to erroneous quantitative measurements if fluctuations in cell numbers are not taken into consideration. Plasma may be preferable in neutropenic patients who may have inadequate numbers of leukocytes for testing. For the CMV antigenemia assay, a total of 4 to 7 ml of whole blood is usually recommended for collection, but at least 10 ml of blood may be required for patients with severe neutropenia (e.g., absolute neutrophil counts of less than 200/mm^3). Any type of anticoagulated blood can be used, including blood collected in heparin, EDTA, sodium citrate, or acid citrate dextrose, although the most extensive experience has been with using heparin or EDTA. The blood should be kept at 4°C during storage and transport and should be processed within 6 to 8 h of collection for accurate and reliable quantification of the viral load and within 24 h and no later than 48 h for qualitative testing (69). A decrease in quantitative antigenemia levels after storage of blood specimens for 24 h to 48 h has been described, although most positive specimens remain positive after this time when held at 4°C (15, 69). Specimens for molecular amplification should be stored at 4°C immediately after collection and then promptly transported to the laboratory for processing. Single-use aliquots of processed specimens should be placed in multiple cryovials for testing and storage. By processing in this manner, specimens are not frozen and thawed repeatedly and are never returned to the original specimen cryovial, thereby avoiding possible degradation of the DNA and cross-contamination of specimens, respectively. If not tested immediately, specimens should be promptly frozen and stored at −70°C. Impression smears, frozen sections, or formaldehyde-fixed and paraffin-embedded material can be used for in situ hybridization or histopathologic examination of tissue specimens obtained from patients with pneumonia, gastrointestinal disease, hepatitis, myocarditis, retinitis, pancreatitis, nephritis, cystitis, or central nervous system disease. For prenatal diagnosis of congenital CMV infection, collection of amniotic fluid has largely replaced chorionic villus sampling or cordocentesis to collect fetal blood. Amniotic fluid should be collected after 21 to 23 weeks of fetal gestation for best sensitivity (64). Neonatal blood collected at birth and dried on paper (e.g., Guthrie cards) has recently been described for neonatal screening and for retrospective diagnosis in patients beyond the neonatal period with a clinical suspicion of congenital CMV infection (9, 129).

Specimens for Virus Isolation

CMV can be isolated from a variety of body fluids; however, urine, respiratory secretions (e.g., saliva, throat washings, and bronchoalveolar lavage fluid), and anticoagulated whole blood (leukocytes) are most common for diagnostic purposes. Urine specimens should be clean-voided specimens. Because excretion of CMV in urine is intermittent, increased recovery of the virus is possible by processing more than one specimen. Adjustment of urine specimens to pH 7.0 with 0.1 N NaOH or 0.1 N HCl is recommended to reduce toxicity to cell cultures. Centrifuging urine specimens to obtain sediment-enriched samples has been advocated but is usually unnecessary and may produce toxicity more frequently than do uncentrifuged urine samples. In the evaluation of immunocompromised patients, blood leukocyte cultures are particularly useful. Detection of CMV in leukocytes is often a better indicator of symptomatic CMV infection than is shedding of virus in urine or respiratory secretions. Fresh blood collected in the presence of heparin, sodium citrate, acid citrate dextrose, or EDTA may be used. A number of procedures for obtaining peripheral blood leukocytes have been described. However, density gradient centrifugation with either Ficoll-Hypaque or a mixture of sodium metrizoate and dextran 500 is most suitable for a clinical laboratory. Both mononuclear cells and granulocytes are efficiently separated from erythrocytes in a single step. The procedure is rapid and easy to perform, and the reagents are commercially available. Compared with traditional sedimentation methods, the technique results in a greater number of virus isolates and an increased yield of infectious foci or plaques. Alternatively, the direct lysis procedure described below may be used, although a reduced ability to culture CMV following direct erythrocyte lysis has been reported (66). Bronchial washings and tissue biopsy and autopsy specimens, particularly of lungs, kidneys, spleen, liver, brain, the gastrointestinal tract, and retinas, also can be processed for virus isolation. Recovery of CMV from tissues is strong evidence for organ involvement. All tissue specimens should be placed in a suitable viral transport medium immediately after collection. The details of specimen collection and processing are given in chapter 76. Since CMV loses infectivity when subjected to freezing and thawing, specimens for virus isolation should be kept at 4°C in an ice-water bath or refrigerator until they can be used to inoculate cultures, preferably within a few hours after collection. When prolonged transport times are unavoidable, infectivity is reasonably well preserved for at least 48 h at 4°C. In general, it is never a good idea to hold specimens for CMV isolation at room temperature and specimens should be transported to the laboratory as quickly as possible after collection to maintain viability of the virus. If freezing the specimen is necessary, an equal volume of 0.4 M sucrose-phosphate added to the specimen helps preserve viral infectivity. All frozen specimens should be stored at −60 to −80°C or in liquid nitrogen. Loss of virus infectivity occurs if specimens are stored at −20°C. All specimens are treated with antibiotics before inoculation of cell cultures.

Specimens for Serologic Testing

Single serum specimens for immunoglobulin G (IgG) antibody are useful in screening for evidence of past infection with CMV and for identifying individuals at risk for CMV infection. This approach is especially helpful in testing sera from organ transplant donors and recipients and from donors of blood products that are to be administered to premature infants or bone marrow transplant patients. Also, knowing the immune status of women prior to conception may be helpful in identifying those individuals who may be most susceptible to primary CMV infection following pregnancy. For serologic diagnosis of recent CMV infection, detection of IgM in a single serum specimen may be beneficial or paired sera should be obtained at least 2 weeks apart when testing for IgG antibody. The acute-phase serum sample should be collected as soon as possible after onset of illness and tested simultaneously with the convalescent-phase serum sample. If congenital infection is suspected, specimens from mother, fetus, and newborn can be submitted for the evaluation of IgG and IgM antibodies for the detection of prenatal, natal, and postnatal CMV infections. When testing for IgM in the fetus, blood should be collected after 22 weeks of gestation since fetal synthesis of antibodies starts at 20 weeks of gestation and may not reach detectable levels for 1 to 2 more weeks. Testing saliva or oral fluids for CMV-specific antibodies has been suggested as a noninvasive alternative to the collection of blood from children (2). In patients with CMV neurologic disease, CSF may be tested for viral antibody if paired with a serum specimen collected on or close to the same date. However, the yield of such testing is low and limited by delays in intrathecal production of virus-specific antibody and passive transfer of serum antibodies across a damaged blood-brain barrier.

DIRECT EXAMINATION

Histopathologic Testing

Histologic examination of Wright-Giemsa-, hematoxylin and eosin-, or Papanicolaou-stained biopsy specimens can be useful in the diagnosis of localized CMV organ disease. Characteristic large cells (cytomegalic cells) with basophilic intranuclear inclusions and, on occasion, eosinophilic cytoplasmic inclusions can be seen in routine sections of biopsy or autopsy material (Fig. 1). The nuclear inclusion has the appearance of an "owl's eye" because it has marginated chromatin that is typically surrounded by a clear halo that extends to the nuclear membrane. The presence of characteristic cytologic changes suggests CMV infection and correlates with active disease in most cases, although additional virologic or serologic confirmation is suggested. Overall, histopathologic diagnosis of CMV disease involves time and labor and is relatively insensitive, and since CMV can infect tissues without producing morphologic changes,

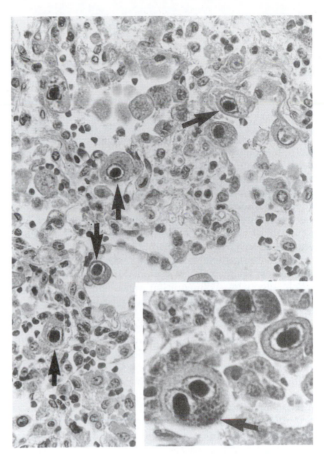

FIGURE 1 Fixed hematoxylin-eosin-stained lung tissue from a patient with interstitial pneumonia. Note the numerous giant cells that possess large intranuclear inclusions surrounded by characteristically clear halos (arrows). Less pronounced granular inclusions may also be present in the cytoplasm (inset). (Courtesy of Eduardo Ruchelli.)

failure to find typical cytomegalic cells does not exclude the possibility of CMV infection. The sensitivity of histopathologic testing can be increased somewhat by using immunohistochemical staining to detect CMV antigens or in situ hybridization to detect CMV nucleic acids. A major obstacle to tissue diagnosis of CMV is the need to perform invasive procedures to obtain specimens for testing.

Antigenemia Assay

The CMV antigenemia assay has been widely used for the direct detection and quantification of CMV from blood leukocytes in recipients of solid-organ and hematopoietic stem cell transplants and individuals infected with HIV. There have been numerous studies comparing the performance of this assay to conventional and shell vial culture isolation of CMV from blood (for a review, see references 14 and 121). The antigenemia assay is a sensitive, specific, and rapid method for the early diagnosis of CMV infection and can be used for routine monitoring of patients at high risk for severe CMV disease. The test is relatively simple to perform and is based on immunocytochemical detection of the 65-kDa lower-matrix phosphoprotein (pp65) in the nuclei of peripheral blood leukocytes. By using this assay, CMV can be detected before the onset of symptoms and the viral load can be quantified to assist in predicting and differentiating CMV disease from asymptomatic infection (41, 68). The procedure has also been used to evaluate the efficacy of antiviral therapy and to predict treatment failure and the development of viral resistance (44, 124), to prompt the institution of preemptive therapy (6, 118), to detect CMV in leukocytes of CSF from AIDS patients with infections of the central nervous system (104), and for diagnosis of congenital CMV infection (4), CMV gastrointestinal disease (61), and CMV infection in the immunocompetent host (89). The pp65 protein has also been found in endothelial cells circulating in the blood of immunocompromised patients, and some investigators have suggested that infection of these cells is associated with organ involvement and more advanced disease (42, 105). The results of the antigenemia assay correlate well with the quantitative detection of CMV DNA in whole blood, leukocytes, or plasma in molecular amplification assays (24, 35, 38, 82, 107).

In the antigenemia assay, leukocytes (mainly polymorphonuclear leukocytes) are enriched from freshly collected whole blood by sedimentation with dextran. A method for direct lysis of erythrocytes and subsequent isolation of leukocytes from whole blood has been described (56) and is now routinely used by many laboratories. This modification allows for a shorter total assay time and the capability of processing more specimens. Following sedimentation, the remaining erythrocytes are lysed with ammonium chloride, the granulocytes are counted in a hemocytometer or automated cell-counting instrument, and a known number of cells (usually 2×10^5, although variations of 5×10^4 to 10^6 cells have been used) are cytocentrifuged onto microscope slides. The cells are fixed with formaldehyde or paraformaldehyde and then permeabilized with the nonionic detergent Nonidet P-40 and stained with suitable monoclonal antibodies directed against CMV pp65. These processes are followed by incubation of the cells with a fluorescein isothiocyanate-labeled secondary antibody diluted in a counterstain. Slides are read by microscopy at $\times 200$ to $\times 400$ magnification. Positive results are viewed as homogeneous apple green fluorescence within the nuclei of infected cells (Fig. 2). Quantitative results are usually expressed as the number of antigen-positive cells per total number of leukocytes evaluated. Absolute CMV antigenemia values or specific thresholds to predict symptomatic disease or prompt administration of preemptive antiviral therapy have not been fully established for interpretation of quantitative testing, and they appear to be different between patient populations. Therefore, it is more important to monitor patients and trend relative rises and/or falls in the level of antigen-positive cells in multiple blood specimens collected over time than it is to rely on a single test result. The presence of small numbers of antigen-positive cells generally indicates asymptomatic infection, whereas increasingly larger numbers are more strongly associated with clinically significant disease. In patients with severe immunosuppression (e.g., after allogeneic hematopoietic stem cell transplantation), however, even very small numbers of antigen-positive cells may be significant. For transplant recipients, the frequency and extent of monitoring vary with the institution and from one transplant population to another and depend on the medical approach taken to manage CMV infection and disease (for a review, see reference 102).

The major advantages of the antigenemia assay are that it is more sensitive than either conventional tube or shell vial cultures for the detection of CMV from blood; it can be completed in 2 to 4 h, providing same-day turnaround of results;

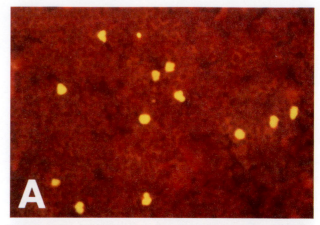

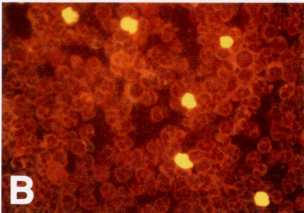

FIGURE 2 CMV antigen-positive polymorphonuclear leukocytes. Note the nuclear staining when a monoclonal antibody directed against pp65 is used. (A) Magnification, $\times 100$; (B) magnification, $\times 400$.

and the procedure can be readily modified for quantitative measure of the viral load. The assay has the disadvantages of being labor-intensive and time-consuming, particularly when large numbers of specimens are being processed; and it should be performed by personnel with experience in immunocytochemical techniques due to the subjective nature of the interpretation. Large volumes of blood are required to perform the assay, and the blood must be processed in a timely manner for accurate results. Considerable time, effort, and expertise are needed in isolating and counting cells, adjusting the cell concentration to 10^6/ml before preparing the slides for staining, and then reading the stained slides. Also, interlaboratory variability exists with regard to the exact procedures used to perform the antigenemia assay and there is a definite need for assay standardization (40, 120, 125). Commercial kits containing monoclonal antibodies and other reagents needed to perform the antigenemia assay are available (Table 1). Several of these assays have been licensed by the FDA, and comparative studies have demonstrated equivalent performance. Because of the low throughput, the antigenemia assay is best suited for laboratories processing small numbers of specimens.

Molecular Amplification

Molecular amplification assays are progressively replacing nonmolecular assays for the diagnosis and monitoring of

TABLE 1 Available commercial CMV antigenemia assays

Manufacturer[a]	Product name	Recommended blood collection and processing			Cell separation technique	No. of cells per slide	Monoclonal antibody used	Total assay time (h)	Reference(s)
		Amt (ml)	Anticoagulant used	Storage conditions					
Biotest Diagnostics, Rockaway, NJ	CMV Brite	5–10	Heparin or EDTA	20–25°C for 6–8 h	Dextran sedimentation	1.5×10^5	C10/C11	4–5	70, 117
	CMV Brite Turbo	3–5	EDTA	20–25°C for 6–8 h	Direct erythrocyte lysis with NH$_4$Cl	2.0×10^5	C10/C11	2	67, 117, 126
Argene, North Massapequa, NY	CINAkit Rapid Antigenemia	7	Heparin or EDTA	2–8°C for up to 24 h	Dextran sedimentation or direct erythrocyte lysis with NH$_4$Cl	2.0×10^5	1C3 + AYM-1	4–5 or 2	77, 117
Millipore Corp., Temecula, CA	Light Diagnostics CMV pp65 Antigenemia	5–10	Heparin or EDTA	20–25°C for up to 24 h	Dextran sedimentation or direct erythrocyte lysis with NH$_4$Cl	2.0×10^5	Proprietary	4–5 or 2	94

[a]CMV Brite, CMV Brite Turbo, and CINAkit are FDA licensed for qualitative testing only; Light Diagnostics kit is not FDA licensed.

CMV infections. PCR is currently the most widely used molecular method for the detection of CMV DNA and mRNAs, and the sensitivity and specificity of PCR for diagnosis of active CMV infection have been evaluated (29, 59, 87, 110, 133). Amplification has been performed with a variety of primer pairs from gene regions of the immediate-early antigen (UL122–123 locus), the major immediate-early antigen (UL122–123 locus), the DNA polymerase (UL54), glycoproteins B (UL55) and H (UL75), pp65 (UL83), pp67 (UL65), US17, HXFL4, the EcoRI D fragment, the HindIII X fragment, the pp150 tegument protein (UL32), the major capsid protein (UL86), and the junction between glycoprotein B and the major immediate-early antigen. Based on published literature, the most common targets for CMV PCR include glycoprotein B, the immediate-early antigen, the major immediate-early antigen, and US17 followed by the pp65 and polymerase genes. Not all primers are equally sensitive in amplifying CMV DNA, and in several studies the sensitivity of the assay was increased by amplifying genomic regions from both the immediate-early and the late CMV genes or by using nested primers to a single gene fragment. The use of both gene fragments enabled the detection of a variety of clinical isolates, indicating that strain variability is not a limiting factor for PCR diagnosis of CMV. PCR has been used successfully to detect CMV DNA in a variety of clinical specimens from organ transplant recipients, patients with AIDS, and infants with congenital infection. It also has been used for the continued surveillance of immunocompromised patients and for evaluation of the therapeutic efficacy of antiviral drugs (43, 44, 122).

Of concern with PCR for CMV diagnosis is whether the test can distinguish between active disease and asymptomatic infection or latency. CMV viremia is considered to be the best predictor of CMV disease, and CMV DNA has been successfully detected in whole blood, purified peripheral blood leukocytes, plasma, and serum by PCR (43, 110, 115, 122). However, PCR is extremely sensitive and the qualitative detection of CMV DNA in these specimens has limited value in predicting symptomatic disease and in monitoring the success of antiviral therapy in immunocompromised patients. CMV DNA can be detected in blood by PCR in the absence of disease and can be found for weeks or months after successful therapy of symptomatic patients (11, 44, 116). However, there are clinical settings in which qualitative PCR appears to be useful, including in the diagnosis of less common forms of CMV infection, such as detection of CMV in CSF of patients with encephalitis or polyradiculomyelitis; in urine, tissue, amniotic fluid, or fetal blood for diagnosis of congenital CMV infection; in the aqueous or vitreous humor in patients with CMV retinitis; and in the blood of patients at high risk of severe infection, such as CMV donor-positive, recipient-negative transplant patients, so that antiviral therapy can be started early in the course of infection. Also, a negative result from qualitative PCR of blood has a high negative predictive value for excluding systemic CMV disease. Qualitative PCR can also be used on tissue specimens from immunocompromised patients with suspected end-organ disease. However, careful consideration should be given to whether detection of CMV by highly sensitive molecular methods truly represents infection of the organ or possible contamination with the virus from infected extracellular fluids that bathe the tissue. While negative PCR results would suggest absence of CMV tissue-invasive infection, positive results may not be significant and should be correlated with clinical and histopathologic findings. In this regard, in situ hybridization or immunohistochemical staining may be helpful in localizing the virus within the tissue.

Similar to the antigenemia assay, measuring the level of CMV DNA in blood appears necessary to predict and diagnose CMV disease in immunocompromised hosts (7, 39). Consequently, a number of quantitative and semiquantitative molecular assays have been developed over the years and have included target and signal amplification methods. The first assays involved conventional end-point PCR, branched-chain DNA technology, and a solution hybridization antibody capture assay (14, 58, 114). More recently, quantitative real-time PCR assays have been introduced (26, 36, 50, 53, 54, 74, 75, 80, 108) and have largely replaced most other methods. As a result, commercial signal amplification and hybrid capture assays are no longer in clinical use. Real-time PCR is most promising because it allows for detection of amplified nucleic acids as they accumulate and technological advances have provided for rapid and accurate quantification over a dynamic range of orders of magnitude, using a variety of different chemistries and platforms. Also, assays for CMV can be multiplexed with tests for other herpesviruses for simultaneous monitoring following transplantation (88, 128). The performances of individual PCR assays have been compared to the antigenemia assay and culture as well as to each other (10, 13, 24, 82, 93, 100, 107, 123, 130). Overall, these molecular methods provide quantitative results comparable to those obtained by the antigenemia assay; they are also more sensitive than culture for detecting CMV infection and can detect CMV before the onset of clinical symptoms. It has been shown that transplant recipients and AIDS patients with active CMV disease have higher levels of CMV DNA and that a rapid rise in the CMV DNA copy number correlates with the presence of symptoms and drug failure during treatment (30, 37, 38, 136). Also, Rasmussen et al. (99) have determined that quantification of CMV DNA from peripheral blood leukocytes can be used to identify HIV-infected patients at risk for development of symptomatic CMV retinitis. It has also been determined that immunocompromised patients with CMV disease have more CMV DNA in either whole blood, plasma, or leukocyte fractions than do patients without disease but that the level of CMV DNA in whole blood or leukocytes is higher than that in plasma (38, 137). Quantification of CMV in plasma, therefore, may be less sensitive for monitoring CMV infection, although a positive result may correlate better with active disease. Although there is general agreement between PCR and antigenemia assays, the quantitative numerical relationship is not exact and differences should be expected since these assays measure different biological features of CMV replication and infection. PCR is extremely sensitive and may detect CMV earlier than the antigenemia assay and may continue to be positive after antigen testing is negative. Conversely, negative PCR results have been reported for patients with low numbers of positive cells in the antigenemia assay (107). Therefore, depending on the test and parameters used, these assays may be more or less sensitive when compared to one another and may have higher or lower positive predictive values for CMV disease. As in the antigenemia assay, absolute CMV DNA levels or threshold values for predicting symptomatic disease and initiating preemptive therapy have not been determined and may differ by specimen type and testing platform selected and from one laboratory and patient population to another. It is currently more important to monitor the relative changes in DNA levels from serial blood specimens collected over time and tested using the same assay. If desired, specific cutoff levels should be prospectively determined based on the assay and specimen used and the type of patients being followed. Because of the high sensitivity of PCR and depending upon the cutoff value selected, the positive predictive value for symptomatic CMV disease may vary and may affect clinical decision making and the length of antiviral therapy. Quantitative PCR methods for the estimation of CMV DNA levels in CSF, amniotic fluid, tissue, and urine of CMV-infected patients have been described (4, 10, 34, 103, 104, 111), but more research is needed to assess the clinical relevance of quantifying CMV DNA from these specimens. It has been shown that the prognosis of congenital CMV infection may be directly related to the amount of CMV in the urine of an infected neonate and that quantifying CMV DNA in the CSF of AIDS patients may help determine if disorders of the central nervous system are attributed more to CMV than to the direct effects of HIV or other opportunistic pathogens.

As an alternative to using quantitative tests, reverse transcriptase PCR assays have been used to demonstrate that qualitative amplification of specific CMV mRNA transcripts that are expressed only during active infection may make it possible to identify the patients at greatest risk for developing symptomatic infection (12, 51, 63, 84). Assays used to detect CMV mRNA have a high specificity for diagnosing CMV disease but are usually less sensitive than other methods. As such, a commercial nucleic acid sequence-based amplification kit developed to monitor the expression of CMV immediate-early and late pp67 mRNA has recently been removed from the worldwide market.

In general, real-time PCR assays for the detection and quantification of CMV DNA are sensitive, specific, and reproducible and significantly reduce the time necessary to report results that may have an impact on the care and management of patients. The method offers the distinct advantages of being less technically demanding and cheaper to perform than more conventional assays, and quality reagents and automated instruments for nucleic acid extraction and amplification and detection are readily available and greatly improve the potential for standardization and increased accuracy of results. The assays also require less specimen volume for testing and can be easily performed on neutropenic patients with low leukocyte counts, the DNA is stable during extended transport and storage times, and large numbers of specimens can be efficiently processed. Furthermore, the overall risk of amplicon contamination has been minimized, as real-time platforms are closed systems. Various commercial real-time and end-point PCR assays are available as either analyte-specific reagents or packaged as complete kits (Table 2). However, most real-time PCR assays are developed in the laboratory by the end user and differ in the types of specimens used, the nucleic acid target selected, the choice and design of suitable oligonucleotide primers and probes, optimization of specimen extraction and PCR amplification conditions, the controls and calibration standards used, the method chosen to detect and/or quantify the amplified product, and the quantitative units of measure and vial loads reported from one laboratory and method to another. Many of the assays require additional validation, and there is a definite need for traceable and commutable international reference materials that include both standards and controls for institutional comparison of results since significant variability in CMV quantification has been observed between laboratories (22, 90, 134). Ultimately, the clinical utility of these assays will

TABLE 2 Available commercial molecular assays for CMV[a]

Manufacturer	Assay	Method	Target	Measurement	Availability	Reference(s)
Roche Diagnostics, Indianapolis, IN	COBAS Amplicor CMV Monitor	End-point PCR	UL54 pol gene	Quantitative	RUO in United States; CE marked in Europe	16, 21, 23, 112
	Light Cycler CMV	Real-time PCR	UL54 pol gene	Qualitative and quantitative	ASR in United States; CE-marked kit in Europe	55, 119
Argene, Verniolle, France	CMV R-gene	Real-time PCR	UL83 pp65 gene	Quantitative	RUO in United States; CE-marked kit in Europe	49
	CMV HHV6,7,8 R-gene	Real-time PCR	CMV UL83 pp65 gene	Quantitative		
Abbott Molecular, Des Plaines, IL	Artus CMV PCR	Real-time PCR	UL123 MIE gene	Quantitative	ASR in United States; CE-marked kit in Europe	20, 45
Qiagen, Valencia, CA	Artus and EASY artus CMV PCR	Real-time PCR	UL123 MIE gene	Quantitative	ASR in United States; CE-marked kit in Europe	20, 55, 83
Nanogen, Milan, Italy	Alert Q-CMV Real Time Complete	Real-time PCR	UL123 MIE gene	Quantitative	Not available in United States; CE-marked kit in Europe	3
	Alert CMV Early Complete	Nested end-point PCR	UL123 MIE gene	Qualitative		
Nanogen, San Diego, CA	MGB Alert CMV Primers and Probes	Real-time PCR	UL123 IE 1 gene	Qualitative and quantitative	ASR for laboratory-developed assays	
Cepheid AB, Bromma, Sweden	CMV Trender	Real-time PCR	Proprietary	Quantitative	Not available in Unitd States; CE-marked kit in Europe	1

[a]Abbreviations: pol, polymerase; pp65, phosphoprotein 65; MIE, major immediate early; IE1, immediate early 1; ASR, analyte-specific reagent; RUO, research use only.

depend on their accuracy, reproducibility, precision, ease of use, cost, availability, and predictive value. Molecular methods, however, are proving to be valuable additions to the analytical tools already being used to provide a rapid diagnosis of established disease, identify patients at risk of developing disease, assess the progression of disease and the risk of relapse, direct the initiation of preemptive therapy, monitor the response to therapy, and predict viral resistance and treatment failure.

VIRUS ISOLATION

Cell Cultures

Human fibroblasts best support the growth of CMV and therefore are used for diagnostic purposes. Acceptable fibroblast cultures include those prepared from human embryonic tissues or foreskins and serially passaged diploid human fetal lung strains such as WI-38, MRC-5, or IMR-90. Diploid fibroblast cells should be used at a low passage number, since they may become less susceptible to CMV infection with increasing cell generations. Several of these fibroblast cell lines are commercially available. CMV can infect and replicate in certain human epithelial cells, but its growth is limited. CMV infection of nonhuman cells can occur but leads to abortive replication with expression of only immediate-early genes and proteins.

Conventional Tube Culture

Specimens to be tested are added in a volume of 0.2 ml to tubes of confluent fibroblasts maintained in Eagle minimal essential medium with 2% fetal bovine serum. Alternatively, the tubes are drained of medium, the inocula are absorbed for 1 h in a stationary position or by centrifugation at 700 × g for 45 min at 30 to 33°C, and then fresh medium is added. After inoculation, the tubes can be rolled or kept stationary at 37°C. At 24 h later, the medium is changed in tubes inoculated with urine or leukocyte specimens. Thereafter, and for other types of specimens, the medium is changed once a week or more frequently as the pH of the culture medium changes or if toxicity appears. When toxicity necessitates passage of the culture, cells rather than culture medium should be passaged, since CMV remains mostly cell associated. Cells are removed by addition of 0.25% trypsin–0.1% EDTA to the monolayers and incubation at 37°C for approximately 1 min. When the cells detach, Eagle minimal essential medium with 2% fetal bovine serum is added, and the cells are used to inoculate fresh tubes. Tubes are examined for cytopathic effect (CPE) for at least 4 weeks for most specimens (6 weeks for leukocyte specimens). Control, uninoculated cultures are handled in the same manner as those inoculated with clinical specimens.

The time of appearance and the extent of CPE depend on the amounts of virus present in specimens. In cultures inoculated with urine from a congenitally infected newborn, CPE may develop by 24 h and progress rapidly to involve most of the monolayer if the virus titer in the urine is extremely high. More commonly, foci of CPE, consisting of enlarged, rounded, refractile cells, appear during the first week, and progression of CPE to surrounding cells proceeds slowly (Fig. 3). In cultures inoculated with urine or respiratory specimens from older individuals, CPE usually appears within 2 weeks. Leukocyte cultures may not become positive until after 3 to 6 weeks. The usual slow progression of CPE in cultures inoculated with clinical specimens is due, at least in part, to limited release of virus into extracellular fluid.

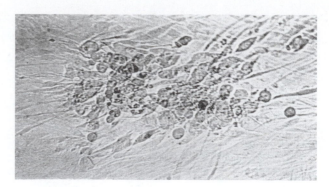

FIGURE 3 CPE produced by a CMV isolate in human skin fibroblasts 10 days postinoculation. Unstained preparation; magnification, ×100. (Courtesy of Sergio Stagno.)

With strains of CMV that have been serially passaged, including laboratory-adapted strains, greater amounts of extracellular virus are released and CPE progresses more rapidly.

For storage of fresh isolates, monolayers exhibiting CPE are treated with trypsin-EDTA and the cells obtained are suspended in Eagle minimal essential medium with 10% fetal bovine serum and 10% dimethyl sulfoxide and then frozen at −70°C. Infectivity can be better maintained for long periods by storage in liquid nitrogen.

Virus Identification

In many laboratories, CMV isolates are identified solely on the basis of characteristic CPE and host cell range. However, viruses such as adenovirus and varicella-zoster virus occasionally produce CPE indistinguishable from that of CMV. Thus, suspected CMV isolates are best confirmed by an immunofluorescence assay (IFA) using monoclonal or polyclonal antibodies that are available from various commercial sources. The appearance of typical nuclear fluorescence of infected cells indicates the presence of CMV. PCR or other molecular amplification methods also can be used for confirmation of suspected isolates.

Spin-Amplification Shell Vial Assay

The spin-amplification shell vial assay as described by Gleaves et al. (47) has been used extensively as a rapid culture method for the detection of CMV in clinical specimens. The technique is based on the amplification of virus in cell cultures after low-speed centrifugation and detects viral antigens produced early in the replication of CMV, before the development of CPE. Even low titers of virus present in specimens are easily amplified and rapidly detected within 24 h. Monoclonal antibodies are commercially available and are used for the detection of CMV early antigens. In situ hybridization with DNA probes to CMV has also been used.

MRC-5 fibroblast cells are grown to confluency on 12-mm-diameter round coverslips in 1-dram (3.7-ml) shell vials and inoculated with 0.2 ml of specimen. Shell vials of MRC-5 cells can be obtained commercially or prepared in the laboratory. Monolayers should be inoculated within 1 week after preparation, since older monolayers demonstrate decreased sensitivity to CMV and increased toxicity (33). Pretreatment of the monolayers with dexamethasone, dimethyl sulfoxide, or these agents plus calcium may increase the sensitivity of the cells to CMV infection (131, 132), although other investigators have been unable to confirm these results (32). Two vials should be inoculated for urine, tissue, and bronchoalveolar lavage fluid specimens, and three vials should be inoculated for blood specimens (92). Alternatively, disruption of purified leukocytes by sonication before their use in the shell vial assay may increase the sensitivity of CMV detection from blood (135). Increasing the frequency of blood collection and the volume of blood obtained also may enhance the diagnostic yield of the shell vial assay from this specimen (91). After inoculation, the vials are centrifuged at 700 × g for 40 min at 25°C, and then 2.0 ml of Eagle minimum essential medium containing 2% fetal bovine serum and antibiotics is added. The cultures are incubated at 37°C for 16 to 24 h, fixed with acetone, and stained. A longer incubation time may be used, but the time should be determined by each laboratory on the basis of individual experience, reagents, staining technique used, and whether monolayers are purchased or prepared in the laboratory. Uninfected and CMV-infected monolayers are included as negative and positive controls, respectively. Mink lung (ML) cells, a nonhuman continuous cell line, are comparable to MRC-5 fibroblasts for the detection of CMV in clinical specimens by shell vial culture (46, 76). A distinct advantage in using ML cells is that this cell line can be propagated and passaged in the laboratory for a long time without a decrease in susceptibility to CMV. Significantly less toxicity and an increase in the number of CMV-positive nuclei were also observed with ML cells. Coverslips are scanned at ×200 to ×250 magnification, and specific staining is confirmed at ×400 to ×630. Positive cells contain apple green fluorescent nuclei against a red cytoplasmic background. Staining of immediate-early antigen appears as an even matte green fluorescence with specks of brighter green (Fig. 4A). Viral inclusions ("owl's eyes") may be visible in the nuclei (Fig. 4B).

The spin-amplification shell vial assay has been a valuable adjunct to conventional virus isolation. It has the important features of being rapid, sensitive, and specific. However, skilled technical personnel and close attention to the quality of specimens, monolayers, and reagents are required for optimum performance.

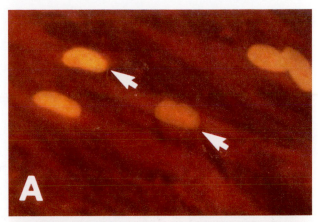
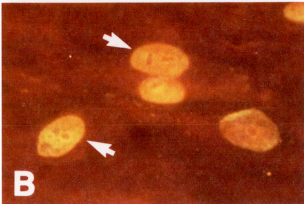

FIGURE 4 Demonstration of CMV early antigens in the nuclei (arrows) of infected MRC-5 cells following shell vial culture and IFA staining. (A) Staining of immediate-early antigen appears as an even matte green fluorescence with specks of brighter green. (B) Viral inclusions (owl's eyes) may be visible in the nuclei. Magnification, ×400.

SEROLOGIC TESTS

A variety of tests with high sensitivities and specificities are available for the detection of either IgM or IgG antibodies to CMV (for an overview, see reference 57). In deciding which test to perform, one should consider such factors as the number of specimens to be tested, the patient population, cost, turnaround time, equipment needs, and ease of performance. The method that is chosen depends on the needs of individual laboratories. For small-volume laboratories, IFA may be more cost-effective and practical, while enzyme immunoassays (EIAs) may be more suitable for laboratories with higher volumes of specimens. Overall, detection of CMV-specific IgM or determination of a seroconversion from a negative to a positive IgG antibody response can be useful for the diagnosis of primary CMV infection in certain clinical settings, and the screening of blood and organ donors and recipients plays an important role in preventing the transmission of latent CMV to patients at high risk for severe CMV disease.

Enzyme Immunoassays

Over the years, EIAs have largely replaced other traditional methods for detecting antibodies to CMV. The main advantages of the EIA are that it is rapid, sensitive, and specific (78, 79, 95). In addition, multiple specimens can be handled daily at a relatively low cost. Kits that detect CMV IgG are available from a number of commercial sources. The kits are easy to use, and the manufacturers have provided detailed instructions. All the materials necessary to perform the assay are included, and the reagents are stable with time. Some companies also provide a spectrophotometer and automated plate washer, which otherwise must be purchased separately at considerable expense. The development of robotics technology has led to the commercial availability of both fully automated and semiautomated EIA instruments that include sample dispensers, diluters, washers, and spectrophotometers with complete computer programming and generation of electronic and written reports. More recently, an EIA that uses the envelope glycoproteins B and H to distinguish CMV strain-specific antibody responses has been developed (85). This assay may be useful for identifying strain diversity in different patient populations and may provide a better understanding of the implications of infection with multiple CMV strains and the role of strain-specific antibody in the protective immune response against CMV.

Immunofluorescence Assays

Indirect and anticomplement IFAs are commonly used methods for detecting CMV antibodies. In the indirect IFA, dilutions of test serum are incubated with virus-infected cells that have been fixed to a glass microscope slide. Specific antibody-antigen complexes are detected using an anti-human antibody conjugated with fluorescein isothiocyanate and fluorescence microscopy. Anticomplement immunofluorescence is similar to the indirect IFA. It differs, however, in that the test serum is first heat inactivated to remove endogenous complement activity and then incubated with virus-infected cells on glass slides. An exogenous source of complement is added and bound by any specific antigen-antibody complexes that have formed. A fluorescein-labeled anticomplement antibody is then added; it binds to the C3 component of complement, and the slides are read with a fluorescence microscope. Anticomplement IFA amplifies the fluorescent signal above what can be seen using an indirect IFA, allowing for the detection of small amounts of antibody or antibodies of low avidity. IFAs are useful and inexpensive methods that offer the advantages of speed and simplicity for the qualitative and quantitative detection of CMV antibodies. Commercial kits are readily available, or antigen-coated slides and labeled secondary antibodies can be purchased separately. The major disadvantages of IFA systems are that they require a fluorescence microscope and darkroom for examining slides and that extensive training is needed to read and interpret the test results.

CMV IgM Antibody Measurements

Commercial reagents and complete EIA and IFA diagnostic kits are available for measuring CMV IgM antibodies. The procedures are essentially the same as those used to detect IgG antibodies, except that anti-human IgM antibodies labeled with suitable markers are used to detect CMV-specific IgM bound to viral antigens on the solid phase. A recognized pitfall of CMV IgM assays is the occurrence of false-positive and false-negative reactions. False-positive reactions occur when sera contain unusually high levels of rheumatoid factor in the presence of specific CMV IgG (27). Rheumatoid factor is an immunoglobulin, usually of the IgM class, that reacts with IgG. It is produced in some rheumatologic, vasculitic, and viral diseases, including CMV infection. IgM rheumatoid factor forms a complex with IgG that may contain CMV-specific IgG. The CMV IgG binds to CMV antigen, carrying nonviral IgM with it; in this setting, a test designed to detect IgM will produce a false-positive result. False-negative reactions occur if high levels of specific IgG antibodies competitively block the binding of IgM to CMV antigen. Therefore, it is highly recommended to separate IgM and IgG fractions before testing to decrease the incidence of both false-positive and false-negative IgM test results.

Rapid and simple methods for the removal of interfering rheumatoid factor and IgG molecules from serum have been developed. These include selective absorption of IgM to a solid phase and removal of IgG by using hyperimmune anti-human IgG, staphylococcal protein A, or recombinant protein G from group G streptococci. Serum pretreatment methods are now readily available and are incorporated in the procedures of commercially available IFA and EIA kits, which have resulted in more-reliable IgM tests. More recently, reverse capture solid-phase IgM assays have been used as an alternative approach to avoiding false-positive or false-negative results. This method uses a solid phase coated with an anti-human IgM antibody to capture the IgM from a serum specimen, after which competing IgG antibody and immune complexes are removed by washing.

The bound IgM antibody is then exposed to specific CMV antigen, and an enzyme-conjugated second antibody and substrate are added. The development and use of recombinantly derived CMV proteins as a source of antigenic substrate also have greatly improved the performance of IgM assays (65, 127).

Although the detection of CMV-specific IgM may be useful in the determination of recent or active infection, the results should be interpreted with caution. Because IgM does not cross the placenta, a positive result from a single serum specimen from an infected newborn is diagnostic. However, there may be a lack of or delay in production of IgM in the newborn. Testing for the presence of CMV-specific IgM antibody beyond the newborn period is usually not recommended since IgM antibody can appear in both primary and reactivated CMV infections and can persist for extended periods after a primary infection. This complicates the interpretation of test results, particularly for pregnant women or immunocompromised patients, and may not be predictive of recent or active infection. Like newborns, immunocompromised individuals also may have a delay in IgM production or may be unable to mount a significant IgM antibody response. Lastly, patients with Epstein-Barr virus-induced infectious mononucleosis may produce heterotypic IgM responses, resulting in false-positive CMV IgM test results.

IgG Avidity Assay

Measurements of CMV-specific IgG avidity have proven useful for distinguishing primary from nonprimary infections in women suspected of having CMV during pregnancy and in solid organ transplant recipients. CMV-specific IgG of low avidity is produced during the first weeks to months following primary infection, while IgG antibody of increasingly higher avidity is produced with past or nonprimary infections. The detection of CMV-specific IgM in maternal serum is not predictive of virus transmission to the fetus, since fewer than 10% of pregnant women who are positive for CMV IgM actually give birth to a congenitally infected infant. More recently, it has been suggested that finding low-avidity CMV-specific IgG antibody in CMV-IgM positive pregnant women may improve the diagnosis of recent primary CMV infection and may have prognostic value with regard to fetal infection (52, 72). In solid organ transplant recipients, it has also been shown that a delay in the development of high-avidity CMV-specific IgG antibody correlates with prolonged antigenemia and a poor prognosis (73). Both commercial and user-developed CMV-specific IgG avidity assays are available, and the tests are performed by making simple modifications to conventional EIA protocols to effectively separate and differentiate antibodies of low and high avidity (28, 97).

Other Serologic Tests

Complement fixation, immune adherence hemagglutination, indirect hemagglutination, and the neutralization test are other serologic tests used to measure CMV antibody. These methods are currently performed in only a limited number of diagnostic laboratories; some of the procedures have the disadvantages of being insensitive, poorly standardized, and relatively labor-intensive and time-consuming. The recent development of a luciferase immunoprecipitation assay has allowed for sensitive and highly quantitative measurements of antibody titers to four different CMV protein fragments (19). This approach may be useful for better understanding host immune responses in different CMV diseases and for monitoring the immune response following administration of a CMV vaccine.

ANTIVIRAL SUSCEPTIBILITY TESTING

Resistance of CMV to ganciclovir has been reported in immunocompromised patients, particularly patients with AIDS receiving long-term ganciclovir treatment for CMV retinitis. Ganciclovir-resistant clinical isolates have also been recovered from bone marrow and solid organ transplant recipients and a patient with chronic lymphocytic leukemia. Although foscarnet is the alternative therapy for ganciclovir-resistant CMV infections, clinical CMV isolates resistant to foscarnet alone or to foscarnet in combination with ganciclovir have been described. The mechanisms of resistance to ganciclovir in CMV include mutations in the catalytic domain of the UL97 phosphotransferase gene, leading to a deficiency in drug phosphorylation, and alterations in the UL54 viral DNA polymerase gene; the latter is also responsible for resistance to foscarnet (for a review, see reference 31). Ganciclovir-resistant CMV isolates with mutations in the UL54 gene are generally cross-resistant to cidofovir, and isolates resistant to ganciclovir, foscarnet, and cidofovir have also been reported.

The described emergence of antiviral drug resistance has led to a definite need for in vitro antiviral susceptibility testing. Laboratory confirmation of drug resistance is essential for defining the mechanisms of antiviral resistance, for determining the frequency with which drug-resistant CMV mutants emerge in clinical practice, for predicting treatment failure and identifying cross-resistance to other antiviral agents, for instituting the most appropriate alternative therapy, and when evaluating new antiviral agents. A number of phenotypic and genotypic assays have been described for testing the susceptibility of CMV to antiviral agents (for an overview, see reference 5). Phenotypic assays measure the ability of CMV to grow in cell culture in the presence of various concentrations of antiviral drug, and they generally require isolation and passage of the virus in cell culture before testing begins. The activity of the antiviral agent against the replication of the virus is measured by one of many methods, including the inhibition of viral plaque formation or virus-induced CPE; a decrease in the production of viral antigens, enzyme activities, or total virus yield; and a reduction in viral nucleic acid synthesis. With each method, results are expressed as the drug concentration that causes a 50% inhibition in the growth of the virus. Genotypic assays have been used to screen CMV isolates for the identification of mutations in the CMV UL97 phosphotransferase gene and the UL54 DNA polymerase gene that confer resistance to ganciclovir and/or foscarnet (8, 25, 113). These assays normally involve using PCR for amplification of specific viral genes and direct sequencing of the amplified products; some assays use specific probes to detect selected mutations or use restriction endonuclease digestion of amplified products to identify alterations in the viral genome known to be associated with viral resistance to a given viral agent. Phenotypic assays offer the distinct advantage of being a direct measure of CMV susceptibility to any antiviral drug and can provide data on the concentration of drug needed to inhibit viral replication. However, phenotypic assays for CMV are cumbersome, labor-intensive, and expensive and have long turnaround times. Genotypic assays offer speed and efficiency in analyzing large numbers of CMV isolates and may allow an earlier detection of the emergence of drug resistance

than phenotypic assays. Current genotypic assays, however, detect only known drug-resistant mutations, and the results may be confounded by the presence of mutations that have no bearing on drug resistance. Phenotypic assays are still required to identify drug-resistant viruses with novel mutations for antiviral resistance. The overall complexities of phenotypic and genotypic assays make either method less than routine for most clinical laboratories.

EVALUATION, INTERPRETATION, AND REPORTING OF RESULTS

There are a number of points to consider when choosing which tests to perform for the detection of CMV. Conventional tube cultures are highly specific and can detect unexpected viruses but are generally too slow and insensitive to have an impact on clinical decision making when considering CMV as the primary pathogen. Shell vial cultures decrease the time required for detecting CMV in culture, but the sensitivity varies by specimen type and from laboratory to laboratory. Cultures also are often positive in the absence of true CMV disease; this is particularly true when screening urine or respiratory specimens for CMV, where shedding of CMV is common during asymptomatic infection and is usually not suggestive of more-severe illness. Isolation of CMV in culture may be useful for postpartum and in utero diagnosis of congenital CMV infection and tissue invasive disease, and CMV isolates are also needed for phenotypic antiviral susceptibility assays.

In the immunocompromised host, the use of direct detection methods to diagnose CMV disease is most beneficial for patient care. Virologic or serologic detection of CMV indicates infection but does not establish whether the infection is responsible for symptomatic illness. CMV is ubiquitous, and asymptomatic excretion is high in patients who never progress to disease. Reactivation of latent virus is also common, and other pathogens may be simultaneously present in patients with overt disease. To implicate CMV as the cause of an illness, laboratory confirmation of active disease in an appropriate clinical setting is required. In this regard, most clinical virology laboratories have largely replaced their conventional tube and shell vial culture systems with CMV antigenemia assays or molecular methods for accurate CMV detection and/or quantification from blood. Quantitative measures of CMV pp65 antigen or CMV DNA or qualitative detection of CMV mRNA can provide a rapid diagnosis of established disease, identify patients at risk of developing disease, assess the progression of disease and the risk of relapse, direct the initiation of preemptive therapy, monitor the response to antiviral therapy, and predict treatment failure and the emergence of drug-resistant virus. Evaluating trends in viral loads over time is currently more useful than interpreting a single test result in relation to a defined cutoff value since the initial viral load, the rate at which it rises, and its persistence with time may predict the risk of CMV disease and possible relapse and aid in establishing treatment failure. Interpretation should be done with caution, as not all changes in quantitative CMV DNA levels may reflect a substantial biological or clinical difference, especially if the changes are small and fall within the expected range of variability for the assay used. Also, an isolated result for CMV viremia may not be predictive of disease and the need for immediate antiviral treatment. Lastly, negative viral load results do not always exclude CMV disease in symptomatic patients; end-organ involvement, particularly in the gastrointestinal tract and lungs, may occur in the absence of detectable levels of CMV viremia. Histopathologic examination and/or PCR can be useful in immunocompromised hosts for the diagnosis of specific organ invasive diseases. However, detection of CMV in tissue specimens must be interpreted with caution, particularly when infections with more than one organism are documented, as the relative importance of each pathogen in producing clinical illness may be difficult to determine.

The isolation of CMV from urine, respiratory secretions, or other body fluids within the first 3 weeks of life is the traditional means of confirming the diagnosis of congenital infection in newborns. Urine is the preferred specimen because it contains greater amounts of virus, and the virus therefore grows quickly in culture. PCR has also been used to find CMV DNA in urine of congenitally infected infants, and viremia in infants with congenital infection has been detected by the antigenemia assay and PCR. Attempts to isolate or detect virus from maternal blood leukocytes and from amniotic fluid and fetal blood and tissue by molecular- and/or antigen-based tests may provide useful information for prenatal diagnosis of congenital CMV infection (for a review, see references 64 and 71). While such prenatal testing is a sensitive indicator of maternal or fetal CMV infection, positive results do not predict which infants will have disease. In this regard, quantitative measures of viral load in congenital CMV infection may prove beneficial for predicting symptomatic outcome and for guiding patient management (4). It has been demonstrated that elevated levels of CMV DNA in blood during early infancy is associated with hearing loss in newborns with symptomatic and asymptomatic congenital CMV infection (17, 18). Also, quantitative real-time PCR has been used to quantify CMV DNA from amniotic fluid samples to predict fetal and neonatal outcomes (48) and to test umbilical cord blood to screen for neonatal CMV infection at delivery (122). Infants not previously tested but found to be excreting virus after 3 weeks of age may have either congenital or acquired infection. Standard serologic or virologic tests do not differentiate between these possibilities.

In general, serologic tests for CMV-specific IgG antibody have limited value for the diagnosis of acute infection since the results are obtained retrospectively and are not predictive of disease. Also, the transplacental passage of maternal IgG antibody begins at 18 weeks of gestation and confounds the diagnosis of CMV infection in the neonate, and immunocompromised hosts may not mount a normal immune response, or they may have been given blood transfusions or intravenous immunoglobulins that contain detectable CMV IgG antibodies. Nonetheless, a history of seroconversion from a negative to a positive IgG antibody response to CMV is diagnostic of primary infection and may be beneficial in evaluating a pregnant woman with symptoms of viral disease. For pregnant women with preexisting CMV-specific IgG and/or IgM antibody, however, IgG avidity testing may be more helpful in distinguishing primary from nonprimary infections and for predicting CMV transmission to the fetus. Use of the IgG avidity assay in immunocompromised hosts may have value in detecting those at highest risk for CMV disease. Whenever possible, serologic diagnoses of CMV infection should be confirmed by other virologic methods. CMV-specific IgG serologic assays play a more important role in the determination of an individual's immune status to CMV. Detection of CMV-specific IgG in a single serum specimen indicates exposure to CMV at some time in the past. Negative serum antibody titers may exclude CMV infection. In the evaluation of an organ donor and recipient, a seronegative recipient who receives an organ or blood products from a seropositive donor is at increased risk for developing primary CMV infection and serious disease. Knowing the serostatus of the donor and recipient is therefore important in determining the treatment or prophylaxis to be used and in considering the type of donor and blood products to be given.

The application of virologic methods, including conventional and shell vial culture, rapid direct-detection assays, and serologic testing, should be combined with clinical assessment of the patient to provide an accurate, reliable diagnosis of CMV infection and disease and to allow subsequent prompt, appropriate patient management and timely intervention with specific antiviral therapy. There is a particular need to differentiate CMV infection from graft rejection in transplant patients, since the administration of potent immunosuppressive antirejection drugs during active CMV infection can result in life-threatening disease.

REFERENCES

1. **Abbate, I., N. Finnstrom, S. Zaniratti, M. C. Solmone, S. Selvaggini, E. Bennici, S. Neri, C. Brega, M. Paterno, and M. R. Capobianchi.** 2008. Evaluation of an automated extraction system in combination with Affigene CMV Trender for CMV DNA quantitative determination: comparison with nested PCR and pp65 antigen test. *J. Virol. Methods* **151:**61–65.

2. **Adler, S. P., and J. B. Wang.** 1996. Salivary antibodies to cytomegalovirus (CMV) glycoprotein B accurately predict CMV infections among preschool children. *J. Clin. Microbiol.* **34:**2632–2634.

3. **Allice, T., F. Cerutti, F. Pittaluga, S. Varetto, A. Franchello, M. Salizzoni, and V. Ghisetti.** 2008. Evaluation of a novel real-time PCR system for cytomegalovirus DNA quantitation on whole blood and correlation with pp65-antigen test in guiding pre-emptive antiviral treatment. *J. Virol. Methods* **148:**9–16.

4. **Arav-Boger, R., and R. Pass.** 2007. Viral load in congenital cytomegalovirus infection. *Herpes* **14:**17–22.

5. **Arens, M. Q., and E. M. Swierkosz.** 2007. Susceptibility test methods, p. 1705–1718. *In* P. R. Murray, E. J. Baron, J. H. Jorgensen, M. L. Landry, and M. A. Pfaller (ed.), *Manual of Clinical Microbiology*, 9th ed. ASM Press, Washington, DC.

6. **Baldanti, F., D. Lilleri, and G. Gerna.** 2008. Human cytomegalovirus load measurement and its applications for preemptive therapy in patients undergoing hematopoietic stem cell transplantation. *Hematol. Oncol.* **26:**123–130.

7. **Baldanti, F., D. Lilleri, and G. Gerna.** 2008. Monitoring human cytomegalovirus infection in transplant recipients. *J. Clin. Virol.* **41:**237–241.

8. **Baldanti, F., A. Sarasini, E. Silini, M. Barbi, A. Lazzarin, K. K. Biron, and G. Gerna.** 1995. Four dually resistant human cytomegalovirus strains from AIDS patients: single mutations in UL97 and UL54 open reading frames are responsible for ganciclovir- and foscarnet-specific resistance, respectively. *Scand. J. Infect. Dis. Suppl.* **99:**103–104.

9. **Barbi, M., S. Binda, and S. Caroppo.** 2006. Diagnosis of congenital CMV infection via dried blood spots. *Rev. Med. Virol.* **16:**385–392.

10. **Bestetti, A., C. Pierotti, M. Terreni, A. Zappa, L. Vago, A. Lazzarin, and P. Cinque.** 2001. Comparison of three nucleic acid amplification assays of cerebrospinal fluid for diagnosis of cytomegalovirus encephalitis. *J. Clin. Microbiol.* **39:**1148–1151.

11. **Bitsch, A., H. Kirchner, R. Dennin, J. Hoyer, L. Fricke, J. Steinhoff, K. Sack, and G. Bein.** 1993. Long persistence of CMV DNA in the blood of renal transplant patients after recovery from CMV infection. *Transplantation* **56:**108–113.

12. **Bitsch, A., H. Kirchner, R. Dupke, and G. Bein.** 1992. Cytomegalovirus transcripts in peripheral blood leukocytes of actively infected transplant patients detected by reverse transcription-polymerase chain reaction. *J. Infect. Dis.* **167:**740–743.

13. **Blank, B. S., P. L. Meenhorst, J. W. Mulder, G. J. Weverling, H. Putter, W. Pauw, W. C. van Dijk, P. Smits, S. Lie-A-Ling, P. Reiss, and J. M. Lange.** 2000. Value of different assays for detection of human cytomegalovirus (HCMV) in predicting the development of HCMV disease in human immunodeficiency virus-infected patients. *J. Clin. Microbiol.* **38:**563–569.

14. **Boeckh, M., and G. Boivin.** 1998. Quantitation of cytomegalovirus: methodologic aspects and clinical applications. *Clin. Microbiol. Rev.* **11:**533–554.

15. **Boeckh, M., P., P. M. Woogerd, T. Stevens-Ayers, C. G. Ray, and R. A. Bowden.** 1994. Factors influencing detection of quantitative cytomegalovirus antigenemia. *J. Clin. Microbiol.* **32:**832–834.

16. **Boivin, G., R. Belanger, R. Delage, C. Beliveau, C. Demers, N. Goyette, and J. Roy.** 2000. Quantitative analysis of cytomegalovirus (CMV) viremia using the pp65 antigenemia assay and the COBAS AMPLICOR CMV MONITOR PCR Test after blood and marrow allogeneic transplantation. *J. Clin. Microbiol.* **38:**4356–4360.

17. **Boppana, S. B., K. B. Fowler, R. F. Pass, L. B. Rivera, R. D. Bradford, F. D. Lakeman, and W. J. Britt.** 2005. Congenital cytomegalovirus infection: association between virus burden in infancy and hearing loss. *J. Pediatr.* **146:**817–823.

18. **Bradford, R. D., G. Cloud, A. D. Lakeman, S. Boppana, D. W. Kimberlin, R. Jacobs, G. Demmler, P. Sanchez, W. Britt, S.-J. Soong, R. J. Whitley, and the National Institute of Allergy and Infectious Diseases Collaborative Antiviral Study Group.** 2005. Detection of cytomegalovirus (CMV) DNA by polymerase chain reaction is associated with hearing loss in newborns with symptomatic congenital CMV infection involving the central nervous system. *J. Infect. Dis.* **191:**227–233.

19. **Burbelo, P. D., A. T. Issa, K. H. Ching, M. Exner, W. L. Drew, H. J. Alter, and M. J. Iadarola.** 2009. Highly quantitative serological detection of anti-cytomegalovirus (CMV) antibody. *Virol. J.* **6:**45. doi:10.1186/1743-422X-6-45.

20. **Caliendo, A. M., J. Ingersoll, A. M. Fox-Canale, S. Pargman, T. Bythwood, M. K. Hayden, J. W. Bremer, and N. S. Lurain.** 2007. Evaluation of real-time PCR laboratory-developed tests using analyte specific reagents for cytomegalovirus quantification. *J. Clin. Microbiol.* **45:**1723–1727.

21. **Caliendo, A. M., B. Schuurman, B. Yen-Lieberman, S. A. Spector, J. Andersen, R. Manjiry, C. Crumpacker, N. S. Lurain, and A. Erice for the CMV Working Group of the Complications of HIV Disease RAC, AIDS Clinical Trials Group.** 2001. Comparison of quantitative and qualitative PCR assays for cytomegalovirus DNA in plasma. *J. Clin. Microbiol.* **39:**1334–1338.

22. **Caliendo, A. M., M. D. Shahbazian, C. Schaper, J. Ingersoll, D. Abdul-Ali, J. Boonyaratanakornkit, X.-L. Pang, J. Fox, J. Preiksaitis, and E. R. Schonbrunner.** 2009. A commutable cytomegalovirus calibrator is required to improve the agreement of viral load values between laboratories. *Clin. Chem.* **55:**9. doi:10.1373/clinchem.2009.124743.

23. **Caliendo, A. M., K. St. George, J. Allega, A. C. Bullotta, L. Gilbane, and C. R. Rinaldo.** 2002. Distinguishing cytomegalovirus (CMV) infection and disease with CMV nucleic acid assays. *J. Clin. Microbiol.* **40:**1581–1586.

24. **Cariani, E., C. P. Pollara, B. Valloncini, F. Perandin, C. Bonfanti, and N. Manca.** 2007. Relationship between pp65 antigenemia levels and real-time quantitative DNA PCR for human cytomegalovirus (HCMV) management in immunocompromised patients. *BMC Infect. Dis.* **7:**138. doi:10.1186/1471-23334-7-138.

25. **Chou, S., S. Guentzel, K. R. Michels, R. C. Miner, and W. L. Drew.** 1995. Frequency of UL97 phosphotransferase mutations related to ganciclovir resistance in clinical cytomegalovirus isolates. *J. Infect. Dis.* **172:**239–242.

26. **Cortez, K. J., S. H. Fischer, G. A. Fahle, L. B. Calhoun, R. W. Childs, A. J. Barrett, and J. E. Bennett.** 2003. Clinical trial of quantitative real-time polymerase chain reaction for detection of cytomegalovirus in peripheral blood of allogeneic

27. **Cremer, N. E., M. Hoffman, and E. H. Lennette.** 1978. Role of rheumatoid factor in complement fixation and indirect hemagglutination tests for immunoglobulin M antibody to cytomegalovirus. *J. Clin. Microbiol.* **8:**160–165.

28. **Curdt, I., G. Praast, E. Sickinger, J. Schultess, I. Herold, H. B. Braun, S.Bernhardt, G. T. Maine, D. D. Smith, S. Hsu, H. M. Christ, D. Pucci, M. Hausmann, and J. Herzogenrath.** 2009. Development of fully automated determination of marker specific immunoglobulin G (IgG) avidity based on the avidity competition assay format: application for Abbott Architect CMV and Toxo IgG avidity assays. *J. Clin. Microbiol.* **47:**603–613.

29. **Demmler, G. J., G. J. Buffone, C. M. Schimbor, and R. A. May.** 1988. Detection of cytomegalovirus in urine from newborns by using polymerase chain reaction DNA amplification. *J. Infect. Dis.* **158:**1177–1184.

30. **Drouet, E., R. Colimon, S. Michelson, N. Fourcade, A. Niveleau, C. Ducerf, A. Boibieux, M. Chevallier, and G. Denoyel.** 1995. Monitoring levels of human cytomegalovirus DNA in blood after liver transplantation. *J. Clin. Microbiol.* **33:**389–394.

31. **Erice, A.** 1999. Resistance of human cytomegalovirus to antiviral drugs. *Clin. Microbiol. Rev.* **12:**286–297.

32. **Espy, M. J., A. D. Wold, D. M. Ilstrup, and T. F. Smith.** 1988. Effect of treatment of shell vial cell cultures with dimethyl sulfoxide and dexamethasone for detection of cytomegalovirus. *J. Clin. Microbiol.* **26:**1091–1093.

33. **Fedorko, D. P., D. M. Ilstrup, and T. F. Smith.** 1989. Effect of age of shell vial monolayers on detection of cytomegalovirus from urine specimens. *J. Clin. Microbiol.* **27:**2107–2109.

34. **Fox, J. C., P. D. Griffiths, and V. C. Emery.** 1992. Quantification of human cytomegalovirus DNA using the polymerase chain reaction. *J. Gen. Virol.* **73:**2405–2408.

35. **Garrigue, I., S. Boucher, L. Couzi, A. Caumont, C. Dromer, M. Neau-Cransac, R. Tabrizi, M.-H. Schrive, H. Fleury, and M.-E. Lafon.** 2006. Whole blood real-time quantitative PCR for cytomegalovirus infection follow-up in transplant recipients. *J. Clin. Virol.* **36:**72–75.

36. **Gault, E. Y. Michael, A. Dehee, C. Belabani, J. C. Nicolas, and A, Garbarg-Chenon.** 2001. Quantitation of human cytomegalovirus DNA by real-time PCR. *J. Clin. Microbiol.* **39:**772–775.

37. **Gerdes, J. C., E. K. Spees, K. Fitting, J. Hiraki, M. Sheehan, D. Duda, T. Jarvi, C. Roehl, and A. D. Robertson.** 1993. Prospective study utilizing a quantitative polymerase chain reaction for detection of cytomegalovirus DNA in the blood of renal transplant patients. *Transplant. Proc.* **25:**1411–1413.

38. **Gerna, G., M. Furione, F. Baldanti, and A. Sarasini.** 1994. Comparative quantitation of human cytomegalovirus DNA in blood leukocytes and plasma of transplant and AIDS patients. *J. Clin. Microbiol.* **32:**2709–2717.

39. **Gerna, G., and D. Lilleri.** 2006. Monitoring transplant patients for human cytomegalovirus: diagnostic update. *Herpes* **13:**4–11.

40. **Gerna, G., E. Percivalle, M. Torsellini, and M. G. Revello.** 1998. Standardization of the human cytomegalovirus antigenemia assay by means of in vitro-generated pp65-positive peripheral blood polymorphonuclear leukocytes. *J. Clin. Microbiol.* **36:**3585–3589.

41. **Gerna, G., M. G. Revello, E. Percivalle, M. Zavattoni, M. Parea, and M. Battaglia.** 1990. Quantitation of human cytomegalovirus viremia by using monoclonal antibodies to different viral proteins. *J. Clin. Microbiol.* **28:**2681–2688.

42. **Gerna, G., M. Zavattoni, F. Baldanti, M. Furione, L. Chezzi, M. G. Revello, and E. Percivalle.** 1998. Circulating cytomegalic endothelial cells are associated with high human cytomegalovirus (HCMV) load in AIDS patients with late-stage disseminated HCMV disease. *J. Med. Virol.* **55:**64–74.

43. **Gerna, G., D. Zipeto, M. Parea, E. Percivalle, M. Zavattoni, A. Gaballo, and G. Milanesi.** 1991. Early virus isolation, early structural antigen detection and DNA amplification by the

polymerase chain reaction in polymorphonuclear leukocytes from AIDS patients with human cytomegalovirus viraemia. *Mol. Cell. Probes* **5:**365–374.

44. **Gerna, G., D. Zipeto, M. Parea, M. G. Revello, E. Silini, E. Percivalle, M. Zavattoni, P. Grossi, and G. Milanesi.** 1991. Monitoring of human cytomegalovirus infections and ganciclovir treatment in heart transplant recipients by determination of viremia, antigenemia, and DNAemia. *J. Infect. Dis.* **164:**488–498.

45. **Gimeno, C., C. Solano, J. C. Latorre, J. C. Hernandez-Boluda, M. A. Clari, M. J. Remigia, S. Furio, M. Calabuig, N. Tormo, and D. Navarro.** 2008. Quantification of DNA in plasma by an automated real-time PCR assay (cytomegalovirus PCR kit) for surveillance of active cytomegalovirus infection and guidance of preemptive therapy for allogeneic hematopoietic stem cell transplant recipients. *J. Clin. Microbiol.* **46:**3311–3318.

46. **Gleaves, C. A., D. A. Hursh, and J. D. Meyers.** 1992. Detection of human cytomegalovirus in clinical specimens by centrifugation culture with a nonhuman cell line. *J. Clin. Microbiol.* **30:**1045–1048.

47. **Gleaves, C. A., T. F. Smith, E. A. Shuster, and G. R. Pearson.** 1984. Rapid detection of cytomegalovirus in MRC-5 cells inoculated with urine specimens by using low-speed centrifugation and monoclonal antibody to an early antigen. *J. Clin. Microbiol.* **19:**917–919.

48. **Goegebuer, T., B. Van Meensel, K. Beuselinck, V. Cossey, M. Van Ranst, M. Hanssens, and K. Lagrou.** 2009. Clinical predictive value of real-time PCR quantification of human cytomegalovirus DNA in amniotic fluid samples. *J. Clin. Microbiol.* **47:**660–665.

49. **Gouarin, S., A. Vabret, C. Scieux, F. Agbalika, J. Cherot, C. Mengelle, C. Deback, J. Petitjean, J. Dina, and F. Freymuth.** 2007. Multicentric evaluation of a new commercial cytomegalovirus real-time PCR quantitation assay. *J. Virol. Methods* **146:**147–154.

50. **Gourlain, K., D. Salmon, E. Gault, C. Leport, C. Katlama, S. Matheron, D. Costagliola, M.-C. Mazeron, A.-M. Fillet, and the Predivir Study Group and CMV AC11 Study Group.** 2003. Quantitation of cytomegalovirus (CMV) DNA by real-time PCR for occurrence of CMV disease in HIV-infected patients receiving highly active antiretroviral therapy. *J. Med. Virol.* **69:**401–407.

51. **Gozlan, J., J.-M. Saloed, C. Chouaid, C. Duvivier, O. Picard, M.-C. Meyohas, and J.-C. Petit.** 1993. Human cytomegalovirus (HCMV) late-mRNA detection in peripheral blood of AIDS patients: diagnostic value for HCMV disease compared with those of viral culture and HCMV DNA detection. *J. Clin. Microbiol.* **31:**1943–1945.

52. **Grangeot-Keros, L., M. J. Mayaux, P. Lebon, F. Freymuth, G. Eugene, R. Stricker, and E. Dussaix.** 1997. Value of cytomegalovirus (CMV) IgG avidity index for the diagnosis of primary CMV infection in pregnant women. *J. Infect. Dis.* **175:**944–946.

53. **Griscelli, F., M. Barrois, S. Chauvin, S. Lastere, D. Bellet, and J.-H. Bourhis.** 2001. Quantification of human cytomegalovirus DNA in bone marrow transplant recipients by real-time PCR. *J. Clin. Microbiol.* **39:**4362–4369.

54. **Guiver, M., A. J. Fox, K. Mutton, N. Mogulkoc, and J. Egan.** 2001. Evaluation of CMV viral load using TaqMan CMV quantitative PCR and comparison with CMV antigenemia in heart and lung transplant recipients. *Transplantation* **71:**1609–1615.

55. **Hanson, K. E., L. B. Reller, J. Kurtzberg, M. Horwitz, G. Long, and B. D. Alexander.** 2007. Comparison of the Digen Hybrid Capture System Cytomegalovirus (CMV) DNA (Version 2.0), Roche CMV UL54 analyte-specific reagent, and QIAGEN RealArt CMV LightCycler PCR reagent tests using AcroMetrix OptiQuant CMV DNA quantification panels and specimens from allogeneic-stem-cell transplant recipients. *J. Clin. Microbiol.* **45:**1972–1973.

56. **Ho, S. K. N., C.-Y. Lo, I. K. P. Cheng, and T.-M. Chan.** 1998. Rapid cytomegalovirus pp65 antigenemia assay by direct erythrocyte lysis and immunofluorescence staining. *J. Clin. Microbiol.* **36:**638–640.

57. **Hodinka, R. L.** 1999. Serological tests in clinical virology, p. 195–211. *In* E. H. Lennette and T. F. Smith (ed.), *Laboratory Diagnosis of Viral Infections*, 3rd ed. Marcel Dekker, New York, NY.

58. **Hodinka, R. L.** 1998. The clinical utility of viral quantitation using molecular methods. *Clin. Diagn. Virol.* **10:**25–47.

59. **Hsia, K., D. H. Spector, J. Lawrie, and S. A. Spector.** 1989. Enzymatic amplification of human cytomegalovirus sequences by polymerase chain reaction. *J. Clin. Microbiol.* **27:**1802–1809.

60. **Husain, S., C. E. Pietrangeli, and A. Zeevi.** 2009. Delayed onset CMV disease in solid organ transplant recipients. *Transplant Immunol.* **21:**1–9. doi:10.1016/j.trim.2008.12.004.

61. **Jang, E. Y., S. Y. Park, E. J. Lee, E. H. Song, Y. P. Chong, S.-O. Lee, S.-O. Choi, J. H. Woo, Y. S. Kim, and S.-H. Kim.** 2009. Diagnostic performance of the cytomegalovirus (CMV) antigenemia assay in patients with CMV gastrointestinal disease. *Clin. Infect. Dis.* **48:**e121–e124.

62. **Koidl, C., M. Bozic, E. Marth, and H. H. Kessler.** 2008. Detection of CMV DNA: is EDTA whole blood superior to EDTA plasma? *J. Virol. Methods* **154:**210–212.

63. **Lam, K. M., N. Oldenburg, M. A. Khan, V. Gaylore, G. W. Mikhail, P. D. Strouhal, J. M. Middeldorp, N. Banner, and M. Yacoub.** 1998. Significance of reverse transcription polymerase chain reaction in the detection of human cytomegalovirus gene transcripts in thoracic organ transplant recipients. *J. Heart Lung Transplant.* **17:**555–565.

64. **Landini, M. P., and T. Lazzarotto.** 1999. Prenatal diagnosis of congenital cytomegalovirus infection: light and shade. *Herpes* **6:**45–49.

65. **Landini, M. P., T. Lazzarotto, G. T. Maine, A. Ripalti, and R. Flanders.** 1995. Recombinant mono- and polyantigens to detect cytomegalovirus-specific immunoglobulin M in human sera by enzyme immunoassay. *J. Clin. Microbiol.* **33:**2535–2542.

66. **Landry, M. L., and D. Ferguson.** 2000. Reduced ability to culture cytomegalovirus from peripheral blood leukocytes isolated by direct erythrocyte lysis. *J. Clin. Microbiol.* **38:**3906.

67. **Landry, M. L., and D. Ferguson.** 2000. Two-hour cytomegalovirus pp65 antigenemia assay for rapid quantitation of cytomegalovirus in blood samples. *J. Clin. Microbiol.* **38:**427–428.

68. **Landry, M. L., and D. Ferguson.** 1993. Comparison of quantitative cytomegalovirus antigenemia assay with culture methods and correlation with clinical disease. *J. Clin. Microbiol.* **31:**2851–2856.

69. **Landry, M. L., D. Ferguson, S. Cohen, K. Huber, and P. Wetherill.** 1995. Effect of delayed specimen processing on cytomegalovirus antigenemia test results. *J. Clin. Microbiol.* **33:**257–259.

70. **Landry, M. L., D. Ferguson, T. Stevens-Ayers, M. W. A. de Jonge, and M. Boeckh.** 1996. Evaluation of CMV Brite kit for detection of cytomegalovirus pp65 antigenemia in peripheral blood leukocytes by immunofluorescence. *J. Clin. Microbiol.* **34:**1337–1339.

71. **Lazzarotto, T., B. Guerra, M. Lanari, L. Gabrielli, M. P. Landini.** 2008. New advances in the diagnosis of congenital cytomegalovirus infection. *J. Clin. Virol.* **41:**192–197.

72. **Lazzarotto, T., P. Spezzacatena, P. Pradelli, D. A. Abate, S. Varani, and M. P. Landini.** 1997. Avidity of immunoglobulin G directed against human cytomegalovirus during primary and secondary infections in immunocompetent and immunocompromised subjects. *Clin. Diagn. Lab. Immunol.* **4:**469–473.

73. **Lazzarotto, T., S. Varani, P. Spezzacatena, P. Pradelli, L. Potena, A. Lombardi, V. Ghisetti, L. Gabrielli, D. A. Abate, C. Magelli, and M. P. Landini.** 1998. Delayed acquisition of high-avidity anti-cytomegalovirus antibody is correlated with prolonged antigenemia in solid organ transplant recipients. *J. Infect. Dis.* **178:**1145–1149.

74. **Leruez-Ville, M., M. Ouachee, R. Delarue, A.-S. Sauget, S. Blanche, A. Buzyn, and C. Rouzioux.** 2003. Monitoring cytomegalovirus infection in adult and pediatric bone marrow

transplant recipients by a real-time PCR assay performed with blood plasma. *J. Clin. Microbiol.* **41:**2040–2026.

75. **Machida, U., M. Kami, T. Fukui, Y. Kazuyama, M. Kinoshita, Y. Tanaka, Y, Kanda, S. Ogawa, H. Honda, S. Chiba, K. Mitani, Y. Muto, K. Osumi, S. Kimura, and H. Hirai.** 2000. Real-time automated PCR for early diagnosis and monitoring of cytomegalovirus infection after bone marrow transplantation. *J. Clin. Microbiol.* **38:**2536–2542.

76. **MacKenzie, D., and L. C. McLaren.** 1989. Increased sensitivity for rapid detection of cytomegalovirus by shell vial centrifugation assay using mink lung cell cultures. *J. Virol. Methods* **26:**183–188.

77. **May, G., J. E. Kuhn, and B. R. Eing.** 2006. Comparison of two commercially available pp65 antigenemia tests and COBAS Amplicor CMV Monitor for early detection and quantification of episodes of human CMV-viremia in transplant recipients. *Intervirology* **49:**261–265.

78. **Mayo, D. R., T. Brennan, S. P. Sirpenski, and C. Seymour.** 1985. Cytomegalovirus antibody detection by three commercially available assays and complement fixation. *Diagn. Microbiol. Infect. Dis.* **3:**455–459.

79. **McHugh, T. M., C. H. Casavant, J. C. Wilber, and D. P. Stites.** 1985. Comparison of six methods for the detection of antibody to cytomegalovirus. *J. Clin. Microbiol.* **22:**1014–1019.

80. **Mengelle, C., C. Pasquier, L. Rostaing, K. Sandres-Saune, J. Puel, L. Berges, L. Righi, C. Bouquies, and J. Izopet.** 2003. Quantitation of human cytomegalovirus in recipients of solid organ transplants by real-time quantitative PCR and pp65 antigenemia. *J. Med. Virol.* **69:**225–231.

81. **Mengelle, C., K. Sandres-Saune, C. Pasquier, L. Rostaing, J.-M. Mansuy, M. Marty, I. Da Silva, M. Attal, P. Massip, and J. Izopet.** 2003. Automated extraction and quantitation of human cytomegalovirus DNA in whole blood by real-time PCR assay. *J. Clin. Microbiol.* **41:**3840–3845.

82. **Mengoli, C., R. Cusinato, M. A. Biasolo, S. Cesaro, C. Parolin, and G. Palu.** 2004. Assessment of CMV load in solid organ trnasplant recipients by pp65 antigenemia and real-time quantitative DNA PCR assay: correlation with pp67 RNA detection. *J. Med. Virol.* **74:**78–84.

83. **Michelin, B. D. A., I. Hadzisejdic, M. Bozic, M. Grahovac, M. Hess, B. Grahovac, E. Marth, and H. H. Kessler.** 2008. Detection of cytomegalovirus (CMV) DNA in EDTA whole-blood samples: evaluation of the quantitative *artus* CMV LightCycler PCR kit in conjunction with automated sample preparation. *J. Clin. Microbiol.* **46:**1241–1245.

84. **Nelson, P. N., B. K. Rawal, Y. S. Boriskin, K. E. Mathers, R. L. Powles, H. M. Steel, Y. S. Tryhorn, P. D. Butcher, and J. C. Booth.** 1996. A polymerase chain reaction to detect a spliced late transcript of human cytomegalovirus in the blood of bone marrow transplant recipients. *J. Virol. Methods* **56:**139–148.

85. **Novak, Z., S. A. Ross, R. K. Patro, S. K. Pati, M. K. Reddy, M. Purser, W. J. Britt, and S. B. Boppana.** 2009. Enzyme-linked immunosorbent assay method for detection of cytomegalovirus strain-specific antibody responses. *Clin. Vaccine Immunol.* **16:**288–290.

86. **O'Connor, S., C. Taylor, L. A. Campbell, S. Epstein, and P. Libby.** 2001. Potential infectious etiologies of atherosclerosis: a multifactorial perspective. *Emerg. Infect. Dis.* **7:**780–788.

87. **Olive, D. M., M. Simsek, and S. Al-Mufti.** 1989. Polymerase chain reaction assay for detection of human cytomegalovirus. *J. Clin. Microbiol.* **27:**1238–1242.

88. **Ono, Y., Y. Ito, K. Kaneko, Y. Shibata-Watanabe, T. Tainaka, W. Sumida, T. Nakamura, H. Kamei, T. Kiuchi, H. Ando, and H. Kimura.** 2008. Simultaneous monitoring by real-time polymerase chain reaction of Epstein-Barr virus, human cytomegalovirus, and human herpesvirus-6 in juvenile and adult liver transplant recipients. *Transplant. Proc.* **40:**3578–3582.

89. **Osawa, R., and N. Singh.** 2009. Cytomegalovirus infection in critically ill patients: a systematic review. *Crit. Care* **13:**R68. doi:10.1186/cc7875.

90. **Pang, X. L., J. D. Fox, J. M. Fenton, G. G. Miller, A. M. Caliendo, and J. K. Preiksaitis for the American Society of Transplantation Infectious Diseases Community of Practice and the Canadian Society of Transplantation.** 2009. Interlaboratory comparison of cytomegalovirus viral load assays. *Am. J. Transplant.* **9:**258–268.

91. **Patel, R., D. W. Klein, M. J. Espy, W. S. Harmsen, D. M. Ilstrup, C. V. Paya, and T. F. Smith.** 1995. Optimization of detection of cytomegalovirus viremia in transplantation recipients by shell vial assay. *J. Clin. Microbiol.* **33:**2984–2986.

92. **Paya, C. V., A. D. Wold, D. M. Ilstrup, and T. F. Smith.** 1988. Evaluation of number of shell vial cell cultures per clinical specimen for rapid diagnosis of cytomegalovirus infection. *J. Clin. Microbiol.* **26:**198–200.

93. **Pellegrin, I., I. Garrigue, D. Ekouevi, L. Couzi, P. Merville, P. Merel, G. Chene, M. H. Schrive, P. Trimoulet, M. E. Lafon, and H. Fleury.** 2000. New molecular assays to predict occurrence of cytomegalovirus disease in renal transplant recipients. *J. Infect. Dis.* **182:**36–42.

94. **Percivalle, E., E. Genini, A. Chiesa, and G. Gerna.** 2008. Comparison of a new Light Diagnostics and the CMV Brite to an in-house developed human cytomegalovirus antigenemia assay. *J. Clin. Virol.* **43:**13–17.

95. **Phipps, P. H., L. Gregoire, E. Rossier, and E. Perry.** 1983. Comparison of five methods of cytomegalovirus antibody screening of blood donors. *J. Clin. Microbiol.* **18:**1296–1300.

96. **Pignatelli, S., P. Dal Monte, G. Rossini, and M. P. Landini.** 2004. Genetic polymorphisms among human cytomegalovirus (HCMV) wild-type strains. *Rev. Med. Virol.* **14:**383–410.

97. **Prince, H. E., and A. L. Leber.** 2002. Validation of an in-house assay for cytomegalovirus immunoglobulin G (CMV IgG) avidity and relationship of avidity to CMV IgM levels. *Clin. Diagn. Lab. Immunol.* **9:**824–827.

98. **Rafailidis, P. I., E. G. Mourtzoukou, I. C. Varbobitis, and M. E. Falagas.** 2008. Severe cytomegalovirus infection in apparently immunocompetent patients: a systematic review. *Virol. J.* **5:**47. doi:10.1186/1743-422X-5-47.

99. **Rasmussen, L., S. Morris, D. Zipeto, J. Fessel, R. Wolitz, A. Dowling, and T. C. Merigan.** 1995. Quantitation of human cytomegalovirus DNA from peripheral blood cells of human immunodeficiency virus-infected patients could predict cytomegalovirus retinitis. *J. Infect. Dis.* **171:**177–182.

100. **Razonable, R. R., R. A. Brown, M. J. Espy, A. Rivero, W. Kremers, J. Wilson, C. Groettum, T. F. Smith, and C. V. Paya.** 2001. Comparative quantitation of cytomegalovirus (CMV) DNA in solid organ transplant recipients with CMV infection by using two high-throughput automated systems. *J. Clin. Microbiol.* **39:**4472–4476.

101. **Razonable, R. R., R. A. Brown, J. Wilson, C. Groettum, W. Kremers, M. Espy, T. F. Smith, and C. Paya.** 2002. The clinical use of various blood compartments for cytomegalovirus (CMV) DNA quantitation in transplant recipients with CMV disease. *Transplantation* **73:**968–973.

102. **Razonable, R. R., and V. C. Emery.** 2004. Management of CMV infection and disease in transplant patients. *Herpes* **11:**77–86.

103. **Revello, M. G., and G. Gerna.** 2002. Diagnosis and management of human cytomegalovirus infection in the mother, fetus, and newborn infant. *Clin. Microbiol. Rev.* **15:**680–715.

104. **Revello, M. G., E. Percivalle, A. Sarasini, F. Baldanti, M. Furione, and G. Gerna.** 1994. Diagnosis of human cytomegalovirus infection of the nervous system by pp65 detection in polymorphonuclear leukocytes of cerebrospinal fluid from AIDS patients. *J. Infect. Dis.* **170:**1275–1279.

105. **Salzberger, B., D. Myerson, and M. Boeckh.** 1997. Circulating cytomegalovirus (CMV)-infected endothelial cells in marrow transplant patients with CMV disease and CMV infection. *J. Infect. Dis.* **176:**778–781.

106. **Sanchez, J. L., and G. A. Storch.** 2002. Multiplex, quantitative, real-time PCR assay for cytomegalovirus and human DNA. *J. Clin. Microbiol.* **40:**2381–2386.

107. Sanghavi, S. K., K. Abu-Elmagd, M. C. Keightley, K. St. George, K. Lewandowski, S. S. Boes, A. Bullotta, R. Dare, M. Lassak, S. Jusain, E. J. Kwak, D. L. Paterson, C. R. Rinaldo. 2008. Relationship of cytomegalovirus load assessed by real-time PCR to pp65 antigenemia in organ transplant recipients. *J. Clin. Virol.* **42:**335–342.

108. Schaade, L., P. Kockelkorn, K. Ritter, and M. Kleines. 2000. Detection of cytomegalovirus DNA in human specimens by LightCycler PCR. *J. Clin. Microbiol.* **38:**4006–4009.

109. Schleiss, M. R., and T. C. Heineman. 2005. Progress toward an elusive goal: current status of cytomegalovirus vaccines. *Expert Rev. Vaccines* **4:**381–406.

110. Shibata, D., W. J. Martin, M. D. Appelman, D. M. Causey, J. M. Leedom, and N. Arnheim. 1988. Detection of cytomegalovirus DNA in peripheral blood of patients with human immunodeficiency virus. *J. Infect. Dis.* **158:**1185–1192.

111. Shinkai, M., and S. Spector. 1995. Quantitation of human cytomegalovirus (HCMV) DNA in cerebrospinal fluid by competitive PCR in AIDS patients with different HCMV central nervous system diseases. *Scand. J. Infect. Dis.* **27:**559–561.

112. Sia, I. G., J. A. Wilson, M. J. Espy, C. V. Paya, and T. F. Smith. 2000. Evaluation of the COBAS AMPLICOR CMV MONITOR Test for detection of viral DNA in specimens taken from patients after liver transplantation. *J. Clin. Microbiol.* **38:**600–606.

113. Smith, I. L., J. M. Cherrington, R. E. Jiles, M. D. Fuller, W. R. Freeman, and S. A. Spector. 1997. High-level resistance of cytomegalovirus to ganciclovir is associated with alterations in both the UL97 and DNA polymerase genes. *J. Infect. Dis.* **176:**69–77.

114. Smith, T. F., M. J. Espy, J. Mandrekar, M. F. Jones, F. R. Cockerill, and R. Patel. 2007. Quantitative real-time polymerase chain reaction for evaluating DNAemia due to cytomegalovirus, Epstein-Barr virus, and BK virus in solid-organ transplant recipients. *Clin. Infect. Dis.* **45:**1056–1061.

115. Spector, S. A., R. Merrill, D. Wolf, and W. M. Dankner. 1992. Detection of human cytomegalovirus in plasma of AIDS patients during acute visceral disease by DNA amplification. *J. Clin. Microbiol.* **30:**2359–2365.

116. Stanier, P., D. L. Taylor, A. D. Kitchen, N. Wales, Y. Tryhorn, and A. S. Tyms. 1989. Persistence of cytomegalovirus in mononuclear cells in peripheral blood from blood donors. *Br. Med. J.* **299:**897–898.

117. St. George, K., M. J. Boyd, S. M. Lipson, D. Ferguson, G. F. Cartmell, L. H. Falk, C. R. Rinaldo, and M. L. Landry. 2000. A multisite trial comparing two cytomegalovirus (CMV) pp65 antigenemia test kits, Biotest CMV Brite and Bartels/Argene CMV antigenemia. *J. Clin. Microbiol.* **38:**1430–1433.

118. Tan, B. H., N. L. Chlebicka, J. G. Hong Low, T. Y. R. Chong, K. P. Chan, and Y. T. Goh. 2008. Use of the cytomegalovirus pp65 antigenemia assay for preemptive therapy in allogeneic hematopoietic stem cell transplantation: a real-world review. *Transpl. Infect. Dis.* **10:**325–332.

119. Tang, W., S. H. Elmore, H. Fan, L. B. Thorne, and M. L. Gulley. 2008. Cytomegalovirus DNA measurement in blood and plasma using Roche LightCycler CMV quantitative reagents. *Diagn. Mol. Pathol.* **17:**166–173.

120. The, T. H., A. P. van den Berg, M. C. Harmsen, W. van der Bij, and W. J. van Son. 1995. The cytomegalovirus antigenemia assay: a plea for standardization. *Scand. J. Infect. Dis.* **99**(Suppl.):25–29.

121. The, T. H., M. van der Ploeg, A. P. van den Berg, A. M. Vlieger, M. van der Giessen, and W. J. van Son. 1992. Direct detection of cytomegalovirus in peripheral blood leukocytes—a review of the antigenemia assay and polymerase chain reaction. *Transplantation* **54:**193–198.

122. Theiler, R. N., A. M.Caliendo, S. Pargman, B. D. Raynor, S. Berga, M. McPheeters, and D. J. Jamieson. 2006. Umbilical cord blood screening for cytomegalovirus DNA by quantitative PCR. *J. Clin. Virol.* **37:**313–316.

123. Tong, C. Y., L. E. Cuevas, H. Williams, and A. Bakran. 2000. Comparison of two commercial methods for measurement of cytomegalovirus load in blood samples after renal transplantation. *J. Clin. Microbiol.* **38:**1209–1213.

124. van den Berg, A. P., A. M. Tegzess, A. Scholten-Sampson, J. Schirm, M. van der Giessen, T. H. The, and W. J. van Son. 1992. Monitoring antigenemia is useful in guiding treatment of severe cytomegalovirus disease after organ transplantation. *Transpl. Int.* **5:**101–107.

125. Verschuuren, E. A., M. C. Harmsen, P. C. Limburg, W. van der Bij, A. P. van den Berg, A. M. Kas-Deelen, B. Meedendorp, W. J. van Son, and T. H. The. 1999. Toward standardization of the human cytomegalovirus antigenemia assay. *Intervirology* **42:**382–389.

126. Visser, C. E., C. J. van Zeijl, E. P. de Klerk, B. M. Schillizi, M. F. Beersma, and A. C. Kroes. 2000. First experiences with an accelerated CMV antigenemia test: CMV Brite Turbo assay. *J. Clin. Virol.* **17:**65–68.

127. Vornhagen, R., B. Plachter, W. Hinderer, T. H. The, J. van Zanten, L. Matter, C. A. Schmidt, H.-H. Sonneborn, and G. Jahn. 1994. Early serodiagnosis of acute human cytomegalovirus infection by enzyme-linked immunosorbent assay using recombinant antigens. *J. Clin. Microbiol.* **32:**981–986.

128. Wada, K., N. Kubota, Y. Ito, H. Yagasaki, K. Kato, T. Yoshikawa, Y. Ono, H. Ando, Y. Fujimoto, T. Kiuchi, S. Kojima, Y. Nishiyama, and H. Kimura. 2007. Simultaneous quantification of Epstein-Barr virus, cytomegalovirus, and human herpesvirus 6 DNA in samples from transplant recipients by multiplex real-time PCR assay. *J. Clin. Microbiol.* **45:**1426–1432.

129. Walter, S., C. Atkinson, M. Sharland, P. Rice, E. Raglan, V. C. Emery, and P. D. Griffiths. 2009. Congenital cytomegalovirus: association between dired blood spot viral load and hearing loss. *Arch. Dis. Child Fetal Neonatal Ed.* **93:**F280–F285.

130. Wattanamano, P., J. L. Clayton, J. J. Kopicko, P. Kissinger, S. Elliot, C. Jarrott, S. Rangan, and M. A. Beilke. 2000. Comparison of three assays for cytomegalovirus detection in AIDS patients at risk for retinitis. *J. Clin. Microbiol.* **38:**727–732.

131. West, P. G., B. Aldrich, R. Hartwig, and G. J. Haller. 1988. Enhanced detection of cytomegalovirus in confluent MRC-5 cells treated with dexamethasone and dimethyl sulfoxide. *J. Clin. Microbiol.* **26:**2510–2514.

132. West, P. G., and W. W. Baker. 1990. Enhancement by calcium of the detection of cytomegalovirus in cells treated with dexamethasone and dimethyl sulfoxide. *J. Clin. Microbiol.* **28:**1708–1710.

133. Wolf, D. G., and S. A. Spector. 1992. Diagnosis of human cytomegalovirus central nervous system disease in AIDS patients by DNA amplification from cerebrospinal fluid. *J. Infect. Dis.* **166:**1412–1415.

134. Wolff, D. J., D. L. Heaney, P. D. Neuwald, K. A. Stellrecht, and R. D. Press. 2009. Multi-site PCR-based CMV viral load assessment-assays demonstrate linearity and precision, but lack numeric standardization. *J. Mol. Diagn.* **11:**87–92.

135. Wunderli, W., M. K. Kagi, E. Gruter, and J. D. Auracher. 1989. Detection of cytomegalovirus in peripheral leukocytes by different methods. *J. Clin. Microbiol.* **27:**1916–1917.

136. Zipeto, D., F. Baldanti, D. Zella, M. Furione, A. Cavicchini, G. Milanesi, and G. Gerna. 1993. Quantification of human cytomegalovirus DNA in peripheral blood polymorphonuclear leukocytes of immunocompromised patients by the polymerase chain reaction. *J. Virol. Methods* **44:**45–56.

137. Zipeto, D., S. Morris, C. Hong, A. Dowling, R. Wolitz, T. C. Merigan, and L. Rasmussen. 1995. Human cytomegalovirus (CMV) DNA in plasma reflects quantity of CMV DNA present in leukocytes. *J. Clin. Microbiol.* **33:**2607–2611.

Epstein-Barr Virus*

BARBARA C. GÄRTNER

99

TAXONOMY

Epstein-Barr virus (EBV) is a member of the *Herpesviridae* and belongs to the subfamily *Gammaherpesvirinae*, replicating in epithelial cells and establishing long-term latency in lymphocytes like its closest human-pathogenic relative, human herpesvirus 8. EBV is subclassified into the genus *Lymphocryptovirus* and is its only human-pathogenic member, whereas human herpesvirus 8 belongs to the genus *Rhadinovirus*.

DESCRIPTION OF THE AGENT

EBV is a morphologically typical herpesvirus, with 162 capsomeres in an icosahedral arrangement surrounded by a lipid-rich envelope. The virus has a double-stranded, 172-kbp DNA genome, linear in the mature virion and circular episomal in latently infected cells. The genome consists of a series of unique sequences alternating with internal repeats, all sandwiched between two terminal repeat elements which are joined during circularization. Integration of viral DNA into host chromosomal DNA has been shown in rare cases, mainly in lymphoblastoid cell lines (43).

EBV primarily infects B cells, which carry CD21, the complement receptor and also the receptor for EBV. It has the ability to transform precursor and mature human B cells to lymphoblastoid cell lines. B cells are the site of latency, but epithelial cells are the main producers of progeny virus. Monocytes may also be productively infected by EBV (31, 67). EBV nuclear antigen 1 (EBNA1), EBNA2, EBNA3 (also referred to as EBNA3a), EBNA4 (EBNA3b), EBNA5 (EBNALP), EBNA6 (EBNA3c), and latent membrane proteins (LMP1, -2A, and -2B) may be expressed in B cells. Four types of B-cell latency have been defined, based on various levels of expression of the latency-associated proteins (32, 57). In latency type 0, only EBV-encoded RNAs (EBERs) and rightward transcripts from the BamHIA gene are expressed. EBER1 and EBER2 are nonpolyadenylated RNAs, are therefore not translated to a protein, and act to inhibit antiviral effects by interferon as well as apoptosis.

EBERs are present in high copy numbers (10^6 to 10^7 copies) in virtually all EBV-infected cells. In latency type I, in addition to type 0 expression profile, EBNA1 and LMP2 are also detectable. In latency type II, LMP1 is expressed in addition to gene products of latency type I. Finally, in latency type III, all EBNA proteins are detectable.

EBV has been propagated in vitro only in B cells from humans and nonhuman primates (43). In a healthy individual, about 1 to 50 B cells per million are infected (82). During lytic replication more than 70 proteins are expressed, including the virus capsid antigens (VCA) and the early antigens (EA) used in diagnostics.

EPIDEMIOLOGY AND TRANSMISSION

Virtually everyone becomes infected with EBV at some time during their life. Under poor hygiene conditions, EBV infection occurs mainly during the first years of life. However, in developed countries about 60% of the population are infected before puberty. By the age of 20 years around 90% of individuals are seropositive, and by the age of 40 almost 100% of the population have seroconverted.

Transmission of EBV occurs mainly by salivary or sexual contact (13, 18, 66). Infectious virus and viral genomes can be detected in oropharyngeal washings from the majority of seropositive individuals (~80%), not only those with infectious mononucleosis (IM) (19). Thus, use of saliva for diagnostics is discouraged. Other, less common routes of transmission include transplanted organs or blood products, which can be problematic in immunosuppressed individuals.

EBV strains may be classified into types A and B (sometimes referred to as types 1 and 2, respectively) based on the polymorphism of their EBNA genes. Prototypic viruses differ mainly in their nucleotide sequences for EBNA2 and, to a lower extent, in other EBNA proteins not routinely used in diagnostics. Since current enzyme immunoassays (EIAs) predominantly use EBNA1, the strain differences might not be relevant for routine diagnostics. Both EBV types have a worldwide distribution, though they predominate in different geographical areas. Dual infections with both types are not uncommon. In immunosuppressed individuals, coinfection with multiple strains of EBV has also been demonstrated (29).

---

*This chapter contains information presented in chapter 103 by Annika Linde and Kerstin I. Falk in the ninth edition of this *Manual*.

CLINICAL SIGNIFICANCE

EBV is associated with different diseases in immunocompetent and immunosuppressed individuals. Primary EBV infections are mostly asymptomatic. With increasing age the rate of symptomatic infections increases, reaching around 50% in young adults. The clinical manifestations of primary EBV infections are largely immune mediated (40).

IM is a self-limiting, lymphoproliferative illness which can be mild or severe (38, 61). The condition is characterized by fever, pharyngitis, tonsillitis, lymphadenophathy, hepatitis, splenomegaly, and lymphocytosis with atypical lymphocytes. The incubation time is relatively long, at 30 to 50 days (37), and the clinical disease generally persists for 1 to 4 weeks; however, protracted illness and postinfectious fatigue and/or depression for up to a year are not uncommon (62). Complications are frequent and may be the only sign of IM. Hematological complications such as anemia, thrombocytopenia, or hemophagocytic lymphohistiocytosis are typical, as is neurological involvement leading to conditions such as meningoencephalitis, radiculitis, or mononeuritis. Exanthema following administration of antibiotics is typical. When visceral organs are affected, almost any symptom resulting from inflammation in the affected organ may be expected. Very rare fatalities can occur due to spleen rupture, overwhelming infection, or hemophagocytic lymphohistiocytosis (39). Treatment of IM with antiviral agents results in termination of viral shedding but does not affect the symptoms (75, 79). EBV is often reactivated in healthy individuals, accompanied by shedding of the virus. At present, no symptoms are known to be associated with reactivation in healthy individuals. It should also be noted that primary EBV infections account for only approximately 50 to 90% of IM cases (38). Aside from noninfectious causes (e.g., malignant diseases), IM also may be caused by other infectious agents, such as acute cytomegalovirus, adenovirus, *Toxoplasma gondii*, or human immunodeficiency virus (HIV) infection. Lymphoma or autoimmune diseases can also mimic mononucleosis.

Chronic active EBV infection is a rare, severe condition, often ending in EBV-associated malignancies or other diseases with a lethal outcome (44). It is characterized by a clonal expansion of EBV-infected T cells and natural killer (NK) cells and a high viral load. Patients often show atypical patterns of EA antibodies (11, 45).

EBV is associated with a variety of tumors, not related to obvious immunosuppression. EBV genomes have been found in tumor cells in >95% of endemic Burkitt's lymphomas and nasopharyngeal carcinomas, <5 to 70% of Hodgkin's disease (depending on the subtype), 2 to 16% of gastric adenocarcinomas, 40 to >90% of T/NK cell lymphomas (depending on the subtype), and 40 to 95% of lymphoepithelioma-like carcinomas.

In immunocompromised patients, both primary infection and EBV reactivation are most commonly associated with lymphoproliferative disorders. Posttransplant lymphoproliferative disorder (PTLD) is defined as lymphoproliferation following transplantation ranging from IM to lymphoma similar to that seen in immunocompetent individuals. Lymphomas are frequently localized to the intestine or brain, particularly in organ transplant recipients. Principal risk factors are (i) EBV primary infection after transplantation and (ii) severe T-cell depletion (e.g., after administration of T-cell antibodies) (9, 47, 84).

EBV-related lymphomas are also a major cause of tumors in AIDS patients. Lymphomas of the central nervous system (CNS), lymphoma, and smooth muscle tumors are strongly associated with EBV (~95%) (15, 41, 46). In oral hairy leukoplakia, lesions appear as white patches at the border of the tongue (78).

X-linked lymphoproliferative syndrome is a rare hereditary immunodeficiency primarily involving T cells and NK cells (27). Affected boys become symptomatic after exposure to EBV, developing acute fatal IM or lymphoproliferative disorders and/or dysgammaglobulinemia. The gene responsible for the syndrome codes for an SH2 (src homology 2) domain (59, 72). Untreated, the disease is ultimately lethal.

Treatment options for EBV-associated malignancies are EBV-specific cytotoxic T lymphocytes (34, 56), monoclonal anti-CD20 antibodies (rituximab) in cases with B-cell involvement (3, 10, 58), chemotherapy (17, 77), or stem cell transplantation.

There is no approved vaccine against EBV. Two studies involving different vaccine prototypes showed that these vaccines failed to prevent EBV infection but were effective in preventing symptomatic disease (16, 68).

COLLECTION, TRANSPORT, AND STORAGE OF SPECIMENS

For the rare cases where excreted virus is to be isolated, 5 to 10 ml of throat gargle, collected in serum-free tissue culture medium or Hanks' balanced salt solution, is sufficient. Approximately 5 to 10 ml of heparinized blood is required either for cell culture and detection of EBV-transformed B cells or for antigen detection in B cells by immunostaining. Blood specimens should be processed as soon as possible, although refrigeration for up to 24 h is acceptable for antigen detection. Fresh biopsy samples or thin cryosections (5 μm) are preferable to formalin-fixed material for antigen detection in other tissues.

Nucleic acid detection techniques (NAT) might be applied to blood, cerebrospinal fluid (CSF), or biopsy samples.

The choice of sample matrix depends on the clinical condition of the patient (Table 1). There is currently no agreement on whether leukocytes, whole blood (in EDTA; heparin may inhibit the PCR), or serum or plasma should be used for monitoring PTLD. Leukocytes and whole blood show a high sensitivity but lower specificity for PTLD, whereas the opposite holds true for cell-free specimens like serum or plasma. Since specificity is more important for a disease with low prevalence, a cell-free sample matrix is likely to be advantageous. For monitoring, it is particularly important that the sample matrix is not varied. The sample quantity required varies, but it is advisable to provide at least 1 ml. Blood specimens used as source for serum, plasma, or peripheral blood mononuclear cells should be processed as soon as possible. If transport time is less than 24 h, samples may be kept at room temperature until separated. Separated materials can thereafter be stored at 5°C for a few days or frozen. Whole blood can be stored for a few days at room temperature or frozen without further processing. For long-term storage, freezing at −70°C is recommended. For detection of EBV by DNA hybridization in peripheral blood lymphocytes, 5 to 10 ml of blood collected in heparin or EDTA is required.

CSF is useful for diagnosis of EBV-associated CNS disease. Sterile CSF without additives should be sent and can be stored as serum. It is advisable to provide at least 0.5 ml. Tissues (e.g., nasopharyngeal brushings for nasopharyngeal carcinoma) and biopsy samples to be examined for viral

TABLE 1 Materials and methods used for diagnosis and monitoring of disease caused by EBV, for indication of EBV-associated malignancies, or for verification of EBV association in diagnosed tumors[a]

Suspected EBV-associated condition	First-choice method	Suitable specimen	Approx value for clinical significance (NAAT)	Units (NAAT)	Second-choice method	Suitable specimen
IM	Serology	Serum			PCR	Plasma or serum
PTLD	Quantitative NAAT	Plasma or serum (whole blood)	$\sim 10^2$–10^4 $\sim 10^3$–10^5	geq/ml geq/ml	In situ hybridization and/or antigen detection	Biopsy sample
Lymphoma in HIV-positive patients	Quantitative NAAT	Plasma or serum (whole blood)	Not defined	geq/ml	In situ hybridization and/or antigen detection	Biopsy sample
Nasopharyngeal carcinoma	Quantitative NAAT (BARF 1 RNA)	Plasma or serum Nasopharyngeal brushings	$\sim 10^2$ Not defined	geq/ml geq/μg of DNA	Serology (IgA)	Serum
Chronic active EBV infection	Quantitative NAAT	Mononuclear cells Plasma or serum	$\sim 10^{2.5}$ $\sim 10^3$–10^4	geq/μg of DNA geq/ml		
Neurological involvement	Quantitative or qualitative NAAT	CSF	Positive	geq/ml	In situ hybridization and/or antigen detection	Biopsy sample
XLP	Genetic analysis	Cells			Quantitative NAAT	Plasma or serum (whole blood)
Other EBV-associated tumors	In situ hybridization and/or antigen detection	Biopsy sample			Quantitative or qualitative NAAT	Plasma or serum

[a]gEq, genome equivalents; XLP, X-linked lymphoproliferative syndrome.

nucleic acids or antigens should be collected and refrigerated in saline or balanced salt solution. Fresh, frozen samples are preferred.

For heterophile antibodies whole blood, serum or capillary fingertip blood may be used for most point-of-care case tests. For EBV-specific tests, 50 μl of acute-phase serum or even less may be sufficient; however, it is advisable to provide 1 to 5 ml. Convalescent-phase serum collected 1 to 2 months after onset may occasionally be required in cases of ambiguous results from the first sample. Plasma can be used, but serum is preferable. Serum can be stored at 5°C for several months. For long-term storage, freezing at −20 or −70°C is recommended.

DIRECT DETECTION

Electron microscopy, virus isolation, and antigen detection by immunohistochemistry are primarily research tools. Routine detection of EBV is restricted to NAT.

Microscopy

Electron microscopy is not an appropriate diagnostic technique for EBV, since latency is the norm and virions are rarely present in sufficient quantity in infected tissues.

Antigen Detection

Antibodies specific to a wide range of EBV antigens are used in immunohistochemistry, such as antibodies specific to EBNA1, EBNA2, LMP1, LMP2, BamHI H right frame 1 protein (BHRF1), BamHI Z left frame 1 protein (BZLF1), and Bam M right frame 1 protein (BMRF1) (12, 28, 32, 60). Although EBNA1 is the only antigen expressed in all EBV-infected cells, sensitivity using currently available antibodies is insufficient compared with EBER in situ hybridization (32).

Since nucleic acid detection is more sensitive for diagnostic purposes (i.e., addressing the simple presence or absence of virus), in situ immunohistochemical techniques are rarely applicable in a diagnostic setting. However, in situ and cytohybridization techniques are ideally suited for the detection of EBV in individual tumor cells. EBER detection was found to be highly sensitive in detecting latent infection in tissues and tumors (65) and is considered the "gold standard" for detection of intracellular EBV, although some authors report to have found EBER-negative EBV-positive cells (42).

Nucleic Acid Detection

Molecular techniques are important tools for detection of EBV in clinical specimens. The choices of method and sample matrix are dependent upon the clinical question to be addressed (Table 1).

A wide variety of detection methods are available, ranging from in situ hybridization on frozen or paraffin sections through cytohybridization on cell suspensions, dot blot hybridization, Southern blot hybridization, and nucleic acid amplification techniques (NAAT) (32, 66). The most commonly used clinical diagnostic tools for direct detection of EBV are NAAT. These can be performed on a range of clinical specimens following DNA extraction. A variety of primers, probes, and techniques have been presented previously. In general, quantitative viral load assessment is superior to qualitative detection. Although some commercial assays are available, many laboratories continue to use in-house assays.

Assessment of viral load can be broken down into two basic strategies based upon the genomic region being targeted. (i) The conserved BamHI W region, coding for a long internal repeat sequence of EBNA1, is present in multiple copies (7 to 11 copies) in EBV-infected cells. NAAT targeting this region have maximal sensitivity in clinical samples. (ii) The genes for LMP1 and thymidine kinase or other parts of the EBNA1 gene are often targeted for quantitative PCRs since these are single-copy regions (B. C. Gärtner, E. MacMahon, and E. Puchhammer-Stöckl, unpublished data). Small amplicons may be more applicable when measuring viral DNA from plasma samples, since EBV DNA in plasma is often free DNA, i.e., not encapsidated, and so may be highly fragmented (69).

Quantitative real-time PCR is the most popular method today for EBV monitoring in patients at risk for EBV-associated disorders (22, 32). External standards are used in most real-time assays. As quantitative standards, the best choices are Namalwa cells containing two integrated EBV copies per cell or Raji cells with approximately 50 copies per cell, as they more accurately reflect clinical samples (Gärtner et al., unpublished). Plasmids represent a second-best choice. For accurate quantitation, the standards should be extracted together with the clinical samples, in a matrix resembling the clinical sample (e.g., EBV-negative cells); they should not be diluted in buffer. Since viral load in EBV-associated diseases is routinely elevated, sensitivity is not as important as specificity. For more details on sample matrix, method, and trigger points, see Table 1.

Results should be reported at least in copies per milliliter. Normalization of viral load by cell number or by microgram of DNA is generally unnecessary in routine diagnostics on blood or CSF samples. A recent study with whole blood showed a close correlation between copies per milliliter and copies per microgram of DNA, with similar intrapatient dynamic trends using both reporting formats, suggesting that normalization to cell number or genomic DNA in cellular specimens may also be unnecessary (33). Only when biopsy samples are evaluated should the results be reported in copies per microgram of DNA, or when coamplification of a cellular single-copy gene is performed should results be presented in copies per number of cells.

Appropriate controls for extraction, contamination, and inhibition should always be included in the assays. Participation in external quality control programs is a must (refer, for example, to http://www.cap.org or http://www.QCMD.org). Proficiency panel studies have demonstrated significant variability (4 $\log_{10}$) in both qualitative and quantitative reporting of EBV viral load results between centers, limiting the validity of interinstitutional result comparison (64). Proficiency panel results in both Europe (Quality Control for Molecular Diagnostics) and North America (College of American Pathologists) have illustrated that for analytes assayed by nucleic acid testing and reported quantitatively, interlaboratory variability is significantly reduced when an international reference standard is available and commercial assays are used calibrated to this standard. A World Health Organization international reference standard for EBV DNA employing an EBV-infected cell line is currently under evaluation and at the time of this writing was expected to be available by the end of 2011. For both commercial and in-house assays it is hoped that the use of calibrators referenced to this international standard will reduce intercenter variability and allow quality improvement processes addressing other variables to proceed more rapidly.

ISOLATION AND IDENTIFICATION PROCEDURES

For EBV isolation, freshly fractionated human cord blood lymphocytes are inoculated with cell-free, filtered saliva or throat gargle specimens and monitored for 4 weeks (35).

Individual viral isolates can be characterized by molecular techniques on the basis of polymorphism of the EBNA1 and EBNA3 genes. In addition, the sizes of many of the EBNA proteins (EBNA1 to -6) are strain dependent. Each isolate induces a distinctive banding profile in Western blotting, thus allowing the fingerprinting or "EBNo-typing" of each virus (29). However, this is not a routine method.

SEROLOGIC TESTS

Heterophile Antibodies

Heterophile antibodies are not EBV specific. Testing relies on polyclonal B-cell stimulation, an epiphenomenon often appearing together with IM: the production of antibodies reacting with erythrocytes of nonhuman animals. Historically, sheep erythrocytes were used (Paul-Bunnell test) but lacked sensitivity (5). Later, horse erythrocytes were used in conjunction with the Davidsohn differential test. Since agglutination of sheep or horse erythrocytes might be due to heterophile antibodies against the non-EBV Forssman antigen, these heterophile antibodies were removed by adsorption of serum with guinea pig kidney cells expressing Forssman antigen. As an additional control, serum was also adsorbed with bovine erythrocytes not expressing the IM antigen. When the two adsorbed sera were then mixed with sheep or horse erythrocytes, a positive result was indicated by stronger agglutination in the guinea pig adsorbed serum.

Latex agglutination tests using erythrocyte antigens are currently used and show a high degree of sensitivity (5). Although they are all intended for laboratory and point-of-care use, the agglutination assays may be unsuitable for persons without laboratory training. Evaluation of a true-positive agglutination result requires experience, since spontaneous agglutination will inevitably develop after some time. Immunochromatographic methods may therefore be easier to read and perform better than agglutination assays (5).

EBV-Specific Antibodies

Serologic testing with EBV-specific assays is still the method of choice for the diagnosis or exclusion of EBV infection (36, 66) (Table 2). The tests differ in methods, antigens, and antibody isotypes used. Most frequently, EIAs are used, although immunofluorescence assays (IFAs) and blot techniques seem to be more reliable. At present, flow cytometry-based assays are generally used to detect EBV antibodies to different antigens (i.e., VCA, EA, and EBNA1) at the same time, in a multiplex approach. In the case of unclear results, any of these methods may be supplemented by avidity testing. Traditionally, antibodies to three antigen complexes are measured, including VCA, EA, and EBNA. In addition, different immunoglobulin (Ig) isotypes (IgG, IgM, and sometimes IgA) are detected. The large numbers of assays can lead to complex antibody patterns, making results difficult to interpret. As far as possible when using EBV assays for different parameters, kits should be from the same manufacturer. The antibody profile for a patient with suspected mononucleosis is presented in Fig. 1.

Immunofluorescence is still the gold standard in EBV serology, but it is labor-intensive and interpretation is subjective. On the whole, IFAs have fairly uniform performance characteristics, principally because the cell substrates are similar among suppliers. The performance of EIAs is much more variable, due to the plethora of antigen preparations used in the different kits. They range from cell extracts to recombinant or fusion proteins and synthetic peptides (36). This means that reference criteria established for interpretation

TABLE 2 Overview of commercial products for EBV diagnosis

Method	No. of products	Difference(s) between kits	Advantage(s)	Limitations
Heterophile antibodies				
Slide agglutination tests	~40 kits	Mostly latex particles; rarely, bovine, horse, or sheep erythrocytes	Very rapid (<15 min), inexpensive	Measures heterophile antibodies; can be positive for 1 yr after IM
Immunochromatographic strip tests			Very rapid (<15 min), inexpensive; easier to read than agglutination tests	Not specific for EBV; can be positive with lymphoma, acute HIV, or other infectious agents
EBV-specific antibodies				
Immunochromatographic strip or paddle tests	~2 kits	Different antigens	Rapid (<25 min)	Depending on the kit, the spectrum of antigens may not be sufficient
EIA: ELISA	~15 kits	Different antigens and antigen preparations	Might be combined with avidity testing for atypical results	Turnaround time of ~2–3 h; interpretation schema of some manufacturers include diagnoses that are not clinically relevant
EIA: dot technique	1 kit		Combined with CMV, *Toxoplasma gondii*	Turnaround time of ~2–3 h
EIA: CLIA	~2 kits	Different antigens and antigen preparations	Rapid (<1 h); random-access avidity testing commercially available	Specific instruments needed
Flow cytometry based, with microparticles	~3 kits	Combined with CMV or combined with heterophile antibodies	Rapid (<1 h); reaction to specific antigens similar to blot assay	Specific instruments needed; variable quality of antigens
Immunofluorescence	3 kits	With EBNA (ACIF) or without	Gold standard, high specificity; might be combined with avidity testing	EBNA ACIF detects IgG not only against EBNA1 but also against EBNA2; must be combined with a non-IFA method to detect only EBNA1 IgG; labor-intensive; turnaround time of ~2–3 h
Immunoblotting	~10 kits	Western blot or line blots	Line blots are easier to read; excellent as confirmation for atypical results; can be combined with avidity testing	Expensive, labor intensive; turnaround time of ~2–3 h
NAAT				
Real-time PCR	~3 kits	Different gene targets, different amplicon lengths	High sensitivity and specificity	NAAT is not standardized; different kits are not comparable; expensive

ᵃELISA, enzyme-linked immunosorbent assay; CLIA, chemiluminescent immunoassay; CMV, cytomegalovirus.

of IFAs may not apply to all EIAs, even when the antigens are referred to by the same name. For example, EBNA is a complex of several large, native proteins detected in Raji cells by anticomplement immunofluorescence (ACIF); in EIAs, the same designation may be given to a single oligopeptide derived from EBNA1 or an EBNA1 recombinant protein. Recombinant proteins and peptides, however, are easier to standardize than cell-grown antigens, and possibly assays using synthetic antigens will be more widely used in the future.

Recently, flow cytometry-based microparticle assays have become more popular, since they allow parallel detection of different antigens. In theory, up to 100 uniquely identifiable fluorescently labeled microspheres can be detected with this technique, each particle coated with a different antigen (30, 86). This approach combines the advantages of a complete antibody profile, like that of a blot, with a turnaround time of 1 to 2 h and random access. In addition to EBV-specific antigens, some assays also include heterophile antibodies or non-EBV antigens. However, specialized instruments are often necessary for signal detection (e.g., Luminex).

Moreover, rapid tests using immunochromatography (e.g., on strips) have been developed for EBV, enabling a fast diagnosis (~20 min) from a single sample. These tests are particularly suited to point-of-care use.

Avidity testing, measuring the strength of antibody-antigen binding, is available for all methods, not only for EIA. It can be applied to differentiate between a primary infection (low avidity) and a past infection (high avidity). Avidity is calculated as the percentage of signal loss resulting from pretreatment of the serum with urea compared with a regular assay. These assays are primarily used in Europe and not in the United States.

The main VCA is a 150-kDa protein, but the p18 and p23 proteins are also included in the VCA complex of proteins expressed in P3HR1 cells, and all three are used for serology (36, 66). VCA EIAs using antigens from infected cells have been available for a long time, and assays using affinity-purified antigen still perform better than EIAs using recombinant or synthetic antigens (24). EIAs and line blots using recombinant VCA (p23-p18) and peptide p18 reportedly give mixed results compared with IFA (7, 23, 24, 76).

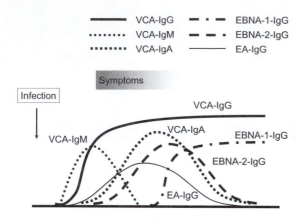

FIGURE 1 Development of antibodies to EBV antigens following primary infection. While there is marked interpatient and interlaboratory variation in titers, the typical relative development of titers by antibody class and antigen specificity is given.

Anti-EA/D (diffuse distribution in cells) and anti-EA/R (restricted to cytoplasm) are antibodies traditionally measured with Raji cells activated to enter the lytic phase by phorbol ester or sodium butyrate. Ethanol fixation eliminates the EA/R complex; cells fixed in ethanol are used for studies of EA/D antibodies. Nowadays, separation of EA antibodies is rarely used for diagnostic applications. Tests using cell-derived and recombinant EA proteins are available but are often somewhat lacking in both specificity and sensitivity (5, 73). Due to their high heterogeneity and their (consequently) low comparability, EA assays are only rarely useful in IM cases. Furthermore, EA antibodies are present in a significant proportion of healthy blood donors and may thus be more problematic than helpful for diagnosing IM (25).

ACIF or assays with equally high sensitivity are necessary to detect the low concentration of EBNA antibodies by IFA. ACIF detects not only EBNA1 but also EBNA2. It should be kept in mind that EBNA2 antibodies occur earlier in the course of infection than EBNA1 antibodies, and therefore the ratios of titers of antibodies to EBNA1 and EBNA2 were used for some time to verify chronic or complicated EBV infections (49, 85). However, no clear association can be made between this ratio and clinical illness, and the significance of antibodies to other EBNA components is still not firmly settled.

The complement-fixing antibodies detected by ACIF may be of almost any Ig isotype and should be referred to as "EBNA Ig." The EBNA staining pattern is nuclear and should be present in all infected cells. The preparations should contain cells from an EBV-negative lymphoblastoid cell line, or EBV-negative cells could be incubated and stained in parallel, to ensure that the nuclear staining does not result from antinuclear factors present in the patients' serum. Commercial EIAs containing cell-derived EBNA or, even better, recombinant EBNA1 (p72) are available and demonstrate high sensitivity (≥95%).

For serologic diagnosis of EBV infection in the United States, EBV antibody panels of two, three, or four markers are commonly performed using EIA and, much less frequently, IFA. Antibody panels can include VCA IgG and VCA IgM only; VCA IgG, VCA IgM, and EBNA IgG; or the last three antibodies plus antibody to EA. If an atypical pattern is observed (see Table 3), testing may be repeated using EIA, the antibody panel could be tested by IFA, or collection of a second blood sample in 1 to 2 weeks could be recommended.

An alternative algorithm used in Europe for serologic diagnosis is provided in Fig. 2. In this cost-effective approach, stepwise analysis and data interpretation features testing for EBNA in serum as the key initial step. This schema is feasible for assays with short incubation times and random access (i.e., microparticle multiplex assays). EBNA1 IgG antibodies normally appear between 6 weeks and 7 months after onset of IM and should be negative in acute IM. They are maintained for life and are therefore a good marker of prior infection. However, in about 5 to 10% of patients, EBNA1 IgG may be present in low titers or even undetectable (71). Increasing age, severe immunosuppression, or rheumatic disorders are often reasons for a reduction or loss of EBNA1 IgG titers. Diagnosis of primary EBV infections should not rely solely on the detection of VCA IgM, since both false-positive and false-negative results are possible. False positives result mainly from the presence of rheumatoid factor cross-reacting with other herpesvirus infections and antinuclear factors (52). False negatives may result from late collection of serum samples due to the long incubation period or from insufficiently sensitive assays.

In rare cases, immunoblotting including VCA p23, VCA p18, and EBNA1 p72 may be performed (2). VCA p18 may be important since antibodies of the IgM class are detectable quite early during infection, whereas IgG antibodies are produced late (similar to EBNA1 IgG) (36, 80). If EBNA1 IgG and p18 IgG are negative, an avidity test of VCA IgG can be informative (2).

In serology for nasopharyngeal carcinoma, different isotypes (IgG and IgA) to a great variety of antigens, e.g., VCA and LMP2 (50), LMP1 (87), thymidine kinase (12), ZEBRA (14), EBNA1 (6, 8), zta (6), and EA (21), have been identified.

TABLE 3 Typical EBV serologic profiles using the most frequently employed antigens and Ig isotypes[a]

Antigen/Ig isotype condition	VCA IgG	VCA IgM	VCA IgA	EA/D IgG	EA/R IgG	EBNA Ig
Seronegative	−	−	−	−	−	−
Primary infection	+ +	+ + +	+	+	±	−
Past infection	+	−	±	−	±	+
Chronic active EBV infection	+ + +	+	+ +	+ +	+	±
Nasopharyngeal carcinoma	+ + +	−	+ + +	+ + +	+	+ + +
X-linked lymphoproliferative syndrome	±	−	−	−	−	−

[a]Atypical patterns include VCA IgM positive only, EBNA positive only, or VCA IgM and EBNA positive but VCA IgG negative. Atypical patterns merit repeat testing, testing of a follow-up sample, or testing by alternate methods. ±, antibodies absent or present in low titers; +, antibodies present; + +, antibodies present in elevated titers; + + +, antibodies present in strongly elevated titers.

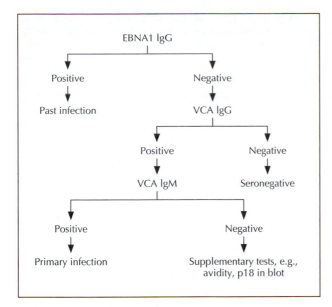

FIGURE 2 Diagnostic algorithm and interpretation scheme based on EBNA1 used with microparticle multiplex assays or rapid tests with random access in Europe. Diagnostic procedures and interpretation may start with EBNA1 IgG. If this parameter is positive, a past infection is proven; if EBNA1 IgG is negative, a negative VCA IgG results in the diagnosis of seronegative and a positive VCA IgM in the diagnosis of a primary infection. If VCA IgG is positive and the other parameters are negative, supplementary tests should be applied, e.g., avidity testing or blots using p18 antigen.

EVALUATION, INTERPRETATION, AND REPORTING OF RESULTS

Antibody assays are the method of choice for diagnosing IM. NAAT is discouraged in IM, since EBV DNA may also be detected in healthy individuals (19, 54, 55), and due to the long incubation period, EBV DNA may even be negative in some patients with IM.

Heterophile antibodies are a marker of IM but not necessarily of EBV. High levels of heterophile antibodies are seen during the first month of IM, normally followed by a rapid decrease. Low but persisting heterophile antibody titers can be found after primary EBV for up to 1 year, which can be misleading, and more importantly, heterophile antibodies may also indicate an acute HIV infection, lymphoma, or infection with another infectious agent (e.g., cytomegalovirus, rubella virus, or *Toxoplasma gondii*) (81, 83). Thus, an EBV-specific serology should always be performed where other causes of IM cannot be ruled out. False negatives (15 to 20%) are the rule among young children (5, 53, 71) but also occur for adolescents and adults. Especially in clinically atypical cases, patients often lack heterophile antibodies. Thus, a negative heterophile antibody test should be supplemented with EBV-specific serology.

Due to the long incubation period, almost all IM patients have peak titers of IgG to various lytic-phase EBV antigens (VCA and EA) but lack antibodies to EBNAs (for details, see Fig. 1). The patient's EBV status can generally be ascertained from a single serum sample by measuring VCA IgG, VCA IgM, and EBNA1 IgG. In at least 90 to 95% of cases, the antibody profile is sufficiently distinct

to determine whether the patient (i) is still susceptible to EBV, (ii) has a current primary infection, or (iii) has a past infection (Table 3). It is discouraged to use other interpretations such as "recent," "convalescent," or "reactivated" infection, as suggested by some manufacturers, since as these diagnoses correspond to a healthy individual, they are of limited clinical relevance. The exact antibody titers and the time needed to develop a full antibody spectrum vary widely among individuals and do not correlate with severity of disease. Thus, quantitative measurement of antibodies is of minor importance in routine diagnostics (88).

In nasopharyngeal carcinoma, serology and viral load are established diagnostic and prognostic markers and also serve as screening parameters in high-risk patients. Viral load and serologic markers are elevated in patients prior to tumor manifestation, during disease, and during recurrence. Reductions in viral load or antibody titers are a marker of effective therapy. Viral load measurement is superior to serology in its diagnostic value, especially for tumor recurrence (20, 51). For example, DNA becomes rapidly undetectable within a few hours of tumor surgery (74), whereas serology follows the slower kinetics of antibody production and half-life.

Monitoring for PTLD is not indicated for all patients, only for those at high risk. The EBV serostatus should always be clarified before transplantation, since EBV primary infection via transplantation is a major risk factor; serology is of little value thereafter (25). Monitoring of viral load by quantitative NAAT is the method of choice (22). Clinical cutoff levels for pathological reactions are not yet clearly defined and must be established for each patient group and for each specimen type (for approximate values, see Table 1). Along with the absolute viral load, the kinetics of viral load increase plays an important role. An increase of 2 log points within a week appears to be a marker for development of PTLD. Nonetheless, it is noteworthy that some patients with high viral load do not develop PTLD and others have manifest PTLD despite low-level or even undetectable EBV DNA in peripheral blood (26).

At present there is no clinical or diagnostic marker to functionally characterize and monitor immunosuppression in patients after transplantation. An increased EBV viral load could, however, indicate excessive immunosuppression even without development of PTLD (1, 48). Immunosuppression may be reduced in patients when EBV viral load increases over a previously defined cutoff. Standardization of viral load measurement is a prerequisite to define cutoffs for this approach.

A high EBV viral load in whole blood or plasma is generally a marker for EBV-related lymphoma; however, CNS lymphomas show high viral loads normally only in CSF and not in blood (4, 20). On the other hand, EBV DNA in CSF is not proof of EBV lymphoma, since it is found in immunosuppressed patients without lymphoma as well (63, 70). Moreover, patients with chronic inflammation in the CNS may also show EBV DNA in CSF, possibly due to latently infected B cells in the CSF (K. Ruprecht, C. Klahr, and B. C. Gärtner, unpublished data). For unambiguous laboratory diagnosis, detection of EBV DNA by amplification should be complemented by other methods, such as in situ immunohistochemical detection of LMP 1 or EBER in tissue.

Patients with X-linked lymphoproliferative syndrome have typically a high viral load and do not develop EBNA antibodies. The ultimate diagnosis, however, is based on genetic analysis for a variety of mutations in the SH2D1A gene domain.

REFERENCES

1. Bakker, N. A., E. A. Verschuuren, M. E. Erasmus, B. G. Hepkema, N. J. Veeger, C. G. Kallenberg, and W. van der Bij. 2007. Epstein-Barr virus-DNA load monitoring late after lung transplantation: a surrogate marker of the degree of immunosuppression and a safe guide to reduce immunosuppression. *Transplantation* **83:**433–438.

2. Bauer, G. 2001. Simplicity through complexity: immunoblot with recombinant antigens as the new gold standard in Epstein-Barr virus serology. *Clin. Lab.* **47:**223–230.

3. Blaes, A. H., B. A. Peterson, N. Bartlett, D. L. Dunn, and V. A. Morrison. 2005. Rituximab therapy is effective for posttransplant lymphoproliferative disorders after solid organ transplantation: results of a phase II trial. *Cancer* **104:**1661–1667.

4. Bonnet, F., A. C. Jouvencel, M. Parrens, M. J. Leon, E. Cotto, I. Garrigue, P. Morlat, J. Beylot, H. Fleury, and M. E. Lafon. 2006. A longitudinal and prospective study of Epstein-Barr virus load in AIDS-related non-Hodgkin lymphoma. *J. Clin. Virol.* **36:**258–263.

5. Bruu, A. L., R. Hjetland, E. Holter, L. Mortensen, O. Natas, W. Petterson, A. G. Skar, T. Skarpaas, T. Tjade, and B. Asjo. 2000. Evaluation of 12 commercial tests for detection of Epstein-Barr virus-specific and heterophile antibodies. *Clin. Diagn. Lab. Immunol.* **7:**451–456.

6. Chan, K. H., Y. L. Gu, F. Ng, P. S. Ng, W. H. Seto, J. S. Sham, D. Chua, W. Wei, Y. L. Chen, W. Luk, Y. S. Zong, and M. H. Ng. 2003. EBV specific antibody-based and DNA-based assays in serologic diagnosis of nasopharyngeal carcinoma. *Int. J. Cancer* **105:**706–709.

7. Chan, K. H., R. X. Luo, H. L. Chen, M. H. Ng, W. H. Seto, and J. S. Peiris. 1998. Development and evaluation of an Epstein-Barr virus (EBV) immunoglobulin M enzyme-linked immunosorbent assay based on the 18-kilodalton matrix protein for diagnosis of primary EBV infection. *J. Clin. Microbiol.* **36:**3359–3361.

8. Chen, M. R., M. Y. Liu, S. M. Hsu, C. C. Fong, C. J. Chen, I. H. Chen, M. M. Hsu, C. S. Yang, and J. Y. Chen. 2001. Use of bacterially expressed EBNA-1 protein cloned from a nasopharyngeal carcinoma (NPC) biopsy as a screening test for NPC patients. *J. Med. Virol.* **64:**51–57.

9. Cherikh, W. S., H. M. Kauffman, M. A. McBride, J. Maghirang, L. J. Swinnen, and D. W. Hanto. 2003. Association of the type of induction immunosuppression with posttransplant lymphoproliferative disorder, graft survival, and patient survival after primary kidney transplantation. *Transplantation* **76:**1289–1293.

10. Choquet, S., V. Leblond, R. Herbrecht, G. Socie, A. M. Stoppa, P. Vandenberghe, A. Fischer, F. Morschhauser, G. Salles, W. Feremans, E. Vilmer, M. N. Peraldi, P. Lang, Y. Lebranchu, E. Oksenhendler, J. L. Garnier, T. Lamy, A. Jaccard, A. Ferrant, F. Offner, O. Hermine, A. Moreau, S. Fafi-Kremer, P. Morand, L. Chatenoud, N. Berriot-Varoqueaux, L. Bergougnoux, and N. Milpied. 2006. Efficacy and safety of rituximab in B-cell posttransplantation lymphoproliferative disorders: results of a prospective multicenter phase 2 study. *Blood* **107:**3053–3057.

11. Cohen, J. I., H. Kimura, S. Nakamura, Y. H. Ko, and E. S. Jaffe. 2009. Epstein-Barr virus-associated lymphoproliferative disease in non-immunocompromised hosts: a status report and summary of an international meeting, 8–9 September 2008. *Ann. Oncol.* **20:**1472–1482.

12. Connolly, Y., E. Littler, N. Sun, X. Chen, P. C. Huang, S. N. Stacey, and J. R. Arrand. 2001. Antibodies to Epstein-Barr virus thymidine kinase: a characteristic marker for the serological detection of nasopharyngeal carcinoma. *Int. J. Cancer* **91:**692–697.

13. Crawford, D. H., A. J. Swerdlow, C. Higgins, K. McAulay, N. Harrison, H. Williams, K. Britton, and K. F. Macsween. 2002. Sexual history and Epstein-Barr virus infection. *J. Infect. Dis.* **186:**731–736.

14. Dardari, R., M. Khyatti, A. Benider, H. Jouhadi, A. Kahlain, C. Cochet, A. Mansouri, B. El Gueddari, A. Benslimane, and I. Joab. 2000. Antibodies to the Epstein-Barr virus transactivator protein (ZEBRA) as a valuable biomarker in young patients with nasopharyngeal carcinoma. *Int. J. Cancer* **86:**71–75.

15. Deyrup, A. T., V. K. Lee, C. E. Hill, W. Cheuk, H. C. Toh, S. Kesavan, E. W. Chan, and S. W. Weiss. 2006. Epstein-Barr virus-associated smooth muscle tumors are distinctive mesenchymal tumors reflecting multiple infection events: a clinicopathologic and molecular analysis of 29 tumors from 19 patients. *Am. J. Surg. Pathol.* **30:**75–82.

16. Elliott, S. L., A. Suhrbier, J. J. Miles, G. Lawrence, S. J. Pye, T. T. Le, A. Rosenstengel, T. Nguyen, A. Allworth, S. R. Burrows, J. Cox, D. Pye, D. J. Moss, and M. Bharadwaj. 2008. Phase I trial of a CD8$^+$ T-cell peptide epitope-based vaccine for infectious mononucleosis. *J. Virol.* **82:**1448–1457.

17. Elstrom, R. L., C. Andreadis, N. A. Aqui, V. N. Ahya, R. D. Bloom, S. C. Brozena, K. M. Olthoff, S. J. Schuster, S. D. Nasta, E. A. Stadtmauer, and D. E. Tsai. 2006. Treatment of PTLD with rituximab or chemotherapy. *Am. J. Transplant.* **6:**569–576.

18. Enbom, M., A. Strand, K. I. Falk, and A. Linde. 2001. Detection of Epstein-Barr virus, but not human herpesvirus 8, DNA in cervical secretions from Swedish women by real-time polymerase chain reaction. *Sex. Transm. Dis.* **28:**300–306.

19. Fafi-Kremer, S., P. Morand, R. Germi, M. Ballout, J. P. Brion, O. Genoulaz, S. Nicod, J. P. Stahl, R. W. Ruigrok, and J. M. Seigneurin. 2005. A prospective follow-up of Epstein-Barr virus LMP1 genotypes in saliva and blood during infectious mononucleosis. *J. Infect. Dis.* **192:**2108–2111.

20. Fan, H., S. C. Kim, C. O. Chima, B. F. Israel, K. M. Lawless, P. A. Eagan, S. Elmore, D. T. Moore, S. A. Schichman, L. J. Swinnen, and M. L. Gulley. 2005. Epstein-Barr viral load as a marker of lymphoma in AIDS patients. *J. Med. Virol.* **75:**59–69.

21. Fan, H., J. Nicholls, D. Chua, K. H. Chan, J. Sham, S. Lee, and M. L. Gulley. 2004. Laboratory markers of tumor burden in nasopharyngeal carcinoma: a comparison of viral load and serologic tests for Epstein-Barr virus. *Int. J. Cancer* **112:**1036–1041.

22. Gärtner, B., and J. K. Preiksaitis. 2010. EBV viral load detection in clinical virology. *J. Clin. Virol.* **48:**82–90.

23. Gärtner, B. C., J. M. Fischinger, K. Roemer, M. Mak, B. Fleurent, and N. Mueller-Lantzsch. 2001. Evaluation of a recombinant line blot for diagnosis of Epstein-Barr virus compared with ELISA, using immunofluorescence as reference method. *J. Virol. Methods* **93:**89–96.

24. Gärtner, B. C., R. D. Hess, D. Bandt, A. Kruse, A. Rethwilm, K. Roemer, and N. Mueller-Lantzsch. 2003. Evaluation of four commercially available Epstein-Barr virus enzyme immunoassays with an immunofluorescence assay as the reference method. *Clin. Diagn. Lab. Immunol.* **10:**78–82.

25. Gärtner, B. C., K. Kortmann, M. Schafer, N. Mueller-Lantzsch, U. Sester, H. Kaul, and H. Pees. 2000. No correlation in Epstein-Barr virus reactivation between serological parameters and viral load. *J. Clin. Microbiol.* **38:**2458.

26. Gärtner, B. C., H. Schafer, K. Marggraff, G. Eisele, M. Schafer, D. Dilloo, K. Roemer, H. J. Laws, M. Sester, U. Sester, H. Einsele, and N. Mueller-Lantzsch. 2002. Evaluation of use of Epstein-Barr viral load in patients after allogeneic stem cell transplantation to diagnose and monitor posttransplant lymphoproliferative disease. *J. Clin. Microbiol.* **40:**351–358.

27. Gaspar, H. B., R. Sharifi, K. C. Gilmour, and A. J. Thrasher. 2002. X-linked lymphoproliferative disease: clinical, diagnostic and molecular perspective. *Br. J. Haematol.* **119:**585–595.

28. Grasser, F. A., P. G. Murray, E. Kremmer, K. Klein, K. Remberger, W. Feiden, G. Reynolds, G. Niedobitek, L. S. Young, and N. Mueller-Lantzsch. 1994. Monoclonal antibodies directed against the Epstein-Barr virus-encoded nuclear antigen 1 (EBNA1): immunohistologic detection of EBNA1 in the malignant cells of Hodgkin's disease. *Blood* **84:**3792–3798.

29. Gratama, J. W., M. A. Oosterveer, W. Weimar, K. Sintnicolaas, W. Sizoo, R. L. Bolhuis, and I. Ernberg. 1994. Detection of multiple 'Ebnotypes' in individual Epstein-Barr virus carriers following lymphocyte transformation by virus derived from peripheral blood and oropharynx. *J. Gen. Virol.* **75(Pt. 1):**85–94.

30. Gu, A. D., H. Y. Mo, Y. B. Xie, R. J. Peng, J. X. Bei, J. Peng, M. Y. Li, L. Z. Chen, Q. S. Feng, W. H. Jia, and Y. X. Zeng. 2008. Evaluation of a multianalyte profiling assay and an enzyme-linked immunosorbent assay for serological examination of Epstein-Barr virus-specific antibody responses in diagnosis of nasopharyngeal carcinoma. Clin. Vaccine Immunol. 15:1684–1688.

31. Guerreiro-Cacais, A. O., L. Li, D. Donati, M. T. Bejarano, A. Morgan, M. G. Masucci, L. Hutt-Fletcher, and V. Levitsky. 2004. Capacity of Epstein-Barr virus to infect monocytes and inhibit their development into dendritic cells is affected by the cell type supporting virus replication. J. Gen. Virol. 85:2767–2778.

32. Gulley, M. L., and W. Tang. 2008. Laboratory assays for Epstein-Barr virus-related disease. J. Mol. Diagn. 10:279–292.

33. Hakim, H., C. Gibson, J. Pan, K. Srivastava, Z. Gu, M. J. Bankowski, and R. T. Hayden. 2007. Comparison of various blood compartments and reporting units for the detection and quantification of Epstein-Barr virus in peripheral blood. J. Clin. Microbiol. 45:2151–2155.

34. Haque, T., G. M. Wilkie, M. M. Jones, C. D. Higgins, G. Urquhart, P. Wingate, D. Burns, K. McAulay, M. Turner, C. Bellamy, P. L. Amlot, D. Kelly, A. MacGilchrist, M. K. Gandhi, A. J. Swerdlow, and D. H. Crawford. 2007. Allogeneic cytotoxic T-cell therapy for EBV-positive posttransplantation lymphoproliferative disease: results of a phase 2 multicenter clinical trial. Blood 110:1123–1131.

35. Henle, W., G. Henle, J. Andersson, I. Ernberg, G. Klein, C. A. Horwitz, G. Marklund, L. Rymo, C. Wellinder, and S. E. Straus. 1987. Antibody responses to Epstein-Barr virus-determined nuclear antigen (EBNA)-1 and EBNA-2 in acute and chronic Epstein-Barr virus infection. Proc. Natl. Acad. Sci. USA 84:570–574.

36. Hess, R. D. 2004. Routine Epstein-Barr virus diagnostics from the laboratory perspective: still challenging after 35 years. J. Clin. Microbiol. 42:3381–3387.

37. Hoagland, R. J. 1964. The incubation period of infectious mononucleosis. Am. J. Public Health Nations Health 54:1699–1705.

38. Hurt, C., and D. Tammaro. 2007. Diagnostic evaluation of mononucleosis-like illnesses. Am. J. Med. 120:911 e1–911 e8.

39. Imashuku, S. 2002. Clinical features and treatment strategies of Epstein-Barr virus-associated hemophagocytic lymphohistiocytosis. Crit. Rev. Oncol. Hematol. 44:259–272.

40. Iwatsuki, K., T. Yamamoto, K. Tsuji, D. Suzuki, K. Fujii, H. Matsuura, and T. Oono. 2004. A spectrum of clinical manifestations caused by host immune responses against Epstein-Barr virus infections. Acta Med. Okayama 58:169–180.

41. Jenson, H. B., C. T. Leach, K. L. McClain, V. V. Joshi, B. H. Pollock, R. T. Parmley, E. G. Chadwick, and S. B. Murphy. 1997. Benign and malignant smooth muscle tumors containing Epstein-Barr virus in children with AIDS. Leuk. Lymphoma 27:303–314.

42. Junying, J., K. Herrmann, G. Davies, D. Lissauer, A. Bell, J. Timms, G. M. Reynolds, S. G. Hubscher, L. S. Young, G. Niedobitek, and P. G. Murray. 2003. Absence of Epstein-Barr virus DNA in the tumor cells of European hepatocellular carcinoma. Virology 306:236–243.

43. Kieff, E., and A. B. Rickinson. 2007. Epstein-Barr virus and its replication, p. 2603–2654. In D. M. Knipe, P. M. Howley, D. E. Griffin, R. A. Lamb, M. A. Martin, B. Roizman, and S. E. Straus (ed.), Fields Virology, 5th ed., vol. 2. Lippincott Williams & Wilkins, Philadelphia, PA.

44. Kimura, H. 2006. Pathogenesis of chronic active Epstein-Barr virus infection: is this an infectious disease, lymphoproliferative disorder, or immunodeficiency? Rev. Med. Virol. 16:251–261.

45. Kimura, H., T. Morishima, H. Kanegane, S. Ohga, Y. Hoshino, A. Maeda, S. Imai, M. Okano, T. Morio, S. Yokota, S. Tsuchiya, A. Yachie, S. Imashuku, K. Kawa, and H. Wakiguchi. 2003. Prognostic factors for chronic active Epstein-Barr virus infection. J. Infect. Dis. 187:527–533.

46. Knowles, D. M. 1997. Molecular pathology of acquired immunodeficiency syndrome-related non-Hodgkin's lymphoma. Semin. Diagn. Pathol. 14:67–82.

47. Landgren, O., E. S. Gilbert, J. D. Rizzo, G. Socie, P. M. Banks, K. A. Sobocinski, M. M. Horowitz, E. S. Jaffe, D. W. Kingma, L. B. Travis, M. E. Flowers, P. J. Martin, H. J. Deeg, and R. E. Curtis. 2009. Risk factors for lymphoproliferative disorders after allogeneic hematopoietic cell transplantation. Blood 113:4992–5001.

48. Lee, T. C., B. Savoldo, C. M. Rooney, H. E. Heslop, A. P. Gee, Y. Caldwell, N. R. Barshes, J. D. Scott, L. J. Bristow, C. A. O'Mahony, and J. A. Goss. 2005. Quantitative EBV viral loads and immunosuppression alterations can decrease PTLD incidence in pediatric liver transplant recipients. Am. J. Transplant. 5:2222–2228.

49. Lennette, E. T., L. Rymo, M. Yadav, G. Masucci, K. Merk, L. Timar, and G. Klein. 1993. Disease-related differences in antibody patterns against EBV-encoded nuclear antigens EBNA 1, EBNA 2 and EBNA 6. Eur. J. Cancer 29A:1584–1589.

50. Lennette, E. T., G. Winberg, M. Yadav, G. Enblad, and G. Klein. 1995. Antibodies to LMP2A/2B in EBV-carrying malignancies. Eur. J. Cancer 31A:1875–1878.

51. Lin, J. C., W. Y. Wang, W. M. Liang, H. Y. Chou, J. S. Jan, R. S. Jiang, J. Y. Wang, C. W. Twu, K. L. Liang, J. Chao, and W. C. Shen. 2007. Long-term prognostic effects of plasma Epstein-Barr virus DNA by minor groove binder-probe real-time quantitative PCR on nasopharyngeal carcinoma patients receiving concurrent chemoradiotherapy. Int. J. Radiat. Oncol. Biol. Phys. 68:1342–1348.

52. Linde, A., B. Kallin, J. Dillner, J. Andersson, L. Jagdahl, A. Lindvall, and B. Wahren. 1990. Evaluation of enzyme-linked immunosorbent assays with two synthetic peptides of Epstein-Barr virus for diagnosis of infectious mononucleosis. J. Infect. Dis. 161:903–909.

53. Linderholm, M., J. Boman, P. Juto, and A. Linde. 1994. Comparative evaluation of nine kits for rapid diagnosis of infectious mononucleosis and Epstein-Barr virus-specific serology. J. Clin. Microbiol. 32:259–261.

54. Ling, P. D., J. A. Lednicky, W. A. Keitel, D. G. Poston, Z. S. White, R. Peng, Z. Liu, S. K. Mehta, D. L. Pierson, C. M. Rooney, R. A. Vilchez, E. O. Smith, and J. S. Butel. 2003. The dynamics of herpesvirus and polyomavirus reactivation and shedding in healthy adults: a 14-month longitudinal study. J. Infect. Dis. 187:1571–1580.

55. Maurmann, S., L. Fricke, H. J. Wagner, P. Schlenke, H. Hennig, J. Steinhoff, and W. J. Jabs. 2003. Molecular parameters for precise diagnosis of asymptomatic Epstein-Barr virus reactivation in healthy carriers. J. Clin. Microbiol. 41:5419–5428.

56. Merlo, A., R. Turrini, R. Dolcetti, P. Zanovello, A. Amadori, and A. Rosato. 2008. Adoptive cell therapy against EBV-related malignancies: a survey of clinical results. Expert Opin. Biol. Ther. 8:1265–1294.

57. Middeldorp, J. M., A. A. Brink, A. J. van den Brule, and C. J. Meijer. 2003. Pathogenic roles for Epstein-Barr virus (EBV) gene products in EBV-associated proliferative disorders. Crit. Rev. Oncol. Hematol. 45:1–36.

58. Milone, M. C., D. E. Tsai, R. L. Hodinka, L. B. Silverman, A. Malbran, M. A. Wasik, and K. E. Nichols. 2005. Treatment of primary Epstein-Barr virus infection in patients with X-linked lymphoproliferative disease using B-cell-directed therapy. Blood 105:994–996.

59. Morra, M., D. Howie, M. S. Grande, J. Sayos, N. Wang, C. Wu, P. Engel, and C. Terhorst. 2001. X-linked lymphoproliferative disease: a progressive immunodeficiency. Annu. Rev. Immunol. 19:657–682.

60. Niedobitek, G., and H. Herbst. 2006. In situ detection of Epstein-Barr virus and phenotype determination of EBV-infected cells. Methods Mol. Biol. 326:115–137.

61. Papesch, M., and R. Watkins. 2001. Epstein-Barr virus infectious mononucleosis. Clin. Otolaryngol. Allied Sci. 26:3–8.

62. Petersen, I., J. M. Thomas, W. T. Hamilton, and P. D. White. 2006. Risk and predictors of fatigue after infectious mononucleosis in a large primary-care cohort. QJM 99:49–55.

63. Plentz, A., W. Jilg, B. Kochanowski, B. Ibach, and A. Knoll. 2008. Detection of herpesvirus DNA in cerebrospinal fluid and correlation with clinical symptoms. Infection 36:158–162.

64. Preiksaitis, J. K., X. L. Pang, J. D. Fox, J. M. Fenton, A. M. Caliendo, and G. G. Miller. 2009. Interlaboratory comparison of Epstein-Barr virus viral load assays. *Am. J. Transplant.* **9:**269–279.

65. Randhawa, P. S., R. Jaffe, A. J. Demetris, M. Nalesnik, T. E. Starzl, Y. Y. Chen, and L. M. Weiss. 1992. Expression of Epstein-Barr virus-encoded small RNA (by the EBER-1 gene) in liver specimens from transplant recipients with posttransplantation lymphoproliferative disease. *N. Engl. J. Med.* **327:**1710–1714.

66. Rickinson, A. B., and E. Kieff. 2007. Epstein-Barr virus, p. 2656–2700. *In* D. M. Knipe, P. M. Howley, D. E. Griffin, R. A. Lamb, M. A. Martin, B. Roizman, and S. E. Straus (ed.), *Fields Virology,* 5th ed., vol. 2. Lippincott Williams & Wilkins, Philadelphia, PA.

67. Savard, M., C. Belanger, M. Tardif, P. Gourde, L. Flamand, and J. Gosselin. 2000. Infection of primary human monocytes by Epstein-Barr virus. *J. Virol.* **74:**2612–2619.

68. Sokal, E. M., K. Hoppenbrouwers, C. Vandermeulen, M. Moutschen, P. Leonard, A. Moreels, M. Haumont, A. Bollen, F. Smets, and M. Denis. 2007. Recombinant gp350 vaccine for infectious mononucleosis: a phase 2, randomized, double-blind, placebo-controlled trial to evaluate the safety, immunogenicity, and efficacy of an Epstein-Barr virus vaccine in healthy young adults. *J. Infect. Dis.* **196:**1749–1753.

69. Stevens, S. J., S. A. Verkuijlen, B. Hariwiyanto, Harijadi, J. Fachiroh, D. K. Paramita, I. B. Tan, S. M. Haryana, and J. M. Middeldorp. 2005. Diagnostic value of measuring Epstein-Barr virus (EBV) DNA load and carcinoma-specific viral mRNA in relation to anti-EBV immunoglobulin A (IgA) and IgG antibody levels in blood of nasopharyngeal carcinoma patients from Indonesia. *J. Clin. Microbiol.* **43:**3066–3073.

70. Studahl, M., L. Hagberg, E. Rekabdar, and T. Bergstrom. 2000. Herpesvirus DNA detection in cerebral spinal fluid: differences in clinical presentation between alpha-, beta-, and gamma-herpesviruses. *Scand. J. Infect. Dis.* **32:**237–248.

71. Sumaya, C. V., and Y. Ench. 1985. Epstein-Barr virus infectious mononucleosis in children. II. Heterophil antibody and viral-specific responses. *Pediatrics* **75:**1011–1019.

72. Sumegi, J., T. A. Seemayer, D. Huang, J. R. Davis, M. Morra, T. G. Gross, L. Yin, G. Romco, E. Klein, C. Terhorst, and A. Lanyi. 2002. A spectrum of mutations in SH2D1A that causes X-linked lymphoproliferative disease and other Epstein-Barr virus-associated illnesses. *Leuk. Lymphoma* **43:**1189–1201.

73. Svahn, A., M. Magnusson, L. Jagdahl, L. Schloss, G. Kahlmeter, and A. Linde. 1997. Evaluation of three commercial enzyme-linked immunosorbent assays and two latex agglutination assays for diagnosis of primary Epstein-Barr virus infection. *J. Clin. Microbiol.* **35:**2728–2732.

74. To, E. W., K. C. Chan, S. F. Leung, L. Y. Chan, K. F. To, A. T. Chan, P. J. Johnson, and Y. M. Lo. 2003. Rapid clearance of plasma Epstein-Barr virus DNA after surgical treatment of nasopharyngeal carcinoma. *Clin. Cancer Res.* **9:**3254–3259.

75. Torre, D., and R. Tambini. 1999. Acyclovir for treatment of infectious mononucleosis: a meta-analysis. *Scand. J. Infect. Dis.* **31:**543–547.

76. Tranchand-Bunel, D., H. Gras-Masse, B. Bourez, L. Dedecker, and C. Auriault. 1999. Evaluation of an Epstein-Barr virus (EBV) immunoglobulin M enzyme-linked immunosorbent assay using a synthetic convergent peptide library, or mixotope, for diagnosis of primary EBV infection. *J. Clin. Microbiol.* **37:**2366–2368.

77. Trappe, R., H. Riess, N. Babel, M. Hummel, H. Lehmkuhl, S. Jonas, I. Anagnostopoulos, M. Papp-Vary, P. Reinke, R. Hetzer, B. Dorken, and S. Oertel. 2007. Salvage chemotherapy for refractory and relapsed posttransplant lymphoproliferative disorders (PTLD) after treatment with single-agent rituximab. *Transplantation* **83:**912–918.

78. Triantos, D., S. R. Porter, C. Scully, and C. G. Teo. 1997. Oral hairy leukoplakia: clinicopathologic features, pathogenesis, diagnosis, and clinical significance. *Clin. Infect. Dis.* **25:**1392–1396.

79. Tynell, E., E. Aurelius, A. Brandell, I. Julander, M. Wood, Q. Y. Yao, A. Rickinson, B. Akerlund, and J. Andersson. 1996. Acyclovir and prednisolone treatment of acute infectious mononucleosis: a multicenter, double-blind, placebo-controlled study. *J. Infect. Dis.* **174:**324–331.

80. van Grunsven, W. M., W. J. Spaan, and J. M. Middeldorp. 1994. Localization and diagnostic application of immunodominant domains of the BFRF3-encoded Epstein-Barr virus capsid protein. *J. Infect. Dis.* **170:**13–19.

81. Vidrih, J. A., R. P. Walensky, P. E. Sax, and K. A. Freedberg. 2001. Positive Epstein-Barr virus heterophile antibody tests in patients with primary human immunodeficiency virus infection. *Am. J. Med.* **111:**192–194.

82. Wagner, H. J., G. Bein, A. Bitsch, and H. Kirchner. 1992. Detection and quantification of latently infected B lymphocytes in Epstein-Barr virus-seropositive, healthy individuals by polymerase chain reaction. *J. Clin. Microbiol.* **30:**2826–2829.

83. Walensky, R. P., E. S. Rosenberg, M. J. Ferraro, E. Losina, B. D. Walker, and K. A. Freedberg. 2001. Investigation of primary human immunodeficiency virus infection in patients who test positive for heterophile antibody. *Clin. Infect. Dis.* **33:**570–572.

84. Walker, R. C., W. F. Marshall, J. G. Strickler, R. H. Wiesner, J. A. Velosa, T. M. Habermann, C. G. McGregor, and C. V. Paya. 1995. Pretransplantation assessment of the risk of lymphoproliferative disorder. *Clin. Infect. Dis.* **20:**1346–1353.

85. Winkelspecht, B., F. Grasser, H. W. Pees, and N. Mueller-Lantzsch. 1996. Anti-EBNA1/anti-EBNA2 ratio decreases significantly in patients with progression of HIV infection. *Arch. Virol.* **141:**857–864.

86. Wong, J., S. Sibani, N. N. Lokko, J. LaBaer, and K. S. Anderson. 2009. Rapid detection of antibodies in sera using multiplexed self-assembling bead arrays. *J. Immunol. Methods* **350:**171–182.

87. Xu, J., A. Ahmad, M. D'Addario, L. Knafo, J. F. Jones, U. Prasad, R. Dolcetti, E. Vaccher, and J. Menezes. 2000. Analysis and significance of anti-latent membrane protein-1 antibodies in the sera of patients with EBV-associated diseases. *J. Immunol.* **164:**2815–2822.

88. Yao, Q. Y., A. B. Rickinson, and M. A. Epstein. 1985. A reexamination of the Epstein-Barr virus carrier state in healthy seropositive individuals. *Int. J. Cancer* **35:**35–42.

Human Herpesviruses 6, 7, and 8

PHILIP E. PELLETT AND GRAHAM TIPPLES

100

The viruses discussed in this chapter are *Human herpesvirus 6* variants A and B (HHV-6A and HHV-6B), *Human herpesvirus 7* (HHV-7), and *Human herpesvirus 8* (HHV-8; Kaposi's sarcoma [KS]-associated herpesvirus). These viruses cause diseases that are clinically significant primarily in small children and in immunocompromised patients (Table 1).

HHV-6

Taxonomy

HHV-6A and HHV-6B, along with HHV-7, comprise the *Roseolovirus* genus of the betaherpesvirus subfamily (97). Roseoloviruses share many features of their genomic architecture and genetic content, the ability to replicate and establish latent infections in lymphocytes, and associations with febrile rash illnesses in young children, and they are opportunistic pathogens in immunocompromised patients. For convenience, in this chapter we frequently refer to HHV-6A and HHV-6B collectively as HHV-6.

Description of the Agent

Like all herpesviruses, HHV-6 virions consist of four concentrically arranged major components: a double-stranded DNA genome (160 to 170 kb) that is contained in the core of an icosahedral capsid, which is surrounded by a proteinaceous tegument, all of which is surrounded by a lipid bilayer envelope that is studded with a variety of virally encoded proteins and a sprinkling of cellular proteins. The viral genomes encode approximately 100 unique genes.

Epidemiology and Transmission

Epidemiology

Collectively, HHV-6A and HHV-6B are highly prevalent, with seroprevalences in many populations exceeding 90% (38). Most individuals become infected by the age of 2 to 3 years (100). In the United States, Japan, and Europe, HHV-6B is the main source of the nearly universal early childhood HHV-6 infections and HHV-6A prevalence in these areas may exceed 50% by adulthood. In Zambia, HHV-6A was detected in >85% of asymptomatic infants, suggesting significant international differences in the epidemiology of the HHV-6 variants (6).

Tissue Distribution

The cell surface receptor for HHV-6 is CD46, a widespread cell surface antigen. HHV-6B DNA has been detected in as many as 90% of peripheral blood mononuclear cell (PBMC) specimens, >80% of brains, >90% of tonsils (in epithelial cells of tonsillar crypts), and 40 to 90% of saliva or oral fluid specimens; it has been detected less frequently in skin, lungs, endomyocardial biopsy specimens, goblet cells and histiocytes in the large intestine, and cervical fluids. During primary infection in young children in the United States, HHV-6A was found by PCR in 2.5% of PBMC and 17% of cerebrospinal fluid (CSF) specimens, while HHV-6B was found in 99% of PBMC and 86% of CSF specimens (some specimens were coinfected) (51). The median salivary viral level of HHV-6 increased from approximately 10^3 copies of HHV-6/ml at 1 week postinfection to 10^5 copies of HHV-6/ml by 8 weeks postinfection (100). HHV-6A DNA has been detected in over half of lung and skin specimens, mostly in conjunction with HHV-6B. In a study of adult brains, 28% were positive for HHV-6A and 75% for HHV-6B (some were dually positive) (28). In bone marrow transplant (BMT) recipients, HHV-6A and HHV-6B were both detected in plasma, while HHV-6B was the variant detected in PBMC (73).

Latency, Persistence, and Transmission

Other than during the acute phase of roseola, HHV-6 can seldom be detected by culture, even though its DNA can be intermittently detected in most children by PCR, and transcripts can be occasionally detected in asymptomatic children (~1% of specimens) (22). This suggests that a true latent infection is established in PBMC. Latent HHV-6 has been detected in monocytes, their CD34$^+$ bone marrow progenitors, and PBMC-derived dendritic cells. HHV-6 DNA is more frequently detected in salivary glands than in saliva, in contrast to HHV-7, which is frequently detected in both the gland and the fluid. HHV-6B primary infection typically occurs within a matter of months of the waning of maternal antibody, with transmission likely being via saliva (81). Breast milk is not a significant vehicle for transmission. Little is known of HHV-6A transmission.

A small percentage of individuals (0.5 to 1%) harbor germ line-integrated HHV-6A or HHV-6B genomes; thus, all of their cells are positive for viral DNA, which may be a

TABLE 1 Disease associations

Virus	Age at primary infection	Principal disease associations	
		Primary infection	Immunocompromised patients
HHV-6A	Unknown	Occasional roseola	Disseminated infections, HCMV-like and HCMV-associated disease, pneumonitis, graft loss
HHV-6B	Before 2 yr	Most roseola, related febrile/rash illness	Disseminated infections, HCMV-like and HCMV-associated disease, pneumonitis, graft loss
HHV-7	>50% by 2 yr	Occasional roseola	HCMV-like and HCMV-associated disease
HHV-8	During childhood in Africa; post-adolescence in the United States and Europe	Unknown	KS, MCD, PEL, acute bone marrow failure in transplant recipients

source for the occasionally detected persistence of high levels of HHV-6 DNA in serum (94) as well as a major source of congenital transmission of HHV-6 (49, 61). Fluorescent in situ hybridization studies have shown that HHV-6 can be integrated into telomeric regions of chromosomes (70).

Clinical Significance

Infections with HHV-6 are generally mild or subclinical in immunocompetent individuals but can be severe in immunocompromised persons.

Primary Infection

HHV-6 primary infection causes roseola (roseola infantum, sixth disease, exanthem subitum) in approximately one-quarter of children. While HHV-6B is the predominant etiologic agent of roseola, rare cases of HHV-6A-associated roseola or febrile illness have been reported. About 90% of children are symptomatic at the time of primary infection, with specifically associated symptoms including fever (58%), fussiness (70%), rhinorrhea (66%), diarrhea (26%), rash (31%), and roseola (24%) (100).

Classic roseola symptoms include an abrupt rise in temperature (39 to 40°C), which persists for 2 to 5 days. Fever abatement coincides with the onset of a maculopapular rash (only rarely vesicular) (Fig. 1) which resolves in 1 to 3 days. The initial appearance of the rash is on the neck, behind the ears, and on the back, followed by spread to the rest of the body, usually excluding the face and distal extremities. The illness lasts 2 to 7 days, usually with no sequelae. Other clinical symptoms may include palpebral edema and suboccipital, postauricular, and cervical lymphadenopathy prior to rash onset.

Primary HHV-6 infection may also present as fever without rash or rash without fever. Less common but more severe forms of primary HHV-6 infection may include fever of >40°C, respiratory tract distress, tympanic inflammation, diarrhea, and convulsions. Although seizures are rare for HHV-6 primary infections (89), such infections with or without clinical roseola account for a significant proportion of febrile seizures in young children (92). Other serious but rare complications reported for HHV-6 primary infections include hepatosplenomegaly, Gianotti-Crosti syndrome (an acrodermatitis of childhood that has also been associated with hepatitis B virus and Epstein-Barr virus [EBV] infections), bulging fontanels, aseptic meningitis, encephalitis (perhaps 1% of meningitis and encephalitis cases) (92), seizures and poor neurologic outcome following congenital infection, or disseminated fatal infection.

Primary HHV-6 infection in adults is rare but can be severe. Clinical presentation in these cases may include mononucleosis-like illness, prolonged lymphadenopathy, and fulminant hepatitis.

Immunocompromised Patients

Under immunocompromised conditions, such as in the transplantation setting or in AIDS patients, HHV-6 can reactivate, sometimes causing disease.

Transplant Recipients

HHV-6 reactivation occurs in approximately one-half of BMT recipients and one-third of solid organ transplant (SOT) recipients (38). There appears to be a temporal pattern of HHV-6, HHV-7, and human cytomegalovirus (HCMV) reactivation for SOT, with the median times

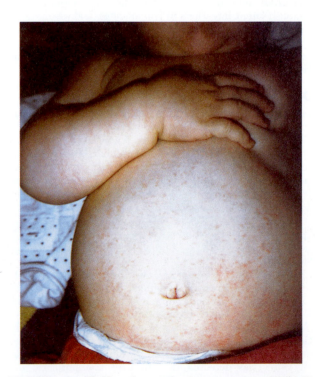

FIGURE 1 Child with roseola during primary HHV-6B infection. Photo courtesy of Stephen Dewhurst, University of Rochester. Previously published in reference 44.

posttransplantation being 20 days, 27 days, and 36 days, respectively (38).

HHV-6 is a consistent, low-to-moderate frequency contributor to posttransplant illness that can sometimes be severe, and its activity might be both a marker of and a contributor to immune suppression (89). In BMT and stem cell transplant recipients, HHV-6 has been associated with encephalitis/encephalopathy, pneumonitis, delayed engraftment, erythematous papular rash, fever, CMV-like disease, graft-versus-host disease, seizures, hepatitis, diarrhea, and bone marrow suppression (reviewed in references 18, 38, and 98). In SOT patients, HHV-6 has been associated with encephalitis, pneumonitis, graft-versus-host disease, fungal disease, and bone marrow suppression. HHV-6B is detected more frequently than HHV-6A in transplant patients. In one study, HHV-6A partitioned into plasma and HHV-6B partitioned into both plasma and circulating lymphocytes (73). This suggests that diagnostics for HHV-6A or HHV-6B may be influenced by the specimen type and that studies focused on one or the other of these compartments may have missed part of the story.

Human Immunodeficiency Virus (HIV)-Infected Patients

Although HHV-6 infects and replicates in CD4$^+$ T cells, no specific role has been established for HHV-6 in AIDS; some interesting data suggest possible pathogenic interactions (47, 58, 64).

Infections in the Brain

HHV-6 can grow in neuronal cells, and neurological symptoms are clearly associated with primary infection. The involvement of HHV-6 in multiple sclerosis is not conclusive (32). However, the more precisely linked the specimens have been to diseased tissue (e.g., microdissected lesions versus CSF versus serum), the stronger the associations have been. Improved and standardized assays and validated controls are needed to allow proper comparison of research results and, potentially, for monitoring patients. There are conflicting data with respect to the association of HHV-6 with progressive multifocal leukoencephalopathy (35, 69).

Other

Drug Hypersensitivity Syndrome

Exposure to various drugs occasionally results in a severe and sometimes fatal reaction variously known as drug hypersensitivity syndrome, drug rash with eosinophilia and systemic symptoms, and anticonvulsant hypersensitivity syndrome. HHV-6 reactivations have been identified in a number of drug rash with eosinophilia and systemic symptoms cases (95), but it remains to be seen whether HHV-6 contributes to either initiation or exacerbation of the events.

Rosai-Dorfman Disease

Rosai-Dorfman disease (histiocytosis with massive lymphadenopathy) patients have had increased HHV-6 antibody titers, HHV-6 DNA detected by in situ hybridization, and strong immunohistochemical staining for HHV-6 antigen in abnormal histiocytes.

Other Diseases

There is no conclusive evidence for causal associations between HHV-6 and malignancy or chronic fatigue syndrome.

Therapy

Antiviral treatment of HHV-6 has been reviewed in depth (38). The clinical circumstances for which antiviral intervention for HHV-6 might be appropriate include HHV-6 reactivation in immunocompromised individuals. There are presently no antivirals licensed for specific treatment of HHV-6; however, an approach similar to that for HCMV has been used.

Collection, Transport, and Storage of Specimens

For virus isolation, blood should be collected in an anticoagulant (such as heparin) and processed through a Ficoll gradient within 24 h; cells for virus isolation should not be frozen. After isolation, HHV-6-infected cells can be stored in standard cryopreservation media. Saliva specimens can be collected for virus detection by various methods, including filter paper strips (99), oral swabs, throat swabs, and expectorated saliva. Serum, plasma, and cells intended for PCR can be shipped frozen.

Direct Examination

Direct detection of HHV-6 can be done by immunohistochemistry (IHC) (59, 72), in situ hybridization, and in situ PCR (15, 76). While those methods have their niches, the most common method of direct detection is PCR.

Nucleic Acid

The sensitivity of PCR is of particular value for the detection of HHV-6, given that even during periods of viral activity, viral DNA can be at a relatively low concentration relative to cellular DNA. A multitude of PCR strategies have been published that utilize numerous HHV-6 genomic targets. The optimal viral target has not yet been determined. Although not necessarily clinically informative, HHV-6A and HHV-6B can be readily distinguished by using variant-specific PCR primers, amplimer size differences, variant-specific hybridization probes, restriction enzyme analysis of PCR amplimers, or by melting curve analysis using real-time PCR.

PCR for HHV-6 in the clinical laboratory can be set up as a component of a herpesvirus multiplex PCR assay that enables simultaneous analysis for multiple human herpesviruses (37, 88). When multiplex assays are used, it is important to consider the clinical management implications and clinical significance (or lack thereof) of positive results for viruses that would not normally be included in the differential diagnosis.

Quantitative PCR (from whole blood or PBMCs) is particularly useful for the determination of baseline viral load levels in transplant patients, with significant increases above the baseline indicating active infection. Although many laboratories use plasma for HCMV and EBV PCR testing, plasma is not as sensitive as whole blood or PBMCs for HHV-6 testing. Optimal samples for quantitative PCR (i.e., whole blood, PBMCs, or plasma) have not been established (1).

We suggest the use of quantitative real-time assays that incorporate a coamplified positive control and allow the HHV-6 variants to be distinguished. Nested PCR strategies are to be avoided because of the problem of contamination control. Important variables that need to be carefully standardized and then incorporated into the sensitivity calculation and interpretation are the amount of material initially lysed to prepare the template (e.g., volume of fluid or number of cells), and then the amount of this material that is included in each reaction mixture (48, 67). Sources

TABLE 2 Commercial sources of reagents and assays[a]

Supplier(s) (location)	HHV-6			HHV-7			HHV-8		
	Serology	IHC	PCR	Serology	IHC	PCR	Serology	IHC	PCR
Advanced Biotechnologies (Columbia, MD)	IFA, ELISA	MAb	DNA, qDNA qPCR	IFA		qDNA qPCR	IFA, ELISA	MAb	DNA, qDNA qPCR
Argene (Verniolle, France)		MAb					IFA, ELISA		
Biotrin (Dublin, Ireland)	IFA (IgG and IgM), ELISA								
Bion Enterprises (Des Plaines, IL)	IFA								
Panbio (Sinnamon Park, Queensland, Australia)	ELISA (IgG and IgM)								
Antibodies-online (Atlanta, GA), Genway (San Diego, CA), Lifespan Biosciences (Seattle, WA), Millipore (Billerica, MA), Santa Cruz Biotechnology (Santa Cruz, CA)		MAb						MAb	
Abcam (Cambridge, MA), AbD Serotec (Raleigh, NC), Meridian Life Sciences (Saco, ME), Raybiotech (Norcross, GA), Thermo Scientific (Waltham, MA)		MAb							

[a]DNA, purified DNA; qDNA, DNA for use as quantitative reference; qPCR, kit for quantitative PCR. No FDA-approved tests are available for any of these viruses.

of reagents, assays, and commercial PCR testing are listed in Tables 2 and 3. Thorough evaluations of HHV-6 PCR assays are essential (37), as are ongoing comparisons and proficiency testing to improve the standardization of quantitative assays (46).

Isolation Procedures

Although HHV-6 can be isolated from PBMC by cocultivation of patient PBMC with stimulated human umbilical cord blood lymphocytes (CBL) (11, 39), primary isolation from clinical specimens is not routinely done in the clinical diagnostic laboratory. Primary cell culture medium consists of RPMI 1640, 10% fetal bovine serum, 100 U of penicillin/ml, 100 μg of streptomycin/ml, and 0.29 mg of L-glutamine/ml. Cells are cultured at starting densities of 10^6 cells per ml. Ficoll-purified primary CBL are first stimulated for 2 to 3 days at 37°C and 5% CO_2 in cell culture media containing 0.01 mg of hydrocortisone/ml and 2 μg of phytohemagglutinin/ml. Stimulated CBLs are then cocultured with an equal volume of Ficoll-purified patient PBMCs in the media described above, except the phytohemagglutinin is replaced with recombinant interleukin-2; interleukin-2 concentrations used in various laboratories range from 0.1 to 5 U/ml. Cultures are monitored daily for cytopathic effect (CPE). Typical HHV-6 CPE consists of loss of CBL clumping, the appearance of large balloon-like cells, and syncytium formation. After 7 to 10 days, the culture is passaged into freshly stimulated CBL. Cultures that remain healthy after another 7 to 10 days are considered negative. HHV-6 infection should be confirmed by immunofluorescence or PCR, as described below.

Isolates from primary CBL cultures can be adapted for propagation in continuous cell lines: HHV-6A isolates in HSB-2 or J-JHAN cells and HHV-6B isolates in Molt-3 cells. HHV-6B strain Z29 grows well in Molt-3 cells of the NIH lineage but not in Molt-3 cells from the ATCC lineage. Culture conditions are similar to those used for propagation in primary cells. Propagation of HHV-6 can be moderately tricky; more extensive procedural details are provided elsewhere (11, 12, 77). It is important to monitor cultures by an immunofluorescence assay (IFA) in addition to CPE. Nonoptimal culture conditions can lead to extensive CPE but little virus production.

Identification

HHV-6 virions have typical herpesvirus morphology by electron microscopy: approximately 200-nm spherical enveloped virions containing a 90- to 110-nm icosahedral capsid with an electron-dense core surrounded by an amorphous tegument (97). Numerous monoclonal antibodies (MAbs) are available (both commercially and from research laboratories) that react with both HHV-6A and/or HHV-6B. MAbs are useful for confirming cell culture CPE for HHV-6 infection, for antigen detection assays, flow cytometry, and immunohistochemical analyses. A comprehensive list of published antibodies, their targets, variant specificity, and commercial sources is provided in reference 3. Sources are also listed in Table 2.

Typing Systems

HHV-6A and HHV-6B can be typed through the use of variant-specific MAbs and variant-specific PCR assays (described above).

Serologic Tests

Numerous serologic methods for detecting HHV-6 antibodies have been described including both enzyme-linked

TABLE 3 Some commercial sources for HHV-6, HHV-7, and HHV-8 testing

Manufacturer (location)	URL	Serology			PCR[a]		
		HHV-6	HHV-7	HHV-8	HHV-6	HHV-7	HHV-8
ARUP Laboratories (Salt Lake City, UT)	aruplab.com	IgG			Q		q
Focus Diagnostics (Cypress, CA)	focusdx.com	IgG IgM	IgG IgM	IgG	Q	Q	Q
LabCorp (Burlington, NC)	labcorp.com	IgG IgM			q		
Medical Diagnostic Laboratories (Hamilton, NJ)	mdlab.com	IgG			q	q	q
Specialty Labs (Valencia, CA)	specialtylabs.com	IgG IgM					
Viracor (Lee's Summit, MO)	viracor.com				Q	Q	Q
North Shore-LIJ Health System Labs (Lake Success, NY)					q		

[a]Q, quantitative PCR; q, qualitative PCR.

immunosorbent assay (ELISA) and IFA formats; commercially available FDA-approved assays are not available. Recent versus past infections can be discriminated through the use of IFA-based antibody avidity tests. Maturation from low- to high-avidity HHV-6 antibody following primary HHV-6 infection takes approximately 5 months. Antibody avidity testing can also be used to differentiate between HHV-6 and HHV-7 primary infections (91). Neutralizing antibodies typically become detectable 3 to 8 days following the onset of fever during primary infection. Sources for commercial serologic testing are listed in Table 3.

Specificity issues for HHV-6 serological methods involve cross-reactivity between HHV-6A, HHV-6B, HHV-7, and CMV (18, 91). Current serological methods based on the use of whole infected cells as antigens do not differentiate between HHV-6A and HHV-6B antibody responses. Although adsorption studies have demonstrated the presence of cross-reactive antibodies to HHV-6 and CMV, the cross-reactivity is generally not sufficient to confound methods based on HHV-6 whole-cell lysates. The simultaneous rise in antibodies to both HHV-6 and CMV seen in some patients is not fully understood; it may be due to varying combinations of simultaneous activity of both viruses and some individuals responding to cross-reactive antigens. Limited cross-reactivity has also been found between HHV-6 and HHV-7 antibody responses; adsorption methods and antibody avidity can be used for differentiation (91).

Antiviral Susceptibilities

The best in vitro antiviral sensitivities and selectivities have consistently been for foscarnet, cidofovir, and ganciclovir. In vitro and in vivo evidence indicates that mutations in the HHV-6 U69-encoded protein kinase or the HHV-6 DNA polymerase gene can cause HHV-6 resistance to these drugs (16, 17). HHV-6 antiviral susceptibility testing can be accomplished by quantitative PCR and by PCR with quenching probes (54). Such testing is available only in research laboratories.

Evaluation, Interpretation, and Reporting of Results

Methods used in the clinical virology laboratory must be thoroughly evaluated in the relevant clinical context (e.g., febrile and/or rash illness in children under 3 years of age and specific forms of disease in immunocompromised individuals such as transplantation patients) to assess sensitivity, specificity, and positive and negative predictive values.

Laboratory diagnosis of HHV-6 is challenging given the many biological and molecular similarities between HHV-6A, HHV-6B, and HHV-7, the association between CMV and HHV-6 reactivation, the need to differentiate between primary and reactivation disease, and the issue of chromosomal integration of HHV-6. Diagnostic tests and their applications are summarized in Table 4. We also refer the reader to the elegant treatment of this issue by Ward (91).

For the purposes of routine testing, serology is only of value for the diagnosis of primary HHV-6 infections in children under 3 years of age with symptoms characteristic of roseola. In such situations, (i) immunoglobulin M (IgM) positive serology, (ii) low-avidity IgG serology, or (iii) IgG seroconversion with a significant rise in titer between acute- and convalescent-phase sera can be considered confirmatory for primary HHV-6 infections. Quantitative PCR-based approaches can be used for detection of both primary infections and reactivation of HHV-6. Serology is of limited value for detection of HHV-6 reactivation. However, HHV-6 PCR diagnostics are confounded by that fact that approximately 1% of individuals harbor exceptionally high HHV-6 loads in their PBMCs (~1 copy per cell equivalent of DNA) due to germ line HHV-6 integration. Although no HHV-6-linked immunologic deficiency, disease, or unusual virologic activity has yet been observed in such individuals, their constitutively high viral loads make diagnostics challenging (61). Quantitative PCR-based assays can be useful to help differentiate between latent, reactivated, and chromosomally integrated HHV-6. Chromosomally integrated HHV-6 cases have viral loads of 5 $\log_{10}$ HHV-6 genomes per ml in serum and >6 log 10 HHV-6 genomes/ml in whole blood, whereas lower viral loads are seen in active and reactivated HHV-6 scenarios (34, 93). Determination of optimal samples for quantitative PCR (i.e., whole blood/PBMCs or plasma) still requires further study, as it has been shown that the presence of HHV-6 DNA in plasma may at least partially reflect DNA from lysed blood PBMCs rather than circulating HHV-6 virus indicative of active infection (1).

Confirmation of HHV-6 in encephalitis cases requires detection of HHV-6 in the CSF and low levels of viral

TABLE 4 Diagnostic methods for HHV-6, -7, and -8^a

Virus	Method	Approach	Advantage(s)	Limitation(s)	Clinical availability	Key reference(s)
HHV-6	Virus isolation	Cocultivate PBMC with stimulated primary CBL	Gold standard for active infection	Slow, need for ongoing access to umbilical cord blood	Not practical in clinical labs	11, 39, 77
	Antigen detection	Use of HHV-6A, -6B variant-common and variant-specific MAb against p41/p38, gp116/54/64, gp82/105, 101K for IHC and culture confirmation	Specific, readily available reagents, precise localization in tissues	Specialized interpretation required; lower throughput than PCR	MAb commercially available	3
	Serology	IgM and IgG by neutralization, immunoblot, IFA, ACIF, ELISA		Single IgG-positive results are uninformative; need paired acute- and convalescent-phase specimens to document disease-linked seroconversion	Kits and reagents commercially available	14, 18
		Antibody avidity	Clear identification of primary infections	Clinical significance of IgM in individuals >3 yr of age is questionable	Avidity test not commercially available	91
	PCR	major antigen: p100/101K Qualitative and quantitative from PBMC, plasma/serum, and CSF		Optimal target not determined; assays not standardized with respect to viral gene target and specimen type; clinically relevant quantitation threshold not standardized; nor able to differentiate active infections from chromosomally integrated high-level HHV-6 expression	Practical for clinical labs; assay and testing commercially available	Numerous methods reported in the literature; 14, 30, 33, 93
		RT-PCR from PBMC to detect active infections	Confirms active infection	Not standardized	No commercially available kit	37, 88
		Herpesvirus multiplex	Convenient for the lab	Clinicians may not want testing done for multiple herpesviruses because of interpretation and clinical utility issues		
HHV-7	Virus isolation	Cocultivation of PBMC with stimulated primary CBL; inoculation of CBLs with saliva from healthy and ill patients	Gold standard for active infections	Not practical in clinical labs	Rare	11
	Antigen detection	Several MAb available from research laboratories, including against pp85	Useful for IHC and culture confirmation	MAb no longer commercially available	Rare	10
	Serology	IgM and IgG NT, immunoblot, IFA, ELISA		Uncertain reliability of IgM for identifying recent infections; need paired acute- and convalescent-phase specimens to document disease-linked seroconversion	Commercially available	10, 13, 85

Method	Test	Use/indication	Comment	Availability	Reference(s)
	Antibody avidity	Identification of primary infections		Commercially available testing	91
PCR	Major antigen: pp85			Commercially available kit	9
	Qualitative and quantitative PCR from PBMCs or plasma/serum	Convenient			37, 88
	Herpesvirus multiplex		Clinicians may not want testing done for multiple herpesviruses because of interpretation and clinical utility issues		
HHV-8					
Virus isolation	Not available				
Antigen detection	MAb against K8.1, ORF59, LANA; for IHC	Identification HHV-8 in tissues from suspected KS, PEL, and MCD; distinguish KS from clinical mimickers	Lower throughput than PCR	MAb are commercially available	52
Serology	IgG IFA based on unstimulated (latent) or stimulated (lytic) PEL cells	Identification HHV-8 infected individuals	Not specific for a particular disease	Reagents, kits, and testing are commercially available	80, 82
	ELISA based on synthetic peptides, purified virions, and expressed proteins				80, 82
	Neutralization assay				57
	Immunoprecipitation with chemiluminescence detection				20
	Major lytic antigens: ORF65 and K8.1				
	Major latent antigen: LANA-1				
PCR	Qualitative and quantitative	Verification of presence of HHV-8 in tissues from suspected KS, PEL, and MCD	PCR from blood is insensitive for detecting infection in the absence of disease	Commercially available reagents and testing	29, 57, 79
	Herpesvirus multiplex		Clinicians may not want testing done for multiple herpesviruses because of interpretation and clinical utility issues	Commercially available kit	37

aACIF, anticomplement immunofluorescence; NT, neutralization test; RT-PCR, reverse transcriptase PCR. No FDA-approved tests are available for these viruses.

DNA in serum or whole blood. Detection of HHV-6 in CSF and high levels of viral DNA in serum or whole blood may be indicative of HHV-6 chromosomal integration and is not diagnostic for HHV-6 encephalitis (91). Rising levels of HHV-6 DNA in CSF or blood, however, suggest acute infection.

Clinical testing for HHV-6 should be limited to circumstances for which there has been a well-characterized association between the disease and HHV-6 infection and when the results of a given test will be diagnostically informative. For example, HHV-6 IgG or IgM serology in an adult done at a single time point is of limited diagnostic value. Clinical scenarios where HHV-6 testing could be considered include primary infection in children under 3 years of age, primary infection or reactivation in immunocompromised individuals such as AIDS patients or transplantation patients, in mononucleosis-like syndromes, and in meningitis/encephalitis cases. Ljungman et al. (62) provide useful recommendations for HHV-6 diagnostics post-stem cell transplantation, including HHV-6 encephalitis. Still relevant in some parts of the world, HHV-6 has been identified as the cause of rash illness incorrectly diagnosed as measles infection. The possibility of primary HHV-6 or HHV-7 infection should be considered when febrile and/or neurologic illness occurs shortly following routine immunizations; such illness may be incorrectly attributed to the vaccine (91). Further studies are needed to improve our understanding of the associations between HHV-6 and disease and to improve the quality of HHV-6 diagnostic testing.

HHV-7

Taxonomy and Description of the Agent
Because of the relative similarity of its nucleotide sequences, genomic architecture, and biology with those of HHV-6A and HHV-6B, HHV-7 is included as a member of the *Roseolovirus* genus of the betaherpesvirus subfamily (97). Like all herpesviruses, HHV-7 virions consist of four concentrically arranged major components: a double-stranded DNA genome (145 kb) contained in the core of an icosahedral capsid, which is surrounded by a proteinaceous tegument, all of which is surrounded by a lipid bilayer envelope that is studded with a variety of virally encoded proteins and a sprinkling of cellular proteins. HHV-7 genomes encode approximately 100 unique genes.

Epidemiology and Transmission

Epidemiology
HHV-7 seroprevalence in healthy adults in Europe, Japan, and the United States ranges from 60 to 90%. Following waning of maternal antibody, HHV-7 seroprevalence rapidly increases to over 50% by 2 years of age and then progresses toward the adult level over the remaining years of childhood.

Tissue Distribution
Although its in vitro host range is restricted to lymphocytes, HHV-7 has a broad cellular host range in vivo. One of its cellular receptors is the lymphocyte antigen, CD4; other receptors must be involved in the infection of other cell types. HHV-7 lytic antigens have been detected in salivary gland acini, lungs, skin, and mammary glands and, more sporadically, in liver, kidney, and tonsils (56). HHV-7 DNA has been detected by PCR in PBMC, salivary glands,

gastric mucosa, skin, and cervical swabs. The virus has seldom been detected in brain tissues. Infectious HHV-7 has been occasionally isolated from PBMC during roseola and is easily isolated from the saliva of healthy adults. The ability to detect HHV-7 DNA in uncultured lymphocytes by PCR, along with the inability to detect infectious virus in the absence of T-cell activation, suggests that the virus is latent in PBMC. Macrophages represent another potential reservoir (101).

Transmission
HHV-7 can be cultured from the saliva of ~75% of healthy adults, with viral loads frequently exceeding 10^6 genomes per ml. While the most plausible route of transmission is via saliva, HHV-7 has also been detected in breast milk, urine, and cervical secretions. In contrast to HHV-6, congenital transmission of HHV-7 has not been documented (50).

Clinical Significance

Primary Infection
HHV-7 causes perhaps 5% of roseola cases as well as other febrile illnesses in children. In one small study, HHV-7 appeared to cause milder roseola than HHV-6 in terms of mean and maximum fever, fever duration, and duration of rash. However, other studies suggest an equal or higher rate of central nervous system complications during HHV-7 primary infections compared with HHV-6 (92). HHV-7 neurologic involvement includes hemiplegia and febrile seizures.

Immunocompromised Patients
HHV-7 becomes latent in lymphocytes following primary infection and can reactivate in immunocompromised hosts such as transplantation recipients and AIDS patients. In bone marrow, liver, and renal transplant patients, simultaneous CMV and HHV-7 activity have sometimes been associated with clinical events (see corresponding HHV-6 section above), and a case of fatal HHV-7-associated encephalitis has been reported, but overall, HHV-7 infections are not frequent contributors to posttransplant illness.

Like HIV, HHV-7 uses CD4 as its major cellular receptor. In vitro, HHV-7 can inhibit HIV infection, possibly due to receptor interference. There is no clear evidence of a role for HHV-7 in AIDS progression.

Interstitial Pneumonia
HHV-7 DNA was detected more frequently and at higher loads in affected tissues from nonimmunocompromised patients with interstitial pneumonia (36, 96). Further study will be required to fully evaluate the significance of this observation.

Pityriasis Rosea
Data are not consistent for an association between HHV-7 and pityriasis rosea (19, 31).

Therapy
HHV-7 antiviral sensitivities are similar to those for HHV-6 and CMV, with ganciclovir, foscarnet, and cidofovir being much more inhibitory than acyclovir (40). Drug-resistant HHV-7 has not been identified, but given the widespread use of ganciclovir for therapy of CMV and "CMV disease," it will likely occasionally emerge. Therapeutic regimens have not been defined; in transplant recipients, they may ultimately be linked to strategies for dealing generically with betaherpesvirus activity.

Collection, Transport, and Storage of Specimens

The methods described above for HHV-6 are appropriate for HHV-7.

Direct Examination

By electron microscopy, HHV-7 virions have appearances typical of herpesviruses. MAbs are available upon request from some research laboratories (10). The most widely used qualitative PCR primer set for HHV-7 was described by Berneman et al. (9). Others have also been described, but their performances have not been compared. Real-time PCR methods for HHV-7 have been described (8, 88), including multiplex assays for multiple herpesviruses (37, 88). Sources of reagents and commercial PCR testing for HHV-7 are listed in Tables 2 and 3.

Isolation Procedures

HHV-7 isolation can be accomplished using the methods described above for HHV-6, but it is not used for routine clinical diagnosis. HHV-7 isolates initially propagated in primary cell culture or previously adapted HHV-7 strains (e.g., strain SB) can be grown in SupT1 cells in a manner similar to propagation of HHV-6 in continuous cells (11).

Identification

MAbs can be useful for confirming cell culture CPE when attempting virus isolation, especially to rule out CPE due to HHV-6, for IHC, and for immunoelectron microscopy. The PCR methods described above provide sensitive, specific, and rapid ways to unambiguously identify the virus. Biologically meaningful subtypes of HHV-7 have not been identified.

Typing Systems

Biologically meaningful subtypes of HHV-7 have not been identified.

Serologic Tests

HHV-7 serologic assays include neutralization tests, immunoblotting, immunoprecipition, IFA (commercially available reagents), and ELISA (reviewed in reference 10). In one comparison of IFA, immunoblotting, and ELISA, the overall performances of the three assays were quite similar, with a small sensitivity advantage for the ELISA and a specificity advantage for the immunoblot assay (13). As described above, antibody avidity testing for both HHV-6 and HHV-7 allows differentiation between HHV-6 and HHV-7 primary infections as well as recent and past HHV-7 infections (91). Table 3 lists commercial sources of HHV-7 reagents.

Antiviral Susceptibilities

Antiviral susceptibility has been evaluated by measuring the inhibition of viral replication by immunofluorescence, by antigen slot blots, and by inhibition of virus-induced cytotoxicity (40).

Evaluation, Interpretation, and Reporting of Results

There are no circumstances that warrant routine single-agent monitoring for HHV-7 activity, but its inclusion in multiplex assays may prove to be of value in monitoring children with suspected encephalitis and/or febrile convulsions (especially in association with recent vaccination) (92) and transplant recipients. Diagnostic tests and their applications are summarized in Table 4. The main issues for HHV-7 diagnostic testing are distinguishing HHV-6 from HHV-7, differentiation of primary HHV-7 infection from reactivation, and distinguishing latent and active infections. Differentiating HHV-6 from HHV-7 can be done both by molecular diagnostics (e.g., PCR) and through the use of specific antibodies.

HHV-8

Taxonomy

HHV-8 is a member of the *Rhadinovirus* genus of the gammaherpesvirus subfamily. Gammaherpesviruses, which include EBV, are characterized by being able to replicate and establish latency in lymphoblastoid cells.

Description of the Agent

HHV-8 virions consist of four concentrically arranged major components: a double-stranded 165-kb DNA genome that is contained in the core of an icosahedral capsid, which is surrounded by a proteinaceous tegument, all of which is surrounded by a lipid bilayer envelope that is studded with a variety of virally encoded proteins and a sprinkling of cellular proteins. HHV-8 genomes encode ~80 proteins and 12 micro-RNAs (47).

Epidemiology and Transmission

Epidemiology

The global distribution of HHV-8 is uneven (42). In much of Africa, HHV-8 seroprevalence is >50%, whereas it is <10% in most of Europe, the United States, and Japan. Seroprevalence is ~30% to 50% in men who have sex with men (MSM) in the United States and Europe. Population-based disparities are likely due to differences in child-rearing and family practices, sexual behaviors, and possibly viral and/or host genotypes. In Africa, the virus is frequently acquired early in life, in a maternally linked manner. In the United States, prevalence rises after adolescence. At least four major HHV-8 genotypes are in global circulation (102).

Tissue Distribution

In the absence of KS, HHV-8 DNA or antigens are seldom detected in seropositive immunocompetent individuals, and they are most frequently detected in the saliva of HIV-negative MSM (24). In HIV-positive MSM, viral DNA can be detected in essentially all KS lesions, >50% of saliva or oral fluid specimens, ~30% of PBMC specimens, ~10% of semen specimens, and less frequently in other types of specimens. The virus is capable of replicating in many cell types, including CD19-positive B cells in AIDS patients, placental tissues (43), and circulating endothelial progenitors during classic KS (41).

Latency and Persistence

HHV-8 DNA has been detected in a variety of tissues but generally with methods that cannot discriminate between latent and lytic infections. Evidence for persistence of HHV-8 in immunocompetent individuals comes from seropositive organ transplant recipients who subsequently developed KS (26). HHV-8 latency has been extensively studied in cell culture systems that employ primary effusion lymphoma (PEL) cell lines that harbor HHV-8. The virus is in a latent state in >95% of cultured PEL cells, with the remainder being in a lytic state. Lytic replication can be induced by agents such as a phorbol ester or the HHV-8 lytic inducer gene encoded by open reading frame

50 (ORF50). A subset of HHV-8 genes is transcribed during latency, including the ORF73 gene that encodes the major latency-associated nuclear antigen 1 (LANA-1), v-cyclin, and the highly expressed K12 (kaposin, also known as *nut-1* and T0.7) (47).

Transmission

Most HHV-8 transmission is probably via oral fluids but may also occur via breast milk and semen. In Africa, the virus is typically acquired in a maternally linked manner early in life, possibly via practices such as premastication of food or use of saliva to soothe bites from blood-sucking arthropods. Although sexual transmission is not the major route, HHV-8 seropositivity is linked to a variety of sexual risk factors among adolescents with high-risk sexual behaviors and MSM (7, 25). HHV-8 can be transmitted via injection drug use and by blood transfusion (in Uganda but not in the United States) (21, 53); screening of blood products does not appear to be imminent.

Clinical Significance

Primary Infection

Little is known of primary HHV-8 infection. There are likely to be significant differences between healthy children, immunocompetent adults, and immunocompromised patients. HHV-8 DNA has been detected in febrile children in areas of virus endemicity. Among 15 HIV-negative MSM who seroconverted to HHV-8, diarrhea, fatigue, localized rash, and lymphadenopathy were sometimes noted in association with primary infection (90). In immunocompromised patients, acute illness associated with HHV-8 primary infection included KS, fever, arthralgia, lymphadenopathy, splenomegaly, and cytopenia (63, 75).

KS

The four major forms of KS are all associated with HHV-8: (i) African endemic KS, which primarily affects children with or without HIV infection; (ii) Mediterranean or classic KS, which affects older men from Mediterranean Europe who have no known immunologic dysfunction; (iii) transplant-associated or idiopathic KS, which affects approximately 1% of SOT recipients in the United States; and (iv) AIDS-associated KS, which is the most common AIDS-associated neoplasm and the most aggressive form of the disease. KS incidence has declined but has not been eliminated since the advent of highly active antiretroviral therapy.

KS is a reactive angioproliferative disease characterized by reddish-brown plaque or nodular lesions on the skin of the trunk or the extremities, in the oral cavity (oral KS), as well as on internal organs (visceral KS). The disease can be disfiguring, disabling, and life-threatening. KS lesions are characterized by networks of vascular slits, spindle-shaped cells of endothelial origin, extravasated red blood cells, and purplish deposits of hemosiderin. HHV-8 is present in the spindle cells, lytically in a small percentage and latently in the remainder.

PEL

PEL is a rare (approximately 3% of AIDS-non-Hodgkin's lymphomas) but frequently aggressive subset of a class of lymphomas known as body-cavity-based lymphomas. PELs occur as lymphomatous effusions in body cavities, seldom disseminate beyond the cavity of origin, and have cell morphologies between those of large-cell immunoblastic lymphoma and anaplastic lymphoma. PELs express CD45 and associated antigens and have clonal immunoglobulin rearrangements suggesting B cell origin but seldom express B cell antigens. PELs have infrequent c-*myc* rearrangements or alterations in other cellular oncogenes, are frequently infected with EBV, and harbor HHV-8 in every cell (27). These lymphomas have a poor prognosis.

MCD

Multicentric Castleman's disease (MCD) is a multicentric angiofollicular B-cell hyperplasia that occurs in germinal centers of lymph nodes (74). The disease has systemic manifestations that include fever, fatigue, recurrent lymphadenopathy, hepatosplenomegaly, bone marrow plasmacytosis, and polyclonal hypergammaglobulinemia. HHV-8-associated MCD occurs predominantly in HIV-infected individuals. HHV-8 is present in scattered B cells in the mantle zone of germinal centers. HHV-8-associated MCD has a poor prognosis. Plasmablastic lymphoma has developed in patients who have the plasmablastic form of MCD.

Disease in Transplant Recipients

Organ transplant recipients are at risk for developing KS (60), with the risk being highest in regions of high HHV-8 seroprevalence. In most cases, the disease is from reactivated prior infection, but graft-derived infections occur (5, 26, 63, 78). In renal transplant recipients, in addition to cutaneous KS, parenchymal KS infiltration has led directly to marrow aplasia with plasmacytosis, fever, splenomegaly, cytopenia, marrow failure, graft failure, and disseminated KS (63, 66). PELs (one in association with KS) have been reported following cardiac transplants (45, 55), as has donor-derived fatal disseminated KS in liver transplant recipients (65).

Other Diseases

Multiple HHV-8-associated cellular proliferations can occur simultaneously in the same individual (e.g., KS plus MCD plus PEL), even in the same lymph node. HHV-8 has been associated with several other diseases. For some (e.g., angioimmunoblastic lymphoproliferative disease, oral plasmablastic lymphomas, prostate cancer, and some cutaneous disease), further work will be required to firmly establish an etiologic association. Initial linkages between HHV-8 and multiple myeloma and primary pulmonary hypertension were not confirmed (47).

Therapy

An important aspect of KS therapy in immune compromised patients is immune reconstitution: highly active retroviral therapy for patients infected with HIV and tapering or modifying immune suppressive regimens in organ transplant recipients. In instances where such approaches are not possible or are ineffective, therapeutic approaches include local and systemic cytotoxic and tissue-destructive regimens and immune enhancement by alpha interferon (2, 23, 60). In cell culture, HHV-8 is exquisitely sensitive to cidofovir and is also sensitive to ganciclovir and foscarnet. Although oral valganciclovir can suppress oral shedding of the virus, the therapeutic effect of these agents has been equivocal in small trials. Nonetheless, in large retrospective analyses, foscarnet or ganciclovir used for controlling other herpesvirus infections has been associated with lower KS risk, possibly due to these agents being more effective for prevention than for treatment of KS.

Because cases of PEL and MCD are so rare, there have been no controlled therapeutic trials. Case reports suggest potential utility of anti-CD20 MAb therapy for both diseases (which may exacerbate KS), valganciclovir for MCD, and cidofovir plus alpha interferon for PEL. Positron emission tomography/computed tomography with fluorodeoxyglucose can be useful for guiding MCD biopsies and for monitoring therapy (4).

Collection, Transport, and Storage of Specimens

Conventional methods can be used for collection and storage of serum or plasma for serology. For preparation of lymphocyte DNA for PCR, blood should be collected in anticoagulant (not heparin) and PBMCs purified on a Ficoll gradient. Oral fluids can be collected for PCR by the methods described above for HHV-6. Biopsies are used for pathologic analyses that may include standard hematoxylin- and eosin-stained cytopathic examination, PCR on total DNA extracted from a section, in situ PCR, or IHC. Standard methods can be used for the preparation of such specimens.

Direct Detection

KS can be readily distinguished from its mimickers such as benign vasculoproliferative lesions and tumors that have a prominent spindle cell component by IHC employing a MAb to the HHV-8 LANA-1 encoded by orf73 (52). Antigen retrieval methods can influence sensitivity.

The PCR primer sets described in the initial description of HHV-8 remain in wide use for qualitative PCR on specimens of all types (29). Nested PCR has been used, but the potential for false positives is higher and outweighs the possible sensitivity increase. Numerous systems have been described for quantitative PCR. Because of the low frequency of circulating HHV-8-infected lymphocytes and low viral copy number in latently infected cells, important variables for PCR from blood specimens include the number of cells in the initial lysis and the total quantity of resulting DNA included in the PCR mixture (67). Plasma and serum are both suitable for evaluating viremia in patients with HHV-8-associated lymphoproliferative diseases (87). Commercial sources of reagents and kits are listed in Table 2, and sources for PCR testing are listed in Table 3. A kit for simultaneous detection and quantification of HCMV and HHV-6, -7, and -8 (Argene, Verniolle, France) had a sensitivity of 96% compared to in-house assays (37).

Isolation Procedures

Reliable systems have not been developed for primary culture of HHV-8 from KS lesions. Ascitic fluids from PEL patients have been used to derive PEL cell lines.

Identification

HHV-8 is readily identified by PCR, hybridization with nucleic acid probes that target abundant transcripts (84, 86), and MAbs (Tables 2 and 4). By electron microscopy, HHV-8 virions have morphology similar to that of other herpesviruses.

Typing Systems

HHV-8 genotyping is based predominantly on the sequence of the highly variable K1 gene sequence (102). HHV-8 genotypes have been associated with the global migration of the virus in association with human migration but have not been specifically associated with any of the major forms of the disease or conclusively associated with pathogenic variation.

Serologic Tests

Serologic testing is the best way to identify HHV-8-infected individuals from single specimens. Commercial sources of reagents and kits are listed in Table 2, testing sources are listed in Table 3, and applications are listed in Table 4.

Latent versus Lytic Antigens

EBV and HHV-8 share two biologic properties relevant to their serodiagnosis: (i) in vivo, they maintain their latent state in circulating lymphocytes and (ii) in vitro, they are propagated in cell lines in which the virus is present in a latent form in >95% of cells but in which the lytic cycle can be induced by treatment with an inducer such as a phorbol ester. Latency is regulated in part by chromatin-associated proteins that are significant antigens: EBNA in the case of EBV and LANA-1 for HHV-8. Other useful antigens include the latently expressed viral cyclin encoded by ORF72 and the lytically expressed antigens encoded by ORF65 and K8.1.

Serologic Assays

The two main varieties of IFA in use for detection of HHV-8 antibodies are based on (i) uninduced PEL cell lines that target LANA-1 and (ii) lytically induced PEL cell lines. Latent fluorescence is restricted to the nucleus, while lytic fluorescence is predominantly cytoplasmic. Most laboratories use serum dilutions in the range of 1:40 to 1:100 for IFA. In addition to PEL cell lines that express complex mixtures of HHV-8 antigens, IFAs have been developed based on single defined antigens expressed via recombinant Semliki Forest viruses as well as multiple defined antigens expressed via baculoviruses (68). The most widely used HHV-8 ELISAs are based on purified virions, purified bacterially expressed ORF65, and synthetic peptides based on ORF65 and K8.1 sequences (80, 82). These assays enable high throughput and objective evaluation of individual specimens relative to a defined cutoff but are less sensitive than lytic IFA. A system has been described that employs transfection of mammalian cells with luciferase-linked antigens, with detection based on chemiluminescence from immune precipitates (20). A neutralizing antibody assay based on inhibiting infectivity of a recombinant HHV-8 that has been engineered to express green fluorescent protein in infected cells was used to demonstrate the potential importance of neutralizing antibody titers in preventing KS (57). Little attention has been paid to serologic methods for identifying and discriminating recent from past infection, such as detection of IgM or antibody avidity.

Sensitivity, Specificity, and Interassay Agreement

Establishing assay cutoffs and assessment of the specificity and sensitivity of HHV-8 serologic assays have been complicated by several issues that revolve around the problem of unambiguously identifying individuals who are truly positive or negative for the virus. Healthy blood donors are often defined as HHV-8 negative, although some of them are likely to be positive for the virus, and KS patients are frequently regarded as true positives, even though some may be seronegative. Most tests identify >95% of specimens from KS patients as being positive, and most identify >90% of European and U.S. blood donors as being negative. In comparison, in-house assays have often performed well compared to commercial tests and there has been little agreement about which blood donor specimens are positive (71, 80); this remains a challenging problem.

Antiviral Susceptibilities

The antiviral susceptibility of HHV-8 is commonly measured as a function of the extent of DNA replication inhibition, for example, through the use of quantitative PCR (83).

Evaluation, Interpretation, and Reporting of Results

We anticipate an expanded role for clinical microbiology and pathology laboratories in the management of HHV-8-related illness. Many individuals at risk for HHV-8 infection and associated disease are under ongoing clinical scrutiny related to their HIV infection, and our understanding of the utility of various virologic and immunologic markers as prognostic indicators is rapidly expanding. In addition, consideration is being given to whether donors and recipients should be matched with respect to HHV-8 status or whether the HHV-8 status of the transplant recipients should be monitored to allow for heightened surveillance for KS and other HHV-8-associated disease.

KS

While KS is often diagnosed on the basis of clinical or histologic presentation, as mentioned above, LANA-1-based IHC is of value in establishing a definitive diagnosis of KS. An area of active research is identification of markers for progression to KS. The major risk identified thus far is being dually positive for HHV-8 and HIV. Quantitative PCR can be used to monitor saliva and blood for the appearance of viral DNA as a harbinger of KS. This has not risen to the level of being a practice guideline.

PEL and MCD

PCR can be useful for initial screening of suspected cases. More definitive diagnosis requires analysis of biopsy specimens or cell smears with a method such as virus-specific IHC.

FUTURE DIRECTIONS

HHV-6, -7, and -8 cause clinically relevant infections that require accurate clinical and laboratory diagnosis. However, this need is generally confined to restricted populations, such as organ transplant recipients or individuals infected with HIV, and occurs at frequencies that have limited the development of licensed convenient commercial assays. Thus, we anticipate continued use of in-house assays that are offered only in reference laboratories, some medical centers, or research settings. In such an environment, standardization of practices can be improved through the use of shared reference materials and interlaboratory comparisons. Multiplex PCR systems that include testing for these viruses are coming into wider use. This places an additional responsibility on clinical virologists to ensure that test interpretation is done in the context of what is known of the biology of these viruses.

REFERENCES

1. **Achour, A., D. Boutolleau, A. Slim, H. Agut, and A. Gautheret-Dejean.** 2007. Human herpesvirus-6 (HHV-6) DNA in plasma reflects the presence of infected blood cells rather than circulating viral particles. *J. Clin. Virol.* **38:**280–285.
2. **Arav-Boger, R.** 2009. Treatment for Kaposi sarcoma herpesvirus: great challenges with promising accomplishments. *Virus Genes* **38:**195–203.
3. **Arsenault, S., A. Gravel, J. Gosselin, and L. Flamand.** 2003. Generation and characterization of a monoclonal antibody specific for human herpesvirus 6 variant A immediate-early 2 protein. *J. Clin. Virol.* **28:**284–290.
4. **Barker, R., F. Kazmi, J. Stebbing, S. Ngan, R. Chinn, M. Nelson, M. O'Doherty, and M. Bower.** 2009. FDG-PET/CT imaging in the management of HIV-associated multicentric Castleman's disease. *Eur. J. Nucl. Med. Mol. Imaging* **36:**648–652.
5. **Barozzi, B., M. Luppi, F. Facchetti, C. Mecucci, M. Alu, R. Sarid, V. Rasini, L. Ravazzini, E. Rossi, S. Festa, B. Crescenzi, D. Wolf, T. Schulz, and G. Torelli.** 2003. Posttransplant Kaposi sarcoma originates from the seeding of donor-derived progenitors. *Nat. Med.* **9:**554–561.
6. **Bates, M., M. Monze, H. Bima, M. Kapambwe, D. Clark, F. C. Kasolo, and U. A. Gompels.** 2009. Predominant human herpesvirus 6 variant A infant infections in an HIV-1 endemic region of Sub-Saharan Africa. *J. Med. Virol.* **81:**779–789.
7. **Batista, M. D., S. Ferreira, M. M. Sauer, H. Tomiyama, M. T. Giret, C. S. Pannuti, R. S. Diaz, E. C. Sabino, and E. G. Kallas.** 2009. High human herpesvirus 8 (HHV-8) prevalence, clinical correlates and high incidence among recently HIV-1-infected subjects in Sao Paulo, Brazil. *PLoS One* **4:**e5613.
8. **Bergallo, M., C. Costa, M. E. Terlizzi, F. Sidoti, S. Margio, S. Astegiano, R. Ponti, and R. Cavallo.** 2009. Development of a LUX real-time PCR for the detection and quantification of human herpesvirus 7. *Can. J. Microbiol.* **55:**319–325.
9. **Berneman, Z. N., D. V. Ablashi, G. Li, M. Eger-Fletcher, M. S. Reitz, Jr., C. L. Hung, I. Brus, A. L. Komaroff, and R. C. Gallo.** 1992. Human herpesvirus 7 is a T-lymphotropic virus and is related to, but significantly different from, human herpesvirus 6 and human cytomegalovirus. *Proc. Natl. Acad. Sci. USA* **89:**10552–10556.
10. **Black, J. B., and P. E. Pellett.** 1999. Human herpesvirus 7. *Rev. Med. Virol.* **9:**245–262.
11. **Black, J. B., and P. E. Pellett.** 2000. Antiviral assays for human herpesviruses 6 and 7, p. 129–138. *In* D. Kinchington and R. F. Schinazi (ed.), *Antiviral Methods and Protocols.* Humana Press, Totowa, NJ.
12. **Black, J. B., K. C. Sanderlin, C. S. Goldsmith, H. E. Gary, C. Lopez, and P. E. Pellett.** 1989. Growth properties of human herpesvirus-6 strain Z29. *J. Virol. Methods* **26:**133–145.
13. **Black, J. B., T. F. Schwarz, J. L. Patton, K. Kite-Powell, P. E. Pellett, S. Wiersbitzky, R. Bruns, C. Muller, G. Jager, and J. Stewart.** 1996. Evaluation of immunoassays for detection of antibodies to human herpesvirus 7. *Clin. Diagn. Lab. Immunol.* **3:**79–83.
14. **Bland, R. M., P. L. Mackie, T. Shorts, S. Pate, and J. Y. Paton.** 1998. The rapid diagnosis and clinical features of human herpesvirus 6. *J. Infect.* **36:**161–165.
15. **Blumberg, B. M., D. J. Mock, J. M. Powers, M. Ito, J. G. Assouline, J. V. Baker, B. Chen, and A. D. Goodman.** 2000. The HHV6 paradox: ubiquitous commensal or insidious pathogen? A two-step in situ PCR approach. *J. Clin. Virol.* **16:**159–178.
16. **Bonnafous, P., D. Boutolleau, L. Naesens, C. Deback, A. Gautheret-Dejean, and H. Agut.** 2008. Characterization of a cidofovir-resistant HHV-6 mutant obtained by in vitro selection. *Antivir. Res.* **77:**237–240.
17. **Bonnafous, P., L. Naesens, S. Petrella, A. Gautheret-Dejean, D. Boutolleau, W. Sougakoff, and H. Agut.** 2007. Different mutations in the HHV-6 DNA polymerase gene accounting for resistance to foscarnet. *Antivir. Ther.* **12:**877–888.
18. **Braun, D. K., G. Dominguez, and P. E. Pellett.** 1997. Human herpesvirus 6. *Clin. Microbiol. Rev.* **10:**521–567.
19. **Broccolo, F., F. Drago, A. M. Careddu, C. Foglieni, L. Turbino, C. E. Cocuzza, C. Gelmetti, P. Lusso, A. E. Rebora, and M. S. Malnati.** 2005. Additional evidence that pityriasis rosea is associated with reactivation of human herpesvirus-6 and -7. *J. Investig. Dermatol.* **124:**1234–1240.
20. **Burbelo, P. D., H. P. Leahy, S. Groot, L. R. Bishop, W. Miley, M. J. Iadarola, D. Whitby, and J. A. Kovacs.** 2009. Four-antigen mixture containing v-cyclin for serological screening of human herpesvirus 8 infection. *Clin. Vaccine Immunol.* **16:**621–627.

21. **Cannon, M. J., E. A. Operskalski, J. W. Mosley, K. Radford, and S. C. Dollard.** 2009. Lack of evidence for human herpesvirus-8 transmission via blood transfusion in a historical US cohort. *J. Infect. Dis.* **199:**1592–1598.

22. **Caserta, M. T., M. P. McDermott, S. Dewhurst, K. Schnabel, J. A. Carnahan, L. Gilbert, G. Lathan, G. K. Lofthus, and C. B. Hall.** 2004. Human herpesvirus 6 (HHV6) DNA persistence and reactivation in healthy children. *J. Pediatr.* **145:**478–484.

23. **Casper, C.** 2008. New approaches to the treatment of human herpesvirus 8-associated disease. *Rev. Med. Virol.* **18:**321–329.

24. **Casper, C., E. Krantz, S. Selke, S. R. Kuntz, J. Wang, M. L. Huang, J. S. Pauk, L. Corey, and A. Wald.** 2007. Frequent and asymptomatic oropharyngeal shedding of human herpesvirus 8 among immunocompetent men. *J. Infect. Dis.* **195:**30–36.

25. **Casper, C., A. S. Meier, A. Wald, R. A. Morrow, L. Corey, and A. B. Moscicki.** 2006. Human herpesvirus 8 infection among adolescents in the REACH cohort. *Arch. Pediatr. Adolesc. Med.* **160:**937–942.

26. **Cattani, P., M. Capuano, R. Graffeo, R. Ricci, F. Cerimele, D. Cerimele, G. Nanni, and G. Fadda.** 2001. Kaposi's sarcoma associated with previous human herpesvirus 8 infection in kidney transplant recipients. *J. Clin. Microbiol.* **39:**506–508.

27. **Cesarman, E., and D. M. Knowles.** 1999. The role of Kaposi's sarcoma-associated herpesvirus (KSHV/HHV-8) in lymphoproliferative diseases. *Semin. Cancer Biol.* **9:**165–174.

28. **Chan, P. K., H. K. Ng, M. Hui, and A. F. Cheng.** 2001. Prevalence and distribution of human herpesvirus 6 variants A and B in adult human brain. *J. Med. Virol.* **64:**42–46.

29. **Chang, Y., E. Cesarman, M. S. Pessin, F. Lee, J. Culpepper, D. M. Knowles, and P. S. Moore.** 1994. Identification of herpesvirus-like DNA sequences in AIDS-associated Kaposi's sarcoma. *Science* **266:**1865–1869.

30. **Chiu, S. S., C. Y. Cheung, C. Y. Tse, and M. Peiris.** 1998. Early diagnosis of primary human herpesvirus 6 infection in childhood: serology, polymerase chain reaction, and virus load. *J. Infect. Dis.* **178:**1250–1256.

31. **Chuh, A. A., H. H. Chan, and V. Zawar.** 2004. Is human herpesvirus 7 the causative agent of pityriasis rosea?—A critical review. *Int. J. Dermatol.* **43:**870–875.

32. **Clark, D.** 2004. Human herpesvirus type 6 and multiple sclerosis. *Herpes* **11**(Suppl. 2):112A–119A.

33. **Clark, D. A., I. M. Kidd, K. E. Collingham, M. Tarlow, T. Aueni, A. Riordan, P. D. Griffiths, V. C. Emery, and D. Pillay.** 1997. Diagnosis of primary human herpesvirus 6 and 7 infections in febrile infants by polymerase chain reaction. *Arch. Dis. Child.* **77:**42–45.

34. **Clark, D. A., and K. N. Ward.** 2008. Importance of chromosomally integrated HHV-6A and -6B in the diagnosis of active HHV-6 infection. *Herpes* **15:**28–32.

35. **Corral, I., C. Quereda, M. J. Perez-Elias, and S. Moreno.** 2003. Search for human herpesvirus 6 DNA in cerebrospinal fluid from AIDS patients with progressive multifocal leukoencephalopathy. *J. Neurovirol.* **9:**136–137.

36. **Costa, C., M. Bergallo, L. Delsedime, P. Solidoro, P. Donadio, and R. Cavallo.** 2009. Acute respiratory distress syndrome associated with HHV-7 infection in an immunocompetent patient: a case report. *New Microbiol.* **32:**315–316.

37. **Deback, C., F. Agbalika, C. Scieux, A. G. Marcelin, A. Gautheret-Dejean, J. Cherot, L. Hermet, O. Roger, and H. Agut.** 2008. Detection of human herpesviruses HHV-6, HHV-7 and HHV-8 in whole blood by real-time PCR using the new CMV, HHV-6, 7, 8 R-gene kit. *J. Virol. Methods* **149:**285–291.

38. **De Bolle, L., L. Naesens, and E. De Clercq.** 2005. Update on human herpesvirus 6 biology, clinical features, and therapy. *Clin. Microbiol. Rev.* **18:**217–245.

39. **De Bolle, L., J. Van Loon, E. De Clercq, and L. Naesens.** 2005. Quantitative analysis of human herpesvirus 6 cell tropism. *J. Med. Virol.* **75:**76–85.

40. **De Clercq, E., L. Naesens, L. De Bolle, D. Schols, Y. Zhang, and J. Neyts.** 2001. Antiviral agents active against human herpesviruses HHV-6, HHV-7 and HHV-8. *Rev. Med. Virol.* **11:**381–395.

41. **Della Bella, S., A. Taddeo, M. L. Calabrò, L. Brambilla, M. Bellinvia, E. Bergamo, M. Clerici, and M. L. Villa.** 2008. Peripheral blood endothelial progenitors as potential reservoirs of Kaposi's sarcoma-associated herpesvirus. *PLoS One* **3:**e1520.

42. **de Sanjose, S., G. Mbisa, S. Perez-Alvarez, Y. Benavente, S. Sukvirach, N. T. Hieu, H. R. Shin, P. T. Anh, J. Thomas, E. Lazcano, E. Matos, R. Herrero, N. Muñoz, M. Molano, S. Franceschi, and D. Whitby.** 2009. Geographic variation in the prevalence of Kaposi sarcoma-associated herpesvirus and risk factors for transmission. *J. Infect. Dis.* **199:**1449–1456.

43. **Di Stefano, M., M. L. Calabrò, I. M. Di Gangi, S. Cantatore, M. Barbierato, E. Bergamo, A. J. Kfutwah, M. Neri, L. Chieco-Bianchi, P. Greco, L. Gesualdo, A. Ayouba, E. Menu, and J. R. Fiore.** 2008. In vitro and in vivo human herpesvirus 8 infection of placenta. *PLoS One* **3:**e4073.

44. **Dollard, S. C., and P. E. Pellett.** 2000. Human herpesviruses 6, 7 and 8. *Rev. Med. Microbiol.* **11:**1–13.

45. **Dotti, G., R. Fiocchi, T. Motta, B. Facchinetti, B. Chiodini, G. M. Borleri, G. Gavazzeni, T. Barbui, and A. Rambaldi.** 1999. Primary effusion lymphoma after heart transplantation: a new entity associated with human herpesvirus-8. *Leukemia* **13:**664–670.

46. **Flamand, L., A. Gravel, D. Boutolleau, R. Alvarez-Lafuente, S. Jacobson, M. S. Malnati, D. Kohn, Y. W. Tang, T. Yoshikawa, and D. Ablashi.** 2008. Multicenter comparison of PCR assays for detection of human herpesvirus 6 DNA in serum. *J. Clin. Microbiol.* **46:**2700–2706.

47. **Ganem, D.** 2007. Kaposi's sarcoma-associated herpesvirus, p. 2847–2888. *In* D. M. Knipe, P. M. Howley, D. E. Griffin, R. A. Lamb, M. A. Martin, B. Roizman, and S. E. Straus (ed.), *Fields Virology*, 5th ed. Lippincott Williams & Wilkins, Philadelphia, PA.

48. **Gautheret-Dejean, A., C. Henquell, F. Mousnier, D. Boutolleau, P. Bonnafous, N. Dhedin, C. Settegrana, and H. Agut.** 2009. Different expression of human herpesvirus-6 (HHV-6) load in whole blood may have a significant impact on the diagnosis of active infection. *J. Clin. Virol.* **46:**33–36.

49. **Hall, C. B., M. T. Caserta, K. Schnabel, L. M. Shelley, A. S. Marino, J. A. Carnahan, C. Yoo, G. K. Lofthus, and M. P. McDermott.** 2008. Chromosomal integration of human herpesvirus 6 is the major mode of congenital human herpesvirus 6 infection. *Pediatrics* **122:**513–520.

50. **Hall, C. B., M. T. Caserta, K. C. Schnabel, C. Boettrich, M. P. McDermott, G. K. Lofthus, J. A. Carnahan, and S. Dewhurst.** 2004. Congenital infections with human herpesvirus 6 (HHV6) and human herpesvirus 7 (HHV7). *J. Pediatr.* **145:**472–477.

51. **Hall, C. B., M. T. Caserta, K. C. Schnabel, C. Long, L. G. Epstein, R. A. Insel, and S. Dewhurst.** 1998. Persistence of human herpesvirus 6 according to site and variant: possible greater neurotropism of variant A. *Clin. Infect. Dis.* **26:**132–137.

52. **Hammock, L., A. Reisenauer, W. Wang, C. Cohen, G. Birdsong, and A. L. Folpe.** 2005. Latency-associated nuclear antigen expression and human herpesvirus-8 polymerase chain reaction in the evaluation of Kaposi sarcoma and other vascular tumors in HIV-positive patients. *Mod. Pathol.* **18:**463–468.

53. **Hladik, W., S. C. Dollard, J. Mermin, A. L. Fowlkes, R. Downing, M. M. Amin, F. Banage, E. Nzaro, P. Kataaha, T. J. Dondero, P. E. Pellett, and E. M. Lackritz.** 2006. Transmission of human herpesvirus 8 by blood transfusion. *N. Engl. J. Med.* **355:**1331–1338.

54. **Isegawa, Y., C. Matsumoto, K. Nishinaka, K. Nakano, T. Tanaka, N. Sugimoto, and A. Ohshima.** 2010. PCR with quenching probes enables the rapid detection and identification of ganciclovir-resistance-causing U69 gene mutations in human herpesvirus 6. *Mol. Cell. Probes* **24:**167–173.

55. **Jones, D., M. E. Ballestas, K. M. Kaye, J. M. Gulizia, G. L. Winters, J. Fletcher, D. T. Scadden, and J. C. Aster.** 1998. Primary-effusion lymphoma and Kaposi's sarcoma in a cardiac-transplant recipient. *N. Engl. J. Med.* **339:**444–449.

56. Kempf, W., V. Adams, P. Mirandola, L. Menotti, D. Di Luca, N. Wey, B. Muller, and G. Campadelli-Fiume. 1998. Persistence of human herpesvirus 7 in normal tissues detected by expression of a structural antigen. *J. Infect. Dis.* 178:841–845.

57. Kimball, L. E., C. Casper, D. M. Koelle, R. Morrow, L. Corey, and J. Vieira. 2004. Reduced levels of neutralizing antibodies to Kaposi sarcoma-associated herpesvirus in persons with a history of Kaposi sarcoma. *J. Infect. Dis.* 189:2016–2022.

58. Kositanont, U., C. Wasi, N. Wanprapar, P. Bowonkiratikachorn, K. Chokephaibulkit, S. Chearskul, K. Chimabutra, R. Sutthent, S. Foongladda, R. Inagi, T. Kurata, and K. Yamanishi. 1999. Primary infection of human herpesvirus 6 in children with vertical infection of human immunodeficiency virus type 1. *J. Infect. Dis.* 180:50–55.

59. Lautenschlager, I., K. Linnavuori, and K. Hockerstedt. 2000. Human herpesvirus-6 antigenemia after liver transplantation. *Transplantation* 69:2561–2566.

60. Lebbe, C., C. Legendre, and C. Frances. 2008. Kaposi sarcoma in transplantation. *Transplant. Rev.* 22:252–261.

61. Leong, H. N., P. W. Tuke, R. S. Tedder, A. B. Khanom, R. P. Eglin, C. E. Atkinson, K. N. Ward, P. D. Griffiths, and D. A. Clark. 2007. The prevalence of chromosomally integrated human herpesvirus 6 genomes in the blood of UK blood donors. *J. Med. Virol.* 79:45–51.

62. Ljungman, P., R. de la Camara, C. Cordonnier, H. Einsele, D. Engelhard, P. Reusser, J. Styczynski, K. Ward, and European Conference on Infections in Leukemia. 2008. Management of CMV, HHV-6, HHV-7 and Kaposi-sarcoma herpesvirus (HHV-8) infections in patients with hematological malignancies and after SCT. *Bone Marrow Transplant.* 42:227–240.

63. Luppi, M., P. Barozzi, T. F. Schulz, G. Setti, K. Staskus, R. Trovato, F. Narni, A. Donelli, A. Maiorana, R. Marasca, S. Sandrini, G. Torelli, and J. Sheldon. 2000. Bone marrow failure associated with human herpesvirus 8 infection after transplantation. *N. Engl. J. Med.* 343:1378–1385.

64. Lusso, P., R. W. Crowley, M. S. Malnati, C. Di Serio, M. Ponzoni, A. Biancotto, P. D. Markham, and R. C. Gallo. 2007. Human herpesvirus 6A accelerates AIDS progression in macaques. *Proc. Natl. Acad. Sci. USA* 104:5067–5072.

65. Marcelin, A. G., A. M. Roque-Afonso, M. Hurtova, N. Dupin, M. Tulliez, M. Sebagh, Z. A. Arkoub, C. Guettier, D. Samuel, V. Calvez, and E. Dussaix. 2004. Fatal disseminated Kaposi's sarcoma following human herpesvirus 8 primary infections in liver-transplant recipients. *Liver Transpl.* 10:295–300.

66. Markowitz, G. S., G. S. Williams, Y. Chang, M. A. Hardy, R. Saouaf, and V. D. D'Agati. 2001. A novel etiology of renal allograft dysfunction. *Am. J. Kidney Dis.* 38:658–663.

67. Martro, E., M. J. Cannon, S. C. Dollard, T. J. Spira, A. S. Laney, C. Y. Ou, and P. E. Pellett. 2004. Evidence for both lytic replication and tightly regulated human herpesvirus 8 latency in circulating mononuclear cells, with virus loads frequently below common thresholds of detection. *J. Virol.* 78:11707–11714.

68. Minhas, V., L. N. Crosby, K. L. Crabtree, S. Phiri, T. J. M'soka, C. Kankasa, W. J. Harrington, C. D. Mitchell, and C. Wood. 2008. Development of an immunofluorescence assay using recombinant proteins expressed in insect cells to screen and confirm presence of human herpesvirus 8-specific antibodies. *Clin. Vaccine Immunol.* 15:1259–1264.

69. Mock, D. J., J. M. Powers, A. D. Goodman, S. R. Blumenthal, N. Ergin, J. V. Baker, D. H. Mattson, J. G. Assouline, E. J. Bergey, B. Chen, L. G. Epstein, and B. M. Blumberg. 1999. Association of human herpesvirus 6 with the demyelinative lesions of progressive multifocal leukoencephalopathy. *J. Neurovirol.* 5:363–373.

70. Nacheva, E. P., K. N. Ward, D. Brazma, A. Virgili, J. Howard, H. N. Leong, and D. A. Clark. 2008. Human herpesvirus 6 integrates within telomeric regions as evidenced by five different chromosomal sites. *J. Med. Virol.* 80:1952–1958.

71. Nascimento, M. C., V. A. de Souza, L. M. Sumita, W. Freire, F. Munoz, J. Kim, C. S. Pannuti, and P. Mayaud. 2007. Comparative study of Kaposi's sarcoma-associated herpesvirus serological assays using clinically and serologically defined reference standards and latent class analysis. *J. Clin. Microbiol.* 45:715–720.

72. Nishimura, N., T. Yoshikawa, T. Ozaki, H. Sun, F. Goshima, Y. Nishiyama, Y. Asano, T. Kurata, and T. Iwasaki. 2005. In vitro and in vivo analysis of human herpesvirus-6 U90 protein expression. *J. Med. Virol.* 75:86–92.

73. Nitsche, A., C. W. Muller, A. Radonic, O. Landt, H. Ellerbrok, G. Pauli, and W. Siegert. 2001. Human herpesvirus 6A DNA is detected frequently in plasma but rarely in peripheral blood leukocytes of patients after bone marrow transplantation. *J. Infect. Dis.* 183:130–133.

74. Oksenhendler, E. 2009. HIV-associated multicentric Castleman disease. *Curr. Opin. HIV AIDS* 4:16–21.

75. Oksenhendler, E., D. Cazals-Hatem, T. F. Schulz, V. Barateau, L. Grollet, J. Sheldon, J. P. Clauvel, F. Sigaux, and F. Agbalika. 1998. Transient angiolymphoid hyperplasia and Kaposi's sarcoma after primary infection with human herpesvirus 8 in a patient with human immunodeficiency virus infection. *N. Engl. J. Med.* 338:1585–1590.

76. Opsahl, M. L., and P. G. Kennedy. 2005. Early and late HHV-6 gene transcripts in multiple sclerosis lesions and normal appearing white matter. *Brain* 128:516–527.

77. Osman, H. K., C. Wells, C. Baboonian, and H. O. Kangro. 1993. Growth characteristics of human herpesvirus-6: comparison of antigen production in two cell lines. *J. Med. Virol.* 39:303–311.

78. Parravicini, C., S. J. Olsen, M. Capra, F. Poli, G. Sirchia, S. J. Gao, E. Berti, A. Nocera, E. Rossi, G. Bestetti, M. Pizzuto, M. Galli, M. Moroni, P. S. Moore, and M. Corbellino. 1997. Risk of Kaposi's sarcoma-associated herpes virus transmission from donor allografts among Italian post-transplant Kaposi's sarcoma patients. *Blood* 90:2826–2829.

79. Pellett, P. E., T. J. Spira, O. Bagasra, C. Boshoff, L. Corey, L. de Lellis, M. L. Huang, J. C. Lin, S. Matthews, P. Monini, P. Rimessi, C. Sosa, C. Wood, and J. A. Stewart. 1999. Multicenter comparison of PCR assays for detection of human herpesvirus 8 DNA in semen. *J. Clin. Microbiol.* 37:1298–1301.

80. Pellett, P. E., D. J. Wright, E. A. Engels, D. V. Ablashi, S. C. Dollard, B. Forghani, S. A. Glynn, J. J. Goedert, F. J. Jenkins, T. H. Lee, F. Neipel, D. S. Todd, D. Whitby, G. J. Nemo, and M. P. Busch. 2003. Multicenter comparison of serologic assays and estimation of *Human herpesvirus* 8 seroprevalence among US blood donors. *Transfusion* 43:1260–1268.

81. Rhoads, M. P., A. S. Magaret, and D. M. Zerr. 2007. Family saliva sharing behaviors and age of human herpesvirus-6B infection. *J. Infect.* 54:623–626.

82. Schatz, O., P. Monini, R. Bugarini, F. Neipel, T. F. Schulz, M. Andreoni, P. Erb, M. Eggers, J. Haas, S. Butto, M. Lukwiya, J. R. Bogner, S. Yaguboglu, J. Sheldon, L. Sarmati, F. D. Goebel, R. Hintermaier, G. Enders, N. Regamey, M. Wernli, M. Sturzl, G. Rezza, and B. Ensoli. 2001. Kaposi's sarcoma-associated herpesvirus serology in Europe and Uganda: multicentre study with multiple and novel assays. *J. Med. Virol.* 65:123–132.

83. Sergerie, Y., and G. Boivin. 2003. Evaluation of susceptibility of human herpesvirus 8 to antiviral drugs by quantitative real-time PCR. *J. Clin. Microbiol.* 41:3897–3900.

84. Staskus, K. A., W. Zhong, K. Gebhard, B. Herndier, H. Wang, R. Renne, J. Beneke, J. Pudney, D. J. Anderson, D. Ganem, and A. T. Haase. 1997. Kaposi's sarcoma-associated herpesvirus gene expression in endothelial (spindle) tumor cells. *J. Virol.* 71:715–719.

85. Stefan, A., M. De Lillo, G. Frascaroli, P. Secchiero, F. Neipel, and G. Campadelli-Fiume. 1999. Development of recombinant diagnostic reagents based on pp85(U14) and p86(U11) proteins to detect the human immune response to human herpesvirus 7 infection. *J. Clin. Microbiol.* 37:3980–3985.

86. Sturzl, M., A. Wunderlich, G. Ascherl, C. Hohenadl, P. Monini, C. Zietz, P. J. Browning, F. Neipel, P. Biberfeld, and B. Ensoli. 1999. Human herpesvirus-8 (HHV-8) gene expression in Kaposi's sarcoma (KS) primary lesions: an in situ hybridization study. *Leukemia* **13**(Suppl. 1):S110–S112.

87. Tedeschi, R., A. Marus, E. Bidoli, C. Simonelli, and P. De Paoli. 2008. Human herpesvirus 8 DNA quantification in matched plasma and PBMCs samples of patients with HHV8-related lymphoproliferative diseases. *J. Clin. Virol.* **43**:255–259.

88. Wada, K., S. Mizoguchi, Y. Ito, J. Kawada, Y. Yamauchi, T. Morishima, Y. Nishiyama, and H. Kimura. 2009. Multiplex real-time PCR for the simultaneous detection of herpes simplex virus, human herpesvirus 6, and human herpesvirus 7. *Microbiol. Immunol.* **53**:22–29.

89. Wang, F. Z., and P. E. Pellett. 2006. Human herpesviruses 6A, 6B, and 7: immunobiology and host response, p. 850–874. *In* A. Arvin, G. Campadelli-Fiume, E. S. Mocarski, B. Roizman, R. J. Whitley, and K. Yamanishi (ed.), *Human Herpesviruses: Biology, Therapy, and Immunoprophylaxis.* Cambridge University Press, Cambridge, United Kingdom.

90. Wang, Q. J., F. J. Jenkins, L. P. Jacobson, L. A. Kingsley, R. D. Day, Z. W. Zhang, Y. X. Meng, P. E. Pellett, K. G. Kousoulas, A. Baghian, and C. R. Rinaldo, Jr. 2001. Primary human herpesvirus 8 infection generates a broadly specific CD8(+) T-cell response to viral lytic cycle proteins. *Blood* **97**:2366–2373.

91. Ward, K. N. 2005. The natural history and laboratory diagnosis of human herpesviruses-6 and -7 infections in the immunocompetent. *J. Clin. Virol.* **32**:183–193.

92. Ward, K. N., N. J. Andrews, C. M. Verity, E. Miller, and E. M. Ross. 2005. Human herpesviruses-6 and -7 each cause significant neurological morbidity in Britain and Ireland. *Arch. Dis. Child.* **90**:619–623.

93. Ward, K. N., H. N. Leong, A. D. Thiruchelvam, C. E. Atkinson, and D. A. Clark. 2007. Human herpesvirus 6 DNA levels in cerebrospinal fluid due to primary infection differ from those due to chromosomal viral integration and have implications for diagnosis of encephalitis. *J. Clin. Microbiol.* **45**:1298–1304.

94. Ward, K. N., A. D. Thiruchelvam, and X. Couto-Parada. 2005. Unexpected occasional persistence of high levels of HHV-6 DNA in sera: detection of variants A and B. *J. Med. Virol.* **76**:563–570.

95. Wong, G. A., and N. H. Shear. 2004. Is a drug alone sufficient to cause the drug hypersensitivity syndrome? *Arch. Dermatol.* **140**:226–230.

96. Yamamoto, K., T. Yoshikawa, S. Okamoto, K. Yamaki, K. Shimokata, and Y. Nishiyama. 2005. HHV-6 and 7 DNA loads in lung tissues collected from patients with interstitial pneumonia. *J. Med. Virol.* **75**:70–75.

97. Yamanishi, K., M. Mori, and P. E. Pellett. 2007. Human herpesviruses 6 and 7, p. 2819–2845. *In* D. M. Knipe, P. M. Howley, D. E. Griffin, R. A. Lamb, M. A. Martin, B. Roizman, and S. E. Straus (ed.), *Fields Virology*, 5th ed. Lippincott Williams & Wilkins, Philadelphia, PA.

98. Yoshikawa, T. 2003. Human herpesvirus-6 and -7 infections in transplantation. *Pediatr. Transplant.* **7**:11–17.

99. Zerr, D. M., M. L. Huang, L. Corey, M. Erickson, H. L. Parker, and L. M. Frenkel. 2000. Sensitive methods for detection of human herpesviruses 6 and 7 in saliva collected in field studies. *J. Clin. Microbiol.* **38**:1981–1983.

100. Zerr, D. M., A. S. Meier, S. S. Selke, L. M. Frenkel, M. L. Huang, A. Wald, M. P. Rhoads, L. Nguy, R. Bornemann, R. A. Morrow, and L. Corey. 2005. A population-based study of primary human herpesvirus 6 infection. *N. Engl. J. Med.* **352**:768–776.

101. Zhang, Y., L. De Bolle, S. Aquaro, A. van Lommel, E. De Clercq, and D. Schols. 2001. Productive infection of primary macrophages with human herpesvirus 7. *J. Virol.* **75**:10511–10514.

102. Zong, J., D. M. Ciufo, R. Viscidi, L. Alagiozoglou, S. Tyring, P. Rady, J. Orenstein, W. Boto, H. Kalumbuja, N. Romano, M. Melbye, G. H. Kang, C. Boshoff, and G. S. Hayward. 2002. Genotypic analysis at multiple loci across Kaposi's sarcoma herpesvirus (KSHV) DNA molecules: clustering patterns, novel variants and chimerism. *J. Clin. Virol.* **23**:119–148.

Adenoviruses

CHRISTINE ROBINSON AND MARCELA ECHAVARRIA

101

In 1953, Rowe and colleagues described an "adenoid degeneration agent" that induced spontaneous deterioration of tissue cultures prepared from adenoids of children (68). In 1954, Hilleman and Werner cultivated a similar agent from military recruits with respiratory illnesses and called it RI-67 (33). The two viruses were subsequently shown to be related, and in 1956 the term "adenovirus" was proposed to acknowledge their initial source. Epidemiologic studies soon identified the virus as a major cause of acute respiratory disease (ARD) and ocular and gastrointestinal disease. In the mid-1960s, adenoviruses were found to cause tumors in rodents, prompting studies that revealed fundamental processes of molecular biology but failed to link the virus convincingly to human cancer. Once again, adenoviruses are of considerable interest as vectors for gene delivery and as emerging human pathogens.

TAXONOMY

Human adenoviruses belong to the *Adenoviridae* family and *Mastadenovirus* genus. Seven species (A through G) are now recognized based on immunologic, biologic, and genetic properties (Table 1). Species B is further subdivided into species B1 and B2. Within each species there are many serotypes which are defined by neutralization using specific antisera. To date, 52 serotypes are accepted (37). New candidates are recognized, but their classification remains under discussion. The use of phylogenetic analysis as the sole means of classifying a new serotype is controversial. Genome types within serotypes are designated by lowercase letters to distinguish them from the reference prototype denoted by the letter "p" (e.g., adenovirus serotype 7h or 7p). Genome types result from variations in DNA and do not have different serologic properties (10). Intraspecies recombination resulting in intermediate strains with hexon sequences of one serotype and fiber sequences of another serotype can occur (38) but is uncommon.

DESCRIPTION OF THE AGENT

Adenoviruses are large, nonenveloped, icosahedral viruses 70 to 90 nm in diameter (Fig. 1). Each particle consists of a single linear, double-stranded DNA molecule of about 36 kb that encodes approximately 40 genes. The DNA is covalently attached to a terminal protein at both 5′ ends and encased by core proteins. A viral protease is also present. Seven structural proteins form the capsid. The major capsid proteins are the hexon, penton base, and fiber. The capsid is formed primarily by 252 capsomeres consisting of the 240 hexons that form the 20 triangular faces and 12 pentons, one at each of the 12 vertices. Each penton consists of a base and a fiber, a rod-like projection of variable length with a terminal knob which interacts with cellular receptors. The hexon has antigenic sites common to all human adenoviruses, but these sites reside within the capsid, so neutralizing antibodies are not induced. Hexons also contain the ε determinant, which induces serotype-specific neutralizing antibodies. The fiber has mostly serotype-specific antigenic determinants and some species specificity. The knob region of the fiber includes the γ determinant, which is responsible for hemagglutination (HA) in vitro.

Productive infection begins by attachment of the viral fiber knobs to cell surface molecules, such as the coxsackie-adenovirus receptor, although most species B viruses and certain species D viruses use CD46 or sialic acid. The specificity of this interaction is an important determinant of tissue tropism. Following secondary interaction of capsids with integrins, particles are internalized by endocytosis and are transported to the nucleus, where viral transcription and DNA replication initiate. Viral structural proteins synthesized in the cytoplasm likewise migrate to the nucleus, where the particles assemble and aggregate, forming large crystalline arrays (Fig. 2A). Productive infection results in 10,000 to over a million viral particles per cell, only 1 to 5% of which are infectious.

Latent infection is not well understood. To date, latency has been documented mostly with species C adenoviruses in the mucosal T lymphocytes of tonsils and adenoids of asymptomatic young children. Similar reservoirs may exist elsewhere in the body. In tonsils and adenoids, low levels of viral DNA can be detected, but no infectious virus is demonstrable until the tissues are placed in explant culture. The highest quantities of viral DNA are detectable in the tissues of young children, suggesting that virus stores may decline with age (23). By contrast, little or no viral DNA is detectable in the circulating white blood cells of healthy individuals (21, 71).

TABLE 1 Properties of the 51 human adenovirus serotypes by species characteristics[a]

| Species | Serotypes | Oncogenic potential | % G+C | HA | | Fiber length (nm) |
				Rhesus	Rat	
A	12, 18, 31	High	47–49	−	±	28–31
B1	3, 7, 16, 21, 50	Weak	50–52	+	−	9–11
B2	11, 14, 34, 35	Weak	50–52	+	−	9–11
C	1, 2, 5, 6	None	57–59	−	±	23–31
D	8–10, 13, 15, 17, 19, 20, 22–30, 32, 33, 36–39, 42–49, 51	None	57–60	±	+	12–13
E	4	None	58	−	±	17
F	40, 41	None	52	−	±	~29
G	52	ND	51	ND	ND	ND

[a]Modified from reference 32 with permission of the publisher. ND, not yet determined.

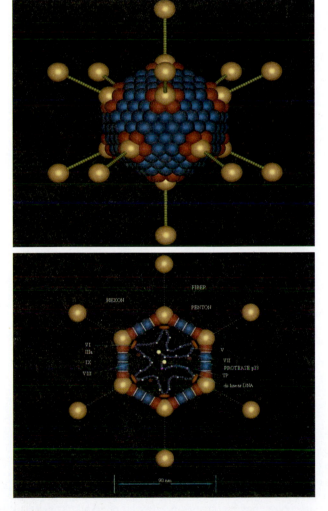

FIGURE 1 Model of an adenovirus particle. (Top) Exterior; (bottom) interior.

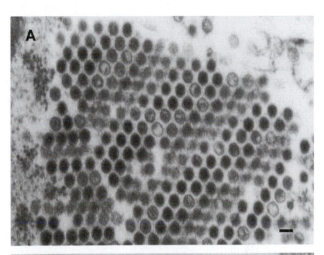

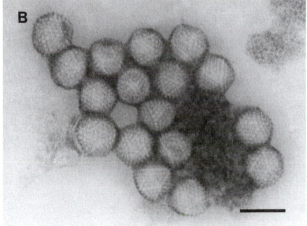

FIGURE 2 Ultrastructure of adenovirus particles. (A) Transmission EM of hepatocyte nucleus containing complete (dark) and empty (clear) adenovirus particles; (B) direct EM of a cluster of adenovirus particles in stool from a child with diarrhea. Bar = 100 nm.

EPIDEMIOLOGY AND TRANSMISSION

Adenovirus infections are common and ubiquitous. About half of the known serotypes cause disease. Adenoviruses are responsible for 1 to 5% of respiratory infections overall but induce 2 to 24% of all respiratory infections and 5 to 15% of all acute diarrheal illnesses in children and 30 to 70% of all respiratory illnesses in unvaccinated new military recruits. Most infections occur in the first few years of life and about half are asymptomatic. By the age of 10, most children have been infected with one or more serotypes. Coinfection with different serotypes and different species is documented, especially when different body sites are sampled (18). The incidence of infection is highest in crowded closed settings, such as day care centers, boarding schools, geriatric facilities, military training camps, and hospitals. Intrafamilial infections are common. There is no obvious difference in susceptibility by gender or ethnic group. Infections occur worldwide, with some differences in serotypes associated with various syndromes in other parts of the world.

Adenovirus infections can be epidemic, endemic, or sporadic, with the pattern of circulation, specific syndrome, and severity varying by serotype, population, and route of exposure. Sporadic infections occur year-round. Respiratory infections are most often associated with species B, C, and E, with serotypes 1, 2, 5, and 6 causing endemic infections and serotypes 4, 7, 14, and 21 causing small epidemics mostly in winter to early summer. A recent survey of U.S. isolates conducted in 2004 to 2006 identified the most common serotypes in civilians as 3, 2, 1, and 5, with an increasing amount of serotype 21 (26). Epidemics of severe respiratory disease in U.S. military recruits typically occur in the winter and spring. Historically, serotypes 4 and 7 were the most common cause. Serotype 4 now predominates, with lesser amounts of species B serotypes 2, 7, and 21 detected. The emerging serotype 14 was also identified (26, 56). Serotype 14 has also caused clusters of severe disease and fatalities among civilians in several states (7). A novel genome type (serotype 14a) is the apparent cause (52). Large epidemics of keratoconjunctivitis are caused mostly by serotypes 8, 9, and 37. Smaller outbreaks of serotypes 3, 4, and 7 occur in the summertime and are associated with contaminated swimming pool water. Adenovirus-associated gastroenteritis is caused primarily by serotypes 40 and 41, which are also known as the "enteric adenoviruses." These infections are endemic globally and occur year-round (76).

Adenovirus infections in persons with primary or acquired immunodeficiencies are increasingly reported (16). Severe infections are reported for individuals with congenital deficiencies, but the most frequent and severe infections are associated with hematopoietic cell transplantation (HCT) and solid organ transplantation (SOT). HCT recipients have the highest incidence of infection (5 to 47%) and highest morality rates (30 to 50%). Risk factors for serious disease in this population include young age, allogeneic transplantation, T-cell depletion, graft mismatch, and total body irradiation. Infection with species A to F viruses are described, and mixed or sequential infections with different serotypes are common (40). Data for SOT recipients are more limited, but this group generally experiences fewer and milder infections than HCT recipients. The lowest incidence is for renal transplant patients, who tend to acquire species B adenoviruses of serotypes 7, 11, 34, and 35. Adenovirus infections can be problematic in lung, small bowel, or liver transplant recipients and lead to graft dysfunction or loss, and fatalities. In the preantiviral era, mortality rates as high as 53% were reported for young liver transplant patients with adenovirus disease. Most infections are with species C viruses, and serotypes 1, 2, or 5 are the most common. Sources of adenovirus in transplant patients can be endogenous reactivation from recipient or donor tissue, as well as community or hospital acquisition (46). Transplantation of adenovirus-positive donor tissue into a negative recipient confers a higher risk than if both parties are either negative or positive. Adenoviruses once caused many serious infections in human immunodeficiency virus/AIDS patients, mostly with species D serotypes rarely identified or problematic in other settings (13). The introduction of highly active antiretroviral therapy has dramatically reduced the incidence of such infections in this population.

Transmission is primarily by the respiratory or fecal-oral route. Airborne transmission occurs by small droplets and, to a lesser extent, large droplet aerosols. Fecal-oral spread probably accounts for the majority of enteric adenovirus infections. Adenoviruses are also spread by contaminated fomites, fingers, and liquids, such as ophthalmic solutions and sewage. Preceding eye trauma facilitates infection and spread of keratoconjunctivitis in environments with high levels of airborne particulates. Spread among new military recruits may involve direct contact as well as aerosol exposure via ventilation systems. Stress and fatigue may be contributory host factors in this setting. The mean incubation period for most respiratory tract infections is 5.6 days and 3 to 10 days for gastroenteritis (48).

Transmission is facilitated by adenoviral resistance to chemical decontaminants and physical treatments. Stability of particles in gastric secretions, bile, and pancreatic proteases also permits passage through the stomach, followed by replication in the intestine. The prolonged period of virus shedding from various body sites aids transmission as well. Length of shedding varies by serotype, body site, patient age, and immune status. In general, nonenteric adenoviruses are shed for several days by adults with upper respiratory tract infections, for a few weeks after ocular infections, and for 3 to 6 weeks from the throat or stool of children with respiratory or generalized illness. Infected children may excrete the virus initially from the respiratory tract and later from the gastrointestinal tract. Excretion in stool can be intermittent and prolonged for 18 months or longer after recovery. In contrast, enteric adenoviruses are shed for only a few days after recovery. Immunocompromised individuals shed adenovirus longer than immunocompetent individuals.

CLINICAL SIGNIFICANCE

The spectrum of adenovirus-associated disease is broad due to the many serotypes and their tissue tropisms (Table 2). Clinical manifestations also depend on age and immune status of the infected person. Most infections affect the respiratory tract, eye, and gastrointestinal tract, with lesser involvement of the urinary tract, heart, central nervous system, liver, pancreas, and genital tract. Disseminated disease is also reported.

Most respiratory tract infections occur early in life and are self-limited and mild. Usual signs and symptoms are fever, nasal congestion, coryza, pharyngitis, cervical adenopathy, and cough, with or without otitis media. An exudative tonsillitis clinically indistinguishable from infection with group A streptococcus has been described. A pertussis-like syndrome has been reported, although adenoviruses are more likely to be copathogens or reactivate in this syndrome than to be a significant cause. The role of

TABLE 2 Adenovirus diseases, associated serotypes, hosts, and suitable specimens[a]

Disease	Associated serotype(s)		Frequent host(s)	Specimen(s)
	Frequent	Infrequent		
URI[b]	1–3, 5, 7	4, 6, 11, 14, 15, 18, 21, 29, 31	Infants, children	NP[c] aspirate or swab, throat swab
LRI[d]	3, 4, 7, 21	1, 2, 5, 7, 8, 11, 35, 14	Infants, children, IP[e]	NP aspirate or swab, BAL, lung tissue
Pertussis syndrome	5	1, 2, 3, 12, 19	Children	Throat swab
ARD	4, 7	2, 3, 5, 8, 11, 14, 21, 35	Military recruits	Throat swab, BAL, lung tissue, NP aspirate or swab
Acute conjunctivitis	1–4, 7	6, 9, 10, 11, 15–17, 19, 20, 22, 37	Children	Conjunctival swab or scraping
Acute hemorrhagic conjunctivitis	11	2–8, 14, 15, 19, 37	Children	Conjunctival swab or scraping
Pharyngoconjunctival fever	3, 4, 7	1, 2, 5, 6, 8, 11–17, 19–21, 29, 37	Children	NP aspirate or swab, throat swab, conjunctival swab or scraping
Epidemic keratoconjunctivitis	8, 9, 37	2, 3, 4, 5, 7, 10, 11, 13–17, 19, 21, 23, 29	Any age	Conjunctival swab or scraping
Gastroenteritis	40, 41	1, 2, 3, 5, 7, 12–18, 21, 25, 26, 29, 31, 52	Children	Stool
HC	11	7, 21, 34, 35	Children, IP	Urine
Hepatitis	1–3, 5, 7	4, 31	Infants, children, IP	Liver tissue, blood
Myocarditis	7, 21		Children	Heart tissue, blood
Meningoencephalitis	7	1–3, 5, 6, 11, 12, 26, 32	Children, IP	Brain tissue, CSF
Sexually transmitted disease	2, 37	1, 4, 5, 7, 9, 11, 18, 19, 31, 49	Teens, adults	Lesion swab
Disseminated disease	1, 2, 5, 11, 34, 35	3, 6, 7, 14, 21, 29, 31, 32, 37–39, 43, 45	IP, newborns	Blood, BAL, urine, involved tissue

[a]Modified from reference 32 with permission of the publisher.
[b]URI, upper respiratory illness.
[c]NP, nasopharyngeal.
[d]LRI, lower respiratory illness.
[e]IP, immunocompromised persons.

adenoviruses in asthma remains controversial (74). Adenoviral lower respiratory tract infections, such as bronchitis, bronchiolitis, croup, and pneumonia, can be severe and sometimes fatal, particularly in young children less than 2 years of age. Long-term sequelae of these lower respiratory tract infections are frequent in some populations (60). Higher mortality is reported for serotypes 5 and 21 and novel genome types, such as 4a and 7h, and when extrapulmonary manifestations occur (6, 26, 52).

Although adenovirus-associated ARD is uncommon in civilian adults, frequent outbreaks in young military recruits were noted beginning in 1953. Symptoms included febrile cold-like illness, pharyngitis with tonsillitis, bronchitis, and pneumonia. Hospitalization rates were as high as 50%, and some fatalities occurred. Live, oral adenovirus vaccines directed against serotypes 4 and 7, the most common serotypes involved at the time, were introduced for this population in 1980 and significantly reduced disease. In 1996, vaccine production lapsed, and the problem recurred. Although the current outbreaks in military facilities are not as severe as in the prevaccine era, they continue be problematic and involve a broader array of serotypes (26). Reintroduction of vaccine to the military is planned. Interestingly, serotype 4 is an uncommon cause of respiratory disease in civilians.

Ocular adenovirus infections are common. The most frequent manifestation is acute follicular conjunctivitis, which is usually superficial and resolves without consequence in a few weeks. Pharyngoconjunctival fever is a follicular conjunctivitis accompanied by upper respiratory tract symptoms, fever, and occasionally lymphadenopathy, pharyngitis, and malaise. Epidemic keratoconjunctivitis is a more serious infection that starts with conjunctivitis but progresses to painful edema of the eyelids, sometimes followed by corneal erosions and infiltrates. Symptoms may resolve in 2 weeks, although reduced vision, photophobia, and foreign body sensation may persist for months to years. Epidemics of acute hemorrhagic conjunctivitis similar to those caused by enterovirus are also described.

The enteric adenoviruses 40 and 41 are a common cause of viral gastroenteritis in children less than 2 years old (Table 2). Diarrhea is usually watery and nonbloody, lacks fecal leukocytosis, and lasts a mean of 10 days, which is somewhat longer than diarrhea due to rotavirus (76). Mild fever, vomiting, and abdominal pain can occur, and respiratory symptoms are sometimes present. Most immunocompetent patients recover uneventfully, although infants with ileostomies or colostomies can have prolonged symptoms, and rare fatalities have been reported for immunocompetent patients. Gastrointestinal syndromes associated with nonenteric adenovirus infections include intussusception, acute mesenteric lymphadenitis, and appendicitis.

Clinical manifestations of adenovirus in immunocompromised patients depend on the individual's underlying disease or transplanted organ, patient age, and serotype involved (16). Infections in transplant patients can involve the graft or other organ systems. Presentations in HCT patients most often include hemorrhagic cystitis (HC), pneumonia, hepatitis, enteritis, and disseminated disease. Fatalities are most frequent in patients with pneumonia or disseminated disease. In liver transplant patients, infections are most often associated with jaundice, hepatomegaly, and hepatitis, with pneumonia and diarrhea in some patients. Enterocolitis with occasional spread to the liver occurs in intestinal transplant recipients. The major clinical presentation in renal transplant patients is acute HC and, to a lesser extent, pneumonia. Infections of the graft in lung transplant recipients can result in necrotizing pneumonitis, leading to respiratory failure and progressive graft loss. Bronchiolitis obliterans can be a late consequence. In the post-highly active antiretroviral therapy era, clinical manifestations in patients with human immunodeficiency virus/AIDS are uncommon until the immune system deteriorates. AIDS patients have presented with adenovirus-associated pneumonia, meningoencephalitis, and hepatitis as well as generalized disease. Symptoms of HC in immunocompromised patients can be especially severe and may signal the start of disseminated disease (19).

Less common clinical manifestations include exanthems, neonatal disease which can be severe and frequently fatal, neurologic manifestations such as meningoencephalitis and encephalitis, acute myocarditis in otherwise normal persons or associated with graft rejection in cardiac transplant patients, macrophage activation syndrome, and venereal disease, including genital lesions and urethritis. The role of adenoviruses in fetal demise remains unclear. An association of adenovirus infections and celiac disease has been noted. Adenovirus type 36 has recently been linked to obesity. Some adenovirus infections resemble Kawasaki disease.

Antivirals have been used to treat some adenovirus-associated clinical entities. Several antivirals, including ganciclovir, ribavirin, and cidofovir, as well as the antiretroviral drugs zalcitabine, alovudine, and stavudine, have in vitro activity against adenovirus. Ribavirin was initially reported to have in vitro activity only against species C serotypes but is now said to be active against most isolates of species A, B, and D and all isolates of species C (58). In vitro studies suggest that cidofovir may be effective against severe lower respiratory tract infection caused by the emerging adenovirus serotype 14a, whereas ribavirin may not (12).

The most common drugs utilized in patient care have been ganciclovir, ribavirin, or cidofovir. Early reports were anecdotal or small in scale and yielded conflicting results. Larger trials are now reported, but none is controlled, serotypes or strains of virus involved are rarely reported, and the effect of treatment on immune reconstitution is infrequently given. Ganciclovir has only a moderate effect in vivo and is no longer recommended for clinical use. Ribavirin has been used with somewhat greater success, but many failures and fatalities are reported. Ribavirin may be somewhat effective against HC, probably due the high drug concentrations achievable in urine.

The most promising antiviral treatment is cidofovir, an acyclic nucleoside phosphonate analogue and broad-spectrum antiviral agent. All adenovirus serotypes are susceptible to cidofovir in vitro. Although resistance can develop with serial passage, little resistance is so far detected in isolates from cidofovir-treated patients (58). Despite its significant side effects of nephrotoxicity, myelosuppression, and uveitis, cidofovir is increasingly used to treat a variety of clinical presentations, mostly in immunocompromised patients. In HCT patients, efficacies up to 98% are reported, and regimes with acceptable levels of toxicity have been

developed (81). Some transplant centers now advocate weekly surveillance of viremia for their high-risk patients in the first few months posttransplantation, followed by pre-emptive cidofovir treatment if results are positive or rising. This strategy still does not completely eliminate adenovirus disease, however, and some pediatric patients clear their viremia spontaneously without treatment (81). A clinical algorithm that recommends treatment only of HCT patients at high risk (as defined by host factors, transplant type, and viremia) was recently proposed and evaluated in a small retrospective series (79). All six low-risk patients cleared their adenovirus infection without treatment, whereas 1 of 10 high-risk patients died. Prospective studies of this approach with additional HCT patients and other populations are warranted.

Other promising strategies include reduction of immunosuppressive therapy or immunotherapy using donor lymphocyte infusion. Both approaches, with or without concomitantly administered antivirals, have improved outcomes for HCT patients in some studies. To avoid inducing graft-versus-host disease with donor lymphocyte infusion, adenovirus-specific cytotoxic lymphocytes have been produced in vitro. A new strategy to expand naive cord blood T cells in vitro with efficacy against adenovirus, Epstein-Barr virus, and cytomegalovirus infections is proposed (8). Combination approaches using intravenous immunoglobulin, antivirals, and reduced immunosuppression have also met with some success. Randomized trials using multiple prevention strategies are eagerly awaited.

COLLECTION, TRANSPORT, AND STORAGE OF SPECIMENS

Adenoviruses are best detected from affected sites early in the course of illness. Suitable specimens vary with the clinical syndrome and test requirements (Table 2). Collection of cell-rich specimens usually results in the highest sensitivity. The new flocked nylon swabs (Copan Diagnostics, Murrieta, CA) are yet to be systematically studied for adenovirus detection, but preliminary results are promising (78). When a deep-seated infection is suspected and tissue from the affected site is unavailable, collection from multiple sites (e.g. respiratory, stool, and urine) or blood is recommended. To demonstrate seroconversion, paired blood specimens should be collected, the first one during the acute illness and the second one 2 to 4 weeks later.

Recovery is optimal if specimens are kept cold (2 to 8°C), transported, and processed as described in earlier chapters. Suitable viral transport media can be laboratory prepared or purchased from commercial sources. Some commercial formulations, such as MicroTest multimicrobe medium M4RT (Remel, Lenexa, KS) or universal transport medium UTM (Copan), preserve infectivity for prolonged periods at room temperature and are also suitable for detection of viral antigen or DNA (67). Plasma or serum should be separated within several hours of collection. Specimens, virus isolates, or DNA extracts can be frozen at −70°C indefinitely with minimal loss of activity. Long-term storage in self-defrosting freezers and repeated freeze-thaw cycles ultimately reduce infectivity and degrade adenovirus DNA.

Adenoviruses are highly resistant to inactivation by chemical and physical treatment. Most serotypes are stable at 36°C for a week, at room temperature for several weeks, and for several months at 4°C. Infectivity is retained for several weeks on paper or in saline and for over a month on nonporous surfaces. Strict adherence to conventional safety practices, such as use of personal protective equipment, biologic safety cabinets, disinfection of work surfaces, and hand-washing, minimizes laboratory infections. Avoid hand-to-eye or hand-to-mouth contact due to the affinity of adenoviruses for mucosal and ocular tissue. Treatments that eliminate infectivity include 1:5 dilution of household bleach for 1 minute, heating to 56°C for 30 minutes or 60°C for 2 minutes, and autoclaving. Serotype 4 is especially heat resistant. Alcohol-based hand gels can destroy infectivity, although several minutes of contact may be required for some products. Variable disinfection is achieved with povidone-iodine, formaldehyde, and UV light. Viral DNA can be detected long after loss of infectivity.

DIRECT DETECTION

Microscopy

Adenovirus-infected cells can be visualized by light microscopy as "smudge cells" in hematoxylin-and-eosin- or Wright-Giemsa-stained tissues, fluid sediments, or cultures. Smudge cells are large late-stage-infected cells containing solitary, central, basophilic nuclear inclusions composed of adenoviral particles (Fig. 2A). Other types of inclusions are described as well (4). Adenoviral inclusions can be mistaken for those of cytomegalovirus, herpes simplex virus, or polyomavirus. Further identification by immunohistochemistry or in situ hybridization is recommended to avoid misdiagnosis (44). The characteristic morphology of adenovirus particles permits their detection by electron microscopy (EM) without need for further identification. Particles, often in large crystalline arrays, can be visualized in the infected cells by transmission EM (Fig. 2A). The large quantity of virus (10^6 to 10^9 particles/ml) in the stools of children with acute diarrhea (Fig. 2B) also permits detection by direct EM (5). The sensitivity of direct EM can be increased by ultracentrifugation, by immunoelectron microscopy using anti-hexon antibodies, or by a special ultracentrifuge rotor (Airfuge; Beckman Coulter, Inc., Fullerton, CA) that permits concentration of virus onto grids prior to examination (29). Few clinical laboratories have access to EM facilities, so other methods are typically used.

Antigen Detection

Antigen detection can be used for the rapid detection of adenoviruses in respiratory, ocular, and gastrointestinal tract specimens. Sensitivity, however, may not be optimal, particularly when testing adults or immunocompromised patients. Most antigen assays target conserved regions of the adenovirus hexon protein and utilize monoclonal antibodies (MAbs). Immunofluorescence (IF), enzyme immunoassay (EIA), and lateral-flow immunochromatography (IC) are the most common formats.

The major application of IF is detection of respiratory tract infections. Suitable specimens are washes, aspirates, or swabs containing exfoliated ciliated columnar epithelial cells from the posterior nasopharynx or mid-turbinate. Touch preparations of fresh tissue or frozen or formalin-fixed tissue sections can be tested as well. General techniques for IF are described in an earlier chapter. High-quality staining reagents are commercially available (Table 3). Positive cells usually display condensed nuclear or granular cytoplasmic staining (Fig. 3). Although indirect IF is highly sensitive and specific, direct IF can provide satisfactory and rapid results (43). Labeled MAbs directed solely against adenovirus or pools of MAbs labeled with different fluorochromes directed against adenoviruses and other respiratory viruses can be used. Pools may be most economical for laboratories with a low prevalence of adenovirus. The reported sensitivity of IF for adenovirus detection in respiratory specimens is 40 to 60% compared to culture, which is lower than the detection rate of most other respiratory viruses. Higher sensitivity (60 to 80%) compared to culture is achievable using

TABLE 3 Representative commercial products available in the U.S. for detection of adenovirus infection

Analyte	Method	Products
Antigen	IF	Argene: Anti-Adenovirus,[b] Anti-Adenovirus, Influenza Virus, Parainfluenza & RSV Group[b]
		Diagnostic Hybrids—D3 Ultra DFA Respiratory Virus Screening & Identification Kit,[a] D3 FastPoint L-DFA Respiratory Virus Identification Kit[a]
		Millipore: Light Diagnostics Respiratory Viral Screen & Identification DFA Kit,[a] Adenovirus Direct DFA[a]
		Trinity Biotech: Bartels Anti-Adenovirus Antibody,[a] Bartels Viral Respiratory Kit[a]
	EIA	Meridian Bioscience: Premier Adenoclone,[a] Premier Adenoclone Type 40/41[a]
		Microgen Bioproducts: Adenoscreen EIA[a]
	IC	Rapid Pathogen Screening, Inc.: RPS Adeno Detector[a]
		SA Scientific: Sure-Vue Adeno Test[a]
	LA	Microgen Bioproducts: Adenoscreen Latex Agglutination Test[a]
		Orion Diagnostica: Diarlex Rota-Adeno,[b] Diarlex Adeno[b]
DNA	In situ hybridization	Enzo Life Sciences: Adenovirus Bioprobe[b]
	PCR	American Type Culture Collection: Adenovirus DNA[b]
		Argene: Adenovirus R-Gene Quantification Complete Kit,[b] Adenovirus Consensus Kit[b]
		Luminex Molecular Diagnostics: Xtag Respiratory Virus Panel[a]
Virus	Neutralization	American Type Culture Collection: Adenovirus,[b] Anti-Adenovirus[b]
Antibody	IF	MBL-Bion Enterprises: Adenovirus IF Control Slides[b]
	EIA	RightChoice: Adenovirus IgG/IgM enzyme-linked immunoassay[b]
		Virion Serion: Adenovirus IgG/IgA EIA[b]
	CF	Virion Serion: Adenovirus CF Reagents[b]

[a]In vitro diagnostic use.
[b]Research use only.

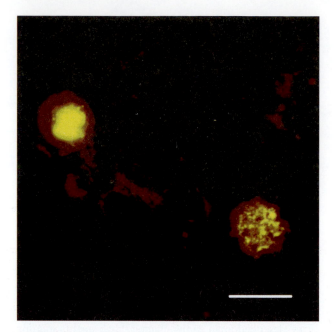

FIGURE 3 Adenovirus antigen demonstrated in two cells of a nasopharyngeal aspirate by direct IF using a rhodamine-conjugated antibody (yellow). Bar = 40 μm.

cytocentrifugation (43) and specimens from pediatric patients. Specificity of IF for adenovirus is excellent (>99%) in most studies. A new system of fixation and staining in liquid phase prior to deposition of cells onto slides is commercially available but is yet to be systematically studied for adenovirus detection.

Antigen detection can also be performed by EIA, IC, or latex agglutination (LA). These technologies are fully described in other chapters. Two types of EIA are available, a serotype 40- and 41-specific EIA and a generic EIA to detect all serotypes (2, 31). Both assays utilize microtiter plates and adenovirus-specific MAbs as capture and detector regents. This format is most economical for large laboratories which test in batch mode. The sensitivity of the serotype 40/41 assay compared to that of 293 cell culture or EM is >90% in most studies, although sensitivity can be lower with some variants (57). Specificity is >97%. The generic EIA detects species F and other species in a single reaction. Sensitivity is high (>95%) when stool is tested, but only 65 to 75% when testing other specimen types. Urine gives the lowest value, and occasional false-positive reactions occur (2, 24). Other formats used less frequently include time-resolved fluoroimmunoassay and radioimmunoassay.

The IC format is attractive for smaller laboratories because tests can be run individually, and results are usually available in less than 30 minutes. The SAS rapid adeno test (SA Scientific, San Antonio, TX) is a commercial assay for testing of eye swabs, nasopharyngeal secretions, and fecal material. Initial reports suggested good sensitivity (84 to 95%) compared to those of culture and PCR on nasopharyngeal specimens, but sensitivity was only 55% when a broader array of specimen types were evaluated (22, 49). Performance is best with specimens from young children. The RPS adeno detector (Rapid Pathogen Screening Inc., South Williamsport, PA) is available for testing of eye swabs. Sensitivity and specificity were 89%

and 94%, respectively, compared to those for PCR in a recent study (69). The assay is insensitive if swabs are placed in viral transport medium prior to testing (72). A generic LA assay for stool specimens is available but infrequently used. Sensitivity is only moderate, and false positives are reported with control latex and neonatal stools (25).

Nucleic Acid Detection

Detection of the genome is increasingly used for sensitive and rapid virus detection for specimens which cannot be tested by conventional methods, and for quantification. Adenoviruses in virtually all specimen types have been detected by PCR or other molecular methods, so the appropriate specimen depends largely on the associated disease (Table 2). Amplification is necessary for detection in most sample types, although viral DNA can be directly detected in some stools by gel electrophoresis and viral DNA can be demonstrated without PCR in infected tissues by in situ hybridization.

Both conventional PCR and real-time amplification are in current use. Degenerate or nondegenerate primers and probes in the hexon or fiber gene or the VA RNA I and II regions are usually selected due to the extensive homology of these regions among serotypes. Assays that utilize multiple primer and probe sets are preferred by many laboratories for uniform detection or quantification of all serotypes (9, 11, 15, 27, 30, 35). Reagents that can aid assay development and verification have recently become available. For example, external adenovirus controls can be procured from the American Type Culture Collection (http://www.atcc.org) and Zeptometrix (http://www.zeptometrix.com). Proficiency testing samples can also be accessed through the College of American Pathologists (http://www.cap.org) and the Quality Control in Molecular Diagnostics (QCMD) program of the European Union (http://www.qcmd.org). Testing of local isolates if available is also advisable to detect unanticipated genetic polymorphisms that can produce false-negative results.

Conventional PCR assays to detect adenovirus species A to G individually or together are described. Detection formats include gel electrophoresis, Southern blot or liquid hybridization and capture onto microtiter plates, or fluidic or solid-phase microarrays (63). Conventional assays that detect all adenoviruses as well as multiplex PCRs for adenoviruses, herpesviruses, and other respiratory viruses are reported (18, 39, 59). One multiplex PCR panel for respiratory virus detection (xTag RVP; Luminex Molecular Diagnostics, Toronto, Canada) is commercially available and captures the products of amplification onto tagged microbeads in solution (54). In clinical trials of this system, sensitivity of adenovirus detection was slightly lower (73%) than those of other respiratory viruses compared to IF and culture, and detection of serotypes 1, 2, 5, 6, 7a, and 41 was limited. Sensitivity was 52% for IF-negative specimens compared to that for a reference PCR (62). A second generation assay with increased sensitivity for adenovirus detection may soon be available.

Real-time PCR is most often used, as it is more rapid and less prone to contamination than conventional PCR and can provide quantitative results. Many real-time generic assays are described, most of which use the same gene regions as conventional PCR (9, 11, 15, 27, 30, 35). In almost all reports, sensitivity of real-time PCR approaches or exceeds that of antigen detection or culture (41). One real-time assay (Adenovirus R-gene; Argene, Verniolle, France) is commercially available and

CE marked in Europe for detection and quantification of adenovirus DNA in many types of specimens, including blood. Results obtained with this assay correlate well with those of other real-time PCR systems (36a). The major application of real-time PCR is detection and quantification of viremia to predict current or incipient localized or disseminated adenovirus disease in immunocompromised patients (17, 50). A multiplex, real-time assay that detects adenovirus, cytomegalovirus, Epstein-Barr virus, and herpes simplex virus in a single reaction may prove valuable in the transplant setting (28). Detection and quantification of viremia can be performed using plasma, peripheral blood mononuclear cells, or whole blood. No significant differences in qualitative sensitivity have been observed among these specimen types, although viral load values were slightly higher for whole blood and plasma than for PBMCs in one recent report (64).

Conventional or real-time generic virus detection assays should be carefully assessed to ensure uniform and sensitive detection of all virus serotypes prior to reporting results. Clinical specificity should also be determined whenever possible because adenovirus DNA can be found in some specimens from healthy control subjects. On average, less than 2% of specimens from healthy individuals contain detectable adenovirus DNA, although values can vary significantly depending on the patient population and specimen type (21, 30, 36, 71). Somewhat higher detection rates are reported for chronic conditions such as asthma, for tonsil and adenoid tissue, or for gastrointestinal biopsies with negative pathology (23, 42, 74). Each laboratory should therefore define the clinical significance of positive PCR results in its patient population and sample types.

Many transplant centers now assess viremia on a weekly basis in their HCT and SOT patients for several months after transplantation or when symptoms appear. Changing viral load values are used to assess clinical response to antivirals and predict outcomes (47). Due to differences in assay characteristics and patient populations, and the lack of universal calibration standards, there is also no single threshold value of viremia that can be recommended to initiate antiviral treatment or preemptive therapy in these patients. Some experts follow in vivo dynamic changes by repeat testing in 2 or 3 days after a single low viral load to identify patients with a rapid increase before initiating treatment.

ISOLATION PROCEDURES

Isolation of virus is the historic "gold standard." Viral culture is slower than antigen or DNA assays and can be less sensitive with some specimen types compared to PCR, yet it remains useful to detect serotypes that might be missed by direct methods and yields infectious progeny for further identification and serotyping. Most specimens are suitable for culture (Table 2). Exceptions are blood and cerebrospinal fluid (CSF), which may contain insufficient virus to be cultivated. For these specimens, DNA amplification is often preferred.

Adenoviruses grow best in human epithelial cells. Primary human embryo or neonatal kidney cells are most sensitive but are rarely available, so human epithelial cell lines, such as A549, Hep2, or sometimes HeLa or KB, are used. Human fibroblasts and nonhuman cells, such as Vero and primary monkey kidney cells that contain endogenous simian virus 40, may support adenovirus replication, but the yield is low. Enteric adenoviruses are often termed "fastidious" because they are noncultivatable or grow slowly in routine cell lines. Cultivation of enteric adenoviruses is most successful in Graham 293 cells (76).

Adenoviruses can be isolated by conventional tube culture or shell vial centrifugation culture (SVCC). These methods are detailed in earlier chapters. Although SVCC is popular because it produces rapid results, tube culture remains useful to detect low inocula or slow-growing serotypes, particularly of species A or D, which may not be evident for 3 or 4 weeks. Holding tubes for 2 weeks is customary for routine diagnostic work. If tubes are held for longer periods, cells should be subpassaged at least once to maintain health of the monolayer. Typical cytopathic effects (CPE) consist of grape-like aggregates of swollen, refractile cells (Fig. 4B). Aggregates may not develop with species D, and a web-like flattening is described for serotypes 3 and 7 (51). CPE is usually evident in 2 to 7 days in A549 cells but may be less characteristic and slower to appear in other cell types. As infection progresses, cells can become highly granular and detach completely from the surface. Most infectious virus remains cell associated so that high-titered preparations can be produced by several freeze-thaw cycles of harvested cells. CPE that develops within hours after inoculation with concentrated preparations is known as "lysis from without" and is due to free penton base. It is prevented by using a lower concentration of inoculum.

A significant proportion of culture-positive specimens can be detected in A549 or Hep2 SVCC after 1 to 5 days of incubation, using fluorophore-conjugated MAbs directed

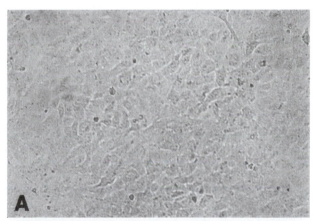
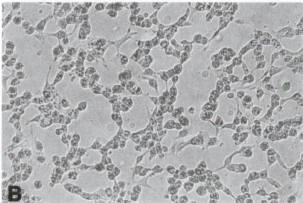

FIGURE 4 Adenovirus CPE in A549 cells. (A) Uninfected cells; (B) advanced adenovirus CPE. Magnification, × 100.

against the adenovirus hexon protein. Often the MAb preparations used to identifiy viral antigen in direct specimens can be used in SVCC. Maximum detection of fluorescent foci requires at least 30 minutes of centrifugation at $700 \times g$ (20). The sensitivity of SVCC compared to that of tube culture under these conditions is approximately 50% at 24 hours, increases somewhat at 2 days, and can approach 100% by 5 days (2, 20, 53, 61, 65). Similar results can be achieved using 24-well microtiter plates. Lower detection rates are reported if human fibroblast or monkey cells are used (77). Dexamethasone, which enhances identification of some viruses in SVCC, does not improve adenovirus detection in SVCC (80). Recovery of adenoviruses from respiratory sources in R-Mix (Diagnostic Hybrids Inc., Athens, OH), a mixture of A549 and mink lung cells, is lower than that for parainfluenza or influenza viruses (45). A recently developed combination called R-Mix Too which consists of A549 and MDCK cells has not been systematically evaluated for adenovirus recovery. Enteric adenoviruses can be detected in SVCC if appropriate cells lines are used (14), but other approaches are more sensitive and convenient.

IDENTIFICATION

Isolates should be definitively identified before a report is generated. For diagnostic work, genus-specific identification is usually sufficient. Most immunologic or molecular methods for direct detection of adenoviruses are suitable for this purpose. Identification by IF is most often used because the technique is simple and rapid. For IF, cells that appear to contain adenovirus should be harvested when at least 20% of the monolayer shows CPE. Other methods that can be used for identification are LA, IC, or PCR. On occasion, CPE-positive variants or new serotypes emerge which cannot be identified by these methods. In these circumstances, EM of infected cells, HA of the isolate, or DNA sequencing may aid identification.

TYPING SYSTEMS

Typing of adenoviruses into species or serotypes is used primarily for epidemiology or studies of pathogenesis or to reveal the cause of an unusual or especially severe infection. Traditional and molecular typing methods are available. Traditional typing requires a viral isolate and detects serologically recognized differences in fiber and hexon epitopes. Molecular typing can be performed with isolates or directly on PCR-positive specimens. The most valuable regions for sequencing are in the fiber or hexon gene, but whole-genome sequencing has been used as well. Typing by serology or molecular methods are usually in agreement, although discrepant results can be obtained on occasion. The two approaches are different in that serology measures a biologic property, whereas genotyping queries DNA.

Traditional typing is performed by provisionally determining the species of an isolate by HA (Table 1) or, if the isolate is from stools, by a species F (serotype 40/41) EIA. Serotyping by HA inhibition (HAI) or serum neutralization (SN) is then performed, utilizing specific antisera that define the serotypes of that species. HAI is the easier assay, but SN is the primary arbiter of serotype. Modified SN procedures are preferred for speed and simplicity over the conventional 7-day test with human epithelial cells (or 293 cells for stool isolates). Intersecting pools of antibody mixtures reduce the number of individual reactions. Modified SN tests include a 3-day test with monkey kidney cells and

a 5-day microneutralization test with Vero cells (32). Interpretation of traditional typing is not always straightforward, especially with intermediate strains, but it remains the gold standard to validate new systems and classify novel viruses.

Molecular typing is increasingly performed. Direct methods use extracted viral DNA from an isolate or specimen. Restriction endonuclease analysis (REA) is the classic direct typing method (1), but some genome types in current circulation do not retain the cleavage patterns of the prototypes, so interpretation can be challenging. REA is still used, however, for presumptive identification of new serotypes, identification of new genome types associated with severe disease, or to confirm results obtained by other means (6, 13, 26, 52). Single-stranded confirmation polymorphism and heteroduplex mobility assays are other direct approaches. Sequence-based typing is rapid and highly accurate. Some assays can be performed directly with clinical material, but isolates are often preferred because of their higher amount of viral DNA. Amplification is then performed by generic or multiplex PCR, or sometimes by nested PCR, to obtain sufficient DNA for analysis (70). Methods of analysis can include measurement of product length, REA, DNA sequencing, REA followed by DNA sequencing, or mass spectrometry. Common regions sequenced are the hypervariable regions 1 to 6 or 7 of the hexon gene or the fiber gene, although other regions, such as E3, can be analyzed. The presence of intermediate strains or coinfections can often be detected by sequence analysis (55). Sequence analysis of polymorphisms in long nucleotide repeats (microsatellites) is proposed to track strains (34). Some molecular typing systems identify only the species or serotypes recovered from a single body site, whereas others are more comprehensive (3, 63, 70).

SEROLOGIC TESTS

Most primary adenovirus infections are accompanied by a diagnostic rise in virus-specific immunoglobulin G (IgG), a less-predictable IgA response, and an IgM response in 20 to 50% of cases. Neutralizing antibodies can persist a decade or more in a relatively undiminished titer, probably maintained by periodic reinfection, reactivation, and heterotypic anamnestic antibody responses. The IgG response can be delayed in many children for months after infection and may not appear in immunocompromised individuals. An IgM response occasionally occurs when virus reactivates.

In recent years, serodiagnosis of adenovirus infections has largely been superseded by other methods of virus detection. Its current use is for epidemiologic investigations, to confirm associations between virus detection and unusual clinical outcome, and to study the immune response. The value of serology for patient care is limited due to the retrospective nature of demonstrating seroconversion, false-negative results due to the delay of the IgG response in children, the insensitivity of IgM assays, persistent infections, and the lack of antibody responses in immunocompromised individuals. False positives also occur due to heterotypic responses or late antibody rises in children unrelated to their current problem.

Serology is typically performed by documenting at least a fourfold rise in virus-specific IgG (seroconversion) or detecting an IgM response in the right setting. For clinical work, it is usually sufficient to know that adenovirus caused the infection, so a genus-specific EIA to detect IgG or IgM antibodies against the hexon protein is adequate. Formats with a viral antigen preparation or a "capture" immunoglobulin on the solid phase are commercially available and sensitive.

Serotype-specific antibody tests are infrequently used for diagnosis but can pinpoint serotypes responsible for a cluster of infection when other specimens are unavailable. HAI and SN are the serotype-specific assays of choice. SN is the standard, with the 3-day monkey kidney test or microneutralization preferred (32). Complement fixation, indirect IF, LA, and radioimmunoassay are rarely used. Assays utilizing genetically modified cells and fluorescent reporter molecules as surrogates for SN activity are increasingly used for serosurveys (73).

EVALUATION, INTERPRETATION, AND REPORTING OF RESULTS

The clinical spectrum of adenoviral disease is broad, so laboratory testing is usually required for accurate diagnosis. Selection of tests should be guided by the patient's symptoms and immune status, interval between disease onset and specimen collection, and laboratory expertise. A majority of adenovirus infections can now be detected within hours or a few days of sampling by direct antigen assays, centrifugation culture, or PCR. Tube culture and serology rarely provide results rapidly enough for clinical decision-making.

Interpretation of positive results can be challenging since many adenovirus infections are asymptomatic or due to reactivation of endogenous virus. Accurate interpretation should consider patient and specimen characteristics, test method, and in some circumstances, the viral serotype or quantity detected. This requires close communication between the laboratory and the clinician. In general, detection of virus from the involved organ or large quantities in a patient with an illness that is epidemiologically associated with adenovirus is evidence that adenovirus is the actual cause of the disease.

Many adenoviral respiratory tract infections can be rapidly detected by IF. This assay is usually more sensitive with children because virus is shed at higher titers and for longer periods than in adults. Adenovirus IF or IC test results provided within a few hours of specimen collection can have a positive impact on patient and fiscal outcomes (66, 75). The following specimens with negative antigen results should be further tested by culture or PCR: specimens from patients who remain hospitalized (e.g., intensive-care patients); lower respiratory tract specimens, such as bronchoalveolar lavage (BAL) or lung tissue; specimens from high-risk patients (e.g., neonates and transplant patients); and specimens from patients with especially severe or unusual presentations. Assessment of viremia may be a useful adjunct for the diagnosis of severe adenoviral disease in immunocompetent children (71). Positive PCR results for respiratory tract specimens and other tissues should be interpreted carefully, however. Low viral DNA loads have been detected in some specimens from asymptomatic subjects and tissues that lack adenovirus pathology.

Adenovirus gastroenteritis is best detected by a serotype 40/41-specific immunoassay or PCR of stools. Interpretation is usually straightforward because these infections are usually mild and self-limited in immunocompetent hosts, with virus shedding infrequent past the symptomatic period. In contrast, nonenteric adenoviruses can be detected in stools of asymptomatic immunocompetent and immunocompromised patients for prolonged periods. Severe or fatal gastrointestinal disease can result in the latter group. Detection of nonenteric adenoviruses in stools of immunocompromised patients can be achieved by generic EIA, generic PCR, or culture. Detection of adenovirus in the stools of transplant recipients does not rule out graft-versus-host disease because adenovirus can be associated with rejection.

Detection of adenoviruses from sites other than the respiratory and gastrointestinal tracts is more straightforward for interpretation because virus is infrequently detected in the absence of disease. Ocular adenovirus infections can be detected by EIA or IC, but culture or PCR may be needed for optimum recovery. In adenovirus-associated HC, PCR is more sensitive than culture. Adenovirus encephalitis and meningitis occur infrequently, so studies comparing traditional to newer methods of detection are lacking, although PCR of CSF is likely to be the optimum approach.

Diagnosis of adenovirus disease in immunocompromised patients is challenging due the many copathogens, high rates of asymptomatic virus shedding, and the protean manifestations of adenovirus infections in this population. HCT and SOT recipients are at highest risk of severe disease and are the usual focus of testing. Some centers utilize surveillance cultures or PCR studies of multiple body sites to detect virus in temporal association with onset of new symptoms. Involvement is then classified as infection, probable disease, or definite disease, depending on the number of virus-positive sites, symptoms, or histologic confirmation. Detection of adenovirus viremia by PCR is increasingly used instead of culture for surveillance. Viremia is usually present during severe or fatal adenovirus infection and often precedes the development of disease, although not all PCR-positive patients become symptomatic. Values then decline following successful treatment. Therefore, many centers now monitor weekly viremia in high-risk transplant patients, treat preemptively based on single high-positive results or dynamic increases from low baselines, and reevaluate viremia to assess response to treatment. Similar approaches may be useful to assess the clinical effectiveness of new treatment modalities for adenovirus disease.

REFERENCES

1. **Adrian, T., G. Wadell, J. C. Hierholzer, and R. Wigand.** 1986. DNA restriction analysis of adenovirus prototypes 1 to 41. *Arch. Virol.* **91:**277–290.
2. **August, M. J., and A. L. Warford.** 1987. Evaluation of a commercial monoclonal antibody for detection of adenovirus antigen. *J. Clin. Microbiol.* **25:**2233–2235.
3. **Banik, U., A. K. Adhikary, E. Suzuki, T. Inada, and N. Okabe.** 2005. Multiplex PCR assay for rapid identification of oculopathogenic adenoviruses by amplification of the fiber and hexon genes. *J. Clin. Microbiol.* **43:**1064–1068.
4. **Bayon, M. N., and R. Drut.** 1991. Cytologic diagnosis of adenovirus bronchopneumonia. *Acta Cytol.* **35:**181–182.
5. **Brown, M.** 1990. Laboratory identification of adenoviruses associated with gastroenteritis in Canada from 1983 to 1986. *J. Clin. Microbiol.* **28:**1525–1529.
6. **Carballal, G., C. Videla, A. Misirlian, P. V. Requeijo, and M. C. Aguilar.** 2002. Adenovirus type 7 associated with severe and fatal acute lower respiratory infections in Argentine children. *BMC Pediatr.* **2:**6.
7. **Centers for Disease Control and Prevention.** 1998. Civilian outbreak of adenovirus acute respiratory disease—South Dakota, 1997. *JAMA* **280:**596.
8. **Childs, R. W., and C. S. Zerbe.** 2009. Expanding multiviral reactive T cells from cord blood. *Blood* **114:**1725–1726.
9. **Claas, E. C., M. W. Schilham, C. S. de Brouwer, P. Hubacek, M. Echavarria, A. C. Lankester, M. J. van Tol, and A. C. Kroes.** 2005. Internally controlled real-time PCR monitoring of adenovirus DNA load in serum or plasma of transplant recipients. *J. Clin. Microbiol.* **43:**1738–1744.
10. **Crawford-Miksza, L. K., and D. P. Schnurr.** 1996. Adenovirus serotype evolution is driven by illegitimate recombination in the hypervariable regions of the hexon protein. *Virology* **224:**357–367.

11. **Damen, M., R. Minnaar, P. Glasius, A. van der Ham, G. Koen, P. Wertheim, and M. Beld.** 2008. Real-time PCR with an internal control for detection of all known human adenovirus serotypes. *J. Clin. Microbiol.* **46**:3997–4003.

12. **Darr, S., I. Madisch, and A. Heim.** 2008. Antiviral activity of cidofovir and ribavirin against the new human adenovirus subtype 14a that is associated with severe pneumonia. *Clin. Infect. Dis.* **47**:731–732.

13. **de Jong, J. C., A. G. Wermenbol, M. W. Verweij-Uijterwaal, K. W. Slaterus, D. P. Wertheim-Van, G. J. van Doornum, S. H. Khoo, and J. C. Hierholzer.** 1999. Adenoviruses from human immunodeficiency virus-infected individuals, including two strains that represent new candidate serotypes Ad50 and Ad51 of species B1 and D, respectively. *J. Clin. Microbiol.* **37**:3940–3945.

14. **Durepaire, N., S. Ranger-Rogez, and F. Denis.** 1996. Evaluation of rapid culture centrifugation method for adenovirus detection in stools. *Diagn. Microbiol. Infect. Dis.* **24**:25–29.

15. **Ebner, K., M. Suda, F. Watzinger, and T. Lion.** 2005. Molecular detection and quantitative analysis of the entire spectrum of human adenoviruses by a two-reaction real-time PCR assay. *J. Clin. Microbiol* **43**:3049–3053.

16. **Echavarria, M.** 2008. Adenoviruses in immunocompromised hosts. *Clin. Microbiol. Rev.* **21**:704–715.

17. **Echavarria, M., M. Forman, M. J. van Tol, J. M. Vossen, P. Charache, and A. C. Kroes.** 2001. Prediction of severe disseminated adenovirus infection by serum PCR. *Lancet* **358**:384–385.

18. **Echavarria, M., D. Maldonado, G. Elbert, C. Videla, R. Rappaport, and G. Carballal.** 2006. Use of PCR to demonstrate presence of adenovirus species B, C, or F as well as coinfection with two adenovirus species in children with flu-like symptoms. *J. Clin. Microbiol.* **44**:625–627.

19. **Echavarria, M. S., S. C. Ray, R. Ambinder, J. S. Dumler, and P. Charache.** 1999. PCR detection of adenovirus in a bone marrow transplant recipient: hemorrhagic cystitis as a presenting manifestation of disseminated disease. *J. Clin. Microbiol.* **37**:686–689.

20. **Espy, M. J., J. C. Hierholzer, and T. F. Smith.** 1987. The effect of centrifugation on the rapid detection of adenovirus in shell vials. *Am. J. Clin. Pathol.* **88**:358–360.

21. **Flomenberg, P., E. Gutierrez, V. Piaskowski, and J. T. Casper.** 1997. Detection of adenovirus DNA in peripheral blood mononuclear cells by polymerase chain reaction assay. *J. Med. Virol.* **51**:182–188.

22. **Fujimoto, T., T. Okafuji, T. Okafuji, M. Ito, S. Nukuzuma, M. Chikahira, and O. Nishio.** 2004. Evaluation of a bedside immunochromatographic test for detection of adenovirus in respiratory samples, by comparison to virus isolation, PCR, and real-time PCR. *J. Clin. Microbiol.* **42**:5489–5492.

23. **Garnett, C. T., G. Talekar, J. A. Mahr, W. Huang, Y. Zhang, D. A. Ornelles, and L. R. Gooding.** 2009. Latent species C adenoviruses in human tonsil tissues. *J. Virol.* **83**:2417–2428.

24. **Gleaves, C. A., J. Militoni, and R. L. Ashley.** 1993. An enzyme immunoassay for the direct detection of adenovirus in clinical specimens. *Diagn. Microbiol. Infect. Dis.* **17**:57–59.

25. **Grandien, M., C. A. Pettersson, L. Svensson, and I. Uhnoo.** 1987. Latex agglutination test for adenovirus diagnosis in diarrheal disease. *J. Med. Virol.* **23**:311–316.

26. **Gray, G. C., T. McCarthy, M. G. Lebeck, D. P. Schnurr, K. L. Russell, A. E. Kajon, M. L. Landry, D. S. Leland, G. A. Storch, C. C. Ginocchio, C. C. Robinson, G. J. Demmler, M. A. Saubolle, S. C. Kehl, R. Selvarangan, M. B. Miller, J. D. Chappell, D. M. Zerr, D. L. Kiska, D. C. Halstead, A. W. Capuano, S. F. Setterquist, M. L. Chorazy, J. D. Dawson, and D. D. Erdman.** 2007. Genotype prevalence and risk factors for severe clinical adenovirus infection, United States 2004-2006. *Clin. Infect. Dis.* **45**:1120–1131.

27. **Gu, Z., S. W. Belzer, C. S. Gibson, M. J. Bankowski, and R. T. Hayden.** 2003. Multiplexed, real-time PCR for quantitative detection of human adenovirus. *J. Clin. Microbiol.* **41**:4636–4641.

28. **Gunson, R. N., A. R. Maclean, S. J. Shepherd, and W. F. Carman.** 2009. Simultaneous detection and quantitation of cytomegalovirus, Epstein-Barr virus, and adenovirus by use of real-time PCR and pooled standards. *J. Clin. Microbiol.* **47**:765–770.

29. **Hammond, G. W., P. R. Hazelton, I. Chuang, and B. Klisko.** 1981. Improved detection of viruses by electron microscopy after direct ultracentrifuge preparation of specimens. *J. Clin. Microbiol.* **14**:210–221.

30. **Heim, A., C. Ebnet, G. Harste, and P. Pring-Akerblom.** 2003. Rapid and quantitative detection of human adenovirus DNA by real-time PCR. *J. Med. Virol.* **70**:228–239.

31. **Herrmann, J. E., D. M. Perron-Henry, and N. R. Blacklow.** 1987. Antigen detection with monoclonal antibodies for the diagnosis of adenovirus gastroenteritis. *J. Infect. Dis.* **155**:1167–1171.

32. **Hierholzer, J.** 1995. Adenoviruses, p. 169–188. *In* E. H. Lennette, D. A. Lennette, and E. T. Lennette (ed.), *Diagnostic Procedures for Viral, Rickettsial, and Chlamydial Infections.* American Public Health Association, Washington, DC.

33. **Hilleman, M. R., and J. Werner.** 1954. Recovery of a new agent from patients with acute respiratory illness. *Proc. Soc. Exp. Biol. Med.* **85**:183–188.

34. **Houng, H. S., L. Lott, H. Gong, R. A. Kuschner, J. A. Lynch, and D. Metzgar.** 2009. Adenovirus microsatellite reveals dynamics of transmission during a recent epidemic of human adenovirus serotype 14 infection. *J. Clin. Microbiol.* **47**:2243–2248.

35. **Huang, M. L., L. Nguy, J. Ferrenberg, M. Boeckh, A. Cent, and L. Corey.** 2008. Development of multiplexed real-time quantitative polymerase chain reaction assay for detecting human adenoviruses. *Diagn. Microbiol. Infect. Dis.* **62**:263–271.

36. **Jartti, T., L. Jartti, V. Peltola, M. Waris, and O. Ruuskanen.** 2008. Identification of respiratory viruses in asymptomatic subjects: asymptomatic respiratory viral infections. *Pediatr. Infect. Dis. J.* **27**:1103–1107.

36a. **Jeulin, H., A. Salmon, P. Bordigoni, and V. Venard.** 2010. Comparison of in-house real-time quantitative PCR to the Adenovirus R-Gene kit for determination of adenovirus load in clinical samples. *J. Clin. Microbiol.* **48**:3132–3137.

37. **Jones, M. S., B. Harrach, R. D. Ganac, M. M. Gozum, W. P. la Cruz, B. Riedel, C. Pan, E. L. Delwart, and D. P. Schnurr.** 2007. New adenovirus species found in a patient presenting with gastroenteritis. *J. Virol.* **81**:5978–5984.

38. **Kajon, A. E., L. M. Dickson, P. Murtagh, D. Viale, G. Carballal, and M. Echavarria.** 2010. Molecular characterization of an adenovirus 3/16 intertypic recombinant isolated in Argentina from an infant hospitalized with acute respiratory infection. *J. Clin. Microbiol.* **48**:1494–1496.

39. **Kim, S. R., C. S. Ki, and N. Y. Lee.** 2009. Rapid detection and identification of 12 respiratory viruses using a dual priming oligonucleotide system-based multiplex PCR assay. *J. Virol. Methods* **156**:111–116.

40. **Kroes, A. C., E. P. de Klerk, A. C. Lankester, C. Malipaard, C. S. de Brouwer, E. C. Claas, E. C. Jol-van der Zijde, and M. J. van Tol.** 2007. Sequential emergence of multiple adenovirus serotypes after pediatric stem cell transplantation. *J. Clin. Virol.* **38**:341–347.

41. **Kuypers, J., A. P. Campbell, A. Cent, L. Corey, and M. Boeckh.** 2009. Comparison of conventional and molecular detection of respiratory viruses in hematopoietic cell transplant recipients. *Transpl. Infect. Dis.* **11**:298–303.

42. **Landry, M. L., and D. Ferguson.** 2009. Polymerase chain reaction and the diagnosis of viral gastrointestinal disease due to cytomegalovirus, herpes simplex virus and adenovirus. *J. Clin. Virol.* **45**:83–84.

43. **Landry, M. L., and D. Ferguson.** 2000. SimulFluor respiratory screen for rapid detection of multiple respiratory viruses in clinical specimens by immunofluorescence staining. *J. Clin. Microbiol.* **38**:708–711.

44. **Landry, M. L., C. K. Fong, K. Neddermann, L. Solomon, and G. D. Hsiung.** 1987. Disseminated adenovirus infection in an immunocompromised host. Pitfalls in diagnosis. *Am. J. Med.* **83**:555–559.

45. **LaSala, P. R., K. K. Bufton, N. Ismail, and M. B. Smith.** 2007. Prospective comparison of R-mix shell vial system with direct antigen tests and conventional cell culture for respiratory virus detection. *J. Clin. Virol.* **38**:210–216.

46. **Leruez-Ville, M., M. Chardin-Ouachee, B. Neven, C. Picard, I. Le Guinche, A. Fischer, C. Rouzioux, and S. Blanche.**

2006. Description of an adenovirus A31 outbreak in a paediatric haematology unit. *Bone Marrow Transplant.* **38:**23–28.

47. **Leruez-Ville, M., V. Minard, F. Lacaille, A. Buzyn, E. Abachin, S. Blanche, F. Freymuth, and C. Rouzioux.** 2004. Real-time blood plasma polymerase chain reaction for management of disseminated adenovirus infection. *Clin. Infect. Dis.* **38:**45–52.

48. **Lessler, J., N. G. Reich, R. Brookmeyer, T. M. Perl, K. E. Nelson, and D. A. Cummings.** 2009. Incubation periods of acute respiratory viral infections: a systematic review. *Lancet Infect. Dis.* **9:**291–300.

49. **Levent, F., J. M. Greer, M. Snider, and G. J. Demmler-Harrison.** 2009. Performance of a new immunochromatographic assay for detection of adenoviruses in children. *J. Clin. Virol.* **44:**173–175.

50. **Lion, T., R. Baumgartinger, F. Watzinger, S. Matthes-Martin, M. Suda, S. Preuner, B. Futterknecht, A. Lawitschka, C. Peters, U. Potschger, and H. Gadner.** 2003. Molecular monitoring of adenovirus in peripheral blood after allogeneic bone marrow transplantation permits early diagnosis of disseminated disease. *Blood* **102:**1114–1120.

51. **Lipson, S. M., I. A. Poshni, R. L. Ashley, L. J. Grady, Z. Ciamician, and S. Teichberg.** 1993. Presumptive identification of common adenovirus serotypes by the development of differential cytopathic effects in the human lung carcinoma (A549) cell culture. *FEMS Microbiol. Lett.* **113:**175–182.

52. **Louie, J. K., A. E. Kajon, M. Holodniy, L. Guardia-LaBar, B. Lee, A. M. Petru, J. K. Hacker, and D. P. Schnurr.** 2008. Severe pneumonia due to adenovirus serotype 14: a new respiratory threat? *Clin. Infect. Dis.* **46:**421–425.

53. **Mahafzah, A. M., and M. L. Landry.** 1989. Evaluation of immunofluorescent reagents, centrifugation, and conventional cultures for the diagnosis of adenovirus infection. *Diagn. Microbiol. Infect. Dis.* **12:**407–411.

54. **Mahony, J., S. Chong, F. Merante, S. Yaghoubian, T. Sinha, C. Lisle, and R. Janeczko.** 2007. Development of a respiratory virus panel test for detection of twenty human respiratory viruses by use of multiplex PCR and a fluid microbead-based assay. *J. Clin. Microbiol.* **45:**2965–2970.

55. **McCarthy, T., M. G. Lebeck, A. W. Capuano, D. P. Schnurr, and G. C. Gray.** 2009. Molecular typing of clinical adenovirus specimens by an algorithm which permits detection of adenovirus coinfections and intermediate adenovirus strains. *J. Clin. Virol.* **46:**80–84.

56. **Metzgar, D., M. Osuna, A. E. Kajon, A. W. Hawksworth, M. Irvine, and K. L. Russell.** 2007. Abrupt emergence of diverse species B adenoviruses at US military recruit training centers. *J. Infect. Dis.* **196:**1465–1473.

57. **Moore, P., A. D. Steele, G. Lecatsas, and J. J. Alexander.** 1998. Characterisation of gastro-enteritis-associated adenoviruses in South Africa. *S. Afr. Med. J.* **88:**1587–1592.

58. **Morfin, F., S. Dupuis-Girod, E. Frobert, S. Mundweiler, D. Carrington, P. Sedlacek, M. Bierings, P. Cetkovsky, A. C. Kroes, M. J. van Tol, and D. Thouvenot.** 2009. Differential susceptibility of adenovirus clinical isolates to cidofovir and ribavirin is not related to species alone. *Antivir. Ther.* **14:**55–61.

59. **Muller, R., A. Ditzen, K. Hille, M. Stichling, R. Ehricht, T. Illmer, G. Ehninger, and J. Rohayem.** 2009. Detection of herpesvirus and adenovirus co-infections with diagnostic DNA-microarrays. *J. Virol. Methods* **155:**161–166.

60. **Murtagh, P., V. Giubergia, D. Viale, G. Bauer, and H. G. Pena.** 2009. Lower respiratory infections by adenovirus in children. Clinical features and risk factors for bronchiolitis obliterans and mortality. *Pediatr. Pulmonol.* **44:**450–456.

61. **Olsen, M. A., K. M. Shuck, A. R. Sambol, S. M. Flor, J. O'Brien, and B. J. Cabrera.** 1993. Isolation of seven respiratory viruses in shell vials: a practical and highly sensitive method. *J. Clin. Microbiol* **31:**422–425.

62. **Pabbaraju, K., K. L. Tokaryk, S. Wong, and J. D. Fox.** 2008. Comparison of the Luminex xTAG respiratory viral panel with in-house nucleic acid amplification tests for diagnosis of respiratory virus infections. *J. Clin. Microbiol.* **46:**3056–3062.

63. **Pehler-Harrington, K., M. Khanna, C. R. Waters, and K. J. Henrickson.** 2004. Rapid detection and identification of human adenovirus species by adenoplex, a multiplex PCR-enzyme hybridization assay. *J. Clin. Microbiol.* **42:**4072–4076.

64. **Perlman, J., C. Gibson, S. B. Pounds, Z. Gu, M. J. Bankowski, and R. T. Hayden.** 2007. Quantitative real-time PCR detection of adenovirus in clinical blood specimens: a comparison of plasma, whole blood and peripheral blood mononuclear cells. *J. Clin. Virol.* **40:**295–300.

65. **Rabalais, G. P., G. G. Stout, K. L. Ladd, and K. M. Cost.** 1992. Rapid diagnosis of respiratory viral infections by using a shell vial assay and monoclonal antibody pool. *J. Clin. Microbiol.* **30:**1505–1508.

66. **Rocholl, C., K. Gerber, J. Daly, A. T. Pavia, and C. L. Byington.** 2004. Adenoviral infections in children: the impact of rapid diagnosis. *Pediatrics* **113:**e51–e56.

67. **Romanowski, E. G., S. P. Bartels, R. Vogel, N. T. Wetherall, C. Hodges-Savola, R. P. Kowalski, K. A. Yates, P. R. Kinchington, and Y. J. Gordon.** 2004. Feasibility of an antiviral clinical trial requiring cross-country shipment of conjunctival adenovirus cultures and recovery of infectious virus. *Curr. Eye Res.* **29:**195–199.

68. **Rowe, W. P., R. Heubner, L. Gilmore, R. Parrot, and T. Ward.** 1953. Isolation of a cytopathogenic agent from human adenoids undergoing spontaneous degeneration in tissue culture. *Proc. Soc. Exp. Biol. Med.* **84:**570–573.

69. **Sambursky, R., S. Tauber, F. Schirra, K. Kozich, R. Davidson, and E. J. Cohen.** 2006. The RPS adeno detector for diagnosing adenoviral conjunctivitis. *Ophthalmology* **113:**1758–1764.6:10

70. **Sarantis, H., G. Johnson, M. Brown, M. Petric, and R. Tellier.** 2004. Comprehensive detection and serotyping of human adenoviruses by PCR and sequencing. *J. Clin. Microbiol.* **42:**3963–3969.

71. **Shike, H., C. Shimizu, J. Kanegaye, J. L. Foley, and J. C. Burns.** 2005. Quantitation of adenovirus genome during acute infection in normal children. *Pediatr. Infect. Dis. J.* **24:**29–33.

72. **Siamak, N. M., R. P. Kowalski, P. P. Thompson, E. G. Romanowski, R. M. Shanks, and Y. J. Gordon.** 2009. RPS Adeno Detector. *Ophthalmology* **116:**591.

73. **Sprangers, M. C., W. Lakhai, W. Koudstaal, M. Verhoeven, B. F. Koel, R. Vogels, J. Goudsmit, M. J. Havenga, and S. Kostense.** 2003. Quantifying adenovirus-neutralizing antibodies by luciferase transgene detection: addressing preexisting immunity to vaccine and gene therapy vectors. *J. Clin. Microbiol.* **41:**5046–5052.

74. **Thavagnanam, S., S. N. Christie, G. M. Doherty, P. V. Coyle, M. D. Shields, and L. G. Heaney.** 2010. Respiratory viral infection in lower airways of asymptomatic children. *Acta Paediatr.* **99:**394–398.

75. **Udeh, B. L., J. E. Schneider, and R. L. Ohsfeldt.** 2008. Cost effectiveness of a point-of-care test for adenoviral conjunctivitis. *Am. J. Med. Sci.* **336:**254–264.

76. **Uhnoo, I., L. Svensson, and G. Wadell.** 1990. Enteric adenoviruses. *Baillieres Clin. Gastroenterol.* **4:**627–642.

77. **Van Doornum, G. J., and J. C. de Jong.** 1998. Rapid shell vial culture technique for detection of enteroviruses and adenoviruses in fecal specimens: comparison with conventional virus isolation method. *J. Clin. Microbiol* **36:**2865–2868.

78. **Walsh, P., C. L. Overmyer, K. Pham, S. Michaelson, L. Gofman, L. DeSalvia, T. Tran, D. Gonzalez, J. Pusavat, M. Feola, K. T. Iacono, E. Mordechai, and M. E. Adelson.** 2008. Comparison of respiratory virus detection rates for infants and toddlers by use of flocked swabs, saline aspirates, and saline aspirates mixed in universal transport medium for room temperature storage and shipping. *J. Clin. Microbiol.* **46:**2374–2376.

79. **Williams, K. M., A. L. Agwu, A. A. Dabb, M. A. Higman, D. M. Loeb, A. Valsamakis, and A. R. Chen.** 2009. A clinical algorithm identifies high risk pediatric oncology and bone marrow transplant patients likely to benefit from treatment of adenoviral infection. *J. Pediatr. Hematol. Oncol.* **31:**825–831.

80. **Woods, G. L., M. Yamamoto, and A. Young.** 1988. Detection of adenovirus by rapid 24-well plate centrifugation and conventional cell culture with dexamethasone. *J. Virol. Methods* **20:**109–114.

81. **Yusuf, U., G. A. Hale, J. Carr, Z. Gu, E. Benaim, P. Woodard, K. A. Kasow, E. M., Horwitz, W. Leung, D. K. Srivastava, R. Handgretinger, and R. T. Hayden.** 2006. Cidofovir for the treatment of adenoviral infection in pediatric hematopoietic stem cell transplant patients. *Transplantation* **81:**1398–1404.

Human Papillomaviruses

PATTI E. GRAVITT AND CHRISTINE C. GINOCCHIO

102

TAXONOMY

Papillomaviruses (PVs) are small (55 nm in diameter), nonenveloped DNA viruses. PVs are classified according to nucleic acid sequence homology into genus, species, type, subtype, and variant (6). Members of the same genus share at least 60% nucleic acid sequence homology. Species are defined by sequence homology of 60 to 70%, with types in the same species having 71 to 89% homology. Subtypes are rare, exhibiting 90 to 98% homology, while variants are more common and show >98% homology. The genus and species groupings based on genotypic variation reflect key phenotypic differences, including species specificity, epithelial tropism (e.g., cutaneous versus mucosal), and oncogenic potential. Human PVs (HPVs) are clustered in five genera: *Alphapapillomavirus, Betapapillomavirus, Gammapapillomavirus, Mupapillomavirus,* and *Nupapillomavirus.* The majority of identified HPVs with clinical significance are found in the genus *Alphapapillomavirus,* which includes types infecting the genital and nongenital mucosal and genital cutaneous surfaces as well as the genotypes associated with human cancers. Table 1 summarizes the clinical manifestations of the genotypes, including oncogenic potential, in the alpha species group. The beta, gamma, mu, and nu types tend to infect nongenital epithelium.

DESCRIPTION OF THE AGENT

PVs contain a circular (or episomal) double-stranded genome and an icosahedral capsid structure consisting of 72 pentamers. The ~8,000-bp viral DNA has eight open reading frames encoding six early (E) proteins and two late structural proteins. DNA transcription is controlled by the long control region (also known as the upstream regulatory region), which contains binding sites for many human transcription factors and regulatory elements, including steroid hormones reviewed in reference 5. Viral gene expression is dependent on the differentiation state of the infected epithelium, with early gene expression occurring predominantly in the suprabasal epithelial cells, while late gene expression is limited to the terminally differentiated keratinocytes. The precise mechanisms of differentiation-dependent viral gene expression have not been elucidated, though recent data suggest a potential role for epigenetic mechanisms, including viral DNA methylation (3, 4). The early viral proteins have pleiotropic roles which generally involve viral DNA replication and transcription (E1 and E2) and interaction with key host regulator proteins (E6 and E7). Two particular interactions between high-risk (HR) virus and host proteins result in loss of major tumor suppressor function. Specifically, the E6 protein from HR genotypes interacts with the human E6-associated protein (E6AP) to target p53 for ubiquitination and proteosomal degradation (38, 55), thereby impairing appropriate cell cycle arrest in response to genomic damage. The E7 protein from HR genotypes binds with pRB (the retinoblastoma protein) (20, 49) to uncouple cyclin-dependent cell division, allowing for dysregulated cell cycle progression. In self-limiting HPV infections, the expression of E6/E7 is tightly regulated and limited to the middle layers of the epithelium to facilitate viral DNA replication in quiescent cells but is downregulated upon terminal differentiation. The dedifferentiation of the epithelium characteristic of high-grade neoplasia is associated with dysregulated expression of E6/E7 in the upper layers of the epithelium (19). Dysregulated E6/E7 expression can occur via loss of E2 regulatory protein expression due to integration of the HPV DNA into the host genome. While integration occurs in high-grade lesions and cancers, it is not a prerequisite and varies by genotype (69). Data remain conflicting as to whether integration is a cause or consequence of the tumorigenic process (52, 53).

EPIDEMIOLOGY AND TRANSMISSION

PVs are strictly species specific, with no animal reservoir. HPVs have been shown to infect both cutaneous and mucosal epithelium of the skin, oral cavity, conjunctiva, anus, and lower genital tract of men and women, with no systemic, or blood-borne, phase. Consequently, transmission occurs via direct epithelium-to-epithelium contact and not exposure to bodily fluids as in the case of hepatitis and human immunodeficiency virus (HIV) infections. Infection is thought to occur only in basal epithelial cells, which are presumably accessed through microtrauma incurred during sexual activity, which can occur through both penetrative and nonpenetrative epithelial abrasive contact. Infection of the skin with the *Betapapillomavirus* species is thought to be nearly ubiquitous (reviewed in reference 23). However, transmission between cohabiting adults has been difficult to demonstrate (16), suggesting that infection occurs early

TABLE 1 Human alphapapillomavirus genotype diversity and clinical manifestations[a]

Species (common use)	Species (ICTV)	HPV genotype(s)	Cancer risk	Common epithelial type infection and clinical manifestations
1	HPV32	32, 42	Low	Mucosal
2	HPV10	3, 10, 28, 29, 77, 78, 94, 117	Low	Cutaneous > mucosal
3	HPV61	61, 62, 72, 81, 83, 89, 84, 86, 87, 102, 114	Low	Mucosal
4	HPV2	2, 27, 57	Low	Cutaneous warts of skin; genital lesions of children
5	HPV26	26, 51, 69, 82	Low and high	Mucosal
6	HPV53	30, 53, 56, 66	Low and high	Mucosal
7	HPV18	18, 45, 39, 59, 68, 70, 85, 97	High	Mucosal; HPV18 is the second most common type in invasive cervical cancers, particularly AdCa
8	HPV7	7, 40, 43, 91	Low	Mucosal and cutaneous; HPV7 causes butcher's warts; often found in HIV-positive patients
9	HPV16	16, 31, 33, 35, 52, 58, 67	High	HPV16 most common type in invasive cancers
10	HPV6	6, 11, 13, 44, 74	Low	Common in benign genital warts; associated with recurrent respiratory papillomatosis; HPV6 may be associated with verrucous carcinoma
11	HPV34	34, 73	Possibly high	Mucosal
13	MMPV1	54	Low	Mucosal
14	HPV90	71, 90, 16	Low	Mucosal

[a]HPVs were recently reclassified by the International Committee on Taxonomy of Viruses (ICTV). The new classification (species, ICTV) and the historical classification (species, common use) are both represented. MMPV, *Macaca mulatta* PV. Species are listed by type; e.g., HPV32 is HPV type 32.

in childhood (1) and persists throughout life. Data have shown the same HPV genotypes infecting multiple skin sites in the same individual (43), somewhat consistent with this hypothesis.

Transmission of anogenital HPV in both men and women is predominantly sexual, though evidence also supports the possibility of autoinoculation between sites and digital/fomite transmission. For example, a study of 240 college-aged men demonstrated a cumulative incidence of 31.9% of detectable HPV DNA under their fingernails (51). It should be particularly noted that a high concordance between anal and cervical HPV infection has been observed, even among women who report no history of receptive anal intercourse (36). Condoms, which do not cover external epithelial sites harboring HPV, offer only partial protection from infection (73).

Sexually active individuals are exposed to and can acquire any one or more of the >40 HPV types known to infect the anogenital tract. Concurrent, multiple-type HPV infections at the same anogenital site is common, particularly among young individuals and those with a compromised immune system (e.g., HIV-positive individuals and organ transplant recipients). These infections can be a combination of both low-risk (LR) and HR viruses.

While direct estimates of per-sex-act transmission probabilities of HPV infection are not available, models using natural history data suggest a very high probability of transmission in a single sex act, 40% (7). It is impossible to know the accuracy of this estimate, but the modeling data do strongly support the ease of transmission of HPV relative to other viruses, such as HIV. The high transmissibility is further reflected in the remarkable cumulative incidence of anogenital HPV in both men and women. It is estimated that at least 80% of sexually active adults will have acquired at least one anogenital HPV infection in their lifetime. Studies of college-aged men and women observed a 24-month cumulative incidence of any HPV infection of 38.8% in women and 62.4% in men (51, 74). Importantly, nearly 50% of newly sexually active women were found to

acquire HPV within 3 years of sexual debut with their first male sexual partner (72). These data highlight the impossibility of any risk stratification to select individuals at high risk of HPV infection.

The average duration of HPV infection in women is 6 to 12 months, with approximately 90% of women becoming HPV DNA negative within 24 months of infection. Because HPV is a largely asymptomatic infection, these natural history estimates are limited by long-interval censored study designs that rarely test for HPV at intervals of <3 to 4 months. Therefore, it is still unknown whether there may be a substantial fraction of HPV which is detectable and clears very quickly. Of more practical concern is the probability that HPV detected during a routine screening will persist or clear. A large study from Costa Rica suggests that most infections clear rapidly (54). Unfortunately, it remains unknown whether an absence of detectable HPV DNA from exfoliated cell samples represents complete eradication of virus, suppression of viral load to undetectable levels, or establishment of virologic latency. Suppression of HPV viral load to undetectable levels and reemergence of replicative virus upon immunosuppression, however, have been well documented for other animal PVs (75). Similarly, it is currently not clear whether prior infection induces type-specific immunity and protection from exposures to the same type (68, 70), though epidemiological data do not fully support repeated reinfections from dually infected partners.

The natural history of anal and penile HPV in men is less well studied. Recent data from a large international cohort examining male genital HPV infection (combined glans/coronal sulcus, shaft, and scrotum exfoliated epithelial samples) reported an overall HPV prevalence of 65.1% for any type of infection and a prevalence of 29.7% for carcinogenic HPV infection (30). These estimates did not differ significantly by age, in contrast to the age-specific patterns of HPV infection observed in women from the same countries. Smaller studies of incident HPV infection in young men have similarly observed a higher risk than that for women of the same age, with a 2-year cumulative incidence of 62.4%, which was significantly associated with a new sex partner in the previous 8 months and a history of cigarette smoking (51). Circumcised men appear more likely to clear HPV infection (45), and data from a randomized controlled trial in Uganda demonstrated that adult male circumcision reduced the prevalence of HPV infection at the coronal sulcus within 2 years (65).

Similarly, the natural history of oral HPV less is only beginning to be evaluated, though it is clear that while HR HPV infection (particularly with HPV type 16) is associated with a subset of head and neck squamous cell cancers, the prevalence of oral HPV infection in the general population is substantially lower than the HPV prevalence in the genital tracts of men and women. Current estimates place oral HPV prevalence from 1.5 to 14% (reviewed in reference 28). Risk factors for oral HPV infection include increasing age (in contrast to younger age for female cervical HPV infection), male gender, HIV infection, iatrogenic immunosuppression, history of a sexually transmitted infection, and number of oral sex partners (reviewed in reference 28).

CLINICAL SIGNIFICANCE

The vast majority of HPV infections at all sites are subclinical and asymptomatic. Most individuals who acquire HPV never know that they have been infected. These infections are characteristically noninflammatory; therefore, they do not result in any of the classic features of an inflammatory response, such as edema and erythema. Because the viruses utilize natural cell death in terminally differentiated keratinocytes to complete their viral life cycle, no tissue destruction or ulceration results from HPV infections. However, despite the abundance of subclinical and self-limited infections in most cases, both HR and LR HPV infections can cause clinical disease in their hosts.

Clinical Manifestations of Female Anogenital Infection

LR HPV infection of the anus, cervix, vagina, and vulva can result in benign warts caused predominantly by HPV types 6 and 11. All LR HPV types can also result in the diagnosis of low-grade squamous intraepithelial lesions (LSILs) on Pap smears. These lesions are characterized by high nuclear/cytoplasmic ratios and the presence of koilocytotic atypia (KA). KA is defined as the presence of nuclear atypia as well as a clearly defined perinuclear halo in cervical epithelial cells (Fig. 1). KA is considered the hallmark of HPV infection.

HR HPV infection can cause both high-grade squamous intraepithelial lesions (HSILs) and invasive cancer at all female anogenital sites, though HR HPV cancers occur at

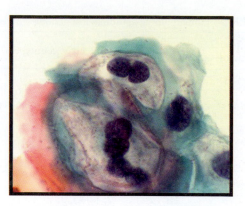

FIGURE 1 Photograph of KA. LSILs on Pap smears are characterized by high nuclear/cytoplasmic ratios and the presence of KA, which is defined as the presence of nuclear atypia as well as a clearly defined perinuclear halo in cervical epithelial cells. Photograph courtesy of Patricia Wasserman, Division of Cytopathology, Department of Pathology and Laboratory Medicine, North Shore-LIJ Health System, Lake Success, NY.

a much higher frequency at the cervix than at the other sites. HSIL is considered a true cancer precursor lesion, in contrast to LSIL, which is generally thought to represent nothing more than viral infection. HSILs are differentiated from LSILs by diminished differentiation, with basaloid cells with a high nuclear/cytoplasmic ratio present close to the epithelial surface. HSILs have been found to contain a higher frequency of genomic abnormalities and are therefore at high risk of progression to invasive cancer. Cervical cancers occur predominantly at the transformation zone, or squamocolumnar junction. The most common treatment for preinvasive neoplasia (cervical intraepithelial neoplasia grade 2 [CIN2] or CIN3) is the loop electrosurgical excision procedure or cold knife cone, which removes the entire cervical transformation zone. Other treatments include laser therapy or cryotherapy; however, the loop electrosurgical excision procedure and cone procedures have the advantage of intact tissue specimens for histopathological review for the presence of lesion margins and have been shown to result in lower recurrence rates (48). The residual presence of HR HPV following excisional therapy is a predictor of disease recurrence (12, 44).

HPV testing for HR types 16, 18, 31, 33, 35, 39, 45, 51, 52, 56, 58, 59, 66, and 68 has become an increasingly integral component of cervical cancer screening programs. Table 2 lists the current recommendations for use of HPV DNA testing in the context of screening (60).

TABLE 2 Clinical indications for appropriate use of HPV tests[a]

Indication	Age restriction
Routine cervical cancer screening in conjunction with cervical cytology (dual testing or cotesting)	30 yr and older
Initial triage management of women with a cytologic result of ASC-US	21 yr and older
Initial triage management of postmenopausal women with cytologic result of LSIL	Postmenopausal
Postcolposcopy management of women of any age with initial cytologic result of AGC or ASC-H (when initial workup does not identify a high-grade lesion)	None
Postcolposcopy management of women 21 yrs and older with initial cytologic results of ASC-US or LSIL (when initial colposcopy does not identify a high-grade lesion)	21 yr and older
Posttreatment surveillance	None

[a]Adapted from reference 60. ASC-US: atypical squamous cells of undetermined significance; AGC, atypical glandular cells; ASC-H, atypical squamous cells, cannot exclude a high-grade SIL.

Clinical Manifestations of Male Anogenital Infection

HPV infection in the anogenital tract of men is more likely to remain undetected, since routine screening for detection of subclinical lesions is not performed in men. Benign warts and flat lesions can occur in all areas of the male lower genital tract, and HR HPV infection may rarely result in the development of anal and penile cancers. Men who have sex with men and HIV-positive men are at a particularly high risk of anal cancer, and anal HPV infection in these men is nearly ubiquitous (17).

Clinical Manifestations of Male and Female Oral Infection

Oral infection is also rarely symptomatic. A very rare syndrome, recurrent respiratory papillomatosis, is caused by infection with LR HPV types that are typically found in genital warts (e.g., HPV types 6 and 11). The juvenile onset form of recurrent respiratory papillomatosis likely is the result of laryngeal HPV acquired from the birth canal of the infected mother. HR HPV, particularly type 16, is also associated with a subset of head and neck cancers, especially cancers of the larynx and oropharynx. Diagnosis of HPV in head and neck tumors yields important prognostic information, as the survival rate for patients with HPV-positive tumors is significantly higher than that for patients with HPV-negative tumors (22).

Primary prevention of up to 90% of genital warts and 70% of invasive cervical cancers is now theoretically possible with the introduction of a highly efficacious vaccine. Gardasil (Merck, West Point, PA) targets HPV types 6, 11, 16, and 18 and prevents external genital lesions and CIN associated with these HPV types in both men (30a) and women (25, 26). An alternative vaccine, Cervarix (GlaxoSmithKline, Research Triangle Park, NC), targets HPV types 16 and 18 and has demonstrated a similar efficacy (50). Both are approved currently in the United States for use in females aged 9 to 26 years, and Gardasil is approved for prevention of genital warts in males aged 9 to 26 years. Both vaccines are based on a recombinant construct of the major capsid protein which is expressed and self-assembled in yeast or insect cell systems into a virus-like particle, which is both morphologically and immunologically indistinguishable from the native virus. The virus-like particle, however, carries no viral nucleic acid and therefore confers no risk of inadvertent HPV infection in vaccine recipients. While these vaccines are nearly 100% efficacious in preventing lesions due to the vaccine types, they offer absolutely no therapeutic benefit to women already exposed to or infected with these types. Therefore, Gardasil and Cervarix are most beneficial when offered prior to sexual debut.

COLLECTION, TRANSPORT, AND STORAGE OF SPECIMENS

Sample collection, transport, and storage recommendations vary based on the purpose and method of HPV testing. Collection of serum follows standard procedures and therefore is not detailed here.

HPV Screening Applications

The use of liquid-based cytology (LBC) facilitates a single sample collection that allows for both Pap smear cytology and HPV testing/genotyping from the same vial. The Hybrid Capture 2 (hc2) test (Qiagen, Gaithersburg, MD) and Cervista HPV HR test (Hologic, Madison, WI) have

U.S. Food and Drug Administration (FDA) approval for testing from residual ThinPrep LBC samples (Hologic, Bedford, MA). Exfoliated cell samples are collected from the endo- and ectocervix using a cervical brush or spatula-endocervical brush combination and rinsed into the LBC media. Specimens are transported at room temperature and stored at 2 to 30°C. The validated stability of the residual ThinPrep sample varies by manufacturer: Cervista reports stability for up to 18 weeks at room temperature, and hc2 reports stability for up to 12 weeks at temperatures between 2 and 30°C. Qiagen also manufactures a standard transport medium (STM) with both brush and Dacron swab collection devices. STM specimens are stable for up to 2 weeks at room temperature, up to 3 weeks at 2 to 8°C, and up to 12 weeks at −20°C.

The use of non-FDA-cleared collection and transport media, including alternative LBC media, such as BD Sure-Path (Becton Dickinson-Tripath, Burlington, NC), viral transport media (M4), Tris-EDTA buffer, and phosphate-buffered saline, would require rigorous validation before manufacturer-determined performance standards for the HPV tests are assumed.

HPV tests from oral, penile, and anal swab samples are not standard clinical tests. Penile and anal swab samples are collected using a saline-moistened Dacron swab, can be placed in the same buffers (e.g., ThinPrep LBC medium and STM) as cervical swabs, and likely have similar stability. Exfoliated oral cells are best sampled using a 30-s oral rinse and gargle with saline or Scope mouthwash. These samples should be stored at −80°C.

HPV Diagnostic Applications

HPV testing from diagnostic tissue specimens is not routine in cervical cancer screening applications, as it is assumed that all CINs are HPV positive. However, it has been found to be useful in the differentiation of primary versus metastatic tumors and HPV type attribution in vaccine trials. In contrast, HPV testing from oropharyngeal cancers provides important prognostic information, as survival is significantly improved in HPV-positive cancers. Fresh biopsy tissue or resected tissue snap frozen in liquid nitrogen is ideal and allows for flexibility in detection of DNA, mRNA, and protein. Paraffin-embedded tissue can be used, although the risk of DNA degradation, and especially RNA degradation, with increasing time in fixation is high. Fixation with 10% buffered neutral formalin is recommended for future PCR testing.

DIRECT DETECTION

Microscopy

Direct visualization of HPV infectious particles is not possible using standard light microscopy. The morphological cellular changes characteristic of HPV infection and associated neoplasia are the basis for standard cervical cytology and are classified based on the Bethesda system (59). Conventional cytology, in which exfoliated cells are smeared onto a glass slide and fixed, has been criticized as suffering from inaccurate readings resulting from obscuring blood and inflammatory cells and poor fixation or air drying. LBC alternatives were developed to prevent these problems and offer the added benefit of residual material for DNA-based tests. A recent large randomized trial compared conventional cytology and LBC and found a modest reduction in smear inadequacy using LBC methods (57), but no benefit in disease detected or positive predictive value (58).

Antigen Detection

At present, immunohistochemical detection of HPV proteins has not been validated for clinically relevant diagnostic applications. However, immunohistochemical or immunocytochemical detection of p16^{INK} tumor suppressor protein is a good biomarker of HR HPV infection and oncogene expression, since there is measurable upregulation of p16 expression in cells expressing HPV E7 (42). p16 staining can be quite useful for differentiating HPV-positive versus HPV-negative oropharyngeal samples (22) and reducing false-negative and false-positive cervical biopsy histological interpretation (41). When using a combination of quantitative p16 immunocytochemistry staining and morphology to exclude false-positive staining of endometrial and other cells, p16 appears in some studies to be useful for differentiation of atypical squamous cells of undetermined significance/LSILs from HSILs (62, 71). However, at present, the lack of standardization of slide interpretation, which remains subjective, limits the reproducibility of this method (66). Commercially available assays for the detection of p16 include the Dako CINtec cytology kit (Dako Cytomation, Glostrup, Denmark) (62, 71) and an enzyme-linked immunosorbent assay (ELISA) (MTM Laboratories AG, Heidelberg, Germany) that does not require microscopic subjective interpretation of staining. One study reported comparable sensitivity and slightly improved specificity of the ELISA for the detection of CIN3 or more severe disease (46), suggesting diagnostic utility if the preliminary performance is validated in larger clinical trials.

Nucleic Acid (NA)-Based Identification and Typing Methods

HPV is not culturable, and therefore, the detection and genotyping of HPV are predominantly dependent on molecular tests that target either HPV DNA or mRNA.

NA Extraction

The appropriate method for HPV NA isolation is a function of the sample type (e.g., fresh tissue, formalin-fixed paraffin-embedded [FFPE] tissue, and exfoliated cells), the collection medium (e.g., STM, PreservCyt LBC medium or SurePath LBC medium), the type of NA target (e.g., mRNA or DNA), the HPV detection assay used, and the purpose of generating the test result.

Fresh Frozen Tissue

NA purification from human tissue samples requires standard methods using organic solvents (e.g., phenol, chloroform, or isoamyl alcohol). Generally, extraction with phenol, chloroform, or isoamyl alcohol and ethanol precipitation can be used. Utilization of commercially available phase-separating microcentrifuge tubes (e.g., Qiagen MaxExtract) may help in reproducible recovery of HPV DNA by minimizing operator error. If RNA targets are detected by the HPV assay, NA isolation should begin with a standard Trizol method.

FFPE Tissue

HPV DNA tests are typically performed on one to three 10-μm sections of FFPE tissue. Extreme caution must be given to preparation of sections to avoid specimen-to-specimen contamination, *particularly for use in PCR assays.* Precautions include use of disposable microtome blades, thorough cleaning of the microtome between specimens with 70% ethanol (EtOH), and changing gloves between each specimen. HPV-negative tissues (e.g., fallopian tubes) should be sectioned periodically as a negative control. Sections are deparaffinized with octane and digested with a buffer containing proteinase K and a nonionic detergent. Large sections can be further purified with organic extraction and EtOH precipitation. DNA from very small tissue biopsy specimens can be lost during organic purification; HPV amplification directly from a crude lysate (after heating at 95°C for 10 min to inactivate the protease) has been demonstrated to be sufficient (32).

Exfoliated Cells

LBC samples are likely to be the most frequently encountered sample type for HPV testing in the clinical laboratory. Manufacturers of most commercial assays provide validated methods for DNA/RNA purification. Most samples in transport media do not require organic purification, and NA extraction is based on precipitation methods. A sample conversion step, provided by the manufacturer, is required for LBC samples to render them compatible with the hc2 test. The Cervista test recommends purification of DNA from PreservCyt samples using the Genfind DNA extraction kit (Hologic). When possible, the recommended protocol should be utilized to ensure that test performance is consistent with that validated by the manufacturers.

Alternative Methods

Numerous NA isolation systems are commercially available, several with high-throughput biorobotic capabilities. Laboratory validation of these methods against the manufacturer's method is necessary before claims of performance equivalent to that reported in the assay trials can be made. Sample transport medium composition will determine what level of purification is required, particularly for enzyme-dependent assays. Additionally, test sensitivity will reflect the volume of the original sample used for purification, any concentration or dilution steps, and the fraction of purified material used in the final assay. To claim comparable performance with an alternative procedure, the final proportion of sample tested should be similar to that used in the manufacturer's performance validation. Finally, it is critical to note that the validation of NA purification methods has primarily been conducted using uterine cervix samples and that comparable performance when using other specimen types cannot be guaranteed.

Detection of HPV

The number of commercially available assays for HPV detection has increased dramatically in recent years (Table 3). In this section, only assays designed to detect the presence or absence of HR HPV infection are discussed, with preference given to those having FDA approval at press time. Standardized protocols are provided with the assay; therefore, details are omitted here. While modifications to these protocols may be warranted, laboratories should understand that performance standards are inextricably linked to the use of the validated protocol. Deviations from the recommended protocol run the risk of compromising performance. Therefore, if deviations are warranted, parallel comparisons are essential to confirm that the deviations do not affect the established performance standards.

HPV Detection Systems

The hc2 test is FDA approved for use as described in Table 2. hc2 is based on hybrid capture signal amplification technology, where full-length RNA probes against 13 HR HPV genotypes (Table 3) are hybridized to denatured target DNA. HPV RNA:DNA hybrids are detected using a sandwich ELISA-type reaction. Hybrids are initially captured onto a

TABLE 3 Commercially available HPV assays[a]

HPV diagnostic test (manufacturer)	NA target	Internal control	Genotypes targeted	Regulatory status	Limit of detection	Method and intended use
hc2 (Qiagen, Inc. [formerly Digene Diagnostics])	DNA	No	16, 18, 31, 33, 35, 39, 45, 51, 52, 56, 58, 59, 68	FDA approved CE marked	5,000 HPV DNA copies	Signal amplification using hybrid capture technology. ASC-US or greater reflex and adjunctive screening for women ≥30 yr old. Well-characterized clinical performance (2). Does not provide specific genotype information
Cervista HPV HR (Hologic, Inc.)	DNA	Yes (human histone 2 gene)	16, 18, 31, 33, 35, 39, 45, 51, 52, 56, 58, 59, 66, 68	FDA approved CE marked	1,250–7,500 HPV DNA copies, depending on genotype	Signal amplification using the Invader chemistry. ASC-US or greater reflex and adjunctive screening for women ≥30 yr old. Minimal clinical validation reported (35). Does not provide specific genotype information
Cervista HPV 16/18 (Hologic, Inc.)	DNA	Yes (human histone 2 gene)	16, 18	FDA approved CE marked		Signal amplification using the Invader chemistry; reflex test for samples positive with the Cervista HPV assay
Roche Amplicor HPV Test (Roche Molecular Diagnostics, Indianapolis, IN)	DNA	Yes (beta-globin)	16, 18, 31, 33, 35, 39, 45, 51, 52, 56, 58, 59, 66, 68	Not FDA approved CE marked		PCR with microwell plate detection. Reported as high risk positive or not high risk positive
Abbott RealTime High Risk HPV Test (Abbott Molecular, Inc.)	DNA	Yes (beta-globin)	16, 18, 31, 33, 35, 39, 45, 51, 52, 56, 58, 59, 66, 68	Not FDA approved CE marked	500–5,000 HPV DNA copies, depending on the type	PCR with TaqMan probe cleavage detection. Reported as high risk positive or not high risk positive. Able to report HPV types 16 and 18
GenProbe Aptima HPV Test (Gen-Probe, Inc.)	mRNA	No	16, 18, 31, 33, 35, 39, 45, 51, 52, 56, 58, 59, 66, 68	Not FDA approved CE marked	38–488 HPV mRNA copies per reaction, depending on genotype	TMA and chemiluminescent probe detection. Reported as high risk positive or negative. Clinical specificity appears to be higher than that of hc2 (18, 62)
PreTect HPV-Proofer (NorChip)	mRNA	Yes (U1A RNA)	16, 18, 31, 33, 45	Not FDA approved CE marked	1–100 HPV+ cells	NASBA amplification with molecular beacon detection. Reported as type-specific result. Clinical specificity higher than for DNA tests, but detects limited types
NucliSENS EasyQ HPV v1 Test (bioMérieux)	mRNA	Yes (U1A RNA)	16, 18, 31, 33, 45	Not FDA approved CE marked	230–30,000 mRNA copies/ml	NASBA amplification with molecular beacon detection. Reported as type-specific result. Little clinical performance information available

[a]NASBA, nucleic acid sequence-based amplification; TMA, transcription-mediated amplification; ASC-US, atypical squamous cells of undetermined significance.

solid-surface microwell by anti-RNA:DNA hybrid antibodies, and signal amplification is achieved by the binding of multiple enzyme-labeled anti-RNA:DNA hybrid antibodies to the captured target hybrid. Addition of substrate produces light, which is measured by a manufacturer-supplied luminometer. Readout of the assay is in relative light units (RLUs), and patient sample results are compared to the internal positive control calibrator. For samples collected in STM, the sample RLU/positive control RLU ratio of ≥1.0 is considered positive for detection of the HR HPV types included in the assay. LBC samples with a ratio of >2.5 are considered positive. Samples with RLU ratios between 1.0 and 2.5 are recommended for repeat testing, though reproducibility will be inherently poor due to stochastic sampling error in samples with low concentrations of HPV DNA. A positive result is indicative of ≥5,000 HPV copies/milliliter in the original sample.

The hc2 test has been extensively evaluated in multiple population-based screening studies and randomized clinical trials (reviewed in reference 13) and has been shown to have a very high sensitivity (pooled sensitivity = 99.4% [13]). While the hc2 test targets only 13 HR HPV types, the probe pool cross-reacts with several LR HPV genotypes (10, 11) and HR type 66. The cross-reactivity affects analytic specificity (34) but has only a modest impact on the clinical specificity and may increase the sensitivity compared to less cross-reactive tests, specifically if cases are defined as CIN2 or more severe (34). The hc2 test does not contain an internal control for specimen adequacy, increasing the risk for false-negative results. However, the rate of false negatives in cervical samples

tested by assays which include a human DNA control is usually reported as <1%. Qiagen has recently reported a next-generation diagnostic system (NextGen) which addresses the LR HPV type cross-reactivity and includes automation to increase the clinical throughput, with a target of processing >2,000 specimens per 8-h shift (21).

The Cervista HR HPV test received FDA approval in 2009 and detects 14 HR HPV DNA targets (Table 3). Cervista is based on signal amplification with the use of Invader chemistry (see Fig. 2). Early results suggest analytic performance and clinical performance comparable to that of hc2 (35) (Cervista product insert; Hologic), though larger population-based studies of screened populations will be required to confirm these results. The test includes an internal control for human histone DNA.

Several other commercial assays are under development, many of which are Conformité Européenne (CE) marked for clinical use in Europe (Table 3). In the interest of space, the details of these assays are not described here. Comparative effectiveness studies are necessary to determine if the newer assays will meet or surpass the clinical performance demonstrated using the hc2 test (2). One large split-sample study compared the performance of some of the assays described in Table 3 to detect CIN2/3 or cancer and reported similar clinical performance for most of the assays targeting HPV DNA (62). Further analyses also demonstrated the ability to optimize clinical sensitivity and specificity by varying the analytic cut point of the assay. Two of the assays target viral E6/E7 mRNA, rather than DNA. The APTIMA HPV assay

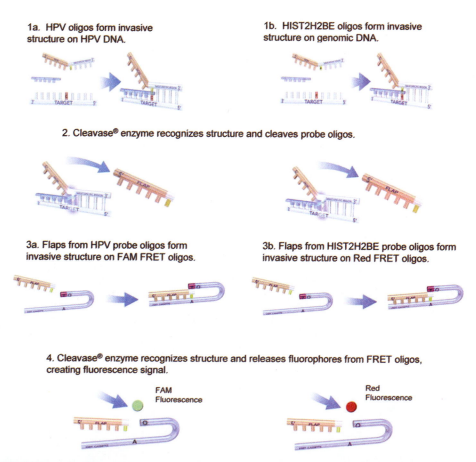

1a. HPV oligos form invasive structure on HPV DNA.

1b. HIST2H2BE oligos form invasive structure on genomic DNA.

2. Cleavase® enzyme recognizes structure and cleaves probe oligos.

3a. Flaps from HPV probe oligos form invasive structure on FAM FRET oligos.

3b. Flaps from HIST2H2BE probe oligos form invasive structure on Red FRET oligos.

4. Cleavase® enzyme recognizes structure and releases fluorophores from FRET oligos, creating fluorescence signal.

FAM Fluorescence

Red Fluorescence

FIGURE 2 Graphic representation of the Invader chemistry in the Cervista HR HPV test. Courtesy of Hologic, Inc., and affiliates.

(Gen-Probe, San Diego, CA) targets E6/E7 mRNA from 14 HR types (types 16, 18, 31, 33, 35, 39, 45, 51, 52, 56, 58, 59, 66, and 68), and PreTect HPV-Proofer (NorChip, Klokkarstua, Norway) targets E6/E7 mRNA of HR types 16, 18, 31, 33, and 45. Theoretically, the detection of early viral transcripts in the upper epithelial layers typically sampled through screening may be a more specific marker of disease, since E6/E7 transcription is confined to the lower third of epithelium in benign infections but is highly expressed in surface epithelial cells in CIN2/3 and cancer lesions (31). In the split-sample comparison, both mRNA-based assays reported a higher specificity than DNA testing; however, the PreTect HPV-Proofer assay demonstrated a lower sensitivity, since the assay detects only 5 of the 14 carcinogenic HPV types (types 16, 18, 31, 33, and 45). A third mRNA-based assay, the NucliSENS EasyQ HPV test (bioMérieux, Grenoble, France), targets E6/E7 mRNA of HR types 16, 18, 31, 33, and 45 (39). Larger population-based comparative studies will be required to determine whether a significant gain in specificity is achieved by using mRNA-based assays.

HPV Genotyping Systems

One of the most characteristic features of HPV infection is the multiplicity of genotypes known to infect the anogenital tract and oral cavity. Complete genotyping has been incredibly useful as a research tool to evaluate the natural history of all genotypes in epidemiological studies; however, the clinical utility is limited. Presently, the American Society for Colposcopy and Cervical Pathology provides recommendations for genotyping only HPV types 16, 18, and 45 (Fig. 3).

Clinical Genotyping for HPV Types 16, 18, and 45

The utility of discriminating genotypes 16, 18, and 45 stems from long-term population-based screening studies which have found that HPV type 16 or 18 detection confers a significant increased risk for progression to CIN2+ within the subsequent 2 to 3 years compared to the other carcinogenic HPV types (40). In addition, HPV types 16, 18, and 45 account for the majority of adenocarcinomas (AdCa), which are located internally and often missed by cytologic screening, whereas the HPV DNA is frequently detected years prior to the AdCa diagnosis. These data led to the current guidelines for reflex HPV type 16/18/45 genotyping of HR HPV DNA test results among cytologically normal women (Fig. 3).

At this time, only the Cervista HPV16/18 (Hologic) is FDA approved for clinical use as a reflex test for samples positive with the Cervista HR HPV test. Genotyping tests are also under development using the hybrid capture technology (Qiagen) (64), consensus PCR, and either chip- or bead-based array detection (Qiagen) (27). The Abbott RealTime High Risk HPV test (Abbott Molecular, Des Plaines, IL) is a real-time PCR test that detects the DNA of 14 HR HPV types (types 16, 18, 31, 33, 35, 39, 45, 51, 52, 56, 58, 59, 66, and 68) and differentially identifies HPV types 16 and 18 (63).

Research-Use-Only Genotyping Systems

Three complete systems are available: the Roche HPV Linear Array (LA) test (Roche Molecular Diagnostics, Basel, Switzerland), the INNO-LiPA HPV Genotyping Extra

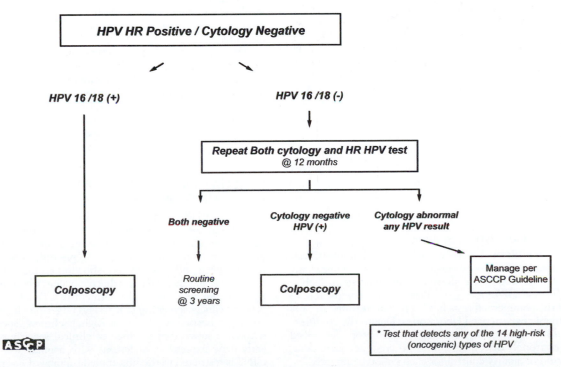

Use of HPV Genotyping to Manage HPV HR * Positive / Cytology negative Women 30 years and Older

FIGURE 3 American Society for Colposcopy and Cervical Pathology 2006 consensus conference recommendations for HPV type 16 or 18 detection (from http://www.asccp.org/pdfs/consensus/clinical_update_20090408.pdf).

(Innogenetics, Ghent, Belgium), and the Papillocheck HPV screening test (Grenier-Bio One, Frickenhausen, Germany). The systems are based on consensus PCR amplification of a broad spectrum of HPV genotypes in a single reaction using an HPV pooled primer cocktail, and genotype discrimination by either reverse hybridization of labeled PCR products to a spectrum of strip-immobilized type-specific probes (LA and INNO-LiPA) or DNA arrays (Papillocheck).

The LA test amplifies over 40 genital HPV genotypes using the PGMY09/11 consensus primer pool (33), allows direct determination of 37 genotypes, and includes a human beta-globin gene amplification as an internal control. Due to intellectual property restrictions, the LA test does not contain a probe for HPV type 52, a common HR genotype, but rather includes a mixed probe which detects HPV types 33, 35, 58, and 52. Hybridization to the mixed probe without hybridization to HPV type 33, 35, and 58 probes implies the presence of HPV type 52. HPV type 52 status in samples positive for HPV types 33, 35, and 58 cannot be determined. However, real-time PCR assays are available for confirmatory testing (47).

The INNO-LiPA HPV Genotyping Extra test is based on the proprietary SPF10 primers which amplify a broad spectrum of HPV genotypes, with direct determination of 28 genotypes by reverse hybridization (67). The INNO-LiPA test also includes an internal amplification control. A single cross-reactive probe detects HPV types 68, 73, and 97 such that infection with these types cannot be discriminated.

The Papillocheck HPV screening test (Greiner-Bio One) is based on amplification and hybridization of E1 gene fragments to a DNA chip spotted with DNA probes specific for 6 LR and 18 HR HPV types (14). Included in the assay is an internal amplification control targeted against the adenosine deaminase 1 gene.

The LA and SPF10/LiPA25 genotyping systems have been directly compared, and performance has been found to be reasonably similar for the detection of one or more HR HPV genotypes. Therefore, for diagnostic purposes, the tests can be considered to perform equivalently. Some type-specific differences in amplification efficiency have been noted for these tests (9, 31), and comparison studies suggest that the LA test detects more genotypes present in HPV infections due to multiple HPV types. Because ~30% of HPV-positive women will have ≥2 genotypes present in a single sample, the LA test may generate more realistic type-specific prevalence estimates for population-based surveys and post-HPV vaccine surveillance. In contrast, the large fragment amplified by the LA test (450 bp) prohibits its utility for HPV typing from fragmented DNA, such as that found in FFPE tissues. The small fragments amplified using the INNO-LiPA SPF10 primers are ideally suited for typing from the fixed tissues.

Alternative Genotyping Systems

Early natural history studies of HPV utilized quite successfully laboratory-developed versions of the now commercially available assays, as well as alternative primer systems such as MY09/11 and GP5+/6+ (31). Performance comparable to that of the commercial tests has been demonstrated in only a few highly experienced laboratories. Due to the complexity of HPV genotyping, the use of laboratory-developed assays is strongly discouraged unless there is adequate demonstration of quality control for each genotype targeted.

Alternative methods for type-specific discrimination following consensus primer amplification are under development. Because of the high degree of similarity among the

HPV genotypes, assays utilizing target-specific probes are likely to be more specific than those based on SYBR green dye intercalation. The Luminex-based bead array hybridization may prove easily automatable and be more suitable for higher-throughput clinical diagnostic laboratories, assuming a clinical indication for complete genotyping. Additional methods describe type-specific detection and quantification of the common HR HPV genotypes, especially HPV types 16 and 18 (31). While HPV viral load is an interesting biomarker in research settings, it has not proven to demonstrate significant diagnostic or prognostic utility. Direct sequencing of consensus primer PCR products is limited in utility to samples with a single type infection (29). Discrimination of HPV sequences from infections with multiple HPV types, which are common, is not possible by standard sequencing technologies.

ISOLATION PROCEDURES

HPV is not culturable, and therefore, the detection and genotyping of HPV are predominantly dependent on molecular tests that target either HPV DNA or mRNA.

SEROLOGIC TESTS

Serologic detection of HPV antibodies is a marker of cumulative exposure and thus cannot determine site of infection or time of infection. Research assays demonstrated limited sensitivity, only detecting antibodies in ~60% of women with DNA from the same type of HPV (8). Therefore, the utility of serologic detection of HPV in clinical practice is extremely limited. With the availability of type-specific prophylactic HPV vaccines that lack therapeutic benefit, both patients and some providers may wish to use antibody testing to evaluate susceptibility prior to making a choice to vaccinate. Because of the described problems with HPV serology, particularly in the context of low-titer antibodies produced during natural infection, this practice is strongly discouraged.

There are currently no commercially available serologic tests for the detection of HPV-specific antibodies. However, the use of prophylactic HPV vaccines has precipitated standardization of serologic assays for immunogenicity testing by the vaccine manufacturers. The relative strengths and weaknesses of the three most common assays used to measure serum HPV antibodies (i.e., ELISA, competitive Luminex immunoassay, and neutralization) have been recently reviewed (56).

EVALUATION, INTERPRETATION, AND REPORTING OF RESULTS

The goal of HPV testing is to identify individuals at high risk of CIN2+ lesions, as part of either routine cervical cancer screening or posttreatment management for prevention of recurrent disease. At present, only the hc2 test has been widely validated, showing reproducibly high sensitivity and negative predictive value when used for the ultimate detection and treatment of CIN2+ disease in cervical cancer screening (2). Assays targeting viral mRNA are hypothesized to have a higher clinical specificity, without a substantial sacrifice of clinical sensitivity, since early gene expression in lesions with a grade lower than CIN2 is restricted to the unsampled suprabasal layers of the epithelium but highly expressed in the outer epithelial cells in true neoplastic lesions (19). While many of the newer DNA or mRNA assays have reported seemingly comparable analytic sensitivity and specificity to hc2 (15, 18, 35, 37), these assays should not be considered to have comparable clinical performance until peer-reviewed clinical validation studies have determined the sensitivity and specificity for detection of CIN2/3 and cancer (61).

Detection of the presence or absence of a pool of HR HPV genotypes is sufficient for the currently approved clinical indications (60). The exception is the possible added positive predictive value in identifying the presence of HPV types 16, 18, and 45 from other HR HPV types. The detection and reporting of LR HPV genotype data have no clinical value. Broad-spectrum genotyping assays are primarily useful for research purposes, including postvaccination genotype distribution surveillance.

REFERENCES

1. Antonsson, A., S. Karanfilovska, P. G. Lindqvist, and B. G. Hansson. 2003. General acquisition of human papillomavirus infections of skin occurs in early infancy. J. Clin. Microbiol. 41:2509–2514.
2. Arbyn, M., P. Sasieni, C. J. Meijer, C. Clavel, G. Koliopoulos, and J. Dillner. 2006. Chapter 9: clinical applications of HPV testing: a summary of meta-analyses. Vaccine 24(Suppl. 3):S78–S89.
3. Badal, S., V. Badal, I. E. Calleja-Macias, M. Kalantari, L. S. Chuang, B. F. Li, and H. U. Bernard. 2004. The human papillomavirus-18 genome is efficiently targeted by cellular DNA methylation. Virology 324:483–492.
4. Badal, V., L. S. Chuang, E. H. Tan, S. Badal, L. L. Villa, C. M. Wheeler, B. F. Li, and H. U. Bernard. 2003. CpG methylation of human papillomavirus type 16 DNA in cervical cancer cell lines and in clinical specimens: genomic hypomethylation correlates with carcinogenic progression. J. Virol. 77:6227–6234.
5. Bernard, H. U. 2002. Gene expression of genital human papillomaviruses and considerations on potential antiviral approaches. Antivir. Ther. 7:219–237.
6. Bernard, H. U., R. D. Burk, Z. Chen, K. van Doorslaer, H. Z. Hausen, and E. M. de Villiers. 2010. Classification of papillomaviruses (PVs) based on 189 PV types and proposal of taxonomic amendments. Virology 401:70–79.
7. Burchell, A. N., H. Richardson, S. M. Mahmud, H. Trottier, P. P. Tellier, J. Hanley, F. Coutlee, and E. L. Franco. 2006. Modeling the sexual transmissibility of human papillomavirus infection using stochastic computer simulation and empirical data from a cohort study of young women in Montreal, Canada. Am. J. Epidemiol. 163:534–543.
8. Carter, J. J., L. A. Koutsky, J. P. Hughes, S. K. Lee, J. Kuypers, N. Kiviat, and D. A. Galloway. 2000. Comparison of human papillomavirus types 16, 18, and 6 capsid antibody responses following incident infection. J. Infect. Dis. 181:1911–1919.
9. Castle, P. E., C. Porras, W. G. Quint, A. C. Rodriguez, M. Schiffman, P. E. Gravitt, P. Gonzalez, H. A. Katki, S. Silva, E. Freer, L. J. Van Doorn, S. Jimenez, R. Herrero, and A. Hildesheim. 2008. Comparison of two PCR-based human papillomavirus genotyping methods. J. Clin. Microbiol. 46:3437–3445.
10. Castle, P. E., M. Schiffman, R. D. Burk, S. Wacholder, A. Hildesheim, R. Herrero, M. C. Bratti, M. E. Sherman, and A. Lorincz. 2002. Restricted cross-reactivity of hybrid capture 2 with nononcogenic human papillomavirus types. Cancer Epidemiol. Biomarkers Prev. 11:1394–1399.
11. Castle, P. E., D. Solomon, C. M. Wheeler, P. E. Gravitt, S. Wacholder, and M. Schiffman. 2008. Human papillomavirus genotype specificity of Hybrid Capture 2. J. Clin. Microbiol. 46:2595–2604.
12. Chan, B. K., J. Melnikow, C. A. Slee, R. Arellanes, and G. F. Sawaya. 2009. Posttreatment human papillomavirus testing for recurrent cervical intraepithelial neoplasia: a systematic review. Am. J. Obstet. Gynecol. 200:422.e1–422.e9.
13. Cuzick, J., M. Arbyn, R. Sankaranarayanan, V. Tsu, G. Ronco, M.-H. Mayrand, J. Dillner, and C. J. L. M. Meijer. 2008. Overview of human papillomavirus-based and other novel options for cervical cancer screening in developed and developing countries. Vaccine 26:K29–K41.
14. Dalstein, V., S. Merlin, C. Bali, M. Saunier, R. Dachez, and C. Ronsin. 2009. Analytical evaluation of the PapilloCheck test, a new commercial DNA chip for detection and genotyping of human papillomavirus. J. Virol. Methods 156:77–83.
15. Day, S. P., A. Hudson, A. Mast, T. Sander, M. Curtis, S. Olson, L. Chehak, N. Quigley, J. Ledford, B. Yen-Lieberman, D. Kohn, D. I. Quigley, and M. Olson. 2009. Analytical performance of the Investigational Use Only Cervista HPV HR test as determined by a multi-center study. J. Clin. Virol. 45(Suppl. 1):S63–S72.
16. de Koning, M. N., L. Struijk, J. N. Bavinck, B. Kleter, J. ter Schegget, W. G. Quint, and M. C. Feltkamp. 2007. Betapapillomaviruses frequently persist in the skin of healthy individuals. J. Gen. Virol. 88:1489–1495.
17. de Pokomandy, A., D. Rouleau, G. Ghattas, S. Vezina, P. Cote, J. Macleod, G. Allaire, E. L. Franco, and F. Coutlee. 2009. Prevalence, clearance, and incidence of anal human papillomavirus infection in HIV-infected men: the HIPVIRG cohort study. J. Infect. Dis. 199:965–973.
18. Dockter, J., A. Schroder, C. Hill, L. Guzenski, J. Monsonego, and C. Giachetti. 2009. Clinical performance of the APTIMA HPV assay for the detection of high-risk HPV and high-grade cervical lesions. J. Clin. Virol. 45(Suppl. 1):S55–S61.
19. Doorbar, J. 2006. Molecular biology of human papillomavirus infection and cervical cancer. Clin. Sci. (London) 110:525–541.
20. Dyson, N., P. M. Howley, K. Munger, and E. Harlow. 1989. The human papilloma virus-16 E7 oncoprotein is able to bind to the retinoblastoma gene product. Science 243:934–937.
21. Eder, P. S., J. Lou, J. Huff, and J. Macioszek. 2009. The next-generation Hybrid Capture High-Risk HPV DNA assay on a fully automated platform. J. Clin. Virol. 45(Suppl. 1):S85–S92.
22. Fakhry, C., W. H. Westra, S. Li, A. Cmelak, J. A. Ridge, H. Pinto, A. Forastiere, and M. L. Gillison. 2008. Improved survival of patients with human papillomavirus-positive head and neck squamous cell carcinoma in a prospective clinical trial. J. Natl. Cancer Inst. 100:261–269.
23. Feltkamp, M. C., M. N. de Koning, J. N. Bavinck, and J. Ter Schegget. 2008. Betapapillomaviruses: innocent bystanders or causes of skin cancer. J. Clin. Virol. 43:353–360.
24. Reference deleted.
25. The Future II Study Group. 2007. Quadrivalent vaccine against human papillomavirus to prevent high-grade cervical lesions. N. Engl. J. Med. 356:1915–1927.
26. Garland, S. M., M. Hernandez-Avila, C. M. Wheeler, G. Perez, D. M. Harper, S. Leodolter, G. W. Tang, D. G. Ferris, M. Steben, J. Bryan, F. J. Taddeo, R. Railkar, M. T. Esser, H. L. Sings, M. Nelson, J. Boslego, C. Sattler, E. Barr, and L. A. Koutsky. 2007. Quadrivalent vaccine against human papillomavirus to prevent anogenital diseases. N. Engl. J. Med. 356:1928–1943.
27. Geraets, D. T., D. A. Heideman, M. N. de Koning, P. J. Snijders, D. C. van Alewijk, C. J. Meijer, L. J. van Doorn, and W. G. Quint. 2009. High-throughput genotyping of high-risk HPV by the Digene HPV Genotyping LQ Test using GP5+/6+-PCR and xMAP technology. J. Clin. Virol. 46(Suppl. 3):S21–S26.
28. Gillison, M. L. 2008. Human papillomavirus-related diseases: oropharynx cancers and potential implications for adolescent HPV vaccination. J. Adolesc. Health 43:S52–S60.
29. Giuliani, L., A. Coletti, K. Syrjanen, C. Favalli, and M. Ciotti. 2006. Comparison of DNA sequencing and Roche Linear Array in human papillomavirus (HPV) genotyping. Anticancer Res. 26:3939–3941.
30. Giuliano, A. R., B. Lu, C. M. Nielson, R. Flores, M. R. Papenfuss, J. H. Lee, M. Abrahamsen, and R. B. Harris. 2008. Age-specific prevalence, incidence, and duration of human papillomavirus infections in a cohort of 290 US men. J. Infect. Dis. 198:827–835.

30a. Giuliano, A. R., J. M. Palefsky, S. Goldstone, E. D. Moreira, Jr., M. E. Penny, C. Aranda, E. Vardas, H. Moi, H. Jessen, R. Hillman, Y. H. Chang, D. Ferris, D. Rouleau, J. Bryan, J. B. Marshall, S. Vuocolo, E. Barr, D. Radley, R. M. Haupt, and D. Guris. 2011. Efficacy of quadrivalent HPV vaccine against HPV infection and disease in males. *N. Engl. J. Med.* 364:401–411.

31. Gravitt, P. E., F. Coutlee, T. Iftner, J. W. Sellors, W. G. Quint, and C. M. Wheeler. 2008. New technologies in cervical cancer screening. *Vaccine* 26(Suppl. 10):K42–K52.

32. Gravitt, P. E., M. B. Kovacic, R. Herrero, M. Schiffman, C. Bratti, A. Hildesheim, J. Morales, M. Alfaro, M. E. Sherman, S. Wacholder, A. C. Rodriguez, and R. D. Burk. 2007. High load for most high risk human papillomavirus genotypes is associated with prevalent cervical cancer precursors but only HPV16 load predicts the development of incident disease. *Int. J. Cancer* 121:2787–2793.

33. Gravitt, P. E., C. L. Peyton, T. Q. Alessi, C. M. Wheeler, F. Coutlee, A. Hildesheim, M. H. Schiffman, D. R. Scott, and R. J. Apple. 2000. Improved amplification of genital human papillomaviruses. *J. Clin. Microbiol.* 38:357–361.

34. Gravitt, P. E., M. Schiffman, D. Solomon, C. M. Wheeler, and P. E. Castle. 2008. A comparison of Linear Array and Hybrid Capture 2 for detection of carcinogenic human papillomavirus and cervical precancer in ASCUS-LSIL triage study. *Cancer Epidemiol. Biomarkers Prev.* 17:1248–1254.

35. Harvey, M., S. Stout, C. R. Starkey, R. Hendren, S. Holt, and G. C. Miller. 2009. The clinical performance of Invader technology and SurePath when detecting the presence of high-risk HPV cervical infection. *J. Clin. Virol.* 45(Suppl. 1):S79–S83.

36. Hernandez, B. Y., K. McDuffie, X. Zhu, L. R. Wilkens, J. Killeen, B. Kessel, M. T. Wakabayashi, C. C. Bertram, D. Easa, L. Ning, J. Boyd, C. Sunoo, L. Kamemoto, and M. T. Goodman. 2005. Anal human papillomavirus infection in women and its relationship with cervical infection. *Cancer Epidemiol. Biomarkers Prev.* 14:2550–2556.

37. Huang, S., B. Erickson, N. Tang, W. B. Mak, J. Salituro, J. Robinson, and K. Abravaya. 2009. Clinical performance of Abbott RealTime High Risk HPV test for detection of high-grade cervical intraepithelial neoplasia in women with abnormal cytology. *J. Clin. Virol.* 45(Suppl. 1):S19–S23.

38. Huibregtse, J. M., M. Scheffner, and P. M. Howley. 1993. Localization of the E6-AP regions that direct human papillomavirus E6 binding, association with p53, and ubiquitination of associated proteins. *Mol. Cell. Biol.* 13:4918–4927.

39. Jeantet, D., F. Schwarzmann, J. Tromp, W. J. Melchers, A. A. van der Wurff, T. Oosterlaken, M. Jacobs, and A. Troesch. 2009. NucliSENS EasyQ HPV v1 test—testing for oncogenic activity of human papillomaviruses. *J. Clin. Virol.* 45(Suppl. 1):S29–S37.

40. Khan, M. J., P. E. Castle, A. T. Lorincz, S. Wacholder, M. Sherman, D. R. Scott, B. B. Rush, A. G. Glass, and M. Schiffman. 2005. The elevated 10-year risk of cervical precancer and cancer in women with human papillomavirus (HPV) type 16 or 18 and the possible utility of type-specific HPV testing in clinical practice. *J. Natl. Cancer Inst.* 97:1072–1079.

41. Klaes, R., A. Benner, T. Friedrich, R. Ridder, S. Herrington, D. Jenkins, R. J. Kurman, D. Schmidt, M. Stoler, and M. von Knebel Doeberitz. 2002. p16INK4a immunohistochemistry improves interobserver agreement in the diagnosis of cervical intraepithelial neoplasia. *Am. J. Surg. Pathol.* 26:1389–1399.

42. Klaes, R., T. Friedrich, D. Spitkovsky, R. Ridder, W. Rudy, U. Petry, G. Dallenbach-Hellweg, D. Schmidt, and M. von Knebel Doeberitz. 2001. Overexpression of p16(INK4A) as a specific marker for dysplastic and neoplastic epithelial cells of the cervix uteri. *Int. J. Cancer* 92:276–284.

43. Kohler, A., T. Forschner, T. Meyer, C. Ulrich, M. Gottschling, E. Stockfleth, and I. Nindl. 2007. Multifocal distribution of cutaneous human papillomavirus types in hairs from different skin areas. *Br. J. Dermatol.* 156:1078–1080.

44. Kreimer, A. R., R. S. Guido, D. Solomon, M. Schiffman, S. Wacholder, J. Jeronimo, C. M. Wheeler, and P. E. Castle. 2006. Human papillomavirus testing following loop

electrosurgical excision procedure identifies women at risk for posttreatment cervical intraepithelial neoplasia grade 2 or 3 disease. *Cancer Epidemiol. Biomarkers Prev.* 15:908–914.

45. Lu, B., Y. Wu, C. M. Nielson, R. Flores, M. Abrahamsen, M. Papenfuss, R. B. Harris, and A. R. Giuliano. 2009. Factors associated with acquisition and clearance of human papillomavirus infection in a cohort of US men: a prospective study. *J. Infect. Dis.* 199:362–371.

46. Mao, C., A. Balasubramanian, M. Yu, N. Kiviat, R. Ridder, A. Reichert, M. Herkert, M. von Knebel Doeberitz, and L. A. Koutsky. 2007. Evaluation of a new p16(INK4A) ELISA test and a high-risk HPV DNA test for cervical cancer screening: results from proof-of-concept study. *Int. J. Cancer* 120:2435–2438.

47. Marks, M., S. B. Gupta, K. L. Liaw, E. Kim, A. Tadesse, F. Coutlee, S. Sriplienchan, D. D. Celentano, and P. E. Gravitt. 2009. Confirmation and quantitation of human papillomavirus type 52 by Roche Linear Array using HPV52-specific TaqMan E6/E7 quantitative real-time PCR. *J. Virol. Methods* 156:152–156.

48. Melnikow, J., C. McGahan, G. F. Sawaya, T. Ehlen, and A. Coldman. 2009. Cervical intraepithelial neoplasia outcomes after treatment: long-term follow-up from the British Columbia Cohort Study. *J. Natl. Cancer Inst.* 101:721–728.

49. Munger, K., B. A. Werness, N. Dyson, W. C. Phelps, E. Harlow, and P. M. Howley. 1989. Complex formation of human papillomavirus E7 proteins with the retinoblastoma tumor suppressor gene product. *EMBO J.* 8:4099–4105.

50. Paavonen, J., P. Naud, J. Salmeron, C. M. Wheeler, S. N. Chow, D. Apter, H. Kitchener, X. Castellsague, J. C. Teixeira, S. R. Skinner, J. Hedrick, U. Jaisamrarn, G. Limson, S. Garland, A. Szarewski, B. Romanowski, F. Y. Aoki, T. F. Schwarz, W. A. Poppe, F. X. Bosch, D. Jenkins, K. Hardt, T. Zahaf, D. Descamps, F. Struyf, M. Lehtinen, G. Dubin, and M. Greenacre. 2009. Efficacy of human papillomavirus (HPV)-16/18 AS04-adjuvanted vaccine against cervical infection and precancer caused by oncogenic HPV types (PATRICIA): final analysis of a double-blind, randomised study in young women. *Lancet* 374:301–314.

51. Partridge, J. M., J. P. Hughes, Q. Feng, R. L. Winer, B. A. Weaver, L. F. Xi, M. E. Stern, S. K. Lee, S. F. O'Reilly, S. E. Hawes, N. B. Kiviat, and L. A. Koutsky. 2007. Genital human papillomavirus infection in men: incidence and risk factors in a cohort of university students. *J. Infect. Dis.* 196:1128–1136.

52. Pett, M., and N. Coleman. 2007. Integration of high-risk human papillomavirus: a key event in cervical carcinogenesis? *J. Pathol.* 212:356–367.

53. Pett, M. R., W. O. Alazawi, I. Roberts, S. Dowen, D. I. Smith, M. A. Stanley, and N. Coleman. 2004. Acquisition of high-level chromosomal instability is associated with integration of human papillomavirus type 16 in cervical keratinocytes. *Cancer Res.* 64:1359–1368.

54. Rodriguez, A. C., M. Schiffman, R. Herrero, S. Wacholder, A. Hildesheim, P. E. Castle, D. Solomon, and R. Burk. 2008. Rapid clearance of human papillomavirus and implications for clinical focus on persistent infections. *J. Natl. Cancer Inst.* 100:513–517.

55. Scheffner, M., B. A. Werness, J. M. Huibregtse, A. J. Levine, and P. M. Howley. 1990. The E6 oncoprotein encoded by human papillomavirus types 16 and 18 promotes the degradation of p53. *Cell* 63:1129–1136.

56. Schiller, J. T., and D. R. Lowy. 2009. Immunogenicity testing in human papillomavirus virus-like-particle vaccine trials. *J. Infect. Dis.* 200:166–171.

57. Siebers, A. G., P. J. Klinkhamer, M. Arbyn, A. O. Raifu, L. F. Massuger, and J. Bulten. 2008. Cytologic detection of cervical abnormalities using liquid-based compared with conventional cytology: a randomized controlled trial. *Obstet. Gynecol.* 112:1327–1334.

58. Siebers, A. G., P. J. Klinkhamer, J. M. Grefte, L. F. Massuger, J. E. Vedder, A. Beijers-Broos, J. Bulten, and M. Arbyn. 2009. Comparison of liquid-based cytology with conventional cytology for detection of cervical cancer precursors: a randomized controlled trial. *JAMA* 302:1757–1764.

59. **Solomon, D., D. Davey, R. Kurman, A. Moriarty, D. O'Connor, M. Prey, S. Raab, M. Sherman, D. Wilbur, T. Wright, Jr., and N. Young.** 2002. The 2001 Bethesda System: terminology for reporting results of cervical cytology. *JAMA* **287:**2114–2119.

60. **Solomon, D., J. L. Papillo, and D. D. Davey.** 2009. Statement on HPV DNA test utilization. *Am. J. Clin. Pathol.* **131:**768–769; discussion, 770–773.

61. **Stoler, M. H., P. E. Castle, D. Solomon, and M. Schiffman.** 2007. The expanded use of HPV testing in gynecologic practice per ASCCP-guided management requires the use of well-validated assays. *Am. J. Clin. Pathol.* **127:**335–337.

62. **Szarewski, A., L. Ambroisine, L. Cadman, J. Austin, L. Ho, G. Terry, S. Liddle, R. Dina, J. McCarthy, H. Buckley, C. Bergeron, P. Soutter, D. Lyons, and J. Cuzick.** 2008. Comparison of predictors for high-grade cervical intraepithelial neoplasia in women with abnormal smears. *Cancer Epidemiol. Biomarkers Prev.* **17:**3033–3042.

63. **Tang, N., S. Huang, B. Erickson, W. B. Mak, J. Salituro, J. Robinson, and K. Abravaya.** 2009. High-risk HPV detection and concurrent HPV 16 and 18 typing with Abbott RealTime High Risk HPV test. *J. Clin. Virol.* **45**(Suppl. 1):S25–S28.

64. **Thai, H., S. Rangwala, T. Gay, K. Keating, S. McLeod, I. Nazarenko, D. O'Neil, D. Pfister, and D. Loeffert.** 2009. An HPV 16, 18, and 45 genotyping test based on Hybrid Capture technology. *J. Clin. Virol.* **45**(Suppl. 1):S93–S97.

65. **Tobian, A. A., D. Serwadda, T. C. Quinn, G. Kigozi, P. E. Gravitt, O. Laeyendecker, B. Charvat, V. Ssempijja, M. Riedesel, A. E. Oliver, R. G. Nowak, L. H. Moulton, M. Z. Chen, S. J. Reynolds, M. J. Wawer, and R. H. Gray.** 2009. Male circumcision for the prevention of HSV-2 and HPV infections and syphilis. *N. Engl. J. Med.* **360:**1298–1309.

66. **Tsoumpou, I., M. Arbyn, M. Kyrgiou, N. Wentzensen, G. Koliopoulos, P. Martin-Hirsch, V. Malamou-Mitsi, and E. Paraskevaidis.** 2009. p16(INK4a) immunostaining in cytological and histological specimens from the uterine cervix: a systematic review and meta-analysis. *Cancer Treat. Rev.* **35:**210–220.

67. **van Hamont, D., M. A. van Ham, J. M. Bakkers, L. F. Massuger, and W. J. Melchers.** 2006. Evaluation of the SPF10-INNO LiPA human papillomavirus (HPV) genotyping test and the Roche linear array HPV genotyping test. *J. Clin. Microbiol.* **44:**3122–3129.

68. **Velicer, C., X. Zhu, S. Vuocolo, K. L. Liaw, and A. Saah.** 2009. Prevalence and incidence of HPV genital infection in women. *Sex. Transm. Dis.* **36:**696–703.

69. **Vinokurova, S., N. Wentzensen, I. Kraus, R. Klaes, C. Driesch, P. Melsheimer, F. Kisseljov, M. Durst, A. Schneider, and M. von Knebel Doeberitz.** 2008. Type-dependent integration frequency of human papillomavirus genomes in cervical lesions. *Cancer Res.* **68:**307–313.

70. **Viscidi, R. P., M. Schiffman, A. Hildesheim, R. Herrero, P. E. Castle, M. C. Bratti, A. C. Rodriguez, M. E. Sherman, S. Wang, B. Clayman, and R. D. Burk.** 2004. Seroreactivity to human papillomavirus (HPV) types 16, 18, or 31 and risk of subsequent HPV infection: results from a population-based study in Costa Rica. *Cancer Epidemiol. Biomarkers Prev.* **13:**324–327.

71. **Wentzensen, N., C. Bergeron, F. Cas, D. Eschenbach, S. Vinokurova, and M. von Knebel Doeberitz.** 2005. Evaluation of a nuclear score for p16INK4a-stained cervical squamous cells in liquid-based cytology samples. *Cancer* **105:**461–467.

72. **Winer, R. L., Q. Feng, J. P. Hughes, S. O'Reilly, N. B. Kiviat, and L. A. Koutsky.** 2008. Risk of female human papillomavirus acquisition associated with first male sex partner. *J. Infect. Dis.* **197:**279–282.

73. **Winer, R. L., J. P. Hughes, Q. Feng, S. O'Reilly, N. B. Kiviat, K. K. Holmes, and L. A. Koutsky.** 2006. Condom use and the risk of genital human papillomavirus infection in young women. *N. Engl. J. Med.* **354:**2645–2654.

74. **Winer, R. L., S. K. Lee, J. P. Hughes, D. E. Adam, N. B. Kiviat, and L. A. Koutsky.** 2003. Genital human papillomavirus infection: incidence and risk factors in a cohort of female university students. *Am. J. Epidemiol.* **157:**218–226.

75. **Zhang, P., M. Nouri, J. L. Brandsma, T. Iftner, and B. M. Steinberg.** 1999. Induction of E6/E7 expression in cottontail rabbit papillomavirus latency following UV activation. *Virology* **263:**388–394.

Human Polyomaviruses

RICHARD S. BULLER

103

TAXONOMY

The polyomaviruses were formerly members of the *Papovaviridae* family but have been reclassified into the *Polyomaviridae*. The recognized human species *BK polyomavirus* (BKPyV) and *JC polyomavirus* (JCPyV) and the primate virus *Simian virus 40* (SV40) reside in the single genus *Polyomavirus* within the family. Lymphotropic polyomavirus (LPyV), a nonhuman primate polyomavirus, is classified as a strain of *African green monkey polyomavirus*. The newly identified putative human polyomaviruses (HPyV) WU polyomavirus (WUPyV), KI polyomavirus (KIPyV), and Merkel cell polyomavirus (MCPyV) have yet to be formally classified, although all current data suggest they are indeed polyomaviruses. Phylogenetic analyses indicate that WUPyV and KIPyV are closely related to each other and form a group distinct from but related to that of BKPyV, JCPyV, and SV40. MCPyV is more closely related to the African green monkey virus (LPyV) than it is to the other HPyV.

DESCRIPTION OF THE AGENTS

The polyomaviruses are small (40- to 45-nm diameter), icosahedral, nonenveloped viruses with a circular double-stranded DNA genome. The size of the genome is relatively small, with all of the human viruses, including the newly identified members and SV40, falling within the range of approximately 5,000 to 5,400 bp. JCPyV, BKPyV, and SV40 have been extensively characterized. The newly characterized viruses have been less well studied.

The genome is organized into an early region that is transcribed prior to DNA replication and a late region transcribed after DNA replication. The noncoding control region (NCCR) separates the early and late regions and includes the origin of replication (63).

Early region transcripts code for the large and small T antigens, nonstructural proteins that regulate viral replication, control of viral transcription, induction of host cell division, and transformation. Late gene transcripts code for viral capsid proteins VP1, VP2, and VP3, of which VP1 is the major capsid protein, comprising approximately 80% of the capsid and being the only surface-exposed protein (63). The late regions of JCPyV, BKPyV, and SV40 also code for a fourth late protein termed the agnoprotein, the function of which is incompletely understood, which appears to be a nonstructural protein involved in viral assembly and release from infected cells (63).

The genomic organization of the newly identified polyomaviruses, KIPyV, WUPyV, and MCPyV, appears to be similar to those previously described, with open reading frames identified for the T antigens and VP1, VP2, and VP3 (4, 48, 53). However, these viruses appear to differ from the previously known human viruses in that there is no agnoprotein open reading frame, at least for KIPyV and WUPyV (4, 53).

The NCCRs of the human viruses BKPyV and JCPyV are hypervariable sequences of approximately 300 to 500 bp in length. The NCCR contains the origin of replication and promoters for early and late gene transcription. The variable nature of the NCCR is apparent when sequences of this region are compared between viruses obtained from different anatomical sites. The NCCR sequence from kidney and urine isolates is referred to as the archetype. Viruses with archetype NCCR sequences do not replicate well in cell cultures and may be the infectious form of the virus.

EPIDEMIOLOGY AND TRANSMISSION

Both BKPyV and JCPyV appear to infect the majority of human beings by adulthood. Seroepidemiology studies reveal that 50% of children acquire anti-BKPyV antibodies by the age of 3 years, with the 50% prevalence for JCPyV being reached by age 6 years (115). For all age groups, the seroprevalence for BKPyV ranges from 55 to 85%, with similar numbers for JCPyV, although there is more variability in the age of seroconversion for JCPyV relative to BKPyV (68). The mechanism of BKPyV and JCPyV transmission is largely speculative, in part due to the fact that primary infection does not appear to cause clinical illness, although there are reports of signs and symptoms such as fever or respiratory illness accompanying seroconversion (68). Respiratory and oral transmission has been hypothesized, since JCPyV can infect tonsillar cells (84) and has been detected in tonsillar tissue (85). However, studies of oral and respiratory specimens have failed to detect BKPyV and JCPyV (11, 114). Uro-oral transmission has been hypothesized, and circumstantial evidence consists of intermittent BKPyV and JCPyV excretion in the urine of immunocompetent and immunocompromised individuals

TABLE 1 Diseases associated with HPV

Virus(es)	Disease association (references)	Comment(s) (reference[s])
BKPyV	PVAN	Seen primarily in kidney transplant recipients (90)
	Hemorrhagic cystitis	Observed primarily in BMT recipients with a prevalence of 10–25% in this population (43)
JCPyV	PML	Observed in patients with compromised cellular immunity (HIV/AIDS, malignancy, and immunomodulatory therapies used to treat multiple sclerosis and psoriasis) (46, 67, 72, 118)
	PVAN	Associated with rare cases of BKPyV-negative PVAN (41, 65, 125)
LPyV	None identified	Primate virus; grows in human B lymphocytes; LPyV sequences found by PCR in PBMC^a of HIV patients with leukoencephalopathies (37)
MCPyV	Merkel cell carcinoma	Associated with 75–88% of Merkel cell carcinoma tumors (7, 48, 50); MCPyV has also been detected in respiratory specimens, suggesting a mode of acquisition (13, 54)
SV40	No firm disease association (95, 102, 107, 120)	Primate virus found to contaminate polio vaccine
WUPyV and KIPyV	No firm disease association	Detected in respiratory secretions and stool specimens (1, 2, 4, 15, 16, 53, 74, 88, 100)

^{a}PBMC, peripheral blood mononuclear cells.

(68, 130), detection of BKPyV and JCPyV in sewage samples (21–23), and the stability of these nonenveloped viruses. Even less is known about the epidemiology and transmission of the newly identified HPyV. WUPyV and KIPyV are found in respiratory secretions and are widely distributed around the globe (1, 2, 4, 15, 16, 53, 74, 77, 94). WUPyV has been detected in respiratory secretions of a 1-day-old infant, raising the possibility of in utero or intrapartum infection (74). Two recent studies have also detected WUPyV in small numbers of serum and stool specimens (88, 100). MCPyV is also found in respiratory specimens (13, 54), and seroprevalences of 50% and 80% in children and adults have been documented, suggesting that infection is common (117).

Human beings were exposed to the nonhuman primate polyomavirus SV40 between 1955 and 1963 when some incompletely formalin-inactivated lots of polio vaccine were found to be contaminated. Monkey kidney cell cultures used to prepare the vaccine were found to be the source of contamination. About 200 cases of paralytic polio occurred due to the presence of infectious poliovirus in the vaccine. Although approximately 100 million Americans were vaccinated during this period, it is not known how many of the lots contained infectious SV40 or how many people became infected with SV40 as the result of this accident (108).

CLINICAL SIGNIFICANCE

Polyomaviruses cause a number of diseases in different patient populations (Table 1). Progressive multifocal leukoencephalopathy (PML) is a rare disease of the central nervous system caused by infection and destruction of myelin-producing oligodendrocytes by JCPyV. Focal demyelination in white matter can be visualized by neuroimaging studies such as magnetic resonance (MR) imaging (Fig. 1). Neurological signs/symptoms include gait or other motor disturbances and cognitive abnormalities (124). Prognosis is poor, with long-term survival defined as greater than 12 months (63).

Polyomavirus-associated nephropathy (PVAN) is the result of BKPyV replication in, and the destruction of, renal tubular epithelial cells in renal transplant patients (90). Increasing levels of virus are initially found in urine, followed by viremia and then development of PVAN (25). Without clinical

intervention, PVAN can result in renal graft dysfunction and, ultimately, graft loss (97). In a prospective study of 78 renal transplant recipients, the probability of developing PVAN was 8% (61). Renal transplant patients may have a propensity to develop PVAN due to the use of more aggressive immunosuppression regimens (97), BKPyV acquisition from the donor kidney, or HLA-mediated predisposition (26, 119). PVAN is treated by reducing immunosuppression; certain antiviral compounds have also been used (25, 27, 36). JCPyV has also been reported to rarely cause PVAN (65, 125).

Other pathological conditions associated with BKPyV include hematuria, urethral stenosis, and hemorrhagic cystitis. Hemorrhagic cystitis is due to BKPyV infection

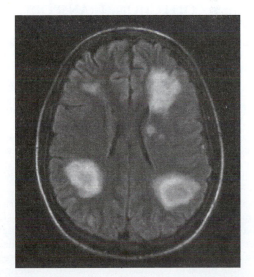

FIGURE 1 MR image showing the brain of a patient with lesions of advanced PML. Lesions are seen bilaterally in frontal lobes and in parieto-occipital subcortical regions. Note that the cortex is spared, with lesions primarily in the white matter, consistent with the pathology of demyelination of white matter tracts (fluid-attenuated inversion recovery T2-weighted MR). Reprinted from *Neurology* (113) with permission of the publisher.

of the bladder epithelium. It is associated with significant morbidity but is rarely fatal (43). The risk of developing the disease has been shown to correlate with increased levels of BKPyV viruria (75) and viremia (47). Treatment is supportive, although the use of select antiviral drugs has been attempted (43).

Attempts to link the newly identified HPyV with specific human diseases are in their infancy. KIPyV and WUPyV have not been firmly associated with human disease. WUPyV DNA and antigens were found in a 2-year-old bone marrow transplant (BMT) patient who died of multiorgan disease (18); a definitive link between virus infection and disease awaits further study. LPyV DNA has been found in human immunodeficiency virus (HIV) patients with leukoencephalopathies (37); this disease association also awaits corroboration.

Merkel cell carcinoma is a rare, highly aggressive neuroepithelial tumor of the skin noted for its high mortality. The recent association of a novel polyomavirus with this cancer is intriguing (48) (Table 1).

Lastly, because of the known ability of polyomaviruses to cause cancer, there have long been concerns that these viruses could be a potential cause of some human cancers. Over the years, there have been many attempts to link SV40 with human cancers, with some of the attempts being reported as successful. However, there has been an inability to reproduce the results of some studies linking particular cancers to this virus due to factors such as contamination with plasmids and serological cross-reactions between SV40 and BKPyV and JCPyV (108). Although debatable, the consensus today is that, other than the recent case of MCPyV, there is currently no convincing evidence that either human or animal polyomaviruses are a significant cause of human cancers. Readers interested in this subject are referred to several excellent reviews on this topic (95, 102, 108, 120).

SPECIMEN COLLECTION, TRANSPORT, AND STORAGE

Although systematic studies of clinical specimens have not been reported for polyomaviruses, as one would expect for these nonenveloped DNA viruses, polyomaviruses appear to be quite stable. A study of JCPyV stability in sewage at 20°C found a t_{90} value (time required for a reduction of 90% of the viral concentration as measured by quantitative PCR) of 64 days and a t_{99} of 127 days, with a greater t_{90} value obtained when the virus was suspended in phosphate-buffered saline (111 days) (20). These data suggest that standard guidelines for the collection, transport, and storage of specimens for viral diagnostics (see chapter 76) should be sufficient for polyomaviruses.

Specimens commonly submitted for the detection of polyomaviruses include blood, cerebrospinal fluid (CSF), urine, respiratory specimens, and tissue. Polyomaviruses can be recovered from peripheral blood mononuclear cells, usually for research purposes. This cell fraction can be prepared from whole blood as outlined in chapter 76. Guidelines for collection and transport of specimens are generally those that apply to molecular testing (see chapter 76 and reference 34). Since nucleic acid detection methods are the primary means by which polyomaviruses are detected in clinical specimens, extracted DNA should be stored in tightly sealed low-binding plastic tubes to prevent evaporation and binding of DNA to the walls of the tubes (34). DNA can be stored in Tris-EDTA buffer at room temperature for up

26 weeks, at 2 to 8°C for up to 1 year, at −20°C for up to 7 years, or at −70°C or lower for at least 7 years (34).

In the event that a commercial kit is used for polyomavirus testing, follow all manufacturer directions for collection, transport, and storage of specimens.

DIRECT EXAMINATION

Microscopy

Histologic assessment of renal biopsy material is the gold standard for the diagnosis of PVAN (25). PVAN is a tubulo-interstitial nephritis that resembles the pathology associated with rejection (40, 42, 90, 99). In contrast to rejection, characteristic basophilic, intranuclear viral inclusions are observed in PVAN (Fig. 2) (40, 90, 99). At least two tissue biopsy specimens must be examined prior to ruling out PVAN due to its patchy nature (25, 42). Papanicolaou stain of urine sediment from patients with PVAN reveals abnormal inclusion-bearing cells referred to as "decoy cells" due to their resemblance to malignant cancer cells (Fig. 2) (112).

Antemortem direct microscopic examination of tissue is performed less commonly for PML than for PVAN due to the risks involved in obtaining brain biopsy material. In brain biopsy specimens, PML appears as foci of demyelination containing macrophages, enlarged oligodendrocytes with basophilic or eosinophilic nuclear inclusions, and enlarged bizarre astrocytes with pleomorphic nuclei, typically in the subcortical white matter (Fig. 3) (3, 66).

Electron microscopy (EM) can be used in the diagnosis of PVAN and PML. Polyomaviruses appear as 40-nm-diameter virions packed in paracrystalline arrays or so-called "stick and ball" or "spaghetti and meatballs" structures (Fig. 2 and 3) (58, 73, 83). BKPyV virions are found by EM in aggregates called "Haufen" in urine of BMT patients (17) and PVAN patients (111). EM may be useful in the diagnosis of Merkel cell carcinoma, as polyomavirus particles have been observed in some cases (126).

Antigen Detection

Immunohistochemical staining of tissue sections using antibodies reactive with polyomavirus antigens has been employed as an adjunct to histopathological examination of tissue for the diagnosis of PVAN (60, 73, 78, 90) and PML (64, 83) (Fig. 2 and 3). In the case of PVAN, the demonstration of polyomavirus antigen can help in determining whether PVAN or rejection is the cause of renal pathology. Commercially available antibodies raised against the SV40 large T antigen that are cross-reactive with JCPyV and BKPyV antigens are most commonly used for this purpose (see http://www.biocompare.com for suppliers), although JCPyV- and BKPyV-specific antibodies have been reported.

Nucleic Acid Detection

ISH

In situ hybridization (ISH) using probes specific for BKPyV or JCPyV is an adjunct histopathologic method sometimes employed for the laboratory diagnosis of PVAN and PML (Fig. 3) (27, 60, 96, 123, 129). The addition of a PCR step may increase sensitivity (123). In the case of PVAN, as is the case for immunohistochemical staining, ISH can aid in discriminating PVAN from rejection by, in this case, localizing the presence of BKPyV nucleic acid to the site of pathology. Biotin- and digoxigenin-labeled BKPyV and

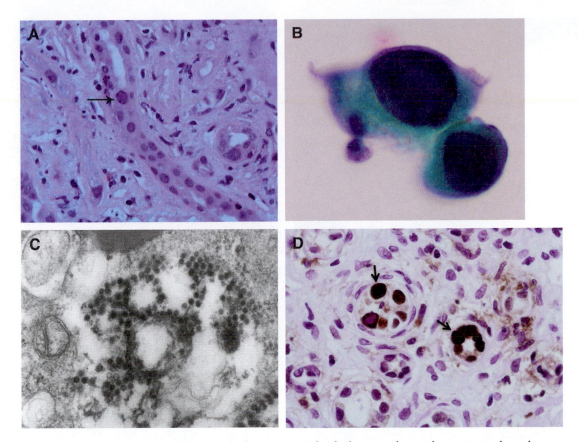

FIGURE 2   PVAN pathology. (A) Photomicrograph of a hematoxylin- and eosin-stained renal biopsy specimen showing nuclear inclusion (arrow) in an epithelial cell in a collecting duct (magnification, ×200). (B) Photomicrograph of Papanicolaou-stained decoy cells from the urine of a patient with PVAN demonstrating the typical enlarged basophilic nuclei (magnification, ×400). (C) Electron micrograph of a renal biopsy specimen showing arrays of typical 40- to 45-nm-diameter polyomavirus virions (magnification, ×12,000). (D) Photomicrograph of an immunostained renal biopsy specimen showing staining of homogenous type 1 nuclear inclusions (arrows) in epithelial cells of distal tubes. (Images courtesy of Helen Liapis, Washington University.)

JCPyV probes suitable for ISH are commercially available (Enzo Life Sciences, Plymouth Meeting, PA).

Southern Blotting

Although Southern blotting is primarily a research tool, the monoclonal integration of MCPyV in Merkel cell tumors can be demonstrated in genomic DNA extracted from Merkel cell tumors by standard Southern blotting techniques followed by hybridization with MCPyV probes (48, 110).

NAATs

There are currently no FDA-approved assays for the detection or quantification of polyomaviruses. Laboratories are therefore left to develop their own tests and confront various issues, including selecting suitable extraction methods, controlling for various biochemical steps in testing, and choosing amplification method/reagents. Information specific to polyomavirus nucleic acid amplification tests (NAATs) addressing these issues is provided below.

Template Extraction

The ideal performance characteristics for BKPyV and JCPyV NAATs are different. Monitoring for PVAN is usually performed with quantitative NAATs for BKPyV that must be reproducible (yielding results with low coefficients of variation) but not necessarily exquisitely sensitive, as low virus concentrations are not considered significant in most instances. In contrast, extremely sensitive assays for the detection of JCPyV in CSF are desirable for use in the diagnosis of PML. The nucleic acid extraction method should be selected to help meet these different performance criteria.

There exist in the peer-reviewed literature several evaluations of extraction methods that examine the ability of different methods to extract and purify BKPyV DNA from clinical specimens (9, 35, 45, 116). In general, there were minimal differences between the automated and manual methods examined for BKPyV-containing specimens, although at times differences were observed in the relative amounts of hands-on or turnaround time for the different methods.

Cross-contamination between specimens due to the extremely high levels of viruria that can occur is a major concern in BKPyV DNA extraction. No evidence of cross-contamination was observed with an automated extractor, suggesting that instrumentation is a viable option (12). Extraction may not be necessary if small sample volumes can be used in NAATs. Two microliters of unprocessed urine added to a 20-μl PCR mixture produced qualitative and quantitative BKPyV results that were not significantly different from those with samples extracted using a manual spin column method (93). A larger sample volume (5 μl) resulted in inhibition.

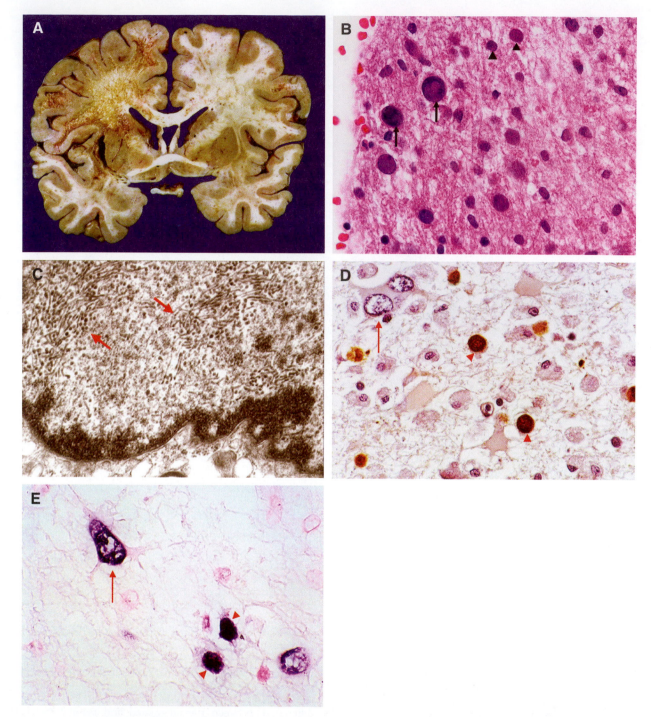

FIGURE 3 PML pathology. (A) Gross section of the brain from a patient with PML demonstrating asymmetric focal patches of involvement mostly confined to the white matter. (B) Photomicrograph of a hematoxylin- and eosin-stained section of the brain from a patient with PML showing "plum-colored" oligodendroglial nuclei (arrows), some with marginated chromatin and inclusions. Infected oligodendrocytes are markedly enlarged compared to more normal sized oligodendroglia (arrowheads) (magnification, ×400). (C) Electron micrograph of the brain from a patient with PML showing the "stick and ball" or "spaghetti and meatballs" (arrows) appearance of JCPyV in an oligodendrocyte (magnification, ×58,000). (D) Photomicrograph of an immunostained brain section demonstrating JCPyV proteins in enlarged immunoreactive oligodendroglial nuclei (arrowhead) but little involvement of atypical astrocytes (arrow) (magnification, ×600). (E) Photomicrograph of in situ hybridization using a labeled JCPyV probe showing a positive signal in oligodendrocytes (arrowheads) and an atypical labeled astrocyte (arrow) (magnification, ×1,000). (Images courtesy of Robert Schmidt, Washington University.)

Internal Controls

Internal controls are particularly important when testing urine specimens for polyomaviruses. Such controls can be used to detect, but cannot distinguish between, problems that arise during extraction, such as incomplete elimination of amplification inhibitors (the primary concern with urine specimens) or poor nucleic acid extraction efficiency. Bacteriophage-based amplification and extraction controls are commercially available (ZeptoMetrix, Buffalo, NY). A seven-member inhibition panel consisting of quantified substances recognized as being NAAT inhibitors of reactions is also available (AcroMetrix, Benicia, CA) and can be used during test validation to assess assay robustness in the presence of known inhibitors.

Positive Controls and Standards

All NAAT reactions require the use of positive and negative controls, while quantitative NAATs require an additional set of quantitated standards for use in constructing a standard curve. There are several options available for laboratories seeking controls and standards for use in NAATs for polyomaviruses. There are no commercially available materials for the newly identified polyomaviruses WUPyV, KIPyV, and MCPyV. For these viruses, laboratories can either identify positive specimens that can be used to clone viral DNA and produce controls/standards or contact researchers in the field for materials. BKPyV and JCPyV control materials are commercially available (whole virus and plasmids encoding entire virus genomes [American Type Culture Collection, Manassas, VA], quantified viral DNA [Advanced Biotechnologies, Inc., Columbia, MD], and quantitated inactivated BKPyV virions [Zepto-metrix]). It is worth noting here that there are currently no international reference quantitation standards for any of the HPyV.

Nucleic Acid Amplification Methods

Conventional laboratory methods for viral diagnosis such as cell culture, rapid antigen detection, and serology have significant drawbacks for the laboratory diagnosis of HPyV, while other methods such as immunohistochemical stains, electron microscopy and ISH are traditionally not performed in microbiology laboratories. Therefore, for the majority of diagnostic microbiology laboratories, nucleic acid amplification will be the method of choice for the detection and/or quantitation of HPyV in clinical specimens.

PCR has been used almost exclusively as a NAAT for the amplification of HPyV from clinical specimens, although alternative amplification formats have been described.

PCR methods can be classified as having either conventional or real-time formats. With conventional PCR assays, oligonucleotide primers amplify a specific DNA sequence, the products of which are then resolved by agarose gel electrophoresis, Southern hybridization, or microplate hybridization. In the case of real-time PCR, the assay usually includes some type of dye-labeled oligonucleotide which emits a characteristic fluorescence upon binding to the specifically amplified amplicon. Although both conventional and real-time PCR methods are capable of producing qualitative or quantitative results, real-time methods are much better suited for performing quantitative assays through the use of quantitation standards and instrument software. This feature, along with other advantages such as rapidity of results, less hands-on time, and a closed system less prone to contamination issues, has made real-time PCR the method of choice for many laboratories.

PCR assays detecting BKPyV and/or JCPyV using different formats have been described in the literature, including conventional assays with either gel detection (5, 89) or microplate colorimetric hybridization detection (86) of amplified products. Real-time PCR assays performed on the Roche Lightcycler platform (6, 44, 92, 106) as well as TaqMan probe-based assays (76, 82, 104) have also been described. A novel NAAT employing loop-mediated isothermal amplification has also been described for BKPyV (19). In the United States at this time, there are relatively few commercial NAAT products available for the detection of BKPyV and JCPyV (Table 2).

NAATs for BKPyV and JCPyV are challenging to design due in part to species-specific sequence variation. A recent study of seven different assays employing two different calibrators reported significant variability in quantification related to the calibrators employed and, more importantly, to primer and probe designs. The most important cause of error was nucleotide mismatch between viruses and amplification/detection oligonucleotides, particularly in the case of BKPyV subtypes III and IV (62). An assay using two modified primer/probe sets was better able to accurately quantify all subtypes detected in the study. Another study found significant nucleotide mismatches in up to 31% of the BKPyV strains when primers and probes from five published real-time PCR assays were aligned against 716 sequences, with subtypes IVa, IVb, and IVc being the most problematic (79). Sequence variability may also affect JCPyV NAATs. False-negative NAAT results (proved by amplification of an alternate target) have been reported in an individual with progressive central nervous system illness and polyomavirus-like particles by EM in brain biopsy

TABLE 2 Commercial nucleic acid amplification products for the detection of JCPyV and BKPyV

Virus(es)	Product (manufacturer)	Comment(s) (regulatory status)[a]
BKPyV	BK virus r-gene primers/probe (Argene, North Massapequa, NY)	Primer/probes for 5′ nuclease real-time assay targeting a sequence in the large T antigen (RUO)
	MGB Alert BK virus primers and probe (Nanogen, San Diego, CA)	Separate set of primers and MGB probe, capable of performing a melt curve analysis, targeting a sequence in the VP1 region (ASR)
	MultiCode-RTx BK virus primer mix (EraGen Biosciences, Madison, WI)	Set of primers targeting VP2 and VP3; combined with use of synthetic bases, allows for amplification and real-time detection (RUO)
JCPyV	JC virus r-gene primers/probe (Argene, North Massapequa, NY)	Primer/probes for 5′ nuclease real-time assay targeting a sequence in the large T antigen (RUO)
JCPyV/BKPyV	JC/BK consensus assay (Argene, North Massapequa, NY)	Amplification and differentiation of JCPyV and BKPyV through PCR and product hybridization to probes in a microwell plate (RUO)

[a]RUO, research use only; MGB, minor groove binder; ASR, analyte-specific reagent.

material (71). Attention to this issue in the assay design phase is important; broadly reactive real-time PCR reagents and less-variable target sequences have been described (62, 79, 92). Additionally, laboratories should align their primers and probes against new sequences at regular intervals to ensure detection of these viruses.

PCR methods have also been published for the newly identified HPyV, although due to the novelty of these agents relative to JCPyV and BKPyV, much less information is available regarding sequence variation. Conventional PCR methods are available (4, 53, 91) and real-time PCR assays employing TaqMan probes (14, 74, 87, 88) have been reported for WUPyV and KIPyV. Conventional PCR assays (48) and real-time PCR assays employing TaqMan probes have also been published (13, 54) for MCPyV. Conventional PCR primers for the detection of LPyV in human specimens have been described (37).

ISOLATION AND CULTURE PROCEDURES

JCPyV and BKPyV can be isolated and propagated in cell culture (8, 105, 107), although currently there is no role for these methods in the laboratory diagnosis of HPyV infections. JCPyV demonstrates restricted host range (human cells only) and can be grown in primary embryonic cells, human brain-derived cells (particularly astrocytes and oligodendrocyte precursors), and the permanent cell line SVG. BKPyV has an expanded host range compared to JCPyV and can grow in similar primary cell cultures, primary human embryonic kidney and lung cells, human foreskin fibroblasts, and continuous cell lines (HeLa and monkey cell lines such as CV-1 and Vero). The cytopathic effect of both viruses includes cellular translucency, nuclear enlargement, and gradual loss of the monolayer. Successful propagation often requires weeks and multiple rounds of blind passage. Most virus remains cell associated.

SEROLOGIC TESTS

Serologic tests for HPyV are primarily investigational tools with little role in the routine diagnosis of HPyV disease. The majority of assays are laboratory developed. For JCPyV and BKPyV, two types of serological tests have been described, including hemagglutination inhibition (HAI) and enzyme immunoassays (EIAs) employing either crude antigens or the use of virus-like particles (VLPs). Detection of an antibody response by HAI is based on the capacity of specific antiviral antibodies to inhibit the agglutination of human erythrocytes mediated by the viral structural VP1 proteins of JCPyV and BKPyV (107). The development of EIAs for the detection of antibodies to both BKPyV and JCPyV was made possible when engineered cell lines capable of producing adequate amounts of JCPyV antigen were developed (51). A comparison of EIA and HAI demonstrated that antibody titers measured by the two assay formats were significantly statistically correlated, although EIA titers were higher (57). More recently, VLPs have been used as antigens in EIAs for the detection of antibodies. VLPs are empty particles that retain the full antigenicity of intact virions. They form spontaneously when viral capsid proteins are expressed in certain systems and are preferred as antigen sources for EIAs because they contain native conformational epitopes that may be missing when other forms of viral antigens are employed (121).

Serologic tests for HPyV are used primarily for seroepidemiological studies and not for diagnosis of infection, although

a study has demonstrated a correlation between kidney donor BKPyV antibody titers and infection in the transplant recipient (26). Despite the fact that JCPyV and BKPyV are closely related, it appears that the antigenic epitopes responsible for the human antibody response are not cross-reactive and antibody tests can discriminate between infections by these two viruses (57). In contrast, it appears that seroreactivity to SV40 is due largely to cross-reactivity with BKPyV (69, 121, 122). Seroreactivity to LPyV does not appear to be due to cross-reactivity with BKPyV or JCPyV (121). A VLP system for detecting seroreactivity to MCPyV has been reported (117). Seroepidemiological studies for WUPyV and KIPyV have not yet been performed. Data from HPyV seroepidemiological studies may need to be reexamined in light of the newly identified HPyV to understand potential serological cross-reactions between these agents.

ANTIVIRAL SUSCEPTIBILITIES

For PML, a number of antiviral agents have been examined, including cidofovir, an acyclic nucleoside phosphonate; topotecan, an inhibitor of DNA topoisomerase I; leflunomide, an immunosuppressive agent with antiviral properties; vidarabine (ARA-A) and cytarabine (ARA-C), synthetic nucleosides that inhibit viral DNA polymerases; and alpha interferon (103). Following evidence that JCPyV uses the serotonin 2A receptor to infect cells in the central nervous system, interest has been shown in investigating drugs, such as risperidone, which bind to this receptor and are approved for treatment of certain neuropsychiatric diseases (49), although another study reported that infection of cells by JCPyV was independent of the serotonin receptor (31). More recently, a study that examined a collection of 2,000 currently approved drugs found evidence that the antimalarial drug mefloquine had activity against JCPyV in vitro, with the authors reporting that a clinical trial of the drug for treatment of PML was ongoing (30). For some of these agents, antiviral activity against JCPyV has been demonstrated in vitro, and encouraging results have at times been reported in case reports. However, studies have been hampered by the fact that PML is a rare disease and the majority of patients are HIV infected and receiving potentially confounding anti-HIV therapy, making it difficult to evaluate the effect of the drug being studied. Unfortunately, most clinical studies of antiviral treatments for PML have failed to demonstrate a consistent benefit (10, 39, 52, 56, 80) and there are no currently FDA-approved drugs for the treatment of this devastating disease. Current approaches to therapy include having optimal highly active antiretroviral therapy (HAART) for HIV-infected patients, with the aim of increasing CD4 cell counts and decreasing the HIV RNA level (124). For non-HIV-infected individuals, reversal or amelioration of the immunosuppressed state ultimately responsible for the disease is recommended (10).

Many of the same agents studied as possible antiviral treatments for PML have also been investigated for the treatment of BKPyV PVAN and, less commonly, hemorrhagic cystitis. In addition to these compounds, fluoroquinolone antibiotics and intravenous immunoglobulin have also been studied. Similar to the situation with the development of antiviral drugs for the treatment of PML, there are currently no FDA-approved agents for the treatment of BKPyV diseases. The lack of antivirals can be attributed to several factors, including the need for prospective randomized controlled studies, the nephrotoxicity exhibited by a number of the drugs, and the confounding variable of the near universal approach of improving immune function in transplant recipients showing signs of BKPyV disease by some form of reduction in the level of immunosuppression. A recent review of the literature for antiviral treatment of PVAN found a total of only 184 patients in 27 published studies examining the use of cidofovir, 189 patients in 18 studies of the use of leflunomide, and 14 patients in 2 studies of the use of fluoroquinolones, with the authors concluding that there was no consensus on the use of antivirals for PVAN (59). Other reviews have come to similar conclusions and underscore the fact that, until larger clinical studies are performed, the mainstay of current therapy for PVAN is the reduction of immunosuppression, although in cases where a patient is in danger of losing a graft to PVAN, a course of an antiviral may be of benefit (98, 101, 127).

EVALUATION, INTERPRETATION, AND REPORTING OF RESULTS

The current trend in laboratory testing for PVAN is to monitor levels of the BKPyV in urine and blood and to reduce immunosuppression when viruria or viremia reaches levels that predict progression to disease. Guidelines published in 2005 for monitoring BKPyV viruria and viremia in renal transplant recipients recommended that (i) patients be screened for viruria every 3 months for the first 2 years after the transplant and (ii) if viruria is detected, then a quantitative NAAT should be employed to monitor urine or plasma, with sustained high levels of viruria ($>10^7$ copies/ml) or viremia ($>10^4$ copies/ml) triggering a renal biopsy (60). Testing for BKPyV viruria has a high negative predictive value and a variable positive predictive value for the development of PVAN, with sustained high levels of viruria ($>10^7$ copies/ml) having a positive predictive value of up to 67% (127). Sustained high levels of BKPyV viruria are frequently followed by the appearance of viremia. The majority of individuals with PVAN have been found to have BKPyV viremia, with the positive predictive value for viremia being about 60% for the development of PVAN (127).

These recommendations are helpful in directing NAAT use and interpretation of NAAT results. However, implementing them is complicated by interlaboratory variability in BKPyV quantification due to the lack of internationally recognized standards that can serve as calibrators and by the use of assays that may not optimally detect and quantify all BKPyV strains. For example, in 2008, the College of American Pathologists sent four proficiency samples to laboratories performing quantitative BKPyV. All 48 laboratories (38 using user-developed assays and 10 using commercial tests) that tested the BKPyV DNA-negative sample reported a negative result. When BKPyV-positive specimens were tested, the results were less encouraging. The sample producing the most variation was tested by 41 laboratories with the following results: mean, 700,946 copies/ml; standard deviation (SD), 1,729,692 copies/ml; coefficient of variation (CV), 246.8%; range, 129 to 10,400,000 copies/ml. For 35 laboratories that also reported log-transformed data on this specimen, the results were as follows: mean, 4.806; SD, 1.231; range, 1.02 to 6.51. The BKPyV-positive specimen with the lowest CV produced the following results: mean, 277,288 copies/ml; SD, 284,990; CV, 102.8%; range, 7,800 to 945,000 copies/ml. Obviously, there is a significant amount of interlaboratory variation in quantitative BKPyV results.

Until the problems of assay variation are resolved, laboratories should work toward the consistent intralaboratory

performance of their own assays. Careful coordination between physicians and the laboratory can result in the establishment of in-house viruria and viremia thresholds for adjusting immunosuppression regimens. The additional effort this requires is clearly worthwhile, since successful implementation of testing algorithms has been shown to significantly reduce PVAN incidence (29, 98).

To draw accurate conclusions regarding the course of infection, patients should be monitored at one site if possible. Sequential measurements by different laboratories will be difficult to interpret given the likelihood of interlaboratory differences in BKPyV quantification. The laboratory should educate physicians and transplant coordinators about this issue.

In cases where PVAN is suspected and BKPyV titers are negative or low, the possibility of a false negative should be considered, due potentially to sequence mismatches between the virus and real-time PCR primers or probe. Alternatively, it may be possible that JCPyV is responsible, in which case it may be best to try to identify this virus either in biopsy material by histological methods or in plasma. Shedding of this virus is common in the urine and may not indicate the presence of a causative organism. Unfortunately, guidelines for interpreting JCPyV levels in peripheral blood are not available.

Quantitative NAATs of urine from BMT recipients to either predict the development of or diagnose hemorrhagic cystitis may be useful. High levels of viruria ($>1 \times 10^9$/ml) can be seen in hemorrhagic cystitis due to BKPyV (24, 75); a negative result suggests another cause of this condition. The interpretation of BKPyV viruria is complicated by the fact that BMT recipients frequently excrete BKPyV in their urine and by the lack of guidelines for thresholds that can be applied to predicting or diagnosing disease. Studies have yielded variable data. One report suggested that viruria of 10^9 to 10^{10} or more copies/ml or an increase of ≥ 3 $\log_{10}$ relative to baseline levels may help implicate BKPyV as the cause (43). Another found that levels of BKPyV viremia of $>10^4$ copies/ml were associated with hemorrhagic cystitis (43); however, this relationship was not observed in a similar study (75).

Serology and culture have little role in the diagnosis of PML. Most individuals are seropositive for JCPyV by adulthood; culture requires special cells and prolonged incubation and is insensitive. Therefore, the preferred diagnostic test for PML is JCPyV-specific NAAT. The detection of JCPyV DNA in CSF is distinctly abnormal. In combination with appropriate imaging studies and patient history, it is strongly suggestive of PML. JCPyV NAAT sensitivities in CSF range from 42 to 100%, with most between 70 and 80%; specificities range from 92 to 100% (32). False-negative JCPyV PCR results in patients with PML, possibly due to mismatches between primers and probes and target sequences (71, 109), have been observed. Additionally, decreased PCR sensitivity has been reported in the HAART era (89.5% pre-HAART versus 57.5% HAART, with the negative predictive value falling from 98 to 89%) (81). These findings underscore the fact that a negative JCPyV result cannot rule out the presence of PML. It may be advantageous to retest CSF with a different NAAT if the initial result is negative in a presumptive case of PML.

Because of the devastating nature of PML, laboratory testing methods have been explored either to help identify patients at increased risk for developing PML or to provide a prognosis for those patients who have already been diagnosed. A single qualitative test for JCPyV DNA in urine and blood does not appear to be useful for the identification of patients at risk of PML, as demonstrated by studies of individuals with HIV and those with immunosuppression unrelated to HIV (including immunomodulatory therapy with natalizumab) (33, 70), and is therefore not recommended. Persistent viruria and rising urine viral loads have been found to be associated with the development of PML in HIV-positive patients (55). The utility of these approaches awaits confirmation by further studies.

Quantitative PCR for the determination of the JCPyV load in the CSF of PML patients has been reported to be potentially useful as a prognostic measure for disease progression. However, because of small study sizes and the lack of standardized quantitative JCPyV NAATs, it has been difficult to formulate guidelines for threshold CSF viral loads. Different reports have indicated, roughly, that JCPyV CSF viral loads of between 10^4 and 10^5 copies/ml separate those PML patients whose disease progresses quickly from those whose illness is stable or progressing more slowly (28, 38, 70, 128).

Laboratory testing for the newly identified HPyV WUPyV, KIPyV, and MCPyV, as well as SV40 and LPyV, is considered investigational at this time, so it is not possible to offer meaningful interpretations for test results for these agents.

REFERENCES

1. **Abed, Y., D. Wang, and G. Boivin.** 2007. WU polyomavirus in children, Canada. *Emerg. Infect. Dis.* **13:**1939–1941.
2. **Abedi Kiasari, B., P. J. Vallely, C. E. Corless, M. Al-Hammadi, and P. E. Klapper.** 2008. Age-related pattern of KI and WU polyomavirus infection. *J. Clin. Virol.* **43:**123–125.
3. **Ahsan, N., and K. V. Shah.** 2006. Polyomaviruses and human diseases. *Adv. Exp. Med. Biol.* **577:**1–18.
4. **Allander, T., K. Andreasson, S. Gupta, A. Bjerkner, G. Bogdanovic, M. A. Persson, T. Dalianis, T. Ramqvist, and B. Andersson.** 2007. Identification of a third human polyomavirus. *J. Virol.* **81:**4130–4136.
5. **Arthur, R. R., S. Dagostin, and K. V. Shah.** 1989. Detection of BK virus and JC virus in urine and brain tissue by the polymerase chain reaction. *J. Clin. Microbiol.* **27:**1174–1179.
6. **Beck, R. C., D. J. Kohn, M. J. Tuohy, R. A. Prayson, B. Yen-Lieberman, and G. W. Procop.** 2004. Detection of polyoma virus in brain tissue of patients with progressive multifocal leukoencephalopathy by real-time PCR and pyrosequencing. *Diagn. Mol. Pathol.* **13:**15–21.
7. **Becker, J. C., R. Houben, S. Ugurel, U. Trefzer, C. Pfohler, and D. Schrama.** 2009. MC polyomavirus is frequently present in Merkel cell carcinoma of European patients. *J. Investig. Dermatol.* **129:**248–250.
8. **Beckmann, A. M., and K. V. Shah.** 1983. Propagation and primary isolation of JCV and BKV in urinary epithelial cell cultures. *Prog. Clin. Biol. Res.* **105:**3–14.
9. **Bergallo, M., C. Costa, G. Gribaudo, S. Tarallo, S. Baro, A. Negro Ponzi, and R. Cavallo.** 2006. Evaluation of six methods for extraction and purification of viral DNA from urine and serum samples. *New Microbiol.* **29:**111–119.
10. **Berger, J. R.** 2000. Progressive multifocal leukoencephalopathy. *Curr. Treat. Options Neurol.* **2:**361–368.
11. **Berger, J. R., C. S. Miller, Y. Mootoor, S. A. Avdiushko, R. J. Kryscio, and H. Zhu.** 2006. JC virus detection in bodily fluids: clues to transmission. *Clin. Infect. Dis.* **43:**e9–e12.
12. **Beuselinck, K., M. van Ranst, and J. van Eldere.** 2005. Automated extraction of viral-pathogen RNA and DNA for high-throughput quantitative real-time PCR. *J. Clin. Microbiol.* **43:**5541–5546.
13. **Bialasiewicz, S., S. B. Lambert, D. M. Whiley, M. D. Nissen, and T. P. Sloots.** 2009. Merkel cell polyomavirus DNA in respiratory specimens from children and adults. *Emerg. Infect. Dis.* **15:**492–494.
14. **Bialasiewicz, S., D. M. Whiley, S. B. Lambert, A. Gould, M. D. Nissen, and T. P. Sloots.** 2007. Development and evaluation of real-time PCR assays for the detection of the newly identified KI and WU polyomaviruses. *J. Clin. Virol.* **40:**9–14.
15. **Bialasiewicz, S., D. M. Whiley, S. B. Lambert, K. Jacob, C. Bletchly, D. Wang, M. D. Nissen, and T. P. Sloots.** 2008. Presence of the newly discovered human polyomaviruses KI and WU in Australian patients with acute respiratory tract infection. *J. Clin. Virol.* **41:**63–68.
16. **Bialasiewicz, S., D. M. Whiley, S. B. Lambert, D. Wang, M. D. Nissen, and T. P. Sloots.** 2007. A newly reported human polyomavirus, KI virus, is present in the respiratory tract of Australian children. *J. Clin. Virol.* **40:**15–18.
17. **Biel, S. S., A. Nitsche, A. Kurth, W. Siegert, M. Ozel, and H. R. Gelderblom.** 2004. Detection of human polyomaviruses in urine from bone marrow transplant patients: comparison of electron microscopy with PCR. *Clin. Chem.* **50:**306–312.
18. **Bijol, V., M. Willby, D. Erdman, C. Paddock, S. Zaki, C. Goldsmith, M. DeLeon-Carnes, B. Batten, T. Jones, W.-J. Shieh, and M. Menegus.** 2009. WU polyomavirus infection in an immunocompromised host: histological, ultrastructural and molecular evidence of multi-organ involvement, abstr. T58. *In Twenty-Fifth Annual Clinical Virology Symposium.* Daytona Beach, FL.
19. **Bista, B. R., C. Ishwad, R. M. Wadowsky, P. Manna, P. S. Randhawa, G. Gupta, M. Adhikari, R. Tyagi, G. Gasper, and A. Vats.** 2007. Development of a loop-mediated isothermal amplification assay for rapid detection of BK virus. *J. Clin. Microbiol.* **45:**1581–1587.
20. **Bofill-Mas, S., N. Albinana-Gimenez, P. Clemente-Casares, A. Hundesa, J. Rodriguez-Manzano, A. Allard, M. Calvo, and R. Girones.** 2006. Quantification and stability of human adenoviruses and polyomavirus JCPyV in wastewater matrices. *Appl. Environ. Microbiol.* **72:**7894–7896.
21. **Bofill-Mas, S., M. Formiga-Cruz, P. Clemente-Casares, F. Calafell, and R. Girones.** 2001. Potential transmission of human polyomaviruses through the gastrointestinal tract after exposure to virions or viral DNA. *J. Virol.* **75:**10290–10299.
22. **Bofill-Mas, S., and R. Girones.** 2003. Role of the environment in the transmission of JC virus. *J. Neurovirol.* **9**(Suppl. 1):54–58.
23. **Bofill-Mas, S., S. Pina, and R. Girones.** 2000. Documenting the epidemiologic patterns of polyomaviruses in human populations by studying their presence in urban sewage. *Appl. Environ. Microbiol.* **66:**238–245.
24. **Bogdanovic, G., P. Priftakis, G. Giraud, M. Kuzniar, R. Ferraldeschi, P. Kokhaei, H. Mellstedt, M. Remberger, P. Ljungman, J. Winiarski, and T. Dalianis.** 2004. Association between a high BK virus load in urine samples of patients with graft-versus-host disease and development of hemorrhagic cystitis after hematopoietic stem cell transplantation. *J. Clin. Microbiol.* **42:**5394–5396.
25. **Bohl, D. L., and D. C. Brennan.** 2007. BK virus nephropathy and kidney transplantation. *Clin. J. Am. Soc. Nephrol.* **2**(Suppl. 1):S36–S46.
26. **Bohl, D. L., G. A. Storch, C. Ryschkewitsch, M. Gaudreault-Keener, M. A. Schnitzler, E. O. Major, and D. C. Brennan.** 2005. Donor origin of BK virus in renal transplantation and role of HLA C7 in susceptibility to sustained BK viremia. *Am. J. Transplant.* **5:**2213–2221.
27. **Bonvoisin, C., L. Weekers, P. Xhignesse, S. Grosch, M. Milicevic, and J. M. Krzesinski.** 2008. Polyomavirus in renal transplantation: a hot problem. *Transplantation* **85:**S42–S48.
28. **Bossolasco, S., G. Calori, F. Moretti, A. Boschini, D. Bertelli, M. Mena, S. Gerevini, A. Bestetti, R. Pedale, S. Sala, A. Lazzarin, and P. Cinque.** 2005. Prognostic significance of JC virus DNA levels in cerebrospinal fluid of patients with HIV-associated progressive multifocal leukoencephalopathy. *Clin. Infect. Dis.* **40:**738–744.
29. **Brennan, D. C., I. Agha, D. L. Bohl, M. A. Schnitzler, K. L. Hardinger, M. Lockwood, S. Torrence, R. Schuessler, T. Roby, M. Gaudreault-Keener, and G. A. Storch.** 2005. Incidence of BK with tacrolimus versus cyclosporine and impact of preemptive immunosuppression reduction. *Am. J. Transplant.* **5:**582–594.
30. **Brickelmaier, M., A. Lugovskoy, R. Kartikeyan, M. M. Reviriego-Mendoza, N. Allaire, K. Simon, R. J. Frisque,**

and L. Gorelik. 2009. Identification and characterization of mefloquine efficacy against JC virus in vitro. *Antimicrob. Agents Chemother.* **53**:1840–1849.

31. Chapagain, M. L., S. Verma, F. Mercier, R. Yanagihara, and V. R. Nerurkar. 2007. Polyomavirus JC infects human brain microvascular endothelial cells independent of serotonin receptor 2A. *Virology* **364**:55–63.

32. Cinque, P., P. Scarpellini, L. Vago, A. Linde, and A. Lazzarin. 1997. Diagnosis of central nervous system complications in HIV-infected patients: cerebrospinal fluid analysis by the polymerase chain reaction. *AIDS* **11**:1–17.

33. Clifford, D. B. 2008. Natalizumab and PML: a risky business? *Gut* **57**:1347–1349.

34. Clinical and Laboratory Standards Institute. 2005. *Collection, Transport, Preparation, and Storage of Specimens for Molecular Methods: Approved Guideline. CLSI document MM13-A, vol. 25.* Clinical and Laboratory Standards Institute, Wayne, PA.

35. Cook, L., E. E. Atienza, A. Bagabag, R. M. Obrigewitch, and K. R. Jerome. 2009. Comparison of methods for extraction of viral DNA from cellular specimens. *Diagn. Microbiol. Infect. Dis.* **64**:45–50.

36. Dall, A., and S. Hariharan. 2008. BK virus nephritis after renal transplantation. *Clin. J. Am. Soc. Nephrol.* **3**(Suppl. 2):S68–S75.

37. Delbue, S., S. Tremolada, E. Branchetti, F. Elia, E. Gualco, E. Marchioni, R. Maserati, and P. Ferrante. 2008. First identification and molecular characterization of lymphotropic polyomavirus in peripheral blood from patients with leukoencephalopathies. *J. Clin. Microbiol.* **46**:2461–2462.

38. Delbue, S., S. Tremolada, and P. Ferrante. 2008. Application of molecular tools for the diagnosis of central nervous system infections. *Neurol. Sci.* **29**(Suppl. 2):S283–S285.

39. De Luca, A., A. Ammassari, P. Pezzotti, P. Cinque, J. Gasnault, J. Berenguer, S. Di Giambenedetto, A. Cingolani, Y. Taoufik, P. Miralles, C. M. Marra, and A. Antinori. 2008. Cidofovir in addition to antiretroviral treatment is not effective for AIDS-associated progressive multifocal leukoencephalopathy: a multicohort analysis. *AIDS* **22**:1759–1767.

40. Drachenberg, C. B., C. O. Beskow, C. B. Cangro, P. M. Bourquin, A. Simsir, J. Fink, M. R. Weir, D. K. Klassen, S. T. Bartlett, and J. C. Papadimitriou. 1999. Human polyoma virus in renal allograft biopsies: morphological findings and correlation with urine cytology. *Hum. Pathol.* **30**:970–977.

41. Drachenberg, C. B., H. H. Hirsch, J. C. Papadimitriou, R. Gosert, R. K. Wali, R. Munivenkatappa, J. Nogueira, C. B. Cangro, A. Haririan, S. Mendley, and E. Ramos. 2007. Polyomavirus BK versus JC replication and nephropathy in renal transplant recipients: a prospective evaluation. *Transplantation* **84**:323–330.

42. Drachenberg, C. B., J. C. Papadimitriou, H. H. Hirsch, R. Wali, C. Crowder, J. Nogueira, C. B. Cangro, S. Mendley, A. Mian, and E. Ramos. 2004. Histological patterns of polyomavirus nephropathy: correlation with graft outcome and viral load. *Am. J. Transplant.* **4**:2082–2092.

43. Dropulic, L. K., and R. J. Jones. 2008. Polyomavirus BK infection in blood and marrow transplant recipients. *Bone Marrow Transplant.* **41**:11–18.

44. Dumonceaux, T. J., C. Mesa, and A. Severini. 2008. Internally controlled triplex quantitative PCR assay for human polyomaviruses JC and BK. *J. Clin. Microbiol.* **46**:2829–2836.

45. Dundas, N., N. K. Leos, M. Mitui, P. Revell, and B. B. Rogers. 2008. Comparison of automated nucleic acid extraction methods with manual extraction. *J. Mol. Diagn.* **10**:311–316.

46. Eng, P. M., B. R. Turnbull, S. F. Cook, J. E. Davidson, T. Kurth, and J. D. Seeger. 2006. Characteristics and antecedents of progressive multifocal leukoencephalopathy in an insured population. *Neurology* **67**:884–886.

47. Erard, V., H. W. Kim, L. Corey, A. Limaye, M. L. Huang, D. Myerson, C. Davis, and M. Boeckh. 2005. BK DNA viral load in plasma: evidence for an association with hemorrhagic cystitis in allogeneic hematopoietic cell transplant recipients. *Blood* **106**:1130–1132.

48. Feng, H., M. Shuda, Y. Chang, and P. S. Moore. 2008. Clonal integration of a polyomavirus in human Merkel cell carcinoma. *Science* **319**:1096–1100.

49. Focosi, D., R. Fazzi, D. Montanaro, M. Emdin, and M. Petrini. 2007. Progressive multifocal leukoencephalopathy in a haploidentical stem cell transplant recipient: a clinical, neuroradiological and virological response after treatment with risperidone. *Antivir. Res.* **74**:156–158.

50. Foulongne, V., N. Kluger, O. Dereure, N. Brieu, B. Guillot, and M. Segondy. 2008. Merkel cell polyomavirus and Merkel cell carcinoma, France. *Emerg. Infect. Dis.* **14**:1491–1493.

51. Frye, S., C. Trebst, U. Dittmer, H. Petry, M. Bodemer, G. Hunsmann, T. Weber, and W. Luke. 1997. Efficient production of JC virus in SVG cells and the use of purified viral antigens for analysis of specific humoral and cellular immune response. *J. Virol. Methods* **63**:81–92.

52. Gasnault, J., Y. Taoufik, C. Goujard, P. Kousignian, K. Abbed, F. Boue, E. Dussaix, and J. F. Delfraissy. 1999. Prolonged survival without neurological improvement in patients with AIDS-related progressive multifocal leukoencephalopathy on potent combined antiretroviral therapy. *J. Neurovirol.* **5**:421–429.

53. Gaynor, A. M., M. D. Nissen, D. M. Whiley, I. M. Mackay, S. B. Lambert, G. Wu, D. C. Brennan, G. A. Storch, T. P. Sloots, and D. Wang. 2007. Identification of a novel polyomavirus from patients with acute respiratory tract infections. *PLoS Pathog.* **3**:e64.

54. Goh, S., C. Lindau, A. Tiveljung-Lindell, and T. Allander. 2009. Merkel cell polyomavirus in respiratory tract secretions. *Emerg. Infect. Dis.* **15**:489–491.

55. Grabowski, M. K., R. P. Viscidi, J. B. Margolick, L. P. Jacobson, and K. V. Shah. 2009. Investigation of pre-diagnostic virological markers for progressive multifocal leukoencephalopathy in human immunodeficiency virus-infected patients. *J. Med. Virol.* **81**:1140–1150.

56. Hall, C. D., U. Dafni, D. Simpson, D. Clifford, P. E. Wetherill, B. Cohen, J. McArthur, H. Hollander, C. Yainnoutsos, E. Major, L. Millar, J. Timpone, et al. 1998. Failure of cytarabine in progressive multifocal leukoencephalopathy associated with human immunodeficiency virus infection. *N. Engl. J. Med.* **338**:1345–1351.

57. Hamilton, R. S., M. Gravell, and E. O. Major. 2000. Comparison of antibody titers determined by hemagglutination inhibition and enzyme immunoassay for JC virus and BK virus. *J. Clin. Microbiol.* **38**:105–109.

58. Herrera, G. A., R. Veeramachaneni, and E. A. Turbat-Herrera. 2005. Electron microscopy in the diagnosis of BK-polyoma virus infection in the transplanted kidney. *Ultrastruct. Pathol.* **29**:469–474.

59. Hilton, R., and C. Y. Tong. 2008. Antiviral therapy for polyomavirus-associated nephropathy after renal transplantation. *J. Antimicrob. Chemother.* **62**:855–859.

60. Hirsch, H. H., D. C. Brennan, C. B. Drachenberg, F. Ginevri, J. Gordon, A. P. Limaye, M. J. Mihatsch, V. Nickeleit, E. Ramos, P. Randhawa, R. Shapiro, J. Steiger, M. Suthanthiran, and J. Trofe. 2005. Polyomavirus-associated nephropathy in renal transplantation: interdisciplinary analyses and recommendations. *Transplantation* **79**:1277–1286.

61. Hirsch, H. H., W. Knowles, M. Dickenmann, J. Passweg, T. Klimkait, M. J. Mihatsch, and J. Steiger. 2002. Prospective study of polyomavirus type BK replication and nephropathy in renal-transplant recipients. *N. Engl. J. Med.* **347**:488–496.

62. Hoffman, N. G., L. Cook, E. E. Atienza, A. P. Limaye, and K. R. Jerome. 2008. Marked variability of BK virus load measurement using quantitative real-time PCR among commonly used assays. *J. Clin. Microbiol.* **46**:2671–2680.

63. Imperiale, M. J., and E. O. Major. 2007. Polyomaviruses, p. 2263–2298. *In* D. M. Knipe, P. M. Howley, D. E. Griffin, M. A. Martin, R. A. Lamb, B. Roizman, and S. E. Straus (ed.), *Fields Virology*, 5th ed., vol. 2. Lippincott Williams & Wilkins, Philadelphia, PA.

64. Jochum, W., T. Weber, S. Frye, G. Hunsmann, W. Luke, and A. Aguzzi. 1997. Detection of JC virus by anti-VP1

immunohistochemistry in brains with progressive multifocal leukoencephalopathy. *Acta Neuropathol.* **94:**226–231.

65. **Kazory, A., D. Ducloux, J. M. Chalopin, R. Angonin, B. Fontaniere, and H. Moret.** 2003. The first case of JC virus allograft nephropathy. *Transplantation* **76:**1653–1655.

66. **Khalili, K., J. Gordon, and M. K. White.** 2006. The polyomavirus, JCV and its involvement in human disease. *Adv. Exp. Med. Biol.* **577:**274–287.

67. **Kleinschmidt-DeMasters, B. K., and K. L. Tyler.** 2005. Progressive multifocal leukoencephalopathy complicating treatment with natalizumab and interferon beta-1a for multiple sclerosis. *N. Engl. J. Med.* **353:**369–374.

68. **Knowles, W. A.** 2006. Discovery and epidemiology of the human polyomaviruses BK virus (BKV) and JC virus (JCV). *Adv. Exp. Med. Biol.* **577:**19–45.

69. **Knowles, W. A., P. Pipkin, N. Andrews, A. Vyse, P. Minor, D. W. Brown, and E. Miller.** 2003. Population-based study of antibody to the human polyomaviruses BKV and JCV and the simian polyomavirus SV40. *J. Med. Virol.* **71:**115–123.

70. **Koralnik, I. J., D. Boden, V. X. Mai, C. I. Lord, and N. L. Letvin.** 1999. JC virus DNA load in patients with and without progressive multifocal leukoencephalopathy. *Neurology* **52:**253–260.

71. **Landry, M. L., T. Eid, S. Bannykh, and E. Major.** 2008. False negative PCR despite high levels of JC virus DNA in spinal fluid: implications for diagnostic testing. *J. Clin. Virol.* **43:**247–249.

72. **Langer-Gould, A., S. W. Atlas, A. J. Green, A. W. Bollen, and D. Pelletier.** 2005. Progressive multifocal leukoencephalopathy in a patient treated with natalizumab. *N. Engl. J. Med.* **353:**375–381.

73. **Latif, S., F. Zaman, R. Veeramachaneni, L. Jones, N. Uribe-Uribe, E. A. Turbat-Herrera, and G. A. Herrera.** 2007. BK polyomavirus in renal transplants: role of electron microscopy and immunostaining in detecting early infection. *Ultrastruct. Pathol.* **31:**199–207.

74. **Le, B. M., L. M. Demertzis, G. Wu, R. J. Tibbets, R. Buller, M. Q. Arens, A. M. Gaynor, G. A. Storch, and D. Wang.** 2007. Clinical and epidemiologic characterization of WU polyomavirus infection, St. Louis, Missouri. *Emerg. Infect. Dis.* **13:**1936–1938.

75. **Leung, A. Y., C. K. Suen, A. K. Lie, R. H. Liang, K. Y. Yuen, and Y. L. Kwong.** 2001. Quantification of polyoma BK viruria in hemorrhagic cystitis complicating bone marrow transplantation. *Blood* **98:**1971–1978.

76. **Limaye, A. P., K. R. Jerome, C. S. Kuhr, J. Ferrenberg, M. L. Huang, C. L. Davis, L. Corey, and C. L. Marsh.** 2001. Quantitation of BK virus load in serum for the diagnosis of BK virus-associated nephropathy in renal transplant recipients. *J. Infect. Dis.* **183:**1669–1672.

77. **Lin, F., M. Zheng, H. Li, C. Zheng, X. Li, G. Rao, F. Wu, and A. Zeng.** 2008. WU polyomavirus in children with acute lower respiratory tract infections, China. *J. Clin. Virol.* **42:**94–102.

78. **Liptak, P., E. Kemeny, and B. Ivanyi.** 2006. Primer: histopathology of polyomavirus-associated nephropathy in renal allografts. *Nat. Clin. Pract. Nephrol.* **2:**631–636.

79. **Luo, C., M. Bueno, J. Kant, and P. Randhawa.** 2008. Biologic diversity of polyomavirus BK genomic sequences: implications for molecular diagnostic laboratories. *J. Med. Virol.* **80:**1850–1857.

80. **Marra, C. M., N. Rajicic, D. E. Barker, B. A. Cohen, D. Clifford, M. J. Donovan Post, A. Ruiz, B. C. Bowen, M. L. Huang, J. Queen-Baker, J. Andersen, S. Kelly, and S. Shriver.** 2002. A pilot study of cidofovir for progressive multifocal leukoencephalopathy in AIDS. *AIDS* **16:**1791–1797.

81. **Marzocchetti, A., S. Di Giambenedetto, A. Cingolani, A. Ammassari, R. Cauda, and A. De Luca.** 2005. Reduced rate of diagnostic positive detection of JC virus DNA in cerebrospinal fluid in cases of suspected progressive multifocal leukoencephalopathy in the era of potent antiretroviral therapy. *J. Clin. Microbiol.* **43:**4175–4177.

82. **McNees, A. L., Z. S. White, P. Zanwar, R. A. Vilchez, and J. S. Butel.** 2005. Specific and quantitative detection of human polyomaviruses BKV, JCV, and SV40 by real time PCR. *J. Clin. Virol.* **34:**52–62.

83. **Mesquita, R., M. Bjorkholm, M. Ekman, G. Bogdanovic, and P. Biberfeld.** 1996. Polyomavirus-infected oligodendrocytes and macrophages within astrocytes in progressive multifocal leukoencephalopathy (PML). *APMIS* **104:**153–160.

84. **Monaco, M. C., W. J. Atwood, M. Gravell, C. S. Tornatore, and E. O. Major.** 1996. JC virus infection of hematopoietic progenitor cells, primary B lymphocytes, and tonsillar stromal cells: implications for viral latency. *J. Virol.* **70:**7004–7012.

85. **Monaco, M. C., P. N. Jensen, J. Hou, L. C. Durham, and E. O. Major.** 1998. Detection of JC virus DNA in human tonsil tissue: evidence for site of initial viral infection. *J. Virol.* **72:**9918–9923.

86. **Moret, H., V. Brodard, C. Barranger, N. Jovenin, M. Joannes, and L. Andreoletti.** 2006. New commercially available PCR and microplate hybridization assay for detection and differentiation of human polyomaviruses JC and BK in cerebrospinal fluid, serum, and urine samples. *J. Clin. Microbiol.* **44:**1305–1309.

87. **Mourez, T., A. Bergeron, P. Ribaud, C. Scieux, R. P. de Latour, A. Tazi, G. Socie, F. Simon, and J. LeGoff.** 2009. Polyomaviruses KI and WU in immunocompromised patients with respiratory disease. *Emerg. Infect. Dis.* **15:**107–109.

88. **Neske, F., K. Blessing, A. Prottel, F. Ullrich, H. W. Kreth, and B. Weissbrich.** 2009. Detection of WU polyomavirus DNA by real-time PCR in nasopharyngeal aspirates, serum, and stool samples. *J. Clin. Virol.* **44:**115–118.

89. **Nickeleit, V., H. H. Hirsch, I. F. Binet, F. Gudat, O. Prince, P. Dalquen, G. Thiel, and M. J. Mihatsch.** 1999. Polyomavirus infection of renal allograft recipients: from latent infection to manifest disease. *J. Am. Soc. Nephrol.* **10:**1080–1089.

90. **Nickeleit, V., H. K. Singh, and M. J. Mihatsch.** 2003. Polyomavirus nephropathy: morphology, pathophysiology, and clinical management. *Curr. Opin. Nephrol. Hypertens.* **12:**599–605.

91. **Norja, P., I. Ubillos, K. Templeton, and P. Simmonds.** 2007. No evidence for an association between infections with WU and KI polyomaviruses and respiratory disease. *J. Clin. Virol.* **40:**307–311.

92. **Pang, X. L., K. Doucette, B. LeBlanc, S. M. Cockfield, and J. K. Preiksaitis.** 2007. Monitoring of polyomavirus BK virus viruria and viremia in renal allograft recipients by use of a quantitative real-time PCR assay: one-year prospective study. *J. Clin. Microbiol.* **45:**3568–3573.

93. **Pang, X. L., K. Martin, and J. K. Preiksaitis.** 2008. The use of unprocessed urine samples for detecting and monitoring BK viruses in renal transplant recipients by a quantitative real-time PCR assay. *J. Virol. Methods* **149:**118–122.

94. **Payungporn, S., T. Chieochansin, C. Thongmee, R. Samransamruajkit, A. Theamboolers, and Y. Poovorawan.** 2008. Prevalence and molecular characterization of WU/KI polyomaviruses isolated from pediatric patients with respiratory disease in Thailand. *Virus Res.* **135:**230–236.

95. **Poulin, D. L., and J. A. DeCaprio.** 2006. Is there a role for SV40 in human cancer? *J. Clin. Oncol.* **24:**4356–4365.

96. **Procop, G. W., R. C. Beck, J. D. Pettay, D. J. Kohn, M. J. Tuohy, B. Yen-Lieberman, R. A. Prayson, and R. R. Tubbs.** 2006. JC virus chromogenic in situ hybridization in brain biopsies from patients with and without PML. *Diagn. Mol. Pathol.* **15:**70–73.

97. **Ramos, E., C. B. Drachenberg, J. C. Papadimitriou, O. Hamze, J. C. Fink, D. K. Klassen, R. C. Drachenberg, A. Wiland, R. Wali, C. B. Cangro, E. Schweitzer, S. T. Bartlett, and M. R. Weir.** 2002. Clinical course of polyoma virus nephropathy in 67 renal transplant patients. *J. Am. Soc. Nephrol.* **13:**2145–2151.

98. **Ramos, E., C. B. Drachenberg, R. Wali, and H. H. Hirsch.** 2009. The decade of polyomavirus BK-associated nephropathy: state of affairs. *Transplantation* **87:**621–630.

99. **Randhawa, P. S., S. Finkelstein, V. Scantlebury, R. Shapiro, C. Vivas, M. Jordan, M. M. Picken, and A. J. Demetris.** 1999. Human polyoma virus-associated interstitial nephritis in the allograft kidney. *Transplantation* **67:**103–109.

100. **Ren, L., R. Gonzalez, X. Xu, J. Li, J. Zhang, G. Vernet, G. Paranhos-Baccala, Q. Jin, and J. Wang.** 2009. WU polyomavirus in fecal specimens of children with acute gastroenteritis, China. *Emerg. Infect. Dis.* **15:**134–135.

101. **Rinaldo, C. H., and H. H. Hirsch.** 2007. Antivirals for the treatment of polyomavirus BK replication. *Expert Rev. Anti Infect. Ther.* **5:**105–115.

102. **Rollison, D. E.** 2006. Epidemiologic studies of polyomaviruses and cancer: previous findings, methodologic challenges and future directions. *Adv. Exp. Med. Biol.* **577:**342–356.

103. **Roskopf, J., J. Trofe, R. J. Stratta, and N. Ahsan.** 2006. Pharmacotherapeutic options for the management of human polyomaviruses. *Adv. Exp. Med. Biol.* **577:**228–254.

104. **Ryschkewitsch, C., P. Jensen, J. Hou, G. Fahle, S. Fischer, and E. O. Major.** 2004. Comparison of PCR-southern hybridization and quantitative real-time PCR for the detection of JC and BK viral nucleotide sequences in urine and cerebrospinal fluid. *J. Virol. Methods* **121:**217–221.

105. **Sack, G. H., J. S. Felix, and A. A. Lanahan.** 1980. Plaque formation and purification of BK virus in cultured human urinary cells. *J. Gen. Virol.* **50:**185–189.

106. **Sehbani, L., B. Kabamba-Mukadi, A. T. Vandenbroucke, M. Bodeus, and P. Goubau.** 2006. Specific and quantitative detection of human polyomaviruses BKV and JCV by LightCycler real-time PCR. *J. Clin. Virol.* **36:**159–162.

107. **Shah, K. V.** 1995. Polyomaviruses, p. 505–510. *In* E. H. Lennette, D. A. Lennette, and E. T. Lennette (ed.), *Diagnostic Procedures for Viral, Rickettsial, and Chlamydial Infections,* 7th ed. American Public Health Association, Washington, DC.

108. **Shah, K. V.** 2007. SV40 and human cancer: a review of recent data. *Int. J. Cancer* **120:**215–223.

109. **Sheikh, S. I., A. Stemmer-Rachamimov, and E. C. Attar.** 2009. Autopsy diagnosis of progressive multifocal leukoencephalopathy with JC virus-negative CSF after cord blood stem-cell transplantation. *J. Clin. Oncol.* **27:**e46–e47.

110. **Shuda, M., H. Feng, H. J. Kwun, S. T. Rosen, O. Gjoerup, P. S. Moore, and Y. Chang.** 2008. T antigen mutations are a human tumor-specific signature for Merkel cell polyomavirus. *Proc. Natl. Acad. Sci. USA* **105:**16272–16277.

111. **Singh, H. K., K. A. Andreoni, V. Madden, K. True, R. Detwiler, K. Weck, and V. Nickeleit.** 2009. Presence of urinary Haufen accurately predicts polyomavirus nephropathy. *J. Am. Soc. Nephrol.* **20:**416–427.

112. **Singh, H. K., L. Bubendorf, M. J. Mihatsch, C. B. Drachenberg, and V. Nickeleit.** 2006. Urine cytology findings of polyomavirus infections. *Adv. Exp. Med. Biol.* **577:**201–212.

113. **Snyder, M. D., G. A. Storch, and D. B. Clifford.** 2005. Atypical PML leading to a diagnosis of common variable immunodeficiency. *Neurology* **64:**1661.

114. **Sundsfjord, A., A. R. Spein, E. Lucht, T. Flaegstad, O. M. Seternes, and T. Traavik.** 1994. Detection of BK virus DNA in nasopharyngeal aspirates from children with respiratory infections but not in saliva from immunedeficient and immunocompetent adult patients. *J. Clin. Microbiol.* **32:**1390–1394.

115. **Taguchi, F., J. Kajioka, and T. Miyamura.** 1982. Prevalence rate and age of acquisition of antibodies against JC virus and BK virus in human sera. *Microbiol. Immunol.* **26:**1057–1064.

116. **Tang, Y. W., S. E. Sefers, H. Li, D. J. Kohn, and G. W. Procop.** 2005. Comparative evaluation of three commercial systems for nucleic acid extraction from urine specimens. *J. Clin. Microbiol.* **43:**4830–4833.

117. **Tolstov, Y. L., D. V. Pastrana, H. Feng, J. C. Becker, F. J. Jenkins, S. Moschos, Y. Chang, C. B. Buck, and P. S. Moore.** 2009. Human Merkel cell polyomavirus infection. II. MCV is a common human infection that can be detected by conformational capsid epitope immunoassays. *Int. J. Cancer* **125:**1250–1256.

118. **Van Assche, G., M. Van Ranst, R. Sciot, B. Dubois, S. Vermeire, M. Noman, J. Verbeeck, K. Geboes, W. Robberecht, and P. Rutgeerts.** 2005. Progressive multifocal leukoencephalopathy after natalizumab therapy for Crohn's disease. *N. Engl. J. Med.* **353:**362–368.

119. **Vera-Sempere, F. J., L. Rubio, V. Felipe-Ponce, A. Garcia, M. J. Sanahuja, I. Zamora, D. Ramos, I. Beneyto, and J. Sanchez-Plumed.** 2006. Renal donor implication in the origin of BK infection: analysis of genomic viral subtypes. *Transplant. Proc.* **38:**2378–2381.

120. **Vilchez, R. A., and J. S. Butel.** 2004. Emergent human pathogen simian virus 40 and its role in cancer. *Clin. Microbiol. Rev.* **17:**495–508.

121. **Viscidi, R. P., and B. Clayman.** 2006. Serological cross reactivity between polyomavirus capsids. *Adv. Exp. Med. Biol.* **577:**73–84.

122. **Viscidi, R. P., D. E. Rollison, E. Viscidi, B. Clayman, E. Rubalcaba, R. Daniel, E. O. Major, and K. V. Shah.** 2003. Serological cross-reactivities between antibodies to simian virus 40, BK virus, and JC virus assessed by virus-like-particle-based enzyme immunoassays. *Clin. Diagn. Lab. Immunol.* **10:**278–285.

123. **von Einsiedel, R. W., I. W. Samorei, M. Pawlita, B. Zwissler, M. Deubel, and H. V. Vinters.** 2004. New JC virus infection patterns by in situ polymerase chain reaction in brains of acquired immunodeficiency syndrome patients with progressive multifocal leukoencephalopathy. *J. Neurovirol.* **10:**1–11.

124. **Weber, T.** 2008. Progressive multifocal leukoencephalopathy. *Neurol. Clin.* **26:**833–854.

125. **Wen, M. C., C. L. Wang, M. Wang, C. H. Cheng, M. J. Wu, C. H. Chen, K. H. Shu, and D. Chang.** 2004. Association of JC virus with tubulointerstitial nephritis in a renal allograft recipient. *J. Med. Virol.* **72:**675–678.

126. **Wetzels, C. T., J. G. Hoefnagel, J. M. Bakkers, H. B. Dijkman, W. A. Blokx, and W. J. Melchers.** 2009. Ultrastructural proof of polyomavirus in merkel cell carcinoma tumour cells and its absence in small cell carcinoma of the lung. *PLoS One* **4:**e4958.

127. **Wiseman, A. C.** 2009. Polyomavirus nephropathy: a current perspective and clinical considerations. *Am. J. Kidney Dis.* **54:**131–142.

128. **Yiannoutsos, C. T., E. O. Major, B. Curfman, P. N. Jensen, M. Gravell, J. Hou, D. B. Clifford, and C. D. Hall.** 1999. Relation of JC virus DNA in the cerebrospinal fluid to survival in acquired immunodeficiency syndrome patients with biopsy-proven progressive multifocal leukoencephalopathy. *Ann. Neurol.* **45:**816–821.

129. **Zheng, H., Y. Murai, M. Hong, Y. Nakanishi, K. Nomoto, S. Masuda, K. Tsuneyama, and Y. Takano.** 2007. JC [corrected] virus detection in human tissue specimens. *J. Clin. Pathol.* **60:**787–793.

130. **Zhong, S., H. Y. Zheng, M. Suzuki, Q. Chen, H. Ikegaya, N. Aoki, S. Usuku, N. Kobayashi, S. Nukuzuma, Y. Yasuda, N. Kuniyoshi, Y. Yogo, and T. Kitamura.** 2007. Age-related urinary excretion of BK polyomavirus by nonimmunocompromised individuals. *J. Clin. Microbiol.* **45:**193–198.

Human Parvoviruses*

JEANNE A. JORDAN

104

TAXONOMY

The *Parvoviridae* family includes the *Parvovirinae*, members of which infect vertebrates, and the *Densovirinae*, members of which infect insects. The *Parvoviridae* family consists of small, nonenveloped, single-stranded DNA viruses. The current classification of parvoviruses is based upon their host range and dependence on other viruses for their replication. The *Parvovirinae* subfamily includes five genera: *Erythrovirus*, *Dependovirus*, *Parvovirus*, *Amdovirus*, and *Bocavirus* (3, 4, 114, 124). This chapter focuses primarily on *Erythrovirus* but does contain brief updates on human bocavirus (HBoV) and the newly described human parvovirus 4 (PARV4).

Erythrovirus replicates autonomously in erythroid progenitor cells. There are three genotypes within the erythroviruses. Genotype 1 consists of human parvovirus B19 (prototype strain, Au), while genotype 2 (prototype strains LaLi and A6) and genotype 3 (prototype strain, V9) are geographically more restricted and found at lower prevalences than genotype 1 (22, 30, 94, 96). The greatest nucleotide divergence is found when genotype 1 (B19) is compared with genotypes 2 and 3 (>11%), with slightly less divergence between genotypes 2 and 3 (~8%) (45, 93, 111). The transmission and epidemiology of genotypes 2 and 3 are much less well understood than those of genotype 1.

Cossart and colleagues first reported their discovery of B19 in 1975 after screening sera of blood donors for hepatitis B virus surface antigen using an Ouchterlony immunodiffusion technique (affected serum; number 19 in panel B) (32). Subsequent evaluation of this blood unit, using immune electron microscopy, revealed viral particles consistent in size and morphology with parvovirus. B19 is the predominant parvovirus pathogen in humans.

HBoV appears to be the second parvovirus associated with disease in humans (3). Allander successfully cloned this virus out of respiratory tract samples from symptomatic individuals using random PCR amplification, sequencing, and bioinformatics. The closest relatives of HBoV are the bovine parvovirus (BPV-1) and canine minute virus (CnMV) bocaviruses (4), and its name reflects this similarity, with "bo" coming from the bovine parvovirus and "ca" from the canine parvovirus. To date, three species of HBoV have been described and include HBoV1, HBoV2, and HBoV3, with more being known about the first than about the last two viruses (7).

PARV4, another human parvovirus, was recently described after it was cloned by sequence-independent PCR amplification from a plasma sample from a symptomatic intravenous-drug user (71). PARV4 has also been detected in pooled plasma and plasma-derived blood products and in autopsy samples of lymphoid tissue, bone marrow, and liver tissue (39). PARV4 is not closely related to any other known human or animal parvovirus and may constitute a new group within the family of parvoviruses. To date, PARV4 includes at least two, if not three, genotypes (39, 40, 71, 76, 77, 114). The pathogenicity of PARV4 remains to be determined.

DESCRIPTION OF THE AGENT

Most of what we know about the nature of erythroviruses has come from the study of human parvovirus B19 (genotype 1). Many important observations regarding the B19 virion have been made using electron microscopy and X-ray crystallography (2, 25, 62). The structure of recombinant B19-like particles has been studied at an ~3.5-Å resolution using the latter technology; the major virus capsid protein, VP2, has a structure like a jelly roll, with a β barrel motif similar to that present in other icosahedral viruses. (62). The diameter of the virus is approximately 26 nm. The complete virion has a molecular mass between 5.5×10^6 and 6.2×10^6 Da and a buoyant density in cesium chloride between 1.39 and 1.42 g/cm^3. The viral particle lacks an envelope, which contributes to the virus's tenacity to resist heat, solvents and detergent treatments, an important consideration when approaching the issue of virus inactivation in blood or blood products (28). The virion does not contain lipids or carbohydrates but does contain phospholipase A_2-like activity, which is required during host cell entry (21, 136).

The B19 capsid is comprised of two structural proteins: VP1, the minor capsid protein (83 kDa), and VP2, the major capsid protein (58 kDa), representing about 4 and 96% of the capsid, respectively (95). The major nonstructural protein is NS1 (71 kDa), a DNA binding protein involved

---

*This chapter contains information presented in chapter 101 by Marialuisa Zerbini and Monica Musiani in the eighth edition of this *Manual*.

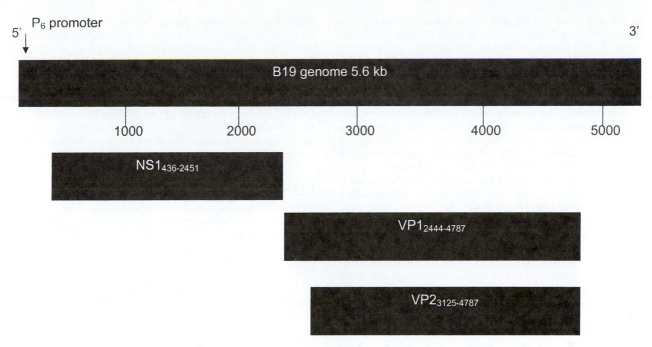

FIGURE 1 Schematic representation of human parvovirus B19 genome and the transcription map with the unique region of VP1 comprising bp 2444 to 3124.

in viral replication. The NS1 protein transactivates P_6, the single promoter present on the genome (102), and induces cellular apoptosis and activates the inflammatory cytokine gene, the interleukin-6 gene (80, 81, 83).

The B19 genome consists of a single-stranded 5.6-kb DNA genome; the 5' and 3' ends contain identical 365-nucleotide repeats (120), and there exists two large and two small open reading frames (ORFs) (112) (Fig. 1). The major left-hand ORF is translated into NS1, an early viral protein, while the major right-hand ORF is translated into the VP1 and VP2 structural proteins, which are expressed later in infection. The antigenic domains of NS1 are located at its carboxy terminus (127). The VP1 and VP2 capsid proteins originate from the same ORF and are identical in sequence, except for an additional 227 amino acids at the amino terminus of VP1. Structurally, this unique region of VP1 is located on the exterior of the virion capsid and contains several neutralizing epitopes, most of which are linear in nature (88). In contrast, most neutralizing epitopes of VP2 are conformational (106). During replication, equal numbers of the plus and minus strands of DNA are packaged into separate virion particles, so that during DNA extraction, under the appropriate salt concentration, the complementary strands hybridize to form a double-stranded DNA structure (10). Zhi and colleagues have constructed an infectious clone of B19 (138).

B19 has an extremely limited cell tropism, replicating only in the nuclei of erythroid progenitor cells of the burst-forming unit and colony-forming unit (31, 119). B19 infection can have a profound effect on an individual, resulting in reticulocytopenia and an abnormally low hematocrit. The cellular receptor that B19 binds to is the blood group P antigen, or globoside (13, 16). Resistance in individuals to B19 infection can be attributed to a lack of the P antigen receptor on erythroid cells (15). The globoside receptor can also be found on other cell types, including cardiac myocytes, white blood cells, platelets, and trophoblasts, and may play a role in pathogenesis in these cell types (55, 129). A coreceptor

has been identified that is necessary for virus entry into target cells, a process mediated by α5β1 integrins (130). A permissive erythroid progenitor cell expresses high levels of both globoside and α5β1 integrins, while the nonpermissive mature erythrocyte contains only globoside, lacking both α5β1 integrins and a nucleus. Therefore, although globoside is necessary for infection, it is not sufficient for a cell to be permissive for B19 infection (131). The Ku80 autoantigen has also been described as a potential cellular coreceptor for human parvovirus B19 infection (86). Another key molecule required for B19 infectivity is phospholipase A_2, which is present in the VP1 unique region (21, 136). The enzyme cleaves phospholipids into arachidonic acid, a molecule used to synthesize both prostaglandins and leukotrienes, which play important roles in the inflammatory process.

Like those of BPV-1 and CnMV, the HBoV genome has three ORFs and contains two nonstructural genes, the NS1 and NP-1 genes, and two overlapping structural genes, the VP1 and VP2 genes (4). The target cell(s) used by HBoV for replication has not yet been identified, so successful propagation in cell culture has not been described.

EPIDEMIOLOGY AND TRANSMISSION

B19 infection is common worldwide. In temperate climates, epidemic manifestations occur more commonly in late winter, spring, or early summer. Epidemic peaks of B19 infection occur in cycles every 3 to 5 years. B19 infection is most common in young children and manifests itself as erythema infectiosum (EI) (fifth disease or slapped cheek syndrome) (101). In individuals who have disorders that shorten their red cell half-life, B19 infection results in transient aplastic crisis (TAC). Both EI and TAC manifestations are usually self-limiting illnesses. The incubation period for B19 infection is approximately 6 to 10 days.

B19 transmission most often occurs by the respiratory route through respiratory secretions and saliva that are expelled or released when an infected individual sneezes or coughs. Transmission of B19 is much more likely to occur among individuals in a household, day care, or crowded environment; this scenario places women with young children at high risk for acquiring infection, which can be problematic for the susceptible woman who becomes infected with B19 while pregnant. Vertical transmission of B19 occurs at a rate of approximately 30%. However, viral transmission to the infant is not synonymous with poor pregnancy outcome or adverse consequences to the infant. In the general population, the seroprevalence of B19-specific immunoglobulin G (IgG) rises steadily from 37% in children aged 1 to 5 years to 87% in individuals who are greater than 50 years old (23). Between 50 and 60% of women in their reproductive years have circulating B19 IgG, leaving a significant percentage who do not (51).

B19 can also be transmitted parenterally from blood or blood products obtained from viremic donors (50, 105). The incidence of B19 in the blood of healthy donors ranges from 1 in 20,000 to 1 in 50,000 donors (50, 79). The risk of transmission is greater when the blood components are made from pooled units than when they are made from single units, placing those individuals requiring repeated doses of any of these blood products at risk of becoming infected with B19 over time, including hemophiliacs, who require lifelong administration of clotting factor concentrate (17, 69, 105). Using nucleic acid amplification testing (NAT), B19 DNA has been detected in numerous batches of albumin, factor VIII, factor IX, clotting factor concentrates, and immunoglobulin (11, 69). Observations in healthy volunteers suggest that acute B19 infection can occur from administration of blood components that contain $\geq 10^7$ genome equivalents/ml (geq/ml) of B19 DNA. In contrast, patients receiving $<10^4$ geq/ml have not shown evidence of virus transmission (17, 132). A recent study linking donors and recipients was undertaken to assess the risk of transmission from B19 DNA-positive units containing $<10^6$ IU/ml into B19-susceptible recipients (B19 IgG negative). In this study 105 B19 DNA-positive donations resulted in the transfusion of 112 B19-positive components into 107 recipients. None of the 24 susceptible cases resulted in a B19 infection (66). The Food and Drug Administration (FDA) does not currently mandate screening of the blood supply for B19. In Europe, screening of blood donations for B19 DNA is not routine, but many manufacturers now perform B19 PCR on plasma pools. The FDA is proposing that manufactured pools contain plasma B19 DNA levels consistently below 10^4 genome copies/ml (17). A similar recommendation in which 10^4 genome copies/ml is considered the maximum permissible limit has been made by the Health Council of The Netherlands (http://www.gezondheidsraad.nl/sites/default/files/02@07E.pdf). This council has also recommended that a high-risk group approach be adopted for cellular blood products containing B19 DNA. In Europe, no official guideline has been published for plasma pools. The presence of neutralizing activity in all of these pools may help to explain the lack of infectivity in pools with lower viral loads (17, 50). Like B19, PARV4 has been readily detectable in pooled plasma products with viral loads ranging from $<10^2$ to $\sim 10^6$ copies per milliliter of plasma, levels well below (1,000-fold lower) the average parvovirus B19 levels found in pooled plasma products (40).

The epidemiology and prevalence of HBoV are similar to those of respiratory syncytial virus, and HBoV appears to be the third most common viral respiratory pathogen affecting infants and young children. HBoV has been detected in respiratory specimens, sera, and feces of symptomatic individuals with lower respiratory tract infection (4, 7). Since its discovery, HBoV has been found in individuals worldwide, with growing evidence that it plays an etiologic role in severe lower respiratory tract infections in hospitalized infants and young children (76). Many studies have described high rates of coinfection with HBoV and other respiratory viruses (128). It is unclear whether HBoV infection has a seasonal pattern or can be found year-round, and the prevalence of HBoV appears to vary depending upon in which country or geographical area the studies have been performed (9, 76).

CLINICAL SIGNIFICANCE

Symptoms associated with B19 infection can vary considerably, from being absent to being life threatening. In immunocompetent individuals, B19 infection is usually an acute self-limiting disease, while in those who are immunocompromised or who have red cells with shortened half-lives, B19 infection can become chronic.

Much of what we first learned about B19 infection in the immunocompetent individual came from two studies out of the United Kingdom that were conducted using healthy adult volunteers (5, 100). These volunteers were infected intranasally with sera known to contain B19 particles. The infection in the B19-seronegative volunteers had two distinct phases: a nonspecific phase occurring at the end of the first week postinoculation and consisting of fever, headache, myalgia, chills, and/or itching, and a more specific phase occurring around day 17 or 18 postinoculation with symptoms including the absence of reticulocytes, followed by a significant drop in hemoglobin, along with a transient decrease in neutrophil, lymphocyte, and/or platelet counts. Viremia became detectable 6 days postinoculation, peaking on days 8 and 9. Viral levels rose to approximately 10^{10} to 10^{12} genome copies/ml of blood. B19-specific IgM antibodies became detectable 2 weeks postinoculation, while IgG antibodies appeared within days of detectable IgM antibodies (Fig. 2).

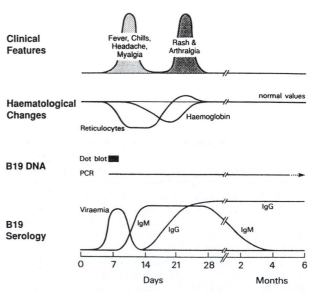

FIGURE 2 Clinical features, hematologic changes, B19 DNA presence, and serologic findings associated with B19 infection in a healthy individual. Reprinted from reference 16.

Anderson and colleagues first described EI in 1983 during an outbreak in a primary school in London, United Kingdom (6). EI has a mean incubation period of approximately 17 to 19 days. Prodromal symptoms may include low-grade fever, headache, and one or more of the following: conjunctivitis, upper respiratory tract complaints, cough, myalgia, nausea, and diarrhea. The specific rash associated with B19 infection first appears on the face as a confluent maculopapular erythema on the cheeks, with relative perioral pallor. This manifestation provides the characteristic slapped-cheek appearance on the individual. The rash may appear next in a bilaterally symmetric fashion on the arms, legs, and trunk. Rarely are the palms of the hands and soles of the feet involved. The rash can wax and wane for an extended period, up to 3 weeks; a rise in body temperature, caused by fever, heat, exercise, or exposure to sunlight, can induce its reappearance.

Patients with acute B19 viremia can also present with a gloves-and-socks syndrome. Bagot and Revuz were the first investigators to link this characteristic papular purpuric gloves-and-socks syndrome (PPGSS) to B19 infection (8). Although most cases of PPGSS involve measurable B19-specific antibodies, a few cases have been shown to lack any evidence of detectable B19-specific IgM antibodies (115).

TAC is an acute, self-limited cessation of the regenerative process within the erythropoietic cell lineage and is characterized by the abrupt onset of severe anemia that is associated with a dramatic decline in circulating reticulocytes. TAC was first described in 1981 as a clinical manifestation associated with B19 infection in children with sickle cell anemia and since then has been described to occur in a wide range of patients with underlying chronic hemolytic anemia or shortened red blood cell half-lives (6, 97).

One of the most important complications of B19 infection is its association with pregnancy loss (35, 123). Brown and colleagues first reported on the association of intrauterine B19 infection and fetal demise in 1984 (18). In a susceptible woman, infection with B19 during pregnancy can result in spontaneous abortion, stillbirth, severe fetal anemia, nonimmune hydrops fetalis, transfusion-dependent congenital anemia, hepatomegaly, or fetal death (14, 121). An inflammatory-mediated immune response and trophoblast apoptosis have been reported to occur in placentas from pregnancies with poor outcome due to B19 infection (54, 57). Although the rate of viral transmission across the placenta is relatively high, between 24 and 51% (134), the risk of fetal death is relatively low, between 1 and 10%, with the greatest risk being associated with infection occurring on or before the 20th week of gestation. B19 is responsible for 16 to 18% of all cases of idiopathic nonimmune hydrops fetalis (53). Although most cases of B19-induced fetal hydrops resolve spontaneously, the presentation can occur rapidly, within a few days, to result in fetal death. Weekly fetal ultrasonography monitoring for hydrops, for up to 14 weeks, is recommended for women who seroconvert to B19 during pregnancy. The fetus is particularly vulnerable to B19 infection and developing hydrops during the second trimester, as this time correlates to the rapid expansion of red blood cells, including the erythrocyte precursor cell, the target cell for B19 infection.

B19 infection can be problematic for the immunocompromised patient: one with congenital or acquired immunodeficiency syndrome, a recipient of a solid-organ or bone marrow transplant, or one with a lymphoproliferative disorder or other malignancy, especially when receiving chemotherapy (41, 67). B19 is the leading cause of pure red cell aplasia in AIDS patients. An immunocompromised patient can present with acute B19 infection that does not resolve but becomes chronic; low- to medium-level viremia can persist for several months or even years, which can lead to selective aplasia of red blood cell precursors within the bone marrow, and occasionally to pancytopenia (90). Chronic infection can lead to persistent and severe anemia, due most likely to the patient's inability to mount an adequate immune response to clear the viremia. In these patients, clinical response to intravenous immunoglobulin (IVIg) is usually quite effective in eliminating the viremia (85).

In 1985, results from two large-scale studies were published describing the association between B19 infection and arthropathy (103, 133). A symmetric, polyarticular involvement of the joints can occur as a consequence of B19 infection in the presence or absence of the specific skin rash. Joint symptoms can occur in up to 33% of adults, being found more commonly in women than in men. Joint involvement is uncommon in children, occurring less than 10% of the time. The involved joints include the proximal interphalangeal joints of the hands and feet and, less frequently, the wrists, elbows, knees, and ankles. Swelling, warmth, redness, and stiffness can accompany the joint pain. These symptoms are usually self-limiting, remaining for a few weeks, but can persist for months or even years (91). The role of B19 in the etiopathogenesis of rheumatoid arthritis and chronic juvenile arthritis remains a source of disagreement (20, 63).

The role of B19 has been firmly established for EI, TAC, nonimmune hydrops fetalis, chronic pure red cell aplasia, and arthropathy syndromes. However, less commonly recognized clinical manifestations have also been associated with B19; these include glomerulonephritis, vasculitis, myocarditis, meningitis, encephalitis, hepatobiliary disease, rheumatic disease, hematologic disorders, and cutaneous eruptions apart from EI (109, 122). The mechanism(s) for these various atypical clinical manifestations remains unknown but has become a priority to elucidate.

HBoV was first described in 2005 and found in young children with respiratory tract infections (4). Since then, HBoV has been associated primarily with acute respiratory tract infections, especially lower respiratory tract infections, in infants and children under the age of 2 or 3 years (26, 59, 76). However, up to 15% of cases of HBoV-associated respiratory tract infection can be found in older children and adults, especially if the individual is immunosuppressed (26). In addition, there can be a high rate of coinfection with other respiratory viral pathogens. Individuals with higher viral loads of HBoV in respiratory tract specimens are often found to be viremic compared to those with lower viral loads in respiratory tract specimens (26). However, HBoV has been found to persist in the respiratory tract far longer than other respiratory viruses, making it unclear as to the relevance of detecting low viral loads in respiratory specimens. It has been suggested that HBoV may be associated with prolonged viral shedding, persistence, or reactivation (110).

All three HBoVs, HBoV1, HBoV2, and HBoV3, have been found in stool samples. However, it is not yet clear that HBoVs cause acute gastroenteritis, as a significant number of these cases also involved copathogens that can cause enteric illness (7, 27, 116). Lastly, unlike with B19, BPV-1, and CnMV, there does not appear to be any association of HBoV with adverse pregnancy outcome (104).

Treatment and Prevention

Infection with B19 is usually a mild, self-limiting febrile illness and as such does not require specific therapy or treatment. Nonsteroidal anti-inflammatory drugs can provide relief to the symptomatic individual with arthritis or arthropathy. In cases where B19 infection is life threatening, treatment will vary with the clinical manifestations presented and the immune status of the patient (135). For instance, blood transfusion therapy can be used to provide temporary relief in patients with acute anemia. Severe fetal anemia, as a result of B19 infection, can be treated with one or more intrauterine transfusions of packed red blood cells. However, this treatment is not without its risks. Fetal anemia can be monitored noninvasively using Doppler measurements, which eliminates the need for funicentesis, fetal transfusion, and their associated risks if anemia is found to be absent (34, 84). IVIg therapy is generally limited to those patients suffering with chronic anemia due to B19 and has been used with much success in relieving anemia in these patients (85). Success with IVIg therapy has also been reported for treatment of juvenile polyarticular arthritis and in a limited number of cases has been used successfully to eliminate B19 viremia in individuals with a history of chronic fatigue syndrome (64, 78, 125). However, it should be noted that as a pooled blood product, IVIg can contain B19 and consequently puts the susceptible patient at risk for acquiring B19 infection (36, 38, 43, 107). Other complications of using IVIg to treat B19 anemia include acute myocardial infarction, acute renal failure, and, more rarely, thrombotic events (24, 126).

COLLECTION, TRANSPORT, AND STORAGE OF SPECIMENS

Serum from whole blood, collected in a sterile tube lacking anticoagulant, is most suitable for serologic testing, although plasma, containing either EDTA or sodium citrate, can also be used. Whole-blood samples being transported to the laboratory should be maintained at 2 to 8°C; temperatures at or below freezing should be avoided during transport and storage to minimize red cell lysis. Serum or plasma, once separated from the cellular components of whole blood, can be stored for short periods at 2 to 8°C, or at −20 or −70°C for much more extended periods, before testing is performed.

Bone marrow aspirates, cord blood, amniotic fluid, and biopsy specimens of placenta and/or fetal tissues (liver, lung, and heart) are suitable for B19 DNA detection using in situ hybridization or NAT, or for antigen detection using immunocytochemistry or immunohistochemistry. Bone marrow and cord blood samples should be collected in sterile tubes containing EDTA or sodium citrate. Heparin should be avoided for NAT because of its inhibitory effect on the *Taq* polymerase unless DNA purification is included in the sample processing protocol. Amniotic fluid should be collected in a sterile tube lacking anticoagulant. Placental and fetal tissues can be placed directly into viral transport media or fixed using 10% buffered formalin. Cellular and fresh tissue samples should be maintained at 2 to 8°C for transport to the laboratory. Once again, freezing temperatures should be avoided for transport or storage prior to sample processing.

DIRECT DETECTION

Microscopy

Electron microscopy can be used to visualize parvoviruses (33). Although this approach is not used routinely in the clinical laboratory for diagnosis, it is a common practice to stain bone marrow smears with hematoxylin and eosin to look for the presence of giant pronormoblasts, which, if present, are pathognomonic for B19 infection (58).

Antigen

Immunocytochemical or Immunohistochemical Analyses

Cytospin preparations of bone marrow aspirates, cord blood, or amniotic fluid specimens can be analyzed by immunocytochemistry for the presence of B19-specific capsid antigen(s) using commercially available antibodies (58). These antibodies can also be used in an immunohistochemical analysis of formalin-fixed, paraffin-embedded placental or fetal tissues for viral antigens (58). However, these procedures are usually performed in an anatomical pathology laboratory or research laboratory, but not a clinical pathology laboratory.

Nucleic Acid

DNA In Situ Hybridization

The specimen types analyzed by immunocytochemistry or immunohistochemistry for viral antigen can be analyzed by in situ hybridization for B19 DNA (53). The DNA probes used for in situ hybridization can consist of either short stretches of B19-specific oligonucleotides or a cloned plasmid containing a nearly full-length genome. Probes are most often labeled with either biotin or digoxigenin to avoid using a radioisotope. A colorimetric substrate is commonly used in conjunction with either alkaline phosphatase or peroxidase, whose products can be visualized using a light microscope. Increased analytical sensitivity can be achieved using a chemiluminescent stubstrate, but this strategy requires a high-performance luminometer and computer to be used in conjunction with an optical microscope.

NAT

At present, NAT is the most sensitive choice for detecting human parvovirus-specific DNA within a specimen, and it is considered the test of choice for diagnosing infection in the immunocompromised or immunosuppressed individual, or in the fetus or neonate for whom using serologic tests would not be advisable. DNA extraction and purification are recommended when analyzing samples for viral DNA by NAT; these include serum, plasma, bone marrow aspirates, cord blood, amniotic fluid, or tissue specimens (fresh or formalin fixed) (137).

Numerous PCR-based primer and probe sets have been described for detecting B19-specific DNA (56, 87). It is important to note that that most of these targets were designed at a time when only genotype 1 had been described and may not necessarily detect genotype 2 or 3 (Table 1). The earliest detection platforms consisted of agarose gel electrophoresis and Southern blot hybridization, or dot blot hybridization techniques, or enzyme immunoassay (EIA). More recently, real-time PCR platforms have been developed in conjunction with fluorescence-labeled probes such as TaqMan, molecular beacons, or fluorescence resonance energy transfer (FRET) probes (1, 42). This approach has many benefits, including speed, reduced risk of contamination, and estimating viral load. Real-time PCR is readily adapted to either qualitative (end point analysis) or quantitative (viral load) detection. A quantitative assay for B19 DNA must demonstrate linearity over a wide range, as viral load can reach levels of 10^{12} geq/ml of blood during

TABLE 1 Diagnostic methods used to detect human parvovirus B19 infections

Approach	Method	Uses	Limitations	Reagents and suppliers
Serology	EIA IFA Immunoblotting	IgM: acute and recent infection IgG: past infection IgG avidity: distinguishes between recent and past infections	Antibodies made to linear antigens decline over time relative to antibodies made against conformational antigens.	Baculovirus-expressed conformational VP2 (DiaSorin [formerly Biotrin Inc.]) *E. coli*-expressed linear VP1 (Focus Diagnostics) *E. coli*-expressed linear VP1 and VP2 (R-Biopharm Inc.)
NAT	Qualitative PCR Quantitative PCR	Detects viral DNA Provides viral load	Primers may or may not recognize genotypes 2 and 3.	Detects genotype 1: LightCycler-Parvovirus 819 assay (Roche) Detect genotypes 1–3: Parvo B19 PCR Kit (Abbott Molecular; CE mark[a]); RealArt Parvo B19 (Qiagen [formerly Artus]; CE mark)

[a] "CE mark" certifies that a product has met European Union health, safety, and environmental requirements (an abbreviation for the French "Conformité Européenne").

the acute phase of infection but rapidly declines with the onset of a robust antibody production (89).

An FDA-cleared NAT assay is not currently available, although several manufacturers offer analyte-specific reagents for detecting B19 DNA. The LightCycler-Parvovirus B19 quantification kit (Roche Diagnostics, Indianapolis, IN) is highly sensitive for genotype 1 but is not suitable for detecting genotype 2 or one of the genotype 3 strains (47). In contrast, the RealArt Parvo B19 LC PCR (Qiagen Sciences Inc., Germantown, MD) has been found to be suitable for detection, quantification, and differentiation of all three genotypes by some investigators but not by others; lower sensitivities have been reported for certain strains (12, 30, 47). Because serology is insufficient for diagnosing B19 infection in the immunocompromised patient, NAT assays being used clinically should be evaluated for the ability to detect the three genotypes. Investigator-designed real-time PCR assays targeting the NS1 gene or VP1 unique region have been successful in detecting genotypes 1 to 3 at similar sensitivities; these approaches use either consensus primer-based PCR followed by restriction fragment length polymorphism digest or DNA sequencing, nested PCR, or multiplex PCR using genotype specific primers and probes (47, 70, 108, 111). However, it is important to keep in mind that the clinical significance, prevalence, and geographical distribution of erythrovirus variants remain largely unknown.

Quantitative real-time PCR assays have been described that are useful for determining viral load in patient specimens or screening blood and blood products for their safety (118). The World Health Organization (WHO) B19 DNA international standard, 99/800, containing 5×10^5 IU of B19 DNA/vial for nucleic acid testing, is now available for use through the National Institute for Biological Standards and Control (NIBSC; Potters Bar, Hertfordshire, United Kingdom) (92).

PCR has also been used successfully to detect HBoV DNA in respiratory specimens, sera, and feces (68). Selected targets include the NS1, NP-1, and VP1/2 genes (4, 76, 77). It should be noted that many of the studies published to date describing the association of HBoV with respiratory or gastrointestinal tract infections have used nested PCR to detect virus from clinical specimens. Additional studies are needed to determine which sample type(s) is best to collect for detecting the virus.

ISOLATION PROCEDURES

Although isolation of parvovirus in culture is possible, successful replication of B19 requires infection of undifferentiated, actively replicating erythroid cells such as freshly harvested bone marrow or fetal cord blood samples. Consequently, it is a protocol that is confined to research laboratories, being impractical to use routinely in the clinical laboratory.

IDENTIFICATION

This virus is identified not in the conventional sense using tissue culture, but through molecular techniques that detect specific DNA sequences and by immunologic methods using antibodies that recognize specific viral capsid proteins.

TYPING SYSTEMS

DNA sequence analysis of the VP1 unique region or the NS1 gene can be used to differentiate among genotypes (47, 70, 108, 111).

SEROLOGIC TESTS

Serologic testing to detect B19-specific antibodies to viral capsid antigen remains the cornerstone in determining the immune status in immunocompetent individuals. In the practice of obstetrics, it is considered the standard of care for the physician to request B19-specific IgM and IgG serologic testing in the case of a pregnant woman with a history of exposure to a B19-infected individual. However, this approach would not be chosen when attempting to diagnose B19 infection in an immunocompromised or immunosuppressed individual, or in a fetus or neonate, due to the patient's limited ability to produce antibodies; instead, NAT should be chosen for this purpose.

Most B19-specific serologic assays incorporate viral antigen(s) generated from recombinant expression vectors due to the limited availability of native B19 capsids. Both prokaryotic and eukaryotic expression systems have been used to produce viral capsid protein(s) (82) or self-assembled empty viral capsids (60). Most B19-specific serologic testing done in the United States is performed using one of two commercially available assays (19, 29). DiaSorin (formerly Biotrin International Inc.) manufactures B19-specific IgM and IgG EIAs for sale and distribution that have been cleared by the FDA; these kits use a μ capture EIA for B19-specific IgM antibody and a baculovirus-expressed conformational VP2 antigen for the B19-specific IgG EIA. The μ capture format is designed to minimize false-negative IgM results; microtiter wells are coated with anti-human IgM antisera, a process that allows for the binding of total IgM antibody in serum or plasma to the solid phase and thus reduces competition from IgG antibodies that can occur due to differences in concentration (Table 1).

Focus Diagnostics Laboratory (Cypress, CA) is the other manufacturer of B19-specific IgM and IgG serologic tests, which are proprietary in nature but are known to incorporate a linear (denatured) VP1 antigen purified from an *Escherichia coli* expression vector; these B19-specific IgM and IgG assays have not been FDA cleared (Table 1).

It is well established that for better accuracy the B19-specific IgG EIA should incorporate a conformational capsid antigen (51, 65, 75). This is based on the fact that circulating IgG antibodies directed against linear epitopes of VP1 and VP2 gradually decline postinfection but that the IgG directed against conformational epitopes of those antigens are maintained long term.

EIAs measuring IgG avidity have also been developed. These assays are helpful in discriminating between primary and secondary infections but are not yet commercially available (99, 117). Standardizing B19 IgG results among laboratories and test systems can be achieved using the WHO international standard (The Second International Standard for Anti-Parvovirus B19 plasma, human NIBSC code 01/602; 77 IU per ampoule) (37). Unfortunately, no such standard exists for B19 IgM determinations.

Commercially available indirect immunofluorescent-antibody (IFA) and Western blot assays can also be used to detect B19-specific IgM or IgG antibodies (74, 98). In the former, the antigen consists of a conformational VP1 protein expressed in insect cells using a recombinant baculovirus expression vector. Sera for IFA B19-specific IgM antibody testing should be pretreated with a suitable adsorbent reagent to prevent interference from rheumatoid factors (which generates a false-positive result) and reduce IgG competition (which produces a false-negative result). These assays can be used as a confirmatory assay in conjunction with an EIA that utilizes the linear, denatured VP1 antigen. In the latter assay, VP1, VP2, and NS1 antigens are used (46). However, this approach has its limitations, as the antigens are denatured, which may limit their diagnostic value.

Assay design and antigen type(s) incorporated into a kit are important features to note when evaluating a commercial assay (52, 72). Capture enzyme immunoassays employing native or recombinant antigens are excellent choices for detecting B19-specific immunoglobulin (51). Systems consisting of either *Escherichia coli*-expressed or baculovirus-expressed B19 capsid antigens or both in combination have been described. Capture EIAs incorporating conformational antigens (nondenatured) only, or in combination with linear antigens (denatured), are superior to those utilizing linear antigens (denatured) alone (65). Several studies have demonstrated differences in B19 IgM and IgG reactivity against conformational and linear epitopes of VP1 and VP2 (65, 73, 75). Accurate B19 serologic diagnosis requires the presence of nondenatured,

conformational antigens. Recombinant B19 nonstructural protein NS1 can also be expressed using either a prokaryotic or eukaryotic expression system. The presence of antibodies to NS1 is associated with persistent B19 infection and chronic arthritis (48).

To date, for HBoV infection, there are no commercially available diagnostic tests that can distinguish between a primary infection and viral shedding, persistence, or reactivation. Recently, enzyme-linked immunosorbent assay-, Western blot-, and/or IFA-based HBoV-specific IgM and IgG serology tests have been described, and these could be used for such purposes (61, 111). Baculovirus-expressed HBoV-specific VP1, VP2, NP-1, and NS1 antigens have been synthesized for use in IFAs, with the VP1 IFA demonstrating the highest sensitivity for detecting IgG antibody (113). To date, no such serology assay has been described for PARV4 antibody detection.

ANTIVIRAL SUSCEPTIBILITIES

To date, there are no antiviral agents described for the treatment of B19, HBoV, or PARV 4 infections.

EVALUATION, INTERPRETATION, AND REPORTING OF RESULTS

Laboratory tests are essential when attempting to diagnose B19 infection due to its wide range of clinical presentations and patients affected. Determining whether to use serologic tests and/or NAT is largely dependent upon the patient's immune status; serologic tests should be used in diagnosing infection of or assessing immune status in the healthy, immunocompetent individual or the individual suffering from TAC. In contrast, NAT is the test of choice for screening the immunocompromised or immunosuppressed individual or diagnosing congenital or neonatal infections, as serologic screening would be unreliable. Quantitative PCR may be useful for monitoring viral loads in patients with chronic infection, as IVIg therapy has been found to relieve their anemia.

Unlike serologic testing, where only serum or plasma samples are acceptable, NAT for B19 DNA can be performed using a wide range of specimen types. The choice of specimen(s) is largely dependent upon the clinical manifestations of the patient, with each specimen type requiring validation before testing can be implemented clinically. Testing sera for the presence of B19-specific IgM antibodies is the most common approach for diagnosing acute infection in the immunocompetent individual (44). Detectable levels of B19-specific IgM can be found within 7 to 10 days of exposure to the virus; IgM antibodies remain measurable for 2 to 3 months before diminishing. Occasionally, IgM antibodies can persist for longer periods, 6 months or more. Therefore, their presence, especially at low levels for an extended period, is suggestive but not conclusive proof of recent infection. Acute infection can also be diagnosed by demonstrating a ≥4-fold rise in B19-specific IgG antibody titer in a patient's sera. However, this procedure requires two separate time points for sample collection and is considered impractical in most clinical situations.

Testing sera for the presence of B19-specific IgG antibodies can determine past or previous infection in the immunocompetent individual. Detecting the presence of IgG antibody, without IgM antibody, implies immunity in the patient. The antibody response to linear or denatured viral capsid proteins diminishes with time. In contrast, the antibody response to conformational capsid proteins persists for years.

Unlike the significant variation in genomic sequence that exists among the three genotypes of *Erythrovirus*, there is a high degree of homology in the VP2 capsid protein for these three genotypes (111). This is expected to result in a high level of immunologic cross-reactivity with IgM and IgG. Therefore, choosing an EIA that incorporates a conformational VP2 antigen would be desirable for detecting all three genotypes of *Erythrovirus*.

REFERENCES

1. **Aberham, C., C. Pendl, P. Gross, G. Zerlauth, and M. Gessner.** 2001. A quantitative, internally controlled real-time PCR assay for the detection of parvovirus B19 DNA. *J. Virol. Methods* **92:**183–191.
2. **Agbandje, M., S. Kajigaya, R. McKenna, N. S. Young, and M. G. Rossmann.** 1994. The structure of human parvovirus B19 at 8 A resolution. *Virology* **203:**106–115.
3. **Allander, T.** 2008. Human bocavirus. *J. Clin. Virol.* **41:**29–33.
4. **Allander, T., M. T. Tammi, M. Eriksson, A. Bjerkner, A. Tiveljung-Lindell, and B. Andersson.** 2005. Cloning of human parvovirus by molecular screening of respiratory tract samples. *Proc. Natl. Acad. Sci. USA* **102:**12891–12896.
5. **Anderson, M. J., P. G. Higgins, L. R. Davis, J. S. Willman, S. E. Jones, I. M. Kidd, J. R. Pattison, and D. A. Tyrrell.** 1985. Experimental parvoviral infection in humans. *J. Infect. Dis.* **152:**257–265.
6. **Anderson, M. J., S. E. Jones, S. P. Fisher-Hoch, E. Lewis, S. M. Hall, C. L. Bartlett, B. J. Cohen, P. P. Mortimer, and M. S. Pereira.** 1983. Human parvovirus, the cause of erythema infectiosum (fifth disease)? *Lancet* **i:**1378.
7. **Arthur, J. L., G. D. Higgins, G. P. Davidson, R. C. Givney, and R. M. Ratcliff.** 2009. A novel bocavirus associated with acute gastroenteritis in Australian children. *PLoS Pathog.* **5(4):**1–11.
8. **Bagot, M., and J. Revuz.** 1991. Papular-purpuric 'gloves and socks' syndrome: primary infection with parvovirus B19? *J. Am. Acad. Dermatol.* **25:**341. (Letter.)
9. **Bastien, N., N. Chui, J. L. Robinson, B. E. Lee, K. Dust, L. Hart, and Y. Li.** 2007. Detection of human bocavirus in Canadian children in a 1-year study. *J. Clin. Microbiol.* **45:**610–613.
10. **Berns, K. I.** 1996. Parvoviridae: the viruses and their replication, p. 2173–2197. *In* B. N. Fields, D. M. Knipe, and P. M. Howley (ed.), *Fields Virology*, 3rd ed. Lippincott-Raven, Philadelphia, PA.
11. **Bonvicini, F., G. Gallinella, M. Cricca, S. Ambretti, S. Delbarba, M. Musiani, and M. Zerbini.** 2004. Molecular testing for detection of in vitro infectivity of plasma pools contaminated with B19 virus. *J. Med. Virol.* **74:**272–276.
12. **Braham, S., J. Gandhi, S. Beard, and B. Cohen.** 2004. Evaluation of the Roche LightCycler parvovirus B19 quantification kit for the diagnosis of parvovirus B19 infections. *J. Clin. Virol.* **31:**5–10.
13. **Brown, K. E., S. M. Anderson, and N. S. Young.** 1993. Erythrocyte P antigen: cellular receptor for B19 parvovirus. *Science* **262:**114–117.
14. **Brown, K. E., S. W. Green, J. Antunez de Mayolo, J. A. Bellanti, S. D. Smith, T. J. Smith, and N. S. Yound.** 1994. Congenital anaemia after transplacental B19 parvovirus infection. *Lancet* **343:**895–896.
15. **Brown, K. E., J. R. Hibbs, G. Gallinella, S. M. Anderson, E. D. Lehman, P. McCarthy, and N. S. Young.** 1994. Resistance to parvovirus B19 infection due to lack of virus receptor (erythrocyte P antigen). *N. Engl. J. Med.* **330:**1192–1196.
16. **Brown, K. E., and N. S. Young.** 1995. Parvovirus B19 infection and hematopoiesis. *Blood Rev.* **9:**176–182.
17. **Brown, K. E., N. S. Young, B. M. Alving, and L. H. Barbosa.** 2001. Parvovirus B19: implications for transfusion medicine. Summary of a workshop. *Transfusion* **41:**130–135.
18. **Brown, T., A. Anand, L. D. Ritchie, J. P. Clewley, and T. M. Reid.** 1984. Intrauterine parvovirus infection associated with hydrops fetalis. *Lancet* **ii:**1033–1034.
19. **Butchko, A. R., and J. A. Jordan.** 2004. Comparison of three commercially available serologic assays used to detect human parvovirus B19-specific immunoglobulin M (IgM) and IgG antibodies in sera of pregnant women. *J. Clin. Microbiol.* **42:**3191–3195.
20. **Caliskan, R., S. Masatlioglu, M. Aslan, S. Altun, S. Saribas, S. Erigin, E. Uckan, V. Koksal, V. Oz, K. Altas, I. Fresko, and B. Kocazeybeck.** 2005. The relationship between arthritis and human parvovirus B19 infection. *Rheumatol. Int.* **26:**7–11. [Epub ahead of print.]
21. **Canaan, S., Z. Zadori, F. Ghomashchi, J. Bollinger, M. Sadilek, M. E. Moreau, P. Tijssen, and M. H. Gelb.** 2004. Interfacial enzymology of parvovirus phospholipases A2. *J. Biol. Chem.* **279:**14502–14508.
22. **Candotti, D., N. Etiz, A. Parsyan, and J. P. Allain.** 2004. Identification and characterization of persistent human erythrovirus infection in blood donor samples. *J. Virol.* **78:**12169–12178.
23. **Centers for Disease Control.** 1989. Risks associated with human parvovirus B19 infection. *MMWR Morb. Mortal. Wkly. Rep.* **38:**81–97.
24. **Chapman, S. A., K. L. Gelkerson, T. D. Davin, and M. R. Pritzker.** 2004. Acute renal failure and intravenous immune globulin: occurs with sucrose-stabilized, but not with D-sorbitol-stabilized, formulation. *Ann. Pharmacother.* **38:** 2059–2067.
25. **Chipman, P. R., M. Agbandje-McKenna, S. Kajigaya, K. E. Brown, N. S. Young, T. S. Baker, and M. G. Rossmann.** 1996. Cryo-electron microscopy studies of empty capsids of human parvovirus B19 complexed with its cellular receptor. *Proc. Natl. Acad. Sci. USA* **93:**7502–7506.
26. **Chow, B. D., Y. T. Huang, and F. P. Esper.** 2008. Evidence of human bocavirus circulating in children and adults, Cleveland, Ohio. *J. Clin. Virol.* **43:**302–306.
27. **Chow, B. D. W., Z. Ou, and F. P. Esper.** 2010. Newly recognized bocaviruses (HBoV, HBoV2) in children and adults with gastrointestinal illness in the United States. *J. Clin. Virol.* **47:**143–147. [Epub ahead of print.]
28. **Clewley, J. P.** 1984. Biochemical characterization of a human parvovirus. *J. Gen. Virol.* **65:**241–245.
29. **Cohen, B. J., and C. M. Bates.** 1995. Evaluation of 4 commercial test kits for parvovirus B19-specific IgM. *J. Virol. Methods* **55:**11–25.
30. **Cohen, B. J., J. Gandhi, and J. P. Clewley.** 2006. Genetic variants of parvovirus B19 identified in the United Kingdom: implications for diagnostic testing. *J. Clin. Virol.* **36:**152–155.
31. **Cooling, L. L., T. A. Koerner, and S. J. Naides.** 1995. Multiple glycosphingolipids determine the tissue tropism of parvovirus B19. *J. Infect. Dis.* **172:**1198–1205.
32. **Cossart, Y. E., A. M. Field, B. Cant, and D. Widdows.** 1975. Parvovirus-like particles in human sera. *Lancet* **i:**72–73.
33. **Curry, A., H. Appleton, and B. Dowsett.** 2006. Application of transmission electron microscopy to the clinical study of viral and bacterial infections: present and future. *Micron* **37(2):**91–106.
34. **Delle Chiaie, L., G. Buck, D. Grab, and R. Terinde.** 2001. Prediction of fetal anemia with Doppler measurement of the middle cerebral artery peak systolic velocity in pregnancies complicated by maternal blood group alloimmunization or parvovirus B19 infection. *Ultrasound Obstet. Gynecol.* **18:**232–236.
35. **Devine, P. A.** 2002. Parvovirus infection in women. *Prim. Care Update Ob/Gyns* **9:**149–153.
36. **Erdman, D. D., B. C. Anderson, T. J. Torok, T. H. Finkel, and L. J. Anderson.** 1997. Possible transmission of parvovirus B19 from intravenous immune globulin. *J. Med. Virol.* **53:** 233–236.
37. **Ferguson, M., and A. Heath.** 2004. Report of a collaborative study to calibrate the Second International Standard for parvovirus B19 antibody. *Biologicals* **32:**207–212.

38. French, A. L., L. Sacks, and G. P. Schechter. 1996. Fifth disease after immunoglobulin administration in an AIDS patient with parvovirus-induced red cell aplasia. *Am. J. Med.* **101**:108–109.

39. Fryer, J. F., E. Delwart, F. M. Hecht, F. Bernardin, M. S. Jones, N. Shah, and S. A. Baylis. 2007. Frequent detection of the parvoviruses, PARV4 and PARV5, in plasma from blood donors and symptomatic individuals. *Transfusion* **47**:1054–1061.

40. Fryer, J. F., A. R. Hubbard, and S. A. Baylis. 2007. Human parvovirus PARV4 in clotting factor VIII concentrates. *Vox Sang.* **93**:341–347.

41. Gallinella, G., E. Manaresi, S. Venturoli, G. L. Grazi, M. Musiani, and M. Zerbini. 1999. Occurrence and clinical role of active parvovirus B19 infection in transplant recipients. *Eur. J. Clin. Microbiol. Infect. Dis.* **18**:811–813.

42. Harder, T. C., M. Hufnagel, K. Zahn, K. Beutel, H. J. Schmitt, U. Ullmann, and P. Rautenberg. 2001. New Light-Cycler PCR for rapid and sensitive quantification of parvovirus B19 DNA guides therapeutic decision-making in relapsing infections. *J. Clin. Microbiol.* **39**:4413–4419.

43. Hayakawa, F., K. Imada, M. Towatari, and H. Saito. 2002. Life-threatening human parvovirus B19 infection transmitted by intravenous immune globulin. *Br. J. Haematol.* **118**:1187–1189.

44. Heegaard, E. D., and K. E. Brown. 2002. Human parvovirus B19. *Clin. Microbiol. Rev.* **15**:485–505.

45. Heegaard, E. D., I. Panum Jensen, and J. Christensen. 2001. Novel PCR assay for differential detection and screening of erythrovirus B19 and erythrovirus V9. *J. Med. Virol.* **65**:362–367.

46. Heegaard, E. D., C. J. Rasksen, and J. Christensen. 2000. Detection of parvovirus B19 NS1-specific antibodies by ELISA and Western blotting employing recombinant NS1 protein as antigen. *FEMS Immunol. Med. Microbiol.* **27**:9–15.

47. Hokynar, K., P. Norja, H. Laitinen, P. Palomaki, A. Garbarg-Chenon, A. Ranki, K. Hedman, and M. Soderlund-Venermo. 2004. Detection and differentiation of human parvovirus variants by commercial quantitative real-time PCR tests. *J. Clin. Microbiol.* **42**:2013–2019.

48. Jones, L. P., D. D. Erdman, and L. J. Anderson. 1999. Prevalence of antibodies to human parvovirus B19 nonstructural protein in persons with various clinical outcomes following B19 infection. *J. Infect. Dis.* **180**:500–504.

49. Jones, M. S., A. Kapoor, V. V. Lukashow, P. Simmonds, F. Hecht, and E. Delwart. 2005. New DNA viruses identified in patients with acute viral infection syndrome. *J. Virol.* **79**:8230–8236.

50. Jordan, J., B. Tiangco, J. Kiss, and W. Koch. 1998. Human parvovirus B19: prevalence of viral DNA in volunteer blood donors and clinical outcomes of transfusion recipients. *Vox Sang.* **75**:97–102.

51. Jordan, J. A. 2000. Comparison of a baculovirus-based VP2 enzyme immunoassay (EIA) to an *Escherichia coli*-based VP1 EIA for detection of human parvovirus B19 immunoglobulin M and immunoglobulin G in sera of pregnant women. *J. Clin. Microbiol.* **38**:1472–1475.

52. Jordan, J. A. 2001. Diagnosing human parvovirus B19 infection: guidelines for test selection. *Mol. Diagn.* **6**:307–312.

53. Jordan, J. A. 1996. Identification of human parvovirus B19 infection in idiopathic nonimmune hydrops fetalis. *Am. J. Obstet. Gynecol.* **174**:37–42.

54. Jordan, J. A., and A. R. Butchko. 2002. Apoptotic activity in villous trophoblast cells during B19 infection correlates with clinical outcome: assessment by the caspase-related M30 Cytodeath antibody. *Placenta* **23**:547–553.

55. Jordan, J. A., and J. A. DeLoia. 1999. Globoside expression within the human placenta. *Placenta* **20**:103–108.

56. Jordan, J. A., S. J. Faas, E. R. Braun, and M. Trucco. 1996. Exonuclease-released fluorescence detection of human parvovirus B19 DNA. *Mol. Diagn.* **1**:321–328.

57. Jordan, J. A., D. Huff, and J. A. DeLoia. 2001. Placental cellular immune response in women infected with human parvovirus B19 during pregnancy. *Clin. Diagn. Lab. Immunol.* **8**:288–292.

58. Jordan, J. A., and L. Penchansky. 1995. Diagnosis of human parvovirus B19-induced anemia: correlation of bone marrow morphology with molecular diagnosis using PCR and immunocytochemistry. *Cell Vision* **2**:279–282.

59. Kahn, J. 2008. Human bocavirus: clinical significance and implications. *Curr. Opin. Pediatr.* **20**:62–66.

60. Kajigaya, S., H. Fujii, A. Field, S. Anderson, S. Rosenfeld, L. J. Anderson, T. Shimada, and N. S. Young. 1991. Self-assembled B19 parvovirus capsids, produced in a baculovirus system, are antigenically and immunogenically similar to native virions. *Proc. Natl. Acad. Sci. USA* **88**:4646–4650.

61. Kantola, K., L. Hedman, T. Allander, T. Jartti, P. Lehtinen, O. Ruuskanen, K. Hedman, and M. Söderlund-Venermo. 2008. Serodiagnosis of human bocavirus infection. *Clin. Infect. Dis.* **46**:540–546.

62. Kaufmann, B., A. A. Simpson, and M. G. Rossmann. 2004. The structure of human parvovirus B19. *Proc. Natl. Acad. Sci. USA* **101**:11628–11633.

63. Kerr, J. R. 2000. Pathogenesis of human parvovirus B19 in rheumatic disease. *Ann. Rheum. Dis.* **59**:672–683.

64. Kerr, J. R., V. S. Cunniffe, P. Kelleher, R. M. Bernstein, and I. N. Bruce. 2003. Successful intravenous immunoglobulin therapy in 3 cases of parvovirus B19-associated chronic fatigue syndrome. *Clin. Infect. Dis.* **36**:100–106.

65. Kerr, S., G. O'Keeffe, C. Kilty, and S. Doyle. 1999. Undenatured parvovirus B19 antigens are essential for the accurate detection of parvovirus B19 IgG. *J. Med. Virol.* **57**:179–185.

66. Kleinman, S. H., S. A. Glynn, T. H. Lee, L. H. Tobler, K. S. Schlumpf, D. S. Todd, H. Qiao, M. Y. Yu, and M. P. Busch. 2009. A linked donor-recipient study to evaluate parvovirus B19 transmission by blood component transfusion. *Blood* **114**(17):3677–3683.

67. Kuo, S. H., L. I. Lin, C. J. Chang, Y. R. Liu, K. S. Lin, and A. L. Cheng. 2002. Increased risk of parvovirus B19 infection in young adult cancer patients receiving multiple courses of chemotherapy. *J. Clin. Microbiol.* **40**:3909–3912.

68. Lau, S. K. P., C. C. Y. Yip, T. I. Que, R. A. Less, R. K. H. Au-Yeung, B. Zhou, L. So, Y. Lau, K. Chan, P. C. Y. Woo, and K. Yuen. 2007. Clinical and molecular epidemiology of human bocavirus in respiratory and fecal samples from children in Hong Kong. *J. Infect. Dis.* **196**:986–993.

69. Lefrere, J. J., M. Mariotti, and M. Thauvin. 1994. B19 parvovirus DNA in solvent/detergent-treated anti-haemophilia concentrates. *Lancet* **343**:211–212.

70. Liefeldt, L., A. Plentz, B. Klempa, O. Kershaw, A. S. Endres, U. Raab, H. H. Neumayer, H. Meisel, and S. Modrow. 2005. Recurrent high level parvovirus B19/genotype 2 viremia in a renal transplant recipient analyzed by real-time PCR for simultaneous detection of genotypes 1 to 3. *J. Med. Virol.* **75**:161–169.

71. Lurcharchaiwong, W., T. Chieochansin, S. Payungporn, A. Theamboonlers, and Y. Poovorawan. 2008. Parvovirus 4 (PARV4) in serum of intravenous drug users and blood donors. *Infection* **36**:144–146.

72. Manaresi, E., G. Gallinella, S. Venturoli, M. Zerbini, and M. Musiani. 2004. Detection of parvovirus B19 IgG: choice of antigens and serological tests. *J. Clin. Virol.* **29**:51–53.

73. Manaresi, E., G. Gallinella, M. Zerbini, S. Venturoli, G. Gentilomi, and M. Musiani. 1999. IgG immune response to B19 parvovirus VP1 and VP2 linear epitopes by immunoblot assay. *J. Med. Virol.* **57**:174–178.

74. Manaresi, E., P. Pasini, G. Gallinella, G. Gentilomi, S. Venturoli, A. Roda, M. Zerbini, and M. Musiani. 1999. Chemiluminescence Western blot assay for the detection of immunity against parvovirus B19 VP1 and VP2 linear epitopes using a videocamera based luminograph. *J. Virol. Methods* **81**:91–99.

75. Manaresi, E., E. Zuffi, G. Gallinella, G. Gentilomi, M. Zerbini, and M. Musiani. 2001. Differential IgM response to conformational and linear epitopes of parvovirus B19 VP1 and VP2 structural proteins. *J. Med. Virol.* **64**:67–73.

76. **Manning, A., V. Russell, K. Eastick, G. H. Leadbetter, N. Hallam, K. Templeton, P. Simmonds.** 2006. Epidemiological profile and clinical associations of human bocavirus and other human parvoviruses. *J. Infect. Dis.* **194:**1283–1290.

77. **Manning, A., S. J. Willey, J. E. Bell, and P. Simmonds.** 2007. Comparison of tissue distribution, persistence, and molecular epidemiology of parvovirus B19 and novel human parvoviruses PARV4 and human bocavirus. *J. Infect Dis.* **195:**1345–1352.

78. **McGhee, S. A., B. Kaska, M. Liebhaber, and E. R. Stiehm.** 2005. Persistent parvovirus associated chronic fatigue treated with high dose intravenous immunoglobulin. *Pediatr. Infect. Dis. J.* **24:**272–274.

79. **McOmish, F., P. L. Yap, A. Jordan, H. Hart, B. J. Cohen, and P. Simmonds.** 1993. Detection of parvovirus B19 in donated blood: a model system for screening by polymerase chain reaction. *J. Clin. Microbiol.* **31:**323–328.

80. **Moffatt, S., N. Tanaka, K. Tada, M. Nose, M. Nakamura, O. Muraoka, T. Hirano, and K. Sugamura.** 1996. A cytotoxic nonstructural protein, NS1, of human parvovirus B19 induces activation of interleukin-6 gene expression. *J. Virol.* **70:**8485–8491.

81. **Moffatt, S., N. Yaegashi, K. Tada, N. Tanaka, and K. Sugamura.** 1998. Human parvovirus B19 nonstructural (NS1) protein induces apoptosis in erythroid lineage cells. *J. Virol.* **72:**3018–3028.

82. **Morinet, F., L. D'Auriol, J. D. Tratschin, and F. Galibert.** 1989. Expression of the human parvovirus B19 protein fused to protein A in Escherichia coli: recognition by IgM and IgG antibodies in human sera. *J. Gen. Virol.* **70:**3091–3097.

83. **Morita, E., A. Nakashima, H. Asao, H. Sato, and K. Sugamura.** 2003. Human parvovirus B19 nonstructural protein (NS1) induces cell cycle arrest at G_1 phase. *J. Virol.* **77:**2915–2921.

84. **Mostello, D., W. L. Holcomb, Jr., J. M. Talsky, and H. N. Winn.** 2004. Fetal parvovirus B19 infection: Doppler studies allow noninvasive treatment of ascites. *J. Ultrasound Med.* **23:**557–560.

85. **Mouthon, L., L. Guillevin, and Z. Tellier.** 2005. Intravenous immunoglobulins in autoimmune- or parvovirus B19-mediated pure red-cell aplasia. *Autoimmun. Rev.* **4:**264–269.

86. **Munakata, Y., T. Saito-Ito, K. Kumura-Ishii, J. Huang, T. Kodra, T. Ishii, Y. Hirabayashi, Y. Koyanagi, and T. Sasaki.** 2005. Ku80 autoantigen as a cellular coreceptor for human parvovirus B19 infection. *Blood* **106:**3449–3456.

87. **Musiani, M., A. Azzi, M. Zerbini, D. Gibellini, S. Venturoli, K. Zakrzewska, M. C. Re, G. Gentilomi, G. Gallinella, and M. La Placa.** 1993. Nested polymerase chain reaction assay for the detection of B19 parvovirus DNA in human immunodeficiency virus patients. *J. Med. Virol.* **40:**157–160.

88. **Musiani, M., E. Manaresi, G. Gallinella, S. Venturoli, E. Zuffi, and M. Zerbini.** 2000. Immunoreactivity against linear epitopes of parvovirus B19 structural proteins. Immunodominance of the amino-terminal half of the unique region of VP1. *J. Med. Virol.* **60:**347–352.

89. **Musiani, M., M. Zerbini, G. Gentilomi, M. Plazzi, G. Gallinella, and S. Venturoli.** 1995. Parvovirus B19 clearance from peripheral blood after acute infection. *J. Infect. Dis.* **172:**1360–1363.

90. **Musiani, M., M. Zerbini, G. Gentilomi, G. Rodorigo, V. De Rosa, D. Gibellini, S. Venturoli, and G. Gallinella.** 1995. Persistent B19 parvovirus infections in haemophilic HIV-1 infected patients. *J. Med. Virol.* **46:**103–108.

91. **Naides, S. J., L. L. Scharosch, F. Foto, and E. J. Howard.** 1990. Rheumatologic manifestations of human parvovirus B19 infection in adults. Initial two-year clinical experience. *Arthritis Rheum.* **33:**1297–1309.

92. **National Institute for Biological Standards and Control (NIBSC).** 2004. *WHO International Standard for Parvovirus B19 DNA for Nucleic Acid Amplification (NAT) Assays. NIBSC Code 99/800. Instructions for Use (17 February 2004, version.5).* National Institute for Biological Standards and Control, Potters Bar, Hertfordshire, United Kingdom.

93. **Nguyen, Q. T., S. Wong, E. D. Heegaard, and K. E. Brown.** 2002. Identification and characterization of a second novel human erythrovirus variant, A6. *Virology* **301:**374–380.

94. **Norja, P., A. M. Eis-Hübinger, M. Söderlund-Veremo, K. Hedman, and P. Simmonds.** 2008. Rapid sequence change and geographical spread of human parvovirus B19: comparison of B19 virus evolution in acute and persistent infections. *J. Virol.* **82:**6427–6433.

95. **Ozawa, K., and N. Young.** 1987. Characterization of capsid and noncapsid proteins of B19 parvovirus propagated in human erythroid bone marrow cell cultures. *J. Virol.* **61:**2627–2630.

96. **Parsyan, A., C. Szmaragd, J. P. Allain, and D. Candotti.** 2007. Identification and genetic diversity of two human parvovirus B19 genotype 3 subtypes. *J. Gen. Virol.* **88:**428–431.

97. **Pattison, J. R., S. E. Jones, J. Hodgson, L. R. Davis, J. M. White, C. E. Stroud, and L. Murtaza.** 1981. Parvovirus infections and hypoplastic crisis in sickle-cell anaemia. *Lancet* **i:**664–665.

98. **Pereira, R. F., W. N. Paula, C. Cubel Rde, and J. P. Nascimento.** 2001. Anti-VP1 and anti-VP2 antibodies detected by immunofluorescence assays in patients with acute human parvovirus B19 infection. *Mem. Instit. Oswaldo Cruz* **96:**507–513.

99. **Pfrepper, K. I., M. Enders, and M. Motz.** 2005. Human parvovirus B19 serology and avidity using a combination of recombinant antigens enables a differentiated picture of the current state of infection. *J. Vet. Med. B* **52:**362–365.

100. **Potter, C. G., A. C. Potter, C. S. Hatton, H. M. Chapel, M. J. Anderson, J. R. Pattison, D. A. Tyrrell, P. G. Higgins, J. S. Willman, H. F. Parry, et al.** 1987. Variation of erythroid and myeloid precursors in the marrow and peripheral blood of volunteer subjects infected with human parvovirus (B19). *J. Clin. Investig.* **79:**1486–1492.

101. **Public Health Laboratory Service Working Party on Fifth Disease.** 1990. Prospective study of human parvovirus (B19) infection in pregnancy. *Br. Med. J.* **300:**1166–1170.

102. **Raab, U., K. Beckenlehner, T. Lowin, H. H. Niller, S. Doyle, and S. Modrow.** 2002. NS1 protein of parvovirus B19 interacts directly with DNA sequences of the p6 promoter and with the cellular transcription factors Sp1/Sp3. *Virology* **293:**86–93.

103. **Reid, D. M., T. M. Reid, T. Brown, J. A. Rennie, and C. J. Eastmond.** 1985. Human parvovirus-associated arthritis: a clinical and laboratory description. *Lancet* **i:**422–425.

104. **Riipinen, A., E. Väisänen, A. Lahtinen, R. Karikoski, M. Nuutila, H. M. Surcel, H. Taskinen, K. Hedman, and M. Söderlund-Venermo.** 2010. Absence of human bocavirus from deceased fetuses and their mothers. *J. Clin. Virol.* **47:**186–188. [Epub ahead of print.]

105. **Robertson, B. H., and D. D. Erdman.** 2000. Non-enveloped viruses transmitted by blood and blood products. *Dev. Biol. Stand.* **102:**29–35.

106. **Saikawa, T., S. Anderson, M. Momoeda, S. Kajigaya, and N. S. Young.** 1993. Neutralizing linear epitopes of B19 parvovirus cluster in the VP1 unique and VP1-VP2 junction regions. *J. Virol.* **67:**3004–3009.

107. **Saldanha, J., and P. Minor.** 1996. Detection of human parvovirus B19 DNA in plasma pools and blood products derived from these pools: implications for efficiency and consistency of removal of B19 DNA during manufacture. *Br. J. Haematol.* **93:**714–719.

108. **Sanabani, S., W. K. Neto, J. Pereira, and E. C. Sabino.** 2006. Sequence variability of human erythroviruses present in bone marrow of Brazilian patients with various parvovirus B19-related hematological symptoms. *J. Clin. Microbiol.* **44:**604–606.

109. **Schenk, T., M. Enders, S. Pollak, R. Hahn, and D. Huzly.** 2009. High prevalence of human parvovirus B19 DNA in myocardial autopsy samples from subjects without myocarditis or dilative cardiomyopathy. *J. Clin. Microbiol.* **47:**106–110.

110. Schildgen, O., A. Müller, T. Allander, I. M. Mackay, S. Völz, B. Kupfer, and A. Simon. 2008. Human bocavirus: passenger or pathogen in acute respiratory tract infections? *Clin. Microbiol. Rev.* **21:**291–304.

111. Servant, A., S. Laperche, F. Lallemand, V. Marinho, G. De Saint Maur, J. F. Meritet, and A. Garbarg-Chenon. 2002. Genetic diversity within human erythroviruses: identification of three genotypes. *J. Virol.* **76:**9124–9134.

112. Shade, R. O., M. C. Blundell, S. F. Cotmore, P. Tattersall, and C. R. Astell. 1986. Nucleotide sequence and genome organization of human parvovirus B19 isolated from the serum of a child during aplastic crisis. *J. Virol.* **58:**921–936.

113. Shirkoohi, R., R. Endo, N. Ishiguro, S. Teramoto, H. Kikuta, and T. Ariga. 2010. Antibodies against structural and nonstructural proteins of human bocavirus in human sera. *Clin. Vaccine Immunol.* **17:**190–193.

114. Simmonds, P., J. Douglas, G. Bestetti, E. Longhi, S. Antinori, C. Parravicini, and M. Corbellino. 2008. A third genotype of the human parvovirus PARV4 in sub-Saharan Africa. *J. Gen. Virol.* **89:**2299–2302.

115. Sklavounou-Andrikopoulou, A., M. Iakovou, S. Paikos, V. Papanikolaou, D. Loukeris, and M. Voulgarelis. 2004. Oral manifestations of papular-purpuric 'gloves and socks' syndrome due to parvovirus B19 infection: the first case presented in Greece and review of the literature. *Oral Dis.* **10:**118–122.

116. Sloots, T. P., P. McErlean, D. J. Speicher, K. E. Arden, M. D. Nissen, and I. M. Mackay. 2006. Evidence of human coronavirus HKU1 and human bocavirus in Australian children. *J. Clin. Virol.* **35:**99–102.

117. Soderlund, M., C. S. Brown, B. J. Cohen, and K. Hedman. 1995. Accurate serodiagnosis of B19 parvovirus infections by measurement of IgG avidity. *J. Infect. Dis.* **171:**710–713.

118. Tabor, E., and J. S. Epstein. 2002. NAT screening of blood and plasma donations: evolution of technology and regulatory policy. *Transfusion* **42:**1230–1237.

119. Takahashi, T., K. Ozawa, K. Takahashi, S. Asano, and F. Takaku. 1990. Susceptibility of human erythropoietic cells to B19 parvovirus in vitro increases with differentiation. *Blood* **75:**603–610.

120. Tattersall, P., and S. F. Cotmore. 1990. Reproduction of autonomous parvovirus DNA, p. 123–140. *In* P. Tijssen (ed.), *Handbook of Parvoviruses*, vol. 1. CRC Press, Boca Raton, FL.

121. Tolfvenstam, T., N. Papadogiannakis, O. Norbeck, K. Petersson, and K. Broliden. 2001. Frequency of human parvovirus B19 infection in intrauterine fetal death. *Lancet* **357:**1494–1497.

122. Torok, T. H. 1997. Unusual clinical manifestations reported in patients with parvovirus B19 infection. *Monogr. Virol.* **20:**61–92.

123. Valeur-Jensen, A. K., C. B. Pedersen, T. Westergaard, I. P. Jensen, M. Lebech, P. K. Andersen, P. Aaby, B. N. Pedersen, and M. Melbye. 1999. Risk factors for parvovirus B19 infection in pregnancy. *JAMA* **281:**1099–1105.

124. van Regenmortel, M. H. V., C. M. Fauquet, D. H. L. Bishop, E. B. Carstens, M. K. Estes, S. M. Lemon, J. Maniloff, M. A. Mayo, D. J. McGeoch, C. R. Pringle, and R. B. Wickner (ed.). 2000. *Virus Taxonomy: Classification and Nomenclature of Viruses. Seventh Report of the International Committee on Taxonomy of Viruses.* Academic Press, San Diego, CA.

125. Viguier, M., L. Guillevin, and L. Laroche. 2001. Treatment of parvovirus B19-associated polyarteritis nodosa with intravenous immune globulin. *N. Eng. J. Med.* **344:**1481–1482.

126. Vo, A. A., V. Cam, M. Toyoda, D. P. Puliyanda, M. Lukovsky, and S. C. Jordan. 2006. Safety and adverse events profiles of intravenous gammaglobulin products used for immunomodulation: a single-center experience. *Clin. J. Am. Soc. Nephrol.* **1:**844–852.

127. von Poblotzki, A., A. Gigler, B. Lang, H. Wolf, and S. Modrow. 1995. Antibodies to parvovirus B19 NS-1 protein in infected individuals. *J. Gen. Virol.* **76:**519–527.

128. Wang, K., W. Wang, H. Yan, P, Ren, J. Zhang, J. Shen, and V. Deubel. 2010. Correlation between bocavirus infection and humoral response, and co-infection with other respiratory viruses in children with acute respiratory infection. *J. Clin. Virol.* **47:**148–155.

129. Wegner, C. C., and J. A. Jordan. 2004. Human parvovirus B19 VP2 empty capsids bind to human villous trophoblast cells in vitro via the globoside receptor. *Infect. Obstet. Gynecol.* **12:**69–78.

130. Weigel-Kelley, K. A., M. C. Yoder, and A. Srivastava. 2003. α5β1 integrin as a cellular coreceptor for human parvovirus B19: requirement of functional activation of β1 integrin for viral entry. *Blood* **102:**3927–3933.

131. Weigel-Kelley, K. A., M. C. Yoder, and A. Srivastava. 2001. Recombinant human parvovirus B19 vectors: erythrocyte P antigen is necessary but not sufficient for successful transduction of human hematopoietic cells. *J. Virol.* **75:**4110–4116.

132. Weimer, T., S. Streichert, C. Watson, and A. Groner. 2001. High-titer screening PCR: a successful strategy for reducing the parvovirus B19 load in plasma pools for fractionation. *Transfusion* **41:**1500–1504.

133. White, D. G., A. D. Woolf, P. P. Mortimer, B. J. Cohen, D. R. Blake, and P. A. Bacon. 1985. Human parvovirus arthropathy. *Lancet* **i:**419–421.

134. Yaegashi, N., T. Niinuma, H. Chisaka, T. Watanabe, S. Uehara, K. Okamura, S. Moffatt, K. Sugamura, and A. Yajima. 1998. The incidence of, and factors leading to, parvovirus B19-related hydrops fetalis following maternal infection; report of 10 cases and meta-analysis. *J. Infect.* **37:**28–35.

135. Young, N. S. 1996. Parvovirus infection and its treatment. *Clin. Exp. Immunol.* **104**(Suppl. 1):26–30.

136. Zadori, Z., J. Szelei, M. C. Lacoste, Y. Li, S. Gariepy, P. Raymond, M. Allaire, I. R. Nabi, and P. Tijssen. 2001. A viral phospholipase A2 is required for parvovirus infectivity. *Dev. Cell* **1:**291–302.

137. Zerbini, M., G. Gallinella, E. Manaresi, M. Musiani, G. Gentilomi, and S. Venturoli. 1999. Standardization of a PCR-ELISA in serum samples: diagnosis of active parvovirus B19 infection. *J. Med. Virol.* **59:**239–244.

138. Zhi, N., Z. Zadori, K. E. Brown, and P. Tijssen. 2004. Construction and sequencing of an infectious clone of the human parvovirus B19. *Virology* **318:**142–152.

Poxviruses

INGER K. DAMON

105

TAXONOMY

All poxviruses described in this chapter belong to the family *Poxviridae* and subfamily *Chordopoxvirinae* (see chapter 75). The genera and species of the viruses discussed in this chapter are shown in Table 1. DNA-based assays, including DNA sequencing, are the most precise methods for poxvirus genus, species, strain, and variant identification and differentiation. The G+C contents of orthopoxviruses, yatapoxviruses, *Molluscum contagiosum virus* (MCV), and parapoxviruses are ~33, ~32, ~60, and ~63%, respectively.

DESCRIPTION OF THE AGENTS

Virions are large and brick shaped (orthopoxviruses, yatapoxviruses, and molluscipoxvirus) or ovoid (parapoxviruses). Virions range in length from 220 to 450 nm and in width and depth from 140 to 260 nm. The appearances of virions under an electron microscope vary somewhat with sample preparation. By cryoelectron microscopy, in unstained, unfixed vitrified specimens, vaccinia virus appears as smooth, rounded rectangles; a uniform core is surrounded by a 30-nm-thick membrane. In conventional negatively stained thin sections, the core appears dumbbell shaped and is surrounded by a complex series of membranes. Lateral bodies of undefined function occupy the space between the outer membrane and the bar of the dumbbell. This feature may be a dehydration effect of negative staining.

Virus particles contain about half of the approximately 200 potential virus genome-encoded proteins. Virions consist of structural proteins and enzymes, including a virtually complete RNA polymerase system for primary transcription of viral genes (57). The genome is a 130- to 375-kbp (depending upon the genus) double-stranded DNA molecule that is encapsidated in a nucleoprotein complex (nucleosome) inside the core. The genome is covalently closed at each end, and its ends are hairpin-like telomeres. Complete genome DNA sequences have been reported for several different poxviruses. GenBank entries are compiled at a dedicated website (http://www.poxvirus.org).

During virus replication (57), virion morphogenesis begins in the cytoplasm in areas known as cytoplasmic factories, where cellular organelles are largely absent. Thin-section electron microscopy observations of cells early after infection show crescent-shaped membrane structures, which progress to ovoid structures, called immature virions, which enclose a dense nucleoprotein complex. Primary transcription precedes the production of the crescents (cup-shaped in three dimensions) and the immature virions. Brick-shaped, membrane-covered mature virions (MVs; also known as intracellular MVs [IMVs]) form as the viral core condenses. These are features that aid the electron microscopist in the identification of poxviruses in clinical materials (73).

A small portion of MVs may be further transported on microtubules from the viral factory and processed to acquire a bilayer tegument (envelope) of Golgi intermediate compartment membrane that contains specific viral proteins. The intracellular enveloped MV then moves along cellular microtubules to the cell surface, where the outermost membrane fuses with the cellular membrane to reveal a cell-associated enveloped virus on the cell surface. The cell-associated enveloped virus can prompt actin polymerization behind the virion, which may facilitate cell-to-cell infection with virus. Enveloped virions can also exit the cell to spread more distantly.

A virus receptor has not been identified. Enveloped and nonenveloped forms attach to cells differently; however, recent studies suggest that the nonenveloped particle (IMV) is the particle which enters, via fusion, into the host cell. A complex of viral proteins is believed to act as a fusion complex. The common result of entry is uncoating of the particle, release of viral contents into the cell, and initiation of virus-controlled transcription of early-class proteins. Recent reviews of virion entry, morphogenesis, and exiting processes have been published (58, 84–86).

EPIDEMIOLOGY AND TRANSMISSION

All current, naturally occurring poxviruses that infect humans are sporadic zoonotic agents, except the *Molluscipoxvirus* species MCV, which is transmitted strictly between humans. The zoonotic poxviruses include members of the genera *Orthopoxvirus* (monkeypox virus, cowpox virus, and the vaccinia virus subspecies, including buffalopox virus), *Parapoxvirus* (orf, pseudocowpox, sealpox, and papulosa stomatitis viruses), and *Yatapoxvirus* (tanapox virus [TPV], Yaba monkey tumor virus [YMTV], and Yaba-like disease virus [YLDV]). Orf virus and MCV infections are the most common poxvirus infections worldwide. These dermatologic lesions often can be readily identified, and laboratory confirmation of clinical diagnosis is often not utilized (19, 70, 71).

TABLE 1 Taxonomy of poxviruses that infect humans

Genus	Species
Orthopoxvirus	Variola virus, vaccinia virus, cowpox virus, monkeypox virus
Parapoxvirus	Orf virus, pseudocowpox virus,[a] bovine papulosa stomatitis virus, sealpox virus
Yatapoxvirus	Tanapox virus, Yaba-like disease virus, Yaba monkey tumor virus
Molluscipoxvirus	Molluscum contagiosum virus

[a]Causes milker's nodule in humans.

Orthopoxviruses

Variola Virus

Variola virus, the cause of smallpox, had a strict human host range and no known animal reservoir. The virus was most often transmitted between humans by large-droplet respiratory particles inhaled by susceptible persons who had close, face-to-face contact with an infectious person. It was spread less commonly by aerosol, by direct contact with a rash lesion, or by sloughed crust material from a scab (27).

Monkeypox Virus

Human monkeypox was first reported in 1970 in the Democratic Republic of the Congo (DRC). Since 1970, the disease has been seen in Liberia, the Ivory Coast, Sierra Leone, Nigeria, Benin, Cameroon, and Gabon, but most cases have been in the DRC. In the 1980s, serosurveys and virologic investigations in the DRC by the World Health Organization (WHO) indicated that (i) monkeys are sporadically infected, as are humans; (ii) three-fourths of cases, mainly those in children under 15 years of age, were from animal contact; (iii) the protective efficacy of vaccinia vaccination is about 85%; (iv) monkeypox virus has a broad host range, including squirrels (*Funisciurus* spp. and *Heliosciurus* spp.); and (v) human monkeypox has a secondary attack rate of 9% among unvaccinated contacts within households (i.e., it is much less transmissible than smallpox). In an outbreak in the DRC, about 250 serosubstantiated cases of monkeypox occurred among 0.5 million people in 78 villages from February 1996 to October 1997. Unlike those in the earlier outbreak, about three-fourths of the cases appeared to result from human-to-human transmission; however, the secondary attack rate of 8% among unvaccinated contacts within households appeared to be about the same as that found in the 1981-to-1986 surveillance (5, 7, 8, 35). More-recent case series have been reported from the DRC (53, 62), and disease with a sustained chain of human-to-human transmission was reported in the Republic of the Congo in 2003 (44).

The emergence of monkeypox in the United States provides another example of the ability of this zoonotic disease to exploit new ecologic niches. The North American prairie dog, diseased after exposure to an infected West African rodent(s), subsequently infected and caused illness in U.S. human populations (9). The characterization of human disease in the United States, caused by a West African virus variant, and its comparison with that classically described in the Congo Basin in the 1980s, enabled clinical and epidemiologic descriptions of distinct monkeypox viral diseases (13, 48).

Vaccinia Virus

Certain strains of vaccinia virus were used for human vaccination to globally eradicate smallpox (27, 29). Since the early 1980s, vaccinia and certain other poxviruses have been used as recombinant vectors for the expression of a variety of proteins, including vaccine immunogens. Infection can be transmitted to laboratory workers by accidental exposure, and significant pathology has been observed in unvaccinated individuals (45). Vaccination is therefore currently recommended for personnel working with live, replicative orthopoxviruses, including vaccinia virus.

The origin of vaccinia virus is uncertain. Vaccinia virus infections are not generally regarded as naturally occurring, although vaccinee-to-cattle and cattle-to-human transmissions occurred on farms during the smallpox eradication campaign. Sporadic outbreaks of infection caused by the vaccinia virus subspecies buffalopox virus that involve transmission between milking buffalo, cattle, and people have been reported, mainly in India but also in Egypt, Bangladesh, Pakistan, and Indonesia. Vaccinia-like lesions have been observed on the animals' teats and the milkers' hands; milk is infectious. Biological data and limited DNA analyses of isolates from an outbreak in India in 1985 suggest that buffalopox virus may be derived from vaccinia virus strains transmitted from humans to livestock during the smallpox vaccination era (22, 52).

Quite interestingly, multiple distinct vaccinia viruses, possibly related to the vaccine strain used during smallpox eradication in Brazil, were recently described for cattle and their farm worker handlers in rural Rio de Janeiro (18, 79) as well as various locales within the Minas Gerais state (18, 51, 59, 92). Historic collections, when reevaluated with additional techniques, suggest that vaccinia-like viruses were previously isolated in the 1960s and 1970s (17). Inadvertent exposure to a vaccinia virus-vectored recombinant rabies virus vaccine dispersed to control rabies in wildlife has resulted in at least two instances of human infection; in both cases the bait was encountered via the family dog (12, 77).

Cowpox Virus

Cowpox, sometimes a rare occupational infection of humans, can be acquired by contact with infected cows. Other animals, e.g., infected rats, pet cats, and zoo and circus elephants, have more often been sources of the disease. Cowpox virus is a rather diverse species and has been isolated from humans and a variety of animals in Europe and adjoining regions of Asia (2, 4). A serosurvey of wild animals in Great Britain found orthopoxvirus antibodies in a portion of bank and field voles and wood mice, which is consistent with small rodents being reservoir hosts (3).

Yatapoxviruses

The epidemiology and natural history of yatapoxviruses are poorly understood. YMTV and YLDV infections have occurred in animal handlers (76); however, TPV is the main naturally occurring human pathogen in the *Yatapoxvirus* genus (28). Tanapox is an endemic zoonosis of equatorial Africa that is thought to be transmitted mechanically to humans by biting insects, especially during the rainy season (39). Recent reports have demonstrated that travelers in regions where the disease is endemic can be infected (20, 88).

Parapoxviruses

Many different parapoxvirus diseases occur in humans (28, 74), generally as occupational infections: milker's nodule (for dairy cattle, the disease is termed pseudocowpox or paravaccinia), orf (for sheep and goats, the disease has been referred to as orf, contagious ecthyma, contagious pustular dermatitis, contagious pustular stomatitis, and sore mouth), and papulosa stomatitis (in calves and beef cattle, the disease is termed bovine papular stomatitis). Parapoxvirus infections are transmitted to humans by direct contact with infected livestock through abraded skin on the hands and fingers, and ocular autoinoculation sometimes occurs (28, 74). Sealpox parapoxvirus infections have been transmitted to humans from pinnipeds (14).

Molluscipoxvirus

MCV is the sole member of the genus *Molluscipoxvirus*. MCV appears to have a human-restricted host range, and it does not grow readily in culture. Molluscum contagiosum occurs worldwide. In children, it is transmitted by direct skin contact, and sexual transmission occurs in adults (28).

CLINICAL SIGNIFICANCE

Orthopoxviruses

A global commission of the WHO declared smallpox eradicated in December 1979, and the declaration was sanctioned by the World Health Assembly in May 1980 (27). Human monkeypox, an emerging zoonotic smallpox-like disease caused by monkeypox virus, with recurrent (and likely endemic) disease in the Congo Basin countries of Africa, is now regarded as the most serious naturally occurring human poxvirus infection (5, 38, 48, 62). The emergence of monkeypox virus as a human pathogen in the United States in 2003 is a classic example of a pathogen exploiting new ecologic niches and hosts.

Variola Virus

Variola major virus strains produced "variola major," a syndrome consisting of a severe prodrome, fever, prostration, and a rash. Toxemia or other forms of systemic shock led to case fatality rates of up to 30%, with secondary attack rates of 30 to 80% among unvaccinated contacts within households. Variola minor virus strains (alastrim, amass, and kaffir viruses) produced "variola minor," a less severe infection with case fatality rates of less than 1%, although secondary attack rates among unvaccinated contacts were as high as those observed with variola major virus infections. DNA and biological data have indicated that alastrim variola minor viruses obtained from Europe and South America are similar to each other but distinct from the so-called African variola minor viruses, which appear to be variola major virus variants (19, 21). Epidemiologically, the disease syndromes were discriminated by case fatality rates; current sequence data indicate that the genetic distinctions between strains causing major or minor disease manifestations are multiple and varied. The last naturally occurring smallpox case occurred in Somalia in October 1977, although a fatal laboratory-associated infection with variola major virus occurred at the University of Birmingham, Birmingham, England, in August 1978 (27).

Naturally acquired variola virus infection caused a systemic febrile rash illness. For ordinary smallpox, the most common clinical presentation, after an asymptomatic incubation period of 10 to 14 days (range, 7 to 17 days), was fever, quickly rising to about 103°F, sometimes with dermal petechiae. Associated constitutional symptoms included backache, headache, vomiting, and prostration. Within a day or two after incubation, a systemic rash appeared that was characteristically centrifugally distributed (i.e., lesions

were present in greater numbers on the oral mucosa, face, and extremities than on the trunk). Initially, the rash lesions appeared macular and then papular, enlarging and progressing to a vesicle by day 4 or 5 and a pustule by day 7; lesions were encrusted and scabby by day 14 and sloughed off. Skin lesions were deep seated and were in the same stage of development on any one area of the body. Milder and more severe forms of the rash were also documented. Less-severe manifestations (modified smallpox or variola sine eruptione) occurred in some vaccinated individuals, whereas hemorrhagic or flat-pox types of smallpox occurred in patients with impaired immune responses.

Variola major smallpox was differentiated into four main clinical types: (i) ordinary smallpox (~90% of cases) produced viremia, fever, prostration, and rash; (ii) modified smallpox (5% of cases) produced a mild prodrome with few skin lesions in previously vaccinated people; (iii) flat smallpox (5% of cases) produced slowly developing focal lesions with generalized infection and an ~50% fatality rate; and (iv) hemorrhagic smallpox (<1% of cases) induced bleeding into the skin and the mucous membranes and was invariably fatal within a week of onset. A discrete type of the ordinary form resulted from alastrim variola minor infection (27).

Before its eradication, smallpox as a clinical entity was relatively easy to recognize, but other exanthematous illnesses were mistaken for this disease (27). For example, the rash of severe chicken pox, caused by varicella-zoster virus, was often misdiagnosed as that of smallpox. However, chicken pox produces a centripetally distributed rash and rarely appears on the palms and soles. In addition, in the case of chicken pox, prodromal fever and systemic manifestations are mild, if present at all. Chicken pox lesions are superficial in nature, and lesions in different developmental stages may be present on the same area of the body. Other diseases confused with vesicular-stage smallpox included monkeypox, generalized vaccinia, disseminated herpes zoster, disseminated herpes simplex virus infection, drug reactions (eruptions), erythema multiforme, enteroviral infections, scabies, insect bites, impetigo, and molluscum contagiosum. Diseases confused with hemorrhagic smallpox included acute leukemia, meningococcemia, and idiopathic thrombocytopenic purpura. The Centers for Disease Control and Prevention (CDC), in collaboration with numerous professional organizations, has developed an algorithm for evaluating patients for smallpox. The algorithm and additional information are available at http://emergency.cdc.gov/agent/smallpox/diagnosis/ and http://www.bt.cdc.gov/EmContact/index.asp. Experience with the algorithm has been summarized previously (81).

Monkeypox Virus

Reviews of human monkeypox infection are available (5, 38). Monkeypox was first recognized by Von Magnus in Copenhagen in 1958 as an exanthem of primates in captivity. Later, the disease was seen in other captive animals, including primates in zoos and animal import centers.

The clinical appearance of human monkeypox, typified by the Congo Basin variant, is much like that of smallpox, with fever, a centrifugally distributed vesiculopustular rash (appearing also on the palms and soles), respiratory distress, and in some cases, death from systemic shock. Like variola virus, monkeypox virus appears to enter through skin abrasions or the mucosa of the upper respiratory tract, where it produces an enanthem and cough. During the primary viremia, the virus then migrates to regional lymph nodes, and during secondary viremia, it is disseminated throughout the body and the skin rash appears. During the prodrome, lymphadenopathy (generally inguinal) with fever and headache is common. Individual skin lesions develop through stages of macule, papule, vesicle, and pustule. Sequelae involve secondary infections, permanent scarring and pitting at the sites of the lesions, and sometimes alopecia and corneal opacities. Acute illness in the United States in 2003, caused by the "West African" variant, appeared generally more mild (13, 48); genomic sequence analyses and comparative epidemiologic and clinical data support the existence of two distinct clades of monkeypox virus. Additional information on clinical manifestations of disease (34) is also available.

Vaccinia Virus

Humans have historically encountered vaccinia virus most commonly in the form of smallpox vaccine (now called vaccinia vaccine), a live-virus preparation that is cross-protective against other orthopoxvirus infections. The most recent recommendations of the Advisory Committee on Immunization Practices (ACIP) on vaccinia vaccination are available at http://www.cdc.gov/mmwr//preview/mmwrhtml/rr5010a1.htm (10). The ACIP recommends vaccination as a safeguard for laboratory and health care workers who are at high risk of orthopoxvirus infection. In the United States, the CDC Drug Service provides the vaccine after CDC approval of a formal request for this purpose by the administering physician. Vaccinia immunoglobulin is available to treat possible postvaccination complications, which can be severe.

Vaccination is done by using a multiple-puncture technique that causes a local lesion, which develops and recedes in a distinctive manner in primary vaccinees during a 3-week period. At the site of percutaneous vaccination, a papule forms within 2 to 5 days, and the lesion reaches maximum size (about 1 cm in diameter) by 8 to 10 days postvaccination after evolving through vesicle and pustule stages; an areola may encircle the site. The pustule dries into a scab, which usually separates by 14 to 21 days after vaccination. In some vaccinated children, fevers with temperatures as high as about 100°F have occurred but have been uncommon in adults, and a regional lymphadenopathy has been observed.

Because of an increased risk for serious adverse events, such as eczema vaccinatum or vaccinia necrosum, the ACIP has stated that the vaccine is contraindicated for persons with eczema or immunocompromising conditions. The possible complications of vaccinia vaccination are described in the ACIP report (10). Despite attempts to prescreen potential vaccinees for contraindications, instances of generalized vaccinia rash, which may arise 10 to 14 days postvaccination, continue to be reported (40). On a clinical basis alone, it is often difficult to distinguish between generalized vaccinia, which represents virus presumably spread hematogenously, and a form of erythema multiforme, which may be immunologically mediated. Laboratory identification of virus within the disseminated rash may differentiate these conditions (40).

Cowpox Virus

In humans, cowpox lesions occur mainly on the fingers, with reddening and swelling. Autoinoculation of other parts of the body may occur, and severe systemic infections have been reported. Skin lesions are likened to those from a primary vaccinia virus vaccination. The site becomes papular, and a vesicle develops in 4 or 5 days. Healing takes about 3 weeks (2).

Yatapoxviruses

The three members of the genus *Yatapoxvirus*, TPV, YLDV of monkeys, and YMTV, are serologically related (76). DNA maps of TPV and YLDV are extremely similar, suggesting that they are the same agent. However, these DNA maps are markedly different from YMTV DNA maps, even though the DNA from the three viruses cross-hybridizes extensively (41, 43).

TPV and YLDV infections in humans consist of a brief fever, followed by development of firm, elevated, round, maculopapular nodules which become necrotic and are distinct from the vesiculopustular lesions of orthopoxvirus infections. Generally, few lesions develop, and these occur primarily on the skin of the upper arms, face, neck, or trunk (37). Symptoms that occur prior to the appearance of lesions include fever, backache, and headache. Lesions umbilicate without pustulation during recovery from infection. They usually heal in 2 to 4 weeks. YMTV produces epidermal histiocytomas, tumor-like masses of histiocytic polygonal mononuclear cell infiltrates that advance to suppurative inflammation.

Parapoxviruses

Milker's nodule occurs as a reddened hemispheric papule that matures into a purplish, smooth, firm nodule varying up to 2 cm in diameter. The lesions usually are not painful and can persist for about 6 weeks. Human orf virus infection is usually found on the fingers, hands, and arms but may also be found on the face and neck. Fever and swelling of draining lymph nodes may be present, and the lesions often ulcerate and are painful. Autoinoculation of the eye may lead to serious sequelae (70). Contact with (e.g., skinning of) certain wild animals, including deer, reindeer, chamois, and Japanese serow, has also been a source of human parapoxvirus infection. Technicians handling gray seals have contracted sealpox virus (14, 74).

Molluscipoxvirus

In children and teenagers, molluscum contagiosum lesions generally appear on the trunk, limbs (except the palms and soles), and face, where there may be ocular involvement. Infection is usually transmitted by direct skin contact. When MCV infection is transmitted sexually among teenagers and adults, the lesions are mostly on the lower abdomen, pubis, inner thighs, and genitalia. Lesions are pearly, flesh-colored, raised, firm, umbilicated nodules, about 5 mm in diameter. The lesions tend to disseminate by autoinoculation. Prior to highly active antiretroviral therapy, MCV was an opportunistic pathogen in approximately 15% of patients with AIDS in the United States. Restriction endonuclease mapping of isolates suggests that there are at least three MCV subtypes (71). Two predominant MCV subtypes, MCVI and MCVII, have been detected in a limited number of samples examined by restriction pattern and base sequence analyses, but no correlation of subtype with disease syndrome or geographic distribution has been confirmed (70, 71). A rapid PCR and restriction fragment length polymorphism analysis using skin lesion material has been described previously for differentiating the MCV subtypes (67).

ANTIVIRAL THERAPY

Currently there are no drugs approved for use in the treatment of poxvirus infections; this is an area of active research and development (83). The experimental drug ST-246, an inhibitor of poxvirus egress, appears to be effective against orthopoxviruses, including variola virus and monkeypoxvirus infections of nonhuman primates (33), and has been used investigationally in the treatment of human smallpox vaccine adverse events (93). The DNA polymerase inhibitor cidofovir and orally bioavailable derivative CMX-001 similarly have in vitro and in vivo data to support antiorthopoxvirus activity and have been used as investigational agents in the treatment of vaccine adverse events (11). Vaccinia immune globulin is licensed for use as a treatment for severe adverse events associated with vaccination and can be obtained from the CDC.

COLLECTION, HANDLING, AND STORAGE OF SPECIMENS

A suspected case of smallpox should be immediately reported to the appropriate local or state health department. After review by the health department, the case should be immediately reported to the CDC if the diagnosis of smallpox is still suspected. Current international recommendations advise that work with variola virus be done using WHO-sanctioned biosafety level 4 laboratories. Two WHO collaborating centers (WHOCCs) currently have the capability to handle smallpox specimens: one at the CDC in Atlanta and the other at the State Center for Virology and Biotechnology, Koltsovo, Russia. The WHOCC at the CDC also has containment facilities appropriate to work with monkeypox virus and other exotic poxviruses (e.g., TPV). Generally, clinical specimens suspected of containing other poxviruses (e.g., parapoxviruses and MCV) can be tested by experienced local staff using biosafety level 2 containment facilities and equipment. Additionally, laboratories testing samples from laboratory workers with potential occupational exposures to vaccinia virus may wish to consider vaccination of staff, in addition to the use of biosafety level 3 containment facilities, equipment, and work practices.

Suitable specimens for laboratory testing of most suspected poxvirus infections are at least two to four scabs and/or material from vesicular lesions. Scabs can be separated from the underlying intact skin with a scalpel or a 26-gauge needle, and each specimen should be stored in a separate container to avoid cross-contamination. Coexistent infectious rash illnesses, including simultaneous chicken pox and monkeypox infections, have been noted (35).

Lesions should be sampled so that both the vesicle fluid and the overlying skin are collected. Once the overlying skin is lifted off and placed in a specimen container, the base of the vesicle should be vigorously swabbed with a wooden applicator or polyester or cotton swab. The viscous material can be applied onto a clean glass microscope slide

and air dried. A "touch prep" can be prepared by pressing a clean slide onto the opened lesion by using a gradual pressing motion. If available, three electron microscope grids can be applied in succession (shiny side to the unroofed vesicle) to the lesion by using minimal, moderate, and moderate pressure. The glass slides and electron microscope grids should be allowed to air dry for about 10 min and then placed in a slide holder or a grid carrier box for transport to a laboratory.

Alternative lesion sampling processes, including storing material on appropriate filter paper types, are being evaluated. Sample storage in transport medium (as done, for example, with herpesviruses) is discouraged, since specimen dilution decreases the sensitivity of direct evaluation by electron microscopy. Specific recommendations for electron microscopy sampling and specimen processing can be found on the Internet (http://www.bt.cdc.gov/agent/smallpox/lab-testing/pdf/em-rash-protocol.pdf). A biopsy of lesions may also provide material suitable for direct viral evaluation or immunohistochemistry. A 3- or 4-mm punch biopsy specimen can be made, and the specimen can be bisected, with half placed in formalin for immunohistochemical testing and the remainder placed in a specimen collection container. Blood and throat swabs obtained from suspected smallpox patients during the prodromal febrile phase and early in the rash phase were also a potential source of virus during the smallpox era (66).

Patient serum can also be obtained for serology to substantiate viral infection diagnoses or to infer a retrospective diagnosis. Paired acute- and convalescent-phase serum specimens can be of great value for diagnosis of infection. In this case, serum should be obtained as early as possible in the disease course and then 3 to 4 weeks later.

Most virus-containing specimens should be stored frozen at −20°C or on dry ice until samples reach their transport destination. Storage at standard refrigerator temperatures is acceptable for less than 7 days. Electron microscopy grids and formalin-fixed tissues should be kept at room temperature.

CLINICAL UTILITY OF LABORATORY TESTS FOR POXVIRUS DIAGNOSIS

Poxvirus infections can often be distinguished by the appearances of rashes and associated dermatopathologies (56). In addition, multiple different clinical laboratory tests can be useful for identifying and differentiating poxviruses, including electron microscopy, antigenic testing, nucleic acid detection, determination of virus growth features, and serology. The utility of these test methods for the diagnosis of poxvirus infections is shown in Table 2.

TABLE 2 Diagnostic tests for poxviruses[a]

Virus(es)	HP	EM	HA	NAT	Isolation	Serology
Orthopoxviruses	X	X	X	X	X[b]	X
Parapoxviruses	X	X		X	X[c]	X
Yatapoxviruses	X	X		X	X[c]	X
MCV	X	X		X		

[a]Abbreviations: HP, histopathology; EM, electron microscopy; HA, hemagglutination; NAT, nucleic acid test. X's indicate the utility of the tests for the specified viruses.
[b]Pock formation on CAM and tissue culture isolation are useful.
[c]Isolation in tissue culture only; viruses do not produce pocks on CAM.

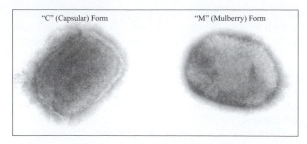

"C" (Capsular) Form   "M" (Mulberry) Form

FIGURE 1 A negative-stain electron micrograph demonstrates the two forms of the brick-shaped monkeypox virus from a cell culture. The surfaces of M (mulberry) virions are covered with short, whorled filaments, while C (capsular)-form virions penetrated by stain present as a sharply defined, dense core surrounded by several laminated zones of differing densities. (Image 3945 from the CDC Public Health Image Library; courtesy of C. Goldsmith, I. Damon, and S. Zaki.)

DIRECT DETECTION

Microscopy

Electron microscopy is a first-line method for laboratory diagnosis of poxvirus infections. Negative-stain electron microscopy of lesion samples was widely used during the smallpox eradication era. Because the clinical diagnosis of poxvirus infection is now infrequent, electron microscopy observations may provide one of the first clues into the cause of an unknown rash illness. Although electron microscopy can distinguish between orthopoxvirus and parapoxvirus morphologies, it cannot differentiate between species; selected serologic, biologic, and DNA-based assays must be used.

Orthopoxviruses have a distinctive brick-shaped, knobby morphology when examined with sodium phosphotungstate or other heavy-metal negative stains (Fig. 1). Parapoxviruses appear ovoid with a spiraling criss-cross surface. The relative sensitivity of the negative-stain method was about 95% for detecting variola virus in smallpox lesions and about 75% for detecting vaccinia virus (60, 61). Sensitivity may be improved by directly pressing a prepared grid into the base of an unroofed skin lesion, as described above (31). Descriptions of methods for negative-stain evaluation and pictures of negative-stained particles are available on the Internet (http://www.bt.cdc.gov/agent/smallpox/lab-testing/pdf/emrash-protocol.pdf) and elsewhere (49, 61).

Poxviruses produce inclusions that have characteristic appearances when stained with May-Grunwald Giemsa and hematoxylin-eosin stains. Perinuclear basophilic or B-type cytoplasmic inclusions (virus factories or viroplasm) are observed with cells infected with any of the poxviruses and represent sites of virus replication. Certain species (e.g., the orthopoxvirus cowpox virus) produce acidophilic inclusions or A-type inclusions. Depending on the strain, A-type inclusions may (V^+) or may not (V^-) contain virions.

Antigen Detection

Orthopoxvirus is the only genus whose members produce a hemagglutinin (HA) antigen, which is detectable by hemadsorption or hemagglutination assays using chicken erythrocytes that are pretested to be suitable for such tests. Direct detection of poxvirus antigens in clinical specimens is not routinely performed in many laboratories as a diagnostic assay.

Nucleic Acid Detection

PCR analysis is used by the WHOCC at the CDC to detect poxvirus DNA in samples. A recent development is the validation of a "pan-poxvirus" PCR assay, which can screen specimens for the presence of poxviruses other than avipoxviruses (47). Multiple single-gene PCR assays, followed by restriction fragment length polymorphism analysis or sequence analysis of the amplicon, permits species identification of orthopoxviruses. A number of different targets are used, including the HA gene, which is unique for the genus *Orthopoxvirus*, the gene for the B cytokine response modifier (CrmB, one of several different tumor necrosis factor receptor homologs produced by orthopoxviruses), and the gene for the A-type inclusion body protein. In these assays, DNA that is present in any orthopoxvirus is amplified (Table 3). The amplicon is digested with the appropriate restriction endonuclease, and digested fragments are electrophoresed. Fragment sizes are compared to reference restriction fragment length polymorphism profiles to discriminate species. Conventional PCR tests for other poxvirus genera have also been reported (89). Other nucleic acid diagnostic approaches include random amplified polymorphic DNA fragment length polymorphism for orthopoxvirus species and strain discrimination (82, 87) discernment of PCR-amplified, fluorescence-labeled DNA fragments by hybridization to orthopoxvirus species-specific DNA immobilized on a microchip.

The high sensitivity of and rapid results from real-time PCR assays make them attractive for laboratory clinical diagnostic use (26). In the United States, many national reference laboratories, as well as the Laboratory Response Network laboratories, use this format of nucleic acid testing for rapid response to diagnose suspected orthopoxvirus infections and/or to rule out smallpox infections. The use of a probe or probes in this type of assay allows for the specificity; however, the extreme sensitivity of the assays can lead to false-positive contaminants from specimen carryover. Many of these methods for detection of orthopoxviruses and other poxviruses are summarized in Table 4. These types of assays are performed primarily at specific reference centers, including the CDC Poxvirus Program/WHOCC for Smallpox and Other Poxvirus Infections.

TABLE 3 Conventional PCR assays for orthopoxvirus detection

Target	Primers (amplicon size, [bp])	Detection method[a]	Reference(s)
HA	Old World viruses: EACP1/EACP2 (900)	TaqI	75
	New World viruses: NACP1/NACP2 (600)	RsaI	
CrmB	VL2N/VL33 (vaccinia, 1200; monkeypox, variola, cowpox, 1300)	NlaIII[b]	50
A-type inclusion body protein	ATI-low-1/ATI-up-1 (1500–1700)	BglII or XbaI	54, 55

[a]Amplicons are digested with specified restriction enzymes to distinguish different viruses.
[b]To distinguish monkeypox, variola, and cowpox viruses.

TABLE 4 Real-time PCR assays for poxvirus detection

Genus, species	Genetic target[a]	Platform or method	Comments	Limitations	Reference
Orthopoxvirus	HA/A56R	LightCycler with hybridization probes	Melting curve analysis differentiates variola virus from other orthopoxviruses	Several cowpox and camelpox virus strains have melting temperature identical to that of variola virus	24
Orthopoxvirus, variola virus	HA/A56R	TaqMAN	Variola virus specific probe cleavage		36
Orthopoxvirus, variola virus	HA/A56R	LightCycler with hybridization probes	Melting curve analysis differentiates variola virus from other orthopoxviruses	Several cowpox virus strains have melting temperature identical to that of variola virus	69
Orthopoxvirus, variola virus	Assay 1: Rpo 18 Assay 2: VETF Assay 3: A13L (VAR) Assay 4: A13L (nVAR-OPX)	LightCycler with hybridization probes	Melting curve analysis differentiates variola virus from other orthopoxviruses		64
Orthopoxvirus, variola virus	Assay 1: B10R Assay 2: B9R Assay 3: HA/A56R	TaqMan		Assay 1 and 2: some cowpox virus strains are amplified Assay 3 is identical to the assay described in reference 36, with a slightly shortened probe	42
Orthopoxvirus, variola virus	14-kD/A27L	LightCycler with hybridization probes	Melting curve analysis differentiates variola virus from other orthopoxviruses		68
Orthopoxvirus, variola virus	crmB	LightCycler with hybridization probes	Melting curve analysis differentiates variola virus from other orthopoxviruses	Specific identification of variola virus has to be performed by restriction enzyme analysis of PCR amplicons	6
Orthopoxvirus, variola virus	crmB	Two TaqMan probes	One probe is variola virus-specific		25
Orthopoxvirus, monkeypox virus	B5R, E9L		Monkeypox virus specific assay (MGB probe) Orthopoxvirus-non-variola detection assay (TaqMan)		46
Orthopoxvirus, variola virus	14kD/A27L	TaqMan	Two probes; one probe is variola virus-specific		78
Orthopoxvirus, variola virus	HA/A56R	TaqMan	Two probes; one probe is variola virus-specific		1
Orthopoxvirus, variola virus	HA/A56R	LightCycler with hybridization probes	Melting curve analysis differentiates variola virus from other orthopoxviruses		72
Orthopoxvirus, vaccinia virus	B8R	TaqMan			65
Yatapoxvirus	101 nt of PstIL fragment	TaqMan		Detects YLDV and tanapox virus, not YMTV	96
Parapoxvirus, Orf virus	B2L	TaqMan			30
Parapoxvirus	B2L	TaqMan			66
Molluscum contagiosum virus	P43K MC080R	TaqMan	Pyrosequencing of the p43K product differentiates MCV1 and MCV2		91

[a]Orthopoxvirus assays use the target's Vaccinia-Copenhagen nomenclature. YLDV, Yaba-like disease virus; YMTV, Yaba monkey tumor virus; nt, nucleotides.

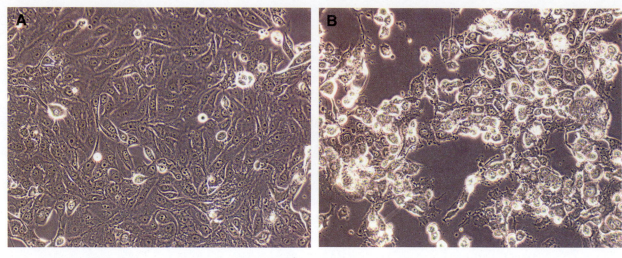

FIGURE 2 Vaccinia virus ("Dryvax") CPE in FHRK-4 cells. (A) Early CPE; (B) mature CPE. (Courtesy of V. Olson.)

ISOLATION AND IDENTIFICATION

Orthopoxviruses can be grown in a variety of established cell culture lines, including Vero, BS-C-1, CV-1, LLCMK-2 monkey kidney cells, human embryonic lung fibroblast cells, HeLa cells, chicken embryo fibroblast cells, and MRC-5 human diploid fibroblast cells, as well as in fetal rhesus monkey kidney (FHRK-4) cells. Cytopathic effects (CPEs) appear as cell rounding with long cytoplasmic extensions (Fig. 2). In some cases, syncytium formation can also be seen, especially with monkeypox virus (Fig. 3). The timing of CPEs varies with the virus inoculum, is often apparent within 24 hours, and progresses more rapidly with vaccinia than with monkeypox. Most laboratories confirm the presence of a specific orthopoxvirus via PCR (see above). Methods for growing and discriminating the morphologies of orthopoxviruses on the chorioallantoic membranes (CAMs) of 12-day-old chicken embryos have been described previously (60, 61, 94, 95). Orthopoxviruses are the only human poxviruses that produce pocks (94, 95) on the CAMs of fertile chicken eggs; pock morphology is useful for biologic species and variant differentiation. Parapoxviruses, yatapoxviruses, and MCV do not form pocks on the CAM, although avipoxviruses, leporipoxviruses, and capripoxviruses do so. Poxvirus genera can usually be identified and differentiated by virus neutralization testing with hyperimmune reference sera (15, 22, 28, 60, 61). However, it can be difficult to identify the infecting species since poxviruses are antigenically closely related within a given genus.

SEROLOGIC TESTS

Orthopoxviruses

When virus-containing clinical specimens are not available, antibody detection may be the only way to define the etiology of the disease. Serologic methods currently used to detect antibodies against human orthopoxviruses include enzyme-linked immunosorbent assays (ELISAs), the virus

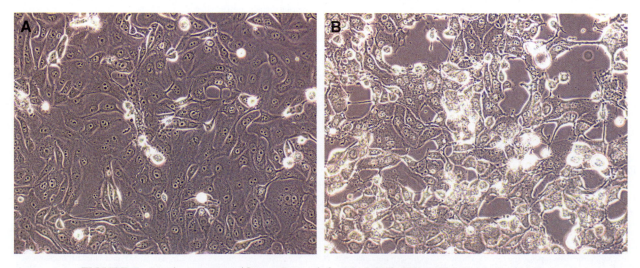

FIGURE 3 Monkeypox virus (Congo Basin clade, v79-I-005) CPE in FRHK-4 cells. (A) Early CPE; (B) mature CPE with syncytia. (Courtesy of V. Olson.)

neutralization test (NT), Western blotting, and hemagglutination inhibition. Various protocols for poxvirus serologic testing used at the CDC are detailed elsewhere (39).

The description of an orthopoxvirus immunoglobulin M (IgM) assay offers great promise to enhance investigations of orthopoxvirus infection outbreaks, often semiretrospective in nature (39). This technique offers the advantage that it measures recent infection or illness with an orthopoxvirus. It is useful for evaluating disease incidence in epidemiologic surveillance studies. For example, during the 2003 U.S. monkeypox outbreak, the IgM capture assay demonstrated ~95% sensitivity and ~95% specificity for epidemiologically linked and laboratory test-confirmed patients when sera were obtained between days 4 and 56 post-rash onset. A low-grade response, termed "equivocal," awaits further research. This assay was also used to detect antiorthopoxvirus IgM in the cerebrospinal fluid of an encephalitic patient with monkeypox (80). A peptide-based ELISA for the identification of monkeypox virus-specific antibodies has been reported (32). It remains an investigational tool rather than a clinical test since its clinical utility has not been further established. In the current state of bioterrorism response awareness, tests to evaluate residual protection from previous vaccination are being requested. It is important to note that there is no one routine immunologic test that defines a person's degree of protection against a poxvirus infection. Protection is genetically defined and requires a concert of cell-mediated and humoral immune responses. Studies (23) suggest that humoral responses may be the critical component of recovery from and survival of a systemic orthopoxvirus infection. The presence of neutralizing antibodies generally indicates recovery from an infection, not always protracted protection from future infection. Neutralizing antibodies against variola, monkeypox, cowpox, or vaccinia viruses may be detectable as early as 6 days after infection or vaccination. Neutralizing antibodies have been detected as long as 20 years after vaccinia vaccination or natural infection with other human orthopoxviruses.

In the virus NT, a fourfold rise in antibody titer between serum samples drawn during the acute and convalescent phases is usually considered diagnostic of poxvirus infection. When only one serum specimen is available from one phase of infection, confirmation of a clinical diagnosis may be difficult or impossible. Because orthopoxviruses are closely related, serum cross-absorption tests, such as those performed in immunofluorescent-antibody or immunodiffusion methods, have been used with variable success with patient and animal sera. Orthopoxvirus antigen cross-absorption assays have been performed using hyperimmune animal sera and have been utilized in serosurveys for animal or human monkeypox infection (60, 61). False-positive results should be ruled out by using appropriate control sets of sera of known provenance.

The Western blot assay is performed essentially as described by Towbin et al. (90) and uses various antigens, including purified virus and sometimes the concentrate of culture fluid from infected cells maintained under medium that contains 1% or no serum supplement. Few laboratories are using this method, as reliable standardization has not been achieved.

Pseudocowpox Virus Orf, Tanapox, and MCV

Serologic methods used to help confirm parapoxvirus infections (milker's nodule and orf) have included ELISAs (16) and Western blot assays that use various antigen preparations. Serologic testing for TPV infection by standard ELISA (16) with antigens obtained from concentrates of infected cell culture, by an indirect immunofluorescent antibody test, and by NT has been moderately effective. Optimally, sera should be collected at the time of actual disease and 3 to 5 weeks or later after the presumed onset date. Because MCV cannot be readily grown in culture, no routine serologic test is available. Molluscum contagiosum is readily diagnosed clinically, often with the aid of electron microscopy and histopathologic testing performed by a local diagnostic facility.

EVALUATION, INTERPRETATION, AND REPORTING OF RESULTS

For confirmation of an infectious agent, cell culture or another mechanism for demonstrating viable virus should be regarded as the gold standard. Absent readily available or feasible tissue culture methods, the use of multiple diagnostic assays or techniques improves the specificity of a diagnosis. Nucleic acid amplification tests, while sensitive, can result in false-positive results. A proficiency survey of nucleic acid amplification tests performed by 33 labs spanning three geographic areas (Europe, Australasia, and the United States) found a substantial rate of false-positive results (~12%) emanating from the small number of laboratories ($n = 5$), highlighting the need for sound molecular practices, which becomes even more critical when testing for potential bio-threat agents (63). The use of multiple nucleic acid tests, with different detection targets, can improve the specificity of a diagnosis. Electron microscopy can be used to evaluate generically for the presence of a poxvirus and can be used to infer the viable agent if multiple virus forms are present but cannot be used to make a specific genus diagnosis except in the case of parapoxvirus infections. Serologic assays are available at a few reference laboratories worldwide but only rarely can be used to make a specific species diagnosis. Histochemistry, combined with immunologic analysis, can be used to identify poxvirus genera in a few reference centers worldwide. A combination of nucleic acid amplification, growth of agent in culture, serology, electron microscopy, and/or immunohistochemistry techniques improves the sensitivity and specificity of a diagnosis.

REFERENCES

1. **Aitichou, M., S. Javorschi, and M. S. Ibrahim.** 2005. Two-color multiplex assay for the identification of orthopox viruses with real-time LUX-PCR. *Mol. Cell. Probes* **19:**323–328.
2. **Baxby, D., M. Bennett, and B. Getty.** 1994. Human cowpox 1969–93: a review based on 54 cases. *Br. J. Dermatol.* **131:**598–607.
3. **Bennett, M., A. J. Crouch, M. Begon, B. Duffy, S. Feore, R. M. Gaskell, D. F. Kelly, C. M. McCracken, L. Vicary, and D. Baxby.** 1997. Cowpox in British voles and mice. *J. Comp. Pathol.* **116:**35–44.
4. **Bennett, M., C. J. Gaskill, D. Baxby, R. M. Gaskill, D. F. Kelly, and J. Naidoo.** 1990. Feline cowpox virus infection. A review. *J. Small Anim. Pract.* **14:**167–173.
5. **Breman, J. G.** 2000. Monkeypox: an emerging infection for humans?, p. 45–67. *In* W. M. Scheld, W. A. Craig, and J. M. Hughes (ed.), *Emerging Infections 4.* ASM Press, Washington, DC.
6. **Carletti F., A. Di Caro, S. Calcaterra, A. Grolla, M. Czub, G. Ippolito, M. R. Capobianchi, and D. Horejsh.** 2005. Rapid, differential diagnosis of orthopox- and herpesviruses based upon real-time PCR product melting temperature and restriction enzyme analysis of amplicons. *J. Virol. Methods* **129:**97–100.

7. **Centers for Disease Control and Prevention.** 1997. Human monkeypox—Kasai Oriental, Democratic Republic of Congo, February 1996–October 1997. *MMWR Morb. Mortal. Wkly. Rep.* **46:**1168–1171.

8. **Centers for Disease Control and Prevention.** 1997. Human monkeypox—Kasai Oriental, Zaire, 1996–1997. *MMWR Morb. Mortal. Wkly. Rep.* **46:**304–307.

9. **Centers for Disease Control and Prevention.** 2003. Update: multistate outbreak of monkeypox—Illinois, Indiana, Kansas, Missouri, Ohio, and Wisconsin, 2003. *MMWR Morb. Mortal. Wkly. Rep.* **52:**642–646.

10. **Centers for Disease Control and Prevention.** 2001. Vaccinia (smallpox) vaccination: recommendations of the Advisory Committee on Immunization Practices (ACIP). *MMWR Morb. Mortal. Wkly. Rep.* **50:**1–22.

11. **Centers for Disease Control and Prevention.** 2009. Progressive vaccinia in a military smallpox vaccinee—United States, 2009. *MMWR Morb. Mortal. Wkly. Rep.* **58:**532–536.

12. **Centers for Disease Control and Prevention.** 2009. Human vaccinia infection after contact with a raccoon rabies vaccine bait—Pennsylvania, 2009. *MMWR Morb. Mortal. Wkly. Rep.* **58:**1204–1207.

13. **Chen, N., G. Li, M. K. Liszewski, J. P. Atkinson, P. B. Jahrling, Z. Feng, J. Schriewer, C. Buck, C. Wang, E. J. Lefkowitz, J. J. Esposito, T. Harms, I. K. Damon, R. L. Roper, C. Upton, and R. M. Buller.** 2005. Virulence differences between monkeypox virus isolates from West Africa and the Congo basin. *Virology* **340:**46–63.

14. **Clark, C., P. G. McIntyre, A. Evans, C. J. McInnes, and S. Lewis-Jones.** 2005. Human sealpox resulting from a seal bite: confirmation that sealpox virus is zoonotic. *Br. J. Dermatol.* **152:**791–793.

15. **Cole, G. A., and R. V. Blanden.** 1982. Immunology of poxviruses, p. 1–19. *In* A. J. Nahmias and R. J. O'Reilly (ed.), *Comprehensive Immunology*, vol. 9. Plenum Press, New York, NY.

16. **Conroy, J. M., R. W. Stevens, and K. E. Hechemy.** 1991. Enzyme immunoassays, p. 87–92. *In* A. Balows, W. J. Hausler, K. L. Herrmann, H. D. Isenberg, and H. J. Shadomy (ed.), *Manual of Clinical Microbiology*, 5th ed. American Society for Microbiology, Washington, DC.

17. **da Fonseca, F. G., G. S. Trindade, R. L. Silva, C. A. Bonjardim, P. C. Ferreira, and E. G. Kroon.** 2002. Characterization of a vaccinia-like virus isolated in a Brazilian forest. *J. Gen. Virol.* **83:**223–228.

18. **Damaso, C. R., J. J. Esposito, R. C. Condit, and N. Moussatche.** 2000. An emergent poxvirus from humans and cattle in Rio de Janeiro State: Cantagalo virus may derive from Brazilian smallpox vaccine. *Virology* **277:**439–449.

19. **Damon, I.** 2007. Poxviruses, p. 2947–2977. *In* D. M. Knipe, P. M. Howley, et al. (ed.), *Fields Virology*, 5th ed. Lippincott Williams and Wilkins, New York, NY.

20. **Dhar, A. D., A. E. Werchniak, Y. Li, J. B. Brennick, C. S. Goldsmith, R. Kline, I. Damon, and S. N. Klaus.** 2004. Tanapox infection in a college student. *N. Engl. J. Med.* **350:**361–366.

21. **Dumbell, K. R., and F. Huq.** 1986. The virology of variola minor. Correlation of laboratory tests with the geographic distribution and human virulence of variola isolates. *Am. J. Epidemiol.* **123:**403–415.

22. **Dumbell, K. R., and M. Richardson.** 1993. Virological investigations of specimens from buffaloes affected by buffalopox in Maharashtra State, India between 1985 and 1987. *Arch. Virol.* **128:**257–267.

23. **Edghill-Smith, Y., H. Golding, J. Manischewitz, L. R. King, D. Scott, M. Bray, A. Nalca, J. W. Hooper, C. A. Whitehouse, J. E. Schmitz, K. A. Reimann, and G. Franchini.** 2005. Smallpox vaccine-induced antibodies are necessary and sufficient for protection against monkeypox virus. *Nat. Med.* **11:**740–747.

24. **Espy, M. J., F. R. Cockerill III, R. F. Meyer, M. D. Bowen, G. A. Poland, T. L. Hadfield, and T. F. Smith.** 2002. Detection of smallpox virus DNA by LightCycler PCR. *J. Clin. Microbiol.* **40:**1985–1988.

25. **Fedele, C. G., A. Negredo, F. Molero, M. P. Sánchez-Seco, and A. Tenorio.** 2006. Use of internally controlled real-time genome amplification for detection of variola virus and other orthopoxviruses infecting humans. *J. Clin. Microbiol.* **44:**4464–4470.

26. **Fedorko, D. P., J. C. Preuss, G. A. Fahle, L. Li, S. H. Fischer, P. Hohman, and J. I. Cohen.** 2005. Comparison of methods for detection of vaccinia virus in patient specimens. *J. Clin. Microbiol.* **43:**4602–4606.

27. **Fenner, F., D. A. Henderson, I. Arita, Z. Jezek, and I. Ladnyi.** 1988. *Smallpox and Its Eradication.* World Health Organization, Geneva, Switzerland.

28. **Fenner, F., and J. H. Nakano.** 1988. Poxviridae: the poxviruses, p. 177–207. *In* E. H. Lennette, P. Halonen, and F. A. Murphy (ed.), *Laboratory Diagnosis of Infectious Diseases*, vol. 2. *Viral, Rickettsial, and Chlamydial Diseases.* Springer-Verlag, New York, NY.

29. **Fenner, F., R. Wittek, and K. R. Dumbell.** 1989. *The Orthopoxviruses.* Academic Press, Inc., New York, NY.

30. **Gallina, L., F. Dal Pozzo, C. J. Mc Innes, G. Cardeti, A. Guercio, M. Battilani, S. Ciulli, and A. Scagliarini.** 2006. Orf virus detection by real time PCR. *J. Virol. Methods* **134:**140–145.

31. **Gelderblom, H. R., and P. R. Hazelton.** 2000. Specimen collection for electron microscopy. *Emerg. Infect. Dis.* **6:**433–434.

32. **Hammarlund, E., M. W. Lewis, S. V. Carter, I. Amanna, S. G. Hansen, L. I. Strelow, S. W. Wong, P. Yoshihara, J. M. Hanifin, and M. K. Slifka.** 2005. Multiple diagnostic techniques identify previously vaccinated individuals with protective immunity against monkeypox. *Nat. Med.* **11:**105–111.

33. **Huggins, J., A. Goff, L. Hensley, E. Mucker, J. Shamblin, C. Wlazlowski, W. Johnson, J. Chapman, T. Larsen, N. Twenhafel, K. Karem, I. K. Damon, C. M. Byrd, T. C. Bolken, R. Jordan, and D. Hruby.** 2009. Nonhuman primates are protected from smallpox virus or monkeypox virus challenges by the antiviral drug ST-246. *Antimicrob. Agents Chemother.* **53:**2620–2625.

34. **Huhn, G. D., A. M. Bauer, K. Yorita, M. B. Graham, J. Sejvar, A. Likos, I. K. Damon, M. G. Reynolds, and M. J. Kuehnert.** 2005. Clinical characteristics of human monkeypox, and risk factors for severe disease. *Clin. Infect. Dis.* **41:**1742–1751.

35. **Hutin, Y. J., R. J. Williams, P. Malfait, R. Pebody, V. N. Loparev, S. L. Ropp, M. Rodriguez, J. C. Knight, F. K. Tshioko, A. S. Khan, M. V. Szczeniowski, and J. J. Esposito.** 2001. Outbreak of human monkeypox, Democratic Republic of Congo, 1996 to 1997. *Emerg. Infect. Dis.* **7:**434–438.

36. **Ibrahim, M. S., D. A. Kulesh, S. S. Saleh, I. K. Damon, J. J. Esposito, A. L. Schmaljohn, and P. B. Jahrling.** 2003. Real-time PCR assay to detect smallpox virus. *J. Clin. Microbiol.* **41:**3835–3839.

37. **Jezek, Z., I. Arita, M. Szczeniowski, K. M. Paluku, K. Ruti, and J. H. Nakano.** 1985. Human tanapox in Zaire: clinical and epidemiological observations on cases confirmed by laboratory studies. *Bull. W. H. O.* **63:**1027–1035.

38. **Jezek, Z., and F. Fenner.** 1988. Human monkeypox. *Monogr. Virol.* **17:**1–140.

39. **Karem, K. L., M. Reynolds, Z. Braden, G. Lou, N. Bernard, J. Patton, and I. K. Damon.** 2005. Characterization of acute-phase humoral immunity to monkeypox: use of immunoglobulin M enzyme-linked immunosorbent assay for detection of monkeypox infection during the 2003 North American outbreak. *Clin. Diagn. Lab. Immunol.* **12:**867–872.

40. **Kelly, C. D., C. Egan, S. W. Davis, W. A. Samsonoff, K. A. Musser, P. Drabkin, J. R. Miller, J. Taylor, and N. M. Cirino.** 2004. Laboratory confirmation of generalized vaccinia following smallpox vaccination. *J. Clin. Microbiol.* **42:**1373–1375.

41. **Knight, J. C., F. J. Novembre, D. R. Brown, C. S. Goldsmith, and J. J. Esposito.** 1989. Studies on tanapox virus. *Virology* **172:**116–124.

42. **Kulesh, D. A., R. O. Baker, B. M. Loveless, D. Norwood, S. H. Zwiers, E. Mucker, C. Hartmann, R. Herrera, D. Miller, D. Christensen, L. P. Wasieloski, Jr., J. Huggins,**

and P. B. Jahrling. 2004. Smallpox and pan-orthopox virus detection by real-time 3′-minor groove binder TaqMan assays on the Roche LightCycler and the Cepheid smart Cycler platforms. *J. Clin. Microbiol.* **42:**601–609.

43. Lapa, S., M. Mikheev, S. Shchelkunov, V. Mikhailovich, A. Sobolev, V. Blinov, I. Babkin, A. Guskov, E. Sokunova, A. Zasedatelev, L. Sandakhchiev, and A. Mirzabekov. 2002. Species-level identification of orthopoxviruses with an oligonucleotide microchip. *J. Clin. Microbiol.* **40:**753–757.

44. Learned, L. A., M. G. Reynolds, D. W. Wassa, Y. Li, V. A. Olson, K. Karem, L. L. Stempora, Z. H. Braden, R. Kline, A. Likos, F. Libama, H. Moudzeo, J. D. Bolanda, P. Tarangonia, P. Boumandoki, P. Formenty, J. M. Harvey, and I. K. Damon. 2005. Extended interhuman transmission of monkeypox in a hospital community in the Republic of the Congo, 2003. *Am. J. Trop. Med. Hyg.* **73:**428–434.

45. Lewis, F. M. T., E. Chernak, E. Goldmann, Y. Li, K. Karem, I. K. Damon, R. Henkel, E. C. Newbern, P. Ross, and C. C. Johnson. 2006. Ocular vaccinia infection in laboratory worker, Philadelphia, 2004. *Emerg. Infect. Dis.* **12:**134–137.

46. Li, Y., V. A. Olson, T. Laue, M. T. Laker, and I. K. Damon. 2006. Detection of monkeypoxvirus with real time PCR assays. *J. Clin. Virol.* **36:**194–203.

47. Li, Y., H. Meyer, H. Zhao, and I. K. Damon. 2010. GC content-based universal PCR assays for poxvirus detection. *J. Clin. Microbiol.* **48:**268–276.

48. Likos, A. M., S. A. Sammons, V. A. Olson, A. M. Frace, Y. Li, M. Olsen-Rasmussen, W. Davidson, R. Galloway, M. L. Khristova, M. G. Reynolds, H. Zhao, D.S. Carroll, A. Curns, P. Formenty, J. J. Esposito, R. L. Regnery, and I. K. Damon. 2005. A tale of two clades: monkeypox viruses. *J. Gen. Virol.* **86:**2661–2672.

49. Long, G. W., J. Nobel, Jr., F. A. Murphy, K. L. Herrmann, and B. Lourie. 1970. Experience with electron microscopy in the differential diagnosis of smallpox. *Appl. Microbiol.* **20:** 497–504.

50. Loparev, V. N., R. F. Massung, J. J. Esposito, and H. Meyer. 2001. Detection and differentiation of Old World orthopoxviruses: restriction fragment length polymorphism of the *crmB* gene region. *J. Clin. Microbiol.* **39:**94–100.

51. Marques, J. T., G. D. Trindade, F. G. Da Fonseca, J. R. Dos Santos, C. A. Bonjardim, P. C. Ferreira, and E. G. Kroon. 2001. Characterization of ATI, TK and IFN-alpha/betaR genes in the genome of the BeAn 58058 virus, a naturally attenuated wild orthopoxvirus. *Virus Genes* **23:**291–301.

52. Mathew, T. 1987. *Advances in Medical and Veterinary Virology, Immunology and Epidemiology: Cultivation and Immunological Studies on Pox Group of Viruses with Special Reference to Buffalo Pox Virus.* Thajema Publishers, New Delhi, India.

53. Meyer, H., M. Perrichot, M. Stemmler, P. Emmerich, H. Schmitz, F. Varaine, R. Shungu, F. Tshioko, and P. Formenty. 2002. Outbreaks of disease suspected of being due to human monkeypox virus infection in the Democratic Republic of Congo in 2001. *J. Clin. Microbiol.* **40:**2919–2921.

54. Meyer, H., S. L. Ropp, and J. J. Esposito. 1997. Gene for A-type inclusion body protein is useful for a polymerase chain reaction assay to differentiate orthopoxviruses. *J. Virol. Methods* **64:**217–221.

55. Meyer, H., S. L. Ropp, and J. J. Esposito. 1998. Poxviruses, p. 199–211. *In* A. Warnes and J. Stephenson (ed.), *Methods in Molecular Medicine: Diagnostic Virology Protocols.* Humana Press, Totowa, NJ.

56. Moriello, K. A., and J. Cooley. 2001. Difficult dermatologic diagnosis. Contagious viral pustular dermatitis (orf), goatpox, dermatophilosis, dermatophytosis, bacterial pyoderma, and mange. *J. Am. Vet. Med. Assoc.* **218:**19–20.

57. Moss, B. 2007. Poxviridae and their replication, p. 2905–2947. *In* D. M. Knipe, P. M. Howley, et al. (ed.), *Fields Virology*, 5th ed. Lippincott Williams & Wilkins, New York, NY.

58. Moss, B. 2006. Poxvirus entry and membrane fusion. *Virology* **344:**48–54.

59. Nagasse-Sugahara, T. K., J. J. Kisielius, M. Ueda-Ito, S. P. Curti, C. A. Figueiredo, A. S. Cruz, M. M. Silva, C. H. Ramos, M. C. Silva, T. Sakurai, and L. F. Salles-Gomes. 2004. Human vaccinia-like virus outbreaks in Sao Paulo and Goias States, Brazil: virus detection, isolation and identification. *Rev. Inst. Med. Trop. Sao Paulo* **46:**315–322.

60. Nakano, J. H. 1978. Comparative diagnosis of poxvirus diseases, p. 267–339. *In* E. Kurstak and C. Kurstak (ed.), *Comparative Diagnosis of Viral Diseases*, vol. 1. Academic Press, Inc., New York, NY.

61. Nakano, J. H. 1979. Poxviruses, p. 257–308. *In* E. H. Lennette and N. J. Schmidt (ed.), *Diagnostic Procedures for Viral, Rickettsial, and Chlamydial Infections*, 5th ed. American Public Health Association, Inc., Washington, DC.

62. Nalca, A., A. W. Rimoin, S. Bavari, and C. A. Whitehouse. 2005. Reemergence of monkeypox: prevalence, diagnostics, and countermeasures. *Clin. Infect. Dis.* **41:**1765–1771.

63. Niedrig, M., H. Meyer, M. Panning, and C. Drosten. 2006. Follow-up on diagnostic proficiency of laboratories equipped to perform orthopoxvirus detection and quantification by PCR: the second international external quality assurance study. *J. Clin. Microbiol.* **44:**1283–1287.

64. Nitsche, A., H. Ellerbrok, and G. Pauli. 2004. Detection of orthopoxvirus DNA by real-time PCR and identification of variola virus DNA by melting analysis. *J. Clin. Microbiol.* **42:**1207–1213.

65. Nitsche, A., B. Steger, H. Ellerbrok, and G. Pauli. 2005. Detection of vaccinia virus DNA on the LightCycler by fluorescence melting curve analysis. *J. Virol. Methods* **126:**187–195.

66. Nitsche, A., M. Büttner, S. Wilhelm, G. Pauli, and H. Meyer. 2006. Real-time PCR detection of parapoxvirus DNA. *Clin. Chem.* **52:**316-319.

67. Nunez, A., J. M. Funes, M. Agromayor, M. Moratilla, A. J. Varas, J. L. Lopez-Estebaranz, M. Esteban, and A. Martin-Gallardo. 1996. Detection and typing of molluscum contagiosum virus in skin lesions by using a simple lysis method and polymerase chain reaction. *J. Med. Virol.* **50:**342–349.

68. Olson, V. A., T. Laue, M. T. Laker, I. V. Babkin, C. Drosten, S. N. Shchelkunov, M. Niedrig, I. K. Damon, and H. Meyer. 2004. Real-time PCR system for detection of orthopoxviruses and simultaneous identification of smallpox virus. *J. Clin. Microbiol.* **42:**1940–1946.

69. Panning, M., M. Asper, S. Kramme, H. Schmitz, and C. Drosten. 2004. Rapid detection and differentiation of human pathogenic orthopox viruses by a fluorescence resonance energy transfer real-time PCR assay. *Clin. Chem.* **50:**702–708.

70. Pepose, J. S., and J. J. Esposito. 1996. Molluscum contagiosum, Orf, and vaccinia virus ocular infections in humans, p. 846–856. *In* J. S. Pepose, G. N. Holland, and K. R. Wilhelmus (ed.), *Ocular Infections and Immunity.* Mosby Year Book, Inc., St. Louis, MO.

71. Porter, C. D., N. W. Blake, J. J. Cream, and L. C. Archard. 1992. Molluscum contagiosum virus, p. 233–257. *In* D. Wright and L. C. Archard (ed.), *Molecular and Cellular Biology of Sexually Transmitted Diseases.* Chapman and Hall, London, England.

72. Putkuri, N., H. Piiparinen, A. Vaheri, and O. Vapalahti. 2009. Detection of human orthopoxvirus infections and differentiation of smallpox virus with real time PCR. *J. Med. Virol.* **81:**146–152.

73. Reed, K. D., J. W. Melski, M. B. Graham, R. L. Regnery, M. J. Sotir, M. V. Wegner, J. J. Kazmierczak, E. J. Stratman, Y. Li, J. A. Fairley, G. R. Swain, V. A. Olson, E. K. Sargent, S. C. Kehl, M. A. Frace, R. Kline, S. L. Foldy, J. P. Davis, and I. K. Damon. 2004. The detection of monkeypox in humans in the Western Hemisphere. *N. Engl. J. Med.* **350:**342–350.

74. Robinson, A. J., and D. J. Lyttle. 1992. Parapoxviruses: their biology and potential as recombinant vaccine vectors, p. 285–327. *In* M. M. Binns and G. L. Smith (ed.), *Recombinant Poxviruses.* CRC Press, Inc., Boca Raton, FL.

75. Ropp, S. L., Q. Jin, J. C. Knight, R. F. Massung, and J. J. Esposito. 1995. PCR strategy for identification and differentiation of small pox and other orthopoxviruses. *J. Clin. Microbiol.* **33:**2069–2076.

76. **Rouhandeh, H.** 1988. Yaba virus, p. 1–15. *In* G. Darai (ed.), *Virus Diseases in Laboratory and Captive Animals.* Martinus Nijhoff, Boston, MA.

77. **Rupprecht, C. E., L. Blass, K. Smith, L. A. Orciari, M. Niezgoda, S. G. Whitfield, R. V. Gibbons, M. Guerra, and C. A. Hanlon.** 2001. Human infection due to recombinant vaccinia-rabies glycoprotein virus. *N. Engl. J. Med.* **345:**582–586.

78. **Scaramozzino, N., A. Ferrier-Rembert, A. L. Favier, C. Rothlisberger, S. Richard, J. M. Crance, H. Meyer, and D. Garin.** 2007. Real-time PCR to identify variola virus or other human pathogenic orthopox viruses. *Clin. Chem.* **53:**606–613.

79. **Schatzmayr, H. G., E. R. Lemos, C. Mazur, A. Schubach, S. Majerowicz, T. Rozental, T. M. Schubach, M. C. Bustamante, and O. M. Barth.** 2000. Detection of poxvirus in cattle associated with human cases in the State of Rio de Janeiro: preliminary report. *Mem. Inst. Oswaldo Cruz* **95:**625–627.

80. **Sejvar, J. J., Y. Chowdary, M. Schomogyi, J. Stevens, J. Patel, K. Karem, M. Fischer, M. J. Kuehnert, S. R. Zaki, C. D. Paddock, J. Guarner, W. J. Shieh, J. L. Patton, N. Bernard, Y. Li, V. A. Olson, R. L. Kline, V. N. Loparev, D. S. Schmid, B. Beard, R. R. Regnery, and I. K. Damon.** 2004. Human monkeypox infection: a family cluster in the midwestern United States. *J. Infect. Dis.* **190:**1833–1840.

81. **Seward, J. F., K. Galil, I. Damon, S. A. Norton, L. Rotz, S. Schmid, R. Harpaz, J. Cono, M. Marin, S. Hutchins, S. S. Chaves, and M. M. McCauley.** 2004. Development and experience with an algorithm to evaluate suspected smallpox cases in the United States, 2002–2004. *Clin. Infect. Dis.* **39:**1477–1483.

82. **Shchelkunov, S. N., E. V. Gavrilova, and I. V. Babkin.** 2005. Multiplex PCR detection and species differentiation of orthopoxviruses pathogenic to humans. *Mol. Cell. Probes* **19:**1–8.

83. **Smee, D. F.** 2008. Progress in the discovery of compounds inhibiting orthopoxviruses in animal models. *Antivir. Chem. Chemother.* **19:**115–124.

84. **Smith, G. L., and M. Law.** 2004. The exit of vaccinia virus from infected cells. *Virus Res.* **106:**189–197.

85. **Smith, G. L., B. J. Murphy, and M. Law.** 2003. Vaccinia virus motility. *Annu. Rev. Microbiol.* **57:**323–342.

86. **Smith, G. L., A. Vanderplasschen, and M. Law.** 2002. The formation and function of extracellular enveloped vaccinia virus. *J. Gen. Virol.* **83:**2915–2931.

87. **Stemmler, M., H. Neubauer, and H. Meyer.** 2001. Comparison of closely related orthopoxvirus isolates by random amplified polymorphic DNA and restriction fragment length polymorphism analysis. *J. Vet. Med. B* **48:**647–654.

88. **Stich, A., H. Meyer, B. Kohler, and K. Fleischer.** 2002. Tanapox: first report in a European traveller and identification by PCR. *Trans. R. Soc. Trop. Med. Hyg.* **96:**178–179.

89. **Torfason, E. G., and S. Gunadottir.** 2002. Polymerase chain reaction for laboratory diagnosis of orf virus infections. *J. Clin. Virol.* **24:**79–84.

90. **Towbin, H., T. Staehelin, and J. Gordon.** 1979. Electrophoretic transfer of proteins from polyacrylamide gels to nitrocellulose sheets: procedure and some applications. *Proc. Natl. Acad. Sci. USA* **76:**4350–4354.

91. **Trama, J. P., M. E. Adelson, and E. Mordechai.** 2007. Identification and genotyping of molluscum contagiosum virus from genital swab samples by real-time PCR and Pyrosequencing. *J. Clin. Virol.* **40:**325–329.

92. **Trindade, G. S., F. G. da Fonseca, J. T. Marques, S. Diniz, J. A. Leite, S. De Bodt, Y. Van der Peer, C. A. Bonjardim, P. C. Ferreira, and E. G. Kroon.** 2004. Belo Horizonte virus: a vaccinia-like virus lacking the A-type inclusion body gene isolated from infected mice. *J. Gen. Virol.* **85:**2015–2021.

93. **Vora, S., I. Damon, V. Fulginiti, S. G. Weber, M. Kahana, S. L. Stein, S. I. Gerber, S. Garcia-Houchins, E. Lederman, D. Hruby, L. Collins, D. Scott, K. Thompson, J. V. Barson, R. Regnery, C. Hughes, R. S. Daum, Y. Li, H. Zhao, S. Smith, Z. Braden, K. Karem, V. Olson, W. Davidson, G. Trindade, T. Bolken, R. Jordan, D. Tien, and J. Marcinak.** 2008. Severe eczema vaccinatum in a household contact of a smallpox vaccinee. *Clin. Infect. Dis.* **46:**1555–1561.

94. **Westwood, J. C., P. H. Phipps, and E. A. Boulter.** 1957. The titration of vaccinia virus on the chorioallantoic membrane of the developing chick embryo. *J. Hyg. Lond.* **55:**123–139.

95. **World Health Organization.** 1960. *Guide to the Laboratory Diagnosis of Smallpox for Smallpox Eradication Programmes.* World Health Organization, Geneva, Switzerland.

96. **Zimmermann, P., I. Thordsen, D. Frangoulidis, and H. Meyer.** 2005. Real-time PCR assay for the detection of tanapox virus and yaba-like disease virus. *J. Virol. Methods* **130:**149–153.

Hepatitis B and D Viruses

REBECCA T. HORVAT AND GARY E. TEGTMEIER

106

HEPATITIS B VIRUS

Introduction

Epidemic hepatitis was first described in the 5th century B.C.E. The earliest documented blood-borne outbreak of hepatitis occurred in Bremen, Germany, in 1883 among shipyard workers who received a smallpox vaccine stabilized with human serum. In 1947, MacCallum and Bauer introduced the term hepatitis A for infectious hepatitis and hepatitis B for "serum" hepatitis based on the different epidemiologic characteristics of the diseases (66a). This terminology was adopted by the World Health Organization (WHO) in 1973 to distinguish the two agents of hepatitis. Hepatitis B virus (HBV) was identified and characterized after the discovery of the Australia antigen by Blumberg and colleagues in 1965 (3, 14). The Australia antigen, now designated hepatitis B surface antigen (HBsAg), is detected in the sera of patients with both acute and chronic HBV. This discovery also revealed that not all posttransfusion hepatitis was associated with HBV and that an additional agent, hepatitis C virus, was responsible for nearly all of the remaining cases (4).

This discovery led to a more complete understanding of HBV which now allows for a more accurate diagnosis with the use of diagnostic assays that detect HBV infection. It is now apparent that HBV is a global health issue associated with approximately 600,000 deaths per year. There is also an abundant amount of information on the natural history of HBV, including its pathogenesis and epidemiology. This has led to safe and effective vaccines, therapeutic agents, and diagnostic assays. Given the tremendous burden of this disease, the laboratory tests used to diagnose and monitor disease progression have become central to the control of the disease.

Taxonomy

HBV is an enveloped DNA virus which is an agent of the *Hepadnaviridae* family. As with other viruses in this family, the HBV genome is a partially double-stranded, circular DNA molecule that replicates via an RNA intermediate (23). The replication of HBV DNA by reverse transcription is unique for human DNA viruses. This mechanism is also found in nonprimate hepadnaviruses and the cauliflower mosaic virus, which have some relatedness to HBV.

Description of the Agent

The HBV virion is composed of the HBsAg in a lipid membrane from the host cell and surrounds a nucleocapsid core. This complete viral particle is also known as the Dane particle (28). The viral core is surrounded by the HBV core antigen (HBcAg) and contains a single molecule of partially double-stranded DNA, hepatitis B e antigen (HBeAg), and a DNA-dependent polymerase (Fig. 1A). The various antigens and antibodies associated with HBV as they appear at different stages of infection are given in Table 1.

HBV particles found in the sera of patients with active HBV infection reveal three distinct morphologic entities in various proportions (Fig. 1A and B). The most abundant forms (by a factor of 10^4 to 10^6) are the small, pleomorphic, spherical, noninfectious particles (17 to 25 nm in diameter) (38). Less numerous are the tubular or filamentous forms, which have diameters similar to those of the small particles. The third and least numerous particle is the complete HBV virion, with a diameter of approximately 42 to 47 nm (28).

The HBV genome is approximately 3,200 bases long and contains overlapping genes (Fig. 1C). There are four open reading frames (ORFs) in the complete minus strand. These ORFs encode the structural proteins (HBsAg, HBcAg, and HBeAg) and proteins needed for replication and regulation (polymerase and X protein). The genome is compact, and most sequences are essential for productive infection (23, 30, 61).

After binding to hepatocytes, the HBV virion is taken up and uncoated. The partially double-stranded, relaxed circular DNA is converted by the host polymerase to a covalently closed circular DNA (cccDNA) template in the cell nucleus. This cccDNA form is used as a template for transcription of the pregenomic RNA (pgRNA) and messenger RNA (23, 61). The pgRNA that is transcribed from the cccDNA in the nucleus moves into the cytoplasm of the host cell. In the cytoplasm, the pgRNA serves as the template for the HBV reverse transcription enzyme as well as the core protein. At the same time, the polymerase converts the pgRNA to a new circular DNA molecule. Early in infection, some newly synthesized genomes from the cytoplasm will circulate back to the nucleus to build up and maintain the pool of cccDNA (88).

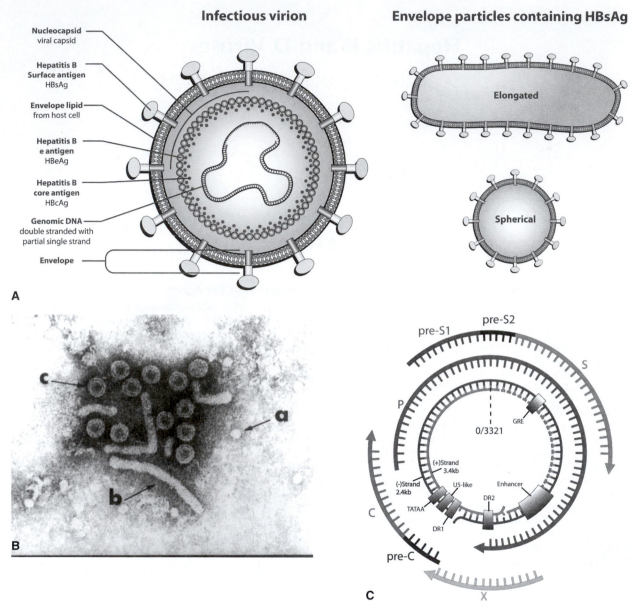

FIGURE 1 (A) The intact infectious HBV virion and the empty particles are shown. The two HBV particles (right) comprised of HBsAg are shown as elongated or tubular and as spherical particles. These particles vastly outnumber the virions. (Designed by University of Kansas Graphic Design Department.) (B) Electron micrograph of serum showing the presence of three distinct morphologic entities: 17- to 25-nm-diameter, pleomorphic, spherical particles (a); tubular or filamentous forms with diameters similar to those of the small particles (b); and 42- to 47-nm-diameter, double-shelled, spherical particles representing the hepatitis B virion (Dane particle) (c). Magnification, ×10⁵. (C) Diagrammatic representation of HBV coding regions. The functioning genome is a double-stranded circular DNA molecule shown in the middle. RNA transcripts (arrows) are generated using both the plus-strand [(+)Strand] and minus-strand [(−)Strand] DNA templates. The largest transcript codes for the viral polymerase shown around the genome as the P transcript. The transcript for surface antigen (S) is produced as three separate transcripts, pre-S1, pre-S2, and S. The core protein is translated from the C transcript. HBeAg is coded within the HBc gene. The transactivating protein is encoded by the X transcript. (Designed by University of Kansas Graphic Design Department.)

TABLE 1 HBV markers in different stages of infection and convalescence

Stage of infection	Molecular marker: HBV DNA	Protein antigen marker		HBV-specific antibody marker			
		HBsAg	HBeAg	Anti-HBc		Anti-HBe	Anti-HBs
				IgM	Total		
Susceptible	−	−	−	−	−	−	−
Early incubation	+	−	−	−	−	−	−
Late incubation	+	+	−/+	−	−	−	−
Acute infection	+	+	+	+	+	−	−
Recent infection[a]	− / +	−	−	++	+	+	+++
Remote infection[b]	− or very low	−	−	−	+	+/−	+
HBsAg-negative acute infection	− ($<10^3$ IU/ml)	−	−	+	+	−	−
HBsAg variant infection	− / +	−	−/+	+/−	+	−	−
Immune-active carrier	++ ($>10^5$ IU/ml)	+	−/+	−/+	+++	−	−
Inactive HBsAg carrier	− ($<10^3$ IU/ml)	+	−	−	+	+	−
Immune-tolerant carrier	+++	+	+	−	+	−	−
Vaccination response	−	−	−	−	−	−	+

[a]This description can be applied to early convalescence and to individuals who remain HBV DNA positive for prolonged periods in the absence of HBsAg.

[b]Remote infection can be applied to individuals with anti-HBc in the absence of other serological markers, including DNA. These patients may or may not have anti-HBs. There is evidence that these patients may reactivate HBV during immunosuppression. HBsAg, complex antigen found on the surface of HBV and on 20-nm-diameter particles and tubular forms; HBcAg, antigen associated with the 27-nm-diameter core of HBV; HBeAg, protein that results from the proteolytic cleavage of the precore/core protein by cellular proteases and that is secreted as soluble protein in serum.

The HBV genome is efficient and uses every nucleotide in a coding region. More than half of the genome is transcribed in more than one ORF. Four viral mRNA transcripts are translated into HBV proteins. The mRNAs are transcribed from various promoter regions on the cccDNA template (Fig. 1C). The longest mRNA acts as the template for genome replication (pgRNA) as well as the translation of the precore, core (HBcAg), and polymerase proteins (61). The second transcript encodes the pre-S1 protein (39 kb), pre-S2 protein (33 kDa), and S protein (24 kDa). A third transcript encodes the pre-S2 protein and the S protein. The smallest mRNA encodes the X protein, which transactivates transcription. Mature virions are produced by transcription of HBV RNA into a circular DNA molecule. The long RNA transcript and the polymerase protein are packaged into HBcAgs, and the reverse transcriptase synthesizes a new viral DNA genome. These particles are then transported to the HBsAg in the endoplasmic reticulum (ER) of the host cell and exported from the cell (21).

The envelope proteins of HBsAg are made up of three polypeptides coded by the S/pre-S region of the HBV genome (Fig. 1C). The major protein is the smallest peptide. It is encoded by the S region and consists of a 226-amino-acid glycosylated polypeptide. The medium-sized S protein is encoded by the S and the pre-S2 regions, which translate into a 281-amino-acid peptide with an additional glycosylation site. The large S protein consists of 389 to 400 amino acids encoded by the pre-S1, pre-S2, and S regions but lacks the pre-S2 glycosylation site. HBsAg is produced in excess of what is needed for virion production, and this excess antigen circulates in the blood of infected individuals as spherical and tubular particles devoid of HBV genomes or core proteins (Fig. 1A and B) (88). Particle counts of 10^{13} per ml have been detected in some sera. HBsAg may persist in serum for variable periods after initial infection. Thus, the HBsAg protein in serum is a diagnostic marker of active viral replication (21).

Two additional HBV-specific proteins play a key role in diagnostic testing, the HBcAg and HBeAg. Both proteins have different antigenic specificities and can be distinguished from HBsAg. The HBcAg is a polypeptide encoded by the C gene of HBV and is translated from the pregenomic mRNA (Fig. 1C). The precore sequence within the C gene contains the start codon for HBeAg translation (88). Because of the different start codons, the two proteins are not antigenically related. In addition, the HBeAg lacks the viral DNA binding domain. The first 29 amino acid residues of the HBeAg are coded within the precore region of the C gene. This part of the HBeAg directs the protein to the host ER. In the ER, this portion of the protein is cleaved off and the HBeAg is released from the host cell into the blood. In the blood, HBeAg is a soluble protein or is bound to albumin, α1-antitrypsin, or immunoglobulin. It is a reliable marker for the presence of intact virions and indicates high infectivity. A mutation at the end of the precore region of the C gene results in a stop codon, which prevents the translation of the HBeAg (19, 24). These precore mutants contribute to the pathogenesis of chronic HBV disease, often leading to acute exacerbation of chronic infections (59). Other HBV gene mutations have been observed in the core, core promoter, envelope, and polymerase regions. The envelope protein variants become relevant if the change results in viruses that escape vaccine-induced immunity. These mutants may not induce detectable antibody to HBsAg used in diagnostic testing and/or may lead to failure of HBV immunoglobulin (HBIG) therapy (107).

Epidemiology and Transmission

HBV infection is prevalent worldwide, representing a global public health problem (67). The WHO estimates that >2 billion people are infected with HBV, and approximately 600,000 people die each year due to acute or chronic HBV. The majority of these individuals live in Asia or Africa, as shown in Fig. 2. Approximately one-fourth of infected children will die as adults from liver cirrhosis or hepatocellular carcinoma (HCC) linked to chronic HBV (27). The Centers for Disease Control and Prevention (CDC) estimates that 800,000 to 1.4 million individuals in the United States are chronically infected with HBV despite a decline in the number of new infections during the last 20 years (http://www.cdc.gov/hepatitis/Statistics.htm, accessed October 2009). In the United States, most infections are in young adults, in whom the risk of chronic infection is lower. In comparison, outside the United States,

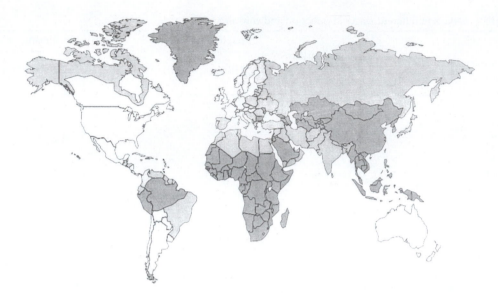

FIGURE 2 Worldwide distribution of chronic hepatitis B in 2006. Dark shading, ≥8% of the population (high HBsAg prevalence); medium shading, 2 to 7% of the population (intermediate HBsAg prevalence); light shading, <2% of the population (low HBsAg prevalence). For multiple countries, estimates of prevalence of HBsAg, a marker of chronic HBV infection, are based on limited data, and they might not reflect the current prevalence in countries that have implemented childhood hepatitis B vaccination. In addition, the prevalence of HBsAg might vary within countries by subpopulation and locality. The source for this figure is reference 22a.

perinatal exposure is more common and leads to chronic infections (27, 104). In the United States, the rate of new HBV infections has declined by 80% since 1991 due to the routine vaccination of children.

The most common modes of HBV transmission are vertical (mother to child perinatally), close contact with infected individuals during early childhood, sexual activity (both heterosexual and male homosexual), and injection drug use or other physical contact with infected bodily fluids (occupational exposure and contaminated blood products, etc.) (9, 63, 69). HBV cannot be transmitted by casual activities, such as talking, hand-holding, or hugging, nor can it be acquired by ingestion of food and water or from a cough or sneeze.

In most countries, HBV infections are reportable to the public health authorities. HBV remains a public health concern that can be addressed by accurate diagnostic detection, infection control, and effective vaccinations (93).

Clinical Significance

HBV infects hepatocytes, leading to an acute infection that resolves or a chronic infection lasting years. In infected individuals, subclinical hepatitis presents as a mild disease without symptoms or jaundice. Symptomatic patients may have abdominal pain, nausea without jaundice (anicteric hepatitis), or nausea with jaundice (icteric hepatitis). Infection may result in complete recovery, fulminant hepatitis with mortality, or a chronic infection. Three phases of chronic disease are now recognized as (i) the immune tolerant phase, (ii) the immune clearance phase, and (iii) the inactive carrier phase (94).

The incubation period of acute HBV infection ranges from 6 weeks to 6 months. The clinical symptoms of acute HBV infection are often mild, but sometimes physical signs such as jaundice, dark urine, clay-colored stools, and hepatomegaly are evident (61). Some patients experience

weight loss, right upper quadrant pain, and a tender enlarged liver (30, 68). Acute HBV infections are usually self-limited, and most patients recover completely after specific antibodies (anti-HBs) clear the virus (11, 42, 68).

The disease outcome of HBV is age dependent, and most patients with acute disease are adults. The acute liver damage associated with HBV infection is caused by the host immune response to infected hepatocytes (71, 84). This immune reaction results in massive necrosis, which can cause permanent damage to the liver. Mortality associated with fulminant hepatic failure is high without liver transplantation. After transplantation, HBV reinfection of the "new" liver is common, resulting in injury to the new liver in some patients. HBIG or antiviral therapy appears to alter this outcome (93). Pathologic features of acute HBV include both degenerative and regenerative parenchymal liver changes that lead to lobular disarray. Cytotoxic T lymphocytes play a role in facilitating viral clearance during acute infection as well as during the pathogenesis of hepatocellular injury (71).

The majority of newborns infected with HBV develop chronic, asymptomatic infections (63, 68). They are immune tolerant to HBV antigens, resulting in the absence of severe liver disease despite high levels of virus (8, 10, 15). Patients who continue to have detectable HBsAg or HBV DNA for at least 6 months after infection have chronic HBV infections (94). Chronic HBV symptoms are nonspecific and go unrecognized for years. Some patients remain positive for HBsAg indefinitely, while other patients convert to HBsAg negativity with the appearance of anti-HBs (10, 63). Interestingly, some of these patients continue to have detectable HBV DNA (63, 84).

The National Institutes of Health (NIH) sponsored a consensus conference on chronic HBV infections (94). The conference defined three phases of chronic HBV infection, the immune tolerant phase, the immune active phase, and the inactive carrier phase. The immune tolerant phase usually occurs in children infected with HBV early in life. It is characterized by high levels of HBV DNA, with little damage in the liver (Table 1). This immune tolerant stage lasts for a few years to several decades (63, 94).

Most individuals progress to the immune active phase, in which the liver shows inflammation with fibrosis, thus the term "active." This pathology results from an immune response to the HBV proteins on infected hepatocytes. The last phase of chronic HBV infection is the inactive carrier phase, characterized by less inflammation in liver biopsy specimens and normal liver enzyme levels. These patients have a lower risk for HCC (61, 69).

Chronic HBV infection is associated with a risk for HCC (27, 69). During HBV infection, the viral DNA randomly integrates into the hepatocyte genome. Since the virus DNA integrates randomly, the number of integration sites increases over time (94). This integrated viral DNA can activate cellular proto-oncogenes or suppress growth regulation genes (50, 69, 102). Some HBV proteins, such as the X protein and the truncated pre-S/S protein, are potent transactivators of cellular genes (50, 102).

Safe and effective vaccines against HBV have been available since 1982. The vaccine efficacy has been proven worldwide (31, 64). The complete HBV vaccination series is protective in >95% of infants, children, and adults (64, 73). Vaccine-induced protection lasts at least 20 years and is likely to be lifelong (73). Currently, there are two single-antigen vaccines for HBV and three different combination vaccines that contain HBsAg. The immune responses induced by vaccines made by different manufacturers are not significantly different. Persons with a known or suspected exposure to HBV should be given HBV vaccine and HBIG as soon as possible after the exposure (6, 9).

There is no specific therapy for acute HBV infections. However, chronic HBV infections are routinely treated with antiviral drugs. The primary goal of treating chronic HBV is to suppress viral replication and slow the progression of liver damage (7, 91, 94). At present, seven therapeutic agents have been approved for use by the FDA. These drugs are classified into two categories: the interferons and nucleoside/nucleotide analogs. The first nucleoside analog approved for treating chronic HBV infection was lamivudine (91, 94). Recently, several additional agents for the treatment of chronic HBV have been approved (adefovir, entecavir, tenofovir, emtricitabine, and telbivudine) (7, 30, 91, 94).

Collection, Transport, and Storage of Specimens

HBV infection is diagnosed by serological and molecular markers using serum or plasma. All commercial assays with FDA clearance have specific requirements defined in their package inserts for specimen types, specimen processing, and storage (Table 2). All laboratories performing HBV assays should follow these requirements. In general, HBV antigens and antibodies are stable at room temperature for several hours to days, can be stored at 4°C for months, and can be frozen at −20°C to −70°C for many years. Although HBV serologic markers are stable at −70°C, repetitive freezing and thawing can lead to their degradation. The use of hemolyzed samples should be avoided because of the possible interference with detection signals.

Plasma recovered from blood collected in tubes containing EDTA (lavender-top tubes) or tubes containing the anticoagulant citrate dextrose (ACD; yellow-top tubes) is used for nucleic acid analysis. Plasma should be separated from red cells within 6 hours and stored at 4°C. The EDTA in the plasma stabilizes the viral nucleic acid, which can then be stored at 4°C for up to 5 days without significantly affecting the results (13, 52). For long-term storage, plasma should be stored at −70°C. Heparinized plasma is unacceptable for nucleic acid analysis because heparin interferes with Taq polymerase-mediated PCR (46, 52). Published data indicate that HBV DNA can be detected without a loss of sensitivity after at least eight freeze-thaw cycles (56, 57).

The HBV virion remains infectious for >7 days outside the host (22). Thus, spills or splashes should be cleaned using absorbent material and disinfected with a 1:10 dilution of household bleach in water. Decontamination should be carried out while wearing gloves. Laboratory personnel should regard all specimens as potentially dangerous. The Occupational Safety and Health Administration (OSHA) standards for occupational exposure to blood-borne pathogens (75) are designed to protect employees exposed to blood and other potentially infectious materials. OSHA mandates that all employees whose job requirements put them at risk for blood-borne pathogens be offered HBV vaccine at no cost. OSHA standards and additional safety recommendations can be found in the literature (35, 86).

Direct Detection

The laboratory diagnosis of HBV uses a combination of tests that detect virus-specific protein and nucleic acid as well as the host immune response to infection. The assays that detect specific HBV proteins and nucleic acid usually indicate an active viral process in the patient (Table 1).

Microscopy

Microscopic detection of HBV does not play a specific role in the diagnosis of disease. However, a liver biopsy is typically used to assess the extent of histologic involvement and damage as well as a response to therapy. Histologic examination is useful for distinguishing among acute viral hepatitis, chronic hepatitis, and cirrhosis (5, 23, 30, 102).

Antigen

Several HBV-specific proteins can be detected in patient serum after infection. A marker of active viral replication is the detection of HBsAg and/or HBeAg during primary infection and during chronic HBV infection (Table 1). The HBsAg is located on the outer surfaces of HBV particles, while the HBeAg is translated from the precore mRNA of the HBcAg (Fig. 1C). The function of the HBeAg has not been clearly identified; however, the detection of this protein in serum is an indication of high viral replication. Both HBsAg and HBeAg are made in large excess by infected host cells and are released into the serum during active infection.

Diagnostic assays with high sensitivity and specificity are available to detect these HBV antigens. Table 1 shows the stage of HBV disease in which these antigens are detected. Table 2 lists the details of specific laboratory assays used to detect the antigens in human serum. In general, HBV antigens are detected using both solid-phase assays and microparticles to capture the protein. The antigen is then detected with well-defined monoclonal antibodies specific for the major immunodominant region of the proteins. These assays vary in the methods used to detect and measure the specific antigens. These vary from the use of automated instruments to completely manual methods (51, 66, 70, 100). The detection methods use colorimetric means, chemiluminescence,

TABLE 2 Commercial systems for serological testing of HBV antigens and antibodies

Name of assay (manufacturer)	Detection method[a]	Type(s) of specimens[a]	Reportable range[b]	Approved use(s)[c]
HBsAg[d]				
Architect HBsAg (Abbott Laboratories)	CMIA	Serum, plasma[e]	Qualitative	A
AxSYM HBsAg (Abbott Laboratories)	MEIA	Serum, plasma[e]	Qualitative	A
Prism HBsAg (Abbott Laboratories)	CIA	Serum, plasma[e] (also ACD)	Qualitative	A
Advia Centaur HBsAg (Siemens Healthcare Diagnostics)	CEIA	Serum, plasma[e]	Qualitative	A
Immulite 2000 (Siemens Healthcare Diagnostics)	CIA	Serum, plasma[e]	Qualitative	A
Genetic Systems HBsAg 3.0 (Bio-Rad Laboratories)	EIA	Serum, plasma[e] (also ACD)	Qualitative	A
ETI-MAK-2 Plus (DiaSorin)	EIA	Serum, plasma[e]	Qualitative	A
Vitros HBsAg (Ortho-Clinical Diagnostics)	CEIA	Serum, plasma[e]	Qualitative	A
Elecsys HBsAg, Cobas HBsAg (Roche Diagnostics)	ECL	Serum, plasma[e] (lithium heparin not validated)	Qualitative	A
HBeAg[d]				
ETI-EBK Plus (DiaSorin)	EIA	Serum, plasma[e]	Qualitative	A
Anti-HBs total[d]				
Architect AUSAB (Abbott Laboratories)	CMIA	Serum, plasma[e]	Quantitative (range, 8 to >1,000 mIU/ml)	A, D
AxSYM AUSAB (Abbott Laboratories)	MEIA	Serum, plasma[e] (Na heparin only)	>12 mIU/ml (reactive), <8 mIU/ml (nonreactive),[d] 12–8 mIU/ml (indeterminate)	A, D
Advia Centaur (Siemens Healthcare Diagnostics)	CMIA	Serum, plasma[e] (note that Na and Li heparin plasma can have high background)	Qualitative; <1, negative; ≥1, positive; ≥0.75–<1.25, retest	A, D
Monolisa anti-HBs (Bio-Rad Laboratories)	EIA	Serum, EDTA, or citrated plasma	Qualitative and quantitative; LOD = 4.14 mIU/ml; results of signal/assay cutoff >1 are positive	A, D
Immulite 2000 (Siemens Healthcare Diagnostics)	CEIA	Serum, EDTA, or heparinized plasma	Qualitative only; positive, >10 mIU/ml; negative, <10 mIU/ml	A, D
ETI-AB-AUK Plus (DiaSorin)	EIA	Serum, plasma[e]	Qualitative only; positive, >10 mIU/ml; negative, <10 mIU/ml	A, D
Vitros anti-HBs (Ortho-Clinical Diagnostics)	CIA	Serum	>12 mIU/ml, positive; <5 mIU/ml, negative; values between >5 and <12, indeterminate	A, D
Monolisa HBsAg 3.0 (Bio-Rad Laboratories)	EIA	Serum, plasma[e] (also ACD), cadaveric serum	Qualitative; cutoff = mean OD of 10 mIU/ml (calibrator)	B, D
Prism HBsAg (Abbott Laboratories)	CIA	Serum, plasma[e] (also ACD) (do not use heparin)	Semiquantitative	C

	Method[a,b]	Specimen[e]	Interpretation	Use[c,d]
Anti-HBc total (IgM and IgG)				
Architect Core (Abbott Laboratories)	CMIA	Serum, plasma[e]	Qualitative (nonreactive, gray zone,[f] reactive)	A
AxSYM Core 2.0 (Abbott Laboratories)	MEIA	Serum, plasma[e]	Qualitative (nonreactive, gray zone,[f] reactive)	A
Prism HBcore assay (Abbott Laboratories)	CIA	Serum, plasma[e] (also ACD) (do not use heparin)	Qualitative (nonreactive, reactive) (note that reactive specimens must be retested in duplicate)	C
Advia Centaur HBc (Siemens Healthcare Diagnostics)	CMIA	Serum, plasma[e]	Qualitative (nonreactive, reactive)	A
Immulite 2000 Anti-HBc (Siemens Healthcare Diagnostics)	CMIA	Serum, plasma[e]	Qualitative (negative, positive)	A
ETI-AB-Corek Plus (DiaSorin)	EIA	Serum, plasma[e]	Qualitative (negative, equivocal,[f] positive)	A
Monolisa anti-HBc	EIA	Serum, plasma[e]	Qualitative (nonreactive, borderline,[f] reactive)	A
Vitros anti-HBc (Ortho-Clinical Diagnostics)	CIA	Serum, plasma[e]	Qualitative (negative, indeterminate,[f] reactive)	A
Anti-HBc IgM				
Archit ct Core-M (Abott Laboratories)	CMIA	Serum, plasma[e]	Qualitative (nonreactive, gray zone, reactive)	A
AxSYM Core-M (Abbott Laboratories)	MEIA	Serum, plasma[e]	Qualitative (nonreactive, gray zone,[f] reactive)	A
Advia Centaur HBc IgM (Siemens Healthcare Diagnostics)	CMIA	Serum, plasma[e]	Qualitative (nonreactive, gray zone,[f] reactive)	A
Immulite 2000 HBc IgM (Siemens Healthcare Diagnostics)	CEIA	Serum, plasma[e]	Qualitative (reactive, equivocal,[f] or nonreactive)	A
ETI-Core-IgMK Plus (DiaSorin)	EIA	Serum, plasma[e]	Qualitative (negative, equivocal,[f] positive)	A
Monolisa HBc IgM (Bio-Rad Laboratories)	EIA	Serum, plasma[e]	Qualitative (nonreactive, borderline,[f] reactive)	A
Vitros HBc IgM (Ortho-Clinical Diagnostics)	CEIA	Serum, plasma[e]	Qualitative (negative, indeterminate,[f] reactive)	A
Anti-HBe				
ETI-AB-EBK Plus (anti-HBe) (DiaSorin)	EIA	Serum, plasma[e]	Qualitative (negative, equivocal,[f] positive)	A

[a]CMIA, chemiluminescent microparticle immunoassay; CIA, chemiluminescent immunoassay; CEIA, chemiluminescent enzyme immunoassay; EIA, enzyme immunoassay; ELFA, enzyme-linked fluorescent assay; ECL-EIA, electrochemiluminescence enzyme immunoassay; MEIA, microparticle enzyme immunoassay.

[b]All information on methods are derived from FDA submissions and manufacturers' information, when available. LOD, limit of detection; OD, optical density.

[c]A, diagnostic use only; not for use in the evaluation of blood, blood products, or tissue/blood donors; B, diagnostic use and screening of blood, blood products, and/or tissue/blood donors; C, screening of blood, blood products, and/or tissue/blood donors only; D, evaluate postvaccination response.

[d]All assays require positive results to be repeated and confirmed with a separate confirmation assay specific for each kit.

[e]Serum includes specimens collected in serum separator tubes; plasma includes collections in potassium EDTA, sodium citrate, sodium heparin, lithium heparin, and/or plasma separator tubes unless otherwise stated for a specific test.

[f]Some reactive and/or gray zone/indeterminate results are repeated in duplicate or with a new specimen before results are reported. See package insert for specific instructions.

or fluorescence to measure the detection of the antigens. Useful information about many diagnostic tests can be found by consulting the FDA website http://www.fda.gov/Medical Devices/ProductsandMedicalProcedures/DeviceApprovalsand Clearances/Recently-ApprovedDevices/default.htm (accessed January 2010).

HBsAg

The detection of HBsAg in serum plays a central role in establishing the diagnosis of HBV infection. Each HBsAg assay is approved by the FDA for diagnostic use only. Such assays should not be used for testing donors of blood, organs, or tissue.

The presence of HBsAg in the serum of a patient indicates high infectivity. Patients who resolve an acute infection eventually produce anti-HBs (see "Serologic Tests" below). However, when HBsAg is present, anti-HBs may be masked due to binding with HBsAg.

For all commercial diagnostic assays, any specimens nonreactive for HBsAg are considered negative and do not require further confirmation. In contrast, testing of specimens reactive for HBsAg must be repeated to verify the positive result. These repeatedly HBsAg-positive specimens must be confirmed by a neutralization assay specific for each manufacturer (Table 2). If the HBsAg-reactive serum is neutralized by the specific anti-HBs antibodies used in the confirmation assay, then the specimen is considered positive for HBsAg. Conversely, if the anti-HBs antibody does not neutralize the positive HBsAg reaction, then the HBsAg test must be considered nonconfirmed. In this situation, a new specimen should be requested and/or a recommendation that the patient be tested for other markers of infections, such as immunoglobulin M (IgM) anti-HBc or anti-HBc total, should be made.

All HBsAg assays are capable of detecting subnanogram amounts of protein, with no loss of specificity (12). For diagnostic applications, this level of sensitivity is sufficient to detect the HBsAg, which is usually abundant in the sera of individuals with actively replicating virus. However, a recent concern is that these assays may not detect certain HBsAg variants that contain mutations within the major antigenic region of the protein. It has been shown that some mutant HBsAg can be missed by commercial assays (20, 26, 32, 51, 53).

The major antigenic determinant on the HBsAg is designated the "a" determinant. This antigenic site is formed by a conformational structure containing a disulfide bond that results in a specific three-dimensional epitope. The region is between amino acids 124 and 147 and is found within the major hydrophilic loop of the protein (38, 81). There is a concern that current diagnostic assays will not detect HBsAg with alterations within this major antigenic epitope, since most HBsAg assays use antibodies that capture the HBsAg using this immunodominant epitope. The first escape mutant was described for a child born to an HBV-positive mother who transmitted HBV to the child despite vaccination and HBIG (39). This virus had a substitution in the HBsAg at amino acid position 145, resulting in a change from glycine to arginine. A single amino acid change altered the antigenic portion of the protein enough such that vaccine-induced antibody no longer recognized the antigen, allowing the altered virus to persist in the infant. Subsequently, the patient remained positive for HBV DNA and HBsAg (with mutation) for longer than 12 years (20). Since that time, other substitution mutants within the "a" determinant region of HBsAg have been recognized

(18, 26, 65, 77). Recent studies have evaluated HBsAg assays to determine their ability to detect well-defined HBsAg mutants and have found that some mutations in the HBsAg continue to be missed by current assays (26, 32, 66, 77, 100).

In response to the concern that blood donors with an HBsAg mutant will not be detected, most countries screen blood donors for anti-HBc in addition to HBsAg. Blood donors in the United States are now tested for the presence of HBV DNA (4). Individuals with positive tests for HBV DNA and anti-HBc and/or patients with positive results for HBeAg and/or HBV DNA but negative results for HBsAg should be checked for infection with an escape mutant.

HBeAg

The detection of HBeAg in serum is a sign of rapid viral replication usually associated with high HBV DNA levels. HBeAg-positive patients are highly infectious. However, some HBV strains do not make the HBeAg due to a precore mutation (18, 19). Patients infected with these mutant strains may have high HBV DNA levels in the absence of detectable HBeAg (24, 61). At the current time, only a single commercial assay is available in the Unites States for the detection of HBeAg in serum. If a test is initially positive, the same principles as those of the HBsAg detection system apply; i.e., specimens should be retested and confirmed with neutralization.

Nucleic Acid Detection

Molecular assays to quantitate HBV DNA are useful for the initial evaluation of HBV infections and the monitoring of patients with chronic infections. In addition, U.S. blood donors are routinely screened for HBV DNA by qualitative tests to detect donors in the early stage of HBV infection.

A number of quantitative assays have been developed to detect and monitor HBV DNA levels in infected patients (16, 97). Regular monitoring of HBV DNA levels provides information on the need for antiviral treatment or a change in the antiviral regimen. Several assays which use a variety of different methods are available for these purposes (5, 97). Most of the available assays have a lower limit of detection (between 5 and 50 copies/ml) and can quantify levels up to 1 million copies/ml (Table 2). This wide range allows for monitoring HBV DNA early after infection and identifying HBV infections resistant to antiviral therapy (97). Several studies show that the persistent suppression of HBV DNA is the primary measure of therapeutic success (80, 94, 102). A high level of HBV DNA following resolution of clinical hepatitis indicates a failure to control viral replication (63).

Commercially available HBV DNA assays differ in their limits of detection, in their dynamic ranges, and in the methods used to measure DNA levels (Table 3). An international HBV DNA standard was established in 2001 by the WHO in response to the need to standardize HBV DNA quantification (45, 87). The standard WHO virus preparation is high-titer genotype A (code 97/746), which has been assigned a potency of 10^6 IU/ml. The standard has established that 1 IU of HBV is equivalent to 5.4 genome equivalents or copies (45). The WHO standard has allowed results for different HBV DNA assays to be reported in IU/ml.

However, despite the availability of this standard, the various quantitative assays usually have different conversion factors, demonstrating their variability (Table 3). Thus, the best practice is the consistent monitoring of patients using the same manufacturer's assay in the same laboratory (97).

TABLE 3 Molecular assays used to detect HBV nucleic acid

Assay name	Method	Quantitative range[a]	Sensitivity[a]	Genotype detection (reference)[a]
Cobas TaqMan HBV test[b,c]	Target DNA amplification with HBV-specific primers	29×10^8 to $>1.1 \times 10^8$ IU/ml 1 IU = 5.82 copies	4–10 IU/ml	A–G; HBV and several precore mutations
Versant HBV DNA 3.0[d]	Binding of target to solid-phase probe; amplification of probe by binding of branched DNA chains	2×10^3 to 1×10^8 genome copies/ml 1 IU = 5.7 copies	2,000 copies/ml	A–G
artus HBV PCR[b,c]	Various real-time PCR instruments (Roto-Gene, ABI Prism, and Lightcycler)[c]	2×10^1 to 10^9 IU/ml[4] 1 IU = 6 copies	3.8 IU/ml	A–H
Abbott real-time PCR[b]	Amplification of target gene within a segment of the surface gene	10 to 10^9 IU/ml 1 IU = 6 copies	10–15 IU/ml	A–G and several polymerase gene variants (101)
Affigene HBV[b]	Amplification and detection of target by Scorpion probe/primer technology used on various instruments (Stratagene Mx3000P/3005P, iCycler iQ/iQ5, Rotor-Gene 3000/6000, ABI 7300[b])	172×10^8 to 1.72×10^8 IU/ml	3.4–51 IU/ml	A–H

[a]Data from manufacturers' literature and websites.
[b]CE-IVD, European Conformity In Vitro Diagnostic Medical Devices.
[c]FDA-IVD, Food and Drug Administration In Vitro Diagnostic Product.
[d]Verify instrumentation use with manufacturer's kit. Evaluated on the Roto-Gene instrument.

Some of the variability of HBV DNA quantification may occur during collection and processing of the specimen. Most assays use serum or plasma (EDTA or ACD) as the specimen of choice. Regardless of the collection tube, the specimen should be separated from the clotted blood within 4 to 6 hours after collection. As with all FDA-approved diagnostic assays, the instructions of the package insert should be followed for specimen type, processing, and storage.

A number of different methods are available to extract HBV DNA (78, 97). Some are labor-intensive and may be prone to variability and contamination. A variety of automated extraction instruments are now available for the isolation of HBV DNA (33, 41, 56, 78, 97).

Current assays quantitate HBV DNA by amplification of target nucleic acid and use a series of known standards to estimate amounts of HBV DNA (Table 2). These assays usually cover a 7- to 8-$\log_{10}$ range, which permits the accurate evaluation of HBV levels that are above a million down to very low levels that occur during treatment or in inactive carriers (97). A variety of studies have shown that a reduction of 1 $\log_{10}$ in HBV DNA levels in the first 6 months of antiviral therapy indicates treatment efficacy (5, 80, 85, 94, 97, 102).

Many of these assays use oligonucleotide primers that recognize a conserved sequence within the HBV precore/core gene (97). Different enzymatic reactions are used to make multiple copies of the HBV target nucleic acid. The assays quantitate HBV DNA with the use of a series of standards containing a known copy number of the target nucleic acid. These standards provide a validation curve that correlates results from each patient sample. Amplification of the target is usually monitored by fluorescent signals by using a variety of dyes. From these data, the viral load is determined by computerized analysis of individual results, which are compared to the standard curve (85, 97).

One commercial assay does not use target amplification. This assay uses nucleic acid capture systems combined with a signal amplification technique, with labeled branched DNA as a signal amplifier in a sandwich assay to quantitate HBV DNA in serum (54).

Isolation Procedures
Although HBV can infect hepatocytes in vitro, culture of HBV is not used for the diagnosis of infection.

Identification
The methods for identification of HBV infection use a combination of molecular, antigenic, and serological methods described in the "Direct Detection" and "Serologic Tests" sections herein.

Typing Systems
Antigenic variation occurs naturally in HBV due to genetic heterogeneity. These various genetic differences are used to classify HBV into eight distinct genotypes, designated A thru H (Table 4). They are distinguished by a genetic divergence of 8% or more within the complete nucleotide sequence (24, 61, 63, 69). The HBV genotypes can also be identified by reverse hybridization assays or with amplification methods such as PCR using genotype-specific primers. At this time, all of the assays are individually developed or available for research use only.

Serologic Tests
Serologic tests for HBV-specific antibodies are used to determine the stage of disease and to establish immunity due to vaccination. As the host mounts an immune response, the first antibodies to appear are IgM anti-HBc and then anti-HBc total, anti-HBe, and finally anti-HBs. Several commercial assays are available for diagnostic testing, as is blood and tissue donor screening for specific HBV antibodies (Table 2).

IgM Anti-HBc
IgM antibody to HBcAg (IgM anti-HBc) persists for several weeks to months. The detection of IgM anti-HBc indicates recent, acute infection of less than 6 months' duration (Table 1). During this stage of disease, the patient's liver enzymes may be elevated. A negative IgM anti-HBc excludes a recent, acute infection, but it does not rule out chronic infection (55, 71, 84). IgM anti-HBc in chronic carriers can occur briefly in patients who move from an

TABLE 4 HBV genotypes and geographic circulation[a]

Genotype	Subtypes and serotypes	Genome size (nucleotides)	Geographic connection(s)	Disease relationship
A	Subtypes A1, A2, A3; serotypes adw2, ayw1	3,221	Northwestern Europe, Spain, Poland, United States, Central Africa, India, Brazil	HCC and cirrhosis in older patients; core promoter mutations (A1762T, G1764A) have been detected
B	Subtypes B1–B6; serotypes adw2, ayw1	3,215	Southeast Asia, Taiwan, Japan, Indonesia, China	HCC and cirrhosis in both younger and older patients; precore mutations (G1896A) have been detected
C	Subtypes C1–C4; serotypes adw2, adrq+, adrq−, ayr	3,215	Asia, Indonesia, India, Australia, United States, Brazil	Higher risk of HCC and chirrhosis than genotype B; precore mutations (G1896A) and core promoter mutations (A1762T, G1764A) have been detected
D	Subtypes D1–D4; serotypes ayw2, ayw3	3,182	Mediterranean area, Middle East, India, Spain, United States, Brazil (generally found worldwide)	Chronic HBV, cirrhosis in older patients; precore mutations (G1896A) and core promoter mutations (A1762T, G1764A) have been detected
E	Subtypes unknown; serotype ayw4	3,212	West Africa	Unknown
F	Subtypes D1–D4; serotypes adw4q−, adw2, ayw4	3,215	Central and South America, Bolivia, Venezuela, Polynesia, Alaska	HCC in young children and adults
G	Subtypes unknown; serotype adw2	3,248	Australia, France, Germany, United States	Almost always is a coinfection with other HBV types
H	Subtypes unknown; serotype adw4	3,215	Central and South America, United States	Unknown

[a]Information derived from references 18, 22a, 62, and 68.

inactive carrier phase to an active HBV replication. In this phase, HBV DNA levels may increase transiently and then decline due to suppression of viral replication. (55, 61)

Total Antibody to Anti-HBc

A negative anti-HBc indicates that a person has not been infected with HBV. A positive result may indicate an acute (HBsAg-positive, IgM anti-HBc-positive), resolved (HBsAg-negative), or chronic (HBsAg-positive) infection (Table 1) (11, 16, 55). Anti-HBc total antibodies remain positive indefinitely after IgM anti-HBc disappears. They can be detected for many years and persist longer than anti-HBs. Anti-HBc total is the best marker for documenting prior exposure to HBV. Anti-HBc should not be present in vaccinated individuals unless they were infected with HBV prior to vaccination. In some patients, the detection of anti-HBc may be the only serological marker for the detection of past infection in a patient with chronic inactive HBV. This may be due to a remote, inactive HBV infection with loss over time of anti-HBs or may be due to an infection with an HBsAg variant in which anti-HBs is not detected (30, 55, 61). The laboratory investigation of these results could be resolved by measuring HBV DNA in both types of patients (10, 24, 30, 61).

Commercial kits for detections of anti-HBc total are available and use a variety of different methods and instrumentation (Table 2). All use recombinant HBcAg for capture of antibody. In competitive tests, if anti-HBc is present in the sample, it competes with a known amount of added labeled human anti-HBc. Samples with anti-HBc lead to signal suppression that is proportional over a limited range to the amount of anti-HBc present. Values generated by positive and negative kit controls are required to calculate assay cutoff and to establish validity. Each assay should be calibrated on a regular basis by following instructions in each kit.

Anti-HBsAg

A negative result for anti-HBs in the absence of any other HBV-specific antigen or antibody indicates that a person has not been infected with HBV or vaccinated against HBV. A positive result is consistent with immunity to HBV due to a resolved infection or from effective vaccination (Table 1).

Assays for anti-HBs are solid-phase tests based on the sandwich principle. Both quantitative and qualitative assays are available (Table 2). These assays have specific indications for diagnostic testing, screening blood and tissue donors, or both. Some anti-HBs assays report quantitative values in IU/ml, while other assays report qualitative results. See Table 2 for specific information. In most assays, an initially reactive result for anti-HBs requires repeat testing in duplicate in an independent run. Anti-HBs quantitation panels are commercially available and useful when validating anti-HBs assays.

Anti-HBs is a key serological marker for both vaccine-induced immunity and immunity due to infection. As HBV vaccination has become more widespread, the use of this serological marker to monitor vaccine success has increased. Both the WHO and the CDC recognize levels of 10 mIU/ml of anti-HBs as protective (6, 22).

Postvaccination testing for the presence of anti-HBs is not recommended for infants, children, or most adults. The CDC lists exceptions to this rule, namely, infants born to mothers who are HBsAg positive, immunocompromised patients, dialysis patients, and health care workers whose successful vaccination needs to be confirmed (22). Infants born to HBV-positive mothers should be tested for anti-HBs after reaching 2 years of age due to passive antibody from the mother (69).

The CDC also made recommendations on the use of detecting anti-HBs after vaccination to prevent the transmission of HBV in the health care setting (9, 22).

HBV "escape" mutants in which the HBsAg is altered can result in HBV infections without detectable anti-HBs (24, 39). Any conformational changes in the major antigenic determinant of HBsAg results in reduced detection of the anti-HBsAg by diagnostic assays (20, 24, 40, 48).

Anti-HBeAg

A positive test for anti-HBe indicates the resolution of acute infection and is associated with a decrease in viral replication (Table 1). Patients who have recovered from acute HBV infection will have detectable anti-HBe, anti-HBc, and anti-HBs.

Generally anti-HBe assays use competitive binding by adding the patient sample to a measured amount of recombinant HBeAg. If anti-HBe is present in the patient's sample, it competes with solid-phase anti-HBe for the limited number of binding sites on the added HBeAg.

Test algorithms for HBeAg/anti-HBe kits vary. Initially reactive samples in the anti-HBe assays are often repeated. If the repeat test is reactive, the sample is reported as positive. The enzyme immunoassays use an indeterminate zone or gray zones around the assay cutoffs. If the samples repeatedly yield values in this zone, additional testing should be performed with a new specimen.

Interestingly, patients infected with HBeAg-negative strains of HBV will still make anti-HBe (18, 19). This finding is likely due to the selection of HBV strains with HBeAg mutations after the development of anti-HBe (18). It has been postulated that the development of immunity to HBeAg may select for HBeAg mutations (19).

Antiviral Susceptibility

Therapy for chronic HBV can require long-term therapy with nucleoside or nucleotide analogs. A disadvantage of long-term therapy is the development of antiviral resistance. As noted above, HBV replicates through an RNA intermediate. The HBV RNA-dependent DNA polymerase is not precise during rapid replication cycles, and proofreading of final copies is not always corrected. This can lead to frequent errors. Some of these errors lead to resistant mutants, which are selected in the presence of antiviral agents (37, 72, 89, 92, 101). Over time, the HBV strains with antiviral resistance become the major viral species (5, 91, 101, 108, 109). Currently, when a patient has a 1-$\log_{10}$ increase from the lowest HBV DNA level, he or she should be evaluated for the development of antiviral resistance (7, 80, 101).

Recently, the nomenclature of HBV antiviral resistance was standardized in order to track nucleotide changes associated with drug resistance and to recognize new mutations (Table 5) (5, 29, 30). Antiviral resistance mutations can

be detected by molecular methods that recognize known mutations associated with resistance (1, 5, 17, 24, 101). Methods used to detect these mutations are available; however, the interpretation of results is not always straightforward. Some mutations will predict resistance to multiple drugs. For example, a single mutation at A181T is associated with resistance to lamivudine, adefovir, tenofovir, and telbivudine (Table 4) (26, 37). In other situations genetic sequence changes may not confer resistance when present alone but will contribute to the resistance when additional mutations are present (7, 92). For example, lamivudine resistance does not occur due to a single mutation at L180M, but with the addition of a mutation such as A181T, resistance to lamivudine occurs. Thus, the detection of an L180M, A181T double mutation, which alters the position of a critical residue in the nucleotide binding pocket, is required for resistance to be apparent (7, 92, 103). Other concerns are that patients treated with multiple drugs will have a combination of sequence changes that represent drug resistance mutations in addition to mutations that occur in order to balance the fitness of these drug-treated HBVs. Many of these single nucleotide changes have no recognized phenotype (7, 85, 91).

Commercial assays are available to detect antiviral resistance mutations in HBV. One assay employs biotinylated amplicons that hybridize to membrane-bound oligonucleotides that represent mutation sequences (INNO-LiPA HBV; Innogenetics). The first generation of this assay detects several lamivudine resistance mutations at amino acid locations 180, 204, and 207 (2, 85). The second-generation assay detects additional resistance sequences, including those associated with lamivudine resistance at amino acid locations 80, 173, 180, and 204, as well as changes at codons 181 and 236 associated with adefovir resistance (2, 76, 85). This version detects HBV resistance mutations in specimens that contain both wild-type HBV and mutant virus. However, these assays are designated "research use only" in the United States and Europe. Some disadvantages with these assays are difficulty in reading the reaction lines of the strip (up to 34 lines per strip), faint bands that are difficult to interpret, and the absence of bands in viral preparations with known mutations (1, 2, 76).

A second assay (Trugene HBV genotyping kit; Siemens Medical Solutions Diagnostics) is available as a research-use-only kit. This assay detects antiviral mutations by direct sequencing from specimens, including specimens with low HBV levels (41). A comparison between the sequence assay and the hybridization assay shows a high concordance. However, the hybridization-based assay was able to detect more of the mixed viral populations (41, 85).

TABLE 5 Antiviral agents and HBV mutations associated with resistance[a]

Antiviral agent	Description of drug	Mutations associated with resistance
IFN-α	Immune modulation	None known
Pegylated IFN-α2a	Immune modulation	
Lamivudine	Nucleoside analog (cytidine)	(L180M + M204V/I/S), A181V/T, S202G/I
Telbivudine	Nucleoside analog (dTTP)	M204I, A181T/V
Entecavir	Nucleoside analog (2-deoxyguanosine)	T184S/C/G/A/I/L/F/M, S202G/C/I, M250V/I/L
Emtricitabine	Nucleoside analog (cytidine)	M204V/I
Adefovir	Nucleotide analog (dATP)	A181V/T, N236T
Tenofovir	Nucleotide analog (dATP)	A194T, N236T, A181V/T

[a]Resistance is defined as virologic breakthrough confirmed by an increase on two consecutive occasions of HBV DNA levels by >1 $\log_{10}$ copies/ml during therapy. Data are derived from references 7, 37, 101, and 109.

A number of laboratory-developed assays have been used to detect antiviral mutations in HBV. These assays use a variety of different techniques to detect the known resistance mutations in HBV (1, 17, 44, 47, 80, 89). One of these methods is to use direct DNA sequencing to detect known resistance mutations. The advantages of DNA sequencing are that it is accurate and mutations can be identified in any part of the HBV genome (89). However, a serious disadvantage is that these methods lack sensitivity since they detect mutants present in 10 to 30% of the viral population. This level of detection does not always meet the goal of consistently identifying resistance mutants that make up at least 10% of the virus population (109). This limits its use clinically. Additionally, it tends to be a time-consuming, labor-intensive method and the reagents can be costly.

Several studies have described the use of individually developed PCR methods to detect HBV-resistant variants using melting temperature to detect mutations (17, 103). However, the sequence variability that naturally occurs in HBV can lead to a change in melting temperature that is not associated with a resistance mutation. Thus, it lacks specificity (103). Another method uses a combination of PCR, hybridization, and sequencing that involves the extension of multiple oligonucleotide primers with fluorescent dideoxynucleoside triphosphates using a DNA polymerase (80).

Several sophisticated methods that use technologies such as matrix-assisted laser adsorption/ionization time-of-flight mass spectrometry and microarray assays are being investigated for the detection of HBV antiviral resistance (44, 47). This new technology offers a highly sensitive means to detect unidentified HBV variants, even when they are present in a small percentage of wild-type/mutant mixtures. While being fast and accurate, these methods require the use of expensive equipment and have not been optimized or extensively validated for clinical use.

The HBV viral load is often used for monitoring and confirming the development of resistance to antiviral therapy. Indeed, resistance to antiviral agents is still generally defined clinically by a 1-log increase in serum HBV DNA levels during antiviral therapy (5, 78). The disadvantage of using the HBV DNA levels to detect antiviral resistance is that other factors, such as compliance and drug metabolism, may also be responsible for increasing HBV DNA levels. Therefore, the combined use of a genotyping assay for mutation detection and quantitative detection of HBV DNA with a reliable and sensitive assay is warranted for optimal monitoring of HBV antiviral therapy (5, 85).

Phenotypic testing has been used to detect HBV antiviral resistance in research and development laboratories. These methods detect drug resistance based on the use of molecular or cellular techniques or animal models (5, 80, 85, 109). However, phenotypic testing is not practical for clinical monitoring, since it is labor-intensive and requires long testing periods.

Evaluation, Interpretation, and Reporting of Results

HBV infection leads to a wide range of disease presentations, from acute hepatitis with fulminant hepatic failure to chronic hepatitis leading to cirrhosis and/or HCC (29, 42, 63, 69). The initial laboratory assessment for suspected viral hepatitis should include laboratory tests that measure serum transaminases, direct and total bilirubin, albumin, and total protein; a complete blood count; coagulation tests; and an alpha fetoprotein test (42). The specific laboratory tests to detect and monitor HBV infection are a mix of viral-antigen detection and molecular measurements of HBV DNA and serological markers. The tests to diagnose new HBV infection use anti-HBc IgM, HBsAg, and HBV DNA (Table 1).

During acute HBV disease, IgM anti-HBc tests are usually positive when serum transaminases are elevated. In a typical acute HBV infection, HBV DNA can be detected 3 to 4 weeks before HBsAg but long before the onset of symptoms and thus is usually not tested (16). The level of IgM anti-HBc declines as disease resolves or becomes chronic. Most patients with an active HBV infection which resolves have detectable anti-HBs shortly after the disappearance of HBsAg. Figure 3 illustrates the typical serologic pattern that occurs in a patient with an acute HBV infection.

Patients who are chronically infected with HBV may present as immune tolerant, may be HBeAg positive, or may be an inactive HBsAg carrier or have HBeAg-negative chronic hepatitis. Chronic HBV stages can be distinguished using a combination of laboratory tests and clinical signs (Table 1 and Fig. 4).

The immune-tolerant phase usually occurs when the patient acquires HBV infection at birth or during early childhood. Infection in this phase is associated with a high level of viral production and the presence of HBeAg. These markers indicate a high rate of viral replication (63, 68). There is an absence of liver disease despite high levels of HBV replication. This is a consequence of immune tolerance, but its underlying pathology is poorly understood (5, 63, 94).

As the host's immune system matures, the patient may move to the immune-active phase also referred to as the HBeAg-positive chronic-hepatitis phase, during which HBV-specific epitopes are recognized by the host immune system, leading to immune-mediated injury in the liver (63). Individuals who acquire HBV perinatally often transition from the immune-tolerant phase to the HBeAg-positive chronic-hepatitis phase between 20 and 30 years of age (10). The liver biopsy specimen in this stage shows active inflammation accompanied by fibrosis. Patients who remain HBeAg positive have a higher risk of progressing to liver disease due to high rates of HBV replication inducing a chronically active immune response (69, 84). Such patients have high HBV DNA levels and increased levels of serum transaminases. However, as these individuals develop anti-HBe, they will revert to HBeAg negativity and move to the inactive carrier phase (Table 1) (21, 69, 84). The transition from the immune-tolerant phase is often not

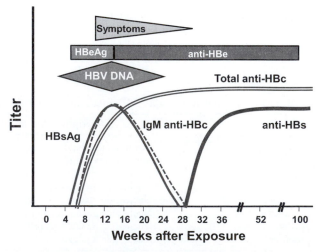

FIGURE 3 Typical sequence of serologic markers in patients with acute HBV infection and with resolution of symptoms.

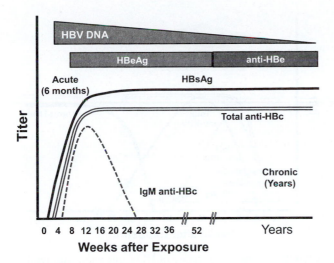

FIGURE 4 Typical sequence of serologic markers in patients with HBV infection that progresses to chronicity. In patients with chronic HBV infection, both HBsAg and IgG anti-HBc remain persistently detectable, generally for life. HBeAg is variably present in these patients.

recognized, since patients with HBeAg-positive, chronic hepatitis often remain asymptomatic (21).

The inactive carrier phase is characterized by the seroconversion to anti-HBe, and patients in this phase alternate between low and undetectable levels of HBV DNA (21, 30). The seroconversion to anti-HBe is associated with a decrease in liver damage and the normalization of serum transaminase levels. Mild hepatitis may be noted on biopsy (84). Many patients remain in this phase for years, if not indefinitely. Patients in the inactive carrier phase that have detectable HBV DNA in serum at intermittent or low levels usually have normal serum transaminases levels.

A portion of inactive HBsAg carriers will develop chronic hepatitis, which recurs in the absence of HBeAg in their serum (HBeAg-negative chronic hepatitis). These patients have a HBV variant that cannot express HBeAg due to mutations in the precore or core-promoter regions of the HBV core gene (24, 25). Patients with chronic hepatitis that are HBeAg negative are more likely to have more advanced liver disease in spite of lower serum HBV DNA levels (24, 30, 104).

Patients who are negative for HBsAg, anti-HBc, and HBV DNA are not infected with HBV. In some individuals, the presence of anti-HBc alone may be the only evidence of an active, occult HBV infection of remote origin. Patients infected with an HBsAg escape mutant will test negative for HBsAg but will be positive when tested for anti-HBc and HBV DNA (79).

Anti-HBs without anti-HBc develops in persons who receive hepatitis B vaccine, and levels anti-HBs of ≥10 mIU/ ml are considered protective (6, 22). Due to the prevalence of vaccinated individuals, the detection of anti-HBc, not anti-HBs, is used to evaluate prior or current HBV infection and the need for HBV vaccination. Passive transfer of anti-HBs or anti-HBc may be observed in neonates of mothers with current or past HBV infections (22). Since blood donations are tested for total anti-HBc and HBV DNA, passive transfer of these makers following blood transfusions is unlikely. Recognition of these possibilities will avoid an erroneous diagnosis

of HBV exposure or infection. Passive antibody levels decline gradually over 3 to 6 months, while levels of antibody induced by infection are stable over many years (22, 64).

The majority of individuals vaccinated for HBV have detectable levels of anti-HBs, but some test negative due to waning levels of anti-HBs. They do, however, respond to a challenge dose of HBsAg vaccine with an anamnestic response in approximately 2 weeks (22, 64). Studies of vaccinated individuals without detectable anti-HBs show that subclinical infection can occur but is blunted by the anamnestic anti-HBs response, such that liver damage is minimal and symptoms do not occur (6, 22).

A small number of vaccinated individuals (<1%) have become infected with HBV isolates that escape vaccine-induced immunity (20, 39, 77). These HBV isolates have mutations in the HBsAg which are not recognized by vaccine-induced immunity (24, 26, 53). Currently, these occurrences are few; however, it is important for laboratories to be vigilant in recognizing the potential of new HBV mutants to cause disease in vaccinated individuals. Additionally, laboratories should offer testing options that detect such infections, such as HBV DNA and anti-HBc, even when the patient has been vaccinated.

Testing for the HBV genotype is usually not required but should be used in selected patients from regions that have variability in HBV genotypes (Table 4). Testing for mutations associated with antiviral resistance is not useful in the initial evaluation of patients (5, 29, 72, 94). The "gold standard" for assessing inflammatory activity (grade) and degree of fibrosis (stage) is the liver. The result of the biopsy is a useful baseline for future follow-up (85).

Molecular assays are used to determine HBV DNA levels and to establish the stage of disease in newly diagnosed patients. They are also used to monitor patients on therapy. The reduction of HBV DNA greater than 1 $\log_{10}$ during antiviral therapy is a measure of treatment response and predicts histological improvement. Increasing HBV DNA levels are associated with chronic liver disease and cirrhosis (69, 94, 104).

Antiviral therapy is given to patients with chronic HBV to prevent progression of liver disease (42, 63, 104). During the course of therapy, treatment response is monitored using biochemical, virologic, serologic, and histologic results. Currently, the most accurate monitor of virologic activity is the HBV DNA level, determined using an assay with a wide dynamic range (5, 78, 84). The loss of HBsAg and seroconversion to anti-HBs with long-lasting suppression of HBV DNA indicates a successful response to therapy (84, 94). Patients who appear to have suppressed HBV DNA levels are monitored periodically because relapse due to antiviral resistance is possible. The most reliable measure of a successful long-term treatment response is the sustained suppression of HBV DNA (5, 84, 94).

When HBV DNA levels increase by 1 $\log_{10}$ in a patient taking antiviral treatment, it may indicate antiviral resistance (5, 84, 92). It is not recommended that resistance testing be performed before the start of therapy, even if the patient has a very high viral level (5, 94). Resistance detection is useful only after a patient has been treated for several months and fails to show a 1-$\log_{10}$ reduction in HBV DNA. These patients are classified as primary nonresponders. They should be tested for the presence of resistant mutants to assist in selecting a new treatment regimen (5, 29, 94). For successfully treated patients who show a virological and/ or biochemical breakthrough, testing for resistance is also helpful (24, 72).

Genotyping of HBV is usually not required to establish therapy for chronic disease. However, there is some evidence that in chronic HBV infections genotype may predict outcome (18, 23, 30). For example, genotype B is associated with less-active liver disease and a decreased rate of cirrhosis compared with genotype C (30, 69). Other studies show an association between HBV genotypes and precore and core promoter mutations (18, 25, 76). The reason why HBV genotype is related to clinical outcomes is not completely obvious, but additional studies should help in our understanding how it effects disease presentation.

HEPATITIS D VIRUS

Introduction

Hepatitis D virus (HDV) is a defective RNA virus that requires the presence of HBV for its replication. HDV has a single-stranded, circular, negative-sense RNA genome that is completely nonhomologous with HBV DNA. The agent was first described in 1977 from Italian patients with chronic HBV, who developed episodes of serious, acute disease (83).

Taxonomy

HDV is unable to replicate without the presence of the host virus, HBV; thus, it is a subviral particle rather than a true virus. The HDV particle is similar to plant subviral agents (36). However, there are some major differences between the plant viroids and HDV. The plant viroids do not encode a specific protein and do not utilize a host or helper virus as HDV does with HBV (95).

Description of the Agent

HDV is generally spherical, with an average diameter ranging from 36 to 43 nm, which is slightly smaller than the HBV particle (83). The 1.7-kb RNA genome of HDV encodes only a single protein, the HDV nucleocapsid protein known as the hepatitis delta antigen (HDAg). It is nonglycosylated and produced in two forms, a short peptide consisting of a 195-amino-acid, 24-kDa protein (HDAg-S) and a larger peptide consisting of a 214-amino-acid, 27-kDa protein (HDAg-L) (49). The protein cannot assemble into viral particles without the presence of HBsAg (60, 95). The HDV RNA genome is surrounded by HDAg, which is then surrounded by the HBsAg. Consequently, HDAg is undetectable on the complete HDV particle. In spite of this, infected individuals produce antibody to the HDV antigen (anti-HDV). However, anti-HDV does not neutralize HDV, whereas anti-HBs has neutralizing activity (95).

The HDV genome has a high degree of complementarity, creating a three-dimensional, double-stranded structure that resists dry heat for long periods of time. The extensive internal complementarity of the HDV genome results in a rod-like structure like that of plant RNA satellite viruses. Not surprisingly, the mode of replication of this virus is unusual. The HDV genome replicates using the host's RNA polymerase II rather than an HDV- or HBV-encoded RNA polymerase (95). The only enzymatic activity inherent to HDV is mediated by RNA elements termed ribozymes, which cleave the newly synthesized, circular RNA genomes, producing linear molecules. After that cleavage, replication of the HDV genome occurs by a rolling-circle mechanism with self-cleavage (58). Synthesis of the HDV particles suppresses HBV viral production. A unique, indispensable relationship exists between HDV and HBV (82).

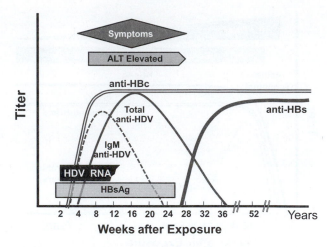

FIGURE 5 Serologic course of HDV infection, with resolution when the virus is acquired as a coinfection with HBV.

Epidemiology and Transmission

It is estimated that around 20 million people worldwide are chronically infected with HDV (83). Several areas of the world have a high prevalence of HDV-infected individuals, including countries bordering the Mediterranean, the Middle East, Central Asia, West Africa, the Amazon Basin, and the South Pacific Islands (83, 90). In these areas of endemicity, HDV appears to be transmitted by close person-to-person spread, such as household contact. Additionally, many of these individuals acquire HDV through exposure to blood-contaminated needles and blood products. Sustained epidemics of clinically severe acute HDV have been observed in these populations, which, not surprisingly, have high HBV carrier rates (90).

Clinical Significance

HDV can be transmitted only to individuals who are infected with HBV already or when both viral agents are transmitted together. A coinfection occurs when a naive individual is infected simultaneously with both viruses (Fig. 5) (95). A superinfection occurs when an individual chronically infected with HBV is infected with HDV (Fig. 6) (95). Acute HDV

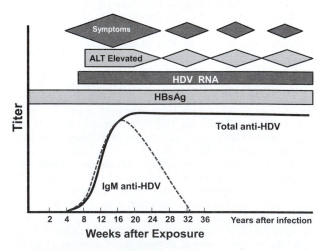

FIGURE 6 Serologic course of HDV infection when the virus is acquired as a superinfection with HBV. Symptoms and ALT levels are shown to indicate the intermittent nature of symptoms and liver involvement.

superinfection has a greater risk of fulminant hepatitis and liver failure than HBV infection alone. Likewise, chronic HDV infections are associated with more rapidly progressing liver damage than infection with HBV alone (34).

Rates of fulminant hepatitis can be as high as 5% in patients with HBV and HDV coinfection (83, 95). A biphasic clinical course is sometimes observed during coinfection. HDV infection does not increase the rate of chronicity of acute HBV but may convert an asymptomatic or mild, chronic HBV infection into a rapidly progressive, fulminant or severe disease (83, 95). Limited success has been achieved in treating chronic HDV patients with gamma interferon (IFN-γ). High-dose, long-term therapy is required, and relapses are common after therapy is stopped (34, 83, 105). Patients with HDV who have hepatic decompensation are candidates for liver transplantation and in general have had favorable outcomes (83). Treatments with antiviral agents known to reduce HBV titers have been studied. However, it appears that therapy with IFN-α in combination with either ribavirin or lamivudine is not useful in treating chronic HDV infections (74, 106). Successful vaccination for HBV also prevents HDV infection, since HDV cannot replicate in the absence of a concurrent HBV infection.

Collection, Transport, and Storage of Specimens

HDV infection is diagnosed by serological and molecular markers using serum or plasma and is suspected only in those patients who are HBV infected from countries in which HDV is prevalent.

Direct Detection

The laboratory diagnosis of HDV depends on the detection of specific antibodies, HDAg, and HDV RNA. HDV infections may also be diagnosed by detecting HDV RNA directly in liver tissue (58, 60, 96, 99). The most current method for the detection of HDV RNA is reverse transcription and amplification (96, 98).

Typing

Based on sequence similarity, the HDV genomes have been classified into three genotypes. Genotype I is the most common and found worldwide. Genotype II has been identified primarily in Japan and Taiwan, while genotype III is typically found in South America. It is unclear whether these differences play a role in disease presentation (43, 60).

Serologic Tests

The diagnosis of HDV infection relies on the detection of anti-HDV using either commercial or laboratory-developed enzyme immunoassays. A positive result for total anti-HDV may indicate either acute or chronic HDV infection. IgM anti-HDV can be detected during either a coinfection or a superinfection. All of the serologic and molecular assays are available from selected reference laboratories (82, 83).

Evaluation, Interpretation, and Reporting of Results

Diagnosis of a coinfection with HBV and HDV relies on the detection of HBsAg, HBeAg, HBV DNA, and IgM anti-HBc in the same serum sample, one that is positive for HDAg, anti-HDV IgM, and HDV RNA (Fig. 5). Anti-HDV appears during acute infection and usually disappears with resolution. A superinfection occurs when HDV infects a patient with chronic HBV, a circumstance usually leading to chronic HDV infection. The diagnosis of HDV superinfection is made when anti-HDV is found simultaneously with HBsAg and anti-HBc in the absence of IgM anti-HBc. Anti-HDV is present indefinitely in patients with chronic HDV infection (95) (Fig. 6).

REFERENCES

1. Aberle, S. W., J. Kletzmayr, B. Watschinger, B. Schmied, N. Vetter, and E. Puchhammer-Stöckl. 2001. Comparison of sequence analysis and the INNO-LiPA HBV DR line probe assay for detection of lamivudine-resistant hepatitis B virus strains in patients under various clinical conditions. *J. Clin. Microbiol.* **39:**1972–1974.
2. Akarsu, M., A. Sengonul, E. Tankurt, A. A. Sayiner, O. Topalak, H. Akpinar, and Y. H. Abacioglu. 2006. YMDD motif variants in inactive hepatitis B carriers detected by Inno-Lipa HBV DR assay. *J. Gastroenterol. Hepatol.* **21:**1783–1788.
3. Alter, H. J., and B. S. Blumberg. 1966. Further studies on a "new" human isoprecipitin system (Australia antigen). *Blood* **27:**297–309.
4. Alter, H. J., and H. G. Klein. 2008. The hazards of blood transfusion in historical perspective. *Blood* **112:**2617–2626.
5. Andersson, K. L., and R. T. Chung. 2009. Monitoring during and after antiviral therapy for hepatitis B. *Hepatology* **49:**S166–S173.
6. Anomymous. 2000. Consensus statements on the prevention and management of hepatitis B and hepatitis C in the Asia-Pacific region. Core Working Party for Asia-Pacific Consensus on Hepatitis B and C. *J. Gastroenterol. Hepatol.* **15:**825–841.
7. Ayoub, W. S., and E. B. Keeffe. 2008. Review article: current antiviral therapy of chronic hepatitis B. *Aliment. Pharmacol. Ther.* **28:**167–177.
8. Barboza, L., S. Salmen, D. L. Peterson, H. Montes, M. Colmenares, M. Hernandez, L. E. Berrueta-Carrillo, and L. Berrueta. 2009. Altered T cell costimulation during chronic hepatitis B infection. *Cell. Immunol.* **257:**61–68.
9. Beltrami, E. M., I. T. Williams, C. N. Shapiro, and M. E. Chamberland. 2000. Risk and management of blood-borne infections in health care workers. *Clin. Microbiol. Rev.* **13:**385–407.
10. Bertoletti, A., and A. Gehring. 2007. Immune response and tolerance during chronic hepatitis B virus infection. *Hepatol. Res.* **37**(Suppl. 3)**:**S331–S338.
11. Bertoletti, A., and A. J. Gehring. 2006. The immune response during hepatitis B virus infection. *J. Gen. Virol.* **87:**1439–1449.
12. Biswas, R., E. Tabor, C. C. Hsia, D. J. Wright, M. E. Laycock, E. W. Fiebig, L. Peddada, R. Smith, G. B. Schreiber, J. S. Epstein, G. J. Nemo, and M. P. Busch. 2003. Comparative sensitivity of HBV NATs and HBsAg assays for detection of acute HBV infection. *Transfusion* **43:**788–798.
13. Blow, J. A., C. N. Mores, J. Dyer, and D. J. Dohm. 2008. Viral nucleic acid stabilization by RNA extraction reagent. *J. Virol. Methods* **150:**41–44.
14. Blumberg, B. S., H. J. Alter, and S. Visnich. 1965. A "new" antigen in leukemia sera. *JAMA* **191:**541–546.
15. Boni, C., P. Fisicaro, C. Valdatta, B. Amadei, V. P. Di, T. Giuberti, D. Laccabue, A. Zerbini, A. Cavalli, G. Missale, A. Bertoletti, and C. Ferrari. 2007. Characterization of hepatitis B virus (HBV)-specific T-cell dysfunction in chronic HBV infection. *J. Virol.* **81:**4215–4225.
16. Bowden, S. 2006. Serological and molecular diagnosis. *Semin. Liver Dis.* **26:**97–103.
17. Cane, P. A., P. Cook, D. Ratcliffe, D. Mutimer, and D. Pillay. 1999. Use of real-time PCR and fluorimetry to detect lamivudine resistance-associated mutations in hepatitis B virus. *Antimicrob. Agents Chemother.* **43:**1600–1608.
18. Carman, W. F. 1996. Molecular variants of hepatitis B virus. *Clin. Lab. Med.* **16:**407–428.
19. Carman, W. F., M. Thursz, S. Hadziyannis, G. McIntyre, K. Colman, A. Gioustoz, G. Fattovich, A. Alberti, and H. C. Thomas. 1995. Hepatitis B e antigen negative chronic

active hepatitis: hepatitis B virus core mutations occur predominantly in known antigenic determinants. *J. Viral Hepat.* **2:**77–84.

20. **Carman, W. F., A. R. Zanetti, P. Karayiannis, J. Waters, G. Manzillo, E. Tanzi, A. J. Zuckerman, and H. C. Thomas.** 1990. Vaccine-induced escape mutant of hepatitis B virus. *Lancet* **336:**325–329.

21. **Caspari, G., and W. H. Gerlich.** 2007. The serologic markers of hepatitis B virus infection—proper selection and standardized interpretation. *Clin. Lab.* **53:**335–400.

22. **Centers for Disease Control.** 1991. Recommendations for preventing transmission of human immunodeficiency virus and hepatitis B virus to patients during exposure-prone invasive procedures. *MMWR Recomm. Rep.* **40:**1–9.

22a. **Chaves, S. S.** 2010. Hepatitis B. *In CDC Health Information for International Travel.* Centers for Disease Control and Prevention, Atlanta, GA. http://wwwnc.cdc.gov/travel/yellowbook/2010/chapter-2/hepatitis-b.aspx.

23. **Chisari, F. V.** 1992. Hepatitis B virus biology and pathogenesis. *Mol. Genet. Med.* **2:**67–104.

24. **Chotiyaputta, W., and A. S. Lok.** 2009. Hepatitis B virus variants. *Nat. Rev. Gastroenterol. Hepatol.* **6:**453–462.

25. **Chu, C. J., E. B. Keeffe, S. H. Han, R. P. Perrillo, A. D. Min, C. Soldevila-Pico, W. Carey, R. S. Brown, Jr., V. A. Luketic, N. Terrault, and A. S. Lok.** 2003. Prevalence of HBV precore/core promoter variants in the United States. *Hepatology* **38:**619–628.

26. **Coleman, P. F.** 2006. Detecting hepatitis B surface antigen mutants. *Emerg. Infect. Dis.* **12:**198–203.

27. **Custer, B., S. D. Sullivan, T. K. Hazlet, U. Iloeje, D. L. Veenstra, and K. V. Kowdley.** 2004. Global epidemiology of hepatitis B virus. *J. Clin. Gastroenterol.* **38:**S158–S168.

28. **Dane, D. S., C. H. Cameron, and M. Briggs.** 1970. Virus-like particles in serum of patients with Australia-antigen-associated hepatitis. *Lancet* **i:**695–698.

29. **Degertekin, B., and A. S. Lok.** 2009. Indications for therapy in hepatitis B. *Hepatology* **49:**S129–S137.

30. **Degertekin, B., and A. S. Lok.** 2009. Update on viral hepatitis: 2008. *Curr. Opin. Gastroenterol.* **25:**180–185.

31. **Doherty, R., S. Garland, M. Wright, M. Bulotsky, C. Liss, H. Lakkis, A. Nikas, and W. Straus.** 2009. Effectiveness of a bivalent Haemophilus influenzae type B-hepatitis B vaccine in preventing hepatitis B virus infection among children born to hepatitis B e antigen-positive carrier mothers. *Pediatr. Infect. Dis. J.* **28:**777–781.

32. **Echevarria, J. M., and A. Avellon.** 2008. Improved detection of natural hepatitis B virus surface antigen (HBsAg) mutants by a new version of the VITROS HBsAg assay. *J. Med. Virol.* **80:**598–602.

33. **Elbeik, T., P. Nassos, P. Kipnis, B. Haller, and V. L. Ng.** 2005. Evaluation of the VACUTAINER PPT plasma preparation tube for use with the Bayer VERSANT assay for quantification of human immunodeficiency virus type 1 RNA. *J. Clin. Microbiol.* **43:**3769–3771.

34. **Farci, P., L. Chessa, C. Balestrieri, G. Serra, and M. E. Lai.** 2007. Treatment of chronic hepatitis D. *J. Viral Hepat.* **14**(Suppl. 1):58–63.

35. **FitzSimons, D., G. Francois, C. G. De, D. Shouval, A. Pruss-Ustun, V. Puro, I. Williams, D. Lavanchy, S. A. De, A. Kopka, F. Ncube, G. Ippolito, and D. P. Van.** 2008. Hepatitis B virus, hepatitis C virus and other blood-borne infections in healthcare workers: guidelines for prevention and management in industrialised countries. *Occup. Environ. Med.* **65:**446–451.

36. **Flores, R.** 2001. A naked plant-specific RNA ten-fold smaller than the smallest known viral RNA: the viroid. *C. R. Acad. Sci. III* **324:**943–952.

37. **Fung, S. K., H. B. Chae, R. J. Fontana, H. Conjeevaram, J. Marrero, K. Oberhelman, M. Hussain, and A. S. Lok.** 2006. Virologic response and resistance to adefovir in patients with chronic hepatitis B. *J. Hepatol.* **44:**283–290.

38. **Gavilanes, F., J. M. Gonzalez-Ros, and D. L. Peterson.** 1982. Structure of hepatitis B surface antigen. Characterization of the lipid components and their association with the viral proteins. *J. Biol. Chem.* **257:**7770–7777.

39. **Gerlich, W. H.** 2006. Breakthrough of hepatitis B virus escape mutants after vaccination and virus reactivation. *J. Clin. Virol.* **36**(Suppl. 1):S18–S22.

40. **Gerlich, W. H., D. Glebe, and C. G. Schuttler.** 2007. Deficiencies in the standardization and sensitivity of diagnostic tests for hepatitis B virus. *J. Viral Hepat.* **14**(Suppl. 1):16–21.

41. **Gintowt, A. A., J. J. Germer, P. S. Mitchell, and J. D. Yao.** 2005. Evaluation of the MagNA Pure LC used with the TRUGENE HBV genotyping kit. *J. Clin. Virol.* **34:**155–157.

42. **Guidotti, L. G., and F. V. Chisari.** 2006. Immunobiology and pathogenesis of viral hepatitis. *Annu. Rev. Pathol.* **1:**23–61.

43. **Hadziyannis, S. J.** 1997. Review: hepatitis delta. *J. Gastroenterol. Hepatol.* **12:**289–298.

44. **Hall, J. G., P. S. Eis, S. M. Law, L. P. Reynaldo, J. R. Prudent, D. J. Marshall, H. T. Allawi, A. L. Mast, J. E. Dahlberg, R. W. Kwiatkowski, M. de Arruda, B. P. Neri, and V. I. Lyamichev.** 2000. Sensitive detection of DNA polymorphisms by the serial invasive signal amplification reaction. *Proc. Natl. Acad. Sci. USA* **97:**8272–8277.

45. **Heermann, K. H., W. H. Gerlich, M. Chudy, S. Schaefer, R. Thomssen, and the Eurohep Pathobiology Group.** 1999. Quantitative detection of hepatitis B virus DNA in two international reference plasma preparations. *J. Clin. Microbiol.* **37:**68–73.

46. **Hess, G., and M. Reuschling.** 1993. Toward routine diagnosis of hepatitis B virus desoxyribonucleic acid. *Clin. Biochem.* **26:**289–293.

47. **Hong, S. P., N. K. Kim, S. G. Hwang, H. J. Chung, S. Kim, J. H. Han, H. T. Kim, K. S. Rim, M. S. Kang, W. Yoo, and S. O. Kim.** 2004. Detection of hepatitis B virus YMDD variants using mass spectrometric analysis of oligonucleotide fragments. *J. Hepatol.* **40:**837–844.

48. **Hsu, C. W., C. T. Yeh, M. L. Chang, and Y. F. Liaw.** 2007. Identification of a hepatitis B virus S gene mutant in lamivudine-treated patients experiencing HBsAg seroclearance. *Gastroenterology* **132:**543–550.

49. **Huang, W. H., C. W. Chen, H. L. Wu, and P. J. Chen.** 2006. Post-translational modification of delta antigen of hepatitis D virus. *Curr. Top. Microbiol. Immunol.* **307:**91–112.

50. **Hussain, S. P., J. Schwank, F. Staib, X. W. Wang, and C. C. Harris.** 2007. TP53 mutations and hepatocellular carcinoma: insights into the etiology and pathogenesis of liver cancer. *Oncogene* **26:**2166–2176.

51. **Huzly, D., T. Schenk, W. Jilg, and D. Neumann-Haefelin.** 2008. Comparison of nine commercially available assays for quantification of antibody response to hepatitis B virus surface antigen. *J. Clin. Microbiol.* **46:**1298–1306.

52. **Jose, M., R. Gajardo, and J. I. Jorquera.** 2005. Stability of HCV, HIV-1 and HBV nucleic acids in plasma samples under long-term storage. *Biologicals* **33:**9–16.

53. **Kajiwara, E., Y. Tanaka, T. Ohashi, K. Uchimura, S. Sadoshima, M. Kinjo, and M. Mizokami.** 2008. Hepatitis B caused by a hepatitis B surface antigen escape mutant. *J. Gastroenterol.* **43:**243–247.

54. **Krajden, M., L. Comanor, O. Rifkin, A. Grigoriew, J. M. Minor, and G. F. Kapke.** 1998. Assessment of hepatitis B virus DNA stability in serum by the Chiron Quantiplex branched-DNA assay. *J. Clin. Microbiol.* **36:**382–386.

55. **Krajden, M., G. McNabb, and M. Petric.** 2005. The laboratory diagnosis of hepatitis B virus. *Can. J. Infect. Dis. Med. Microbiol.* **16:**65–72.

56. **Krajden, M., J. Minor, L. Cork, and L. Comanor.** 1998. Multi-measurement method comparison of three commercial hepatitis B virus DNA quantification assays. *J. Viral Hepat.* **5:**415–422.

57. **Krajden, M., J. M. Minor, O. Rifkin, and L. Comanor.** 1999. Effect of multiple freeze-thaw cycles on hepatitis B virus DNA and hepatitis C virus RNA quantification as measured with branched-DNA technology. *J. Clin. Microbiol.* **37:**1683–1686.

58. Kuo, M. Y., L. Sharmeen, G. Dinter-Gottlieb, and J. Taylor. 1988. Characterization of self-cleaving RNA sequences on the genome and antigenome of human hepatitis delta virus. *J. Virol.* **62:**4439–4444.

59. Kusumoto, K., H. Yatsuhashi, R. Nakao, R. Hamada, M. Fukuda, Y. Tamada, N. Taura, A. Komori, M. Daikoku, K. Hamasaki, K. Nakao, H. Ishibashi, Y. Miyakawa, and K. Eguchi. 2008. Detection of HBV core promoter and precore mutations helps distinguish flares of chronic hepatitis from acute hepatitis B. *J. Gastroenterol. Hepatol.* **23:**790–793.

60. Lai, M. M. 1995. Molecular biologic and pathogenetic analysis of hepatitis delta virus. *J. Hepatol.* **22:**127–131.

61. Liang, T. J. 2009. Hepatitis B: the virus and disease. *Hepatology* **49:**S13–S21.

62. Liu, W. C., M. Lindh, M. Buti, P. H. Phiet, M. Mizokami, H. H. Li, K. T. Sun, K. C. Young, P. N. Cheng, I. C. Wu, and T. T. Chang. 2008. Genotyping of hepatitis B virus—genotypes a to g by multiplex polymerase chain reaction. *Intervirology* **51:**247–252.

63. Lok, A. S., and B. J. McMahon. 2007. Chronic hepatitis B. *Hepatology* **45:**507–539.

64. Lu, C. Y., Y. H. Ni, B. L. Chiang, P. J. Chen, M. H. Chang, L. Y. Chang, I. J. Su, H. S. Kuo, L. M. Huang, D. S. Chen, and C. Y. Lee. 2008. Humoral and cellular immune responses to a hepatitis B vaccine booster 15–18 years after neonatal immunization. *J. Infect. Dis.* **197:**1419–1426.

65. Lu, H. Y., Z. Zeng, X. Y. Xu, N. L. Zhang, M. Yu, and W. B. Gong. 2006. Mutations in surface and polymerase gene of chronic hepatitis B patients with coexisting HBsAg and anti-HBs. *World J. Gastroenterol.* **12:**4219–4223.

66. Ly, T. D., A. Servant-Delmas, S. Bagot, S. Gonzalo, M. P. Ferey, A. Ebel, E. Dussaix, S. Laperche, and A. M. Roque-Afonso. 2006. Sensitivities of four new commercial hepatitis B virus surface antigen (HBsAg) assays in detection of HBsAg mutant forms. *J. Clin. Microbiol.* **44:**2321–2326.

66a. MacCallum, F. O., and D. J. Bauer. 1947. Homologous serum hepatitis. *Lancet.* **ii:**691–692.

67. Maddrey, W. C. 2000. Hepatitis B: an important public health issue. *J. Med Virol.* **61:**362–366.

68. McMahon, B. J. 2005. Epidemiology and natural history of hepatitis B. *Semin. Liver Dis.* **25**(Suppl. 1):3–8.

69. McMahon, B. J. 2009. The natural history of chronic hepatitis B virus infection. *Hepatology* **49:**S45–S55.

70. Mizuochi, T., Y. Okada, K. Umemori, S. Mizusawa, and K. Yamaguchi. 2006. Evaluation of 10 commercial diagnostic kits for in vitro expressed hepatitis B virus (HBV) surface antigens encoded by HBV of genotypes A to H. *J. Virol. Methods* **136:**254–256.

71. Nayersina, R., P. Fowler, S. Guilhot, G. Missale, A. Cerny, H. J. Schlicht, A. Vitiello, R. Chesnut, J. L. Person, A. G. Redeker, and F. V. Chisari. 1993. HLA A2 restricted cytotoxic T lymphocyte responses to multiple hepatitis B surface antigen epitopes during hepatitis B virus infection. *J. Immunol.* **150:**4659–4671.

72. Nguyen, M. H., and E. B. Keeffe. 2009. Chronic hepatitis B: early viral suppression and long-term outcomes of therapy with oral nucleos(t)ides *J. Viral Hepat.* **16:**149–155.

73. Ni, Y. H., L. M. Huang, M. H. Chang, C. J. Yen, C. Y. Lu, S. L. You, J. H. Kao, Y. C. Lin, H. L. Chen, H. Y. Hsu, and D. S. Chen. 2007. Two decades of universal hepatitis B vaccination in Taiwan: impact and implication for future strategies. *Gastroenterology* **132:**1287–1293.

74. Niro, G. A., F. Rosina, and M. Rizzetto. 2005. Treatment of hepatitis D. *J. Viral Hepat.* **12:**2–9.

75. Occupational Safety and Health Administration, U.S. Department of Labor. 2009. Bloodborne pathogens. 29 *Code of Federal Regulations* 1910.1030. Occupational Safety and Health Administration, U.S. Department of Labor, Washington, DC.

76. Olivero, A., A. Ciancio, M. L. Abate, S. Gaia, A. Smedile, and M. Rizzetto. 2006. Performance of sequence analysis, INNO-LiPA line probe assays and AFFIGENE assays in the detection of hepatitis B virus polymerase and precore/core promoter mutations. *J. Viral Hepat.* **13:**355–362.

77. Osiowy, C. 2006. Detection of HBsAg mutants. *J. Med. Virol.* **78**(Suppl. 1):S48–S51.

78. Pawlotsky, J. M., G. Dusheiko, A. Hatzakis, D. Lau, G. Lau, T. J. Liang, S. Locarnini, P. Martin, D. D. Richman, and F. Zoulim. 2008. Virologic monitoring of hepatitis B virus therapy in clinical trials and practice: recommendations for a standardized approach. *Gastroenterology* **134:**405–415.

79. Peters, M. G. 2009. Special populations with hepatitis B virus infection. *Hepatology* **49:**S146–S155.

80. Punia, P., P. Cane, C. G. Teo, and N. Saunders. 2004. Quantitation of hepatitis B lamivudine resistant mutants by real-time amplification refractory mutation system PCR. *J. Hepatol.* **40:**986–992.

81. Qiu, X., P. Schroeder, and D. Bridon. 1996. Identification and characterization of a C(K/R)TC motif as a common epitope present in all subtypes of hepatitis B surface antigen. *J. Immunol.* **156:**3350–3356.

82. Rizzetto, M. 2009. Hepatitis D: the comeback? *Liver Int.* **29**(Suppl. 1):140–142.

83. Rizzetto, M. 2009. Hepatitis D: thirty years after. *J. Hepatol.* **50:**1043–1050.

84. Rotman, Y., T. A. Brown, and J. H. Hoofnagle. 2009. Evaluation of the patient with hepatitis B. *Hepatology* **49:**S22–S27.

85. Sablon, E., and F. Shapiro. 2005. Advances in molecular diagnosis of HBV infection and drug resistance. *Int. J. Med. Sci.* **2:**8–16.

86. Safadi, R., Y. Greenboim, and M. Donchin. 2000. Impact of standard vaccination of health care workers with hepatitis B vaccine on reducing the occupational risk of infection. *J. Hosp. Infect.* **45:**250–251.

87. Saldanha, J., W. Gerlich, N. Lelie, P. Dawson, K. Heermann, and A. Heath. 2001. An international collaborative study to establish a World Health Organization international standard for hepatitis B virus DNA nucleic acid amplification techniques. *Vox Sang.* **80:**63–71.

88. Seeger, C., and W. S. Mason. 2000. Hepatitis B virus biology. *Microbiol. Mol. Biol. Rev.* **64:**51–68.

89. Selabe, S. G., E. Song, R. J. Burnett, and M. J. Mphahlele. 2009. Frequent detection of hepatitis B virus variants associated with lamivudine resistance in treated South African patients infected chronically with different HBV genotypes. *J. Med. Virol.* **81:**996–1001.

90. Shakil, A. O., S. Hadziyannis, J. H. Hoofnagle, A. M. Di Bisceglie, J. L. Gerin, and J. L. Casey. 1997. Geographic distribution and genetic variability of hepatitis delta virus genotype. *Virology* **234:**160–167.

91. Shamliyan, T. A., R. MacDonald, A. Shaukat, B. C. Taylor, J. M. Yuan, J. R. Johnson, J. Tacklind, I. Rutks, R. L. Kane, and T. J. Wilt. 2009. Antiviral therapy for adults with chronic hepatitis B: a systematic review for a National Institutes of Health Consensus Development Conference. *Ann. Intern. Med.* **150:**111–124.

92. Shaw, T., A. Bartholomeusz, and S. Locarnini. 2006. HBV drug resistance: mechanisms, detection and interpretation. *J. Hepatol.* **44:**593–606.

93. Shepard, C. W., E. P. Simard, L. Finelli, A. E. Fiore, and B. P. Bell. 2006. Hepatitis B virus infection: epidemiology and vaccination. *Epidemiol. Rev.* **28:**112–125.

94. Sorrell, M. F., E. A. Belongia, J. Costa, I. F. Gareen, J. L. Grem, J. M. Inadomi, E. R. Kern, J. A. McHugh, G. M. Petersen, M. F. Rein, D. B. Strader, and H. T. Trotter. 2009. National Institutes of Health Consensus Development Conference statement: management of hepatitis B. *Ann. Intern. Med.* **150:**104–110.

95. Taylor, J. M. 2006. Hepatitis delta virus. *Virology* **344:**71–76.

96. Tseng, C. H., K. S. Jeng, and M. M. Lai. 2008. Transcription of subgenomic mRNA of hepatitis delta virus requires a modified hepatitis delta antigen that is distinct from antigenomic RNA synthesis. *J. Virol.* **82:**9409–9416.

97. Valsamakis, A. 2007. Molecular testing in the diagnosis and management of chronic hepatitis B. *Clin. Microbiol. Rev.* **20:**426–439.

98. Wang, T. C., and M. Chao. 2003. Molecular cloning and expression of the hepatitis delta virus genotype IIb genome. *Biochem. Biophys. Res.Commun.* **303:**357–363.

99. Wang, X. W., S. P. Hussain, T. I. Huo, C. G. Wu, M. Forgues, L. J. Hofseth, C. Brechot, and C. C. Harris. 2002. Molecular pathogenesis of human hepatocellular carcinoma. *Toxicology* **181–182:**43–47.

100. Weber, B., T. Dengler, A. Berger, H. W. Doerr, and H. Rabenau. 2003. Evaluation of two new automated assays for hepatitis B virus surface antigen (HBsAg) detection: IMMULITE HBsAg and IMMULITE 2000 HBsAg. *J. Clin. Microbiol.* **41:**135–143.

101. Whalley, S. A., D. Brown, C. G. Teo, G. M. Dusheiko, and N. A. Saunders. 2001. Monitoring the emergence of hepatitis B virus polymerase gene variants during lamivudine therapy using the LightCycler. *J. Clin. Microbiol.* **39:**1456–1459.

102. Wursthorn, K., M. P. Manns, and H. Wedemeyer. 2008. Natural history: the importance of viral load, liver damage and HCC. *Best Pract. Res. Clin. Gastroenterol.* **22:**1063–1079.

103. Yeon, J. E. 2008. Technique for the early detection of drug-resistant HBV DNA during antiviral therapy. *Intervirology* **51**(Suppl. 1):7–10.

104. Yim, H. J., and A. S. Lok. 2006. Natural history of chronic hepatitis B virus infection: what we knew in 1981 and what we know in 2005. *Hepatology* **43:**S173–S181.

105. Yurdaydin, C., H. Bozkaya, H. Karaaslan, F. O. Onder, O. E. Erkan, K. Yalcin, H. Degertekin, A. M. Bozdayi, and O. Uzunalimoglu. 2007. A pilot study of 2 years of interferon treatment in patients with chronic delta hepatitis. *J. Viral Hepat.* **14:**812–816.

106. Yurdaydin, C., H. Bozkaya, F. O. Onder, H. Senturk, H. Karaaslan, M. Akdogan, H. Cetinkaya, E. Erden, O. Erkan-Esin, K. Yalcin, A. M. Bozdayi, R. F. Schinazi, J. L. Gerin, O. Uzunalimoglu, and A. Ozden. 2008. Treatment of chronic delta hepatitis with lamivudine vs lamivudine + interferon vs interferon. *J. Viral Hepat.* **15:**314–321.

107. Zheng, X., K. M. Weinberger, R. Gehrke, M. Isogawa, G. Hilken, T. Kemper, Y. Xu, D. Yang, W. Jilg, M. Roggendorf, and M. Lu. 2004. Mutant hepatitis B virus surface antigens (HBsAg) are immunogenic but may have a changed specificity. *Virology* **329:**454–464.

108. Zoulim, F. 2006. In vitro models for studying hepatitis B virus drug resistance. *Semin. Liver Dis.* **26:**171–180.

109. Zoulim, F., M. Buti, and A. S. Lok. 2007. Antiviral-resistant hepatitis B virus: can we prevent this monster from growing? *J. Viral Hepat.* **14**(Suppl. 1):29–36.

Transmissible Spongiform Encephalopathies

ADRIANO AGUZZI AND MARKUS GLATZEL

107

TAXONOMY

Prions

The most widely accepted hypothesis on the nature of the infectious agent causing transmissible spongiform encephalopathies (TSEs), which is termed a prion (for proteinaceous infectious particle), predicates that it consists of a scrapie-like prion protein (PrP^{Sc}), an abnormally folded, protease-resistant, beta-sheet-rich isoform of a normal cellular prion protein (PrP^{C}) (30). According to this theory, the prion does not contain any informational nucleic acids, and its infectivity propagates simply by recruitment and "autocatalytic" conformational conversion of cellular prion protein into disease-associated PrP^{Sc} (1). The size of the minimal infectious unit of PrP^{Sc} is still a matter of debate; recent studies indicate that oligomeric PrP^{Sc} consisting of 14 to 28 PrP^{Sc} molecules harbors the highest converting activity (34).

A large body of experimental and epidemiological evidence is compatible with the protein-only hypothesis, and very stringently designed experiments have failed to disprove it. It would go well beyond the scope of this chapter to review all the efforts that have been undertaken to this effect. Perhaps most impressively, knockout mice carrying a homozygous deletion of the murine *Prnp* gene that encodes PrP^{C} ($Prnp^{0/0}$ mice) fail to develop disease upon inoculation with infectious brain homogenate, nor does their brain carry prion infectivity (33). Reintroduction of *Prnp* by transgenesis, even in a shortened, redacted form, restores infectibility and prion replication in $Prnp^{0/0}$ mice (14, 15). In addition, all familial cases of human TSEs are characterized by mutations in the human PrP^{C} gene (designated *PRNP*) (13, 22). Numerous studies demonstrating that infectious prions may be synthesized in cell-free systems and consist exclusively of PrP^{Sc} go a long way towards settling the score as to the proteinaceous nature of the infectious agent (3, 8, 24).

DESCRIPTION OF THE AGENT

As outlined above, the evidence that the abnormal form of PrP^{C}, PrP^{Sc}, represents the infectious agent is overwhelming. The three-dimensional structure of PrP^{C} has been solved by nuclear magnetic resonance spectroscopy, but similar analyses have not been possible for PrP^{Sc} (21, 31). Studies employing Fourier transform infrared spectroscopy or electron crystallography have demonstrated that PrP^{Sc} is rich in beta-sheets possibly arranged in parallel beta-helices (40, 41).

EPIDEMIOLOGY AND TRANSMISSION

Human prion diseases manifest as sporadic, genetic, and acquired disorders. They are referred to as sporadic Creutzfeldt-Jakob disease (sCJD), genetic CJD (gCJD), variant CJD (vCJD), and iatrogenic CJD (iCJD).

Sporadic CJD

sCJD is a rapidly progressive dementia, usually leading to death within 6 months of disease onset (18). The cause of sCJD remains enigmatic. To date no obvious risk factors have been identified (32). Because of the short mean duration of this disease, incidence and mortality rates for sCJD are similar; thus, mortality rates are routinely used to describe the epidemiology of this disease (12). Mortality rates are fairly constant both over time and between countries, oscillating around 1.5 cases per million per year (http://www.eurocjd.ed.ac.uk/allcjd.htm). Unlike other dementias such as Alzheimer's and Parkinson's diseases, whose incidence rises with age, the peak incidence is between 55 and 65 years of age (11).

Genetic CJD

gCJD can be subdivided into three phenotypes: hereditary CJD, Gerstmann-Sträussler-Scheinker syndrome (GSS), and fatal familial insomnia (FFI). The mode of inheritance in all of these diseases, which cosegregate with mutations in *PRNP*, is autosomal dominant (22). Incidences of gCJD vary from country to country with Slovakia reaching the highest incidence of more than one case per million for the time period 1999 to 2002 (39).

Variant CJD

vCJD, a relatively new member of human prion diseases, was first reported in 1996 (40). Biochemical, neuropathological, epidemiological, and transmission studies indicate that vCJD represents transmission of bovine spongiform encephalopathy (BSE) prions to humans (6, 19). The incidence of vCJD in the United Kingdom rose each year from 1996 to 2001, evoking fears of a large upcoming epidemic (1). Since 2001 the incidence of vCJD in the United

Kingdom has dropped; however, other countries such as France and Spain have reported a significant number of vCJD cases (http://www.eurocjd.ed.ac.uk). Predictions on the future of the vCJD epidemic indicate that the total number of vCJD victims will be limited (36). vCJD has a distinct clinicopathological profile including young age of onset (median age at death, 29 years) (4).

Iatrogenic CJD

iCJD is caused by accidental prion exposure during medical or neurosurgical procedures such as implantation of human dura mater, treatment with human cadaveric pituitary extracts, or blood transfusion (2, 18). iCJD is rare, with fewer than 300 published cases (5). The majority of cases were caused by implantation of dura mater and injection of pituitary growth hormone. Recent epidemiological data confirm the observation that iCJD mainly affects individuals younger than 39 years (23).

CLINICAL SIGNIFICANCE

Initial symptoms of sCJD include rapid cognitive decline, sleep disturbances, and behavioral abnormalities. As the disease progresses, other clinical features such as extrapyramidal symptoms (i.e., akinesia, which is the inability to initiate movement), pyramidal symptoms (i.e., loss of fine motor skills), ataxia, and visual disturbances appear and patients usually develop myoclonus (involuntary twitching of a muscle) (16). Terminally affected sCJD patients typically develop a state of akinetic mutism prior to death. The disease course is usually short, the mean duration of the illness being 4 to 5 months (Table 1).

The clinical presentation of gCJD varies with the underlying mutation. Some mutations present with a clinical picture that is similar to that of sCJD (Table 2). The age at onset tends to be younger and the disease duration longer than for sCJD. FFI and GSS represent exceptions. FFI has a unique clinical course characterized by profound disruption of the normal sleep-wake cycle, insomnia, and sympathetic overactivity such as accelerated heart rate or perspiration, whereas GSS presents with a progressive cerebellar ataxia (10).

In iCJD, the site of prion exposure seems to dictate the incubation time from exposure to onset of prion disease-related symptoms. Direct intracerebral exposure to prions and implantation of prion-contaminated dura, for example, are associated with short incubation periods (16 to 28 months), whereas exposure to prions at sites outside the central nervous system (CNS) results in long incubation times ranging from 5 to 30 years (9). Furthermore, there is evidence that the route of prion exposure influences the clinical presentation. Dura mater- or growth hormone-related cases of iCJD present with a predominantly ataxic phenotype, whereas dementia was the initial symptom in cases in which prions were directly introduced into the CNS.

The fact that vCJD carries a distinct clinical profile has facilitated the formulation of diagnostic criteria. vCJD victims are much younger than sCJD patients (median age at death, 29 years). Furthermore, initial features and illness duration are relatively specific with initial psychiatric symptoms and median illness duration of 14 months (Table 1). It has been hard to estimate incubation times for vCJD due to the fact that the exact time points of prion exposure are not defined.

The diagnosis of human prion diseases is based on the evaluation of clinical signs and auxiliary examinations (9). Electroencephalography (EEG) has historically been used to substantiate the diagnosis of a human prion disease. The usefulness of EEG has been questioned due to its limited sensitivity (43). Recent advances in neuroimaging, especially in magnetic resonance imaging (MRI), have revealed that different human prion diseases have specific patterns. For vCJD, the "pulvinar sign," a high T2 MRI signal in the posterior thalamus, seems to be pathognomonic (37). For sCJD, a high T2 MRI signal in the striatum and a high MRI signal in the cortex in fluid-attenuated inversion recovery sequences (a pulse sequence used in brain imaging to suppress cerebrospinal fluid [CSF] effects on the image) are classical findings (37).

COLLECTION, STORAGE, AND TRANSPORT OF SPECIMENS

Safety and Security

Human prions are classified as biosafety level 2 (BSL-2) or BSL-3 agents depending on the source of the infectious material and the level of infectivity of the source specimen. Unfixed samples of brain or spinal cord, as well as other tissues such as lymphoid tissue specimen from vCJD-diseased individuals known to contain high amounts of infectious prions should be handled at BSL-3 (28). In clinical laboratories, personal protective clothing such as disposable gowns, gloves, and barrier protection for mucous membranes (eye protection or full face visor) are recommended when working with potentially contaminated specimens. In addition, strict adherence to standard working procedures aimed at minimizing the chance of penetrating injuries is essential. Prions are not inactivated by formalin. A procedure recommended by the College of American Pathologists (http//:www.cap.org) for safe handling of tissues is adequate formalin fixation, followed by agitation in sufficient amount of formic acid (95 to 100% [vol/vol]; the sample should be entirely immersed in formic acid) for 1 h, and subsequent formalin fixation for 2 days prior to embedding. Formic acid inactivates formalin-treated prions but has minimal effect on the quality of histology. Disposable histologic equipment should be used whenever possible.

Blood and bone marrow are presumed to contain low levels of infectivity (http://www.advisorybodies.doh.gov.uk/acdp/tseguidance/). These specimens can be handled safely under BSL-2 conditions by adhering to universal precautions for prevention of transmission of bloodborne pathogens. These specimens can be tested in automated analyzers found throughout clinical laboratories if instruments are enclosed and can contain spillage and waste can be disposed of safely. Maintenance and emergency procedures that protect the user from exposure should be outlined in laboratory standard operating procedures and implemented. Manual processing (specimen decanting, for example) should be performed inside a negative-pressure laminar flow hood in a contained environment.

Prions can be substantially but not completely inactivated by physical exposure to steam or dry heat at high temperatures. Disposable laboratory equipment should be used whenever possible. Potentially contaminated laboratory waste should be autoclaved (at 134 to 137°C for 20 min) and then incinerated (http://www.advisorybodies.doh.gov.uk/acdp/tseguidance/). Chemical exposure to high concentrations of either sodium hypochlorite (>5.25% solution, freshly prepared) or sodium hydroxide (1 N solution) for 1 h is effective against prions and can be used to disinfect spills. Reusable laboratory material should be immersed in a freshly prepared >5.25% solution of sodium hypochlorite or a 1 N solution of sodium hydroxide for 1 h and then rinsed with water before being packaged for

TABLE 1 Clinical, diagnostic, and neuropathological features of human prion diseases

Human prion disease	Clinical features			Diagnostic tests				Genetics		Postmortem neuropathological examination	
	Age at onset (yr)	Disease duration (mean)	Leading clinical symptoms	CSF 14-3-3	EEG	MRI	Biopsy	Codon 129	PRNP mutation	Histopathological features	Biochemical tests
sCJD	60–70	6 mo (1–35 mo)	Progressive dementia and neurological signs (e.g., myoclonus, cerebellar ataxia, visual problems, extra pyramidal symptoms)	Positive in >90%	PSWC[a] 60–70%	Brain atrophy hyperintensities in basal ganglia and/or cortical 67%	Brain, muscle	MM 70%, MV 14%, VV 16%	Not observed	Spongiform changes, neuronal loss, astrogliosis, PrP deposition (various patterns)	PrP^{Sc} typing (WB[b])
Inherited CJD											
gCJD	50–60	6 mo (2–41 mo)	Clinical symptoms similar to sCJD	Positive in >90%	PSWC 75%	Similar to sCJD			Over 25 disease-associated mutations, e.g., E200K	Similar to sCJD	PrP^{Sc} typing (WB)
GSS	50–60	5–6 yr (3 mo–13 yr)	Cerebellar dysfunction (ataxia, nystagmus, dysarthria)	Usually negative	Nonspecific alterations	Normal or non-specific cerebral or cerebellar atrophy			P102L (plus 11 less common mutations)	Spongiform changes, neuronal loss, astrogliosis, P-P deposition (multicentric plaques)	PrP^{Sc} typing (WB)
FFI	50 (20–63)	13–15 mo (6–42 mo)	Insomnia autonomic dysfunction	Negative	Nonspecific alterations	Normal or non-specific cerebral or cerebellar atrophy		M (on the mutated allele)	D178N	Involvement of thalami	PrP^{Sc} typing (WB)
Acquired CJD											
vCJD	26 (12–74)	14 mo (6–24 mo)	Early psychiatric symptoms (depression, anxiety, social withdrawal), dysesthesia; later neurological deficits and cognitive decline	Positive in 50%	Nonspecific alterations, no PSWC	Hyperintensities in the posterior thalamus ("pulvinar sign") 78%	Brain, muscle, tonsils	MM 100%	Not observed	Spongiform changes, neuronal loss, astrogliosis, PrP deposition (florid plaques)	PrP^{Sc} typing (WB)
iCJD	—[c]	Similar to sCJD	Clinical symptoms similar to sCJD	Positive in 77%	Similar to sCJD	Similar to sCJD		MM 57%, MV 20%, VV 23%	Not observed	Similar to sCJD	PrP^{Sc} typing (WB)

[a]PSWC, periodic sharp wave complexes.
[b]WB, Western blotting.
[c]—, age at onset depending on iatrogenic exposure: incubation period, 1 to 30 years.

TABLE 2 Disease-causing mutations in *PRNP*

Mutations that cause GSS	Mutations that cause a disease that is clinically similar to sCJD	Mutations that cause FFI	Mutations that cause nonclassifiable neuropsychiatric symptoms
P102L (codon 129V)	P105S	D178N (codon 129M)	G114V
P105K (codon 129V)	I138M		Q160stop (codon 129M)
A117V (codon 129V)	G124S		N171S
G131V (codon 129M)	D178N (codon 129V)		T183A
Y145stop (codon 129M)	V180I		H187R
H187R (codon 129V)	V180I + M232R		
F198S (codon 129V)	T188R		
D202N (codon 129V)	T188A		
Q121P	T188K		
Q217R (codon 129M)	E196K		
M232T	E200K		
192-bp insertion	V203I		
	R208H		
	V120I		
	E211Q		
	M232R		
	P238S		
	24-,48-, 96-, 120-, 144-, 168-, and 216-bp insertions		

autoclave sterilization at 134°C for at least 20 min (http://www.advisorybodies.doh.gov.uk/acdp/tseguidance/). The guidelines for the reprocessing of instruments may vary between countries; therefore, readers should also refer to their country's specific guidelines.

Specimen Collection

Whole blood may be used for isolation of DNA for genetic analysis (exclusion of gCJD). Blood should be shipped in a chilled container. Currently, an approved blood-based screening test for human prion diseases is not available. CSF is routinely used to monitor elevation of nonspecific neuronal injury markers. CSF should be shipped at 4°C. Tissue may be used for histopathology and biochemical examination. Brain biopsies can only be recommended in order to exclude the diagnosis of diseases for which therapeutic options are available. Nonneural tissues (lymphatic tissue or muscle) may be useful in order to confirm the suspicion of vCJD. Tissue should be fixed in formalin for histologic assessment as described above and snap-frozen for Western blotting. Formalin-fixed material may be shipped at room temperature, whereas snap-frozen material must be shipped on dry ice.

Shipping

Shipping of infectious material via water, land (road or train), and air must comply with the "Recommendations of the United Nations Committee of Experts on the Transport of Dangerous Goods." In these guidelines, human prions are listed in category 6 (Toxic and Infectious Substances), division 2 (Infectious Substances). The code numbers UN 2900 apply for this type of pathogen. Certified shipping containers must be used.

DIRECT DETECTION

Microscopy

Although it is not routinely recommended for the diagnosis of human prion diseases, histologic examination of CNS tissue can be diagnostically helpful premortem.

Routine hematoxylin and eosin stains are used to interpret the vacuolization patterns, whereas immunohistochemical demonstration of PrP is necessary in order to determine PrP deposition patterns (Fig. 1). Postmortem, defined regions within the CNS (cerebellum and thalamus) and nonneuronal tissues can be sampled to demonstrate distinct PrP deposition patterns (7). Histologically, prion diseases are characterized by spongiform changes, astrogliosis, and neuronal loss. These changes are most evident in the cerebral cortex and in the cerebellum. The prominent cerebellar involvement is typical for prion diseases and clearly separates this group of diseases from other dementing illnesses such as Alzheimer's disease and diffuse Lewy body disease (34). In vCJD and in about 10 to 20% of sCJD patients prion plaques are a prominent feature and may be demonstrated by Congo red staining or immunohistochemistry. Birefringence, an indication of proteins assuming beta-pleated sheet conformation under polarized light, usually a characteristic feature of amyloid plaques, may be absent due to harsh pretreatment of fixed tissue.

Antigen Detection

Western blotting is routinely performed on unfixed tissue originating from the CNS. Generally, this test is undertaken in a postmortem setting. In rare cases where a brain biopsy is justified, a biopsy specimen may be used for this test.

The basis of biochemical characterization of PrP^{Sc} resides in the relative resistance of PrP^{Sc} to proteolytic degradation. Whereas PrP^C is entirely digested by proteinase K, identical treatment of PrP^{Sc} leads to removal of a variable number of N-terminal amino acids. Western blotting of digested PrP^{Sc} reveals three distinct bands, corresponding to di-, mono-, and unglycosylated forms (26). The molecular classification of PrP^{Sc} takes two parameters into account: molecular weight of unglycosylated PrP^{Sc} and the relative amounts of PrP^{Sc} di-, mono-, and unglycosylated forms. The resulting information is then used to establish the "type" of PrP^{Sc} according to proposed schemes (20, 26, 27) (Fig. 2). Depending on the exact conditions under which

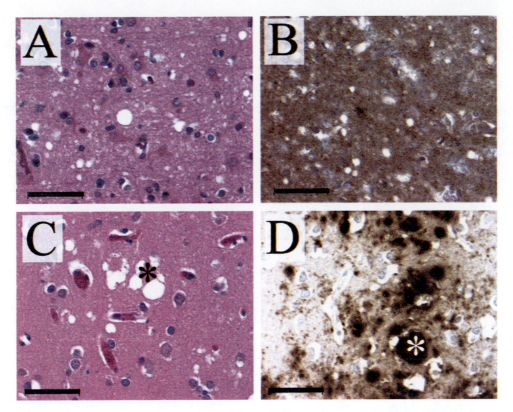

FIGURE 1 Histological features of prion diseases. CNS parenchyma of sCJD (A and B) and vCJD (C and D) shows astrogliosis and widespread spongiform changes. PrP depositions are synaptic (A and B) and in the form of florid plaques (asterisk, C and D). Panels A and C are hematoxylin and eosin stains, and panels B and D are immunohistochemical stains for PrP (scale bar = 50 μm).

the protease digestion and the Western blotting procedure are performed, between three and six different PrP^{Sc} types can be distinguished. Distinct PrP^{Sc} types are thought to represent the molecular correlates of distinct prion strains. The fact that the PrP^{Sc} types found in vCJD patients and in BSE-diseased cattle are identical is one of the main argu-

ments supporting the theory that BSE prions are responsible for the vCJD epidemic in humans (19). Novel anti-PrP antibodies are able to discriminate PrP^{Sc} types and have thus facilitated diagnostic procedures (29).

In addition to Western blotting, sandwich enzyme-linked immunosorbent assays are available to detect PrP^{Sc} partially resistant to proteinase K. Although these tests do not give exact information on PrP^{Sc} types, recent studies propagate their use in a diagnostic setting for human prion diseases (38).

Nucleic Acid Analysis: Genetic Testing

For genetic testing, routinely DNA is extracted from whole blood. The entire open reading frame may be amplified for sequencing, using PCR (17).

Sequencing of *PRNP* allows for the exclusion of gCJD (42). More than 30 disease-causing insertional or point mutations in *PRNP* have been identified to date (Table 2).

In addition, there are several *PRNP* polymorphisms, one of which (codon 129M/V) may have a disease-modifying function (18). Homozygosity for methionine at codon 129 constitutes a risk factor for the development of prion disease: methionine homozygotes are overrepresented among sCJD patients, and all clinically diseased vCJD patients are homozygous for methionine at codon 129.

CSF Analysis

To date there are no serologic screening or confirmatory tests for prion diseases. Rather, several studies have evaluated the usefulness of surrogate markers, such as 14-3-3 and tau

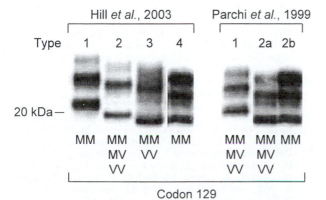

FIGURE 2 Western blot analysis of PrP^{Sc}. Depicted are PrP^{Sc} types according to two proposed schemes (20, 26) which discriminate PrP^{Sc} types based on the mobility of the unglycosylated band of PrP^{Sc} and the signal intensity of PrP^{Sc} di-, mono-, and unglycosylated forms. One scheme (20) differentiates four principal PrP^{Sc} types (1 through 4). Three principal PrP^{Sc} types (1, 2a, and 2b) are proposed in the second scheme (22).

proteins, that are found in CSF as a consequence of neuronal death. These proteins are ubiquitously expressed. The 14-3-3 protein participates in protein kinase signaling and is involved in neuronal migration. Tau is a phosphoprotein that promotes assembly and stability of axons by binding to microtubules. Elevation of these protein levels is relatively nonspecific and can be seen in other conditions such as encephalitis, cerebral infarction, and paraneoplastic neurological disorders. Satisfactory sensitivity and specificity (over 90%) can only be achieved in selected cohorts (42). Results from these tests, in combination with clinical data, may help at best to strengthen the diagnosis of a probable human prion disease. While 14-3-3 is routinely tested with a Western blot, tau may be measured in an enzyme-linked immunosorbent assay format (43). Recent data indicate that measurement of the serine proteinase inhibitor alpha1-antichymotrypsin in urine may constitute a sensitive and easily assessable biomarker for sCJD (2, 25).

EVALUATION, REPORTING, AND INTERPRETATION OF RESULTS

The diagnosis of human prion disorders can be difficult to establish but is best approached through careful consideration of clinical presentation, and other clinical studies such as neuroimaging, brain biopsy, and histological assessment can be performed to rule out treatable disorders. Detection of spongiform changes and deposition of PrP^{Sc} in affected areas can help establish the diagnosis of prion disorders. The absence of these changes (for example, due to sampling bias) is not helpful in the exclusion of these disorders. Less invasive tests such as detection of surrogate markers (tau and 14-3-3) in the CSF can be helpful when interpreted in the context of clinical and neuroimaging data. Genetic testing can be performed to establish the diagnosis of gCJD. The constellation of tests that can be helpful in the diagnosis of each of these disorders is shown in Table 2. All testing other than detection of surrogate markers in the CSF, sequencing of *PRNP*, and neuropathology is usually performed on a research basis.

REFERENCES

1. Aguzzi, A., F. Baumann, and J. Bremer. 2008. The prion's elusive reason for being. *Annu. Rev. Neurosci.* **31:**439–477.
2. Aguzzi, A., and M. Glatzel. 2006. Prion infections, blood and transfusions. *Nat. Clin. Pract. Neurol.* **2:**321–329.
3. Atarashi, R., R. A. Moore, V. L. Sim, A. G. Hughson, D. W. Dorward, H. A. Onwubiko, S. A. Priola, and B. Caughey. 2007. Ultrasensitive detection of scrapie prion protein using seeded conversion of recombinant prion protein. *Nat. Methods* **4:**645–650.
4. Beisel, C. E., and D. M. Morens. 2004. Variant Creutzfeldt-Jakob disease and the acquired and transmissible spongiform encephalopathies. *Clin. Infect. Dis.* **38:**697–704.
5. Brown, P., M. Preece, J. P. Brandel, T. Sato, L. McShane, I. Zerr, A. Fletcher, R. G. Will, M. Pocchiari, N. R. Cashman, J. H. d'Aignaux, L. Cervenakova, J. Fradkin, L. B. Schonberger, and S. J. Collins. 2000. Iatrogenic Creutzfeldt-Jakob disease at the millennium. *Neurology* **55:**1075–1081.
6. Bruce, M. E., R. G. Will, J. W. Ironside, I. McConnell, D. Drummond, A. Suttie, L. McCardle, A. Chree, J. Hope, C. Birkett, S. Cousens, H. Fraser, and C. J. Bostock. 1997. Transmissions to mice indicate that 'new variant' CJD is caused by the BSE agent. *Nature* **389:**498–501.
7. Budka, H., A. Aguzzi, P. Brown, J. M. Brucher, O. Bugiani, F. Gullotta, M. Haltia, J. J. Hauw, J. W. Ironside, K. Jellinger, et al. 1995. Neuropathological diagnostic criteria for Creutzfeldt-Jakob Disease (CJD) and other human spongiform encephalopathies (prion diseases). *Brain Pathol.* **5:**459–466.

8. Castilla, J., P. Saa, C. Hetz, and C. Soto. 2005. In vitro generation of infectious scrapie prions. *Cell* **121:**195–206.
9. Collins, P. S., V. A. Lawson, and P. C. Masters. 2004. Transmissible spongiform encephalopathies. *Lancet* **363:**51–61.
10. Collins, S., C. A. McLean, and C. L. Masters. 2001. Gerstmann-Straussler-Scheinker syndrome, fatal familial insomnia, and kuru: a review of these less common human transmissible spongiform encephalopathies. *J. Clin. Neurosci.* **8:**387–397.
11. Debatin, L., J. Streffer, M. Geissen, J. Matschke, A. Aguzzi, and M. Glatzel. 2008. Association between deposition of beta-amyloid and pathological prion protein in sporadic Creutzfeldt-Jakob disease. *Neurodegener. Dis.* **5:**347–354.
12. de Pedro-Cuesta, J., M. Glatzel, J. Almazan, K. Stoeck, V. Mellina, M. Puopolo, M. Pocchiari, I. Zerr, H. A. Kretzschmar, J. P. Brandel, N. Delasnerie-Laupretre, A. Alperovitch, C. van Duijn, P. Sanchez-Juan, S. Collins, V. Lewis, G. H. Jansen, M. B. Coulthart, E. Gelpi, H. Budka, and E. Mitrova. 2006. Human transmissible spongiform encephalopathies in eleven countries: diagnostic pattern across time, 1993–2002. *BMC Public Health* **6:**278.
13. Dossena, S., L. Imeri, M. Mangieri, A. Garofoli, L. Ferrari, A. Senatore, E. Restelli, C. Balducci, F. Fiordaliso, M. Salio, S. Bianchi, L. Fioriti, M. Morbin, A. Pincherle, G. Marcon, F. Villani, M. Carli, F. Tagliavini, G. Forloni, and R. Chiesa. 2008. Mutant prion protein expression causes motor and memory deficits and abnormal sleep patterns in a transgenic mouse model. *Neuron* **60:**598–609.
14. Fischer, M., T. Rülicke, A. Raeber, A. Sailer, M. Moser, B. Oesch, S. Brandner, A. Aguzzi, and C. Weissmann. 1996. Prion protein (PrP) with amino-proximal deletions restoring susceptibility of PrP knockout mice to scrapie. *EMBO J.* **15:**1255–1264.
15. Flechsig, E., D. Shmerling, I. Hegyi, A. J. Raeber, M. Fischer, A. Cozzio, C. von Mering, A. Aguzzi, and C. Weissmann. 2000. Prion protein devoid of the octapeptide repeat region restores susceptibility to scrapie in prp knockout mice. *Neuron* **27:**399–408.
16. Gambetti, P., Q. Kong, W. Zou, P. Parchi, and S. G. Chen. 2003. Sporadic and familial CJD: classification and characterisation. *Br. Med. Bull.* **66:**213–239.
17. Glatzel, M., E. Abela, M. Maissen, and A. Aguzzi. 2003. Extraneural pathologic prion protein in sporadic Creutzfeldt-Jakob disease. *N. Engl. J. Med.* **349:**1812–1820.
18. Glatzel, M., K. Stoeck, H. Seeger, T. Luhrs, and A. Aguzzi. 2005. Human prion diseases: molecular and clinical aspects. *Arch. Neurol.* **62:**545–552.
19. Hill, A. F., M. Desbruslais, S. Joiner, K. C. Sidle, I. Gowland, J. Collinge, L. J. Doey, and P. Lantos. 1997. The same prion strain causes VCJD and BSE. *Nature* **389:**448–450. (Letter.)
20. Hill, A. F., S. Joiner, J. D. Wadsworth, K. C. Sidle, J. E. Bell, H. Budka, J. W. Ironside, and J. Collinge. 2003. Molecular classification of sporadic Creutzfeldt-Jakob disease. *Brain* **126:**1333–1346.
21. Hornemann, S., C. Korth, B. Oesch, R. Riek, G. Wider, K. Wuthrich, and R. Glockshuber. 1997. Recombinant full-length murine prion protein, mPrP(23-231): purification and spectroscopic characterization. *FEBS Lett.* **413:**277–281.
22. Kovacs, G. G., M. Puopolo, A. Ladogana, M. Pocchiari, H. Budka, C. van Duijn, S. J. Collins, A. Boyd, A. Giulivi, M. Coulthart, N. Delasnerie-Laupretre, J. P. Brandel, I. Zerr, H. A. Kretzschmar, J. de Pedro-Cuesta, M. Calero-Lara, M. Glatzel, A. Aguzzi, M. Bishop, R. Knight, G. Belay, R. Will, and E. Mitrova. 2005. Genetic prion disease: the EUROCJD experience. *Hum. Genet.* **118:**166–174.
23. Ladogana, A., M. Puopolo, E. A. Croes, H. Budka, C. Jarius, S. Collins, G. M. Klug, T. Sutcliffe, A. Giulivi, A. Alperovitch, N. Delasnerie-Laupretre, J. P. Brandel, S. Poser, H. Kretzschmar, I. Rietveld, E. Mitrova, P. Cuesta Jde, P. Martinez-Martin, M. Glatzel, A. Aguzzi, R. Knight, H. Ward, M. Pocchiari, C. M. van Duijn, R. G. Will, and I. Zerr. 2005. Mortality from Creutzfeldt-Jakob disease and related disorders in Europe, Australia, and Canada. *Neurology* **64:**1586–1591.

24. Legname, G., I. V. Baskakov, H. O. Nguyen, D. Riesner, F. E. Cohen, S. J. DeArmond, and S. B. Prusiner. 2004. Synthetic mammalian prions. *Science* **305**:673–676.

25. Miele, G., H. Seeger, D. Marino, R. Eberhard, M. Heikenwalder, K. Stoeck, M. Basagni, R. Knight, A. Green, F. Chianini, R. P. Wuthrich, C. Hock, I. Zerr, and A. Aguzzi. 2008. Urinary alpha1-antichymotrypsin: a biomarker of prion infection. *PLoS ONE* **3**:e3870.

26. Parchi, P., R. Castellani, S. Capellari, B. Ghetti, K. Young, S. G. Chen, M. Farlow, D. W. Dickson, A. A. F. Sima, J. Q. Trojanowski, R. B. Petersen, and P. Gambetti. 1996. Molecular basis of phenotypic variability in sporadic Creutzfeldt-Jakob disease. *Ann. Neurol.* **39**:767–778.

27. Parchi, P., A. Giese, S. Capellari, P. Brown, W. Schulz-Schaeffer, O. Windl, I. Zerr, H. Budka, N. Kopp, P. Piccardo, S. Poser, A. Rojiani, N. Streichemberger, J. Julien, C. Vital, B. Ghetti, P. Gambetti, and H. Kretzschmar. 1999. Classification of sporadic Creutzfeldt-Jakob disease based on molecular and phenotypic analysis of 300 subjects. *Ann. Neurol.* **46**:224–233.

28. Pauli, G. 2005. Tissue safety in view of CJD and variant CJD. *Cell Tissue Bank* **6**:191–200.

29. Polymenidou, M., R. Moos, M. Scott, C. Sigurdson, Y. Z. Shi, B. Yajima, I. Hafner-Bratkovic, R. Jerala, S. Hornemann, K. Wuthrich, A. Bellon, M. Vey, G. Garen, M. N. James, N. Kav, and A. Aguzzi. 2008. The Pom monoclonals: a comprehensive set of antibodies to non-overlapping prion protein epitopes. *PLoS ONE* **3**:e3872.

30. Prusiner, S. B. 1998. Prions. *Proc. Natl. Acad. Sci. USA* **95**:13363–13383.

31. Riek, R., S. Hornemann, G. Wider, M. Billeter, R. Glockshuber, and K. Wuthrich. 1996. NMR structure of the mouse prion protein domain PrP(121-321). *Nature* **382**:180–182.

32. Ruegger, J., K. Stoeck, L. Amsler, T. Blaettler, M. Zwahlen, A. Aguzzi, M. Glatzel, K. Hess, and T. Eckert. 2009. A case-control study of sporadic Creutzfeldt-Jakob disease in Switzerland: analysis of potential risk factors with regard to an increased CJD incidence in the years 2001–2004. *BMC Public Health* **9**:18.

33. Sailer, A., H. Büeler, M. Fischer, A. Aguzzi, and C. Weissmann. 1994. No propagation of prions in mice devoid of PrP. *Cell* **77**:967–968.

34. Schoch, G., H. Seeger, J. Bogousslavsky, M. Tolnay, R. C. Janzer, A. Aguzzi, and M. Glatzel. 2005. Analysis of prion strains by PrP(Sc) profiling in sporadic Creutzfeldt-Jakob disease. *PLoS Med.* **3**:e14.

35. Reference deleted.

36. Sneath, P. H. 2004. Estimation of the size of the VCJD epidemic. *Antonie van Leeuwenhoek* **86**:93–103.

37. Tschampa, H. J., I. Zerr, and H. Urbach. 2007. Radiological assessment of Creutzfeldt-Jakob disease. *Eur. Radiol.* **17**:1200–1211.

38. Uro-Coste, E., H. Cassard, S. Simon, S. Lugan, J. M. Bilheude, A. Perret-Liaudet, J. W. Ironside, S. Haik, C. Basset-Leobon, C. Lacroux, K. Peoch, N. Streichenberger, J. Langeveld, M. W. Head, J. Grassi, J. J. Hauw, F. Schelcher, M. B. Delisle, and O. Andreoletti. 2008. Beyond Prp res type 1/type 2 dichotomy in Creutzfeldt-Jakob disease. *PLoS Pathog.* **4**:e1000029.

39. Will, R. G., A. Alperovitch, S. Poser, M. Pocchiari, A. Hofman, E. Mitrova, R. de Silva, M. D'Alessandro, N. Delasnerie-Laupretre, I. Zerr, C. van Duijn, et al. 1998. Descriptive epidemiology of Creutzfeldt-Jakob disease in six European countries, 1993–1995. *Ann. Neurol.* **43**:763–767.

40. Will, R. G., J. W. Ironside, M. Zeidler, S. N. Cousens, K. Estibeiro, A. Alperovitch, S. Poser, M. Pocchiari, A. Hofman, and P. G. Smith. 1996. A new variant of Creutzfeldt-Jakob disease in the UK. *Lancet* **347**:921–925.

41. Wille, H., M. D. Michelitsch, V. Guenebaut, S. Supattapone, A. Serban, F. E. Cohen, D. A. Agard, and S. B. Prusiner. 2002. Structural studies of the scrapie prion protein by electron crystallography. *Proc. Natl. Acad. Sci. USA* **99**:3563–3568.

42. Windl, O., M. Dempster, J. P. Estibeiro, R. Lathe, R. Desilva, T. Esmonde, R. Will, A. Springbett, T. A. Campbell, K. C. L. Sidle, M. S. Palmer, and J. Collinge. 1996. Genetic basis of Creutzfeldt-Jakob disease in the United Kingdom—a systematic analysis of predisposing mutations and allelic variation in the PRNP gene. *Hum. Genet.* **98**:259–264.

43. Zerr, I., M. Pocchiari, S. Collins, J. P. Brandel, J. de Pedro Cuesta, R. S. Knight, H. Bernheimer, F. Cardone, N. Delasnerie-Laupretre, N. Cuadrado Corrales, A. Ladogana, M. Bodemer, A. Fletcher, T. Awan, A. Ruiz Bremon, H. Budka, J. L. Laplanche, R. G. Will, and S. Poser. 2000. Analysis of EEG and CSF 14-3-3 proteins as aids to the diagnosis of Creutzfeldt-Jakob disease. *Neurology* **55**:811–815.

section V ANTIVIRAL AGENTS AND SUSCEPTIBILITY TEST METHODS

VOLUME EDITOR: MARIE LOUISE LANDRY

SECTION EDITORS: ANGELA M. CALIENDO, CHRISTINE C. GINOCCHIO, AND ALEXANDRA VALSAMAKIS

Antiviral Agents

NELL S. LURAIN AND KENNETH D. THOMPSON

108

The use of antiviral agents for the treatment of viral diseases continues to expand. Most of the agents currently approved by the Food and Drug Administration (FDA) are active against one or more of the following viruses: human immunodeficiency virus types 1 and 2 (HIV-1 and HIV-2), hepatitis B and C viruses (HBV and HCV, respectively), the human herpesviruses, and influenza A and B viruses. This chapter is organized according to these virus groups, with cross-referencing for agents with activity against more than one group of viruses. The major targets of these agents are viral replication enzymes, proteases, and entry/exit pathways (28, 32, 60, 74, 98, 104, 126). In a few cases, approved drugs for the above families of viruses have also been used to treat viruses in other families. The expanded spectrum of drug usage is discussed in the individual drug sections.

AGENTS AGAINST HUMAN IMMUNODEFICIENCY VIRUS TYPES 1 AND 2

There are now five classes of antiviral agents for treatment of HIV-1: (i) nucleoside and nucleotide reverse transcriptase inhibitors (NRTIs and NtRTIs), (ii) nonnucleoside reverse transcriptase inhibitors (NNRTIs), (iii) protease inhibitors (PIs), (iv) entry/fusion inhibitors, and (v) integrase strand transfer inhibitors (INSTIs). Current information on each drug is available through the AIDSinfo website (http://AIDSinfo.nih.gov), which has separate guidelines for the use of approved antiretroviral agents in (i) adolescents and adults, (ii) pediatric patients, and (iii) pregnant HIV-1-infected women (113, 116, 155). These guidelines describe the agents, along with dosage, adverse effects, and drug interactions. Working groups for each of these patient populations regularly update the guidelines. Additional information can be obtained from the package inserts available from pharmaceutical company websites. Changes in recommended drug doses, as well as observed adverse effects and drug interactions, occur frequently, making it necessary to consult the most up-to-date sources.

Antiretroviral agents are administered in combinations of different drug classes termed highly active antiretroviral therapy (HAART) to maximize efficacy and to minimize the induction of drug resistance. HAART is now generally regarded as any combination regimen designed to achieve the goal of complete virus suppression. These regimens comprise a minimum of three drugs, which are usually NNRTI based (two NRTIs and/or NtRTIs plus one NNRTI), PI based (two NRTIs and/or NtRTIs plus one or more PIs), or, more recently, INSTI based (two NRTIs and/or NtRTIs plus one INSTI) (113). Monotherapy is restricted to prevention of perinatal transmission of HIV (116).

There are currently 25 approved antiretroviral drugs (32), with numerous possible combinations for treatment regimens. Recommended regimens for adults and adolescents are given in the guidelines (113) for treatment-naïve and treatment-experienced patients. The large number of drugs creates a tremendous potential for drug interactions among the different classes as well as for interactions with other types of drugs prescribed for conditions associated with HIV infection. Close monitoring of these complex interactions is required to avoid detrimental changes in drug levels and/or toxicity.

Table 1 summarizes the structures, mechanisms of action, and major adverse effects of the individual drugs and drug combinations approved by the FDA. Drug interactions described below for each drug are only highlights of potential interactions. Frequent updates and more-comprehensive information can be obtained from the AIDSinfo website listed above.

Nucleoside and Nucleotide Reverse Transcriptase Inhibitors

The NRTIs and NtRTIs are not active as administered but must be phosphorylated by cellular kinases to the nucleoside triphosphate form, which lacks a 3'-hydroxyl group for DNA chain elongation. The NRTIs require triphosphorylation, while the NtRTIs require diphosphorylation (32). These antiviral agents act as competitive inhibitors of the viral reverse transcriptase (RT), which results in chain termination. They are active against both the HIV-1 and HIV-2 RTs, and they are used as dual combination backbones in regimens with NNRTIs, PIs, and INSTIs (113). Several of them are also active against the HBV DNA polymerase, which has RT activity (see "Agents against Hepatitis B Virus" below) (159). Lactic acidosis with hepatic steatosis is a rare but very serious adverse effect associated with all members of this class. These toxic effects of NRTIs and NtRTIs appear to be the result of inhibition of the mitochondrial DNA polymerase γ (11, 25).

TABLE 1 Antiviral agents for HIV therapy

Antiviral agent (abbreviation)	Trade name (pharmaceutical company[a])	Structure	Mechanism of action, route of administration	Major adverse effects[b]
NRTIs and NtRTIs				
Abacavir (ABC)	Ziagen (GSK)	Carbocyclic guanosine analogue (NRTI)	Converted to triphosphate analogue of dGTP by cellular kinases, competitive inhibitor of RT, viral DNA chain terminator; oral administration	Hypersensitivity reaction associated with HLA-B*5701, lactic acidosis and severe hepatomegaly with steatosis
Didanosine (ddI)	Videx (BMS)	2′,3′-Dideoxyinosine (adenosine analogue; NRTI)	Converted to dideoxy triphosphate analogue of dATP by cellular kinases; activity and administration similar to those of ABC	Pancreatitis, peripheral neuropathy, nausea, diarrhea, lactic acidosis and severe hepatomegaly with steatosis
Emtricitabine (FTC)	Emtriva (Gilead)	Thio, 5-fluorocytosine analogue (NRTI)	Converted to triphosphate analogue of dCTP by cellular kinases; activity and administration similar to those of ABC	Minimal toxicity, skin hyper-pigmentation, lactic acidosis and severe hepatomegaly with steatosis, posttreatment exacerbation of HBV coinfection
Lamivudine (3TC)	Epivir (GSK)	Dideoxycytidine analogue (NRTI)	Converted to triphosphate analogue of dCTP by cellular kinases; activity and administration similar to those of ABC	Minimal toxicity, lactic acidosis and severe hepatomegaly with steatosis, posttreatment exacerbation of HBV coinfection
Stavudine (d4T)	Zerit (BMS)	2′,3′-Didehydro-2′,3′-dideoxythymidine (NRTI)	Converted to triphosphate analogue of dTTP by cellular kinases; activity and administration similar to those of ABC	Peripheral neuropathy, lipodystrophy, motor weakness, lactic acidosis and severe hepatomegaly with steatosis
Tenofovir disoproxil fumarate (TDF)	Viread (Gilead)	Acyclic diester prodrug; acyclic analogue of adenosine monophosphate (NtRTI)	Diester hydrolysis required for conversion to tenofovir, monophosphate analogue requires diphosphorylation by cellular kinases; activity and administration similar to those of ABC	Asthenia, headache, GI symptoms, lactic acidosis and severe hepatomegaly with steatosis, posttreatment exacerbation of HBV coinfection
Zidovudine (AZT or ZDV)	Retrovir (GSK)	3′-Azido-2′,3′-dideoxythymidine (NRTI)	Converted to triphosphate analogue of dTTP by cellular kinases; activity and administration similar to those of ABC	Bone marrow suppression, GI symptoms, headache, insomnia, lactic acidosis and severe hepatomegaly with steatosis
NRTI-NtRTI combinations				
Abacavir + lamivudine	Epzicom (GSK)	ABC + 3TC	See individual NRTIs above	See individual NRTIs above
Abacavir + zidovudine + lamivudine	Trizivir (GSK)	ABC + AZT + 3TC	See individual NRTIs above	See individual NRTIs above
Emtricitibine + tenofovir + efavirenz	Atripla (Gilead and BMS)	FTC + TDF + EFV	See individual NRTI and NtRTI above and individual NNRTI below	See individual NRTI and NtRTI above and individual NNRTI below
Tenofovir + emtricitabine	Truvada (Gilead)	TDF + FTC	See individual NRTI and NtRTI above	See individual NRTI and NtRTI above
Zidovudine + lamivudine	Combivir (GSK)	AZT + 3TC	See individual NRTIs above	See individual NRTIs above
NNRTIs				
Delavirdine (DLV)	Rescriptor (Pfizer)	Nonnucleoside inhibitor of HIV-1 RT	Noncompetitive inhibitor binds to HIV-1 RT, close to catalytic site, and disrupts normal polymerization function; oral administration	Skin rash (Stevens-Johnson syndrome), headache, elevated transaminases

(Continued on next page)

TABLE 1 (*Continued*)

Antiviral agent (abbreviation)	Trade name (pharmaceutical company[a])	Structure	Mechanism of action, route of administration	Major adverse effects[b]
Efavirenz (EFV)	Sustiva (BMS)	Similar to DLV, but structurally unrelated	Activity and administration similar to those of DLV	Skin rash (Stevens-Johnson syndrome), psychiatric symptoms, CNS symptoms (e.g., dizziness, insomnia, and confusion), elevated transaminases, teratogenic effects
Etravirine (ETR)	Intelence (Tibotec)	Similar to DLV, but structurally unrelated	Activity and administration similar to those of DLV	Skin rash (Stevens-Johnson syndrome), GI symptoms
Nevirapine (NVP)	Viramune (BI)	Similar to DLV, but structurally unrelated	Activity and administration similar to those of DLV	Severe hepatotoxicity, skin rashes (Stevens-Johnson syndrome)
PIs Atazanavir (ATV)	Reyataz (BMS)	Azapeptide aspartyl peptidomimetic substrate analogue of HIV-1 and HIV-2 proteases	Binds competitively to active site of HIV protease, prevents cleavage of viral polyprotein precursors, produces immature, noninfectious viral particles; oral administration	Indirect hyperbilirubinemia, prolonged PR interval, hyperglycemia, fat redistribution, increased bleeding episodes with hemophilia, nephrolithiasis
Darunavir (DRV)	Prezista (Tibotec)	Nonpeptidic PI	Inhibits protease dimerization, prevents cleavage of viral polyprotein; oral administration	Skin rash (Stevens-Johnson syndrome), hepatotoxicity, hyperglycemia, fat redistribution, GI symptoms, elevated transaminases, increased bleeding episodes with hemophilia, nephrolithiasis
Fosamprenavir (FPV)	Lexiva (GSK)	Phosphorylated prodrug of amprenavir, similar to ATV	Converted to amprenavir by cellular phosphatases; activity and administration similar to those of ATV	Skin rash, GI symptoms, headache, hyperlipidemia, fat redistribution, elevated transaminases, hyperglycemia, increased bleeding episodes with hemophilia
Indinavir (IDV)	Crixivan (Merck)	Peptidomimetic substrate similar to ATV	Activity and administration similar to those of ATV	Nephrolithiasis and urolithiasis, GI symptoms, indirect hyperbilirubinemia, hyperlipidemia, hemolytic anemia, headache, hyperglycemia, fat redistribution, increased bleeding episodes with hemophilia
Lopinavir (LPV) + ritonavir (RTV)	Kaletra (Abbott)	Coformulation of LPV and RTV (4:1 ratio); peptidomimetic substrate similar to ATV	Activity and administration similar to those of ATV	GI symptoms, asthenia, hyperlipidemia, elevated transaminases, hyperglycemia, hyperlipidemia, fat redistribution, increased bleeding episodes with hemophilia
Nelfinavir (NFV)	Viracept (Pfizer)	Monomethane sulfonate salt of protease substrate analogue similar to ATV	Activity and administration similar to those of ATV	Diarrhea, hyperlipidemia, hyperglycemia, fat redistribution, elevated transaminases, increased bleeding episodes with hemophilia
Ritonavir (RTV)	Norvir (Abbott)	Peptidomimetic substrate similar to IDV	Activity and administration similar to those of ATV	Severe GI symptoms, circumoral paresthesias, hyperlipidemia, hepatitis, asthenia, taste disturbance, hyperglycemia, fat redistribution, increased bleeding episodes with hemophilia

(*Continued on next page*)

TABLE 1 Antiviral agents for HIV therapy (*Continued*)

Antiviral agent (abbreviation)	Trade name (pharmaceutical company[a])	Structure	Mechanism of action, route of administration	Major adverse effects[b]
Saquinavir (SQV)	Invirase (Roche)	Hard gel formulation, peptidomimetic substrate similar to ATV	Activity and administration similar to those of ATV	GI symptoms, hyperlipidemia, elevated transaminases, headache, hyperglycemia, fat redistribution, increased bleeding episodes with hemophilia
Tipranavir (TPV)	Aptivus (BI)	Nonpeptidic protease inhibitor, coadministered with RTV	Activity and administration similar to those of DRV	Hepatotoxicity, hyperglycemia, sulfa allergy skin rash, hyperlipidemia, fat redistribution, increased bleeding episodes with hemophilia, rare intracranial hemorrhage
Entry inhibitors				
Enfuvirtide (T20)	Fuzeon (Roche)	36-Amino-acid synthetic peptide (residues 127 to 162 of gp41), N terminus is acetylated, C terminus is carboxamide	Binds to first heptad repeat in gp41, prevents conformational changes required for fusion of viral and cellular membranes; administered by injection	Local injection site reactions, pneumonia, hypersensitivity reactions
Maraviroc (MVC)	Selzentry (Pfizer)	Allosteric binding to coreceptor CCR5 alters conformation, prevents gp120 binding	CCR5 coreceptor antagonist; oral administration	Upper respiratory tract infections, cough, pyrexia, rash, dizziness
INSTI				
Raltegravir (RAL)	Isentress (Merck)	Integrase strand transfer inhibitor	Prevents formation of covalent bond between unintegrated HIV DNA and host DNA, preventing formation of provirus; oral administration	Headache, GI symptoms, asthenia, fatigue, pyrexia, CPK elevation

[a]Pharmaceutical companies: Abbott Laboratories, North Chicago, IL; BI, Boehringer Ingelheim Pharmaceuticals, Ridgefield, CT; BMS, Bristol-Myers Squibb, Princeton, NJ; Gilead Sciences, Foster City, CA; GSK, GlaxoSmithKline, Research Triangle Park, NC; Merck & Co., Whitehouse Station, NJ; Pfizer, New York, NY; Roche Pharmaceuticals, Nutley, NJ; Tibotec Therapeutics, Division of Ortho Biotech Products, L.P., Raritan, NJ.

[b]Gastrointestinal (GI) symptoms include nausea, vomiting, and diarrhea.

Abacavir

Pharmacology

The oral bioavailability of abacavir (ABC) is 83%. The half-life in plasma is 1.5 h, and the intracellular half-life is 12 to 26 h. ABC can be administered with or without food. It is metabolized by alcohol dehydrogenase and glucuronyl transferase, and 82% of the metabolites are excreted by the kidneys. Placental passage has been demonstrated in animal studies (116). ABC penetration of the central nervous system (CNS) is adequate to inhibit HIV replication (14). ABC is recommended as an alternative drug in dual-NRTI backbones, although recent studies suggest that ABC is associated with an increased risk of cardiovascular disease (62, 138). ABC is contraindicated as an alternative drug in dual-NRTI or -NtRTI backbones in combination with an NNRTI or with PIs for patients who are positive for the HLA-B*5701 major histocompatibility complex class I allele, which is associated with a hypersensitivity reaction to the drug (94, 113). Combination formulations of two and three NRTIs and/or NtRTIs containing ABC are commercially available (Table 1).

Drug Interactions

ABC decreases the level of methadone. Ethanol increases the concentration of ABC in plasma through common metabolic pathways (113).

Didanosine

Pharmacology

The oral bioavailability of didanosine (ddI) is 30 to 40%. The half-life in serum is 1.5 h, and the intracellular half-life is >20 h. It should be administered without food. Half of the drug is excreted by the kidneys. There is little penetration of the CNS, but ddI has been shown to cross the human placenta (116). ddI is recommended only as an alternative therapy with another NRTI (except for stavudine [d4T] or tenofovir [TDF]) in either NNRTI-based or PI-based drug regimens (113).

Drug Interactions

Administration of ddI with either d4T or TDF can increase the rate and severity of toxicities associated with each individual drug. Ganciclovir (GCV), valganciclovir (val-GCV), ribavirin (RBV), and allopurinol also increase ddI exposure, leading to increased ddI toxicity (113, 123, 124).

Emtricitabine

Pharmacology

The oral bioavailability of emtricitabine (FTC) is 93%. The half-life in plasma is 10 h, and the intracellular half-life is >20 h. FTC can be administered with or without food. It is excreted mostly unchanged (86%) by the kidneys, and the remainder is eliminated in the feces. It shows intermediate penetration of cells of the CNS (144), but it is not known whether FTC crosses the human placenta (116). FTC is recommended as a preferred drug in combination with TDF in either NNRTI-based or PI-based regimens for treatment-naïve patients. Coadministration with lamivudine (3TC) is not recommended, because both drugs have similar resistance patterns and there is no therapeutic advantage for the combination (113).

Drug Interactions

No significant interactions with other antiretroviral agents have been reported (113, 118).

Lamivudine

Pharmacology

The oral bioavailability of 3TC is 86%. The half-life in serum is 5 to 7 h, and the intracellular half-life is 18 to 22 h. The drug can be administered with or without food, and 71% is excreted by the kidney. 3TC crosses the human placenta (116) and shows intermediate penetration of the CNS (144). 3TC is recommended for use in alternative dual-NRTI regimens with ABC, ddI, or zidovudine (ZDV) combined with either an NNRTI or with PIs for treatment-naïve patients (113). Coadministration of 3TC with FTC is not recommended (see "Emtricitabine").

Drug Interactions

3TC is actively excreted by the kidney via the organic cationic transport system, and possible interactions should therefore be considered for other drugs which use the same pathway, such as trimethoprim-sulfamethoxazole (113).

Stavudine

Pharmacology

The oral bioavailability of d4T is 86%. The half-life in serum is 1.0 h, and the intracellular half-life is 7.5 h. d4T can be administered with or without food. Fifty percent of the drug is excreted by the kidneys. Placental passage occurs in animals, and d4T shows intermediate penetration of the CNS (45, 116). d4T is used as an alternative drug in dual-NRTI or -NtRTI backbones in combination with an NNRTI or PIs (113).

Drug Interactions

d4T combined with ddI can increase the rate and severity of toxicities associated with each individual drug. ZDV and RBV inhibit the phosphorylation of d4T (55, 120).

Tenofovir

Pharmacology

The oral bioavailability of TDF is 25% without food and 39% with a high-fat meal, although the drug is administered without regard to meals. The half-life in serum is 17 h, and the intracellular half-life is >60 h. The drug is excreted mostly unchanged (70 to 80%) by the kidneys. TDF has been shown to cross the placenta in animal studies, but it has a low level of penetration of the CNS (116, 144). It is less likely than other NRTIs and NtRTIs to be associated with mitochondrial toxicity. TDF is recommended as a preferred NRTI or NtRTI in dual combination backbones with FTC (48, 113).

Drug Interactions

TDF increases the concentration of ddI in plasma, leading to increased toxicity (123, 124). There may be increased toxicity associated with coadministration with GCV, val-GCV, acyclovir (ACV), or cidofovir (CDV) (113).

Zalcitabine

The sale of zalcitabine (Hivid) was suspended by Roche Pharmaceuticals in December 2006 because it was no longer recommended by treatment guidelines (www .fda.gov/downloads/Drugs/DrugSafety/DrugShortages/ ucm086099.pdf).

Zidovudine

Pharmacology

ZDV was the first agent used for antiretroviral therapy (42). The oral bioavailability is 60%, the half-life in serum is 1.1 h, and the intracellular half-life is 7 h. ZDV can be administered without regard to meals. It is metabolized to the glucuronide, which is excreted by the kidneys.

ZDV crosses the blood-brain barrier to achieve effective concentrations in the CNS (144), and it also crosses the placenta. ZDV with 3TC is the preferred dual-NRTI backbone for combination regimens in pregnant women (116). It can be given as standard monotherapy that is administered intravenously to pregnant women during labor to prevent maternal-fetal transmission and can be administered orally to the child at birth (35, 116). For adults and adolescents, ZDV is recommended with 3TC as an alternative dual-NRTI backbone with NNRTI-based and PI-based regimens (113).

Drug Interactions

ZDV inhibits the phosphorylation of d4T by thymidine kinase (TK) (55). RBV inhibits phosphorylation of ZDV (120). GCV and alpha interferon (IFN-α) may enhance the hematologic toxicity associated with ZDV (18, 22).

NRTI-NtRTI Combination Formulations

There are five fixed-dose double and triple combinations involving the NRTIs and NtRTIs, which are available as the following commercial formulations for convenience of administration: ABC-3TC-ZDV (Trizivir), ABC-3TC (Epzicom), FTC-TDF (Truvada), 3TC-ZDV (Combivir), and FTC-TDF-efavirenz (EFV) (Atripla). The triple combination ABC-3TC-ZDV is not recommended except when preferred or alternative NNRTI- or PI-based regimens cannot be used because of potential drug interactions, toxicity, or complexity of the drug regimen. Clinical trials have shown the ABC-3TC-ZDV combination to be equivalent to PI-based regimens but inferior to NNRTI-based regimens in reducing HIV RNA loads in plasma to below detectable levels (52, 113). The dual combinations are used as NRTI or NtRTI backbones in combination with an NNRTI or with PIs in triple- or quadruple-drug therapy. The triple coformulation FTC-TDF-EFV contains the preferred drugs for NNRTI-based regimens. A quadruple NRTI-NtRTI regimen of ZDV-3TC-ABC-TDF, which is not a commercial formulation, has been studied in clinical trials and was found to have inferior virologic efficacy and increased toxicity, and therefore it is not recommended (113).

Nonnucleoside Reverse Transcriptase Inhibitors

Drugs in the NNRTI class do not require intracellular anabolism for activation. There is no common structure, but they bind noncompetitively to the HIV-1 RT, close to the catalytic site. Disruption of DNA polymerization activity leads to premature DNA chain termination. The HIV-2 RT is resistant to this class of drugs (32).

There are currently four FDA-approved NNRTIs: nevirapine (NVP), delavirdine (DLV), EFV, and etravirine (ETR). All are metabolized by the cytochrome P450 (CYP450) system, which also metabolizes the PIs (see below) and other drugs used to treat conditions associated with HIV infection. The common pathway can lead to serious interactions, which either induce or inhibit individual drug metabolism.

NNRTIs are often preferred for first-line therapeutic regimens with two NRTIs and/or NtRTIs, for the following reasons: (i) there is a low incidence of gastrointestinal symptoms, (ii) NNRTIs have a long half-life that allows tolerance of missed doses, and (iii) use of NNRTIs saves PIs for future regimens. The disadvantages of the NNRTIs are (i) the relatively small number of mutations required to confer cross-resistance to the first-generation drugs in this class, (ii) side effects related to the CNS, and (iii) the teratogenic effects associated with the preferred NNRTI, EFV (113, 148).

Delavirdine

Pharmacology

The bioavailability of DLV is 85%, and the half-life in plasma is 5.8 h. DLV can be administered with or without food. The protein binding level in plasma is 98%, and there is little CNS penetration (144). DLV is metabolized primarily in the liver by the CYP450 system and is an inhibitor of CYP3A4. The metabolites are excreted in the urine (51%) and eliminated in the feces (44%). DLV is not recommended for use in combination regimens for treatment-naïve patients or pregnant women, because it has lower antiviral activity and requires more frequent dosing than the other NNRTIs (113).

Drug Interactions

Dose modification or cautious use is indicated for patients receiving the antifungal agents itraconazole and voriconazole, oral contraceptives, methadone, or erectile dysfunction drugs. Coadministration of the following drugs with DLV is contraindicated: the lipid-lowering agents simvastatin and lovastatin, the gastrointestinal motility agent cisapride, the anticonvulsants phenobarbital and phenytoin, the benzodiazepines midazolam and triazolam, ergot derivatives, the antimycobacterial drugs rifampin and rifabutin, the herb St. John's wort, and the PI fosamprenavir (FPV) (113, 120).

Efavirenz

Pharmacology

The oral bioavailability of EFV is undetermined. The half-life in serum is 40 to 55 h. The drug should be administered without food. EFV is 99.5% protein bound in the plasma, mainly to albumin. CNS penetration is intermediate (144), but EFV has been shown to cross the placenta in animals (116). EFV is metabolized by CYP3A4 and CYP2B6 and is an inducer and inhibitor of CYP3A4. Glucuronidated metabolites are excreted in the urine (14 to 34%) and eliminated in the feces (16 to 61%). EFV is the preferred NNRTI in triple regimens with two NRTIs and/ or NtRTIs, except in pregnant women, because teratogenic effects have been observed in cynomolgus monkeys during the first trimester of pregnancy (116).

Drug Interactions

Dose modifications may be necessary for potential drug interactions between EFV and the following: indinavir (IDV), lopinavir/ritonavir (LPV/r), FPV, nelfinavir (NFV), saquinavir (SQV), clarithromycin, rifabutin, rifampin, simvastatin, lovastatin, methadone, itraconazole, anticonvulsants, and oral contraceptives (113, 120). Contraindicated drugs are rifapentine, cisapride, midazolam, triazolam, ergot derivatives, St. John's wort, voriconazole, and atazanavir (ATV) (in treatment-experienced patients).

Etravirine

Pharmacology

The oral bioavailability of ETR is unknown. The half-life in serum is 41 h ± 21 h. Drug levels are reduced under fasting conditions, so ETR should be taken with meals. ETR is 99.9% protein bound in plasma, mainly to albumin. It is not known whether ETR penetrates the CNS or crosses the placenta. ETR is metabolized by CYP3A4, CYP2C9, and CYP2C19. It induces CYP3A4 and inhibits CYP2C9 and CYP2C19. ETR is eliminated in the feces (93.7%) and excreted in the urine (1.2%) (70). ETR is the first of the second-generation NNRTIs, but it has not been studied in large trials of treatment-naïve patients, and therefore it is not yet recommended for treatment of this population. ETR is reported to be active against HIV-1 strains that are resistant to other NNRTIs, including HIV-1 group O strains (12), so it is currently used in regimens for treatment-experienced patients who have failed therapy (70).

Drug Interactions

Because ETR is the most recently approved NNRTI, the list of drug-drug interactions continues to grow, and there are conflicting recommendations that will likely be resolved as the use of ETR increases. Dose modifications may be required for coadministration with the following: LPV/r, SQV, antiarrhythmics, dexamethasone, erectile dysfunction drugs, warfarin, lipid-lowering drugs, diazepam, voriconazole, ketoconazole, and itraconazole. ETR should not be coadministered with the following drugs: EFV, NPV, ATV, FPV, tipranavir (TPV), hormonal contraceptives, St. John's wort, clarithromycin, rifampin, rifapentine, rifabutin (if coadministered with a ritonavir [RTV]-boosted PI), and phenobarbital (70, 113).

Nevirapine

Pharmacology

The oral bioavailability of NVP is >90%, and the half-life in serum is 25 to 30 h. NVP is 60% protein bound, the concentration in the cerebrospinal fluid (CSF) is 45% of the concentration in plasma, and penetration into the CNS is high (144). NVP can be administered with or without food. It is metabolized in the liver by CYP450 isoenzymes and is a CYP3A4 inducer. Glucuronidated metabolites are excreted in the urine (80%) and feces (10%). NVP is known to cross the human placenta (116). It has been used in resource-limited regions as a single agent which can be administered orally in an intrapartum or newborn prophylaxis regimen to prevent mother-to-child transmission (100, 116). NVP is recommended in NNRTI-based combination regimens with NRTIs or NtRTIs for pregnant women with CD4$^+$ T-cell counts of ≤250 cells/mm^3 or as an alternative to EFV for males with counts of ≤400 cells/mm^3. NVP is not recommended for patients with moderate to severe hepatic impairment (Child-Pugh class B or C) (113).

Drug Interactions

NVP reduces the concentrations in plasma of IDV, SQV, oral contraceptives, fluconazole, ketoconazole, clarithromycin, and methadone (120). Coadministration of ATV, ETR, rifampin, rifapentine, or St. John's wort with NVP is contraindicated (113).

Protease Inhibitors

The PIs, like the NNRTIs, require no intracellular anabolism for antiviral activity. The target is the HIV-encoded protease, which is required for posttranslational processing of the precursor Gag polyprotein (38). Most PIs are peptidomimetic, as they mimic the peptide bond normally cleaved by the protease (32). TPV and darunavir (DRV) are nonpeptidic molecules that are reported to inhibit protease dimerization as well as normal enzymatic activity (75). Inhibition of this activity by PIs results in production of immature, noninfectious viral particles. The relative activities of PIs against the HIV-1 versus HIV-2 protease vary among the drugs and are dependent on the amino acid sequences of the target binding sites (98).

PIs are commonly used in HAART regimens in combination with NRTIs or NtRTIs for maximum antiretroviral activity and to minimize the development of resistance. PI-based regimens introduced initially led to treatment failure related to limited bioavailability, frequent dosing, and toxicity. There are several characteristics of these drugs that lead to these treatment-related problems. They are highly bound to plasma protein, mainly alpha-1 acid glycoprotein (AAG) (44). The low concentration of unbound drug is responsible for the therapeutic activity as well as for toxicity. PIs are substrates for P-glycoprotein and multidrug resistance-associated protein (MRP). These are efflux transporters, which enhance elimination of the drugs from cells in the intestine, liver, and kidneys and reduce intracellular drug concentrations (160). All of the PIs are metabolized in the intestine and liver by enzymes of the CYP450 system (8), mainly by CYP3A, CYP2C9, and CYP2C19. An individual PI can induce and/or inhibit specific CYP450 isoenzymes, which can enhance or reduce its own metabolism or that of other PIs. As noted above, the CYP450 system metabolizes the NNRTIs and numerous other drugs that may be used for conditions associated with HIV infection. Thus, the choice of treatment regimens is complicated by multiple potential drug-drug interactions, which may enhance toxicity and/or require dose modifications of coadministered drugs (113).

Although most PIs are inhibitors of CYP3A4, RTV is the most inhibitory. For this reason, RTV is used in boosting regimens to improve the pharmacokinetic profile of a second PI (158, 160). Subtherapeutic concentrations of RTV increase the systemic exposure of a second PI by reducing the rate of metabolism and increasing the half-life (8), which lowers dosing requirements and food effects for the second drug. An example is LPV, which alone has very little bioavailability and a very short half-life but is used therapeutically in combination with RTV both for treatment-naïve patients and for salvage therapy (23, 158, 160). The effect of RTV on the pharmacokinetics of other PIs varies as a result of differences in interactions with components of the CYP450 system that determine bioavailability (160). Specific recommendations are described below for each drug.

Atazanavir

Pharmacology

ATV is an azapeptide PI that differs structurally from other peptidomimetic PIs. The bioavailability is undetermined, and the half-life in serum is 7 h. The bioavailability, however, is increased by administration with food. ATV is 86% protein bound and penetrates the CNS (111). It is metabolized in the liver by CYP3A4, and it is also an inhibitor of this enzyme. The metabolites are eliminated in the feces (79%) and urine (13%). ATV crosses the placenta at minimal levels (116).

ATV has the advantage of once-daily dosing and a low pill burden, and the drug exposure can be increased by boosting with RTV (54). ATV boosted with RTV is a preferred PI for use in regimens with two NRTIs and/or NtRTIs. TDF or ddI combined with 3TC is not recommended for regimens with unboosted ATV (113).

Drug Interactions

Drugs that may require dose modifications or cautious use with ATV include antifungal agents, rifabutin, clarithromycin, oral contraceptives, atorvastatin, the anticonvulsants carbamazepine, phenobarbital, and phenytoin, methadone (RTV boosted), erectile dysfunction agents, H2 receptor antagonists, proton pump inhibitors, antacids, and buffered medications. Drugs that are contraindicated for coadministration with ATV include IDV, NVP, ETR, EFV (in treatment-experienced patients), the antihistamines astemizole and terfenadine, the calcium channel blocker bepridil, simvastatin, lovastatin, rifampin, rifapentine, cisapride, proton pump inhibitors, pimozide, midazolam, triazolam, ergot derivatives, St. John's wort, and irinotecan (113).

Darunavir

Pharmacology

The bioavailability of DRV is 37% for DRV alone and 82% for DRV boosted with RTV, and the half-life in serum is 15 h when the drug is boosted. It should be administered with food. The protein binding level in plasma is 95%, mainly to AAG. DRV is metabolized in the liver by CYP3A4, for which it is an inhibitor. It is eliminated in the feces (79.5%) and the urine (13.9%). It is not known whether it crosses the placenta (116). DRV boosted with RTV is recommended for use in preferred PI-based regimens with two NRTIs for treatment-naïve patients (113).

Drug Interactions

Drugs that may require dose modifications are the antidepressants paroxetine and sertraline, erectile dysfunction drugs, methadone (RTV boosted), atorvastatin, and rosuvastatin. Drugs that are contraindicated are LPV/r, SQV, TDF, lovastatin, simvastatin, midazolam, trizolam, ergot derivatives, St. John's wort, rifampin, rifapentine, astemizole, terfenadine, cisapride, pimozide, carbamazepine, phenobarbitol, phenytoin, and fluticasone.

Fosamprenavir

Pharmacology

FPV is a prodrug with no antiviral activity and must be converted to amprenavir (APV) by cellular phosphatases (153). The bioavailability of APV is undetermined, and the half-life in serum is 7.7 h. It can be administered with or without food. The protein binding level in plasma is 90%. APV is metabolized in the liver by CYP3A4, for which it is an inhibitor and inducer (40). It is eliminated in the feces (75%) and urine (14%). It is not known whether APV crosses the placenta (116). FPV boosted with RTV has a high level of penetration into the CNS (144) and is recommended as a preferred drug for use in PI-based regimens with two NRTIs and/or NtRTIs for treatment of naïve patients. Unboosted FPV is recommended in similar regimens as an alternative PI (113).

Drug Interactions

Drugs that may require dose modifications or cautious use with FPV include erectile dysfunction drugs, atorvastatin, and methadone. Drugs that are contraindicated for coadministration with FPV include ETR, DLV, TPV, simvastatin, lovastatin, rifampin, rifapentine, cisapride, pimozide, midazolam, triazolam, antihistamines, ergot derivatives, St. John's wort, and oral contraceptives (113, 120).

Indinavir

Pharmacology

The bioavailability of IDV is 65%, and the half-life in serum is 1.5 to 2.0 h. IDV should be administered with low-calorie, low-fat food. It is 60% protein bound in plasma, mainly to AAG (44). IDV is an inhibitor of CYP3A4. The majority of the drug (83%) is eliminated as metabolites in the feces. There is minimal passage of IDV across the placenta (116), but RTV-boosted IDV penetrates the CNS (64, 144).

RTV-boosted and unboosted IDV forms are not recommended as components of PI-based regimens for treatment-naïve patients because of inconvenient dosing (unboosted form) and the adverse complication of nephrolithiasis (RTV-boosted form) (113).

Drug Interactions

Coadministered drugs that may require dose modifications or cautious use include antifungal agents, anticonvulsants, calcium channel blockers, atorvastatin, erectile dysfunction drugs, methadone (RTV boosted), and vitamin C, especially grapefruit juice. Drugs that are contraindicated for coadministration with IDV include ATV, TPV, amiodarone, simvastatin, lovastatin, rifampin, rifapentine, ergot derivatives, midazolam, triazolam, cisapride, pimozide, and St. John's wort (113, 120).

Lopinavir/Ritonavir

Pharmacology

LPV is administered only in combination with low-dose RTV (LPV/r), and the combined formulation (Kaletra) is commercially available. The bioavailability of LPV/r is undetermined, and the half-life is 5 to 6 h. The oral tablet formulation can be taken with or without food; the oral solution should be taken with food of moderate fat content. The protein binding level in plasma is 99%, mainly to AAG. LPV/r inhibits CYP3A4 and, to a lesser extent, CYP2D6. It is eliminated mainly in the feces (82.6%) and in the urine (10.4%), as metabolites. LPV crosses the placenta (116).

LPV/r has a high level of penetration of the CNS (144) and is a preferred drug in PI-based regimens with two NRTIs and/or NtRTIs for treatment-naïve patients (113).

Drug Interactions

Drugs that may require dose modifications when coadministered with LPV/r include erectile dysfunction drugs, rosuvastatin, atorvastatin, calcium channel blockers, and methadone (113, 120). Drugs that are contraindicated for coadministration include DRV, FPV, TPV, simvastatin, lovastatin, oral contraceptives, midazolam, triazolam, flecainide, propafenone, rifampin, rifapentine, astemizole, terfenadine, cisapride, pimozide, ergot derivatives, fluticazone, and St. John's wort (113, 120).

Nelfinavir

Pharmacology

The bioavailability of NFV is 20 to 80%, and the half-life in serum is 3.5 to 5 h. NFV shows the greatest accumulation in cells compared to the other PIs, but the protein binding level is >98% (44). It should be administered with food. NFV is both an inhibitor and an inducer of CYP3A4 (40). The majority of the drug (87%) is eliminated in the feces. There is minimal placental passage (116) and little penetration of the CNS (144). NFV is not recommended for use in PI-based regimens with two NRTIs and/or NtRTIs for treatment-naïve patients because of lower antiretroviral efficacy (113). Boosting with RTV does not affect exposure. NFV is recommended as an alternative PI for pregnant women for perinatal prophylaxis (116, 158).

Drug Interactions

Drugs that require dose modifications or cautious use include rifabutin, atorvastatin, anticonvulsants, methadone, and erectile dysfunction agents. Drugs that are contraindicated for coadministration with NFV include TPV, the antiarrhythmics amiodarone and quinidine, simvastatin, lovastatin, rifampin, rifapentine, cisapride, pimozide, midazolam, triazolam, astemizole, terfenadine, ergot derivatives, St. John's wort, proton pump inhibitors, and oral contraceptives (113, 120).

Ritonavir

Pharmacology

The oral bioavailability of RTV is undetermined, and the half-life in serum is 3 to 5 h. RTV should be administered with food. It is 98% protein bound in plasma and is metabolized by CYP3A. The major metabolite is isopropylthiazole, which has the same antiviral activity as the parent drug. RTV is eliminated in the feces (86.4%) and urine (11.3%) (113). Passage across the placenta is minimal (116).

The main role of RTV in current HIV therapeutics is to enhance the pharmacokinetics of a second PI (158), because RTV is such a strong inhibitor of CYP3A4. Low-dose RTV is a pharmacoenhancer of IDV, FPV, SQV, LPV, ATV, TPV, and DRV. The use of RTV alone in PI-based regimens is not recommended because of gastrointestinal intolerance (113). RTV-boosted PIs are recommended in combination with two NRTIs and/or NtRTIs in PI-based regimens for treatment-naïve and treatment-experienced patients (113, 158).

Drug Interactions

In general, RTV is a very strong inhibitor of CYP3A4 that has numerous potential drug interactions requiring close monitoring (113, 120). Coadministered drugs that may require dose modifications or cautious use include ketoconazole, itraconazole, rifampin, rifabutin, clarithromycin, atorvastatin, pravastatin, carbamazepine, clonazepam, ethosuximide, methadone, erectile dysfunction drugs, atovaquone, quinine, rosuvastatin, desipramine, trazadone, and theophylline. Drugs that are contraindicated for coadministration with RTV include ETR, bepridil, amiodarone, flecainide, propafenone, quinidine, simvastatin, lovastatin, rifapentine, cisapride, pimozide, midazolam, triazolam, ergot derivatives, oral contraceptives, and St. John's wort.

Saquinavir

Pharmacology

The oral bioavailability of SQV is approximately 4%. The half-life in serum is 1 to 2 h. SQV is a CYP3A4 inhibitor. It should be administered with food. SQV is 97% bound to plasma proteins and is eliminated mainly in the feces (81%) (113). There is minimal passage of SQV across the placenta (116) and very little penetration of the CNS (144).

RTV-boosted regimens of SQV with two NRTIs and/or NtRTIs are recommended as alternative therapy for treatment-naïve patients. Unboosted SQV is not recommended for use in PI-based regimens because of low oral bioavailability, the need for multiple dosing, and a high pill burden (113).

Drug Interactions

Coadministered drugs that require dose modifications or cautious use include antifungal agents, dihydropyridine, diltiazem, atorvastatin, rosuvastatin, anticonvulsants, methadone, erectile dysfunction agents, proton pump inhibitors, and grapefruit juice. Drugs that are contraindicated for coadministration with SQV include TPV, DRV, amiodarone, bepridil, flecainide, propafenone, quinidine, astemizole, terfenadine, fluticasone, simvastatin, lovastatin, rifampin, rifapentine, cisapride, pimozide, oral contraceptives, midazolam, triazolam, ergot derivatives, St. John's wort, garlic supplements, and dexamethasone (113, 120).

Tipranavir

Pharmacology

TPV is a nonpeptidic protease inhibitor (157). The oral bioavailability is undetermined, and the half-life is 6 h. It can be administered with or without food. TPV is >99.9% protein bound in plasma, to both albumin and AAG. Metabolism is mainly through CYP3A4. TPV is eliminated in the feces (82.3%) and urine (4.4%). It is not known whether TPV crosses the placenta (116), and penetration of the CNS is low (144). TPV requires coadministration with RTV to reach effective levels in plasma (8, 74). TPV is not recommended for use in PI-based regimens for treatment-naïve patients. The current indicated use is for patients who are highly treatment experienced or who are infected with virus strains resistant to multiple PIs.

Drug Interactions

Coadministration of TPV with the following drugs may require dose modification: rosuvastatin, atorvastatin, methadone, and erectile dysfunction agents. Coadministration of the following drugs is contraindicated: ATV, ETR, FPV, LPV, NFV, SQV, bepridil, amiodarone, flecainide, propafenone, quinidine, rifampin, rifapentine, lovastatin, simvastatin, midazolam, triazolam, ergot derivatives,

cisapride, pimozide, astemizole, terfenadine, oral contraceptives, St. John's wort, and fluticasone (8, 74, 113).

Entry Inhibitors

Newer classes of antiretroviral agents have been developed that target the entry of HIV into the host cell. Enfuvirtide (T20), a fusion inhibitor, was the first of these drugs to be approved. It is a linear synthetic peptide of 36 L-amino acids that binds to the first heptad repeat in the gp41 subunit of the HIV-1 envelope glycoprotein. The sequence of the peptide was derived from that of HIV-1$_{LAI}$, a subtype B strain (26). Binding prevents conformational changes that are required for fusion between the virus envelope and the cell membrane (104). Entry is inhibited, thereby preventing infection of the target cell.

Maraviroc (MVC), a CCR5 antagonist, is the second drug targeting viral entry. The use of this drug is dependent on the prior determination of the viral tropism, because only virus strains utilizing the CCR5 coreceptor (R5) are susceptible. The rationale for this novel antiviral target is that coreceptor tropism of primary HIV-1 infection is most commonly CCR5, and the switch to CXCR4 or dual tropism occurs much later in the course of infection. Allosteric binding of MVC to the CCR5 coreceptor results in a conformational change, which inhibits HIV-1 gp120 binding and viral entry into the target cell (146).

Enfuvirtide

Pharmacology

The bioavailability of T20 by subcutaneous injection is 84% (104), and the half-life in serum is 3.8 h. T20 is 92% protein bound in plasma. It is assumed that the metabolism of the drug produces the constituent amino acids, which enter the amino acid pool in the body and are recycled. It is not active against HIV-2, but there are recent data that suggest that it is active against HIV-1 non-B subtypes, and possibly group O as well (121). Limited data indicate that T20 does not cross the placenta (116), and it does not penetrate the CNS (144). T20 is not recommended for use in NNRTI- or PI-based regimens for treatment-naïve patients because there are no data from clinical trials and it requires injection for delivery. It is presently used in salvage therapy regimens for treatment-experienced patients who have not responded to their current antiretroviral therapy (39, 116).

Drug Interactions

There is no evidence that T20 induces or inhibits any of the CYP450 isoenzymes, so it is unlikely to interact with any of the drugs that are metabolized by the CYP450 system. No significant interactions with other antiretroviral drugs have been identified (104).

Maraviroc

Pharmacology

MVC is a CCR5 coreceptor antagonist that prevents HIV-1 binding of R5 strains to this coreceptor, but it has no activity against X4 strains. The bioavailability is 33%, and the half-life in serum is 14 to 18 h. It is 76% protein bound in the plasma, to both albumin and AAG. It can be administered with or without food. MVC is metabolized by CYP3A4 and eliminated in the feces (76%) and urine (20%). It is not known whether it crosses the placenta (116). MVC is approved for use only in treatment-experienced patients, because there are not yet sufficient data for use in treatment-naïve patients. In addition, testing for tropism is required prior to administration to ensure that only R5 virus is detectable (39, 74, 113, 146).

Drug Interactions

Coadministration of MVC with the following drugs may require dose modification: itraconazole, ketoconazole, voriconazole, carbamazepine, phenobarbital, phenytoin, clarithromycin, rifabutin, rifampin, EFV, and all PIs except TPV. Coadministration with rifapentine or St. John's wort is contraindicated.

Integrase Strand Transfer Inhibitors

A new class of antiretroviral drugs targets the HIV-1 integrase enzyme that mediates transfer of the reverse-transcribed HIV-1 DNA into the host chromosome. The activity of this enzyme includes 3′ processing of the reverse-transcribed DNA to generate hydroxyls at the 3′ ends of both strands, followed by strand transfer that joins viral and host DNAs. The integrase inhibitors that are approved or are currently in phase III trials target the strand transfer activity of the enzyme (32, 60).

Raltegravir

Pharmacology

Raltegravir (RAL) is the first approved INSTI. It is reportedly active against HIV-1 group O isolates (12) as well as HIV-1 group M and HIV-2 isolates (60). The bioavailability has not been established, and the half-life in serum is 9 h. It is 83% protein bound in plasma. RAL can be administered with or without food. It is eliminated in the feces (51%) and urine (32%). Clearance is by UDP-glucuronosyltransferase glucuronidation. RAL with TDF or FTC is now recommended as an INSTI-based preferred regimen for treatment-naïve patients (24, 60, 82, 113).

Drug Interactions

Coadministration of the following drugs may require dose modification: rifampin, phenytoin, phenobarbital, ATZ, TPV, EFV, ETR, and TDF. RAL is not an inducer or inhibitor of CYP450 enzymes, and therefore it does not affect the pharmacokinetics of most of the drugs that interact with the other classes of antiretroviral agents (60).

AGENTS AGAINST HEPATITIS C VIRUS

The only antiviral agents that have shown any activity in achieving a sustained virologic response against chronic HCV infection are standard IFN-α 2a and 2b, pegylated IFN-α (PEG-IFN) 2a and 2b, and combinations of these IFNs with RBV (Table 2). RBV monotherapy is not effective against HCV infection. Numerous studies have led to the current standard of care, which is combined therapy with pegylated IFN-α and RBV (46, 95, 142).

Another factor that plays a role in the virologic response is the HCV genotype. Of the six HCV genotypes, genotypes 2 and 3 are the most responsive, while the rates of sustained virologic response are lower for genotypes 1, 4, 5, and 6 (77, 81, 132).

Interferons

IFN-α is a type I IFN naturally secreted by hematopoietic cells. There are multiple members of the IFN-α family, with broad biological effects, including antiviral, antiproliferative, and immunomodulatory activities (129).

Pegylated IFN-α 2a and 2b

The IFN-α agents are produced through recombinant DNA technology from cloned human leukocyte IFN genes expressed in *Escherichia coli*. PEG-IFNs are covalent conjugates of standard IFN with a single branched (IFN-α 2a) or straight (IFN-α 2b) polyethylene glycol (PEG) chain. The molecular masses are 60,000 (2a) and 31,000 (2b) Da, respectively. Pegylation reduces clearance of the drug, which in turn prolongs the half-life compared to that of standard IFN (46, 95).

Pharmacology

Both PEG-IFN 2a and 2b are administered by subcutaneous injection. For HCV antiviral therapy, PEG-IFN 2a

TABLE 2 Antiviral agents for HCV therapy

Antiviral agent	Trade name (pharmaceutical company[a])	Structure	Mechanism of action, route of administration	Major adverse effects
PEG-IFN 2a	Pegasys (Roche)	IFN-α 2a covalent conjugate with branched PEG chains; molecular mass of 60,000 Da	Binds to cell receptors, inducer of innate immune response, stimulation of IFN response genes, inhibition of viral replication in infected cells, broad biological effects on noninfected cells; administered by subcutaneous injection	Fever, myalgia, headache, fatigue, neuropsychiatric disorders, infections, cytopenias, cerebral vascular disorders, hypersensitivity, autoimmune disorders, pancreatitis
PEG-IFN 2b	Peg-Intron (S-P)	IFN-α 2b covalent conjugate with straight PEG chains; molecular mass of 31,000 Da	Same as PEG-IFN 2a	Same as PEG-IFN 2a
Ribavirin	Copegus (Roche), Rebetol (S-P)	Synthetic nucleoside analogue	Mechanism not established; oral administration	Hemolytic anemia, myocardial infarction, teratogenic effects, anemia, hypersensitivity, impairment of pulmonary function, GI symptoms[b]

[a]Pharmaceutical companies: Roche Pharmaceuticals, Nutley, NJ; S-P, Schering-Plough, Kenilworth, NJ.
[b]Gastrointestinal (GI) symptoms include nausea, vomiting, and diarrhea.

and 2b are always administered with RBV. Absorption of coadministered RBV is increased with food, so the IFNs and RBV are administered with meals. PEG-IFN has decreased renal clearance and an extended half-life of 160 h (2a) or 40 h (2b), which allows for once-weekly dosing (50). PEG-IFN is eliminated in part (30%) by the kidneys.

Drug Interactions
The potential interaction of PEG-IFN with drugs metabolized by CYP2C8/9 (e.g., warfarin or phenytoin) or CYP2D6 (e.g., flecainide) may require dose modification. PEG-IFN may also affect the metabolism of theophylline and methadone.

Other Approved Agents

Ribavirin

Pharmacology
The bioavailability of RBV is reported to be 52% (122) and is increased by a high-fat meal, and therefore RBV should be administered with food. The half-life in plasma is 120 to 170 h, and the drug may persist in other body compartments for up to 6 months. The pathway for elimination has not been determined. RBV appears not to be a substrate for the CYP450 isoenzymes. RBV is used as standard therapy, always in combination with PEG-IFN 2a or 2b, for the treatment of HCV.

RBV has also been used as monotherapy to treat other RNA viruses, including respiratory syncytial virus (RSV), Lassa fever virus, influenza virus, parainfluenza virus, and hantavirus, but there are no conclusive data demonstrating RBV treatment efficacy (9, 27, 86, 88, 99, 108, 114, 134). An aerosolized formulation of RBV (Virazole; Valeant Pharmaceuticals, Costa Mesa, CA) has been approved for treatment of hospitalized infants and young children with severe RSV lower respiratory tract infections.

Drug Interactions
Coadministration of ddI or d4T with RBV is contraindicated. The use of ZDV plus RBV is linked to higher rates of anemia (113, 117).

Specifically Targeted Antiviral Therapies for HCV
Because the IFNs do not act directly on the virus, the development of other agents that target the viral replication cycle is of great current interest. These new drugs are collectively referred to as specifically targeted antiviral therapies for HCV (STAT-Cs) or direct-acting antiviral (DAA) agents. Among those in later stages of development are inhibitors of the NS3-encoded serine protease and the NS5B-encoded RNA polymerase (89, 125a, 135). Although these inhibitors have demonstrated effective anti-HCV activity, rapid emergence of drug resistance is a problem. As a result, the most effective regimens appear to be triple combinations of each drug with PEG-IFN and RBV (125a, 135). These drugs in combination appear to be most useful for treatment of genotype 1 infections, because this genotype is more refractory to PEG-IFN–RBV therapy than genotypes 2 and 3 (89, 125a, 135).

AGENTS AGAINST HEPATITIS B VIRUS
There are two major classes of drugs available to treat HBV: nucleoside and nucleotide analogues and IFNs. Because a large percentage of patients are coinfected with HIV, these agents are categorized by whether they have activity against both viruses or only HBV. Of the drugs that are specifically approved for HBV, PEG-IFN 2a or 2b, adefovir (ADV),

entecavir (ETV), and telbivudine (LdT) are active only against HBV, while 3TC and TDF are active against both HBV and HIV (Table 3). FTC is approved only for HIV, but it has been shown to have activity against HBV (51, 113). The common target for antiviral drugs active against both viruses is the RT function of the HIV and HBV replication enzymes (43, 136, 159).

Chronic HBV infection plays an important role in the morbidity and mortality of HIV-infected patients (137). The strategy for selecting antiviral therapy regimens for coinfected patients is based on the need to treat one or both viruses. If only HIV requires treatment, drugs with activity against both HIV and HBV, such as 3TC or TDF, should be withheld. If only HBV needs to be treated, drugs without HIV activity, such as PEG-IFN 2a/2b, ADV, or LdT, can be used. If both viruses require treatment, HAART regimens with dual NRTIs or NtRTIs that suppress replication of both viruses, such as TDF with 3TC or FTC, should be considered (113, 137). 3TC monotherapy rapidly selects for HBV resistance (101), so combination therapy with one NRTI (3TC or FTC) and one NtRTI (TDF or ADV) is required. PEG-IFN is used to treat HBV infection, but the side effects limit the length of therapy, and the response appears to be lower in HIV-HBV-coinfected patients (137). There is some evidence that individual HBV genotypes (A to H) may have different responses to therapy. Genotype A appears to have the best response (1, 68, 137). It should be noted, however, that PEG-IFN is the only drug that can eliminate covalently closed circular HBV DNA to cure chronic HBV infection (85).

Nucleoside and Nucleotide Analogues

Adefovir dipivoxil

Pharmacology
ADV-dipivoxil is a diester prodrug that is converted to the active drug ADV. ADV-dipivoxil is administered without regard to food, and the bioavailability is 59%. The half-life of ADV is 7.5 h, and it is excreted by the kidneys. There are no data on placental passage of the drug.

ADV was originally developed as an antiretroviral drug, but the high dose required for HIV therapy is associated with nephrotoxicity (159). A much lower dosage is effective against HBV (43, 137). ADV is effective for treatment of chronic HBV infection. The rate of viral load decline is lower, but development of drug resistance is delayed compared to that for other NRTIs or NtRTIs (71) that are active against HBV. ADV is recommended as dual therapy with 3TC for patients with 3TC-resistant HBV. Studies have shown that monotherapy selects ADV-resistant virus, while administration of both drugs appears to control the development of ADV resistance (71, 78).

Drug Interactions
ADV is not a substrate, inhibitor, or inducer of any of the CYP450 isoenzymes. There is no interaction with 3TC, ETV, or TDF. It is possible that drugs that reduce renal function or compete for active tubular secretion could increase the concentration of ADV and/or the coadministered drug in serum.

Emtricitabine

Pharmacology
See the information on HIV antiviral agents above, and also see Table 1. FTC is approved for antiviral therapy in

TABLE 3 Antiviral agents for HBV therapy

Antiviral agent (abbreviation)	Trade name, (pharmaceutical company[a])	Structure	Mechanism of action, route of administration	Major adverse effects
Adefovir (ADV) dipivoxil	Hepsera (Gilead)	Diester prodrug, nucleotide analogue	Diester hydrolysis required for conversion to the monophosphate analogue adefovir, requires diphosphorylation by cellular kinases, inhibitor of HBV RT, viral DNA chain terminator; oral administration	Headache, asthenia, gastrointestinal symptoms, severe acute exacerbations of hepatitis B on discontinuation of treatment, nephrotoxicity, lactic acidosis, severe hepatomegaly with steatosis
Entecavir (ETV)	Baraclude (BMS)	2′-Deoxyguanosine nucleoside analogue	Inhibitor of HBV DNA polymerase (RT) functions (priming, reverse transcription, plus-strand DNA synthesis); oral administration	Headache, fatigue, dizziness, severe acute exacerbations of hepatitis B on discontinuation of treatment, lactic acidosis, severe hepatomegaly with steatosis
Lamivudine (3TC)	See Table 1		Inhibitor of HBV DNA polymerase (RT), viral DNA chain terminator (see Table 1)	Additional adverse reaction for HBV-infected patients: severe acute exacerbations of hepatitis on discontinuation of treatment
Telbivudine (LdT)	Tyzeka (Novartis)	β-L enantiomer of thymidine nucleoside analogue (L-deoxythymidine)	Same as 3TC	Fatigue, increased creatine kinase, headache, myopathy, cough, gastrointestinal symptoms, severe acute exacerbations of hepatitis B on discontinuation of treatment, lactic acidosis, severe hepatomegaly with steatosis
Tenofovir (TDF) PEG-IFN 2a and 2b	See Table 1 See Table 2		Same as 3TC	Same as 3TC

[a]Pharmaceutical companies: BMS, Bristol-Myers Squibb, Princeton, NJ; Gilead Sciences, Foster City, CA; Novartis Pharmaceuticals Corporation, East Hanover, NJ.

HIV-infected patients. It has activity against HBV but has not yet been licensed for HBV antiviral therapy. FTC and 3TC are biochemically similar and appear to be interchangeable for potential use in treatment of HIV-HBV-coinfected patients. However, they also share the same HBV resistance mutations, so combined therapy with these two drugs is not recommended (137, 159). In addition, as with 3TC, severe acute exacerbations of HBV can occur once therapy is discontinued (113).

Drug Interactions
See the discussion on HIV antiviral agents.

Entecavir

Pharmacology
The bioavailability of ETV is approximately 100%, and the half-life is 24 h. ETV should be administered without food. It is excreted by the kidney (62 to 73%), mainly as unmetabolized drug. ETV has shown low activity against HIV, but there is evidence that resistance mutations are selected. For this reason, it is recommended that ETV be used in HIV-coinfected patients only if they are receiving effective antiretroviral therapy (43, 97, 137).

Drug Interactions
ETV is not a substrate, inhibitor, or inducer of any of the CYP450 isoenzymes. There is no interaction with 3TC, ADV, or TDF. It is possible that drugs that reduce renal

function or compete for active tubular secretion could increase the concentration of ETV and/or the coadministered drug in serum.

Lamivudine

Pharmacology
See the information on HIV antiviral agents above, and also see Table 1. 3TC was the first nucleoside analogue that was approved for treatment of chronic HBV infection. Because it has activity against both HIV and HBV, it has been effective in reducing loads in plasma for both viruses as part of HAART regimens. However, HBV-specific drug resistance mutations are selected over long-term therapy at a higher rate (20% per year) in coinfected patients than in those that are HIV negative (43). Selection of HBV drug resistance mutations eventually decreases efficacy for treatment of chronic hepatitis. Discontinuation of 3TC in HBV-infected patients can produce severe flare-ups of liver transaminases, which are usually self-limited but have been fatal in a few cases. Another common problem is the rebound viremia that occurs when therapy is terminated (113). This is thought to be derived from the viral covalently closed circular DNA, which is not affected by nucleoside or nucleotide therapy and remains in the infected hepatocytes (159). For coinfected patients, recent recommendations suggest using combination dual-NTRI or -NtRTI therapy that includes TDF to reduce the rate of selection of 3TC-resistant HBV strains (67, 137).

Drug Interactions
See the discussion on HIV antiviral agents.

Telbivudine

Pharmacology
The bioavailability of LdT is 68%, and it can be administered with or without food. The half-life is 40 to 50 h, and the drug is excreted mainly by the kidneys. LdT has a relatively low genetic barrier to resistance, and therefore it is not recommended as a first-line drug for treatment of chronic HBV infection (107).

Drug Interactions
LdT does not alter the pharmacokinetics of other nucleoside or nucleotide analogues used in the treatment of HBV (e.g., 3TC, ADV, or TDF). Coadministration with PEG-IFN 2a may be associated with increased risk of peripheral neuropathy (43).

Tenofovir disoproxil fumarate

Pharmacology
See the information on HIV antiviral agents above, and also see Table 1. TDF is approved for treatment of both HBV- and HIV-infected patients. It does not show cross-resistance with 3TC-resistant HBV mutants, and it appears to have a lower potential for selection of resistance mutations. For this reason, TDF and FTC or TDF and 3TC are recommended as dual-nucleoside backbones in therapeutic regimens to reduce the possibility of selection of drug-resistant HBV strains in coinfected patients who are on antiretroviral therapy (43, 67, 113, 137).

Drug Interactions
See the discussion on HIV antiviral drugs.

Pegylated IFN-α 2a and 2b
See the information on HCV. In recent studies of HBV-infected patients who were not coinfected with HIV, combination therapy with PEG-IFN and 3TC did not produce a better response than that with PEG-IFN alone (79, 96). There is some evidence that HBV genotypes may affect the response to treatment (1). PEG-IFN is contraindicated for use in patients who (i) are HIV coinfected, (ii) are hypersensitive to PEG-IFN, (iii) have autoimmune hepatitis, or (iv) have hepatic decompensation. Therefore, the recommended use of the drug for HBV infection is limited to compensated HBe antigen-negative or antigen-positive cirrhotic patients who do not require antiretroviral therapy (79, 96, 137).

AGENTS AGAINST HERPESVIRUSES
Most of the antiviral compounds that are approved to treat the eight human herpesviruses are nucleoside or nucleotide analogues which inhibit DNA replication. Several of these compounds require phosphorylation by a virus-encoded enzyme as well as cellular kinases for activation. The ultimate target of most of these drugs is the viral DNA polymerase, although other enzymatic steps in DNA synthesis also may be inhibited (33). In addition to the nucleoside and nucleotide analogues, the antiherpesvirus compounds include a pyrophosphate analogue (foscarnet [FOS]) that targets the viral DNA polymerase directly, an antisense oligonucleotide (fomivirsen), and an entry inhibitor (n-docosanol). The structure, mode of action, route of administration, and adverse effects of each drug are summarized in Table 4.

Acyclovir and Valacyclovir
ACV was one of the first effective antiviral compounds available clinically and has been in general use for the past 30 years. Valacyclovir (val-ACV), the L-valyl ester prodrug, is rapidly converted to ACV after oral administration (109). ACV is phosphorylated by the viral TKs of herpes simplex virus types 1 and 2 (HSV-1 and HSV-2) and varicella-zoster virus (VZV) and by the UL97 kinase of human cytomegalovirus (HCMV) (141).

Spectrum of Activity
ACV and val-ACV are active against HSV-1, HSV-2, and VZV (92), and both drugs have been used prophylactically to prevent HCMV disease in some patients following transplantation (59, 125).

Pharmacology
The pharmacokinetics of ACV after oral administration has been evaluated in healthy volunteers and in immunocompromised patients with HSV and VZV infection. The protein binding level for val-ACV in plasma is 13.5 to 17.9%, and that for ACV is 22 to 33%. The bioavailability of ACV administered as val-ACV is 54%, while the bioavailability resulting from oral ACV is 12 to 20%. The ACV half-life is 2.5 to 3.3 h in patients with normal renal function but increases to 14 h in patients with end-stage renal disease (109). ACV may be administered with or without food.

ACV is excreted by the kidneys. Two inactive metabolites are excreted: 9-[(carboxymethoxy)methyl] guanine and 8-hydroxy-9-[2-(hydroxyethoxy)methyl] guanine. A dosage adjustment is recommended for patients with reduced renal function (109).

Drug Interactions
There are no clinically significant drug-drug interactions in patients with normal renal function.

Cidofovir
CDV is a nucleotide analogue of dCMP which does not require a virus-encoded enzyme for activation. After phosphorylation by cellular kinases, CDV diphosphate becomes the active nucleotide triphosphate, which inhibits the HCMV DNA polymerase. In HCMV, two successive CDV molecules must be incorporated for complete chain termination (156).

Spectrum of Activity
CDV is active against several herpesviruses, including HCMV, HSV, and VZV (73). CDV also has antiviral activity against poxviruses (93), adenovirus (106), polyomaviruses (76), and human papillomavirus (47, 131).

Pharmacology
CDV must be administered with probenecid (29, 154). Approximately 90% of the CDV dose administered is recovered unchanged in the urine within 24 h. The half-life is 2.4 to 3.2 h. When CDV is administered with probenecid, the renal clearance of CDV is reduced to a level consistent with creatinine clearance, suggesting that probenecid blocks active renal tubular secretion of CDV (29). In vitro, CDV is <6% bound to plasma or serum proteins.

Drug Interactions
No clinically significant interactions have been identified for CDV. However, the required administration of

TABLE 4 Antiviral agents for herpesviruses

Antiviral agent (abbreviation)	Trade name (pharmaceutical company)[a]	Structure	Mode of action, route of administration	Major adverse effects[b]	Viruses targeted
DNA polymerase inhibitors					
Acyclovir (ACV)	Zovirax (GSK)	2-Amino-1,9-dihydro-9-[(2-hydroxyethoxy)methyl]-6H-purine-6-one	Converted to monophosphate by viral TK or HCMV UL97 kinase, converted to triphosphate by cellular kinases, DNA chain terminator; oral or i.v. formulations	Minimal toxicity, GI symptoms, headache, nephrotoxicity precipitation in renal tubules if maximum solubility exceeded	HSV-1, HSV-2, VZV
Valacyclovir (val-ACV)	Valtrex (GSK)	L-Valyl ester of acyclovir	Mode of action, same as that of ACV; oral formulation with increased bioavailability	GI symptoms, headache, dizziness, abdominal pain, nephrotoxicity, thrombotic thrombocytopenia, hemolytic-uremic syndrome (high dosage)	HSV-1, HSV-2, VZV, HCMV[c]
Cidofovir (CDV)	Vistide (Gilead)	1-[(S)-3-hydroxy-2-(phosphonomethoxy)propyl] cytosine dihydrate	Converted to di- and triphosphate by cellular kinases, DNA chain terminator (two successive molecules required); i.v. administration with probenecid	CDV effects: renal toxicity, decreased intraocular pressure, neutropenia, fever; probenecid effects: headache, GI symptoms, rash	HCMV,[d] HSV-1, HSV-2, VZV
Foscarnet (FOS)	Foscavir (AstraZeneca)	Trisodium phosphonoformate	Pyrophosphate analogue, noncompetitive inhibitor of DNA polymerase pyrophosphate binding site; i.v. formulation only	Renal impairment, fever, nausea, anemia, diarrhea, vomiting, headache, seizures, altered serum electrolytes	HCMV, HSV-1, HSV-2, EBV
Ganciclovir (GCV)	Cytovene (Roche)	9-[2-Hydroxy-1-(hydroxymethyl) ethoxymethyl] guanine	Converted to monophosphate by HCMV UL97 kinase or HSV or VZV TK, converted to triphosphate by cellular kinases, DNA chain terminator; oral and i.v. formulations	Fever, neutropenia, anemia, thrombocytopenia, impaired renal function, diarrhea	HCMV,[e] HSV-1, HSV-2
Valganciclovir (val-GCV)	Valcyte (Roche)	L-Valyl ester of ganciclovir	Oral prodrug of GCV with increased bioavailability; activity same as that of GCV	Diarrhea, neutropenia, nausea, headache, anemia	HCMV[e]

Penciclovir (PCV)	Denavir (Novartis)	9-[4-Hydroxy-3-(hydroxymethyl) butyl] guanine	Mode of action similar to that of ACV, limited DNA chain elongation; topical formulation only	Headache and application site reaction no different from placebo effects	HSV-1[f]
Famciclovir (FCV)	Famvir (Novartis)	Diacetyl 6-deoxy analog of penciclovir	Mode of action same as that of PCV; oral prodrug of penciclovir	Headache, GI symptoms, anorexia	HSV-1, HSV-2, VZV
Vidarabine (Ara-A) (no longer available in United States)	VIRA-A	9H-purin-6-amino-9-β-D-arabinofuranosyl monohydrate	Mode of action not established, likely inhibits viral DNA synthesis; ophthalmic ointment for topical use	Lacrimation, conjunctival pain, keratitis, photophobia	HSV-1, HSV-2[g]
Trifluridine	Viroptic (Monarch)	α,α,α-Trifluorothymidine	Mode of action not established, may inhibit viral DNA synthesis; ophthalmic aqueous solution for topical use	Burning on instillation and palpebral edema, punctate keratopathy, hypersensitivity reaction, stromal edema, keratitis sicca, hyperemia, increased ocular pressure	HSV-1[h]
Drugs with other antiviral mechanisms					
n-Docosanol	Abreva (GSK)	Saturated 22-carbon aliphatic alcohol	Prevents HSV entry into cells by inhibition of fusion between HSV envelope and cell membrane; nonprescription topical cream formulation	Headache and skin rash	Oral HSV
Fomivirsen	Vitravene (no longer available in United States)	Oligonucleotide complementary to IE2 transcript of HCMV	Binding of the oligonucleotide to mRNA blocks translation of IE2 gene product and virus replication; administered by ophthalmic injection	Uveitis, iritis, and vitritis	HCMV

[a]Pharmaceutical companies: AstraZeneca, Wilmington, DE; BMS, Gilead Sciences, Foster City, CA; GSK, GlaxoSmithKline, Research Triangle Park, NC; Monarch Pharmaceutical, Bristol, TN; Novartis, East Hanover, NJ; Roche Pharmaceuticals, Nutley, NJ.

[b]Gastrointestinal (GI) symptoms include nausea, vomiting, and diarrhea.

[c]Valacyclovir is used in some transplant settings for HCMV prophylaxis.

[d]Cidofovir also has reported activity against human papillomavirus, polyomavirus, adenovirus, and poxvirus.

[e]Ganciclovir and valganciclovir also have in vitro activity against EBV, HHV-6, HHV-7, and HHV-8.

[f]Penciclovir is used to treat herpes labialis but also has activity against HSV-2 and VZV.

[g]Vidarabine has in vitro activity against vaccinia virus and VZV.

[h]Trifluridine is used to treat herpes keratitis but also has activity against HSV-2 and VZV.

probenecid with CDV may produce drug-drug interactions resulting from the potential block of acidic drug transport in the kidneys (29).

Foscarnet

Spectrum of Activity
Although FOS is active against several herpesviruses, including HSV, HCMV, VZV, and Epstein-Barr virus (EBV), it is most commonly used to treat drug-resistant HSV and HCMV.

Pharmacology
Pharmacokinetic data indicate that FOS undergoes negligible metabolism, appears to be distributed widely from the circulation, and is eliminated via the renal route. The available data, however, indicate that the pharmacokinetics of the drug varies among patients and within individual patients, particularly with regard to FOS levels in plasma (87). The FOS terminal half-life determined by urinary excretion is 87.5 ± 41.8 h, possibly due to release of FOS from bone (21). Approximately 90% of FOS is excreted as unchanged drug in urine. Systemic clearance of FOS decreases and the half-life increases with diminishing renal function, which may require FOS dosage modification (4).

Drug Interactions
Because FOS is reported to decrease calcium concentrations in serum, caution is advised for patients receiving other agents known to affect calcium levels in serum, such as intravenous pentamidine. Renal impairment is a major adverse effect of FOS, and therefore the use of FOS should be avoided in combination with other potentially nephrotoxic drugs, such as aminoglycosides, amphotericin B, and intravenous pentamidine (128).

Ganciclovir and Valganciclovir
GCV was the first effective anti-HCMV drug developed for clinical use. GCV is an acyclic nucleoside analogue of 2′-deoxyguanosine, which requires phosphorylation by a viral kinase to become active. GCV monophosphate is subsequently phosphorylated to the di- and triphosphate form by cellular kinases (28).

Spectrum of Activity
GCV is active against HCMV as well as HSV-1, HSV-2, VZV, EBV, human herpesvirus 6 (HHV-6), HHV-7, and HHV-8 (16, 31, 139, 143).

Pharmacology
Val-GCV, the L-valyl ester prodrug of GCV, is rapidly converted to GCV after oral administration (30). The bioavailability of val-GCV is 60.9%, compared to 5.6% for the oral formulation of GCV. The half-life of GCV is 4 h in healthy volunteers and 6.5 h in transplant recipients (119, 151). GCV is only 1 to 2% protein bound. Renal excretion of unchanged drug by glomerular filtration and active tubular secretion is the major route of elimination of GCV (91%). Val-GCV should be administered with food.

Drug Interactions
Coadministration of GCV with ddI results in significantly increased levels of ddI (31, 124). Coadministration of GCV with ZDV requires dose modifications of both drugs because of their common adverse hematological effects of neutropenia and anemia. Dosage modifications may also be required with drugs that inhibit renal tubular secretion,

such as probenecid. Imipenem-cilastatin should not be administered with GCV (31).

Penciclovir and Famciclovir
Famciclovir (FCV), an oral prodrug, is the diacetyl 6-deoxy analogue of penciclovir (PCV) (147) which undergoes rapid conversion to the active compound, PCV. PCV is only available as a 1% cream for the topical treatment of herpes labialis (127). FCV was developed to improve the bioavailability of the parent compound (90).

Spectrum of Activity
PCV and FCV are active against HSV-1, HSV-2, and VZV (36). Neither of these compounds is active against other human herpesviruses.

Pharmacology
The bioavailability of PCV is 77%, and the half-life is 2 h. It can be given with or without food. PCV is <20% protein bound and is eliminated in the urine (73%) and feces (27%) (133). Although PCV is structurally related to ACV, it has a higher affinity for the HSV TK than that of ACV. However, ACV triphosphate has a higher affinity for the HSV DNA polymerase than that of PCV triphosphate. As a result, the two compounds have similar anti-HSV potencies (5).

Drug Interactions
No clinically significant drug interactions have been identified for PCV.

Vidarabine

Spectrum of Activity
Vidarabine (Ara-A) was the first anti-HSV compound shown to reduce the mortality of proven HSV encephalitis (150). It has antiviral activity against HSV-1, HSV-2, VZV, HCMV, and vaccinia virus. It is approved for topical treatment of acute keratoconjunctivitis caused by HSV.

Pharmacology
Ara-A is a purine nucleoside analogue that is rapidly deaminated to arabinosylhypoxanthine, the main metabolite, which has much lower antiviral activity (6) but may act synergistically with the parent drug to inhibit DNA replication. Because of low solubility, systemic absorption of Ara-A should not be expected to occur following ocular administration. Trace amounts of the metabolite are found in the aqueous humor.

Drug Interactions
Coadministration of Ara-A with corticosteroids is contraindicated.

Trifluridine

Spectrum of Activity
Trifluridine is a fluorinated pyrimidine nucleoside approved for the topical treatment of epithelial keratitis caused by HSV (20). It has activity against HSV-1, HSV-2, and vaccinia virus (115).

Pharmacology
Intraocular penetration of trifluridine occurs after topical instillation into the eye. Decreased corneal integrity or stromal or uveal inflammation may enhance the penetration of trifluridine into the aqueous humor. Systemic

absorption following therapeutic dosing with trifluridine appears to be negligible (15).

Drug Interactions
There are no reported drug interactions by the topical route of administration.

Fomivirsen
Fomivirsen is a phosphorothioate oligonucleotide which is complementary (antisense) to the HCMV immediate-early 2 transcript with the following sequence: 5'-GCG TTT GCT CTT CTT CTT GCG-3' (110).

Spectrum of Activity
Fomivirsen is approved only for the treatment of retinitis caused by HCMV (66), but the brand-name form Vitravene (Isis Pharmaceuticals) is no longer available in the United States.

Pharmacology
Hybridization of the oligonucleotide with the mRNA target leads to inhibition of specific protein synthesis and thus viral replication. Fomivirsen is cleared from the vitreous over the course of 7 to 10 days (49). The long intravitreal residence time provides a pharmacokinetic basis for treatment intervals (80).

Fomivirsen is metabolized by exonucleases, which sequentially remove residues from the terminal ends of the oligonucleotide. It is assumed that mononucleotide metabolites are further catabolized, similar to endogenous nucleotides, and are excreted as low-molecular-weight metabolites.

Drug Interactions
There are no reported drug interactions.

n-Docosanol

Spectrum of Activity
n-Docosanol exhibits in vitro antiviral activity against several lipid-enveloped viruses, including HSV-1, HSV-2, and RSV (72).

Pharmacology
A topical preparation of n-docosanol is available without prescription as a 10% cream for the treatment of herpes labialis.

Drug Interactions
There are no reported drug interactions with topical administration.

Other Antiherpesvirus Drugs
There are several antiviral agents that are undergoing clinical trials or that are approved for conditions other than antiviral therapy. Among these, maribavir is a novel antiviral agent in the benzimidazole drug class (145), but its in vivo efficacy has not yet been established. Unlike GCV, which is phosphorylated by the UL97 kinase, maribavir inhibits UL97 kinase activity directly. Importantly, maribavir has also been found to be effective in vitro against GCV-resistant strains of HCMV. Maribavir is not associated with nephrotoxicity or hematologic toxicities but has been associated with taste disturbances (91).

Two other drugs that are approved for other medical conditions have also been reported to have antiviral activity against HCMV, although no clinical trials have been conducted. These are leflunomide, which is approved for treatment of rheumatoid arthritis (3, 84), and artesunate, which is an antimalarial agent (37, 130).

AGENTS AGAINST INFLUENZA VIRUSES
The two classes of antiviral agents for the treatment of influenza are M2 protein inhibitors and neuraminidase inhibitors (NAIs). The M2 inhibitors are active only against type A influenza viruses, while the NAIs have activity against both type A and B viruses (2, 102, 112). The structure, mode of action, route of administration, and adverse effects of each drug are summarized in Table 5. Recommendations for use of these antivirals for influenza prevention and therapy are available from the Centers

TABLE 5 Antiviral agents for influenza viruses

Antiviral agent	Trade name (pharmaceutical company[a])	Structure	Mode of action, route of administration	Major adverse effects[b]
Amantadine	Symmetrel (Endo)	1-Adamantanamine hydrochloride	Prevents release of nucleic acid by interfering with viral M2 protein; oral administration	CNS symptoms, GI symptoms
Rimantadine	Flumadine (Forrest)	Methyl-1-adamantanemethyl amine hydrochloride	Same as amantadine	GI symptoms, CNS symptoms
Oseltamivir	Tamiflu (Roche, Gilead)	Sialic acid analogue	Competitive inhibitor of NA affecting release of influenza virus particles from host cells; oral administration	GI symptoms (usually mild), transient neuropsychiatric symptoms
Zanamivir	Relenza (GSK)	5-(Acetylamino)-4-[(aminoiminomethyl)amino]-2,6-anhydro-3,4,5-trideoxy-D-glycerol-D-galacto-non-2-enonic acid	Same as oseltamivir; administered by oral inhalation	Respiratory function deterioration after inhalation

[a]Pharmaceutical companies: Endo Pharmaceuticals Inc., Chadds Ford, PA; Forrest Laboratories, Inc., St. Louis, MO; Roche Laboratories Inc., Nutley, NJ (licensor, Gilead Sciences, Inc., Foster City, CA); GSK, GlaxoSmithKline, Research Triangle Park, NC.
[b]CNS symptoms include confusion, anxiety, insomnia, difficulty concentrating, dizziness, hallucinations, and seizures; gastrointestinal (GI) symptoms include nausea, vomiting, and anorexia; neuropsychiatric symptoms include self-injury and delirium.

for Disease Control and Prevention (CDC) website (http://www.cdc.gov/h1n1flu/recommendations.htm).

M2 Protein Inhibitors

The virus-encoded M2 protein facilitates the hydrogen ion-mediated dissociation of the matrix protein-ribonucleoprotein complex within the endosome and the release of the viral ribonucleoprotein into the cytoplasm of the host cell. The M2 inhibitors block the passage of H^+ ions through the M2 ion channel, which prevents uncoating of the virus (33, 69, 102, 105).

Amantadine and Rimantadine

Amantadine was the first anti-influenza virus agent discovered and was licensed in 1966 for therapy and prophylaxis of influenza A virus infections (126). Rimantadine was licensed in 1993 (103). These adamantanes differ in their metabolism and adverse effects, but they have similar antiviral activities against influenza A viruses. Neither drug has activity against influenza B viruses. Recent reports indicate that both seasonal influenza virus (H3N2 virus) and the current pandemic virus (H1N1 virus) have a high incidence of resistance to both drugs (63, 140), and therefore the adamantanes are no longer recommended for influenza prophylaxis and empiric therapy.

Pharmacology

After oral administration of amantadine or rimantadine, the maximum nasal concentrations of the two drugs are similar (58). Both compounds have nearly complete oral bioavailability. The half-life in plasma is 12 to 18 h for amantadine and 24 to 36 h for rimantadine. Amantadine is primarily excreted unchanged in the urine by glomerular filtration and tubular secretion, while rimantadine is metabolized by the liver (102).

When these compounds are started within 48 h of the onset of influenza symptoms, there has been an associated 1-day reduction of clinical symptoms, including fever, systemic complaints, and virus shedding. Efficacy rates of up to 85% have been shown for preventing influenza illness (152). Of the adverse effects listed in Table 5, CNS symptoms are associated more frequently with amantadine than with rimantadine (53).

Drug Interactions

Drugs that may interact with amantadine include anticholinergic medications and antihistamines (53). No clinically significant drug interactions have been reported for rimantadine, although the manufacturer's package insert indicates that the chronic use of cimetidine may reduce drug clearance and that coadministration with acetaminophen or aspirin may reduce the peak concentration of rimantadine.

Neuraminidase Inhibitors

The influenza virus neuraminidase (NA) is an envelope glycoprotein that cleaves the terminal sialic acid residues, releasing the virion from the infected cell. The virus-encoded NA allows the influenza virus to spread from cell to cell. Two NAIs are approved for the treatment of influenza A and B virus infections, namely, oseltamivir and zanamivir (34). Of these two NAIs, oseltamivir is the most widely used. However, it was recently reported that a very high percentage of seasonal H1N1 influenza virus isolates are resistant to oseltamivir as the result of a single amino acid substitution, but they remain sensitive to zanamivir (19, 63). The pandemic H1N1 strain is largely sensitive to both NAIs, but there have been a few reports of oseltamivir-resistant isolates (63, 83). The potential rapid development of resistance to antiviral drugs by influenza virus strains should be noted, as treatment guidelines will likely change in the near future. For this reason, a new investigational NAI, peramivir, is included in this section.

Oseltamivir

Pharmacology

Oseltamivir phosphate is an ethyl ester prodrug requiring ester hydrolysis for conversion to the active form, oseltamivir carboxylate. After oral administration, oseltamivir phosphate is readily absorbed from the gastrointestinal tract and is extensively converted to oseltamivir carboxylate, predominantly by hepatic esterases (61). At least 75% of an oral dose reaches the systemic circulation as oseltamivir carboxylate. The binding of oseltamivir carboxylate to plasma proteins is low. The half-life in plasma is 6 to 10 h. There are fewer side effects if it is administered with food. Oseltamivir carboxylate is not further metabolized and is eliminated in the urine (41). The efficacy of oseltamivir in preventing naturally occurring influenza illness has been demonstrated in treatment and prophylaxis studies (10, 57, 149).

Drug Interactions

Studies of oseltamivir suggest that clinically significant drug interactions are unlikely, because neither the drug nor the metabolite oseltamivir carboxylate is a substrate for the CYP450 isoenzymes or for glucuronyl transferases. The potential exists for interaction with other agents, such as probenecid, that are excreted in the urine by the same pathways (41). Oseltamivir should not be administered in the period 2 weeks before and 48 h after administration of live influenza vaccine.

Zanamivir

Zanamivir treatment has been shown to reduce the severity and duration of naturally occurring, uncomplicated influenza illness in adults (13). Zanamivir is administered only to the respiratory tract by oral inhalation, using a blister pack (65). The contents of each blister are inhaled by use of a specially designed breath-activated plastic device for the inhaling powder. This route rapidly provides high local concentrations at the site of delivery. Because of the respiratory route of administration, zanamivir is contraindicated for patients with underlying airway disease, such as asthma. As noted above, the H1N1 strains that have become resistant to oseltamivir remain sensitive to zanamivir.

Pharmacology

The absolute oral bioavailability of zanamivir is low, averaging 2%. After intranasal or oral inhaled administration, a median of 10 to 20% of the dose is systemically absorbed, with maximum concentrations in serum generally reached within 1 to 2 h. The remaining 70 to 80% is left in the oropharynx and is eliminated in the feces. The median half-life in serum ranges from 2.5 to 5.5 h, and the systemically absorbed drug is excreted unchanged in the urine. The low level of absorption of the drug after inhalation produces low concentrations in serum, with only modest systemic zanamivir exposure (41).

Drug Interactions

Zanamivir is not metabolized, and therefore there is a very low potential for drug-drug interaction (17).

Peramivir

Peramivir (BioCryst Pharmaceuticals) is an unapproved investigational NAI that is currently being evaluated in clinical trials (56). The FDA issued an emergency use authorization for the treatment of hospitalized patients with pandemic 2009 H1N1 influenza who have potentially life-threatening disease. This emergency use authorization was canceled in June 2010. Peramivir is presently available in the United States only through participation in ongoing phase III clinical trials. The drug is administered intravenously and is active against both influenza A and B viruses, including strains that may be resistant to approved NAIs. Reported adverse effects include diarrhea, nausea, vomiting, and neutropenia (7).

REFERENCES

1. **Akuta, N., and H. Kumada.** 2005. Influence of hepatitis B virus genotypes on the response to antiviral therapies. *J. Antimicrob. Chemother.* **55:**139–142.
2. **American Academy of Pediatrics Committee on Infectious Diseases.** 2007. Antiviral therapy and prophylaxis for influenza in children. *Pediatrics* **119:**852–860.
3. **Avery, R. K., B. J. Bolwell, B. Yen-Lieberman, N. Lurain, W. J. Waldman, D. L. Longworth, A. J. Taege, S. B. Mossad, D. Kohn, J. R. Long, J. Curtis, M. Kalaycio, B. Pohlman, and J. W. Williams.** 2004. Use of leflunomide in an allogeneic bone marrow transplant recipient with refractory cytomegalovirus infection. *Bone Marrow Transplant.* **34:**1071–1075.
4. **Aweeka, F., J. Gambertoglio, J. Mills, and M. A. Jacobson.** 1989. Pharmacokinetics of intermittently administered intravenous foscarnet in the treatment of acquired immunodeficiency syndrome patients with serious cytomegalovirus retinitis. *Antimicrob. Agents Chemother.* **33:**742–745.
5. **Bacon, T. H., M. J. Levin, J. J. Leary, R. T. Sarisky, and D. Sutton.** 2003. Herpes simplex virus resistance to acyclovir and penciclovir after two decades of antiviral therapy. *Clin. Microbiol. Rev.* **16:**114–128.
6. **Bean, B.** 1992. Antiviral therapy: current concepts and practices. *Clin. Microbiol. Rev.* **5:**146–182.
7. **Birnkrant, D., and E. Cox.** 2009. The emergency use authorization of peramivir for treatment of 2009 H1N1 influenza. *N. Engl. J. Med.* **361:**2204–2207.
8. **Boffito, M., D. Maitland, Y. Samarasinghe, and A. Pozniak.** 2005. The pharmacokinetics of HIV protease inhibitor combinations. *Curr. Opin. Infect. Dis.* **18:**1–7.
9. **Bonney, D., H. Razali, A. Turner, and A. Will.** 2009. Successful treatment of human metapneumovirus pneumonia using combination therapy with intravenous ribavirin and immune globulin. *Br. J. Haematol.* **145:**667–669.
10. **Bowles, S. K., W. Lee, A. E. Simor, M. Vearncombe, M. Loeb, S. Tamblyn, M. Fearon, Y. Li, and A. McGeer.** 2002. Use of oseltamivir during influenza outbreaks in Ontario nursing homes, 1999–2000. *J. Am. Geriatr. Soc.* **50:**608–616.
11. **Brinkman, K., J. A. Smeitink, J. A. Romijn, and P. Reiss.** 1999. Mitochondrial toxicity induced by nucleoside-analogue reverse-transcriptase inhibitors is a key factor in the pathogenesis of antiretroviral-therapy-related lipodystrophy. *Lancet* **354:**1112–1115.
12. **Briz, V., C. Garrido, E. Poveda, J. Morello, P. Barreiro, C. de Mendoza, and V. Soriano.** 2009. Raltegravir and etravirine are active against HIV type 1 group O. *AIDS Res. Hum. Retrovir.* **25:**225–227.
13. **Calfee, D. P., and F. G. Hayden.** 1998. New approaches to influenza chemotherapy. Neuraminidase inhibitors. *Drugs* **56:**537–553.
14. **Capparelli, E. V., S. L. Letendre, R. J. Ellis, P. Patel, D. Holland, and J. A. McCutchan.** 2005. Population pharmacokinetics of abacavir in plasma and cerebrospinal fluid. *Antimicrob. Agents Chemother.* **49:**2504–2506.
15. **Carmine, A. A., R. N. Brogden, R. C. Heel, T. M. Speight, and G. S. Avery.** 1982. Trifluridine: a review of its antiviral activity and therapeutic use in the topical treatment of viral eye infections. *Drugs* **23:**329–353.
16. **Casper, C., E. M. Krantz, L. Corey, S. R. Kuntz, J. Wang, S. Selke, S. Hamilton, M. L. Huang, and A. Wald.** 2008. Valganciclovir for suppression of human herpesvirus-8 replication: a randomized, double-blind, placebo-controlled, crossover trial. *J. Infect. Dis.* **198:**23–30.
17. **Cass, L. M., C. Efthymiopoulos, and A. Bye.** 1999. Pharmacokinetics of zanamivir after intravenous, oral, inhaled or intranasal administration to healthy volunteers. *Clin. Pharmacokinet.* **36**(Suppl. 1)**:**1–11.
18. **Castello, G., G. Mela, A. Cerruti, M. Mencoboni, and R. Lerza.** 1995. Azidothymidine and interferon-alpha in vitro effects on hematopoiesis: protective in vitro activity of IL-1 and GM-CSF. *Exp. Hematol.* **23:**1367–1371.
19. **Cheng, P. K., A. P. To, T. W. Leung, P. C. Leung, C. W. Lee, and W. W. Lim.** 2010. Oseltamivir- and amantadine-resistant influenza virus A (H1N1). *Emerg. Infect. Dis.* **16:**155–156.
20. **Chilukuri, S., and T. Rosen.** 2003. Management of acyclovir-resistant herpes simplex virus. *Dermatol. Clin.* **21:**311–320.
21. **Chrisp, P., and S. P. Clissold.** 1991. Foscarnet. A review of its antiviral activity, pharmacokinetic properties and therapeutic use in immunocompromised patients with cytomegalovirus retinitis. *Drugs* **41:**104–129.
22. **Cimoch, P. J., J. Lavelle, R. Pollard, K. G. Griffy, R. Wong, T. L. Tarnowski, S. Casserella, and D. Jung.** 1998. Pharmacokinetics of oral ganciclovir alone and in combination with zidovudine, didanosine, and probenecid in HIV-infected subjects. *J. Acquir. Immune Defic. Syndr. Hum. Retrovirol.* **17:**227–234.
23. **Cooper, C. L., R. P. van Heeswijk, K. Gallicano, and D. W. Cameron.** 2003. A review of low-dose ritonavir in protease inhibitor combination therapy. *Clin. Infect. Dis.* **36:**1585–1592.
24. **Cooper, D. A., R. T. Steigbigel, J. M. Gatell, J. K. Rockstroh, C. Katlama, P. Yeni, A. Lazzarin, B. Clotet, P. N. Kumar, J. E. Eron, M. Schechter, M. Markowitz, M. R. Loutfy, J. L. Lennox, J. Zhao, J. Chen, D. M. Ryan, R. R. Rhodes, J. A. Killar, L. R. Gilde, K. M. Strohmaier, A. R. Meibohm, M. D. Miller, D. J. Hazuda, M. L. Nessly, M. J. DiNubile, R. D. Isaacs, H. Teppler, and B. Y. Nguyen.** 2008. Subgroup and resistance analyses of raltegravir for resistant HIV-1 infection. *N. Engl. J. Med.* **359:**355–365.
25. **Cote, H. C., Z. L. Brumme, K. J. Craib, C. S. Alexander, B. Wynhoven, L. Ting, H. Wong, M. Harris, P. R. Harrigan, M. V. O'Shaughnessy, and J. S. Montaner.** 2002. Changes in mitochondrial DNA as a marker of nucleoside toxicity in HIV-infected patients. *N. Engl. J. Med.* **346:**811–820.
26. **Covens, K., K. Kabeya, Y. Schrooten, N. Dekeersmaeker, E. Van Wijngaerden, A. M. Vandamme, S. De Wit, and K. Van Laethem.** 2009. Evolution of genotypic resistance to enfuvirtide in HIV-1 isolates from different group M subtypes. *J. Clin. Virol.* **44:**325–328.
27. **Crotty, S., D. Maag, J. J. Arnold, W. Zhong, J. Y. Lau, Z. Hong, R. Andino, and C. E. Cameron.** 2000. The broad-spectrum antiviral ribonucleoside ribavirin is an RNA virus mutagen. *Nat. Med.* **6:**1375–1379.
28. **Crumpacker, C. S.** 1996. Ganciclovir. *N. Engl. J. Med.* **335:**721–729.
29. **Cundy, K. C., B. G. Petty, J. Flaherty, P. E. Fisher, M. A. Polis, M. Wachsman, P. S. Lietman, J. P. Lalezari, M. J. Hitchcock, and H. S. Jaffe.** 1995. Clinical pharmacokinetics of cidofovir in human immunodeficiency virus-infected patients. *Antimicrob. Agents Chemother.* **39:**1247–1252.
30. **Curran, M., and S. Noble.** 2001. Valganciclovir. *Drugs* **61:**1145–1150.
31. **Cvetkovic, R. S., and K. Wellington.** 2005. Valganciclovir: a review of its use in the management of CMV infection and disease in immunocompromised patients. *Drugs* **65:**859–878.
32. **De Clercq, E.** 2009. Anti-HIV drugs: 25 compounds approved within 25 years after the discovery of HIV. *Int. J. Antimicrob. Agents* **33:**307–320.
33. **De Clercq, E.** 2004. Antiviral drugs in current clinical use. *J. Clin. Virol.* **30:**115–133.
34. **Dreitlein, W. B., J. Maratos, and J. Brocavich.** 2001. Zanamivir and oseltamivir: two new options for the treatment and prevention of influenza. *Clin. Ther.* **23:**327–355.

35. **Durand-Gasselin, L., A. Pruvost, A. Dehee, G. Vaudre, M. D. Tabone, J. Grassi, G. Leverger, A. Garbarg-Chenon, H. Benech, and C. Dollfus.** 2008. High levels of zidovudine (AZT) and its intracellular phosphate metabolites in AZT- and AZT-lamivudine-treated newborns of human immunodeficiency virus-infected mothers. *Antimicrob. Agents Chemother.* **52:**2555–2563.

36. **Earnshaw, D. L., T. H. Bacon, S. J. Darlison, K. Edmonds, R. M. Perkins, and R. A. Vere Hodge.** 1992. Mode of antiviral action of penciclovir in MRC-5 cells infected with herpes simplex virus type 1 (HSV-1), HSV-2, and varicella-zoster virus. *Antimicrob. Agents Chemother.* **36:**2747–2757.

37. **Efferth, T., M. R. Romero, D. G. Wolf, T. Stamminger, J. J. Marin, and M. Marschall.** 2008. The antiviral activities of artemisinin and artesunate. *Clin. Infect. Dis.* **47:**804–811.

38. **Eron, J. J., Jr.** 2000. HIV-1 protease inhibitors. *Clin. Infect. Dis.* 30(Suppl. 2):S160–S170.

39. **Este, J. A., and A. Telenti.** 2007. HIV entry inhibitors. *Lancet* **370:**81–88.

40. **Fellay, J., C. Marzolini, L. Decosterd, K. P. Golay, P. Baumann, T. Buclin, A. Telenti, and C. B. Eap.** 2005. Variations of CYP3A activity induced by antiretroviral treatment in HIV-1 infected patients. *Eur. J. Clin. Pharmacol.* **60:**865–873.

41. **Fiore, A. E., D. K. Shay, K. Broder, J. K. Iskander, T. M. Uyeki, G. Mootrey, J. S. Bresee, and N. S. Cox.** 2008. Prevention and control of influenza: recommendations of the Advisory Committee on Immunization Practices (ACIP), 2008. *MMWR Recomm. Rep.* **57:**1–60.

42. **Fischl, M. A., D. D. Richman, M. H. Grieco, M. S. Gottlieb, P. A. Volberding, O. L. Laskin, J. M. Leedom, J. E. Groopman, D. Mildvan, R. T. Schooley, et al.** 1987. The efficacy of azidothymidine (AZT) in the treatment of patients with AIDS and AIDS-related complex. A double-blind, placebo-controlled trial. *N. Engl. J. Med.* **317:**185–191.

43. **Fontana, R. J.** 2009. Side effects of long-term oral antiviral therapy for hepatitis B. *Hepatology* **49:**S185–S195.

44. **Ford, J., S. H. Khoo, and D. J. Back.** 2004. The intracellular pharmacology of antiretroviral protease inhibitors. *J. Antimicrob. Chemother.* **54:**982–990.

45. **Foudraine, N. A., R. M. Hoetelmans, J. M. Lange, F. de Wolf, B. H. van Benthem, J. J. Maas, I. P. Keet, and P. Portegies.** 1998. Cerebrospinal-fluid HIV-1 RNA and drug concentrations after treatment with lamivudine plus zidovudine or stavudine. *Lancet* **351:**1547–1551.

46. **Fried, M. W., M. L. Shiffman, K. R. Reddy, C. Smith, G. Marinos, F. L. Goncales, Jr., D. Haussinger, M. Diago, G. Carosi, D. Dhumeaux, A. Craxi, A. Lin, J. Hoffman, and J. Yu.** 2002. Peginterferon alfa-2a plus ribavirin for chronic hepatitis C virus infection. *N. Engl. J. Med.* **347:**975–982.

47. **Gallagher, T. Q., and C. S. Derkay.** 2008. Recurrent respiratory papillomatosis: update 2008. *Curr. Opin. Otolaryngol. Head Neck Surg.* **16:**536–542.

48. **Gallant, J. E., E. DeJesus, J. R. Arribas, A. L. Pozniak, B. Gazzard, R. E. Campo, B. Lu, D. McColl, S. Chuck, J. Enejosa, J. J. Toole, and A. K. Cheng.** 2006. Tenofovir DF, emtricitabine, and efavirenz vs. zidovudine, lamivudine, and efavirenz for HIV. *N. Engl. J. Med.* **354:**251–260.

49. **Geary, R. S., S. P. Henry, and L. R. Grillone.** 2002. Fomivirsen: clinical pharmacology and potential drug interactions. *Clin. Pharmacokinet.* **41:**255–260.

50. **Ghany, M. G., D. B. Strader, D. L. Thomas, and L. B. Seeff.** 2009. Diagnosis, management, and treatment of hepatitis C: an update. *Hepatology* **49:**1335–1374.

51. **Gish, R. G., H. Trinh, N. Leung, F. K. Chan, M. W. Fried, T. L. Wright, C. Wang, J. Anderson, E. Mondou, A. Snow, J. Sorbel, F. Rousseau, and L. Corey.** 2005. Safety and antiviral activity of emtricitabine (FTC) for the treatment of chronic hepatitis B infection: a two-year study. *J. Hepatol.* **43:**60–66.

52. **Gulick, R. M., H. J. Ribaudo, C. M. Shikuma, S. Lustgarten, K. E. Squires, W. A. Meyer III, E. P. Acosta, B. R. Schackman, C. D. Pilcher, R. L. Murphy, W. E. Maher, M. D. Witt, R. C. Reichman, S. Snyder, K. L. Klingman, and D. R. Kuritzkes.** 2004. Triple-nucleoside regimens versus efavirenz-containing regimens for the initial treatment of HIV-1 infection. *N. Engl. J. Med.* **350:**1850–1861.

53. **Harper, S. A., K. Fukuda, T. M. Uyeki, N. J. Cox, and C. B. Bridges.** 2004. Prevention and control of influenza: recommendations of the Advisory Committee on Immunization Practices (ACIP). *MMWR Recomm. Rep.* **53:**1–40.

54. **Havlir, D. V., and S. D. O'Marro.** 2004. Atazanavir: new option for treatment of HIV infection. *Clin. Infect. Dis.* **38:**1599–1604.

55. **Havlir, D. V., C. Tierney, G. H. Friedland, R. B. Pollard, L. Smeaton, J. P. Sommadossi, L. Fox, H. Kessler, K. H. Fife, and D. D. Richman.** 2000. In vivo antagonism with zidovudine plus stavudine combination therapy. *J. Infect. Dis.* **182:**321–325.

56. **Hayden, F.** 2009. Developing new antiviral agents for influenza treatment: what does the future hold? *Clin. Infect. Dis.* **48**(Suppl. 1):S3–S13.

57. **Hayden, F. G., R. Belshe, C. Villanueva, R. Lanno, C. Hughes, I. Small, R. Dutkowski, P. Ward, and J. Carr.** 2004. Management of influenza in households: a prospective, randomized comparison of oseltamivir treatment with or without postexposure prophylaxis. *J. Infect. Dis.* **189:**440–449.

58. **Hayden, F. G., A. Minocha, D. A. Spyker, and H. E. Hoffman.** 1985. Comparative single-dose pharmacokinetics of amantadine hydrochloride and rimantadine hydrochloride in young and elderly adults. *Antimicrob. Agents Chemother.* **28:**216–221.

59. **Hazar, V., S. Kansoy, A. Kupesiz, M. Aksoylar, M. Kantar, and A. Yesilipek.** 2004. High-dose acyclovir and pre-emptive ganciclovir in prevention of cytomegalovirus disease in pediatric patients following peripheral blood stem cell transplantation. *Bone Marrow Transplant.* **33:**931–935.

60. **Hicks, C., and R. M. Gulick.** 2009. Raltegravir: the first HIV type 1 integrase inhibitor. *Clin. Infect. Dis.* **48:**931–939.

61. **Hill, G., T. Cihlar, C. Oo, E. S. Ho, K. Prior, H. Wiltshire, J. Barrett, B. Liu, and P. Ward.** 2002. The anti-influenza drug oseltamivir exhibits low potential to induce pharmacokinetic drug interactions via renal secretion—correlation of in vivo and in vitro studies. *Drug Metab. Dispos.* **30:**13–19.

62. **Hsue, P. Y., P. W. Hunt, Y. Wu, A. Schnell, J. E. Ho, H. Hatano, Y. Xie, J. N. Martin, P. Ganz, and S. G. Deeks.** 2009. Association of abacavir and impaired endothelial function in treated and suppressed HIV-infected patients. *AIDS* **23:**2021–2027.

63. **Hurt, A. C., J. K. Holien, M. W. Parker, and I. G. Barr.** 2009. Oseltamivir resistance and the H274Y neuraminidase mutation in seasonal, pandemic and highly pathogenic influenza viruses. *Drugs* **69:**2523–2531.

64. **Isaac, A., S. Taylor, P. Cane, E. Smit, S. E. Gibbons, D. J. White, S. M. Drake, S. Khoo, and D. J. Back.** 2004. Lopinavir/ritonavir combined with twice-daily 400 mg indinavir: pharmacokinetics and pharmacodynamics in blood, CSF and semen. *J. Antimicrob. Chemother.* **54:**498–502.

65. **Ison, M. G., J. W. Gnann, Jr., S. Nagy-Agren, J. Treannor, C. Paya, R. Steigbigel, M. Elliott, H. L. Weiss, and F. G. Hayden.** 2003. Safety and efficacy of nebulized zanamivir in hospitalized patients with serious influenza. *Antivir. Ther.* **8:**183–190.

66. **Jabs, D. A., and P. D. Griffiths.** 2002. Fomivirsen for the treatment of cytomegalovirus retinitis. *Am. J. Ophthalmol.* **133:**552–556.

67. **Jain, M. K., L. Comanor, C. White, P. Kipnis, C. Elkin, K. Leung, A. Ocampo, N. Attar, P. Keiser, and W. M. Lee.** 2007. Treatment of hepatitis B with lamivudine and tenofovir in HIV/HBV-coinfected patients: factors associated with response. *J. Viral Hepat.* **14:**176–182.

68. **Janssen, H. L., M. van Zonneveld, H. Senturk, S. Zeuzem, U. S. Akarca, Y. Cakaloglu, C. Simon, T. M. So, G. Gerken, R. A. de Man, H. G. Niesters, P. Zondervan, B. Hansen, and S. W. Schalm.** 2005. Pegylated interferon alfa-2b alone or in combination with lamivudine for HBeAg-positive chronic hepatitis B: a randomised trial. *Lancet* **365:**123–129.

69. Jing, X., C. Ma, Y. Ohigashi, F. A. Oliveira, T. S. Jardetzky, L. H. Pinto, and R. A. Lamb. 2008. Functional studies indicate amantadine binds to the pore of the influenza A virus M2 proton-selective ion channel. *Proc. Natl. Acad. Sci. USA* **105:**10967–10972.

70. Johnson, L. B., and L. D. Saravolatz. 2009. Etravirine, a next-generation nonnucleoside reverse-transcriptase inhibitor. *Clin. Infect. Dis.* **48:**1123–1128.

71. Kaplan, J. E., C. Benson, K. H. Holmes, J. T. Brooks, A. Pau, and H. Masur. 2009. Guidelines for prevention and treatment of opportunistic infections in HIV-infected adults and adolescents: recommendations from CDC, the National Institutes of Health, and the HIV Medicine Association of the Infectious Diseases Society of America. *MMWR Recomm. Rep.* **58:**1–207.

72. Katz, D. H., J. F. Marcelletti, M. H. Khalil, L. E. Pope, and L. R. Katz. 1991. Antiviral activity of 1-docosanol, an inhibitor of lipid-enveloped viruses including herpes simplex. *Proc. Natl. Acad. Sci. USA* **88:**10825–10829.

73. Kim, C. U., B. Y. Luh, and J. C. Martin. 1990. Synthesis and antiviral activity of (S)-9-[4-hydroxy-3-(phosphonomethoxy) butyl]guanine. *J. Med. Chem.* **33:**1797–1800.

74. Kiser, J. J. 2008. Pharmacologic characteristics of investigational and recently approved agents for the treatment of HIV. *Curr. Opin. HIV AIDS* **3:**330–341.

75. Koh, Y., S. Matsumi, D. Das, M. Amano, D. A. Davis, J. Li, S. Leschenko, A. Baldridge, T. Shioda, R. Yarchoan, A. K. Ghosh, and H. Mitsuya. 2007. Potent inhibition of HIV-1 replication by novel non-peptidyl small molecule inhibitors of protease dimerization. *J. Biol. Chem.* **282:** 28709–28720.

76. Kuypers, D. R., A. K. Vandooren, E. Lerut, P. Evenepoel, K. Claes, R. Snoeck, L. Naesens, and Y. Vanrenterghem. 2005. Adjuvant low-dose cidofovir therapy for BK polyomavirus interstitial nephritis in renal transplant recipients. *Am. J. Transplant.* **5:**1997–2004.

77. Laguno, M., C. Cifuentes, J. Murillas, S. Veloso, M. Larrousse, A. Payeras, L. Bonet, F. Vidal, A. Milinkovic, A. Bassa, C. Villalonga, I. Perez, C. Tural, M. Martinez-Rebollar, M. Calvo, J. L. Blanco, E. Martinez, J. M. Sanchez-Tapias, J. M. Gatell, and J. Mallolas. 2009. Randomized trial comparing pegylated interferon alpha-2b versus pegylated interferon alpha-2a, both plus ribavirin, to treat chronic hepatitis C in human immunodeficiency virus patients. *Hepatology* **49:**22–31.

78. Lampertico, P., M. Vigano, E. Manenti, M. Iavarone, E. Sablon, and M. Colombo. 2007. Low resistance to adefovir combined with lamivudine: a 3-year study of 145 lamivudine-resistant hepatitis B patients. *Gastroenterology* **133:**1445–1451.

79. Lau, G. K., T. Piratvisuth, K. X. Luo, P. Marcellin, S. Thongsawat, G. Cooksley, E. Gane, M. W. Fried, W. C. Chow, S. W. Paik, W. Y. Chang, T. Berg, R. Flisiak, P. McCloud, and N. Pluck. 2005. Peginterferon alfa-2a, lamivudine, and the combination for HBeAg-positive chronic hepatitis B. *N. Engl. J. Med.* **352:**2682–2695.

80. Leeds, J. M., S. P. Henry, S. Bistner, S. Scherrill, K. Williams, and A. A. Levin. 1998. Pharmacokinetics of an antisense oligonucleotide injected intravitreally in monkeys. *Drug Metab. Dispos.* **26:**670–675.

81. Legrand-Abravanel, F., F. Nicot, A. Boulestin, K. Sandres-Saune, J. P. Vinel, L. Alric, and J. Izopet. 2005. Pegylated interferon and ribavirin therapy for chronic hepatitis C virus genotype 4 infection. *J. Med. Virol.* **77:**66–69.

82. Lennox, J. L., E. DeJesus, A. Lazzarin, R. B. Pollard, J. V. Madruga, D. S. Berger, J. Zhao, X. Xu, A. Williams-Diaz, A. J. Rodgers, R. J. Barnard, M. D. Miller, M. J. DiNubile, B. Y. Nguyen, R. Leavitt, and P. Sklar. 2009. Safety and efficacy of raltegravir-based versus efavirenz-based combination therapy in treatment-naive patients with HIV-1 infection: a multicentre, double-blind randomised controlled trial. *Lancet* **374:**796–806.

83. Leung, T. W., A. L. Tai, P. K. Cheng, M. S. Kong, and W. Lim. 2009. Detection of an oseltamivir-resistant pandemic influenza A/H1N1 virus in Hong Kong. *J. Clin. Virol.* **46:** 298–299.

84. Levi, M. E., N. Mandava, L. K. Chan, A. Weinberg, and J. L. Olson. 2006. Treatment of multidrug-resistant cytomegalovirus retinitis with systemically administered leflunomide. *Transpl. Infect. Dis.* **8:**38–43.

85. Levrero, M., T. Pollicino, J. Petersen, L. Belloni, G. Raimondo, and M. Dandri. 2009. Control of cccDNA function in hepatitis B virus infection. *J. Hepatol.* **51:**581–592.

86. Leyssen, P., J. Balzarini, E. De Clercq, and J. Neyts. 2005. The predominant mechanism by which ribavirin exerts its antiviral activity in vitro against flaviviruses and paramyxoviruses is mediated by inhibition of IMP dehydrogenase. *J. Virol.* **79:**1943–1947.

87. Lietman, P. S. 1992. Clinical pharmacology: foscarnet. *Am. J. Med.* **92:**8S–11S.

88. Liu, V., G. S. Dhillon, and D. Weill. 2010. A multi-drug regimen for respiratory syncytial virus and parainfluenza virus infections in adult lung and heart-lung transplant recipients. *Transpl. Infect. Dis.* **12:**38–44.

89. Liu-Young, G., and M. J. Kozal. 2008. Hepatitis C protease and polymerase inhibitors in development. *AIDS Patient Care STDS* **22:**449–457.

90. Luber, A. D., and J. F. Flaherty, Jr. 1996. Famciclovir for treatment of herpesvirus infections. *Ann. Pharmacother.* **30:**978–985.

91. Ma, J. D., A. N. Nafziger, S. A. Villano, A. Gaedigk, and J. S. Bertino, Jr. 2006. Maribavir pharmacokinetics and the effects of multiple-dose maribavir on cytochrome P450 (CYP) 1A2, CYP 2C9, CYP 2C19, CYP 2D6, CYP 3A, N-acetyltransferase-2, and xanthine oxidase activities in healthy adults. *Antimicrob. Agents Chemother.* **50:**1130–1135.

92. Machida, H. 1986. Comparison of susceptibilities of varicella-zoster virus and herpes simplex viruses to nucleoside analogs. *Antimicrob. Agents Chemother.* **29:**524–526.

93. Magee, W. C., K. Y. Hostetler, and D. H. Evans. 2005. Mechanism of inhibition of vaccinia virus DNA polymerase by cidofovir diphosphate. *Antimicrob. Agents Chemother.* **49:**3153–3162.

94. Mallal, S., E. Phillips, G. Carosi, J. M. Molina, C. Workman, J. Tomazic, E. Jagel-Guedes, S. Rugina, O. Kozyrev, J. F. Cid, P. Hay, D. Nolan, S. Hughes, A. Hughes, S. Ryan, N. Fitch, D. Thorborn, and A. Benbow. 2008. HLA-B*5701 screening for hypersensitivity to abacavir. *N. Engl. J. Med.* **358:**568–579.

95. Manns, M. P., J. G. McHutchison, S. C. Gordon, V. K. Rustgi, M. Shiffman, R. Reindollar, Z. D. Goodman, K. Koury, M. Ling, and J. K. Albrecht. 2001. Peginterferon alfa-2b plus ribavirin compared with interferon alfa-2b plus ribavirin for initial treatment of chronic hepatitis C: a randomised trial. *Lancet* **358:**958–965.

96. Marcellin, P., G. K. Lau, F. Bonino, P. Farci, S. Hadziyannis, R. Jin, Z. M. Lu, T. Piratvisuth, G. Germanidis, C. Yurdaydin, M. Diago, S. Gurel, M. Y. Lai, P. Button, and N. Pluck. 2004. Peginterferon alfa-2a alone, lamivudine alone, and the two in combination in patients with HBeAg-negative chronic hepatitis B. *N. Engl. J. Med.* **351:**1206–1217.

97. McMahon, M. A., B. L. Jilek, T. P. Brennan, L. Shen, Y. Zhou, M. Wind-Rotolo, S. Xing, S. Bhat, B. Hale, R. Hegarty, C. R. Chong, J. O. Liu, R. F. Siliciano, and C. L. Thio. 2007. The HBV drug entecavir—effects on HIV-1 replication and resistance. *N. Engl. J. Med.* **356:**2614–2621.

98. Menendez-Arias, L., and J. Tozser. 2008. HIV-1 protease inhibitors: effects on HIV-2 replication and resistance. *Trends Pharmacol. Sci.* **29:**42–49.

99. Mertz, G. J., L. Miedzinski, D. Goade, A. T. Pavia, B. Hjelle, C. O. Hansbarger, H. Levy, F. T. Koster, K. Baum, A. Lindemulder, W. Wang, L. Riser, H. Fernandez, and R. J. Whitley. 2004. Placebo-controlled, double-blind trial of intravenous ribavirin for the treatment of hantavirus cardiopulmonary syndrome in North America. *Clin. Infect. Dis.* **39:**1307–1313.

100. **Mmiro, F. A., J. Aizire, A. K. Mwatha, S. H. Eshleman, D. Donnell, M. G. Fowler, C. Nakabiito, P. M. Musoke, J. B. Jackson, and L. A. Guay.** 2009. Predictors of early and late mother-to-child transmission of HIV in a breastfeeding population: HIV Network for Prevention Trials 012 experience, Kampala, Uganda. *J. Acquir. Immune Defic. Syndr.* **52:**32–39.

101. **Mohanty, S. R., and S. J. Cotler.** 2005. Management of hepatitis B in liver transplant patients. *J. Clin. Gastroenterol.* **39:**58–63.

102. **Monto, A. S.** 2003. The role of antivirals in the control of influenza. *Vaccine* **21:**1796–1800.

103. **Monto, A. S., S. E. Ohmit, K. Hornbuckle, and C. L. Pearce.** 1995. Safety and efficacy of long-term use of rimantadine for prophylaxis of type A influenza in nursing homes. *Antimicrob. Agents Chemother.* **39:**2224–2228.

104. **Mould, D. R., X. Zhang, K. Nieforth, M. Salgo, N. Buss, and I. H. Patel.** 2005. Population pharmacokinetics and exposure-response relationship of enfuvirtide in treatment-experienced human immunodeficiency virus type 1-infected patients. *Clin. Pharmacol. Ther.* **77:**515–528.

105. **Mould, J. A., J. E. Drury, S. M. Frings, U. B. Kaupp, A. Pekosz, R. A. Lamb, and L. H. Pinto.** 2000. Permeation and activation of the M2 ion channel of influenza A virus. *J. Biol. Chem.* **275:**31038–31050.

106. **Naesens, L., L. Lenaerts, G. Andrei, R. Snoeck, D. Van Beers, A. Holy, J. Balzarini, and E. De Clercq.** 2005. Antiadenovirus activities of several classes of nucleoside and nucleotide analogues. *Antimicrob. Agents Chemother.* **49:**1010–1016.

107. **Nash, K.** 2009. Telbivudine in the treatment of chronic hepatitis B. *Adv. Ther.* **26:**155–169.

108. **Nguyen, J. T., J. D. Hoopes, D. F. Smee, M. N. Prichard, E. M. Driebe, D. M. Engelthaler, M. H. Le, P. S. Keim, R. P. Spence, and G. T. Went.** 2009. Triple combination of oseltamivir, amantadine, and ribavirin displays synergistic activity against multiple influenza virus strains in vitro. *Antimicrob. Agents Chemother.* **53:**4115–4126.

109. **Ormrod, D., L. J. Scott, and C. M. Perry.** 2000. Valaciclovir: a review of its long term utility in the management of genital herpes simplex virus and cytomegalovirus infections. *Drugs* **59:**839–863.

110. **Orr, R. M.** 2001. Technology evaluation: fomivirsen, Isis Pharmaceuticals Inc./CIBA Vision. *Curr. Opin. Mol. Ther.* **3:**288–294.

111. **Orrick, J. J., and C. R. Steinhart.** 2004. Atazanavir. *Ann. Pharmacother.* **38:**1664–1674.

112. **Oxford, J. S.** 2007. Antivirals for the treatment and prevention of epidemic and pandemic influenza. *Influenza Other Respi. Viruses* **1:**27–34.

113. **Panel on Antiretroviral Guidelines for Adults and Adolescents.** 1 December 2009, posting date. *Guidelines for the Use of Antiretroviral Agents in HIV-1-Infected Adults and Adolescents,* p. 1–161. U.S. Department of Health and Human Services, Washington, DC. http://www.aidsinfo.nih.gov/ContentFiles/AdultandAdolescentGL.pdf.

114. **Patterson, J. L., and R. Fernandez-Larsson.** 1990. Molecular mechanisms of action of ribavirin. *Rev. Infect. Dis.* **12:** 1139–1146.

115. **Pepose, J. S., T. P. Margolis, P. LaRussa, and D. Pavan-Langston.** 2003. Ocular complications of smallpox vaccination. *Am. J. Ophthalmol.* **136:**343–352.

116. **Perinatal HIV Guidelines Working Group. Public Health Service Task Force.** 29 April 2009, posting date. *Recommendations for Use of Antiretroviral Drugs in Pregnant HIV-Infected Women for Maternal Health and Interventions To Reduce Perinatal HIV Transmission in the United States,* p. 1–90. U.S. Department of Health and Human Services, Washington, DC. http://aidsinfo.nih.gov/ContentFiles/PerinatalGL.pdf.

117. **Perronne, C.** 2006. Antiviral hepatitis and antiretroviral drug interactions. *J. Hepatol.* **44:**S119–S125.

118. **Perry, C. M.** 2009. Emtricitabine/tenofovir disoproxil fumarate: in combination with a protease inhibitor in HIV-1 infection. *Drugs* **69:**843–857.

119. **Pescovitz, M. D., J. Rabkin, R. M. Merion, C. V. Paya, J. Pirsch, R. B. Freeman, J. O'Grady, C. Robinson, Z. To,** K. Wren, L. Banken, W. Buhles, and F. Brown. 2000. Valganciclovir results in improved oral absorption of ganciclovir in liver transplant recipients. *Antimicrob. Agents Chemother.* **44:**2811–2815.

120. **Piscitelli, S. C., and K. D. Gallicano.** 2001. Interactions among drugs for HIV and opportunistic infections. *N. Engl. J. Med.* **344:**984–996.

121. **Poveda, E., P. Barreiro, B. Rodes, and V. Soriano.** 2005. Enfuvirtide is active against HIV type 1 group O. *AIDS Res. Hum. Retrovir.* **21:**583–585.

122. **Preston, S. L., G. L. Drusano, P. Glue, J. Nash, S. K. Gupta, and P. McNamara.** 1999. Pharmacokinetics and absolute bioavailability of ribavirin in healthy volunteers as determined by stable-isotope methodology. *Antimicrob. Agents Chemother.* **43:**2451–2456.

123. **Pruvost, A., E. Negredo, H. Benech, F. Theodoro, J. Puig, E. Grau, E. Garcia, J. Molto, J. Grassi, and B. Clotet.** 2005. Measurement of intracellular didanosine and tenofovir phosphorylated metabolites and possible interaction of the two drugs in human immunodeficiency virus-infected patients. *Antimicrob. Agents Chemother.* **49:**1907–1914.

124. **Ray, A. S., L. Olson, and A. Fridland.** 2004. Role of purine nucleoside phosphorylase in interactions between 2′,3′-dideoxyinosine and allopurinol, ganciclovir, or tenofovir. *Antimicrob. Agents Chemother.* **48:**1089–1095.

125. **Reischig, T., P. Jindra, J. Mares, M. Cechura, M. Svecova, O. Hes, K. Opatrny, Jr., and V. Treska.** 2005. Valacyclovir for cytomegalovirus prophylaxis reduces the risk of acute renal allograft rejection. *Transplantation* **79:**317–324.

125a. **Sarrazin, C., and S. Zeuzem.** 2010. Resistance to direct antiviral agents in patients with hepatitis C virus infection. *Gastroenterology* **138:**447–462.

126. **Schmidt, A. C.** 2004. Antiviral therapy for influenza: a clinical and economic comparative review. *Drugs* **64:**2031–2046.

127. **Schmid-Wendtner, M. H., and H. C. Korting.** 2004. Penciclovir cream—improved topical treatment for herpes simplex infections. *Skin Pharmacol. Physiol.* **17:**214–218.

128. **Schwarz, A., and A. Perez-Canto.** 1998. Nephrotoxicity of antiinfective drugs. *Int. J. Clin. Pharmacol. Ther.* **36:**164–167.

129. **Sen, G. C.** 2001. Viruses and interferons. *Annu. Rev. Microbiol.* **55:**255–281.

130. **Shapira, M. Y., I. B. Resnick, S. Chou, A. U. Neumann, N. S. Lurain, T. Stamminger, O. Caplan, N. Saleh, T. Efferth, M. Marschall, and D. G. Wolf.** 2008. Artesunate as a potent antiviral agent in a patient with late drug-resistant cytomegalovirus infection after hematopoietic stem cell transplantation. *Clin. Infect. Dis.* **46:**1455–1457.

131. **Shehab, N., B. V. Sweet, and N. D. Hogikyan.** 2005. Cidofovir for the treatment of recurrent respiratory papillomatosis: a review of the literature. *Pharmacotherapy* **25:**977–989.

132. **Shire, N. J., and K. E. Sherman.** 2005. Clinical trials of treatment for hepatitis C virus infection in HIV-infected patients: past, present, and future. *Clin. Infect. Dis.* **41**(Suppl. 1): S63–S68.

133. **Simpson, D., and K. A. Lyseng-Williamson.** 2006. Famciclovir: a review of its use in herpes zoster and genital and orolabial herpes. *Drugs* **66:**2397–2416.

134. **Smee, D. F., B. L. Hurst, M. H. Wong, K. W. Bailey, and J. D. Morrey.** 2009. Effects of double combinations of amantadine, oseltamivir, and ribavirin on influenza A (H5N1) virus infections in cell culture and in mice. *Antimicrob. Agents Chemother.* **53:**2120–2128.

135. **Soriano, V., M. G. Peters, and S. Zeuzem.** 2009. New therapies for hepatitis C virus infection. *Clin. Infect. Dis.* **48:**313–320.

136. **Soriano, V., M. Puoti, M. Bonacini, G. Brook, A. Cargnel, J. Rockstroh, C. Thio, and Y. Benhamou.** 2005. Care of patients with chronic hepatitis B and HIV co-infection: recommendations from an HIV-HBV international panel. *AIDS* **19:**221–240.

137. **Soriano, V., M. Puoti, M. Peters, Y. Benhamou, M. Sulkowski, F. Zoulim, S. Mauss, and J. Rockstroh.** 2008. Care of HIV patients with chronic hepatitis B: updated recommendations from the HIV-Hepatitis B Virus International Panel. *AIDS* **22:**1399–1410.

138. **Strategies for Management of Anti-Retroviral Therapy/ INSIGHT and DAD Study Groups.** 2008. Use of nucleoside reverse transcriptase inhibitors and risk of myocardial infarction in HIV-infected patients. *AIDS* **22:**F17–F24.

139. **Sun, H. Y., M. M. Wagener, and N. Singh.** 2008. Prevention of posttransplant cytomegalovirus disease and related outcomes with valganciclovir: a systematic review. *Am. J. Transplant.* **8:**2111–2118.

140. **Suzuki, Y., R. Saito, H. Zaraket, C. Dapat, I. Caperig-Dapat, and H. Suzuki.** 2010. Rapid and specific detection of amantadine-resistant influenza A viruses with a Ser31Asn mutation by the cycling probe method. *J. Clin. Microbiol.* **48:**57–63.

141. **Talarico, C. L., T. C. Burnette, W. H. Miller, S. L. Smith, M. G. Davis, S. C. Stanat, T. I. Ng, Z. He, D. M. Coen, B. Roizman, and K. K. Biron.** 1999. Acyclovir is phosphorylated by the human cytomegalovirus UL97 protein. *Antimicrob. Agents Chemother.* **43:**1941–1946.

142. **Teo, M., and P. Hayes.** 2004. Management of hepatitis C. *Br. Med. Bull.* **70:**51–69.

143. **Torres-Madriz, G., and H. W. Boucher.** 2008. Immunocompromised hosts: perspectives in the treatment and prophylaxis of cytomegalovirus disease in solid-organ transplant recipients. *Clin. Infect. Dis.* **47:**702–711.

144. **Tozzi, V., P. Balestra, M. F. Salvatori, C. Vlassi, G. Liuzzi, M. L. Giancola, M. Giulianelli, P. Narciso, and A. Antinori.** 2009. Changes in cognition during antiretroviral therapy: comparison of 2 different ranking systems to measure antiretroviral drug efficacy on HIV-associated neurocognitive disorders. *J. Acquir. Immune Defic. Syndr.* **52:**56–63.

145. **Trofe, J., L. Pote, E. Wade, E. Blumberg, and R. D. Bloom.** 2008. Maribavir: a novel antiviral agent with activity against cytomegalovirus. *Ann. Pharmacother.* **42:**1447–1457.

146. **Vandekerckhove, L., C. Verhofstede, and D. Vogelaers.** 2009. Maraviroc: perspectives for use in antiretroviral-naive HIV-1-infected patients. *J. Antimicrob. Chemother.* **63:**1087–1096.

147. **Vere Hodge, R. A., D. Sutton, M. R. Boyd, M. R. Harnden, and R. L. Jarvest.** 1989. Selection of an oral prodrug (BRL 42810; famciclovir) for the antiherpesvirus agent BRL 39123 [9-(4-hydroxy-3-hydroxymethylbut-l-yl)guanine; penciclovir]. *Antimicrob. Agents Chemother.* **33:**1765–1773.

148. **Walmsley, S., A. Avihingsanon, J. Slim, D. J. Ward, K. Ruxrungtham, J. Brunetta, U. F. Bredeek, D. Jayaweera, C. J. Guittari, P. Larson, M. Schutz, and F. Raffi.** 2009. Gemini: a noninferiority study of saquinavir/ritonavir versus lopinavir/ritonavir as initial HIV-1 therapy in adults. *J. Acquir. Immune Defic. Syndr.* **50:**367–374.

149. **Whitley, R. J.** 2007. The role of oseltamivir in the treatment and prevention of influenza in children. *Expert Opin. Drug Metab. Toxicol.* **3:**755–767.

150. **Whitley, R. J., S. J. Soong, R. Dolin, G. J. Galasso, L. T. Ch'ien, and C. A. Alford.** 1977. Adenine arabinoside therapy of biopsy-proved herpes simplex encephalitis. National Institute of Allergy and Infectious Diseases collaborative antiviral study. *N. Engl. J. Med.* **297:**289–294.

151. **Wiltshire, H., C. V. Paya, M. D. Pescovitz, A. Humar, E. Dominguez, K. Washburn, E. Blumberg, B. Alexander, R. Freeman, N. Heaton, and K. P. Zuideveld.** 2005. Pharmacodynamics of oral ganciclovir and valganciclovir in solid organ transplant recipients. *Transplantation* **79:**1477–1483.

152. **Wintermeyer, S. M., and M. C. Nahata.** 1995. Rimantadine: a clinical perspective. *Ann. Pharmacother.* **29:**299–310.

153. **Wire, M. B., M. J. Shelton, and S. Studenberg.** 2006. Fosamprenavir: clinical pharmacokinetics and drug interactions of the amprenavir prodrug. *Clin. Pharmacokinet.* **45:**137–168.

154. **Wolf, D. L., C. A. Rodriguez, M. Mucci, A. Ingrosso, B. A. Duncan, and D. J. Nickens.** 2003. Pharmacokinetics and renal effects of cidofovir with a reduced dose of probenecid in HIV-infected patients with cytomegalovirus retinitis. *J. Clin. Pharmacol.* **43:**43–51.

155. **Working Group on Antiretroviral Therapy and Medical Management of HIV-Infected Children.** 23 February 2009, posting date. *Guidelines for the Use of Antiretroviral Agents in Pediatric HIV Infection.* U.S. Department of Health and Human Services, Washington, DC. http://aidsinfo.nih.gov/ ContentFiles/PediatricGuidelines.pdf.

156. **Xiong, X., J. L. Smith, and M. S. Chen.** 1997. Effect of incorporation of cidofovir into DNA by human cytomegalovirus DNA polymerase on DNA elongation. *Antimicrob. Agents Chemother.* **41:**594–599.

157. **Yeni, P.** 2003. Tipranavir: a protease inhibitor from a new class with distinct antiviral activity. *J. Acquir. Immune Defic. Syndr.* **34**(Suppl. 1)**:**S91–S94.

158. **Youle, M.** 2007. Overview of boosted protease inhibitors in treatment-experienced HIV-infected patients. *J. Antimicrob. Chemother.* **60:**1195–1205.

159. **Younger, H. M., A. J. Bathgate, and P. C. Hayes.** 2004. Nucleoside analogues for the treatment of chronic hepatitis B. *Aliment. Pharmacol. Ther.* **20:**1211–1230.

160. **Zeldin, R. K., and R. A. Petruschke.** 2004. Pharmacological and therapeutic properties of ritonavir-boosted protease inhibitor therapy in HIV-infected patients. *J. Antimicrob. Chemother.* **53:**4–9.

Mechanisms of Resistance to Antiviral Agents*

ROBERT W. SHAFER, ISABEL NAJERA, AND SUNWEN CHOU

109

Understanding the mechanisms of viral drug resistance is critical to the clinical management of individuals receiving antiviral therapy, the development of new antiviral drugs, and the surveillance of drug resistance. This chapter reviews the mechanisms of resistance to antiviral drugs used to treat seven common viral infections, i.e., infections with herpes simplex virus (HSV), cytomegalovirus (CMV), varicella-zoster virus (VZV), human immunodeficiency virus types 1 and 2 (HIV-1 and HIV-2), influenza A and B viruses, hepatitis B virus (HBV), and hepatitis C virus (HCV).

Antiviral drug resistance is usually mediated by mutations in the molecular targets of drug therapy, and the development of drug resistance is the most compelling evidence that an antiviral drug acts by specifically inhibiting a virus rather than its cellular host. Drug-resistant virus subpopulations may exist at low levels in clinical isolates or may arise only during drug exposure. The error-prone polymerase enzymes in RNA viruses cause these viruses to develop resistance more frequently than DNA viruses.

Drug-resistant viruses are identified by in vitro passage experiments with increasing concentrations of an inhibitory drug and by ex vivo analysis of virus isolates obtained from individuals receiving antiviral therapy. In vitro drug susceptibility is most commonly quantified as the drug concentration required to inhibit virus replication by 50%. The clinical significance of reduced drug susceptibility is determined by studying the treatment responses of individuals harboring those viruses.

HERPESVIRUSES

All currently licensed systemic drugs for the herpesviruses target the viral DNA polymerase. Nucleoside analogs that are selectively phosphorylated by viral enzymes are commonly used as initial therapy. Oral bioavailability is improved by the use of prodrugs that are metabolized to the parent drug. Acyclovir (ACV) and its prodrug, valacyclovir (VCV), and famciclovir (FCV)—the prodrug of penciclovir (PCV)—have been used to successfully treat genital HSV infections, VZV infections, and mucocutaneous HSV infections in immunocompromised hosts.

Ganciclovir (GCV) and its prodrug, valganciclovir, are used to treat CMV infection. These selective nucleoside analogs are supplemented by the drugs foscarnet (phosphonoformate [FOS])—a pyrophosphate analog—and cidofovir (CDV)—a phosphomethoxycytosine nucleotide analog—which inhibit viral DNA polymerase without prior activation by viral enzymes. FOS and CDV are generally used as second- and third-line drugs when there is a lack of response to initial therapy. Table 1 summarizes the antiviral agents, mechanisms of resistance, and mutations involved in drug resistance in herpesviruses.

Herpes Simplex Virus

Both ACV and PCV are initially monophosphorylated by the HSV thymidine kinase (TK) and then converted to triphosphates by cellular enzymes. In their active form, these drugs inhibit viral DNA polymerase by competing with GTP for incorporation into newly synthesized DNA chains, where they cause chain termination. Because the viral TK enzyme is not essential for HSV replication, many TK drug resistance mutations act by decreasing the phosphorylation of nucleoside analogs. This is by far the most common mechanism of ACV and PCV resistance in HSV (75).

Most TK mutants are classified as TK negative, usually arising from frameshift or stop mutations that delete important functional domains, or TK partial, when a mutation reduces the phosphorylation of both natural nucleosides and antiviral drugs (147). Mutants with frameshifting nucleotide insertion or deletion mutations at homopolymeric TK loci (e.g., runs of G bases) are among the most common (75). TK-altered mutants, which selectively reduce the phosphorylation of antiviral nucleosides without affecting the phosphorylation of natural nucleosides, occur less commonly. Although the TK mutations selected by PCV often differ from those selected by ACV, cross-resistance is expected (174). The effects of specific substitutions on TK activity and drug susceptibility can be defined by site-directed mutagenesis of control strains (67). Although TK mutations can be used to diagnose ACV resistance in HSV clinical isolates (66), phenotypic assays are well established (118) and continue to be standard practice, in part due to the diversity of TK mutations and sequence polymorphisms.

TK-negative HSV mutants are attenuated in mouse models with respect to virulence, latency, and reactivation potential (32). However, animal studies (80) and

---

*This chapter contains information presented in chapter 113 by Robert W. Shafer, Shirit Einav, and Sunwen Chou in the ninth edition of this *Manual*.

TABLE 1 Mechanisms of resistance to HSV, VZV, and CMV inhibitors

Virus	Antiviral agent(s)	Mechanism(s) of resistance	Mutations
HSV	Acyclovir (ACV), valacyclovir (VCV), penciclovir (PCV), famciclovir (FCV)	TK and/or DNA polymerase mutations	TK frameshift or substitution mutations causing a TK-deficient phenotype and cross-resistance among the four drugs; less commonly, TK-altered or DNA polymerase mutations
	Foscarnet (FOS)	DNA polymerase mutations	Mutations clustering in regions II, III, and VI (probable pyrophosphate-binding regions)
	Cidofovir (CDV)	DNA polymerase mutations	Mutations in regions δC and II (based on limited data from laboratory strains)
VZV	ACV, VCV, PCV, FCV	TK and/or DNA polymerase mutations	TK frameshift or substitution mutations causing a TK-deficient phenotype and cross-resistance among the four drugs; less commonly, TK-altered or DNA polymerase mutations
	FOS	DNA polymerase mutations	Mutations clustering in regions II, III, and VI (probable pyrophosphate-binding regions)
	CDV	DNA polymerase mutations	No VZV-specific data are available
CMV	Ganciclovir (GCV)	UL97 kinase mutations and/or DNA polymerase mutations	Usually, UL97 mutations at residues 460, 520, 592, 594, 595, and 603; less frequently, other mutations at codons 590 to 607; DNA polymerase mutations (regions exo, IV, δC, and V) sometimes confer resistance, usually along with UL97 mutations
	FOS	DNA polymerase mutations	Mutations in regions II, III, and VI; some mutants may also have decreased GCV susceptibility
	CDV	DNA polymerase mutations	Regions exo, IV, δC, and V, resulting in cross-resistance to GCV

clinical case reports (146, 170) show that resistant viruses cause overt disease and recurrent infection. Even isolates with frameshift mutations that are predicted to be TK negative may in fact express some TK activity—through mechanisms such as ribosomal frameshifting and genetic reversion (81)—that enables reactivation from latency (80). Although drug-resistant HSV TK mutants can easily be selected in cell culture, in most reports the prevalence of ACV-resistant HSV in clinical practice has remained stable, at about 0.3% in immunocompetent hosts and 7% in immunocompromised hosts (189). An exception is the report of ACV-resistant corneal HSV isolates in 11 (6.4%) of 173 immunocompetent patients with keratitis (60); four of these isolates contained a TK frameshift mutation and were cross-resistant to GCV.

HSV TK mutants are expected to remain susceptible to drugs that do not depend on virally mediated phosphorylation, including FOS, which is currently the main alternative therapy for ACV-resistant HSV infection, and CDV. DNA polymerase (pol) mutations are occasionally responsible for HSV resistance to ACV, PCV, FOS, and CDV. Because the viral DNA polymerase is essential for replication, mutations are more selective and usually consist of single amino acid changes in functional domains of the enzyme. The resistance and cross-resistance properties vary depending on the mutation and are best evaluated by site-directed mutagenesis or recombinant phenotyping (14). These analyses show that pol mutations conferring ACV or FOS resistance are distributed among several conserved regions, with some clustering of mutations in regions II, III, and VI. A few mutations confer resistance to both ACV and FOS (75). Little is known about the range of CDV resistance mutations in clinical isolates, but available information suggests that there is no consistent cross-resistance with ACV or FOS (14).

Varicella-Zoster Virus

Because VZV also carries a TK, the antiviral drugs in use and the mechanisms of resistance are similar to those for HSV. ACV is less potent against VZV than against HSV, and either intravenous ACV or oral prodrugs (VCV or FCV) are needed to obtain reliable antiviral activity (156). VZV treatment efficacy depends more on the prompt initiation of adequately bioavailable therapy than on loss of drug susceptibility (44). Notable exceptions include AIDS patients, who may develop chronic, spreading, verrucous skin lesions in which prolonged viral replication selects for resistant strains (152).

Analogous to HSV, most ACV-resistant VZV strains contain mutations that result in TK deficiency or substitutions that alter substrate specificity (75). A tendency has been reported for resistance mutations to cluster at certain TK gene loci (75, 148). Although the available database of resistance mutations is limited, known TK resistance mutations, as well as those predicted to result in the loss of TK activity, may be used for genotypic resistance assays (90). However, like the case when an Oka VZV vaccine strain infection became ACV resistant (22), the interpretation of uncharacterized TK mutations must be aided by phenotypic assays.

ACV-resistant VZV is treated with FOS (22, 90) and CDV. FOS resistance maps to codons in conserved functional domains II and III of the VZV DNA polymerase (75), similar to the case for FOS-resistant HSV and CMV mutants. Some mutants selected by FOS treatment in cell culture grow more slowly than the wild type (205), with unknown clinical implications. DNA polymerase mutations conferring resistance to these alternative drugs and to ACV are mostly distinct, although specific information relating to FOS or CDV resistance in clinical isolates is limited and not validated by mutagenesis studies (75).

Cytomegalovirus

CMV lacks a TK but carries another kinase, encoded by the UL97 gene, which is essential for the production of normal amounts of infectious virus in cell culture and is a potential antiviral drug target (166). GCV, the standard initial therapy for CMV disease, is monophosphorylated by the UL97 kinase and subsequently converted to the active triphosphate form in infected cells (193). Risk factors for CMV resistance include high levels of ongoing viral replication—such as those seen in immunocompromised hosts—coupled with antiviral drug exposure of a few months or more (76). Since the advent of combination antiretroviral therapy, there has been a marked decrease in drug-resistant CMV infection in HIV-infected persons. However, the routine use of anti-CMV therapy in transplant recipients has caused an increase in drug resistance, particularly in patients with posttransplant primary CMV infection and lung transplantation (76).

More than 90% of GCV-resistant CMV isolates contain UL97 mutations (37) that are proven or presumed to impair GCV phosphorylation. To preserve the important functions of UL97 in the viral life cycle, these mutations are preferentially localized to codons 460, 520, and 590 to 607, with the most common being M460VI, H520Q, C592G, A594V, L595S, and C603W (37). Various other point mutations and in-frame deletion mutations conferring resistance have been observed at codons 590 to 607, while others in this region may confer little or no drug resistance (37). Occasionally, GCV resistance is caused instead by mutations in the UL54 DNA polymerase gene (*pol*), in the absence of UL97 mutations (62). Genotypic resistance testing is the standard clinical diagnostic practice for CMV because of the limited number of UL97 codons involved and the technical difficulty of phenotypic testing. UL97 is not known or expected to be involved in resistance to FOS or CDV.

After continued exposure to GCV, mutations in the UL54 *pol* gene may accumulate, usually in the presence of preexisting UL97 mutations, and may contribute to an increased level of resistance to the drug (40, 187). Recombinant phenotyping confirms that a combination of UL97 and *pol* mutations confers high-level GCV resistance (42). GCV and CDV resistance mutations in UL54 have been reported for codons 301, 408 to 413, and 501 to 545, corresponding to the exonuclease IV and δC regions of *pol*, and for codons 978 to 988 (region V) (39).

FOS resistance mutations in CMV *pol* often involve conserved regions II (e.g., codons 700 and 715), III (e.g., codons 802 and 809), and VI (e.g., codon 781), as well as some nonconserved loci (e.g., codon 756) (76). Some FOS resistance mutations in region III confer low-grade cross-resistance to GCV (41). The nonviability of an L845P *pol* mutant indicates that this region of *pol* is likely essential in the recognition of the incoming nucleotide triphosphate and in pyrophosphate exchange (41). Very occasionally, single *pol* mutations are sufficient to confer resistance to all three of the above drugs, i.e., GCV, CDV, and FOS (42, 178). Finally, some CMV *pol* mutations have been associated with a slow-growth phenotype (76).

The wide distribution of known and potential CMV *pol* resistance mutations means that genotypic resistance testing requires sequencing from codons 300 to 1000. Furthermore, the interpretation of results is more complicated than that for UL97. Despite a fairly extensive database, there remain many sequence changes in *pol* that are indeterminate for drug resistance and require further analysis by recombinant phenotyping (76).

Maribavir, a benzimidazole L-riboside that inhibits the viral UL97 kinase, is an investigational CMV drug that has entered late-stage clinical trials (16). Maribavir-resistant laboratory CMV mutants have been isolated that contain mutations in UL97 (37) or UL27 (38). Another class of experimental drugs with clinical promise targets viral DNA

cleavage and processing; resistant strains have mutations in UL56, UL89, or UL104 (6).

HUMAN IMMUNODEFICIENCY VIRUS

Twenty-four antiretroviral drugs belonging to six mechanistic classes have been licensed for HIV-1 treatment, including seven nucleoside and one nucleotide reverse transcriptase inhibitor (NRTI), nine protease inhibitors (PIs), four nonnucleoside RT inhibitors (NNRTIs), one fusion inhibitor, one integrase inhibitor (INI), and one CCR5 inhibitor. Among these 24 inhibitors, the NRTI dideoxycytidine and the NNRTI delavirdine are rarely, if ever, used, and the PI ritonavir (RTV) is used solely to inhibit the metabolism of other PIs, thereby increasing their levels. One NNRTI, one INI, and one CCR5 inhibitor are in phase III clinical trials. Table 2 summarizes the antiviral agents, mechanisms of resistance, and mutations involved in drug resistance in HIV-1.

HIV-1 genetic variability results from the high rate of RT enzyme errors, the high rate of virus replication in vivo, recombination when viruses with different sequences infect the same cell, and the accumulation of proviral variants during the course of infection (43). The virus population within an individual does not consist of a single genotype but is instead an ensemble of innumerable related genotypes or quasispecies. The selection of drug-resistant variants depends on the extent to which virus replication continues during incompletely suppressive therapy, the ease of acquisition of a particular mutation (or set of mutations), and the effect of drug resistance mutations on drug susceptibility and virus replication.

In previously untreated individuals with drug-susceptible HIV-1, combinations of three drugs from two drug classes lead to prolonged virus suppression and, in most patients, immune reconstitution. Once complete HIV-1 suppression is achieved, it usually persists indefinitely as long as therapy is not interrupted. However, because antiretroviral therapy does not inhibit proviral HIV-1 DNA, viral eradication is not possible. Recurrent viremia and immunological decline ensue whenever therapy is discontinued, regardless of the previous duration of virological suppression.

HIV-1 drug resistance may be acquired or transmitted. Drug resistance is acquired in patients in whom ongoing virus replication occurs in the presence of suboptimal antiviral therapy. Whereas suboptimal virus therapy was once a consequence of an insufficient number of active drugs, it is now usually a consequence of treatment interruptions or incomplete adherence. Transmitted drug resistance accounts for about 15% of new infections in the United States, 10% of new infections in Europe, 5% of new infections in South and Central America, and <5% of new infections in most parts of sub-Saharan Africa and South and Southeast Asia (30, 73, 202).

The presence of either acquired or transmitted drug resistance prior to starting a new antiretroviral treatment regimen is an independent predictor of the virological response to that regimen (93, 111, 130). In addition, prospective clinical trials have shown that drug resistance testing, particularly genotypic testing, provides clinical benefit in selecting treatment for infected individuals (94).

Nucleoside/Nucleotide RT Inhibitor Resistance

The NRTIs are prodrugs that must be triphosphorylated, or diphosphorylated in the case of the nucleotide tenofovir (TDF), to achieve their active form. This dependence

TABLE 2 Mechanisms of resistance to HIV-1 inhibitors

Drug(s)	Mechanism of resistance	Drug resistance mutations
NRTIs (abacavir [ABC], didanosine [ddI], emtricitabine [FTC], lamivudine [3TC], stavudine [d4T], zidovudine [ZDV], tenofovir [TDF])	RT mutations that allow the enzyme to discriminate between NRTIs and naturally occurring nucleosides	M184V mutation confers high-level resistance to 3TC and FTC; K65R mutation confers high-level resistance to ddI, ABC, and TDF, intermediate resistance to 3TC and FTC, low-level resistance to d4T, and increased susceptibility to ZDV; L74V mutation confers resistance to ddI and ABC; Q151M mutation occurs in association with A62V, V75I, F77L, and F116Y mutations and confers high-level resistance to ZDV, d4T, ddI, and ABC and intermediate resistance to TDF, 3TC, and FTC
	RT mutations that promote ATP-dependent hydrolytic removal of chain-terminating nucleotide monophosphates (selected by thymidine analogs and also referred to as TAMs)	M41L, D67N, K70R, L210W, T215FY, and K219QE mutations develop in viruses from patients receiving ZDV and d4T but confer cross-resistance with the other NRTIs, except for 3TC and FTC; T69SS mutation is an uncommon double-amino-acid insertion that confers resistance to each of the NRTIs when it occurs in combination with multiple TAMs; E44D and V118I mutations are among the many accessory NRTI resistance mutations that usually occur in combination with TAMs
NNRTIs (efavirenz [EFV], etravirine [ETR], nevirapine [NVP], rilpivirine[a])	Mutations in the HIV-1 RT NNRTI-binding pocket	K103N, V106AM, Y188L, and G190AS mutations are associated with high-level resistance to NVP and EFV; Y181C mutation is associated with high-level resistance to NVP, intermediate resistance to ETR, and low-level resistance to EFV; Y181C (and particularly Y181IV) mutation, in combination with additional mutations, such as L100I, K101P, V179F, and M230L, is associated with high-level resistance to all NNRTIs; A98G, K101E, V106I, V108I, E138AK, V179D/E, H221Y, P225H, F227L, and K238T mutations are accessory NNRTI resistance mutations
PIs (atazanavir [ATV], darunavir [DRV], fosamprenavir [FPV], indinavir [IDV], lopinavir plus ribavirin [LPV/r], nelfinavir [NFV], saquinavir [SQV], tipranavir [TPV])	Protease mutations interfere with inhibitor binding or compensate for the decreased replication associated with other mutations	Substrate cleft mutations: L23I, D30N, V32I, I47VA, G48VMA, I50VL, V82AFSTMC, and I84VAC; flap mutations: M46IL, F53L, and I54VMTLAS; mutations at other generally conserved positions: L10IVFR, V11I, K20IT, L24IF, L33F, K43T, Q58E, A71VTIL, G73SCTA, T74P, L76V, N88DSTG, L89I, and L90M; although several of the major mutations are strongly linked to individual PIs, the extent of cross-resistance among PIs is complicated when multiple PI-resistant mutations occur in combination
INIs (raltegravir [RAL], elvitegravir[a])	Mutations in residues surrounding the enzyme's active site	Q148HKR mutation, with or without G140S mutation, confers high-level resistance to RAL and elvitegravir; N155H-plus-E92Q mutation confers high-level resistance to RAL and elvitegravir; Y143CR-plus-T97A mutation confers high-level resistance to RAL; T66I and S147G mutations have been selected for only by elvitegravir and appear to have a minimal effect on RAL; F121Y mutation is a RAL and elvitegravir resistance mutation that has not been observed in vivo; multiple accessory INI resistance mutations have also been reported
Fusion inhibitor (enfuvirtide [ENF])	Mutations in the first heptad repeat region (HR1) of the gp41 transmembrane protein	ENF is a peptide mimetic of the HR2 region of gp41; drug resistance mutations in the HR1 region interfere with the association of the HR1 and HR2 domains necessary for virus-cell fusion; in vitro and in vivo, mutations occur in a highly conserved region between gp41 residues 36 and 45
CCR5 inhibitors (maraviroc [MVC], vicriviroc[a])	In clinical settings, virological failure and resistance are usually caused by the expansion of a preexisting CXCR4-tropic variant that was not detected at the start of therapy; in vitro and, occasionally, in vivo resistance is caused by gp120 mutations that facilitate binding to an inhibitor-bound CCR5 molecule	There are many reports of specific mutations, mutational profiles, and algorithms, such as position-specific scoring matrices, for predicting tropism based on HIV-1 gp120 V3 sequences; no consistent pattern of gp120 mutations has been identified to be associated with virus binding to an inhibitor-bound CCR5 receptor

[a]Rilpivirine, elvitegravir, and vicriviroc are in phase III clinical trials. An up-to-date summary linking individual RT, protease, and integrase mutations to NRTIs, NNRTIs, PIs, and INIs can be found at http://hivdb.stanford.edu/pages/drugSummaries.html.

on intracellular phosphorylation complicates the in vitro assessment of both NRTI activity and NRTI resistance, because phosphorylation occurs at different rates in different cell types and leads to marked discordances between in vitro and in vivo NRTI potencies. Specifically, differences between the highly activated lymphocytes used for susceptibility testing and the wider variety of cells that are infected in vivo likely explain why the NRTIs differ in their dynamic susceptibility ranges and in their clinically significant levels of in vitro resistance (140). Clinical isolates from persons failing NRTI therapy may have several-hundred-fold reductions in susceptibility to zidovudine (ZDV), lamivudine (3TC), and emtricitabine (FTC) but will rarely have more than fivefold reductions in susceptibility to didanosine (ddI), stavudine (d4T), and TDF. However, even very slight reductions in susceptibility to the second category of drugs—as low as 1.5-fold—are clinically significant (216).

There are two biochemical mechanisms of NRTI resistance. One mechanism is mediated by discriminatory mutations that reduce the affinity of RT for an NRTI, preventing its addition to the growing DNA chain (173). Another mechanism is mediated by primer-unblocking mutations that favor the hydrolytic removal of an NRTI that has been incorporated into the HIV-1 primer chain (8, 140). Primer-unblocking mutations, because they are selected by the thymidine analog inhibitors ZDV and d4T, are also referred to as thymidine analog mutations (TAMs).

All recommended first-line treatment regimens include one of the cytosine analogs—3TC or FTC—because they have been found to be essential to the success of most NRTI-containing first-line regimens. Although 3TC and FTC are highly potent, they each have a low genetic barrier to resistance, in that a single mutation—M184V (or, less commonly, M184I)—confers a >200-fold decrease in susceptibility to these drugs. Indeed, M184V is the most common mutation to emerge in patients developing virological failure on a first-line regimen. Although the M184V mutation limits the effectiveness of 3TC and FTC in salvage therapy, these drugs retain some benefit even in the presence of the M184V mutation, possibly because this mutation reduces HIV-1 replication and increases HIV-1 susceptibility to ZDV, d4T, and TDF (216). Although the M184V mutation decreases ddI and abacavir (ABC) susceptibility, about 1.5-fold and 3-fold, respectively, these inhibitors retain moderate activity against viruses containing this mutation alone (216).

The most common primer-unblocking mutations, or TAMs, include M41L, D67N, K70R, L210W, T215Y/F, and K219Q/E. A subset of these mutations—M41L, L210W, and T215Y—is particularly important for causing cross-resistance to ddI, ABC, and TDF (114, 141, 143). In patients receiving regimens without thymidine analogs, the K65R and L74V mutations have replaced the TAMs as the mutations that occur most commonly in combination with the M184V mutation. The K65R mutation causes low-level resistance to d4T, intermediate resistance to 3TC and FTC, and high-level resistance to ABC, ddI, and TDF; however, it increases susceptibility to ZDV (157).

The T69SSS and Q151M mutations are multi-NRTI resistance mutations. The T69SSS mutation is a double-amino-acid insertion at HIV-1 RT position 69. It nearly always occurs with multiple TAMs, and in this setting it causes intermediate resistance to 3TC and FTC and high-level resistance to the remaining NRTIs (135). The Q151M mutation usually occurs in combination with several otherwise uncommon mutations (A62V, V75I, F77L,

and F116Y). It causes intermediate resistance to TDF, 3TC, and FTC and high-level resistance to the remaining NRTIs (179, 185).

Nonnucleoside RT Inhibitor Resistance

Efavirenz (EFV), nevirapine (NVP), and etravirine (ETR) are the most commonly used NNRTIs. The NNRTIs inhibit HIV-1 RT allosterically by binding to a hydrophobic pocket close to the enzyme's active site. This hydrophobic "NNRTI-binding" pocket is less well conserved than the enzyme's active deoxynucleoside triphosphate-binding site. Indeed, HIV-2 and HIV-1 group O viruses are intrinsically resistant to most NNRTIs (218), and HIV-1 group M viruses have greater interisolate variability in their susceptibility to NNRTIs than to NRTIs (158).

Resistance emerges rapidly when NNRTIs are administered as monotherapy or in the presence of incomplete virus suppression, suggesting that NNRTI resistance is caused by the selection of rare preexisting populations of mutant viruses within an individual. NVP and EFV have low genetic barriers to resistance, in that a single mutation in the NNRTI-binding pocket may result in high-level resistance to one or more NNRTIs. ETR has a higher genetic barrier to resistance, and a minimum of two mutations are required to significantly reduce its activity in vivo (204). ETR's increased genetic barrier to resistance is a result of its ability to rearrange itself, thereby adopting multiple binding modes within the NNRTI-binding pocket (51).

The NRTIs and NNRTIs are often synergistic. Several NNRTI resistance mutations increase susceptibility to certain NRTIs (115), and combinations of certain NRTI resistance mutations increase NNRTI susceptibility (215).

Protease Inhibitor Resistance

There are nine FDA-licensed PIs: atazanavir (ATV), darunavir (DRV), fosamprenavir (FPV), indinavir (IDV), lopinavir (LPV), nelfinavir (NVP), RTV, saquinavir (SQV), and tipranavir (TPV). NFV and IDV, although once commonly used, are rarely clinically indicated because of their poor pharmacokinetic properties when administered alone and their toxicity when administered with RTV. Of the remaining PIs, LPV (which is coformulated with RTV), DRV, SQV, and TPV are licensed for use with RTV boosting (denoted by "/r" following the PI name); ATV and FPV are licensed for use with and without RTV boosting.

Mutations in the substrate cleft reduce the binding affinity between PIs and mutant protease enzymes. Mutations elsewhere in the enzyme either compensate for the decreased kinetics of enzymes with active-site mutations or cause resistance by altering enzyme catalysis, dimer stability, or inhibitor binding kinetics or by reshaping the active site through long-range structural perturbations (63). Mutations at several of the protease cleavage sites are also selected during PI treatment, improving the kinetics of protease enzymes with PI resistance mutations (49, 108).

More than 80 nonpolymorphic, PI-selected mutations have been reported (180), and most of these contribute to decreased in vitro susceptibility to one or more PIs (169). The mutations with the greatest impact on susceptibility are in the substrate cleft, such as D30N, V32I, I47VA, G48VM, I50VL, V82ATLFS, and I84VAC. However, several mutations in the enzyme flap, including M46IL and I54VMLTSA, and in the enzyme core, such as L76V and N88S, can also profoundly influence susceptibility. At several positions, different mutations can have greatly different effects on PI susceptibility (169).

RTV-boosted PIs, particularly LPV/r and DRV/r, have a high genetic barrier to resistance, and multiple mutations are required to compromise antiviral activity (56, 103). Several proof-of-concept studies have shown that LPV/r alone is effective at fully suppressing HIV-1 RNA levels to below detectable levels for 48 weeks in more than two-thirds of patients (15). In addition, viruses from patients with virological failure on an initial boosted PI-containing regimen rarely contain PI resistance mutations. A large proportion of such patients experience resuppression of virus levels without a change in therapy, suggesting that virological failure of an initial boosted PI-containing regimen is often a result of nonadherence (15).

Integrase Inhibitor Resistance

Following reverse transcription and the generation of double-stranded viral DNA, HIV-1 integrase catalyzes the cleavage of the conserved 3′ dinucleotide CA (3′ processing) and the ligation of the viral 3′-OH ends to the 5′ DNA of host chromosomal DNA (strand transfer). HIV-1 integrase is composed of three functional domains: the N-terminal domain, encompassing amino acids 1 to 50; the catalytic core domain (CCD), which encompasses amino acids 51 to 212 and contains the catalytic triad D64, D116, and E152; and the C-terminal domain, which encompasses amino acids 213 to 288 and is involved in nonspecific binding to host chromosomal DNA. The catalytic triad requires divalent metal cations to catalyze the strand transfer reaction.

Crystal structures of the CCD plus the C-terminal domain (31) and the CCD plus the N-terminal domain (207) have been solved, but the relative conformations of the three domains of the active multimeric form of the enzyme are not known. There is one published crystal structure of the CCD bound to an early prototype diketo acid inhibitor, 5CITEP (77), but there are none of the CCD domain bound to the one approved INI, raltegravir (RAL), or to any of the INIs in clinical development. However, based on the 5CITEP structure and several modeling studies, it has been shown that HIV-1 integrase strand transfer inhibitors bind within the CCD active site and chelate the divalent metal ions critical for enzymatic function (33, 207).

Three genetic mechanisms of RAL resistance have been identified: (i) G140S-plus-Q148HKR mutation, (ii) N155H-plus-E92Q mutation, and (iii) Y143CR-plus-T97A mutation (65). Each of these combinations of mutations confers a >100-fold-decreased RAL susceptibility and causes a loss of virological suppression in patients receiving RAL. Q148 interacts with a 5′-terminal cytosine of viral DNA and likely forms a hydrogen bond with most INIs (33). N155 points into the active site and forms a hydrogen bond with D116, one of the three catalytic aspartate residues (137). Y143 is part of the highly flexible active-site loop that participates in DNA and INI binding (4). The Q148 mutations and the N155H and E92Q mutations are each associated with high-level cross-resistance to the investigational INI elvitegravir. Y143 mutations do not appear to reduce elvitegravir susceptibility. Likewise, elvitegravir resistance mutations, such as T66I and S147G, have not been associated with RAL cross-resistance (184).

Fusion Inhibitor Resistance

The HIV-1 envelope consists of surface (gp120) and transmembrane (gp41) glycoproteins. gp120 binds to the CD4 receptor and to one of the chemokine coreceptors (CCR5 or CXCR4) on target cells. After gp120-CD4 coreceptor binding, gp41 undergoes a conformational change that promotes fusion of viral and cellular membranes. Two heptad repeat regions (HR1 and HR2) of gp41 form a helical bundle of HR1 and HR2 trimers. Enfuvirtide (ENF) is a highly active synthetic peptide that inhibits fusion by binding to HR1 and preventing it from bundling with HR2 (106).

ENF-resistant isolates contain either single or double mutations between positions 36 and 45 of gp41 HR1 (142). Single mutants typically have on the order of 10-fold-decreased susceptibility to ENF, whereas double mutants are about 100-fold less susceptible. Despite its being one of the most potent antiretroviral drugs, the genetic barrier to ENF resistance is low, and virological rebound emerges rapidly if ENF is not administered with a sufficient number of other active inhibitors (128).

CCR5 Inhibitor Resistance

Maraviroc (MVC) allosterically inhibits the binding of HIV-1 gp120 to the seven-transmembrane-domain G protein-coupled CCR5 receptor (89). Whereas HIV-1 gp120 binds to the N terminus and the second extracellular loop region of CCR5, MVC binds to a pocket formed by the transmembrane helices (131). Despite the high variability in gp120, there are minimal differences in the susceptibilities of wild-type viruses to MVC and other CCR5 inhibitors, suggesting that these inhibitors disrupt a highly conserved protein-protein interaction (59, 190).

CCR5 inhibitor resistance develops during in vitro passage experiments via gp120 mutations that enable HIV-1 to bind to the CCR5–CCR5-inhibitor complex (212). Resistance via this mechanism, however, does not occur rapidly, nor does it occur by a consistent pattern of gp120 mutations. In patients receiving CCR5 inhibitors, the most common mechanism of virological failure is the expansion of preexisting CXCR4-tropic viruses that are intrinsically insensitive to CCR5 inhibitors (211). Less commonly, virological failure emerges via mutations that allow HIV-1 to bind to the CCR5–CCR5-inhibitor complex (145).

Intersubtype Variation

During its spread among humans, group M HIV-1 has evolved into multiple subtypes that differ from one another by 10 to 30% along their genomes (109). Antiretroviral drugs used to treat HIV-1 were developed by use of subtype B isolates—the predominant subtype in North America and Western Europe—and the vast majority of data on the genetic mechanisms of HIV-1 drug resistance were generated from observations on subtype B viruses. However, HIV-1 subtype B viruses account for only ~10% of the global HIV pandemic.

HIV-1 protease and RT genes belonging to different subtypes differ from one another by 10 to 12% of their nucleotides and 5 to 6% of their amino acids. Naturally occurring polymorphisms differ between subtypes but are not responsible for clinically significant effects on drug susceptibility (159). Although the drug resistance mutations observed in subtype B viruses are also the main drug resistance mutations in non-B subtypes (100), several studies have reported differences in the frequencies with which specific mutations occur in different subtype viruses subjected to the same antiretroviral drugs (19, 26, 27, 82, 192). Of most clinical relevance are the data suggesting that the multi-NRTI-resistant mutation K65R may occur more frequently in certain non-B subtypes, particularly subtype C (95, 98).

HEPATITIS B VIRUS

HBV is a partially double-stranded DNA virus of about 3.2 kb. Following infection, its genome localizes to the nucleus, where it is converted to a covalently closed circular DNA (cccDNA) form that serves as the template for transcription of mRNA and genomic RNA. Genomic RNA is reverse transcribed to viral DNA, and the resulting viral cores either bud into the endoplasmic reticulum and are exported from the cell or return to the nucleus for conversion back to cccDNA (71). HBV cccDNA is highly stable and can be eliminated by cell turnover but not by drug therapy (210). Therefore, complete cure or eradication of infection is highly unusual with current antiviral therapy.

HBV replicates at a high rate and produces an estimated 10^{11} virions per day (153). In the absence of therapy, HBV DNA levels are often as high as 10^8 to 10^{10} copies/ml. The HBV polymerase is considered an RT because of the prominent role of reverse transcription in HBV replication. HBV RT is functionally and structurally similar to HIV-1 RT and has an error rate similar to that of other retroviral polymerases (87). However, the overlapping arrangement of open reading frames in the HBV genome limits the viability of many spontaneous mutants (221). For example, the nucleotides encoding the HBV RT also encode the HBV envelope, in a different reading frame. Therefore, the rate at which mutations become fixed is estimated to be considerably lower than that for HIV-1 (24). HBV is classified into eight genotypes differing from one another by about 10% of their nucleotides; although several small studies suggest that viruses belonging to different genotypes may respond differently to interferon (IFN), there is no evidence that viral genotype influences the response to nucleoside analogs (125, 150).

Anti-HBV Drug Therapy

During the past 5 years, three new nucleoside analog inhibitors (NRTIs) have been licensed by the FDA, highly sensitive quantitative PCR assays have become the standard for monitoring HBV therapy, and new guidelines recommend genotypic resistance testing for patients who experience primary or secondary virological failure while receiving NRTIs (101, 102, 126, 127). The most recent generation of real-time PCR assays have a wide dynamic range and are sensitive enough to detect HBV DNA levels in plasma of as low as about 10 to 15 WHO IU/ml (about 50 to 100 HBV DNA copies/ml) (171). Although in vitro phenotypic testing is the gold standard used to confirm genotypic antiviral

resistance, it cannot be performed routinely because of the lack of a convenient standardized cell culture system (127).

There are two forms of IFN and five nucleoside or nucleotide analogs (NRTIs) licensed for the treatment of chronic HBV infection. IFN-α was licensed in 1992, and pegylated IFN-α 2a was licensed in 2005. The five licensed nucleosides include 3TC (licensed in 1998), adefovir (ADV) (licensed in 2002), entecavir (ETV) (licensed in 2005), telbivudine (β-L-2′-deoxythymidine [LdT]) (licensed in 2006), and TDF (licensed in 2008). FTC, which is structurally similar to 3TC, is also active against HBV and is frequently used to treat HBV because it is coformulated with TDF (as Truvada) for HIV treatment. 3TC, FTC, and LdT are L-nucleoside analogs. ADV and TDF are acylic nucleotide analogs, and ETV is a deoxyguanosine analog. Table 3 summarizes the antiviral agents, mechanisms of resistance, and mutations involved in drug resistance in HBV.

IFN-α, particularly pegylated IFN-α, remains an important treatment option for HBV infection. Used in combination with NRTIs, it has proven highly effective at suppressing virus levels (163) and at inducing sustained remissions and HBsAg seroconversion in some patients (149). A lack of response to IFN-α, however, is not associated with specific HBV changes, suggesting that IFN-α resistance, although it may be partly genotype dependent, generally reflects host rather than viral factors.

HBV RT and Nucleoside Analog Resistance

The three-dimensional structure of HBV RT has not been solved because of difficulty in obtaining sufficient amounts of highly purified active protein. However, homology modeling with other polymerases, including HIV-1 RT, has provided insight into the role of many of its residues (10, 52). In 2001, a standardized numbering system for mutations was established for the RT part of the HBV *pol* gene (191).

3TC, the first licensed NRTI, is no longer recommended for use as monotherapy because of the high incidence of drug resistance associated with its use: 15% to 30% of individuals treated for 1 year, 40% to 50% of those treated for 3 years, and 70% of those treated for 5 years developed 3TC resistance (113, 133). High-level (>1,000-fold) 3TC resistance is caused by the M204VI mutation, which is in the YMDD motif adjacent to two of the RT enzyme's catalytic aspartates (199). Modeling studies suggest that the M204VI mutation sterically inhibits HBV RT binding to 3TC (52). M204 mutations are also frequently

TABLE 3 Mechanisms of resistance to HBV inhibitors

Antiviral agent(s)	Mechanism of resistance	Mutations[b]
IFN-α	Unknown	Unknown
Ribavirin	Unknown	Unknown
L-Nucleoside analogs (lamivudine [3TC], telbivudine [LdT], emtricitabine [FTC][a]) acyclic nucleotide analogs (adefovir [ADV], tenofovir [TDF]), and a deoxyguanosine analog (entecavir [ETV])	RT mutations that interfere with nucleotide triphosphate binding; whether any of these mutations also facilitate primer unblocking is not known	M204VI, L180M, V173L, and L80M mutations emerge during 3TC treatment and confer cross-resistance to LdT and FTC and partial cross-resistance to ETV; M204VI mutation also emerges during LdT therapy; N236T mutation emerges during therapy with ADV and causes partial cross-resistance to TDF; A181VT mutation emerges during therapy with ADV and, less commonly, with 3TC, and causes partial resistance to TDF but not to ETV; I169T, T184G, S202I, and M250V mutations emerge during therapy with ETV, particularly when ETV is used for the treatment of 3TC-resistant viruses

[a] FTC is not licensed for HBV treatment. However, it is frequently used in combination with TDF for salvage therapy because there is a coformulation of the two drugs (Truvada).

[b] Several mutations are not shown because they are either extremely rare (e.g., M204S and A181S) or because their association with resistance is controversial (e.g., A233V for ADV and A194T for TDF).

accompanied by compensatory mutations, particularly L180M and, less commonly, V173L and/or L80I (5, 55, 155, 209). M204VI and its accompanying mutations cause high-level cross-resistance to FTC and LdT and a lower level of cross-resistance to ETV. Although LdT is associated with a decreased incidence of drug resistance after 2 years compared with that for 3TC (11% versus 26%), it is also not a preferred option for initial therapy (124, 126).

The emergence of ETV resistance is exceedingly uncommon when it is used for the treatment of NRTI-naive patients (198). Although ETV retains considerable antiviral activity against 3TC-resistant variants (181), the risk of virological failure and emergence of high-level ETV resistance is much higher in patients with 3TC resistance than in NRTI-naive patients. The presence of M204VI-plus-L180M mutation and two or three of the following additional mutations—I169T, T184G, S202I, and M250V—leads to high-level ETV resistance (36, 181, 196–198).

ADV and TDF retain activity against viruses with the 3TC resistance mutations M204VI, L180M, V173L, and L80M (162, 214). However, TDF's increased potency likely renders it the preferred option for treating 3TC-resistant viruses (102, 127, 132). When ADV is used in patients with 3TC resistance, it is more effective in combination with 3TC than it is alone, possibly because ADV may be more active against 3TC-resistant than wild-type viruses (102, 126, 127, 167).

ADV resistance emerges more slowly than 3TC resistance, occurring in about 10% and 30% of individuals after 2 and 5 years, respectively (88, 133, 213). The N236T and A181VT mutations, which are close to the HBV active site, reduce ADV susceptibility (7, 18, 68, 88, 172). Although the levels of reduced susceptibility associated with these mutations—3- to 10-fold—are much lower than the level of 3TC resistance conferred by M204VI mutation, these reductions in ADV susceptibility are associated with virologic breakthrough (7, 68).

The HBV RT A181VT mutation is unique in that it confers resistance to both L-nucleosides and acyclic nucleotides and has been reported to emerge in individuals receiving 3TC as well as ADV (18, 203, 220). The A181T mutation is of particular interest because it causes a stop codon in the reading frame coding for the surface protein, potentially allowing for ongoing hepatocellular replication without accompanying viral load rebound (208). The N236T mutation causes partial cross-resistance to TDF but not to 3TC, ETV, or LdT (219).

Virological and clinical resistance to TDF is exceedingly uncommon in NRTI-naive individuals. However, the ADV resistance mutations N236T and A181VT confer partial cross-resistance to TDF (195, 200, 225), and in such patients, ETV or TDF plus an L-nucleoside is recommended (102).

HEPATITIS C VIRUS

HCV is a positive-sense, single-stranded, enveloped virus with a genome of about 9.5 kb. The six major HCV genotypes differ from each other by more than 35% along their genomes (186, 223). Like HIV-1, HCV exists in vivo as a complex quasispecies consisting of an ensemble of viral genomes differing from one another by up to 10% (134). Although the combination of pegylated IFN-α and ribavirin is currently the only approved treatment for HCV (74), many HCV-specific inhibitors are in advanced clinical development. Table 4

TABLE 4 Mechanisms of resistance to HCV inhibitors

Antiviral agent(s)	Mechanism of resistance	Mutations
IFN-α	Unknown	Genotype 1 isolates respond less well than genotype 2 or 3 isolates, but the molecular basis for this is not known
Ribavirin	Unknown; ribavirin's mechanism of action most likely involves inhibition of IMP dehydrogenase; it may also involve direct RdRp inhibition, lethal mutagenesis, or modulation of immune responses	Unknown
PIs[a] (telaprevir [phase III], boceprevir [phase III], macrocylic inhibitors [TMC435, BI201335, ITMN-191, MK-7009])	Substrate cleft mutations that interfere with inhibitor binding	V36AM, T54A, V55A, R155KT, A156SVT, and V170AT mutations are selected by and associated with decreased susceptibility to telaprevir and boceprevir; in clinical trials, combinations of mutations at positions 36 and 155 or 156 have been associated with high-level telaprevir resistance; preliminary data suggest that mutations at positions 155 and 168 may be the most important mutations conferring macrocyclic inhibitor resistance
Nucleoside inhibitors[a] (NM203 [withdrawn], R1626 [withdrawn], R7128 [phase II])	Steric hindrance of nucleoside analog incorporation	S282T mutation in combination with compensatory mutations has been selected both in vitro and in vivo by 2'-C-methyl-modified nucleoside analogs, including valopcitabine (NM203; an oral prodrug of the nucleoside analog 2'-C-methylcytidine) and R7128 (a prodrug of PSI-6130); S96T mutation, with or without N142T mutation, was selected in vitro by R1626 (a prodrug of R1479 [4'-azidocytidine]) but was not observed in a clinical trial in which R1626 was used in combination with pegylated IFN-α 2a and ribavirin
Nonnucleoside inhibitors[a]	Interference with binding to each of the four allosteric binding pockets that have been identified	Multiple mutations have emerged during in vitro passage with each of the nonnucleoside inhibitors in development; these mutations are localized to the known allosteric RdRp sites

[a] All directly acting small-molecule inhibitors of HCV are in clinical development.

summarizes the antiviral agents, mechanisms of resistance, and mutations involved in drug resistance in HCV.

Interferon and Ribavirin

Pegylated IFN-α plus ribavirin for 6 to 12 months is the standard treatment for HCV. A dose-response relationship exists between the nucleoside analog ribavirin and the likelihood of virus suppression, but the mechanism by which ribavirin acts is not known. The leading hypothesis is that ribavirin interferes with deoxynucleoside triphosphate metabolism by inhibiting cellular IMP dehydrogenase (116, 183). Additional hypotheses include a role for ribavirin in directly inhibiting HCV RNA polymerase (129), increasing HCV mutagenesis (35, 50), or modulating the T-cell immune response to HCV (183).

Several findings suggest that viral factors influence the response to therapy with IFN. First, HCV genotype 2 and 3 viruses are significantly more likely than genotype 1 viruses to respond to IFN (sustained virological response rates of about 70% versus 30%) (74, 119). Second, therapy is more successful in acutely infected persons, possibly because they harbor less-complex mixtures of quasispecies than persons who are chronically infected (64). Finally, and most controversially, several authors have proposed that a 40-amino-acid region of NS5A influences IFN responsiveness (61). However, no specific mutations have been shown to be selected by or cause resistance to either IFN or ribavirin.

Investigational Direct-Acting Antivirals

Protease Inhibitors

Small-molecule inhibitors targeting the NS3 serine protease and the NS5B RNA-dependent RNA polymerase (RdRp) are the subject of intense drug discovery efforts. At least 12 compounds are in phase II or III trials, and at least 12 more are in phase I trials (23, 177). Five additional investigational inhibitors are no longer being developed because of toxicities observed in clinical trials. Many of the small-molecule inhibitors have been designed to inhibit HCV genotype 1 viruses because genotype 1 viruses are the most common HCVs in the United States and Europe and are the most difficult to treat with IFN plus ribavirin.

The NS3 serine protease comprises the 189 N-terminal amino acids of NS3. NS3 forms a heterodimer with the 54-amino-acid NS4A protein (NS3/4A), and together they cleave four sites in the HCV polypeptide precursor to generate the N termini of NS4A, NS4B, NS5A, and NS5B. NS3/4A also appears to take part in host immune evasion by cleaving several critical intracellular immune mediators (70). NS3/4A serine protease is a challenging drug target because it has a shallow substrate-binding pocket that normally binds a long peptide substrate with which it forms multiple weak interactions (112). Several three-dimensional structures of NS3/4A, with and without inhibitors, have been determined (161).

Inhibitors targeting the NS3/4A complex include peptidomimetics, such as telaprevir (92) and boceprevir (13), which are in phase III clinical trials, and several macrocyclic inhibitors, which are at earlier stages of clinical development (175). Telaprevir and boceprevir monotherapies each produce marked but transient reductions in HCV levels in plasma that are followed by virological rebound and drug resistance (194). However, in phase II trials, these inhibitors have been used in combination with pegylated IFN-α and ribavirin and have led to rates of sustained virological suppression that are about 20% higher than the rates observed with standard therapy (92, 138).

The mutations associated with telaprevir and boceprevir resistance are similar and are generally in the protease substrate cleft, and they include V36AM, T54A, V55A, R155KT, A156SVT, and V170AT mutations (105, 176, 177, 194). In clinical trials, a combination of two telaprevir mutations, usually mutations at positions 36 and 155 or 156, is required for high-level telaprevir resistance. Preliminary data suggest that mutations at positions 155 and 168 may also be important mutations associated with resistance to the investigational macrocyclic inhibitors (104, 177).

Although the mutations associated with HCV PI resistance are for the most part conserved in HCV sequences from genotype 1 viruses, sporadic mutations at these positions have been reported both as majority variants detectable by standard sequencing and as variants detected by deep sequencing methods (9, 110). Of greater clinical significance, however, is the observation that the PIs appear to have different activities against viruses belonging to different genotypes. For example, telaprevir monotherapy produced median 4.4-, 3.9-, 0.5-, and 0.9-log$_{10}$ IU/ml reductions in virus levels in patients with genotype 1, 2, 3, and 4 viruses, respectively (177).

Polymerase Inhibitors

HCV RdRp is comprised of the 530 N-terminal amino acids encoded by the NS5B gene. A C-terminal extension of NS5B anchors the catalytic domain to the endoplasmic reticulum as part of a larger viral replication complex that includes the NS3 RNA helicase. HCV RdRp, like other polymerases, contains palm, thumb, and finger subdomains that enclose the RNA template groove and a GDD catalytic triad (161). HCV RdRp inhibitors include chain-terminating nucleoside analogs and nonnucleoside analogs that target NS5B allosterically.

Nucleoside analog RdRp inhibitors appear to be equally active against the different HCV genotypes. The genetic barrier to nucleoside analog resistance also appears to be higher than that for the other two main classes of HCV inhibitors. Prolonged passage in vitro is required for the emergence of resistance, and the mutations associated with nucleoside analog resistance generally reduce viral fitness (3). Two non-cross-resistant mutational patterns associated with nucleoside analog resistance have been described. The S282T mutation in combination with compensatory mutations was selected both in vitro and in vivo by 2′-C-methyl-modified nucleoside analogs, including valopcitabine (NM283; a prodrug of the nucleoside analog 2′-C-methylcytidine), R7128 (a prodrug of PSI-6130), and MK-0608 (3, 177). The S96T mutation, with or without the N142T mutation, was selected in vitro by R1626 (a prodrug of R1479 [4′-azidocytidine]) (121), but these mutations were not observed in a phase II trial of R1626 in combination with pegylated IFN-α and ribavirin which led to complete virological suppression in 75% of participants (165). Although valopcitabine and R1626 have been withdrawn from further clinical evaluation because of gastrointestinal and hematologic toxicities (23), clinical experience with these inhibitors demonstrates the potential of HCV RdRp nucleoside analogs.

Investigational nonnucleoside inhibitors targeting four allosteric binding sites are in early clinical development (23). Mutations associated with resistance to each of the four allosteric sites have been selected in vitro and/or in vivo (177). Cross-resistance between nonnucleoside inhibitors targeting different sites or between nonnucleoside and nucleoside inhibitors has not been described. However, nonnucleoside inhibitors have displayed a low genetic barrier to resistance (122, 160), and several nonnucleoside inhibitor resistance mutations have been reported to occur in previously untreated individuals, either as dominant variants detected by standard sequencing or as minor variants detected by more sensitive methods (110, 123).

INFLUENZA VIRUSES

Influenza A, B, and C viruses have segmented, encapsidated, minus-strand RNA genomes, each associated with a polymerase complex. The RNA particles are located inside a shell of M1 protein that lines the viral lipid membrane. Embedded in the membranes of influenza A and B viruses are three proteins: two spiked glycoproteins—hemagglutinin (HA) and neuraminidase (NA)—and the membrane channel protein M2 (matrix 2). Influenza C virus does not have an NA but instead has a single surface glycoprotein with both HA- and NA-like activities. There are four licensed anti-influenza drugs belonging to two mechanistic classes: M2 channel blockers, including the adamantane derivatives amantadine and rimantadine, and the NA inhibitors zanamivir (ZMV) and oseltamivir (OMV). Peramivir (PMV) is a third NA inhibitor in clinical development. M2 channel blockers are active only against influenza A virus. NA inhibitors are active against influenza A and B viruses but not against influenza C virus. Table 5 summarizes the antiviral agents, mechanisms of resistance, and mutations involved in drug resistance in influenza virus.

The most clinically relevant influenza A viruses currently include the seasonal H3N2 and H1N1 strains (introduced in 1968 and 1977, respectively); H5N1 avian influenza virus, which is widely disseminated in waterfowl and has caused sporadic human infections in Southeast Asia since 1997 (1); and a pandemic H1N1 swine-origin influenza virus (H1N1-SOIV) which emerged in 2009 (53,

72). The incidence, prevalence, and mechanisms of antiviral resistance differ among these four influenza A viruses.

M2 Channel Blockers

The M2 protein is a tetrameric pH-activated proton-selective channel that plays a role in virus uncoating and possibly in regulating the HA activity of newly formed viruses (25). The passage of hydrogen ions through the M2 channel into the virion following endocytosis promotes the dissociation of the matrix M1 protein from the ribonucleoprotein complex and allows the ribonucleoprotein to enter the cell nucleus and initiate replication. By controlling the pH within trans-Golgi vesicles during virus egress, M2 also prevents the exposure of the acid-sensitive HA to an adversely low pH (79). Amantadine and rimantadine interfere with the penetration of hydrogen ions through the M2 channel and prevent transport of the ribonucleoprotein complex to the nucleus (79, 164).

Cross-resistance to both drugs results from single amino acid substitutions at positions 26, 27, 30, 31, and 34 within the M2 transmembrane domain (11, 12). Adamantane resistance develops rapidly during in vitro passage experiments and in about 30% of persons receiving amantadine or rimantadine (12, 91). Amantadine- and rimantadine-resistant variants maintain normal infectivity and virulence in animal models and cause typical disease in humans (11, 91).

Although fewer than 2% of H3N2 viruses sampled globally between 1995 and 2002 were adamantane resistant, sharp increases in resistance caused almost entirely by the M2 S31N mutation appeared following this period, first in Asia and then worldwide (20, 224). By the 2005–2006 season, 92% of H3N2 viruses in the United States were adamantane resistant (21). Molecular phylogenetic studies suggest that selective drug pressure resulting from amantadine and rimantadine use, particularly in Southeast Asia, where these drugs are often available without a prescription, was responsible for multiple independent S31N mutation-containing H3N2

TABLE 5 Mechanisms of resistance to influenza virus inhibitors

Antiviral agent(s)	Mechanism of resistance	Mutations
M2 channel blockers (amantadine, rimantadine)	M2 transmembrane domain substitutions, which interfere with transfer of hydrogen ions	Mutations at residues 26, 27, 30, 31, and 34, particularly A30V and S31N mutations; since 2005, nearly all seasonal H3N2 viruses have contained the S31N mutation and have become intrinsically resistant to amantadine and rimantadine; H5N1 and H1N1-SOIV also contain the S31N mutation and are intrinsically resistant to amantadine and rimantadine
NA inhibitors (oseltamivir [OMV], zanamivir [ZMV], peramivir [PMV][a])	NA mutations in the receptor-binding site decrease inhibitor binding; most of these mutations are highly conserved framework mutations; two of these mutations directly contact sialic acid receptors; in animal models and in vitro, HA mutations that reduce the affinity of HA for its receptor—and thus the need for NA—have been described	H274Y mutation is the most commonly occurring OMV resistance mutation, conferring cross-resistance to PMV but not to ZMV; since 2008, nearly all seasonal H1N1 viruses have contained this mutation and are intrinsically resistant to OMV; this mutation also emerges commonly in patients with H5N1 and H1N1-SOIV who receive OMV
		R152K and R292K mutations confer high-level resistance to each of the NA inhibitors; together with mutations at position 119, these mutations are the most common mutations associated with resistance among H3N2 viruses
		Several accessory NA inhibitor resistance mutations have been observed with increased frequency in H1N1 and H5N1 viruses from treated and untreated patients, including I222M, N294S, and Q136K mutations
		D198N mutation causes intermediate resistant to OMV and ZMV but not to PMV; it has been reported to emerge in influenza B viruses

[a] Peramivir is undergoing clinical investigation. Although it has a resistance profile similar to that of OMV, it has the advantage of having an intravenous formulation.

lineages (69). However, the worldwide dissemination of adamantane resistance appears to be due to the "hitchhiking" of the S31N mutation on a variant containing a novel HA that first appeared in Hong Kong in 2005 and then spread worldwide (151). Although seasonal H1N1 strains are generally adamantane susceptible, H5N1 strains (34) and H1N1-SOIV (29) harbor the S31N mutation and are intrinsically adamantane resistant.

Neuraminidase Inhibitors

HA binds to sialic (*N*-acetylneuraminic) acid-containing cellular receptors and initiates viral infection. NA cleaves the alpha-ketosidic bonds linking terminal sialic acid residues to adjacent oligosaccharide moieties, preventing the formation of aggregates between HA and cell surface sialic acids and allowing newly formed viruses to be released from the surfaces of infected cells (47, 201). NA may also promote viral spread within mucosal secretions in the respiratory tract (47, 201). Because HA binds to cellular receptors to initiate infection, whereas NA destroys cellular receptors to allow virus release from cells, a balance between these two activities is required for efficient infection. Indeed, mutations that decrease the affinity of HA for its cellular receptor allow the virus to exit infected cells without the need for significant NA activity (83). However, HA mutations are not selected in vivo during NA inhibitor therapy and do not cause clinically relevant NA inhibitor resistance (85).

The three-dimensional structures of NAs from multiple influenza A virus subtypes and from influenza B viruses have been solved by X-ray crystallography (46, 47, 201). NA is a homotetramer containing 470 amino acids. A hydrophobic stalk peptide at its N terminus is responsible for membrane anchoring. A globular head contains the enzyme active site, a pocket into which sialic acid and substrate analogs bind (201). Among influenza A viruses, NAs differ by about 50%, and influenza B virus NAs differ from those of influenza A viruses by about 70% (48). Nonetheless, the folded structure of the polypeptide brings into proximity a number of amino acids that are nearly invariant in all influenza virus strains. Eight of these strain-invariant amino acids—R118, D151, R152, R224, E276, R292, R371, and Y406 (according to the N2 numbering system)—contact sialic acid directly, and 10—E119, R156, W178, S179, D/N198, I222, E227, H274, N294, and E425—provide a supporting framework (48, 206).

ZMV and OMV are sialic acid analogs that competitively inhibit NA (206). ZMV and OMV are active against a wide range of strains, including each of the nine identified avian virus NA subtypes (84). Although OMV and ZMV appear to be less active against influenza B virus in vitro, the clinical significance of this finding is uncertain (84). ZMV, which is administered by aerosol, has a guanidine group at position 4 of the transition-state analog of sialic acid. OMV, which is administered orally, is a carbocyclic analog of sialic acid and has a bulky side chain necessitating a conformational change in NA to allow binding (46). Because ZMV is administered solely as an aerosol and because its structure is more similar to that of the natural sialic acid than that of OMV is (96), the emergence of ZMV resistance has occurred primarily in vitro; there has been only a single case report of ZMV resistance arising during therapy (86).

There is no standard method for assessing phenotypic influenza virus susceptibility. NA inhibitor activity can be measured in enzymatic assays, in cell culture, and in animal models (mice and ferrets). However, NA inhibitor activity in cell culture is variable because different clinical isolates have different degrees of dependence on HA activity and because

the cells used for in vitro assays have different concentrations of glycoconjugate receptors (136, 222). Moreover, the effects of different NA inhibitor resistance mutations on susceptibility and viral fitness depend on the viral subtype and genetic context in which these mutations occur (2).

During the first few years of its use, OMV resistance was initially reported to occur in about 1% to 4% of treated adults (85) and in a larger proportion of treated children (107, 217). There was no evidence of naturally occurring OMV resistance, and there were no reports of transmitted resistance (139, 144). In the 2007–2008 season, a significant proportion of seasonal H1N1 infections worldwide were caused by a strain containing the OMV resistance mutation H274Y (58, 182). By the 2008–2009 season, >95% of seasonal H1N1 strains in the United States were OMV resistant (58).

The H274Y mutation reduces OMV susceptibility several hundred- to several thousandfold and causes high-level cross-resistance to PMV but not to ZMV (2, 83, 96, 139). Epidemiologic and molecular phylogenetic data suggest that the fixation of the H274Y mutation in H1N1 strains was not a result of selective drug pressure. The H274Y mutation emerged in the dominant circulating seasonal 2007–2008 H1N1 virus possibly because it complemented one or more other mutations in the dominant clade (45). In contrast to predictions based on in vitro studies and animal models (99), the H274Y mutation-containing H1N1 viruses that have emerged since 2007 retain their transmissibility and pathogenicity (78).

Although H5N1 viruses and H1N1-SOIVs are intrinsically susceptible to OMV and ZMV (120), virological failure resulting from the H274Y mutation appears to occur more frequently in patients treated with OMV for these infections than for the pre-2007 seasonal H1N1 viruses (2, 54, 57, 96). It also appears that H274Y mutation-containing H1N1-SOIVs may be more easily transmissible than the pre-2007 seasonal H1N1 viruses (28). Among H3N2 viruses, the E119V framework mutation and the R292K catalytic mutation have been responsible for resistance in patients receiving OMV (168, 188). The E119GAD framework mutation causes high-level ZMV resistance and low-level OMV resistance. The E119V mutation causes high-level OMV resistance, but its effect on ZMV and PMV susceptibility has been variable (2, 83, 139).

Other NA inhibitor resistance mutations that have been reported for H1N1, H5N1, and H3N2 viruses obtained from patients receiving OMV include the I222M and N294S framework mutations (1, 45, 96, 107, 117). Recent surveillance studies have reported several less-well-characterized H1N1 and H5N1 mutations that confer moderately decreased susceptibility to ZMV and PMV (17, 97, 154).

REFERENCES

1. **Abdel-Ghafar, A. N., T. Chotpitayasunondh, Z. Gao, F. G. Hayden, D. H. Nguyen, M. D. de Jong, A. Naghdaliyev, J. S. Peiris, N. Shindo, S. Soeroso, and T. M. Uyeki.** 2008. Update on avian influenza A (H5N1) virus infection in humans. *N. Engl. J. Med.* **358:**261–273.
2. **Abed, Y., M. Baz, and G. Boivin.** 2006. Impact of neuraminidase mutations conferring influenza resistance to neuraminidase inhibitors in the N1 and N2 genetic backgrounds. *Antivir. Ther.* **11:**971–976.
3. **Ali, S., V. Leveque, S. Le Pogam, H. Ma, F. Philipp, N. Inocencio, M. Smith, A. Alker, H. Kang, I. Najera, K. Klumpp, J. Symons, N. Cammack, and W. R. Jiang.** 2008. Selected replicon variants with low-level in vitro resistance to the hepatitis C virus NS5B polymerase inhibitor PSI-6130 lack cross-resistance with R1479. *Antimicrob. Agents Chemother.* **52:**4356–4369.

4. Alian, A., S. L. Griner, V. Chiang, M. Tsiang, G. Jones, G. Birkus, R. Geleziunas, A. D. Leavitt, and R. M. Stroud. 2009. Catalytically-active complex of HIV-1 integrase with a viral DNA substrate binds anti-integrase drugs. *Proc. Natl. Acad. Sci. USA* **106:**8192–8197.

5. Allen, M. I., M. Deslauriers, C. W. Andrews, G. A. Tipples, K. A. Walters, D. L. Tyrrell, N. Brown, and L. D. Condreay. 1998. Identification and characterization of mutations in hepatitis B virus resistant to lamivudine. *Hepatology* **27:**1670–1677.

6. Andrei, G., E. De Clercq, and R. Snoeck. 2008. Novel inhibitors of human CMV. *Curr. Opin. Investig. Drugs* **9:**132–145.

7. Angus, P., R. Vaughan, S. Xiong, H. Yang, W. Delaney, C. Gibbs, C. Brosgart, D. Colledge, R. Edwards, A. Ayres, A. Bartholomeusz, and S. Locarnini. 2003. Resistance to adefovir dipivoxil therapy associated with the selection of a novel mutation in the HBV polymerase. *Gastroenterology* **125:**292–297.

8. Arion, D., N. Sluis-Cremer, and M. A. Parniak. 2000. Mechanism by which phosphonoformic acid resistance mutations restore 3′-azido-3′-deoxythymidine (AZT) sensitivity to AZT-resistant HIV-1 reverse transcriptase. *J. Biol. Chem.* **275:**9251–9255.

9. Bartels, D. J., Y. Zhou, E. Z. Zhang, M. Marcial, R. A. Byrn, T. Pfeiffer, A. M. Tigges, B. S. Adiwijaya, C. Lin, A. D. Kwong, and T. L. Kieffer. 2008. Natural prevalence of hepatitis C virus variants with decreased sensitivity to NS3.4A protease inhibitors in treatment-naive subjects. *J. Infect. Dis.* **198:**800–807.

10. Bartholomeusz, A., B. G. Tehan, and D. K. Chalmers. 2004. Comparisons of the HBV and HIV polymerase, and antiviral resistance mutations. *Antivir. Ther.* **9:**149–160.

11. Belshe, R. B., B. Burk, F. Newman, R. L. Cerruti, and I. S. Sim. 1989. Resistance of influenza A virus to amantadine and rimantadine: results of one decade of surveillance. *J. Infect. Dis.* **159:**430–435.

12. Belshe, R. B., M. H. Smith, C. B. Hall, R. Betts, and A. J. Hay. 1988. Genetic basis of resistance to rimantadine emerging during treatment of influenza virus infection. *J. Virol.* **62:**1508–1512.

13. Berman, K., and P. Y. Kwo. 2009. Boceprevir, an NS3 protease inhibitor of HCV. *Clin. Liver Dis.* **13:**429–439.

14. Bestman-Smith, J., and G. Boivin. 2003. Drug resistance patterns of recombinant herpes simplex virus DNA polymerase mutants generated with a set of overlapping cosmids and plasmids. *J. Virol.* **77:**7820–7829.

15. Bierman, W. F., M. A. van Agtmael, M. Nijhuis, S. A. Danner, and C. A. Boucher. 2009. HIV monotherapy with ritonavir-boosted protease inhibitors: a systematic review. *AIDS* **23:**279–291.

16. Biron, K. K., R. J. Harvey, S. C. Chamberlain, S. S. Good, A. A. Smith III, M. G. Davis, C. L. Talarico, W. H. Miller, R. Ferris, R. E. Dornsife, S. C. Stanat, J. C. Drach, L. B. Townsend, and G. W. Koszalka. 2002. Potent and selective inhibition of human cytomegalovirus replication by 1263W94, a benzimidazole L-riboside with a unique mode of action. *Antimicrob. Agents Chemother.* **46:**2365–2372.

17. Boltz, D. A., B. Douangngeun, P. Phommachanh, S. Sinthasak, R. Mondry, C. A. Obert, P. Seiler, R. Keating, Y. Suzuki, H. Hiramatsu, E. Govorkova, and R. G. Webster. 2010. Emergence of H5N1 avian influenza viruses with reduced sensitivity to neuraminidase inhibitors and novel reassortants in Lao People's Democratic Republic. *J. Gen. Virol.* **91:**949–959.

18. Borroto-Esoda, K., M. D. Miller, and S. Arterburn. 2007. Pooled analysis of amino acid changes in the HBV polymerase in patients from four major adefovir dipivoxil clinical trials. *J. Hepatol.* **47:**492–498.

19. Brenner, B., D. Turner, M. Oliveira, D. Moisi, M. Detorio, M. Carobene, R. G. Marlink, J. Schapiro, M. Roger, and M. A. Wainberg. 2003. A V106M mutation in HIV-1 clade C viruses exposed to efavirenz confers cross-resistance to non-nucleoside reverse transcriptase inhibitors. *AIDS* **17:**F1–F5.

20. Bright, R. A., M. J. Medina, X. Xu, G. Perez-Oronoz, T. R. Wallis, X. M. Davis, L. Povinelli, N. J. Cox, and A. I. Klimov. 2005. Incidence of adamantane resistance among influenza A (H3N2) viruses isolated worldwide from 1994 to 2005: a cause for concern. *Lancet* **366:**1175–1181.

21. Bright, R. A., D. K. Shay, B. Shu, N. J. Cox, and A. I. Klimov. 2006. Adamantane resistance among influenza A viruses isolated early during the 2005–2006 influenza season in the United States. *JAMA* **295:**891–894.

22. Bryan, C. J., M. N. Prichard, S. Daily, G. Jefferson, C. Hartline, K. A. Cassady, L. Hilliard, and M. Shimamura. 2008. Acyclovir-resistant chronic verrucous vaccine strain varicella in a patient with neuroblastoma. *Pediatr. Infect. Dis. J.* **27:**946–948.

23. Burton, J. R., Jr., and G. T. Everson. 2009. HCV NS5B polymerase inhibitors. *Clin. Liver Dis.* **13:**453–465.

24. Buti, M., F. Rodriguez-Frias, R. Jardi, and R. Esteban. 2005. Hepatitis B virus genome variability and disease progression: the impact of pre-core mutants and HBV genotypes. *J. Clin. Virol.* **34**(Suppl. 1):S79–S82.

25. Cady, S. D., W. Luo, F. Hu, and M. Hong. 2009. Structure and function of the influenza A M2 proton channel. *Biochemistry* **48:**7356–7364.

26. Camacho, R., A. Godinho, P. Gomes, A. Abecasis, A.-M. Vandamme, C. Palma, A. P. Carvalho, J. Cabanas, and J. Goncalves. 2005. Different substitutions under drug pressure at protease codon 82 in HIV-1 subtype G compared to subtype B infected individuals including a novel I82M resistance mutations. *Antivir. Ther.* **10:**S151.

27. Cane, P. A., A. de Ruiter, P. Rice, M. Wiselka, R. Fox, and D. Pillay. 2001. Resistance-associated mutations in the human immunodeficiency virus type 1 subtype C protease gene from treated and untreated patients in the United Kingdom. *J. Clin. Microbiol.* **39:**2652–2654.

28. Centers for Disease Control and Prevention. 2009. Oseltamivir-resistant 2009 pandemic influenza A (H1N1) virus infection in two summer campers receiving prophylaxis—North Carolina, 2009. *MMWR Morb. Mortal. Wkly. Rep.* **58:**969–972.

29. Centers for Disease Control and Prevention. 2009. Update: drug susceptibility of swine-origin influenza A (H1N1) viruses, April 2009. *MMWR Morb. Mortal. Wkly. Rep.* **58:**433–435.

30. Chan, P., and R. Kantor. 2009. Transmitted drug resistance in nonsubtype B HIV-1 infection. *HIV Ther.* **3:**447–465.

31. Chen, J. C., J. Krucinski, L. J. Miercke, J. S. Finer-Moore, A. H. Tang, A. D. Leavitt, and R. M. Stroud. 2000. Crystal structure of the HIV-1 integrase catalytic core and C-terminal domains: a model for viral DNA binding. *Proc. Natl. Acad. Sci. USA* **97:**8233–8238.

32. Chen, S. H., A. Pearson, D. M. Coen, and S. H. Chen. 2004. Failure of thymidine kinase-negative herpes simplex virus to reactivate from latency following efficient establishment. *J. Virol.* **78:**520–523.

33. Chen, X., M. Tsiang, F. Yu, M. Hung, G. S. Jones, A. Zeynalzadegan, X. Qi, H. Jin, C. U. Kim, S. Swaminathan, and J. M. Chen. 2008. Modeling, analysis, and validation of a novel HIV integrase structure provide insights into the binding modes of potent integrase inhibitors. *J. Mol. Biol.* **380:**504–519.

34. Cheung, C. L., J. M. Rayner, G. J. Smith, P. Wang, T. S. Naipospos, J. Zhang, K. Y. Yuen, R. G. Webster, J. S. Peiris, Y. Guan, and H. Chen. 2006. Distribution of amantadine-resistant H5N1 avian influenza variants in Asia. *J. Infect. Dis.* **193:**1626–1629.

35. Chevaliez, S., R. Brillet, E. Lazaro, C. Hezode, and J. M. Pawlotsky. 2007. Analysis of ribavirin mutagenicity in human hepatitis C virus infection. *J. Virol.* **81:**7732–7741.

36. Choe, W. H., S. P. Hong, B. K. Kim, S. Y. Ko, Y. K. Jung, J. H. Kim, J. E. Yeon, K. S. Byun, K. H. Kim, S. I. Ji, S. O. Kim, C. H. Lee, and S. Y. Kwon. 2009. Evolution of hepatitis B virus mutation during entecavir rescue therapy in patients with antiviral resistance to lamivudine and adefovir. *Antivir. Ther.* **14:**985–993.

37. Chou, S. 2008. Cytomegalovirus UL97 mutations in the era of ganciclovir and maribavir. *Rev. Med. Virol.* **18:**233–246.

38. **Chou, S.** 2009. Diverse cytomegalovirus UL27 mutations adapt to loss of viral UL97 kinase activity under maribavir. *Antimicrob. Agents Chemother.* **53:**81–85.

39. **Chou, S., N. S. Lurain, K. D. Thompson, R. C. Miner, and W. L. Drew.** 2003. Viral DNA polymerase mutations associated with drug resistance in human cytomegalovirus. *J. Infect. Dis.* **188:**32–39.

40. **Chou, S., G. Marousek, S. Guentzel, S. E. Follansbee, M. E. Poscher, J. P. Lalezari, R. C. Miner, and W. L. Drew.** 1997. Evolution of mutations conferring multidrug resistance during prophylaxis and therapy for cytomegalovirus disease. *J. Infect. Dis.* **176:**786–789.

41. **Chou, S., G. I. Marousek, L. C. Van Wechel, S. Li, and A. Weinberg.** 2007. Growth and drug resistance phenotypes resulting from cytomegalovirus DNA polymerase region III mutations observed in clinical specimens. *Antimicrob. Agents Chemother.* **51:**4160–4162.

42. **Chou, S., L. C. Van Wechel, H. M. Lichy, and G. I. Marousek.** 2005. Phenotyping of cytomegalovirus drug resistance mutations by using recombinant viruses incorporating a reporter gene. *Antimicrob. Agents Chemother.* **49:**2710–2715.

43. **Coffin, J. M.** 1995. HIV population dynamics in vivo: implications for genetic variation, pathogenesis, and therapy. *Science* **267:**483–489.

44. **Cohen, J. I., P. A. Brunell, S. E. Straus, and P. R. Krause.** 1999. Recent advances in varicella-zoster virus infection. *Ann. Intern. Med.* **130:**922–932.

45. **Collins, P. J., L. F. Haire, Y. P. Lin, J. Liu, R. J. Russell, P. A. Walker, S. R. Martin, R. S. Daniels, V. Gregory, J. J. Skehel, S. J. Gamblin, and A. J. Hay.** 2009. Structural basis for oseltamivir resistance of influenza viruses. *Vaccine* **27:**6317–6323.

46. **Collins, P. J., L. F. Haire, Y. P. Lin, J. Liu, R. J. Russell, P. A. Walker, J. J. Skehel, S. R. Martin, A. J. Hay, and S. J. Gamblin.** 2008. Crystal structures of oseltamivir-resistant influenza virus neuraminidase mutants. *Nature* **453:**1258–1261.

47. **Colman, P. M.** 1994. Influenza virus neuraminidase: structure, antibodies, and inhibitors. *Protein Sci.* **3:**1687–1696.

48. **Colman, P. M., P. A. Hoyne, and M. C. Lawrence.** 1993. Sequence and structure alignment of paramyxovirus hemagglutinin-neuraminidase with influenza virus neuraminidase. *J. Virol.* **67:**2972–2980.

49. **Cote, H. C., Z. L. Brumme, and P. R. Harrigan.** 2001. Human immunodeficiency virus type 1 protease cleavage site mutations associated with protease inhibitor cross-resistance selected by indinavir, ritonavir, and/or saquinavir. *J. Virol.* **75:**589–594.

50. **Crotty, S., D. Maag, J. J. Arnold, W. Zhong, J. Y. Lau, Z. Hong, R. Andino, and C. E. Cameron.** 2000. The broad-spectrum antiviral ribonucleoside ribavirin is an RNA virus mutagen. *Nat. Med.* **6:**1375–1379.

51. **Das, K., A. D. Clark, Jr., P. J. Lewi, J. Heeres, M. R. De Jonge, L. M. Koymans, H. M. Vinkers, F. Daeyaert, D. W. Ludovici, M. J. Kukla, B. De Corte, R. W. Kavash, C. Y. Ho, H. Ye, M. A. Lichtenstein, K. Andries, R. Pauwels, M. P. De Bethune, P. L. Boyer, P. Clark, S. H. Hughes, P. A. Janssen, and E. Arnold.** 2004. Roles of conformational and positional adaptability in structure-based design of TMC125-R165335 (etravirine) and related non-nucleoside reverse transcriptase inhibitors that are highly potent and effective against wild-type and drug-resistant HIV-1 variants. *J. Med. Chem.* **47:**2550–2560.

52. **Das, K., X. Xiong, H. Yang, C. E. Westland, C. S. Gibbs, S. G. Sarafianos, and E. Arnold.** 2001. Molecular modeling and biochemical characterization reveal the mechanism of hepatitis B virus polymerase resistance to lamivudine and emtricitabine. *J. Virol.* **75:**4771–4779.

53. **Dawood, F. S., S. Jain, L. Finelli, M. W. Shaw, S. Lindstrom, R. J. Garten, L. V. Gubareva, X. Xu, C. B. Bridges, and T. M. Uyeki.** 2009. Emergence of a novel swine-origin influenza A (H1N1) virus in humans. *N. Engl. J. Med.* **360:**2605–2615.

54. **de Jong, M. D., T. T. Tran, H. K. Truong, M. H. Vo, G. J. Smith, V. C. Nguyen, V. C. Bach, T. Q. Phan, Q. H. Do, Y. Guan, J. S. Peiris, T. H. Tran, and J. Farrar.** 2005. Oseltamivir resistance during treatment of influenza A (H5N1) infection. *N. Engl. J. Med.* **353:**2667–2672.

55. **Delaney, W. E., IV, H. Yang, C. E. Westland, K. Das, E. Arnold, C. S. Gibbs, M. D. Miller, and S. Xiong.** 2003. The hepatitis B virus polymerase mutation rtV173L is selected during lamivudine therapy and enhances viral replication in vitro. *J. Virol.* **77:**11833–11841.

56. **De Meyer, S., H. Azijn, D. Surleraux, D. Jochmans, A. Tahri, R. Pauwels, P. Wigerinck, and M. P. de Bethune.** 2005. TMC114, a novel human immunodeficiency virus type 1 protease inhibitor active against protease inhibitor-resistant viruses, including a broad range of clinical isolates. *Antimicrob. Agents Chemother.* **49:**2314–2321.

57. **Deyde, V. M., T. G. Sheu, A. A. Trujillo, M. Okomo-Adhiambo, R. Garten, A. I. Klimov, and L. V. Gubareva.** 2010. Detection of molecular markers of drug resistance in the 2009 pandemic influenza A (H1N1) viruses using pyrosequencing. *Antimicrob. Agents Chemother.* **54:**1102–1110.

58. **Dharan, N. J., L. V. Gubareva, J. J. Meyer, M. Okomo-Adhiambo, R. C. McClinton, S. A. Marshall, K. St. George, S. Epperson, L. Brammer, A. I. Klimov, J. S. Bresee, and A. M. Fry.** 2009. Infections with oseltamivir-resistant influenza A (H1N1) virus in the United States. *JAMA* **301:**1034–1041.

59. **Dorr, P., M. Westby, S. Dobbs, P. Griffin, B. Irvine, M. Macartney, J. Mori, G. Rickett, C. Smith-Burchnell, C. Napier, R. Webster, D. Armour, D. Price, B. Stammen, A. Wood, and M. Perros.** 2005. Maraviroc (UK-427,857), a potent, orally bioavailable, and selective small-molecule inhibitor of chemokine receptor CCR5 with broad-spectrum anti-human immunodeficiency virus type 1 activity. *Antimicrob. Agents Chemother.* **49:**4721–4732.

60. **Duan, R., R. D. de Vries, A. D. Osterhaus, L. Remeijer, and G. M. Verjans.** 2008. Acyclovir-resistant corneal HSV-1 isolates from patients with herpetic keratitis. *J. Infect. Dis.* **198:**659–663.

61. **Enomoto, N., I. Sakuma, Y. Asahina, M. Kurosaki, T. Murakami, C. Yamamoto, Y. Ogura, N. Izumi, F. Marumo, and C. Sato.** 1996. Mutations in the nonstructural protein 5A gene and response to interferon in patients with chronic hepatitis C virus 1b infection. *N. Engl. J. Med.* **334:**77–81.

62. **Erice, A., C. Gil-Roda, J. L. Perez, H. H. Balfour, Jr., K. J. Sannerud, M. N. Hanson, G. Boivin, and S. Chou.** 1997. Antiviral susceptibilities and analysis of UL97 and DNA polymerase sequences of clinical cytomegalovirus isolates from immunocompromised patients. *J. Infect. Dis.* **175:**1087–1092.

63. **Erickson, J. W., S. V. Gulnik, and M. Markowitz.** 1999. Protease inhibitors: resistance, cross-resistance, fitness and the choice of initial and salvage therapies. *AIDS* **13**(Suppl. A):S189–S204.

64. **Farci, P., R. Strazzera, H. J. Alter, S. Farci, D. Degioannis, A. Coiana, G. Peddis, F. Usai, G. Serra, L. Chessa, G. Diaz, A. Balestrieri, and R. H. Purcell.** 2002. Early changes in hepatitis C viral quasispecies during interferon therapy predict the therapeutic outcome. *Proc. Natl. Acad. Sci. USA* **99:**3081–3086.

65. **Fransen, S., M. Karmochkine, W. Huang, L. Weiss, C. J. Petropoulos, and C. Charpentier.** 2009. Longitudinal analysis of raltegravir susceptibility and integrase replication capacity of HIV-1 during virologic failure. *Antimicrob. Agents Chemother.* **53:**4522–4524.

66. **Frobert, E., J. C. Cortay, T. Ooka, F. Najioullah, D. Thouvenot, B. Lina, and F. Morfin.** 2008. Genotypic detection of acyclovir-resistant HSV-1: characterization of 67 ACV-sensitive and 14 ACV-resistant viruses. *Antivir. Res.* **79:**28–36.

67. **Frobert, E., T. Ooka, J. C. Cortay, B. Lina, D. Thouvenot, and F. Morfin.** 2005. Herpes simplex virus thymidine kinase mutations associated with resistance to acyclovir: a site-directed mutagenesis study. *Antimicrob. Agents Chemother.* **49:**1055–1059.

68. **Fung, S. K., H. B. Chae, R. J. Fontana, H. Conjeevaram, J. Marrero, K. Oberhelman, M. Hussain, and A. S. Lok.** 2006. Virologic response and resistance to adefovir in patients with chronic hepatitis B. *J. Hepatol.* **44:**283–290.

69. Furuse, Y., A. Suzuki, and H. Oshitani. 2009. Large-scale sequence analysis of M gene of influenza A viruses from different species: mechanisms for emergence and spread of amantadine resistance. *Antimicrob. Agents Chemother.* **53:**4457–4463.

70. Gale, M., Jr., and E. M. Foy. 2005. Evasion of intracellular host defence by hepatitis C virus. *Nature* **436:**939–945.

71. Ganem, D., and A. M. Prince. 2004. Hepatitis B virus infection—natural history and clinical consequences. *N. Engl. J. Med.* **350:**1118–1129.

72. Garten, R. J., C. T. Davis, C. A. Russell, B. Shu, S. Lindstrom, A. Balish, W. M. Sessions, X. Xu, E. Skepner, V. Deyde, M. Okomo-Adhiambo, L. Gubareva, J. Barnes, C. B. Smith, S. L. Emery, M. J. Hillman, P. Rivailler, J. Smagala, M. de Graaf, D. F. Burke, R. A. Fouchier, C. Pappas, C. M. Alpuche-Aranda, H. Lopez-Gatell, H. Olivera, I. Lopez, C. A. Myers, D. Faix, P. J. Blair, C. Yu, K. M. Keene, P. D. Dotson, Jr., D. Boxrud, A. R. Sambol, S. H. Abid, K. St. George, T. Bannerman, A. L. Moore, D. J. Stringer, P. Blevins, G. J. Demmler-Harrison, M. Ginsberg, P. Kriner, S. Waterman, S. Smole, H. F. Guevara, E. A. Belongia, P. A. Clark, S. T. Beatrice, R. Donis, J. Katz, L. Finelli, C. B. Bridges, M. Shaw, D. B. Jernigan, T. M. Uyeki, D. J. Smith, A. I. Klimov, and N. J. Cox. 2009. Antigenic and genetic characteristics of swine-origin 2009 A(H1N1) influenza viruses circulating in humans. *Science* **325:**197–201.

73. Geretti, A. M. 2007. Epidemiology of antiretroviral drug resistance in drug-naive persons. *Curr. Opin. Infect. Dis.* **20:**22–32.

74. Ghany, M. G., D. B. Strader, D. L. Thomas, and L. B. Seeff. 2009. Diagnosis, management, and treatment of hepatitis C: an update. *Hepatology* **49:**1335–1374.

75. Gilbert, C., J. Bestman-Smith, and G. Boivin. 2002. Resistance of herpesviruses to antiviral drugs: clinical impacts and molecular mechanisms. *Drug Resist. Updat.* **5:**88–114.

76. Gilbert, C., and G. Boivin. 2005. Human cytomegalovirus resistance to antiviral drugs. *Antimicrob. Agents Chemother.* **49:**873–883.

77. Goldgur, Y., R. Craigie, G. H. Cohen, T. Fujiwara, T. Yoshinaga, T. Fujishita, H. Sugimoto, T. Endo, H. Murai, and D. R. Davies. 1999. Structure of the HIV-1 integrase catalytic domain complexed with an inhibitor: a platform for antiviral drug design. *Proc. Natl. Acad. Sci. USA* **96:**13040–13043.

78. Gooskens, J., M. Jonges, E. C. Claas, A. Meijer, P. J. van den Broek, and A. M. Kroes. 2009. Morbidity and mortality associated with nosocomial transmission of oseltamivir-resistant influenza A(H1N1) virus. *JAMA* **301:**1042–1046.

79. Grambas, S., M. S. Bennett, and A. J. Hay. 1992. Influence of amantadine resistance mutations on the pH regulatory function of the M2 protein of influenza A viruses. *Virology* **191:**541–549.

80. Grey, F., M. Sowa, P. Collins, R. J. Fenton, W. Harris, W. Snowden, S. Efstathiou, and G. Darby. 2003. Characterization of a neurovirulent aciclovir-resistant variant of herpes simplex virus. *J. Gen. Virol.* **84:**1403–1410.

81. Griffiths, A., M. A. Link, C. L. Furness, and D. M. Coen. 2006. Low-level expression and reversion both contribute to reactivation of herpes simplex virus drug-resistant mutants with mutations on homopolymeric sequences in thymidine kinase. *J. Virol.* **80:**6568–6574.

82. Grossman, Z., V. Istomin, D. Averbuch, M. Lorber, K. Risenberg, I. Levi, M. Chowers, M. Burke, N. Bar Yaacov, and J. M. Schapiro. 2004. Genetic variation at NNRTI resistance-associated positions in patients infected with HIV-1 subtype C. *AIDS* **18:**909–915.

83. Gubareva, L. V. 2004. Molecular mechanisms of influenza virus resistance to neuraminidase inhibitors. *Virus Res.* **103:**199–203.

84. Gubareva, L. V., L. Kaiser, and F. G. Hayden. 2000. Influenza virus neuraminidase inhibitors. *Lancet* **355:**827–835.

85. Gubareva, L. V., L. Kaiser, M. N. Matrosovich, Y. Soo-Hoo, and F. G. Hayden. 2001. Selection of influenza virus mutants in experimentally infected volunteers treated with oseltamivir. *J. Infect. Dis.* **183:**523–531.

86. Gubareva, L. V., M. N. Matrosovich, M. K. Brenner, R. C. Bethell, and R. G. Webster. 1998. Evidence for zanamivir resistance in an immunocompromised child infected with influenza B virus. *J. Infect. Dis.* **178:**1257–1262.

87. Gunther, S., L. Fischer, I. Pult, M. Sterneck, and H. Will. 1999. Naturally occurring variants of hepatitis B virus. *Adv. Virus Res.* **52:**25–137.

88. Hadziyannis, S. J., N. C. Tassopoulos, E. J. Heathcote, T. T. Chang, G. Kitis, M. Rizzetto, P. Marcellin, S. G. Lim, Z. Goodman, J. Ma, C. L. Brosgart, K. Borroto-Esoda, S. Arterburn, and S. L. Chuck. 2006. Long-term therapy with adefovir dipivoxil for HBeAg-negative chronic hepatitis B for up to 5 years. *Gastroenterology* **131:**1743–1751.

89. Hartley, O., P. Klasse, Q. Sattentau, and J. P. Moore. 2005. V3: HIV's switch hitter. *AIDS Res. Hum. Retrovir.* **21:**171–189.

90. Hatchette, T., G. A. Tipples, G. Peters, A. Alsuwaidi, J. Zhou, and T. L. Mailman. 2008. Foscarnet salvage therapy for acyclovir-resistant varicella zoster: report of a novel thymidine kinase mutation and review of the literature. *Pediatr. Infect. Dis. J.* **27:**75–77.

91. Hayden, F. G., R. B. Belshe, R. D. Clover, A. J. Hay, M. G. Oakes, and W. Soo. 1989. Emergence and apparent transmission of rimantadine-resistant influenza A virus in families. *N. Engl. J. Med.* **321:**1696–1702.

92. Hezode, C., N. Forestier, G. Dusheiko, P. Ferenci, S. Pol, T. Goeser, J. P. Bronowicki, M. Bourliere, S. Gharakhanian, L. Bengtsson, L. McNair, S. George, T. Kieffer, A. Kwong, R. S. Kauffman, J. Alam, J. M. Pawlotsky, and S. Zeuzem. 2009. Telaprevir and peginterferon with or without ribavirin for chronic HCV infection. *N. Engl. J. Med.* **360:**1839–1850.

93. Hicks, C. B., P. Cahn, D. A. Cooper, S. L. Walmsley, C. Katlama, B. Clotet, A. Lazzarin, M. A. Johnson, D. Neubacher, D. Mayers, and H. Valdez. 2006. Durable efficacy of tipranavir-ritonavir in combination with an optimised background regimen of antiretroviral drugs for treatment-experienced HIV-1-infected patients at 48 weeks in the Randomized Evaluation of Strategic Intervention in Multi-Drug Resistant Patients with Tipranavir (RESIST) studies: an analysis of combined data from two randomised open-label trials. *Lancet* **368:**466–475.

94. Hirsch, M. S., H. F. Gunthard, J. M. Schapiro, F. Brun-Vezinet, B. Clotet, S. M. Hammer, V. A. Johnson, D. R. Kuritzkes, J. W. Mellors, D. Pillay, P. G. Yeni, D. M. Jacobsen, and D. D. Richman. 2008. Antiretroviral drug resistance testing in adult HIV-1 infection: 2008 recommendations of an International AIDS Society-USA panel. *Clin. Infect. Dis.* **47:**266–285.

95. Hosseinipour, M. C., J. J. van Oosterhout, R. Weigel, S. Phiri, D. Kamwendo, N. Parkin, S. A. Fiscus, J. A. Nelson, J. J. Eron, and J. Kumwenda. 2009. The public health approach to identify antiretroviral therapy failure: high-level nucleoside reverse transcriptase inhibitor resistance among Malawians failing first-line antiretroviral therapy. *AIDS* **23:**1127–1134.

96. Hurt, A. C., J. K. Holien, and I. G. Barr. 2009. In vitro generation of neuraminidase inhibitor resistance in A(H5N1) influenza viruses. *Antimicrob. Agents Chemother.* **53:**4433–4440.

97. Hurt, A. C., J. K. Holien, M. Parker, A. Kelso, and I. G. Barr. 2009. Zanamivir-resistant influenza viruses with a novel neuraminidase mutation. *J. Virol.* **83:**10366–10373.

98. Invernizzi, C. F., D. Coutsinos, M. Oliveira, D. Moisi, B. G. Brenner, and M. A. Wainberg. 2009. Signature nucleotide polymorphisms at positions 64 and 65 in reverse transcriptase favor the selection of the K65R resistance mutation in HIV-1 subtype C. *J. Infect. Dis.* **200:**1202–1206.

99. Ives, J. A., J. A. Carr, D. B. Mendel, C. Y. Tai, R. Lambkin, L. Kelly, J. S. Oxford, F. G. Hayden, and N. A. Roberts. 2002. The H274Y mutation in the influenza A/H1N1 neuraminidase active site following oseltamivir phosphate treatment leaves virus severely compromised both in vitro and in vivo. *Antivir. Res.* **55:**307–317.

100. Kantor, R., D. A. Katzenstein, B. Efron, A. P. Carvalho, B. Wynhoven, P. Cane, J. Clarke, S. Sirivichayakul, M. A. Soares, J. Snoeck, C. Pillay, H. Rudich, R. Rodrigues, A. Holguin, K. Ariyoshi, M. B. Bouzas, P. Cahn, W. Sugiura, V. Soriano, L. F. Brigido, J. Grossman, L. Morris, A. M. Vandamme, A. Tanuri, P. Phanuphak, J. N. Weber, D. Pillay, P. R. Harrigan, R. Camacho, J. M. Schapiro, and R. W. Shafer. 2005. Impact of HIV-1 subtype and antiretroviral therapy on protease and reverse transcriptase genotype: results of a global collaboration. *PLoS Med.* **2:**e112.

101. Keeffe, E. B., D. T. Dieterich, S. H. Han, I. M. Jacobson, P. Martin, E. R. Schiff, and H. Tobias. 2008. A treatment algorithm for the management of chronic hepatitis B virus infection in the United States: 2008 update. *Clin. Gastroenterol. Hepatol.* **6:**1315–1341.

102. Keeffe, E. B., D. T. Dieterich, J. M. Pawlotsky, and Y. Benhamou. 2008. Chronic hepatitis B: preventing, detecting, and managing viral resistance. *Clin. Gastroenterol. Hepatol.* **6:**268–274.

103. Kempf, D. J., J. D. Isaacson, M. S. King, S. C. Brun, Y. Xu, K. Real, B. M. Bernstein, A. J. Japour, E. Sun, and R. A. Rode. 2001. Identification of genotypic changes in human immunodeficiency virus protease that correlate with reduced susceptibility to the protease inhibitor lopinavir among viral isolates from protease inhibitor-experienced patients. *J. Virol.* **75:**7462–7469.

104. Kieffer, T. L., A. D. Kwong, and G. R. Picchio. 2010. Viral resistance to specifically targeted antiviral therapies for hepatitis C (STAT-Cs). *J. Antimicrob. Chemother.* **65:**202–212.

105. Kieffer, T. L., C. Sarrazin, J. S. Miller, M. W. Welker, N. Forestier, H. W. Reesink, A. D. Kwong, and S. Zeuzem. 2007. Telaprevir and pegylated interferon-alpha-2a inhibit wild-type and resistant genotype 1 hepatitis C virus replication in patients. *Hepatology* **46:**631–639.

106. Kilby, J. M., and J. J. Eron. 2003. Novel therapies based on mechanisms of HIV-1 cell entry. *N. Engl. J. Med.* **348:**2228–2238.

107. Kiso, M., K. Mitamura, Y. Sakai-Tagawa, K. Shiraishi, C. Kawakami, K. Kimura, F. G. Hayden, N. Sugaya, and Y. Kawaoka. 2004. Resistant influenza A viruses in children treated with oseltamivir: descriptive study. *Lancet* **364:**759–765.

108. Kolli, M., S. Lastere, and C. A. Schiffer. 2006. Coevolution of nelfinavir-resistant HIV-1 protease and the p1-p6 substrate. *Virology* **347:**405–409.

109. Korber, B., M. Muldoon, J. Theiler, F. Gao, R. Gupta, A. Lapedes, B. H. Hahn, S. Wolinsky, and T. Bhattacharya. 2000. Timing the ancestor of the HIV-1 pandemic strains. *Science* **288:**1789–1796.

110. Kuntzen, T., J. Timm, A. Berical, N. Lennon, A. M. Berlin, S. K. Young, B. Lee, D. Heckerman, J. Carlson, L. L. Reyor, M. Kleyman, C. M. McMahon, C. Birch, J. Schulze Zur Wiesch, T. Ledlie, M. Koehrsen, C. Kodira, A. D. Roberts, G. M. Lauer, H. R. Rosen, F. Bihl, A. Cerny, U. Spengler, Z. Liu, A. Y. Kim, Y. Xing, A. Schneidewind, M. A. Madey, J. F. Fleckenstein, V. M. Park, J. E. Galagan, C. Nusbaum, B. D. Walker, G. V. Lake-Bakaar, E. S. Daar, I. M. Jacobson, E. D. Gomperts, B. R. Edlin, S. M. Donfield, R. T. Chung, A. H. Talal, T. Marion, B. W. Birren, M. R. Henn, and T. M. Allen. 2008. Naturally occurring dominant resistance mutations to hepatitis C virus protease and polymerase inhibitors in treatment-naive patients. *Hepatology* **48:**1769–1778.

111. Kuritzkes, D. R., C. M. Lalama, H. J. Ribaudo, M. Marcial, W. A. Meyer III, C. Shikuma, V. A. Johnson, S. A. Fiscus, R. T. D'Aquila, B. R. Schackman, E. P. Acosta, and R. M. Gulick. 2008. Preexisting resistance to non-nucleoside reverse-transcriptase inhibitors predicts virologic failure of an efavirenz-based regimen in treatment-naive HIV-1-infected subjects. *J. Infect. Dis.* **197:**867–870.

112. Kwong, A. D., J. L. Kim, G. Rao, D. Lipovsek, and S. A. Raybuck. 1999. Hepatitis C virus NS3/4A protease. *Antivir. Res.* **41:**67–84.

113. Lai, C. L., J. Dienstag, E. Schiff, N. W. Leung, M. Atkins, C. Hunt, N. Brown, M. Woessner, R. Boehme, and L. Condreay. 2003. Prevalence and clinical correlates of YMDD variants during lamivudine therapy for patients with chronic hepatitis B. *Clin. Infect. Dis.* **36:**687–696.

114. Lanier, E. R., M. Ait-Khaled, J. Scott, C. Stone, T. Melby, G. Sturge, M. St. Clair, H. Steel, S. Hetherington, G. Pearce, W. Spreen, and S. Lafon. 2004. Antiviral efficacy of abacavir in antiretroviral therapy-experienced adults harbouring HIV-1 with specific patterns of resistance to nucleoside reverse transcriptase inhibitors. *Antivir. Ther.* **9:**37–45.

115. Larder, B. A. 1994. Interactions between drug resistance mutations in human immunodeficiency virus type 1 reverse transcriptase. *J. Gen. Virol.* **75:**951–957.

116. Lau, J. Y., R. C. Tam, T. J. Liang, and Z. Hong. 2002. Mechanism of action of ribavirin in the combination treatment of chronic HCV infection. *Hepatology* **35:**1002–1009.

117. Le, Q. M., M. Kiso, K. Someya, Y. T. Sakai, T. H. Nguyen, K. H. Nguyen, N. D. Pham, H. H. Ngyen, S. Yamada, Y. Muramoto, T. Horimoto, A. Takada, H. Goto, T. Suzuki, Y. Suzuki, and Y. Kawaoka. 2005. Avian flu: isolation of drug-resistant H5N1 virus. *Nature* **437:**1108.

118. Leary, J. J., R. Wittrock, R. T. Sarisky, A. Weinberg, and M. J. Levin. 2002. Susceptibilities of herpes simplex viruses to penciclovir and acyclovir in eight cell lines. *Antimicrob. Agents Chemother.* **46:**762–768.

119. Legrand-Abravanel, F., P. Colson, H. Leguillou-Guillemette, L. Alric, I. Ravaux, F. Lunel-Fabiani, M. Bouviers-Alias, P. Trimoulet, M. L. Chaix, C. Hezode, J. Foucher, H. Fontaine, A. M. Roque-Afonso, M. Gassin, E. Schvoerer, C. Gaudy, B. Roche, M. Doffoel, L. D'Alteroche, S. Vallet, Y. Baazia, B. Pozzetto, V. Thibault, J. B. Nousbaum, D. Roulot, H. Coppere, T. Poinard, C. Payan, and J. Izopet. 2009. Influence of the HCV subtype on the virological response to pegylated interferon and ribavirin therapy. *J. Med. Virol.* **81:**2029–2035.

120. Leneva, I. A., N. Roberts, E. A. Govorkova, O. G. Goloubeva, and R. G. Webster. 2000. The neuraminidase inhibitor GS4104 (oseltamivir phosphate) is efficacious against A/Hong Kong/156/97 (H5N1) and A/Hong Kong/1074/99 (H9N2) influenza viruses. *Antivir. Res.* **48:**101–115.

121. Le Pogam, S., W. R. Jiang, V. Leveque, S. Rajyaguru, H. Ma, H. Kang, S. Jiang, M. Singer, S. Ali, K. Klumpp, D. Smith, J. Symons, N. Cammack, and I. Najera. 2006. In vitro selected Con1 subgenomic replicons resistant to 2'-C-methyl-cytidine or to R1479 show lack of cross resistance. *Virology* **351:**349–359.

122. Le Pogam, S., H. Kang, S. F. Harris, V. Leveque, A. M. Giannetti, S. Ali, W. R. Jiang, S. Rajyaguru, G. Tavares, C. Oshiro, T. Hendricks, K. Klumpp, J. Symons, M. F. Browner, N. Cammack, and I. Najera. 2006. Selection and characterization of replicon variants dually resistant to thumb- and palm-binding nonnucleoside polymerase inhibitors of the hepatitis C virus. *J. Virol.* **80:**6146–6154.

123. Le Pogam, S., A. Seshaadri, A. Kosaka, S. Chiu, H. Kang, S. Hu, S. Rajyaguru, J. Symons, N. Cammack, and I. Najera. 2008. Existence of hepatitis C virus NS5B variants naturally resistant to non-nucleoside, but not to nucleoside, polymerase inhibitors among untreated patients. *J. Antimicrob. Chemother.* **61:**1205–1216.

124. Liaw, Y. F., E. Gane, N. Leung, S. Zeuzem, Y. Wang, C. L. Lai, E. J. Heathcote, M. Manns, N. Bzowej, J. Niu, S. H. Han, S. G. Hwang, Y. Cakaloglu, M. J. Tong, G. Papatheodoridis, Y. Chen, N. A. Brown, E. Albanis, K. Galil, and N. V. Naoumov. 2009. 2-Year GLOBE trial results: telbivudine is superior to lamivudine in patients with chronic hepatitis B. *Gastroenterology* **136:**486–495.

125. Liu, C. J., and J. H. Kao. 2008. Genetic variability of hepatitis B virus and response to antiviral therapy. *Antivir. Ther.* **13:**613–624.

126. Lok, A. S., and B. J. McMahon. 2009. Chronic hepatitis B: update 2009. *Hepatology* **50:**661–662.

127. Lok, A. S., F. Zoulim, S. Locarnini, A. Bartholomeusz, M. G. Ghany, J. M. Pawlotsky, Y. F. Liaw, M. Mizokami, and C. Kuiken. 2007. Antiviral drug-resistant HBV: standardization of nomenclature and assays and recommendations for management. *Hepatology* **46:**254–265.

128. Lu, J., S. G. Deeks, R. Hoh, G. Beatty, B. A. Kuritzkes, J. N. Martin, and D. R. Kuritzkes. 2006. Rapid emergence of enfuvirtide resistance in HIV-1-infected patients: results of a clonal analysis. *J. Acquir. Immune Defic. Syndr.* **43:**60–64.

129. Maag, D., C. Castro, Z. Hong, and C. E. Cameron. 2001. Hepatitis C virus RNA-dependent RNA polymerase (NS5B) as a mediator of the antiviral activity of ribavirin. *J. Biol. Chem.* **276:**46094–46098.

130. Madruga, J. V., P. Cahn, B. Grinsztejn, R. Haubrich, J. Lalezari, A. Mills, G. Pialoux, T. Wilkin, M. Peeters, J. Vingerhoets, G. de Smedt, L. Leopold, R. Trefiglio, and B. Woodfall. 2007. Efficacy and safety of TMC125 (etravirine) in treatment-experienced HIV-1-infected patients in DUET-1: 24-week results from a randomised, double-blind, placebo-controlled trial. *Lancet* **370:**29–38.

131. Maeda, K., D. Das, H. Ogata-Aoki, H. Nakata, T. Miyakawa, Y. Tojo, R. Norman, Y. Takaoka, J. Ding, G. F. Arnold, E. Arnold, and H. Mitsuya. 2006. Structural and molecular interactions of CCR5 inhibitors with CCR5. *J. Biol. Chem.* **281:**12688–12698.

132. Marcellin, P., E. J. Heathcote, M. Buti, E. Gane, R. A. de Man, Z. Krastev, G. Germanidis, S. S. Lee, R. Flisiak, K. Kaita, M. Manns, I. Kotzev, K. Tchernev, P. Buggisch, F. Weilert, O. O. Kurdas, M. L. Shiffman, H. Trinh, M. K. Washington, J. Sorbel, J. Anderson, A. Snow-Lampart, E. Mondou, J. Quinn, and F. Rousseau. 2008. Tenofovir disoproxil fumarate versus adefovir dipivoxil for chronic hepatitis B. *N. Engl. J. Med.* **359:**2442–2455.

133. Marcellin, P., G. K. Lau, F. Bonino, P. Farci, S. Hadziyannis, R. Jin, Z. M. Lu, T. Piratvisuth, G. Germanidis, C. Yurdaydin, M. Diago, S. Gurel, M. Y. Lai, P. Button, and N. Pluck. 2004. Peginterferon alfa-2a alone, lamivudine alone, and the two in combination in patients with HBeAg-negative chronic hepatitis B. *N. Engl. J. Med.* **351:**1206–1217.

134. Martell, M., J. I. Esteban, J. Quer, J. Genesca, A. Weiner, R. Esteban, J. Guardia, and J. Gomez. 1992. Hepatitis C virus (HCV) circulates as a population of different but closely related genomes: quasispecies nature of HCV genome distribution. *J. Virol.* **66:**3225–3229.

135. Masquelier, B., E. Race, C. Tamalet, D. Descamps, J. Izopet, C. Buffet-Janvresse, A. Ruffault, A. S. Mohammed, J. Cottalorda, A. Schmuck, V. Calvez, E. Dam, H. Fleury, and F. Brun-Vezinet. 2001. Genotypic and phenotypic resistance patterns of human immunodeficiency virus type 1 variants with insertions or deletions in the reverse transcriptase (RT): multicenter study of patients treated with RT inhibitors. *Antimicrob. Agents Chemother.* **45:**1836–1842.

136. Matrosovich, M. N., T. Y. Matrosovich, T. Gray, N. A. Roberts, and H. D. Klenk. 2004. Human and avian influenza viruses target different cell types in cultures of human airway epithelium. *Proc. Natl. Acad. Sci. USA* **101:**4620–4624.

137. McColl, D. J., and X. Chen. 2010. Strand transfer inhibitors of HIV-1 integrase: bringing IN a new era of antiretroviral therapy. *Antivir. Res.* **85:**101–118.

138. McHutchison, J. G., G. T. Everson, S. C. Gordon, I. M. Jacobson, M. Sulkowski, R. Kauffman, L. McNair, J. Alam, and A. J. Muir. 2009. Telaprevir with peginterferon and ribavirin for chronic HCV genotype 1 infection. *N. Engl. J. Med.* **360:**1827–1838.

139. McKimm-Breschkin, J., T. Trivedi, A. Hampson, A. Hay, A. Klimov, M. Tashiro, F. Hayden, and M. Zambon. 2003. Neuraminidase sequence analysis and susceptibilities of influenza virus clinical isolates to zanamivir and oseltamivir. *Antimicrob. Agents Chemother.* **47:**2264–2272.

140. Meyer, P. R., S. E. Matsuura, R. F. Schinazi, A. G. So, and W. A. Scott. 2000. Differential removal of thymidine nucleotide analogues from blocked DNA chains by human immunodeficiency virus reverse transcriptase in the presence of

physiological concentrations of 2′-deoxynucleoside triphosphates. *Antimicrob. Agents Chemother.* **44:**3465–3472.

141. Miller, M. D., N. Margot, B. Lu, L. Zhong, S. S. Chen, A. Cheng, and M. Wulfsohn. 2004. Genotypic and phenotypic predictors of the magnitude of response to tenofovir disoproxil fumarate treatment in antiretroviral-experienced patients. *J. Infect. Dis.* **189:**837–846.

142. Mink, M., S. M. Mosier, S. Janumpalli, D. Davison, L. Jin, T. Melby, P. Sista, J. Erickson, D. Lambert, S. A. Stanfield-Oakley, M. Salgo, N. Cammack, T. Matthews, and M. L. Greenberg. 2005. Impact of human immunodeficiency virus type 1 gp41 amino acid substitutions selected during enfuvirtide treatment on gp41 binding and antiviral potency of enfuvirtide in vitro. *J. Virol.* **79:**12447–12454.

143. Molina, J. M., A. G. Marcelin, J. Pavie, L. Heripret, C. M. De Boever, M. Troccaz, G. Leleu, and V. Calvez. 2005. Didanosine in HIV-1-infected patients experiencing failure of antiretroviral therapy: a randomized placebo-controlled trial. *J. Infect. Dis.* **191:**840–847.

144. Monto, A. S., J. L. McKimm-Breschkin, C. Macken, A. W. Hampson, A. Hay, A. Klimov, M. Tashiro, R. G. Webster, M. Aymard, F. G. Hayden, and M. Zambon. 2006. Detection of influenza viruses resistant to neuraminidase inhibitors in global surveillance during the first 3 years of their use. *Antimicrob. Agents Chemother.* **50:**2395–2402.

145. Moore, J. P., and D. R. Kuritzkes. 2009. A piece de resistance: how HIV-1 escapes small molecule CCR5 inhibitors. *Curr. Opin. HIV AIDS* **4:**118–124.

146. Morfin, F., G. Souillet, K. Bilger, T. Ooka, M. Aymard, and D. Thouvenot. 2000. Genetic characterization of thymidine kinase from acyclovir-resistant and -susceptible herpes simplex virus type 1 isolated from bone marrow transplant recipients. *J. Infect. Dis.* **182:**290–293.

147. Morfin, F., and D. Thouvenot. 2003. Herpes simplex virus resistance to antiviral drugs. *J. Clin. Virol.* **26:**29–37.

148. Morfin, F., D. Thouvenot, M. De Turenne-Tessier, B. Lina, M. Aymard, and T. Ooka. 1999. Phenotypic and genetic characterization of thymidine kinase from clinical strains of varicella-zoster virus resistant to acyclovir. *Antimicrob. Agents Chemother.* **43:**2412–2416.

149. Moucari, R., A. Korevaar, O. Lada, N. Martinot-Peignoux, N. Boyer, V. Mackiewicz, A. Dauvergne, A. C. Cardoso, T. Asselah, M. H. Nicolas-Chanoine, M. Vidaud, D. Valla, P. Bedossa, and P. Marcellin. 2009. High rates of HBsAg seroconversion in HBeAg-positive chronic hepatitis B patients responding to interferon: a long-term follow-up study. *J. Hepatol.* **50:**1084–1092.

150. Moucari, R., M. Martinot-Peignoux, V. Mackiewicz, N. Boyer, M. P. Ripault, C. Castelnau, L. Leclere, A. Dauvergne, D. Valla, M. Vidaud, M. H. Nicolas-Chanoine, and P. Marcellin. 2009. Influence of genotype on hepatitis B surface antigen kinetics in hepatitis B e antigen-negative patients treated with pegylated interferon-alpha2a. *Antivir. Ther.* **14:**1183–1188.

151. Nelson, M. I., L. Simonsen, C. Viboud, M. A. Miller, and E. C. Holmes. 2009. The origin and global emergence of adamantane resistant A/H3N2 influenza viruses. *Virology* **388:**270–278.

152. Nikkels, A. F., R. Snoeck, B. Rentier, and G. E. Pierard. 1999. Chronic verrucous varicella zoster virus skin lesions: clinical, histological, molecular and therapeutic aspects. *Clin. Exp. Dermatol.* **24:**346–353.

153. Nowak, M. A., S. Bonhoeffer, A. M. Hill, R. Boehme, H. C. Thomas, and H. McDade. 1996. Viral dynamics in hepatitis B virus infection. *Proc. Natl. Acad. Sci. USA* **93:**4398–4402.

154. Okomo-Adhiambo, M., H. T. Nguyen, K. Sleeman, T. G. Sheu, V. M. Deyde, R. J. Garten, X. Xu, M. W. Shaw, A. I. Klimov, and L. V. Gubareva. 2010. Host cell selection of influenza neuraminidase variants: implications for drug resistance monitoring in A(H1N1) viruses. *Antivir. Res.* **85:**381–388.

155. Ono, S. K., N. Kato, Y. Shiratori, J. Kato, T. Goto, R. F. Schinazi, F. J. Carrilho, and M. Omata. 2001. The polymerase L528M mutation cooperates with nucleotide binding-site mutations, increasing hepatitis B virus replication and drug resistance. *J. Clin. Investig.* **107:**449–455.

156. Ormrod, D., and K. Goa. 2000. Valaciclovir: a review of its use in the management of herpes zoster. *Drugs* **59:**1317–1340.

157. Parikh, U. M., D. L. Koontz, C. K. Chu, R. F. Schinazi, and J. W. Mellors. 2005. In vitro activity of structurally diverse nucleoside analogs against human immunodeficiency virus type 1 with the K65R mutation in reverse transcriptase. *Antimicrob. Agents Chemother.* **49:**1139–1144.

158. Parkin, N. T., N. S. Hellmann, J. M. Whitcomb, L. Kiss, C. Chappey, and C. J. Petropoulos. 2004. Natural variation of drug susceptibility in wild-type HIV-1. *Antimicrob. Agents Chemother.* **48:**437–443.

159. Parkin, N. T., and J. M. Schapiro. 2004. Antiretroviral drug resistance in non-subtype B HIV-1, HIV-2 and SIV. *Antivir. Ther.* **9:**3–12.

160. Pauwels, F., W. Mostmans, L. M. Quirynen, L. van der Helm, C. W. Boutton, A. S. Rueff, E. Cleiren, P. Raboisson, D. Surleraux, O. Nyanguile, and K. A. Simmen. 2007. Binding-site identification and genotypic profiling of hepatitis C virus polymerase inhibitors. *J. Virol.* **81:**6909–6919.

161. Penin, F., J. Dubuisson, F. A. Rey, D. Moradpour, and J. M. Pawlotsky. 2004. Structural biology of hepatitis C virus. *Hepatology* **39:**5–19.

162. Peters, M. G., H. Hann Hw, P. Martin, E. J. Heathcote, P. Buggisch, R. Rubin, M. Bourliere, K. Kowdley, C. Trepo, D. Gray Df, M. Sullivan, K. Kleber, R. Ebrahimi, S. Xiong, and C. L. Brosgart. 2004. Adefovir dipivoxil alone or in combination with lamivudine in patients with lamivudine-resistant chronic hepatitis B. *Gastroenterology* **126:**91–101.

163. Piccolo, P., I. Lenci, L. Demelia, F. Bandiera, M. R. Piras, G. Antonucci, L. Nosotti, T. Mari, A. De Santis, M. L. Ponti, O. Sorbello, F. Iacomi, and M. Angelico. 2009. A randomized controlled trial of pegylated interferon-alpha2a plus adefovir dipivoxil for hepatitis B e antigen-negative chronic hepatitis B. *Antivir. Ther.* **14:**1165–1174.

164. Pielak, R. M., J. R. Schnell, and J. J. Chou. 2009. Mechanism of drug inhibition and drug resistance of influenza A M2 channel. *Proc. Natl. Acad. Sci. USA* **106:**7379–7384.

165. Pockros, P. J., D. Nelson, E. Godofsky, M. Rodriguez-Torres, G. T. Everson, M. W. Fried, R. Ghalib, S. Harrison, L. Nyberg, M. L. Shiffman, I. Najera, A. Chan, and G. Hill. 2008. R1626 plus peginterferon alfa-2a provides potent suppression of hepatitis C virus RNA and significant antiviral synergy in combination with ribavirin. *Hepatology* **48:**385–397.

166. Prichard, M. N. 2009. Function of human cytomegalovirus UL97 kinase in viral infection and its inhibition by maribavir. *Rev. Med. Virol.* **19:**215–229.

167. Rapti, I., E. Dimou, P. Mitsoula, and S. J. Hadziyannis. 2007. Adding-on versus switching-to adefovir therapy in lamivudine-resistant HBeAg-negative chronic hepatitis B. *Hepatology* **45:**307–313.

168. Reece, P. A. 2007. Neuraminidase inhibitor resistance in influenza viruses. *J. Med. Virol.* **79:**1577–1586.

169. Rhee, S. Y., J. Taylor, G. Wadhera, A. Ben-Hur, D. L. Brutlag, and R. W. Shafer. 2006. Genotypic predictors of human immunodeficiency virus type 1 drug resistance. *Proc. Natl. Acad. Sci. USA* **103:**17355–17360.

170. Saijo, M., T. Suzutani, K. Itoh, Y. Hirano, K. Murono, M. Nagamine, K. Mizuta, M. Niikura, and S. Morikawa. 1999. Nucleotide sequence of thymidine kinase gene of sequential acyclovir-resistant herpes simplex virus type 1 isolates recovered from a child with Wiskott-Aldrich syndrome: evidence for reactivation of acyclovir-resistant herpes simplex virus. *J. Med. Virol.* **58:**387–393.

171. Saldanha, J., W. Gerlich, N. Lelie, P. Dawson, K. Heermann, and A. Heath. 2001. An international collaborative study to establish a World Health Organization international standard for hepatitis B virus DNA nucleic acid amplification techniques. *Vox Sang.* **80:**63–71.

172. Santantonio, T., M. Fasano, S. Durantel, L. Barraud, M. Heichen, A. Guastadisegni, G. Pastore, and F. Zoulim. 2009. Adefovir dipivoxil resistance patterns in patients with lamivudine-resistant chronic hepatitis B. *Antivir. Ther.* **14:**557–565.

173. Sarafianos, S. G., K. Das, S. H. Hughes, and E. Arnold. 2004. Taking aim at a moving target: designing drugs to inhibit drug-resistant HIV-1 reverse transcriptases. *Curr. Opin. Struct. Biol.* **14:**716–730.

174. Sarisky, R. T., M. R. Quail, P. E. Clark, T. T. Nguyen, W. S. Halsey, R. J. Wittrock, J. O'Leary Bartus, M. M. Van Horn, G. M. Sathe, S. Van Horn, M. D. Kelly, T. H. Bacon, and J. J. Leary. 2001. Characterization of herpes simplex viruses selected in culture for resistance to penciclovir or acyclovir. *J. Virol.* **75:**1761–1769.

175. Sarrazin, C., J. Hong, S. Lim, Z. Qin, S. Susser, B. Bradford, S. Porter, et al. 2009. Incidence of virologic escape observed during ITMN-191 (R7227) monotherapy is genotpe dependent, associated with specific NS3 substitution, and suppressed upon combination with peginterferon alfa-2A/ribavirin. *J. Hepatol.* **50**(Suppl. 1):S350.

176. Sarrazin, C., T. L. Kieffer, D. Bartels, B. Hanzelka, U. Muh, M. Welker, D. Wincheringer, Y. Zhou, H. M. Chu, C. Lin, C. Weegink, H. Reesink, S. Zeuzem, and A. D. Kwong. 2007. Dynamic hepatitis C virus genotypic and phenotypic changes in patients treated with the protease inhibitor telaprevir. *Gastroenterology* **132:**1767–1777.

177. Sarrazin, C., and S. Zeuzem. 2010. Resistance to direct antiviral agents in patients with hepatitis C virus infection. *Gastroenterology* **138:**447–462.

178. Scott, G. M., A. Weinberg, W. D. Rawlinson, and S. Chou. 2007. Multidrug resistance conferred by novel DNA polymerase mutations in human cytomegalovirus isolates. *Antimicrob. Agents Chemother.* **51:**89–94.

179. Shafer, R. W., M. J. Kozal, M. A. Winters, A. K. Iversen, D. A. Katzenstein, M. V. Ragni, W. A. Meyer, P. Gupta, S. Rasheed, R. Coombs, and T. C. Merigan. 1994. Combination therapy with zidovudine and didanosine selects for drug-resistant human immunodeficiency virus type 1 strains with unique patterns of pol gene mutations. *J. Infect. Dis.* **169:**722–729.

180. Shahriar, R., S. Y. Rhee, T. F. Liu, W. J. Fessel, A. Scarsella, W. Towner, S. P. Holmes, A. R. Zolopa, and R. W. Shafer. 2009. Nonpolymorphic human immunodeficiency virus type 1 protease and reverse transcriptase treatment-selected mutations. *Antimicrob. Agents Chemother.* **53:**4869–4878.

181. Sherman, M., C. Yurdaydin, H. Simsek, M. Silva, Y. F. Liaw, V. K. Rustgi, H. Sette, N. Tsai, D. J. Tenney, J. Vaughan, B. Kreter, and R. Hindes. 2008. Entecavir therapy for lamivudine-refractory chronic hepatitis B: improved virologic, biochemical, and serology outcomes through 96 weeks. *Hepatology* **48:**99–108.

182. Sheu, T. G., V. M. Deyde, M. Okomo-Adhiambo, R. J. Garten, X. Xu, R. A. Bright, E. N. Butler, T. R. Wallis, A. I. Klimov, and L. V. Gubareva. 2008. Surveillance for neuraminidase inhibitor resistance among human influenza A and B viruses circulating worldwide from 2004 to 2008. *Antimicrob. Agents Chemother.* **52:**3284–3292.

183. Shields, W. W., and P. J. Pockros. 2009. Ribavirin analogs. *Clin. Liver Dis.* **13:**419–427.

184. Shimura, K., E. Kodama, Y. Sakagami, Y. Matsuzaki, W. Watanabe, K. Yamataka, Y. Watanabe, Y. Ohata, S. Doi, M. Sato, M. Kano, S. Ikeda, and M. Matsuoka. 2008. Broad antiretroviral activity and resistance profile of the novel human immunodeficiency virus integrase inhibitor elvitegravir (JTK-303/GS-9137). *J. Virol.* **82:**764–774.

185. Shirasaka, T., M. F. Kavlick, T. Ueno, W. Y. Gao, E. Kojima, M. L. Alcaide, S. Chokekijchai, B. M. Roy, E. Arnold, R. Yarchoan, and H. Mitsuya. 1995. Emergence of human immunodeficiency virus type 1 variants with resistance to multiple dideoxynucleosides in patients receiving therapy with dideoxynucleosides. *Proc. Natl. Acad. Sci. USA* **92:**2398–2402.

186. **Simmonds, P., J. Bukh, C. Combet, G. Deleage, N. Enomoto, S. Feinstone, P. Halfon, G. Inchauspe, C. Kuiken, G. Maertens, M. Mizokami, D. G. Murphy, H. Okamoto, J. M. Pawlotsky, F. Penin, E. Sablon, I. T. Shin, L. J. Stuyver, H. J. Thiel, S. Viazov, A. J. Weiner, and A. Widell.** 2005. Consensus proposals for a unified system of nomenclature of hepatitis C virus genotypes. *Hepatology* **42:**962–973.

187. **Smith, I. L., J. M. Cherrington, R. E. Jiles, M. D. Fuller, W. R. Freeman, and S. A. Spector.** 1997. High-level resistance of cytomegalovirus to ganciclovir is associated with alterations in both the UL97 and DNA polymerase genes. *J. Infect. Dis.* **176:**69–77.

188. **Stephenson, I., J. Democratis, A. Lackenby, T. McNally, J. Smith, M. Pareek, J. Ellis, A. Bermingham, K. Nicholson, and M. Zambon.** 2009. Neuraminidase inhibitor resistance after oseltamivir treatment of acute influenza A and B in children. *Clin. Infect. Dis.* **48:**389–396.

189. **Stranska, R., R. Schuurman, E. Nienhuis, I. W. Goedegebuure, M. Polman, J. F. Weel, P. M. Wertheim-Van Dillen, R. J. Berkhout, and A. M. van Loon.** 2005. Survey of acyclovir-resistant herpes simplex virus in the Netherlands: prevalence and characterization. *J. Clin. Virol.* **32:**7–18.

190. **Strizki, J. M., C. Tremblay, S. Xu, L. Wojcik, N. Wagner, W. Gonsiorek, R. W. Hipkin, C. C. Chou, C. Pugliese-Sivo, Y. Xiao, J. R. Tagat, K. Cox, T. Priestley, S. Sorota, W. Huang, M. Hirsch, G. R. Reyes, and B. M. Baroudy.** 2005. Discovery and characterization of vicriviroc (SCH 417690), a CCR5 antagonist with potent activity against human immunodeficiency virus type 1. *Antimicrob. Agents Chemother.* **49:**4911–4919.

191. **Stuyver, L. J., S. A. Locarnini, A. Lok, D. D. Richman, W. F. Carman, J. L. Dienstag, and R. F. Schinazi.** 2001. Nomenclature for antiviral-resistant human hepatitis B virus mutations in the polymerase region. *Hepatology* **33:**751–757.

192. **Sugiura, W., Z. Matsuda, Y. Yokomaku, K. Hertogs, B. Larder, T. Oishi, A. Okano, T. Shiino, M. Tatsumi, M. Matsuda, H. Abumi, N. Takata, S. Shirahata, K. Yamada, H. Yoshikura, and Y. Nagai.** 2002. Interference between D30N and L90M in selection and development of protease inhibitor-resistant human immunodeficiency virus type 1. *Antimicrob. Agents Chemother.* **46:**708–715.

193. **Sullivan, V., C. L. Talarico, S. C. Stanat, M. Davis, D. M. Coen, and K. K. Biron.** 1992. A protein kinase homologue controls phosphorylation of ganciclovir in human cytomegalovirus-infected cells. *Nature* **358:**162–164.

194. **Susser, S., C. Welsch, Y. Wang, M. Zettler, F. S. Domingues, U. Karey, E. Hughes, R. Ralston, X. Tong, E. Herrmann, S. Zeuzem, and C. Sarrazin.** 2009. Characterization of resistance to the protease inhibitor boceprevir in hepatitis C virus-infected patients. *Hepatology* **50:**1709–1718.

195. **Tan, J., B. Degertekin, S. N. Wong, M. Husain, K. Oberhelman, and A. S. Lok.** 2008. Tenofovir monotherapy is effective in hepatitis B patients with antiviral treatment failure to adefovir in the absence of adefovir-resistant mutations. *J. Hepatol.* **48:**391–398.

196. **Tenney, D. J., S. M. Levine, R. E. Rose, A. W. Walsh, S. P. Weinheimer, L. Discotto, M. Plym, K. Pokornowski, C. F. Yu, P. Angus, A. Ayres, A. Bartholomeusz, W. Sievert, G. Thompson, N. Warner, S. Locarnini, and R. J. Colonno.** 2004. Clinical emergence of entecavir-resistant hepatitis B virus requires additional substitutions in virus already resistant to lamivudine. *Antimicrob. Agents Chemother.* **48:**3498–3507.

197. **Tenney, D. J., R. E. Rose, C. J. Baldick, S. M. Levine, K. A. Pokornowski, A. W. Walsh, J. Fang, C. F. Yu, S. Zhang, C. E. Mazzucco, B. Eggers, M. Hsu, M. J. Plym, P. Poundstone, J. Yang, and R. J. Colonno.** 2007. Two-year assessment of entecavir resistance in lamivudine-refractory hepatitis B virus patients reveals different clinical outcomes depending on the resistance substitutions present. *Antimicrob. Agents Chemother.* **51:**902–911.

198. **Tenney, D. J., R. E. Rose, C. J. Baldick, K. A. Pokornowski, B. J. Eggers, J. Fang, M. J. Wichroski, D. Xu, J. Yang, R.**

B. Wilber, and R. J. Colonno. 2009. Long-term monitoring shows hepatitis B virus resistance to entecavir in nucleoside-naive patients is rare through 5 years of therapy. *Hepatology* **49:**1503–1514.

199. **Tipples, G. A., M. M. Ma, K. P. Fischer, V. G. Bain, N. M. Kneteman, and D. L. Tyrrell.** 1996. Mutation in HBV RNA-dependent DNA polymerase confers resistance to lamivudine in vivo. *Hepatology* **24:**714–717.

200. **van Bommel, F., R. A. de Man, H. Wedemeyer, K. Deterding, J. Petersen, P. Buggisch, A. Erhardt, D. Huppe, K. Stein, J. Trojan, C. Sarrazin, W. O. Bocher, U. Spengler, H. E. Wasmuth, J. G. Reinders, B. Moller, P. Rhode, H. H. Feucht, B. Wiedenmann, and T. Berg.** 2010. Long-term efficacy of tenofovir monotherapy for hepatitis B virus-monoinfected patients after failure of nucleoside/nucleotide analogues. *Hepatology* **51:**73–80.

201. **Varghese, J. N., J. L. McKimm-Breschkin, J. B. Caldwell, A. A. Kortt, and P. M. Colman.** 1992. The structure of the complex between influenza virus neuraminidase and sialic acid, the viral receptor. *Proteins* **14:**327–332.

202. **Vercauteren, J., A. M. Wensing, D. A. van de Vijver, J. Albert, C. Balotta, O. Hamouda, C. Kucherer, D. Struck, J. C. Schmit, B. Asjo, M. Bruckova, R. J. Camacho, B. Clotet, S. Coughlan, Z. Grossman, A. Horban, K. Korn, L. Kostrikis, C. Nielsen, D. Paraskevis, M. Poljak, E. Puchhammer-Stockl, C. Riva, L. Ruiz, M. Salminen, R. Schuurman, A. Sonnerborg, D. Stanekova, M. Stanojevic, A. M. Vandamme, and C. A. Boucher.** 2009. Transmission of drug-resistant HIV-1 is stabilizing in Europe. *J. Infect. Dis.* **200:**1503–1508.

203. **Villet, S., C. Pichoud, G. Billioud, L. Barraud, S. Durantel, C. Trepo, and F. Zoulim.** 2008. Impact of hepatitis B virus rtA181V/T mutants on hepatitis B treatment failure. *J. Hepatol.* **48:**747–755.

204. **Vingerhoets, J., H. Azijn, E. Fransen, I. De Baere, L. Smeulders, D. Jochmans, K. Andries, R. Pauwels, and M. P. de Bethune.** 2005. TMC125 displays a high genetic barrier to the development of resistance: evidence from in vitro selection experiments. *J. Virol.* **79:**12773–12782.

205. **Visse, B., J. M. Huraux, and A. M. Fillet.** 1999. Point mutations in the varicella-zoster virus DNA polymerase gene confer resistance to foscarnet and slow growth phenotype. *J. Med. Virol.* **59:**84–90.

206. **von Itzstein, M.** 2007. The war against influenza: discovery and development of sialidase inhibitors. *Nat. Rev. Drug Discov.* **6:**967–974.

207. **Wang, J. Y., H. Ling, W. Yang, and R. Craigie.** 2001. Structure of a two-domain fragment of HIV-1 integrase: implications for domain organization in the intact protein. *EMBO J.* **20:**7333–7343.

208. **Warner, N., and S. Locarnini.** 2008. The antiviral drug selected hepatitis B virus rtA181T/sW172* mutant has a dominant negative secretion defect and alters the typical profile of viral rebound. *Hepatology* **48:**88–98.

209. **Warner, N., S. Locarnini, M. Kuiper, A. Bartholomeusz, A. Ayres, L. Yuen, and T. Shaw.** 2007. The L80I substitution in the reverse transcriptase domain of the hepatitis B virus polymerase is associated with lamivudine resistance and enhanced viral replication in vitro. *Antimicrob. Agents Chemother.* **51:**2285–2292.

210. **Werle-Lapostolle, B., S. Bowden, S. Locarnini, K. Wursthorn, J. Petersen, G. Lau, C. Trepo, P. Marcellin, Z. Goodman, W. E. Delaney IV, S. Xiong, C. L. Brosgart, S. S. Chen, C. S. Gibbs, and F. Zoulim.** 2004. Persistence of cccDNA during the natural history of chronic hepatitis B and decline during adefovir dipivoxil therapy. *Gastroenterology* **126:**1750–1758.

211. **Westby, M., M. Lewis, J. Whitcomb, M. Youle, A. L. Pozniak, I. T. James, T. M. Jenkins, M. Perros, and E. van der Ryst.** 2006. Emergence of CXCR4-using human immunodeficiency virus type 1 (HIV-1) variants in a minority of HIV-1-infected patients following treatment with the CCR5 antagonist maraviroc is from a pretreatment CXCR4-using virus reservoir. *J. Virol.* **80:**4909–4920.

212. Westby, M., C. Smith-Burchnell, J. Mori, M. Lewis, M. Mosley, M. Stockdale, P. Dorr, G. Ciaramella, and M. Perros. 2007. Reduced maximal inhibition in phenotypic susceptibility assays indicates that viral strains resistant to the CCR5 antagonist maraviroc utilize inhibitor-bound receptor for entry. *J. Virol.* **81:**2359–2371.

213. Westland, C. E., H. Yang, W. E. Delaney IV, C. S. Gibbs, M. D. Miller, M. Wulfsohn, J. Fry, C. L. Brosgart, and S. Xiong. 2003. Week 48 resistance surveillance in two phase 3 clinical studies of adefovir dipivoxil for chronic hepatitis B. *Hepatology* **38:**96–103.

214. Westland, C. E., H. Yang, W. E. Delaney IV, M. Wulfsohn, N. Lama, C. S. Gibbs, M. D. Miller, J. Fry, C. L. Brosgart, E. R. Schiff, and S. Xiong. 2005. Activity of adefovir dipivoxil against all patterns of lamivudine-resistant hepatitis B viruses in patients. *J. Viral Hepat.* **12:**67–73.

215. Whitcomb, J. M., W. Huang, K. Limoli, E. Paxinos, T. Wrin, G. Skowron, S. G. Deeks, M. Bates, N. S. Hellmann, and C. J. Petropoulos. 2002. Hypersusceptibility to non-nucleoside reverse transcriptase inhibitors in HIV-1: clinical, phenotypic and genotypic correlates. *AIDS* **16:**F41–F47.

216. Whitcomb, J. M., N. T. Parkin, C. Chappey, N. S. Hellmann, and C. J. Petropoulos. 2003. Broad nucleoside reverse-transcriptase inhibitor cross-resistance in human immunodeficiency virus type 1 clinical isolates. *J. Infect. Dis.* **188:**992–1000.

217. Whitley, R. J., F. G. Hayden, K. S. Reisinger, N. Young, R. Dutkowski, D. Ipe, R. G. Mills, and P. Ward. 2001. Oral oseltamivir treatment of influenza in children. *Pediatr. Infect. Dis. J.* **20:**127–133.

218. Yang, G., Q. Song, M. Charles, W. C. Drosopoulos, E. Arnold, and V. R. Prasad. 1996. Use of chimeric human immunodeficiency virus types 1 and 2 reverse transcriptases for structure-function analysis and for mapping susceptibility to nonnucleoside inhibitors. *J. Acquir. Immune Defic. Syndr. Hum. Retrovirol.* **11:**326–333.

219. Yang, H., C. Westland, S. Xiong, and W. E. Delaney IV. 2004. In vitro antiviral susceptibility of full-length clinical hepatitis B virus isolates cloned with a novel expression vector. *Antivir. Res.* **61:**27–36.

220. Yeh, C. T., R. N. Chien, C. M. Chu, and Y. F. Liaw. 2000. Clearance of the original hepatitis B virus YMDD-motif mutants with emergence of distinct lamivudine-resistant mutants during prolonged lamivudine therapy. *Hepatology* **31:**1318–1326.

221. Zaaijer, H. L., F. J. van Hemert, M. H. Koppelman, and V. V. Lukashov. 2007. Independent evolution of overlapping polymerase and surface protein genes of hepatitis B virus. *J. Gen. Virol.* **88:**2137–2143.

222. Zambon, M., and F. G. Hayden. 2001. Position statement: global neuraminidase inhibitor susceptibility network. *Antivir. Res.* **49:**147–156.

223. Zein, N. N. 2000. Clinical significance of hepatitis C virus genotypes. *Clin. Microbiol. Rev.* **13:**223–235.

224. Ziegler, T., M. L. Hemphill, M. L. Ziegler, G. Perez-Oronoz, A. I. Klimov, A. W. Hampson, H. L. Regnery, and N. J. Cox. 1999. Low incidence of rimantadine resistance in field isolates of influenza A viruses. *J. Infect. Dis.* **180:**935–939.

225. Zoulim, F., and S. Locarnini. 2009. Hepatitis B virus resistance to nucleos(t)ide analogues. *Gastroenterology* **137:**1593–1608.

Susceptibility Test Methods: Viruses*

MAX Q. ARENS AND ELLA M. SWIERKOSZ

110

During the past decades, safe and effective antiviral therapy has been developed for treatment of a number of viral infections (11, 28, 29). Great strides have been made most notably in development of antiviral agents for treatment of human immunodeficiency virus (HIV). While the overwhelming majority of clinical virus isolates from drug-naive patients are susceptible to antiviral agents, widespread use of some antiviral agents has led to the emergence of drug-resistant strains, particularly in immunocompromised hosts (6, 8, 9, 10 12, 42, 83). Diagnostic virology laboratories are increasingly asked to perform in vitro testing of antiviral agents when patients fail to clinically respond to antiviral therapy. This chapter discusses the clinical situations in which antiviral resistance has emerged, thus necessitating in vitro susceptibility testing, and provides an overview of the phenotypic and genotypic susceptibility testing methods that have been employed to detect resistance.

CLINICAL INDICATIONS FOR ANTIVIRAL SUSCEPTIBILITY TESTING

Antiviral susceptibility testing is essential for defining mechanisms of antiviral resistance, for determining the frequency with which drug-resistant viral mutants emerge in clinical practice, for testing for cross-resistance to alternative agents, and for evaluating new antiviral agents. Because clinical deterioration of patients undergoing antiviral therapy can be associated with resistant virus, antiviral susceptibility testing may be helpful in certain clinical situations. Persistent or worsening herpes simplex virus type 1 (HSV-1) or varicella zoster virus (VZV) infection while on acyclovir (ACV) may indicate drug resistance. Alternative therapy, such as foscarnet and cidofovir, are available. Furthermore, HSV or VZV causing recurrent infection is often thymidine kinase (TK) competent and therefore susceptible to ACV, which has minimal toxicity compared to foscarnet. Persistent or worsening human cytomegalovirus (HCMV) retinitis, pneumonitis, or colitis unresponsive to ganciclovir may also

indicate drug-resistant virus. Cidofovir and foscarnet can be used as alternative agents. Influenza A isolates resistant to amantadine and rimantadine readily emerged during clinical trials of these drugs; therefore, continuous shedding or transmission of influenza A virus in a population which is being prophylaxed or treated with these agents may be due to drug resistance. Prolonged influenza virus shedding during therapy with a neuraminidase (NA) inhibitor (NI) may be due to emergence of NI-resistant virus. Due to the emergence of resistance to adamantanes and NIs, ongoing monitoring of influenza viruses is essential for determining effective chemoprophylaxis and treatment (http://www.cdc.gov/H1N1flu/recommendations.htm).

Monitoring for HIV type 1 (HIV-1) antiretroviral resistance is essential when beginning antiretroviral therapy (ART), for assessing failure of a particular regimen to suppress HIV replication and to test for cross-resistance to alternative antiretroviral drugs to aid in selection of appropriate salvage therapy. Guidelines developed by the U.S. Department of Health and Human Services (available at http://www.aidsinfo.nih.gov/Guidelines/, accessed 21 September 2009) have recommended that resistance testing be performed for persons with acute and chronic HIV infection at entry into care, whether or not treatment is to be initiated, prior to initiation of therapy, and when changing antiretroviral regimens in cases of virologic failure, drug intolerance, or suboptimal suppression of viral load. A viral tropism assay should be performed prior to the initiation of a CC chemokine receptor type 5 (CCR5) antagonist. Baseline resistance testing is recommended because transmission of drug-resistant HIV strains has been documented and has been associated with suboptimal response to therapy (82). A genotypic assay is recommended when testing antiretroviral-naïve persons because of its more rapid turnaround time. Plasma HIV RNA (viral load) is the most important indicator of response to ART and should be measured in all patients upon entry into care, upon initiation or change of therapy, within 2 to 8 weeks after initiation or change of therapy. Repeat viral load testing should be performed at 4- to 8-week intervals until the level falls below the assay's limit of detection and at regular intervals thereafter (http://www.aidsinfo.nih.gov/Guidelines/). In cases of suboptimal viral load reduction, there may be resistance to only one component of the combination therapy; substitution of an

---

*This chapter contains information presented in chapter 114 by Max Q. Arens and Ella M. Swierkosz in the ninth edition of this *Manual* and in chapter 12 by Max Q. Arens and Ella M. Swierkosz in the fourth edition of the *Clinical Virology Manual* (S. Specter et al. [ed.], ASM Press, Washington, DC, 2009).

alternative drug may provide clinical benefits, although, in general, at least two fully active agents should be added to a failing regimen. Prolonged treatment of chronic hepatitis B virus (HBV) infections selects for antiviral resistance at various rates, depending upon the particular agent used. Resistance testing of treated patients with HBV virologic breakthrough after treatment with nucleoside/nucleotide analogs is recommended (83, 84).

DEFINITION OF ANTIVIRAL RESISTANCE

Antiviral resistance is a decrease in susceptibility to an antiviral drug that can be clearly established by in vitro testing and can be confirmed by genetic analysis of the virus and biochemical study of the altered enzymes. In vitro drug resistance must be distinguished from clinical resistance, in which the viral infection fails to respond to therapy. Clinical failures may or may not be due to the presence of a drug-resistant virus. Failure to achieve clinical response also hinges on other factors such as the patient's immunologic status and the pharmacokinetics of the drug in that individual patient. For example, limited penetration of drug into the central nervous system may allow escape of HIV-1 despite suppression of virus at other sites. Poor oral absorption and binding to plasma proteins may limit bioavailability of certain drugs. Furthermore, administration of certain antiretroviral drugs in combination may interfere with absorption or stimulate elimination of one or more of the coadministered drugs. Patient-specific factors, such as nonadherence, intolerance to an antiretroviral drug, or an intercurrent infection, can also lead to increases in HIV-1 plasma viremia despite in vitro susceptibility.

VARIABLES OF ANTIVIRAL SUSCEPTIBILITY TESTING

To date, few standards exist for antiviral susceptibility testing. The Clinical and Laboratory Standards Institute (CLSI; formerly National Committee for Clinical Laboratory Standards or NCCLS) published an approved standard for susceptibility testing of HSV as a first step in developing consensus protocols for antiviral susceptibility testing (97). The major obstacle to standardization of antiviral susceptibility testing is that many variables influence the final result. These include (i) cell line, (ii) viral inoculum titer, (iii) incubation time, (iv) concentration range of the antiviral agent tested, (v) reference strains, (vi) assay method, (vii) end-point criteria, (viii) calculation of endpoint, and (ix) interpretation of endpoint. Testing of a single virus isolate may lead to greatly different endpoints, depending on the type of cell culture used (33, 59, 80). For example, the activity of ACV appeared greater than that of penciclovir (PCV) when a plaque reduction assay (PRA) was performed with Vero cells; the converse was true when the assay was performed with WI-38 VA-13 and WISH cell lines. Both drugs had comparable activity levels when tested with A549 cells (80). The titer of the virus inoculum is also critical; too large an inoculum can make a susceptible isolate appear resistant; too small an inoculum can make all isolates appear susceptible (59). The length of time that virus incubates in the presence of drug must be sufficient to allow detection of small plaques, in the case of a PRA, or to allow growth of a subpopulation of resistant virus, which may replicate at a slower rate than that of wild-type virus (4). The prolonged incubation time of peripheral blood mononuclear cell (PBMC)-based assays for HIV-1 susceptibility testing have

been shown to select for subpopulations of HIV-1 variants not present in the starting inoculum (76). Moreover, different assay methods can produce different results. For example, the dye uptake (DU) assay for HSV susceptibility testing produces 50% inhibitory concentrations (IC$_{50}$s) higher than those produced by PRA (64). The concentration range of the drug tested affects the quality of the dose-response curve and therefore the validity of end-point calculations. Susceptibility results are usually expressed as IC$_{50}$s because of the greater mathematical precision of the 50% endpoint than of a 90 or 99% endpoint. (Synonyms for IC$_{50}$ are 50% inhibitory concentration and 50% effective concentration.) However, debate continues concerning the appropriate endpoint, i.e., 50% versus 90 or 99% inhibition. IC$_{50}$s are more precise and reproducible, but IC$_{90}$s may correlate better with clinical response and are better at detecting subpopulations of drug-resistant strains among sensitive ones (35, 97). Moreover, few studies have correlated in vitro results with clinical response (6, 46, 70, 81, 108, 127).

Another critical variable is the heterogeneity within the population of a virus "isolate." A single clinical isolate actually represents a mixture of drug-susceptible and drug-resistant phenotypes (5, 65, 109, 128). A virus population that has never encountered an antiviral agent is predominantly drug susceptible; resistant virus may be present at low levels. The presence of low levels of resistant virus in a population that is predominantly drug susceptible might not be reflected in the IC$_{50}$ but would manifest its presence in higher IC$_{90}$s or IC$_{99}$s. At this time it is unknown whether a small fraction of drug-resistant virus is important to the behavior of the virus in vivo or how such a fraction might affect the response of the infection to therapy in an otherwise healthy host. However, in immunocompromised patients, under the continued selective pressure of antiviral therapy, resistant virus can emerge, and its presence can often be correlated with progressive viral disease (6, 23, 40, 42, 46, 70, 102, 110, 111, 112, 123).

The genetic locus at which a mutation occurs also affects susceptibility testing endpoints. For example, DNA polymerase mutations of HSV, VZV, and HCMV usually confer relatively smaller increases in in vitro resistance than do TK mutations, which could go undetected in a mixed population of wild-type and mutant virus. In HIV-1, the level of in vitro resistance to protease (PR) inhibitors (PIs) increased as the number of PR gene mutations increased (63). A good definition of such mixtures can be obtained only by testing appropriate concentrations of drug and a sufficiently large fraction of the population to detect resistant strains.

TESTING METHODS

Phenotypic versus Genotypic Assays

Phenotypic assays are in vitro susceptibility assays that measure the inhibitory effect of antiviral agents on the entire virus population in a patient isolate. A variety of endpoint measurements have been utilized and include a reduction in the number of plaques; inhibition of viral DNA synthesis; reduction in the yield of a viral structural protein, e.g., hemagglutinin of influenza or p24 antigen of HIV; and reduction in the enzymatic activity of a functional protein, e.g., HIV-1 reverse transcriptase (RT) and influenza virus NA. Phenotypic assays in use include PRA, DU, DNA hybridization, enzyme immunoassay (EIA), NA inhibition, and yield reduction assays for herpes group and influenza A viruses, and PBMC cocultivation and recombinant virus assays (RVAs) for HIV-1. Genotypic assays analyze viral nucleic acid to detect specific mutations that cause antiviral drug resistance. Genotyping has been applied primarily to HBV, HCMV, and HIV-1. Genotypic assays include DNA sequencing by automated sequencers, PCR amplification and restriction enzyme digestion of the products, and hybridization to microarrays of oligonucleotide probes. Phenotypic and genotypic assays have unique features that complement each other. Phenotypic assays are better suited to assess the combined effect of multiple resistance mutations on drug susceptibility. This is especially important for viruses such as HBV, HCMV, and HIV-1, which acquire resistance-associated mutations in multiple genes that may be manifest as new patterns of resistance, cross-resistance, multidrug resistance, or even reversal of resistance (63, 69, 120, 124, 128). However, most phenotypic assays are labor-intensive and expensive and have a long turnaround time. Genotypic assays are relatively inexpensive and have shorter turnaround times but cannot detect mutations outside the selected target. Interpretation of genotypic assays is problematic due to the complex interactions of resistance mutations, which result in a particular drug-resistance phenotype. The major phenotypic and genotypic assays in use are discussed below.

Control Strains

Simultaneous testing of control strains is crucial when antiviral susceptibility testing is being done. Reference strains should include genetically and phenotypically well-characterized drug-susceptible and drug-resistant isolates. Drug-resistant strains chosen for reference should include those with drug resistance phenotypes relevant to the mode of action of the drug to be tested. For example, for testing nucleoside analogs, which require phosphorylation by viral TK, e.g., ACV versus HSV and VZV, TK-negative or -deficient strains should be included. Susceptibility testing of HCMV should include both UL97 and UL54 mutants. For HIV-1 testing, mutants resistant to both nucleoside analog and nonnucleoside analog inhibitors of RT, and mutants resistant to PIs should be used. The National Institute of Allergy and Infectious Diseases (NIAID) AIDS Research and Reference Reagent Program (Bethesda, MD) provides upon request a number of reference strains of HSV, VZV, and HCMV, including the drug-resistant strains mentioned above and laboratory control strains HCMV AD169 and VZV Oka. For susceptibility testing of HIV-1, the NIAID AIDS Research and Reference Reagent Program has a repository of strains with various resistance phenotypes. Pharmaceutical companies and the American Type Culture Collection are also a source of control strains.

PHENOTYPIC ASSAYS

PRA for CMV, HSV, and VZV

The PRA has classically been the "standard" method of antiviral susceptibility testing to which new methods are compared (13, 15, 62, 64, 93). Because many variations of the PRA have been reported, the CLSI developed a standard for PRA testing of HSV (97). Likewise, the HCMV Resistance Working Group of the AIDS Clinical Trials Groups has formulated a standardized PRA for HCMV susceptibility testing (78). The challenges associated with HCMV susceptibility testing by PRA became apparent when, despite adherence to a consensus PRA protocol, some collaborating laboratories had difficulty distinguishing drug-susceptible and drug-resistant HCMV isolates.

The principle of the PRA is the inhibition of viral plaque formation in the presence of antiviral agent. The concentration of antiviral agent inhibiting plaque formation by 50% is considered the IC_{50}. Although the PRA is tedious and consumes more reagents than other methods, it is appropriate for small-scale testing of isolates. Prior to performing the antiviral susceptibility assay per se, titers of HSV isolates must be determined to ensure an inoculum appropriate for the surface area of the assay wells or plates (i.e., approximately 100 PFU/60-mm-wide tissue culture plate). Because clinical strains of HCMV and VZV are cell associated and because low-titer cell-free stocks are less stable during storage, infected cell suspensions (obtained by trypsin treatment of the infected monolayer) can be conveniently used for these viruses. Two or three passages of clinical strains of HCMV and VZV in cell culture are usually necessary to obtain a sufficient titer of virus. Low-passage isolates should be used because they are more likely to be representative of the original mixed population of the clinical isolate than a higher-passage stock would be. Well-characterized drug-susceptible and drug-resistant strains of HSV, HCMV AD169, and VZV Oka or Ellen serve as reference strains. Stepwise instructions for performance of the PRA for HSV, VZV, and HCMV have been published elsewhere (64, 97, 129, 130)

A modified PRA has been described that utilizes Vero or CV-1 cells that have stably been transformed with the *Escherichia coli lacZ* gene under the control of an HSV-1 early promoter which expresses beta-galactosidase only after infection with HSV. Plaques were visualized after histochemical staining for beta-galactosidase (132, 133). Proposed susceptibility breakpoints determined by the PRA are listed in Table 1.

DU Assay

The DU assay has been used for many years for susceptibility testing of HSV (64, 93). This assay is based on the preferential uptake of a vital dye (neutral red) by viable cells but not by nonviable cells. The extent of viral lytic activity is determined by the relative amount of dye bound to viable cells after infection with HSV compared with the amount bound to uninfected cells. The dye bound by viable cells is eluted by ethanol and measured colorimetrically. The drug concentration inhibiting viral lytic activity by 50% is considered the IC_{50}.

The DU assay consistently gives IC_{50}s of ACV that are three to five times greater than those given by PRA. This difference is most likely due to the higher inoculum used in the DU assay (500 PFU/ml) and to the use of a liquid overlay, which allows drug-resistant virus to "amplify," thus resulting in a more sensitive detection of small amounts of drug-resistant virus. Therefore, the DU assay uses a cutoff IC_{50} of >3 μg/ml to denote ACV resistance (Table 1).

Advantages of the DU method include its ability to be semiautomated, allowing for efficient testing of large numbers of isolates and its ability to detect smaller amounts of resistant virus than the PRA can detect. Disadvantages are the relatively high cost of automated equipment and the technical problems caused by overseeding of cells into the culture wells and precipitation of neutral red onto the monolayer. The stepwise procedure for the DU assay has been published previously (64, 93).

DNA Hybridization

DNA hybridization assays have been used to measure the effect of different antiviral compounds on DNA synthesis. These methods semiquantitatively measure the amount of

TABLE 1 Proposed guidelines for antiviral susceptibility results of herpes group and influenza A viruses

Virus	Antiviral agent	Method	IC$_{50}$ denoting resistance	Reference(s)
HSV	Acyclovir	PRA	≥2 µg/ml	93
		DNA hybridization	≥2 µg/ml	42, 131
		DU	≥3 µg/ml	64, 93
	Famciclovir (active metabolite = penciclovir)	PRA and DNA hybridization	Definitive breakpoints cannot be established	80, 128
	Foscarnet	PRA	>100 µg/ml	110
	Vidarabine	PRA	≥2-fold increase of IC$_{50}$ compared to control or pretherapy isolate	112
HCMV	Cidofovir	PRA and DNA hybridization	>2 µM	25, 47, 124
	Foscarnet	PRA and DNA hybridization	>400 µM	25, 47
			>324 µM	124
	Ganciclovir	PRA and DNA hybridization	≥3–4 fold increase of IC$_{50}$ compared to pretherapy isolate or control strain (≈3 µg/ml)	40, 45, 103
			>6 µM	26, 47
			>8 µM	124
Influenza A virus	Amantadine/rimantadine	EIA	>0.1 µg/ml	8, 9
Influenza A and B viruses	Oseltamivir and zanamivir	NI assay	>8-fold decrease in NA activity	55, 56
VZV	Acyclovir	PRA and DNA hybridization	≥3–4 fold increase of IC$_{50}$ compared to pretherapy isolate or to control strain	13, 70, 111
	Famciclovir	PRA and DNA hybridization	Definitive breakpoints cannot be established	128
	Foscarnet	Late antigen reduction assay	300 µM	111

viral DNA produced in the absence and presence of antiviral drug, and IC$_{50}$s are calculated from these data. Good correlation between the PRA and a dot blot hybridization assay has been demonstrated (14, 51). The stepwise procedure has been detailed previously (130). DNA-DNA hybridization test kits previously commercially available (Hybriwix Probe Systems, Diagnostic Hybrids, Inc., Athens, OH) have been used successfully for susceptibility testing of HSV, HCMV, and VZV (24, 25, 26, 32, 42, 70, 110, 111, 112, 124, 131). The Hybriwix assays are no longer commercially available.

EIAs

EIAs have been developed for susceptibility testing of HSV, VZV, and influenza A virus (8, 10, 106, 113). The EIA permits quantitative measurement of viral activity by spectrophotometric analysis; IC$_{50}$s are calculated as the concentrations of antiviral agent that reduce the absorbance to 50% of that of the virus control. Susceptibility results for HSV and VZV determined by this method have correlated well with those obtained by PRA.

Susceptibility testing of influenza A virus by PRA is tedious and labor intensive. The EIA is technically easier and is more suitable for the testing of multiple isolates (8). The EIA utilizes antibodies to influenza A virus hemagglutinins (H1 or H3); viral hemagglutinin expression correlates with viral growth. Amantadine and rimantadine activities are measured by inhibition of hemagglutinin expression. Amantadine- or rimantadine-susceptible and -resistant isolates, whose M2

gene sequences are known, serve as controls and must be tested in parallel with patient isolates. A protocol for the EIA for susceptibility testing of influenza A virus has been published (129). No commercial EIAs are available.

NIAs

Two inhibitors of influenza virus NA, oseltamivir and zanamivir, are approved for treatment of influenza A and B virus infections (21). Susceptibility studies to date have indicated that an assay of NA activity was the best predictor of in vivo response to NI (55). NA activity is assayed using solubilized supernatant from viral culture as the source of viral NA. After incubation of the viral NA with various concentrations of NI, a fluorogenic substrate is added. Fluorescence is quantitated by a fluorimeter, and the IC$_{50}$ is calculated relative to the activity of viral NA in the control reaction (no NI) (55). A commercially available chemiluminescent NA inhibition assay (NIA), NA-Star, is available (Applied Biosystems, Foster City, CA) and has been used to monitor susceptibility of novel influenza A (H1N1) to NIs (22). A zanamivir-resistant influenza B isolate from an immunocompromised child that was cross-resistant to oseltamivir showed a 1,000-fold increase in the IC$_{50}$ for zanamivir by the NIA (55, 56).

YRAs

The yield reduction assays (YRAs) reflect the ability of an antiviral agent to inhibit the production of infectious virus rather than the formation of a plaque. For the testing of the susceptibility of HSV to PCV and ACV, cell monolayers are infected with virus, incubated in the presence of antiviral compound, and then lysed. Cell-free virus titers are subsequently determined by plaque assay. The endpoint is defined as the concentration of antiviral agent that reduces virus yield by 50% in comparison with that of untreated control cultures. When used for testing the susceptibility of HSV to PCV and ACV, the IC_{50}s for PCV were equivalent to or lower than those for ACV (17, 80). The greater activity of PCV is postulated to be the result of the extended half-life of PCV-triphosphate (17). For susceptibility testing of influenza A virus to rimantadine, cell monolayers are infected with virus in the presence or absence of rimantadine, and virus replication is assessed by measuring hemagglutinin titers. A virus is considered drug susceptible if the hemagglutinin titer is reduced at least fourfold compared to that of untreated virus (20, 39).

Measurement of HSV and VZV TK Activity by Plaque Autoradiography

Functional viral TK is required for initial phosphorylation of ACV. To determine whether resistance to ACV is due to diminished or altered viral TK, two plaque autoradiograph methods are used (90). Incorporation of [^{125}I]iododeoxycytidine (IdC), a pyrimidine analog selectively phosphorylated by the VZV- or HSV-specific TK, correlates well with the ACV phosphorylating potential of HSV and VZV isolates. Incorporation of [^{14}C]thymidine (deoxyribosylthymine [dT]) specifically assesses the thymidine phosphorylating activity of these isolates and is useful for analyzing resistance to pyrimidine nucleoside analogs (ACV is a purine nucleoside analog). Most ACV-resistant HSV and VZV fail to incorporate both substrates due to diminished TK activity (TK$^-$); occasionally, strains with altered substrate (TK^a) activity are seen that fail to incorporate IdC but are able to incorporate dT. For IdC incorporation, Vero cells (HSV) and MRC-5 cells (VZV) are used. For dT incorporation, LMTK$^-$ TK$^-$ mouse LM cells (Roswell Park Memorial Institute, Buffalo, NY) are used for HSV; the TK$^-$ cell line 143B is used for VZV dT incorporation. These assays provide both quantitative and qualitative evaluations of the TK status of a mixed population of TK$^+$ and TK$^-$. The IdC and dT plaque autoradiograph methods have been detailed elsewhere (90, 130).

Assays for HIV

A number of phenotypic assays are in use for testing of HIV-1 isolate susceptibility to nucleoside analog RT inhibitors (63, 72, 75, 79, 92, 105, 122, 128, 138, 140). A serious limitation of some of these procedures is that not all clinical isolates grow in the cell culture lines used in these assays. The AIDS Clinical Trials Group developed an assay performed with PBMCs that allowed growth of almost all clinical isolates of HIV-1 (72). Viral activity is quantitated by measurement of the p24 antigen of HIV-1. The PBMC assay, however, is labor intensive, costly, and difficult to control because of the many variables of the assay and has a long turnaround time (weeks). Moreover, this assay requires cocultivation of infected PBMCs with uninfected donor PBMCs to produce a stock of the clinical isolate being tested, which has been shown to select for subpopulations of HIV-1 not present in the original isolate (76).

A new generation of phenotypic assays, RVAs, have been developed to circumvent these problems (63, 75, 92, 105, 122). The RVA involves RT-PCR amplification of complete RT and PR gene coding sequences directly from the patient's plasma. The amplified RT and PR gene sequences from the patient strain are ligated into a viral vector and then cotransfected along with a plasmid that expresses murine leukemia virus envelope proteins into a suitable receptive cell line. These cells then contain the patient's RT and PR gene-coding sequences in a background of an HIV-1 strain from which the original RT and PR sequences had been deleted. The susceptibilities of the chimeric pseudotyped viruses to all clinically available RT and PR inhibitors are subsequently determined in a single assay in which the ability of virus particles to replicate in the presence of various levels of antiretroviral drug is measured. Two RVAs are commercially available: the Antivirogram assay (developed by Virco, Mechelen, Belgium, and available in the United States from the Laboratory Corporation of America) (63) and the PhenoSense assay (Monogram Biosciences, South San Francisco, CA) (105). Detection of resistance is accomplished by measurement of luciferase activity (the luciferase gene is in the viral vector) in the target cells in one assay (Monogram) or by use of the HeLa-CD4 plaque reduction method in the other assay (Virco). RVAs thus allow determination of the phenotypic resistance patterns of circulating virus in vivo and circumvent the problem of selection of nonrepresentative variants during cultivation. The RVA can be completed in approximately 10 days from the time of cotransfection (63, 75, 92, 105, 122). Zhang et al. (145) compared these two phenotypic assays and concluded that the PhenoSense results are more precise (i.e., show lower variability) and that the PhenoSense assay is more likely to detect resistance to abacavir, didanosine, and stavudine. Limitations of RVAs are the necessity for a minimum of 500 to 1,000 copies of HIV-1 RNA/ml plasma, a lack of consensus as to the appropriate increase in the IC_{50} for each drug that correlates with clinical resistance, and uncertainty about the proportion of the total population of virus that a subpopulation of resistant virus must achieve to be detectable by these assays (57, 63).

Maraviroc is an entry inhibitor recently approved for treatment of adult patients with HIV-1 strains resistant to multiple antiretroviral agents. It exploits the requirement for HIV-1 to bind a coreceptor, in addition to the CD4 receptor, for viral entry into the host cell. The two major coreceptors for HIV-1 are CXC chemokine receptor type 4 (CXCR4) and CCR5, expressed on T lymphocytes and macrophages, respectively. Maraviroc is a noncompetitive inhibitor of the chemokine coreceptor CCR5; it selectively binds to CCR5, preventing fusion between HIV-1 viral and cellular membranes and thus entry into cells (88). Because some HIV-1 strains are also tropic for CXCR4 and some strains are "dual-tropic," using both CXCR4 and CCR5, patient isolates must be characterized, prior to initiation of maraviroc therapy, by means of a "tropism" assay to determine the identity of the required receptor. Three coreceptor tropism assays are available commercially: the Phenoscript assay [VIRalliance, Paris, France] (19); the Trofile assay [Monogram Biosciences, San Francisco, CA]; and the Sensitrop II molecular HIV co-receptor tropism assay, developed by Pathway Diagnostics (Malibu, CA) and offered exclusively through Quest Diagnostics. An enhanced-sensitivity, second-generation, commercially available HIV tropism assay is offered by Monogram Biosciences, Inc. (107); it replaced the original Trofile assay in June 2008. In the Trofile assay, recombinant "pseudoviruses" are generated that express patient-derived envelope proteins and a luciferase reporter gene, which are then used to infect target cell lines expressing either CCR5 or CXCR4 in the presence and absence of maraviroc. Infection is measured by the amount of luciferase activity present in the target cells. Virologic failure with maraviroc therapy is associated with outgrowth of a preexisting minority population of CXCR4 virus not initially detectable by the Trofile assay and by selection of variants with mutations in the V3 loop region of the gp120 gene, allowing virus to utilize maraviroc-CCR5 complexes for entry (94).

Monogram Biosciences also has a different specific phenotypic assay for detection of resistance to the integrase inhibitors (e.g., raltegravir) called PhenoSense Integrase. The assay is based on the same recombinant virus technology as described above, but in this case, the patient's viral integrase gene is amplified and inserted into the viral vector containing luciferase and transfected into cells for growth in the presence of integrase inhibitors. The integrase gene, although contiguous with the PR and RT genes, is not currently included in any commercial genotype assays, so the phenotype is the only commercial method available to demonstrate resistance to integrase inhibitors. The mutations that confer resistance to integrase inhibitors are known and include two different genetic pathways with a major mutation at either Q148H/K/R or N155H. Thus, laboratory-developed genotypic assays to detect resistance are possible for labs that have the interest and capability.

GENOTYPIC ASSAYS

The genetic basis for antiviral resistance has been studied extensively for HBV, HCMV, and HIV-1 and more recently for influenza viruses. Although not all resistance-associated mutations are known, the majority have been elucidated, allowing the application of molecular diagnostic methods. The major advantage of genotypic assays is the relatively rapid turnaround time compared to phenotypic assays.

Human Cytomegalovirus

Genotypic assays have been used to screen HCMV isolates for mutations associated with ganciclovir resistance. Both UL97 (phosphotransferase) and UL54 (DNA polymerase) mutations can be detected; UL97 mutations are responsible for most ganciclovir resistance found to date (124). A number of approaches have been applied successfully to genotyping HCMV.

PCR amplification of short fragments of the UL97 gene followed by restriction endonuclease digestion has been used to detect mutations at positions 460, 520, 594, and 595 (24, 25, 44, 45). In one study, this assay detected 78% of ganciclovir-resistant UL97 mutants (25). PCR amplification followed by restriction digestion could recognize mutant virus when present at 10% of the total virus population (124). The major advantage of this PCR-restriction endonuclease method is the speed with which UL97 mutations can be identified, since HCMV sequences can be directly amplified from many clinical samples. However, the absence of mutations at these key codons in UL97 does not necessarily exclude ganciclovir resistance, as it has been shown that resistance can be attributed to other mutations in UL97 or to mutations in UL54 alone (47).

PCR amplification and sequencing of nearly the entire UL54 gene and the fragment of the UL97 gene spanning the conserved domains of the phosphotransferase should theoretically detect all the mutations currently known to confer resistance to ganciclovir (4, 25, 47, 124). Wolf et al. (141) identified a complete set of overlapping primers to be used for sequencing the full UL97 gene. UL97-associated ganciclovir

resistance mutations also have been detected directly in patient blood and cerebrospinal fluid (16, 125, 141).

Sequencing of the UL54 gene for genotypic detection of resistance to ganciclovir, foscarnet, and cidofovir is a large task not generally undertaken by the routine clinical virology laboratory. The UL54 codons that confer resistance to all three anti-HCMV drugs are between codons 408 and 841, inclusively (44, 86). Thus, one must amplify a fragment of about 1,500 bp and use 3 or 4 sequencing primers in each direction to obtain a reliable sequence. In a study by Smith et al. (124), UL97 mutations could be detected in 89% of ganciclovir-resistant isolates, whereas UL54 mutations were present in all high-level ganciclovir-resistant isolates. A caveat that applies to genotypic analysis is that not every mutation is a cause of antiviral resistance. Marker transfer experiments must be performed to definitively determine that a particular mutation is associated with drug resistance. For this purpose, PCR-amplified UL97 and UL54 fragments containing resistance-associated mutations were cotransfected with HCMV strain AD169 (drug susceptible). The resulting recombinant plaques were assayed for antiviral susceptibility by PRA. To further verify transfer of the mutations in question, sequencing was performed across the transfected fragment (4, 26).

The field of HCMV genotyping for detection of drug resistance is still evolving. A standardized protocol for sequencing of the UL97 gene was developed by members of the AIDS Clinical Trials Group HCMV Laboratories and published several years ago (87). Nevertheless, the discovery of new mutations that confer drug resistance is ongoing, as evidenced by the recent description of a deletion at UL97 codon 601 that was responsible for the early development of ganciclovir resistance in a renal transplant recipient (58). A recent review has provided an updated synopsis of the current state of knowledge of drugs for and resistance to HCMV (53).

Human Immunodeficiency Virus

The development of antiretroviral drug resistance is currently a significant cause of treatment failures with HIV-infected patients (66, 67). Genotyping for detection of mutations that confer resistance has become a routine component of management of HIV-infected individuals. (The International AIDS Society—USA maintains a list of mutations associated with antiretroviral drug resistance, which is periodically updated [http://www.iasusa.org/resistance_mutations/index.html].) Because of the lack of proofreading activity in the RT enzyme that copies the genome of HIV, the virus exists in infected individuals as a population of variants or quasispecies (36). This results in the random appearance and subsequent selection of resistant mutants in the presence of a selection pressure such as an inhibitory drug. Initially, a single mutation may occur, confer a low level of resistance, and then grow to predominance in the population. With ongoing replication, additional mutations that confer high-level resistance appear, and the population as a whole becomes highly resistant (91). For some drugs, such as lamivudine (3TC) and nevirapine, a single mutation confers high-level resistance (117).

Genotypic methods that have been used for detection of mutations in HIV, including sequencing, selective PCR, oligonucleotide-specific hybridization, microarray hybridization (GeneChip; Affymetrix, Inc., Santa Clara, CA), and reverse-hybridization (line probe assay [LiPA]; Bayer Diagnostics NAD, Norwood, MA). The LiPA for detection of mutations in HIV is currently not commercially available. Sequencing methods have been developed by several noncommercial laboratories and by two commercial companies, Abbott Diagnostics (Abbott Park, IL; formerly available from Applied Biosystems, Inc.) and Siemens Health Care Diagnostics, Inc. (Deerfield, IL). Shafer (117) has reviewed the various assays available for genotypic analysis of HIV-1.

Dideoxynucleotide sequencing is the most commonly used method of HIV-1 PR and RT gene sequence analysis (37, 117). Two commercially available systems have been used successfully for this purpose: the Trugene HIV-1 genotyping kit and the OpenGene DNA sequencing system (Siemens Medical Solutions Diagnostics, Tarrytown, NY) and the ViroSeq HIV-1 genotyping system (Celera/Abbott Diagnostics) (27, 31, 43, 96, 135). Both systems have been approved for in vitro diagnostic use. The sequencing systems rely on initial extraction of viral RNA from patient plasma, RT-PCR of the extracted RNA to amplify about 1,500 bp of PR and RT, and then a sequencing reaction with dye terminators (ViroSeq) or dye-labeled primers (Trugene). Both companies make sequencing instruments for electrophoresis of the samples, and both provide software to assemble the segments and align the assembled patient sequence with a reference sequence to aid in the identification of mutant codons. With the primers for PCR and the sequencing primers, the ViroSeq system provides double coverage at a minimum for the entire 1.5-kb sequence of interest, and quadruple coverage may be obtained for certain regions. The ViroSeq software combines the functions of several previously available software packages to trim the sequence segments, generate a contiguous consensus sequence that is generated by assemblage of the overlapping individual segments, and align the consensus sequence with a reference sequence. The operator must manually toggle through the entire sequence, edit (confirm or override) the computer base calls, and also make the final decision about polymorphic sites where a mutant base might constitute a minor proportion in the background of the wild-type base. The ABI software prints a complete mutation report that identifies "reported" and "novel" mutations based on the Los Alamos National Laboratory HIV database, which is available online at http://hiv-web.lanl.gov. The ViroSeq system has been used to successfully detect RT and PR gene mutations in pediatric samples and in non-subtype B HIV-1 samples (31, 96).

The Trugene genotyping kit may be used in conjunction with a number of extraction procedures. The purified viral RNA is amplified in a single-tube RT-PCR step, the product of which can be used directly in the subsequent sequencing reactions. It employs a proprietary methodology using 4 pairs of sequencing primers; the upstream primer of each pair is labeled with one dye, and the downstream primer of each pair is labeled with another dye. Each primer pair is present in each of 4 dideoxy-terminator reactions, one reaction for each of the four dideoxy bases. Thus, this arrangement requires 16 different reactions and 16 lanes on the sequencing gel in order to cover the HIV PR and RT genes in both directions. The data are analyzed with the Trugene software and interpreted to provide a resistance report. Two studies have demonstrated improved virological outcome when genotyping information is considered in patient management decisions (27, 135).

A number of studies have compared the various laboratory-developed and commercial sequencing methods. An interlaboratory study compared the ability of 13 laboratories to detect RT mutations in cultured PBMC pellets. Highly concordant results were obtained overall, with some

difficulty encountered with a clinical isolate that contained a mixture of wild-type and mutant codons. A mutant codon which was present at less than 50% of a mixed population of resistant and susceptible genotypes was not consistently detected (37). Two large multicenter studies compared sequencing results among participating laboratories for detection of RT mutations in either coded plasmid mixtures or spiked plasma samples. Laboratories had difficulty in detecting mutations for which the mutants represented 25% or less of the total DNA population at that codon (115, 116). Even the editing process can contribute variability to the overall HIV genotype determination, as shown by Huang et al. (68). In this study, sequence concordance was high, even though different editing strategies were used by different labs, but 12% of the resistance mutations present in the 10 electronic files that were distributed and analyzed were not identified in some labs.

The LiPA was manufactured by Innogenetics but marketed by Bayer Diagnostics NAD as the Versant HIV-1 RT resistance assay and Versant HIV-1 PR resistance assay. It has been withdrawn from the market.

The Virtual Phenotype assay (Virco) utilizes a proprietary algorithm to compare a virus genotype to a large database of known genotypes and phenotypes to predict a phenotype based on sequence data (57, 117). Two RT and PR gene sequence analysis programs are available online from Stanford University at http://hivdb.stanford.edu (accessed 7 August 2007). One program compares an HIV-1 sequence submitted by the investigator to a consensus reference sequence, ultimately linking RT and PR gene sequence variations to the antiretroviral therapy history of the patient from whom the sequences were obtained (118). In the second sequence analysis program, Drug Resistance Interpretation, PR and RT gene sequences are entered by the user, and the program produces a phenotypic interpretation based on correlations of genotypes and accumulated information on clinical outcome (117).

Monogram Biosciences, Inc., offers a genotyping assay, GeneSeq HIV, using the dideoxynucleotide chain termination method of DNA sequencing. Based upon the mutations detected, an interpretation algorithm is applied to predict a resistance profile. PhenoSense GT (Monogram Biosciences) combines the results of PhenoSense HIV with GeneSeq HIV, providing a "net assessment" of drug resistance as well as a listing of mutations detected. Other genotype interpretation systems are available commercially or publicly (137).

A concern with each of the genotypic methods is that mutant variants present at low frequencies may not be detectable and that mixtures of HIV-1 strains with minor sequence variations may not be distinguishable (57, 117). Genotypic assays do allow more rapid and efficient detection of resistance than phenotypic assays and may allow earlier detection of emerging resistance than phenotypic assays. Also, because of the complex interactions among different combinations of resistance mutations, predictions of phenotype based on genotype alone may not be accurate (18, 117). Moreover, genotypic assays can detect only known resistance-associated mutations. The complexity of these tests makes them impractical for many diagnostic virology laboratories. Measurement of plasma HIV-1 RNA levels (viral load) reflects the extent of virus replication in an infected individual and remains the strongest predictor of clinical outcome. Declining HIV-1 RNA levels during treatment indicates response to therapy, while a significant rise in RNA levels indicates treatment failure (89) (http://www.aidsinfo.nih.gov).

Documentation of resistance to enfuvirtide (T-20) is problematic. It is a synthetic peptide inhibitor that interferes with viral entry by blocking formation of a hairpin structure that is necessary for fusion of the viral membrane with the cell membrane. Resistance to enfuvirtide is conferred rather quickly (within weeks) and is the result of a single mutation or a combination of mutations within the *env* HR1 domain; the substitutions most frequently associated with enfuvirtide resistance occur in codons 36 to 43 (85). However, mutations in other regions of the *env* gene and coreceptor usage and density may play a role in development of resistance (73).

Of recent concern with respect to the now greater availability of antiretrovirals in resource-limited countries is the question of whether the genotyping methods that have been developed for use in Western countries, mainly with HIV group M subtype B virus, will work on non-B subtypes. This concern is significant since subtype B accounts for only about 12% of the global AIDS pandemic. In a set of 35 HIV isolates from group M subtypes A to J, full-length sequences were created with the ViroSeq reagents in 84% of the specimens tested and with the TrueGene in 53% of the specimens tested (7). Both methods amplified RNA from plasma levels of about 100 to 1,000 copies/ml. Eshelman et al. (48) employed the ViroSeq system to genotype 126 samples (114 of which were non-B subtypes) and successfully sequenced 124 of these. Genotypes performed in a second lab with the same 126 samples were 98 to 100% identical to the primary lab results. Thus, it appears that the two commercially available genotyping systems work tolerably well on subtypes other than B and should be generally usable in geographic regions where non-B subtypes predominate.

Aside from the mechanics of performing HIV genotypes on non-B subtypes, there is the question of whether these subtypes exhibit drug-resistant mutation patterns in the same way and at the same locations as the subtype B strains. In an authoritative recent paper on this topic, Kantor et al. (74) looked at the correlation between antiretroviral treatment and the distribution of mutations in HIV sequences from 3,686 individuals infected with non-B subtypes and compared the data with mutations in HIV sequences from 4,769 patients with subtype B. All of the known subtype B resistance mutations occurred in the non-B subtypes, and 80% were correlated with antiretroviral treatment of the patients with the non-B subtypes. The authors concluded that it is reasonable for global monitoring of resistance to continue to focus on the known subtype B resistance mutations, as there are apparently no unique or previously unrecognized mutations in non-B subtypes.

Hepatitis B Virus

Five nucleoside analogs, 3TC, adefovir dipivoxil (ADV), telbivudine, tenofovir, and entecavir are approved for treatment of chronic HBV and act at the level of the HBV DNA polymerase. Alpha-2b interferon (IFN-α2b) and pegylated IFN-α2a (PegIFN) are approved for treatment and have both antiviral and immunomodulating activity (119, 121). However, PegIFN has replaced IFN-α2b due to its more convenient dosing schedule.

Three regions of the HBV genome are relevant to treatment, resistance to the various drugs, and type/subtype determination: (i) the active site of the viral DNA polymerase gene, (ii) mutations in the precore region of the HBV genome, and (iii) mutations in the core (C-gene) and the surface (S-gene) proteins.

3TC was the first clinically useful drug for treatment of HBV and is still widely used today, although resistance is virtually ensured (approximately 20% and 70% of patients develop resistance after 1 and 5 years of 3TC therapy, respectively) if the drug is used long enough with any given patient (84). The active site of the HBV DNA polymerase enzyme is very similar to that of HIV (they both have the same complement of enzymatic activities), and thus, it seemed reasonable that many of the nucleoside analogues that inhibit HIV RT would also inhibit HBV polymerase. The most common locus of 3TC resistance mutations, rtM204V/I/S, is located within the YMDD motif in the C domain of the viral RT gene (the "M" of the YMDD motif). The rtM204I mutation conferring 3TC resistance can occur independently of other mutations; however, rtM204V/S mutations are found only in conjunction with other mutations, such as rtL180M/C (120). rtL180M/C mutations, located in domain B of the RT, are insufficient alone to confer resistance but enhance levels of 3TC resistance and improve the replication fitness of rtM204I/V/S (120). Other, rarer mutations are rtL80V/I, rtI169T, rtV173L, rtA181T, rtT184S, and rtQ215S, many of which are "compensatory mutations," i.e., they enhance the viral fitness of 3TC-resistant mutants (120, 136, 143). ADV, an acyclic analog of dAMP, suppresses HBV replication at a slower rate than 3TC or entecavir but selects for resistance mutations at a much slower rate than 3TC (120, 143). However, adefovir-resistant mutants emerge more rapidly in patients with 3TC-resistant HBV. In addition to primary therapy for chronic HBV, adefovir also has been used as rescue therapy for treatment of 3TC-resistant HBV. Mutations associated with adefovir resistance in vivo are rtN236T and rtA181V/T. Other, less frequently occurring mutations associated with adefovir resistance are L80V/I, V84M, V214A, S85A, Q215S, P237H, and N238T/D (2, 3, 120, 143). Tenofovir is more effective clinically than adefovir because of the higher dosage. To date, no genotypic mutations associated with resistance to tenofovir have been detected. (52).

Entecavir is a carbocyclic deoxyguanosine analog that acts directly on the HBV DNA polymerase to cause delayed or nonobligate chain termination and also blocks priming of the RT reaction (121). It is active against 3TC- and ADV-resistant HBV. Resistance to entecavir is rare, having occurred in only 2 patients of the more than 500 enrolled in phase II and III clinical trials (134). Interestingly, resistance to entecavir alone was not observed; the two patients with resistance to entecavir had preexisting mutations to 3TC (rtL180M/rtM204V) which, in combination with new entecavir-induced mutations (rtM250V/rtI169T and rtT184G/rtS202I), resulted in high-level resistance to both drugs (120, 134). Thus, patients with 3TC resistance due to mutations at codons 180 and 204, when exposed to entecavir, may develop additional RT mutations and be highly resistant to both drugs (134). A fourth nucleoside analogue, telbivudine, approved by the FDA in 2006 for the treatment of chronic HBV infection, inhibits HBV DNA polymerase, causing DNA chain termination resulting in inhibition of HBV replication. Telbivudine resistance was associated with the M204I mutation (77). 3TC-resistant strains with mutations in the YMDD motif are cross resistant to telbivudine (143). Strategies for rescue therapy for patients with antiviral-resistant HBV must take into account prior treatment received, pattern of mutations found, and cross-resistance with alternative agents (83).

As with HIV-1, both genotypic and phenotypic assays have been utilized to detect HBV drug resistance mutations (120). Sequence analysis of the active site of the HBV polymerase is most commonly used for detection of the mutations known to confer resistance to these drugs. Direct sequencing is problematic because it is unable to detect resistant mutants in low concentrations. Cloning of the HBV polymerase region followed by sequence analysis of inserts from single recombinant clones is more sensitive but not amenable to clinical laboratories (120). Two commercial direct sequencing assays, the Trugene HBV genotyping kit (Siemens Medical Solutions Diagnostics) and Affigene HBV DE/3TC assay (Sangtec Molecular Diagnostics AB, Bromma, Sweden), amplify and sequence either a 1.2-kb sequence of the HBV RT gene, encompassing the central portion of the RT domain (Trugene HBV) or codons 180 and 204 (Affigene) (98, 142). Restriction fragment length polymorphism analysis can detect mutants at a level as low as 5% but again is not amenable to a clinical laboratory (120). Various DNA hybridization assays have been described (120) and include a second-generation, commercial, LiPA, INNO-LiPA HBV DR version 2 (Innogenetics N.V., Ghent, Belgium), which detects 3TC resistance mutations at codons 80, 173, 180, and 204 and adefovir resistance mutations at codons 181 and 236 of HBV polymerase (60, 101). Advantages and disadvantages of various genotypic assays for HBV drug resistance have been reviewed by Valsamakis (136).

In addition to genotypic assays, phenotypic assays have been utilized for characterization of HBV drug resistance. A variety of phenotyping methods have been employed and are reviewed by Shaw et al. (120). One method involves generation of point mutations associated with drug resistance by site-directed mutagenesis of "laboratory" strains of HBV followed by transfection of permissive cell lines with plasmid vectors containing the mutation of interest and subsequent exposure to an antiviral drug(s). The phenotype is deduced by comparing replications of cell lines with or without mutations in the presence of drug. Similarly, full-length HBV genomes also have been used for transfection experiments. Another strategy is the use of recombinant baculoviruses to deliver HBV genomes into cell culture systems, such as HepG2 cells, which are then exposed to antiviral agents. Alternatively, "virtual phenotyping" correlates patient clinical data and viral mutational data to assign an antiviral drug phenotype (120). SeqHepB is a combination of an HBV genome sequence analysis program and a relational database containing data from multiple sources (144). The program determines genotype and performs mutational analysis of HBV genomic sequences to generate a resistance profile based on the primary and secondary mutations found in the sequence. The sequence analysis component of SeqHepB (Last Resort Support Pty Ltd., Victoria, Australia) can be accessed by registered users via http://seqhepb.com/index.html (accessed 28 September 2009).

The precore (preC) region of the HBV genome has recently gained significance because there are indications that it may be associated with IFN resistance. There is long-standing evidence (49) that mutations in the preC region have a negative effect on IFN treatment, and more recent in vitro experiments have supported this contention (139). The development of a G1896A (codon 28) mutation results in a termination codon that interrupts translation of the HBeAg precursor and thus initiates an e-antigen-negative chronic hepatitis. Sequencing of this region is a reasonable method for detection of these mutations. Alternatively, Innogenetics has a LiPA assay (INNO-LiPA HBV PreCore) that is capable of detecting this mutation as well as precore promoter mutations that may also be present (codons 1762 and 1764).

Furthermore, classification of HBV into types, A to H, based on the genomic sequence has yielded unexpected correlations with the clinical course of disease. It has long been known that some types, for example, type B, are associated with less active liver disease, slower progression, and more likely spontaneous HBeAg seroconversion than other types, for example, type C (99). Recent studies with PegIFN have yielded the clinically relevant information that the response was type dependent (71). Patients with type A had a 47% response (i.e., loss of HBeAg), patients with type B a 44% response, patients with type C a 28% response, and patients with type D a 25% response. Thus, there is increasing evidence that determination of the HBV type is an important predictive factor in IFN treatment and the overall course of disease (50). The genotype can be determined by sequencing the entire genome, the core region, or the surface protein region. Two commercially available assays, the INNO-LiPA HBV genotyping kit (Innogenetics) and the Trugene HBV genotyping kit (Siemens), identify the HBV genotype based on type-specific sequences in the HBV S gene region (54, 100).

Quantitative HBV DNA testing is used in the initial evaluation of patients with chronic HBV infection and to determine efficacy of antiviral therapy (84). Andersson and Chung (1) recently summarized currently available commercial HBV viral load assays, detailing dynamic range and limit of detection. Recommendations for monitoring of patients on HBV therapy include baseline quantitative HBV DNA levels and additional levels periodically, with the goal of achieving undetectable levels of HBV DNA (84). The first indication of antiviral resistance is an increase in viral load levels of ≥ 1 log10 IU/ml (84). Genotyping for detection of resistance should be performed if resistance is suspected because of rising DNA levels or the appearance of symptoms (83, 84). While studies to date have demonstrated the efficacy of anti-HBV therapy for short-term virologic, biochemical, and histologic markers of infection, long-term studies are needed to determine if anti-HBV therapy prevents cirrhosis, liver failure, and hepatocellular carcinoma (119).

Influenza Virus

Genotypic assays for detection of resistance to the adamantane derivates, amantadine and rimantadine, have largely replaced phenotypic assays. Complete cross-resistance between amantadine and rimantadine has been demonstrated and is associated with amino acid substitution at position 26, 27, 30, 31, or 34 in the transmembrane region of the M2 protein of influenza A viruses (9). Both conventional sequencing and pyrosequencing have been used to identify mutations in the M2 gene sequences associated with resistance (20, 22, 39). In addition to NIAs for detection of resistance to NIs in influenza A virus, pyrosequencing of the NA gene has been employed (38). The most commonly reported mutation seen to date associated with oseltamivir resistance in influenza A (H1N1) viruses is H274Y (95); the E119V, R292K, and N294S mutations were associated with oseltamivir resistance in N2 NA (38). Sequencing of a zanamivir- and oseltamivir-resistant influenza B virus from an immunocompromised child demonstrated an R152K mutation in the NA gene (56).

INTERPRETATION OF ANTIVIRAL SUSCEPTIBILITY RESULTS

Table 1 lists breakpoint IC_{50}s proposed by various investigators for herpes group viruses and influenza viruses. The concentration of antiviral agent by which virus is considered susceptible has generally been based on median susceptibilities of large numbers of clinical isolates from patients prior to, during, and after antiviral therapy. Because of the variables that affect antiviral susceptibility results, the absolute IC_{50} value can vary from assay to assay and from laboratory to laboratory. Moreover, in vitro results indicating susceptibility or resistance may not correlate with the response of the infection to therapy in vivo. The clinical response of the patient depends upon a number of other factors, such as immunological status and pharmacokinetics of the drug in that particular patient (dose or route of administration could be inappropriate). A poor clinical response may occur even though the antiviral susceptibility testing denotes in vitro susceptibility (35). Patients with HSV infections who are immunocompromised may fail to respond to therapy, despite in vitro IC_{50}s indicating susceptibility to vidarabine or ACV (42, 110, 112). Conversely, HSV isolates for which IC_{50}s of ACV are >2 μg/ml can occasionally be recovered from otherwise healthy hosts who have responded to ACV therapy (81). Thus, a high IC_{50} derived by in vitro susceptibility testing is not sufficient to designate a viral strain as resistant. Neither can in vitro susceptibility to a drug a priori predict successful clinical outcome. Whenever possible, evidence of genetic alteration of the virus should be considered as well.

Interpretation of antiviral susceptibility results is further complicated by the variability in the endpoint due to testing methodologies (30, 64, 93, 103). Because endpoints are dependent on test method, each new method and antiviral agent must be correlated with a historic standard that has been used to test large numbers of isolates. Also, the absolute IC_{50} may vary from assay to assay and laboratory to laboratory. Moreover, because small subpopulations of resistant virus may not be reflected in IC_{50}s, IC_{90} values may be more predictive of clinical response. One approach to interpreting susceptibility endpoints is to compare the IC_{50}s of an isolate obtained prior to therapy (or of a well-characterized reference control strain) with that of an isolate obtained during therapy; a significant increase in the ratio of such IC_{50}s denotes resistance. However, pretherapy isolates are often unavailable, and the IC_{50} ratio considered clinically significant is unclear. Large-scale collaborative comparisons of methods with the same viral isolates are necessary to standardize antiviral susceptibility testing and to establish definitive interpretive guidelines. Only when a standardized assay is adopted can prospective studies be performed to correlate in vivo response with in vitro susceptibility. Such studies are essential before definitive interpretive breakpoints are established.

Susceptibility testing of PCV illustrates the effect that cell line and testing method have on endpoint. When ACV and PCV, which is structurally similar to ACV, were tested with HSV isolates in Vero cells by PRA, PCV appeared less active than ACV and HSV-2 isolates appeared to be resistant to PCV. In contrast, PCV appeared more active than ACV against some HSV isolates when SCC25 cells were used. Both drugs appeared to have comparable activities when tested in MRC-5 and A549 cells (80). When clinical isolates of VZV were tested by plaque reduction and DNA hybridization, IC_{50}s for DNA hybridization were significantly lower than those by PRA (126). Variability in endpoint also was seen with VZV, depending on the composition of the inoculum (cell free versus cell associated). Therefore, breakpoints for susceptibility testing of PCV with HSV and VZV cannot be established at this time (80, 126).

A limitation of phenotypic testing for HIV-1 is the lack of consensus as to the absolute IC_{50}s denoting resistance of HIV-1 to antiretroviral drugs. In vitro susceptibility of HIV-1 results are usually expressed as the "fold increase" in the IC_{50} of an isolate obtained during therapy compared to a pretreatment isolate or a drug-susceptible isolate (63, 114). The increase in the IC_{50} considered clinically significant is likely to vary by drug or drug class (57). The Antivirogram assay (Virco) has established cutoffs denoting reduced susceptibility at two standard deviations above the mean value for 1,000 isolates from untreated HIV-positive individuals and for several thousand isolates of genetically wild-type virus. Both Virco and ViroLogic are aware of the importance of clinical cutoff values and are making diligent efforts to ascribe accurate values for use by physicians.

The significance and clinical utility of phenotypic and genotypic analysis of HIV-1 are increasingly being recognized. A report that reanalyzed data from previous studies demonstrated that baseline genotypic and phenotypic drug resistance predicted virological failure (34). Genotypic analysis of the PR gene in patients who were on ART but were PI naive has also been shown to be predictive of virological and immune response to therapy with PIs (104). Prospective studies have demonstrated improved virological outcome when genotyping information is considered in patient management decisions (27, 41, 135). Drug resistance testing is now recommended to help guide selection of salvage therapy after treatment failure and for guiding therapy for pregnant women (66). However, limitations of genotypic testing include the difficulty in interpretation of resistance mutations and inability to detect minority variants.

It is important to remember that ART may fail for reasons other than the emergence of drug-resistant virus, such as drug antagonism; nonadherence; increased clearance of one antiretroviral drug when coadministered with another drug; inadequate penetration of drug into a sequestered site, i.e., central nervous system; or malabsorption of drug from the gastrointestinal tract (57, 63).

FUTURE DIRECTIONS

Both phenotypic and genotypic assays remain valuable tools for determination of antiviral resistance. As new antiviral agents are introduced with novel modes of antiviral activity (61), laboratory assays must be developed to detect the inevitable emergence of resistant virus. Standardization of antiviral susceptibility testing is ongoing. To this end, some progress has been made. A protocol for HSV plaque assays is now published (97) and a standardized procedure for the sequencing of the HCMV UL97 gene (87) has been published. Standardization is hampered by the many variables that affect susceptibility testing results. No single assay method, cell line, or inoculum composition (cell free versus cell associated) appears sufficient for testing all viruses. A major problem with culture-based susceptibility testing of viruses other than HSV is that assays may require weeks to complete, a fact that limits their utility in management of acute cases. Genotypic assays for UL97 and UL54 mutations of HCMV have largely replaced culture-based assays as more resistance-associated mutations are identified. Detection of antiviral resistance in patients with HIV-1 and HBV infections is considered an integral component of patient management and will continue to evolve as newer antiviral agents are approved.

REFERENCES

1. **Andersson, K. L., and R. T. Chung.** 2009. Monitoring during and after antiviral therapy for hepatitis B. *Hepatology* **49:**S166–S173.

2. **Angus, P., R. Vaughan, S. Xiong, H. Yang, W. Delaney, C. Gibbs, C. Brosgart, D. Colledge, R. Edwards, A. Ayres, A. Bartholomeusz, and S. Locarnini.** 2003. Resistance to adefovir dipivoxil therapy associated with the selection of a novel mutation in the HBV polymerase. *Gastroenterology* **125:**292–297.

3. **Arens, M.** 2001. Clinically relevant sequence-based genotyping of HBV, HCV, CMV, and HIV. *J. Clin. Virol.* **22:**11–29.

4. **Baldanti, F., M. R. Underwood, S. C. Stanat, K. K. Biron, S. Chou, A. Sarasini, E. Silini, and G. Gerna.** 1996. Single amino acid changes in the DNA polymerase confer foscarnet resistance and slow-growth phenotype, while mutations in the UL97-encoded phosphotransferase confer ganciclovir resistance in three double-resistant human cytomegalovirus strains recovered from patients with AIDS. *J. Virol.* **70:**1390–1395.

5. **Baldanti, F., M. R. Underwood, C. L. Talarico, L. Simoncini, A. Sarasini, K. K. Biron, and G. Gerna.** 1998. The Cys 607→Tyr change in the UL97 phosphotransferase confers ganciclovir resistance to two human cytomegalovirus strains recovered from two immunocompromised patients. *Antimicrob. Agents Chemother.* **42:**444–446.

6. **Bean, B., C. Fletcher, J. Englund, S. N. Lehrman, and M. N. Ellis.** 1987. Progressive mucocutaneous herpes simplex infection due to acyclovir-resistant virus in an immunocompromised patient: correlation of viral susceptibilities and plasma levels with response to therapy. *Diagn. Microbiol. Infect. Dis.* **7:**199–204.

7. **Beddows, S., S. Galpin, S. H. Kazmi, A. Ashraf, A. Johargy, A. J. Frater, N. White, R. Braganza, J. Clarke, M. McClure, and J. N. Weber.** 2003. Performance of two commercially available sequence-based HIV-1 genotyping systems for the detection of drug resistance against HIV type 1 group M subtypes. *J. Med. Virol.* **70:**337–342.

8. **Belshe, R. B., B. Burk, F. Newman, R. L. Cerruti, and I. S. Sim.** 1989. Resistance of influenza A virus to amantadine and rimantadine: results of one decade of surveillance. *J. Infect. Dis.* **159:**430–435.

9. **Belshe, R. B., M. H. Smith, C. B. Hall, R. Betts, and A. J. Hay.** 1988. Genetic basis of resistance to rimantadine emerging during treatment of influenza virus infection. *J. Virol.* **62:**1508–1512.

10. **Berkowitz, F. E., and M. J. Levin.** 1985. Use of an enzyme-linked immunosorbent assay performed directly on fixed infected cell monolayers for evaluating drugs against varicella-zoster virus. *Antimicrob. Agents Chemother.* **28:**207–210.

11. **Beutner, K. R.** 1995. Valacyclovir: a review of its antiviral activity, pharmacokinetic properties, and clinical efficacy. *Antivir. Res.* **28:**281–290.

12. **Biron, K. K.** 1991. Ganciclovir-resistant human cytomegalovirus isolates; resistance mechanisms and *in vitro* susceptibility to antiviral agents. *Transplant. Proc.* **23**(Suppl. 3):162–167.

13. **Biron, K. K., and G. B. Elion.** 1980. *In vitro* susceptibility of varicella-zoster virus to acyclovir. *Antimicrob. Agents Chemother.* **18:**443–447.

14. **Biron, K. K., J. A. Fyfe, S. C. Stanat, L. K. Leslie, J. B. Sorrell, C. U. Lambe, and D. M. Coen.** 1986. A human cytomegalovirus mutant resistant to the nucleoside analog 9-{[2-hydroxy-1-(hydroxymethyl)ethoxy]methyl}guanine (BW B759U) induces reduced levels of BW B759U triphosphate. *Proc. Natl. Acad. Sci. USA* **83:**8769–8773.

15. **Biron, K. K., S. C. Stanat, J. B. Sorrell, J. A. Fyfe, P. M. Keller, C. U. Lambe, and D. J. Nelson.** 1985. Metabolic activation of the nucleoside analog q-[2-hydroxy-1-(hydroxymethyl)ethoxymethyl] guanine in human diploid fibroblasts infected with human cytomegalovirus. *Proc. Natl. Acad. Sci. USA* **82:**2473–2477.

16. **Boivin, G, S. Chou, M. R. Quirk, A. Erice, and M. C. Jordon.** 1996. Detection of ganciclovir resistance mutations and quantitation of cytomegalovirus (CMV) DNA in leukocytes of patients with fatal disseminated CMV disease. *J. Infect. Dis.* **173:**523–528.

17. **Boyd, M. R., S. Safrin, and E. R. Kern.** 1993. Penciclovir: a review of its spectrum of activity, selectivity, and cross-resistance pattern. *Antivir. Chem. Chemother.* **4**(Suppl. 1):3–11.

18. **Boyer, P. L., H.-Q. Gao, and S. H. Hughes.** 1998. A mutation at position 190 of human immunodeficiency virus type 1 reverse transcriptase interacts with mutations at positions 74 and 75 via the template primer. *Antimicrob. Agents Chemother.* **42:**447–452.

19. **Braun, P. and F. Wiesman.** 2007. Phenotypic assays for the determination of coreceptor tropism in HIV-1 infected individuals. *Eur. J. Med. Res.* **12:**463–471.

20. **Bright, R. A., M.-J. Medina, X. Xu, G. Perez-Oronoz, T. R. Wallis, X. M. Davis, L. Povinelli, N. J. Cox, and A. I. Klimov.** 2005. Incidence of adamantine resistance among influenza A (H3N2) viruses isolated worldwide from 1994–2005: a cause for concern. Lancet **366:**1175–1181.

21. **Centers for Disease Control and Prevention.** 1999. Neuraminidase inhibitors for treatment of influenza A and B infections. *MMWR Morb. Mortal. Wkly. Rep.* **48**(RR14):1–9.

22. **Centers for Disease Control and Prevention.** 2009. Update: drug susceptibility of swine-orgin influenza A (H1N1) viruses, April 2009. *MMWR Morb. Mortal. Wkly Rep.* **58:**433–435.

23. **Chatis, P. A., and C. S. Crumpacker.** 1992. Resistance of herpesviruses to antiviral drugs. *Antimicrob. Agents Chemother.* **36:**1589–1595.

24. **Chou, S., A. Erice, M. C. Jordon, G. M. Vercellotti, K. R. Michels, C. L. Talarico, S. C. Stanat, and K. K. Biron.** 1995. Analysis of the UL97 phosphotransferase coding sequence in clinical cytomegalovirus isolates and identification of mutations conferring ganciclovir resistance. *J. Infect. Dis.* **171:**576–583.

25. **Chou, S., S. Guentzel, K. R. Michels, R. C. Miner, and W. L. Drew.** 1995. Frequency of UL97 phosphotransferase mutations related to ganciclovir resistance in clinical cytomegalovirus isolates. *J. Infect. Dis.* **172:**239–242.

26. **Chou, S., G. Marousek, S. Guentzel, S. E. Follansbee, M. E. Poscher, J. P. Lalezari, R. C. Miner, and W. L. Drew.** 1997. Evolution of mutations conferring multidrug resistance during prophylaxis and therapy for cytomegalovirus disease. *J. Infect. Dis.* **176:**786–789.

27. **Cingolani A., A. Antinori, M. G. Rizzo, R. Murri, A. Ammassari, F. Baldini, S. Di Giambenedetto, R. Cauda, and A. De Luca.** 2002. Usefulness of monitoring HIV drug resistance and adherence in individuals failing highly active antiretroviral therapy: a randomized study (ARGENTA). *AIDS* **16:**369–379.

28. **Cirelli, R., K. Herne, M. McCrary, P. Lee, and S. K. Tyring.** 1996. Famciclovir: review of clinical efficacy and safety. *Antivir. Res.* **29:**141–151.

29. **Coen, D. M. and D. D. Richman.** 2007. Antiviral agents, p. 447–485. *In* D. M. Knipe and P. M. Howley (ed.), *Fields Virology*, 5th ed. Lippincott Williams & Wilkins, Philadelphia, PA.

30. **Cole, N. L., and H. H. Balfour, Jr.** 1987. *In vitro* susceptibility of cytomegalovirus isolates from immunocompromised patients to acyclovir and ganciclovir. *Diagn. Microbiol. Infect. Dis.* **6:**255–261.

31. **Cunningham, S., B. Ank, D. Lewis, W. Lu, M. Wantman, J. Dileanis, J. B. Jackson, P. Palumbo, P. Krogstad, and S. H. Eshelman.** 2001. Performance of the Applied Biosystems ViroSeq human immunodeficiency virus type 1 (HIV-1) genotyping system for sequence- based analysis of HIV-1 in pediatric plasma samples. *J. Clin. Microbiol.* **39:**1254–1257.

32. **Dankner, W. M., D. Scholl, S. C. Stanat, M. Martin, R. L. Sonke, and S. A. Spector.** 1990. Rapid antiviral DNA-DNA hybridization assay for human cytomegalovirus. *J. Virol. Methods* **28:**293–298.

33. **De Clercq, E.** 1982. Comparative efficacy of antiherpes drugs in different cell lines. *Antimicrob. Agents Chemother.* **21:**661–663.

34. **DeGruttola, V., L. Dix, R. D'Aquila, D. Holder, A. Phillips, M. Ait-Kaled, J. Baxter, P. Clevenbergh, S. Hammer, R. Harrigan, D. Katzenstein, R. Lanier, M. Miller, M. Para, S. Yerly, A. Zolopa, J. Murray, A. Patick, V. Miller, S. Castillo, L. Pedneault, and J. Mellors.** 2002. The relation between baseline HIV drug resistance and response to antiretroviral therapy: re-analysis of retrospective and prospective studies using a standardized data analysis plan. *Antivir. Ther.* **5:**41–48.

35. **Dekker, C., M. N. Ellis, C. McLaren, G. Hunter, J. Rogers, and D. W. Barry.** 1983. Virus resistance in clinical practice. *J. Antimicrob. Chemother.* **12:**137–152.

36. **Delwart, E. L., H. Pan, H. W. Sheppard, D. Wolpert, A. U. Neumann, B. Korber, and J. L. Mullins.** 1998. Slower evolution of human immunodeficiency virus type 1 quasispecies during progression to AIDS. *J. Virol.* **71:**7498–7508.

37. **Demeter, L. M., R. D'Aquila, O. Weislow, E. Lorenzo, A. Erice. J. Fitzgibbon, R. Shaker, D. Richman, T. M. Howard, Y. Zhao, E. Fisher, D. Huang, D. Mayers, S. Sylvester, M. Arens, K. Sannerud, S. Rasheed, V. Johnson, D. Kiritzkes, P. Reichelderfer, and A. Japour for the ACTG Sequencing Working Group.** 1998. Interlaboratory concordance of DNA sequence analysis to detect reverse transcriptase mutations in HIV-1 proviral DNA. *J. Virol. Methods* **75:**93–104.

38. **Deyde, V. M., M. Okomo-Adhiambo, T. G. Sheu, T. R. Wallis, A. Fry, N. Dharan, A. I. Klimov, and L. V. Gubareva.** 2009. Pyrosequencing as a tool to detect molecular markers of resistance to neuraminidase inhibitors in seasonal influenza A viruses. *Antivir. Res.* **81:**16–24.

39. **Deyde, V. M., X. Xu, R. A. Bright, M. Shaw, C. B. Smith, Y. Zhang, Y. Shu, L. V. Gubareva, N. J. Cox, and A. I. Klimov.** 2007. Surveillance of resistance to adamantanes among influenza A(H3N2) and A(H1N1) viruses isolated worldwide. *J. Infect. Dis.* **196:**249–257.

40. **Drew, W. L., R. C. Miner, D. F. Busch, S. E. Follansbee, J. Gullett, S. G. Mehalko, S. M. Gordon, W. F. Owen, Jr., T. R. Matthews, W. C. Buhles, and B. DeArmond.** 1991. Prevalence of resistance in patients receiving ganciclovir for serious cytomegalovirus infection. *J. Infect. Dis.* **163:**716–719.

41. **Durant, J., P. Clevenbergh, P. Halfon, P. Delgiudice. S. Porsin, P. Simonet, N. Montagne, C. A. B. Boucher, J. M. Schapiro, and P. Dellamonica.** 1999. Drug-resistance genotyping in HIV-1 therapy: the VIRADAPT randomized controlled trial. *Lancet* **353:**2196–2199.

42. **Englund, J. A., M. E. Zimmerman, E. M. Swierkosz, J. L. Goodman, D. R. Scholl, and H. H. Balfour, Jr.** 1990. Herpes simplex virus resistant to acyclovir. A study in a tertiary care center. *Ann. Intern. Med.* **112:**416–422.

43. **Erali, M., S. Page, L. G. Reimer, and D. R. Hillyard.** 2001. Human immunodeficiency virus type 1 drug resistance test: a comparison of three sequence-based methods. *J. Clin. Microbiol.* **39:**2157–2165.

44. **Erice, A.** 1999. Resistance of human cytomegalovirus to antiviral drugs. *Clin. Microbiol. Rev.* **12:**286–297.

45. **Erice, A.** 2000. Antiviral susceptibility testing, p. 271–289. *In* G. A. Storch (ed.), *Essentials of Diagnostic Virology.* Churchill Livingstone, New York, NY.

46. **Erice, A., S. Chou, K. K. Biron, S. C. Stanat, H. H. Balfour, Jr., and M. C. Jordan.** 1989. Progressive disease due to ganciclovir-resistant cytomegalovirus in immunocompromised patients. *N. Engl. J. Med.* **320:**289–293.

47. **Erice, A., C. Gil-Roda, J.-L. Perez, H. H. Balfour, Jr., K. J. Sannerud, M. N. Hanson, G. Boivin, and S. Chou.** 1997. Antiviral susceptibilities and analysis of UL97 and DNA polymerase sequences of clinical cytomegalovirus isolates from immunocompromised patients. *J. Infect. Dis.* **175:**1087–1092.

48. **Eshelman, S. H., J. Hackett, Jr., P. Swanson, S. P. Cunningham, B. Drews, C. Brennan, S. G. Devare, L. Zekeng, L. Kaptue, and N. Marlowe.** 2004. Performance of the Celera Diagnostics ViroSeq HIV-1 genotyping system for sequence-based analysis of diverse human immunodeficiency virus type 1 strains. *J. Clin. Microbiol.* **42:**2711–2717.

49. **Fattovich, G., G. McIntyre, M. Thursz, K. Coleman, G. Giuliano, A. Alberti, H. C. Thomas, and W. F. Carman.** 1995. Hepatitis B virus precore/core variation and interferon therapy. *Hepatology* **22:**1355–1362.

50. **Fung, S. K. and A. S. F. Lok.** 2004. Hepatitis B virus genotypes: do they play a role in the outcome of HBV infection? *Hepatology* **40:**790–792.

51. **Gadler, H.** 1983. Nucleic acid hybridization for measurement of effects of antiviral compounds on human cytomegalovirus DNA replication. *Antimicrob. Agents Chemother.* **24:**370–374.

52. **Ghany, M. G., and E. C. Doo.** 2009. Antiviral resistance and hepatitis B therapy. *Hepatology* **49:**S174–S184.

53. **Gilbert, C., and G. Boivin.** 2005. Human cytomegalovirus resistance to antiviral drugs. *Antimicrob. Agents Chemother.* **49:**873–883.

54. **Gintowt, A. A., J. J. Germer, P. S. Mitchell, and J. D. C. Yao.** 2005. Evaluation of the MagNA Pure LC used with the TRU-GENE™ HBV Genotyping Kit. *J. Clin. Virol.* **34:**155–157.

55. **Gubareva, L. V., L. Kaiser., M. N. Matrosovich, Y. Soo-Hoo, and F. G. Hayden.** 2001. Selection of influenza virus mutants in experimentally infected volunteers treated with oseltamivir. *J. Infect. Dis.* **183:**523–531.

56. **Gubareva, L. V., M. N. Mastrosovich, M. K. Brenner, R. C. Bethell, and R. G. Webster.** 1998. Evidence for zanamivir resistance in an immunocompromised child infected with influenza B virus. *J. Infect. Dis.* **179:**1257–1262.

57. **Hanna, G. J. and R. T. D'Aquila.** 2001. Clinical use of genotypic and phenotypic drug resistance testing to monitor antiretroviral chemotherapy. *Clin. Infect. Dis.* **32:**774–782.

58. **Hantz, S., D. Michel, A.-M. Fillet, V. Guigonis, G. Champier, M.-C. Mazeron, A. Bensman, F. Denis, T. Mertens, A. Dehee, and S. Alain.** 2005. Early selection of a new UL97 mutant with a severe defect of ganciclovir phosphorylation after valaciclovir prophylaxis and short-term ganciclovir therapy in a renal transplant recipient. *Antimicrob. Agents Chemother.* **49:**1580–1583.

59. **Harmenberg, J., B. Wahren, and B. Oberg.** 1980. Influence of cells and virus multiplicity on the inhibition of herpesviruses with acycloguanosine. *Intervirology* **14:**239–244.

60. **Hassain, M., S. Fung, E. Libbrecht, E. Sablon, C. Cursaro, P. Andreone, and A. S. F. Lok.** 2006. Sensitive line probe assay that simultaneously detects mutations conveying resistance to lamivudine and adefovir. *J. Clin. Microbiol.* **44:**1094–1097.

61. **Hayden, F.** 2009. Developing new antiviral agents for influenza treatment; what does the future hold? *Clin. Infect. Dis.* **48**(Suppl. 1):S3–S13.

62. **Hayden, F. G., K. M. Cote, and G. D. Douglas, Jr.** 1980. Plaque inhibition assay for drug susceptibility testing of influenza viruses. *Antimicrob. Agents Chemother.* **17:**865–870.

63. **Hertogs, K., M.-P. De Bethune, V. Miller, T. Ivens, P. Schel, A. Van Cauwenberge, C. Van Den Eynde, V. Van Gerwen, H. Azijn, M. Van Houtte, F. Peeters, S. Staszewski, M. Conant, S. Bloor, S. Kemp, B. Larder, and R. Pauwels.** 1998. A rapid method for simultaneous detection of phenotypic resistance to inhibitors of protease and reverse transcriptase in recombinant human immunodeficiency virus type 1 isolates from patients treated with antiretroviral drugs. *Antimicrob. Agents Chemother.* **42:**269–276.

64. **Hill, E. L., M. N. Ellis, and P. Nguyen-Dinh.** 1991. Antiviral and antiparasitic susceptibility testing, p.1184–1188. *In* A. Balows, W. J. Hausler, Jr., K. L. Hermann, H. D. Isenberg, and H. J. Shadomy (ed.), *Manual of Clinical Microbiology,* 5th ed. American Society for Microbiology, Washington, DC.

65. **Hill, E. L., G. A. Hunter, and M. N. Ellis.** 1991. *In vitro* and *in vivo* characterization of herpes simplex virus clinical isolates recovered from patients infected with human immunodeficiency virus. *Antimicrob. Agents Chemother.* **35:**2322–2328.

66. **Hirsch, M. S., F. Brun-Vezinet, R. T. D'Aquila, S. M. Hammer, V. A. Johnson, D. R. Kiritzkes, C. Loveday, J. W. Mellors, B. Clotet, B. Conway, L. M. Demeter, S. Vella, D. M. Jacobsen, and D. D. Richman.** 2000. Antiretroviral drug resistance testing in adult HIV-1 infection: recommendations of an International AIDS Society—USA Panel. *JAMA* **283:**2417–2426.

67. **Hirsch, M. S., B. Conway, R. T. D'Aquila, V. A. Johnson, F. Brun-Vezinet, B. Clotet, L. M. Demeter, S. M. Hammer, D. M. Jacobsen, D. R. Kuritzkes, C. Loveday, M. W. Mellors, S. Vella, and D. D. Richman.** 1998. Antiretroviral drug resistance testing in adults with HIV infection: implications for clinical management. International AIDS Society—USA Panel. *JAMA* **279:**1984–1991.

68. **Huang, D. D., S. H. Eshelman, D. J. Brambilla, P. E. Palumbo, and J. W. Bremer.** 2003. Evaluation of the editing process in human immunodeficiency virus type 1 genotyping. *J. Clin. Microbiol.* **41:**3265–3272.

69. Iversen, A. K., R. W. Shafer, K. Wehrly, M. A. Winters, J. I. Mullins, B. Chesebro, and T. C. Merigan. 1996. Multidrug-resistant human immunodeficiency virus type 1 strains resulting from combination antiretroviral therapy. J. Virol. 70:1086–1090.

70. Jacobson, M. A., T. G. Berger, S. Fikrig, P. Cecherer, J. W. Moohr, S. C. Stanat, and K. K. Biron. 1990. Acyclovir-resistant varicella zoster virus infection after chronic oral acyclovir therapy in patients with the acquired immunodeficiency syndrome (AIDS). Ann. Intern. Med. 112:187–191.

71. Janssen, H. L. A., M. vanZonneveld, H. Senturk, S. Zeuzem, U. S. Akarca, Y. Cakaloglu, C. Simon, T. M. K. So, G. Gerken, R. A. deMan, H. G. M. Niesters, P. Zondervan, B. Hansen and S. W. Schalm. 2005. Pegylated interferon alfa-2b alone or in combination with lamivudine for HBeAg-positive chronic hepatitis B: a randomized trial. Lancet 365:123–129.

72. Japour, A. J., D. L. Mayers, V. A. Johnson, D. R. Kuritzkes, L. A. Beckett, J.-M. Arduino, J. Lane, R. J. Black, P. S. Reichelderfer, R. T. D'Aquila, C. S. Crumpacker, the RV-43 Study Group, and the AIDS Clinical Trials Group Virology Committee Resistance Working Group. 1993. Standardized peripheral blood mononuclear cell culture assay for determination of drug susceptibilities of clinical human immunodeficiency virus type 1 isolates. Antimicrob. Agents Chemother. 37:1095–1101.

73. Johnson, V., F. Brun-Vezinet, B. Clotet, H. F. Gunthard, D. R. Kuritzkes, D. Pillay, J. M. Schapiro, and D. D. Richman. 2008. Update of the drug resistance mutations in HIV-1: December 2008. Top. HIV Med. 16:138–145.

74. Kantor, R., D. A. Katzenstein, B. Efron, A. P. Carvalho, B. Wynhoven, P. Cane, J. Clarke, S. Sirivichayakul, M. A. Soares, J. Snoeck, C. Pillay, H. Rudich, R. Rodrigues, A. Holguin, K. Ariyoshi, M. B. Bouzas, P. Cahn, W. Sugiura, V. Soriano, L. F. Brigido, Z. Grossman, L. Morris, A.-M. Vandamme, A. Tanuri, P. Rhanuphak, J. N. Weber, D. Pillay, P. R. Harrigan, R. Camacho, J. M. Schapiro, and R. W. Shafer. 2005. Impact of HIV-1 subtype and antiviral therapy on protease and reverse transcriptase genotype: results of a global collaboration. PLoS Med. 2:325–337.

75. Kellam, P., and B. A. Larder. 1994. A recombinant virus assay: a rapid, phenotypic assay for assessment of drug susceptibility of human immunodeficiency virus type 1 isolates. Antimicrob. Agents. Chemother. 38:23–30.

76. Kusumi, K., B. Conway, S. Cunningham, A. Berson, C. Evans, A. K. N. Iversen, D. Colvin, M. V. Gallo, S. Coutre, E. G. Shpaer, D. V. Faulkner, A. DeRonde, S. Volkman, C. Williams, M. S. Hirsch, and J. I. Mullins. 1992. Human immunodeficiency virus type 1 envelope gene structure and diversity in vivo and after cocultivation in vitro. J. Virol. 66:875–885.

77. Lai, C.-L., N. Leung, E.-K. Teo, M. Tong, F. Wong, H.-W. Hann, S. Han, T. Poynard, M. Myers, G. Chao, D. Lloyd, N. A. Brown, and the Telbivudine Phase II Investigator Group. 2005. A 1-year trial of telbivudine, lamivudine, and the combination in patients with hepatitis B e antigen-positive chronic hepatitis B. Gastroenterology 129:528–536.

78. Landry, M. L., S. Stanat, K. Biron, D. Brambilla, W. Britt, J. Jokela, S. Chou. W. L. Drew, A. Erice, B. Gilliam, N. Lurain, J. Manischewitz, R. Miner, M. Nokta, P. Reichelderfer, S. Spector, A. Weinberg, B. Yen-Lieberman, C. Crumpacker, and the AIDS Clinical Trials Group CMV Resistance Working Group. 2000. A standardized plaque reduction assay for determination of drug susceptibilities of cytomegalovirus clinical isolates. J. Clin. Microbiol. 44:688–692.

79. Larder, B. A., G. Darby, and D. D. Richman. 1989. HIV with reduced sensitivity to zidovudine (AZT) isolated during prolonged therapy. Science 243:1731–1734.

80. Leary, J. J., R. Wittrock, R. T. Sarisky, A. Weinberg, and M. J. Levin. 2002. Susceptibilities of herpes simplex viruses to penciclovir and acyclovir in eight cell lines. Antimicrob. Agents Chemother. 46:762–768.

81. Lehrman, S. N., J. M. Douglas, L. Corey, and D. W. Barry. 1986. Recurrent genital herpes and suppressive oral acyclovir therapy. Relation between clinical outcome and in-vitro drug sensitivity. Ann. Intern. Med. 104:786–790.

82. Little, S. J., S. Holte, J. Routy, E. S. Daar, M. Markowitz, A. C. Collier, R. A. Koup, J. W. Mellors, E. Connick, B. Conway, M. Kilby, L. Wang, J. M. Whitcomb, N. S. Hellmann, and D. D. Richman. 2002. Antiretroviral-drug resistance among patients recently infected with HIV. N. Engl. J. Med. 347:385–394.

83. Lok, A. S. F. 2007. Navigating the maze of hepatitis B treatments. Gastroenterology 132:1586–1594.

84. Lok, A. S. F., and B. J. McMahon. 2007. Chronic hepatitis B: AASLD practice guidelines. Hepatology 45:507–539.

85. Lu, J., S. G. Deeks, R. Hoh, G. Beatty, B. A. Kuritzkes, J. N. Martin, and D. R. Kuritzkes. 2006. Rapid emergence of enfuvirtide resistance in HIV-1-infected patients. J. Acquir. Immune Defic. Syndr. 43:60–64.

86. Lurain, N. S., K. D. Thompson, E. W. Holmes, and G. S. Read. 1992. Point mutations in the DNA polymerase gene of human cytomegalovirus that results in resistance to antiviral agents. J. Virol. 66:7146–7152.

87. Lurain, N. S., A. Weinberg, C. S. Crumpacker, and S. Chou. 2001. Sequencing of cytomegalovirus UL97 gene for genotypic antiviral resistance testing. Antimicrob. Agents Chemother. 45:2775–2780.

88. MacArthur, R. D. and R. M. Novak. 2008. Maraviroc: the first of a new class of antiretroviral agents. Clin. Infect. Dis. 47:236–241.

89. Marschner, I. C., A. C. Collier, R. W. Combs, R. T. D'Aquila, V. DeGruttola, M. A. Fischl, S. M. Hammer, M. D. Hughes, V. A. Johnson, D. A. Katzenstein. D. D. Richman, L. M. Smeaton, S. A. Spector, and M. S. Saag. 1998. Uses of changes in plasma levels of human immunodeficiency virus type 1 RNA to assess the clinical benefit of antiretroviral therapy. J. Infect. Dis. 177:40–47.

90. Martin, J. L., M. N. Ellis, P. M. Keller, K. K. Biron, S. N. Lehrman, D. W. Barry, and P. A. Furman. 1985. Plaque autoradiography assay for the detection and quantitation of thymidine kinase-deficient and thymidine kinase-altered mutants of herpes simplex virus in clinical isolates. Antimicrob. Agents Chemother. 28:181–187.

91. Martinez-Picado, J., A. V. Savara, L. Sutton, and R. T. D'Aquila. 1999. Replicative fitness of protease inhibitor-resistant mutants of human immunodeficiency virus type 1. J. Virol. 73:3744–3752.

92. Martinez-Picado, J., L. Sutton, M. P. De Pasquale, A. V. Savara, and R. T. D'Aquila. 1999. Human immunodeficiency virus type 1 cloning vectors for antiviral resistance testing. J. Clin. Microbiol. 37:2943–2951.

93. McLaren, C., M. N. Ellis, and G. A. Hunter. 1983. A colorimetric assay for the measurement of the sensitivity of herpes simplex viruses to antiviral agents. Antiviral Res. 3:223–224.

94. Moore, J. P., and D. R. Kuritzkes. 2009. A pièce de resistance: how HIV-1 escapes small molecular CCR5 inhibitors. Curr. Opin. HIV AIDS 4:118–124.

95. Moscona, A. 2009. Global transmission of oseltamivir-resistant influenza. N. Engl. J. Med. 360:953–956.

96. Mracna, M., G. Becker-Pergola, J. Dileanis, L. A. Guay, S. Cunningham, J. B. Jackson, and S. H. Eshleman. 2001. Performance of Applied Biosystems ViroSeq HIV-1 genotyping system for sequence-based analysis of non-subtype B human immunodeficiency virus type 1 from Uganda. J. Clin. Microbiol. 39:4323–4327.

97. NCCLS. 2004. Antiviral Susceptibility Testing: Herpes Simplex Virus by Plaque Reduction Assay; Approved standard. NCCLS M33-A. NCCLS, Wayne, PA.

98. Olivero, A., A. Ciancio, M. L. Abate, S. Gaia, A. Smedile, and M. Rizzetto. 2006. Performance of sequence analysis, INNO-LiPA line probe assays and AFFIGENE assays in the detection of hepatitis B virus polymerase and precore/core promoter mutations. J. Viral Hepat. 13:355–362.

99. Orito, E., M. Mizokami, H. Sakugawa, K. Michitaka, K. Ishikawa, and T. Ichida. 2001. A case-controlled study for clinical and molecular biological differences between hepatitis B viruses of genotypes B and C. Hepatology 33:218–223.

100. Osiowy, C., and E. Giles. 2003. Evaluation of the INNO-LiPA HBV Genotyping assay for determination of hepatitis B virus genotype. *J. Clin. Microbiol.* **41**:5473–5477.

101. Osiowy, C., J.-P. Villeneuve, E. J. Heathcote, E. Giles, and J. Borlang. 2006. Detection of the rtN236T and rt181V/T mutations associated with resistance to adefovir dipivoxil in samples from patients with chronic hepatitis B virus infection by the INNO-LiPA HBV DR line probe assay (version 2). *J. Clin. Microbiol.* **44**:1994–1997.

102. Pahwa, S., K. Biron, W. Lim, P. Swenson, M. H. Kaplan, N. Sadick, and R. Pahwa. 1988. Continuous varicella-zoster infection associated with acyclovir resistance in a child with AIDS. *JAMA* **260**:2879–2882.

103. Pepin, J.-M., F. Simon, M. C. Dazza, and F. Brun-Vezinet. 1992. The clinical significance of *in vitro* cytomegalovirus susceptibility to antiviral drugs. *Res. Virol.* **143**:126–128.

104. Perez, E. E., S. L. Rose, B. Peyser, S. L. Lamers. B. Burkhardt, B. M. Dunn, A. D. Hutson, J. W. Sleasman, and M. M. Goodenow. 2001. Human immuno-deficiency virus type 1 protease genotype predicts immune and viral responses to combination therapy with protease inhibitors (PIs) in PI-naive patients. *J. Infect. Dis.* **183**:579–588.

105. Petropoulos, C. J., N. T. Parkin, K. L. Limoli, Y. S. Lie, T. Wrin, W. Huang, H. Tian, D. Smith, G. A. Winslow, D. J. Capon, and J. M. Whitcomb. 2000. A novel phenotypic drug susceptibility assay for human immunodeficiency virus type 1. *Antimicrob. Agents Chemother.* **42**:920–928.

106. Rabalaiss, G. P., M. J. Levin, and F. E. Berkowitz. 1987. Rapid herpes simplex virus susceptibility testing using an enzyme-linked immunosorbent assay performed in situ on fixed virus-infected monolayers. *Antimicrob. Agents Chemother.* **31**:946–948.

107. Reeves, J. D., E. Coakley, C. J. Petropoulos, and J. M. Whitcomb. 2009. An enhanced sensitivity Trofile™ HIV coreceptor tropisms assay for selecting patients for therapy with entry inhibitors targeting CCR5: a review of analytical and clinical studies. *J. Viral Entry* **3**:94–102.

108. Richman, D. D. 1995. Clinical significance of drug resistance in human immunodeficiency virus. *Clin. Infect. Dis.* **21**(Suppl. 2):S166–S169.

109. Richman, D. D., J. C. Guatelli, J. Grimes, A. Tsiatis, and T. R. Gingeras. 1991. Detection of mutations associated with zidovudine resistance in human immunodeficiency virus utilizing the polymerase chain reaction. *J. Infect. Dis.* **164**:1075–1081.

110. Safrin, S., T. Assaykeen, S. Follansbee, and J. Mills. 1990. Foscarnet therapy for acyclovir-resistant mucocutaneous herpes simplex virus infection in 26 AIDS patients: preliminary data. *J. Infect. Dis.* **161**:1078–1084.

111. Safrin, S., T. G. Berger, I. Gilson, P. R. Wolfe, C. B. Wofsy, J. Mills, and K. K. Biron. 1991. Foscarnet therapy in five patients with AIDS and acyclovir-resistant varicella-zoster virus infection. *Ann. Intern. Med.* **115**:19–21.

112. Safrin, S., C. Crumpacker, P. Chatis, R. Davis, R. Hafner, J. Rush, H. A. Kessler, B. Landry, J. Mills, and the AIDS Clinical Trials Group. 1991. A controlled trial comparing foscarnet with vidarabine for acyclovir-resistant mucocutaneous herpes simplex in the acquired immunodeficiency syndrome. *N. Engl. J. Med.* **325**:551–555.

113. Safrin, S., E. Palacios, and B. J. Leahy. 1996. Comparative evaluation of microplate enzyme-linked immunosorbent assay versus plaque reduction assay for antiviral susceptibility testing of herpes simplex virus isolates. *Antimicrob. Agents Chemother.* **40**:1017–1019.

114. Schinazi, R. F., B. A. Larder, and J. W. Mellors. 1997. Mutations in HIV-1 reverse transcriptase and protease associated with drug resistance. *Int. Antiviral News* **5**:129–134.

115. Schuurman, R., D. Brambilia, T. de Groot, D. Huang, S. Land, J. Bremer, I. Benders, and C. A. Boucher. 2002. Underestimation of HIV type 1 drug resistance mutations: results from the ENVA-2 genotyping proficiency program. *AIDS Res. Hum. Retrovir.* **18**:243–248.

116. Schuurman, R., L. Demeter, P. Reichelderfer, J. Tijnagel, T. DeGroot, and C. Boucher. 1999. Worldwide evaluation of DNA sequencing approaches for identification of drug resistance mutations in the human immunodeficiency virus type 1 reverse transcriptase. *J. Clin. Microbiol.* **37**:2291–2296.

117. Shafer, R. W. 2002. Genotypic testing for human immunodeficiency virus type 1 drug resistance. *Clin. Microbiol. Rev.* **15**:247–277.

118. Shafer, R. W., D. R. Jung, and B. J. Betts. 2000. Human immunodeficiency virus type 1 reverse transcriptase and protease mutation search engine for queries. *Nat. Med.* **6**:1290–1292.

119. Shamliyan, T. A., R. MacDonald, A. Shaukat, B. C. Tayor, J.-M. Yuan, J. R. Johnson, J. Tacklind. I. Rutks, R. Kane, and T. J. Wilt. 2009. Antiviral therapy for adults with chronic hepatitis B: a systematic review for a National Institutes of Health Consensus Development Conference. *Ann. Intern. Med.* **150**:111–124.

120. Shaw, T., A. Bartholomeusz, and S. Locarnini. 2006. HBV drug resistance: mechanisms, detection and interpretation. *J. Hepatol.* **44**:593–606.

121. Shaw, T., and S. Locarnini. 2004. Entecavir for the treatment of chronic hepatitis B. *Expert Rev. Anti-infect. Ther.* **2**:853–871.

122. Shi, C., and J. W. Mellors. 1997. A recombinant retroviral system for rapid *in vivo* analysis of human immunodeficiency virus type 1 susceptibility to reverse transcriptase inhibitors. *Antimicrob. Agents Chemother.* **41**:2781–2785.

123. Sibrack, C. D., L. T. Gutman, C. M. Wilfert, C. McLaren, M. H. St. Clair, P. M. Keller, and D. W. Barry. 1982. Pathogenicity of acyclovir-resistant herpes simplex virus type 1 from an immunodeficient child. *J. Infect. Dis.* **146**:673–682.

124. Smith, I. L., J. M. Cherrington, R. E. Jiles, M. D. Fuller, W. R. Freeman, and S. A. Spector. 1997. High-level resistance of cytomegalovirus to ganciclovir is associated with alterations in both the UL97 and DNA polymerase genes. *J. Infect. Dis.* **176**:69–77. (Erratum, **177**:1140–1441, 1998.)

125. Spector, S. A., K. Hsia, D. Wolf, M. Shinkai, and I. Smith. 1995. Molecular detection of human cytomegalovirus and determination of genotypic ganciclovir resistance in clinical specimens. *Clin. Infect. Dis.* **21**(Suppl. 2):S170–S173.

126. Standring-Cox, R., T. H. Bacon, and B. A. Howard. 1996. Comparison of a DNA probe assay with the plaque reduction assay for measuring the sensitivity of herpes simplex virus and varicella-zoster virus to penciclovir and acyclovir. *J. Virol. Methods* **56**:3–11.

127. St. Clair, M. H., P. M. Hartigan, J. C. Andrews, C. L. Vavro, M. S. Simberkoff, J. D. Hamilton, and the VA Cooperative Study Group. 1993. Zidovudine resistance, syncytium-inducing phenotype, and HIV disease progression in a case-control study. *J. Acquir. Immune Defic. Syndr.* **6**:891–897.

128. St. Clair, M. H., J. L. Martin, G. Tudor-Williams, M. C. Bach, C. L. Vavro, D. M. King, P. Kellam, S. D. Kemp, and B. A. Larder. 1991. Resistance to ddI and sensitivity to AZT induced by a mutation in HIV-1 reverse transcriptase. *Science* **253**:1557–1559.

129. Swierkosz, E. M., and K. K. Biron. 1994. Antiviral susceptibility testing, p. 8.26.2–8.26.21. *In* H. D. Isenberg (ed.). *Clinical Microbiology Procedures Handbook*, supplement 1. American Society for Microbiology, Washington, DC.

130. Swierkosz, E. M., and K. K. Biron. 1995. Antiviral susceptibility testing, p. 139–154. *In* E. H. Lennette, D. A. Lennette, and E. T. Lennette (ed.), *Diagnostic Procedures for Viral, Rickettsial and Chlamydial Infections*, 7th ed. American Public Health Association, Washington, DC.

131. Swierkosz, E. M., D. R. Scholl, J. L. Brown, J. D. Jollick, and C. A. Gleaves. 1987. Improved DNA hybridization method for detection of acyclovir-resistant herpes simplex virus. *Antimicrob. Agents Chemother.* **31**:1465–1469.

132. Tebas, P., D. Scholl, J. Jollick, K. McHarg, M. Arens, and P. D. Olivo. 1998. A rapid assay to screen for drug-resistant herpes simplex virus. *J. Infect. Dis.* **177**:217–220.

133. Tebas, P., E. C. Stabel, and P. D. Olivo. 1995. Antiviral susceptibility testing with a cell line which expresses β-galactosidase after infection with herpes simplex virus. *Antimicrob. Agents Chemother.* **39**:1287–1291.

134. Tenney, D. J., S. M. Levine, R. E. Rose, A. W. Walsh, S. P. Weinheimer, L. Discotto, M. Plym, K. Pokornowski, C. F. Yu, P. Angus, A. Ayres, A. Bartholomeusz, W. Sievert, G. Thompson, N. Warner, S. Locarnini, and R. J. Colonno. 2004. Clinical emergence of entecavir-resistant hepatitis B virus requires additional substitutions in virus already resistant to lamivudine. *Antimicrob. Agents and Chemother.* **48:**3498–3507.

135. Tural, C., L. Ruiz, C. Holtzer, J. Schapiro, P. Viciana, J. Gonzalez, P. Domingo, C. Boucher, C. Rey-Joly, and B. Clotet. 2002. Clinical utility of HIV-1 genotyping and expert advice: the Havana trial. *AIDS* **16:**209–218.

136. Valsamakis, A. 2007. Molecular testing in the diagnosis and management of chronic hepatitis B. *Clin. Microbiol. Rev.* **20:**426–439.

137. Van Laethem, K., and A.-M. Vandamme. 2006. Interpreting resistance data for HIV-1 therapy management-know the limitations. *AIDS Rev.* **8:**37–43.

138. Walter, H., B. Schmidt, K. Korn, A. M. Vandamme, T. Harrer, and K. Uberla. 1999. Rapid, phenotypic HIV-1 drug sensitivity assay for protease and reverse transcriptase inhibitors. *J. Clin. Virol.* **13:**71–80.

139. Wang, Y., L. Wei, D. Jiang, X. Cong, R. Fei, J. Xiao, and Y. Wang. 2005. In vitro resistance to interferon of hepatitis B virus with precore mutation. *World J. Gastroenterol.* **11:**649–655.

140. Wilson, J. W., P. Bean, T. Robins, F. Graziano, and D. H. Persing. 2000. Comparative evaluation of three human immunodeficiency virus genotyping systems: the HIV-GenotypR method, the HIV PRT GeneChip assay, and the HIV-1 RT line probe assay. *J. Clin. Microbiol.* **38:**3022–3028.

141. Wolf, D. G., I. L. Smith, D. J. Lee, W. R. Freeman, M. Flores-Aguilar, and S. A. Spector. 1995. Mutations in human cytomegalovirus UL97 gene confer clinical resistance to ganciclovir and can be detected directly in patient plasma. *J. Clin. Investig.* **95:**257–263.

142. Woo, H.-Y., H. Park, B.-I. Kim, W.-K. Jeon, Y. K. Cho, and Y. J. Kim. 2007. Comparison of mass spectrometric analysis and TRUGENE™ HBV genotyping for monitoring lamivudine resistance in chronic hepatitis B patients. *Antivir. Ther.* **12:**7–13.

143. Yuan, H.-J., and W. M. Lee. 2007. Molecular mechanisms of resistance to antiviral therapy in patients with chronic hepatitis B. *Curr. Mol. Med.* **7:**185–197.

144. Yuen, L. K. W., A. Ayres, M. Littlejohn, D. Colledge, A. Edgely, W. J. Maskill, S. A. Locarnini, and A. Bartholomeusz. 2007. SEQHEPB: a sequence analysis program and relational database for chronic hepatitis B. *Antivir. Res.* **75:**64–74.

145. Zhang, J., S.-Y. Rhee, J. Taylor, and R. Shafer. 2005. Comparison of the precision and sensitivity of the Antivirogram and PhenoSense HIV drug susceptibility assays. *J. Acquir. Immune Defic. Syndr.* **38:**439–444.

MYCOLOGY

VOLUME EDITOR: DAVID W. WARNOCK

SECTION EDITORS: MARY E. BRANDT AND ELIZABETH M. JOHNSON

GENERAL

FUNGI

section VI

Taxonomy and Classification of Fungi

MARY E. BRANDT AND DAVID W. WARNOCK

111

There are at least 100,000 named species of fungi. However, it has been estimated that the number of undiscovered species ranges from 1 million to more than 10 million, and it has been calculated that about 1,000 to 1,500 new species are described each year (5, 10). Of the named species of fungi, fewer than 500 have commonly been associated with human or animal disease, and no more than 50 are capable of causing infection in otherwise healthy individuals. On the other hand, an increasing number of ubiquitous environmental molds are now being implicated as opportunistic pathogens, capable of producing serious or lethal disease in hosts that are immunocompromised or debilitated. These molds are organisms whose natural habitat is in the soil or on plants, wood, compost heaps, or decomposing food. Many are familiar to mycologists, plant pathologists, and food microbiologists, but they present problems for clinical microbiologists, who often have had no formal training in the identification of fungi. Fungal identification can be challenging and sometimes frustrating because of the importance placed on the morphological characteristics of the organisms, and the need to become familiar with a range of different structures and terms. Indeed, it is fair to state that obscure mycological terms are one of the major factors that discourage many microbiologists from mastering fungal identification. However, investing time to learn the basic structures and principles of taxonomy, classification, and nomenclature can result in the ability to recognize and identify correctly many medically important fungi.

MORPHOLOGICAL CHARACTERISTICS OF THE FUNGI

Fungi form a separate group of eukaryotic organisms which differ from other groups, such as the plants and animals, in several major respects. Fungal cells are encased within a rigid cell wall, mostly composed of chitin, glucan, chitosan, mannan, and glycoproteins in various combinations. These features contrast with the animals, which have no cell walls, and the plants, which have cellulose as the major cell wall component. As in other eukaryotic organisms, fungal cells have a true nucleus with a surrounding membrane, and cell division is accompanied by meiosis or mitosis.

Fungi are heterotrophic, that is, they lack chlorophyll, and therefore require preformed organic carbon compounds for their nutrition. Fungi live embedded in a food source or medium and obtain their nourishment by secreting enzymes into the external substrate and by absorbing the released nutrients through their cell wall. Fungi are found throughout nature, performing an essential service in returning to the soil nutrients removed by plants.

Fungi can be multicellular or unicellular. In multicellular organisms, the basic structural unit is a chain of multinucleate, tubular, filament-like cells (termed a hypha). In most multicellular fungi the vegetative stage consists of a mass of branching hyphae, termed a mycelium or thallus. Each individual hypha has a rigid cell wall and increases in length as a result of apical growth with mitotic cell division. In the more primitive fungi, the hyphae remain aseptate (without cross walls). In the more advanced groups, however, the hyphae are divided into compartments or cells by the development of more or less frequent cross walls, termed septa. Such hyphae are referred to as being septate. Fungi that exist in the form of microscopic multicellular mycelium are commonly called molds.

Many fungi that exist in the form of independent single cells propagate by budding out similar cells from their surface. The bud may become detached from the parent cell, or it may remain attached and itself produce another bud. In this way, a chain of cells may be produced. Fungi that do not produce hyphae but just consist of a loose arrangement of budding cells are called yeasts. Under certain conditions, continued elongation of the parent cell before it buds results in a chain of elongated cells, termed a pseudohypha. Unlike for a true hypha, the connection between adjacent pseudohyphal cells shows a marked constriction. A few yeast species are able to form true hyphae, and others can form arthroconidia by fragmentation of an existing hypha. Yeasts are neither a natural nor a formal taxonomic group but are a growth form shown in a wide range of unrelated fungi.

Many medically important fungi change their growth form as part of the process of tissue invasion. These so-called dimorphic pathogens usually change from a multicellular mold form in the natural environment to a budding, single-celled yeast form in tissue. *Histoplasma capsulatum*, *Blastomyces dermatitidis*, *Paracoccidioides brasiliensis*, and *Sporothrix schenckii* are the best-known examples of this dimorphic change, but many other fungal pathogens show subtle morphological differences between forms found in tissue and in culture.

Fungi reproduce by means of microscopic propagules called spores. The term conidium is used to describe spores that result from an asexual process (involving mitosis only). Except for the occasional mutation, asexual conidia are identical to the parent. They are generally short-lived propagules that are produced in enormous numbers to ensure dispersion to new habitats. Many fungi are also capable of sexual reproduction (involving meiosis, preceded by fusion of the nuclei of two cells). Some species are self-fertile (homothallic) and able to form sexual structures between different cells within an individual thallus. Most, however, are heterothallic and do not form their sexual structures unless two different isolates come into contact. Once two compatible haploid nuclei have fused, meiosis can occur, and this leads to the production of the sexual spores. In some species the haploid sexual spores are borne singly on specialized generative cells and the whole structure is microscopic in size. In other cases, however, the spores are produced in millions in macroscopic "fruiting bodies" such as mushrooms. Sexual reproduction and its accompanying structures form one scheme for classification of the fungi.

NOMENCLATURE OF FUNGI

The scientific names of fungi are subject to the International Code of Botanical Nomenclature (ICBN) (http://www.bgbm.org/iapt/nomenclature/code/default.htm), a convention that dates from the time when biologists regarded these organisms as "lower plants." The rules of the ICBN must be followed when proposing the name for a new fungal species; otherwise, the name being proposed can be rejected as invalid. The main requirements for valid publication are that the name must be in Latin binomial form, the publication must contain a concise description of the essential and differential characteristics of the fungus in Latin, and a living culture of the specimen on which the author based his original description of the species must be preserved.

Names of fungi may have to be changed for a number of reasons. Many common and widely distributed species of fungi have been described as new many times and thus have come to have more than one name. In general, the correct name for any species is the earliest name published in line with the requirements of the code of nomenclature. The later names are termed synonyms. To avoid confusion, however, the ICBN permits certain exceptions. The most significant of these is when an earlier generic name has been overlooked, a later name is in common use, and a reversion to the earlier name would cause problems.

Another reason for changing the name of a fungus is when new research necessitates the transfer of a species from one genus to another or establishes it as the type of a new genus. Such changes are quite in order, but with the provision that the specific epithet should remain unchanged, except for inflection according to the rules of Latin grammar. However often a species is transferred to a new genus, the correct species epithet is always the first one that was applied to that particular organism. As an example, when *Phialophora parasitica* was moved to a new genus, it became *Phaeoacremonium parasiticum*.

If there is one complication of fungal nomenclature that is confusing to many microbiologists, it is the fact that a large number of fungi appear to bear more than one name. This is an apparent departure from the basic principle of biological classification, in which an organism can only have one correct name. As described in the previous section of this chapter, many fungi have an asexual stage (or anamorph), characterized by the production of asexual conidia, and a sexual stage (or teleomorph), characterized by sexual spores (e.g., ascospores and basidiospores). Many fungi propagate asexually and the teleomorph is unknown or only rarely encountered. Because of this, mycologists have often given separate names to the asexual and sexual stages. Often this is because the anamorph and teleomorph were described and named at different times without the connection between them being recognized. The code of nomenclature permits this practice, and while the name of the teleomorph takes precedence and covers both stages, the name given to an anamorph may be used as appropriate. Thus, it is permissible to refer to a fungus by its asexual designation if this is the stage that is usually obtained in culture. For example, *Blastomyces dermatitidis* is the anamorph of the ascomycete *Ajellomyces dermatitidis*. The anamorph is the stage that is ordinarily encountered in culture, and only under certain special conditions is the sexual stage formed. Although the correct name typified by the teleomorph is *Ajellomyces dermatitidis*, *Blastomyces dermatitidis* remains the name that is most widely recognized and used.

The taxonomy and nomenclature of fungi that have both asexual and sexual stages are challenging. Some teleomorphic fungi can produce more than one asexual form of propagation, the term synanamorph being used to describe each of these different anamorphs. These may bear separate names. As an example, the teleomorphic species *Pseudallescheria boydii* can also exist in two different synanamorphic forms, named *Graphium fructicola* and *Scedosporium boydii*. These three names all refer to one and the same organism (see chapter 118).

TAXONOMY AND CLASSIFICATION OF THE FUNGI

The kingdom Fungi is one of the six kingdoms of life (5, 6). It is organized in a hierarchical manner, each rank being named with, and recognizable by, a particular ending: phylum, -mycota; subphylum, -mycotina; class, -mycetes; order, -ales; and family, -aceae (13). Each family is composed of a number of genera, and these are divided into species. The kingdom Fungi is currently divided into seven phyla, which include the Ascomycota and Basidiomycota (12). The phylum Zygomycota is no longer accepted due to its polyphyletic nature (12). Pending resolution of their relationships, the organisms that have traditionally been placed in the Zygomycota are at this time divided among the phylum Glomeromycota and four subphyla incertae sedis. The subphylum Mucoromycotina has been proposed to accommodate the Mucorales, while the subphylum Entomophthoromycotina has been created for the Entomophthorales (12).

In addition to the true fungi, there are a number of human and animal pathogens, including *Pythium insidiosum* and *Rhinosporidium seeberi*, that are now placed in the kingdoms Protozoa and Stramenopila (formerly Chromista) (see chapter 125). These organisms, while not fungi sensu stricto, are "fungus mimics" or "pseudofungi," protists that have become similar to fungi in one or more respects. Furthermore, molecular studies have established that several organisms long considered protists belong to the kingdom Fungi. These include *Pneumocystis*, now placed in the Ascomycota, and the microsporidians.

Historically, the classification of fungi has largely been based on their morphology, rather than on the physiological and biochemical differences that are of such importance

TABLE 1 Simplified taxonomic scheme illustrating major groups of the kingdom Fungi in which medically important fungi are classified[a]

Taxonomic designation	Representative genus or genera
Subphylum: Mucoromycotina	
Order: Mucorales	*Lichtheimia, Rhizopus*
Subphylum: Entomophthoromycotina	
Order: Entomophthorales	*Basidiobolus, Conidiobolus*
Phylum: Basidiomycota	
Class: Tremellomycetes	
Order: Filobasidiales	*Filobasidium, Filobasidiella* (teleomorphs of *Cryptococcus* species)
Class: Agaricomycetes	
Order: Agaricales	*Schizophyllum*
Phylum: Ascomycota	
Class: Pneumocystidomycetes	
Order: Pneumocystidales	*Pneumocystis*
Class: Saccharomycetes	
Order: Saccharomycetales	*Clavispora, Debaryomyces, Issatchenkia, Kluyveromyces* (teleomorphs of *Candida* species); *Saccharomyces*
Class: Eurotiomycetes	
Order: Onygenales	*Arthroderma* (teleomorphs of *Microsporum* and *Trichophyton* species); *Ajellomyces* (teleomorphs of *Blastomyces* and *Histoplasma* species)
Order: Eurotiales	*Emericella, Eurotium, Neosartorya* (teleomorphs of *Aspergillus* species)
Class: Sordariomycetes	
Order: Hypocreales	*Gibberella, Nectria* (teleomorphs of *Fusarium* species)
Order: Microascales	*Pseudallescheria* (teleomorph of *Scedosporium* species

[a]Modified from reference 12.

in bacterial classification. In recent years, however, the advent of rapid DNA sequencing has ushered in a revolution in fungal taxonomy based on a phylogenetic approach to species recognition (PSR concept). This relies on comparative analysis of variable nucleic acid characters to define fungal species (11, 16). Under the PSR, a species is defined as a group of organisms which share concordance of multiple gene genealogies (DNA sequences at different genetic loci), rather than organisms that share a common morphology or organisms that can mate with one another. Portions of genes are often used to construct the genealogies. Concordant branches among the gene trees are used to connect species. Although the major application of the PSR, defining species, is beyond the scope of the clinical microbiology laboratory, results obtained by PSR can be applied to medically important fungi. Several new species have been recognized within medically important species formerly defined by morphology. For example, *Coccidioides posadasii* has been separated from *Coccidioides immitis* and comprises isolates from outside the state of California (9).

The sexual spores and their mode of production have historically formed the main basis for classification of fungi into the Zygomycota, Ascomycota, and Basidiomycota. In some fungi, however, the asexual stage or anamorph has proved so successful as a means of rapid dispersal to new habitats that the sexual stage or teleomorph has disappeared, or at least has not been discovered. Even in the absence of the teleomorph it is now often possible to assign these fungi to the Ascomycota or Basidiomycota on the basis of DNA sequences of the anamorphs (4). In the past, these asexual fungi were classified in an artificial group, the "Fungi Imperfecti" (also termed the form division Deuteromycota) and were divided into artificial form classes according to the morphological characteristics of their asexual reproductive structures. There is no longer any separate formal grouping for those fungi that appear to be strictly anamorphic, or for which no teleomorph has been discovered. Nonetheless, mycologists continue to employ the asexual reproductive characteristics of molds, at least for routine identification purposes.

A simplified taxonomic scheme illustrating the major groups of medically important fungi is presented in Table 1. These groups are described in the following sections. A simplified key to their identification is provided in Table 2.

Kingdom Fungi

Subphyla Mucoromycotina and Entomophthoromycotina (formerly Zygomycota)

The traditional Zygomycota have been divided among the phylum Glomeromycota and four subphyla pending resolution of further taxonomic questions (12). In these groups of lower fungi, the thallus is aseptate (or possesses few cross walls) and consists of wide, hyaline (colorless) branched hyphal elements. The asexual spores (termed sporangiospores) are nonmotile and are produced inside a closed sac, termed a sporangium, the wall of which ruptures to release them. Sexual reproduction leads to the formation of a single large zygospore with a thickened wall. Most of the medically important species are heterothallic and do not form their sexual structures unless two compatible isolates come into contact.

The subphylum Mucoromycotina contains the order Mucorales, which is the most clinically important and includes the genera *Lichtheimia* (formerly *Absidia*), *Mucor*, *Rhizomucor*, and *Rhizopus*. The subphylum Entomophthoromycotina contains one order of medical importance, the Entomophthorales. The Entomophthorales includes the genera *Basidiobolus* and *Conidiobolus*, agents of subcutaneous infections.

TABLE 2 Simplified key to the main groups of medically important fungi[a]

1a. Fungus not culturable on routine media, occurs as cyst-like cells in tissue	Pneumocystidomycetes
1b. Fungus culturable	2
2a. Colonies consist of budding cells at 30°C	3
2b. Colonies consist of hyphae at 30°C	5
3a. Colonies black	Black yeasts
3b. Colonies white, cream, pink, or red	4
4a. Urease test positive	Basidiomycetous yeasts
4b. Urease test negative	Ascomycetous yeasts
5a. Hyphae septate	6
5b. Hyphae nearly aseptate	9
6a. Clamp connections present	Filamentous basidiomycetes
6b. Clamp connections absent	7
7a. Fruiting bodies absent	Hyphomycetes
7b. Fruiting bodies present	8
8a. Fruiting bodies containing ascospores in asci	Eurotiomycetes
8b. Fruiting bodies containing conidia	Coelomycetes
9a. Sporulation abundant	Glomeromycota
9b. Sporulation absent; zoospores formed in water cultures	Oomycota

[a]In this dichotomous key, the information required for identification is arranged as pairs of contrasted characteristics, the pairs being numbered consecutively on the left. Each member of the pair leads, on the right side of the page, either to the name of a group of fungi or to another higher number, i.e., to a further pair of contrasted characteristics. To use the key, start at point number 1 and follow through in the sequence indicated.

Phylum Basidiomycota

Most members of the phylum Basidiomycota, a group of higher fungi, have a septate, filamentous thallus, but some are typical yeasts. Sexual reproduction leads to the formation of haploid basidiospores on the outside of a generative cell, termed a basidium. Fifteen classes are recognized, but only a few members of this large phylum are of medical importance. The most prominent are the basidiomycetous yeasts with anamorphic stages belonging to the genera *Cryptococcus*, *Malassezia*, and *Trichosporon*. The genus *Cryptococcus*, which contains more than 30 species, has teleomorphs that have been assigned to the genera *Filobasidium* and *Filobasidiella* (3).

In culture, filamentous basidiomycetes often produce fast-growing, nonsporulating (sterile) white colonies with clamp connections. These are hyphal outgrowths which, at cell division, make a connection between the two cells forming a bypass around the septum to allow the migration of a nucleus. The basidia are often produced in macroscopic structures termed basidiomata or basidiocarps, and the basidiospores are often forcibly discharged. Asexual reproduction is variable, with some species producing spores like those of the Ascomycota (see below), but many others are not known to produce spores at all. Most filamentous basidiomycetes are wood-rotting fungi or obligate plant pathogens. The most frequently reported clinically important filamentous basidiomycete is *Schizophyllum commune*.

Phylum Ascomycota

The large phylum Ascomycota contains almost 50% of all named fungal species and accounts for around 80% of fungi of medical importance (10). Sexual reproduction leads to the development of haploid spores, termed ascospores, which are produced in a sac-like structure termed an ascus. The Ascomycota show a gradual transition from primitive forms that produce single asci to species that produce large structures, termed ascocarps or ascomata, containing numerous asci. Variations in ascus structure are of major importance in the classification of these fungi. Asexual reproduction consists of the production of conidia from a generative or conidiogenous cell. In some species the conidiogenous cell cannot be distinguished from the rest of the mycelium. In others, a special structure is produced which bears one or more conidiogenous cells.

The phylum Ascomycota includes four classes of medical importance: the Pneumocystidomycetes, Saccharomycetes, Eurotiomycetes, and Sordariomycetes. The class Pneumocystidomycetes contains the genus *Pneumocystis*, formerly classified as a member of the kingdom Protozoa but now reassigned to the fungi on the basis of small-subunit ribosomal DNA and other gene sequence comparisons (1). The class Saccharomycetes contains the ascomycetous yeasts, while the Eurotiomycetes and the Sordariomycetes contain the filamentous ascomycetes.

The order Saccharomycetales, which belongs to the class Saccharomycetes, is characterized by vegetative yeast cells which proliferate by budding or fission. These fungi do not produce ascomata, the ascus being formed by direct transformation of a budding vegetative cell, by "mother-bud" conjugation, or by conjugation between two independent single cells. Many members of this order have an anamorphic stage belonging to the genus *Candida*. This genus, which consists of around 200 anamorphic species, has teleomorphs in more than 10 different genera, including *Clavispora*, *Debaryomyces*, *Issatchenkia*, *Kluyveromyces*, and *Pichia* (14).

In the class Eurotiomycetes, sexual reproduction leads to the formation of ascomata containing asci with ascospores. This class has seven orders that include species pathogenic to humans. Among the more important are the Onygenales, which contains the teleomorphs of the dermatophytes and a number of dimorphic systemic pathogens (including *Histoplasma capsulatum* and *Blastomyces dermatitidis*) and the Eurotiales, which includes the teleomorphs of the anamorphic genera *Aspergillus* and *Penicillium*. In the class Sordariomycetes, the order Sordariales contains many of the teleomorphs of the anamorphic genus *Fusarium*. In addition, the teleomorphs of numerous melanized fungi of medical importance belong to a number of orders in the classes Eurotiomycetes or Sordariomycetes. These include the Chaetothyriales, Microascales, Hypocreales, and Ophiostomatales.

Although most of the septate molds that are isolated in clinical laboratories belong to one of the classes described above, it is unusual to encounter their sexual reproductive structures in routine cultures. The few species which do produce ascomata in relative abundance include *Pseudallescheria boydii* (anamorph, *Scedosporium boydii*) and *Emericella nidulans* (anamorph, *Aspergillus nidulans*). For the most part, however, routine identification of these molds is based on the form and arrangement of the asexual spore-bearing structures and the manner in which the spores are produced (see below).

Kingdom Protozoa

Microsporidians, some of which are obligate parasites of humans, have long been classified with the protozoa. However, phylogenetic analysis has indicated that these organisms belong among the fungi (17), and the phylum Microsporidia within the kingdom Fungi has been created to accommodate them (12). However, parasitologists have been reluctant to part with this group, while mycologists have been just as reluctant to accept it. For the time being at least, the microsporidia have been retained alongside the Protozoa, while acknowledging that these organisms are, in fact, true fungi (see chapter 140).

Kingdom Stramenopila (formerly Chromista)

Members of the order Pythiales mostly occur in the soil or on plants; one species, *Pythium insidiosum*, is of clinical significance (see chapter 125). Long regarded as fungi, these slime molds are most closely related to some algal groups and are now placed in the kingdom Stramenopila and phylum Oomycota (15).

IDENTIFICATION OF YEASTS

Yeasts are neither a natural nor a formal taxonomic group but are growth forms found in a wide range of unrelated ascomycetous and basidiomycetous fungi. Their identification relies on a combination of morphological, physiological, and biochemical characteristics. Useful morphological characteristics include the color of the colonies, the size and shape of the cells, the presence of a capsule around the cells, the production of hyphae or pseudohyphae, and the production of chlamydospores. Useful biochemical tests include the assimilation and fermentation of sugars and the assimilation of nitrate. Most yeasts of medical importance can be identified using one of the commercial tests systems that are based on sugar assimilation profiles of isolates. However, it is important to remember that microscopic examination of cultures on cornmeal agar is essential to avoid confusion between organisms with identical biochemical profiles (see chapter 115).

The so-called black yeasts are not a formal taxonomic group, but the description is applied to a wide range of unrelated ascomycetous and basidiomycetous fungi that are able to produce melanized budding cells at some stage in their life cycle (8). Because most of these fungi are also able to produce true mycelium, their routine identification is largely based on the morphological characteristics of the asexual spore-bearing structures and the manner in which the spores are produced.

CLASSIFICATION AND IDENTIFICATION OF ANAMORPHIC MOLDS

Most of the septate molds that are isolated in clinical laboratories do not produce their sexual reproductive structures in routine cultures, and their identification is based on the manner in which the asexual spores are produced. Two artificial form classes of anamorphic or "mitosporic" molds are currently recognized, based on the mode of conidium formation. The Hyphomycetes produce their conidia directly on the hyphae or on specialized conidiophores, while the Coelomycetes have more elaborate reproductive structures, termed conidiomata. Although these form classes are no longer formally recognized, they continue to offer a useful framework for identification based on morphology.

Form Class Coelomycetes

Three artificial orders are recognized: the Sphaeropsidales, Melanconiales, and Pycnothyriales. In the Sphaeropsidales, the conidia are produced in conidiomata that are either spherical with an apical opening and with conidiogenous cells lining the inner cavity wall (termed pycnidia) or open and cup shaped, in which case the conidiogenous cells cover the conidiomatal surface (termed acervuli). A few members of this form class are common pathogens of humans. One of the more frequently encountered species is *Neoscytalidium dimidiatum*, a plant pathogen which can also cause infections of the skin and nails. Until recently, this species was known by the synanamorph names *Nattrassia mangiferae* and *Scytalidium dimidiatum*.

Form Class Hyphomycetes

The Hyphomycetes contains a large number of septate anamorphic molds of medical importance, including the genera *Aspergillus*, *Blastomyces*, *Cladophialophora*, *Fusarium*, *Histoplasma*, *Microsporum*, *Penicillium*, *Phialophora*, *Scedosporium*, and *Trichophyton*. In addition, numerous Hyphomycetes have been reported as occasional opportunistic pathogens of humans. For this reason, it is important for clinical microbiologists to be able to recognize and correctly identify this group of fungi.

As mentioned earlier, the process of conidiogenesis is of major importance in the identification of these molds. Two basic methods of conidiogenesis can be distinguished: thallic conidiogenesis, in which an existing hyphal cell is converted into one or more conidia, and blastic conidiogenesis, in which conidia are produced as a result of some form of budding process (for a detailed discussion of this topic, see reference 8).

Thallic Conidiogenesis

In thallic conidiogenesis, the conidia are produced from an existing hyphal cell. Arthroconidia, which are derived from the fragmentation of an existing hypha, represent the simplest form of thallic conidiogenesis and have evolved in many different groups of fungi. The first step in the examination of cultures of these molds should be to ascertain whether another spore form is present. If so, identification should be based upon that form. The few molds of medical importance which produce arthroconidia as their sole means of conidiogenesis include *Coccidioides* species.

Aleurioconidia are formed from the side or tip of an existing hypha and, during the initial stage before a septum is laid down, can resemble short hyphal branches. This form of thallic conidiogenesis is characteristic of the dermatophytes (*Epidermophyton*, *Microsporum*, and *Trichophyton* spp.), as well as a number of dimorphic systemic pathogens, including

Blastomyces dermatitidis, *Histoplasma capsulatum*, and *Paracoccidioides brasiliensis*.

Chlamydospores are formed as a result of the enlargement of an existing hyphal cell to form a thicker-walled resting spore. Many fungi produce chlamydospores, usually in response to adverse conditions, and they are seldom useful for identification purposes.

Blastic Conidiogenesis

Many fungi have evolved some form of repeated budding that allows them to produce large numbers of asexual spores from a single conidiogenous cell. There are two basic forms of blastic conidiogenesis: holoblastic development, in which all layers of the wall of the conidiogenous cell swell out to form the conidium, and enteroblastic development, in which the conidium is produced from within the conidiogenous cell, the outer layers of the cell wall breaking open and an inner layer extending through the opening to become the new spore wall. These two forms of blastic conidiogenesis can be further subdivided according to the details of spore development.

Almost all the molds that produce holoblastic conidia have melanized cell walls and thus are similar in colonial appearance. The morphological characteristics of their conidia and the manner in which the spores are produced serve as the main distinguishing features. Holoblastic conidia range in size from minute unicellular to large thick-walled multicelled conidia. In some species, the first formed conidium buds to produce a second, and the second produces a third, and so on until a chain of conidia is produced with the youngest at its tip. As each spore can produce more than one bud, a branching chain becomes possible (e.g., *Cladophialophora* species). In another group, the conidiogenous cell that produced the first spore then grows past it to produce a second. If this process is repeated, it will result in an elongated conidiogenous cell with numerous lateral single spores along its sides. This is termed sympodial development and is typical of species of *Bipolaris* and *Exserohilum*.

In molds that produce enteroblastic conidia, the wall of the conidium is derived from the inner layer of the wall of the conidiogenous cell. This permits a succession of conidia to be produced from the same point. There are two main forms of enteroblastic conidiogenesis: phialidic, in which the specialized conidiogenous cell from which the conidia are produced is termed a phialide, and annellidic, in which the conidiogenous cell is termed an annellide.

In phialidic conidiogenesis, the first blown-out cell breaks open at its tip and remains as a collarette, from the inside of which conidia are produced in succession. In some species, the collarette is distinct (e.g., *Phialophora* species), but in others it is almost invisible at the tip of the phialide. In some phialidic molds, such as species of *Fusarium* and *Acremonium*, the conidia are not firmly attached to each other and often move aside to accumulate in a wet mass around the phialide, which makes them suited for water dispersal. In other phialidic molds, such as species of *Aspergillus* and *Penicillium*, continuous replenishment of the inner wall of the tip of the phialide results in the formation of an unbranched chain of connected conidia, with the youngest at the base. These dry spores are readily disrupted and are suited for airborne dispersal.

Annellides, like phialides, are conidiogenous cells which produce conidia at their tips in unbranched chains (e.g., *Scopulariopsis* species) or in wet masses (e.g., *Scedosporium* species). In annellidic conidiogenesis the first blown-out cell becomes a conidium but leaves a small amount of wall material around the tip of the annellide. Subsequent conidia are produced through the scar of the previous one, each time leaving some wall material at the tip. Unlike phialides, annellides increase in length each time a new spore is produced. An old annellide that has produced many conidia will have a number of apical scars or annellations at its tip.

IDENTIFICATION OF MOLDS

Most molds can be identified after growth in culture, but the criteria for recognition often differ from the fundamental characteristics that are used as a basis for classification. Macroscopic characteristics, such as colonial form, surface color, pigmentation, and growth rate, are often helpful in mold identification. Although the culture medium, incubation temperature, age of the culture, and amount of inoculum can influence colonial appearance and growth rate, these characteristics remain sufficiently constant to be useful in the process of identification. Molds that fail to sporulate in culture are often impossible to identify to the species level, and it is therefore important to select culture conditions which favor sporulation. Although molds often grow best on rich media, such as Sabouraud's dextrose agar, overproduction of mycelium often results in loss of sporulation.

POLYPHASIC IDENTIFICATION

A frequent problem with the traditional morphological approach to fungal identification is that nonsporulating organisms cannot be identified or given a taxonomic placement. With comparative DNA sequence analysis, many such isolates can now be identified and classified by applying PSR concepts. Interpretive criteria for identification of fungi using DNA sequencing have recently been published (7).

Many clinical laboratories today employ DNA sequencing as part of their routine protocol for fungal identification. In circumstances where morphology-based identification is not helpful, an isolate may be a candidate for DNA-based identification. This approach may be useful when an isolate displays atypical morphology, fails to sporulate, or requires lengthy incubation or incubation on specialized media in order to sporulate or if the phenotypic results are nonspecific or confusing. Precise identification of particular isolates may also be necessary as part of outbreak investigations or during other studies of the epidemiological significance of particular groups of organisms. In these cases, DNA sequencing may be required. A polyphasic approach to fungal identification that combines both morphological and genotypic approaches may be the most useful, practical, and cost-effective way forward for fungal identification at this time (2).

COMMON MYCOLOGICAL TERMS

Acervulus (plural, acervuli): an open or cup-shaped structure on which conidia are formed.

Acropetal: a chain of conidia in which new conidia are formed at the tip of the chain.

Aleurioconidium (plural, aleurioconidia): a thallic conidium that is formed from the end of an undifferentiated hypha or from a short side branch.

Aleuriospore: *see* Aleurioconidium.

Anamorph: the asexual form of a fungus.

Annellide: a specialized conidiogenous cell from which a succession of spores is produced and which has a column of apical scars at its tip.

Annelloconidium (plural, annelloconidia): a blastic conidium that is formed from an annellide.

Annellospore: *see* Annelloconidium.

Apophysis: the enlargement of a sporangium just below the columella.

Appressorium (plural, appressoria): a swelling on a germ tube or hypha, typical of *Colletotrichum* spp.

Arthroconidium (plural, arthroconidia): a thallic conidium produced as a result of fragmentation of an existing hypha into separate cells.

Arthrospore: *see* Arthroconidium.

Ascocarp: a structure that contains asci.

Ascoma (plural, ascomata): *see* Ascocarp.

Ascospore: a haploid spore produced within an ascus following meiosis.

Ascus (plural, asci): a thin-walled sac containing ascospores, characteristic of the Ascomycota.

Aseptate: without cross walls or septa.

Ballistoconidium: a conidium that is forcibly discharged.

Ballistospore: *see* Ballistoconidium.

Basidiocarp: a structure that produces basidia.

Basidioma (plural, basidiomata): *see* Basidiocarp.

Basidiospore: a haploid spore produced on a basidium following meiosis.

Basidium: a cell upon which basidiospores are produced, characteristic of the Basidiomycota.

Basipetal: a chain of conidia in which new conidia are formed at the base of the chain.

Blastic: of or pertaining to one of the two basic forms of conidiogenesis, in which enlargement of the conidial initial occurs before a delimiting septum is laid down.

Blastoconidium (plural, blastoconidia): a blastic conidium produced by the enlargement of a part of a conidiogenous cell before a septum is laid down.

Blastospore: *see* Blastoconidium.

Catenate: in chains.

Cerebriform: having a convoluted surface (a description of colonies).

Chlamydospore: a resting conidium formed as a result of the enlargement of an existing hyphal cell.

Clavate: club-like in shape, narrowing towards the base.

Cleistothecium (plural, cleistothecia): a form of closed ascocarp with no predefined opening, which splits open to release the ascospores.

Coelomycete: an artificial taxonomic grouping referring to anamorphic molds that form conidia within a specialized multihyphal structure, such as an acervulus or pycnidium.

Collarette: a cup-shaped structure at the tip of a conidiogenous cell.

Columella (plural, columellae): the swollen tip of the sporangiophore projecting into the sporangium in some Mucorales.

Conidiogenesis: the process of conidium formation.

Conidiogenous cell: any cell that produces or becomes a conidium.

Conidioma (plural, conidiomata): a specialized conidium-bearing structure.

Conidiophore: a specialized hypha or cell on which, or as part of which, conidia are produced.

Conidium (plural, conidia): an asexual spore.

Cruciate: having septa in the form of a cross (a description of spores).

Cuneiform: thinner at one end than at the other (a description of spores).

Dematiaceous: darkly pigmented.

Denticle: a small tooth-like projection on which a spore is borne.

Distoseptate: of or pertaining to spores in which the individual cells are each surrounded by a sac-like wall distinct from the outer wall.

Echinulate: of or pertaining to spores with small pointed spines.

Endoconidium (plural, endoconidia): a conidium formed inside a hypha.

Enteroblastic: a form of conidiogenesis in which conidia are produced from within a conidiogenous cell.

Euseptate: of or pertaining to spores in which the outer and inner walls of the septum are continuous.

Floccose: having a cotton-like texture (a description of colonies).

Fusiform: of or pertaining to spores with a spindle-like shape.

Geniculate: of or pertaining to an irregular conidiogenous cell formed by some holoblastic molds.

Glabrous: having a wax-like texture (a description of colonies).

Gymnothecium (plural, gymnothecia): an ascocarp in which the asci are distributed within a loose network of hyphae.

Heterothallic: self-sterile; sexual reproduction of a heterothallic fungus cannot take place unless two compatible mating strains are present.

Hilum: a scar at the base of a conidium.

Holoblastic conidiogenesis: a form of conidiogenesis in which both the inner and outer walls of the conidiogenous cell swell out to form the conidium.

Homothallic: self-compatible; sexual reproduction of a homothallic fungus can take place within an individual strain.

Hülle cell: a large, thick-walled, sterile cell found in some *Aspergillus* spp.

Hyaline: colorless, transparent, or translucent.

Hypha (plural, hyphae): one of the individual filaments that make up the mycelium of a fungus.

Hyphomycete: an artificial taxonomic grouping referring to anamorphic molds that form conidia directly on the hyphae or on specialized conidiophores.

Macroconidium (plural, macroconidia): the larger of two different sizes of conidia produced by a fungus in the same manner.

Meristematic: perpetually increasing in biomass in all directions with concordant septum formation.

Merosporangium (plural, merosporangia): a cylindrical outgrowth from the end of a sporangiophore in which a chain-like series of sporangiospores is produced, characteristic of *Syncephalastrum* spp.

Metula (plural, metulae): a conidiophore branch that bears phialides, characteristic of *Aspergillus* and *Penicillium* spp.

Microconidium (plural, microconidia): the smaller of two different sizes of conidia produced by a fungus in the same manner.

Mitosporic: anamorphic.

Mold: a filamentous fungus.

Moniliaceous: hyaline or lightly colored.

Muriform cell: a thick-walled, darkly pigmented cell found in tissues affected by chromoblastomycosis.

Mycelium: a mass of branching filaments which make up the vegetative growth of a fungus.

Oligokaryotic cell: a cell with several nuclei.

Oospore: a sexual spore produced in the Oomycota.

Ostiole: the opening through which spores are released from an ascocarp or pycnidium.

Perithecium (plural, perithecia): a flask-shaped ascocarp with an apical opening (ostiole) through which the ascospores are released.

Phialide: a specialized conidiogenous cell from which a succession of spores is produced.

Pleoanamorphism: term used to describe a fungus that has more than one anamorph.

Pleomorphic: of or pertaining to a nonsporing strain of a fungus.

Pseudohypha (plural, pseudohyphae): a chain of yeast cells which have arisen as a result of budding and have elongated without becoming detached from each other, forming a hypha-like filament.

Punctate: marked with small spots (a description of colonies).

Pycnidiospore: a conidium formed within a pycnidium.

Pycnidium (plural, pycnidia): a flask-shaped structure with an apical opening (ostiole) inside which conidia are produced.

Pyriform: pear-like in shape.

Rhizoid: a short branching hypha that resembles a root.

Sclerotic body: *see* Muriform cell.

Sclerotium (plural, sclerotia): a firm mass of hyphae, normally having no spores in or on it.

Septate: having cross walls or septa.

Septum (plural, septa): a cross wall in a fungal hypha or spore.

Sessile: not having a stem.

Sporangiole: *see* Sporangiolum.

Sporangiolum (plural, sporangiola): a small sporangium, containing a small number of asexual spores, characteristic of the Mucorales.

Sporangiophore: a specialized hypha upon which a sporangium develops.

Sporangiospore: an asexual spore produced in a sporangium, characteristic of the Glomeromycota.

Sporangium (plural, sporangia): a closed sac-like structure containing asexual spores, characteristic of the Glomeromycota.

Sporodochium (plural, sporodochia): a specialized structure in which conidia are borne on a compact mass of short conidiophores.

Stroma (plural, stromata): a solid mass of hyphae, sometimes bearing spores on short conidiophores, or having ascocarps or pycnidia embedded in it.

Sympodial: developing a single conidium at successive sites along a lengthening conidiogenous cell.

Synanamorph: any one of two or more anamorphs which have the same teleomorph.

Synnema (plural, synnemata): a compact group of erect and sometimes fused conidiophores bearing conidia at the tip, along the upper portion of the sides, or both.

Teleomorph: the sexual form of a fungus.

Thallic: of or pertaining to one of the two basic forms of conidiogenesis, in which enlargement of the conidial initial occurs after a delimiting septum has been laid down.

Thallus: the vegetative growth of a fungus.

Vesicle: the swollen tip of the conidiophore in *Aspergillus* spp., or the swollen part of a sporogenous cell in other fungi.

Villose: covered with long hairs (a description of spores).

Yeast: a unicellular, budding fungus.

Zoospore: a motile asexual spore.

Zygospore: a thick-walled, sexual spore produced in the Glomeromycota.

REFERENCES

1. **Alexopoulos, C. J., C. W. Mims, and M. Blackwell.** 1996. *Introductory Mycology*, 4th ed. John Wiley and Sons, Inc., New York, NY.

2. **Balajee, S. A., L. Sigler, and M. E. Brandt.** 2007. DNA and the classical way: identification of medically important molds in the 21st century. *Med. Mycol.* **45:**475–490.

3. **Barnett, J. A., R. W. Payne, and D. Yarrow.** 2000. *Yeasts: Characteristics and Identification*, 3rd ed. Cambridge University Press, Cambridge, United Kingdom.

4. **Blackwell, M.** 1993. Phylogenetic systematics and ascomycetes, p. 93–103. *In* D. R. Reynolds and J. W. Taylor (ed.), *The Fungal Holomorph: Mitotic, Meiotic and Pleomorphic Speciation in Fungal Systematics.* CAB International, Wallingford, United Kingdom.

5. **Buckley, M.** 2008. *The Fungal Kingdom: Diverse and Essential Roles in Earth's Ecosystem.* American Academy of Microbiology, Washington, DC. http://academy.asm.org/images/stories/documents/fungalkingdom.pdf.

6. **Cavalier-Smith, T.** 1998. A revised six-kingdom system of life. *Biol. Rev.* **73:**203–266.

7. **Clinical and Laboratory Standards Institute.** 2007. *Interpretive Criteria for Identification of Bacteria and Fungi by DNA Target Sequencing.* Approved guideline MM18-A. Clinical and Laboratory Standards Institute, Wayne, PA.

8. **de Hoog, G. S., J. Guarro, J. Gené, and M. J. Figueras.** 2000. *Atlas of Clinical Fungi*, 2nd ed. Centraalbureau voor Schimmelcultures, Baarn, The Netherlands.

9. **Fisher, M. C., G. L. Koenig, T. J. White, and J. W. Taylor.** 2002. Molecular and phenotypic description of *Coccidioides posadasii* sp. nov., previously recognized as the non-California population of *Coccidioides immitis. Mycologia* **94:**73–84.

10. **Guarro, J., J. Gené, and A. M. Stchigel.** 1999. Developments in fungal taxonomy. *Clin. Microbiol. Rev.* **12:**454–500.

11. **Hawksworth, D. L.** 2006. Pandora's mycological box: molecular sequences vs. morphology in understanding fungal relationships and biodiversity. *Rev. Iberoam. Micol.* **23:**127–133.

12. **Hibbett, D. S., M. Binder, J. F. Bischoff, M. Blackwell, P. F. Cannon, O. E. Eriksson, S. Huhndorf, T. James, P. M. Kirk, R. Lucking, H. T. Lumbsch, F. Lutzoni, P. B. Matheny, D. J. McLaughlin, M. J. Powell, S. Redhead, C. L. Schoch, J. W. Spatafora, J. A. Stalpers, R. Vilgalys, M. C. Aime,

A. Aptroot, R. Bauer, D. Begerow, G. L. Benny, L. A. Castlebury, P. W. Crous, Y.-C. Dai, W. Gams, D. M. Geiser, G. E. Griffith, C. Gueidan, D. L. Hawksworth, G. Hestmark, K. Hosaka, R. A. Humber, K. D. Hyde, J. E. Ironside, U. Koljalg, C. P. Kurtzman, K.-H. Larsson, R. Lichtwardt, J. Longcore, J. Miadlikowska, A. Miller, J.-M. Moncalvo, S. Mozley-Standridge, F. Oberwinkler, E. Parmasto, V. Reeb, J. D. Rogers, C. Roux, L. Ryvarden, J. P. Sampaio, A. Schussler, J. Sugiyama, R. G. Thorn, L. Tibell, W. A. Untereiner, C. Walker, Z. Wang, A. Weir, M. Weiss, M. M. White, K. Winka, Y.-J. Yao, and N. Zhang. 2007. A higher-level phylogenetic classification of the *Fungi. Mycol. Res.* **111**:509–547.

13. Kirk, P. M., P. F. Cannon, J. C. David, and J. A. Stalpers. 2001. *Dictionary of the Fungi,* 9th ed. CABI Publishing, Wallingford, United Kingdom.

14. Kurtzman, C. P., and J. W. Fell (ed.). 1998. *The Yeasts, a Taxonomic Study,* 4th ed. Elsevier, Amsterdam, The Netherlands.

15. Schurko, A. M., L. Mendoza, C. A. Lévesque, N. L. Désaulniers, A. W. de Cock, and G. R. Klassen. 2003. A molecular phylogeny of *Pythium insidiosum. Mycol. Res.* **107**:537–544.

16. Taylor, J. W., D. J. Jacobson, S. Kroken, T. Kasuga, D. M. Geiser, D. S. Hibbert, and M. C. Fisher. 2000. Phylogenetic species recognition and species concepts in fungi. *Fungal Genet. Biol.* **31**:21–32.

17. Thomarat, F., C. P. Vivares, and M. Gouy. 2004. Phylogenetic analysis of the complete genome sequence of *Encephalitozoon cuniculi* supports the fungal origin of microsporidia and reveals a high frequency of fast-evolving genes. *J. Mol. Evol.* **59**:780–791.

Specimen Collection, Transport, and Processing: Mycology

KARIN L. McGOWAN

112

Successful laboratory diagnosis of fungal infections requires attentiveness on the part of physicians and nurses, proper collection and transport of appropriate specimens, and comprehensive procedures in the laboratory. This chapter offers guidelines for specimen collection and transport, specimen handling, specimen pretreatment and processing in the laboratory, medium selection, and incubation of cultures.

SPECIMEN COLLECTION AND TRANSPORT

As in bacteriology, the goals of a good mycology laboratory are to accurately isolate and identify fungi suspected of causing infection. It is our responsibility to provide the guidelines for proper specimen selection, collection, and transport to the laboratory. Table 1 is a listing of the types of specimens most commonly submitted for fungal culture (20, 34, 50). Once collected properly, all specimens should be transported in leak-proof sterile containers and processed as soon as possible. Anaerobic transport media or anaerobic containers should never be used for fungi. Fungi are quite resilient, but because some fungi can be affected by temperatures above 37°C and below 10°C, transport at room temperature is recommended. Dermatophytes are particularly sensitive to cold temperatures. With the exception of skin, hair, and nails, specimens that contain the normal bacterial biota should be transported as rapidly as possible because bacterial overgrowth can inhibit slower-growing fungi as well as reduce fungal viability. If such specimens cannot be transported to the laboratory within 2 h, they should be stored at 4°C.

As with other infectious diseases, the best specimen for determining the causative agent comes from the active infective site (e.g., cerebrospinal fluid [CSF] for meningitis). For a number of fungal diseases, however, peripheral specimens as well as specimens from the active infective site may also be useful. Table 2 is a listing of the clinical sites associated with recovery of different pathogenic fungi. Laboratories should not hesitate to suggest that peripheral specimens be taken when specific fungal diseases are suspected. Prostate fluid, for example, is an excellent high-yield specimen when endemic mycoses are suspected, but it is a specimen not often submitted to clinical laboratories (32, 41, 48, 55, 58).

Fortunately, many of the specimen collection and transport guidelines for mycology are similar to those used in bacteriology. In those occasions where they differ, it is critical to convey that information to physicians and nurses. One such difference is in specimen volume. The volume of material required for fungal cultures usually exceeds that used in bacteriology because several types of specimens (body fluids, respiratory secretions, etc.) need to be concentrated or pretreated prior to plating to maximize recovery of fungi. In general, except for a few specific sites noted in Table 1, specimens submitted on swabs are not optimal for recovering fungi, and this practice should be discouraged.

Mycology laboratories should be encouraged to offer physicians different types of fungal cultures. The choice of media used for primary isolation as well as the length and temperature of incubation can vary with the culture request. In my laboratory, fungal culture choices include a dermatophyte culture for hair, skin, and nail specimens; a rule-out *Candida* culture for vaginal, urine, skin, and throat specimens; a fungal blood culture (lysis-centrifugation culture); and a complete fungal culture. By choosing the culture type, physicians can signal the laboratory when they suspect a specific pathogen, which can often reduce the time that cultures need to be kept in the laboratory.

SPECIMEN HANDLING, PRETREATMENT, AND SAFETY

If specimens that are unacceptable for any reason are received in the lab, they should be rejected and appropriate physicians should be notified. Poor-quality specimens can result in incorrect information, including false-negative results. As required by the Joint Commission (formerly called JCAHO), a requisition must accompany each specimen and must include the following: patient name, age, sex, and location or address, physician name, specific culture site, date and time of specimen collection, name of person who collected the specimen, clinical diagnosis, and any special culture request. In addition, each specimen must have a firmly attached label indicating the patient name, location, physician, and date and time of collection (23).

Pretreatment of several specimen types is necessary to maximize the recovery of fungi (34, 50). While this takes additional time and effort, it allows the lab to make the

TABLE 1 Specimen collection and transport guidelines[a]

Specimen type	Collection procedure	Processing procedure	Transport time and temp	Comments
Abscess (drainage, exudate, pus, or wound material)	Clean surface with 70% alcohol. Collect from active peripheral edge with sterile needle and syringe. If open, use swab system or aspirate.	If thick, pretreat similarly to sputum specimen.	≤2 h, RT	Examine for grains or granules and note color if present.
Blood	Disinfect skin with iodine tincture or chlorhexidine prior to obtaining specimen (2). Use maximum volume of blood recommended for the system used.	Manual	If ≤2 h, RT; if longer, RT	All systems for bacteria will recover all yeast species, except for *Malassezia* spp., but will not recover molds. Special fungal media for automated systems are best for molds.
		Biphasic (Septi-Chek)	If ≤2 h, RT; if longer, RT	
		Automated systems (BACTEC [BD Diagnostics, Sparks, MD], BacT/ALERT [bioMérieux, Durham, NC], VersaTREK [TREK Diagnostic Systems, Cleveland, OH])	If ≤2 h, RT; if longer, RT	
		Lysis-centrifugation (manual or Isolator system)	If ≤2 h, RT; if longer, RT, but process in ≤16 h	Lysis-centrifugation systems are good for recovery of molds, especially those causing endemic mycoses; they give high contamination and false-positive rates.
Bone marrow	Collect aseptically in a heparinized syringe or lysis-centrifugation tube.	Clotted bone marrow is an unacceptable specimen.	If ≤15 min, RT; if longer, RT	Pediatric Isolator tubes are best.
Catheter tip (intravascular)	Remove distal 3 to 5 cm of line tip and place in sterile container.	Use method of Maki at al. (31) for catheter tips.	If ≤15 min, RT; if longer, 4°C	Avoid media containing cycloheximide.
Cutaneous specimen (hair, skin, nails)	Disinfect all types with 70% alcohol. Hair: hair root is most important, plucking is best; submit 10 to 12 hairs in sterile dry container or envelope. Skin: scrape with dull edge of a scalpel or glass slide or vigorously brush in a circular motion with a soft-bristle toothbrush. Nails: clip or scrape with a scalpel. Material under nail should also be scraped. Submit in sterile container or clean, dry paper envelope.	Only the leading edge of a lesion should be sampled, as centers are often nonviable. All specimens should be pressed gently onto the agar with a sterile swab; do not streak agar plates. If used, toothbrushes should be pressed gently into agar as well.	<72 h, RT (very stable). Never refrigerate, as dermatophytes are sensitive to cold.	Select hairs which fluoresce under Wood's light. Hair and skin can be collected with a soft-bristle toothbrush. For pityriasis versicolor (M. *furfur*), olive oil or a paper disk saturated with olive oil should be placed on the first quadrant of the agar plate.
Eye (corneal scraping, vitreous humor)	Corneal scraping: taken by physicians, with media/ slides inoculated directly. Vitreous humor: taken by needle aspiration	Corneal scraping: inoculate noninhibitory media in X- or C-shaped motion. Vitreous humor: concentrate by centrifugation; use sediment for media and smears.	If ≤15 min, RT; if longer, RT If ≤15 min, RT; if longer, RT	Very little material usually available. Avoid media with cycloheximide.

(Continued on next page)

TABLE 1 *(Continued)*

Specimen type	Collection procedure	Processing procedure	Transport time and temp	Comments
Medical devices	Collect surgically. Transport in a sterile container.	Use sterile scalpel to collect (by scraping) biofilm or vegetative growth.	If ≤15 min, RT; if longer, 4°C.	Avoid media containing cycloheximide. Device material is recovered best by using liquid medium.
Prostate fluid	Have patient empty bladder, and then massage prostate gland to yield fluid.	Inoculate media directly or transport in sterile wide-mouth container.	If ≤15 min, RT; if longer, RT	Fluid should always be examined microscopically. The first urine following massage has a high yield. This fluid is excellent for detection of endemic mycoses.
Respiratory tract, lower (sputum, bronchial aspirate, BAL fluid)	Use first-morning sputum, collected after brushing teeth. Collect brushings and BAL fluid surgically. Place all samples in sterile containers. Inoculate media containing antimicrobial agents, with and without cycloheximide.	Viscous lower respiratory tract specimens should be pretreated and centrifuged to concentrate their contents.	If ≤2 h, RT; if longer, 4°C	Saliva or 24-h sputa are unacceptable specimens. Methods for mycobacterial decontamination are not acceptable.
Respiratory tract, upper (oral, oropharyngeal, and sinus samples)	Swab oral lesions, avoiding tongue. Use thin wire or a flexible swab for oropharynx. Collect sinus contents surgically.	Use swab transport system for oral and oropharyngeal samples. Place sinus contents in sterile container.	Oral: if ≤2 h, RT; if longer, RT Sinus: if ≤15 min, RT; if longer, RT	Selective and chromogenic media are best for recovery of *Candida*.
Sterile body fluids (CSF and pericardial, peritoneal, and synovial fluids)	Collect as for bacteriology. Concentrate by centrifugation, and use sediment for inoculation. Clots should be ground.	Except CSF, put sterile body fluids in sterile Vacutainer tubes with heparin or in lysis-centrifugation tubes to prevent blood clotting. Except for CSF, blood culture bottles can be used for recovery of yeast.	If ≤15 min, RT; if longer, RT (never refrigerate)	Sterile fluid sediment should always be examined microscopically. With specimen volumes ≤2 ml, fluid should be plated directly, using as much fluid on each plate as possible.
Stool	Specimen use should be discouraged.			
Tissue	Collect surgically. A larger volume is needed than that for bacteriology.	Use a sterile container, kept moist (saline drops) to prevent drying. Except with *H. capsulatum*, mincing, not grinding is critical. Tissue pieces should be pressed into the agar so they are partially embedded. Grind tissue for recovery of *H. capsulatum*.	If ≤15 min, RT; if longer, RT	Tissue biopsy is recommended for invasive disease. Examine subcutaneous tissue for granules (see information for abscesses).
Urine	Use first morning clean-catch, suprapubic, or catheterized specimens; 24-h specimens are unacceptable.	Use a sterile container or urine transport system. Concentrate specimens by centrifugation, and use sediment for inoculation.	If ≤2 h, RT; if longer, 4°C; urine transport systems can stay at RT for up to 72 h.	Chromogenic media are best for recovery of *Candida*. Use sediment for microscopic examination.
Vaginal samples	Collect as for bacteriology.	Use swab transport system or sterile container for washings.	If ≤2 h, RT; if longer, RT	Antibacterial media or chromogenic agars are best for recovery of *Candida*

[a]Abbreviations: BAL, bronchoalveolar lavage fluid; CSF, cerebrospinal fluid; RT, room temperature.

TABLE 2 Common clinical sites for laboratory recovery of pathogenic fungi

Disease	Recovery from tissue[a]														
	Blood	Bone	Bone marrow	Brain	CSF	Eye	Hair	Nails	Joint fluid	Prostate fluid	Lower respiratory tract	Sinus/nasal cavity	Skin[b]	Tissue	Urine
Aspergillosis	X			X		X		X			X	X	X	X	X
Blastomycosis	X			X	X				X	X	X	X	X	X	X
Candidiasis	X		X	X	X	X		X	X	X	X	X	X	X	X
Chromoblastomycosis				X								X	X	X	
Coccidioidomycosis	X	X	X	X	X				X	X	X	X	X	X	X
Cryptococcosis	X	X	X	X	X	X					X		X	X	X
Dermatophytosis							X	X					X		
Fusariosis	X			X		X		X	X		X	X	X	X	
Histoplasmosis	X		X	X	X	X			X		X		X	X	X
Mucormycosis				X		X					X	X	X	X	
Paracoccidioidomycosis	X		X	X	X						X	X	X	X	
Penicilliosis	X		X	X					X	X	X		X	X	X
Pneumocystitis			X								X			X	
Scedosporiosis	X		X	X	X	X					X	X	X	X	
Sporotrichosis	X			X	X	X			X		X	X	X	X	
Trichosporonosis	X		X	X	X	X				X	X	X	X	X	
Zygomycosis	X			X							X		X	X	X

[a] X, recovery of fungus from indicated tissue.
[b] Includes skin and mucous membranes.

most out of every specimen submitted, particularly for those that are difficult to obtain from patients. Pretreatment procedures are listed in Table 3 and include centrifugation of urine and sterile body fluids, mincing of nail and tissue specimens, lysis and centrifugation of blood or bone marrow received in Isolator tubes (Wampole Laboratories, Cranbury, NJ), and lysis by mucolytic agents, followed by centrifugation, for respiratory secretions. Such procedures release fungi enclosed within cells, concentrate fungal material in the specimen, and help to reduce or eliminate bacteria present in contaminated specimens because of the action of mucolytic agents, such as N-acetyl-L-cysteine, 5% oxalic acid, or dithiothreitol (Sputolysin).

All work in mycology should be carried out in a certified type 2 laminar-airflow biosafety cabinet whenever possible. There are different biosafety regulations in Europe and other countries, and for this reason, practices may differ. Biosafety level 2 procedures are recommended for personnel working with clinical specimens that may contain dimorphic fungi as well as other potential pathogenic fungi. Gloves should be worn for processing specimens and cultures. A number of techniques are available for examining clinical specimens microscopically, and these are discussed in chapter 114 in this *Manual*.

SPECIMEN PROCESSING AND CULTURE GUIDELINES

Abscess (Drainage, Exudate, Pus, and Wound Material)

Abscess specimens should be collected from the active peripheral edge of open abscesses or aspirated from closed abscesses by use of a syringe. Abscess, pus, or drainage material should be examined for grains or granules by use of a dissecting microscope. The presence of grains or granules is indicative of a mycetoma. If none are present, the material can be inoculated directly onto media. If the specimen is thick, it should be pretreated similarly to a sputum specimen. If present, grains and granules should be teased out of the specimen and washed in sterile distilled water, sterile saline, or either solution plus antibiotics. The color of the granules should be noted and recorded. A portion should be crushed between two glass slides and examined microscopically for the presence of hyphae. Both true fungal hyphae and bacteria (branching gram-positive rods) can be observed with grains. If branching gram-positive rods are seen, a modified acid-fast stain should be performed to look for *Nocardia*. Another portion of the grains and granules should be crushed by using sterile technique (sterile glass rod or mortar and pestle) and then inoculated directly onto media (29).

Blood

Fungemia is a major cause of morbidity and mortality in hospitalized patients, with *Candida* species being the major cause (44, 46). Early detection of organisms in the bloodstream is incredibly important because it is an indicator of disseminated disease. As in bacteriology, the volume of blood, the blood-to-broth ratio, and the number of blood cultures are all critical factors, with the volume of blood being the most important variable. For adults, 20 to 30 ml per culture, divided between 2 bottles, is recommended for the highest recovery rate (9, 30, 54) and the shortest time to detection (7). Studies recommend a 5- to 10-fold dilution of blood in broth, and dilutions of <1:5 may result in reduced

TABLE 3 Pretreatment of clinical specimens prior to plating

Specimen	Pretreatment	Comments
Abscess, drainage, pus, granules	Granules should be washed and crushed; other materials should be centrifuged at 2,000 × g for 10 min.	Essential for best recovery
Blood, bone marrow	Lysis in Isolator tubes and then centrifugation for 30 min at 3,000 × g, using a 35° fixed-angle rotor or swinging bucket	Critical for detection of *H. capsulatum* and other dimorphic fungi
Body fluids	Centrifugation at 2,000 × g for 10 min or membrane filtration	Essential for best recovery with volumes of ≥1 ml; blood clots should be teased apart
Nails	Mince into tiny pieces; push pieces down into agar	Essential for maximum recovery of dermatophytes
Respiratory secretions (bronchoalveolar lavage fluid, sputum)	Lysis with mucolytic agents,[a] followed by centrifugation at 2,000 × g for 10 min	Critical for detection of *Pneumocystis jirovecii*; improves recovery for other mycoses
Tissue	Mince into tiny pieces or grind in a mortar; push pieces down into agar	Essential for best recovery; for zygomycetes and other molds, mincing is best; for *H. capsulatum*, grinding is best
Urine	Centrifugation at 2,000 × g for 10 min	Essential for best recovery, particularly with deep mycoses

[a]N-Acetyl-L-cysteine, 5% oxalic acid, or dithiothreitol (Sputolysin).

recovery of organisms (3, 44). For infants and children, total blood volumes based on the weight of the patient are presently recommended (3, 24, 51). Unlike bacteremia, fungemia is almost always continuous in patients with infectious endocarditis, so the timing of obtaining a blood culture for fungi is not critical (9). Both iodine tincture and chlorhexidine are effective for skin decontamination prior to obtaining the blood culture (2). In a review of 270 cases of fungal endocarditis in the world literature, the organisms responsible were *Candida albicans* (24%), non-*C. albicans Candida* spp. (28%), *Aspergillus* spp. (24%), *Histoplasma* spp. (6%), and other yeasts and molds (17%) (13). In Europe, if blood cultures are negative in patients with suspected *Candida* endocarditis, then a laboratory diagnosis can often be achieved by *Candida* serology testing.

There are presently a wide variety of manual, biphasic, automated, and continuously monitoring systems for blood cultures, but no single commercial system or culture medium can detect all potential blood pathogens. If manual blood cultures are used, a biphasic system is best for fungi (Septi-Chek; Becton Dickinson Diagnostic Systems, Sparks, MD), and the agar slant should be rewashed with the broth-blood mixture each time the bottles are examined. Many automated and continuously monitoring systems are available, and several have medium modifications to enhance fungal growth. These include the BACTEC (BD Diagnostics, Sparks, MD), BacT/ALERT 3D (bioMérieux, Durham, NC), and VersaTREK (Trek Diagnostic Systems, Cleveland, OH) blood culture systems. Studies evaluating all of these systems have shown that they can recover all pathogenic yeast species except for *Malassezia* spp. Even without specific fungal media, automated and continuously monitoring systems are able to recover *Candida*, *Cryptococcus*, *Rhodotorula*, and *Trichosporon* spp., with sensitivities equal to or higher than those of manual or lysis-centrifugation methods (7, 9, 18, 25, 35–38, 42, 56). Automated systems

with routine bacteriology media are not, however, satisfactory for molds and *Nocardia* spp. (56).

Lysis-centrifugation performed either manually (9) or by using the commercially available Isolator collection system is a more sensitive method for recovery of molds and dimorphic fungi such as *Histoplasma capsulatum* (19, 21, 56). Several studies, however, have argued against the routine use of lysis-centrifugation for all fungal blood cultures because of high contamination rates, high false-positivity rates, and equivalent or shorter times to detection of yeasts than those with automated systems (11, 25, 35). If molds are suspected, either a special fungal medium for an automated system, such as BACTEC MYCO/F lytic medium or BacT/ALERT MB, or a lysis-centrifugation system should be considered (10). Blood placed in either adult or pediatric Isolator tubes should be kept at room temperature until it is processed, ideally within 16 h of collection. Sediment from lysis-centrifugation should be streaked onto a variety of enriched media not containing cycloheximide and onto a chocolate agar plate (43). The only yeast species requiring special processing are the *Malassezia* species, which require lipids for growth. This can be achieved by overlaying solid media with a thin layer of olive oil or adding a paper disk saturated with olive oil to a subculture plate or plates containing sediment from a lysis-centrifugation tube (3, 14, 29). Specialized media such as modified Dixon's, Leeming's, and Ushijima's media can also be used to isolate *Malassezia* species, if available.

Bone Marrow

Bone marrow is most useful for the diagnosis of disseminated candidiasis, cryptococcosis, and histoplasmosis. Approximately 0.5 ml (pediatrics) to 3 ml (adults) should be collected aseptically in a heparinized syringe or pediatric Isolator tube. Because lysis-centrifugation enhances the recovery of *H. capsulatum* and other molds, the use of

Isolator tubes is the method of choice for these organisms. Clotted bone marrow is an unacceptable specimen. With the exception of *H. capsulatum*, fungi are rarely seen in bone marrow aspirates from immunocompetent hosts. For immunocompromised patients, however, bone marrow is an excellent specimen, and *Aspergillus* spp., *Candida* spp., *Cryptococcus neoformans*, *H. capsulatum*, and *Penicillium marneffei* can all be observed (1). While it is quite clear that microscopic examination of Giemsa-stained bone marrow can be diagnostic, recent data show that compared with other, less-invasive methods, such as blood cultures, bone marrow aspirate cultures are of limited value and should be performed only selectively (12). Bone marrow should not be placed into blood culture bottles because with many continuously monitoring systems, the specimen will quickly register a false-positive result due to CO_2 from massive numbers of white blood cells.

Catheter Tips (Intravascular)

If performed simultaneously with blood cultures, quantitative bacterial and fungal cultures have been advocated to demonstrate catheter tip colonization. Acceptable specimens are intravenous or intra-arterial catheter tips, with the distal 3 to 5 cm of the line tip being submitted to the laboratory for culture. Specimens should be placed in a sterile container and transported and stored at room temperature. The semiquantitative method of Maki et al. (31) is the most common method used in clinical laboratories, where the catheter tip is rolled across the surface of an agar plate four times and cultures yielding ≥15 CFU are considered positive. The semiquantitative method distinguishes infection (≥15 colonies) from contamination and is considered a more specific method to diagnose catheter-related septicemia than culturing the catheter tip in broth.

Cutaneous Specimens (Hair, Skin, and Nails)

Hair

The hair root is the most important part to culture for detection of fungi, so plucking or pulling rather than cutting hair is recommended. The area should be cleaned with 70% alcohol and allowed to dry. Infected hairs can appear dull, broken, and faded. Hairs which fluoresce under Wood's light should also be selected for culture. Hair should be submitted in a sterile container or clean, dry paper envelope. Hair can also be collected by using a soft-bristle toothbrush and rubbing in a circular motion over margins or patches of alopecia (hair loss) (22).

Skin

The area should be cleaned with 70% alcohol and allowed to dry. The skin should then be scraped with the dull edge of a scalpel or glass slide or vigorously brushed in a circular motion with a soft-bristle toothbrush (22). Only the leading edge of a skin lesion should be sampled, because the centers of lesions are frequently nonviable. Skin can be submitted in a sterile container or clean, dry paper envelope or on a toothbrush.

Nails

Nails should be cleaned with 70% alcohol and then clipped or scraped with a scalpel. If material is present under the leading edge of the nail, it should also be scraped and submitted in a sterile container or paper envelope designed specifically for this purpose. Prior to being plated, nail pieces should be pulverized or minced into tiny pieces by use of a scalpel.

All cutaneous specimens should be inoculated into the agar medium by gently pressing them onto the agar with a sterile swab or scalpel. Distribute the pieces evenly over the agar surface; do not streak the plate with a sterile loop. If a toothbrush is used to collect skin and/or hair specimens, the brush should be pressed gently onto the surface of the agar in four or five places on the plate, leaving an imprint. If organisms are present, growth will occur within the bristle imprint. By nature, cutaneous specimens are usually contaminated with bacteria. For this reason, a plate of inhibitory medium with chloramphenicol and cycloheximide, such as Mycosel, should be used for dermatophytes. Because *Trichosporon* spp., the cause of white piedra, in addition to *Scopulariopsis* and *Fusarium* species, are sensitive to both chloramphenicol and cycloheximide, a noninhibitory medium such as Sabouraud dextrose agar should also be inoculated with nail specimens. For patients suspected of having pityriasis versicolor, caused by *Malassezia furfur*, direct microscopy is normally diagnostic, but a noninhibitory medium such as Sabouraud dextrose agar can be inoculated, and then olive oil or a paper disk saturated with olive oil should be placed on the first quadrant of the plate. *Malassezia furfur* grows best at ≥35°C but can grow at 30°C. Cutaneous specimens should never be refrigerated because dermatophytes are sensitive to low temperatures.

Eye Specimens (Corneal Scrapings and Vitreous Humor)

Several types of eye infections require that corneal scrapings and/or vitreous humor be obtained by an ophthalmologist. These include mycotic or fungal keratitis, fungal endophthalmitis, and extension oculomycosis. Mycotic or fungal keratitis is an infection of the cornea. The most common causes are *Acremonium* spp., *Aspergillus* spp., *C. albicans*, *Candida parapsilosis*, *Candida tropicalis*, *Curvularia* spp., and *Fusarium* spp. (6, 52). Fungal endophthalmitis is a late-stage result of hematogenous dissemination of a systemic fungal infection. It can involve many areas of the eye and surrounding tissues. The most common causes are *Aspergillus* spp., *Blastomyces dermatitidis*, *Candida* spp., *C. neoformans*, *Coccidioides* spp., *H. capsulatum*, *Paracoccidioides brasiliensis*, and *Sporothrix schenckii* (6, 52). Extension oculomycosis is a result of rhinocerebral mucormycosis, and like fungal endophthalmitis, it may involve many areas of the eye and surrounding tissues. The diagnosis of these infections requires attempting to demonstrate the organism on a microscopic exam plus positive culture. Corneal scrapings are taken by physicians, and media are inoculated directly by use of a heat-sterilized platinum spatula (49). Very little material is usually obtained because of the risks of corneal thinning or perforation. Physicians should be instructed to first inoculate the specimen directly onto a noninhibitory medium, such as Sabouraud dextrose agar, and then to place some material on a sterile glass slide (in the center) for staining. The scraping should be placed in two or three places on the plate, using an X- or C-shaped motion (50). The inoculated plate should be kept at room temperature and transported immediately to the laboratory. Vitreous or vitreous humor is the clear, gelatinous material that fills the space between the lens of the eye and the retina. When taken by physicians, vitreous is often diluted with irrigation fluid. For this reason, it should be concentrated by centrifugation, and the sediment should be used to inoculate media and to make smears. Specimens should be placed onto Sabouraud dextrose agar, inhibitory mold agar, and/or brain heart infusion (BHI) agar with 10% sheep blood and incubated at 30°C. Media containing cycloheximide should be avoided (6, 27, 52).

Medical Devices

A wide variety of medical devices (contact lenses, stents, wound-healing dressings, contraceptives, surgical implants, replacement joints, etc.) may be submitted for fungal culture. Most are collected surgically and should be submitted in a sterile container and transported and stored at room temperature. Each should be examined for vegetative growth and biofilms, and if these are present, they should be scraped from the device by use of a sterile scalpel for direct inoculation of agar media and broth (50). Specimens should be placed onto Sabouraud dextrose agar, inhibitory mold agar, and/or BHI agar with 10% sheep blood and incubated at 30°C. Media containing cycloheximide should be avoided. If biofilm or vegetative growth areas are not obvious, portions of the device should be placed in a broth medium such as BHI broth and incubated at 30°C.

Prostate Fluid

Prostate fluid consists of secretions of the testes, seminal vesicles, prostate, and bulbourethral glands. After the bladder is emptied, the prostate gland is massaged to yield pure prostatic fluid. The prostate is frequently seeded when organisms are present in the bloodstream. A key clinical sign in males with endemic mycoses is the complaint of a history of chronic urinary tract infections but negative urine cultures. Prostatic fluid for such patients is frequently positive when cultured for fungi. The secretions should also be examined microscopically. After the prostate fluid is obtained, the next urine specimen should also be obtained and submitted for culture because this urine has a high yield (32, 41, 48, 55, 58).

Lower Respiratory Tract Specimens (Sputum, Bronchial Aspirate, and Bronchoalveolar Lavage Fluid)

After a patient's teeth have been brushed, sputum should be collected as a first morning specimen. Neither saliva nor 24-h sputum specimens are acceptable for fungal culture. Viscous lower respiratory tract specimens should be pretreated before being processed. Lysis with mucolytic agents, such as N-acetyl-L-cysteine, 5% oxalic acid, or dithiothreitol (Sputolysin), followed by centrifugation at 2,000 × g for 10 min and then plating of the sediment, greatly increases the yield and improves the recovery of many fungi. Sodium hydroxide, which is used to concentrate specimens for detection of mycobacteria, should not be used because it inhibits the growth of many fungi. Unfortunately, centrifugation also increases the number of bacteria in the sediment, and for this reason, media containing antimicrobial agents, with and without cycloheximide, should be used. As in bacteriology, lower respiratory tract specimens should be examined for the presence of blood, pus, or necrotic portions, since these have the highest yields (45, 57).

Upper Respiratory Tract Specimens (Oral and Oropharyngeal Specimens)

The mucosal surface of gums, oral lesions, and oropharyngeal specimens submitted for fungal culture are usually screened for candidiasis. When thrush is suspected, lesions should be scraped gently with moist swabs and submitted for microscopy and a rule-out yeast culture. Antibacterial media or chromogenic agars for Candida spp. should be inoculated. While culture is not required to make the diagnosis of candidiasis, it can be useful if microscopy is not available in an outpatient setting or if species other than C. albicans are suspected. On rare occasions, oral lesions can be seen with histoplasmosis or paracoccidioidomycosis, but they do not resemble those seen with Candida spp. If these are suspected, a full fungal culture and microscopic smear should be performed. The use of nasal swabs should be discouraged because of contamination from environmental spores in the nasal cavity making interpretation of culture results difficult. Nasal tissue or sinus washings are better specimens and should be plated on a variety of media containing antibiotics, but not cycloheximide, since significant pathogens recovered from these sites (Aspergillus spp.) are sensitive to cycloheximide (4).

Sterile Body Fluids (CSF and Pericardial, Peritoneal, and Synovial Fluids)

With the exception of CSF, sterile body fluids are often placed in sterile Vacutainer tubes with heparin to prevent blood clotting. Lysis-centrifugation Isolator tubes can also be used for this purpose. With specimen volumes of ≥2 ml, these tubes plus CSF lumbar puncture tubes should be centrifuged at 2,000 × g for 10 min, and the sediment should be used to inoculate media. The supernatant fluid can be used for serologic tests (27). With specimen volumes of ≤2 ml, the specimen should be plated directly, using as much fluid on each plate as possible. Use of a Cytospin centrifuge to prepare microscopic smears is recommended (5, 47). Because sterile fluids are so rarely culture positive for fungi, many laboratories inoculate medium slants with screw-cap lids rather than plates to avoid questions concerning possible contamination. In some countries, a purity plate is placed in the biosafety cabinet when sterile body fluids or tissues are being processed. Growth on the purity plate would signal a contamination event during processing.

Stool

Submission of stool specimens for routine fungal culture should be discouraged. Many Candida spp. are part of the normal stool biota, and anything that disrupts the normal gastrointestinal tract biota, such as diet or use of antibiotics, can yield a predominance of yeast when stool is cultured. Neither colonization with yeast nor a predominance of yeast indicates invasive disease with Candida. If invasive disease of the gastrointestinal tract is suspected, a colonoscopy and tissue biopsy should be performed (8, 26).

Tissue

With one exception (H. capsulatum), fungi present in tissue are best recovered when the tissue is minced, not ground. For the mucoraceous molds, in particular, mincing is critical for the recovery of organisms. Tissues should be minced by use of a scalpel, and the pieces of tissue should be pressed into the agar so they are partially embedded (16). Two to four pieces should be placed onto each piece of media being inoculated. Further streaking of the plate with sterile loops should not be done. When the medium is inoculated this way, fungi grow out directly from the piece of tissue. Laboratories often question if growth on agar plates is contamination. When growth comes directly from the tissue piece, it is unquestionably significant growth. A portion of the specimen can be ground for microscopic examination/ smears.

When H. capsulatum is suspected, the tissue should be ground or homogenized. Because this pathogen is intracellular, organisms need to be released from the cells to be available to grow on media. If needed, a small amount of sterile broth or distilled water can be added to smooth the process of grinding. Subcutaneous tissue should be examined for the presence of granules (as described above, for abscesses). Homogenate or tissue pieces should be inoculated onto enriched media containing antibacterial agents, and for systemic mycoses, enriched media containing both blood and antibacterial agents are best.

Urine

Clean-catch, suprapubic, or catheterized urine specimens should all be obtained as first morning specimens. Large volumes (10 to 50 ml) give the best results and should be centrifuged for maximum recovery, particularly for agents of deep mycoses. Urine should be centrifuged at $2,000 \times g$ for 10 min. The sediment should be used for microscopic smears and inoculation of media. Quantification of organisms, as performed in bacteriology, is not useful (14). Twenty-four-hour urine specimens are not acceptable.

Vaginal Specimens

Vaginal specimens submitted for fungal culture are frequently screened just for vaginal candidiasis. For this reason, having a rule-out *Candida* culture as a culture choice is helpful for clinicians and laboratorians. *Candida* spp. are part of the normal vaginal biota, and their presence alone

TABLE 4 Media suggested for the recovery of fungi from clinical specimens

Medium[a]	Properties	Comments
Primary media without antibacterials or antifungals		
BHI medium	With or without sheep blood	Supports growth of all fungi
Littman oxgall agar	Excellent for primary isolation of fungi and dermatophytes	Supports growth of all fungi; oxgall prevents spreading of colonies
SDA	4% glucose, slightly acid pH	Good for dermatophytes but overgrows with bacteria; poor choice for primary media (46a)
SDA, Emmons modification	2% glucose, near-neutral pH (6.9) is better for fungi	Supports growth of all fungi
Sabhi medium	With or without sheep blood	Supports growth of all fungi, but designed for dimorphics; blood can inhibit sporulation
Primary media with antibacterials or antifungals		
Any of the above media	Choice of chloramphenicol, ciprofloxacin, gentamicin, penicillin, or streptomycin alone or in combination	Inhibits bacteria well; BHI and Sabhi media with blood plus antibiotics are best choices for dimorphics; for isolation of pathogenic fungi other than dermatophytes
IMA	Contains chloramphenicol to inhibit bacteria	Excellent for growth of dermatophytes
Mycosel or Mycobiotic	SAB with chloramphenicol, cycloheximide, and 1% glucose	Inhibits bacteria, but cycloheximide inhibits many pathogenic fungi
Selective/differential media		
DTM or DIM	For diagnosis of dermatophytes, using color change of medium as an indicator; contains antibiotics to inhibit bacteria	Frequent false-positive results for nondermatophyte fungi with DTM
Yeast extract phosphate	Used with chloramphenicol and ammonium hydroxide	Recovery of dimorphics from contaminated specimens
CHROMagar *Candida* or Albicans ID agar	Selective and differential medium for isolation and presumptive identification of *Candida* spp.; includes chromogenic substrates plus antibacterials	Most bacteria inhibited; excellent for detecting mixed cultures of yeast; number of *Candida* species detected is manufacturer dependent
Specialized media		
CMA	With and without Tween 80	Tween 80 addition results in rapid and abundant chlamydospore formation; supports growth of most fungi but has no bacterial inhibitors
PDA or PFA	Stimulates production of spores and sporulating bodies	Often used for slide cultures; PFA is best for these
RSA	Sodium acetate agar	For yeast, induces ascospore production
Niger seed or bird seed and EBM	Contains chloramphenicol; used for selective isolation and identification of *C. neoformans*	*C. neoformans* appears as dark brown colonies

[a]Abbreviations: BHI, brain heart infusion agar; SDA, Sabouraud dextrose agar; Sabhi medium, Sabouraud dextrose and brain heart infusion agar; IMA, inhibitory mold agar; DTM, dermatophyte test medium; DIM, dermatophyte identification medium; CMA, cornmeal agar; PDA, potato dextrose agar; PFA, potato flake agar; RSA, rapid sporulation agar; EBM, esculin base medium.

is not significant. Appropriate clinical symptoms plus a positive microscopic exam or culture are sufficient to diagnose vaginal candidiasis. Culture is not required to confirm vaginal candidiasis, but microscopic exams are not available in all settings, while culture is available. Antibacterial media or chromogenic agars for *Candida* spp. should be inoculated. On rare occasions, vaginal lesions can be seen with histoplasmosis or paracoccidioidomycosis. These lesions do not resemble those seen with *Candida* spp. If these are suspected, a full fungal culture and microscopic smear should be performed.

SELECTION AND INCUBATION OF MEDIA

Table 4 is a listing of various media used for the recovery of fungi from clinical specimens, including primary media, selective and/or differential media, and specialized media. Optimal recovery of fungal pathogens depends upon a number of factors, including the choice of an appropriate specimen(s), collection and transport of a quality specimen, appropriate pretreatment of specimens, the media chosen for inoculation and incubation, a proper incubation temperature, and sufficient time of incubation. A wide variety of media are available for primary isolation, and in many laboratories, the choice is based on personal experience and the technologist's preferences. As with bacteria, a battery of several media needs to be used because no single fungal medium is sufficient for detection of all of the clinically important fungi. Several factors should be considered in selecting a battery of several media, as follows.

- Choices of media should be driven by the type of specimen being processed (20, 34, 50). Media that inhibit bacterial growth but allow for the growth of fungi should be used for nonsterile specimens that may contain large numbers of bacteria (BHI or Sabhi medium plus antibiotics or inhibitory mold agar). The eukaryotic protein synthesis inhibitor cycloheximide should be used in one medium choice, with or without antibiotics. The battery for sterile body sites should include one or two media lacking antibiotics plus one medium with antibiotics.

- Cycloheximide is a component in several primary media and suppresses saprophytic fungi, but it is known to inhibit the growth of some *Aspergillus* spp., some *Candida* spp., *Cryptococcus* species, *Nattrassia mangiferae*, *Pseudallescheria boydii*, *Penicillium marneffei*, most members of the Mucorales, *Scopulariopsis*, *Trichosporon asahii*, and many saprophytic or opportunistic fungi. While cycloheximide prevents fast-growing contaminants from overgrowing slow-growing pathogens such as *H. capsulatum*, it should not be included in all medium choices.

- Chloramphenicol, with or without other antibiotics, is included in several primary media to suppress the growth of bacteria. While these are excellent medium choices for processing of specimens that contain the bacterial biota, they prevent the growth of *Nocardia* and aerobic actinomycetes. Mycology laboratories that are responsible for culturing these organisms must include other media for these pathogens, such as Sabouraud agar.

- Dimorphic fungi which grow endemically grow best on an enriched medium (BHI or Sabhi medium) with antibiotics and 5 to 10% sheep blood. The sheep blood promotes the growth of dimorphic fungi but inhibits sporulation. Molds recovered on this enriched medium should be subcultured immediately to blood-free enriched medium to promote conidiation and for DNA probe testing.

Exceptions to using a battery of media would be for fungal cultures that screen for a specific pathogen, such as a rule-out *Candida* culture, where a chromogenic medium that is selective and differential for yeast can be used, or a rule-out dermatophyte culture, where a single Mycosel or Mycobiotic plate can be used. In attempting to isolate *Malassezia* spp., Sabouraud agar with antibiotics should be supplemented with sterile olive oil by adding 0.5 ml of oil to the surface of the plate after inoculation or dropping an olive oil-saturated paper disk on the first half of the plate. Alternatively, specialized media, such as modified Dixon's, Leeming's, and Ushijima's media, can also be used, if available.

The container used for fungal media is often debated because of safety issues related to fungi which grow endemically (33). Agar plates are considered more dangerous, are easily contaminated, and dehydrate the fastest, but they offer the largest surface area to work from, and colonies are easier to reach on plates. Plates can be sealed individually or placed in plastic bags to avoid environmental contamination and to provide a layer of safety beyond the use of a laminar-airflow biosafety cabinet. Screw-cap flat-sided bottles and agar slants in tubes both reduce contamination and are safer to use, but both have the disadvantage of a narrow opening through which to access colonies. Most clinical laboratories use plated media, but some compromise by using flat-sided bottles or tubes with those specimen types that are rarely culture positive, such as CSF or other sterile fluids, to avoid later questions concerning possible contaminants.

Inoculated media should be incubated aerobically at 30°C, but if a 30°C incubator is not available, then 25°C should be used. *S. schenckii*, a rare exception, grows faster at 27 to 28°C, but it still grows well at 30°C.

The length of incubation depends on the type of fungal culture requested. Cultures that screen for *Candida* spp. need to be incubated for no longer than 72 h, cultures that screen for dermatophytes need to be incubated for only 8 days, and cultures screening for all pathogens, including fungi which grow endemically, should routinely be held for 4 weeks. A single study suggests that 3 weeks of incubation may be sufficient (28). Culture media should be examined every 2 to 3 days for the first 2 weeks and weekly thereafter.

REFERENCES

1. **Bain, B. J., D. M. Clark, I. A. Lampert, and B. S. Wilkins.** 2001. *Bone Marrow Pathology*, 3rd ed., p. 99. Wiley-Blackwell, New York, NY.
2. **Barenfanger, J., C. Drake, J. Lawhorn, and S. J. Verhulst.** 2004. Comparison of chlorhexidine and tincture of iodine for skin antisepsis in preparation for blood culture collection. *J. Clin. Microbiol.* **42:**2216–2217.
3. **Baron, E. J., M. P. Weinstein, W. M. Dunne, Jr., P. Yagupsky, D. F. Welch, and D. M. Wilson.** 2005. *Cumitech 1C, Blood cultures IV.* Coordinating ed., E. J. Baron. ASM Press, Washington, DC.
4. **Carrol, K., and L. Reimer.** 1996. Microbiology and laboratory diagnosis of upper respiratory tract infections. *Clin. Infect. Dis.* **23:**442–448.
5. **Chapin-Robertson, K., S. E. Dahlberg, and S. C. Edberg.** 1992. Clinical and laboratory analyses of cytospin-prepared Gram stains for recovery and diagnosis of bacteria from sterile body fluids. *J. Clin. Microbiol.* **30:**377–380.
6. **Chern, K. C., D. M. Meisler, K. R. Wilhelmus, D. B. Jones, G. A. Stern, and C. Y. Lowder.** 1996. Corneal anesthetic abuse and *Candida* keratitis. *Ophthalmology* **103:**37–40.
7. **Chiarini, A., A. Palmeri, T. Amato, R. Immordino, S. Distefano, and A. Giammanco.** 2008. Detection of bacterial

and yeast species with the Bactec 9120 automated system with routine use of aerobic, anaerobic, and fungal media. *J. Clin. Microbiol.* **46:**4029–4033.

8. Cimbaluk, D., J. Scudiere, J. Butsch, and S. Jakate. 2005. Invasive candidal enterocolitis followed shortly by fatal cerebral hemorrhage in immuno-compromised patients. *J. Clin. Gastroenterol.* **39:**795–797.

9. Cockerill, F. R., III, J. W. Wilson, E. A. Vetter, K. M. Goodman, C. A. Torgerson, W. S. Harmsen, C. D. Schleck, D. M. Illstrup, J. A. Washington III, and W. R. Wilson. 2004. Optimal testing parameters for blood cultures. *Clin. Infect. Dis.* **38:**1724–1730.

10. Cockerill, F. R., III, C. A. Torgerson, G. S. Reed, E. A. Vetter, A. L. Weaver, J. C. Dale, G. D. Roberts, N. K. Henry, D. M. Illstrup, and J. E. Rosenblatt. 1996. Clinical comparison of Difco ESP, Wampole Isolator, and Becton Dickinson Septi-Chek aerobic blood culturing systems. *J. Clin. Microbiol.* **34:**20–24.

11. Creger, R. J., K. E. Weeman, M. R. Jacobs, A. Morrisey, P. Parker, R. M. Fox, and H. M. Lazarus. 1998. Lack of utility of the lysis-centrifugation blood culture method for detection of fungemia in immunocompromised cancer patients. *J. Clin. Microbiol.* **36:**290–293.

12. Duong, S., B. J. Dezube, G. Desai, K. Eichelberger, Q. Qian, and J. E. Kirby. 2009. Limited utility of bone marrow culture: a ten-year retrospective analysis. *Lab. Med.* **40:**37–38.

13. Ellis, M. E., H. Al-Abdely, A. Sandridge, W. Greer, and W. Ventura. 2001. Fungal endocarditis: evidence in the world literature. *Clin. Infect. Dis.* **32:**50–62.

14. Fisher, J. E., C. L. Newman, and J. D. Sobel. 1995. Yeast in the urine: solutions for a budding problem. *Clin. Infect. Dis.* **20:**183–189.

15. Forbes, B. A., D. F. Sahm, and A. S. Weissfeld. 2007. *Bailey & Scott's Diagnostic Microbiology*, 12th ed., p. 778–797. Mosby Elsevier, St. Louis, MO.

16. Forbes, B. A., D. F. Sahm, and A. S. Weissfeld. 2007. *Bailey & Scott's Diagnostic Microbiology*, 12th ed., p. 629–713. Mosby Elsevier, St. Louis, MO.

17. Fraser, V. J., M. Jones, and J. Dunkel. 1992. Candidemia in a tertiary care hospital: epidemiology, risk factors, and predictors of mortality. *Clin. Infect. Dis.* **15:**414–421.

18. Fricker-Hidalgo, H., B. Lebeau, H. Pelloux, and R. Grillot. 2004. Use of the BACTEC 9240 system with mycosis-IC/F blood culture bottles for detection of fungemia. *J. Clin. Microbiol.* **42:**1855–1856.

19. Gaur, A. H., M. A. Giannini, P. M. Flynn, J. W. Boudreaux, M. A. Mestemacher, J. L. Shenep, and T. Hayden. 2003. Optimizing blood culture practices in pediatric immunocompromised patients: evaluation of media types and blood culture volume. *Pediatr. Infect. Dis. J.* **22:**545–552.

20. Hazen, K. C. 1998. Section 6. Mycology and aerobic actinomycetes, p. 255–283. *In* H. D. Isenberg (ed.), *Essential Procedures for Clinical Microbiology*. American Society for Microbiology, Washington, DC.

21. Hellinger, W. C., J. J. Cawley, S. Alvarez, S. F. Hogan, W. S. Harmsen, D. M. Ilstrup, and F. R. Cockerill III. 1995. Clinical comparison of the Isolator and BacT/Alert aerobic blood culture systems. *J. Clin. Microbiol.* **33:**1787–1790.

22. Hubbard, T. W., and J. M. de Triquet. 1992. Brush-culture method for diagnosing tinea capitis. *Pediatrics* **90:**416–418.

23. Joint Commission (JCAHO). 2009. *IM.6.240. Clinical Laboratory Improvement Act Subpart K Sec. 493.1232, Sec. 493.1242, and Sec. 493.1249.* Joint Commission, Oakbrook Terrace, IL.

24. Kellogg, J. A., J. P. Manzella, and D. A. Bankert. 2000. Frequency of low-level bacteremia in children from birth to fifteen years of age. *J. Clin. Microbiol.* **38:**2181–2185.

25. Kosmin, A. R., and T. Fekete. 2008. Use of fungal blood cultures in an academic medical center. *J. Clin. Microbiol.* **46:**3800–3801.

26. Kouklakis, G., S. Dokas, E. Molyvas, P. Vakianis, and A. Efthymiou. 2001. *Candida* colitis in a middle-aged male

27. Kwon-Chung, K. J., and J. Bennett. 1992. *Medical Mycology*, p. 45–46. Lea & Febiger, Philadelphia, PA.

28. Labarca, J. A., E. A. Wagar, A. E. Grasmick, H. M. Kokkinos, and D. A. Bruckner. 1998. Critical evaluation of 4-week incubation for fungal cultures: is the fourth week useful? *J. Clin. Microbiol.* **35:**3683–3685.

29. Larone, D. H. *Medically Important Fungi: a Guide to Identification*, 4th ed. ASM Press, Washington, DC.

30. Lee, A., S. Mirrett, L. B. Reller, and M. P. Weinstein. 2007. Detection of bloodstream infections in adults: how many blood cultures are needed? *J. Clin. Microbiol.* **45:**3546–3548.

31. Maki, D. G., C. D. Weise, and H. W. Sarafin. 1977. A semiquantitative culture method for identifying intravenous-catheter-related infection. *N. Engl. J. Med.* **296:**1305–1309.

32. Mawhorter, S. D., G. V. Curley, E. D. Kursh, and C. E. Farver. 2000. Prostatic and central nervous system histoplasmosis in an immunocompetent host: case report and review of the prostatic histoplasmosis literature. *Clin. Infect. Dis.* **30:**595–598.

33. McGinnis, M. R. 1980. *Laboratory Handbook of Medical Mycology.* Academic Press, New York, NY.

34. Merz, W. G., and G. D. Roberts. 1999. Detection and recovery of fungi from clinical specimens, p. 709–722. *In* P. R. Murray et al. (ed.), *Manual of Clinical Microbiology*, 7th ed. American Society for Microbiology, Washington, DC.

35. Mess, T., and E. S. Daar. 1997. Utility of fungal blood cultures for patients with AIDS. *Clin. Infect. Dis.* **25:**1350–1353.

36. Mirrett, S., L. B. Reller, C. A. Petti, C. W. Woods, B. Vazirani, R. Sivadas, and M. P. Weinstein. 2003. Controlled clinical comparison of BacT/ALERT standard aerobic medium with BACTEC standard aerobic medium for culturing blood. *J. Clin. Microbiol.* **41:**2391–2394.

37. Mirrett, S., K. E. Hanson, and L. B. Reller. 2007. Controlled clinical comparison of VersaTREK and BacT/ALERT blood culture systems. *J. Clin. Microbiol.* **45:**299–302.

38. Morello, J. A., S. M. Matushek, W. M. Dunne, and D. B. Hinds. 1991. Performance of a BACTEC nonradiometric medium for pediatric blood cultures. *J. Clin. Microbiol.* **29:**359–362.

39. Morrell, R. M., B. L. Wasilauskas, and C. H. Steffe. 1996. Performance of fungal blood cultures by using the Isolator collection system: is it cost effective? *J. Clin. Microbiol.* **34:**3040–3043.

40. Musial, C. E., F. R. Cockerill III, and G. D. Roberts. 1988. Fungal infections of the immunocompromised host: clinical and laboratory aspects. *Clin. Microbiol. Rev.* **1:**349–364.

41. Neal, P. M., and A. Nikolai. 2008. Systemic blastomycosis diagnosed by prostate needle biopsy. *Clin. Med. Res.* **6:**24–28.

42. Petti, C. A., A. K. M. Zaidi, S. Mirrett, and L. B. Reller. 1996. Comparison of Isolator 1.5 and BACTEC NR660 aerobic 6A blood culture systems for detection of fungemia in children. *J. Clin. Microbiol.* **34:**1877–1879.

43. Procop, G. W., F. R. Cockerill III, E. A. Vetter, W. S. Harmsen, J. G. Hughes, and G. D. Roberts. 2000. Performance of five agar media for recovery of fungi from Isolator blood cultures. *J. Clin. Microbiol.* **38:**3827–3829.

44. Reimer, L. G., M. L. Wilson, and M. P. Weinstein. 1997. Update on detection of bacteremia and fungemia. *Clin. Microbiol. Rev.* **10:**444–465.

45. Reimer, L. G., and K. C. Carroll. 1998. Role of the microbiology laboratory in the diagnosis of lower respiratory tract infections. *Clin. Infect. Dis.* **26:**742–748.

46. Richardson, M., and C. Lass-Flörl. 2008. Changing epidemiology of systemic fungal infections. *Clin. Microbiol. Infect.* **4**(Suppl.):5–24.

46a. Scognamiglio, T., R. Zinchuk, P. Gumpeni, and D. H. Larone. 2010. Comparison of inhibitory mold agar to Sabouraud dextrose agar as a primary medium for isolation of fungi. *J. Clin. Microbiol.* **48:**1924–1925.

47. **Shanholtzer, C. J., P. J. Schaper, and L. R. Peterson.** 1982. Concentrated Gram stain smears prepared with a cytospin centrifuge. *J. Clin. Microbiol.* **16:**1052–1056.

48. **Sohail, M. R., P. E. Andrews, and J. E. Blair.** 2005. Coccidioidomycosis of the male genital tract. *J. Urol.* **173:** 1978–1982.

49. **Sonntag, H. G.** 2002. Sampling and transport of specimens for microbial diagnosis of ocular infections. *Dev. Ophthalmol.* **33:**362–367.

50. **Sutton, D. A.** 2007. Specimen collection, transport, and processing: mycology, p. 1728–1736. *In* P. R. Murray, E. J. Baron, J. H. Jorgensen, M. L. Landry, and M. A. Pfaller (ed.), *Manual of Clinical Microbiology*, 9th ed. American Society for Microbiology, Washington, DC.

51. **Szymzcak, E. G., J. T. Barr, W. A. Durbin, and D. A. Goldman.** 1979. Evaluation of blood culture procedures in a paediatric hospital. *J. Clin. Microbiol.* **9:**88–92.

52. **Tanure, M. A., E. J. Cohen, S. Sudesh, C. J. Rapuano, and P. R. Laibson.** 2000. Spectrum of fungal keratitis at Wills Eye Hospital, Philadelphia, Pennsylvania. *Cornea* **19:**307–312.

53. **Telenti, A., and G. D. Roberts.** 1989. Fungal blood cultures. *Eur. J. Clin. Microbiol. Infect. Dis.* **8:**825–831.

54. **Washington, J. A., II, and D. M. Illstrup.** 1986. Blood cultures: issues and controversies. *Rev. Infect. Dis.* **8:**792–802.

55. **Watts, B., P. Argekar, S. Saint, and C. A. Kauffman.** 2007. Clinical problem-solving. Building a diagnosis from the ground up—a 49-year-old man came to the clinic with a 1-week history of suprapubic pain and fever. *N. Engl. J. Med.* **356:**1456–1462.

56. **Witebsky, F. G., and V. J. Gill.** 1995. Fungal blood culture systems: which ones and when to use them. *Clin. Microbiol. Newsl.* **17:**161–163.

57. **Wolf, J., and A. Daley.** 2007. Microbiological aspects of bacterial lower respiratory tract illness in children: typical pathogens. *Paediatr. Respir. Rev.* **8:**204–211.

58. **Yurkanin, J. P., F. Ahmann, and B. L. Dalkin.** 2006. Coccidioidomycosis of the prostate: a determination of incidence, report of 4 cases, and treatment recommendations. *J. Infect.* **52:**e19–e25.

Reagents, Stains, and Media: Mycology

JAMES W. SNYDER, RONALD M. ATLAS, AND MARK T. LaROCCO

113

A variety of stains, media, and reagents are available to the mycology laboratory for the detection, isolation, characterization, and identification of yeasts and moulds. Familiarity with the composition and characteristics of these materials is critical to the diagnostic approach when processing specimens from patients with suspected mycotic diseases. The direct microscopic examination of properly stained clinical material is rapid and cost-effective and may denote the presumptive etiologic agent (4, 7, 10). Results of direct examination can also guide the laboratory in the selection of media that best support fungal growth in vitro (4). Stained preparations made from fungal cultures are essential for definitive identification.

Many media are available for the primary inoculation and cultivation of fungi from clinical specimens. No one specific medium or combination of media is adequate for all specimens. Media should be carefully selected based on specimen type and suspected fungal agents. Media can be dispensed into containers such as 25- by 150-mm screw-cap tubes or 100-mm-diameter petri dishes. Petri plates, in contrast to agar tubes (slants/deeps), offer the advantage of a large surface area for isolation and dilution of inhibitory substances in the specimens, but they must be poured thick, with at least 25 ml of medium, in order to resist dehydration during incubation. Because plates are vented, they are more likely to become contaminated during incubation. Plates may be placed in gas-permeable bags or sealed with gas-permeable tape (Shrink Seals; Scientific Device Laboratory, Des Plaines, IL) to offset this disadvantage. It is recommended that plated media be used for cultivating fungi and for safety purposes.

Although it is recommended that fungal cultures be incubated for up to 4 weeks before being regarded as negative, it is important to understand that many cultures can be read after 48 h. For example, most yeasts are detected within 5 or fewer days, dermatophytes are detected within 1 week, and dematiaceous and dimorphic fungi may require 2 to 4 weeks. Therefore, to account for differences in growth rates, fungal cultures should be examined at regular intervals (e.g., daily during the first week, three times the second week, twice at 3 weeks, and once at 4 weeks) rather than being evaluated once at the end of 4 weeks. Plates must be opened inside a certified biological safety cabinet to prevent contamination of the plate and exposure of personnel to potentially dangerous fungi. Tubed media have a smaller surface area but offer maximum safety and resistance to dehydration and contamination. If the specimen is from a contaminated site, it is important to include media that contain inhibitory substances such as chloramphenicol, gentamicin, or cycloheximide. Chloramphenicol or gentamicin inhibits most bacterial contaminants, while cycloheximide inhibits most saprobic moulds. Remember that cycloheximide may also inhibit opportunistic fungi such as some species of *Aspergillus*, *Fusarium*, *Scopulariopsis*, *Pseudallescheria*, mucoraceous fungi, some dematiaceous fungi, and yeasts such as *Cryptococcus* species and some *Candida* species. It is important to use media with and without inhibitory agents. Specimens from normally sterile sites can be inoculated to media without inhibitory substances.

Each new lot of medium, whether purchased or prepared in-house, must be subjected to a quality control protocol that verifies appearance, pH, and performance (12). Both positive and negative control strains need to be included in quality assurance testing protocols. Media for primary isolation should be tested for optimal growth of several fungal pathogens. Selective media should be tested with strains known to be sensitive and resistant to the inhibitory agent in the media, while differential media should be evaluated with fungi that produce both positive and negative reactions. Many media are also commercially available as prepared plates or tubes. Although manufacturers perform quality control testing, clinical laboratories still need to ensure that media meet performance standards. Some widely used commercially prepared media are exempt from routine quality assurance testing. These media include cornmeal agar, inhibitory mould agar, inhibitory mould agar with gentamicin, soy peptone agar with cycloheximide/chloramphenicol without pH indicators, potato dextrose agar, brain heart infusion agar with 5% sheep blood containing chloramphenicol/gentamicin, Sabouraud's dextrose agar, and Sabouraud's dextrose agar with chloramphenicol/gentamicin (12). Nonexempt media that require specific quality assurance testing include cornmeal agar with Tween, brain heart infusion agar with 5% sheep blood and cycloheximide/chloramphenicol, bismuth sulfite-glucose-glycine-yeast (BiGGY) agar, birdseed agar, brain heart infusion with 5% sheep blood and penicillin/streptomycin, dermatophyte test medium, and potato flakes agar with or without cycloheximide/chloramphenicol (12).

Unless stated otherwise, the reagents and media listed in this chapter should be prepared by dissolving the components in the stated liquid with a magnetic stirring bar. The standard sterilization technique of autoclaving at 121°C at 15 lb/in^2 for 15 min should be used when needed. However, certain solutions such as those containing antibiotics or carbohydrates cannot be autoclaved because they will be denatured. These solutions are sterilized by filtration through a 0.22-μm-pore-size filter; *Candida* chromogenic agars can be microwaved.

Storage of prepared reagents in sterile, airtight, screw-cap containers is recommended. Some reagents require storage in dark containers, and some need to be stored refrigerated (2 to 8°C) instead of at room temperature. Special storage instructions are given when appropriate. Standard safety precautions should be taken when preparing the reagents. Follow the safety guidelines for the chemicals being used, in addition to the laboratory safety protocols.

The stains, media, and reagents listed in this chapter include those commonly used and a few specialized items. For more specific information not included here, refer to the literature cited in the chapter.

REAGENTS

■ *N*-Acetyl-L-cysteine (NALC) (0.5%)
NALC (Alpha Tec Systems, Inc.) is a mucolytic agent used for digestion of sputum specimens submitted for detection of *Pneumocystis jirovecii* cysts and/or trophozoites by microscopic examination. This compound can also be used for preparing samples for microscopic examination for a wide range of fungi. Sodium citrate (0.1 M) is included in the mixture to exert a stabilizing effect on the acetyl-L-cysteine.

■ Dithiothreitol (Sputolysin), 0.0065 M
Dithiothreitol is a mucolytic agent that can be purchased commercially and has been used to prepare sputum specimens for detection of *P. jirovecii*. Equal volumes of sputum and dithiothreitol are mixed and incubated at 35°C. The mixture is periodically mixed vigorously until nearly liquefied (complete liquefaction disperses the cells of *P. jirovecii*, making microscopic detection difficult). As with NALC, dithiothreitol can be useful for preparing samples for microscopic examination of a wide range of fungi.

■ Potassium hydroxide (KOH)
Wet mounts prepared in 10% KOH are used to distinguish fungi in thick mucoid specimens or in specimens that contain keratinous material such as skin, hair, and nails. The proteinaceous components of the host cells are partially digested, leaving the fungal cell wall intact and more apparent. An aliquot of specimen is added to a drop of 10% or 20% KOH, which can be preserved with 0.1% thimerosal (Sigma Chemical Co.). The slide is held at room temperature for 5 to 30 min after the addition of KOH, depending on the specimen type, to allow digestion to occur. Digestive capabilities can be enhanced with gentle heating or the addition of 40% dimethyl sulfoxide.

■ Potassium hydroxide (10%) with lactophenol cotton blue (LPCB)
The wet mount with KOH and LPCB is used for the same purpose as the KOH preparation but incorporates LPCB dye (see below). LPCB enhances the visibility of fungi because

aniline blue stains the outer cell wall of fungi, and lactic acid serves as an additional clearing agent. The phenol component in LPCB acts as a fungicide.

■ Sodium hydroxide (10 or 25% with added glycerin)
Solutions of sodium hydroxide may be used as alternatives to potassium hydroxide for the direct microscopic examination of hair, skin, and nails for dermatophyte-mediated infections. Visualization of fungal elements may be enhanced by the addition of glucan-binding fluorescent brighteners such as calcofluor white or Congo red, both of which bind to chitin, a major component of the fungal cell wall.

STAINS

■ Alcian blue stain
Alcian blue and the more commonly used mucicarmine stain (see below) are mucopolysaccharide stains. These are useful for visualizing the polysaccharide capsule produced by *C. neoformans* in histological sections of tissue.

Basic procedure
Deparaffinized sections are stained in Alcian blue (1 g in 100 ml of acetic acid, 3% solution) for 30 min, washing in running tap water, and then rinsing in distilled water. The sections are counterstained in nuclear fast red (0.1 g in 100 ml of aluminum sulfate, 5% solution). After dehydration through 95% and absolute alcohol, the sections are cleared with xylene and mounted in Permount (Fisher Scientific). Capsular polysaccharides stain blue against a pink background.

■ Ascospore stain
Ascomycetous fungi may produce ascospores when grown on media that promote their formation. Visualization of ascospores can be accomplished with a differential staining procedure consisting of malachite green and safranin. Ascospores stain green, while the vegetative portion of the fungus stains red. The Kinyoun acid-fast stain (see chapter 115) may also be used for visualizing ascospores, as these structures tend to be acid-fast.

Basic procedure
A thin smear of growth is applied to a glass slide and heat fixed. The slide is flooded with malachite green (5 g in 100 ml of distilled water) for 3 min, washed with tap water, decolorized with 95% ethyl alcohol for 30 s, and counterstained with aqueous safranin (5%) for 30 s. The slide is washed with tap water, allowed to air dry, and examined at ×400 to ×1,000 magnification.

■ Calcofluor white
Calcofluor white and related compounds such as Uvitex 2B and Blankophor are nonspecific, nonimmunological fluorochromes that bind to β1,3 and β1,4 polysaccharides, specifically cellulose and chitin of fungal cell walls. Like the auramine-rhodamine stain, calcofluor white has become commonplace in microbiology laboratories because of the rapidity with which specimens can be observed. The fluorochrome can be mixed with KOH to clear the specimen for easier observation of fungal elements, including *P. jirovecii*. Fungal elements appear bluish white against a dark background when excited with UV or blue-violet radiation. Optimal fluorescence occurs with UV excitation. A barrier filter such as 510, 520, or 530 should be used for

eye protection. Organisms impart a green fluorescence (4). Typical *P. jirovecii* cysts are generally 5 to 8 μm in diameter, round, and uniform in size, and they exhibit a characteristic peripheral cyst wall staining with an intense "double-parenthesis-like" structure (5, 6). Yeast cells are differentiated from *P. jirovecii* by budding and intense staining. Care must be used in interpreting the calcofluor white staining result because nonspecific reactions may be observed. Cotton fibers fluoresce strongly and must be differentiated from fungal hyphae. Additionally, tissues such as brain biopsy specimens from patients with tumors may fluoresce and resemble hyphae suggestive of *Aspergillus* or other moulds with branching hyphae.

Basic procedure

KOH (10%) is mixed in equal proportion with calcofluor white solution (0.1 g of calcofluor white M2R and 0.05 g of Evans blue in 100 ml of water). The specimen is covered with this mixture, a coverslip is applied, and the preparation is examined with UV light at ×100 to ×400 magnification. For optimal detection, it is recommended that the preparation not be examined with the fluorescence microscope for at least 10 min after preparing the mixture, as some fungi will not be immediately visible (G. Roberts, personal communication).

■ **Colloidal carbon wet mounts (India ink, nigrosin)**

Colloidal carbon wet mounts are used for visualization of encapsulated microorganisms, especially *Cryptococcus neoformans*. The polysaccharide capsule of organisms is refractory to the particles of ink, and capsules appear as clear halos around the organism. Artifacts such as erythrocytes, leukocytes, and talc particles from gloves or bubbles following a myelogram may displace the colloidal suspension and mimic yeast (false positive). These artifacts make it necessary to perform a careful examination of the wet mount for properties consistent with the organisms (e.g., rounded forms with buds of various sizes and double-contoured cell walls). Interpretation can also be hindered if the emulsion with the colloid suspension is too thick, blocking transmission of light.

Basic procedure

Mix equal parts of the patient's cerebrospinal fluid with either Pelikan India ink or nigrosin on a slide. Add a coverslip and examine at ×100 to ×1,000 magnification.

■ **Fontana-Masson stain**

The Fontana-Masson stain was originally developed for demonstrating melanin granules in mammalian tissue. It has a mycological application in detecting dematiaceous (melanin-containing) fungi, and to a lesser extent *Cryptococcus neoformans/gattii*, in histological sections. Fungal elements appear brown to brownish black against a reddish background.

Basic procedure

A silver solution is prepared by adding concentrated ammonium hydroxide to 10% silver nitrate until the precipitated form disappears. Deparaffinized sections of tissue are hydrated and placed in heated silver solution for 30 to 60 min. The slides are then rinsed in distilled water and toned in gold chloride (0.2 g in 100 distilled water) for 10 min followed by fixation in 5% sodium thiosulfate for 5 min. The sections are dehydrated through increasing concentrations of alcohol, cleared in xylene, and mounted with a coverslip.

■ **Giemsa stain**

The Giemsa stain is used for the detection of intracellular yeast forms of *Histoplasma capsulatum* in bone marrow and buffy coat specimens. The fungus is usually seen as small oval yeast cells that stain blue and have a hyaline halo that represents poorly staining cell wall. The stain can also be used to visualize the trophozoite of *P. jirovecii*.

Basic procedure

A thin smear is prepared on a glass slide and placed in 100% methanol for 1 min. The slide is drained and then flooded with freshly prepared Giemsa stain (stock Giemsa stain diluted 1:10 with phosphate-buffered water). After 5 min, the slide is rinsed with distilled water and air dried. Examine at ×100 to ×400 magnification.

■ **Lactophenol cotton blue**

Lactophenol cotton blue is a basic mounting medium for fungi consisting of phenol, lactic acid, glycerol, and aniline (cotton) blue dye. The solution may be filtered to remove precipitated dye and stored at room temperature. It is commonly used for the microscopic examination of fungal cultures by tease or tape preparation. The addition of 10% polyvinyl alcohol (LPCB-PVA) makes an excellent permanent stain or fixative for mounting slide culture preparations (4).

Basic procedure

Concentrated phenol (20% [vol/vol]) is added to a mixture of glycerol (40%), lactic acid (20%), and water (20%), followed by the addition of aniline blue (0.05 g). The solution may be filter sterilized to remove precipitated dye. A drop is added to a glass slide, and tease or tape mount is prepared. Add a coverslip and examine at ×100 to ×400 magnification.

■ **Methenamine silver stain**

Methenamine silver stains are perhaps the most useful stains for visualizing fungi in tissue. Fungal elements are sharply delineated in black against a pale green or yellow background. They are specialized stains that are more often performed in the histology laboratory than in the microbiology laboratory. Grocott's modification of the Gomori methenamine silver stain is commonly used for the histopathological examination of deparaffinized tissues for fungi.

Basic procedure

Stock methenamine silver nitrate solution is prepared by adding 3% methenamine (3 g in 100 ml of distilled water) to 5% silver nitrate (5 g in 100 ml of distilled water) until a white precipitate forms that clears upon shaking. This solution is then diluted 1:2 with distilled water to which 5 ml of 5% photographic-grade borax is added. Prepared slides are oxidized in a solution of chromic acid (5 g in 100 ml of distilled water), neutralized in sodium bisulfite (1 g in 100 ml of distilled water), placed in the diluted methenamine silver nitrate solution, and heated in an oven to 58 to 60°C until the material turns yellowish brown. After being rinsed vigorously in distilled water, the slides are toned in gold chloride (0.1 g in 100 ml of distilled water). Unreduced silver is removed by placing the slides in a sodium thiosulfate solution (2 g in 100 ml of distilled water) and counterstained in 0.03% light green. Rinse, blot dry, and examine at ×100 to ×400 magnification.

■ Mucicarmine stain

The mucicarmine stain is useful for differentiating *C. neoformans/gattii* from other fungi of similar size and shape when found in samples of tissue. The mucopolysaccharide in the capsular material of the fungus stains deep rose to red, whereas the other tissue elements stain yellow.

Basic procedure

Fixed tissue sections on glass slides are stained first with Weigert's iron hematoxylin and then placed in a solution of mucicarmine (1 g of carmine combined with 0.5 g of anhydrous aluminum chloride in 2 ml of distilled water and then diluted in 100 ml of 50% ethanol) for 30 to 60 min. The slides are rinsed in distilled water and then counterstained in mentanil yellow (0.25 g in 100 ml of distilled water). Rinse, blot dry, and examine at ×100 to ×400 magnification.

■ Periodic acid-Schiff (PAS) stain

The periodic acid-Schiff (PAS) stain is used to detect fungi in clinical specimens, especially yeast cells and hyphae in tissues. Fungi stain a bright pink-magenta or purple against an orange background if picric acid is used as the counterstain, or against a green background if light green is used. The procedure is a multistep method combining hydrolysis and staining. The periodic acid step hydrolyzes the cell wall aldehydes, which are then able to combine with the modified Schiff reagent, coloring the cell wall carbohydrates a bright pink-magenta. The PAS stain is an excellent general stain, because most fungi in clinical material take up the stain. However, the PAS staining procedure is rather involved, requiring several different reagents and time-consuming steps, and has been replaced in many laboratories by the calcofluor white staining procedure. The PAS stain cannot be used with undigested respiratory secretions, since mucin also stains bright pink-magenta.

Basic procedure

The prepared slide is fixed in formalin-ethanol for 1 min and is then air dried. The slide is then immersed in 5% periodic acid for 5 min, followed by 2 min in basic fuchsin (0.1 g of dye in 5 ml of 95% alcohol–95 ml of H$_2$O). The slide is rinsed in water and immersed in zinc or sodium hydrosulfite solution for 10 min (1 g of zinc or sodium hydrosulfite in 0.5 g of tartaric acid and 100 ml of H$_2$O). Rinse in water and counterstain with saturated aqueous picric acid for 2 min or with light green stain (1 g of dye in 0.25 ml of acetic acid and 100 ml of 80% alcohol) for 5 s. Rinse, blot dry, and examine at ×100 to ×400 magnification.

■ Toluidine blue O

Toluidine blue O is used primarily for the rapid detection of *P. jirovecii* from lung biopsy specimen imprints and bronchoalveolar lavage (BAL) specimens (15). Toluidine blue O stains the cysts of *P. jirovecii* reddish blue or dark purple against a light blue background. The cysts are often clumped and may be punched in, appearing crescent shaped. Trophozoites are not discernible. Although the silver stain, monoclonal antibody, and calcofluor white stains are also used, the toluidine blue O stain is easy and rapid and yields reliable results with appropriate specimens (e.g., BAL specimens).

Basic procedure

After the slide is air dried, place it in the sulfation reagent (45 ml of glacial acetic acid mixed with 15 ml of concentrated sulfuric acid) for 10 min. Rinse in cold water for 5 min, drain, and place in toluidine blue O (0.3 g of dye in 60 ml of H$_2$O) for 3 min. Rinse in 95% ethanol, followed by absolute ethanol and then xylene. Examine at ×100 to ×1,000 magnification.

MEDIA

■ Acetate ascospore agar

Acetate ascospore agar is used for the cultivation of ascosporogenous yeasts such as *Saccharomyces cerevisiae*. A potassium acetate formulation has been shown to be a better sporulation medium than the previously used formulation with sodium acetate. Ascospores produced on this medium are visible microscopically after staining with Kinyoun carbolfuchsin acid-fast stain.

■ Antifungal susceptibility testing media

Recent advances in methods for antifungal susceptibility testing have resulted in several media that are now used for this type of testing (see chapter 128). The broth dilution method for yeasts and filamentous fungi described in the Clinical and Laboratory Standards Institute (formerly the National Committee for Clinical and Laboratory Standards) M38-A2 and M27-A3 documents (2, 3) uses RPMI 1640 synthetic medium without sodium bicarbonate and supplemented with L-glutamine. The medium is buffered to pH 7.0 with 0.165 M morpholinepropanesulfonic acid (MOPS). Although this medium supports the growth of most fungi, it is not optimal for *Cryptococcus* species (18), nor does it accurately discriminate amphotericin B-resistant *Candida* spp. (17).

The Antifungal Susceptibility Testing Subcommittee of the European Committee on Antibiotic Susceptibility Testing (AFST-EUCAST) has described a proposed standard broth microdilution that is based on the M27-A3 broth microdilution reference procedure. Both procedures utilize RPMI 1640 as the primary assay medium, but that used in the EUCAST procedure differs from the CLSI procedure with the incorporation of 2% glucose (19, 20).

■ Assimilation broth media for yeasts (carbohydrates)

Assimilation broth media for yeasts are used for the detection of assimilation, i.e., carbohydrate utilization by yeasts in the presence of oxygen. The medium uses a yeast nitrogen base, distilled water, and an individual carbohydrate. The assimilation patterns of various carbohydrates help to distinguish among different species of yeast. Since all yeasts assimilate glucose, it acts as a positive control. Usually, the media are prepared as liquids in tubes, and a positive test is growth that is observed as turbidity.

■ Assimilation broth media for yeasts (nitrogen)

Carbon assimilation broth media are used to determine the ability of yeasts to utilize different carbohydrates as a sole source of carbon in a chemically defined growth medium. The growth medium, yeast nitrogen base, contains vitamins required for growth but is insufficient to support growth without supplementation with glucose or other carbohydrates.

■ Birdseed agar

Birdseed agar is a selective and differential medium used for the isolation of *Cryptococcus* species, especially *C. neoformans* and *C. gattii*, which are unique in that they produce the enzyme phenol oxidase. The breakdown of the substrate (*Guizotia abyssinica* seeds or niger seed) produces melanin, which is absorbed into the yeast wall and which imparts a tan to brown pigmentation of the colonies. Colonies of other yeasts are beige or cream in color. Chloramphenicol is the selective agent that inhibits bacteria and some fungi. Creatinine enhances melanization of some strains of *C. neoformans*.

■ **Bismuth sulfite-glucose-glycine yeast (BiGGY) agar**

Bismuth sulfite-glucose-glycine yeast agar is a selective and differential medium used for the isolation and differentiation of *Candida* spp. Peptone, glucose, and yeast extract are the nutritive bases. *Candida* species reduce the bismuth sulfite to bismuth sulfide, which results in pigmentation of the yeast colony and, with some species, the surrounding medium. *Candida albicans* appears as brown to black colonies with no pigment diffusion and no sheen, whereas *Candida tropicalis* appears as dark brown colonies with black centers, black pigment diffusion, and a sheen. Specific colonial morphologies and growth patterns of the different *Candida* species are also detected. The bismuth sulfite also acts as an inhibitor of bacterial growth, making the medium selective.

■ **Blood-glucose-cysteine agar**

Blood-glucose-cysteine agar medium is used to promote the mould-to-yeast conversion of *Histoplasma capsulatum*, *Blastomyces dermatitidis*, *Paracoccidioides brasiliensis*, and *Sporothrix schenckii*. The medium contains tryptose blood agar base, L-cysteine, and defibrinated sheep blood. Penicillin is added to inhibit bacterial contamination.

■ **Brain heart infusion agar (fungal formulation)**

Brain heart infusion agar with sheep blood is a medium used for the cultivation and isolation of all fungi including fastidious dimorphic fungi. The nutritive base is brain heart infusion agar with 10% sheep blood for added enrichment. The antibiotics chloramphenicol and gentamicin are added to make the medium selective by inhibiting bacteria and saprophytic fungi.

■ **Bromcresol purple-milk solids-glucose medium**

Bromcresol purple-milk solids-glucose (Dermatophyte Milk Agar; Hardy Diagnostics) is a differential medium used for the identification of some dermatophytes. The medium's differential capacity is based on the type of growth (profuse versus restricted) and change in the pH indicator due to the production of alkaline by-products.

■ **Canavanine-glycine-bromthymol blue agar**

Canavanine-glycine-bromthymol blue agar is a differential medium for distinguishing *C. neoformans* from *C. gattii*. The medium contains glycine, thiamine, L-canavanine sulfate, and bromthymol blue. A colony of *C. neoformans* is streaked onto the surface of the agar and incubated at 30°C for 1 to 5 days. *C. gattii* (serotypes B and C) turns the medium cobalt blue, whereas *C. neoformans* var. *grubii* (serotype A) and *C. neoformans* var. *neoformans* (serotype D) leave the medium greenish yellow.

■ ***Candida* chromogenic media**

The introduction of chromogenic media has facilitated the direct and rapid identification of yeasts. These media contain chromogenic substrates that are hydrolyzed by species-specific enzymes, e.g., β-N-acetylhexosaminidase and, depending on the medium, a second enzyme, β-glucosidase or phosphatase, resulting in identification of yeasts to the species level based on colonial features and color development (11, 13, 16). Commercially available chromogenic media are summarized in Table 1.

A brief description of selected chromogenic agar products that are FDA approved for use in U.S. laboratories is provided as an overview of how different yeasts react with chromogenic substrates and the resultant characteristic colony color.

■ **CHROMagar (BD Biosciences)**

CHROMagar is a differential and selective medium used for the isolation and differentiation of clinically important yeasts. The nutritive base is peptone and glucose. Chloramphenicol makes the medium selective by inhibiting bacteria. The medium is available with and without fluconazole, the former providing the additional selection of fluconazole-resistant yeasts such as *Candida krusei*. A proprietary chromogenic mixture allows the differentiation of many yeast species. For example, *C. albicans* forms yellow-green to blue-green colonies. Colonial morphology as well as distinctive color patterns have been shown to make the presumptive identification of yeast species very reliable (13, 16). The medium has been shown to be more selective than Sabouraud agar and helpful in identifying mixed cultures of yeasts and may enhance the rapid assimilation of trehalose by *Candida glabrata* (16). The colonies on the medium should be evaluated at 48 h. Although *C. neoformans* and *Geotrichum* species can grow on this medium, definitive identification requires subculture to a nonselective medium followed by utilization of the appropriate biochemical and morphological characterization tools.

TABLE 1 Commercial sources of yeast chromogenic agar media

Medium	Manufacturer
Candida diagnostic agar (CDA)	PPR Diagnostics
Candida Chromogenic Agar	Laboratorios CONDA
CandiSelect	Bio-Rad
CandiSelect 4	Bio-Rad[a]
CHROMagar Candida	CHROMagar Microbiology
CHROMagar	BD Biosciences[b]
chromID Candida agar (CAN2)	bioMérieux[b]
HiCrome Candida agar	HiMedia Laboratories
HiCrome Candida differential agar	HiMedia Laboratories
Oxoid chromogenic Candida medium	Oxoid

[a]510k exempt (medical device, class I: low risk).
[b]FDA approved for use in U.S. laboratories.

■ **chromID Candida Agar (CAN2) (bioMérieux)**

Colonies of *C. albicans* produce a blue color following the hydrolysis of a hexosaminidase chromogenic substrate in the presence of an inducer of the enzyme (bioMérieux patent). The hydrolysis of a second substrate (pink color) differentiates mixed cultures and indicates the need for identification of other species of yeast (bioMérieux patent).

■ **Christensen's urea agar**

The ability to hydrolyze urea is an important phenotypic characteristic for the presumptive identification of *Cryptococcus*, *Trichosporon*, and *Rhodotorula* spp. Urea hydrolysis also facilitates separation of certain dermatophytes, in particular *T. mentagrophytes* and *T. rubrum*. The medium contains 2% urea with phenol red serving as the indicator.

■ **Cornmeal agar with 1% dextrose**

Cornmeal agar with 1% dextrose is used for the cultivation of fungi and the differentiation of *Trichophyton mentagrophytes* from *Trichophyton rubrum* on the basis of pigment production. The replacement of Tween 80 (polysorbate 80) with dextrose promotes the growth and production of a red pigment by *T. rubrum*.

■ **Cornmeal agar with Tween 80**

Cornmeal agar with Tween (polysorbate) 80 is used for the cultivation and differentiation of *Candida* species on the basis of mycelial characteristics. Tween 80, a surfactant, is specifically incorporated in lieu of dextrose for the demonstration of pseudohyphal, chlamydospore, and arthrospore formation. Chlamydospore production is best obtained if the yeast inoculum is placed under a coverslip or following subsurface inoculation creating a microaerophilic environment. The basic nutrients for yeast growth are provided by cornmeal infusion.

■ **Czapek-Dox agar**

Czapek-Dox agar is a medium used for the differentiation of *Aspergillus* spp. (4, 10). Sucrose is the sole carbon source with sodium nitrate serving as the sole nitrogen source. Any bacteria or fungi that can utilize sodium nitrate as a nitrogen source can grow on this medium.

■ **Dermatophyte test medium (DTM)**

Dermatophyte test medium is used as a screening medium for the recovery, selection, and differentiation of dermatophytes (*Microsporum*, *Trichophyton*, and *Epidermophyton*) from cutaneous specimens (hair, skin, and nails). Nitrogenous and carbonaceous compounds are provided by soy peptone. Cycloheximide inhibits saprophytic moulds, chloramphenicol inhibits many gram-positive bacteria, and gentamicin inhibits gram-negative bacteria. The morphology and microscopic characteristics are easily identified with this medium. Pigmentation cannot be discerned because of the presence of phenol red indicator. The medium is yellow and turns red with growth of dermatophytes. *Aspergillus* species and other saprophytic fungi can grow and produce pigment on this medium, which accounts for its recommended use as a screening medium only.

■ **Fermentation broth**

Fermentation broth is used for the differentiation of yeasts based upon carbohydrate fermentation. Yeasts that ferment carbohydrates turn the medium yellow.

Procedure

Dissolve yeast extract (4.5 g) and peptone (7.5 g) in distilled water and mix with bromthymol blue. Adjust medium to pH 7.0 and dispense 2.0-ml aliquots into 16- by 125-mm screw-cap test tubes. Place one Durham tube (upside down) into each test tube and autoclave to 15 min at 121°C. After the medium has cooled, aseptically add 1.0 ml of 6% filter-sterilized aqueous solution of carbon source to be tested.

■ **Inhibitory mould agar**

Inhibitory mould agar is a selective and enriched medium that is used for the general cultivation of cycloheximide-sensitive fungi (e.g., *Cryptococcus*, mucoraceous fungi, and *H. capsulatum*) from contaminated specimens. Casein and animal tissue provide growth nutrients. Yeast extract serves as a source of vitamins. Chloramphenicol inhibits many gram-positive and gram-negative bacteria. Gentamicin is another additive that inhibits some gram-negative bacteria.

■ **Lactrimel agar (Borelli's medium)**

Lactrimel agar (Borelli's medium) is composed of whole-wheat flour, skim milk, and honey, which favors the sporulation of most dermatophytes. The medium may also be used for the morphological examination of dematiaceous fungi.

■ **Leeming and Notman medium**

Leeming and Notman medium is used for the isolation and growth of lipodependent *Malassezia* species. The key components of the medium include ox bile, glycerol monostearate, glycerol, Tween 80, and cows' milk (whole fat) (8). The medium may serve as an alternative to Sabouraud glucose agar, since not all species can grow on this medium, e.g., *M. globosa*, *M. restricta*, and *M. obtusa*, which require more complex media for their isolation.

■ **Littman oxgall agar**

Littman oxgall agar is a selective general-purpose medium used for the isolation of fungi from contaminated specimens. Crystal violet and streptomycin are the selective agents and inhibit bacteria. Oxgall restricts the spreading of fungal colonies. The isolation characteristics of this medium are similar to those of Sabouraud dextrose agar with chloramphenicol and inhibitory mould agar in that it allows the growth of fungi that are sensitive to cycloheximide.

■ **Malt extract (2%) agar**

This medium is used for the cultivation of yeasts and moulds. A variety of formulations have been described but typically include malt extract with agar and are supplemented with peptone, glucose, maltose, and dextrin and/or glycerol.

■ **Mycobiotic or Mycosel agar**

Mycobiotic (Remel) and Mycosel (BD Diagnostic Systems) are trade names for a selective medium principally formulated for the isolation of dermatophytes but also used for the isolation of other pathogenic fungi from specimens contaminated with saprophytic fungi and bacteria. The medium consists primarily of peptones from a pancreatic digest of soybean meal and dextrose. The selective agents are cycloheximide and chloramphenicol. Cycloheximide inhibits the faster-growing saprophytic fungi but is also inhibitory to some clinically relevant species. These inhibited fungi include some *Candida* and *Aspergillus* species, mucoraceous fungi, and *C. neoformans*. Chloramphenicol inhibits gram-negative and gram-positive organisms.

■ **Niger seed agar**

See Birdseed agar.

■ **Potato dextrose agar**

Potato dextrose agar is a medium used to stimulate conidium production by fungi. The medium also stimulates pigment production in some dermatophytes. This medium is most commonly used with the slide culture technique to view morphological characteristics. Infusions from potatoes and dextrose provide nutrient factors for excellent growth. The incorporation of tartaric acid in the medium lowers the pH, thereby inhibiting bacterial growth.

■ **Potato flake agar**

Potato flake agar is a medium useful in the stimulation of conidia by fungi. Its advantages over potato dextrose agar may be preparation and stability. Potato flakes and dextrose provide the nutrient factors that allow excellent growth. The pH is adjusted to 5.6 to enhance growth of fungi and to inhibit bacterial growth. The medium may be made selective by the addition of cycloheximide and chloramphenicol.

■ **Sabouraud-brain heart infusion (SABHI)**

Sabouraud-brain heart infusion agar is a general-purpose medium used for the isolation and cultivation of all fungi. The medium is a combination of brain heart infusion agar and Sabouraud dextrose agar. The combined formulation allows for the recovery of most fungi including the yeast phase of dimorphic fungi. The inclusion of sheep blood provides essential growth factors for the more fastidious fungi and enhances the growth of *H. capsulatum*. Selectivity is attained by the addition of chloramphenicol, cycloheximide, penicillin, and/or streptomycin.

■ **Sabouraud dextrose agar**

Sabouraud dextrose agar was formulated by Sabouraud for cultivating dermatophytes. The medium consists of pancreatic digest of casein, peptic digest of animal tissue, and dextrose at 4% concentration and buffered to a pH of 5.6. Emmons modified the original formulation by reducing the dextrose concentration to 2% and adjusting the pH nearer to neutrality at 6.9 to 7.0. Antibiotic additives in various combinations include cycloheximide, chloramphenicol, gentamicin, ciprofloxacin, penicillin, and/or streptomycin, which inhibit some fungi and gram-positive and gram-negative bacteria to achieve selectivity for this medium. This medium is also available as a broth.

■ **Soil extract agar**

Soil extract agar is a medium composed of garden soil, yeast extract, and glucose. The primary use of this medium is to promote sporulation of some saprobic fungi and for mating strains of *B. dermatitidis* (4).

■ **Tomato juice agar**

Tomato juice agar is a medium containing tomato juice and yeast powder, which is used to promote ascopore formation (4, 10).

■ **Trichophyton agars 1 to 7**

Trichophyton agars are a set of seven media that facilitate the identification of *Trichophyton* species on the basis of their growth factor requirements. The basic ingredients in the media are listed below. Growth in all seven media is then scored on a scale of 1 to 4, and an identification is assigned.

1. Casamino Acids; vitamin-free
2. Casamino Acids plus inositol
3. Casamino Acids plus inositol and thiamine
4. Casamino Acids plus thiamine
5. Casamino Acids plus niacin
6. Ammonium nitrate
7. Ammonium nitrate plus histidine

■ **V8 agar**

V8 agar is a medium consisting of dehydrated potato flakes and tomato juice that induces early sporulation of some environmental fungi. The naturally low pH makes the medium inhibitory to most bacteria.

■ **Water (tap) agar**

This medium is nutritionally deficient (1% water–agar; 1 g of agar, 100 ml of sterile tap water) and promotes the sporulation of dematiaceous fungi, *Apophysomyces elegans*, and *Saksenaea vasiformis* (14; A. Desalvo, personal communication). The medium can be supplemented with sterilized carnation leaves for the identification of *Fusarium* spp. (9).

■ **Yeast carbon agar**

Yeast carbon agar is a solid medium recommended for use in qualitative procedures for the classification of yeasts according to their ability to assimilate nitrogenous compounds. The yeast carbon base provides amino acids, vitamins, trace elements, and salts that are necessary to support growth. The ability to assimilate nitrogen is tested by the addition of various nitrogen sources such as potassium nitrate.

■ **Yeast extract-phosphate agar with ammonia (Smith's medium)**

Yeast extract-phosphate agar with ammonia (Smith's medium) is used for the isolation and sporulation of *H. capsulatum* and *B. dermatitidis* from contaminated specimens. This consists of phosphate buffer (Na_2HPO_4, KH_2PO_4, and distilled water). It should be mixed well with the pH adjusted to 6.0 with 1 N HCl or 1 N NaOH and yeast extract agar solution. Before inoculation of specimens, one drop of ammonium hydroxide is applied to the agar surface and allowed to diffuse into the medium. The combination of ammonium hydroxide and chloramphenicol suppresses bacteria and many moulds and yeasts, thus permitting detection of the slowly growing dimorphic fungi.

Note

Consult reference 1 for additional information regarding specific formulations and preparation of the respective media described in this section.

APPENDIX
Commercial Manufacturers and Supplies of Fungal Media, Stains, and Reagents

Alpha Tec Systems, Inc.
P.O. Box 5435
Vancouver, WA 98668
800-221-6058
http://www.alphatec.com

BD Diagnostic Systems
7 Loveton Circle
Sparks, MD 21152
800-675-0908
http://www.bd.com

bioMérieux, Inc.
100 Rodolphe St.
Durham, NC 27712
800-654-4682

Bio-Rad Laboratories
5500 East Second St.
Benicia, CA 94510
800-224-6723

Biosepar
Munich, Germany
49 (0) 8631 167 48 55
http://www.biosepar.de

CHROMagar
4 Place du 18 Juin 1940
75006 Paris
France
33 1 45 48 07 07
chromagar@chromagar.com

Difco Laboratories, Inc.
920 Henry St.
Detroit, MI 48201
313-442-8800
tech-support@VGDLLC.com

Fisher Scientific
2000 Park Lane Dr.
Pittsburgh, PA 15275
800-766-7000
http://www.fishersci.com

Fluka
Chemika/Biochemika
Industriestrasse 25
9471 Buchs
Switzerland
41 (0) 81 755 25 11
webmaster@sial.com
Flukatec@eurnotes.sial.com

Hardy Diagnostics
1430 West McCoy Lane
Santa Maria, CA 93455
800-266-2222
http://www.hardydiagnostics.com

HiMedia Laboratories Pvt. Ltd.
23 Vadhani Est. LBS marg
Bombay 400086
India
91 22 40951919
info@himedialabs.com

Laboratorios Conda
c/La Forja, 9
28850 Torrejón de Ardoz, Madrid
Spain
Phone: 34 91 761 02 00
Fax: 34 91 761 02 06 or 91 656 82 28
http://www.condalab.com

Oxoid Limited
Wade Road
Basingstoke, Hampshire RG24 8PW
United Kingdom
44 (0) 1256 841144
Fax: 44 (0) 1256 814626
Oxoid.infor@thermofisher.com

PPR Diagnostics Limited
7 Ivory House
East Smithfield, London E1W 1AT

United Kingdom
Technical: 44 (0) 20 7848 4451
Fax: 44 (0) 1442 866 739
http://www.pprdiag.co.uk

Remel
12076 Santa Fe Dr.
Lenexa, KS 66215
800-255-6730
http://www.remel.com

Scientific Device Laboratory
411 Jarvis Ave.
Des Plaines, IL 60018
847-803-9495
http://www.scientificdevice.com

Sigma-Aldrich Corp
3050 Spruce St.
St. Louis, MO 63103
314-771-5765
http://www.sigmaaldrich.com

REFERENCES

1. **Atlas, R. M., and J. W. Snyder.** 2006. *Handbook of Media for Clinical Microbiology*. Taylor & Francis, Boca Raton, FL.
2. **Clinical and Laboratory Standards Institute.** 2008. *Reference Method for Broth Dilution Antifungal Susceptibility Testing of Yeasts.* Approved standard, 3rd ed. CLSI document M27-A3. Clinical and Laboratory Standards Institute, Wayne, PA.
3. **Clinical and Laboratory Standards Institute.** 2008. *Reference Method for Broth Dilution Antifungal Susceptibility Testing of Filamentous Fungi.* Approved standard M38-A2. Clinical and Laboratory Standards Institute, Wayne, PA.
4. **Dismukes, W. E., P. G. Pappas, and J. D. Sobel.** 2003. *Clinical Mycology.* Oxford University Press, Inc., New York, NY.
5. **Hageage, G. J., and B. J. Harrington.** 1984. Use of calcofluor white in clinical mycology. *Lab. Med.* **15:**109–112.
6. **Kim, Y. K., S. Parulekar, P. K. Yu, R. J. Pisani, T. F. Smith, and J. P. Anhault.** 1990. Evaluation of calcofluor white stain for detection of *Pneumocystis carinii*. *Diagn. Microbiol. Infect. Dis.* **13:**307–310.
7. **Larone, D. H.** 2002. *Medically Important Fungi*, 4th ed. ASM Press, Washington, DC.
8. **Leeming, J. P., and F. H. Notman.** 1987. Improved methods for the isolation and enumeration of *Malassezia furfur* from human skin. *J. Clin. Microbiol.* **25:**2017–2019.
9. **Leslie, J. F., and B. A. Summerell.** 2006. *The Fusarium Laboratory Manual.* Blackwell Publishing, Ames, IA.
10. **McGinnis, M.** 1980. *Laboratory Handbook of Medical Mycology.* Academic Press, New York, NY.
11. **Murray, M., R. Zinchuk, and D. Larone.** 2005. CHROMagar Candida as the sole primary medium for isolation of yeasts and as a source medium for rapid-assimilation-of-trehalose test. *J. Clin. Microbiol.* **43:**1210–1212.
12. **National Committee for Clinical Laboratory Standards.** 2004. *Quality Control for Commercially Prepared Microbiological Culture Media.* Standard M22-A3. National Committee for Clinical Laboratory Standards, Wayne, PA.
13. **Odds, F. C., and R. Bernaerts.** 1994. CHROMagar Candida, a new differential isolation medium for presumptive identification of clinically important *Candida* species. *J. Clin. Microbiol.* **32:**1923–1929.
14. **Padhye, A. A., and L. Ajello.** 1988. Simple method of inducing sporulation by *Apophysomyces elegans* and *Saksenaea vasiformis*. *J. Clin. Microbiol.* **26:**1861–1863.
15. **Paradis, I. L., C. Ross, A. Dekker, and J. Dauber.** 1990. A comparison of modified methenamine silver and toluidine blue stains for the detection of *Pneumocystis carinii* in bronchoalveolar lavage specimens from immunosuppressed patients. *Acta Cytol.* **34:**511–518.

16. **Pincus, D. H., S. Orenga, and S. Chatellier.** 2007. Yeast identification—past, present, and future methods. *Med. Mycol.* **45:**97–121.

17. **Rex, J. R., C. R. Cooper, W. Merz, J. Galgiani, and E. Anaissie.** 1995. Detection of amphotericin B-resistant *Candida* isolates in a broth-based system. *Antimicrob. Agents Chemother.* **39:**906 909.

18. **Sanati, H., S. Messer, M. Pfaller, M. Witt, R. Larsen, A. Espinel-Ingroff, and M. Ghannoum.** 1996. Multicenter evaluation of a broth microdilution method for susceptibility testing of *Cryptococcus neoformans*. *J. Clin. Microbiol.* **34:**1280–1282.

19. **Subcommittee on Antifungal Susceptibility Testing (AFST) of the ESCMID European Committee for Antimicrobial Susceptibility Testing (EUCAST).** 2008. EUCAST Definitive Document EDef 7.1: method for the determination of broth dilution MICs of antifungal agents for fermentative yeasts. *Clin. Microbiol. Infect.* **14:**398–405.

20. **Subcommittee on Antifungal Susceptibility Testing (AFST) of the ESCMID European Committee for Antimicrobial Susceptibility Testing (EUCAST).** 2008. EUCAST technical note on the method for the determination of broth dilution minimum inhibitory concentrations of antifungal agents for conidia-forming moulds. *Clin. Microbiol. Infect.* **14:**982–984.

General Approaches for Direct Detection of Fungi*

YVONNE R. SHEA

114

As the number of invasive fungal infections increases, the rapid and accurate diagnosis of the etiologic agent becomes even more vital for the initiation of appropriate antifungal therapy. This chapter is a review of non-culture-based detection methods that can be performed directly with clinical materials in a clinical laboratory. These methods include direct microscopic examination, antigen detection, detection of fungus-specific metabolites, detection of cell wall components, detection of fungus-specific nucleic acids, and serologic diagnosis. All methods discussed should be used as an adjunct to proper culturing, as culture remains the standard for detection and identification of fungi in clinical specimens. Culture methodology for the isolation of fungi is reviewed in chapters 112 and 113.

DIRECT MICROSCOPIC EXAMINATION

Gross examination of clinical material should be performed before specimen processing occurs. Specimens should be examined for areas of caseous necrosis, microabscesses, grains and granules, and firm nodules, which may indicate granulomas. Granulomas and caseous necrosis may indicate histoplasmosis, and microabscesses can be seen with hepatosplenic candidiasis, whereas grains or granules can be seen with mycetoma. Certain fungal organisms are more likely to be recovered from specific body sites (72) (Table 1). The pathology associated with fungal organisms may vary according to the competence of the host immune defenses.

Knowledge of the patient's residence and recent travel history may provide diagnostic clues to fungal disease because some fungal pathogens are more common in certain regions of the world (Table 2). For example, although eumycetoma has been reported worldwide, most cases come from tropical and subtropical regions around the Tropic of Cancer (32). *Madurella mycetomatis*, *Scedosporium apiospermum*, *Leptosphaeria senegalensis*, and *Madurella grisea* account for 95% of eumycetoma infections (8). Grains and granules should be examined for color, size, shape, and consistency because these characteristics can help to identify the etiologic agent (Table 2).

The ability to recognize typical staining characteristics and structures of fungi, such as sclerotic cells or muriform bodies of chromoblastomycosis, can assist in the diagnosis, guide appropriate testing, and facilitate proper antifungal therapy. A number of stains or procedures can be used to detect fungal organisms by direct examination of clinical specimens (Table 3). Stain methodology can be found in chapter 113.

The value of the Gram stain should not be underestimated, as it is the frontline stain in most laboratories and the stain with which most technologists are familiar. Differentiating yeast from mold is important because yeast may represent normal colonization, while mold can indicate a deeper infectious process. Although Gram reactions can vary, yeast cells and pseudohyphae generally stain gram positive and hyphae (septate and aseptate) stain gram negative. The size and shape of budding yeast-like cells can indicate a presumptive species identification. *Cryptococcus* species yeast cells are generally very round and display an amorphous orange-staining material, presumably the capsule.

Examination of smears for specific morphologic patterns can help to establish the identification of the organism. *Aspergillus* species tend to form hyphae of a consistent diameter (4 to 6 μm) and commonly demonstrate 45° branching and less commonly exhibit 90° branching. *Fusarium* and *Scedosporium* species look very similar to *Aspergillus* species in tissue (43). Sporulation in tissue is rare but can be distinctive with certain fungi. Aleurioconidia can be indicative of *Aspergillus terreus* (87), *Fusarium* species can produce micro- and, rarely, macroconidia, and *Scedosporium* species can produce annelloconidia in vivo. The detection of phialides and phialoconidia can assist in the preliminary identification of *Fusarium*, *Paecilomyces*, and *Acremonium* species. When fungal stains show both unicellular forms and filaments that appear to be hyphae or pseudohyphae, infection with *Fusarium*, *Paecilomyces*, or *Acremonium* species should be considered, although filamentous yeast should also be included in the differential diagnosis. (49). Mucoraceous molds exhibit aseptate (or rarely septate) hyphae of irregular diameter that tend to branch at 90°. The lack of regular septations causes an absence of internal support for the hyphae, and the hyphae can become twisted and folded in a ribbon-like manner. The Splendore-Hoeppli phenomenon on hematoxylin and eosin (H&E) sections may be

---

*This chapter contains information presented in chapter 112 by William G. Merz and Glenn D. Roberts in the eighth edition of this *Manual*.

TABLE 1 Selection of clinical specimens for recovery of opportunistic fungal pathogens[a]

Suspected pathogen	Blood	Bone marrow	Brain and CSF	Catheter or catheter exit site	Eye	Respiratory sites	Skin, mucous membranes	Urine	Multiple systemic sites
Yeasts									
Candida spp.	X	X	X	X	X	X	X	X	X
Cryptococcus neoformans	X	X	X		X	X	X	X	X
Malassezia spp.	X			X			X		
Trichosporon spp.	X			X		X	X	X	X
Molds									
Aspergillus spp.			X		X	X	X	X	X
Dematiaceous fungi			X		X	X	X		X
Dermatophytes							X[b]		
Fusarium spp.	X				X	X	X		X
Paecilomyces spp.			X			X	X		X
Scedosporium spp.	X		X		X	X			X
Zygomycetes			X		X	X	X		X
Dimorphic fungi									
Blastomyces dermatitidis			X			X	X	X	X
Coccidioides immitis	X	X	X		X	X	X	X	X
Histoplasma capsulatum	X	X	X		X	X	X	X	X
Paracoccidioides brasiliensis		X	X			X	X		X
Penicillium marneffei	X	X	X			X	X		X
Sporothrix schenckii	X		X			X	X		X
Other									
Pneumocystis jirovecii						X			X

[a]Adapted from reference 52. The anatomic site of the fungal infection can be an indicator of what mycotic agent to suspect, but in an immunocompromised patient population, virtually any fungus can be an opportunistic pathogen.
[b]Dermatophytes usually do not invade tissue but colonize only the outer layer of the skin.

seen with blastomycosis and sporotrichosis as well as with infections caused by *Basidiobolus* and *Conidiobolus* species. Dematiaceous molds may display multiple forms, such as septate hyphae with parallel walls, rounded forms arranged in chains, or muriform bodies. The diagnosis of phaeohyphomycosis can be made only if pigmented hyphae are observed. Sometimes pigmentation can be observed by using a traditional KOH preparation. Some structures can provide definitive diagnosis of the etiologic agent (e.g., spherules of *Coccidioides* spp.). Specimens obtained from patients treated with antifungal drugs may demonstrate uncharacteristic formations, such as variations of hypha size within the same hyphal structure, clearing of septations within the hyphae, or bulb forms within the hyphae or in the hyphal tips.

Artifacts seen in smears can hinder correct diagnosis. Lysed lymphocytes in cerebrospinal fluid (CSF) have been mistaken for *Cryptococcus neoformans*; collagen fibers and swab fibers may be mistaken for hyphae, as each can fluoresce with calcofluor white; and fat droplets may be confused with budding yeast-like cells. A careful smear review in each of these situations should help avoid misinterpretation, but when in doubt, a second reader or second procedure should be employed. Correct interpretation is critical to appropriate patient care.

Detection of fungi in clinical material can be difficult because the specimen may be inadequate, relatively few fungi may be present, or similarly appearing organisms may be indistinguishable on initial examination. With the exception of dermatologic specimens, when specimen volume is minimal, the culture should take precedence over the smear, because direct examinations are less sensitive than culture. For dermatologic samples, direct microscopy is diagnostic and cultures are not always successful. When possible, always perform both smear and culture, given that culture alone may not distinguish between colonization and tissue invasion. Conversely, only nonviable organisms may be present in specimens obtained while the patient is receiving antifungal therapy, and microscopy may be the

TABLE 2 Characteristic fungal elements seen by direct examination of clinical specimens

Morphologic fungal element found	Organism(s)	Diam range (μm)	Characteristic features	Geographic distribution
Yeast forms	*Histoplasma capsulatum*	2–5	Small; oval to round budding cells; often found clustered within histiocytes; difficult to detect when present in small numbers; often intracellular (Fig. 23)	Var. *capsulatum*: worldwide, eastern half of the United States (localized in Ohio and Mississippi River valleys) and throughout Mexico, Central and South America African histoplasmosis: tropical areas of Africa (Gabon, Uganda, Kenya)
	Sporothrix species	2–6	Small; oval to round to cigar shaped; single or multiple buds present; uncommonly seen in clinical specimens (Fig. 21)	Most often reported from Mexico, Central and South America (Brazil), Asia (Japan). More widespread in temperate and tropical zones.
	Cryptococcus spp.	2–15	Cells vary in size; usually spherical but may be football shaped; buds usually single and "pinched off"; capsule may or may not be evident; rarely, pseudohyphal forms with or without capsule may be seen (Fig. 7, 15, and 16)	*Cryptococcus gattii*: tropics and southern hemisphere, Pacific Northwest region of the United States; eucalyptus trees
	Blastomyces dermatitidis	8–15	Cells usually large and spherical, double refractile; buds usually single, but several may remain attached to parent cells; buds connected by broad base (Fig. 22)	Southeast and south-central United States, Great Lakes region, near St. Lawrence River
	Paracoccidioides brasiliensis	5–60	Cell usually large and surrounded by smaller buds around periphery (mariner's wheel appearance); smaller cells (2–5 μm) that resemble *H. capsulatum* may be present; buds have "pinched off" appearance (Fig. 25)	South and Central America
Yeast forms (fission)	*Penicillium marneffei*	3	Fission yeast, not budding, elongated, curved with septa visible (Fig. 26)	Southeast Asia and China
Cysts and trophozoites	*Pneumocystis jirovecii*	1–4 4–5	Trophozoites: small pleomorphic forms Cysts: round to cup shape with up to 8 intracystic bodies (Fig. 18)	Worldwide
Spherules	*Coccidioides immitis, Coccidioides posadasii*	10–200	Spherules vary in size; some contain endospores, others are empty and collapsed; hyphae may be seen in cavitary lesions (Fig. 24)	Southwestern United States, Mexico, Central and South America (*C. posadasii* organisms are non-Californian strains)
Yeast forms and pseudohyphae or true hyphae	*Candida* spp.	3–4 (yeast forms); 5–10 (pseudohyphae)	Cells usually exhibit single budding; pseudohyphae, when present, are constricted at ends and remain attached like links of sausage; true hyphae, when present, have parallel walls and are separated (Fig. 4–6)	Worldwide
Yeast forms and pseudohyphae	*Malassezia* species	3–8 (yeast forms); 5–10 (pseudohyphae)	Short, curved hyphal elements may be present along with round yeast cells that are round at one end and flattened at point of conidiation (Fig. 8)	Worldwide
Wide nonseptate hyphae	Mucoraceous molds	10–30	Hyphae are large, ribbonlike, often fractured or twisted. Occasional septa may be present, branching usually at right angles (Fig.3, 11, and 12). The Splendore-Hoeppli phenomenon on H&E sections may be seen with *Basidiobolus* and *Conidiobolus* species.	Entomophthorales: worldwide *Basidiobolus ranarum*: tropical areas of Asia, Africa, South America (mostly Brazil), Mexico, Australia (children) *Conidiobolus coronatus* and *C. incongruus*: tropical and subtropical regions of Africa and Southeast Asia (adults)
Hyaline septate hyphae	Dermatophytes (skin and nails)	3–15	Hyaline septate hyphae commonly seen; chains of arthroconidia may be present (Fig. 19)	Worldwide
	Dermatophytes (hair)	3–12	Arthroconidia on periphery of hair shaft that produce sheaths indicate ectothrix infection. Arthroconidia formed by fragmentation of hyphae within hair shaft indicate endothrix infection. Long hyphal filaments or channels within hair shaft indicate favus hair infection.	Worldwide

	Organism	Size (µm)	Microscopic appearance	Geographic distribution
Hyaline septate hyphae	*Aspergillus* spp.	4–6	*Aspergillus* spp. are generally septate with consistent diameter throughout; often show repeated dichotomous, 45° angle branching (Fig. 1, 9, 10, 13, and 14)	Worldwide
	Scedosporium spp. (not eumycetoma), *Fusarium* spp., *Paecilomyces* spp.	3–12	Hyphae are septate, difficult to distinguish from other hyaline molds. May exhibit less 45° angle and more 90° angle branching.	
Dematiaceous septate hyphae	Dematiaceous fungi	1.5–6	Dematiaceous polymorphous hyphae, budding cells with single septa and chains of swollen rounded cells may be present. Occasionally, aggregates may be present when infection is caused by *Phialophora* or *Exophiala* spp. (Fig. 2).	*Phaeoannellomyces werneckii*: subtropical coastal locations; *Piedraia hortae*: tropical climates of Central and South America, Southeast Asia, and the South Pacific Islands; *Rhinocladiella mackenziei*: Middle East
Sclerotic bodies (muriform cells)	*Cladophialophora carrionii*, *Fonsecaea compacta*, *Fonsecaea pedrosoi*, *Phialophora verrucosa*, *Rhinocladiella aquaspersa*	5–20	Brown, round to pleomorphic, thick-walled cells with transverse septa. Commonly, cells contain two fission plates that form tetrads of cells. Occasionally, branched septate hyphae may be found in addition to sclerotic bodies (Fig. 20).	Occurs worldwide, although the majority of reported cases are from typical and subtropical regions of the Americas and Africa
Granules (white grain eumycetomas)	*Acremonium* spp. (*A. falciforme*, *A. kiliense*, *A. recifei*)	200–300	White, soft granule; cement-like matrix absent	Asia, North, South and Central America, Oceania, Europe
	Aspergillus nidulans	65–160	White, soft granule; cement-like matrix absent	Africa
	Fusarium spp. (*F. moniliforme*, *F. oxysporum*, *F. solani*)	80–200	White-yellowish color of the grains, edges are entire or lobed; surrounded by an eosinophilic homogeneous material. Hyphae comprising the granules are not embedded in cement.	Europe, South America, Caribbean, Africa, Asia
	Neotestudina rosatii	300–600	White, soft granule with cement-like matrix at periphery	West Africa
	Pseudallescheria boydii	200–300	White-yellow, soft granules composed of hyphae and swollen cells at periphery in cement-like matrix (Fig. 17)	Worldwide, most common in North America
Granules (black grain eumycetomas)	*Curvularia* spp. (*C. geniculata*, *C. lunata*)	500–1,000	Black, hard grains with cement-like matrix at periphery	Worldwide
	Exophiala jeanselmei	200–300	Black, soft granules, vacuolated, cement-like matrix absent, made of dark hyphae and swollen cells	Worldwide
	Leptosphaeria senegalensis, *Leptosphaeria tompkinsii*	400–600	Black, hard granules; cement-like matrix; in tissue sections, the central part consists of hyphae, and a black cement-like substance is seen at the periphery	West Africa (specifically Senegal and Mauritania)
	Madurella grisea	300–600	Black and soft with a brown cement-like material in the periphery of the granules	India, Africa, Central and South America
	Madurella mycetomatis	200–900	Black to brown hard granules of two types: (i) rust, brown, compact, and filled with cement-like matrix and (ii) deep brown, filled with numerous vesicles, 6–14 µm in diameter, cement-like matrix in periphery and central area of light-colored hyphae	India, Africa, and South America
	Pyrenochaeta romeroi, *P. mackinnonii*	40–100 × 50–160	Black, soft granules composed of polygonal swollen cells at periphery, cement-like matrix	Africa, India, and South America

TABLE 3 Methods and stains available for direct microscopic detection of fungi in clinical specimens[a]

Method	Use	Time required (min)	Color of fungus	Comments
Alcian blue	Detection of *C. neoformans* in CSF	2	Capsule stains blue against a pink background	Mucopolysaccharide stain, not commonly used; like India ink, does not detect all cases.
Calcofluor white	Detection of all fungi and cysts of *Pneumocystis jirovecii*	1–2	Depending on which barrier filter is used, fungal elements appear blue-white or bright green against a dark background (Fig. 10 and 12). Cysts have "double parenthesis-like" structure in center.	Requires fluorescence microscope; collagen and swab fibers also fluoresce, fat droplets may look similar to yeast cells. Counterstain minimizes background fluorescence.
Fontana-Masson (FM)	Detection of melanin of dematiaceous fungi and *C. neoformans*	60	Cell walls black. Background pale pink.	Many nondematiaceous fungi (some *Aspergillus*, *Zygomycetes*, and *Trichosporon* species) can be FM positive. If hyaline in H&E, examine morphology carefully.
Giemsa stain	Primarily used for the examination of bone marrow and peripheral blood smears	15	Detects trophozoite stage of *P. jirovecii*	Detects intracellular *H. capsulatum* and fission yeast cells of *P. marneffei* (Fig. 26)
Diff-Quik	Also applied to other speci-mens, such as BAL fluid, CSF	2–3	Yeast cells and trophozoites appear blue-purple (Fig. 15)	Differentiate from *Leishmania*
Wright		7		Also stains other fungi
Gomori meth-enamine silver (GMS) stain	Detection of fungi and *Pneumocystis jirovecii*	5–60	Fungi and *P. jirovecii* cysts stain gray to black. Background is green (Fig. 9, 11, 13, and 21).	Often stains fungi too densely to observe structural details. Yeast cells and cysts of *Pneumocystis* may appear similar in size and shape.
Gram stain	Detection of bacteria and fungi	3	Generally yeast and pseudohyphae stain gram positive and hyphae (septate and aseptate) appear gram negative (Fig. 1–8)	*Cryptococcus* spp. stain weakly in some instances and exhibit only stippling. Often have orange amorphous material around yeast (Fig. 7). Not all fungi are detected.
H&E	General purpose histologic stain	30–60	Stains some fungal elements violet to bluish purple; tissue back-ground is displayed as shades of red. Demonstrates natural pigment of dematiaceous fungi (Fig. 14, 17, and 24).	Permits visualization of host tissue response to the fungus. *Aspergillus* spp. and *Zygomycetes* stain well. The Splendore-Hoeppli phenom-enon may be seen with *Basidiobolus* spp.
India ink, nigrosin	Detection of *C. neoformans* in CSF	1	Capsules around yeast cells clear halos against a black background (Fig. 16)	When positive in CSF, diagnostic of menin-gitis. Negative in many cases of meningitis, not reliable. Cryptococcal antigen testing recommended.
Mucicarmine	Stains mucin	60	Stains capsule of *Cryptococcus* pinkish red	May also stain cell walls of *B. dermatitidis* and *Rhinosporidium seeberi*
Papanicolaou	Cytologic stain used primarily to detect malignant cells	30	Depending on cell type detected, background stains in subtle range of green blue, orange to pink hues. *Candida* stains gold, while other fungi may not stain at all.	Further stains should be performed
PAS	Detection of fungi	20–25	Fungi stain pink, background stains shades of purple	PAS stain-positive artifacts can appear as yeast cells. *B. dermatitidis* appears pleomorphic.
Potassium hydroxide (KOH)	Clearing of speci-men to make fungi more read-ily visible	5–30	Hyaline molds and yeasts appear transparent, while dematiaceous molds may display golden brown hyphae	Addition of lactophenol cotton blue or methylene blue enhances the visibility of fungi
Toluidine blue	Detection of *P. jirovecii* in respiratory specimens	25	Cyst walls are purple (Fig. 18)	The background and other fungi stain the same color

[a]H&E, hematoxylin and eosin; PAS, periodic acid-Schiff.

only method for detecting the etiologic agent. Specimen quantity and quality may be compromised when multiple clinical laboratories process portions of the specimens. Good communication between the pathology and microbiology services, in union with the clinician, can greatly enhance diagnostic accuracy.

Any positive smear result must be reported promptly and clearly convey what has been seen, so that the clinician understands what type of organism has been detected. When possible, additional comments should be entered to clarify the type of structures or possible organism identification. For example, "Budding yeast-like cells seen" can indicate many different species of yeasts, while "Budding yeast-like cells resembling *Malassezia* group" offers a clue to the type and significance of the infection. Figures 1 through 26 illustrate characteristic fungal structures seen in the direct examination of clinical specimens.

ANTIGEN DETECTION

Aspergillus Species

A diagnostic marker for invasive aspergillosis (IA) is galactomannan (GM). GM is a polysaccharide cell wall component that is released into blood by growing hyphae. The Platelia *Aspergillus* GM immunoassay (Bio-Rad, Hercules, CA) has been evaluated in numerous studies as a diagnostic tool for IA, but the reported sensitivities and specificities have been variable. Explanations for this variability include the patient group under investigation (serum GM has a better performance as a diagnostic marker in neutropenic patients with hematological malignancies and allogeneic hematopoietic stem cell transplant recipients than in solid-organ transplant recipients), age of patient population, the number and type of collected specimens (serial samples, single samples, blood, and bronchoalveolar lavage [BAL] fluid), the time the specimen was obtained during the course of the infection, receipt of prophylactic or empirical antifungal therapies (54), and in earlier studies, various test cutoff values (55). The results are expressed as a GM index (GMI) value. The manufacturer's guidelines state that a GMI of 0.5 or higher is positive. Although the sensitivity and specificity in serum and BAL specimens are high with certain patient groups, the GM assay is FDA approved for serum samples only at this time. Its accuracy with BAL and other body fluids (e.g., CSF and urine) is still being validated (13, 36). False positives have been associated with dietary GM; autoantibodies; mycosis with shared antigens; airway colonization with *Aspergillus* spp.; *Penicillium, Alternaria,* and *Paecilomyces* in BAL specimens; Plasmalyte and other fluids containing sodium gluconate; drug therapies with amoxicillin-clavulanic acid (56) or piperacillin-tazobactam (86); the galactoxylomannan component of the *Cryptococcus* capsular polysaccharide (15); and bifidobacterial lipoglycan (61). Additionally, patients undergoing hemodialysis may have falsely high titers because hemodialysis is unable to clear *Aspergillus* antigen from serum (26). Reduced detection of GM may occur with patients with chronic granulomatous disease or Job's syndrome (84), low fungal burdens, or walled-off infections or with those with IA who are receiving antifungal therapy active against molds (85). Despite the known drawbacks associated with the GM assay, GM detection remains a tool in the diagnosis of IA and is a promising marker of the therapeutic response of IA. Boutboul et al. (7) showed that serum GMI values significantly increased in patients with

IA who did not respond to antifungal therapy, whereas no significant change occurred in patients who responded to therapy. Patients with IA that have persistent or increasing serum GMI values eventually died of or with IA (52). The European Organization for Research and Treatment of Cancer/Mycoses Study Group (EORTC/MSG) revised their criteria for proven and probable invasive fungal disease to reflect the importance of antigen tests, including the GM assay (17). Immunodiagnosis, metabolite detection, and molecular techniques for the diagnosis of aspergillosis are further described in chapter 117.

Blastomyces dermatitidis

Antigen detection methods are generally not used for the diagnosis of blastomycosis. A *Blastomyces dermatitidis* enzyme immunoassay (EIA) (MiraVista Diagnostics, Indianapolis, IN) for the detection of antigenuria has been evaluated, demonstrating a sensitivity of 92.9%, specificity of 79.3%, and cross-reactivity with patients with histoplasmosis, paracoccidioidomycosis, penicilliosis marneffei, cryptococcosis, and aspergillosis (21).

Candida Species

Distinguishing colonization from disease complicates the diagnosis of candidiasis by antigen detection (70). To detect candidiasis, diagnostic markers of mannan and mannoproteins have been evaluated. Mannan, which is highly immunogenic, is one of the major cell wall components of *Candida* species and is shed into the blood during infection. Frequent testing is required because mannan is rapidly cleared from the blood. Several kits have been marketed for the detection of mannan.

The Pastorex *Candida* LA test (Bio-Rad, Marnes-La-Coquette, France) and Platelia *Candida* antigen test (Bio-Rad, Munich, Germany) have good specificity but low sensitivity. The Platelia *Candida* antibody and antigen test (Bio-Rad) has been shown to have a higher sensitivity but poor specificity due to the large numbers of false positives obtained when patients are merely colonized with *Candida* (78).

The Cand-Tec latex agglutination (LA) test (Ramco Laboratories, Houston, TX) is designed to detect a heat-sensitive circulating antigen associated with *Candida* species. Studies using the Cand-Tec test have demonstrated extreme variability in both sensitivity and specificity, and thus it is not reliable for the diagnosis of disseminated candidiasis (1, 64, 69, 73).

Coccidioides Species

Antigen testing for coccidioidomycosis is limited. MiraVista Diagnostics (Indianapolis, IN) offers the MVista *Coccidioides* quantitative antigen EIA which uses antibodies to detect *Coccidioides* GM. Urine, serum, plasma, CSF, BAL fluid, and other sterile body fluids are acceptable. Antigen can be detected in the CSF of some patients with *Coccidioides* meningitis and the BAL fluid of those with pulmonary coccidioidomycosis. As with the MVista *Histoplasma* EIA, the MVista *Coccidioides* EIA was modified after studies with EDTA-heat treatment of serum at 100°C. Urine and serum samples (with and without EDTA-heat treatment) were tested from patients with coccidioidomycosis using the MVista *Coccidioides* EIA. Antigenemia was detected in 28.6% of patients whose samples were not EDTA-heat treated and in 73.1% of those whose samples were treated. Antigenuria was detected in 50% of patients. Specificity of 100% was obtained with healthy subjects,

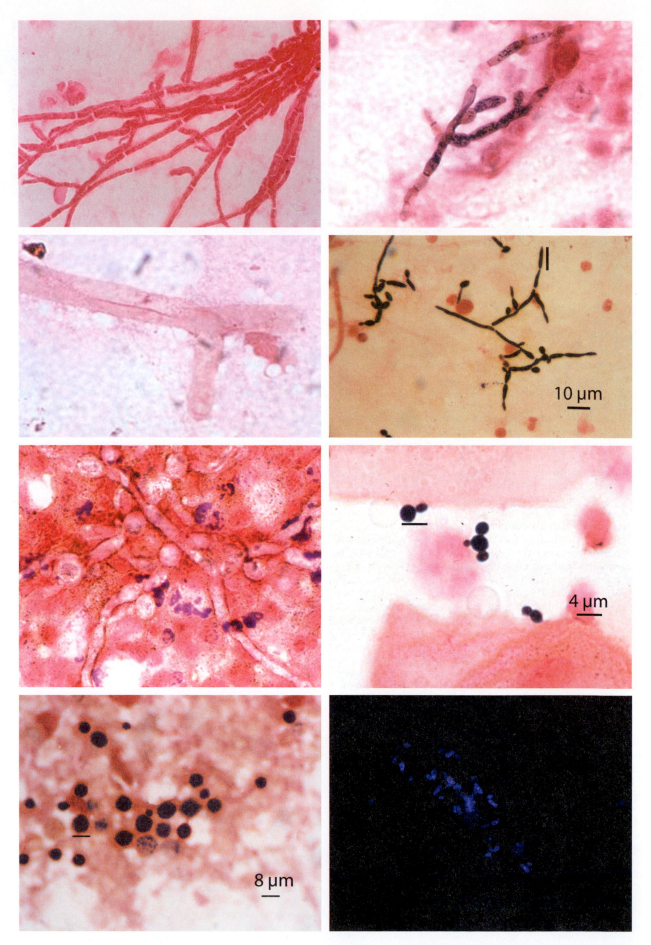

but cross-reactions were seen with 22.2% of patients with histoplasmosis or blastomycosis. Other limitations include false-positive reactions due to anti-rabbit or heterophile antibodies and rheumatoid factor (22).

Cryptococcus neoformans

The glucuronoxylomannan component of the *Cryptococcus neoformans* capsular polysaccharide is used for diagnosis of cryptococcosis. Prior to the molecular era, *C. neoformans* isolates were classified on the basis of antigenic differences in the capsular polysaccharides into five serotypes (A, B, C, D, and AD hybrids). Strains of A, D, and AD serotypes are now classified as *C. neoformans*, while B and C serotype strains are classified as *Cryptococcus gattii*. With the varietal classification, *C. neoformans* var. *grubii* corresponds to serotype A or molecular types VNI and VNII. *C. neoformans* var. *neoformans* corresponds to serotype D and molecular type VNIV. AD strains belong to the *C. neoformans* VNIII molecular type. The prevalence of serotypes varies by geographic region. AD strains amount to about 15% of isolates in Europe. Infections with *C. neoformans* serotype A have a global distribution, while those with serotype D are more prevalent in certain geographical regions, such as France and several other European countries. *C. gattii* serotype B is less prevalent than serotype C, but both serotypes have similar geographic distributions. Although the taxonomy of *Cryptococcus neoformans* is complicated and ongoing, commercially available cryptococcal antigen detection methods detect all serotypes (63). Latex antigen detection methods (Meridian cryptococcal antigen LA system, Meridian Diagnostics, Inc., Cincinnati, OH; Murex Cryptococcus test, Murex Corp., Norcross, GA; Crypto-LA test, Wampole Laboratories, Cranbury, NJ; and latex antigen detection system, Immuno-mycologics, Norman, OK) and the EIA (Premier cryptococcal antigen sandwich EIA; Meridian Diagnostics, Inc.) are sensitive (93 to 100%) and specific (93 to 100%) diagnostic tools (28, 29, 38, 42, 81). All methods are well established for the detection and quantitation of circulating capsular polysaccharide antigen from *C. neoformans* in serum and CSF. Titer determinations resulting from different latex kits should not be used interchangeably because results may vary considerably. When comparing titers between current and previous specimens, titrations should be performed using the same kit at the same time. Studies for the detection of cryptococcal antigen in BAL fluid have met with variable results (2, 44). With both the latex and EIA methodologies, false-negative as well as false-positive results have been described. False-negative results can occur with low titers of cryptococcal antigen,

early infection, poorly encapsulated strains with low production of polysaccharide, and prozone phenomenon (28). False-positive results have been well documented with LA systems (4, 5, 27, 33). Most false-positive reactions have been eliminated through procedural modifications (30, 94) and incorporation of control reagents (3).

The Premier cryptococcal antigen EIA yields few false-positive results, including cross-reaction with *Trichosporon*, *Capnocytophaga canimorsus* sepsis, *Stomatococcus* infection, and unidentified causes (9, 58, 88). EIA titers are not numerically equivalent to latex titers.

Histoplasma capsulatum

The diagnosis of histoplasmosis is usually made by a combination of culture, histopathology, measurement of antibodies, and detection of antigen. In active infections, antigens are released into tissues and enter body fluids adjacent to the sites of the infection. The sensitivity of antigen testing in acute pulmonary, subacute pulmonary, chronic pulmonary, and progressively disseminated histoplasmosis has been reported as 77, 34, 21, and 92%, respectively (80). Although antigen testing and serology have the highest sensitivity, using a range of tests for the diagnosis of histoplasmosis is recommended, as test sensitivity differs with disease presentation.

H. capsulatum antigen can be detected in blood, urine, CSF, or BAL fluid using an EIA (Mira Vista Diagnostics, Indianapolis, IN) in cases of disseminated histoplasmosis. It has been suggested that the antigen EIA should be used as a screening test to be validated by antibody testing by immunodiffusion (ID) and/or complement fixation (CF) when positive; however, the EIA may be negative for patients with positive ID or CF. The sensitivity of urinary antigen detection in disseminated histoplasmosis varies with patients with AIDS (95%), nonimmunosuppressed patients (80%), and immunosuppressed patients (82%) (91). This test may be used to monitor therapy, as antigen concentration declines during effective treatment and increases with relapse. The sensitivity for detection of *Histoplasma* antigen is lower in serum than in urine. Recently, Swartzentruber et al. (79) found that EDTA-heat treatment of serum and other fluids with blood contamination improved the sensitivity for the detection of antigenemia in patients with proven or probable acute pulmonary histoplasmosis. Antigen is detected in CSF specimens from 25 to 50% of patients with *Histoplasma* meningitis (89) and in BAL fluid specimens from 93.5% of patients with histoplasmosis. In 10% of patients with histoplasmosis, antigen was detected in BAL but not in urine or serum (31). Cross-reactions

---

FIGURE 1 (row 1, left)   Gram stain of BAL specimen showing gram-negative branching septate hyphae of *Aspergillus fumigatus*. Magnification, approximately ×1,000.

FIGURE 2 (row 1, right)   Gram stain of skin biopsy with gram-variable branching hyphae of *Exophiala jeanselmei*. Magnification, approximately ×1,000.

FIGURE 3 (row 2, left)   Gram stain of skin biopsy with gram-negative aseptate hyphae of the *Rhizopus microsporus* group. Magnification, approximately ×1,000.

FIGURE 4 (row 2, right)   Gram stain of sputum with *Candida albicans* showing gram-positive budding yeast cells with pseudohyphae.

FIGURE 5 (row 3, left)   Gram stain of spleen demonstrating ghost-like budding yeast-like cells with pseudohyphae. Magnification, approximately ×1,000.

FIGURE 6 (row 3, right)   Gram stain of vaginal secretions with gram-positive budding yeast cells of *Candida glabrata*.

FIGURE 7 (row 4, left)   Gram stain of skin abscess with *Cryptococcus neoformans* showing gram-positive and gram-variable budding yeast cells of variable size surrounded by amorphous orange halos.

FIGURE 8 (row 4, right)   Calcofluor white stain of skin lesion showing typical yeast cells of *Malassezia* spp. Magnification, approximately ×400.

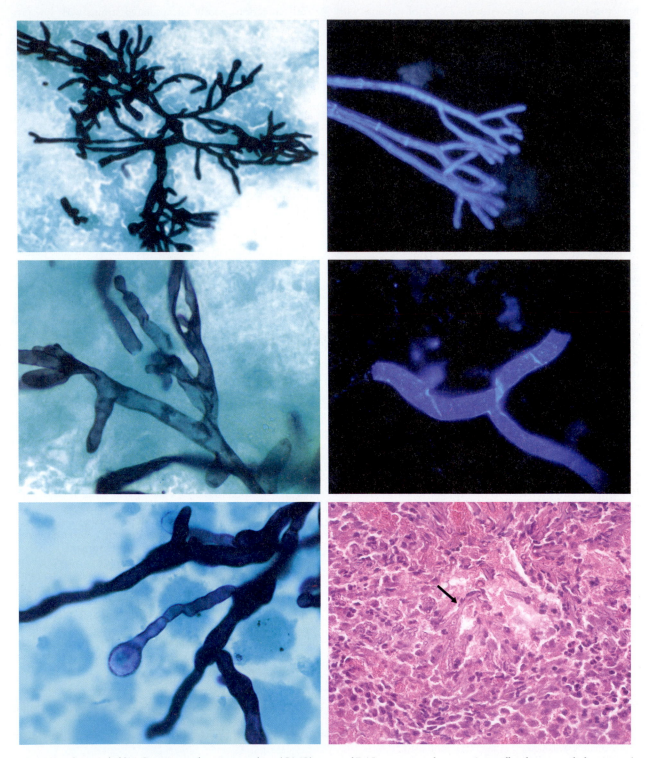

FIGURE 9 (row 1, left)   Gomori methenamine silver (GMS) stain of BAL specimen showing *Aspergillus fumigatus* dichotomously branching septate hyphae. Magnification, approximately ×400.

FIGURE 10 (row 1, right)   Calcofluor white stain of BAL specimen showing *Aspergillus fumigatus* dichotomously branching septate hyphae. Magnification, approximately ×500.

FIGURE 11 (row 2, left)   GMS stain of skin biopsy with *Rhizopus* spp. showing ribbon-like hyphae. Magnification, approximately ×400.

FIGURE 12 (row 2, right)   Calcofluor white stain of *Rhizopus* spp. showing ribbon-like hyphae. Magnification, approximately ×500.

FIGURE 13 (row 3, left)   GMS stain of lung biopsy specimen showing *Aspergillus fumigatus* with bulb formation at hyphal tip. Magnification, approximately ×1,000.

FIGURE 14 (row 3, right)   H&E stain of lung biopsy specimen showing *Aspergillus fumigatus* dichotomously branching septate hyphae (shown at arrow). Magnification, approximately ×400.

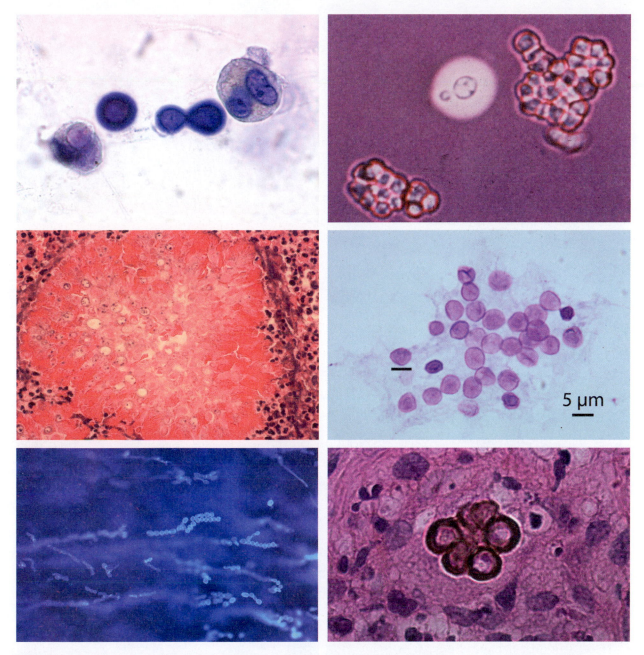

FIGURE 15 (row 1, left)   Diff-Quik stain of CSF with *Cryptococcus neoformans*. Magnification, approximately ×400.
FIGURE 16 (row 1, right)   India ink preparation of CSF showing encapsulated budding yeast cell of *Cryptococcus neoformans*. Magnification, approximately ×400.
FIGURE 17 (row 2, left)   H&E stain of eumycotic mycetoma granule of *Scedosporium apiospermum*. Magnification, approximately ×400.
FIGURE 18 (row 2, right)   Toluidine blue stain of BAL specimen showing cysts of *P. jirovecii*.
FIGURE 19 (row 3, left)   Calcofluor white stain of toenail specimen showing arthroconidia and hyphae of *Trichophyton rubrum*. Magnification, approximately ×200.
FIGURE 20 (row 3, right)   Sclerotic cells (copper penny) in tissue of *Fonsecaea pedrosoi* chromoblastomycosis. Magnification, ×1,000.

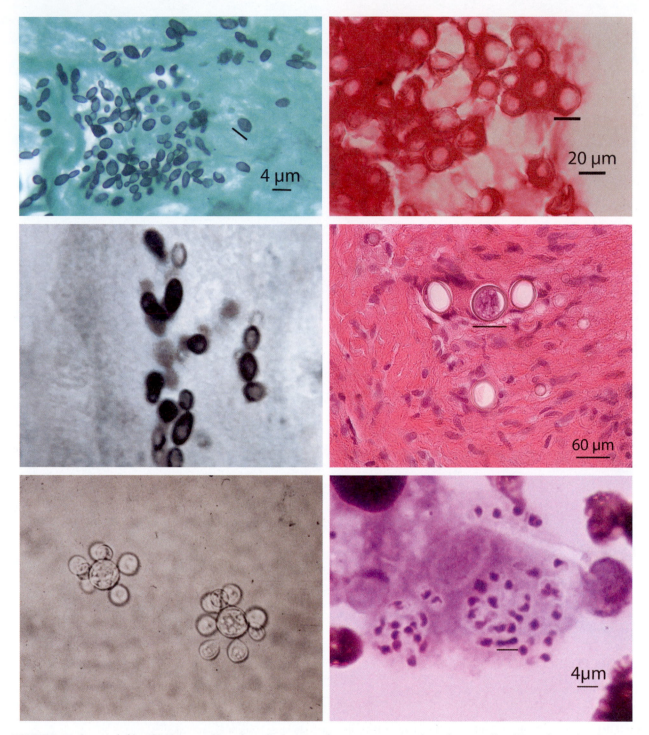

FIGURE 21 (row 1, left)   GMS stain of lymph node showing characteristic cigar-shaped yeast cells of *Sporothrix schenckii*.

FIGURE 22 (row 1, right)   Gram stain of abscess material showing large, broad-based, budding yeast cell with thick refractile wall characteristic of *Blastomyces dermatitidis*.

FIGURE 23 (row 2, left)   GMS stain of lymph node showing blastoconidia of *H. capsulatum*. Magnification, ×625.

FIGURE 24 (row 2, right)   H&E stain of *Coccidioides immitis*. Large, round, thick-walled spherules (10 to 80 μm in diameter) filled with endospores (2 to 5 μm in diameter). Young spherules have a clear center with peripheral cytoplasm and a prominent thick wall.

FIGURE 25 (row 3, left)   Bright-field photomicrograph of *Paracoccidioides brasiliensis*, showing multiple budding yeast cells resembling mariner's wheels. Magnification, ×1,590.

FIGURE 26 (row 3, right)   Wright-Giemsa stain of BAL specimen showing characteristic fission yeast cells of *Penicillium marneffei*.

occur with paracoccidioidomycosis, blastomycosis, *Penicillium marneffei* infection, and African histoplasmosis.

(1→3)-β-D-GLUCAN PANFUNGAL DETECTION

The measurement of (1→3)-β-D-glucan (BG) in blood can be used as a diagnostic marker for invasive fungal infections. BG is a major cell wall polysaccharide component of many fungi, with the exception of the mucoraceous molds, which do not produce BG. *Cryptococcus* species and the yeast form of *Blastomyces dermatitidis* produce low levels of BG.

Several commercial assays for the detection of BG are available (Fungitec G test MK series [Seikagaku Kogyo Corporation, Tokyo, Japan]; Wako β-glucan test [Wako Pure Chemical Industries, Tokyo, Japan]; and Maruha B-G Star [Maruha Corp., Tokyo, Japan]), but there is little experience in the use of these tests outside Japan (34). Comparison of the various BG tests is difficult because each utilizes different reagents and methodologies. The only commercially available test in the United States is the Fungitell (Glucatell) test (Associates of Cape Cod, Falmouth, MA). The Fungitell assay is based upon the ability of fungal BG to activate an enzyme in the clotting cascade of the *Limulus* horseshoe crab. The recommended positive cutoff value is ≥80 pg/ml (Fungitell product insert [October 2004]; Associates of Cape Cod).

Studies have shown that the Fungitell serum BG detection assay is a highly sensitive and specific diagnostic tool for the detection of invasive fungal infections (including aspergillosis, *Fusarium* infection, trichosporonosis, and candidiasis) (41, 67, 68, 71). Difficulties arise when comparing the data from these studies because different cutoff values have been used to interpret the results. Additionally, analysis of the patient population must be considered because test results vary with patient population. The sensitivity and specificity results for the Fungitell BG test also vary with the frequency of sampling. Serial sampling studies tend to report a higher sensitivity than once-a-week or once-per-episode studies (25). Overall, the range of predicted assay accuracy is unsatisfactory (sensitivity of 60 to 100% and specificity of 64 to 99%; positive predictive values, 43 to 100%; negative predictive values, 73 to 100%).

BG is also a component of the *Pneumocystis jirovecii* cell wall. Desmet et al. (18) have shown the sensitivity and specificity of BG detection with the Fungitell assay for *Pneumocystis* infection to be 100 and 96.4%, respectively, using a cutoff value of 100 pg/ml. Other studies of *Pneumocystis* infection have followed the manufacturer's guidelines, using positive BG values of ≥80 pg/ml. (16). Further studies are needed to better define the role of BG determination in the diagnosis of *Pneumocystis* infection.

With all BG tests, false positives occur with patients who are on hemodialysis using cellulose membranes (40, 65), are being treated with certain blood products (such as serum albumin and immunoglobulins), or have been exposed to gauze, cotton, or sponges containing glucan (37, 66). Patients who have bacterial infections have also been found to have false-positive BG tests (74). Sera which are hemolytic or lipemic or contain bilirubin have been shown to give inconsistent results and should not be tested (77). Additionally, cross-reactions occur with β-lactams (amoxicillin-clavulinic acid) (62) and antitumoral polysaccharides (including lentinan, crestin, *Sclerotinia sclerotiorum* glucan, and schizophyllan) (6). All false-positive results generally show similar kinetics, displaying a sudden rise and fall in BG levels in serum. True-positive results generally show a constant rise of BG levels,

which then decrease and become negative if the patient responds to antifungal therapies. Patients not responding to antifungal treatment do not show a decrease in BG levels. BG testing must always be utilized in conjunction with other diagnostic tests (e.g., GM, histopathological diagnosis, culture of samples, and radiological exams) for the conclusive diagnosis of invasive fungal infection.

FUNGUS-SPECIFIC METABOLITE DETECTION

In addition to antigen detection methods, fungus-specific metabolites have been used as markers to detect fungal infections. These included the fungal polyols D-arabinitol and D-mannitol and the ratio of D-arabinitol to L-arabinitol. None of the fungus-specific metabolite detection methods are commercially available (10–12, 23, 35, 46, 59, 76).

MASS SPECTROMETRY

Matrix-assisted laser desorption ionization–time of flight mass spectrometry has been shown to be a rapid, accurate method for identifying bacteria and fungi recovered on agar culture media (53, 75, 83). Studies are in progress to determine the potential of direct identification of fungi in positive blood culture broths and patient samples.

NUCLEIC ACID DETECTION

Molecular amplification techniques offer increased sensitivity over traditional staining and culture methods but may give positive results in asymptomatic individuals because of colonization or subclinical infection. Advantages to molecularly based detection include speed, enhanced sensitivity of detection, wider range of detectable organisms due to DNA sequence-based identification, detection of fungi that appear to be causing disease but cannot be cultured (organisms affected by antifungal agents or hepatosplenic candidiasis), and resistance marker detection (82). Molecular methods have been applied directly to clinical materials or the contents of blood culture bottles. Critical factors influencing fungal DNA detection in clinical samples are the correct processing of specimens, DNA extraction protocol (51), PCR design (target selection and amplicon specification method), and quality control requirements. No universally accepted nucleic acid-based detection system is available due to the lack of standardization in DNA amplification methods.

Clinical materials may require further processing than fungal isolates due to the presence of PCR inhibitors found in specimens or blood culture bottles. Automated DNA extraction methods may significantly reduce contamination rates and may allow for a method of standardization among institutions using molecular detection methods (57). Numerous target genes for fungal detection and identification have been evaluated. With the exception of beta-tubulin and elongation factor 1-alpha genes for the detection of molds, multicopy genes are more sensitive than single-copy genes. In general, universal primers are used to amplify the initial target, and then species-specific primers are used to identify the organism (93). The failure to amplify specific DNA may result from fungal DNA concentrations below detection limits, a focal infection with various amounts of fungal elements within the tissue, or destruction of DNA during formalin fixation.

Numerous methodologies to identify the presence of the amplified target region have been evaluated. These include

DNA probes, platforms enabling high-throughput analyses (e.g., DNA microarrays and Luminex [xMAP] [Luminex Corp., Austin, TX]), fluorescent in situ hybridization, PCR and panfungal PCR assays, reverse-hybridization line probe assays, isothermal systems (nucleic acid sequence-based amplification, loop-mediated isothermal amplification, and rolling circle amplification), and pyrosequencing. Lau et al. provide a comprehensive summary of the advantages and disadvantages for each of these systems (47). Prior to implementation in the clinical laboratory, proper validation must be performed (14).

Real-time PCR methods, such as TaqMan (Perkin-Elmer, Wellesley, MA) and Lightcycler (Roche Molecular Systems, Pleasanton, CA) techniques, enable rapid amplification, hybridization, and amplicon detection in a single reaction. Real-time technology can provide quantitative results because the point at which the PCR enters the log/linear phase is detectable and reflects the amount of target DNA in the original sample.

NASBA is a technique that involves amplification and detection of mRNA. Unlike PCR, NASBA is an isothermal process, uses RNA polymerase, and amplifies mRNA. RNA is generally less stable than DNA in dead cells; therefore, its detection may indicate the viability of the organism. Because thermal denaturation is absent, there is little contaminating background of genomic DNA (50).

Pyrosequencing is a real-time, nonelectrophoretic sequencing method. This method relies on the sequential addition and incorporation of nucleotides in a primer-directed polymerase extension reaction. The pyrophosphate released on incorporation of a base-paired nucleotide is coupled to the enzymes ATP sulfurylase and luciferase to generate detectable light. The light is proportional to the number of nucleotides incorporated, allowing for the sequence to be determined in real time (19). (For detailed illustrations on pyrosequencing, go to http://www.pyrosequencing.com.)

The Luminex (xMAP) technology employs a flow cytometer with a dual-laser system that allows the simultaneous detection of different target sequences in a multiplex and high-throughput format. The assay uses a liquid suspension hybridization design with specific oligonucleotide probes that are covalently bound to the surface of fluorescent color-coded microspheres. Biotinylated target amplicons hybridize to their complementary probe sequences and are quantified. (45)

The use of PCR for the diagnosis of IA illustrates the difficulties with nonstandardized nucleic acid tests. Mengoli et al. (60) identified 7,059 references and selected 141 citations for systematic review and meta-analysis. In their review, it was found that there were too few studies to determine whether the underlying disease or use of antifungal prophylaxis influenced the results and whether the diagnostic yield of PCR differed for different patient populations. It was determined that a single PCR-negative result was sufficient to exclude a diagnosis of proven or probable IA, while two positive tests were required to confirm the diagnosis of IA. Donnelly et al. (20) reviewed the challenges of devising a standard by which different techniques could be assessed for accuracy and precision through the coordination of different working groups (including ISHAM [International Society for Human and Animal Mycology], the Laboratory Working Group, the Clinical Working Group, the Infectious Disease Group of the EORTC, and the Infectious Diseases Working Party of the European Group for Blood and Marrow Transplantation.) White et al. summarizes an update on the *Aspergillus* PCR standardization project

(92). In this review it was found that the efficiency of the *Aspergillus* PCR was limited by the extraction procedures utilized and the compliance of some centers in the study. Recommendations included guidelines for blood collection, volume, extraction, and quality control. *Aspergillus* PCR is promising, as the groundwork for developing a standard approach is underway.

SEROLOGY

Antibody detection tests are often helpful for the diagnosis of fungal infections in immunocompetent hosts but are less useful with immunocompromised patients, as they are less likely to be able to mount a sufficient response. Further information about serologic diagnosis can also be found in chapter 5 as well as the appropriate organism chapters of this *Manual*.

Aspergillus Species

The detection of antibodies against *Aspergillus* for the diagnosis of IA has produced conflicting results (39). Immunoglobulin G (IgG) antibodies are usually positive for patients with aspergilloma and allergic bronchopulmonary aspergillosis. The sensitivity and specificity of the ID and counterimmunoelectrophoresis tests are similar.

Blastomyces dermatitidis

Serologic diagnosis of blastomycosis is generally performed using ID, CF, or an enzyme-linked immunosorbent assay. ID tests are more specific, while enzyme-linked immunosorbent assays are more sensitive. The CF test has poor sensitivity compared with the ID test (48). The yeast form of *B. dermatitidis* releases two surface antigens, A antigen and W1-1. Antibodies directed against W1-1 also recognize the A antigen. W1-1 antibody tests are not currently available commercially. A positive ID test using purified A antigen is specific and diagnostic for blastomycosis. A negative ID test does not rule out a diagnosis of blastomycosis, as this test is reported to be negative for 10% of patients with disseminated infection and over 60% of patients with localized disease.

Candida Species

Antibody assays generally cannot discriminate between systemic candidiasis and colonization (90). Ellepola et al. (24) summarized numerous methods developed to detect *Candida* antibodies and antigens. *Candida* antibody assays generally have poor sensitivity and low specificity. With immunocompetent patients, the determination of the presence and titer of precipitating antibodies to *Candida albicans* in serum may provide supportive evidence for endocarditis, osteomyelitis, endophthalmitis, and systemic candidosis (69).

Coccidioides Species

The serologic diagnosis of coccidioidomycosis is performed using ID, LA, CF, or EIA methods. The ID and LA tests are useful for the initial screening of specimens and can be confirmed by other tests if positive. The LA test detects early IgM antibody responses to coccidioidal infection, while the CF test detects primarily IgG antibodies produced during the convalescent phase of disease or during chronic infection. The ID test can detect both IgM and IgG antibodies, depending on whether unheated (IgG) or heated (IgM) coccidiodin is used as the antigen. Performing both the ID (or LA) and CF tests in parallel provides the highest sensitivity and specificity. The *Coccidioides* EIA (Meridian Diagnostics, Inc.) detects both anti-*Coccidioides* IgG and

IgM antibodies in sera and CSF specimens from patients with coccidioidomycosis. Although the sensitivity (97%) and specificity (94%) are high, confirmation of positive ID results is recommended, as some false-positive results may occur with CSF specimens and IgM detection (95). Commercial kits contain both antigens and positive controls for both types of antibody.

Cryptococcus neoformans

Antibody detection may be useful for the early diagnosis of cryptococcal disease, because antibodies are not yet neutralized by the large amount of capsular antigen released during the progression of the infection (48), but is not widely available due to high false-positive and false-negative rates.

Histoplasma capsulatum

The primary serologic tests for histoplasmosis are the ID and CF tests. The ID test detects precipitins to H and M antigens of *Histoplasma capsulatum*. The ID test is more specific but less sensitive than the CF test. The detection of precipitins to H antigens is specific for active disease, but H bands develop only in 20% of patients tested and usually disappear within the first 6 months of infection. M precipitins can be detected in up to 70% of patients with acute pulmonary histoplasmosis and nearly all patients with chronic pulmonary infection. Serology is usually negative during the first 2 months of acute infection. Cross-reactivity can occur in up to 40% of patients with paracoccidioidomycosis, blastomycosis, and aspergillosis; 16% of patients with coccidioidomycosis; and 8% of patients with candidiasis (80). False-negative results may occur in immunocompromised patients with active infection. Monitoring ID antibody titers is not recommended, as there are no data correlating antibody clearance, treatment failure, or relapse (91).

The CF test, which measures antibodies to heat-killed yeast cells and mycelial filtrate (histoplasmin) antigens, is more sensitive but less specific than the ID test. Antibodies to the yeast antigen are the first to appear and the last to disappear, while antibodies to histoplasmin appear later. Detection of the yeast phase is regarded as more sensitive. Approximately 90 to 95% of cases have positive titers to one or both antigens. Titers to mycelial antigen are higher in chronic infection. CF antibodies generally appear 3 to 6 weeks after infection by *H. capsulatum*, and repeated tests will give positive results for months. The results of CF tests are of greatest diagnostic usefulness when both acute and convalescent serum specimens can be obtained. A high titer (1:32 or higher) or a fourfold increase is indicative of active histoplasmosis. Lower titers (1:8 or 1:16), although less specific, may also provide presumptive evidence of infection, but they can also be detected in the serum of healthy persons from regions where histoplasmosis is endemic. Antibody titers will gradually decline and eventually disappear months to years after a patient recovers.

REFERENCES

1. **Bar, W., and H. Hecker.** 2002. Diagnosis of systemic *Candida* infections in patients of the intensive care unit. Significance of serum antigens and antibodies. *Mycoses* **45:**22–28.
2. **Baughman, R. P., J. C. Rhodes, M. N. Dohn, H. Henderson, and P. T. Frame.** 1992. Detection of cryptococcal antigen in bronchoalveolar lavage fluid: a prospective study of diagnostic utility. *Am. Rev. Respir. Dis.* **145:**1226–1229.
3. **Bennett, J. E., and J. W. Bailey.** 1971. Control for rheumatoid factor in the latex test for cryptococcosis. *Am. J. Clin. Pathol.* **56:**360–365.
4. **Blevins, L. B., J. Fenn, H. Segal, P. Newcomb-Gayman, and K. C. Carroll.** 1995. False-positive cryptococcal antigen latex agglutination caused by disinfectants and soaps. *J. Clin. Microbiol.* **33:**1674–1675.
5. **Boom, W. H., D. J. Piper, K. L. Ruoff, and M. J. Ferraro.** 1985. New cause for false-positive results with the cryptococcal antigen test by latex agglutination. *J. Clin. Microbiol.* **22:**856–857.
6. **Borchers, A. T., C. L. Keen, and M. E. Gershwin.** 2004. Mushrooms, tumors, and immunity: an update. *Exp. Biol. Med.* (Maywood) **229:**393–406.
7. **Boutboul, F., C. Alberti, T. Leblanc, et al.** 2002. Invasive aspergillosis in allogeneic stem cell transplant recipients: increasing antigenemia is associated with progressive disease. *Clin. Infect. Dis.* **34:**939–943.
8. **Bustamante, B., and P. E. Campos.** 2003. Eumycetoma, p. 390–398. *In* W. E. Dismukes, P. G. Pappas, and J. D. Sobel (ed.), *Clinical Mycology*. Oxford University Press, New York, NY.
9. **Chanock, S. J., P. Toltzis, and C. Wilson.** 1993. Cross-reactivity between *Stomatococcus mucilaginosus* and latex agglutination for cryptococcal antigen. *Lancet* **342:**1119–1120.
10. **Chaturvedi, V., B. Wong, and S. L. Newman.** 1996. Oxidative killing of *Cryptococcus neoformans* by human neutrophils. Evidence that fungal mannitol protects by scavenging reactive oxygen intermediates. *J. Immunol.* **15:**3836–3840.
11. **Christensson, B., G. Sigmundsdottir, and L. Larsson.** 1999. D-Arabinitol—a marker for invasive candidiasis. *Med. Mycol.* **37:**391–396.
12. **Christensson, B., T. Wiebe, C. Pehrson, and L. Larsson.** 1997. Diagnosis of invasive candidiasis in neutropenic children with cancer by determination of D-arabinitol/L-arabinitol ratios in urine. *J. Clin. Microbiol.* **35:**636–640.
13. **Clancy, C. J., R. A. Jaber, H. L. Leather, J. R. Wingard, B. Staley, L. J. Wheat, C. L. Cline, K. H. Rand, D. Schain, M. Baz, and M. H. Nguyen.** 2007. Bronchoalveolar lavage galactomannan in diagnosis of invasive pulmonary aspergillosis among solid-organ transplant recipients. *J. Clin. Microbiol.* **45:**1759–1765.
14. **Clinical and Laboratory Standards Institute.** 2006. *Molecular Diagnostic Methods for Infectious Disease; Approved Standard*, 2nd ed. CLSI/NCCLS document MM3-A. Clinical and Laboratory Standards Institute, Wayne, PA.
15. **Dalle, F., P. E. Charles, K. Blanc, D. Caillot, P. Chavanet, F. Dromer, and A. Bonnin.** 2005. *Cryptococcus neoformans* galactoxylomannan contains an epitope(s) that is cross-reactive with *Aspergillus* galactomannan. *J. Clin. Microbiol.* **43:**2929–2931.
16. **Del Bono, V., A. Mularoni, E. Furafo, E. Delfino, L. Rosasco, F. Miletich, and C. Viscoli.** 2009. Clinical evaluation of a (1,3)-beta-D-glucan assay for presumptive diagnosis of Pneumocystis jiroveci pneumonia in immunocompromised patients. *Clin. Vaccine Immunol.* **16:**1524–1526.
17. **De Pauw, B., T. H. Walsh, J. P. Donnelly, D. A. Stevens, J. E. Edwards, T. Calandra, P. G. Pappas, J. Maertens, O. Lortholary, C. A. Kauffman, D. W. Denning, T. F. Patterson, G. Maschmeyer, J. Bille, W. E. Dismukes, R. Herbrecht, W. W. Hope, C. C. Kibbler, B. J. Kullberg, K. A. Marr, P. Muñoz, F. C. Odds, J. R. Perfect, A. Restrepo, M. Ruhnke, B. H. Segal, J. D. Sobel, T. C. Sorrell, C. Viscoli, J. R. Wingard, T. Zaoutis, and J. E. Bennett.** 2008. Revised definitions of invasive fungal disease from the European Organization for Research and Treatment of Cancer/Invasive Fungal Infections Cooperative Group and the National Institute of Allergy and Infections Diseases Mycoses Study Group (EORTC/MSG) Consensus Group. *Clin. Infect. Dis.* **46:**1813–1821.
18. **Desmet, S., E. Wijngaarden, J. Maertens, J. Veraegen, E. Verbeken, P. De Munter, W. Meerssemen, B. Van Meensel, J. Van Eldere, and K. Lagrou.** 2009. Serum (1-3)-beta-D-glucan as a tool for diagnosis of Pneumocystis jirovecii pneumonia in patients with human immunodeficiency virus infection or hematological malignancy. *J. Clin. Microbiol.* **47:**3871–3874.

19. **Diggle, M. A., and S. C. Clarke.** 2004. Pyrosequencing: sequence typing at the speed of light. *Mol. Biotechnol.* **28:**129–137.

20. **Donnelly, J. P., R. A. Barnes, and J. Loeffler.** 2008. Challenges and progress in setting a standard for PCR for invasive aspergillosis. *Curr. Fungal Infect. Rep.* **2:**232–236.

21. **Durkin, M., J. Witt, A. Lemonte, B. Wheat, and P. Connolly.** 2004. Antigen assay with the potential to aid in diagnosis of blastomycosis. *J. Clin. Microbiol.* **42:**4873–4875.

22. **Durkin, M., P. Connolly, T. Kuberski, R. Myers, B. M. Kubak, D. Bruckner, D. Pegues, and L. J. Wheat.** 2008. Diagnosis of coccidioidomycosis with use of the *Coccidioides* antigen enzyme immunoassay. *Clin. Infect. Dis.* **47:**e69–e73.

23. **Eisen, D. P., P. B. Bartley, W. Hope, G. Sigmundsdottir, C. Pehrson, L. Larsson, and B. Christensson.** 2002. Urine D-arabinitol/L-arabinitol ratio in diagnosing *Candida* infection in patients with haematological malignancy and HIV infection. *Diagn. Microbiol. Infect. Dis.* **42:**39–42.

24. **Ellepola, A. N., and C. J. Morrison.** 2005. Laboratory diagnosis of invasive candidiasis. *J. Microbiol.* **43:**65–84.

25. **Ellis, M., B. Al-Ramadi, M. Finkelmaan, U. Hedstrom, J. Kristensen, and H. L. Klingspor.** 2008. Assessment of the clinical utility of serial beta-D-glucan concentrations in patients with persistent neutropenic fever. *J. Med. Microbiol.* **57:**287–295.

26. **El Saleeby, C. M., K. J. Allison, K. M. Knapp, T. J. Walsh, and R. T. Hayden.** 2005. Discordant rise in galactomannan antigenemia in a patient with resolving aspergillosis, renal failure, and ongoing hemodialysis. *J. Clin. Microbiol.* **43:**3560–3563.

27. **Eng, R. H., and A. Person.** 1981. Serum cryptococcal antigen determination in the presence of rheumatoid factor. *J. Clin. Microbiol.* **14:**700–702.

28. **Frank, U. K., S. L. Nishimura, N. C. Li, K. Sugai, D. M. Yajko, W. K. Hadley, V. L. Ng.** 1993. Evaluation of an enzyme immunoassay for detection of cryptococcal capsular polysaccharide antigen in serum and cerebrospinal fluid. *J. Clin. Microbiol.* **31:**97–101.

29. **Gade, W., S. W. Hinnefeld, L. S. Babcock, P. Gilligan, W. Kelly, K. Wait, D. Greer, M. Pinilla, and R. L. Kaplan.** 1991. Comparison of the PREMIER cryptococcal antigen enzyme immunoassay and the latex agglutination assay for detection of cryptococcal antigens. *J. Clin. Microbiol.* **29:**1616–1619.

30. **Gray, L. D., and G. D. Roberts.** 1988. Experience with the use of pronase to eliminate interference factors in the latex agglutination test for cryptococcal antigen. *J. Clin. Microbiol.* **26:**2450–2451.

31. **Hage, C. A., T. E. Davis, D. Fuller, L. Egan, J. R. Witt III, L. J. Wheat, and K. S. Knox.** 2010. Diagnosis of histoplasmosis by antigen detection in BAL fluid. *Chest* **137:**623–628.

32. **Hay, R. J., E. S. Mahgoub, G. Leon, S. al-Sogair, and O. Welsh.** 1992. Mycetoma. *J. Med. Vet. Mycol.* **30**(Suppl. 1):41–49.

33. **Heelan, J. S., L. Corpus, and N. Kessimian.** 1991. False-positive reactions in the latex agglutination test for *Cryptococcus neoformans* antigen. *J. Clin. Microbiol.* **29:**1260–1261.

34. **Hossain, M. A., T. Miyazaki, K. Mitsutake, H. Kakeya, Y. Yamamoto, K. Yanagihara, S. Kawamura, T. Otsubo, Y. Hirakata, T. Tashiro, and S. Kohno.** 1997. Comparison between Wako-WB003 and Fungitec G tests for detection of (1→3)-beta-D-glucan in systemic mycosis. *J. Clin. Lab. Anal.* **11:**73–77.

35. **Hui, M., S. W. Cheung, M. L. Chin, K. C. Chu, R. C. Chan, and A. F. Cheng.** 2004. Development and application of a rapid diagnostic method for invasive candidiasis by the detection of D-/L-arabinitol using gas chromatography/mass spectrometry. *Diagn. Microbiol. Infect. Dis.* **49:**117–123.

36. **Husain, S., C. J. Clancy, M. H. Nguyen, S. Swartzentruber, H. Leather, A. M. LeMonte, M. Durkin, K. S. Knox, C. A. Hage, C. Bentsen, N. Singh, J. R. Wingard, and L. J. Wheat.** 2008. Performance characteristics of the Platelia *Aspergillus* enzyme immunoassay for detection of *Aspergillus* galactomannan antigen in bronchoalveolar lavage fluid. *Clin. Vaccine Immunol.* **15:**1760–1763.

37. **Ikemura, K., K. Ikegami, T. Shimazu, T. Yoshioka, and T. Sugimoto.** 1989. False-positive result in Limulus test caused by Limulus amebocyte lysate-reactive material in immunoglobulin products. *J. Clin. Microbiol.* **27:**1965–1968.

38. **Jaye, D. L., K. B. Waites, B. Parker, S. L. Bragg, and S. A. Moser.** 1998. Comparison of two rapid latex agglutination tests for detection of cryptococcal capsular polysaccharide. *Am. J. Clin. Pathol.* **109:**634–641.

39. **Kappe, R., A. Schulze-Berge, and H. G. Sonntag.** 1996. Evaluation of eight antibody tests and one antigen test for the diagnosis of invasive aspergillosis. *Mycoses* **39:**13–23.

40. **Kato, A., T. Takita, M. Furuhashi, T. Takahashi, Y. Maruyama, and A. Hishida.** 2001. Elevation of blood (1→3)-beta-D-glucan concentrations in hemodialysis patients. *Nephron* **89:**15–19.

41. **Kawazu, M., Y. Kanda, Y. Nannya, K. Aoki, M. Kurokawa, S. Chiba, T. Motokura, H. Hirai, and S. Ogawa.** 2004. Prospective comparison of the diagnostic potential of real-time PCR, double-sandwich enzyme-linked immunosorbent assay for galactomannan, and a (1→3)-beta-D-glucan test in weekly screening for invasive aspergillosis in patients with hematological disorders. *J. Clin. Microbiol.* **42:**2733–2741.

42. **Kiska, D. L., D. R. Orkiszewski, D. Howell, and P. H. Gilligan.** 1994. Evaluation of new monoclonal antibody-based latex agglutination test for detection of cryptococcal polysaccharide antigen in serum and cerebrospinal fluid. *J. Clin. Microbiol.* **32:**2309–2311.

43. **Koneman, E., and G. Roberts.** 2002. The appearance of fungi in tissues. *Lab. Med.* **12:**927–933.

44. **Kralovic, S. M., and J. C. Rhodes.** 1998. Utility of routine testing of bronchoalveolar lavage fluid for cryptococcal antigen. *J. Clin. Microbiol.* **36:**3088–3099.

45. **Landlinger, C., S. Preuner, B. Willinger, B. Haberpursch, Z. Racil, J. Mayer, and T. Lion.** 2009. Species-specific identification of a wide range of clinically relevant fungal pathogens by use of Luminex xMAP technology. *J. Clin. Microbiol.* **47:**1063–1073.

46. **Larsson, L., C. Pehrson, T. Wiebe, and B. Christensson.** 1994. Gas chromatographic determination of D-arabinitol/L-arabinitol ratios in urine: a potential method for diagnosis of disseminated candidiasis. *J. Clin. Microbiol.* **32:**1855–1859.

47. **Lau A., S. Chen, S. Sleiman, and T. Sorrell.** 2009. Current status and future perspectives on molecular and serological methods in diagnostic mycology. *Future Microbiol.* **4:**1185–1222.

48. **Lindsley, M. D., D. W. Warnock, and C. J. Morrison.** 2006. Serological and molecular diagnosis of fungal infections, p. 569–605. *In* B. Detrick, R. G. Hamilton, and J. D. Folds (ed.), *Manual of Molecular and Clinical Laboratory Immunology*, 7th ed. ASM Press, Washington, DC.

49. **Liu, K., D. N. Howell, J. R. Perfect, and W. A. Schell.** 1998. Morphologic criteria for the preliminary identification of *Fusarium, Paecilomyces,* and *Acremonium* species by histopathology. *Am. J. Clin. Pathol.* **109:**45–54.

50. **Loeffler, J., C. Dorn, H. Hebart, P. Cox, S. Magga, and H. Einsele.** 2003. Development and evaluation of the nuclisens basic kit NASBA for the detection of RNA from *Candida* species frequently resistant to antifungal drugs. *Diagn. Microbiol. Infect. Dis.* **45:**217–220.

51. **Loeffler, J., H. Hebart, U. Schumacher, H. Reitze, and H. Einsele.** 1997. Comparison of different methods for extraction of fungal pathogens from cultures and blood. *J. Clin. Microbiol.* **35:**3311–3312.

52. **Maertens, J., I. Raad, G. Petrikkos, M. Boogaerts, D. Selleslag, F. B. Petersen, C. A. Sable, N. A. Kartsonis, A. Ngai, A. Taylor, T. F. Patterson, D. W. Denning, T. J. Walsh, and the Caspofungin Salvage Aspergillosis Study Group.** 2004. Efficacy and safety of caspofungin for treatment of invasive aspergillosis in patients refractory to or intolerant of conventional antifungal therapy. *Clin. Infect. Dis.* **39:**1563–1571.

53. **Marklein, G., M. Josten, U. Klanke, E. Müller, R. Horré, T. Maier, T. Wenzel, M. Kostrzewa, G. Bierbaum, A. Hoerauf,**

and H. G. Sahl. 2009. Matrix-assisted laser desorption ionization–time of flight mass-spectrometry for fast and reliable identification of clinical yeast isolates. *J. Clin. Microbiol.* **47:**2912–2917.

54. Marr, K. A., M. Laverdiere, A. Gugel, and W. Leisenring. 2005. Antifungal therapy decreases sensitivity of the *Aspergillus* galactomannan enzyme immunoassay. *Clin. Infect. Dis.* **40:**1762–1769.

55. Marr, K. A., S. A. Balajee, L. McLaughlin, M. Tabouret, C. Bentsen, and T. J. Walsh. 2004. Detection of galactomannan antigenemia by enzyme immunoassay for the diagnosis of invasive aspergillosis: variables that affect performance. *J. Infect. Dis.* **190:**641–649.

56. Mattei, D., D. Rapezzi, N. Mordini, F. Cuda, C. Lo Nigro, M. Musso, A. Arnelli, S. Cagnassi, and A. Gallamini. 2004. False-positive *Aspergillus* galactomannan enzyme-linked immunosorbent assay results in vivo during amoxicillin-clavulanic acid treatment. *J. Clin. Microbiol.* **42:**5362–5363.

57. McLintock, L. A., and B. L. Jones. 2004. Advances in the molecular and serological diagnosis of invasive fungal infection in haemato-oncology patients. *Br. J. Haematol.* **126:**289–297.

58. McManus, E. J., and J. M. Jones. 1985. Detection of a *Trichosporon beigelii* antigen cross-reactive with *Cryptococcus neoformans* capsular polysaccharide in serum from a patient with disseminated *Trichosporon* infection. *J. Clin. Microbiol.* **21:**681–685.

59. Megson, G. M., D. A. Stevens, J. R. Hamilton, and D. W. Denning. 1996. D-Mannitol in cerebrospinal fluid of patients with AIDS and cryptococcal meningitis. *J. Clin. Microbiol.* **34:**218–221.

60. Mengoli, C., M. Cruciani, R. A. Barnes, J. Loeffler, and J. P. Donnelly. 2009. Use of PCR for diagnosis of invasive aspergillosis: systematic review and meta-analysis. *Lancet Infect. Dis.* **9:**89–96.

61. Mennink-Kersten, M. A., D. Ruegebrink, R. R. Klont, A. Warris, F. Gavini, H. J. Op den Camp, and P. E. Verweij. 2005. Bifidobacterial lipoglycan as a new cause for false-positive platelia *Aspergillus* enzyme-linked immunosorbent assay reactivity. *J. Clin. Microbiol.* **43:**3925–3931.

62. Mennink-Kersten, M. A., A. Warris, and P. E. Verweij. 2006. 1,3-β-D-Glucan in patients receiving intravenous amoxicillin-clavulanic acid. *N. Engl. J. Med.* **354:**2834–2835.

63. Mitchell, T. G., and J. R. Perfect. 1995. Cryptococcosis in the era of AIDS—100 years after the discovery of *Cryptococcus neoformans*. *Clin. Microbiol. Rev.* **8:**515–548.

64. Mitsutake, K., T. Miyazaki, T. Tashiro, Y. Yamamoto, H. Kakeya, T. Otsubo, S. Kawamura, M. A. Hossain, T. Noda, Y. Hirakata, and S. Kohno. 1996. Enolase antigen, mannan antigen, Cand-Tec antigen, and beta-glucan in patients with candidemia. *J. Clin. Microbiol.* **34:**1918–1921.

65. Nagasawa, K., T. Yano, G. Kitabayashi, H. Morimoto, Y. Yamada, A. Ohata, M. Usami, and T. Horiuchi. 2003. Experimental proof of contamination of blood components by (1→3)-beta-D-glucan caused by filtration with cellulose filters in the manufacturing process. *J. Artif. Organs* **6:**49–54.

66. Nakao, A., M. Yasui, T. Kawagoe, H. Tamura, S. Tanaka, and H. Takagi. 1997. False-positive endotoxemia derives from gauze glucan after hepatectomy for hepatocellular carcinoma with cirrhosis. *Hepatogastroenterology* **44:**1413–1418.

67. Odabasi, Z., G. Mattiuzzi, E. Estey, H. Kantarjian, F. Saeki, R. J. Ridge, P. A. Ketchum, M. A. Finkelman, J. H. Rex, and L. Ostrosky-Zeichner. 2004. Beta-D-glucan as a diagnostic adjunct for invasive fungal infections: validation, cutoff development, and performance in patients with acute myelogenous leukemia and myelodysplastic syndrome. *Clin. Infect. Dis.* **15:**199–205.

68. Ostrosky-Zeichner, L., B. D. Alexander, D. H. Keft, J. Vazquez, P. G. Pappas, F. Saeki, P. A. Ketchum, J. Wingard, R. Schiff, H. Tamura, M. A. Finkelman, and J. H. Rex. 2005. Multicenter clinical evaluation of the (1→3) beta-D-glucan assay as an aid to diagnosis of fungal infections in humans. *Clin. Infect. Dis.* **41:**654–659.

69. Pallavicini, F., I. Izzi, M. A. Pennisi, G. Morace, G. G. Portaccio, G. Bello, F. Iodice, D. Godino, C. Del Borgo, and R. Proietti. 1999. Evaluation of the utility of serological tests in the diagnosis of candidemia. *Minerva Anestesiol.* **65:**637–639.

70. Pappas, P. G., J. H. Rex, J. D. Sobel, S. G. Filler, W. E. Dismukes, T. J. Walsh, J. E. Edwards, and the Infectious Diseases Society of America. 2004. Guidelines for treatment of candidiasis. *Clin. Infect.* **38:**161–189.

71. Pazos, C., J. Ponton, and A. Del Palacio. 2005. Contribution of (1→3)-beta-D-glucan chromogenic assay to diagnosis and therapeutic monitoring of invasive aspergillosis in neutropenic adult patients: a comparison with serial screening for circulating galactomannan. *J. Clin. Microbiol.* **43:**299–305.

72. Pfaller, M. A., and M. R. McGinnis. 2003. The laboratory and clinical mycology, p. 67–79. *In* E. J. Anaissie, M. R. McGinnis, and M. A. Pfaller (ed.), *Clinical Mycology.* Churchill Livingstone, Philadelphia, PA.

73. Phillips, P., A. Dowd, P. Jewesson, G. Radigan, M. G. Tweeddale, A. Clarke, I. Geere, and M. Kelly. 1990. Non-value of antigen detection immunoassays for diagnosis of candidemia. *J. Clin. Microbiol.* **28:**2320–2326.

74. Pickering, J. W., H. W. Sant, C. A. Bowles, W. L. Roberts, and G. L. Woods. 2005. Evaluation of a (1→3)-beta-D-glucan assay for diagnosis of invasive fungal infections. *J. Clin. Microbiol.* **43:**5957–5962.

75. Prod'hom, G., A. Bizzini, C. Durussel, J. Bille, and G. Greub. 2010. Matrix-assisted laser desorption ionization–time of flight mass spectrometry for direct bacterial identification from positive blood culture pellets. *J. Clin. Microbiol.* **48:**1481–1483.

76. Roboz, J., E. Nieves, and J. F. Holland. 1990. Separation and quantification by gas chromatography-mass spectrometry of arabinitol enantiomers to aid the differential diagnosis of disseminated candidiasis. *J. Chromatogr.* **500:**413–426.

77. Sant, H. W., J. W. Pickering, and G. L. Woods. 2005. Evaluation of the Fungitell (1→3) β-D-glucan assay for invasive fungal infection, abstr. F-011. *Abstr. 105th Gen. Meet. Am. Soc. Microbiol.* American Society for Microbiology, Washington, DC.

78. Sendid, B., D. Caillot, B. Baccouch-Humbert, L. Klingspor, M. Grandjean, A. Bonnin, and D. Poulain. 2003. Contribution of the Platelia *Candida*-specific antibody and antigen tests to early diagnosis of systemic *Candida tropicalis* infection in neutropenic adults. *J. Clin. Microbiol.* **41:**4551–4558.

79. Swartzentruber, S., A. LeMonte, J. Witt, D. Fuller, T. Davis, C. Hage, P. Connolly, M. Durkin, and L. J. Wheat. 2009. Improved detection of *Histoplasma* antigenemia following dissociation of immune complexes. *Clin. Vaccine Immunol.* **16:**320–322.

80. Swartzentruber S., L. Rhodes, K. Kurkjian, M. Zahn, M. E. Brandt, P. Connolly, and L. J. Wheat. 2009. Diagnosis of acute pulmonary histoplasmosis by antigen detection. *Clin. Infect. Dis.* **49:**1878–1882.

81. Tanner, D. C., M. P. Weinstein, B. Fedorciw, K. L. Joho, J. J. Thorpe, and L. Reller. 1994. Comparison of commercial kits for detection of cryptococcal antigen. *J. Clin. Microbiol.* **32:**1680–1684.

82. Trama, J. P., E. Mordechai, and M. E. Adelson. 2005. Detection of *Aspergillus fumigatus* and a mutation that confers reduced susceptibility to itraconazole and posaconazole by real-time PCR and pyrosequencing. *J. Clin. Microbiol.* **43:**906–908.

83. van Veen, S. Q., E. C. Claas, and E. J. Kuijper. 2010. High-throughput identification of bacteria and yeast by matrix-assisted laser desorption ionization–time of flight mass spectrometry in conventional medical microbiology laboratories. *J. Clin. Microbiol.* **48:**900–907.

84. Verweij, P. E., C. M. Weemaes, J. H. Curfs, S. Bretagne, and J. F. Meis. 2000. Failure to detect circulating *Aspergillus* markers in a patient with chronic granulomatous disease and invasive aspergillosis. *J. Clin. Microbiol.* **38:**3900–3901.

85. **Verweij, P. E., and M. A. S. H. Mennink-Kersten.** 2006. Issues with galactomannan testing. *Med. Mycol.* **44:**S179–S183.

86. **Walsh, T. J., S. Shoham, R. Petraitiene, T. Sein, R. Schaufele, A. Kelaher, H. Murray, C. Mya-San, J. Bacher, and V. Petraitis.** 2004. Detection of galactomannan antigenemia in patients receiving piperacillin-tazobactam and correlations between in vitro, in vivo, and clinical properties of the drug-antigen interaction. *J. Clin. Microbiol.* **42:**4744–4748.

87. **Walsh, T. J., V. Petraitis, R. Petraitiene, A. Field-Ridley, D. Sutton, M. Ghannoum, T. Sein, R. Schaufele, J. Peter, J. Bacher, H. Casler, D. Armstrong, A. Espinel-Ingroff, M. G. Rinaldi, and C. A. Lyman.** 2003. Experimental pulmonary aspergillosis due to *Aspergillus terreus*: pathogenesis and treatment of an emerging fungal pathogen resistant to amphotericin B. *J. Infect. Dis.* **188:**305–319.

88. **Westerink, M. A. J., D. Amsterdam, R. J. Petell, M. N. Stram, and M. A. Apicella.** 1987. Septicemia due to DF-2. Cause of a false-positive cryptococcal latex agglutination result. *Am. J. Med.* **83:**155–158.

89. **Wheat, L. J., C. E. Musial, and E. Jenny-Avital.** 2005. Diagnosis and management of central nervous system histoplasmosis. *Clin. Infect. Dis.* **40:**844–852.

90. **Wheat, L. J.** 2009. Approach to the diagnosis of invasive aspergillosis and candidiasis. *Clin. Chest Med.* **30:**367–377.

91. **Wheat, L. J.** 2009. Approach to the diagnosis of endemic mycoses. *Clin. Chest Med.* **30:**379–389.

92. **White, P. L., S. Bretagne, L. Klingspor, W. J. Melchers, E. McCulloch, B. Schulz, N. Finnstrom, C. Mengoli, R. A. Barnes, J. P. Donnelly, and J. Loeffler on behalf of the European Aspergillus PCR Initiative.** 2010. *Aspergillus* PCR: one step closer to standardization. *J. Clin. Microbiol.* **48:**1231–1240.

93. **White, T. J., T. Bruns, S. Lee, and J. Taylor.** 1990. Amplification and direct sequencing of fungal ribosomal RNA genes for phylogenetics. *In* M. A. Innis, D. H. Gelfand, J. J. Sninsky, and T. J. White (ed.), *PCR Protocols: A Guide to Methods and Applications.* Academic Press, Inc., New York, NY.

94. **Whittier, S., R. L. Hopfer, and P. H. Gilligan.** 1994. Elimination of false-positive serum reactivity in latex agglutination test for cryptococcal antigen in human immunodeficiency virus-infected population. *J. Clin. Microbiol.* **32:**2158–2161.

95. **Zartarian, M., E. M. Peterson, and L. M. de la Maza.** 1997. Detection of antibodies to *Coccidioides immitis* by enzyme immunoassay. *Am. J. Clin. Pathol.* **107:**148–153.

Candida, Cryptococcus, and Other Yeasts of Medical Importance

SUSAN A. HOWELL AND KEVIN C. HAZEN

115

TAXONOMY OF YEASTS

The taxonomy of yeasts is continually evolving, and currently yeasts that are of medical importance (and relevant to this chapter) belong to two classes: the Saccharomycetes (previously Hemiascomycetes or Endomycetes), which contains Candida species, and the Tremellomycetes (previously Heterobasidiomycetes), which contains the basidiomycetous fungi Trichosporon and Cryptococcus. Malassezia species are also basidiomycetous fungi but belong to a different subphylum, the Ustilaginomycetes.

Historically, species have been defined based on genetic similarity (ability to mate), morphology, or biology. Taylor et al. (243) introduced the phylogenetic concept for species identification in fungi, describing isolates of the same species as isolates that share a common evolutionary descent. The phylogenetic concept of species identification is gradually becoming ascendant, particularly because it allows isolates that lack either the ability to mate or demonstrable morphological characteristics to be identified and given a taxonomic placement.

Kurtzman and Robnett (130) examined approximately 500 ascomycetous yeasts for phylogenetic relationships using the sequence of the ~600-nucleotide D1/D2 domain of the large ribosomal subunit. Conspecific strains were found to have less than 1% sequence divergence, usually 1- to 3-nucleotide differences, whereas isolates that belonged to different species were found to have more than 1% nucleotide differences in this region. Fell et al. (82) also examined the D1/D2 and internal transcribed spacer (ITS) ribosomal DNA (rDNA) regions of basidiomycetous yeasts belonging to three classes. Both studies identified some genera that were polyphyletic, for example, species of Candida and Cryptococcus, in which members previously identified as the same species were distributed across different taxonomic classes. Other genera such as Malassezia were monophyletic and remained segregated in the same taxonomic class. The differences between traditional taxonomy and phylogenetics have occurred because too few biological characteristics are available to be compared between some organisms, and those that are shared between species may not reflect a genetic similarity (131).

The laboratorian should be familiar with both anamorph and teleomorph names for organisms. Historically, the teleomorph (sexual stage) name is used for an organism when appropriate sexual structures (such as asci and ascospores) are present. The teleomorph name is also given preference in some DNA sequence databases. The anamorph (asexual stage) name is used when a sexual stage cannot be demonstrated or does not occur. Generally, the anamorphic state is the one recovered from clinical specimens, as mating studies are usually needed to produce the teleomorphic (sexual) form. Lists of anamorph and teleomorph names can be found at http://www.doctorfungus.org and in mycology textbooks.

Genus Blastoschizomyces

Blastoschizomyces capitatus is a taxon derived from the combination of the obsolete taxa Blastoschizomyces pseudotrichosporon and Trichosporon capitatum (218). The teleomorph is Dipodascus capitatus.

Genus Candida

The heterogeneous genus Candida belongs to the order Saccharomycetales within the ascomycetes. The genus contains approximately 200 species. This number is not immutable. Technological advances that affect apparent taxonomic relationships will continually result in reassignments of present species and discovery of new species. These advances may also lead to the designation of new genera.

Teleomorphs encompassing several genera have been demonstrated for different species of Candida. The teleomorphic genera include Clavispora, Debaryomyces, Kluyveromyces, Pichia, and Yarrowia. This large number of teleomorphic relationships demonstrates that the previously designated form genus Candida within the mitosporic fungi (formerly Deuteromycota) was a mixture of phylogenetically unrelated species. One reason for the wide variety of species is the definition of Candida. The genus designation is used for any asexual yeast which does not have one of the following features: (i) acetic acid production; (ii) visually detectable red, pink, or orange pigments; (iii) arthroconidia; (iv) unipolar or bipolar budding on a broad base; (v) blastoconidia formed sympodially; (vi) buds formed on stalks; (vii) needle-shaped terminal conidia; (viii) triangular cells; (ix) enteroblastic-basipetal budding, usually with mucoid colonies and the ability to grow on inositol as a sole carbon source; and (x) ballistoconidia (129).

The genus *Candida* no longer contains species that are diazonium blue B positive, a trait associated with yeasts having a basidiomycetous affinity (such as *Cryptococcus*). Diazonium blue B-positive organisms (e.g., *Candida humicola, Candida curvata, Candida diffluens,* and *Candida scottii*) have been reassigned to either the *Cryptococcus* or *Rhodotorula* genus.

A number of species have been merged into *Candida albicans,* including *Candida claussenii* and *Candida langeronii* (257). *C.albicans* var. *africana* is a germ tube-positive, chlamydospore-negative yeast closely related to *Candida albicans* (216). Recent multilocus sequence typing placed *Candida stellatoidea* type I with *C. africana,* in a group of strains highly distinct from the majority of *C. albicans* strains (120), so the position of this group remains controversial. *C. stellatoidea* type II has been redefined as a sucrose-negative variant of *C. albicans* (133, 213).

Recent phylogenetic studies have suggested that many species are now species complexes, made up of phylogenetically closely related but largely morphologically indistinguishable species. Based on genetic and phenotypic evidence, Tavanti et al. (240) have recommended that *Candida parapsilosis* groups II and III be designated *Candida orthopsilosis* sp. nov. and *Candida metapsilosis* sp. nov. Similarly, *Candida guilliermondii* was found to be a heterogeneous species complex that contained strains indistinguishable by phenotype, but karyotyping and DNA/DNA reassociation studies indicated that there were several species in this complex (248). Sequencing of the D1/D2 domains showed little variance; however, ITS sequencing supported the DNA reassociation data and the new species *Candida fermentati* (teleomorph *Pichia carribica*) and *Candida carpophila* were confirmed. The closely related but phenotypically indistinguishable *Candida bracarensis* (61) and *Candida nivariensis* (3) were detected among isolates of *Candida glabrata.* Although these species can be phylogenetically distinguished from one another, their clinical and epidemiological significance remains to be determined.

Genus *Cryptococcus*

The taxonomy of the *C. neoformans-Cryptococcus gattii* species complex has been reviewed recently (32). Two species and five serotypes have now been formed from *C. neoformans.* Serotype A was proposed by some as *C. neoformans* var. *grubii* and by others as the distinct species *Cryptococcus grubii.* Serotype D was recognized as *C. neoformans* var. *neoformans.* The A/D serotype was recognized as an intervarietal *C. grubii/C. neoformans* hybrid. Serotypes B and C were recognized as the distinct species *C. gattii.* Serotypes A and D were found to produce the teleomorphic state *Filobasidiella neoformans,* and serotypes B and C produce the teleomorph originally named *Filobasidiella bacillispora.*

Genus *Malassezia*

There are currently 13 species of *Malassezia*: *Malassezia dermatis, M. furfur, M. globosa, M. japonica, M. nana, M. obtusa, M. restricta, M. slooffiae, M. sympodialis, M. yamatoensis* (97, 113, 236–238), *M. pachydermatis, M. caprae,* and *M. equina* (37), and the last three species are zoophilic. *Malassezia* species have a basidiomycetous affiliation within the subphylum Ustilaginomycotina (82). Species may be distinguished genetically by karyotyping (25), large-subunit rDNA sequence (97), using PCR (101, 151), using PCR-restriction fragment length polymorphism (166), by amplified fragment length polymorphism and sequence analysis (100), and by phenotype using cell morphology and a series of biochemical tests (97, 99).

Genus *Pichia*

The teleomorphic genus *Pichia* encompasses several species of *Candida* (for example, *C. guilliermondii* var. *guilliermondii* and *Candida norvegensis*). *Pichia anomala* and *Pichia angusta* are the teleomorphs of the obsolete species *Hansenula anomala* (*Candida pelliculosa*) and *Hansenula polymorpha*, respectively. Recently, *P. anomala* was renamed *Wickerhamomyces anomalus* (131) following a phylogenetic reevaluation of some species of the genus. *Kodomaea ohmeri*, previously classified as *Pichia ohmeri*, is the teleomorph of *Candida guilliermondii* var. *membranifaciens*.

Genus *Trichosporon*

Trichosporon beigelii used to be known as the major human pathogen of the genus *Trichosporon*. However, isolates of *T. beigelii* have been described as variable in their morphology and physiology (139). In 1992, this genus underwent a major revision and 19 taxa were recognized, casting doubt on the use of *T. beigelii* as a valid species name (98).

DESCRIPTION OF THE AGENTS

Yeasts are unicellular, eukaryotic, budding cells, generally round to oval or, less often, elongate or irregular in shape. They multiply principally by the production of blastoconidia (buds), such that a typical medically important yeast is composed of a progenitor cell with one or more attached progeny. When blastoconidia are produced one from the other in a linear fashion without separating, a structure termed a pseudohypha is formed. Under certain circumstances, such as growth under reduced-oxygen tension, some yeasts may produce true septate hyphae.

Cultures of yeasts are moist, creamy, or glabrous to membranous in texture. Several produce a capsule which makes the colony mucoid. With rare exceptions, aerial hyphae are not produced. Colonies may be hyaline or brightly colored, or they may be darkly pigmented due to the presence of melanins. The latter group, referred to as phaeoid fungi and belonging to the class Eurotiomycetes, is discussed in chapter 122. Dimorphic fungal pathogens possessing a yeast phase in tissue are discussed in chapters 120 and 122.

Yeasts are generally identified by observing the macroscopic and microscopic features mentioned above. In the routine laboratory, biochemical tests in the forms of manual kits or automated instruments are used to obtain a species identification. However, when organisms that show distinct variations in test results are detected, the phenotypic identification is often of low certainty. These variants may represent separate species not defined by the phenotypic database used by the test instrument. Investigation of phenotype variants by molecular methods has led to the identification of new species, for example, *Candida dubliniensis* and *C. africana*, which were both described as variants of *C. albicans* for some time. Molecular methods offer tremendous promise for facilitating accurate and quick species identification.

Genus *Blastoschizomyces*

Macroscopically, colonies are glabrous with radiating edges, white to cream colored, and shiny. Microscopically, isolates produce true hyphae, pseudohyphae, and annelloconidia resembling arthroconidia (Fig. 1f). Based on morphological features alone, *B. capitatus* can be difficult to separate from *Trichosporon* spp., and physiological tests are needed. *B. capitatus* is nonfermentative and can be separated from *Trichosporon* spp. by growth on Sabouraud dextrose agar at

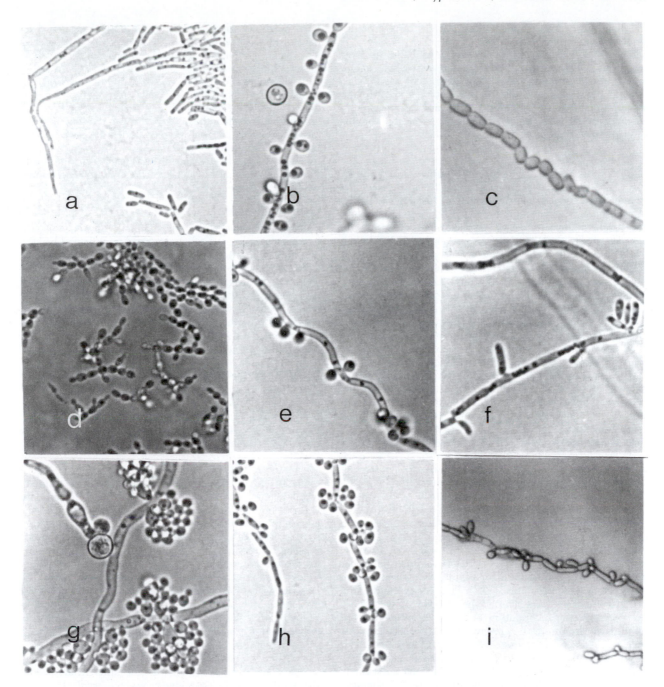

FIGURE 1 Morphological features of some yeast and yeast-like organisms on cornmeal agar at 24 to 48 h and ambient temperature. (a) *Candida krusei*: extremely elongated, rarely branched pseudohyphae; few blastoconidia. (b) *Candida tropicalis*: blastoconidia formed at septa and between septa. (c) *Geotrichum candidum*: arthroconidia. (d) *Candida guilliermondii*: chains of blastoconidia forming sparse pseudohyphae in a young culture. (e) *Candida lusitaniae*: short distinctly curved pseudohyphae with blastoconidia formed at, and occasionally between, septa. (f) *Blastoschizomyces capitatus*: true hyphae and annelloconidia resembling arthroconidia. (g) *Candida albicans*: blastoconidia, chlamydospores, true hyphae, and pseudohyphae. (h) *Candida parapsilosis*: elongated, delicately curved pseudohyphae with blastoconidia at septa. (i) *Trichosporon* spp.: blastoconidia formed at the corners of arthroconidia. Magnification, ×370. (Courtesy of B. A. Davis.)

45°C and on cycloheximide-containing agar at room temperature, and failure to hydrolyze urea.

Dipodascus capitatus is the teleomorph of *Blastoschizomyces capitatus*. *D. capitatus* is heterothallic and asci are round to ellipsoidal, containing hyaline ellipsoidal ascospores. Only glucose, galactose, glycerol, D,L-lactate, and succinate assimilation tests are positive; hyphae, arthroconidia, and clavate conidia with truncated bases may be seen. The organism grows at 37 to 45°C.

Genus *Candida*

Blastoconidia of *Candida* spp. vary in shape, from round to oval to elongate. Occasional initial isolates, especially from patients receiving antimicrobial agents, may be highly pleomorphic. Asexual reproduction is by multilateral budding, and true mycelium may be present. Several species of *Candida*, most notably *C. albicans*, are diploid (182).

Appearance of pseudohyphae and attachment of blastoconidia are important characteristics to observe when identifying *Candida* spp. Figure 1 illustrates these morphological features. Observation of germ tubes and chlamydospores is also helpful in identifying *C. albicans*. Growth on fungal media can be detected as early as 24 h; however, colonies usually are visible in 48 to 72 h as white to cream colored or tan. They are creamy in texture and may become more membranous and convoluted with age. Occasionally, initial isolates of *C. albicans* on Sabouraud dextrose agar are wrinkled or rugose but revert to smooth colonies on subculture. In our experience, many isolates of *C. albicans* produce "colonies with feet" (i.e., colonies with short marginal extensions) on blood agar while most other yeasts do not, with the exception that this might be observed in 25% of isolates of *Candida tropicalis* and *Candida krusei* (35). These colonies should not be used to perform germ tube tests because hyphal or pseudohyphal cells will be present in the inoculum.

Colonies of *C. krusei* tend to spread radially on Sabouraud dextrose agar and blood agar, which can be a useful clue to the identification of the organism. Most *Candida* spp. grow well aerobically at 25 to 30°C, and many grow at 37°C or above.

A reddish colony variant of *C. glabrata*, which would otherwise have been confused with *Rhodotorula*, has been described (192). Bile-dependent strains of *C. glabrata* have also been isolated from urine (110). These isolates either do not grow on routine media or appear as pinpoint colonies on MacConkey agar containing bile. *Candida nivariensis* can be distinguished from the closely related *C. glabrata* by its inability to assimilate trehalose. Although *C. nivariensis* was originally considered less susceptible to azoles and flucytosine than *C. glabrata*, this difference has been questioned (30, 146). *Candida bracarensis* also resembles *C. glabrata*, but it produces a different color on CHROMagar and can ferment trehalose (3, 61).

Distinguishing *C. albicans* from *C. dubliniensis* can be important, especially if the patient has been exposed to fluconazole, because the latter species can be induced to develop resistance under azole pressure (170). Several single tests have been suggested to help differentiate these two species from each other. These include growth at 45°C (positive for *C. albicans*), reduction of 2,3,5-triphenyltetrazolium chloride (positive for *C. dubliniensis*), production of a dark green color on CHROMagar (*C. dubliniensis*), production of β-glucosidase (*C. albicans*), and abundant chlamydoconidia on Staib agar (*C. dubliniensis*) (4, 187, 206, 222, 249). These tests are generally not rapid and are not definitive at separating these species (e.g., some isolates of *C. albicans* do not grow at 45°C). Other differential agar media have

been suggested (5, 122). An agglutination test has been developed that distinguishes between these two species. The Bichro-Dubli test (Fumouze Diagnostics, Levallois-Perret, France) identified 8 isolates of *C. dubliniensis* among 229 isolates recorded as *C. albicans* on the basis of their CHROMagar color (53). Molecular testing is required to obtain a definitive identification.

There is evidence that *C. albicans* var. *africana* may be a new cause of vaginitis that is often misidentified as *C. albicans* on the Vitek 2 ID-YST system (216). This species is germ tube positive but chlamydospore negative, slower to grow than *C. albicans*, and unable to assimilate N-acetylglucosamine, trehalose, or lactate (244).

Genus *Clavispora*

Clavispora lusitaniae is the teleomorph of *Candida lusitaniae*. *C. lusitaniae* cells are oval or elongated, multilateral budding occurs on a narrow base, and pseudohyphae are produced. Colonies are white to cream, smooth, and shiny (or occasionally dull). The organism is heterothallic, and conjugation of opposite mating types produces asci that quickly disintegrate, releasing one or two smooth clavate ascospores. Growth occurs at 42°C. Fermentation reactions are variable, but *C. lusitaniae* grows on a variety of sugars, including sucrose, but not on mannitol or inositol. Nitrate and urease are negative.

Genus *Cryptococcus*

The genus *Cryptococcus* contains many species, six of which are noted in Table 1. *Cryptococcus* is a round to somewhat oval yeast-like fungus ranging greatly in size, from 3.5 to 8 μm or more in diameter, with single budding and a narrow neck between parent and daughter cell (Fig. 2). Unusually large yeast cells (up to 60 μm) have been observed, and this size appears to be associated with higher incubation temperatures (147). Occasionally, several buds may be seen; rarely, pseudohyphae are observed. The cell wall is quite fragile, and it is not unusual to find collapsed or crescent-shaped cells, especially in stained tissue sections. Cells are characterized by the presence of a polysaccharide (galactoxylomannan) capsule varying from a wide halo to a nearly undetectable, lighter zone around the cells, depending upon the strain and the medium used. Colonies typically are mucoid due to the presence of capsular material, become dry and duller with age, and exhibit a wide range of colors (cream, tan, pink, or yellow). The color may darken with age. Strains possessing only a slight capsule may appear similar to colonies of *Candida*. All members of the genus produce urease, utilize various carbohydrates, and are nonfermentative.

Standard laboratory tests do not differentiate among the serotypes of *C. neoformans* and *C. gattii*. However, media have been recommended for separating serotypes A and D from serotypes B and C, but these media (glycine-cycloheximide-phenol red agar and canavanine-glycine-bromthymol blue agar) are not available commercially at this time (134, 219).

All species of *Cryptococcus* are nonfermentative aerobes. Separation of species is based upon assimilation of various carbohydrates and KNO_3 reduction (Table 1). *C. neoformans* and *C. gattii* may be distinguished from other species of *Cryptococcus* by these biochemical studies, as well as growth at 37°C, which may also be seen with *Cryptococcus albidus* and *Cryptococcus laurentii*. *C. neoformans*/*C. gattii* may be differentiated from other yeasts and from other species of *Cryptococcus* by their production of brown colonies on birdseed agar, although with occasional isolates (particularly serotype C) the production of phenol oxidase may have

TABLE 1 Cultural and biochemical characteristics of yeasts frequently isolated from clinical specimens[a]

Species	Growth at 37°C	Pellicle in broth	Pseudo- or true hyphae	Chlamydospores	Germ tubes	Capsule, India ink	Assimilation of: Glucose	Maltose	Sucrose	Lactose	Galactose	Melibiose	Cellobiose	Inositol	Xylose	Raffinose	Trehalose	Dulcitol	Fermentation of: Glucose	Malose	Sucrose	Lactose	Galactose	Trehalose	Urease	KNO₃ utilization	Phenol oxidase	Ascospores
Candida albicans	+	−	+	+[b]	+	−	+	+	+*	−	+	−	−	−	+	−	+	−	F	F	−	−	F	F	−	−	−	−
C. catenulata	+*	−	+	−	−	−	+	+	−	−	+	−	−	−	+	−	+	−	F*	F	−	−	F	F	−	−	−	−
C. dubliniensis	+	−	+	+[b]	+	−	+	+	+	−	+	−	−	−	+*	−	+	−	F	F	−	−	F	F	−	−	−	−
C. famata	+	−	−	−	−	−	+	+	+	+*	+	+	+	−	+	+	+	+*	W	−	W	−	−	W	−	−	−	−*
C. glabrata	+	−	−	−	−	−	+	+	−	−	−	−	−	−	−	−	+	−	F	−	−	−	−	F	−	−	−	−
C. guilliermondii	+	−	+	−	−	−	+	+	+	−	+	+	+	−	+	+	+	+	F	−	F	−	F*	F	−	−	−	−*
C. kefyr	+	−	+	−	−	−	+	−	+	+	+	−	+*	−	+*	+	−*	−	F	−	F	F*	F	−	−	−	−	−
C. krusei[c]	+	+	+	−	−	−	+	−	−	−	−	−	−	−	−	−	−	−	F	−	−	−	−	−	+*	−	−	−*
C. lambica	+*	+	+	−	−	−	+	−	−	−	−	−	−	−	+	−	−	−	F	−	−	−	−	−	−	−	−	−*
C. lipolytica[c]	+	+	+	−	−	−	+	−	−	−	−	−	−	−	−	−	−	−	−	−	−	−	−	−	+	−	−	−*
C. lusitaniae[d]	+	−	+	−	−	−	+	+	+	−	+	−	+	−	+	−	+	−	F	−	F	−	F	F	−	−	−	−*
C. parapsilosis[e]	+	−	+	−	−	−	+	+	+	−	+	−	−	−	+	−	+	−	F	−	−	−	−	−	−	−	−	−
C. pintolopesii[f]	+	−	−	−	−	−	+	−	−	−	−	−	−	−	−	−	−	−	−	−	F	−	−	−	−	−	−	−
C. rugosa	+	−	+	−	−	−	+	−	−	−	+	−	−	−	+*	−	−	−	−	−	−	−	−	−	−	−	−	−
C. tropicalis[d,e]	+	+	+	−[g]	−	−	+	+	+	−	+	−	+	−	+	−	+	−	F	F	F	−	F*	F*	−	−	−	−
C. zeylanoides	−	−*	+	−	−	−	+	−	−	−	−*	−	−*	−	−	−	+	−	−	−	−	−	−	−	−	−	−	−
Cryptococcus neoformans	+	−	R	−	−	+	+	+	+	−	+	−	+	+	+*	+	+	−							+	−	+	−
Cryptococcus albidus	−*	−	−	−	−	+	+	+	+	+*	+*	+	+	+	+	+	+	+*							+	+	−	−
Cryptococcus laurentii	+*	−	−	−	−	+	+	+	+	+	+	+*	+	+	+	+	+*	+							+	−	−	−
Cryptococcus luteolus	−	−	−	−	−	+	+	+	+	−	+	+	+	+	+	+	+	+							+	−	−	−
Cryptococcus terreus	−*	−	−	−	−	+	+	+*	−	+*	+*	−	−	+	+	+	+	−*							+	−	−	−
Cryptococcus uniguttulatus	−	−	−	−	−	+	+	+	+	+	−*	−	−*	+	+	+*	−*	−							+	−	−	−
Rhodotorula mucilaginosa	+	−	−	−	−	−*	+	+	+	−	+*	−	+	−	+	+	+	−							+	+	−	−
R. rubra	+	−	−	−	−	−*	+	+	+	−	+	−	+*	−	+	+	+	−							+	−	−	−
Saccharomyces cerevisiae	+	−	−*	−	−	−	+	+	+	−	+	−	−	−	−	+	+*	−	F	F	F	−	F	F*	−	−	−	+
Pichia anomala	+*	−	−	−	−	−	+	+	+	−	+	−	+	−	+	−	+	−	F	F*	F	−	F	−	−	+	−	+
Geotrichum candidum[h]	−*	+	+	−	−	−	+	−	−	−	+	−	−	−	+	−	−	−							−	−	−	−
Blastoschizomyces capitatus	+	+	+	−	−	−	+	−	−	−	+	−	−	−	−	−	−	−							−	−	−	−
Prototheca wickerhamii[h]	+	−	−	−	−	−	+	−	−	−	+	−	−	−	−	−	+	−							−	−	−	−
Sporobolomyces salmonicolor	+*	+	+*	−	−	−	+	+	+	−	+*	−	+	−	W	−	+	−							+	+	−	−
Trichosporon asahii	+	−	+	−	−	−	+	+	+*	+	+	−	+	+*	+*	−	+*	−							+	−	−	−
Trichosporon mucoides	+	−	+	−	−	−	+	+	+	+	+	+	+	+	+	+	+	+							+	−	−	−
Trichosporon ovoides	+*	−	+	−	−	−	+	+	+	+	+	+	+	+	+	+	+								+	−	−	−

[a]Modified from references 204 and 252. Symbols: +, growth greater than that of the negative control; −, negative reaction; *, some isolates may give the opposite reaction; R, rare; F, the sugar is fermented (i.e., gas is produced); W, weak reaction.

[b]*C. albicans* typically produces single and no more than two terminal chlamydospores, while some isolates of *C. dubliniensis* produce terminal chlamydospore in pairs, triplets, and clusters. See discussion in text for additional methods to differentiate *C. dubliniensis* and *C. albicans*.

[c]*C. lipolytica* assimilates erythritol; *C. krusei* does not. Maximum growth temperatures are 43 to 45°C for *C. krusei* and 33 to 37°C for *C. lipolytica*.

[d]*C. lusitaniae* assimilates rhamnose; *C. tropicalis* usually does not.

[e]*C. parapsilosis* assimilates L-arabinose; *C. tropicalis* usually does not.

[f]*C. pintolopesii* is a thermophilic yeast capable of growth at 40 to 42°C.

[g]Rare strains of *C. tropicalis* produce teardrop-shaped chlamydospores.

[h]Not yeasts but may be confused with several yeast genera.

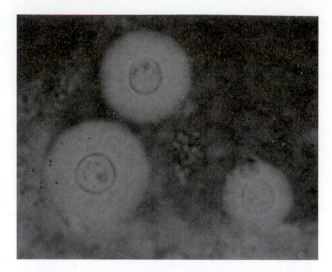

FIGURE 2 India ink preparation of *Cryptococcus neoformans*. Magnification, ×400. (Courtesy of E. S. Jacobson.)

to be induced. Differentiation from the genus *Rhodotorula*, which also occasionally forms a capsule, produces urease, and is nonfermentative, usually is accomplished by noting utilization of inositol (Table 1) and absence of carotenoid pigments characteristically present in *Rhodotorula*.

Genus *Debaryomyces*

Debaryomyces contains at least 15 species that may be found in the environment, in the gastrointestinal (GI) tract of vertebrates, and in processed foods, dairy products, and meat. The species of human importance is *Debaryomyces hansenii*, the teleomorph of *Candida famata*.

On culture the yeast may be grayish white to yellowish, soft, shiny or dull, and smooth or with wrinkles. Budding yeasts and, rarely, pseudohyphae may be seen. Conjugation between mother cell and bud occurs, and asci containing one to four round or oval warty ascospores are formed. Fermentation reactions are variable, urease is negative, nitrate is negative, inositol is negative, and the maximum growth temperature is 35°C. However, growth at 37°C is not a reliable characteristic to distinguish the closely related *D. hansenii* and *Debaryomyces fabryi*, while riboflavin production is more specific to *D. fabryi* and *Debaryomyces subglobosus*

(teleomorph of *Candida famata* var. *flareri*) (180). *D. hansenii* is often misidentified as *Pichia guilliermondii* (teleomorph of *Candida guilliermondii*), but these species can be distinguished by the assimilation of D,L-lactate and lack of pseudohyphal formation in *D. hansenii* and the reverse for *P. guilliermondii* (73), although the production of pseudohyphae may not occur in all strains (M. Brandt, personal communication).

Genus *Malassezia*

Twelve of the thirteen species require lipid for growth; only *M. pachydermatis* can grow independently of lipid supplementation of the media. Van Abbe (247) and Leeming and Notman (140) have designed media optimal for the growth and isolation of all of the *Malassezia* species. These media are not commercially available, and the alternative of overlaying Sabouraud dextrose agar with a few drops of sterile olive oil has been used, but some of the more fastidious species do not survive on this medium (164). The inoculated media should be incubated aerobically at 32 to 35°C in a moist atmosphere for up to 2 weeks to permit development of the slower-growing species. Colonies are cream to beige and smooth to deeply folded, and they have a brittle texture that is frequently difficult to suspend.

Malassezia is distinguished microscopically from other yeasts by the formation of a prominent monopolar bud scar or collarette, resulting from the continued formation of daughter cells at that site (Fig. 3d). These structures are absent from *C. glabrata*, which could otherwise be confused with *Malassezia* species due to its small size and typical unipolar budding. Sympodial budding has been observed in cultures of *M. sympodialis* and *M. japonica*. The species vary in shape from spherical to oval or elongated, have thick cell walls, and range in length from 1.5 to 8 μm. Identification of the individual species is not routinely attempted but can be achieved based on morphology, utilization of certain lipids (including Tween 20, 40, and 80 and Cremophor [castor oil]), and reactions with esculin and catalase (99, 164) (Table 2). Organisms that are identified as *Candida lipolytica* (glucose, glycerol, and sorbitol positive) with the API 20C AUX (bioMérieux SA, Marcy l'Etoile, France) may actually be *M. pachydermatis* (152). In this case, morphology is helpful.

Genus *Pichia*

Variations in colony morphology may cause confusion with *Cryptococcus* and *Candida* spp. Texture may be smooth to wrinkled, and color may be white, cream, or tan.

TABLE 2 *Malassezia* species phenotypic characteristics[a]

Species	Cell shape	Lipid requiring	Tween 20	Tween 40	Tween 60	Tween 80	Cremophor	Catalase	Growth at 37°C	Bud type
M. caprae	Round/oval	+	−	+	+	V	−	+	W	Narrow base
M. dermatis	Oval/round	+	+	+	+	+	W	+	+	ND
M. equina	Oval	+	W	+	+	+	−	+	W	Narrow base
M. furfur	Oval/round	+	+	+	V−	+	V	+	+	Broad base
M. globosa	Round	+	−	−	−	−	−	+	W	Narrow base
M. japonica	Round/oval	+	−	V	+	−	ND	+	+	Sympodial
M. nana	Oval	+	V	+	+	V	−	+	+	Narrow base
M. obtusa	Oval/round	+	−	−	−	−	−	+	W	Broad base
M. pachydermatis	Oval	−	+	+	+	+	V	V	+	Broad base
M. restricta	Round/oval	+	−	−	−	−	−	−	W	Narrow base
M. slooffiae	Oval/round	+	V	+	+	W	−	+	+	Broad base
M. sympodialis	Oval	+	W	+	+	+	W	+	+	Sympodial
M. yamatoensis	Oval	+	+	+	+	+	ND	+	+	Narrow base

[a]Based on references 10 and 37. +, positive; −, negative; W, weak; V, variable; ND, not determined.

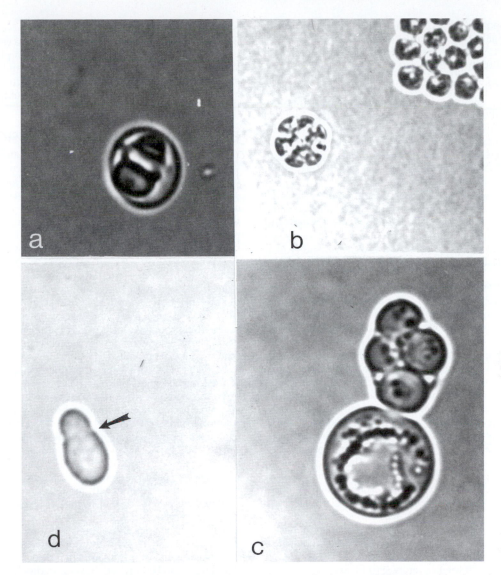

FIGURE 3 Diagnostic features of selected yeasts. (a) Ascus of *Pichia anomala* containing hat-shaped ascospores; (b) sporangium of *Prototheca wickerhamii* containing sporangiospores; (c) *Saccharomyces cerevisiae* with vegetative cell and ascus containing four globose ascospores; (d) bottle-shaped, budding yeast demonstrating annelloconidium and collarette (arrow) of *Malassezia furfur*. Magnification, ×1,000. (Courtesy of B. A. Davis.)

Microscopically, multilateral budding cells are observed; yeasts and pseudohyphae may be seen.

Individual species of *Pichia* are either homothallic or heterothallic. *P. anomala* is heterothallic, but the sporogenous diploid form occurs naturally and is the one usually recovered from clinical specimens. These diploid cells convert to form asci which disintegrate to reveal one to four hat (or saturn)-shaped ascopores (Fig. 3a), a morphology which is characteristic of *Pichia* species. Carbohydrate assimilation and fermentation studies are needed to identify the individual species, although urease is negative, nitrate is positive, inositol is negative, and growth at 37°C can be variable.

Genus *Rhodotorula*

Rhodotorula spp. share many similar physiological and morphological properties with *Cryptococcus* spp. Both are round to oval, multilateral budding yeasts with capsules; produce urease; and fail to ferment carbohydrates. *Rhodotorula* spp.

differ from cryptococci by their inability to assimilate inositol and their obvious carotenoid pigment. When a capsule is present, it is typically small, unlike for *C. neoformans*. The commonest *Rhodotorula* pathogens are *Rhodotorula mucilaginosa* and *Rhodotorula glutinis*. *R. mucilaginosa* can be distinguished from *R. glutinis* by nitrate assimilation, as the former is negative. This is a useful additional test, as occasionally commercial kits fail to distinguish these species (71).

Genus *Saccharomyces*

Saccharomyces cerevisiae is the most common species of the genus recovered in the clinical laboratory. Multilateral budding yeast cells are round to oval, and short rudimentary (occasionally well-developed) pseudohyphae may be formed. Ascospore production can be enhanced easily by growing the yeast on Fowell's acetate agar (87; see chapter 113) for 2 to 5 days at room temperature. Asci contain one to four round, smooth ascospores (Fig. 3c). Other physiological properties are listed in Table 1. Assimilation of raffinose by *S. cerevisiae* is noteworthy. Very few yeasts encountered in the clinical laboratory utilize this carbon source.

Genus *Sporobolomyces*

Sporobolomyces spp. are basidiomycetous yeasts that are environmental organisms. Three species have been isolated from human infection: *Sporobolomyces roseus*, *Sporobolomyces holsaticus*, and *Sporobolomyces salmonicolor*, the last two species having the teleomorphs *Sporidiobolus johnsonii* (homothallic) and *Sporidiobolus salmonicolor* (heterothallic), respectively.

The colonies are soft and shades of salmon pink. Budding oval to ellipsoidal yeasts, pseudohyphae, and ballistoconidia on large sterigmata may be seen. Fermentation is absent and assimilation is variable; colonies are sucrose positive, urease positive, nitrate positive, and inositol negative, and growth at 37°C is variable.

Genus *Trichosporon*

Trichosporon yeasts have no known sexual state, are basidiomycetes, and are closely related to *Cryptococcus*. They grow easily on standard mycological laboratory media, do not ferment carbohydrates, can assimilate various complex sugars, and are urease positive. Colonies form usually within a week on solid media and are cream colored and smooth. They may become dry, moist or shiny, folded, cerebriform, and elevated, with or without marginal zones with age.

They produce blastoconidia of various shapes, well-developed hyphae, pseudohyphae, and arthroconidia (Fig. 1i). *Trichosporon loubieri* also produces one- and two-celled giant cells (189), while *Trichosporon mycotoxinivorans* produces giant cells with up to eight cells depending on the growth medium (K. C. Hazen, C. C. Moore, and D. M. Padgett, unpublished observation). In cases where a *Trichosporon* isolate produces only a few blastoconidia, differentiation from *Geotrichum* spp. may be difficult. Inoculation of malt extract broth at room temperature encourages blastoconidium production in *Trichosporon* spp., usually within 48 to 72 h. These morphological and physiological characteristics have been used to distinguish among the species in the laboratory (96) (Table 3).

Genus *Yarrowia*

The only human-associated pathogen in the genus *Yarrowia* is *Yarrowia lipolytica*, which is the teleomorph of *Candida lipolytica*. *C. lipolytica* is infrequently isolated, although it appears to be an emerging pathogen. It is urease positive, and isolates vary in their susceptibilities to amphotericin B, fluconazole, itraconazole, and caspofungin.

EPIDEMIOLOGY AND TRANSMISSION

Medically important yeasts are found on humans and other warm-blooded animals and in the environments they inhabit (reviewed in reference 184). Some yeasts, such as *Candida albicans*, *Candida glabrata*, and most likely *Candida dubliniensis*, appear to be obligatory saprobes of humans and some other warm-blooded animals. Environmental sampling of foods, plants, potable water, and juices (pasteurized and unpasteurized) has revealed an amazing array of yeast species known as opportunistic pathogens. In all cases, the presence of these yeasts could be attributed to direct and indirect warm-blooded animal contamination. For example, Arias et al. (9) noted the presence of *C. parapsilosis*, *C. tropicalis*, *Clavispora lusitaniae*, *Candida zeylanoides*, and several other yeast species in single-strength orange juice which had been pasteurized but subsequently contaminated. These observations make clear that immunocompromised patients are repeatedly exposed to potential yeast pathogens other than those residing as part of their normal microbiota, and care should be exercised in preparing foods and in monitoring the level of contamination associated with devices or creams which may be applied to the patient (149, 193). Parenteral nutrition fluids and devices are particularly prone to contamination with yeasts, especially *C. parapsilosis* (245). It is also noteworthy that the hospital environment can contribute to the development of colonization with *Candida* species as well as facilitate replacement of colonizing less virulent species with more virulent species (26).

Person-to-person transmission has a negligible impact on disease development, except in nosocomial outbreaks, in which hands or fomites are often the source. Invasive yeast infections are associated with opportunism; thus, the yeasts causing disease must be present when the conditions are such that disease can be initiated. Several studies have shown that

TABLE 3 Characteristics of clinically important *Trichosporon* species[a]

Characteristic	*T. asahii*	*T. asteroides*	*T. cutaneum*	*T. inkin*	*T. loubieri*	*T. mucoides*	*T. mycotoxinivorans*	*T. ovoides*
Assimilation of:								
Melibiose	−	−	+	−	+	+	+	−
Raffinose	−	−	+	−	+	+	+	V
L-Rhamnose	+	−	+	−	V	+	+	+
L-Arabinitol	+	+	+	−	V	+	W	−
Galactitol (dulcitol)	−	−	−	−	−	+	+	−
Ribitol (adonitol)	V	V	+	−	?	+	?	−
Sorbitol	−	V	+	−	V	+	+	−
Xylitol	V	+	+	−	V	+	W[a]	V
Growth at 37°C	+	V	−	+	+	+	+	+
Growth at 42°C	−	−	−	V	+	−	−	−
Urease	+	+	+	+	+	+	+	+
Growth on 0.01% cycloheximide	+	V	−	V	+	+	+	+
Growth on 0.1% cycloheximide	−	V	−	−	+	+	+	−
Appressoria (on slide culture)	−	−	−	+	−	−	−	+
Fusiform giant cells	−	−	−	−	+	−	+	−

[a]Modified from references 96, 167, 189, and 252.
[b]Symbols: +, growth greater than negative control; −, negative; V, variable; W, weakly positive; ?, not reported.

transmission of yeasts through sexual contact (including oral) does occur, but establishment of the transferred organisms in the recipient is affected by a variety of factors, most notably the recipient's current normal microbiota, immunological status, and antifungal status (74, 211). Regarding the last factor, recipients with human immunodeficiency virus (HIV) and on low-dose fluconazole have been documented to develop oral colonization with a partner's fluconazole-resistant isolate through salivary exchange (74).

Genus *Candida*

Candida species are ubiquitous yeasts, being found on many plants and as the normal biota of the alimentary tract of mammals and mucocutaneous membranes of humans (184). Essentially all areas of the GI tract of humans can harbor *Candida.* The most commonly isolated species (50 to 70% of yeast isolates) from the GI tract of humans is *C. albicans,* followed by *C. tropicalis, C. parapsilosis,* and *C. glabrata.*

Candidemia is the fourth commonest cause of hospital-acquired bloodstream infection in the United States and much of the rest of the developed world and accounts for more than half of all episodes of sepsis in nonneutropenic patients in an intensive care unit (ICU) or surgical ward (190). A surveillance study of bloodstream infections in the United States, Canada, Latin America, and Europe from 1997 to 1999 (198) reported that over 55% of bloodstream infections were due to *C. albicans,* 15% were due to *C. glabrata* and *C. parapsilosis,* and 9% were due to *C. tropicalis.* The proportion of non-*C. albicans* species causing candidemia differed according to geographic location, with 45% in the United States and 55% in Latin America. *C. glabrata* accounted for 21% of the non-*C. albicans* species in the United States, and *C. parapsilosis* accounted for 25% in Latin America, 16% in Canada, and 17% in Europe. Similar trends were reported by two of the authors 6 years later (196) and in a recent study of data from Australia, Belgium, Brazil, and Greece (114).

C. albicans infections still predominate, but it is likely that the increase in non-*C. albicans* infections is linked to changes in the populations at risk. Pfaller and Diekema (196) demonstrated that older adults were more likely to be infected with *C. glabrata* than children, and associated risk factors were patient age, severity of underlying disease, use of broad-spectrum antibiotics, use of central venous catheters, and length of stay in ICU, with the link to the use of fluconazole strong only in cancer centers. *C. parapsilosis* has a greater incidence of bloodstream infections in children than in adults (196), but this organism is a known pathogen of the young (149).

A new cause of vaginitis is being reported from centers around the world following genetic characterisation of *C. africana.* In a study in Italy (216), genetic investigations of clinical *C. albicans* isolates revealed that 3% were *C. dubliniensis* isolated from vaginal, oral, and gastric fluid and 7% were *C. albicans* var. *africana* isolated exclusively from vaginal specimens. *C. africana* has been isolated from vaginitis patients from Africa, Spain, Germany, and Italy, suggesting that this variant may have a wide distribution but is associated primarily with vaginal infection. *C. africana* (identified by DNA sequencing) was recently isolated from the urine of a 14-year-old female resident of Virginia with an uncomplicated urinary tract infection, suggesting that the organism may also be in the United States (K. C. Hazen, unpublished observation).

Genus *Cryptococcus*

The organisms comprising the *C. neoformans* species complex have been reviewed (144). *C. neoformans* affects immunocompromised hosts worldwide, with *C. neoformans* var. *grubii* (serotype A) being the most commonly isolated type, although *C. neoformans* var. *neoformans* (serotype D) is more commonly isolated in Europe (32). *C. gattii* predominantly affects immunocompetent hosts in areas of endemicity, although approximately 10% of AIDS cases involve infection with this species in southern California and in parts of sub-Saharan Africa, including Botswana (144).

C. neoformans was first detected in the environment in the late 19th century, when Sanfelice recovered the yeast from peach juice. Since then, however, *C. neoformans* var. *grubii* and *C. neoformans* var. *neoformans* have been most frequently associated with pigeon (and other bird) droppings and soils contaminated with these droppings. The yeast usually is not found in fresh droppings but is most evident in the bird excreta that have accumulated over long periods on window ledges, vacant buildings, and other roosting sites (132). The environmental habitat of *C. gattii* was originally identified as being the gum tree *Eucalyptus camaldulensis;* however, a number of other trees have been indicated as sources, and it has been suggested that soil may be the main reservoir. *C. gattii* has been reported from subtropical areas and from temperate areas of Europe, Australia, Papua New Guinea, New Zealand, Colombia, and Vancouver Island in Canada (32, 144, 231, 234).

CLINICAL SIGNIFICANCE

Genus *Blastoschizomyces*

Blastoschizomyces is recognized as an emerging cause of invasive fungal disease in leukemic patients (51, 154) and those with endocarditis (208) and spondydiscitis and osteomyelitis (43). It is widely distributed in nature, has been recovered as normal skin biota and from the GI tract, and has been associated with onychomycosis (68). Disseminated disease, which is usually diagnosed by blood culture, is often associated with immunosuppressive conditions (12), in particular, neutropenia. The rate of mortality from invasive disease is high in neutropenic patients, and survival is associated with neutrophil count recovery.

Genus *Candida*

Candida spp. can be present in clinical specimens as a result of environmental contamination, colonization, or actual disease processes. An accurate diagnosis requires proper handling of clinical material, ensuring that specimens reach the laboratory in a timely fashion and have been taken and stored in an appropriate manner. *Candida* spp. that are normal biota can invade tissue and produce life-threatening pathology in patients whose immune defenses have been altered by disease or iatrogenic intervention.

C. albicans is the most common species isolated from nearly all forms of candidiasis (184). Contributing to its high association with disease is its high prevalence in the normal population, as described above. In addition, *C. albicans* appears to possess a number of virulence determinants, including proteases, adhesins, surface integrins, and switching, that may promote successful parasitism (38, 117, 177, 265).

Only *C. tropicalis* appears to be more virulent than *C. albicans* when present in patients with leukemia or lymphoreticular malignant disease (262). Other medically important *Candida* spp. include *C. catenulata, C. ciferrii, C. dubliniensis, C. guilliermondii, C. haemulonii, C. kefyr, C. krusei, C. lipolytica, C. lusitaniae, C. norvegensis, C. parapsilosis, C. pulcherrima, C. rugosa, C. utilis, C. viswanathii,* and

C. zeylanoides (108, 215). This list is not exclusive, as other rare agents will certainly be added in the future. The species that are emerging as opportunistic pathogens include *C. (Yarrowia) lipolytica*, *C. lusitaniae*, and *C. krusei*. These three species have been isolated from cases of fungemia. Two other fluconazole-resistant species, *C. inconspicua* and *C. norvegensis*, are rare agents of candidiasis.

C. glabrata is emerging as a significant pathogen, with a relatively high proportion of strains exhibiting reduced susceptibility to fluconazole. *C. glabrata* is regarded as a symbiont of humans and can be isolated routinely from the oral cavity and the genitourinary, alimentary, and respiratory tracts of most individuals. As an agent of serious infection, it has been associated with endocarditis (41), meningitis (7), and multifocal, disseminated disease (112). It is recovered often from urine specimens and has been estimated to account for as much as 20% of *Candida* urinary tract infections (85). As it may be slow growing, routine urine cultures should be incubated for at least 2 days. Two other yeasts that may resemble *C. glabrata* are *C. nivariensis*, which is an emerging cause of deep infection, and *C. bracarensis*, which has been isolated from AIDS patients.

C. dubliniensis is most frequently isolated from the oropharynx of HIV-positive patients but may infrequently be recovered from blood, urine, and vaginal or other specimen sites, especially if the patient is immunocompromised. Acute pseudomembranous oral candidiasis is the presentation seen in patients with compromised cell-mediated immunity. It is most often caused by *C. albicans* and *C. dubliniensis*. It may be present in the prodromal stages of AIDS or accompany late stages of AIDS (CD4 T-cell count of <400 cells/μl) (201, 241). Mucocutaneous forms of candidiasis are often related to defects in cell-mediated immunity, while systemic spread is generally associated with neutropenia (201, 241). Thus, despite the presence of oral or esophageal candidiasis, systemic spread of *Candida* organisms is uncommon in AIDS patients. When it occurs, systemic spread is associated with a drop in the neutrophil count (75).

Genus *Clavispora*

Clavispora lusitaniae is a normal component of the human GI tract but is an emerging opportunist causing fungemia mainly of patients with malignancy. Other occasional infections include peritonitis, urinary tract infection, and meningitis (107).

Genus *Cryptococcus*

Cryptococcus neoformans var. *grubii*, *C. neoformans* var. *neoformans*, and *C. gattii* are considered the only human pathogens in the genus *Cryptococcus*, although *C. albidus* (116, 128) and a few others, including *C. adeliensis*, rarely have been implicated in disease in severely debilitated individuals (103, 214). Differences in disease manifestation among patients from areas where various serotypes are endemic appear to be more dependent on host immune status than on *C. neoformans* variety (48). Serotypes A and D are opportunistic pathogens in that they attack immunocompromised individuals. Serotypes B and C infect immunocompetent as well as immunosuppressed individuals and are therefore primary pathogens.

Initial cryptococcal infection begins by inhalation of the fungus into the lungs, usually followed by hematogenous spread to the brain and meninges. Involvement of the skin, bones, and joints is seen, and *C. neoformans* is often cultured from the urine of patients with disseminated infection. In patients without HIV infection, cryptococcosis, particularly cryptococcal meningitis, usually is seen in association with

underlying conditions such as lupus erythematosus, sarcoidosis, leukemia, lymphomas, and Cushing's syndrome.

In nearly 45% of AIDS patients, cryptococcosis was reported as the first AIDS-defining illness. Because none of the presenting signs or symptoms of cryptococcal meningitis (such as headache, fever, and malaise) are sufficiently characteristic to distinguish it from other infections that occur in patients with AIDS, determining cryptococcal antigen titers and culturing blood and cerebrospinal fluid (CSF) are useful in making a diagnosis (54).

Genus *Debaryomyces*

D. hansenii has been isolated from pigeon droppings (158) and is an infrequent cause of fungemia and endophthalmitis (210, 235).

Genus *Malassezia*

Malassezia yeasts are isolated from the skin of humans and other warm-blooded animals as commensals but can be agents of dermatological diseases. *M. sympodialis*, *M. slooffiae*, *M. globosa*, and *M. restricta* are the most frequent human colonizers (27, 28, 63, 97). The main causative agents of the skin infection pityriasis versicolor are *M. globosa*, *M. sympodialis*, and, occasionally, *M. slooffiae* or *M. furfur* (11, 64, 102, 178). Other dermatological diseases, including seborrhoeic dermatitis and folliculitis, have been associated with *Malassezia* yeasts, often because there was a clinical response following antifungal therapy, with a reduction in yeast numbers. *M. restricta*, *M. globosa*, *M. furfur*, *M. sympodialis*, and *M. obtusa* have all been recovered from patients with seborrhoeic dermatitis, and *M. restricta* and *M. globosa* have been isolated from patients with folliculitis (10). However, as *Malassezia* may be present on the skin in high numbers and there are no other characteristic features to provide laboratory diagnosis, the exact role of the organisms in these diseases remains unclear. There have been reports of onychomycosis caused by *Malassezia* species (52, 65, 229); however, whether these yeasts are true invaders of nail or secondary colonizers is undecided. In addition, *M. furfur* and *M. pachydermatis* may, rarely, cause systemic infections, usually of neonates in ICUs (152, 164).

Genus *Pichia*

Pichia anomala and *Pichia angusta* are the two species in the genus *Pichia* that are most commonly associated with disease in humans. *Pichia anomala* is found mainly in the environment but is an opportunistic pathogen that can colonize human skin and has been a cause of fungemia in neonates (13, 45). It has also been associated with catheter-related infections (6, 126, 179). *Pichia angusta* has been recovered from mediastinal lymph nodes of a child with chronic granulomatous disease (160). *Kodomaea (Pichia) ohmeri* has been increasingly reported as an agent of disease in immunocompromised patients (reviewed in reference 106). There have been a number of reports of human infection caused by *Pichia* species, several of which have been fully identified only by DNA sequencing, as routine microbiological tests were not conclusive: *P. fabianii* was recently described as a cause of endocarditis (105) and *P. farinosa* as a cause of bloodstream infection in a lymphoma patient (1).

Genus *Rhodotorula*

Rhodotorula spp. are normal inhabitants of moist skin and can be recovered from such environmental sources as shower curtains, bathtub grout, and toothbrushes (60). In rare instances, *Rhodotorula* spp. have been reported to cause septicemia (202), meningitis (209), systemic infection (118, 217), peritonitis associated with peritoneal dialysis (77), and sepsis related to complications from indwelling central venous catheters (124).

Genus *Saccharomyces*

Usually thought to be nonpathogenic, *Saccharomyces cerevisiae* has been reported to cause thrush, vulvovaginitis, empyema, and fungemia (60, 79, 108). Person-to-person contact and exposure to commercial strains associated with health foods and baking may contribute to the ability of the organisms to colonize and infect human hosts (159).

Genus *Sporobolomyces*

Sporobolomyces spp. are environmental organisms, some of which have been linked to human diseases, including dermatitis (23), respiratory disease (59, 227), and AIDS (172, 207), and *Sporobolomyces* has been reported as a cause of endophthalmitis (228). Three species have been isolated from human infection: *S. roseus*, *S. holsaticus*, and *S. salmonicolor.*

Genus *Trichosporon*

Trichosporon beigelii used to be known as the major human pathogen in the genus *Trichosporon*, primarily causing the superficial hair infection white piedra and, rarely, causing systemic disease referred to as trichosporonosis. Some mycologists continue to designate *T. beigelii* as the etiologic agent responsible for clinical disease caused by *Trichosporon* yeasts because differentiating among species can be problematic, but this practice is not correct.

Yeasts of this genus may be isolated from soil, animals, and humans, but nearly all systemic human infections are usually caused by one of six species: *T. asahii*, *T. asteroides*, *T. cutaneum*, *T. inkin*, *T. mucoides*, and *T. ovoides*. *T. loubieri* is an apparently rare cause of disseminated trichosporonosis (156, 189), *T. japonicum* has been isolated from the sputum of a neutropenic child (2), and *T. mycotoxinivorans* (167) has also been associated with disseminated disease (Hazen et al., unpublished). White piedra is a superficial infection characterized by nodules of approximately 0.5 mm attached to the hair shafts on the head, axilla, or genital area. Infections in the genital area are usually due to *T. inkin*, and rarely encountered infections of hairs on the head are caused by *T. ovoides*. *T. asteroides* and *T. cutaneum* have been associated with superficial skin lesions, and *T. asahii*, and less often *T. mucoides*, is the cause of disseminated infection mainly associated with neutropenic patients with hematological malignancy or receiving immunosuppressive therapy (76). Others at risk for trichosporonosis include patients with AIDS, extensive burns, or intravenous catheters; those receiving corticosteroids; or those who have undergone heart valve surgery (42, 62, 171). In addition, *T. asahii* and *T. mucoides* are thought to be the major causes of summer-type hypersensitivity pneumonitis in Japan, a condition that results from inhalation of arthroconidia present in the homes of the patients (181).

COLLECTION, TRANSPORT, AND STORAGE OF SPECIMENS

No special practices for collection or transport of specimens from patients with suspected yeast infection need be followed. The reader is referred to chapter 112 of this *Manual* for standard practices for collection, transport, and storage. However, when specimens are collected and sent to the laboratory, consideration should be given to the possibility that a particular fungus is highly infectious (e.g., *Coccidioides*

species) or has unusual growth requirements (e.g., lipids for *Malassezia* species). Such information regarding the suspected etiologic agent should be provided to the laboratory in a manner that precedes manipulation of the specimen.

Transportation of specimens should be accomplished in less than 2 h. If a delay is anticipated, specimens should be stored at 4°C. Yeasts can withstand normal refrigeration temperatures.

DIRECT EXAMINATION

The appropriate examination of a clinical specimen prior to proper processing of the material is essential. Additionally, it often aids the laboratorian and the physician in obtaining a preliminary identification and in either ruling in or ruling out certain pathogenic yeasts. Some methods are universal to the preliminary observation of fungi in a specimen, e.g., Gram stain, calcofluor, and 20% potassium hydroxide (KOH). If 20% KOH is used on a preparation, neither India ink nor Gram stain may be subsequently added. Chapter 113 describes in more detail various stains and examination procedures used in the mycology laboratory.

Microscopy

In performing the microscopic examination of a specimen for yeasts, features may be observed that may aid in identification (Fig. 4): (i) size and shape of the organism, (ii) morphology of the bud attachment site and number of buds, (iii) presence or absence of a capsule, (iv) thickness of the cell wall, (v) presence of pseudohyphae, and (vi) presence of arthroconidia. A great deal of information can be gleaned from careful direct microscopic examination of an appropriately prepared and stained specimen.

KOH

Wet mounts prepared in 10 to 30% KOH solution may be used to distinguish fungi in mucoid secretions or in skin, hair, or nail. The KOH digests the proteinaceous material, leaving the fungal elements intact. Gentle warming may speed this process, but care should be taken when using strong concentrations of KOH, as the KOH rapidly crystallizes if overheated or left for prolonged periods before examination. The specimen is prepared by placing an aliquot onto a slide, adding to it a drop of KOH, and placing a coverslip on top. Ensure that enough KOH is present to completely cover the specimen. For skin and nail the specimen may be gently squashed while removing excess KOH. In these thick materials, this makes visualization of the fungus easier. Hairs should always be viewed without squashing to obtain maximal information about the type of fungal infection. Dimethyl sulfoxide (40% [vol/vol] in distilled water) may be added to the KOH reagent to facilitate clearing without the need for heating or incubation, but the specimen should be examined quickly. Bubbles can be confused with yeast cells. Budding cells with internal heterogeneous material should be seen in order to enhance confidence that the object is a yeast cell. Round and oval objects lacking buds are common in tissue specimens and could be erroneously identified as yeasts.

The calcofluor stain (Blankophore, Uvitex 2B) fluoresces under filtered UV light to enhance detection of fungus as it binds to chitin in the cell wall, showing as bright green (168). A specimen may be prepared as described above, the coverslip removed and a drop of calcofluor added, excess fluid removed, and the specimen viewed. Alternatively, a drop of calcofluor can be added at the time of mounting in KOH.

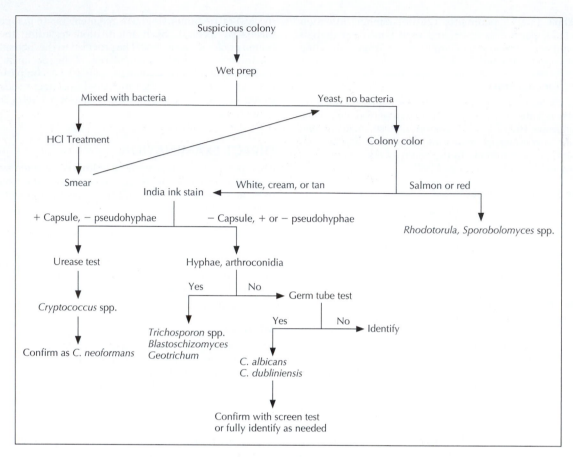

FIGURE 4 Scheme for identification of yeasts from clinical specimens.

However, the stain may fail to penetrate thick nail samples when prepared in this way.

The diagnostic feature of pityriasis versicolor seen by direct microscopic examination of skin scrapings is the presence of short blunt-ended *Malassezia* hyphae among *Malassezia* yeasts ("spaghetti and meatballs"). Visualization of *Malassezia* species can be enhanced by the use of the stain calcofluor white with UV fluorescence.

India Ink

The India ink stain is used to examine specimens of CSF, urine, and other body fluids for the presence of *Cryptococcus* species. It generally is not useful on primary specimens, such as sputum or other highly cellular material, which do not allow even distribution of the ink. India ink is used to visualize capsules which are transparent by bright-field illumination alone, as the ink is excluded from the capsule, showing a clear halo around the yeast. Artifacts such as erythrocytes, lymphocytes, or talc from gloves appear to cause a halo effect; therefore, careful examination for the presence of yeast cells and bud formation is essential. A specimen should be prepared by placing a drop of the centrifuged sediment of a fluid specimen on a slide, adding a drop of Pelikan India ink or nigrosin solution, and placing a coverslip on top. While this method is relatively rapid and is generally satisfactory, a preferred method is to place a coverslip on the specimen and place a drop of ink on the side of the coverslip to allow the ink to diffuse underneath. This provides a gradient of ink which will contain an optimal region to detect a capsule. India ink solution should

be replaced regularly, as it becomes contaminated; alternatively, a solution of 10% nigrosin in 10% formalin (using appropriate safety precautions) can be prepared.

Yeast in Tissue Sections

C. neoformans can be distinguished from other nondematiaceous yeasts in fixed tissue by the use of a Fontana-Masson stain which detects melanin precursors in the cell wall. Mucicarmine stains the capsule, which helps to distinguish *Cryptococcus* spp. from yeasts with similar morphologies. *C. neoformans* yeast cells in tissue are typically rounder than yeasts of *Candida* species and tend to vary in size.

Yeasts can be visualized in tissue using Gomori's silver stain, although they stain blackish and some of the internal detail may be difficult to see. Periodic acid-Schiff stain is also useful, and fungal material stains reddish.

Antigen Detection

Signs and symptoms of invasive yeast infections generally overlap those of bacterial infections, necessitating development of rapid non-culture-based methods for diagnosis. See chapter 114 and reference 137 for a comprehensive review of antigen testing. Non-culture-based tests for discriminating fungal versus bacterial infection and for detection of specific genera have been developed. Of all of these tests, the cryptococcal antigen test has proven the most successful, but recent progress suggests that a similarly successful *Candida* serology test may be available in the near future.

The unique composition of the fungal cell wall makes it particularly well suited as a focus for fungal serologic tests. Many of the more common pathogenic yeasts contain β-1,3-glucan in the wall. β-1,3-Glucan is detected by two commercial kits, Glucatell (Associates of Cape Cod) and Fungitek G (Seikagaku Corp.). Repeat testing for patients with negative results is recommended, as single-test positive results provide generally good sensitivities and specificities (183) and repeatedly negative tests have a high negative predictive value. Repeat testing for patients who tested positive also improves the specificity of the test (183, 250). A positive test, however, does not provide information about the specific etiology, which is a weakness if tailored antifungal therapy is desired.

Genus *Candida*

With the exception of cryptococcal antigen tests for serum and CSF, efforts to develop other genus- or species-specific antigen detection systems have focused primarily on candidemia and disseminated candidiasis. No commercially available tests have been developed for body fluids and tissues other than blood and CSF. Carbohydrate antigens have provided useful targets for several commercial kits for the detection of disseminated candidiasis. Protein antigens have also been investigated. Extracellularly secreted aspartyl proteinases appear promising (173), but no commercial test is available. Another antigen, D-arabinitol, has been under investigation for over a decade and has been incorporated into the COBAS FARA II centrifugal autoanalyzer (Roche Diagnostic Systems) (266). While only a limited number of laboratories have evaluated D-arabinitol as a marker for candidiasis, the antigen appears promising. D-Arabinitol levels appear to correlate with therapeutic success (78).

Another test, the Platelia *Candida* Ag test (Bio-Rad, Marnes La Coquette, France), utilizes monoclonal antibody EB-CA1, which targets an α-1,2-oligomannoside common among multiple species of *Candida*. The test has shown reasonable sensitivity and high specificities, although these vary from study to study. Sendid et al. (224) have recommended that both the antigen and the antibody tests (Platelia *Candida* Ab) be performed to maximize early diagnosis of invasive candidiasis. The specificity of the antigen test can be further enhanced by including a test for a second antigen, β-1,2-oligomannan, which is found in only a limited number of *Candida* species: *C. albicans, C. glabrata,* and *C. tropicalis* (225). *C. dubliniensis* variably expresses the antigen (111).

Genus *Cryptococcus*

Detection of cryptococcal antigen (capsular galactoxylomannan) in serum and CSF has been available for over two decades and detects both *C. neoformans* and *C. gattii.* During this time commercial tests have evolved to overcome early problems with specificity and sensitivity. The chief problem was false positives due to rheumatoid factor. Once this factor is destroyed, the sensitivity and specificity of the current generation of cryptococcal antigen tests are high. Antigen detection kits include the Murex Cryptococcus Test (Remel, Lenexa, KS), the Cryptococcal Antigen LA System (Meridian Bioscience Inc.), the Crypto-LA test (Inverness Medical Professional Diagnostics, Princeton, NJ), and the PREMIER Cryptococcal EIA Antigen assay (Meridian). These tests have been recommended as the primary evaluative tool in lieu of an India ink stain for screening CSF in suspected cases of cryptococcal meningitis. This is because the sensitivity of the India ink stain is low.

False-positive tests due to causes other than rheumatoid factor have been obtained. These have been associated with trichosporonosis, *Capnocytophaga canimorsus* septicemia, malignancy, *Rothia* (formerly *Stomatococcus*) bacteremia, some soaps and disinfectants, and hydroxyethyl starch (used in fluid resuscitation) (24, 46, 115, 150, 161, 165, 254). Interestingly, the cryptococcal galactoxylomannan contains an epitope that cross-reacts with the galactomannan antigen of *Aspergillus* spp., which is the antigen target of the Platelia *Aspergillus* assay (66).

Monitoring a decrease in antigen titer as an indication of effective anticryptococcal therapy has been suggested. However, while the titer may decrease after initiation of therapy in non-HIV patients, it may remain greater than 200 despite microbiological clearance (148). Lu et al. (148) have suggested that a better indicator of successful therapy is the return of CSF glucose and chloride levels and leukocyte count to normal limits. Mycological sterility is also a useful indicator of successful therapy.

Specific Tests for Invasive Infections Caused by Other Yeasts

Not surprisingly, little effort has been undertaken to develop serologic tests for detection of invasive infections caused by yeasts other than *Candida* and *Cryptococcus* species. With the growing awareness of bloodstream infections caused by *Trichosporon* species, specific serologic tests for their detection may be developed. Before this occurs, a possible strategy is to use the serum cryptococcal antigen test in combination with compatible signs and symptoms and underlying disease to suggest a diagnosis of trichosporonosis.

Nucleic Acid Detection

To date, there is no U.S. Food and Drug Administration (FDA)-approved nucleic acid-based assay for the detection and identification of yeasts directly from specimens. However, the FDA has approved several commercially available peptide nucleic acid fluorescent in situ hybridization (PNA FISH) kits (AdvanDx, Woburn, MA) for identification of yeasts directly from positive blood cultures. The probes specifically detect *C. albicans, C. glabrata,* or *C. tropicalis* as individual species or detect a yeast species group (e.g., *C. albicans* and *C. parapsilosis* fluoresce green wth the Yeast Traffic Light PNA FISH kit) in blood cultures by targeting species-specific rRNA sequences. Nucleic acid peptides that mimic 26S rRNA are used to hybridize to target rRNA. The probes are also coupled to a fluorophore which is detectable when the probe binds to its target. Several studies have shown that the *C. albicans* PNA FISH assay is 100% specific (188, 212, 261). In the most comprehensive study, the test was found to have excellent sensitivity (99%), specificity (100%), positive predictive value (100%), and negative predictive value (99.3%) (261). The test can rapidly (1.5 h) indicate whether *C. albicans* is present and can thus indicate whether a non-*C. albicans* yeast is present (188, 212). Other PNA FISH assays are similarly rapid. The test does not replace subculture because blood cultures may contain mixed species; therefore, PNA FISH-positive blood cultures should be subcultured to ensure that no other yeast species is present. *C. dubliniensis* is not detected with the PNA FISH probe. With this test, laboratories can report whether a positive blood culture with a yeast contains *C. albicans* within a few hours after the culture becomes positive (119).

The time required to identify a pathogen could be shortened if more efficient methods of detecting fungal DNA in the specimen were developed. Automated blood culture systems are available, but these may take more than 24 h for a positive specimen to be detected. Apaire-Marchais et al. (8)

have developed a rapid immunomagnetic separation system for *Candida* species from blood that recovers yeasts directly from the specimen so they can be inoculated onto growth media. Meanwhile, real-time PCR has the ability to detect candidemia much earlier than conventional blood culture, but it does not always detect all cases of systemic infection with all species (123, 162, 253). Bennett (22) provides a very balanced discussion on the use of this technique, which is likely to be used alongside blood culture protocols while it is developed further.

Real-time PCR has been used to detect *Candida* species in respiratory samples, blood, and tissue from the maxillary sinus (137, 220). Six *Candida* species were detected with species probes designed against the ITS2 region. Detection in clinical specimens was as good as traditional diagnostic tests, although one specimen grew *C. lusitaniae*, while the PCR recognized *C. glabrata*. Cross-reaction between the species was unlikely, as there were 10 mismatches between the sequences for *C. glabrata* and *C. lusitaniae*, so it is possible that the methods were detecting different yeasts present in the bronchoalveolar lavage specimen. Microarrays have been tested as diagnostic tools for the detection of invasive fungal infection. Samples of blood, bronchoalveolar lavage fluid, and tissue from neutropenic patients were used, and results were concordant with those of other diagnostic tests (culture, histology, imaging, etc.); however, administration of antifungals was found to inhibit detection of the pathogen (233).

ISOLATION PROCEDURES

Processing specimens for fungal recovery is usually performed in conjunction and as an extension of the processing procedure for recovery of bacteria. The primary difference is the selection of media used for primary plating. These media are discussed in chapter 113. Most media used for the recovery of fungi contain an antibacterial such as chloramphenicol or gentamicin; however, incorporation of cycloheximide (Acti-Dione) should be avoided, as only *C. albicans*, some *Trichosporon* species, and *Malassezia* species are able to grow in the presence of this agent. One processing step that has unproven advantages for isolation of yeasts from sputum specimens is the use of mucolytic agents (*N*-acetyl-L-cysteine or sputolysin).

There are, however, yeast infections for which specialized processing steps should be considered. For example, recovery of *C. neoformans* from blood or bone marrow is enhanced if lysis-centrifugation followed by inoculation onto solid media is used (92). If *C. neoformans* is suspected from a respiratory specimen, setting up primary media which include a niger seed or related medium will enhance detection.

For some yeasts, a medium supplement may be needed to either enhance or support growth during primary culture. If *Malassezia* species are suspected, the primary culture plate should be supplemented with an olive oil overlay applied with a swab prior to inoculation. *Malassezia pachydermatis* grows without the overlay, but it is required to grow *M. furfur*. This may not be successful for other *Malassezia* species, as these are more fastidious. The detection of bile-dependent and bile-enhanced isolates of *C. glabrata* is enhanced by the addition of 8 μg of fluconazole/ml to the primary medium. This selects for bile-dependent isolates which have defects in the ergosterol synthesis pathway and are fluconazole resistant (15, 110). This becomes a particularly powerful method when combined with a primary medium containing a chromogenic indicator used for presumptive identification of some yeasts (e.g., CHROMagar) (191).

The appropriate selection of isolation media is essential even though detection of infectious agents using molecular methods is becoming more commonplace in the diagnostic setting. Successful culture is still necessary to perform antifungal susceptibility tests, for preservation in culture collections, and for epidemiological study.

IDENTIFICATION

The use of a sound systematic approach to yeast identification is important. With the numerous yeast identification systems available today, most commonly encountered yeast species can be identified easily; however, repeat testing is sometimes necessary, and observation of morphological characteristics on cornmeal-Tween or similar morphology agars should be mandatory. Isolates that are problematic should be sent for DNA sequence analysis to confirm their identity.

The sections that follow outline the identification tests available, while the section "Description of the Agents" above contains the genus-specific detail. This topic has also previously been reviewed (88, 205).

Macroscopic Characteristics of Yeasts

Most yeasts grow well (*Malassezia* species are an exception) on common mycological and bacteriological media. Growth is usually detected in 48 to 72 h, and subcultures or laboratory-adapted strains may grow more rapidly. Colonies have a smooth to wrinkled, creamy appearance; some pigment may be observed initially or intensify with age. Heavily encapsulated yeasts give a very moist, mucoid appearance.

The ability of yeasts to grow at 37°C is a very important characteristic. Most pathogenic species grow readily at 25 and 37°C, while saprobes usually fail to grow at the higher temperature. Spiking around the edge of a colony grown in CO_2 is indicative of *Candida albicans* and has been reported to be more sensitive than germ tube production (17). This feature is the same as the colonies with feet described in the *Candida* section of "Description of the Agents" above.

Pellicle growth on the surface of liquid media such as Sabouraud dextrose broth or malt extract broth has been used in the past to assist with yeast identification. More recent evidence suggests that this characteristic can be variable; however, as an ancillary test, it may be helpful with identifying *Candida tropicalis* and *Candida krusei*.

Microscopic Characteristics of Yeasts

Upon isolation of a suspected yeast from a clinical specimen, the first examination should be a wet preparation of a colony. This provides an initial clue to the organism's identity. There are several fungi that produce yeast-like colonies that are not yeasts. Observations should include size and shape of the yeast, method of bud attachment, and presence or absence of pseudohyphae, true hyphae, or arthroconidia (Table 4). Any round or slightly oval budding yeast with rare or no pseudohyphae seen in this preparation should be examined further for the presence of a capsule.

The same wet preparation as used for the initial microscopic examination can be used for an India ink examination for the presence of encapsulated yeasts (Fig. 2) (see above). Capsular size cannot be used for identification purposes, as this characteristic may be influenced by culture age, medium composition, and strain variation. The presence of a capsule does not automatically ensure that the yeast is *Cryptococcus neoformans*, as other cryptococci,

TABLE 4 Microscopic appearance of several yeasts and yeast-like fungi on morphology agar

Organism(s)	Pseudohyphae	True hyphae	Blastoconidia	Arthroconidia	Annelloconidia	Chlamydospores	Ascospores
B. capitatus	X	X	X		X		
C. albicans/ C. dubliniensis	X	X	X			X	
Other Candida spp.	X[a]	X[a]	X				X[a]
Cryptococcus spp.			X				
Geotrichum spp.		X		X			
Pichia spp.	X[a]		X				X
Rhodotorula spp.			X				
Saccharomyces spp.	X[a]		X				X
Trichosporon spp.	X	X	X	X			

[a]Strain variation.

Rhodotorula spp., and rare *Candida* spp. produce capsule-like structures. In practice, any nonpigmented, round, encapsulated yeast recovered from CSF should be considered *C. neoformans* until proven otherwise.

Purity of Cultures

Before any additional physiological tests are performed, it is essential to ensure that the culture is pure. A Gram stain of the culture can verify purity, but often bacterial contamination can be detected during the wet preparation examination. If the culture is mixed with bacteria, the isolate should be inoculated to a blood agar plate or Sabouraud dextrose agar containing antibiotics and individual colonies subcultured for purity or treated with hydrochloric acid (Fig. 4). The HCl procedure is performed by inoculating a colony into three tubes of Sabouraud dextrose broth (each containing 5 ml). A capillary pipette is used to add 4 drops of 1 N HCl to the first tube, 2 drops to the second tube, and 1 drop to the third tube. After incubation at 25°C for 24 to 48 h, 0.1 ml of each broth is subcultured onto fresh Sabouraud dextrose agar plates.

It is possible that more than one yeast species will be recovered from a clinical specimen, especially if the specimen is from a normally nonsterile site (264). In addition, multiple yeast species may be responsible for fungemia episodes. Careful attention to colonial morphology and microscopic characteristics can offer clues to a mixed population. Subculturing individual isolates to additional media can be helpful (264), and the use of a chromogenic medium may delineate the presence of more than one yeast species.

Chromogenic Agars

Presumptive identification of one or two yeast species based on colony characteristics can be obtained with chromogenic agar media (reviewed in reference 205). CHROMagar *Candida* (CHROMagar France, Paris, France, distributed in the United States by Becton Dickinson/BBL, Sparks, MD) allows differentiation of over 10 species and is marketed for the presumptive identification of *C. albicans, C. tropicalis,* and *C. krusei.* Colony identification is based on the differential release of chromogenic breakdown products from various substrates following exoenzyme activity. It is important to recognize that identifications are presumptive. Evidence suggests that variation in colony appearance occurs among the species (20, 200). The directions of the manufacturer must be strictly followed, as is the case for any rapid test based on exoenzyme activity. Incubation time and temperature significantly affect the colony appearance. The medium is useful for the detection of mixed yeast infections, especially in blood, and for resolving identification problems. Other chromogenic media are now commercially available (see chapter 113): CandidaID (bioMérieux)

and CandiSelect (Bio-Rad) perform similarly to CHROMagar. No one medium detects all instances of mixed yeast blood cultures (142, 259, 260). Approximately 2 to 10% of *C. albicans* isolates produce white colonies, rather than colored colonies, on these chromogenic media, strongly supporting the concept that these media provide only a presumptive identification. Other chromogenic media, namely, Oxoid Chromogenic Candida Agar (Oxoid, Basingstoke, United Kingdom) and HiCrome (HiMedia Laboratories, Mumbai, India), have been introduced recently, but published papers describing extensive comparative trials against other chromogenic media are not available.

Morphology Studies

While examination of a wet preparation gives a primary indication of the yeast involved, more extensive study of morphology on cornmeal-Tween agar or other similar agars offers the opportunity to correlate morphological characteristics with results of biochemical testing, as these characteristics form part of the identification code for many commercially available kits. Microscopic examination should reveal the thick-walled chlamydospores of *Candida albicans/Candida dubliniensis;* attention should be given to the size and shape of the pseudohyphae and the arrangement of blastoconidia along the pseudohyphae, presence of capsules, etc. (Fig. 1 and Table 4).

Germ Tube Test

One of the most valuable and simple tests for the rapid presumptive identification of *C. albicans* is the germ tube test (Fig. 5a). The test is considered presumptive because not all isolates of *C. albicans* are germ tube positive and false positives

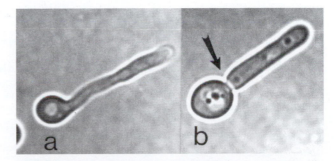

FIGURE 5 Germ tube test. (a) Germ tube formation of *Candida albicans;* (b) blastoconidial germination with constriction (arrow) of *Candida tropicalis* not seen with true germ tubes of *C. albicans.* Magnification, ×400. (Courtesy of B. A. Davis.)

may be obtained, especially with *C. tropicalis*, despite well-trained staff (70). Also, *C. dubliniensis* is germ tube positive, although most isolates do not form germ tubes in a commercial synthetic germination medium (69). Microscopic observation of the preparation reveals that the short hyphal initials produced by *C. albicans* are not constricted at the junction of the blastoconidium and germ tube. *Candida tropicalis* can produce hyphal initials, but the blastoconidia are larger than those of *C. albicans*, and there is a definite constricture where the hyphal initial joins the blastoconidium (Fig. 5b). In addition to using a known culture of *C. albicans* as a positive test control, negative controls using *C. tropicalis* and *C. glabrata* also should be included. Optimum conditions are obtained by using colonies grown on Sabouraud dextrose agar or blood agar at 30°C for 24 to 48 h (unpublished observations). The test is performed by first lightly touching a colony with a bacteriological loop so that a thin film of organism is obtained, then transferring the inoculum into the test substrate (such as fetal bovine serum), followed by incubation at 37°C for up to 3 h. Germ tube tests should be read after 2 to 3 h to prevent clumping of hyphal initials and to reduce the number of false positives. In addition, a heavy inoculum of yeasts and the presence of bacteria can each lead to false-negative results.

Ascospore Formation

Homothallic yeasts recovered from clinical specimens may be present in their teleomorphic (sexual) state. In order to enhance production of ascospores by ascomycetous yeasts, cultures should be inoculated onto media such as Fowell's acetate agar (87), V8 juice agar, or yeast extract-malt extract agar; incubated at room temperature for 2 to 5 days; and examined by wet preparation for the presence of ascospores within asci. Some mycologists prefer to perform special stains to detect ascospores. The Ziehl-Neelsen stain routinely employed in mycobacteriology can be used if needed; however, most ascospores can be detected easily in a drop of sterile distilled water. Ascospore production in *Saccharomyces cerevisiae* is evidenced by the presence of one to four globose spores (Fig. 3c); *Pichia anomala* (*Wickerhamomyces anomalus*) produces one to four hat-shaped spores (Fig. 3a). Ascospore formation is a valuable test to aid in identification when equivocal results are obtained by other identification methods (Table 5).

Phenol Oxidase Test

The phenol oxidase test is a screening procedure that detects the ability of *Cryptococcus neoformans* to produce phenol oxidase on substrates containing caffeic acid. The most frequently used medium is "birdseed" agar (containing niger or thistle seeds), and a number of formulations showing various degrees of success have been described. Test performance is related to the glucose content of the medium; the more glucose in the medium, the less likely a valid test result will be obtained. *C. neoformans* and *C. gattii* colonies turn a dark brown in 2 to 5 days. Because of the wide variation in medium formulations, the test must be subjected constantly to quality control measures. Some laboratories advocate the use of birdseed agar as part of the primary plating for respiratory cultures for early detection of *C. neoformans* isolates. A rapid phenol oxidase test utilizes a caffeic acid disc which is rehydrated, then inoculated with several yeast colonies, and incubated at 35 to 37°C for up

TABLE 5 Appearance of asci or ascospores of ascomycetous yeasts[a]

Anamorphic sp.	Previous synonym or obsolete name	Teleomorph (alternative sp.)	Hetero- or homothallic	Ascospores
Blastoschizomyces capitatus	*Geotrichum capitatum*, *Trichosporon capitatum*	*Clavispora capitatus*	Hetero	4/ascus, hyaline ellipsoidal, with slimy sheath when released
Candida ciferrii		*Stephanoascus ciferrii*	Hetero	1–4/ascus, helmet or hat shaped
Candida famata	*Torulopsis candida*	*Debaryomyces hansenii*	Homo	1–2/ascus, spherical with warts[b]
Candida guilliermondii		*Pichia guilliermondii* (*Yamadazyma guillermondii*)	Hetero	Variable
Candida kefyr	*Candida pseudotropicalis*, *Candida macedoniensis*	*Kluyveromyces marxianus* var. *marxianus*	Homo	1–4/ascus, crescent to reniform, agglutinates on MEA[c]
Candida krusei		*Issatchenkia orientalis* *Pichia kudriavzevii*	Homo	1–2/ascus, spherical[d]
Candida lipolytica		*Yarrowia lipolytica*	Hetero	1–4/ascus, spherical to hat-shaped protuberance on 1 or 2 ends
Candida lusitaniae	*Candida obtusa, Candida parapsilosis* var. *obtusa*	*Clavispora lusitaniae*	Hetero	1–4/ascus, clavate on MEA
Candida norvegensis		*Pichia norvegensis*	Homo	1–4/ascus, hat shaped on acetate agar
Candida pintolopesii	*Candida slooffii*	*Arxiozyma telluris*	Homo	1–2/ascus, spherical to ovoid, rough to spiny
Candida pelliculosa		*Pichia anomala*	Hetero	1–4/ascus, hat shaped
Candida pulcherrima		*Metschnikowia pulcherrima*	Hetero	1–2/ascus, from chlamydospore, spherical with peduncle
Candida utilis		*Pichia jadinii*	Homo	1–4/ascus, hat shaped on MEA
		Saccharomyces cerevisiae	Homo	1–4/ascus, spherical or short ellipsoidal (on acetate agar)

[a]Modified from reference 108.
[b]Difficult to see.
[c]MEA, malt extract agar.
[d]Difficult to induce.

to 4 h. The disc should be examined every 30 min for the production of a brown pigment. If pigment is produced, it is presumptive for *C. neoformans*; if no pigment is detected but *C. neoformans* is suspected, further identification should be conducted.

Urease

The urease test detects a yeast's ability to produce the enzyme urease. In the presence of suitable substrates urease splits urea, producing ammonia, which raises the pH and causes a color shift in the phenol red indicator from amber to pinkish red. The urease test aids in the identification of the urease-positive basidiomycetous yeasts (*Cryptococcus, Malassezia, Rhodotorula,* and *Trichosporon*) from the urease-negative ascomycetous yeasts (*Candida, Saccharomyces, Geotrichum, Blastoschizomyces,* etc.). Nearly all *Candida* spp. encountered in clinical specimens are urease negative, exceptions being *Yarrowia* (*Candida*) *lipolytica* and some strains of *C. krusei,* both of which do not assimilate inositol. A rapid disc test can take from 4 to 72 h for a reaction to develop, while the more definitive urea agar slants can take from 24 to 72 h.

Rapid Trehalose

The rapid trehalose test can provide a presumptive identification of *C. glabrata* within 3 h. The Clinical and Laboratory Standards Institute (CLSI) has approved a rapid test procedure (document M35-A2) for identification of *C. glabrata* based primarily on rapid trehalose assimilation (19, 58a). False positives occur with trehalose tests (84), but these can be reduced if the results are correlated with small cell size and failure to produce germ tubes. Several modifications of the rapid trehalose assay have been introduced. The Glabrata RTT (Fumouze Diagnostics) combines hydrolysis of trehalose and maltose and includes a control (a sugar-free basal medium). *C. glabrata* hydrolyzes the trehalose rapidly, but not the maltose (which other yeasts may hydrolyze). The test provides acceptable sensitivity and specificity, but the choice of growth medium for the test inoculum influences the likelihood of obtaining false positives. Blood agar should be avoided, as both *C. albicans* and *C. tropicalis* cause high false-positive results (89, 260). The most suitable media appear to be CHROMagar and Sabouraud dextrose (4%)

agar. Combining colony color on chromogenic agars with the GLABRATA RTT or the rapid trehalose test could help improve specificity (175, 203). Rapid trehalose and maltose hydrolysis have also been modified into a 30-s dipstick assay. This test provides adequate specificity and sensitivity, but these parameters are affected by the medium used to grow the test inoculum (203).

Phenotypic Systems

A variety of manual and semiautomatic single phenotypic to multiphenotypic assay systems have been made commercially available (Table 6). Most are designed to help identify the most common yeast etiologic agents. The systems vary in ease of use and accuracy. Generally the systems designed to identify multiple genera and their species are less reliable with unusual or rare pathogens (e.g., *C. inconspicua*), although sometimes rare isolates of common species such as *C. parapsilosis, C. guilliermondii,* and *C. krusei* can result in misidentification or poor species discrimination (34, 95).

Carbohydrate Assimilation Tests

The mainstay of yeast identification to the species level is the carbohydrate assimilation test (Table 6), which measures the ability of a yeast to utilize a specific carbohydrate as the sole source of carbon in the presence of oxygen. There are several reliable commercially available kits, such as API 20C AUX (bioMérieux SA), API ID32C (not available in the United States), Auxacolor 2 (Bio-Rad, Hercules, CA), and BBL Minitek Yeast Set (Becton Dickinson/BBL) and automated and semiautomated systems (e.g., ID 32 C and Vitek 2 YST, produced by bioMérieux) on the market today (Table 6) that make the classical Wickerham and Burton method (256) unnecessary for routine clinical isolates. None of these tests are 100% concordant with the Wickerham-Burton method, and they do not uniformly agree with each other. Assimilation reactions provided in reference books, such as those by Barnett et al. (18) and Kurtzman and Fell (129), are based on the Wickerham-Burton method. Because commercial assimilation tests are only similar to the Wickerham-Burton tests, their assimilation reaction profiles may differ from those provided in reference books.

TABLE 6 Rapid tests (<24 h) and semirapid tests (<48 h) available for presumptive or definitive identification of yeasts following colony formation

Group 1 (for single species)		Group 2 (for several species)	Group 3 (for multiple genera)
Test name	Organism identified	Test name	Test name
Albicans-Sure	*C. albicans*	CandiSelect	Vitek-Yeast Biochemical Card
Albicans ID[a]	*C. albicans*	Candida check	Microbial Identification System (MIDI)
Albistrip[a]	*C. albicans*	CHROMagar	Microscan Rapid Yeast ID
BactiCard Candida	*C. albicans*	Fungiscreen H[a]	Quantum II
Bichrolatex Albicans[a]	*C. albicans*		IDS RapID Yeast Plus System
Fluoroplate[a]	*C. albicans*		Uni-Yeast Tek
Germ tube	*C. albicans*		API 20C AUX
Rapidec albicans[a]	*C. albicans*		API ID32C[a]
C. albicans screen (Murex CA 50)	*C. albicans*		API Candida
MUAG test	*C. albicans*		Auxacolor 2
PNA FISH Candida	*C. albicans*		Vitek2 ID-YST
Bichrolate krusei[a]	*C. krusei*		BBL Minitek
Rapid trehalose assimilation	*C. glabrata*		
Caffeic acid disk	*C. neoformans*		

[a] Test not available in the United States.

Carbon assimilation and, occasionally, fermentation studies are needed to differentiate species (Table 1), but rapid confirmation tests for particular species are becoming available (see "Rapid Identification of Yeasts" below and Table 6). Of the *Candida* spp. usually recovered from clinical specimens, *C. guilliermondii* is the only one to assimilate dulcitol (galactitol), and *C. kefyr* (previously *C. pseudotropicalis*) assimilates lactose. The assimilation of rhamnose can be helpful in separating *C. lusitaniae* from the biochemically similar but rhamnose-negative variants of *C. tropicalis* (221). For atypical isolates of *C. lusitaniae*, which can be confused with *C. tropicalis*, good growth on trichophyton agar no. 1 with biotin but weak growth on vitamin-free medium indicates *C. tropicalis* (239). Certain rare strains of *C. tropicalis* may assimilate cellobiose weakly and exhibit an assimilation pattern similar to that of *C. parapsilosis*. The inclusion of arabinose is helpful, since *C. parapsilosis* readily assimilates this carbohydrate, while most strains of *C. tropicalis* do not. Urease generally is not produced, nor is KNO_3 utilized by the *Candida* species listed in Table 1. However, occasional isolates of *C. krusei* may be urease positive.

Nitrate Tests

The nitrate assimilation procedure is similar to that of the carbon assimilation test. It tests the ability of a yeast to utilize nitrate as a sole nitrogen source. The test is most beneficial when trying to identify *Cryptococcus*, *Rhodotorula*, and *Pichia* spp. In order for yeasts to utilize nitrate, they must reduce it. Nitrate reduction assays, however, have limited value for identification of yeasts and are used primarily for discrimination of *Cryptococcus* species.

Carbohydrate Fermentation Tests

Fermentative yeasts recovered from clinical specimens produce carbon dioxide and alcohol; therefore, production of gas is indicative of fermentation. The pH of the medium may not change. Rarely are fermentation studies needed to identify most of the commonly isolated yeasts if the mycologist is familiar with typical morphology on cornmeal agar. The test is most helpful in differentiating the various species of *Candida*; *Cryptococcus* and *Rhodotorula* spp. are nonfermentative.

Rapid Identification of Yeasts

Rapid identification of yeasts has an impact on patient management. This is particularly true given the recognition that various yeast species (such as *C. glabrata*, *C. krusei*, *C. parapsilosis*, *C. lusitaniae*, *C. tropicalis*, and *C. neoformans*) are inherently or potentially resistant to amphotericin B, the newer azole agents, and echinocandins (91, 251).

Rapid tests are divided into those that provide definitive or presumptive identification within the same day (<24 h) of colony formation and either are specific to a single species, are limited to a few species, or apply to multiple genera (Table 6). In general, tests listed within groups 1 and 2 in Table 6 provide presumptive results, and confirmation of the identification is needed.

Tests based on preformed enzymes may be acutely affected by incubation temperature (109) and are effectively limited to the more common yeast species isolated in the clinical laboratory. However, detection of specific exoenzymes can be useful for resolution of the confusion between two or three possible species. In particular, several rapid tests are available for this purpose, particularly for detection of *Candida albicans* (for example, the *Candida albicans* screen [Carr-Scarborough Microbiologicals, Decatur, GA] and

the Albistrip [Lab M Ltd., Bury, United Kingdom]). These tests are excellent for confirmation of a germ tube-positive organism such as *C. albicans* and could be used in place of more long-term identification tests for this purpose. However, similar results are obtained for *C. dubliniensis*. Using these tests for confirmation purposes can provide financial savings to the clinical laboratory. Both tests depend on the production of two enzymes (proline aminopeptidase and β-galactosaminidase) instead of a single enzyme (β-galactosaminidase) which could otherwise lead to spurious results (232).

A rapid test to help distinguish some *Cryptococcus* species uses the ability to reduce nitrate on a rapid nitrate swab test (Remel). This can supplement the results of more comprehensive tests and help to distinguish *C. neoformans* (nitrate negative) from *C. albidus* and *Cryptococcus terreus* (nitrate positive). Molecular tests and serologic tests appear to be promising rapid alternatives with higher sensitivity and specificity.

Molecular Methods

At present, yeasts are not identified in many routine clinical laboratories using nucleic acid technology. The lack of this technology can lead to problems in the identification of unusual species, as characteristic profiles may not be present in the commercially available phenotype databases, resulting in misidentifications. Also, several species have been revealed to be heterogeneous species complexes using genetic identification methods, and these are often not distinguished by kits based on phenotype. As a result, increasing use is being made of rDNA sequencing and comparison to genetic databases for conclusive identification. Two widely used databases are GenBank (http://www.ncbi.nlm.nih.gov/blast) and the CBS yeast database (http://www.cbs.knaw.nl/yeast/biolomics.aspx), with the latter containing databases for strains held in the culture collection. Lau et al. (137) highlight the need to be aware of how the genetic database being used is maintained. GenBank contains unrefereed sequences, and errors are known to occur, whereas the CBS has a curated ITS sequence database. Reference texts such as the *Atlas of Clinical Fungi* (72) have included restriction maps of ribosomal operons for described fungi. Molecular approaches and guidelines to fungal identification are described in CLSI documents MM18-A and MM03-02 (57, 58).

In order to develop a universal genetic identification system for yeasts, the most reproducible, specific, and sensitive sequence for comparison must be identified, and the majority of research has focused on the rDNA regions. The large subunit, specifically the D1/D2 region, was shown to be highly discriminatory for the ascomycetous yeasts (130) and similarly for the basidiomycetous yeasts (83, 223), although differentiation of some closely related species in the latter study (223) was achieved using the ITS and intergenic spacer regions. Other studies have also used the ITS1 and ITS2 regions (49, 246). Chen et al. demonstrated that the ITS2 sequence alone can be sufficient for discriminating *Candida* species (50). Linton et al. (145) conducted a study assessing the value of direct 26S rDNA sequencing using over 3,000 isolates submitted to the United Kingdom Mycology Reference Laboratory. Ciardo et al. (55) compared ITS sequencing to the ID 32C system for yeast strains. Hall et al. (104) used a commercially available MicroSeq D2 large-subunit rDNA sequencing system to identify 131 clinical yeast isolates and compared the results to those obtained by conventional methods, including the API 20C AUX system. Comparisons of 100 isolates representing 19 species of *Candida* using the MicroSeq kit matched 98% with identifications using the API 20C AUX. For the remaining isolates, representing 9 species, there was 81.3% concordance between the systems. Most of the discrepancies were attributed to a lack of available data in the relevant databases.

Recently, pyrosequencing, a novel method for rapid determination of a short stretch of DNA sequence, has been examined as a potentially fast identification method. Montero et al. (169) identified only 69.1% of 133 isolates representing 43 yeast species by comparing the sequences of the hypervariable ITS region to traditional methods, as it was not possible to identify the *Trichosporon* or *Cryptococcus* isolates to the species level. In contrast, Boyanton et al. (33) obtained 100% agreement between pyrosequencing and traditional identification methods for 60 isolates of the species *C. albicans, C. dubliniensis, C. glabrata, C. guilliermondii, C. krusei, C. lusitaniae, C. parapsilosis,* and *C. tropicalis.* Also, Borman et al. demonstrated that pyrosequencing of 25 bp of the ITS2 region correctly identified most clinically important *Candida* species (29).

For organisms that are difficult to grow or require noncommercially available materials, these methods hold great potential. For example, identification of *Malassezia* species otherwise requires both specialized growth media and phenotypic identification tests. However, more research is needed before a universal genetic database can be devised, as the D1/D2 and ITS regions do not appear to identify all yeasts. Using the ribosomal 5.8S ITS sequence, only 6 of 15 *Debaryomyces* species were correctly identified; the remaining species were differentiated using the sequences of the ACT1 (actin) gene (155).

Many laboratories do not possess the equipment or facilities to develop molecular technologies for mycology; however, there are a number of other DNA-based methods available to aid in identification. Restriction enzyme analysis, karyotyping using pulsed-field gel electrophoresis, and species-specific probes have all been used to identify yeast species and have been reviewed (93, 137, 205). However, it must be remembered that these techniques were developed before many of the species complexes were discovered and may not be able to distinguish among them. If the laboratory is not able to provide sequencing, genetic targets can be amplified and compared for size or for structure by digesting the amplicon with a suitable restriction endonuclease (258). However, variations can occur within species due to mutations at the restriction site. The potential of these methods was demonstrated by Massonet et al. (157) when comparing 61 isolates of *Candida, Cryptococcus, Blastoschizomyces,* and *Saccharomyces* by ITS2 fragment length polymorphism with the phenotypic identification systems API ID32C and VITEK 2. The genetic analysis correctly identified 55 or 59 isolates dependent on the method of extraction, the API ID32C identified 58 isolates, and the VITEK 2 (fluorometric card) identified only 41 isolates. Other studies have also used the ITS1 and ITS2 regions (49, 246). Microarrays for fungal identification have been produced using the ITS regions. Leinberger et al. (141) identified *C. albicans, C. dubliniensis, C. krusei, C. tropicalis, C. guilliermondii,* and *C. lusitaniae.* A further modification on this principle was able to distinguish *C. parapsilosis, C. orthopsilosis,* and *C. metapsilosis* among 24 other fungal pathogens, including 10 other *Candida* species (39).

White et al. (255) and Lau et al. (137) have reviewed developments for the rapid diagnosis of invasive candidiasis, including PCR-based methods. New techniques combining enzyme immunoassay formats for the rapid detection of species-specific amplicons and the use of real-time PCR are discussed. Other rapid identification systems developed include the DiversiLab system of automated repetitive sequence-based PCR (Bacterial Barcodes, Athens, GA). This method uses primers against noncoding repetitive sequences, and amplified products are separated on a microfluidic chip to generate a fingerprint of intensity of fluorescence versus migration time. This technique was used to screen 115 clinical isolates of *Candida* species by sequence analysis of the ITS region and obtained 99% concordant results with traditional identification methods (263). Although results can be obtained within 24 h of a pure culture being obtained, identification is dependent on a comprehensive library of species fingerprints for comparison. The Luminex (Austin, TX) multianalyte profiling platform has been used on a number of types of clinical specimens and enables screening of a range of fungal pathogens simultaneously. The method uses a microsphere (bead) suspension array whereby each bead contains an individual probe designed to hybridize to a different amplified fungal DNA sequence. Landlinger et al. (135) used the ITS2 region to design 75 genus- and species-specific hybridization probes to detect fungal infection in blood, pulmonary biopsy specimens, and bronchotracheal secretions. In this study, one blood culture grew *C. albicans* but the Luminex system identified it as *C. dubliniensis.* No further tests seem to have been done to establish which result was in error.

An alternative method to DNA-based technologies is matrix-assisted laser desorption ionization–time-of-flight mass spectrometry. This method requires a pure colony of yeasts and produces a mass spectrum fingerprint characteristic of the organism. As with other fingerprinting techniques, this method requires an adequate database of reference strains for comparison to the test isolate to facilitate rapid routine identification of clinical yeast isolates (153).

The obvious advantage of using molecular methods is speed, as results are often available within 24 h of colony isolation, whereas traditional methods usually take at least 48 h. However, development of molecular databases and standardization remain issues before any of these tests become commonplace (discussed in reference 31), and it is likely that molecular tests will complement the phenotypic methods currently used in the clinical environment.

Troubleshooting Difficult Identifications

Laboratories sometimes encounter yeast isolates that do not fit easily into a specific species, particularly when commercial identification systems are used. There are key features that help separate troublesome organisms from others. For example, urease production separates basidiomycetous yeasts from most ascomycetous yeasts. Maximum growth temperature, cycloheximide resistance, and the ability to assimilate cellobiose, inositol, or trehalose are helpful. For more difficult identifications, use of traditional auxanographic methods but with carbon source-impregnated disks on yeast carbon base agar plates (rather than spotting the sugar on the edge of the plate as done by Beijerinck [21]) may provide the most accurate assimilation information. Differential media such as chromogenic agars or eosin methylene blue agar (*C. glabrata* and *C. kefyr* produce distinct colonies) may sometimes help (174). Fermentation tests should also be considered, as should a second commercial system but one that utilizes a different endpoint (e.g., growth versus exoenzyme production). Isolates that consistently fail to be identified by conventional tests should be sent to a reference laboratory for sequencing.

ORGANISMS RESEMBLING YEASTS

Occasionally, organisms such as moulds or algae grow on mycological media and produce colonies which resemble those produced by yeasts. However, careful attention to morphological characteristics differentiates them. Examples of such organisms which are recovered from clinical specimens and which superficially can be confused with yeasts include *Geotrichum* species (white to cream-colored colonies), *Ustilago* species (white, compact to moist colonies), black yeasts (initially white to tan colonies), and *Prototheca* species (white to cream-colored, dull or moist to mucoid colonies). These organisms are described elsewhere in this *Manual*.

TYPING SYSTEMS

In order to understand the epidemiology of infection, to distinguish between endogenous and exogenous infections (and, in the latter, to locate the source), to examine transmission, or to monitor the spread of drug resistance, it is necessary to be able to distinguish among isolates within a species. Successful strain typing is dependent upon the choice of technique(s) and experimental conditions for maximum discrimination, and this has to be established for each species tested.

DNA-based typing methods began in the 1980s with restriction enzyme analysis, which required careful selection of the enzyme used to maximize discrimination. Other methods quickly followed: Southern blotting using species-specific or generic probes, karyotyping, pulsed-field gel electrophoresis–restriction enzyme analysis, and random amplified polymorphic DNA analysis. These methods are all subject to discrepancies due to mutation or laboratory reproducibility, and they have been reviewed (93, 230, 242). Most of these techniques have been superceded by more accurate and reproducible methods, such as microsatellite typing and multilocus sequence typing (MLST). Gil-Lamaignere et al. (93) and Taylor et al. (242) have critically reviewed the limitations and applications of these techniques.

Microsatellite typing is the amplification of short tandem repeat sequences that are polymorphic, resulting in bands of various lengths related to the number of repeats contained therein. Variation in the number of repeats occurs during DNA replication, and this provides the characteristic fingerprint. This is a fast typing method but cannot be used to estimate isolate relatedness unless the bands are sequenced and the contents compared (see, for example, reference 86). MLST is an accurate and reproducible method of fingerprinting that uses the sequences of six to eight selected housekeeping genes and identifies polymorphic nucleotide sites. The method can be used to establish population structures by assessing variation in sequence for a set number of genes, and this has enabled databases to be developed for interlaboratory comparisons. The method has been used to type a number of yeast species (47, 56, 186), and it recently demonstrated the spread of *Cryptococcus gattii* from Vancouver Island in Canada to the northwest United States (36). MLST has been used to develop a consensus typing scheme for *C. gattii* and for *C. neoformans* (163).

MLST has been used to demonstrate that most patients with *C. albicans* carried the same strain at multiple sites or over a time period, and to confirm that microvariation can be detected over time when some isolates are stored (185). However, while MLST provided detail on the population structure of clinical isolates of *C. glabrata* from Taiwan, greater typing discrimination was achieved using pulsed-field gel electrophoresis–restriction enzyme analysis (143).

SEROLOGIC TESTS

Genus *Candida*

Invasive *Candida* infections are life threatening, but detection by relatively noninvasive methods such as blood culture is problematic. A test for detection of antibody to *Candida* mannan is available, for example, using the Platelia Candida AB EIA kit (Bio-Rad Laboratories), but such tests have poor sensitivity and specificity (137). These poor results are due to the presence of *Candida* species as part of the commensal flora and antibodies against cell wall components that may be found in colonized individuals. The utility of these tests is maximized when combined with detection of antigen levels, as the antibody and antigen levels may show an inverse correlation during disease progression. More detail on antigen testing is found above.

ANTIMICROBIAL SUSCEPTIBILITIES

Details of susceptibility testing methods, antifungal resistance profiles, and mechanisms of yeasts and moulds are described in other chapters of this *Manual*. Table 7 contains the MICs from a number of sources for 36 yeast species. The references used to compile the table all have used CLSI methods, with the following exceptions: Lass-Flörl et al. (136), who followed European Committee on Antimicrobial Susceptibility Testing methodology; the *Atlas of Clinical Fungi* (72); and Ashbee (10), who reports data from published work. The data on *Malassezia* from Ashbee's review have been included because there is little information on the susceptibility of these organisms. Most species of *Candida* are sensitive to the echinocandins, although there is some variation within species with regard to caspofungin (121, 194), while *Cryptococcus* species are resistant to these agents. *Candida krusei* is intrinsically resistant to fluconazole but is susceptible to posaconazole and voriconazole, while some strains of *C. glabrata* may show elevated fluconazole MICs. *C. norvegensis* and *C. inconspicua* are also fluconazole resistant. Few *Candida* species are resistant in vitro to amphotericin B, although *C. lusitaniae* may exhibit secondary resistance to amphotericin B. Therefore, clinical response to this drug may be poor despite in vitro susceptibility tests indicating strains to be sensitive (107, 127). However, clinically relevant breakpoints have not been established for sensitivity testing of yeasts against amphotericin B. Approximately 10% of *C. albicans* isolates are resistant to flucytosine, and 30% develop resistance during the course of treatment (80). MICs for the six common human *Trichosporon* species indicate all species to have resistance to flucytosine (MICs, 12.5 to 50 μg/ml), to have higher fluconazole MICs than those for most *Candida* species (MICs, 0.38 to 25 μg/ml), and to be variably susceptible to amphotericin B (MICs, 0.25 to >4 μg/ml), ketoconazole (MICs, 0.01 to 1.25 μg/ml), and itraconazole (MICs, 0.1 to 0.15 μg/ml) (44, 96). Echinocandins (caspofungin) are considered ineffective against *Trichosporon* species.

EVALUATION, INTERPRETATION, AND REPORTING OF RESULTS

As taxonomic relationships are devised and revised, the names of organisms change. To prevent confusion, it is recommended that clinical reports include the more familiar

TABLE 7 Antifungal susceptibilities

Organism	MIC (μg/ml) of drug[a]								Reference(s)
	AmB	5FC	Flucon	Itra	Vori	Pos	Casp	Terb	
Blastomyces capitatus	0.5–2.0	0.25–0.5	16–32	0.12–0.50	0.25–0.5	0.03–0.25[c]	ND	ND	40,[c] 90
Candida albicans	0.06–1.0	1.0[b]	0.25–64	0.06–4	0.015–1	0.03–0.12[c]	0.015–0.125	0.03–128[b]	40,[c] 94
C. dubliniensis	0.05–0.38	0.12	0.12–64	0.015–0.5	0.008–0.5	0.03[c]	ND	ND	40,[c] 72
C. famata	0.5[b]	1.0[a]	4–8[b]	0.25[b]	0.06[a]	0.03–0.25[c]	ND	>128[b]	40[c]
C. glabrata	0.125–4	ND	1–>64	0.125–4	0.03–1	0.03–1.0[c]	0.015–0.5	>128[b]	40,[c] 94
C. guilliermondii	0.06–32	0.06–4	0.5–>128	0.06–>8	0.06–>8	0.06–8	0.03–>8	0.625–100[b]	195, 199
C. haemulonii	0.5–32	ND	2–128	0.125–4	0.03–2	ND	0.125–0.25	ND	125
C. kefyr	0.5[b]	0.03–16[b]	0.5–1[b]	0.25–0.5[a]	0.03[a]	0.03[c]	ND	0.5–50[b]	40[c]
C. krusei	0.03–16	0.06–64	32–64[b]	0.5[a]	0.5–1.0[a]	0.03	0.03–2.0	8–32[b]	40,[c] 197
C. lusitaniae	1.5–2.0	0.004–>32	0.064–6.0	0.004–0.5	0.003–0.094	0.03[c]	4–8	ND	40,[c] 81, 136
C. parapsilosis	0.125–1	1.0[a]	0.25–8	0.015–2	0.015–1	0.03–0.12[c]	0.06–2	0.125–2[b]	40,[c] 94
C. rugosa	0.5–1.0	0.12–1.0	1–8	0.03–0.12	0.03–0.06	0.03[c]	ND	ND	40,[c] 72
C. tropicalis	0.06–1	1.0[a]	0.05–32	0.03–4	0.03–1	0.03–>16[c]	0.015–0.125	1.0[b]	40,[c] 94
Cryptococcus neoformans	0.5–1[b]	2–8[b]	2–8[b]	0.5[b]	0.25[a]	0.125–0.5	>8	2–8[b]	136
Kodamaea ohmeri	0.25–0.5	ND	2–32	0.125–0.5	0.3–0.5	ND	0.125–0.25	ND	138
Malassezia dermatis	0.03–0.12	ND	2	0.016–0.03	0.12	ND	ND	0.03–4	10
M. furfur	0.12–16	>64	2–32	0.03–25	0.03–16	0.03–32[c]	ND	0.03–50	10
M. globosa	0.10–4	ND	12.5–50	0.016–6.3	0.03–0.12	0.03–0.06[c]	ND	0.06–16	10
M. japonica	ND	ND	ND	0.016	ND	ND	ND	ND	10
M. nana	ND	ND	ND	0.016	ND	ND	ND	ND	10
M. obtusa	0.03–0.06	ND	2	0.016–1.6	0.03–0.06	ND	ND	0.03–64	10
M. pachydermatis	0.12	>64	4–16	0.016–6.3	0.03–0.25	ND	ND	0.03–50	10
M. restricta	4–8	ND	0.5–1	0.0156–6.3	0.03	0.03[c]	ND	0.06–4	10
M. slooffiae	0.5–8	>64	1–4	0.016–0.8	0.03–0.25	0.03[c]	ND	0.03–25	10
M. sympodialis	0.06–0.5	>64	0.25–16	0.016–0.2	0.03–0.125	0.03–0.06	ND	0.03–6.3	10
M. yamatoensis	ND	ND	ND	0.016	ND	ND	ND	ND	10
Pichia anomala	0.12–1	ND	2–16	0.06–1	0.03–0.5	ND	0.03–0.25	ND	67
Rhodotorula glutinis	0.25–0.5	>64	64	2–16	2–16	0.06[c]	ND	ND	40,[c] 226
R. mucilaginosa	0.5–1	ND	0.5–>64	0.25–4	0.25–4	ND	ND	ND	72
Saccharomyces cerevisiae	0.5[b]	0.125[b]	0.25–>64	0.015–>4	0.03[a]	0.015–>4	4–8	0.125[b]	14, 136
Sporobolomyces salmonicolor	0.25–16	ND	8–64	0.25–0.5	0.12–0.25	ND	ND	ND	226
Trichosporon asahii	025–1.0	22.2[d]	1–16	0.12–1	0.12–1	0.03–0.25[c]	>8	ND	40,[c] 72,[d] 136, 226
T. asteroides	0.25–4.0	0.5–64	0.125–1	0.03–0.125	0.03–0.06	ND	2–>16	ND	44
T. cutaneum	0.012	6.25	2.2	0.01	ND	ND	ND	ND	72
T. mucoides	1	50[d]	2–64	0.25–2	0.12–0.16	ND	ND	ND	72,[d] 226
T. ovoides	0.03	35.3	4.4	0.02	ND	ND	ND	ND	72

[a]Abbreviations: AmB, amphotericin B; 5-FC, flucytosine; Flucon, fluconazole; Itra, itraconazole; Vori, voriconazole; Pos, posaconazole; Casp, caspofungin; Terb, terbinafine; ND, not determined.
[b]MICs taken from http://www.mycology.adelaide.edu.au/Laboratory_Methods/Antifungal_Susceptibility_Testing/astrprofiles.html.
[c]MICs taken from reference 40 for posaconazole.
[d]MICs taken from reference 72 for 5FC.

species names alongside any new classification being used. For *Candida* species, rather than change the name of these organisms from names that are deeply entrenched in the literature and in the minds of physicians and laboratorians, the species have retained their *Candida* genus taxon and have been placed within the order mitosporic *Saccharomycetales* in the class Saccharomycetes.

As in clinical bacteriology, the significance of isolating a species known to be a member of the normal microbiota or a common contaminant depends on numerous factors, including, but not limited to, the patient's underlying disease, geographic and hospital environment, specimen site, preceding antimicrobial and device management, specimen collection and quality, and specimen processing. In general, the isolation of yeasts from sterile body sites is suggestive of infection, but the caveat to consider is the influence of the method of collection (e.g., *C. albicans* in CSF collected by lumbar puncture). The more challenging decision about significance is when the yeast is present in specimens obtained from nonsterile body sites.

Review of the literature reveals a surprising lack of evidence-based studies regarding development of criteria for establishing significance in nonsterile body sites. Clinical microbiology laboratories typically apply bacterial criteria to assess specimens for possible fungal infection. An example of this is to not report yeasts unless they predominate (above bacteria). There are several problems with this approach. First, yeasts are not as abundant as bacteria in the normal microbiota, so an increase in relative abundance may reflect yeast infection. Roughly 10 times more bacteria than yeasts can occupy the same volume of tissue. Second, a specimen from a patient who is receiving antibacterial agents may contain more abundant yeasts, the reporting of which may mislead the patient's physician about the yeast's significance. Third, when the abundance of a yeast is considered insufficient to warrant further investigation, the species may not be reported. This could lead to unfortunate consequences because certain yeasts, such as *C. tropicalis*, are considered particularly aggressive in immunocompromised patients.

Two specimens that are particularly problematic are sputum and urine (clean catch, indwelling catheter, and "in and out" catheter). The significance of *Candida* species in sputum regardless of quantity has been questioned (16, 176). The presence of yeasts in sputum has little significance, as the respiratory tract is frequently colonized by *Candida* species in patients receiving ventilatory support. The latest Infectious Diseases Society of America guidelines recommend that antifungal therapy not be initiated on the basis of a positive respiratory tract culture, and in cases where *Candida* pneumonia is suspected, histopathological evidence should be sought (190). Similarly, the presence of a few *C. neoformans* CFU in sputum does not necessarily imply etiologic significance unless there is patient information which is strongly suggestive of cryptococcosis. To prevent unnecessary testing but still provide useful information to physicians, Barenfanger et al. (16) recommend reporting "yeast, not *Cryptococcus*" for all respiratory secretion specimens in which a rapidly growing yeast is obtained, and confining full identification to patients for whom candidal pneumonia was indicated by histopathology. Patients for whom the limited form of identification was used were found to experience a shorter length of stay in hospital, received fewer antifungals, had a lower mortality rate, and incurred fewer expenses. *Cryptococcus* species are ruled out using a rapid urease test. This approach allows

physicians the opportunity to request further identification if desired. A similar approach to rapidly growing yeasts isolated from routine urine specimens (urinary tract infection is the only presentation) could also be used. However, in this situation, differentiation of *C. glabrata* from other common yeast uropathogens could be achieved using one of the simple rapid tests.

The significance of yeasts in urine must be examined in the context of the clinical setting and whether therapy would be desirable. If the patient is asymptomatic and there is no predisposing condition, then the situation should be monitored. If a predisposing condition is identified, then treatment may be justified, but for patients with higher risk factors, such as neonates or immunocompromised patients with fever and risk of candidemia, treatment should be commenced. Fluconazole is the frontline therapy unless *C. krusei* or *C. glabrata* infection is suspected, and in these cases irrigation of the bladder with amphotericin B may be implicated (190).

Although yeast species express different profiles of susceptibility to antifungals, especially to the expanding spectrum of new antifungal agents (Table 7), the most commonly isolated *Candida* species are generally susceptible to the triazoles, the polyenes, and the echinocandins. The two exceptions for the triazoles are *C. glabrata* and *C. krusei* (*C. parapsilosis* isolates are occasionally resistant to the echinocandins). *C. krusei* is relatively rarely isolated from infections. Thus, the need to identify rapidly growing yeasts present in clinically significant quantities from nonsterile sites can be limited to performing a rapid screen for *C. glabrata*. It is more important to obtain a yeast's antifungal susceptibility profile if there is a failure to respond to antifungal therapy or if an azole-resistant isolate is suspected (190).

REFERENCES

1. **Adler, A., C. Hidalgo-Grass, T. Boekhout, B. Theelen, E. Sionov, and I. Polacheck.** 2007. *Pichia farinosa* bloodstream infection in a lymphoma patient. *J. Clin. Microbiol.* **45:**3456–3458.
2. **Agirbasli, H., H. Bilgen, S. K. Ozcan, B. Otlu, G. Sinik, N. Cerikcioglu, R. Durmaz, E. Can, N. Yalman, G. Gedikoglu, and T. Sugita.** 2008. Two possible cases of *Trichosporon* infections in bone-marrow-transplanted children: the first case of *T. japonicum* isolated from clinical specimens. *Jpn. J. Infect. Dis.* **61:**130–132.
3. **Alcoba-Florez, J., S. Mendez-Alvarez, J. Cano, J. Guarro, E. Perez-Roth, and M. del Pilar Arevalo.** 2005. Phenotypic and molecular characterization of *Candida nivariensis* sp. nov., a possible new opportunistic fungus. *J. Clin. Microbiol.* **43:**4107–4111.
4. **Al Mosaid, A., D. Sullivan, I. F. Salkin, D. Shanley, and D. C. Coleman.** 2001. Differentiation of *Candida dubliniensis* from *Candida albicans* on Staib agar and caffeic acid-ferric citrate agar. *J. Clin. Microbiol.* **39:**323–327.
5. **Al Mosaid, A., D. J. Sullivan, and D. C. Coleman.** 2003. Differentiation of *Candida dubliniensis* from *Candida albicans* on Pal's agar. *J. Clin. Microbiol.* **41:**4787–4789.
6. **Alter, S. J., and J. Farley.** 1994. Development of *Hansenula anomala* infection in a child receiving fluconazole therapy. *Pediatr. Infect. Dis. J.* **13:**158–159.
7. **Anhalt, E., J. Alvarez, and R. Bert.** 1986. *Torulopsis glabrata* meningitis. *South. Med. J.* **79:**916.
8. **Apaire-Marchais, V., M. Kempf, C. Lefrancois, A. Marot, P. Licznar, J. Cottin, D. Poulain, and R. Robert.** 2008. Evaluation of an immunomagnetic separation method to capture *Candida* yeasts cells in blood. *BMC Microbiol.* **8:**157–160.
9. **Arias, C. R., J. K. Burns, L. M. Friedrich, R. M. Goodrich, and M. E. Parish.** 2002. Yeast species associated with orange juice: evaluation of different identification methods. *Appl. Environ. Microbiol.* **68:**1955–1961.

10. **Ashbee, H. R.** 2007. Update on the genus *Malassezia*. *Med. Mycol.* **45:**287–303.

11. **Aspiroz, C., M. Ara, M. Varea, A. Rezusta, and C. Rubio.** 2002. Isolation of *Malassezia globosa* and M. *sympodialis* from patients with pityriasis versicolor in Spain. *Mycopathologia* **154:**111–117.

12. **Baird, D. R., M. Harris, R. Menon, and R. Stoddart.** 1985. Systemic infection with *Trichosporon capitatum* in two patients with leukemia. *Eur. J. Clin. Microbiol.* **4:**62–64.

13. **Bakir, M., N. Cerikcioglu, A. Tirtir, S. Berrak, E. Ozek, and C. Canpolat.** 2004. *Pichia anomala* fungaemia in immunocompromised children. *Mycoses* **47:**231–235.

14. **Barchiesi, F., D. Arzeni, A. W. Fothergill, L. F. Di Francesco, F. Caselli, M. G. Rinaldi, and G. Scalise.** 2000. In vitro activities of the new antifungal triazole SCH 56592 against common and emerging yeast pathogens. *Antimicrob. Agents Chemother.* **44:**226–229.

15. **Bard, M., A. M. Sturm, C. A. Pierson, S. Brown, K. M. Rogers, J. Eckstein, R. Barbuch, N. D. Lees, S. A. Howell, and K. C. Hazen.** 2005. Sterol uptake in *Candida glabrata*: rescue of sterol auxotrophic strains. *Diagn. Microbiol. Infect. Dis.* **52:**285–293.

16. **Barenfanger, J., P. Arakere, R. D. Cruz, A. Imran, C. Drake, J. Lawhorn, S. J. Verhulst, and N. Khardori.** 2003. Improved outcomes associated with limiting identification of *Candida* spp. in respiratory secretions. *J. Clin. Microbiol.* **41:**5645–5649.

17. **Barnes, R. A., and L. Vale.** 2005. 'Spiking' as a rapid method for differentiation of *Candida albicans* from other yeast species. *J. Hosp. Infect.* **60:**78–80.

18. **Barnett, J. A., R. W. Payne, and D. Yarrow.** 2000. *Yeasts: Characteristics and Identification*, 3rd ed. Cambridge University Press, Cambridge, United Kingdom.

19. **Baron, E. J.** 2001. Rapid identification of bacteria and yeast: summary of the National Committee for Clinical Laboratory Standards proposed guideline. *Clin. Infect. Dis.* **33:**220–225.

20. **Baumgartner, C., A. Freydiere, and Y. Gille.** 1996. Direct identification and recognition of yeast species from clinical material by using Albicans ID and CHROMagar Candida plates. *J. Clin. Microbiol.* **34:**454–456.

21. **Beijerinck, M. W.** 1889. L'auxanographie, ou la méthode de l'hydrodiffusion dans la gélatine appliqué aux recherches microbiologiques. *Arch. Néerl. Sci. Exactes Nat.* **23:**367–372.

22. **Bennett, J.** 2008. Is real-time polymerase chain reaction ready for real use in detecting candidemia? *Clin. Infect. Dis.* **46:**897–898.

23. **Bergman, A. G., and C. A. Kauffman.** 1984. Dermatitis due to *Sporobolomyces* infection. *Arch. Dermatol.* **120:**1059–1060.

24. **Blevins, L. B., J. Fenn, H. Segal, P. Newcomb-Gayman, and K. C. Carroll.** 1995. False-positive cryptococcal antigen latex agglutination caused by disinfectants and soaps. *J. Clin. Microbiol.* **33:**1674–1675.

25. **Boekhout, T., and R. W. Bosboom.** 1994. Karyotyping of Malassezia yeasts: taxonomic and epidemiological implications. *Syst. Appl. Microbiol.* **17:**146–153.

26. **Bonassoli, L. A., and T. I. Svidzinski.** 2002. Influence of the hospital environment on yeast colonization in nursing students. *Med. Mycol.* **40:**311–313.

27. **Bond, R., R. M. Anthony, M. Dodd, and D. H. Lloyd.** 1996. Isolation of *Malassezia sympodialis* from feline skin. *J. Med. Vet. Mycol.* **34:**145–147.

28. **Bond, R., S. A. Howell, P. J. Haywood, and D. H. Lloyd.** 1997. Isolation of *Malassezia sympodialis* and *Malassezia globosa* from healthy pet cats. *Vet. Rec.* **141:**200–201.

29. **Borman, A. M., C. J. Linton, S. J. Miles, and E. M. Johnson.** 2008. Molecular identification of pathogenic fungi. *J. Antimicrob. Chemother.* **61**(Suppl. 1)**:**i7–i12.

30. **Borman, A. M., R. Petch, C. J. Linton, M. D. Palmer, P. D. Bridge, and E. M. Johnson.** 2008. *Candida nivariensis*, an emerging pathogenic fungus with multidrug resistance to antifungal agents. *J. Clin. Microbiol.* **46:**933–938.

31. **Boudewijns, M., J. M. Bakkers, P. D. Sturm, and W. J. Melchers.** 2006. 16S rRNA gene sequencing and the routine clinical microbiology laboratory: a perfect marriage? *J. Clin. Microbiol.* **44:**3469–3470.

32. **Bovers, M., F. Hagen, and T. Boekhout.** 2008. Diversity of the *Cryptococcus neoformans-Cryptococcus gattii* species complex. *Rev. Iberoam. Micol.* **25:**S4–S12.

33. **Boyanton, B. L., Jr., R. A. Luna, L. R. Fasciano, K. G. Menne, and J. Versalovic.** 2008. DNA pyrosequencing-based identification of pathogenic *Candida* species by using the internal transcribed spacer 2 region. *Arch. Pathol. Lab. Med.* **132:**667–674.

34. **Buchaille, L., A.-M. Freydiere, R. Guinet, and Y. Gille.** 1998. Evaluation of six commercial systems for identification of medically important yeasts. *Eur. J. Clin. Microbiol. Infect. Dis.* **17:**479–488.

35. **Buschelman, B., R. N. Jones, M. A. Pfaller, F. P. Koontz, and G. V. Doern.** 1999. Colony morphology of *Candida* spp. as a guide to species identification. *Diagn. Microbiol. Infect. Dis.* **35:**89–91.

36. **Byrnes, E. J., III, R. J. Bildfell, S. A. Frank, T. G. Mitchell, K. A. Marr, and J. Heitman.** 2009. Molecular evidence that the range of the Vancouver Island outbreak of *Cryptococcus gattii* infection has expanded into the Pacific Northwest in the United States. *J. Infect. Dis.* **199:**1081–1086.

37. **Cabanes, F. J., B. Theelen, G. Castella, and T. Boekhout.** 2007. Two new lipid-dependent *Malassezia* species from domestic animals. *FEMS Yeast Res.* **7:**1064–1076.

38. **Calderone, R. A. (ed.).** 2002. Candida *and Candidiasis*. ASM Press, Washington, DC.

39. **Campa, D., A. Tavanti, F. Gemignani, C. S. Mogavero, I. Bellini, F. Bottari, R. Barale, S. Landi, and S. Senesi.** 2008. DNA microarray based on arrayed-primer extension technique for identification of pathogenic fungi responsible for invasive and superficial mycoses. *J. Clin. Microbiol.* **46:**909–915.

40. **Canton, E., J. Peman, A. Espinel-Ingroff, E. Martin-Mazuelos, A. Carrillo-Munoz, and J. P. Martinez.** 2008. Comparison of disc diffusion assay with the CLSI reference method (M27-A2) for testing in vitro posaconazole activity against common and uncommon yeasts. *J. Antimicrob. Chemother.* **61:**135–138.

41. **Carmody, T. J., and K. K. Kane.** 1986. *Torulopsis (Candida) glabrata* endocarditis involving a bovine pericardial xenograft heart valve. *Heart Lung* **15:**40–42.

42. **Cawley, M. J., G. R. Braxton, L. R. Haith, Jr., K. J. Reilley, R. E. Guilday, and M. L. Patton.** 2000. *Trichosporon beigelii* infection: experience in a regional burn center. *Burns* **26:**482–486.

43. **Celik, A. D., R. Ozaras, S. Kantarcioglu, A. Mert, F. Tabak, and R. Ozturk.** 2009. Spondylodiscitis due to an emergent fungal pathogen: *Blastoschizomyces capitatus*, a case report and review of the literature. *Rheumatol. Int.* **29:**1237–1241.

44. **Chagas-Neto, T. C., G. M. Chaves, A. S. Melo, and A. L. Colombo.** 2009. Bloodstream infections due to *Trichosporon* spp.: species distribution, *Trichosporon asahii* genotypes determined on the basis of ribosomal DNA intergenic spacer 1 sequencing, and antifungal susceptibility testing. *J. Clin. Microbiol.* **47:**1074–1081.

45. **Chakrabarti, A., K. Singh, A. Narang, S. Singhi, R. Batra, K. L. Rao, P. Ray, S. Gopalan, S. Das, V. Gupta, A. K. Gupta, S. M. Bose, and M. M. McNeil.** 2001. Outbreak of *Pichia anomala* infection in the pediatric service of a tertiary-care center in northern India. *J. Clin. Microbiol.* **39:**1702–1706.

46. **Chanock, S. J., P. Toltzis, and C. Wilson.** 1993. Cross-reactivity between *Stomatococcus mucilaginosus* and latex agglutination for cryptococcal antigen. *Lancet* **342:**1119–1120.

47. **Chen, K. W., Y. C. Chen, Y. H. Lin, H. H. Chou, and S. Y. Li.** 2009. The molecular epidemiology of serial *Candida tropicalis* isolates from ICU patients as revealed by multilocus sequence typing and pulsed-field gel electrophoresis. *Infect. Genet. Evol.* **9:**912–920.

48. **Chen, S., T. Sorrell, G. Nimmo, B. Speed, B. Currie, D. Ellis, D. Marriott, T. Pfeiffer, D. Parr, K. Byth, and the Australasian Cryptococcal Study Group.** 2000. Epidemiology and host- and variety-dependent characteristics of infection due to *Cryptococcus neoformans* in Australia and New Zealand. *Clin. Infect. Dis.* **31:**499–508.

49. **Chen, Y. C., J. D. Eisner, M. M. Kattar, S. L. Rassoulian-Barrett, K. Lafe, U. Bui, A. P. Limaye, and B. T. Cookson.** 2001. Polymorphic internal transcribed spacer region 1 DNA

sequences identify medically important yeasts. *J. Clin. Microbiol.* **39:**4042–4051.

50. **Chen, Y. C., J. D. Eisner, M. M. Kattar, S. L. Rassoulian-Barrett, K. LaFe, S. L. Yarfitz, A. P. Limaye, and B. T. Cookson.** 2000. Identification of medically important yeasts using PCR-based detection of DNA sequence polymorphisms in the internal transcribed spacer 2 region of the rRNA genes. *J. Clin. Microbiol.* **38:**2302–2310.

51. **Cheung, M. Y., N. C. Chiu, S. H. Chen, H. C. Liu, C. T. Ou, and D. C. Liang.** 1999. Mandibular osteomyelitis caused by *Blastoschizomyces capitatus* in a child with acute myelogenous leukemia. *J. Formos. Med. Assoc.* **98:**787–789.

52. **Chowdhary, A., H. S. Randhawa, S. Sharma, M. E. Brandt, and S. Kumar.** 2005. *Malassezia furfur* in a case of onychomycosis: colonizer or etiologic agent? *Med. Mycol.* **43:**87–90.

53. **Chryssanthou, E., V. Fernandez, and B. Petrini.** 2007. Performance of commercial latex agglutination tests for the differentiation of *Candida dubliniensis* and *Candida albicans* in routine diagnostics. *APMIS* **115:**1281–1284.

54. **Chuck, S. L., and M. A. Sande.** 1989. Infections with *Cryptococcus neoformans* in the acquired immunodeficiency syndrome. *N. Engl. J. Med.* **321:**794–799.

55. **Ciardo, D. E., G. Schar, E. C. Bottger, M. Altwegg, and P. P. Bosshard.** 2006. Internal transcribed spacer sequencing versus biochemical profiling for identification of medically important yeasts. *J. Clin. Microbiol.* **44:**77–84.

56. **Cliff, P. R., J. A. Sandoe, J. Heritage, and R. C. Barton.** 2008. Use of multilocus sequence typing for the investigation of colonisation by *Candida albicans* in intensive care unit patients. *J. Hosp. Infect.* **69:**24–32.

57. **Clinical and Laboratory Standards Institute.** 2008. *Interpretive Criteria for Identification of Bacteria and Fungi by DNA Target Sequencing; Approved Guideline.* CLSI document MM18-A. Clinical and Laboratory Standards Institute, Wayne, PA.

58. **Clinical and Laboratory Standards Institute.** 2006. *Molecular Diagnostic Methods for Infectious Diseases; Approved Guideline—Second Edition.* CLSI document MM03-02. Clinical and Laboratory Standards Institute, Wayne, PA.

58a. **Clinical and Laboratory Standards Institute/NCCLS.** 2008. *Abbreviated Identification of Bacteria and Yeast; Approved Guideline,* 2nd ed. CLSI document M35-A2. Clinical and Laboratory Standards Institute/NCCLS, Wayne, PA.

59. **Cockcroft, D. W., B. A. Berscheid, I. A. Ramshaw, and J. Dolovich.** 1983. *Sporobolomyces:* a possible cause of extrinsic allergic alveolitis. *J. Allergy Clin. Immunol.* **72:**305–309.

60. **Cooper, B. H., and M. Silva-Hutner.** 1985. Yeasts of medical importance, p. 526–541. *In* E. H. Lennette, A. Balows, W. J. Hausler, Jr., and H. J. Shadomy (ed.), *Manual of Clinical Microbiology,* 4th ed. American Society for Microbiology, Washington, DC.

61. **Correia, A., P. Sampaio, S. James, and C. Pais.** 2006. *Candida bracarensis* sp. nov., a novel anamorphic yeast species phenotypically similar to *Candida glabrata.* *Int. J. Syst. Evol. Microbiol.* **56:**313–317.

62. **Cox, G. M., and J. R. Perfect.** 1998. *Cryptococcus neoformans* var. *neoformans* and *gattii* and *Trichosporon* species, p. 474–484. *In* L. Ajello and R. J. Hay (ed.), *Topley & Wilson's Microbiology and Microbial Infections,* 9th ed., vol. 4. *Medical Mycology.* Arnold, London, United Kingdom.

63. **Crespo, M. J., M. L. Abarca, and F. J. Cabanes.** 1999. Isolation of *Malassezia furfur* from a cat. *J. Clin. Microbiol.* **37:**1573–1574.

64. **Crespo-Erchiga, V., A. Ojeda Martos, A. Vera Casano, A. Crespo-Erchiga, F. Sanchez Fajardo, and E. Gueho.** 1999. Mycology of pityriasis versicolor. *J. Mycol. Med.* **9:**143–148.

65. **Crozier, W. J., and K. A. Wise.** 1993. Onychomycosis due to *Pityrosporum.* *Australas. J. Dermatol.* **34:**109–112.

66. **Dalle, F., P. E. Charles, K. Blanc, D. Caillot, P. Chavanet, F. Dromer, and A. Bonnin.** 2005. *Cryptococcus neoformans* galactoxylomannan contains an epitope(s) that is cross-reactive with *Aspergillus* galactomannan. *J. Clin. Microbiol.* **43:**2929–2931.

67. **da Matta, D. A., L. P. de Almeida, A. M. Machado, A. C. Azevedo, E. J. Kusano, N. F. Travassos, R. Salomao, and A. L. Colombo.** 2007. Antifungal susceptibility of 1000 Candida bloodstream isolates to 5 antifungal drugs: results of a multicenter study conducted in Sao Paulo, Brazil, 1995–2003. *Diagn. Microbiol. Infect. Dis.* **57:**399–404.

68. **D'Antonio, D., F. Romano, A. Iacone, B. Violante, P. Fazii, E. Pontieri, T. Staniscia, C. Caracciolo, S. Bianchini, R. Sferra, A. Vetuschi, E. Gaudio, and G. Carruba.** 1999. Onychomycosis caused by *Blastoschizomyces capitatus.* *J. Clin. Microbiol.* **37:**2927–2930.

69. **Davis, L. E., C. E. Shields, and W. G. Merz.** 2005. Use of a commercial reagent leads to reduced germ tube production by *Candida dubliniensis.* *J. Clin. Microbiol.* **43:**2465–2466.

70. **Dealler, S. F.** 1991. *Candida albicans* colony identification in 5 minutes in a general microbiology laboratory. *J. Clin. Microbiol.* **29:**1081–1082.

71. **De Almeida, G. M., S. F. Costa, M. Melhem, A. L. Motta, M. W. Szeszs, F. Miyashita, L. C. Pierrotti, F. Rossi, and M. N. Burattini.** 2008. *Rhodotorula* spp. isolated from blood cultures: clinical and microbiological aspects. *Med. Mycol.* **46:**547–556.

72. **de Hoog, G. S., J. Guarro, J. Gene, and M. J. Figueras.** 2000. *Atlas of Clinical Fungi,* 2nd ed. Centraalbureau voor Schimmelcultures, Delft, The Netherlands.

73. **Desnos-Ollivier, M., M. Ragon, V. Robert, D. Raoux, J. C. Gantier, and F. Dromer.** 2008. *Debaryomyces hansenii (Candida famata),* a rare human fungal pathogen often misidentified as *Pichia guilliermondii (Candida guilliermondii).* *J. Clin. Microbiol.* **46:**3237–3242.

74. **Dromer, F., L. Improvisi, B. Dupont, M. Eliaszewicz, G. Pialoux, S. Fournier, and V. Feuillie.** 1997. Oral transmission of *Candida albicans* between partners in HIV-infected couples could contribute to dissemination of fluconazole-resistant isolates. *AIDS* **11:**1095–1101.

75. **Drouhet, E., and B. Dupont.** 1991. Candidosis in heroin addicts and AIDS: new immunologic data on chronic mucocutaneous candidosis, p. 61–72. *In* E. Tümbay, H. P. R. Seeliger, and O. Ang (ed.), *Candida and Candidamycosis.* Plenum Press, New York, NY.

76. **Ebright, J. R., M. R. Fairfax, and J. A. Vazquez.** 2001. *Trichosporon asahii,* a non-*Candida* yeast that caused fatal septic shock in a patient without cancer or neutropenia. *Clin. Infect. Dis.* **33:**e28–e30.

77. **Eisenberg, E. S., B. E. Alpert, R. A. Weiss, N. Mittman, and R. Soeiro.** 1983. *Rhodotorula rubra* peritonitis in patients undergoing continuous ambulatory peritoneal dialysis. *Am. J. Med.* **75:**349–352.

78. **Ellepola, A. N., and C. J. Morrison.** 2005. Laboratory diagnosis of invasive candidiasis. *J. Microbiol.* **43**(Spec. No.):65–84.

79. **Eschete, M. L., and B. C. West.** 1980. *Saccharomyces cerevisiae* septicemia. *Arch. Intern. Med.* **140:**1539.

80. **Espinel-Ingroff, A.** 2008. Mechanisms of resistance to antifungal agents: yeasts and filamentous fungi. *Rev. Iberoam. Micol.* **25:**101–106.

81. **Favel, A., A. Michel-Nguyen, A. Datry, S. Challier, F. Leclerc, C. Chastin, K. Fallague, and P. Regli.** 2004. Susceptibility of clinical isolates of *Candida lusitaniae* to five systemic antifungal agents. *J. Antimicrob. Chemother.* **53:**526–529.

82. **Fell, J. W., T. Boekhout, A. Fonseca, G. Scorzetti, and A. Ststzell-Tallman.** 2000. Biodiversity and systematics of basidiomycetous yeasts as determined by large-subunit rDNA D1/D2 domain sequence analysis. *Int. J. Syst. Evol. Microbiol.* **50:**1351–1371.

83. **Fell, J. W., and A. S. Tallman.** 1984. *Sporobolomyces* Kluyver et van Niel, p. 911–920. *In* N. J. W. Kreger-van Rij (ed.), *The Yeasts: a Taxonomic Study,* 3rd ed. Elsevier Science Publishers, Amsterdam, The Netherlands.

84. **Fenn, J. P., E. Billetdeaux, H. Segal, L. Skodack-Jones, P. E. Padilla, M. Bale, and K. Carroll.** 1999. Comparison of four methodologies for rapid and cost-effective identification of *Candida glabrata.* *J. Clin. Microbiol.* **37:**3387–3389.

85. **Fidel, P. L., Jr., J. A. Vazquez, and J. D. Sobel.** 1999. *Candida glabrata:* review of epidemiology, pathogenesis, and clinical disease with comparison to *C. albicans.* *Clin. Microbiol. Rev.* **12:**80–96.

86. Foulet, F., N. Nicolas, O. Eloy, F. Botterel, J. C. Gantier, J. M. Costa, and S. Bretagne. 2005. Microsatellite marker analysis as a typing system for *Candida glabrata. J. Clin. Microbiol.* **43:**4574–4579.

87. Fowell, R. R. 1952. Sodium acetate agar as a sporulation medium for yeast. *Nature* **170:**578.

88. Freydiere, A.-M., R. Guinet, and P. Boiron. 2001. Yeast identification in the clinical microbiology laboratory: phenotypical methods. *Med. Mycol.* **39:**9–33.

89. Freydiere, A. M., J. D. Perry, O. Faure, B. Willinger, A. M. Tortorano, A. Nicholson, J. Peman, and P. E. Verweij. 2004. Routine use of a commercial test, GLABRATA RTT, for rapid identification of *Candida glabrata* in six laboratories. *J. Clin. Microbiol.* **42:**4870–4872.

90. Gadea, I., M. Cuenca-Estrella, E. Prieto, T. M. Diaz-Guerra, J. I. Garcia-Cia, E. Mellado, J. F. Tomas, and J. L. Rodriguez-Tudela. 2004. Genotyping and antifungal susceptibility profile of *Dipodascus capitatus* isolates causing disseminated infection in seven hematological patients of a tertiary hospital. *J. Clin. Microbiol.* **42:**1832–1836.

91. Galgiani, J. N., J. Reiser, C. Brass, A. Espinel-Ingroff, M. A. Gordon, and T. M. Kerkering. 1987. Comparison of relative susceptibilites of *Candida* species to three antifungal agents as determined by unstandardized methods. *Antimicrob. Agents Chemother.* **31:**1343–1347.

92. Geha, D. J., and G. D. Roberts. 1994. Laboratory detection of fungemia. *Clin. Lab. Med.* **14:**83–97.

93. Gil-Lamaignere, C., E. Roilides, J. Hacker, and F. M. Muller. 2003. Molecular typing for fungi—a critical review of the possibilities and limitations of currently [sic] and future methods. *Clin. Microbiol. Infect.* **9:**172–185.

94. Gonzalez, G. M., M. Elizondo, and J. Ayala. 2008. Trends in species distribution and susceptibility of bloodstream isolates of *Candida* collected in Monterrey, Mexico, to seven antifungal agents: results of a 3-year (2004 to 2007) surveillance study. *J. Clin. Microbiol.* **46:**2902–2905.

95. Graf, B., T. Adam, E. Zill, and U. B. Gobel. 2000. Evaluation of the VITEK 2 system for rapid identification of yeasts and yeast-like organisms. *J. Clin. Microbiol.* **38:**1782–1785.

96. Guého, E., L. Improvisi, G. S. de Hoog, and B. Dupont. 1994. *Trichosporon* on humans: a practical account. *Mycoses* **37:**3–10.

97. Gueho, E., G. Midgley, and J. Guillot. 1996. The genus *Malassezia* with description of four new species. *Antonie van Leeuwenhoek J. Microbiol. Serol.* **69:**337–355.

98. Guého, E., M. T. Smith, G. S. de Hoog, G. Billon-Grand, R. Christen, and W. H. Batenburg-van der Vegte. 1992. Contributions to a revision of the genus *Trichosporon.* *Antonie van Leeuwenhoek J. Microbiol. Serol.* **61:**289–316.

99. Guillot, J., E. Guého, M. Lesourd, G. Midgley, G. Chévrier, and B. Dupont. 1996. Identification of *Malassezia* species. *J. Mycol. Med.* **6:**103–110.

100. Gupta, A. K., T. Boekhout, B. Theelen, R. Summerbell, and R. Batra. 2004. Identification and typing of *Malassezia* species by amplified fragment length polymorphism and sequence analyses of the internal transcribed spacer and large-subunit regions of ribosomal DNA. *J. Clin. Microbiol.* **42:**4253–4260.

101. Gupta, A. K., Y. Kohli, and R. C. Summerbell. 2000. Molecular differentiation of seven *Malassezia* species. *J. Clin. Microbiol.* **38:**1869–1875.

102. Gupta, A. K., Y. Kohli, R. C. Summerbell, and J. Faergemann. 2001. Quantitative culture of *Malassezia* species from different body sites of individuals with or without dermatoses. *Med. Mycol.* **39:**243–251.

103. Hajjeh, R. A., M. E. Brandt, and R. W. Pinner. 1995. Emergence of cryptococcal disease: epidemiologic perspectives 100 years after its discovery. *ER* **17:**303–320.

104. Hall, L., S. Wohlfiel, and G. D. Roberts. 2003. Experience with the MicroSeq D2 Large-Subunit Ribosomal DNA Sequencing Kit for identification of commonly encountered, clinically important yeast species. *J. Clin. Microbiol.* **41:**5099–5102.

105. Hamal, P., J. Ostransky, M. Dendis, R. Horvath, F. Ruzicka, V. Buchta, M. Vejsova, P. Sauer, P. Hejnar, and V. Raclavsky. 2008. A case of endocarditis caused by the yeast *Pichia fabianii* with biofilm production and developed in vitro resistance to azoles in the course of antifungal treatment. *Med. Mycol.* **46:**601–605.

106. Han, X. Y., J. J. Tarrand, and E. Escudero. 2004. Infections by the yeast *Kodomaea (Pichia) ohmeri:* two cases and literature review. *Eur. J. Clin. Microbiol. Infect. Dis.* **23:**127.

107. Hawkins, J. L., and L. M. Baddour. 2003. *Candida lusitaniae* infections in the era of fluconazole availability. *Clin. Infect. Dis.* **36:**e14–e18.

108. Hazen, K. C. 1995. New and emerging yeast pathogens. *Clin. Microbiol. Rev.* **8:**462–478.

109. Hazen, K. C., and B. W. Hazen. 1987. Temperature-modulated physiological characteristics of *Candida albicans.* *Microbiol. Immunol.* **31:**497–508.

110. Hazen, K. C., J. Stei, C. Darracott, A. Breathnach, J. May, and S. A. Howell. 2005. Isolation of cholesterol-dependent *Candida glabrata* from clinical specimens. *Diagn. Microbiol. Infect. Dis.* **52:**35–37.

111. Hazen, K. C., J. G. Wu, and J. Masuoka. 2001. Comparison of hydrophobic properties between *Candida albicans* and *Candida dubliniensis. Infect. Immun.* **69:**779–786.

112. Hickey, W. F., L. H. Sommerville, and F. J. Schoen. 1983. Disseminated *Candida glabrata:* report of a uniquely severe infection and a literature review. *Am. J. Clin. Pathol.* **80:**724–727.

113. Hirai, A., R. Kano, K. Makimura, E. R. Duarte, J. S. Hamdan, M. A. Lachance, H. Yamaguchi, and A. Hasegawa. 2004. *Malassezia nana* sp. nov., a novel lipid-dependent yeast species isolated from animals. *Int. J. Syst. Evol. Microbiol.* **54:**623–627.

114. Holley, A., J. Dulhunty, S. Blot, J. Lipman, S. Lobo, C. Dancer, J. Rello, and G. Dimopoulos. 2009. Temporal trends, risk factors and outcomes in *albicans* and non-*albicans* candidaemia: an international epidemiological study in four multidisciplinary intensive care units. *Int. J. Antimicrob. Agents* **33:**554.e1–554.e7.

115. Hopper, R. L., E. V. Perry, and V. Fainstein. 1982. Diagnostic value of cryptococcal antigen in the cerebrospinal fluid of patients with malignant disease. *J. Infect. Dis.* **145:**915.

116. Horowitz, I. D., E. A. Blumburg, and L. Krevolin. 1993. *Cryptococcus albidus* and mucormycosis emphyema in a patient receiving hemodialysis. *South. Med. J.* **86:**1070–1072.

117. Hostetter, M. K. 2008. The iC3b receptor of *Candida albicans* and its roles in pathogenesis. *Vaccine* **26**(Suppl. 8): I108–I112.

118. Huttova, M., K. Kralinsky, J. Horn, I. Marinova, K. Iligova, J. Fric, S. Spanik, J. Filka, J. Uher, J. Kurak, and V. Krcmery, Jr. 1998. Prospective study of nosocomial fungal meningitis in children—report of 10 cases. *Scand. J. Infect. Dis.* **30:**485–487.

119. Jabra-Rizk, M. A., J. K. Johnson, G. Forrest, K. Mankes, T. F. Meiller, and R. A. Venezia. 2005. Prevalence of *Candida dubliniensis* fungemia at a large teaching hospital. *Clin. Infect. Dis.* **41:**1064–1067.

120. Jacobsen, M. D., T. Boekhout, and F. C. Odds. 2008. Multilocus sequence typing confirms synonymy but highlights differences between *Candida albicans* and *Candida stellatoidea. FEMS Yeast Res.* **8:**764–770.

121. Kartsonis, N., J. Killar, L. Mixson, C.-M. Hoe, C. Sable, K. Bartizal, and M. Motyl. 2005. Caspofungin susceptibility testing of isolates from patients with esophageal candidiasis or invasive candidiasis: relationship of MIC to treatment outcome. *Antimicrob. Agents Chemother.* **49:**3616–3623.

122. Khan, Z. U., S. Ahmad, E. Mokaddas, and R. Chandy. 2004. Tobacco agar, a new medium for differentiating *Candida dubliniensis* from *Candida albicans. J. Clin. Microbiol.* **42:**4796–4798.

123. Khlif, M., C. Mary, H. Sellami, A. Sellami, H. Dumon, A. Ayadi, and S. Ranque. 2009. Evaluation of nested and real-time PCR assays in the diagnosis of candidaemia. *Clin. Microbiol. Infect.* **15:**656–661.

124. Kiehn, T. E., E. Gorey, A. E. Brown, F. F. Edwards, and D. Armstrong. 1992. Sepsis due to *Rhodotorula* related to use of indwelling central venous catheters. *Clin. Infect. Dis.* **14:**841–846.

125. **Kim, M. N., J. H. Shin, H. Sung, K. Lee, E. C. Kim, N. Ryoo, J. S. Lee, S. I. Jung, K. H. Park, S. J. Kee, S. H. Kim, M. G. Shin, S. P. Suh, and D. W. Ryang.** 2009. *Candida haemulonii* and closely related species at 5 university hospitals in Korea: identification, antifungal susceptibility, and clinical features. *Clin. Infect. Dis.* **48:**e57–e61.

126. **Klein, A. S., G. T. Tortora, R. Malowitz, and W. H. Green.** 1988. *Hansenula anomala:* a new fungal pathogen. *Ann. Intern. Med.* **148:**1210–1213.

127. **Kollia, K., M. Arabatzis, O. Kostoula, A. Kostourou, A. Velegraki, E. Belessiotou, A. Lazou, and A. Kostourou.** 2003. *Clavispora (Candida) lusitaniae* susceptibility profiles and genetic diversity in three tertiary hospitals (1998–2001). *Int. J. Antimicrob. Agents* **22:**458–460.

128. **Krumholz, R. A.** 1972. Pulmonary cryptococcosis. A case due to *Cryptococcus albidus. Am. Rev. Respir. Dis.* **105:**421–424.

129. **Kurtzman, C. P., and J. W. Fell (ed.).** 1998. *The Yeasts: a Taxonomic Study,* 4th ed. Elsevier, New York, NY.

130. **Kurtzman, C. P., and C. J. Robnett.** 1998. Identification and phylogeny of ascomycetous yeasts from analysis of nuclear large subunit (26S) ribosomal DNA partial sequences. *Antonie van Leeuwenhoek J. Microbiol. Serol.* **73:**331–371.

131. **Kurtzman, C. P., C. J. Robnett, and E. Basehoar-Powers.** 2008. Phylogenetic relationships among species of *Pichia, Issatchenkia* and *Williopsis* determined from multigene sequence analysis, and the proposal of *Barnettozyma* gen. nov., *Lindnera* gen. nov. and *Wickerhamomyces* gen. nov. *FEMS Yeast Res.* **8:**939–954.

132. **Kwon-Chung, K. J., and J. E. Bennett.** 1992. *Medical Mycology.* Lea and Febiger, Philadelphia, PA.

133. **Kwon-Chung, K. J., J. B. Hicks, and P. N. Lipke.** 1990. Evidence that *Candida stellatoidea* type II is a mutant of *Candida albicans* that does not express sucrose-inhibitable α-glucosidase. *Infect. Immun.* **58:**2804–2808.

134. **Kwon-Chung, K. J., I. Polacheck, and J. E. Bennett.** 1982. Improved diagnostic medium for separation of *Cryptococcus neoformans* var. *neoformans* (serotypes A and D) and *Cryptococcus neoformans* var. *gattii* (serotypes B and C). *J. Clin. Microbiol.* **15:**535–537.

135. **Landlinger, C., S. Preuner, B. Willinger, B. Haberpursch, Z. Racil, J. Mayer, and T. Lion.** 2009. Species-specific identification of a wide range of clinically relevant fungal pathogens by use of Luminex xMAP technology. *J. Clin. Microbiol.* **47:**1063–1073.

136. **Lass-Flörl, C., A. Mayr, S. Perkhofer, G. Hinterberger, J. Hausdorfer, C. Speth, and M. Fille.** 2008. Activities of antifungal agents against yeasts and filamentous fungi: assessment according to the methodology of the European Committee on Antimicrobial Susceptibility Testing. *Antimicrob. Agents Chemother.* **52:**3637–3641.

137. **Lau, A., S. Chen, S. Sleiman, and T. Sorrell.** 2009. Current status and future perspectives on molecular and serological methods in diagnostic mycology. *Future Microbiol.* **4:** 1185-1222.

138. **Lee, J. S., J. H. Shin, M. N. Kim, S. I. Jung, K. H. Park, D. Cho, S. J. Kee, M. G. Shin, S. P. Suh, and D. W. Ryang.** 2007. *Kodamaea ohmeri* isolates from patients in a university hospital: identification, antifungal susceptibility, and pulsed-field gel electrophoresis analysis. *J. Clin. Microbiol.* **45:**1005–1010.

139. **Lee, J. W., G. A. Melcher, M. G. Rinaldi, P. A. Pizzo, and T. J. Walsh.** 1990. Patterns of morphologic variation among isolates of *Trichosporon beigelii. J. Clin. Microbiol.* **28:**2823–2827.

140. **Leeming, J. P., and F. H. Notman.** 1987. Improved methods for isolation and enumeration of *Malassezia furfur* from human skin. *J. Clin. Microbiol.* **25:**2017–2019.

141. **Leinberger, D. M., U. Schumacher, I. B. Autenrieth, and T. T. Bachmann.** 2005. Development of a DNA microarray for detection and identification of fungal pathogens involved in invasive mycoses. *J. Clin. Microbiol.* **43:**4943–4953.

142. **Letscher-Bru, V., M.-H. Meyer, A.-C. Galoisy, J. Waller, and E. Candolfi.** 2002. Prospective evaluation of the new chromogenic medium Candida ID, in comparison with Candiselect, for isolation of molds and isolation and presumptive identification of yeast species. *J. Clin. Microbiol.* **40:**1508–1510.

143. **Lin, C. Y., Y. C. Chen, H. J. Lo, K. W. Chen, and S. Y. Li.** 2007. Assessment of *Candida glabrata* strain relatedness by pulsed-field gel electrophoresis and multilocus sequence typing. *J. Clin. Microbiol.* **45:**2452–2459.

144. **Lin, X., and J. Heitman.** 2006. The biology of the *Cryptococcus neoformans* species complex. *Annu. Rev. Microbiol.* **60:**69–105.

145. **Linton, C. J., A. M. Borman, G. Cheung, A. D. Holmes, A. Szekely, M. D. Palmer, P. D. Bridge, C. K. Campbell, and E. M. Johnson.** 2007. Molecular identification of unusual pathogenic yeast isolates by large ribosomal subunit gene sequencing: 2 years of experience at the United Kingdom Mycology Reference Laboratory. *J. Clin. Microbiol.* **45:**1152–1158.

146. **Lockhart, S. R., S. A. Messer, M. Gherna, J. A. Bishop, W. G. Merz, M. A. Pfaller, and D. J. Diekema.** 2009. Identification of *Candida nivariensis* and *Candida bracarensis* in a large global collection of *Candida glabrata* isolates: comparison to the literature. *J. Clin. Microbiol.* **47:**1216–1217.

147. **Love, G. L., G. D. Boyd, and D. L. Greer.** 1985. Large *Cryptococcus neoformans* isolated from brain abscess. *J. Clin. Microbiol.* **22:**1068–1070.

148. **Lu, H., Y. Zhou, Y. Yin, X. Pan, and X. Weng.** 2005. Cryptococcal antigen test revisited: significance for cryptococcal meningitis therapy monitoring in a tertiary Chinese hospital. *J. Clin. Microbiol.* **43:**2989–2990.

149. **Lupetti, A., A. Tavanti, P. Davini, E. Ghelardi, V. Corsini, I. Merusi, A. Boldrini, M. Campa, and S. Senesi.** 2002. Horizontal transmission of *Candida parapsilosis* candidemia in a neonatal intensive care unit. *J. Clin. Microbiol.* **40:**2363–2369.

150. **Lyman, C. A., S. J. N. Devi, J. Nathanson, C. E. Frasch, P. A. Pizzo, and T. J. Walsh.** 1995. Detection and quantitation of the glucuronoxylomannan-like polysaccharide antigen from clinical and nonclinical isolates of *Trichosporon beigelii* and implications for pathogenicity. *J. Clin. Microbiol.* **33:**126–130.

151. **Makimura, K., Y. Tamura, M. Kudo, K. Uchida, and H. Yamaguchi.** 2000. Species identification and strain typing of *Malassezia* species stock strains and clinical isolates based on the DNA sequences of nuclear ribosomal internal transcribed spacer 1 regions. *J. Med. Microbiol.* **49:**29–35.

152. **Marcon, M. J., and D. A. Powell.** 1992. Human infections due to *Malassezia* spp. *Clin. Microbiol. Rev.* **5:**101–119.

153. **Marklein, G., M. Josten, U. Klanke, E. Muller, R. Horre, T. Maier, T. Wenzel, M. Kostrzewa, G. Bierbaum, A. Hoerauf, and H. G. Sahl.** 2009. Matrix-assisted laser desorption ionization–time of flight mass spectrometry for fast and reliable identification of clinical yeast isolates. *J. Clin. Microbiol.* **47:**2912–2917.

154. **Martino, P., M. Venditti, A. Micozzi, G. Morace, L. Polonelli, M. P. Mantovani, M. C. Petti, V. L. Burgio, C. Santini, P. Serra, and F. Mandelli.** 1990. *Blastoschizomyces capitatus:* an emerging cause of invasive fungal disease in leukemia patients. *Rev. Infect. Dis.* **12:**570–582.

155. **Martorell, P., M. T. Fernandez-Espinar, and A. Querol.** 2005. Sequence-based identification of species belonging to the genus *Debaryomyces. FEMS Yeast Res.* **5:**1157–1165.

156. **Marty, F. M., D. H. Barouch, E. P. Coakley, and L. R. Baden.** 2003. Disseminated trichosporonosis caused by *Trichosporon loubieri. J. Clin. Microbiol.* **41:**5317–5320.

157. **Massonet, C., J. Van Eldere, M. Vaneechoutte, T. De Baere, J. Verhaegen, and K. Lagrou.** 2004. Comparison of VITEK 2 with ITS2-fragment length polymorphism analysis for identification of yeast species. *J. Clin. Microbiol.* **42:**2209–2211.

158. **Mattsson, R., P. D. Haemig, and B. Olsen.** 1999. Feral pigeons as carriers of *Cryptococcus laurentii, Cryptococcus unguttulatus* and *Debaryomyces hansenii. Med. Mycol.* **37:**367–369.

159. **McCullough, M. J., K. V. Clemons, C. Farina, J. H. McCuster, and D. A. Stevens.** 1998. Epidemiological in-

vestigation of vaginal *Saccharomyces cerevisiae* isolates by a genotypic method. *J. Clin. Microbiol.* **36**:557–562.

160. **McGinnis, M. R., D. H. Walker, and J. D. Folds.** 1980. *Hansenula polymorpha* infection in a child with chronic granulomatous disease. *Arch. Pathol. Lab. Med.* **104**:290–292.

161. **McManus, E. J., and J. M. Jones.** 1985. Detection of a *Trichosporon beigelii* antigen cross-reactive with *Cryptococcus neoformans* capsular polysaccharide in serum from a patient with disseminated *Trichosporon* infection. *J. Clin. Microbiol.* **21**:681–685.

162. **McMullan, R., L. Metwally, P. V. Coyle, S. Hedderwick, B. McCloskey, H. J. O'Neill, C. C. Patterson, G. Thompson, C. H. Webb, and R. J. Hay.** 2008. A prospective clinical trial of a real-time polymerase chain reaction assay for the diagnosis of candidemia in nonneutropenic, critically ill adults. *Clin. Infect. Dis.* **46**:890–896.

163. **Meyer, W., D. M. Aanensen, T. Boekhout, M. Cogliati, M. R. Diaz, M. C. Esposto, M. Fisher, F. Gilgado, F. Hagen, S. Kaocharoen, A. P. Litvintseva, T. G. Mitchell, S. P. Simwami, L. Trilles, M. A. Viviani, and J. Kwon-Chung.** 2009. Consensus multi-locus sequence typing scheme for *Cryptococcus neoformans* and *Cryptococcus gattii. Med. Mycol.* **47**:561–570.

164. **Midgley, G.** 2000. The lipophilic yeasts: state of the art and prospects. *Med. Mycol.* **38**(Suppl. 1):9–16.

165. **Millon, L., T. Barale, M.-C. Julliot, J. Martinez, and G. Mantion.** 1995. Interference by hydroxyethyl starch used for vascular filling in latex agglutination test for cryptococcal antigen. *J. Clin. Microbiol.* **33**:1917–1919.

166. **Mirhendi, H., K. Makimura, K. Zomorodian, T. Yamada, T. Sugita, and H. Yamaguchi.** 2005. A simple PCR-RFLP method for identification and differentiation of 11 *Malassezia* species. *J. Microbiol. Methods* **61**:281–284.

167. **Molnar, O., G. Schatzmayr, E. Fuchs, and H. Prillinger.** 2004. *Trichosporon mycotoxinivorans* sp. nov., a new yeast species useful in biological detoxification of various mycotoxins. *Syst. Appl. Microbiol.* **27**:661–671.

168. **Monheit, J. E., D. F. Cowan, and D. G. Moore.** 1984. Rapid detection of fungi in tissues using calcofluor white and fluorescence microscopy. *Arch. Pathol. Lab. Med.* **108**:616–618.

169. **Montero, C. I., Y. R. Shea, P. A. Jones, S. M. Harrington, N. E. Tooke, F. G. Witebsky, and P. R. Murray.** 2008. Evaluation of pyrosequencing technology for the identification of clinically relevant non-dematiaceous yeasts and related species. *Eur. J. Clin. Microbiol. Infect. Dis.* **27**:821–830.

170. **Moran, G. P., D. Sangland, S. M. Donnelly, D. B. Shanley, D. Sullivan, and D. C. Coleman.** 1998. Identification and expression of multidrug transporters responsible for fluconazole resistance in *Candida dubliniensis. Antimicrob. Agents Chemother.* **42**:1819–1830.

171. **Moretti-Branchini, M. L., K. Fukushima, A. Z. Schreiber, K. Nishimura, P. M. O. Papaiordanou, P. Trabasso, R. Tanaka, and M. Miyaji.** 2001. *Trichosporon* species infection in bone marrow transplanted patients. *Diagn. Microbiol. Infect. Dis.* **39**:161–164.

172. **Morris, J. T., M. Beckius, and C. K. McAllister.** 1991. *Sporobolomyces* infection in an AIDS patient. *J. Infect. Dis.* **164**:623–624.

173. **Morrison, C. J., S. F. Hurst, and E. Reiss.** 2003. Competitive binding inhibition enzyme-linked immunosorbent assay that uses the secreted aspartyl proteinase of *Candida albicans* as an antigenic marker for diagnosis of disseminated candidiasis. *Clin. Diagn. Lab. Immunol.* **10**:835–848.

174. **Munson, E. L., D. R. Troy, J. K. Weber, S. A. Messer, and M. A. Pfaller.** 2002. Presumptive identification of *Candida kefyr* on Levine formulation of eosin methylene blue agar. *J. Clin. Microbiol.* **40**:4281–4284.

175. **Murray, M. P., R. Zinchuk, and D. H. Larone.** 2005. CHROMagar Candida as the sole primary medium for isolation of yeasts and as a source medium for the rapid-assimilation-of-trehalose test. *J. Clin. Microbiol.* **43**:1210–1212.

176. **Murray, P. R., R. E. Van Scoy, and G. D. Roberts.** 1977. Should yeasts in respiratory secretions be identified? *Mayo Clin. Proc.* **52**:42–45.

177. **Naglik, J., A. Albrecht, O. Bader, and B. Hube.** 2004. *Candida albicans* proteinases and host/pathogen interactions. *Cell. Microbiol.* **6**:915–926.

178. **Nakabayashi, A., Y. Sei, and J. Guillot.** 2000. Identification of *Malassezia* species isolated from patients with seborrhoeic dermatitis, atopic dermatitis, pityriasis versicolor and normal subjects. *Med. Mycol.* **38**:337–341.

179. **Neumeister, B., M. Rockemann, and R. Marre.** 1992. Fungaemia due to *Candida pelliculosa* in a case of acute pancreatitis. *Mycoses* **35**:309–310.

180. **Nguyen, H. V., C. Gaillardin, and C. Neuveglise.** 2009. Differentiation of *Debaryomyces hansenii* and *Candida famata* by rRNA gene intergenic spacer fingerprinting and reassessment of phylogenetic relationships among *D. hansenii, C. famata, D. fabryi, C. flareri* (=*D. subglobosus*) and *D. prosopidis*: description of *D. vietnamensis* sp. nov. closely related to *D. nepalensis. FEMS Yeast Res.* **9**:641–662.

181. **Nishiura, Y., K. Nkagawa-Yoshida, M. Suga, T. Shinoda, E. Guého, and M. Ando.** 1997. Assignment and serotyping of *Trichosporon* species: the causative agents of summer-type hypersensitivity pneumonitis. *J. Med. Vet. Mycol.* **35**:45–52.

182. **Noble, S. M., and A. D. Johnson.** 2007. Genetics of *Candida albicans*, a diploid human fungal pathogen. *Annu. Rev. Genet.* **41**:193–211.

183. **Odabasi, Z., G. Mattiuzzi, E. Estey, H. Kantarjian, F. Saeki, R. J. Ridge, P. A. Ketchum, M. A. Finkelman, J. H. Rex, and L. Ostrosky-Zeichner.** 2004. Beta-D-glucan as a diagnostic adjunct for invasive fungal infections: validation, cutoff development, and performance in patients with acute myelogenous leukemia and myelodysplastic syndrome. *Clin. Infect. Dis.* **39**:199–205.

184. **Odds, F. C.** 1988. *Candida and Candidosis*, 2nd ed. Bailliere Tindall, London, United Kingdom.

185. **Odds, F. C., A. D. Davidson, M. D. Jacobsen, A. Tavanti, J. A. Whyte, C. C. Kibbler, D. H. Ellis, M. C. J. Maiden, D. J. Shaw, and N. A. R. Gow.** 2006. *Candida albicans* strain maintenance, replacement, and microvariation demonstrated by multilocus sequence typing. *J. Clin. Microbiol.* **44**:3647–3658.

186. **Odds, F. C., and M. D. Jacobsen.** 2008. Multilocus sequence typing of pathogenic *Candida* species. *Eukaryot. Cell* **7**:1075–1084.

187. **Odds, F. C., L. Van Nuffel, and G. Dams.** 1998. Prevalence of *Candida dubliniensis* isolates in a yeast stock collection. *J. Clin. Microbiol.* **36**:2869–2873.

188. **Oliveira, K., G. Haase, C. Kurtzman, J. J. Hyldig-Nielsen, and H. Stender.** 2001. Differentiation of *Candida albicans* and *Candida dubliniensis* by fluorescent in situ hybridization with peptide nucleic acid probes. *J. Clin. Microbiol.* **39**:4138–4141.

189. **Padhye, A. A., S. Verghese, P. Ravichandran, G. Balamurugan, L. Hall, P. Padmaja, and M. C. Fernandez.** 2003. *Trichosporon loubieri* infection in a patient with adult polycystic kidney disease. *J. Clin. Microbiol.* **41**:479–482.

190. **Pappas, P. G., C. A. Kauffman, D. Andes, D. K. Benjamin, Jr., T. F. Calandra, J. E. Edwards, Jr., S. G. Filler, J. F. Fisher, B. J. Kullberg, L. Ostrosky-Zeichner, A. C. Reboli, J. H. Rex, T. J. Walsh, and J. D. Sobel.** 2009. Clinical practice guidelines for the management of candidiasis: 2009 update by the Infectious Diseases Society of America. *Clin. Infect. Dis.* **48**:503–535.

191. **Patterson, T. F., S. G. Revankar, W. R. Kirkpatrick, O. Dib, A. W. Fothergill, S. W. Redding, D. A. Sutton, and M. G. Rinaldi.** 1996. Simple method for detecting fluconazole-resistant yeasts with chromogenic agar. *J. Clin. Microbiol.* **34**:1794–1797.

192. **Peltroche-Llacsahuanga, H., S. von Oy, and G. Haase.** 2002. First isolation of reddish-pigmented *Candida (Torulopsis) glabrata* from a clinical specimen. *J. Clin. Microbiol.* **40**:1116–1118.

193. **Pfaller, M. A.** 1996. Nosocomial candidiasis: emerging species, reservoirs, and modes of transmission. *Clin. Infect. Dis.* **22**(S2):S89–S94.

194. **Pfaller, M. A., L. Boyken, R. J. Hollis, S. A. Messer, S. Tendolkar, and D. J. Diekema.** 2006. Global surveillance of in vitro activity of micafungin against *Candida*: a comparison

with caspofungin by CLSI-recommended methods. *J. Clin. Microbiol.* **44:**3533.

195. **Pfaller, M. A., L. Boyken, R. J. Hollis, S. A. Messer, S. Tendolkar, and D. J. Diekema.** 2006. In vitro susceptibilities of *Candida* spp. to caspofungin: four years of global surveillance. *J. Clin. Microbiol.* **44:**760–763.

196. **Pfaller, M. A., and D. J. Diekema.** 2007. Epidemiology of invasive candidiasis: a persistent public health problem. *Clin. Microbiol. Rev.* **20:**133–163.

197. **Pfaller, M. A., D. J. Diekema, D. L. Gibbs, V. A. Newell, E. Nagy, S. Dobiasova, M. Rinaldi, R. Barton, and A. Veselov.** 2008. *Candida krusei*, a multidrug-resistant opportunistic fungal pathogen: geographic and temporal trends from the ARTEMIS DISK Antifungal Surveillance Program, 2001 to 2005. *J. Clin. Microbiol.* **46:**515–521.

198. **Pfaller, M. A., D. J. Diekema, R. N. Jones, H. S. Sader, A. C. Fluit, R. J. Hollis, and S. A. Messer.** 2001. International surveillance of bloodstream infections due to *Candida* species: frequency of occurrence and in vitro susceptibilities to fluconazole, ravuconazole, and voriconazole of isolates collected from 1997 through 1999 in the SENTRY antimicrobial surveillance program. *J. Clin. Microbiol.* **39:**3254–3259.

199. **Pfaller, M. A., D. J. Diekema, S. A. Messer, L. Boyken, R. J. Hollis, and R. N. Jones.** 2003. In vitro activities of voriconazole, posaconazole, and four licensed systemic antifungal agents against *Candida* species infrequently isolated from blood. *J. Clin. Microbiol.* **41:**78–83.

200. **Pfaller, M. A., A. Houston, and S. Coffman.** 1996. Application of CHROMagar Candida for rapid screening of clinical specimens for *Candida albicans*, *Candida tropicalis*, *Candida krusei*, and *Candida (Torulopsis) glabrata*. *J. Clin. Microbiol.* **34:**58–61.

201. **Phelan, J. A., B. R. Saltzman, G. H. Friedland, and R. S. Klein.** 1987. Oral findings in patients with acquired immunodeficiency syndrome. *Oral Surg.* **64:**50–56.

202. **Pien, F. D., R. L. Thompson, D. Deye, and G. D. Roberts.** 1980. *Rhodotorula* septicemia: two cases and a review of the literature. *Mayo Clin. Proc.* **55:**258–260.

203. **Piens, M. A., J. D. Perry, H. Raberin, F. Parant, and A. M. Freydière.** 2003. Routine use of a one minute trehalase and maltase test for the identification of *Candida glabrata* in four laboratories. *J. Clin. Pathol.* **56:**687–689.

204. **Pincus, D. H., D. C. Coleman, W. R. Pruitt, A. A. Padhye, I. F. Salkin, M. Geimer, A. Bassel, D. J. Sullivan, M. Clarke, and V. Hearn.** 1999. Rapid identification of *Candida dubliniensis* with commercial yeast identification systems. *J. Clin. Microbiol.* **37:**3533–3539.

205. **Pincus, D. H., S. Orenga, and S. Chatellier.** 2007. Yeast identification—past, present, and future methods. *Med. Mycol.* **45:**97–121.

206. **Pinjon, E., D. Sullivan, I. Salkin, D. Shanley, and D. Coleman.** 1998. Simple, inexpensive, reliable method for differentiation of *Candida dubliniensis* from *Candida albicans*. *J. Clin. Microbiol.* **36:**2093–2095.

207. **Plazas, J., J. Portilla, V. Boix, and M. Pérez-Mateo.** 1994. *Sporobolomyces salmonicolor* lymphadenitis in an AIDS patient. Pathogen or passenger? *AIDS* **8:**387–398.

208. **Polacheck, I., I. F. Salkin, R. Kitzes-Cohen, and R. Raz.** 1992. Endocarditis caused by *Blastoschizomyces capitatus* and taxonomic review of the genus. *J. Clin. Microbiol.* **30:**2318–2322.

209. **Pore, R. S., and J. Chen.** 1976. Meningitis caused by *Rhodotorula*. *Sabouraudia* **14:**331–335.

210. **Rao, N. A., A. V. Nerenberg, and D. J. Forster.** 1991. *Torulopsis candida* (*Candida famata*) endophthalmitis simulating *Propionibacterium acnes* syndrome. *Arch. Ophthalmol.* **109:**1718–1721.

211. **Reed, B. D., P. Zazove, C. L. Pierson, D. W. Gorenflo, and J. Horrocks.** 2003. *Candida* transmission and sexual behaviors as risks for a repeat episode of *Candida* vulvovaginitis. *J. Womens Health* **12:**979–989.

212. **Rigby, S., G. W. Procop, G. Haase, D. Wilson, G. Hall, C. Kurtzman, K. Oliveira, S. Von Oy, J. J. Hyldig-Nielsen, J. Coull, and H. Stender.** 2002. Fluorescence in situ hybridization with peptide nucleic acid probes for rapid identification

of *Candida albicans* directly from blood culture bottles. *J. Clin. Microbiol.* **40:**2182–2186.

213. **Rikkerink, E. H. A., B. B. Magee, and P. T. Magee.** 1990. Genomic structure of *Candida stellatoidea*: extra chromosomes and gene duplication. *Infect. Immun.* **58:**949–954.

214. **Rimek, D., G. Haase, A. Luck, J. Casper, and A. Podbielski.** 2004. First report of a case of meningitis caused by *Cryptococcus adeliensis* in a patient with acute myeloid leukemia. *J. Clin. Microbiol.* **42:**481–483.

215. **Rinaldi, M. G.** 1993. Biology and pathogenicity of *Candida* species, p. 1–20. *In* G. P. Bodey (ed.), *Candidiasis: Pathogenesis, Diagnosis and Treatment*, 2nd ed. Raven Press, New York, NY.

216. **Romeo, O., and G. Criseo.** 2009. Molecular epidemiology of *Candida albicans* and its closely related yeasts *Candida dubliniensis* and *Candida africana*. *J. Clin. Microbiol.* **47:**212–214.

217. **Rusthoven, J. J., R. Feld, and P. J. Tuffnell.** 1984. Systemic infection by *Rhodotorula* spp. in the immunocompromised host. *J. Infect.* **8:**244–246.

218. **Salkin, I. F., M. A. Gordon, W. M. Samsonoff, and C. L. Rieder.** 1985. *Blastoschizomyces capitatus*, a new combination. *Mycotaxon* **22:**373–380.

219. **Salkin, I. F., and N. J. Hurd.** 1982. New medium for differentiation of *Cryptococcus neoformans* serotype pairs. *J. Clin. Microbiol.* **15:**169–171.

220. **Schabereiter-Gurtner, C., B. Selitsch, M. L. Rotter, A. M. Hirschl, and B. Willinger.** 2007. Development of novel real-time PCR assays for detection and differentiation of eleven medically important *Aspergillus* and *Candida* species in clinical specimens. *J. Clin. Microbiol.* **45:**906–914.

221. **Schlitzer, R. L., and D. G. Ahearn.** 1982. Characterization of atypical *Candida tropicalis* and other uncommon clinical yeast isolates. *J. Clin. Microbiol.* **15:**511–516.

222. **Schoofs, A., F. C. Odds, R. Colebunders, M. Ieven, and H. Goossens.** 1997. Use of specialised isolation media for recognition and identification of *Candida dubliniensis* isolates from HIV-infected patients. *Eur. J. Clin. Microbiol. Infect. Dis.* **16:**296–300.

223. **Scorzetti, G., J. W. Fell, A. Fonseca, and A. Statzell-Tallman.** 2002. Systematics of basidiomycetous yeasts: a comparison of large subunit D1/D2 and internal transcribed spacer rDNA regions. *FEMS Yeast Res.* **2:**495–517.

224. **Sendid, B., D. Caillot, B. Baccouch-Humbert, L. Klingspor, M. Grandjean, A. Bonnin, and D. Poulain.** 2003. Contribution of the Platelia *Candida*-specific antibody and antigen tests to early diagnosis of systemic *Candida tropicalis* infection in neutropenic adults. *J. Clin. Microbiol.* **41:**4551–4558.

225. **Sendid, B., T. Jouault, R. Coudriau, D. Camus, F. Odds, M. Tabouret, and D. Poulain.** 2004. Increased sensitivity of mannanemia detection tests by joint detection of α- and β-linked oligomannosides during experimental and human systemic candidiasis. *J. Clin. Microbiol.* **42:**164–171.

226. **Serena, C., M. Marine, F. J. Pastor, N. Nolard, and J. Guarro.** 2005. In vitro interaction of micafungin with conventional and new antifungals against clinical isolates of *Trichosporon*, *Sporobolomyces* and *Rhodotorula*. *J. Antimicrob. Chemother.* **55:**1020–1023.

227. **Seuri, M., K. Husman, H. Kinnunen, M. Reiman, R. Kreus, P. Kuronen, K. Lehtomaki, and M. Paananen.** 2000. An outbreak of respiratory diseases among workers at a water-damaged building—a case report. *Indoor Air* **10:**138–145.

228. **Sharma, V., J. Shankar, and V. Kotamarthi.** 2005. Endogeneous [sic] endophthalmitis caused by *Sporobolomyces salmonicolor*. *Eye* **20:**945–946.

229. **Silva, V., G. A. Moreno, L. Zaror, E. de-Oliveira, and O. Fischman.** 1997. Isolation of *Malassezia furfur* from patients with onychomycosis. *J. Med. Vet. Mycol.* **35:**73–74.

230. **Soll, D. A.** 2000. The ins and outs of DNA fingerprinting the infectious fungi. *Clin. Microbiol. Rev.* **13:**332–370.

231. **Sorrell, T. C., A. G. Brownlee, P. Ruma, R. Malik, T. J. Pfeiffer, and D. H. Ellis.** 1996. Natural environmental sources of *Cryptococcus neoformans* var. *gattii*. *J. Clin. Microbiol.* **34:**1261–1263.

232. **Spicer, A. D., and K. C. Hazen.** 1992. Rapid confirmation of *Candida albicans* identification by combination of two presumptive tests. *Med. Microbiol. Lett.* **1:**284–289.

233. **Spiess, B., W. Seifarth, M. Hummel, O. Frank, A. Fabarius, C. Zheng, H. Morz, R. Hehlmann, and D. Buchheidt.** 2007. DNA microarray-based detection and identification of fungal pathogens in clinical samples from neutropenic patients. *J. Clin. Microbiol.* **45:**3743–3753.

234. **Stephen, C., S. Lester, W. Black, M. Fyfe, and S. Raverty.** 2002. Multispecies outbreak of cryptococcosis on southern Vancouver Island, British Columbia. *Can. Vet. J.* **43:**792–794.

235. **St-Germain, G., and M. Laverdière.** 1986. *Torulopsis candida,* a new opportunistic pathogen. *J. Clin. Microbiol.* **24:**884–885.

236. **Sugita, T., M. Tajima, M. Takashima, M. Amaya, M. Saito, R. Tsuboi, and A. Nishikawa.** 2004. A new yeast, *Malassezia yamatoensis,* isolated from a patient with seborrheic dermatitis, and its distribution in patients and healthy subjects. *Microbiol. Immunol.* **48:**579–583.

237. **Sugita, T., M. Takashima, M. Kodama, R. Tsuboi, and A. Nishikawa.** 2003. Description of a new yeast species, *Malassezia japonica,* and its detection in patients with atopic dermatitis and healthy subjects. *J. Clin. Microbiol.* **41:**4695–4699.

238. **Sugita, T., M. Takashima, T. Shinoda, H. Suto, T. Unno, R. Tsuboi, H. Ogawa, and A. Nishikawa.** 2002. New yeast species, *Malassezia dermatis,* isolated from patients with atopic dermatitis. *J. Clin. Microbiol.* **40:**1363–1367.

239. **Summerbell, R. C.** 1992. *Candida lusitaniae* confirmed by a simple test. *Abstr. 92nd Annu. Meet. Am. Soc. Microbiol.,* abstr. F-90.

240. **Tavanti, A., A. D. Davidson, N. A. Gow, M. C. Maiden, and F. C. Odds.** 2005. *Candida orthopsilosis* and *Candida metapsilosis* spp. nov. to replace *Candida parapsilosis* groups II and III. *J. Clin. Microbiol.* **43:**284–292.

241. **Tavitian, A., J.-P. Raufman, and L. E. Rosenthal.** 1986. Oral candidiasis as a marker for esophageal candidiasis in the acquired immunodeficiency syndrome. *Ann. Intern. Med.* **104:**54–55.

242. **Taylor, J. W., D. M. Geiser, A. Burt, and V. Koufopanou.** 1999. The evolutionary biology and population genetics underlying fungal strain typing. *Clin. Microbiol. Rev.* **12:**126–146.

243. **Taylor, J. W., D. J. Jacobson, S. Kroken, T. Kasuga, D. M. Geiser, D. S. Hibbett, and M. C. Fisher.** 2000. Phylogenetic species recognition and species concepts in fungi. *Fungal Genet. Biol.* **31:**21–32.

244. **Tietz, H. J., M. Hopp, A. Schmalreck, W. Sterry, and V. Czaika.** 2001. *Candida africana* sp. nov., a new human pathogen or a variant of *Candida albicans? Mycoses* **44:**437–445.

245. **Trofa, D., A. Gacser, and J. D. Nosanchuk.** 2008. *Candida parapsilosis,* an emerging fungal pathogen. *Clin. Microbiol. Rev.* **21:**606–625.

246. **Turenne, C. Y., S. E. Sanche, D. J. Hoban, J. A. Karlowsky, and A. M. Kabani.** 1999. Rapid identification of fungi by using the ITS2 genetic region and an automated fluorescent capillary electrophoresis system. *J. Clin. Microbiol.* **37:**1846–1851.

247. **Van Abbe, N. J.** 1964. The investigation of dandruff. *J. Soc. Cosmet. Chem.* **15:**609–630.

248. **Vaughan-Martini, A., C. P. Kurtzman, S. A. Meyer, and E. B. O'Neill.** 2005. Two new species in the *Pichia guilliermondii* clade: *Pichia caribbica* sp. nov., the ascosporic state of *Candida fermentati,* and *Candida carpophila* comb. nov. *FEMS Yeast Res.* **5:**463–469.

249. **Velegraki, A., and M. Logotheti.** 1998. Presumptive identification of an emerging yeast pathogen: *Candida dubliniensis* (sp. nov.) reduces 2,3,5-triphenyltetrazolium chloride. *FEMS Immunol. Med. Microbiol.* **20:**239–241.

250. **Verweij, P. E., D. Poulain, T. Obayashi, T. F. Patterson, D. W. Denning, and J. Ponton.** 1998. Current trends in the detection of antigenaemia, metabolites and cell wall markers

for the diagnosis and therapeutic monitoring of fungal infections. *Med. Mycol.* **36**(Suppl. 1)**:**146–155.

251. **Walsh, T. J., and A. Pizzo.** 1988. Treatment of systemic fungal infections: recent progress and current problems. *Eur. J. Clin. Microbiol. Infect. Dis.* **7:**460–475.

252. **Warren, N. G., and K. C. Hazen.** 1999. *Candida, Cryptococcus,* and other yeasts of medical importance, p. 1184–1199. *In* P. R. Murray, E. J. Baron, M. A. Pfaller, F. C. Tenover, and R. H. Yolken (ed.), *Manual of Clinical Microbiology,* 7th ed. ASM Press, Washington, DC.

253. **Wellinghausen, N., D. Siegel, J. Winter, and S. Gebert.** 2009. Rapid diagnosis of candidaemia by real-time PCR detection of *Candida* DNA in blood samples. *J. Med. Microbiol.* **58:**1106–1111.

254. **Westerink, M. A., D. Amsterdam, R. J. Petell, M. N. Stram, and M. A. Apicella.** 1987. Septicemia due to DF-2. Cause of a false-positive cryptococcal latex agglutination result. *Am. J. Med.* **83:**155–158.

255. **White, P. L., A. E. Archer, and R. A. Barnes.** 2005. Comparison of non-culture-based methods for detection of systemic fungal infections, with an emphasis on invasive *Candida* infections. *J. Clin. Microbiol.* **43:**2181–2187.

256. **Wickerham, L. J., and K. A. Burton.** 1948. Carbon assimilation tests for the classification of yeasts. *J. Bacteriol.* **56:**363–371.

257. **Wickes, B. L., J. B. Hicks, W. G. Merz, and K. J. Kwon-Chung.** 1992. The molecular analysis of synonymy among medically important yeasts within the genus *Candida. J. Gen. Microbiol.* **138:**901–907.

258. **Williams, D. W., M. J. Wilson, M. A. O. Lewis, and A. J. C. Potts.** 1995. Identification of *Candida* species by PCR and restriction fragment length polymorphism analysis of intergenic spacer regions of ribosomal DNA. *J. Clin. Microbiol.* **33:**2476–2479.

259. **Willinger, B., C. Hillowoth, B. Selitsch, and M. Manafi.** 2001. Performance of Candida ID, a new chromogenic medium for presumptive identification of *Candida* species, in comparison to CHROMagar Candida. *J. Clin. Microbiol.* **39:**3793–3795.

260. **Willinger, B., S. Wein, A. M. Hirschl, M. L. Rotter, and M. Manafi.** 2005. Comparison of a new commercial test, GLABRATA RTT, with a dipstick test for rapid identification of *Candida glabrata. J. Clin. Microbiol.* **43:**499–501.

261. **Wilson, D. A., M. J. Joyce, L. S. Hall, L. B. Reller, G. D. Roberts, G. S. Hall, B. D. Alexander, and G. W. Procop.** 2005. Multicenter evaluation of a *Candida albicans* peptide nucleic acid fluorescent in situ hybridization probe for characterization of yeast isolates from blood cultures. *J. Clin. Microbiol.* **43:**2909–2912.

262. **Wingard, J. R., J. D. Dick, W. G. Merz, G. R. Sandford, R. Saral, and W. H. Burns.** 1982. Differences in virulence of clinical isolates of *Candida tropicalis* and *Candida albicans* in mice. *Infect. Immun.* **37:**833–836.

263. **Wise, M. G., M. Healy, K. Reece, R. Smith, D. Walton, W. Dutch, A. Renwick, J. Huong, S. Young, J. Tarrand, and D. P. Kontoyiannis.** 2007. Species identification and strain differentiation of clinical *Candida* isolates using the DiversiLab system of automated repetitive sequence-based PCR. *J. Med. Microbiol.* **56:**778–787.

264. **Yamane, N., and Y. Saitoh.** 1985. Isolation and detection of multiple yeasts from a single clinical sample by use of Pagano-Levin agar medium. *J. Clin. Microbiol.* **21:**276–277.

265. **Yang, Y. L.** 2003. Virulence factors of *Candida* species. *J. Microbiol. Immunol. Infect.* **36:**223–228.

266. **Yeo, S. F., Y. Zhang, D. Schafer, S. Campbell, and B. Wong.** 2000. A rapid, automated enzymatic fluorometric assay for determination of D-arabinitol in serum. *J. Clin. Microbiol.* **38:**1439–1443.

Pneumocystis

MELANIE T. CUSHION

116

The yeast-like fungi in the genus *Pneumocystis* are extracellular, host-obligate, host-specific, and typically restricted to the lung tissues of mammals, although extrapulmonary manifestations have been reported (95). Once known collectively by the single genus and species, "*Pneumocystis carinii*," it is now understood that distinct species of *Pneumocystis* infect different mammalian hosts. Current evidence suggests *Pneumocystis* can exist with little consequence in hosts with intact immune systems (44, 76), but debilitation of the immune system, induced by various means including infectious or immunosuppressive agents, congenital defects, or malnutrition, can lead to organism proliferation within the lung alveoli and eventually a lethal pneumonia if untreated. No species of *Pneumocystis* can be cultivated continuously outside the mammalian lung, impeding diagnostic capabilities as well as basic scientific research. A recent report of the ability of *Pneumocystis* spp. to form biofilms outside the lung holds promise for development of an in vitro system (12). Limited therapy is available with which to treat the pneumonia, since these fungi are not susceptible to standard antifungal drugs such as amphotericin B and fluconazole.

TAXONOMY

Taxonomic problems have plagued the organisms known as "*Pneumocystis carinii*" since their original description in 1909 by Carlos Chagas, who mistakenly identified the cyst forms as life cycle stages of the protozoan parasite *Trypanosoma cruzi*. In 1914, these organisms were provided an identity of their own and given the binomial epithet that reflected their predilection for the lung, *pneumo*, and characteristic morphological form, *cystis*, and honored the Italian investigator, Antonio Carini, who provided the slides for study, *carinii*. *P. carinii* was presumed to be a protozoan parasite at the time of identification; its potential fungal nature was first raised in the 1950s, and the controversy about its protozoan or fungal nature continued to the late 20th century. A more detailed early history of *Pneumocystis* identification and nomenclature can be found in reference 83.

In the late 1980s, phylogenetic analyses based on the nuclear small subunit rRNA sequence alignments showed that *Pneumocystis carinii* was a member of the fungal kingdom (25, 90). Subsequently, additional gene sequence comparisons and cDNA and genomic sequence data emerging from the *Pneumocystis* Genome Project showed that the closest extant relatives to *P. carinii* were the fission yeast *Schizosaccharomyces pombe* and the plant pathogen *Taphrina deformans* (10, 19). The most recent phylogenetic classification of the fungi places *Pneumocystis carinii* in the phylum Ascomycota, subphylum Taphrinomycotina, class Pneumocystidomycetes, order Pneumocystidales, and genus *Pneumocystis* (38). Within the Taphrinomycotina are the genera *Taphrina* (plant pathogens), *Neolecta* (associated with trees, may be parasitic), *Pneumocystis*, and *Schizosaccharomyces* (fission yeasts).

Pneumocystis species all appear to contain similar life cycle stages, although the clusters of organisms removed from the lungs of the different species can vary in presentation and size. For example, clusters of *Pneumocystis jirovecii* are often much larger than those obtained from rodent lungs, stain more intensely with Wright-Giemsa-like stains, and form multilayered mats comprised of several layers of organisms that hinder identification of individual life cycle stages (for examples, see Fig. 3B, D, and F). Until 1976, "*Pneumocystis carinii*" was thought to represent a single zoonotic species. At that time, Frenkel described serologic differences between human- and rat-derived organisms that he suggested were representative of distinct species (33), but these assertions were largely ignored by the medical community. It is now clear that the organism first identified as "*Pneumocystis carinii*" is actually a collection of many species within the genus *Pneumocystis* that likely number in the hundreds to thousands. Almost every mammal examined to date appears to harbor at least one species of *Pneumocystis* that is not found in any other mammal. Five *Pneumocystis* species have been formally described according to the International Code of Botanical Nomenclature: *Pneumocystis carinii* (33, 34, 83) and *Pneumocystis wakefieldiae* (14) are found in rats, *Pneumocystis murina* is found in the lungs of mice (51), *P. jirovecii* is found in human beings (34, 83), and *Pneumocystis oryctolagi* resides in rabbits (20). The name *P. jirovecii* has not been without controversy but now seems entrenched within the scientific and clinical communities (37).

DESCRIPTION OF THE AGENTS

The terminology used to describe the various life cycle stages of *Pneumocystis* bears remnants of its earlier classification as a protozoan parasite. This discussion introduces

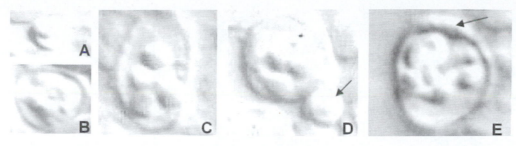

FIGURE 1 Major developmental forms of *Pneumocystis*. (A) Single trophic form; (B) sporocyte (precyst); (C) cyst with 4 visible spores (intracystic bodies); (D) cyst with 3 intracystic spores and a spore that has apparently excysted (arrow); (E) cyst with localized thickening of the cell wall (arrow) and 8 visible spores. Nomarski interference contrast microscopy; magnification, ×1,000.

terms more suitable for its fungal identity but retains those commonly found in the literature for continuity. Three developmental forms are generally recognized: the trophozoite (trophic form), 1 to 4 μm (Fig. 1A); the precyst (sporocyte), 5 to 6 μm (Fig. 1B); and the cyst (ascus), 5 to 8 μm (Fig. 1C to E). *Pneumocystis* spp. reproduce extracellularly within the mammalian lung alveoli. The trophic forms appear amoeboid in structure in electron micrographs, but in freshly prepared specimens, they are ellipsoidal and often occur in clusters with other trophic forms and developmental stages. The nucleus and often the mitochondrion are visible in rapid Wright-Giemsa-stained specimens by light microscopy. The trophic forms do not stain with fungal stains designed to complex with the cell wall, such as methenamine silver. The sporocyte is smaller than the mature cyst and frequently oval in shape. This stage contains a rigid cell wall lacking in the trophic forms and is stained with methenamine and other fungal wall stains. At the sporocyte stage, the nuclei are at varying levels of nuclear division (from 2 to 8 nuclei) but have not yet been compartmentalized into separate spore structures. Aggregates of mitochondrion can also be seen in this stage. The mature cyst is spherical in shape; contains eight spores, although these may not all be visible; has a thick cell wall that excludes stains such as the rapid Wright-Giemsa stain; and can be visualized with cell wall-complexing stains such as methenamine silver. The cyst/ascus is considered the diagnostic morphological form. All developmental forms and various poorly defined intermediate stages are often found in large, multilayered, tightly adherent aggregates or clusters in clinical specimens, making identification of each stage difficult (see Fig. 3B, D, and F).

EPIDEMIOLOGY AND TRANSMISSION

In the late 1970s and early 1980s, Walzer et al. (104) and Hughes (43) conducted a series of animal studies that showed *Pneumocystis* infection was likely transmitted by an airborne route. Immunosuppressed, *Pneumocystis*-free rats could acquire the infection from infected rats housed in the same room or from infected cage mates. Transmission through water, food, or ingestion of infected lungs was not observed in the same experimental studies. The agent of transmission has not yet been definitively identified. However, a recent study using a novel, echinocandin-treated mouse model of *Pneumocystis* infection, which depletes cysts while sparing trophic populations, reported that the treated mice could not transmit the infection, providing strong evidence that the cyst is the transmissive form (15).

Putative Life Cycle

Histochemical and ultrastructural studies form the basis of the current understanding of the life cycle of *Pneumocystis*, due to a historic lack of a long-term cultivation method outside the lung. Thus, any life cycle should be considered presumptive until definitive kinetic analyses are able to be performed. Human- and rat-derived *Pneumocystis* species have been the most extensively studied of the species in this group, and discussion of the life cycle in this chapter is based on these findings (7, 8, 18, 60). There is no evidence for an intracellular phase, although the organisms can be frequently observed within macrophages as a result of the host response to the infection. Despite numerous attempts to find an environmental cycle for *Pneumocystis*, none have been identified. A growing body of evidence suggests that the reservoir for *Pneumocystis* is its mammalian host, a situation similar to other host-dependent pathogens like *Entamoeba histolytica* or *Mycobacterium tuberculosis*. Studies with humans and animal models support a role for neonates and immune-competent hosts as potential reservoirs that are colonized transiently or longer term.

A schematic of a proposed life cycle can be found in Fig. 2, with a detailed description provided in the legend. The various life cycle stages of *Pneumocystis* are most often found together in very large adherent clusters that resemble biofilms in vivo (Fig. 2B). A recent report showing the in vitro formation of biofilms by *P. murina* and *P. carinii* provides support for the formation of these structures in vivo (12). Trophic forms are presumed to be the vegetative stages of the *Pneumocystis* life cycle and reproduce asexually by binary fission, not budding, as do most yeast. It is likely that they also participate in the sexual mode of reproduction using a process similar to yeast mating type systems, although these processes are only now beginning to be defined (86, 100). Several fungal meiosis-specific and mating type gene homologs have been identified in cDNA and genomic *P. carinii* databases, lending credence to the existence of these processes (19). After mating and karyogamy (nuclear fusion), the zygotic nucleus undergoes meiosis and sporogenesis is initiated, resulting in formation of the precyst, or sporocyte. Following meiosis, an additional mitotic replication occurs, with subsequent compartmentalization of the nuclei and organelles into 8 ascospores. The end product of sporogenesis is the spherical cyst, or ascus. The process of spore release has not been described but may involve a localized thickening at one pole of the ascus. It should be noted that, unlike other fungi, all the

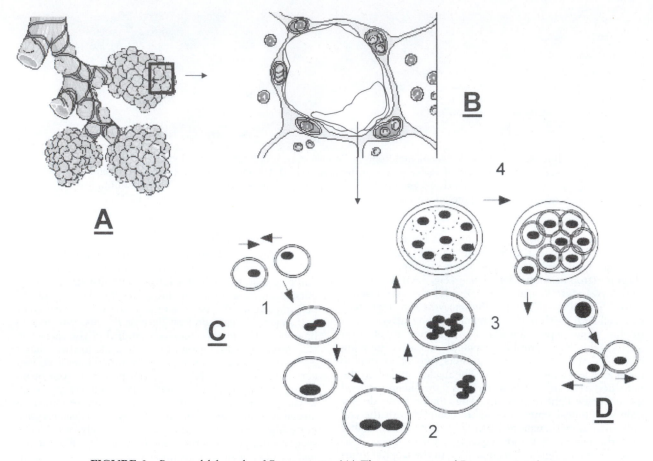

FIGURE 2 Proposed life cycle of *Pneumocystis*. (A) The primary site of *Pneumocystis* infection is the lung alveoli. Three clusters of alveoli are illustrated. An expanded schematic of an alveolus (box) is shown in panel B. (B) Single alveolus with *Pneumocystis* organisms depicted as the shape with an arrow attached to the cells lining the alveoli in some areas (type I pneumocytes) and un-attached to other alveolar cells (type II pneumocytes). (C) Putative sexual cycle of *Pneumocystis* in the lung alveoli: (1) opposite mating types fuse and undergo karyogamy, resulting in a diploid zygote; (2) the zygote then undergoes meiosis, resulting in four nuclei; (3) additional postmeiotic mitosis increases the number of nuclei to eight; (4) the nuclei and mitochondria (not shown) are compartmentalized by invagination of the inner plasma membrane, resulting in eight spores. Spores are released from the ascus (cyst) and presumably enter into the vegetative phase of the cycle. (D) Asexual replication cycle of *Pneumocystis*. Trophic forms undergo binary fission after mitotic replication of the nucleus. (Drawn with SmartDraw Suite, version 7.3.)

developmental stages of *Pneumocystis* contain a double membrane (21).

Transmission and Epidemiology

Evidence from several different studies suggests that (i) *Pneumocystis* is transmitted by an airborne route, (ii) it is likely to be acquired early in life, (iii) it can be transmitted among immunologically intact individuals, (iv) immunosuppressed and infected hosts are able to transmit the infection to immunologically intact hosts, and (v) transmission requires a short period of exposure and low numbers of organisms.

Beard et al. reported that the expansion of *P. jirovecii* carrying a double mutation in the DHPS gene in selected human immunodeficiency virus (HIV)-infected populations provides strong support for transmission of *P. jirovecii* by a person-to-person route as well as a positive selective mechanism (4). Previous and recent epidemiological surveys showing the clustering of *P. jirovecii*-specific genotypes with patients' place of residence is consistent with the

hypothesis of person-to-person transmission of *P. jirovecii* via the airborne route (27, 62). A recent report from Japan documented a *Pneumocystis* pneumonia (PCP) outbreak in a renal transplantation unit with 27 cases in a single year that could be traced by molecular methods back to the outpatient clinic (107). The median incubation time was estimated to be 53 days, with a range of 7 to 188 days. Several such outbreaks have been reported over the past 2 decades, providing a cautionary note for immunosuppressed patients gathering in a community setting as well as for appropriate prophylaxis therapy for susceptible populations. However, a recent report on the epidemiology of *P. jirovecii* colonization in families showed only a 3.3% detection in children of HIV-infected adults, in which their colonization rate was 11.4%, suggesting that merely close contact with potential reservoirs is not sufficient to induce this state (88).

Serologic studies performed in the 1970s and 1980s showed that *P. jirovecii* is acquired early in life (75, 89). Most human beings become seropositive to *P. jirovecii* organisms or antigens by the ages of 2 to 4 years. Vargas et al. detected *P. jirovecii* DNA in nasopharyngeal aspirates in 24/72 infants (32%) suffering from mild respiratory infections (98). Seroconversion developed in 67/79 (85%) of the same cohort of infants by 20 months of age. In the rat model of infection, newborn rats acquired *Pneumocystis*-specific DNA in their oral cavities by 1 to 2 hours after birth (45). No evidence for in utero transmission in rats was found after extensive analysis of fetal tissue by PCR, suggesting that the neonates were infected through close contact with the mother or through the air.

Experimental evidence indicates that very few organisms are required to initiate *Pneumocystis* infection and that the organism is very efficient in its method of transmission. Studies have shown that fewer than 10 *P. carinii* organisms were sufficient to establish a fulminant infection in immunosuppressed rats (16) and a 1-day period of exposure was all that was needed to transmit the infection from an infected *scid/scid* mouse to an uninfected *scid/scid* mouse (87). Likewise, transmission from infected patients to immune-competent health care workers has been reported (23). The widespread prevalence of *Pneumocystis* in commercial colonies housing healthy rats not only supports the very efficient dissemination of the infection throughout the members of a colony but also shows that the organism thrives in the immune-competent host (13, 44, 82). Evidence that healthy human populations may also serve as reservoirs or sources of infection is accumulating. A recent study conducted in humans without underlying lung disease or immunosuppression found that 20% of the oropharyngeal wash samples from 50 persons were positive for *P. jirovecii* by nested PCR targeting the mitochondrial large subunit ribosomal gene (61). In a study of 851 non-HIV-infected patients with pneumonia in China, *P. jirovecii* was detected in 14.5% by methenamine silver staining and in 24% by PCR (92). Further studies employing quantitative PCR should help to resolve the potential use of PCR as a diagnostic tool versus its use as a detection method.

Colonization

Emerging reports of the detection of *P. jirovecii* in populations without underlying immunosuppression and those with chronic underlying diseases that have not been historically associated with its presence may suggest colonization or expansion of host range (49, 53, 65–69, 71, 88, 93). Colonization, carriage, asymptomatic infection, and subclinical infection have all been used to describe the presence of *Pneumocystis* organisms or DNA in the absence of PCP. The effects of the presence of low numbers of *P. jirovecii* on the host have yet to be determined, and the role of carriage in mild respiratory infections, chronic lung disease, and progression to PCP is now being actively investigated. The most common underlying conditions in HIV-negative individuals associated with the presence of *P. jirovecii* include asthma and chronic lung diseases, chronic obstructive pulmonary disease, cystic fibrosis, Epstein-Barr virus infection, lupus erythematosus, high-dose corticosteroid use, rheumatoid arthritis, thyroiditis, ulcerative colitis, and pregnancy. Should the presence of *P. jirovecii* be confirmed as a causal agent in the underlying pathogenesis of any of these diseases, treatment of this cofactor could improve patient outcome.

CLINICAL SIGNIFICANCE

PCP remains the leading opportunistic infection associated with AIDS patients, even in the era of highly active antiretroviral therapy (HAART) (103). The mortality rate associated with PCP prior to and after the era of HAART (1996 forward) has not changed significantly in the United States, with an average of 10 to 13.5% (81, 103). In developing countries and within urban American cities, the mortality is much higher despite the availability of HAART (31, 94). The mortality rate for a medically underserved population in Atlanta, GA, from 1996 to 2006 was 37%, while patients who required aggressive intervention, such as mechanical ventilation, experienced an 80% mortality rate from PCP (94). In patients with cancer and other non-HIV diseases, there has been little improvement in mortality rates, and oftentimes, these patients fared more poorly than those with HIV. In one such study, the mortality of non-HIV-infected patients with PCP was 48% while HIV-infected patients experienced a 17% mortality (64). Although the incidence of PCP in pediatric populations has declined, PCP and its association with immune reconstitution inflammatory syndrome (IRIS) (63) causes significant clinical problems in these populations and vulnerable adult populations worldwide.

Within the mammalian lung, the trophic forms of *Pneumocystis* adhere to the type I pneumocytes presumably through macromolecular bridges (57, 77–79). Type I cells are responsible for the gas exchange between the alveolar capillaries and the alveolar lumen. Besides attachment to the type I cells, the various developmental stages of the parasite adhere to one another, producing large clusters that extend outwardly into the alveolar lumen. In severe, untreated infections, most of the alveoli are filled with organisms. Direct attachment to the cells responsible for gas exchange combined with the accumulation of organisms within the alveoli results in impaired gas exchange and altered lung compliance as well as other physiologic changes associated with the pneumonia, such as hypoxia (39, 96).

Histopathologic findings can be characterized by two traits: (i) alveolar interstitial thickening and (ii) a frothy eosinophilic honeycombed exudate in the lumina of the lung. The interstitial thickening is a result of hyperplasia and hypertrophy of the type II pneumocyte, interstitial edema, mononuclear cell infiltration, and, in some cases, mild fibrosis. The exudate is apparent upon staining with hematoxylin and eosin, which does not stain the organisms but clearly permits visualization of the eosinic exudate. Methenamine silver or another yeast cell wall stain must be used to visualize the cyst form of the organism, considered the diagnostic stage.

Immune Reconstitution Inflammatory Syndrome

Treatment with antiretroviral therapy improves immune function with a concomitant increase of CD4 cells within a few months after the start of therapy. This improvement in immune responses can be accompanied by a paradoxical, exaggerated inflammatory response manifested against infectious or noninfectious agents that often results in clinical worsening, which is referred to as IRIS (63). IRIS occurs more frequently in adults but has been reported in children. In adults, IRIS has been associated with patients harboring mycobacterial infections, PCP, cryptococcal infections, cytomegalovirus, varicella, herpes simplex virus infections, or progressive multifocal leukoencephalopathy.

Presentation in Children

PCP is a common manifestation among HIV-infected children. The highest incidence occurs during the first year of life, peaking at 3 to 6 months (63). Although a significant and dramatic decline in PCP infection rates in U.S. infants has been reported by the CDC and Perinatal AIDS Collaborative Transmission Study *Pneumocystis*, it remains a deadly neonatal disease in Africa, where postmortem analysis showed that 44% of children who died between 2000 and 2001 had PCP (58).

PCP was first described in children and considered a pediatric infection in its early history (35). Prominent epidemics of "interstitial plasma cell pneumonia" in undernourished children housed in suboptimal conditions after World War II were manifestations of the disease that was later identified as *P. jirovecii* pneumonia. The infection in these children was characterized by a plasma cell infiltrate, in contrast to the type II cell hypertrophy and scanty mononuclear infiltrate described in adults with the pneumonia (105). Clinical features of PCP in children include fever, tachypnea, dyspnea, and cough. Onset can be acute or subtle, associated with nonspecific conditions such as mild cough, loss of appetite, diarrhea, and weight loss. Fever may or may not be present, but most children exhibit rapid breathing with short shallow breaths at the time the pneumonia is visible by radiographic methods. Bilateral basilar rales, respiratory distress, and hypoxia are often evident upon physical exam. In HIV-infected children, 4 clinical variables are independently associated with PCP: age of less than 6 months, respiratory rate of greater than 59 breaths per minute, arterial percentage of hemoglobin saturation less than or equal to 92%, and the absence of vomiting (29, 63).

Most children with PCP manifest frank hypoxia with low arterial oxygen pressure and an alveolar-arterial oxygen difference ($[A-a]DO_2$) of greater than 30 mm Hg. The $CD4^+$ count is often less than 200 cells/mm^3 but can be higher. Children older than 5 years have a percent $CD4^+$ of less than 15%. Like adults, children often have bilateral diffuse parenchymal infiltrates with a "ground-glass" appearance, but such manifestations may be altogether lacking or mild.

Presentation in Adults

Adults with PCP frequently present with dyspnea, nonproductive cough, inability to breathe deeply, chest tightness, and night sweats (39). A low-grade fever (e.g., 38.5°C) and tachypnea are often present, while hemoptysis or sputum production is rare. Upon physical examination, few pronounced abnormalities are detected, but various degrees of respiratory distress, small respiratory volumes, and fine basilar rales can be observed. Patients with AIDS often have a more insidious progression to clinical disease than those not infected with HIV but who are immunosuppressed.

The chest radiograph may appear normal or reflect a disease state. Diffuse, symmetrical, interstitial infiltrates are most commonly present, while focal infiltrates, lobar consolidations, cavities, and nodules are less common. Infiltrates in early infection may be widely distributed, but consolidation increases as the disease progresses. Administration of aerosolized pentamidine as a prophylactic measure has been associated with increased frequency of apical infiltrates and pneumothoraces. The severity of abnormalities on the chest radiograph is considered prognostic and can be correlated with higher mortality. If the radiograph is normal or unchanged from a prior radiograph, a diffusing capacity of the lung for carbon monoxide (DL_{CO}) is recommended if the patient's symptoms consist of a nonproductive cough or shortness of breath, with or without fever. If the DL_{CO} (corrected for hemoglobin) is ≤75% of the predicted value or decreased ≥20% from the baseline, the patient should undergo diagnostic evaluation of sputum or bronchoscopy or both (105).

The oxygenation impairment induced by pneumocystosis can be detected in most patients by a widening of the alveolar-arterial oxygen gradient $[(A-a)DO_2]$ correlated with severity of disease and respiratory alkalosis (105). However, it should be noted that a significant number of patients can have a normal $(A-a)DO_2$ gradient at rest. Impaired diffusing capacity, alterations in lung compliance, total lung capacity, and vital capacity and hypoxemia are other physiologic changes that may be associated with *P. jirovecii* infection (39). Abnormalities in surfactant proteins also occur in infected individuals with increases in surfactant protein A and D most notable, since these proteins are considered components of innate immunity (2, 80, 84).

Extrapulmonary Pneumocystosis

The incidence of *Pneumocystis* organisms in sites other than the lung has been reported in 1 to 3% of postmortem examinations of patients with pulmonary *P. jirovecii* infections (22, 73, 95). This is likely an underestimate due to the limited number of autopsies currently performed and the lack of suspicion of extrapulmonary pneumocystosis. Methenamine silver staining or immunofluorescent kits served to identify the cyst stage of *Pneumocystis* in tissue samples and fine-needle aspirates in antemortem cases. The lymph nodes were the most frequent site of extrapulmonary involvement in a series of 52 patients (44%), followed by the spleen, bone marrow, and liver (33%). *P. jirovecii* has been detected in the adrenal glands, gastrointestinal tract, genitourinary tract, thyroid, ear, liver, pancreas, eyes, skin, and other sites. Infection of multiple extrapulmonary sites was associated with a rapidly fatal outcome. Pathological findings correlated with the organ where the infection was present. For example, retinal cotton wool spots were reported in infected eyes and pancytopenia was observed in patients with bone marrow lesions.

COLLECTION, TRANSPORT, AND STORAGE OF SPECIMENS

P. jirovecii pneumonia should be considered in any immunocompromised patient who presents with fever, respiratory symptoms, or infiltrates on chest radiograph. While mostly restricted to the lung, *P. jirovecii* has been found as extrapulmonary masses (e.g., pleura, intra-abdominal) in HIV-positive patients and should be included in a differential diagnosis in such patients. As no symptoms are specific for *P. jirovecii* pneumonia, a definitive diagnosis must be made by morphologic identification of the organism. Algorithms for clinical evaluation and treatment of PCP and differential diagnosis for HIV-associated pneumonias have been recently updated, and the reader is referred to these reviews for further details (40, 105).

The diagnosis of PCP relies on efficient sampling. The organism can be detected in a variety of respiratory specimens including induced sputum, bronchoalveolar lavage fluid (BALF), tracheal aspirate fluid, tissue obtained by transbronchial biopsy, cellular material obtained by bronchial brush, pleural fluid, and tissue obtained by open-thorax lung biopsy. The diagnostic yield is dependent upon the underlying disease state of the patient and the expertise of the staff obtaining the sample. In some hospitals where the staff are trained to obtain sputum samples and there is a large population with AIDS, 80% of diagnoses of PCP were made from induced sputum (36). In contrast, the diagnostic yield from non-AIDS patients can be quite low and bronchoalveolar lavage or other methods may be needed to ensure an appropriate diagnosis (3, 41). It is recommended that multiple slides from non-AIDS patients be examined, especially when there is a high degree of suspicion. Hospitals serving a diverse population often rely on methods other than induced sputum. A notable drawback of using induced sputum as the primary procedure for the diagnosis of PCP is the lack of information concerning other infections or disease processes that may be present in the lung. The diagnosis of extrapulmonary pneumocystosis relies on accurate sampling of the infected organ and subsequent staining of the histological sections. For infants and young children who are unable to produce sputum or in which this method is not warranted, tracheal aspirate fluid, open-thorax lung biopsy, or respiratory specimens must be obtained by a special pediatric bronchoscopy service (6, 98).

Bronchoalveolar Lavage

Fluid obtained by bronchoalveolar lavage is sufficiently liquid and does not require treatment with mucolytic agents. Twenty to 30 ml should be concentrated by centrifugation at $3,000 \times g$ for 15 min. The resultant pellet is reconstituted in 0.5 to 1.0 ml of buffer or saline, and a sterile wooden applicator is used to smear the sediment on glass slides, which are then fixed in absolute methanol, acetone, or a commercial fixative in rapid staining kits. Samples in limited quantities can be concentrated by use of a Cytospin centrifuge (Shandon Southern, Sewickley, PA) or equivalent. The addition of 1 drop of 22% bovine serum albumin to 500 μl of sample aids in adherence to the slide. Slides are air dried and then processed for staining. Morphological criteria for recognition of *P. jirovecii* stained by various procedures are discussed below and summarized in Table 1.

Induced Sputum Collection

Sputum collection is best done in a centralized facility by pulmonary function laboratory technicians, respiratory therapists, or specially trained assistants. Deep inhalation of nebulized 3% sodium chloride solution by the patient results in osmotic accumulation of fluid in and irritation of the respiratory passages with subsequent coughing and expectoration of bronchoalveolar contents. It is important to have the patient vigorously brush the teeth, tongue, and gums with a toothbrush and normal saline for 5 to 10 minutes prior to sputum induction, followed by thorough rinsing, to remove as much cellular debris of oral origin as possible. Toothpaste should not be used, as it can interfere with subsequent processing and staining of the specimen. The induced sputum specimen is usually mucoid and translucent in appearance; only rarely is it purulent. When *P. jirovecii* clusters are present in the unstained sputum, they are typically 0.1 to 0.2 mm in diameter and cream to light tan in color. Smearing sputa directly on slides followed by staining was shown to be a less-sensitive method than treatment with a mucolytic agent followed by concentration of the specimen (72).

Induced sputum is mucolyzed by the addition of an equal volume (at least 2 ml) of freshly prepared 0.0065 M dithiothreitol (Stat-Pak Sputolysin; Caldon-Biotech, Carlsbad, CA) or 0.5% N-acetyl-L-cysteine and incubation on a rotary shaker at 35°C with intermittent vigorous vortexing until the specimen is almost completely liquefied (complete liquefaction leads to dispersal of the *P. jirovecii* clusters, making microscopic detection more difficult). Some protocols require the addition of a clearing reagent for optimal results (e.g., Light Diagnostics *Pneumocystis carinii* DFA kit; Millipore, Billerica, MA). The specimen is then concentrated by centrifugation at $3,000 \times g$ for 5 min, and the sediment is smeared on glass slides, which are air dried and heat fixed by exposure to a heating block (50 to 60°C). Prolonged heat fixation is important in fixing the material to the slide (~30 min), since most of the natural cellular adhesions are removed during mucolysis. Slides containing the fixed material are then stained and examined microscopically (see below). Samples can be concentrated using a Cytospin centrifuge as described for BALF (above).

Open-Thorax Lung Biopsy

Open-thorax lung biopsy is the most invasive of the sampling procedures and is not routinely performed. This technique also suffers from a lack of sensitivity (54). However, should the laboratory receive such a specimen, the tissue should be blotted onto sterile gauze to reduce excess fluid (which would interfere with a diagnostic imprint) and used to make touch imprints by pressing several cut surfaces onto sterile glass slides. The remainder of the tissue can be used for histological sections or microbiological cultures after mincing or grinding. Glass slides with touch imprints should be air dried and then treated with absolute methanol or fixatives included in commercial kits of rapid Wright-Giemsa-like stains, such as Hema 3 (Fisher Scientific, Inc., Cincinnati, OH). Infected tissue stained in this manner reveals the presence of clusters of trophic forms and cysts with reddish purple nuclei and blue cytoplasm; cysts are surrounded by a halo of dye exclusion (see "Microscopy" below for a more detailed description). Slides should be fixed in acetone or a vendor-recommended fixative for immunofluorescent staining. Alternatively, a more concentrated sample can be achieved by maceration of the tissue with sterile scissors followed by homogenization in a lab blender designed to reduce the risk of aerosolization or potential contact by lab personnel (e.g., a Stomacher lab blender; Tekmar, Inc. Cincinnati, OH) for 10 to 20 min in 5 ml of saline or buffer/gram of tissue. After being sieved through sterile gauze to filter out large tissue particulates, the supernatant is concentrated by centrifugation ($3,000 \times g$ for 10 min) and then reconstituted in 1 to 5 ml of saline or buffer. Slides are prepared with 10-μl drops of the homogenate, which are then air dried, fixed, and stained as desired.

Transbronchial Biopsy

Fiber-optic bronchoscopy is the most common invasive technique for collection of tissue, but like open-thorax lung biopsy, this procedure is rarely performed today. Tissue should be handled as described for open-thorax lung biopsy above.

Nasopharyngeal Aspirates and Oropharyngeal Washes

Recent studies of humans reported the ability to detect *P. jirovecii*-specific DNA in nasopharyngeal aspirates (98) and oropharyngeal washes (70, 97) after amplification by PCR with *P. jirovecii*-specific primers. Current studies are exploring the use of oropharyngeal swabs as an additional sampling method. Although further studies addressing the correlation of the presence of *P. jirovecii* in the oral cavities and the disease state of the host are needed, handling and staining of oropharyngeal washes and nasopharyngeal aspirates are presented here, since use of PCR is becoming widespread for the diagnosis of infectious diseases. These methods will be extremely useful for sampling of pediatric populations where more invasive techniques of sampling are problematic or where the yield is low.

TABLE 1 Comparison of stains used to detect *Pneumocystis jirovecii*

Stain	Time to perform stain	Cyst wall	Trophic and other forms	Advantages	Disadvantages
Giemsa	30–60 min	Unstained; cyst wall appears as a clear ring around spores/intracystic bodies	Nuclei stain red-purple; cytoplasm stains light to dark blue, depending on thickness and depth of cluster	Inexpensive; stain simple to perform; stains all life cycle stages of *Pneumocystis*; stains most other pathogens (e.g., bacteria, parasites, fungi) and host cells	Experienced reader required to distinguish *Pneumocystis* clumps from stained host cells
Rapid Giemsa-like stains (e.g., Diff-Quik, Hema 3)	<5 min				
Fluorescein-conjugated monoclonal antibody kits (direct and indirect immuno-fluorescence)	15–30 min	Stains and fluoresces apple green; cyst contents usually unstained (appear black or dull); fold in cyst wall sometimes apparent, giving a crinkled, raisin-like appearance	Stained; appear as small polygons or spheres outlined in apple green; nuclei may stain; clusters can stain with a diffuse green glow	Recommended for less experienced personnel; immunofluorescent staining is sensitive and specific for *Pneumocystis*	Requires fluorescence microscope; reagents are expensive
Methenamine silver (Gomori/Grocott)	30 min (microwave); 1–2 h (rapid); 6–24 h (conventional)	Stains brown to black; cyst wall thickenings (double comma) and fold in the cyst wall stain dark brown to black; does not differentiate empty cysts from those with spores	Unstained	Easy to detect cysts; host cells not stained.	Prolonged staining time for conventional method; moderate costs; strong acids used; only the cyst form is stained; stains other fungi
Toluidine blue O/cresyl echt violet	1–6 h	Stains violet to purple; cyst wall thickenings and folds stain darker violet to purple; does not differentiate empty cysts from those with spores	Unstained	Easy to detect cysts; host cells not stained	Prolonged staining time; moderate costs; strong acids used; only the cyst is stained; stains other fungi
Calcofluor white	<5 min	Stains blue-white or green, depending on filter; cyst wall and thickenings intensely fluorescent	Unstained	Cyst fluoresces brilliantly; simple to perform; inexpensive	Requires fluorescence microscope; strong alkali used; only cyst is stained; stains other fungi; some expertise is required to distinguish *Pneumocystis* cysts from other fungi
Gram-Wiegert	<5 min	Unstained wall; intracystic bodies stain purple	Trophic forms faintly visible	Commonly available in cytopathology laboratories	Faint staining; can be overcome by experienced observer, but better stains are available
Papanicolaou	1–6 h	Unstained wall; intracystic bodies stain purple	Trophic forms faintly visible	Commonly available in cytopathology laboratories	Faint staining; can be overcome by experienced observer, but better stains are available

Oropharyngeal wash samples are obtained by gargling with 10 ml of sterile physiologic saline (0.9% NaCl) for a period of 1 min (61). Samples are then centrifuged at 2,900 × *g* for 5 min and kept frozen at −20°C until DNA is extracted. After digestion with proteinase K at 56°C for 2 h, DNA can be extracted using any number of commercial kits available.

Nasopharyngeal aspirates are collected using a suction catheter and sterile saline (98). If the amount of collected specimen is small or it is highly viscous, sterile saline should be washed through the catheter to dilute the specimen or added to the final collection tube. The sample can then be treated with a mucolytic agent and subsequently stained (as described above) or prepared for PCR by DNA extraction (described below).

DIRECT EXAMINATION AND IDENTIFICATION
Microscopy
A variety of stains have been used for the identification of *P. jirovecii* organisms. One of the most common stains used

by pathologists for tissue sections, hematoxylin and eosin, does not stain the organism but rather the foamy exudates within the lung alveoli, often described as "honeycombed" in appearance. Stains that illustrate the morphology of the organism by microscopic examination are those used for diagnosis in the clinical laboratory.

A common staining procedure used for the diagnosis of PCP is methenamine silver, which also stains other fungi (Table 1; Fig. 3C). Cell wall and membrane polysaccharides of fungi are oxidized to aldehydes by treatment with periodic acid, which in turn reduce the silver ion to metallic silver at alkaline pH. Addition of gold salts stabilizes the complex, and excess silver is removed by a sodium thiosulfate rinse. Variations of the methenamine silver stain (e.g., Grocott's or Gomori's) are used for both tissue sections and bodily fluids such as BALF or induced sputum (9, 59, 85). Disadvantages to use of the silver staining process have been the instability of solutions, the capricious nature of the metal impregnation, and the length of time required for

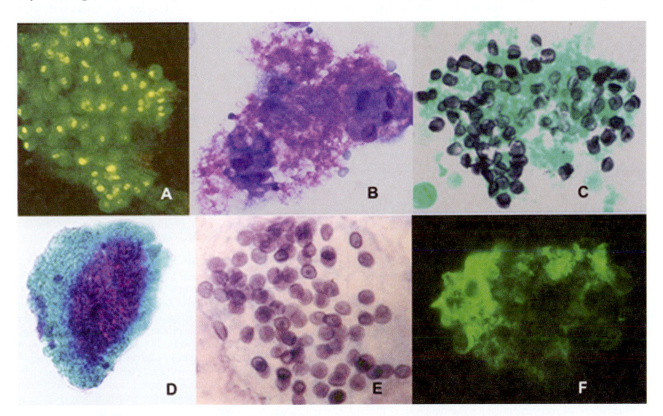

FIGURE 3 Morphology and tinctorial characteristics of *P. jirovecii* in clinical samples stained with various stains (magnification, ~×960 unless stated otherwise). (A) Calcofluor stain of BALF. Cyst walls with internal thickenings (double comma) are highly fluorescent (color varies with barrier filter used). (B) Rapid Giemsa-like (Diff-Quik) stain of BALF. A thick cluster of mostly trophic forms (2 to 3 μm) with small reddish-purple nuclei and light blue to red-violet cytoplasm is shown. Boundaries of trophic forms are rarely discernible with this stain. Trophic forms overlay each other to produce darker-staining blue cytoplasm. Large dark purple host nuclei are admixed in the cluster. (C) Gomori's methenamine silver stain (Grocott) of organisms from BALF. Cyst walls and thickenings (double comma) can be observed as well as collapsed cup shapes and a crinkled raisin-like appearance. Note the lack of budding. Trophic forms are not stained with silver-based stains. (D) Papanicolaou's stain of BALF. Note the distinctive alveolar cast morphology. Magnification, ~×380. (E) Toluidine blue O stain of *P. jirovecii* in BALF. Cyst walls are stained light purple. The crinkled appearances of the cysts are illustrated with this stain as well as the darker-staining central body. Note the lack of budding with this and other cyst wall stains. Trophic forms are not stained. (F) Direct fluorescent antibody stain of an organism cluster from BALF. Note the apple green fluorescence distributed unevenly over the cluster, with accumulation on a cyst wall (lower left of cluster). Structures within the cysts are unstained and appear black.

staining (1 to 2 h or 6 to 24 h [Table 1]). These disadvantages have been largely overcome with kits using standardized laboratory microwave ovens for controlled processing and supplied reagents (e.g., modified Gomori methenamine silver [GMS] microwave staining kit; Sigma-Aldrich, St. Louis, MO). Unlike other pathogenic fungi, *P. jirovecii* does not bud, and this feature can be used to discriminate between these organisms and other fungi found in the lung that bud, e.g., *Histoplasma capsulatum*. Silver-stained cysts have a distinctive, black, cup-shaped morphology against green-colored host cell architecture. In some staining reactions, cyst wall thickenings appear as a "double comma" morphology. More often, the folds in the wall stain a dark brown to black to produce a crinkled, raisin-like appearance (Fig. 3C). Intracystic daughter forms cannot be seen with this stain, and cysts that are empty (nonviable) appear the same as those with the full contingent of eight spores.

Other stains that complex with components of the cyst wall include periodic acid-Schiff, toluidine blue, cresyl echt violet, and calcofluor. The reactions to some of the more commonly used stains are described in Table 1. Cresyl echt violet stain produces results similar to the toluidine blue O (Fig. 2E) and has the same drawbacks, since a mixture of sulfuric acid and glacial acetic acid is necessary for the step prior to staining with the dye. Cysts stained by toluidine blue are similar in appearance to those stained with methenamine silver, except for the light purple color. Staining with calcofluor, whether in commercial kits (e.g., Fungifluor; Polysciences, Inc., Warrington, PA) or prepared in-house, can produce variable effects. Designed to detect only the cysts, excitation at 420 to 490 nm with a suppression filter of 515 nm produces a yellow-green or apple green fluorescence, often with a characteristic "double parentheses" staining body within the cyst (Fig. 3A). Excitation in the ultraviolet range (340 to 380 nm) with a suppression filter of 430 nm produces a fluorescent blue color that is not as intense and sometimes difficult to visualize. Refer to the vendor instructions for optimal filter requirements.

In contrast to the cyst wall stains, Giemsa and rapid Giemsa-like stains do not stain the cyst wall but instead stain the nuclei of all the various life cycle stages a reddish purple and the cytoplasm a light blue (Fig. 2B). The cyst wall excludes the dyes and appears with a circumscribed clear zone surrounding the reddish purple nuclei of the daughter forms within. Note the thick mat type of appearance, characteristic of the human infection. Lung cells are often present, and their nuclei are much larger than those of *Pneumocystis* and stain a deep reddish purple (Fig. 2B). Originally used for quantitation of rat *P. carinii* (17), the rapid variants of the Giemsa stain are recommended for the diagnosis of PCP using BALF, induced sputum, or impression imprints because of the low cost, ease, and rapidity of the staining procedure. Commercial kits such as Hema-Quik (Fisher Scientific Co., Cincinnati, OH) produce similar results. The staining procedure requires less than a minute to perform, and all forms of the organism are detected. Since there are approximately 10-fold-more trophic forms than cysts, the sensitivity of detection is likely to be increased. This stain also permits assessment of specimen quality of BALFs by demonstration of host alveolar macrophages, which should be present in a productive sample. In addition, the distinctive Giemsa-stained morphological appearance of other organisms likely to be encountered in the lung environment, such as *Cryptococcus neoformans* or *Toxoplasma gondii*, permit rapid diagnosis of pulmonary infections caused by these pathogens which may not be detected with other stains. Because background host cells also stain, training and expertise in interpreting cellular elements in the Giemsa-stained preparations is necessary. Laboratories with a lower volume of *P. jirovecii* specimens may prefer to use immunofluorescent staining or one of the other stains described in Table 1.

Direct and indirect fluorescein-conjugated monoclonal anti-*P. jirovecii* antibodies used for immunofluorescent assay (IFA) are targeted to a family of surface glycoproteins that contain both common and distinct epitopes, within and among *Pneumocystis* species (52). Depending on the monoclonal antibody supplied with the kit, staining may target only the cyst form or all forms of the organism. Since trophic forms are more numerous than cysts, kits using those antibodies directed to all forms of the organism (such as 2G2 and 3F6; available from DAKO Corp., Carpinteria, CA, and Chemicon International Inc., Temecula, CA [now under the Millipore brand]) are more sensitive (54). The typical fluorophore conjugated to the antibody or used in an indirect assay is fluorescein isothiocyanate, which produces a brilliant apple green color. The staining reaction shows a diffuse surface pattern distributed over the entire cluster of organisms (Fig. 2F) and often stains the matrix in which the organisms are embedded. Single cysts usually appear with a distinctive rim of fluorescence and duller interior fluorescence. It should be noted that kits using a direct staining procedure may not react with *P. jirovecii* on slides fixed in ethanol (26) and fixation in acetone or vendor recommendations for fixation should be followed.

Papanicolaou's stain, frequently used for cytopathological specimens, stains the clusters of extracellular organisms a greenish color, although thick clusters of organisms can collect the stain and appear bicolored with pink to purple and green/turquoise staining as in Fig. 2D. A diagnostic criterion is the presence of distinctive alveolar casts, as shown in Fig. 2D. Organism architecture is better observed with the Giemsa-like stains. Likewise, Gram's stain produces a negative (pink) reaction with poorly defined organism morphology.

Nucleic Acid Detection

Amplification of *P. jirovecii* DNA is not yet used routinely for the diagnosis of PCP in the clinical laboratory setting. Although more sensitive than conventional methods relying on organism detection by microscopic methods, the presence of a specific *P. jirovecii* PCR product has not been strictly correlated with underlying disease but holds great promise as a highly sensitive clinical test (46). In contrast to conventional microscopic methods of detection, PCR-based methods can be more labor-intensive, expensive, and time-consuming. As the clinical laboratory begins to rely more on these amplification techniques or other molecular modalities in the future, it is likely that *P. jirovecii* detection will be included in the battery of infectious-diseases kits offered by commercial vendors. Significantly, evidence is accumulating for the emergence of drug resistance in human *P. jirovecii*, and PCR can be used for identification of potentially resistant strains or species of the organism. Although the significance of infections with multiple genotypes of *P. jirovecii* is currently unclear, PCR-based detection systems would also be able to detect PCP caused by single or multiple genotypes. Quantitative PCR tests for PCP are being conducted by commercial firms such as ViraCor laboratories (www.viracor.com).

Detection of *P. jirovecii* can be accomplished by targeting the large ribosomal subunit of the mitochondrial rRNA (mtLSU) using direct or nested PCR (1, 24, 28, 30, 42, 91). This gene is present in multiple copies per organism and provides the most sensitive target for detection. DNA

TABLE 2 Suggested primers and conditions for PCR detection of *Pneumocystis*

Gene target	Primer	Sequence (5' to 3')	Expected product size (bp)	Conditions
MtLSU				
Primary[a]	pAZ102-E	GATGGCTGTTTCCAAGCCCA	346	94°C for 1 min, 55°C for 1 min, and 72°C for 2 min for 40 cycles; termination, 72°C for 5 min
	pAZ102-H	GTGTACGTTGCAAAGTACTC		
Nested[b]	pAZ102-X	GTGAAATACAAATCGGACTAGG	267	94°C for 1 min, 55°C for 1 min, and 72°C for 2 min for 35 cycles; termination, 72°C for 5 min
	pAZ102-Y	TCACTTAATATTAATTGGGGAGC		
DHPS[c]				
Round 1	F1	CCTGGTATTAAACCAGTTTTGCC		94°C for 5 min, 92°C for 30 s, 52°C for 30 s, and 72°C for 1 min, for 35 cycles; termination, 72°C for 5 min
	B45	CAATTTAATAAATTTCTTTCCAAATAGCATC		
Round 2	AHUM	GCGCCTACACATATTATGGCCATTTTAAATC	300	94°C for 5 min, 92°C for 30 s, 55°C for 30 s, and 72°C for 1 min for 35 cycles; termination, 72°C for 5 min
	BN	GGAACTTTCAACTTGGCAACCAC		

[a]From reference 101.
[b]From reference 99.
[c]Dihydropteroate synthase gene; from references 4 and 55.

can be isolated from clinical samples using commercial kits such as the PhaseLock system (Eppendorf Scientific, Westbury, NY) or a series of products designed for the clinical laboratory by vendors such as Qiagen (Valencia, CA). The primers targeting the mtLSU and PCR conditions are listed in Table 2. The expected amplicon sizes are approximately 346 bp for the first product and 267 bp for the second. If genotyping of the isolates is desired, the PCR amplicon can be sequenced directly or by cloning and subsequent sequencing of the clones. Cloning permits the assessment of the presence of infections caused by more than a single genotype. Manuals of molecular methods or vendor instructions should be consulted for these procedures.

ISOLATION PROCEDURES

Detection of *Pneumocystis* by growth in artificial media or tissue culture is not a diagnostic option, since no species of the organism can be continuously cultivated outside the mammalian lung.

TYPING SYSTEMS

There is currently only one recognized species of *Pneumocystis* that causes pneumonia in humans, *P. jirovecii*. There is no standard typing system at this time, and in many settings, the diagnosis of PCP is simply made at the genus level as "*Pneumocystis* pneumonia." It may become desirable in the future to track the emergence of *P. jirovecii* organisms that are resistant to trimethoprim-sulfamethoxazole (TMP-SMX), or evaluate the potential for therapeutic response. In anticipation of this goal, the primers targeting the regions of the dihydropteroate gene (DHPS) associated with sulfa resistance in other pathogens are shown in Table 2. The nucleotide positions at which the mutations occur are nucleotides (nt) 165 and 171. Changes at these nucleotide positions result in changes in amino acids. The following are the four genotypes for this target gene: genotype 1, nt 165 (A) and nt 171 (C) (resulting in Thr and Pro); genotype 2, nt 165 (G) and nt 171 (C) (resulting

in Ala and Pro); genotype 3, nt 165 (A) and nt 171 (T) (resulting in Thr and Ser); and genotype 4, 165 (G) and nt 171 (T) (resulting in Ala and Ser). The last genotype, GT, represents a double mutation in the DHPS gene that has been associated with drug resistance and is emerging as the dominant genotype for *P. jirovecii* isolates in some areas (4). Although atovaquone resistance in PCP has been associated with mutations in the mitochondrial cytochrome b_1 gene (50), resistance to TMP-SMX is much more problematic, and identification of mutations in the DHPS gene will likely be the more critical genetic region to evaluate in the clinical setting. In addition to the 4 genotypes at the mtLSU locus, there are over 60 different genotypes using the intertranscribed spacer regions of the nucleus-encoded rRNA locus (56), but such typing is outside the scope of the clinical laboratory at this time.

SEROLOGIC TESTS

Serologic assays to detect anti-*P. jirovecii* antibodies are useful for epidemiological studies but not for diagnosis of PCP. Most human beings become seropositive for *Pneumocystis jirovecii* antibodies early in their childhood at 2 to 4 years of age and likely come in contact with the organism many times over their lifetimes. In some cases, a rise in antibody titer can be detected in some PCP patients over time; in others, antibody titers can just as frequently drop or remain the same. More recently, serologic responses to certain fragments of the major surface glycoprotein of *P. jirovecii* have been shown to be predictive for some clinical outcomes, such as recovery, and hold promise as potential therapeutic monitoring applications (102). Antigen-capture assays for *Pneumocystis jirovecii* antigens have not proven clinically useful.

A number of other laboratory tests have been used for the diagnosis of PCP but do not provide a definitive diagnosis. These include an increased arterial-alveolar gradient, an elevation of serum lactic dehydrogenase levels, and gallium and diethylenetriamine pentaacetic acid scans. The last two tests are not routinely used due to higher costs (105).

ANTIMICROBIAL SUSCEPTIBILITIES

Two drugs comprise the mainstay of therapy for acute PCP, TMP-SMX and pentamidine isethionate (105). Secondary treatments such as atovaquone and clindamycin-primaquine have been used for milder forms of the disease, and treatment with corticosteroids has been used to improve the clinical outcome in some patients. However, there have been significant rates of relapse and recurrence with such second-line therapies (74). TMP-SMX is a drug combination that targets the enzymes dihydrofolate reductase (trimethoprim) and dihydropteroate synthase (sulfamethoxazole), both integral steps in the folic acid pathway. Pentamidine is a cationic diamidine that was first used to treat African trypanosomiasis, "sleeping sickness," and was later found to be efficacious as PCP therapy. The mode of action of this drug is not known but may involve suppression of mitochondrial activity (11) or inhibition of topoisomerases (5). Pentamidine and TMP-SMX have significant side effects, including nephrotoxicity and, in the case of TMP-SMX, severe rash, fever, and neutropenia that often necessitate a change to alternative treatment. In a recent study of HIV type 1-infected patients with a first episode of PCP, only 64% completed TMP-SMX treatment (32). Neither drug is considered pneumocysticidal. Administration of pentamidine via an aerosolized route delivers the drug efficiently to the areas of infection, but it has been shown to be less effective than other drugs in the treatment of PCP (105). Aerosolized-pentamidine administration is typically used for prophylaxis.

PCP remains refractory to most common antifungal drugs such as the azoles or amphotericin B. Echinocandins, which are β-1,3-D-glucan inhibitors, are a relatively new family of antifungal drugs that are fungicidal against candidal infections and fungistatic against *Aspergillus* infections (48). Reports of the efficacy of echinocandins for PCP have been contradictory, due in large part to the anecdotal nature of the reports (47, 106). Systematic studies of the three clinically available echinocandins, caspofungin, anidulafungin, and micafungin, in rodent models of PCP revealed dramatic reductions in cysts, but not trophic forms, suggesting that use as monotherapies would not be efficacious but a combination with TMP-SMX may prove beneficial to some patients (15).

Mutations in the DHPS gene of *Pneumocystis jirovecii* associated with sulfa resistance in other pathogens have been identified in about 50% of the PCP isolates in certain geographic areas (4). The presence of the mutations in the DHPS gene of *P. jirovecii* were associated with previous TMP-SMX therapy, but the impact of the mutations in terms of outcome and response to therapy is not yet clear.

Monitoring of drug efficacy by evaluating organism burdens in clinical specimens, especially BALF, is not practical due to the problems in sampling efficiency. Reasons for the inability to assess organism burdens in response to therapy are: (i) the organisms may colonize discrete regions of the lung not accessible to sputum induction or lavage; (ii) the volume of fluid recovered from individual patients is variable; (iii) with induced sputum collection, patients vary in their efforts to produce the sample; (iv) microscopic enumeration of trophic and cyst forms may be problematic due to the presence of large clusters that preclude accurate quantitation; (v) it is not known to what capacity the organisms obtained by induced sputum or BALF reflect the disease state. With the advent of highly sensitive quantitation techniques such as real-time PCR, which permits detection of very low template numbers, the problems of accurate quan-

titation can be overcome. Experimental studies are being conducted to validate the use of quantitative real-time PCR for diagnostic purposes (42). However, the same questions of sampling efficiency and predictive ability will remain associated with real-time PCR as well as other issues. Assays targeting genomic sequences will have to be interpreted with caution because they do not provide assessment of organism viability or whether the intact organism is present. A more responsive assay would target quantitation of an mRNA present to determine both diagnosis and viability.

EVALUATION, INTERPRETATION, AND REPORTING OF RESULTS

The microscopic demonstration of *P. jirovecii* in tissue and fluids by staining with GMS or a rapid variant of the Wright-Giemsa stain, by IFA, or by other stains such as Papanicolaou should be considered sufficient for diagnosis. In many cases, the fungi are present as large clusters of organisms in which it may be difficult to differentiate the life cycle stages within the dense assemblage using the Wright-Giemsa or Papanicolaou stain. Because of this, it is recommended that a stain which only visualizes the cyst form of *Pneumocystis* (e.g., GMS) is used for diagnosis because it is easier to interpret. The rapid stains can be used as a preliminary diagnostic technique, followed by the definitive cyst stain. IFA can be helpful in laboratories that are less familiar with *P. jirovecii* morphology, but this requires a fluorescence microscope, which may not always be available. The outcome of IFA staining depends on the monoclonal antibody target. Some kits use monoclonal antibodies targeting the surface glycoprotein present on all of the life cycle stages but which also stain the dense matrix in which the *P. jirovecii* organisms are embedded, resulting in a highly fluorescent mass with little detail. Since there are no other species of the genus that are known to cause pneumonia in humans, the presence of these fungi can be reported as *Pneumocystis jirovecii* or *Pneumocystis* spp. "*Pneumocystis carinii*" should not be used, as this species infects rats. Treatment should be initiated upon demonstration of *P. jirovecii* by microscopic methods and based on clinical evaluation of the patient. Moderate-to-severe PCP is treated with a combination of corticosteroids and intravenous TMP-SMX, clindamycin-primaquine, or pentamidine. Mild-to-moderate PCP is treated with TMP-SMX, TMP-dapsone, pentamidine, atovaquone, or clindamycin-primaquine (105).

REFERENCES

1. Alvarez-Martinez, M. J., J. M. Miro, M. E. Valls, A. Moreno, P. V. Rivas, M. Sole, N. Benito, P. Domingo, C. Munoz, E. Rivera, H. J. Zar, G. Wissmann, A. R. Diehl, J. C. Prolla, M. T. de Anta, J. M. Gatell, P. E. Wilson, S. R. Meshnick, and Spanish PCP Working Group. 2006. Sensitivity and specificity of nested and real-time PCR for the detection of *Pneumocystis jiroveci* in clinical specimens. *Diagn. Microbiol. Infect. Dis.* **56:**153–160.
2. Atochina-Vasserman, E. N., A. J. Gow, H. Abramova, C. J. Guo, Y. Tomer, A. M. Preston, J. M. Beck, and M. F. Beers. 2009. Immune reconstitution during Pneumocystis lung infection: disruption of surfactant component expression and function by S-nitrosylation. *J. Immunol.* **182:**2277–2287.
3. Baughman, R. P. 1994. Use of bronchoscopy in the diagnosis of infection in the immunocompromised host. *Thorax* **49:**3–7.
4. Beard, C. B., J. L. Carter, S. P. Keely, L. Huang, N. J. Pieniazek, I. N. Moura, J. M. Roberts, A. W. Hightower, M.

S. Bens, A. R. Freeman, S. Lee, J. R. Stringer, J. S. Duchin, C. Del Rio, D. Rimland, R. P. Baughman, D. A. Levy, V. J. Dietz, P. Simon, and T. R. Navin. 2000. Genetic variation in *Pneumocystis carinii* isolates from different geographic regions: implications for transmission. *Emerg. Infect. Dis.* **6:**265–272.

5. Bell, C. A., C. C. Dykstra, N. A. Naiman, M. Cory, T. A. Fairley, and R. R. Tidwell. 1993. Structure-activity studies of dicationically substituted bis-benzimidazoles against *Giardia lamblia*: correlation of antigiardial activity with DNA binding affinity and giardial topoisomerase II inhibition. *Antimicrob. Agents Chemother.* **37:**2668–2673.

6. Birriel, J. A., Jr., J. A. Adams, M. A. Saldana, K. Mavunda, S. Goldfinger, D. Vernon, B. Holzman, and R. M. McKey, Jr. 1991. Role of flexible bronchoscopy and bronchoalveolar lavage in the diagnosis of pediatric acquired immunodeficiency syndrome-related pulmonary disease. *Pediatrics* **87:**897–899.

7. Campbell, W. G., Jr. 1972. Ultrastructure of Pneumocystis in human lung. Life cycle in human pneumocystosis. *Arch. Pathol.* **93:**312–324.

8. Chandler, F. W., Jr., J. K. Frenkel, and W. G. Campbell, Jr. 1979. Pneumocystis pneumonia. Animal model: *Pneumocystis carinii* pneumonia in the immunosuppressed rat. *Am. J. Pathol.* **95:**571–574.

9. Chandra, P., M. D. Delaney, and C. U. Tuazon. 1988. Role of special stains in the diagnosis of *Pneumocystis carinii* infection from bronchial washing specimens in patients with the acquired immune deficiency syndrome. *Acta Cytol.* **32:**105–108.

10. Cushion, M. T. 2004. Pneumocystis: unraveling the cloak of obscurity. *Trends Microbiol.* **12:**243–249.

11. Cushion, M. T., F. Chen, and N. Kloepfer. 1997. A cytotoxicity assay for evaluation of candidate anti-*Pneumocystis carinii* agents. *Antimicrob. Agents Chemother.* **41:**379–384.

12. Cushion, M. T., M. S. Collins, and M. J. Linke. 2009. Biofilm formation by *Pneumocystis* spp. *Eukaryot. Cell* **8:**197–206.

13. Cushion, M. T., M. Kaselis, S. L. Stringer, and J. R. Stringer. 1993. Genetic stability and diversity of *Pneumocystis carinii* infecting rat colonies. *Infect. Immun.* **61:**4801–4813.

14. Cushion, M. T., S. P. Keely, and J. R. Stringer. 2005. Validation of the name *Pneumocystis wakefieldiae*. *Mycologia* **97:**268.

15. Cushion, M. T., M. J. Linke, A. Ashbaugh, T. Sesterhenn, M. S. Collins, K. Lynch, R. Brubaker, and P. D. Walzer. 2010. Echinocandin treatment of *Pneumocystis* pneumonia in rodent models depletes cysts leaving significant trophic burdens that cannot transmit the infection. *PLoS ONE* **5:**e8524.

16. Cushion, M. T., M. J. Linke, M. Collins, S. P. Keely, and J. R. Stringer. 1999. The minimum number of *Pneumocystis carinii* f. sp. *carinii* organisms required to establish infections is very low. *J. Eukaryot. Microbiol.* **46:**111S.

17. Cushion, M. T., J. J. Ruffolo, M. J. Linke, and P. D. Walzer. 1985. *Pneumocystis carinii*: growth variables and estimates in the A549 and WI-38 VA13 human cell lines. *Exp. Parasitol.* **60:**43–54.

18. Cushion, M. T., J. J. Ruffolo, and P. D. Walzer. 1988. Analysis of the developmental stages of *Pneumocystis carinii*, in vitro. *Lab. Investig.* **58:**324–331.

19. Cushion, M. T., A. G. Smulian, B. E. Slaven, T. Sesterhenn, J. Arnold, C. Staben, A. Porollo, R. Adamczak, and J. Meller. 2007. Transcriptome of *Pneumocystis carinii* during fulminate infection: carbohydrate metabolism and the concept of a compatible parasite. *PLoS ONE* **2:**e423.

20. Dei-Cas, E., M. Chabe, R. Moukhlis, I. Durand-Joly, e. M. Aliouat, J. R. Stringer, M. Cushion, C. Noel, G. S. de Hoog, J. Guillot, and E. Viscogliosi. 2006. *Pneumocystis oryctolagi* sp. nov., an uncultured fungus causing pneumonia in rabbits at weaning: review of current knowledge, and description of a new taxon on genotypic, phylogenetic and phenotypic bases. *FEMS Microbiol. Rev.* **30:**853–871.

21. De Stefano, J. A., M. T. Cushion, R. G. Sleight, and P. D. Walzer. 1990. Analysis of *Pneumocystis carinii* cyst wall. I. Evidence for an outer surface membrane. *J. Protozool.* **37:**428–435.

22. Droste, A., G. Grosse, and F. Niedobitek. 1991. Extrapulmonary manifestations of *Pneumocystis carinii* infection in AIDS. *Verh. Dtsch. Ges. Pathol.* **75:**158–162. (In German.)

23. Dumoulin, A., E. Mazars, N. Seguy, D. Gargallo-Viola, S. Vargas, J. C. Cailliez, E. M. Aliouat, A. E. Wakefield, and E. Dei-Cas. 2000. Transmission of *Pneumocystis carinii* disease from immunocompetent contacts of infected hosts to susceptible hosts. *Eur. J. Clin. Microbiol. Infect. Dis.* **19:**671–678.

24. Durand-Joly, I., M. Chabe, F. Soula, L. Delhaes, D. Camus, and E. Dei-Cas. 2005. Molecular diagnosis of Pneumocystis pneumonia. *FEMS Immunol. Med. Microbiol.* **45:**405–410.

25. Edman, J. C., J. A. Kovacs, H. Masur, D. V. Santi, H. J. Elwood, and M. L. Sogin. 1988. Ribosomal RNA sequence shows *Pneumocystis carinii* to be a member of the fungi. *Nature* **334:**519–522.

26. Elvin, K., and E. Linder. 1993. Application and staining patterns of commercial anti-*Pneumocystis carinii* monoclonal antibodies. *J. Clin. Microbiol.* **31:**2222–2224.

27. Esteves, F., M. A. Montes-Cano, C. de la Horra, M. C. Costa, E. J. Calderon, F. Antunes, and O. Matos. 2008. *Pneumocystis jirovecii* multilocus genotyping profiles in patients from Portugal and Spain. *Clin. Microbiol. Infect.* **14:**356–362.

28. Etoh, K. 2008. Evaluation of a real-time PCR assay for the diagnosis of Pneumocystis pneumonia. *Kurume Med. J.* **55:**55–62.

29. Fatti, G. L., H. J. Zar, and G. H. Swingler. 2006. Clinical indicators of *Pneumocystis jiroveci* pneumonia (PCP) in South African children infected with the human immunodeficiency virus. *Int. J. Infect. Dis.* **10:**282–285.

30. Fillaux, J., S. Malvy, M. Alvarez, R. Fabre, S. Cassaing, B. Marchou, M. D. Linas, and A. Berry. 2008. Accuracy of a routine real-time PCR assay for the diagnosis of *Pneumocystis jirovecii* pneumonia. *J. Microbiol. Methods* **75:**258–261.

31. Fisk, D. T., S. Meshnick, and P. H. Kazanjian. 2003. *Pneumocystis carinii* pneumonia in patients in the developing world who have acquired immunodeficiency syndrome. *Clin. Infect. Dis.* **36:**70–78.

32. Fisk, M., E. K. Sage, S. G. Edwards, J. D. Cartledge, and R. F. Miller. 2009. Outcome from treatment of *Pneumocystis jirovecii* pneumonia with co-trimoxazole. *Int. J. STD AIDS* **20:**652–653.

33. Frenkel, J. K. 1976. *Pneumocystis jiroveci* n. sp. from man: morphology, physiology, and immunology in relation to pathology. *Natl. Cancer Inst. Monogr.* **43:**13–30.

34. Frenkel, J. K. 1999. Pneumocystis pneumonia, an immunodeficiency-dependent disease (IDD): a critical historical overview. *J. Eukaryot. Microbiol.* **46:**89S–92S.

35. Gajdusek, D. C. 1957. *Pneumocystis carinii*; etiologic agent of interstitial plasma cell pneumonia of premature and young infants. *Pediatrics* **19:**543–565.

36. Hadley, W. K., and V. L. Ng. 1999. Pneumocystis, p. 1200–1211. *In* P. M. Murray, E. J. Baron, M. A. Pfaller, F. C. Tenover, and R. H. Yolken (ed.), *Manual of Clinical Microbiology*, 7th ed. ASM Press, Washington, DC.

37. Hawksworth, D. L. 2007. Responsibility in naming pathogens: the case of *Pneumocystis jirovecii*, the causal agent of pneumocystis pneumonia. *Lancet Infect. Dis.* **7:**3–5.

38. Hibbett, D. S., M. Binder, J. F. Bischoff, M. Blackwell, P. F. Cannon, O. E. Eriksson, S. Huhndorf, T. James, P. M. Kirk, R. Lucking, L. H. Thorsten, F. Lutzoni, P. B. Matheny, D. J. McLaughlin, M. J. Powell, S. Redhead, C. L. Schoch, J. W. Spatafora, J. A. Stalpers, R. Vilgalys, M. C. Aime, A. Aptroot, R. Bauer, D. Begerow, G. L. Benny, L. A. Castlebury, P. W. Crous, Y. C. Dai, W. Gams, D. M. Geiser, G. W. Griffith, C. Gueidan, D. L. Hawksworth, G. Hestmark, K. Hosaka, R. A. Humber, K. D. Hyde, J. E. Ironside, U. Koljalg, C. P. Kurtzman, K. H. Larsson, R. Lichtwardt, J. Longcore, J. Miadlikowska, A. Miller, J. M. Moncalvo, S. Mozley-Standridge, F. Oberwinkler, E. Parmasto, V. Reeb, J. D. Rogers, C. Roux, L. Ryvarden, J. P. Sampaio, A. Schussler, J. Sugiyama, R. G. Thorn, L. Tibell, W. A. Untereiner, C. Walker, Z. Wang, A. Weir, M. Weiss, M. M. White, K. Winka, Y. J. Yao, and N. Zhang. 2007. A higher-level phylogenetic classification of the Fungi. *Mycol. Res.* **111:**509–547.

39. **Huang, L.** 2005. Clinical presentation and diagnosis of *Pneumocystis* pneumonia in HIV-infected patients, p. 349–406. *In* P. D. Walzer and M. T. Cushion (ed.), Pneumocystis *Pneumonia*. Marcel-Dekker, New York, NY.

40. **Huang, L., and K. Crothers.** 2009. HIV-associated opportunistic pneumonias. *Respirology* **14:**474–485.

41. **Huang, L., F. M. Hecht, J. D. Stansell, R. Montanti, W. K. Hadley, and P. C. Hopewell.** 1995. Suspected *Pneumocystis carinii* pneumonia with a negative induced sputum examination. Is early bronchoscopy useful? *Am. J. Respir. Crit. Care Med.* **151:**1866–1871.

42. **Huggett, J. F., M. S. Taylor, G. Kocjan, H. E. Evans, S. Morris-Jones, V. Gant, T. Novak, A. M. Costello, A. Zumla, and R. F. Miller.** 2008. Development and evaluation of a real-time PCR assay for detection of *Pneumocystis jirovecii* DNA in bronchoalveolar lavage fluid of HIV-infected patients. *Thorax* **63:**154–159.

43. **Hughes, W. T.** 1982. Natural mode of acquisition for de novo infection with *Pneumocystis carinii. J. Infect. Dis.* **145:**842–848.

44. **Icenhour, C. R., S. L. Rebholz, M. S. Collins, and M. T. Cushion.** 2001. Widespread occurrence of *Pneumocystis carinii* in commercial rat colonies detected using targeted PCR and oral swabs. *J. Clin. Microbiol.* **39:**3437–3441.

45. **Icenhour, C. R., S. L. Rebholz, M. S. Collins, and M. T. Cushion.** 2002. Early acquisition of *Pneumocystis carinii* in neonatal rats as evidenced by PCR and oral swabs. *Eukaryot. Cell* **1:**414–419.

46. **Jarboui, M. A., A. Sellami, H. Sellami, F. Cheikhrouhou, F. Makni, N. Ben Arab, M. Ben Jemaa, and A. Ayadi.** 2010. Molecular diagnosis of *Pneumocystis jiroveci* pneumonia in immunocompromised patients. *Mycoses* **53:**329–333.

47. **Kamboj, M., D. Weinstock, and K. A. Sepkowitz.** 2006. Progression of *Pneumocystis jiroveci* pneumonia in patients receiving echinocandin therapy. *Clin. Infect. Dis.* **43:**e92–e94.

48. **Kauffman, C. A., and P. L. Carver.** 2008. Update on echinocandin antifungals. *Semin. Respir. Crit. Care Med.* **29:**211–219.

49. **Kaur, N., and T. C. Mahl.** 2007. *Pneumocystis jiroveci* (*carinii*) pneumonia after infliximab therapy: a review of 84 cases. *Dig. Dis. Sci.* **52:**1481–1484.

50. **Kazanjian, P., W. Armstrong, P. A. Hossler, C. H. Lee, L. Huang, C. B. Beard, J. Carter, L. Crane, J. Duchin, W. Burman, J. Richardson, and S. R. Meshnick.** 2001. *Pneumocystis carinii* cytochrome b mutations are associated with atovaquone exposure in patients with AIDS. *J. Infect. Dis.* **183:**819–822.

51. **Keely, S. P., J. M. Fischer, M. T. Cushion, and J. R. Stringer.** 2004. Phylogenetic identification of *Pneumocystis murina* sp. nov., a new species in laboratory mice. *Microbiology* **150:**1153–1165.

52. **Keely, S. P., and J. R. Stringer.** 2009. Complexity of the MSG gene family of *Pneumocystis carinii. BMC Genomics* **10:**367.

53. **Komano, Y., M. Harigai, R. Koike, H. Sugiyama, J. Ogawa, K. Saito, N. Sekiguchi, M. Inoo, I. Onishi, H. Ohashi, F. Amamoto, M. Miyata, H. Ohtsubo, K. Hiramatsu, M. Iwamoto, S. Minota, N. Matsuoka, G. Kageyama, K. Imaizumi, H. Tokuda, Y. Okochi, K. Kudo, Y. Tanaka, T. Takeuchi, and N. Miyasaka.** 2009. *Pneumocystis jiroveci* pneumonia in patients with rheumatoid arthritis treated with infliximab: a retrospective review and case-control study of 21 patients. *Arthritis Rheum.* **61:**305–312.

54. **Kovacs, J. A., V. J. Gill, S. Meshnick, and H. Masur.** 2001. New insights into transmission, diagnosis, and drug treatment of *Pneumocystis carinii* pneumonia. *JAMA* **286:**2450–2460.

55. **Lane, B. R., J. C. Ast, P. A. Hossler, D. P. Mindell, M. S. Bartlett, J. W. Smith, and S. R. Meshnick.** 1997. Dihydropteroate synthase polymorphisms in *Pneumocystis carinii. J. Infect. Dis.* **175:**482–485.

56. **Lee, C. H., J. Helweg-Larsen, X. Tang, S. Jin, B. Li, M. S. Bartlett, J. J. Lu, B. Lundgren, J. D. Lundgren, M. Olsson, S. B. Lucas, P. Roux, A. Cargnel, C. Atzori, O. Matos, and J. W. Smith.** 1998. Update on *Pneumocystis carinii* f. sp. *hominis* typing based on nucleotide sequence variations in internal transcribed spacer regions of rRNA genes. *J. Clin. Microbiol.* **36:**734–741.

57. **Limper, A. H., S. T. Pottratz, and W. J. Martin.** 1991. Modulation of *Pneumocystis carinii* adherence to cultured lung cells by a mannose-dependent mechanism. *J. Lab. Clin. Med.* **118:**492–499.

58. **Madhi, S. A., C. Cutland, K. Ismail, C. O'Reilly, A. Mancha, and K. P. Klugman.** 2002. Ineffectiveness of trimethoprim-sulfamethoxazole prophylaxis and the importance of bacterial and viral coinfections in African children with *Pneumocystis carinii* pneumonia. *Clin. Infect. Dis.* **35:**1120–1126.

59. **Mahan, C. T., and G. E. Sale.** 1978. Rapid methenamine silver stain for Pneumocystis and fungi. *Arch. Pathol. Lab. Med.* **102:**351–352.

60. **Matsumoto, Y., and Y. Yoshida.** 1984. Sporogony in *Pneumocystis carinii*: synaptonemal complexes and meiotic nuclear divisions observed in precysts. *J. Protozool.* **31:**420–428.

61. **Medrano, F. J., M. Montes-Cano, M. Conde, C. de la Horra, N. Respaldiza, A. Gasch, M. J. Perez-Lozano, J. M. Varela, and E. J. Calderon.** 2005. *Pneumocystis jirovecii* in general population. *Emerg. Infect. Dis.* **11:**245–250.

62. **Miller, R. F., A. R. Lindley, A. Copas, H. E. Ambrose, R. J. Davies, and A. E. Wakefield.** 2005. Genotypic variation in *Pneumocystis jirovecii* isolates in Britain. *Thorax* **60:**679–682.

63. **Mofenson, L. M., M. T. Brady, S. P. Danner, K. L. Dominguez, R. Hazra, E. Handelsman, P. Havens, S. Nesheim, J. S. Read, L. Serchuck, R. Van Dyke, Centers for Disease Control and Prevention, National Institutes of Health, HIV Medicine Association of the Infectious Diseases Society of America, Pediatric Infectious Diseases Society, and American Academy of Pediatrics.** 2009. Guidelines for the prevention and treatment of opportunistic infections among HIV-exposed and HIV-infected children: recommendations from CDC, the National Institutes of Health, the HIV Medicine Association of the Infectious Diseases Society of America, the Pediatric Infectious Diseases Society, and the American Academy of Pediatrics. *MMWR Recomm. Rep.* **58:**1–166.

64. **Monnet, X., E. Vidal-Petiot, D. Osman, O. Hamzaoui, A. Durrbach, C. Goujard, C. Miceli, P. Bouree, and C. Richard.** 2008. Critical care management and outcome of severe Pneumocystis pneumonia in patients with and without HIV infection. *Crit. Care* **12:**R28.

65. **Mori, S., I. Cho, H. Ichiyasu, and M. Sugimoto.** 2008. Asymptomatic carriage of *Pneumocystis jiroveci* in elderly patients with rheumatoid arthritis in Japan: a possible association between colonization and development of *Pneumocystis jiroveci* pneumonia during low-dose MTX therapy. *Mod. Rheumatol.* **18:**240–246.

66. **Mori, S., I. Cho, and M. Sugimoto.** 2009. A followup study of asymptomatic carriers of *Pneumocystis jiroveci* during immunosuppressive therapy for rheumatoid arthritis. *J. Rheumatol.* **36:**1600–1605.

67. **Morris, A.** 2008. Is there anything new in *Pneumocystis jirovecii* pneumonia? Changes in *P. jirovecii* pneumonia over the course of the AIDS epidemic. *Clin. Infect. Dis.* **46:**634–636.

68. **Morris, A., J. D. Lundgren, H. Masur, P. D. Walzer, D. L. Hanson, T. Frederick, L. Huang, C. B. Beard, and J. E. Kaplan.** 2004. Current epidemiology of Pneumocystis pneumonia. *Emerg. Infect. Dis.* **10:**1713–1720.

69. **Morris, A., M. Netravali, H. M. Kling, T. Shipley, T. Ross, F. C. Sciurba, and K. A. Norris.** 2008. Relationship of pneumocystis antibody response to severity of chronic obstructive pulmonary disease. *Clin. Infect. Dis.* **47:**e64–e68.

70. **Morris, A., F. C. Sciurba, I. P. Lebedeva, A. Githaiga, W. M. Elliott, J. C. Hogg, L. Huang, and K. A. Norris.** 2004. Association of chronic obstructive pulmonary disease severity and Pneumocystis colonization. *Am. J. Respir. Crit. Care Med.* **170:**408–413.

71. **Morris, A., F. C. Sciurba, and K. A. Norris.** 2008. Pneumocystis: a novel pathogen in chronic obstructive pulmonary disease? *COPD* **5:**43–51.

72. **Ng, V. L., I. Gartner, L. A. Weymouth, C. D. Goodman, P. C. Hopewell, and W. K. Hadley.** 1989. The use of mucolysed induced sputum for the identification of pulmonary pathogens

associated with human immunodeficiency virus infection. *Arch. Pathol. Lab. Med.* **113:**488–493.

73. **Ng, V. L., D. M. Yajko, and W. K. Hadley.** 1997. Extrapulmonary pneumocystosis. *Clin. Microbiol. Rev.* **10:**401–418.

74. **Patel, N., and H. Koziel.** 2004. *Pneumocystis jiroveci* pneumonia in adult patients with AIDS: treatment strategies and emerging challenges to antimicrobial therapy. *Treat. Respir. Med.* **3:**381–397.

75. **Peglow, S. L., A. G. Smulian, M. J. Linke, C. L. Pogue, S. Nurre, J. Crisler, J. Phair, J. W. Gold, D. Armstrong, and P. D. Walzer.** 1990. Serologic responses to *Pneumocystis carinii* antigens in health and disease. *J. Infect. Dis.* **161:**296–306.

76. **Peterson, J. C., and M. T. Cushion.** 2005. Pneumocystis: not just pneumonia. *Curr. Opin. Microbiol.* **8:**393–398.

77. **Pottratz, S. T.** 1998. *Pneumocystis carinii* interactions with respiratory epithelium. *Semin. Respir. Infect.* **13:**323–329.

78. **Pottratz, S. T., and W. J. Martin.** 1990. Role of fibronectin in *Pneumocystis carinii* attachment to cultured lung cells. *J. Clin. Investig.* **85:**351–356.

79. **Pottratz, S. T., J. Paulsrud, J. S. Smith, and W. J. Martin.** 1991. *Pneumocystis carinii* attachment to cultured lung cells by pneumocystis gp 120, a fibronectin binding protein. *J. Clin. Investig.* **88:**403–407.

80. **Qu, J., L. He, Z. Rong, J. Pan, X. Chen, D. C. Morrison, and X. Li.** 2001. Alteration of surfactant proteins A and D in bronchoalveolar lavage fluid of *Pneumocystis carinii* pneumonia. *Chin. Med. J.* **114:**1143–1146.

81. **Radhi, S., T. Alexander, M. Ukwu, S. Saleh, and A. Morris.** 2008. Outcome of HIV-associated Pneumocystis pneumonia in hospitalized patients from 2000 through 2003. *BMC Infect. Dis.* **8:**118.

82. **Rebholz, S. L., and M. T. Cushion.** 2001. Three new karyotype forms of *Pneumocystis carinii* f. sp. *carinii* identified by contoured clamped homogeneous electrical field (CHEF) electrophoresis. *J. Eukaryot. Microbiol.* **2001**(Suppl.):109S–110S.

83. **Redhead, S. A., M. T. Cushion, J. K. Frenkel, and J. R. Stringer.** 2006. Pneumocystis and *Trypanosoma cruzi*: nomenclature and typifications. *J. Eukaryot. Microbiol.* **53:**2–11.

84. **Schmidt, R., P. Markart, C. Ruppert, B. Temmesfeld, R. Nass, J. Lohmeyer, W. Seeger, and A. Gunther.** 2006. Pulmonary surfactant in patients with Pneumocystis pneumonia and acquired immunodeficiency syndrome. *Crit. Care Med.* **34:**2370–2376.

85. **Schumann, G. B., and J. J. Swensen.** 1991. Comparison of Papanicolaou's stain with the Gomori methenamine silver (GMS) stain for the cytodiagnosis of *Pneumocystis carinii* in bronchoalveolar lavage (BAL) fluid. *Am. J. Clin. Pathol.* **95:**583–586.

86. **Smulian, A. G., T. Sesterhenn, R. Tanaka, and M. T. Cushion.** 2001. The ste3 pheromone receptor gene of *Pneumocystis carinii* is surrounded by a cluster of signal transduction genes. *Genetics* **157:**991–1002.

87. **Soulez, B., F. Palluault, J. Y. Cesbron, E. Dei-Cas, A. Capron, and D. Camus.** 1991. Introduction of *Pneumocystis carinii* in a colony of SCID mice. *J. Protozool.* **38:**123S–125S.

88. **Spencer, L., M. Ukwu, T. Alexander, K. Valadez, L. Liu, T. Frederick, A. Kovacs, and A. Morris.** 2008. Epidemiology of Pneumocystis colonization in families. *Clin. Infect. Dis.* **46:**1237–1240.

89. **Stagno, S., L. L. Pifer, W. T. Hughes, D. M. Brasfield, and R. E. Tiller.** 1980. *Pneumocystis carinii* pneumonitis in young immunocompetent infants. *Pediatrics* **66:**56–62.

90. **Stringer, J. R., J. C. Edman, M. T. Cushion, F. F. Richards, and J. Watanabe.** 1992. The fungal nature of Pneumocystis. *J. Med. Vet. Mycol.* **30**(Suppl. 1):271–278.

91. **Strutt, M., and M. Smith.** 2005. Development of a real-time probe-based PCR assay for the diagnosis of Pneumocystis pneumonia. *Med. Mycol.* **43:**343–347.

92. **Sun, L., M. J. Huang, Y. J. An, and Z. Z. Guo.** 2009. An epidemiologic study on Pneumocystis pneumonia in non-HIV infected patients in China. *Zhonghua Liu Xing Bing Xue Za Zhi* **30:**348–351.

93. **Teichmann, L. L., M. Woenckhaus, C. Vogel, B. Salzberger, J. Scholmerich, and M. Fleck.** 2008. Fatal Pneumocystis pneumonia following rituximab administration for rheumatoid arthritis. *Rheumatology* (Oxford) **47:**1256–1257.

94. **Tellez, I., M. Barragan, C. Franco-Paredes, P. Petraro, K. Nelson, and C. Del Rio.** 2008. *Pneumocystis jiroveci* pneumonia in patients with AIDS in the inner city: a persistent and deadly opportunistic infection. *Am. J. Med. Sci.* **335:**192–197.

95. **Telzak, E. E., R. J. Cote, J. W. Gold, S. W. Campbell, and D. Armstrong.** 1990. Extrapulmonary *Pneumocystis carinii* infections. *Rev. Infect. Dis.* **12:**380–386.

96. **Thomas, C. F., Jr., and A. H. Limper.** 2007. Current insights into the biology and pathogenesis of Pneumocystis pneumonia. *Nat. Rev. Microbiol.* **5:**298–308.

97. **Tsolaki, A. G., R. F. Miller, and A. E. Wakefield.** 1999. Oropharyngeal samples for genotyping and monitoring response to treatment in AIDS patients with *Pneumocystis carinii* pneumonia. *J. Med. Microbiol.* **48:**897–905.

98. **Vargas, S. L., W. T. Hughes, M. E. Santolaya, A. V. Ulloa, C. A. Ponce, C. E. Cabrera, F. Cumsille, and F. Gigliotti.** 2001. Search for primary infection by *Pneumocystis carinii* in a cohort of normal, healthy infants. *Clin. Infect. Dis.* **32:**855–861.

99. **Vargas, S. L., C. A. Ponce, F. Gigliotti, A. V. Ulloa, S. Prieto, M. P. Munoz, and W. T. Hughes.** 2000. Transmission of *Pneumocystis carinii* DNA from a patient with *P. carinii* pneumonia to immunocompetent contact health care workers. *J. Clin. Microbiol.* **38:**1536–1538.

100. **Vohra, P. K., J. G. Park, B. Sanyal, and C. F. Thomas, Jr.** 2004. Expression analysis of PCSTE3, a putative pheromone receptor from the lung pathogenic fungus *Pneumocystis carinii*. *Biochem. Biophys. Res. Commun.* **319:**193–199.

101. **Wakefield, A. E., F. J. Pixley, S. Banerji, K. Sinclair, R. F. Miller, E. R. Moxon, and J. M. Hopkin.** 1990. Amplification of mitochondrial ribosomal RNA sequences from *Pneumocystis carinii* DNA of rat and human origin. *Mol. Biochem. Parasitol.* **43:**69–76.

102. **Walzer, P. D., K. Djawe, L. Levin, K. R. Daly, J. Koch, L. Kingsley, M. Witt, E. T. Golub, J. H. Bream, B. Taiwo, and A. Morris.** 2009. Long-term serologic responses to the *Pneumocystis jirovecii* major surface glycoprotein in HIV-positive individuals with and without *P. jirovecii* infection. *J. Infect. Dis.* **199:**1335–1344.

103. **Walzer, P. D., H. E. Evans, A. J. Copas, S. G. Edwards, A. D. Grant, and R. F. Miller.** 2008. Early predictors of mortality from *Pneumocystis jirovecii* pneumonia in HIV-infected patients: 1985–2006. *Clin. Infect. Dis.* **46:**625–633.

104. **Walzer, P. D., V. Schnelle, D. Armstrong, and P. P. Rosen.** 1977. Nude mouse: a new experimental model for *Pneumocystis carinii* infection. *Science* **197:**177–179.

105. **Walzer, P. D., and A. G. Smulian.** 2010. Pneumocystis species, p. 3377–3390. *In* G. L. Mandell, J. E. Bennett, and R. Dolin (ed.), *Mandell, Douglas and Bennett's Principles and Practice of Infectious Diseases*. Churchill Livingstone Elsevier, Philadelphia, PA.

106. **Waters, L., and M. Nelson.** 2007. The use of caspofungin in HIV-infected individuals. *Expert Opin. Investig. Drugs* **16:**899–908.

107. **Yazaki, H., N. Goto, K. Uchida, T. Kobayashi, H. Gatanaga, and S. Oka.** 2009. Outbreak of *Pneumocystis jiroveci* pneumonia in renal transplant recipients: *P. jiroveci* is contagious to the susceptible host. *Transplantation* **88:**380–385.

Aspergillus and Penicillium

S. ARUNMOZHI BALAJEE AND MARY E. BRANDT

117

ASPERGILLUS SPECIES

Taxonomy

The genus *Aspergillus* is comprised of anamorphic (asexual) species with known or presumed associations to eight different teleomorph (sexual) genera classified in the family Trichocomaceae of the Ascomycota. The family Trichocomaceae also contains teleomorphs of the genera *Penicillium* and *Paecilomyces* (some species) (121). As members of the class Euascomycetes, aspergilli are distantly related to other ascomycetes, such as dimorphic fungi, dermatophytes, and *Pseudallescheria* species. The taxonomy of *Aspergillus* has been in flux, and this genus has now been subdivided into subgenera and sections (32, 65). Peterson's analysis of large-subunit ribosomal DNA (rDNA) sequences derived from 215 taxa correlated to a large degree with many of the species originally described by Raper and Fennell (115) but demonstrated a need for taxonomic revision (112). Three main branches on the phylogenetic tree were used to define the subgenera *Aspergillus*, *Fumigati*, and *Nidulantes*, and sections formerly recognized were either retained or redisposed. A result of this realignment is that the subgenus *Aspergillus* includes both uniseriate and biseriate species and species of different colors, whereas in prior treatments these were key characters that separated groupings of species. At this time, the genus *Aspergillus* includes seven subgenera: *Aspergillus*, *Fumigati*, *Ornati*, *Clavati*, *Nidulantes*, *Circumdati*, and *Stilbothamnium*. Each subgenus contains several sections, with each section composed of a number of species (64).

In practice, *Aspergillus* species are identified mainly on the basis of phenotypic characteristics of the anamorph (Fig. 1). Early monographic treatments (115) also included descriptions of the teleomorph, although Raper used the anamorphic name *Aspergillus* to refer to these organisms (44). The use of different binomials to represent the same living organism has resulted in confusion; to alleviate this confusion, the concept of one name for one fungus was proposed in 1991. In 2005, the XVII International Botanical Congress established a committee to consider this proposal, and the committee's report is due in 2011 (44).

A list of names in current use for the family Trichocomaceae includes 184 species of *Aspergillus* and 70 associated teleomorphs (121).

Description of the Agent

Aspergillus is a large genus of fungi containing about 184 species whose members reproduce by producing conidia in dry chains on phialides, cells with a terminal opening through which enteroblastic conidia are produced repetitively. Phialides can be produced directly from the vesicle (uniseriate) or from an intermediate series of cells called metulae (biseriate). In general, *Aspergillus* colonies usually grow very rapidly, producing powdery white, green, yellowish, brown, or black colonies. They are ubiquitous in the environment and are found worldwide, in soil, water, foods, and other environmental niches, with the dry conidia being dispersed easily in the air and by birds or insects. Several *Aspergillus* species also produce mycotoxins which are harmful to humans and animals when ingested (see chapter 124 in this *Manual*).

About 40 *Aspergillus* species have been implicated in human or animal infection, but some of these have been recorded only once (25). Some reports have been discounted because the fungus isolated was not reliably demonstrated to be a pathogen or because the description clearly represented another fungus or was inadequate for evaluation (132). *Aspergillus fumigatus* still accounts for most cases of aspergillosis, with A. *flavus* and A. *niger* being the other more common pathogenic species worldwide (72). A. *terreus* is increasingly being reported (56, 75, 99), and A. *lentulus* is the newest species recognized as an agent of human disease (7). There has also been an increase in reports demonstrating the recovery of previously recognized *Aspergillus* species, such as A. *udagawae* and A. *viridinutans*, from human infections. Importantly, these species appear to have different in vitro susceptibility patterns and show differences in clinical disease (1, 141).

Aspergillosis is a general term used to refer to infections caused by members of the genus *Aspergillus*. Invasive pulmonary aspergillosis is the most serious form, occurring in immunocompromised individuals. A classification of *Aspergillus* infections is given in Table 1.

Epidemiology and Transmission

Invasive aspergillosis is most commonly caused by *Aspergillus fumigatus* in humans, but other species, such as A. *flavus*, A. *nidulans*, and A. *terreus*, have also been impli-

---

*This chapter contains information presented in chapter 121 by Paul E. Verweij and Mary E. Brandt in the ninth edition of this *Manual*.

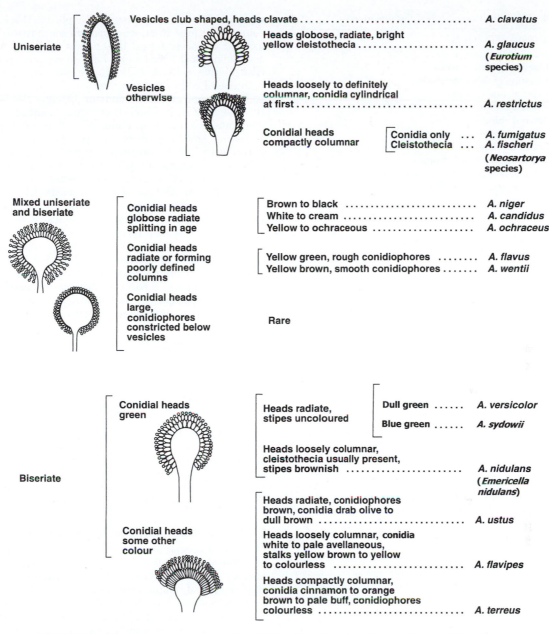

FIGURE 1   Key to representative species of *Aspergillus*. (Reprinted from reference 106 with permission from the publisher.)

cated in causing invasive infection. In some centers, a shift toward *Aspergillus* species other than *A. fumigatus* has been reported, although significant variation exists between centers (80, 99). Inhalation of conidia may lead to a variety of disease entities, ranging from asthma in atopic subjects to invasive infection in patients with severely compromised host defenses. Most invasive infections occur in the lungs, and the incidence of infection largely depends on the risk of the patient population. Typically, the incidence of invasive aspergillosis is around 5% of patients with hematological malignancy, especially acute myeloid leukemia and myelodysplastic syndrome, but may be as high as 15% of patients receiving a hematopoietic stem cell transplant (99).

Because these organisms are ubiquitous in the environment, numerous health care-associated outbreaks have

been described in the published literature. Guidelines from the Centers for Disease Control and Prevention and the Healthcare Infection Control Practices Advisory Committee provide recommendations for health care facilities to prevent such outbreaks (148). Although invasive pulmonary aspergillosis is believed to be acquired primarily by inhalation of airborne conidia, there is some evidence that water may play a role in transmission. *A. fumigatus* has been cultured from hospital water (145) and other sources in a hospital, such as showerheads, and strains recovered from water were found to be highly related to those recovered from patients (146). Patients might be exposed to *Aspergillus* conidia during showering by inhaling droplets contaminated with conidia. Genotyping may help in a further understanding of the significance of waterborne transmission of invasive aspergillosis.

TABLE 1 Classification of *Aspergillus* infection[a]

I. Disease in the normal host
  A. Toxicosis or mycotoxicosis
    1. Ingestion of mycotoxins
    2. Ingestion of other metabolites
  B. Allergic manifestations
    1. Allergic asthma
    2. Allergic rhinitis
    3. Allergic sinusitis
    4. Extrinsic allergic alveolitis
    5. Hypersensitivity pneumonitis
    6. Allergic bronchopulmonary aspergillosis
  C. Superficial or noninvasive infections
    1. Cutaneous infection
    2. Otomycosis
    3. Sinusitis
    4. Saprophytic bronchopulmonary aspergillosis
    5. Tracheobronchitis
  D. Invasive infection
    1. Single organ
    2. Multiple organs (disseminated)
II. Infection associated with tissue damage or foreign body
  A. Keratitis and endophthalmitis
  B. Burn wound infection
  C. Osteomyelitis
  D. Prosthetic valve endocarditis
  E. Vascular graft infection
  F. Aspergilloma (fungus ball)
  G. Empyema and pleural aspergillosis
  H. Peritonitis
III. Infection in the compromised host
  A. Primary cutaneous aspergillosis
  B. Sino-orbital infection
  C. Pulmonary aspergillosis
    1. Invasive tracheobronchitis
    2. Chronic necrotizing pulmonary aspergillosis
    3. Acute invasive pulmonary aspergillosis
  D. Central nervous system aspergillosis
  E. Invasive (disseminated) aspergillosis
  F. Gastrointestinal infarction (rare)

[a] Other fungi discussed in this chapter may present with similar clinical syndromes, and their structures in tissue may resemble those of *Aspergillus* species.

Clinical Significance

Invasive infections caused by *Aspergillus* species are associated with high rates of morbidity and mortality, especially in transplant recipients and immunosuppressed patients. Invasive aspergillosis is now considered the second most common hospital-acquired fungal infection requiring hospitalization in the United States. After *Candida* species, *Aspergillus* species are the second most common genus recovered from positive fungal cultures in hospitalized patients, but positive cultures alone may not indicate a pathogenic process (111).

Recovery of *Aspergillus* species from high-risk patients is associated with invasive infection, although the probability of infection depends on the host group. Assessment of the pathologic importance of any species of *Aspergillus* isolated from clinical specimens can be difficult, even with positive radiological or (high-resolution) computerized tomography (CT) findings, because aspergilli are routinely isolated from respiratory, cutaneous, and other specimens. It is imperative to determine clinical significance by (i) demonstrating hyphae in fresh clinical material, (ii) isolating heavy growth from a single specimen or the same species from multiple

specimens, and (iii) demonstrating hyphae in tissue. Fungal culture of at least three serial sputum specimens is recommended whenever fungal infection is suspected. Clinical and radiological correlations help to separate true from false-positive cultures (52). Consensus definitions have been published by the European Organization for Research and Treatment of Cancer and the Mycoses Study Group (EORTC/MSG), in which host factors, clinical signs and symptoms, and mycology results are used to classify patients as having proven, probable, or possible invasive fungal infection (3, 29). For invasive aspergillosis, the consensus definitions recognize antigen detection and high-resolution CT, but not (yet) nucleic acid detection techniques, as diagnostic tools. The use of the consensus definitions will help to standardize research into performance characteristics of new diagnostic tests and procedures.

Infections may be primary or secondary, and they vary in severity and clinical course (97). The clinical manifestations (Table 1) are determined largely by the local or general immunologic and physiologic state of the host, but various forms of the disease may integrate and overlap (69, 97). The major risk factors for invasive aspergillosis include hematologic malignancy, stem cell or solid-organ transplantation, pulmonary diseases, and glucocorticosteroid or cytotoxic drug therapy (5, 43, 109). Aspergillosis in human immunodeficiency virus (HIV)-infected patients is uncommon and occurs largely among severely leukopenic individuals (48, 101). Invasive pulmonary aspergillosis and cerebral aspergillosis are life-threatening complications in patients with advanced AIDS (42, 98, 101, 150). Modification to antiretroviral therapy, combined with antifungal therapy, results in improved survival of some HIV-infected patients (98, 150), but collectively, aspergilloses are associated with poor survival (48, 98, 101). Because different species of *Aspergillus* vary in their susceptibility to antifungal agents, every effort must be made to identify the fungus to the species level when it is isolated from an at-risk patient.

Collection, Transport, and Storage of Specimens

Methods of collection, transport, and storage of specimens are detailed in chapter 112. Invasive pulmonary aspergillosis is very difficult to diagnose and usually requires a combination of clinical, culture, radiographic, and direct antigen findings. Sputum, bronchoalveolar lavage fluid, and other nonsterile lower respiratory tract specimens can be collected for fungus culture, but it must be appreciated that aspergilli isolated from these sites may reflect contamination or colonization (111). The most convincing evidence of aspergillosis is provided by recovery of organisms from normally sterile sites, such as lung tissue obtained from biopsy, and by histopathologic demonstration of hyphal elements in tissue.

Aspergillus can be recovered from cultures of sinus tissue, other tissue biopsy specimens, skin biopsy specimens, heart valves, and appropriate ophthalmologic samples. Although *Aspergillus* endocarditis can occur in an appropriate patient, blood cultures for *Aspergillus* are usually negative. Conversely, positive blood cultures for *Aspergillus* are frequently indicative of contamination, even in a patient population at risk for aspergillosis (127).

Direct Examination

Microscopy

Hyphal elements and the details of hyphal morphology of aspergilli may be observed readily in routine KOH preparations, with or without a fluorescent compound such as calcfluor white or Blankophor P, or in tissue sections with fungal stains such as the Gomori methenamine silver stain. In hematoxylin-and-eosin-stained tissue, viable hyphae are often basophilic to amphophilic, whereas hyphae in macerated or necrotic tissue tend to be eosinophilic (17). The appearance of *Aspergillus* hyphae may vary with the type of infection. In invasive aspergillosis, aspergilli typically are seen as hyaline, septate hyphae that are 3 to 6 μm in diameter, branch dichotomously at acute (45°) angles (Fig. 2A), and have smooth parallel walls with no or slight constrictions at the septa (17). In invasive aspergillosis, hyphae proliferate extensively throughout the tissue, often in parallel or radial arrays. Aspergilli colonizing pulmonary cavitary lesions grow as tangled masses of hyphae and, in chronic infection, may exhibit atypical hyphal features such as swellings measuring up to 12 μm in diameter and/ or an absence of conspicuous septa. When hyphal elements typical of aspergilli are present in histologic sections, a presumptive diagnosis of invasive fungal infection can be made, but culture or specific immunohistochemical staining is required to identify the pathogen. In particular, hyphae of *Fusarium* or *Scedosporium* species may resemble those of aspergilli both in their propensity to grow in the lumens of blood vessels and in their formation of dichotomously branched hyphae (123). More promising are the molecular biological techniques that allow species identification by use of species-specific probes (45).

The presence of typical conidial heads or ascomata in lung cavities or in the ear canal aids in the diagnosis and may allow a presumptive identification of the fungus. In tissue, *A. terreus* displays distinctive aleurioconidia along the lateral walls of hyphae, thus permitting early clinical recognition of this species in histopathologic specimens (143). Calcium oxalate crystals also may be found in respiratory specimens, especially if *A. niger* is the cause of infection (126). Free conidia may resemble structures such as yeast cells or cysts of *Pneumocystis jirovecii* when stained with Gomori methenamine silver stain, which masks the conidium color, but conidia of the aspergilli are often roughened. Hyphae of the zygomycetes are generally broader (up to 15 μm), have nonparallel walls (which often appear collapsed and twisted), and are infrequently septate (17).

Antigen Detection

In patients with invasive infection, antigen detection may be helpful in establishing an early diagnosis (76, 93). Monitoring levels of circulating antigens also may be useful for management of such patients, especially those with immunosuppression or underlying hematologic malignancies (87, 138). The most widely used antigen assay detects levels of the fungal cell wall carbohydrate galactomannan in blood (serum). The original formulation was a latex agglutination test, the Pastorex *Aspergillus* test (Bio-Rad, Marnes-La-Coquette, France), which was evaluated in several hospital and clinical laboratories (50, 116, 139). Results showed that the test lacked sensitivity and that a low level of false-positive results (~6%) occurred for patients with no evidence of invasive disease. The development of a commercially available enzyme-linked immunosorbent assay (ELISA) format, Platelia *Aspergillus* (Bio-Rad), which employs the same monoclonal antibody as the latex kit, resulted in significantly improved sensitivity of antigen detection. Circulating galactomannan antigen was detected earlier than with the latex kit (140), and several large, prospective, autopsy-controlled clinical studies confirmed the potential of the ELISA to identify patients at high risk for invasive aspergillosis at an early stage of infection (86,

87, 131). In approximately two-thirds of patients, circulating galactomannan antigen was detected before diagnosis was made by other means (86). However, the main clinical evaluations have taken place with neutropenic patients with hematologic malignancies, and studies of other risk groups, such as solid-organ transplant recipients, indicate a less-favorable performance, although the number of studies of solid-organ transplant recipients is limited. Success in detecting antigenemia is directly related to the frequency of monitoring of samples (87). Monitoring of antigen titers in patients with hematologic malignancies has shown that the course of the antigen titer corresponds to the response to treatment (87, 137). Circulating galactomannan can be detected in other body fluids of patients with invasive aspergillosis, including cerebrospinal fluid (137), urine, and bronchoalveolar lavage fluid (66, 100). Although this application is potentially useful, the assay has thus far been validated only for serum and appears to be most useful for neutropenic patients with hematologic malignancies without antifungal therapy (35). A recent study demonstrated that in neutropenic patients with seropositive invasive aspergillosis, serum galactomannan index outcomes strongly correlated with survival, autopsy findings, and response outcomes (84). Conversely, the assay has limited utility for nonneutropenic patients due to low sensitivity.

In addition to the detection of *Aspergillus* galactomannan, assays have been developed to detect $(1{\rightarrow}3)$-β-D-glucan, a characteristic fungal cell wall constituent common to a broad range of fungal pathogens. The commercially available assay is the Fungitell kit (Associates of Cape Cod, East Falmouth, MA) (103). Although $(1{\rightarrow}3)$-β-D-glucan itself is not immunogenic, the detection system is based on the activation of a proteolytic coagulation cascade. Circulating $(1{\rightarrow}3)$-β-D-glucan was detected in patients with systemic fungal infections, including invasive aspergillosis (58, 110); the positivity of this test, particularly when used in a serial fashion, often precedes the microbiological or clinical diagnosis of invasive fungal infection. Both galactomannan and glucan antigen tests have now been added as diagnostic criteria in the recently revised EORTC/MSG definitions of invasive fungal disease (29).

Factors that hamper the use and reliability of these markers in patient management have emerged. Most notably, exposure of high-risk patients to mold-active antifungal agents significantly reduces the sensitivity of galactomannan detection (89, 90), a phenomenon that also appears to apply to detection of circulating fungal DNA (74). In one study, the sensitivity of the ELISA was only 20% for patients on antifungal prophylaxis, as opposed to 80% for those not receiving prophylaxis (89). ELISA reactivity was reported for certain beta-lactam antibacterial agents (2) and, more recently, for patients treated with piperacillin-tazobactam and amoxicillin-clavulanic acid (10, 131, 144). The ELISA reactivity observed in batches of these antibiotics might be due to the use of *Penicillium* fungi for the production of the antibacterial agents. Other exogenous sources of cross-reactivity might include bacteria that are present in the microflora of the intestine. The β-1,5-linked galactofuranosyl chain of the galactomannan molecule, which is the target for the EB-A2 immunoglobulin M (IgM) monoclonal antibody used in the ELISA, was also found to be present as a membrane-associated molecule in *Bifidobacterium* spp. (94, 95). Since these bacteria are present in the human gut and are found in very large numbers in neonates, it was suggested that these bacteria could cause positive galactomannan results in those patient groups with disruption of the integrity of the intestinal barrier (94).

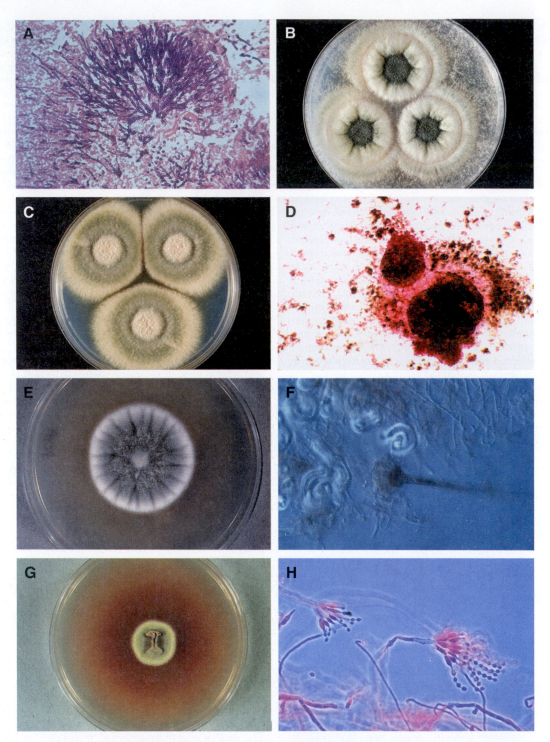

FIGURE 2 (A) Section of lung, stained with hematoxylin and eosin, showing dichotomously branched hyphae of *Aspergillus* in invasive aspergillosis. (B) *Aspergillus lentulus* colony on potato dextrose agar. (C) *Emericella (Aspergillus) nidulans* colony on potato dextrose agar. (D) *Emericella (Aspergillus) nidulans* showing cleistothecia. (E) *Aspergillus ustus* colony on malt extract agar. (F) *Aspergillus ustus* showing biseriate head, brown stipe, and Hülle cells. (G) Colony of *Penicillium marneffei* showing diffusing red pigment on Sabouraud dextrose agar after 7 days. Note that several *Penicillium* species produce diffusible red pigments. (H) Compact biverticillate penicillus of *Penicillium marneffei*.

False-positive reactions of $(1\rightarrow3)$-β-D-glucan are known to occur for some patients. These include subjects experiencing renal failure and undergoing hemodialysis with cellulose membranes (60), subjects treated with certain immunoglobulin products (54), and specimens (or subjects) exposed to glucan-containing gauze or related materials (103). This underscores the need to combine serological $(1\rightarrow3)$-β-D-glucan monitoring with clinical examination of the patient and other diagnostic procedures, such as high-resolution CT, when making a diagnosis.

Nucleic Acid Detection Techniques

The sensitivity and specificity of molecular techniques make them attractive as alternative methods for the early diagnosis of invasive aspergillosis, but they are still experimental. In the absence of a commercial nucleic acid-based system, conclusions with respect to the performance and diagnostic value of molecular techniques cannot be drawn, since comparisons between different in-house systems are extremely difficult to interpret (92). Collectively, molecular techniques appear to be sensitive and specific (34, 151) and can be applied to a broad spectrum of clinical specimens, including respiratory samples (100), tissue biopsy specimens (45, 107), and blood (13, 34, 59). In addition, exposure to antifungal drugs might improve the sensitivity of this assay compared to galactomannan detection, where drug therapy decreases the sensitivity of the assay.

Initially, PCR primers were designed that specifically amplified DNA from *Aspergillus* species (151), but alternative approaches have been evaluated in which a broad range of pathogenic fungi can be detected as the first step and identification to the species level can be achieved as a second step (34). The latter approach has great potential, since severely immunocompromised patients are at risk for infections due to a broad range of fungal pathogens. Automated systems are increasingly being used and have been adapted for lysis of fungal cells in clinical specimens and recovery of fungal DNA (39). Furthermore, technical advances in postamplification analysis have enabled real-time detection and quantification of the fungal DNA load in blood or tissue samples (TaqMan, LightCycler, and molecular beacon technologies) (22, 82).

A recent systematic review and meta-analysis of the use of PCR tests for the diagnosis of invasive aspergillosis from more than 10,000 blood, serum, or plasma samples obtained from 1,618 patients at risk for invasive aspergillosis, retrieved from 16 published studies, revealed that a single PCR-negative result was sufficient to exclude a diagnosis of proven or probable invasive aspergillosis if PCR was used as a screening tool from the start of the risk period, but two positive tests were required to confirm the diagnosis (due to the need for higher specificity). It was also observed that at-risk populations varied, and there was great heterogeneity in the PCR methods used. In recognition of this, an international initiative involving many investigators has been created to devise a standard for *Aspergillus* PCR, which would allow clinical validation and subsequent widespread use of a PCR assay (92).

Isolation

In general, *Aspergillus* species can be cultured on routine mycological media and do not possess specific growth requirements. Most identification schemes utilize specific media and incubation conditions for the descriptions of potentially variable characteristics, such as colony color and diameter (Fig. 1). *Aspergillus* species do not require specific

biohazard precautions in the laboratory, although culture materials frequently are handled in a biosafety cabinet to avoid dispersal of the dry spores throughout the environment and cross contamination of other cultures. The main disadvantages of culture are that it is relatively insensitive and that the culture process requires several days (49).

Identification

Diagnostic features of the more common medically important aspergilli are described in Table 2, and placement of species within sections follows the scheme used by Peterson (112). Species that commonly produce sexual structures (cleistothecia and ascospores) (Fig. 2D) are described under their teleomorph names, namely, *Eurotium*, *Emericella*, and *Neosartorya*. Figure 1 presents a diagrammatic key to several species.

Both macroscopic and microscopic characters are required for identification of *Aspergillus* species. When grown on media such as Sabouraud dextrose agar, aspergilli tend to reproduce in the asexual form. Subculture to standard Czapek-Dox medium, Czapek-Dox medium with added glucose (20 to 30%), 2% malt extract agar (115), or modifications of these media (65) allows comparison of colonial and microscopic features with those given in monographs and taxonomic keys (32, 64, 65, 106, 115, 121). However, standard descriptions are often based on growth after 7 days, and it usually takes longer for development of the teleomorph. Some species are osmophilic and grow poorly on media with low concentrations of sugar. Colony diameters on standard media at 25 and 37°C, obverse and reverse colors, texture, topography, and the presence of exudate droplets or diffusible pigments are recorded after 7 days (Fig. 2B, C, and E) (32, 65, 106). Isolates not immediately identifiable should be retained longer for possible development of ascomata or other structures that may be helpful in their identification.

Important microscopic features include differences in size, shape, color, and wall ornamentation of various structures; the shape and size of vesicles; and the arrangement of metulae and phialides. An upright stipe or conidiophore arises either directly from the vegetative hyphae or from a specialized hyphal cell called a foot cell, is usually nonseptate, and varies in color, length, and wall ornamentation in different species. The stipe terminates in a swollen cell, called a vesicle (Fig. 1 and 2F), which is globose, subglobose, hemispherical, pyriform (pear-shaped), or clavate (club-shaped). Either the entire vesicle or the upper portion of it is covered with phialides, which give rise to the conidia. Phialides arise simultaneously directly from the vesicle (uniseriate), from the intermediate series of cells called metulae (biseriate), or by a combination of both processes, as occurs in A. *flavus* (Fig. 1). Examination of a colony under a dissecting microscope allows observation of conidial chains to determine whether they are borne in a single column (columnar) or whether the columns are split, with some arising at right angles to the stipe (radiate). The conidia are typically ellipsoidal or globose and vary in size, color, and wall markings, depending upon the species. Sclerotia are firm, fruiting-body-like structures composed of swollen hyphal cells but lacking internal spores. Hülle cells are globose or variable in shape and have thick and highly refractive walls (Fig. 2F). They commonly occur immersed in the vegetative mycelium near the center of a colony, where their presence may be indicated by droplets of exudate. Hülle cells are often associated with cleistothecial ascomata, such as in *Emericella* species (*Aspergillus nidulans*) (Fig. 2D and Table 2). Cleistothecia have walls composed of enlarged hyphal cells and interiors filled

TABLE 2 Characteristics of some medically important *Aspergillus* species grown on identification media[a]

Section[b] and species	Seriation		Colony color	Microscopic features[c]	Comments[d]
	Uniseriate	Biseriate			
Fumigati					
A. *fumigatus*	+		Dark blue-green to grayish turquoise; slate gray with age; reverse variable	Conidiophore mostly up to 300 μm long and 5–8 μm wide, smooth, uncolored or greenish; vesicle dome shaped, 20–30 μm in diameter, with phialides on upper half only; head strongly columnar; conidia subglobose to globose, occasionally ellipsoidal, smooth to echinulate, 2–3.5 μm in diameter	Distinguished by blue-green colonies, growth at 45°C, and columnar heads with single layer of phialides. Sterile white fast-growing or glabrous (waxy) cerebriform slow-growing variants may be confirmed by thermotolerance and DNA sequence. Cosmopolitan airborne mold often found in compost piles, soil of potted plants, most common pathogen.
A.*lentulus*	+		Mostly floccose and usually white, interspersed with olive green colonies; reverse yellow in color with no diffusible pigment	Stipes are smooth walled, colorless, and 250–300 μm long; vesicles are diminutive, 8–10 μm wide, hyaline, subclavate in shape, and fertile over only half of the area; few short, flask-shaped, uniseriate phialides give rise to conidia 2.5–3.0 μm in diameter. Conidia number fewer than six or seven per chain, are bluish to olive green in color, and are globose, and the surface is rough with ornamentation (Fig. 2B).	Cryptic new species, has been recovered worldwide; slow-sporulating phenotype, hence the name *lentulus*
Flavi					
A. *flavus*	+	+	Yellow to dark yellowish green	Conidiophore mostly 400–850 μm long and 20 μm wide, roughened, uncolored; vesicle subglobose or globose, 25–45 μm in diameter; loosely radiate or splitting into columns in age; conidia globose or ellipsoidal, roughened, 3–6 μm in diameter	Toxigenic; brown to black sclerotia sometimes present; growth usually enhanced at 37°C; heads vary in size and seriation; colony color may be influenced by culture medium additives, such as yeast extract; second most common human pathogen
Nigri					
A. *niger*		+	Black with white margin and yellow surface mycelium; reverse uncolored or pale yellow	Conidiophore 400–3,000 μm long and 15–20 μm wide, smooth, uncolored to brownish near tip; vesicle globose, 30–75 μm in diameter; radiate, then splitting into columns in age; conidia globose with thick walls, brownish black, roughened, 4–5 μm in diameter	Frequent cause of otomycosis; sometimes associated with intracavitary colonization, especially in diabetics
Versicolores					
A. *versicolor*		+	Green to gray-green or tan with patches of pink or yellow; reverse variable and often deep red	Conidiophore 200 to 400 μm long and 5 μm wide, smooth, uncolored, yellowish or pale brown; vesicle ovate to elliptical, 9–16 μm in diameter; head radiate to loosely columnar; conidia globose, echinulate, 2.5–3 μm in diameter; Hülle cells globose	Toxigenic; distinguished by slow-growing, greenish-tan or variably colored colonies and small biseriate vesicles. Conidial heads of A. *sydowii* are similar, but colonies are blue-green. Reduced structures resembling penicilli sometimes present.

(Continued on next page)

TABLE 2 *(Continued)*

Section[b] and species	Seriation		Colony color	Microscopic features[c]	Comments[d]
	Uniseriate	Biseriate			
Terrei A. *terreus*		+	Tan to cinnamon brown, rarely orange-brown, reverse yellow or tan	Conidiophore 100–250 μm long and 4.5–6 μm wide, smooth, uncolored; vesicle dome shaped, 10–16 μm in diameter, with phialides on upper half; head columnar; conidia globose or subglobose, smooth, 2 μm in diameter; solitary single-celled conidia commonly formed sessile on submerged hyphae	Cinnamon brown colonies, columnar heads, and solitary accessory conidia are highly distinctive
Nidulantes Emericella nidulans (anamorph, A. nidulans)		+	Dark green if mainly conidial; buff to purplish brown if cleistothecial; reverse deep red to purple	Conidiophore 70–150 μm long and 3–6 μm wide, smooth, brown; vesicle hemispherical, 8–12 μm in diameter; phialides on upper part, columnar; conidia globose, rough, 3–4 μm in diameter; cleistothecia reddish brown, globose, 100–250 μm, Hülle cells globose; ascospores lenticular with two longitudinal crests ca. 5 μm long, reddish purple (Fig. 2C and D)	Toxigenic; distinguished by reddish brown cleistothecia, abundant Hülle cells, reddish purple ascospores with two crests, short conidiophores and stout metulae
Emericella quadrilineata		+	Olive green to grayish purple; reverse purple	Conidial heads, ascocarps, and Hülle cells similar to those of E. nidulans; Ascospores also similar but have 2 major and 2 minor equatorial crests.	Distinguished from E. nidulans by 4 crests on ascospores
Flavipedes A. *flavipes*		+	White with patches of yellow or pale grayish buff; reverse yellow to golden brown	Conidiophore 150–400 μm long and 4–8 μm wide, smooth to roughened, uncolored to pale brown, vesicle subglobose, 10–20 μm in diameter; radiate to loosely columnar; conidia globose, smooth, 2–3 μm in diameter; cleistothecia and Hülle cells rarely produced	Distinguished from A. terreus by slower-growing colonies, metulae usually formed over entire vesicle, and radiate to loosely columnar heads
Usti A. *ustus*		+	Brownish gray or olive gray, reverse yellow, dull reddish, or purplish	Conidiophore 75–400 μm long and 4–7 μm wide, smooth, becoming brown; vesicle globose or subglobose, 7–16 μm in diameter, fertile over upper two-thirds; radiate to loosely columnar; conidia globose, rough, 3–4.5 μm in diameter; irregular Hülle cells often present (Fig. 2E and F)	Distinguished by dull gray-green colonies, small vesicles, brown conidiophores and irregularly shaped Hülle cells, when present
A. *deflectus*		+	Slow-growing, becoming mouse gray with pinkish margins or patches of yellow	Conidiophore 40–125 μm long and 2.5–3.5 μm wide, smooth, reddish brown; vesicle hemispherical, 5–7 μm in diameter, typically bent at right angle to stipe; phialides on upper surface, columnar; conidia globose, 3–3.5 μm in diameter, smooth to roughened; Hülle cells sometimes present	Distinguished by vesicle bent almost at right angle to stipe; rarely reported as pathogen in humans and dogs

(Continued on next page)

TABLE 2 Characteristics of some medically important *Aspergillus* species grown on identification media[a] *(Continued)*

Section[b] and species	Seriation		Colony color	Microscopic features[c]	Comments[d]
	Uniseriate	Biseriate			
Aspergillus *Eurotium* spp. (anamorphs, *A. glaucus* and other spp.)	+		Deep green mixed with bright yellow; reverse uncolored or pale yellow	Conidiophore 200–350 μm long and 7–12 μm wide, smooth, uncolored to pale brown; vesicle globose, 15–30 μm in diameter; conidial heads large, radiate; conidia subglobose, echinulate, 5 μm in diameter; cleistothecia thin walled, yellow, globose, 75–150 μm, ascospores smooth or roughened, with furrow and rounded or frilled crests	Formerly called *glaucus* group; osmophilic, reproduction enhanced on high-sugar media; growth poor at 37°C; difficult to distinguish by features of conidial heads but readily identified by ascospore morphology. *E. repens*, *E. ruber*, and *E. amstelodami* rarely reported as pathogens. *E. umbrosus* reported as cause of farmer's lung is another name for *E. herbariorum* (anamorph, *A. glaucus*).
Restricti *A. restrictus*	+		Dull olive green to brownish green, very slow growing	Conidiophore 80–200 μm long and 4–8 μm wide, smooth or roughened, uncolored; vesicle hemispherical, 8–20 μm in diameter, phialides on upper third; head columnar; conidia cylindrical to ellipsoidal, roughened, 4–7 μm long and 3–4 μm wide	May be confused with *A. fumigatus* but differs by very slow growth on routine media, slightly enhanced growth on high-sugar media, no growth at 37°C, cylindrical conidia developing in long, adherent columns
Candidi *A. candidus*	+	+	White to cream	Conidiophore mostly 200–500 μm long and 7–10 μm wide, smooth to roughened, uncolored; vesicle globose or subglobose, 17–35 μm in diameter, fertile over entire surface; radiate; conidia globose, smooth, 3–4 μm in diameter; reddish purple sclerotia sometimes present	Distinguished from all colored aspergilli by white, slow-growing colonies; from *A. niveus* by larger vesicles, metulae covering entire surface, and absence of teleomorph; predominantly biseriate, but sometimes uniseriate on smaller heads

[a]Modified from previous versions of this chapter.
[b]Modern concepts have replaced group names with subgenera and sections.
[c]Refer to "Taxonomy" and "Identification" in the *Aspergillus* section of this chapter for descriptions of terms.
[d]Only species producing potent toxins are noted as toxigenic, but other species may produces toxins of lesser significance.

randomly with asci and ascospores. Shape, color, size, and wall features of both ascomata and ascospores are important characters for differentiating teleomorphs of *Aspergillus* species. Poorly sporulating variants of aspergilli are isolated occasionally, especially from patients with chronic respiratory infections (12). *A. fumigatus* species complex isolates should be considered if a sterile white mold grows at 45°C. Variants sometimes appear highly atypical and present with glabrous (waxy) cerebriform colonies not recognizable as *Aspergillus*. Incubation at 25°C in the presence of light may induce sporulation in some aspergilli (9). Recent studies have also shown that the cryptic species *A. lentulus* (a relative of *A. fumigatus*) (Fig. 2B) may demonstrate a poorly sporulating phenotype (7).

DNA sequencing can be particularly helpful in the identification of nonsporulating isolates or isolates with atypical morphology. The internal transcribed spacer regions (ITS1 and ITS2) of rDNA have been found to be more discriminatory than the 28S ribosomal subunit (D1–D2 region) for identification of 13 clinically important *Aspergillus* species (47). PCR-based assays utilizing these sequences have also been developed (47). Recognizing the growing role of molecular methods in *Aspergillus* species recognition, the recently convened international working group meeting entitled "*Aspergillus* Systematics in the Genomic Era" proposed several recommendations, including the use of the ITS regions for section (species complex)-level identification and use of a protein coding locus (β-tubulin) for identification of individual species within each *Aspergillus* section (8). This *Aspergillus* working group has recommended the use of the term "species complex" to denote each section within the *Aspergillus* subgenera. Since isolates can fairly easily be identified to the section level by use of morphological methods, but molecular methods are required for identification of isolates within each section, the use of the term "species complex" will help to support correct identification in resource-limited clinical microbiology laboratories. For instance, using morphological methods, the laboratory can identify a fungus as "A. *fumigatus* species complex" and indicate that further molecular methods are required if confirmatory identification of the isolate as a species within the A. *fumigatus* complex is required.

Typing Systems

Historically, genetic fingerprinting and epidemiological studies have been hampered by the lack of robust, reproducible typing methods. Increased knowledge of the genetics of aspergilli and the advent of more-user-friendly methods to prepare and manipulate DNA now allow for detailed analyses. Molecular techniques are useful in detection-identification systems and for epidemiological studies, although most techniques have been applied to type A. *fumigatus* strains only. Several methods can be used to genotype aspergilli, including random amplified polymorphic DNA (RAPD) analysis, restriction fragment length polymorphism analysis, use of repetitive element and/or complex probes with Southern blotting (129), amplified fragment length polymorphism analysis, and microsatellite length polymorphism analysis. However, a major problem with pattern-based techniques, such as RAPD, restriction fragment length polymorphism, and amplified fragment length polymorphism analyses, is the low level of concordance between laboratories and limited data-sharing capabilities (11). These limitations can be overcome by using the recently developed microsatellite methods for A. *fumigatus* (31). Employing a panel of nine microsatellites, Balajee and colleagues recently demonstrated the utility of this method in typing epidemiologically related A. *fumigatus* isolates (6). A comparative sequence-based method called CSP typing (typing of a gene encoding a cell surface protein) has also been tested as a genotyping method for A. *fumigatus* but appears to be less discriminatory than the microsatellite-based methods (63).

Regardless of fingerprinting method, A. *fumigatus* shows enormous genetic variability among both clinical and environmental strains, indicating that any A. *fumigatus* strain can cause disease in humans (24, 41). Furthermore, the degree of genetic diversity significantly reduces the potential of genotyping A. *fumigatus* for the purpose of infection control, since a considerable number of environmental isolates would have to be genotyped in order to match the patient strain with an environmental strain. For A. *fumigatus*, genotyping might be useful during clusters of infection in order to establish the presence of a common source. Nevertheless, some studies have shown genetic relatedness between environmental and patient strains, suggesting that aspergillosis has a nosocomial origin in some cases (24, 26, 40, 77, 78). Similar results have been obtained with RAPD typing patterns (4, 14, 72) and Southern blots probed with either rDNA (130) or nonribosomal genomic sequences. Invasive aspergillosis has been linked to a nosocomial origin for A. *fumigatus* (41), A. *flavus* (77), and A. *terreus* (75). By using genotyping, specific niches within the hospital environment could be found, as was the case with A. *terreus*, where genotypes of strains recovered from potted plants in the direct environment of infected patients were indistinguishable from those of strains isolated from patients (75).

Serologic Tests

The detection of antibody in serum or other body fluids and reactivity in skin tests are to some degree dependent upon the purity, chemical nature, and uniqueness of the antigen preparation used (71). Extracts of the whole mycelium, metabolic products secreted into the medium during the growth of *Aspergillus* spp., purified antigens, and, more recently, expressed and purified recombinant antigens have all been used in serologic tests and immunoassays. Although such antigen preparations are available commercially, standardized antigens are still not widely available. As reviewed by Kurup and Kumar (71), two of the major reasons for the lack of standardized antigens are that (i) antigen preparations are highly variable and (ii) antigens show various degrees of cross-reactivity. Work is ongoing to address these issues and to find ways to express, purify, and prepare improved antigen preparations.

Several serologic tests with disparate sensitivities have been developed to detect circulating antibodies. As noted above, these have proven especially valuable in aiding the diagnosis of allergic aspergillosis and aspergilloma but are less useful in the diagnosis of acute invasive disease in patients with little or no humoral response. However, antibody detection might be useful as a diagnostic tool for specific host groups, such as lung transplant recipients (135) and patients with chronic granulomatous disease (120). It has also been suggested that serology could be used as a means of retrospective diagnosis for patients who had undergone immunological reconstitution after an episode of neutropenia (49).

Double immunodiffusion and counterimmunoelectrophoresis remain the most widely used techniques, primarily because they are simple and easy to perform (71, 76). Other tests which have achieved some success for diagnosis of aspergillosis include ELISA, biotin-avidin linked sandwich ELISA (BALISA), radioimmunoassay, and indirect immunofluorescence assay (79, 124). Of these, various ELISAs are the most amenable to the clinical laboratory. While in some cases these assays can be highly sensitive, reliable, and versatile, their routine use in many clinical laboratories has been limited by interlaboratory discrepancies in results and by immunological responses leading to false-positive results for some patient groups (71). The reasons for these problems vary but are due primarily to the ubiquitous nature of aspergilli (leading to high background antibody titers), the lack of ability to mount diagnostic humoral immune responses in immunocompromised patients, cross-reactivities between different fungi and even bacteria, and the selection of *Aspergillus* antigens used (67, 71). Using molecular biological techniques, it is now possible to produce A. *fumigatus* proteins in an expression system that yields large quantities of pure recombinant antigen. These antigens can serve as the basis for the development of ELISA methods to quantify the immune response (76). For example, the presence of antibodies directed against the recombinant protein mitogillin proved to correlate well with clinical disease, especially for patients with aspergilloma, with only 1.3% of healthy volunteers showing detectable antibodies (149). Quantitation of the immunoglobulin isotypes will be important to optimize the diagnostic value of the assay and to understand further the humoral response in patients with aspergillosis.

Antimicrobial Susceptibilities

The number of antifungal agents that are licensed for treatment of patients with invasive aspergillosis has increased. The development of lipid formulations of amphotericin B and the triazoles itraconazole, voriconazole, and posaconazole broadened the therapeutic arsenal. Until recently, the polyenes were considered the gold standard for treatment of invasive aspergillosis, but many treating physicians now use voriconazole as first-line therapy (46, 108). Other antifungal drugs approved for treatment of invasive aspergillosis include the echinocandins caspofungin, micafungin, and anidulafungin. Of the contemporary antifungals, a recent study suggests that the most active agents in vitro against *Aspergillus* spp. are anidulafungin, caspofungin, and posaconazole (96). For a more detailed review of treatment practices for aspergillosis, the reader is directed to the recent Infectious Diseases Society of America guideline document (142).

A reference method for in vitro susceptibility testing of conidium-forming molds has been developed by the Clinical Laboratory Standards Institute (CLSI) (20) (see chapter 128 in this *Manual*). By use of this method, the polyenes and azoles are active in vitro, although no interpretive breakpoints have been established for any drugs with any molds, including *Aspergillus*. Rodriguez-Tudela et al. recently proposed an epidemiological cutoff of <1 mg/liter for itraconazole and voriconazole for wild-type populations of *A. fumigatus* (119). For amphotericin B, however, there is no clear correlation with clinical response because there is a narrow distribution of MICs, with no clear resistance phenotype (57). The exception to this is *A. terreus*, which is considered resistant to amphotericin B, with MICs as high as 16 µg/ml (143). Itraconazole, voriconazole, and posaconazole are active in vitro against *Aspergillus* species, with posaconazole typically showing the lowest MICs (113). There is a good correlation between high MICs and treatment failure, at least in experimental models of invasive aspergillosis (27, 28).

Several mutations in the CYP51 gene, which encodes the target of azole antifungal agents, cytochrome P450 sterol 14α-demethylase, have been identified that correspond to amino acid substitutions and phenotypic resistance of *Aspergillus* against azoles (37, 91). The frequency of resistance against azoles, however, is low, and resistance appears to be found in patients who receive long-term azole prophylaxis or therapy (23, 147) and in patients with aspergilloma or with chronic aspergillosis and prior itraconazole therapy. In addition, resistance has also been reported for patients with acute invasive aspergillosis in the Netherlands, at a rate of 6 to 12.8%, with a single dominant mechanism. Interestingly, this study suggests an environmental mode of acquisition of azole-resistant *A. fumigatus*, with some evidence that resistance might have developed through exposure to azole fungicides in the environment rather than in azole-treated patients in the hospital (128). In contrast to this study, Howard et al. demonstrated that resistant *A. fumigatus* isolates evolved from an originally susceptible clinical *A. fumigatus* isolate exposed to azole therapy rather than via environmentally acquired resistance (53).

Testing the activity of echinocandins against *Aspergillus* is not reliable by the CLSI methodology and reading of MIC endpoints. Exposure of *Aspergillus* to caspofungin results in morphologic changes that can be detected only by microscopic examination. Therefore, the minimal effective concentration (MEC) was suggested as a microscopic endpoint, which enables in vitro testing against this class of antifungal agents (70).

Several commercial kits are available for testing of the in vitro activities of antifungal drugs against molds, including *Aspergillus*. For instance, the Etest employs strips that contain a gradient of antifungal drug concentrations and shows a good correlation with the CLSI reference method (36). Currently, in the United States, Etests have been approved by the U.S. Food and Drug Administration only for yeast susceptibility testing.

Evaluation, Interpretation, and Reporting of Results

In the laboratory, *Aspergillus* isolates should be identified to the species level when they are recovered from patients at risk for *Aspergillus* infections. A particularly important species is *A. terreus*, which is resistant to amphotericin B (143). *A. nidulans* and *A. ustus* (55) have also been reported to be less susceptible to amphotericin B than is *A. fumigatus* (68).

On the other hand, *Aspergillus* species recovered from nonsterile specimens in immunocompetent patients may not be causative agents of disease and may not require identification to the species level (111). Decisions regarding workup of these samples should be discussed between microbiologists and clinicians.

The diagnosis of invasive aspergillosis remains very difficult, and information obtained by various diagnostic tests and procedures, such as clinical symptoms and signs, chest radiograph, high-resolution CT, and, if possible, culture and histology, needs to be considered. The conventional approach to the management of patients at risk for invasive aspergillosis is to administer antifungal agents empirically to neutropenic patients who are persistently febrile despite treatment with broad-spectrum antibacterial agents or to those who develop pulmonary infiltrates during antibacterial therapy. The development of tests that detect circulating surrogate markers, such as fungal antigens or DNA, and the use of high-resolution CT allow for alternative approaches to be evaluated. The optimal use of detection of circulating markers appears to be in prospective monitoring of high-risk patients during the period of increased risk, since circulating markers can be early indicators of infection in most patients. Once the marker is detected, patients may undergo a diagnostic workup that includes high-resolution CT of the chest in order to confirm the presence of the infection. The probability of infection is very high for this group, and early antifungal treatment can then be administered selectively. The above strategy proved to be superior to the conventional approach in a decision analysis (125), and a feasibility study indicated that the preemptive treatment strategy might be an alternative to empiric therapy (85).

It should be appreciated that no MIC breakpoints are available for any molds with any antifungal drug. This prevents a straightforward correlation between MIC value and clinical outcome (117). The interpretation of MIC testing of molds remains problematic (118), with the most potential value from testing of *A. fumigatus* isolates against azoles. In general, the most useful information regarding antifungal susceptibility can be obtained by identifying the fungal agent to the species level.

PENICILLIUM MARNEFFEI

Taxonomy

Like its close relative *Aspergillus*, the genus *Penicillium* comprises anamorphic (asexual) species with connections to the ascomycete family Trichocomaceae (121). About 200 species have been placed into four subgenera according to conidiophore branching (32, 114), but molecular analysis has shown three of these subgenera to be polyphyletic (isolates of different genetic origins are in the same group). The only true pathogen is *Penicillium marneffei*, a member of the subgenus *Biverticillium* (81). The species is unique among the penicillia in being dimorphic, forming a unicellular yeast-like organelle in tissue that reproduces by planate division (division by fission). The thermally regulated growth of this species shows typical features of *Penicillium* at room temperature and shows yeast cells (arthroconidia) at body temperature.

Epidemiology and Transmission

Penicillium marneffei infection is an important emerging public health problem, especially among patients infected with HIV in areas of endemicity in Southeast Asia, with cases being reported from Manipur State, India, Myanmar, Malaysia, southern China, Hong Kong, Taiwan, and northern Thailand (21). Within these regions, *P. marneffei* infection is regarded as an AIDS-defining illness, and the severity of the disease depends on the immunological status of the infected individual.

The natural history and mode of transmission of the organism remain unclear. Soil exposure, especially during the rainy season, has been suggested to be a critical risk factor (18, 33, 88). Even though the fungus was discovered in 1956, in the bamboo rat (*Rhizomys sinensis*) in Vietnam, decaying organic material and soil are most likely its natural habitat. When multilocus microsatellite typing was used to characterize this fungus, several isolates from bamboo rats and humans were shown to share identical multilocus genotypes. These data suggest that either transmission of *P. marneffei* occurs from rodents to humans or, more likely, humans and rodents are coinfected from the same environmental sources (136).

Patients are infected by inhalation of *P. marneffei* conidia. Pulmonary alveolar macrophages are the primary host defense mechanism. The fungus proliferates within phagocytic cells, resulting in granulomas in immunocompetent individuals. In AIDS, the infection typically develops in individuals with CD4$^+$ cell counts under 50 cells/ml and rapidly disseminates.

Clinical Significance

P. marneffei has been reported to be the fourth most common cause of disseminated opportunistic infection in patients with AIDS in areas where it is endemic (18, 33). Infections are more common in immunosuppressed than immunocompetent hosts and are usually disseminated, with multiple-organ involvement, including the lungs, liver, and skin. The fungus can usually be isolated from characteristic skin lesions, which are present in 60% of cases, or from blood or bone marrow (33, 88). Presumptive diagnosis may be made by demonstration of the yeast-like cells of *P. marneffei* in Wright-stained smears from skin lesions or in biopsy specimens from these sites (88).

Collection, Transport, and Storage of Specimens

Methods of collection, transport, and storage of specimens are detailed in chapter 112.

Direct Examination

The yeast-like cells are oval or cylindrical and 3 to 6 μm long, and they may have a cross wall. Yeast cells of *Histoplasma capsulatum* may appear similar, especially when they are within phagocytes, but they may show evidence of budding rather than division by fission. The yeast may be stained in tissue sections by methenamine silver or periodic-acid Schiff stain.

Isolation

P. marneffei can be cultured easily from clinical specimens. The fungus grows well on Sabouraud dextrose agar (Fig. 2G). Culture of bone marrow is the most sensitive culture method (100%), followed by culture of specimens obtained from skin biopsy samples (90%) and blood culture (76%). Handling and culture of specimens possibly containing *P. marneffei* should be performed with care, avoiding inhalation of conidia from sporulating mold cultures or accidental injection into the skin. Biosafety level 2 practices and facilities are recommended for propagating and manipulating cultures known to contain *P. marneffei*. In Europe, *P. marneffei* is classified as a hazard group 3 organism and should be handled within a containment level 3 facility, as should any sample likely to contain this organism. The main drawbacks of fungal culture are the long turnaround time and the need for invasive procedures to obtain tissue.

Identification

Members of the genus *Penicillium* are the ubiquitous blue-green molds that are among the most common of all laboratory contaminants and that can be isolated easily (2 to 5 days) from respiratory specimens and body surfaces. *Penicillium marneffei* is thermally dimorphic, growing as a mold at 25°C. The yeast phase is produced at 37°C on any rich medium, such as brain heart infusion agar. Definitive identification is made by observing the conversion of mold to yeast at 37°C or the reverse at 25°C. Isolates of *P. marneffei* have a distinctive morphology (Fig. 2G and H), with conidiophore-bearing biverticillate penicillia composed of four or five metulae with smooth-walled conidia. A diffusible red pigment produced in culture is one of the first indications that an isolate may be *P. marneffei*. However, red pigment can also be produced by other *Penicillium* species that are not associated with human infection, including *P. citrinum*, *P. janthinellum*, *P. purpurogenum*, and *P. rubrum*. Yeast-like colonies at 37°C are beige and may be glabrous or appear heaped and wrinkled due to the overproduction of arthroconidial forms.

Typing Systems

Exact typing systems, including multilocus microsatellite typing, have been developed to characterize genetic diversity in *P. marneffei* (38). Typing of strains showed clustering into two distinct clades, corresponding to isolates obtained from patients living in the eastern parts of the *P. marneffei* range and in the western sector, including Thailand and India. Potential geographic isolation of populations was also suggested by other investigators (73). Identical multilocus genotypes were found in isolates from bamboo rats and humans, but interpretation in relation to the pathogenesis of the infection remains unclear (136).

Serologic Tests

Serologic methods have been developed and are proving to be important in the early diagnosis of infection, but no commercial tests are available. A number of studies have aimed at detecting fungal antibodies and/or antigens in the sera and body fluids of infected patients. Culture filtrates from *P. marneffei* cultured in liquid media and anti-*P. marneffei* rabbit sera were incorporated into an immunodiffusion test to detect antibody and antigens, respectively. Other assays include an indirect immunofluorescent-antibody test using the yeast hyphae or germinating conidia as antigens (62), a latex agglutination test, and an ELISA (30, 61, 88). Antigens may be detected in urine as well as serum. Specific antibodies against a recombinant cell wall-associated protein (Mp1p) were generated to produce an ELISA-based antibody test. Approximately 80% (14 of 17 patients) of documented HIV-positive penicilliosis patients tested positive for the specific antibody. No false-positive results were found for serum samples from 90 healthy blood donors, 20 patients with typhoid fever, and 55 patients with tuberculosis, indicating a high specificity of the test. Thus, this ELISA-based test for the detection of anti-Mp1p antibody can be of significant value as a diagnostic for penicilliosis (15, 16).

Antimicrobial Susceptibilities

Amphotericin B, voriconazole, and itraconazole are commonly used to treat patients with penicilliosis, with amphotericin B used for seriously ill patients. Although no formal breakpoints have been established, *P. marneffei* appears to be highly susceptible in vitro to itraconazole, voriconazole, and ketoconazole, but less so to fluconazole (105, 134). The echinocandins are active against *P. marneffei*, but in vitro the drugs are more active against the mycelial forms than the yeast-like forms (102, 105).

Other *Penicillium* Species

Penicillium species other than *P. marneffei* have been implicated in human infection, but the validity of some reports has been questioned (132). Although *Penicillium* species grow over a wide range of temperatures, from 5 to 45°C, many species are completely or strongly inhibited at 37°C and thus have low potential for causing human infection. Even repeated isolation of a *Penicillium* species from patient specimens does not necessarily indicate an etiologic role, unless the isolate is accompanied by typical fungal elements in tissue specimens or smears of lesion exudate. Other factors to consider in assessing the significance of repeated isolation include the isolation of any other fungal species, the patient's possible exposure to airborne conidia, and a diagnosis of bronchiectasis, since conidia may remain viable for prolonged periods without invasion or colonization (72). Nonetheless, several species have been reported to cause peritonitis, urinary tract infection, endocarditis, lung infection, fungemia, and disseminated infection (19, 25, 72, 83). The role of penicillia in allergy and hypersensitivity pneumonitis is well established (51). Identification of *Penicillium* species is a complex task, requiring growth of an isolate on several media at different temperatures and careful microscopic examination (32, 114, 122). Czapek yeast extract agar, malt extract agar, and 25% glycerol nitrate agar are used, with incubation at 5, 25, and 37°C. The use of Sabouraud dextrose agar alone is not recommended.

Evaluation and Interpretation of Results

Penicillium marneffei remains the only member of the genus that has been implicated unequivocally as a causative agent of disease. A number of other species can produce red pigment, but they do not display thermal dimorphism, the characteristic of this species. Diagnosis of penicilliosis marneffei should include positive culture, direct smear, and/or serology and an appropriate history of exposure to the area of endemicity in Southeast Asia. Most other species have low potential for causing human infection. It should also be appreciated that no MIC breakpoints are available for any molds with any antifungal drug, so MIC testing is not warranted.

REFERENCES

1. **Alcazar-Fuoli, L., E. Mellado, A. Alastruey-Izquierdo, M. Cuenca-Estrella, and J. L. Rodriguez-Tudela.** 2008. *Aspergillus* section *Fumigati*: antifungal susceptibility patterns and sequence-based identification. *Antimicrob. Agents Chemother.* **52:**1244–1251.

2. **Ansorg, R., R. van den Boom, and R. M. Rath.** 1997. Detection of *Aspergillus* galactomannan antigen in foods and antibiotics. *Mycoses* **40:**353–357.

3. **Ascioglu, S., J. H. Rex, B. de Pauw, J. E. Bennett, J. Bille, F. Crokaert, D. W. Denning, J. P. Donnelly, J. E. Edwards, Z. Erjavec, D. Fiere, O. Lortholary, J. Maertens, J. F. Meis, T. F. Patterson, J. Ritter, D. Selleslag, P. M. Shah, D. A. Stevens, and T. J. Walsh.** 2002. Defining opportunistic invasive fungal infections in immunocompromised patients with cancer and hematopoietic stem cell transplants: an international consensus. *Clin. Infect. Dis.* **34:**7–14.

4. **Aufauvre-Brown, A., J. Cohen, and D. W. Holden.** 1992. Use of randomly amplified polymorphic DNA markers to distinguish isolates of *Aspergillus fumigatus*. *J. Clin. Microbiol.* **30:**2991–2993.

5. **Baddley, J. W., T. P. Stroud, D. Salzman, and P. G. Pappas.** 2001. Invasive mold infections in allogeneic bone marrow transplant recipients. *Clin. Infect. Dis.* **32:**1319–1324.

6. **Balajee, S. A., H. A. de Valk, B. A. Lasker, J. F. Meis, and C. H. Klaassen.** 2008. Utility of a microsatellite assay for identifying clonally related outbreak isolates of *Aspergillus fumigatus*. *J. Microbiol. Methods* **73:**252–256.

7. **Balajee, S. A., J. L. Gribskov, E. Hanley, D. Nickle, and K. A. Marr.** 2005. *Aspergillus lentulus* sp. nov., a new sibling species of *A. fumigatus*. *Eukaryot. Cell* **4:**625–632.

8. **Balajee, S. A., J. Houbraken, P. E. Verweij, S. B. Hong, T. Yaghuchi, J. Varga, and R. A. Samson.** 2007. *Aspergillus* species identification in the clinical setting. *Stud. Mycol.* **59:**39–46.

9. **Balajee, S. A., M. D. Lindsley, N. Iqbal, J. Ito, P. G. Pappas, and M. E. Brandt.** 2007. Nonsporulating clinical isolate identified as *Petromyces alliaceus* (anamorph *Aspergillus alliaceus*) by morphological and sequence-based methods. *J. Clin. Microbiol.* **45:**2701–2703.

10. **Bart-Delabesse, E., M. Basile, A. Al Jijakli, D. Souville, F. Gay, B. Philippe, M. Bossi, M. Danis, J. P. Vernant, and A. Datry.** 2005. Detection of *Aspergillus* galactomannan antigenemia to determine biological and clinical implications of beta-lactam treatments. *J. Clin. Microbiol.* **43:**5214–5220.

11. **Bart-Delabesse, E., J. Sarfati, J. P. Debeaupuis, W. van Leeuwen, A. van Belkum, S. Bretagne, and J. P. Latge.** 2001. Comparison of restriction fragment length polymorphism, microsatellite length polymorphism, and random amplification of polymorphic DNA analyses for fingerprinting *Aspergillus fumigatus* isolates. *J. Clin. Microbiol.* **39:**2683–2686.

12. **Brandt, M. E., L. Gade, C. B. McCloskey, and S. A. Balajee.** 2009. Atypical *Aspergillus flavus* isolates associated with chronic azole therapy. *J. Clin. Microbiol.* **47:**3372–3375.

13. **Buchheidt, D., M. Hummel, D. Schleiermacher, B. Spiess, R. Schwerdtfeger, O. A. Cornely, S. Wilhelm, S. Reuter, W. Kern, T. Sudhoff, H. Morz, and R. Hehlmann.** 2004. Prospective clinical evaluation of a LightCycler-mediated polymerase chain reaction assay, a nested-PCR assay and a galactomannan enzyme-linked immunosorbent assay for detection of invasive aspergillosis in neutropenic cancer patients and haematological stem cell transplant recipients. *Br. J. Haematol.* **125:**196–202.

14. **Buffington, J., R. Reporter, B. A. Lasker, M. M. McNeil, J. M. Lanson, L. A. Ross, L. Mascola, and W. R. Jarvis.** 1994. Investigation of an epidemic of invasive aspergillosis: utility of molecular typing with the use of random amplified polymorphic DNA probes. *Pediatr. Infect. Dis. J.* **13:**386–393.

15. **Cao, L., K. M. Chan, D. Chen, N. Vanittanakom, C. Lee, C. M. Chan, T. Sirisanthana, D. N. Tsang, and K. Y. Yuen.** 1999. Detection of cell wall mannoprotein Mp1p in culture supernatants of *Penicillium marneffei* and in sera of penicilliosis patients. *J. Clin. Microbiol.* **37:**981–986.

16. **Cao, L., D. L. Chen, C. Lee, C. M. Chan, K. M. Chan, N. Vanittanakom, D. N. Tsang, and K. Y. Yuen.** 1998. Detection of specific antibodies to an antigenic mannoprotein for diagnosis of *Penicillium marneffei* penicilliosis. *J. Clin. Microbiol.* **36:**3028–3031.

17. **Chandler, F. W., and J. C. Watts.** 1987. *Pathologic Diagnosis of Fungal Infections.* American Society of Clinical Pathologists, Inc., Chicago, IL.

18. **Chariyalertsak, S., T. Sirisanthana, O. Saengwonloey, and K. E. Nelson.** 2001. Clinical presentation and risk behaviors of patients with acquired immunodeficiency syndrome in Thailand, 1994–1998: regional variation and temporal trends. *Clin. Infect. Dis.* **32:**955–962.

19. **Cimon, B., J. Carrere, J. P. Chazalette, J. F. Vinatier, D. Chabasse, and J. P. Bouchara.** 1999. Chronic airway colonization by *Penicillium emersonii* in a patient with cystic fibrosis. *Med. Mycol.* **37:**291–293.

20. **Clinical and Laboratory Standards Institute.** 2002. *Reference Method for Broth Dilution Antifungal Susceptibility Testing of Conidium-Forming Filamentous Fungi: Approved Standard M38-A.* CLSI, Wayne, PA.

21. **Cooper, C. R., Jr., and M. R. McGinnis.** 1997. Pathology of *Penicillium marneffei*. An emerging acquired immunodeficiency syndrome-related pathogen. *Arch. Pathol. Lab. Med.* **121:**798–804.

22. **Costa, C., D. Vidaud, M. Olivi, E. Bart-Delabesse, M. Vidaud, and S. Bretagne.** 2001. Development of two real-time quantitative TaqMan PCR assays to detect circulating *Aspergillus fumigatus* DNA in serum. *J. Microbiol. Methods* **44:**263–269.

23. **Dannaoui, E., E. Borel, M. F. Monier, M. A. Piens, S. Picot, and F. Persat.** 2001. Acquired itraconazole resistance in *Aspergillus fumigatus*. *J. Antimicrob. Chemother.* **47:**333–340.

24. **Debeaupuis, J. P., J. Sarfati, V. Chazalet, and J. P. Latge.** 1997. Genetic diversity among clinical and environmental isolates of *Aspergillus fumigatus*. *Infect. Immun.* **65:**3080–3085.

25. **De Hoog, G. S., J. Guarro, J. Gene, and M. J. Figueras.** 2000. *Atlas of Clinical Fungi*, 2nd ed. Centraalbureau voor Schimmelcultures, Baarn, The Netherlands.

26. **Denning, D. W., K. V. Clemons, L. H. Hanson, and D. A. Stevens.** 1990. Restriction endonuclease analysis of total cellular DNA of *Aspergillus fumigatus* isolates of geographically and epidemiologically diverse origin. *J. Infect. Dis.* **162:**1151–1158.

27. **Denning, D. W., S. A. Radford, K. L. Oakley, L. Hall, E. M. Johnson, and D. W. Warnock.** 1997. Correlation between in-vitro susceptibility testing to itraconazole and in-vivo outcome of *Aspergillus fumigatus* infection. *J. Antimicrob. Chemother.* **40:**401–414.

28. **Denning, D. W., K. Venkateswarlu, K. L. Oakley, M. J. Anderson, N. J. Manning, D. A. Stevens, D. W. Warnock, and S. L. Kelly.** 1997. Itraconazole resistance in *Aspergillus fumigatus*. *Antimicrob. Agents Chemother.* **41:**1364–1368.

29. **De Pauw, B., T. J. Walsh, J. P. Donnelly, et al.** 2008. Revised definitions of invasive fungal disease from the European Organization for Research and Treatment of Cancer/Invasive Fungal Infections Cooperative Group and the National Institute of Allergy and Infectious Diseases Mycoses Study Group (EORTC/MSG) Consensus Group. *Clin. Infect. Dis.* **46:**1813–1821.

30. **Desakorn, V., M. D. Smith, A. L. Walsh, A. J. Simpson, D. Sahassananda, A. Rajanuwong, V. Wuthiekanun, P. Howe, B. J. Angus, P. Suntharasamai, and N. J. White.** 1999. Diagnosis of *Penicillium marneffei* infection by quantitation of urinary antigen by using an enzyme immunoassay. *J. Clin. Microbiol.* **37:**117–121.

31. **de Valk, H. A., J. F. Meis, I. M. Curfs, K. Muehlethaler, J. W. Mouton, and C. H. Klaassen.** 2005. Use of a novel panel of nine short tandem repeats for exact and high-resolution fingerprinting of *Aspergillus fumigatus* isolates. *J. Clin. Microbiol.* **43:**4112–4120.

32. **Domsch, K. H., W. Gams, and T. H. Anderson.** 1980. *Compendium of Soil Fungi.* IHW-Verlag, Eching, Germany. [Reprint, IHW-Verlag, Eching, Germany, 1993.]

33. **Duong, T. A.** 1996. Infection due to *Penicillium marneffei*, an emerging pathogen: review of 155 reported cases. *Clin. Infect. Dis.* **23:**125–130.

34. **Einsele, H., H. Hebart, G. Roller, J. Loffler, I. Rothenhofer, C. A. Muller, R. A. Bowden, J. van Burik, D. Engelhard, L. Kanz, and U. Schumacher.** 1997. Detection and identification of fungal pathogens in blood by using molecular probes. *J. Clin. Microbiol.* **35:**1353–1360.

35. **Erjavec, Z., H. Kluin-Nelemans, and P. E. Verweij.** 2009. Trends in invasive fungal infections, with emphasis on invasive aspergillosis. *Clin. Microbiol. Infect.* **15:**625–633.

36. **Espinel-Ingroff, A.** 2001. Comparison of the E-test with the NCCLS M38-P method for antifungal susceptibility testing of common and emerging pathogenic filamentous fungi. *J. Clin. Microbiol.* **39:**1360–1367.

37. **Ferreira, M. E., A. L. Colombo, I. Paulsen, Q. Ren, J. Wortman, J. Huang, M. H. Goldman, and G. H. Goldman.** 2005. The ergosterol biosynthesis pathway, transporter genes, and azole resistance in *Aspergillus fumigatus*. *Med. Mycol.* **43**(Suppl. 1)**:**S313–S319.

38. **Fisher, M. C., D. Aanensen, S. de Hoog, and N. Vanittanakom.** 2004. Multilocus microsatellite typing system for *Penicillium marneffei* reveals spatially structured populations. *J. Clin. Microbiol.* **42:**5065–5069.

39. **Fredricks, D. N., C. Smith, and A. Meier.** 2005. Comparison of six DNA extraction methods for recovery of fungal DNA as assessed by quantitative PCR. *J. Clin. Microbiol.* **43:**5122–5128.

40. **Girardin, H., J. P. Latge, T. Srikantha, B. Morrow, and D. R. Soll.** 1993. Development of DNA probes for fingerprinting *Aspergillus fumigatus*. *J. Clin. Microbiol.* **31:**1547–1554.

41. **Girardin, H., J. Sarfati, F. Traore, J. Dupouy Camet, F. Derouin, and J. P. Latge.** 1994. Molecular epidemiology of nosocomial invasive aspergillosis. *J. Clin. Microbiol.* **32:**684–690.

42. **Gradon, J. D., J. G. Timpone, and S. M. Schnittman.** 1992. Emergence of unusual opportunistic pathogens in AIDS: a review. *Clin. Infect. Dis.* **15:**134–157.

43. **Grossi, P., C. Farina, R. Fiocchi, and D. Dalla Gasperina.** 2000. Prevalence and outcome of invasive fungal infections in 1,963 thoracic organ transplant recipients: a multicenter retrospective study. *Transplantation* **70:**112–116.

44. **Hawksworth, D. L.** 2009. Separate name for fungus's sexual stage may cause confusion. *Nature* **458:**29.

45. **Hendolin, P. H., L. Paulin, P. Koukila-Kähkölä, V. J. Anttila, H. Malmberg, M. Richardson, and J. Ylikoski.** 2000. Panfungal PCR and multiplex liquid hybridization for detection of fungi in tissue specimens. *J. Clin. Microbiol.* **38:**4186–4192.

46. **Herbrecht, R., D. W. Denning, T. F. Patterson, J. E. Bennett, R. E. Greene, J. W. Oestmann, W. V. Kern, K. A. Marr, P. Ribaud, O. Lortholary, R. Sylvester, R. H. Rubin, J. R. Wingard, P. Stark, C. Durand, D. Caillot, E. Thiel, P. H. Chandrasekar, M. R. Hodges, H. T. Schlamm, P. F. Troke, and B. de Pauw.** 2002. Voriconazole versus amphotericin B for primary therapy of invasive aspergillosis. *N. Engl. J. Med.* **347:**408–415.

47. **Hinrikson, H. P., S. F. Hurst, L. De Aguirre, and C. J. Morrison.** 2005. Molecular methods for the identification of *Aspergillus* species. *Med. Mycol.* **43**(Suppl. 1)**:**S129–S137.

48. **Holding, K. J., M. S. Dworkin, P. C. Wan, D. L. Hanson, R. M. Klevens, J. L. Jones, and P. S. Sullivan.** 2000. Aspergillosis among people infected with human immunodeficiency virus: incidence and survival. *Clin. Infect. Dis.* **31:**1253–1257.

49. **Hope, W. W., T. J. Walsh, and D. W. Denning.** 2005. Laboratory diagnosis of invasive aspergillosis. *Lancet Infect. Dis.* **5:**609–622.

50. **Hopwood, V., E. M. Johnson, J. M. Cornish, A. B. Foot, E. G. Evans, and D. W. Warnock.** 1995. Use of the Pastorex aspergillus antigen latex agglutination test for the diagnosis of invasive aspergillosis. *J. Clin. Pathol.* **48:**210–213.

51. **Horner, W. E., A. Helbling, J. E. Salvaggio, and S. B. Lehrer.** 1995. Fungal allergens. *Clin. Microbiol. Rev.* **8:**161–179.

52. **Horvath, J. A., and S. Dummer.** 1996. The use of respiratory-tract cultures in the diagnosis of invasive pulmonary aspergillosis. *Am. J. Med.* **100:**171–178.

53. **Howard, S. J., D. Cerar, M. J. Anderson, A. Albarrag, M. C. Fisher, A. C. Pasqualotto, M. Laverdiere, M. C. Arendrup, D. S. Perlin, and D. W. Denning.** 2009. Frequency and evolution of azole resistance in Aspergillus fumigatus associated with treatment failure. *Emerg. Infect. Dis.* **15:**1068–1076.

54. **Ikemura, K., K. Ikegami, T. Shimazu, T. Yoshioka, and T. Sugimoto.** 1989. False-positive result in *Limulus* test caused by *Limulus* amebocyte lysate-reactive material in immunoglobulin products. *J. Clin. Microbiol.* **27**:1965–1968.

55. **Iwen, P. C., M. E. Rupp, M. R. Bishop, M. G. Rinaldi, D. A. Sutton, S. Tarantolo, and S. H. Hinrichs.** 1998. Disseminated aspergillosis caused by *Aspergillus ustus* in a patient following allogeneic peripheral stem cell transplantation. *J. Clin. Microbiol.* **36**:3713–3717.

56. **Iwen, P. C., L. Sigler, S. Tarantolo, D. A. Sutton, M. G. Rinaldi, R. P. Lackner, D. I. McCarthy, and S. H. Hinrichs.** 2000. Pulmonary infection caused by *Gymnascella hyalinospora* in a patient with acute myelogenous leukemia. *J. Clin. Microbiol.* **38**:375–381.

57. **Johnson, E. M., K. L. Oakley, S. A. Radford, C. B. Moore, P. Warn, D. W. Warnock, and D. W. Denning.** 2000. Lack of correlation of in vitro amphotericin B susceptibility testing with outcome in a murine model of *Aspergillus* infection. *J. Antimicrob. Chemother.* **45**:85–93.

58. **Kami, M., Y. Tanaka, Y. Kanda, S. Ogawa, T. Masumoto, K. Ohtomo, T. Matsumura, T. Saito, U. Machida, T. Kashima, and H. Hirai.** 2000. Computed tomographic scan of the chest, latex agglutination test and plasma (1→3)-beta-D-glucan assay in early diagnosis of invasive pulmonary aspergillosis: a prospective study of 215 patients. *Haematologica* **85**:745–752.

59. **Kanda, Y., H. Akiyama, Y. Onozawa, T. Motegi, S. Yamagata-Murayama, and H. Yamaguchi.** 1997. *Aspergillus* endocarditis in a leukemia patient diagnosed by a PCR assay. *Kansenshogaku Zasshi* **71**:269–272.

60. **Kato, A., T. Takita, M. Furuhashi, T. Takahashi, Y. Maruyama, and A. Hishida.** 2001. Elevation of blood (1,3)-beta-D-glucan concentrations in hemodialysis patients. *Nephron* **89**:159.

61. **Kaufman, L., P. G. Standard, M. Jalbert, P. Kantipong, K. Limpakarnjanarat, and T. D. Mastro.** 1996. Diagnostic antigenemia tests for penicilliosis marneffei. *J. Clin. Microbiol.* **34**:2503–2505.

62. **Kaufman, L., P. G. Standard, M. Jalbert, and D. E. Kraft.** 1997. Immunohistologic identification of *Aspergillus* spp. and other hyaline fungi by using polyclonal fluorescent antibodies. *J. Clin. Microbiol.* **35**:2206–2209.

63. **Klaassen, C. H., H. A. de Valk, S. A. Balajee, and J. F. Meis.** 2009. Utility of CSP typing to sub-type clinical *Aspergillus fumigatus* isolates and proposal for a new CSP type nomenclature. *J. Microbiol. Methods* **77**:292–296.

64. **Klich, M. A.** 2002. *Identification of Common* Aspergillus *Species*, 1st ed. Centraalbureau voor Schimmelcultures, Utrecht, The Netherlands.

65. **Klich, M. A., and J. I. Pitt.** 1988. *A Laboratory Guide to Common* Aspergillus *Species and Their Teleomorphs*. Commonwealth Scientific and Industrial Research Organization, North Ryde, Australia.

66. **Klont, R. R., M. A. Mennink-Kersten, and P. E. Verweij.** 2004. Utility of *Aspergillus* antigen detection in specimens other than serum specimens. *Clin. Infect. Dis.* **39**:1467–1474.

67. **Knight, F., and D. W. Mackenzie.** 1992. Aspergillus antigen latex test for diagnosis of invasive aspergillosis. *Lancet* **339**:188.

68. **Kontoyiannis, D. P., R. E. Lewis, G. S. May, N. Osherov, and M. G. Rinaldi.** 2002. *Aspergillus nidulans* is frequently resistant to amphotericin B. *Mycoses* **45**:406–407.

69. **Krasnick, J., R. Patterson, and M. Roberts.** 1995. Allergic bronchopulmonary aspergillosis presenting with cough variant asthma and identifiable source of *Aspergillus fumigatus*. *Ann. Allergy Asthma Immunol.* **75**:344–346.

70. **Kurtz, M. B., I. B. Heath, J. Marrinan, S. Dreikorn, J. Onishi, and C. Douglas.** 1994. Morphological effects of lipopeptides against *Aspergillus fumigatus* correlate with activities against (1,3)-beta-D-glucan synthase. *Antimicrob. Agents Chemother.* **38**:1480–1489.

71. **Kurup, V. P., and A. Kumar.** 1991. Immunodiagnosis of aspergillosis. *Clin. Microbiol. Rev.* **4**:439–456.

72. **Kwon-Chung, K. J., and J. E. Bennett.** 1992. *Medical Mycology.* Lea & Febiger, Philadelphia, PA.

73. **Lasker, B. A., and Y. Ran.** 2004. Analysis of polymorphic microsatellite markers for typing *Penicillium marneffei* isolates. *J. Clin. Microbiol.* **42**:1483–1490.

74. **Lass-Flörl, C., E. Gunsilius, G. Gastl, H. Bonatti, M. C. Freund, A. Gschwendtner, G. Kropshofer, M. P. Dierich, and A. Petzer.** 2004. Diagnosing invasive aspergillosis during antifungal therapy by PCR analysis of blood samples. *J. Clin. Microbiol.* **42**:4154–4157.

75. **Lass-Flörl, C., P. Rath, D. Niederwieser, G. Kofler, R. Würzner, A. Krezy, and M. P. Dierich.** 2000. Aspergillus terreus infections in haematological malignancies: molecular epidemiology suggests association with in-hospital plants. *J. Hosp. Infect.* **46**:31–35.

76. **Latge, J. P.** 1999. *Aspergillus fumigatus* and aspergillosis. *Clin. Microbiol. Rev.* **12**:310–350.

77. **Leenders, A., A. van Belkum, S. Janssen, S. de Marie, J. Kluytmans, J. Wielenga, B. Lowenberg, and H. Verbrugh.** 1996. Molecular epidemiology of apparent outbreak of invasive aspergillosis in a hematology ward. *J. Clin. Microbiol.* **34**:345–351.

78. **Lin, D., P. F. Lehmann, B. H. Hamory, A. A. Padhye, E. Durry, R. W. Pinner, and B. A. Lasker.** 1995. Comparison of three typing methods for clinical and environmental isolates of *Aspergillus fumigatus*. *J. Clin. Microbiol.* **33**:1596–1601.

79. **Lindsley, M. D., D. W. Warnock, and C. J. Morrison.** 2006. Serological and molecular diagnosis of fungal infection, p. 569–605. *In* B. Detrick, R. G. Hamilton, and J. D. Folds (ed.), *Manual of Molecular and Clinical Laboratory Immunology*, 7th ed. ASM Press, Washington, DC.

80. **Lionakis, M. S., and D. P. Kontoyiannis.** 2004. The significance of isolation of saprophytic molds from the lower respiratory tract in patients with cancer. *Cancer* **100**:165–172.

81. **LoBuglio, K. F., and J. W. Taylor.** 1995. Phylogeny and PCR identification of the human pathogenic fungus *Penicillium marneffei*. *J. Clin. Microbiol.* **33**:85–89.

82. **Loeffler, J., K. Kloepfer, H. Hebart, L. Najvar, J. R. Graybill, W. R. Kirkpatrick, T. F. Patterson, R. Dietz, R. Bialek, and H. Einsele.** 2002. Polymerase chain reaction detection of *Aspergillus* DNA in experimental models of invasive aspergillosis. *J. Infect. Dis.* **185**:1203–1206.

83. **Lopez-Martinez, R., L. Neumann, and A. Gonzalez-Mendoza.** 1999. Case report: cutaneous penicilliosis due to *Penicillium chrysogenum*. *Mycoses* **42**:347–349.

84. **Maertens, J., K. Buve, K. Theunissen, W. Meersseman, E. Verbeken, G. Verhoef, J. Van Eldere, and K. Lagrou.** 2009. Galactomannan serves as a surrogate endpoint for outcome of pulmonary invasive aspergillosis in neutropenic hematology patients. *Cancer* **115**:355–362.

85. **Maertens, J., K. Theunissen, G. Verhoef, J. Verschakelen, K. Lagrou, E. Verbeken, A. Wilmer, J. Verhaegen, M. Boogaerts, and J. Van Eldere.** 2005. Galactomannan and computed tomography-based preemptive antifungal therapy in neutropenic patients at high risk for invasive fungal infection: a prospective feasibility study. *Clin. Infect. Dis.* **41**:1242–1250.

86. **Maertens, J., J. Verhaegen, H. Demuynck, P. Brock, G. Verhoef, P. Vandenberghe, J. Van Eldere, L. Verbist, and M. Boogaerts.** 1999. Autopsy-controlled prospective evaluation of serial screening for circulating galactomannan by a sandwich enzyme-linked immunosorbent assay for hematological patients at risk for invasive aspergillosis. *J. Clin. Microbiol.* **37**:3223–3228.

87. **Maertens, J., J. Verhaegen, K. Lagrou, J. Van Eldere, and M. Boogaerts.** 2001. Screening for circulating galactomannan as a noninvasive diagnostic tool for invasive aspergillosis in prolonged neutropenic patients and stem cell transplantation recipients: a prospective validation. *Blood* **97**:1604–1610.

88. **Marques, S. A., A. M. Robles, A. M. Tortorano, M. A. Tuculet, R. Negroni, and R. P. Mendes.** 2000. Mycoses associated with AIDS in the Third World. *Med. Mycol.* **38**(Suppl. 1):269–279.

89. **Marr, K. A., S. A. Balajee, L. McLaughlin, M. Tabouret, C. Bentsen, and T. J. Walsh.** 2004. Detection of galactomannan antigenemia by enzyme immunoassay for the diagnosis of invasive aspergillosis: variables that affect performance. *J. Infect. Dis.* **190**:641–649.

90. **Marr, K. A., M. Laverdiere, A. Gugel, and W. Leisenring.** 2005. Antifungal therapy decreases sensitivity of the Aspergillus galactomannan enzyme immunoassay. *Clin. Infect. Dis.* **40:**1762–1769.

91. **Mellado, E., G. Garcia-Effron, M. J. Buitrago, L. Alcazar-Fuoli, M. Cuenca-Estrella, and J. L. Rodriguez-Tudela.** 2005. Targeted gene disruption of the 14-alpha sterol demethylase (cyp51A) in *Aspergillus fumigatus* and its role in azole drug susceptibility. *Antimicrob. Agents Chemother.* **49:**2536–2538.

92. **Mengoli, C., M. Cruciani, R. A. Barnes, J. Loeffler, and J. P. Donnelly.** 2009. Use of PCR for diagnosis of invasive aspergillosis: systematic review and meta-analysis. *Lancet Infect. Dis.* **9:**89–96.

93. **Mennink-Kersten, M. A., J. P. Donnelly, and P. E. Verweij.** 2004. Detection of circulating galactomannan for the diagnosis and management of invasive aspergillosis. *Lancet Infect. Dis.* **4:**349–357.

94. **Mennink-Kersten, M. A., R. R. Klont, A. Warris, H. J. Op den Camp, and P. E. Verweij.** 2004. Bifidobacterium lipoteichoic acid and false ELISA reactivity in aspergillus antigen detection. *Lancet* **363:**325–327.

95. **Mennink-Kersten, M. A., D. Ruegebrink, R. R. Klont, A. Warris, F. Gavini, H. J. Op den Camp, and P. E. Verweij.** 2005. Bifidobacterial lipoglycan as a new cause for false-positive Platelia *Aspergillus* enzyme-linked immunosorbent assay reactivity. *J. Clin. Microbiol.* **43:**3925–3931.

96. **Messer, S. A., G. J. Moet, J. T. Kirby, and R. N. Jones.** 2009. Activity of contemporary antifungal agents, including the novel echinocandin anidulafungin, tested against *Candida* spp., *Cryptococcus* spp., and *Aspergillus* spp.: report from the SENTRY Antimicrobial Surveillance Program (2006 to 2007). *J. Clin. Microbiol.* **47:**1942–1946.

97. **Miller, W. T.** 1996. Aspergillosis: a disease with many faces. *Semin. Roentgenol.* **31:**52–66.

98. **Moreno, A., M. Perez-Elias, J. Casado, E. Navas, V. Pintado, J. Fortun, C. Quereda, and A. Guerrero.** 2000. Role of antiretroviral therapy in long-term survival of patients with AIDS-related pulmonary aspergillosis. *Eur. J. Clin. Microbiol. Infect. Dis.* **19:**688–693.

99. **Morgan, J., K. A. Wannemuehler, K. A. Marr, S. Hadley, D. P. Kontoyiannis, T. J. Walsh, S. K. Fridkin, P. G. Pappas, and D. W. Warnock.** 2005. Incidence of invasive aspergillosis following hematopoietic stem cell and solid organ transplantation: interim results of a prospective multicenter surveillance program. *Med. Mycol.* **43**(Suppl. 1):S49–S58.

100. **Musher, B., D. Fredricks, W. Leisenring, S. A. Balajee, C. Smith, and K. A. Marr.** 2004. *Aspergillus* galactomannan enzyme immunoassay and quantitative PCR for diagnosis of invasive aspergillosis with bronchoalveolar lavage fluid. *J. Clin. Microbiol.* **42:**5517–5522.

101. **Mylonakis, E., M. Paliou, P. E. Sax, P. R. Skolnik, M. J. Baron, and J. D. Rich.** 2000. Central nervous system aspergillosis in patients with human immunodeficiency virus infection. Report of 6 cases and review. *Medicine* (Baltimore) **79:**269–280.

102. **Nakai, T., J. Uno, F. Ikeda, S. Tawara, K. Nishimura, and M. Miyaji.** 2003. In vitro antifungal activity of micafungin (FK463) against dimorphic fungi: comparison of yeast-like and mycelial forms. *Antimicrob. Agents Chemother.* **47:**1376–1381.

103. **Nakao, A., M. Yasui, T. Kawagoe, H. Tamura, S. Tanaka, and H. Takagi.** 1997. False-positive endotoxemia derives from gauze glucan after hepatectomy for hepatocellular carcinoma with cirrhosis. *Hepatogastroenterology* **44:**1413–1418.

104. **Obayashi, T., M. Yoshida, T. Mori, H. Goto, A. Yasuoka, H. Iwasaki, H. Teshima, S. Kohno, A. Horiuchi, A. Ito, et al.** 1995. Plasma (1→3)-beta-D-glucan measurement in diagnosis of invasive deep mycosis and fungal febrile episodes. *Lancet* **345:**17–20.

105. **Odabasi, Z., V. L. Paetznick, J. R. Rodriguez, E. Chen, and L. Ostrosky-Zeichner.** 2004. In vitro activity of anidulafungin against selected clinically important mold isolates. *Antimicrob. Agents Chemother.* **48:**1912–1915.

106. **Onions, A. H. S., D. Allsopp, and H. O. W. Eggins.** 1981. *Smith's Introduction to Industrial Mycology.* Edward Arnold, London, United Kingdom.

107. **Paterson, P. J., S. Seaton, T. D. McHugh, J. McLaughlin, M. Potter, H. G. Prentice, and C. C. Kibbler.** 2006. Validation and clinical application of molecular methods for the identification of molds in tissue. *Clin. Infect. Dis.* **42:**51–56.

108. **Patterson, T. F.** 2002. New agents for treatment of invasive aspergillosis. *Clin. Infect. Dis.* **35:**367–369.

109. **Patterson, T. F., W. R. Kirkpatrick, M. White, J. W. Hiemenz, J. R. Wingard, B. Dupont, M. G. Rinaldi, D. A. Stevens, and J. R. Graybill.** 2000. Invasive aspergillosis. Disease spectrum, treatment practices, and outcomes. *Medicine* (Baltimore) **79:**250–260.

110. **Pazos, C., J. Ponton, and A. Del Palacio.** 2005. Contribution of (1→3)-beta-D-glucan chromogenic assay to diagnosis and therapeutic monitoring of invasive aspergillosis in neutropenic adult patients: a comparison with serial screening for circulating galactomannan. *J. Clin. Microbiol.* **43:**299–305.

111. **Perfect, J. R., G. M. Cox, J. Y. Lee, C. A. Kauffman, L. de Repentigny, S. W. Chapman, V. A. Morrison, P. Pappas, J. W. Hiemenz, and D. A. Stevens.** 2001. The impact of culture isolation of *Aspergillus* species: a hospital-based survey of aspergillosis. *Clin. Infect. Dis.* **33:**1824–1833.

112. **Peterson, S. W.** 2000. Phylogenetic relationships in *Aspergillus* based upon rDNA sequence analysis, p. 323–355. *In* R. A. Samson and J. I. Pitt (ed.), *Integration of Modern Taxonomic Methods for* Penicillium *and* Aspergillus *Classification.* Harwood Academic Publishers, Amsterdam, The Netherlands.

113. **Pfaller, M. A.** 2000. Antifungal susceptibility testing: progress and future developments. *Braz. J. Infect. Dis.* **4:**55–60.

114. **Pitt, J. I.** 2000. *A Laboratory Guide to Common Penicillium Species,* 3rd ed. Food Science Australia, North Ryde, Australia.

115. **Raper, B. K., and D. I. Fennell.** 1965. *The Genus* Aspergillus. The Williams and Wilkins Company, Baltimore, MD.

116. **Rath, P. M., R. Oeffelke, K. D. Muller, and R. Ansorg.** 1996. Non-value of *Aspergillus* antigen detection in bronchoalveolar lavage fluids of patients undergoing bone marrow transplantation. *Mycoses* **39:**367–370.

117. **Rex, J. H., and M. A. Pfaller.** 2002. Has antifungal susceptibility testing come of age? *Clin. Infect. Dis.* **35:**982–989.

118. **Rex, J. H., M. A. Pfaller, T. J. Walsh, V. Chaturvedi, A. Espinel-Ingroff, M. A. Ghannoum, L. L. Gosey, F. C. Odds, M. G. Rinaldi, D. J. Sheehan, and D. W. Warnock.** 2001. Antifungal susceptibility testing: practical aspects and current challenges. *Clin. Microbiol. Rev.* **14:**643–658.

119. **Rodriguez-Tudela, J. L., L. Alcazar-Fuoli, E. Mellado, A. Alastruey-Izquierdo, A. Monzon, and M. Cuenca-Estrella.** 2008. Epidemiological cutoffs and cross-resistance to azole drugs in *Aspergillus fumigatus. Antimicrob. Agents Chemother.* **52:**2468–2472.

120. **Sambatakou, H., M. Guiver, and D. Denning.** 2003. Pulmonary aspergillosis in a patient with chronic granulomatous disease: confirmation by polymerase chain reaction and serological tests, and successful treatment with voriconazole. *Eur. J. Clin. Microbiol. Infect. Dis.* **22:**681–685.

121. **Samson, R. A., and J. I. Pitt.** 2000. *Integration of Modern Taxonomic Methods for* Penicillium *and* Aspergillus *Classification.* Harwood Scientific Publishers, Amsterdam, The Netherlands.

122. **Samson, R. A., E. S. Hoekstra, J. C. Frisvad, and O. Filtenborg.** 2002. *Introduction to Food and Airborne Fungi,* 6th ed. Centraal Bureau voor Schimmelcultures, Utrecht, The Netherlands.

123. **Sangoi, A. R., W. M. Rogers, T. A. Longacre, J. G. Montoya, E. J. Baron, and N. Banaei.** 2009. Challenges and pitfalls of morphologic identification of fungal infections in histologic and cytologic specimens: a ten-year retrospective review at a single institution. *Am. J. Clin. Pathol.* **131:**364–375.

124. **Schonheyder, H.** 1987. Pathogenetic and serological aspects of pulmonary aspergillosis. *Scand. J. Infect. Dis.* **51**(Suppl.):1–62.

125. **Severens, J. L., J. P. Donnelly, J. F. Meis, P. F. De Vries Robbe, B. E. De Pauw, and P. E. Verweij.** 1997. Two strategies for managing invasive aspergillosis: a decision analysis. *Clin. Infect. Dis.* **25:**1148–1154.

126. **Severo, L. C., G. R. Geyer, N. da Silvo Porto, M. B. Wagner, and A. T. Londero.** 1997. Pulmonary *Aspergillus niger* intracavitary colonization. Report of 23 cases and a review of the literature. *Rev. Iberoam. Micol.* **14:**104–110.

127. **Simoneau, E., M. Kelly, A. C. Labbe, J. Roy, and M. Laverdiere.** 2005. What is the clinical significance of positive blood cultures with Aspergillus sp. in hematopoietic stem cell transplant recipients? A 23 year experience. *Bone Marrow Transplant.* **35:**303–306.

128. **Snelders, E., R. A. Huis In't Veld, A. J. Rijs, G. H. Kema, W. J. Melchers, and P. E. Verweij.** 2009. Possible environmental origin of resistance of *Aspergillus fumigatus* to medical triazoles. *Appl. Environ. Microbiol.* **75:**4053–4057.

129. **Soll, D. R.** 2000. The ins and outs of DNA fingerprinting the infectious fungi. *Clin. Microbiol. Rev.* **13:**332–370.

130. **Spreadbury, C. L., B. W. Bainbridge, and J. Cohen.** 1990. Restriction fragment length polymorphisms in isolates of *Aspergillus fumigatus* probed with part of the intergenic spacer region from the ribosomal RNA gene complex of *Aspergillus nidulans.* *J. Gen. Microbiol.* **136:**1991–1994.

131. **Sulahian, A., F. Boutboul, P. Ribaud, T. Leblanc, C. Lacroix, and F. Derouin.** 2001. Value of antigen detection using an enzyme immunoassay in the diagnosis and prediction of invasive aspergillosis in two adult and pediatric hematology units during a 4-year prospective study. *Cancer* **91:**311–318.

132. **Summerbell, R. C.** 2003. *Aspergillus, Fusarium, Sporothrix, Piedraia,* and their relatives, p. 237–498. *In* D. H. Howard (ed.), *Pathogenic Fungi in Humans and Animals.* Marcel Dekker, Inc., New York, NY.

133. Reference deleted.

134. **Supparatpinyo, K., K. E. Nelson, W. G. Merz, B. J. Breslin, C. R. Cooper, Jr., C. Kamwan, and T. Sirisanthana.** 1993. Response to antifungal therapy by human immunodeficiency virus-infected patients with disseminated *Penicillium marneffei* infections and in vitro susceptibilities of isolates from clinical specimens. *Antimicrob. Agents Chemother.* **37:**2407–2411.

135. **Tomee, J. F., G. P. Mannes, W. van der Bij, T. S. van der Werf, W. J. de Boer, G. H. Koeter, and H. F. Kauffman.** 1996. Serodiagnosis and monitoring of *Aspergillus* infections after lung transplantation. *Ann. Intern. Med.* **125:**197–201.

136. **Vanittanakom, N., C. R. Cooper, Jr., M. C. Fisher, and T. Sirisanthana.** 2006. *Penicillium marneffei* infection and recent advances in the epidemiology and molecular biology aspects. *Clin. Microbiol. Rev.* **19:**95–110.

137. **Verweij, P. E., K. Brinkman, H. P. Kremer, B. J. Kullberg, and J. F. Meis.** 1999. *Aspergillus* meningitis: diagnosis by non-culture-based microbiological methods and management. *J. Clin. Microbiol.* **37:**1186–1189.

138. **Verweij, P. E., E. C. Dompeling, J. P. Donnelly, A. V. Schattenberg, and J. F. Meis.** 1997. Serial monitoring of *Aspergillus* antigen in the early diagnosis of invasive aspergillosis. Preliminary investigations with two examples. *Infection* **25:**86–89.

139. **Verweij, P. E., A. J. Rijs, B. E. De Pauw, A. M. Horrevorts, J. A. Hoogkamp-Korstanje, and J. F. Meis.** 1995. Clinical evaluation and reproducibility of the Pastorex *Aspergillus* antigen latex agglutination test for diagnosing invasive aspergillosis. *J. Clin. Pathol.* **48:**474–476.

140. **Verweij, P. E., D. Stynen, A. J. Rijs, B. E. de Pauw, J. A. Hoogkamp-Korstanje, and J. F. Meis.** 1995. Sandwich enzyme-linked immunosorbent assay compared with Pastorex latex agglutination test for diagnosing invasive aspergillosis in immunocompromised patients. *J. Clin. Microbiol.* **33:**1912–1914.

141. **Vinh, D. C., Y. R. Shea, J. A. Sugui, E. R. Parrilla-Castellar, A. F. Freeman, J. W. Campbell, S. Pittaluga, P. A. Jones, A. Zelazny, D. Kleiner, K. J. Kwon-Chung, and S. M. Holland.** 2009. Invasive aspergillosis due to *Neosartorya udagawae. Clin. Infect. Dis.* **49:**102–111.

142. **Walsh, T. J., E. J. Anaissie, D. W. Denning, R. Herbrecht, D. P. Kontoyiannis, K. A. Marr, V. A. Morrison, B. H. Segal, W. J. Steinbach, D. A. Stevens, J. A. van Burik, J. R. Wingard, and T. F. Patterson.** 2008. Treatment of aspergillosis: clinical practice guidelines of the Infectious Diseases Society of America. *Clin. Infect. Dis.* **46:**327–360.

143. **Walsh, T. J., V. Petraitis, R. Petraitiene, A. Field-Ridley, D. Sutton, M. Ghannoum, T. Sein, R. Schaufele, J. Peter, J. Bacher, H. Casler, D. Armstrong, A. Espinel-Ingroff, M. G. Rinaldi, and C. A. Lyman.** 2003. Experimental pulmonary aspergillosis due to *Aspergillus terreus:* pathogenesis and treatment of an emerging fungal pathogen resistant to amphotericin B. *J. Infect. Dis.* **188:**305–319.

144. **Walsh, T. J., S. Shoham, R. Petraitiene, T. Sein, R. Schaufele, A. Kelaher, H. Murray, C. Mya-San, J. Bacher, and V. Petraitis.** 2004. Detection of galactomannan antigenemia in patients receiving piperacillin-tazobactam and correlations between in vitro, in vivo, and clinical properties of the drug-antigen interaction. *J. Clin. Microbiol.* **42:**4744–4748.

145. **Warris, A., P. Gaustad, J. F. Meis, A. Voss, P. E. Verweij, and T. G. Abrahamsen.** 2001. Recovery of filamentous fungi from water in a paediatric bone marrow transplantation unit. *J. Hosp. Infect.* **47:**143–148.

146. **Warris, A., C. H. Klaassen, J. F. Meis, M. T. De Ruiter, H. A. De Valk, T. G. Abrahamsen, P. Gaustad, and P. E. Verweij.** 2003. Molecular epidemiology of *Aspergillus fumigatus* isolates recovered from water, air, and patients shows two clusters of genetically distinct strains. *J. Clin. Microbiol.* **41:**4101–4106.

147. **Warris, A., C. M. Weemaes, and P. E. Verweij.** 2002. Multidrug resistance in *Aspergillus fumigatus. N. Engl. J. Med.* **347:**2173–2174.

148. **Weber, D. J., A. Peppercorn, M. B. Miller, E. Sickbert-Benett, and W. A. Rutala.** 2009. Preventing healthcare-associated *Aspergillus* infections: review of recent CDC/HICPAC recommendations. *Med. Mycol.* **47**(Suppl. 1):S199–S209.

149. **Weig, M., M. Frosch, K. Tintelnot, A. Haas, U. Gross, B. Linsmeier, and J. Heesemann.** 2001. Use of recombinant mitogillin for improved serodiagnosis of *Aspergillus fumigatus*-associated diseases. *J. Clin. Microbiol.* **39:**1721–1730.

150. **Woitas, R. P., J. K. Rockstroh, A. Theisen, C. Leutner, T. Sauerbruch, and U. Spengler.** 1998. Changing role of invasive aspergillosis in AIDS—a case control study. *J. Infect.* **37:**116–122.

151. **Yamakami, Y., A. Hashimoto, I. Tokimatsu, and M. Nasu.** 1996. PCR detection of DNA specific for *Aspergillus* species in serum of patients with invasive aspergillosis. *J. Clin. Microbiol.* **34:**2464–2468.

Fusarium and Other Opportunistic Hyaline Fungi

DEANNA A. SUTTON AND MARY E. BRANDT

118

The opportunistic hyaline or lightly colored (also referred to as moniliaceous) moulds constitute a phylogenetically diverse group of common to rare anamorphic (asexual) and teleomorphic (sexual) fungi that typically occur as saprobes in soil, in air, or on plant litter or as facultative plant pathogens. Some may be recovered from specimens without having any clinical significance. Others are isolated infrequently enough to challenge the diagnostic proficiency of the laboratory, and critical assessment is required to evaluate the significance of their recovery. While several of the genera treated in this chapter include species having either lightly colored or dark (melanized) conidia, the emphasis is on those fungi that grow in tissue in the form of hyaline or lightly colored, septate hyphal elements.

The term fusariosis is used to define infections caused by species of *Fusarium* (135) (Table 1), but the practice of coining disease names based on the genus of fungus involved is disadvantageous for infections caused by uncommon or rare fungal pathogens. The wide variety of fungi involved makes it difficult to place the organisms into accessible groups, and problems arise when fungus names are changed. To avoid unnecessary name changes for disease names based on the genus of the fungus involved, two major disease groups have been proposed: hyalohyphomycosis and phaeohyphomycosis (5). Although the groups were defined as encompassing similar clinical spectra, they were distinguished by the presence in tissue of septate hyphal filaments without (hyalohyphomycosis) or with (phaeohyphomycosis) pigmentation or melanin in the cell wall. However, some fungi, such as *Scedosporium* species or *Neoscytalidium dimidiatum* (formerly *Scytalidium dimidiatum* [*Nattrassia mangiferae*]) (219), which form darkly pigmented colonies and conidia in vitro, produce hyaline or lightly pigmented hyphae in tissue. The Masson-Fontana silver stain helps to detect melanin pigmentation of fungal elements in tissue, but the results are not always decisive (see also the discussion in chapter 113). Some fungi with variable pigmentation may stain faintly or inconsistently. In practice, the terms for the disease categories have been used to designate infections caused by fungi that are either hyaline or pigmented (melanized, phaeoid, or dematiaceous) in vitro. Although it may be useful to have terms for broad categories of mycotic diseases, there are problems in categorizing fungi by color. A subcommittee of the International Society for Human and Animal Mycology has suggested that fungal diseases be named by providing a specific description of the pathology and naming the causative agent, e.g., subcutaneous cyst caused by fungus X (144, 201).

TAXONOMY AND IDENTIFICATION

The opportunistic hyaline moulds belong to several genera. Most display no teleomorph (meiotic or sexual stage) and comprise genera which are either anamorphs (mitotic or asexual stages) of the Ascomycota and Basidiomycota or genera for which no sexual state has been described (see chapter 111). Today the relationships between many anamorphs and their sexual relatives are known through discovery of teleomorphs or are inferred by comparison of nucleic acids. This knowledge is extremely important in understanding fungal relationships and has allowed for the placement of asexual fungi next to their sexual relatives in fungal phylogenetic trees. Rapid developments in this area have led to significant changes in generic and species concepts, particularly among the fusaria (134, 145–151, 210, 211, 237). Teleomorphs may develop in culture from homothallic species (see chapter 111); however, they may be difficult to obtain without the use of specialized media and extended incubation. In this chapter, the name of the teleomorph is used for species that are identified mainly by their sexual structures.

Most of the pathogenic moulds considered in this chapter are classified in the form-class Hyphomycetes (genera which bear their conidia free) (78, 103). Phenotypic identification of Hyphomycetes is based on morphology of the conidia and the mechanisms by which conidia are formed (conidiogenesis; see chapter 111). Three basic tools are necessary for practical observation of these features. (i) An ocular micrometer is essential for determining sizes of conidia or sexual spores when present. Identification of moulds often requires comparison with published taxonomic descriptions, in which size is often a key criterion for species distinction. (ii) A dissecting microscope with magnification of up to ×60 and basal illumination is useful for the examination of colonies in plates or tubes for the presence of conidia in chains or slimy heads; specialized structures such as Hülle cells, sclerotia, or conidiomata; or sexual fruiting bodies forming under the aerial mycelium or embedded in the agar. (iii) Microscopic mounts which allow observation of how a fungus forms its conidia also are necessary. Slide culture preparations are excellent for many fungi and generally necessary for those with small, delicate conidia (94, 215); however, rapidly

TABLE 1 Classification of *Fusarium* infections[a]

I. Healthy host
  A. Keratitis
    1. Trauma and penetration of cornea
    2. Contamination of soft contact lenses, solutions, or cases
    3. Local immunosuppression by corticosteroid drops
  B. Onychomycosis[b]
    1. Distal subungual lesion in toenails in females
    2. Lateral subungual onychomycosis
    3. Proximal subungual onychomycosis
    4. Paronychia-like reaction in proximal nail fold
  C. Intertrigo[b]
  D. Tinea pedis[b] (interdigital infection)
  E. Hyperkeratotic plantar lesions[b]
  F. Skin infections[b]
  G. Surgical wound infections
  H. Burns
  I. Ulcers
  J. Otitis media
  K. Peritonitis (CAPD[c])
  L. Catheter-associated fungemia
  M. Fungemia with or without organ involvement
  N. Pneumonia
  O. Sinusitis
  P. Septic arthritis
  Q. Thrombophlebitis
  R. Endophthalmitis
  S. Osteomyelitis
II. Immunocompromised host
  A. Endophthalmitis
  B. Sinusitis
  C. Pneumonia
  D. Skin involvement
  E. Fungemia
  F. Disseminated infection
  G. Brain abscess
  H. Peritonitis

[a]Adapted from references 83, 133, 137, and 139. Patients infected with other fungi discussed in this chapter may present with similar clinical syndromes, and fungal structures in tissue may resemble those of *Aspergillus* species.
[b]Patients from whom a dermatophyte has not been isolated.
[c]CAPD, continuous ambulatory peritoneal dialysis.

growing species such as those in the genus *Trichoderma* should be harvested early or examined by tease mounts. Morphological features of importance for identification of conidial fungi include (i) conidium size, shape, and pattern of septation; (ii) color of conidia and conidiophore, whether light (hyaline) or dark (melanized or phaeoid); (iii) developmental aspects of conidiogenesis, including the nature of the conidiogenous cell; (iv) mechanism of conidium liberation or dehiscence; and (v) structure of the conidioma (if present). Differences in conidial shape and septation are useful characters for preliminary distinction and have traditionally been used for grouping conidial fungi (known as Saccardo spore groups). Conidia may be nonseptate or may have one or more septa (amerosporae, didymosporae, and phragmosporae, respectively). Some fungi produce both nonseptate and septate conidia, and these conidia are often referred to as micro- and macroconidia. Conidia also vary in shape. Some are long and narrow (scolecosporae), as in *Fusarium* species. Development of a conidium may occur by conversion of an existing cell or several cells (thallicarthric or arthrosporic) or may involve new wall building or blowing out of a portion of the wall (blastic). Conidiogenesis usually occurs at a

particular location on a conidiogenous cell. If development occurs at a site that remains fixed and gives rise to more than one conidium, then the site is stable or determinate. If development occurs at new points on the conidiogenous cell (or axis), then the site is unstable or indeterminate. New sites may occur on an axis which lengthens (progressive) or shortens (retrogressive). The conidiogenous cell produces a single conidium or multiple conidia. Sympodial development involves the development of a single conidium at successive sites on a lengthening axis. Conidiogenous cells which are specialized to produce multiple conidia include the phialide and annellide. Conidia are produced successively (serially) and develop in slimy masses or in chains, with the youngest at the base of the chain (basipetal). Although it is sometimes difficult to differentiate between the two types of cells, the annellide elongates and sometimes narrows during the formation of each new conidium, leaving an often imperceptible series of rings or scars on the conidiogenous cell. Scrutiny of the cell by use of an oil immersion objective may be necessary to make this distinction. Holoblastic conidiogenesis, in which both inner and outer cell walls are involved, usually results in the formation of acropetal chains, with the youngest conidium at the tip of the chain. The distinction between acropetal and basipetal chains may be revealed by comparison of the size and wall morphologies of the top and bottom conidia of the chain. The youngest conidium is recognizable by its smaller size, its lighter color if the conidia are pigmented, and differences in wall ornamentation if the conidia are roughened. Some conidiogenous cells form multiple conidia simultaneously over the surface of the swollen cell. When mature, conidia detach by fission of a double septum (schizolytic dehiscence) or by sacrifice of a supporting cell (rhexolytic dehiscence), either by fracture of a thin-walled region or by lysis of the supporting cell. Lytic dehiscence typically occurs in the dermatophytes and related fungi.

The presence of different spore states can make identification difficult. Careful examination and sometimes subculture are required to assess whether the spore types represent different states of the same fungus or whether the isolate is contaminated. Moulds having more than one independent stage are called pleomorphic (occasionally polymorphic) fungi. Other conidial forms of the same fungus are called synanamorphs. These may be represented by simple yeast stages or by the formation of complex conidiomatal structures such as sporodochia (conidiophores borne crowded on a compact mass of hyphae or a hyphal stroma), synnemata (conidiophores aggregated into a compound stalk), or pycnidia (conidiogenous cells formed inside a round or oval fruiting body). Expression of a synanamorph may be influenced by the agar medium used and may be lost upon repeated subculture.

The number of hyaline fungal species that have been reported to cause opportunistic infection in humans and animals is increasing, and it is beyond the scope of this chapter to describe them all. Some reports identify the fungus only to the genus level, while others provide the fungus name but without salient details of its colonial and microscopic features. A continuing and vexing problem is that verification of authenticity of reports cannot be done if the fungus is inadequately described and illustrated and if case isolates are not sent for deposit in culture collections. This chapter describes the salient colonial and microscopic features of the medically important species in the genus *Fusarium* (Table 2) and other selected currently recognized hyaline opportunists (Table 3). Detailed descriptions of species listed are found in several reference manuals (47, 48, 52, 53, 57, 94, 187, 194, 195, 207, 210, 215, 225) as well as the current literature.

TABLE 2 Key phenotypic features of clinically significant *Fusarium* species[a]

Complex	Colonial form	Sporodochia[b]	Conidiogenous	Macroconidia[c]	Microconidia	Chlamydospores
FSSC						
F. solani (Fig. 1A)	Mostly cream, occasionally slightly blue-green, reddish, or lavender; floccose; rapid growth	Cream in confluent pionnotes	Long monophialides	Multiseptate, abundant, stout, thick walled; dorsal and ventral surfaces only almost parallel	Abundant, mostly 0-1 septate; oval to kidney shaped in false heads	Present, single and pairs
F. falciforme (formerly Acremonium falciforme)	Cream to pale brown, glabrous to velvety; slow growth; lavender reverse on SDA[d]	Seldom seen on on PDA	Long monophialides	Poor conidial production; mostly lack foot cells	One to three celled	Present, often pale brown
F. lichenicola (formerly Cylindrocarpon lichenicola)	Initially white, then pale yellow to light brown; floccose; rapid growth	Seldom seen	Long monophialides	Straight, multiseptate, rounded at apices, truncate basal cells	Absent	Short chains and clusters, brown, rough
Neocosmospora vasinfecta[e]	Flat, thin, almost transparent, becoming punctate with production of orange to pale brown perithecia	Absent	Long monophialides	Absent on PDA	Similar to those seen in F. solani	As in F. solani
FOSC						
F. oxysporum (Fig. 1B)	White to lavender, salmon tinge, lavender reverse; floccose; rapid growth	Orange, erumpent	Short monophialides	Multiseptate, slightly sickle shaped, thin walled, delicate	Mostly 0-septate, oval to kidney shaped, in false heads only	Present, abundant, single and pairs
GFSC						
F. verticillioides (formerly F. moniliforme) (Fig. 1C)	White to lavender with lavender reverse; floccose; rapid growth	Usually absent on PDA, tan to orange on CLA	Medium-length monophialides	Multiseptate, almost straight	0-1 septate, oval to clavate, truncate, occur in false heads and chains	Absent
F. thapsinum	Morphologically indistinguishable from F. verticillioides except for yellow diffusing pigment on PDA, although not produced by all strains	Same as for F. verticillioides	Same as for F. verticillioides	Same as for F. verticillioides	Same as for F. verticillioides	Same as for F. verticillioides
F. napiforme	White to lavender, lavender reverse	Usually absent on PDA; tan on CLA	Medium-length monophialides	Multiseptate, falcate to almost straight	0-1 septate, ovoid to pyriform (pear shaped) to napiform (beet shaped) in false heads and short chains	Sparse, short chains or clusters

(Continued on next page)

TABLE 2 Key phenotypic features of clinically significant *Fusarium* species[a] (*Continued*)

Complex	Colonial form	Sporodochia[b]	Conidiogenous	Macroconidia[c]	Microconidia	Chlamydospores
F. proliferatum (Fig. 1D)	White to lavender, lavender reverse; floccose; rapid growth	May be absent on PDA; tan on CLA	Monophialides and polyphialides	Multiseptate, falcate to almost straight	Oval to pyriform, truncate; occur in false heads	Absent
F. nygamai	White to lavender, lavender reverse; floccose; rapid growth; orange to violet spore mass common centrally	Orange on CLA	Monophialides and polyphialides; however, polyphialide production variable	Multiseptate, falcate to almost straight, thin walled	Oval to clavate, mostly 0-septate, in false heads and short chains (to 20 conidia in length)	Few to abundant, single, chains, clusters; smooth or rough, hyaline to yellow
FCSC						
F. chlamydosporum	White to pink to carmine, brown centrally with production of chlamydospores; floccose; rapid growth	Uncommon on PDA; tan to orange on CLA	Short monophialides and short polyphialides, often with three openings	Rare except on sporodochia	0-2 septate, fusiform, apiculate; may be slow to form in some strains on PDA	Abundant, brown, rough, in chains and clusters
FDSC						
F. dimerum (Fig. 1E)	Slimy, yeastlike due to conidial masses; aerial mycelium sparse to absent; salmon to light orange, reverse same or pale yellow; slow growth	Orange, well developed on CLA	Monophialides; conidiation on agar surface from lateral phialidic pegs	Abundant; 0-1 septate with septum in middle; curved	Ellipsoidal to ovoidal to curved, mostly one celled	Derived from macroconidia; hyphal chlamydospores rare or absent
F. delphinoides (Fig. 1F)	Similar to *F. dimerum* except for reverse, which may be speckled with red-brown clumps of pigment	Same as for *F. dimerum*	Same as for *F. dimerum*	Can be 2-septate; when 1-septate, septum is off-center	Same as for *F. dimerum*	Same as for *F. dimerum*
FIESC						
F. incarnatum[f]	Buff to light brown, reverse salmon; floc-cose; rapid growth	Orange, produced by some strains on CLA	Monophialides and polyphialides	Those produced in aerial mycelium almost straight; those produced in pionnotes[g] or sporodochia curved	0-septate, sparse or absent	Sparse, intercalary, single or chains

[a]On potato dextrose agar (PDA) after 4 days incubation at 25°C unless otherwise noted. See references cited in the text for a more detailed description of the features noted in this table. List is not all-inclusive.

[b]Cushion-shaped mats of hyphae, conidiophores, and macroconidia.

[c]Most characteristic macroconidia for all species are those formed in sporodochia on carnation leaf agar (CLA); macroconidia, also formed in aerial mycelium on PDA, are often smaller.

[d]SDA, Sabouraud dextrose agar.

[e]Ascomata perithecial, walls of textura angularis type, asci cylindrical, eight spored (30 to 100 by 11 to 15 μm); ascospores one celled, thick walled, roughened, yellow to brown, globose to ellipsoidal (10 to 15 by 7 to 12 μm).

[f]Taxonomy in state of flux; *F. incarnatum* and *F. pallidoroseum* may be separate species.

[g]A flat mass of macroconidia having a greasy or fatty appearance.

TABLE 3 Key phenotypic features of selected hyaline moulds[a]

Genus	Key features	Etiologic agent(s)	Comments
Homothallic ascomycetes[b]			
Achaetomium (Fig. 1G)	Colonies fast growing, white to yellowish with pink diffusible pigment. Conidia formed from minute phialides. Ascomata perithecia bearing thin-walled setae. Ascospores brown, smooth, fusoidal.	A. strumarium	Growth at 42°C, neurotropic; compare with Chaetomium. See also chapter 122.
Aphanoascus	Colonies moderately fast growing, yellowish white, granular; cycloheximide tolerant. Cleistothecia globose, containing roughened ascospores; associated with a Chrysosporium anamorph consisting of terminal one-celled sessile conidia and alternate arthroconidia.	A. fulvescens	Compare with Chrysosporium and dermatophytes
Cephalotheca (Fig. 2D and E)	Colonies moderately fast growing, velvety to lanose, orange-gray with light brown reverse. A homothallic ascomycete forming black, superficial, ciliated cleistothecia and small, brown, kidney-shaped, foveolate (delicately pitted) ascospores; associated with a Phialemonium-like anamorph.	C. foveolata	UV light and extended incubation enhance production of ascomata
Chaetomium	Colonies fast growing, yellowish green to gray. Anamorph absent or conidia formed from phialides. Ascomata perithecia bearing coiled, straight, branched brown or indistinct setae. Ascospores lemon shaped, brown, smooth.	C. atrobrunneum C. globosum C. perlucidum	C. atrobrunneum and C. perlucidum grow at 42°C and are neurotropic. See also chapter 122.
Gymnascella (Fig. 1H and 2A and B)	Colonies yellowish white, becoming bright yellow or yellowish green or orange. Ascospores borne in naked clusters, smooth, pale yellow. Anamorph absent. Ascospores of G. hyalinospora are oblate and yellowish; those of G. dankaliensis are reddish orange and ornamented with a thickened polar band and minute thickenings on the sides.	G. hyalinospora G. dankaliensis	G. hyalinospora also known as Narasimhella hyalinospora; may give positive results for B. dermatitidis with GenProbe DNA probe
Microascus (Fig. 2C)	Colonies moderately fast growing, hyaline, or gray-brown to black. Ascomata perithecia with necks, containing yellowish to reddish orange (straw-colored) ascospores extruded in cirri; associated with a hyaline or phaeoid Scopulariopsis anamorph.	M. cirrosus M. cinereus M. trigonosporus M. manginii	Ascospore shapes for the first three species listed which are dark are heart shaped, wedge shaped, and triangular, respectively
Thermoascus	Colonies yellow-orange to reddish orange, woolly to granular. Thermophilic with growth to 50°C. Ascomata non-ostiolate; ascospores pale yellow, elliptical, thick walled, rough. Paecilomyces anamorphs, P. crustaceous and P. taitungiacus, have conidia that are initially rectangular, becoming elliptical to subglobose.	T. crustaceus T. taitungiacus	T. taitungiacus fails to grow at 20°C and has irregularly verrucose ascospores. T. crustaceus has finely echinulate ascospores.
Filamentous basidiomycetes			
Inonotus (Fig. 3A)	Colonies fast growing, woolly, yellowish-orange; cycloheximide and benomyl resistant. Thick-walled setal hyphae and hyphal swellings present; conidia absent. Confirm with sequencing.	I. tropicalis	Syn. Phellinus tropicalis; wood-destroying poroid basidiomycete
Hormographiella	Colonies fast growing, white, amber to tan, woolly; cycloheximide sensitive, benomyl resistant. Conidiophores short, bearing short fertile branches. Arthroconidia schizolytic, thin walled, single celled, often adherent around the conidiophores. Sclerotia sometimes present. Basidiomycete anamorph.	H. aspergillata (anamorph of Coprinus cinereus) H. verticillata	Differs from A. kalrae by cycloheximide sensitivity, fast growth
Oxyporus	Colonies moderately fast growing at 35°C but with poor growth at 25°C; white and woolly. Conidia absent. Confirm with sequencing.	O. corticola	White-rot decay fungus of woody angiosperms and gymnosperms

(Continued on next page)

TABLE 3 Key phenotypic features of selected hyaline moulds[a] (Continued)

Genus	Key features	Etiologic agent(s)	Comments
Schizophyllum (Fig. 2F to H)	Colonies fast growing, growth enhanced at 37°C. White, woolly or cottony, cycloheximide sensitive. Conidia absent. Hyphae bearing clamp connections and short, thin pegs or spicules, but both may be absent. Clamped isolates usually develop fan shaped, gilled basidiocarps (mushrooms) on sporulation media after 3–6 wks.	*S. commune*	Clinical picture resembles aspergillosis, and clampless isolates resemble aspergilli by histopathology
Sporotrichum	Colonies fast growing, white to buff to beige, woolly. Conidiophores with profuse branching, each branch terminating with a conidium. Conidia ellipsoidal, truncate, thick walled, smooth. Large (20- to 60-μm) globose chlamydospores and arthroconidia also present. Basidiomycete anamorph.	*S. pruinosum* (anamorph of *Phanerchaete chrysosporium*)	Large globose chlamydospores similar to those produced by *Emmonsia parva* can be seen in sputum
Quambalaria	Colonies moderately fast growing, white to lavender red diffusible pigment often present; cycloheximide sensitive. Conidiophores solitary, forming conidia sympodially on small denticles on sides or at tips. Primary conidia bear one to three secondary conidia.	*Q. cyanescens*	Synonyms include *Fugomyces cyanescens*, *Sporothrix cyanescens*, and *Cerinosterus cyanescens*
Hyphomycetes *Acremonium*	Colonies slow growing (usually <3 cm in 10 days), often white, cottony, fasciculate (spiky), glabrous or moist and pink or salmon colored. Conidiogenous cells solitary, slender (ca. 2 μm wide), mostly unbranched, awl (needle)-shaped phialides. Conidia one celled, straight or curved, in slimy masses.	*A. alabamense* *A. kiliense* *A. potronii* *A. recifei* *A. curvulum* *A. strictum* *Acremonium* spp.	Differs from *Fusarium* by low growth rate, narrower hyphae (mostly <2 μm wide), and more slender and needle-like phialides. Compare with *Lecythophora* and *Phialemonium*.
Acrophialophora	Colonies fast growing, white, darkening to grayish brown centrally. Conidiophores brown, long, seta-like, echinulate. Conidiogenous cells, flask-shaped phialides borne near the tip of conidiophores or on vegetative hyphae. Conidia in long chains, one celled, lemon shaped, smooth or rough; distinct spiral bands may be visible.	*A. fusispora*	Growth at 40°C. Potentially neurotropic species. Compare with *Paecilomyces* spp., *Scedosporium prolificans*, and *Phialosimplex*.
Arthrographis	Colonies slow growing, growth enhanced at 37°C, initially white and yeastlike, becoming hyphal and buff, with a yellow reverse. Cycloheximide tolerant. Conidiophores dendritic (tree-like), bearing lateral branches. Arthroconidia formed by fragmentation of branches or from undifferentiated hyphae.	*A. kalrae*	Compare with *Onychocola* and *Hormographiella*
Beauveria	Colonies slow to moderately fast growing, yellowish white. Conidiogenous cells solitary, in whorls, or in sporodochia, basally swollen, proliferating sympodially at the tip in a zigzag (geniculate) fashion. Conidia one celled, subglobose.	*B. bassiana*	Compare with *Engyodontium album* and *Sporothrix*. Biological control agent for insects.
Chrysosporium (Fig. 3B and C)	Colonies slow to moderately fast growing, yellowish white. Conidia single celled, smooth to roughened; aleurioconidia formed sessile or at the ends or on the sides of unswollen stalks. Arthroconidia sometimes present. (See *Aphanoascus* and *Emmonsia*.)	*C. zonatum* *C. ophiodiicola* (anamorph of *Nannizziopsis vriesii*)	Reports of infection by unnamed species are difficult to evaluate because isolates are not adequately described to confirm etiology
Cylindrocarpon	Colonies fast growing; felty or cottony; yellowish white, tan, orange, or purple (sometimes diffusing pigments). Conidiogenous cells, awl-shaped phialides with a single opening, solitary, in branched structures or in sporodochia (conidiophores borne crowded in a compact mass of hyphae). Macroconidia straight or slightly curved with rounded ends, multicelled; microconidia not clearly distinguished from macroconidia. Chlamydospores sometimes present.	*C. destructans* *C. cyanescens*	Distinguished from *Fusarium* by rounded apical cells and absence of foot cells

(Continued on next page)

TABLE 3 (Continued)

Genus	Key features	Etiologic agent(s)	Comments
Engyodontium	Colonies slow to moderately fast growing, yellowish white. Conidiogenous cells solitary or borne in whorls, basally swollen, tapering at the tip and proliferating sympodially in a zigzag (geniculate) fashion. Conidia one celled, subglobose.	*E. album*	Compare with *Beauveria*
Geosmithia (Fig. 3D)	Colonies moderately fast growing with enhanced growth at 35°C. Cream to buff colored. Stipes and metulae rough. Cuneiform (wedge-shaped) to ellipsoidal conidia borne from rough-walled phialides lacking narrow necks as in *Penicillium* or *Paecilomyces*.	*G. argillacea* (anamorph of *Talaromyces eburneus*)	Syn. *Penicillium argillaceum*. Compare conidia with those of *P. crustaceus*.
Lecythophora	Colonies white to salmon, moist or fasciculate (spiky), or tan, darkening to black in patches. Conidiogenous cells, adelophialides (short, stumpy phialides without a basal septum), as well as awl-shaped phialides. *L. mutabilis* forms brown chlamydospores, while *L. hoffmannii* does not.	*L. hoffmannii* *L. mutabilis*	Differs from *Acremonium* by predominance of adelophialides. Hyphal elements usually reported as hyaline. See also chapter 122.
Metarhizium	Colonies moderately fast growing, becoming olivaceous green or buff. Conidiogenous cells, cylindrical phialides borne on verticillately or irregularly branched conidiophores formed on sporodochia. Conidia cylindrical, smooth, yellowish green, forming in adherent columns. Irregularly shaped appressoria may be present.	*M. anisopliae*	Biological control agent for insects
Myceliophthora (Fig. 3E)	Colonies fast growing, thermophilic (up to 50°C); cinnamon brown. One to three conidia formed on small denticles borne on the sides or at the ends of short, swollen stalks. Conidia initially smooth and hyaline; brown and rough at maturity.	*M. thermophila*	Differs from *Chrysosporium* by swollen stalks
Myriodontium	Colonies moderately fast growing, yellowish white, often zonate, powdery. Conidia formed at the ends of narrow stalks borne at right angles to the fertile hyphae.	*M. keratinophilum*	Differs from *Chrysosporium* by stalks borne at right angles
Onychocola (Fig. 3F and G)	Colonies restricted, raised, yellowish white to grayish white, cycloheximide tolerant. One- or two-celled cylindrical or swollen arthroconidia forming in adherent chains, detaching by schizolysis or lysis of thin-walled cells. Brown knobby setae often present.	*O. canadensis*	Differs from *Neoscytalidium dimidiatum* (see chapter 122) and *Hormographiella* by adherent chains, slow growth, and cycloheximide tolerance
Paecilomyces (Fig. 3H and 4A and B)	About 40 species grouped into two sections. Section *Paecilomyces* includes the thermotolerant *P. variotii* and anamorphs of *Byssochlamys* and *Thermoascus* with fast growing yellowish brown, buff, or orange colonies. Section *Isarioidea* includes *P. lilacinus* and species that are mostly reddish gray or violet. Conidiogenous cells, phialides formed on verticillately branched condiophores. Conidia single celled, in chains.	*P. variotii* *P. lilacinus* *P. javanicus* *P. fumosoroseus*	See *Thermoascus* for additional anamorphic species
Phialemonium (Fig. 4C)	Colonies slow growing, white to grayish or yellowish. Conidiogenous cells, adelophialides (short, stumpy phialides without a basal septum), as well as awl-shaped phialides. *P. ovobatum* produces a green diffusible pigment; *P. curvatum* may produce sporodochia.	*P. obovatum* *P. curvatum* (syn. *P. chlamydosporum*)	Compare with *Acremonium* and *Lecythophora*. Also see chapter 122.
Phialosimplex gen. nov. (Fig. 4D and E)	Colonies are moderately fast growing, pale, white, cream to yellowish white, sometimes fasciculate centrally with occasional sectoring. Some species produce diffusible yellow pigment. Inhibited by cycloheximide. Conidiogenous cells, mostly monophialides, narrow, swollen at base. Conidia borne in long chains or heads, hyaline, subglobose, pyriform, obovoid or ovoid, truncate. Chlamydospores and sclerotia present or absent.	*P. caninus* *P. chlamydosporus* (syn. *Sagenomella chlamydospora*) *P. sclerotialis*	Compare with *Acrophialophora fusispora*

(Continued on next page)

TABLE 3 Key phenotypic features of selected hyaline moulds[a] (Continued)

Genus	Key features	Etiologic agent(s)	Comments
Scopulariopsis (Fig. 4F)	Colonies white, buff, gray-brown to black. Conidiogenous cells, annellides formed on branched conidiophores with one or two levels of branching. Conidia one celled, globose, or ellipsoidal, in chains. *S. brevicaulis* has buff or tan granular colonies, thick-walled smooth to coarsely roughened conidia that are truncate at the base and rounded or pointed at the tip. *S. candida* has white colonies and smooth conidia.	*S. brevicaulis* *S. candida* *S. acremonium*	See also *Microascus* and chapter 122 for phaeoid species
Trichoderma (Fig. 4G and H)	Colonies fast growing, cottony or woolly, white becoming yellowish green to dark green, sometimes with a yellow diffusing pigment. Conidiogenous cells, flask-shaped or cylindrical phialides, single or in whorls; conidia green, smooth, ellipsoidal to subglobose.	*T. longibrachiatum* *T. citrinoviride* *T. harzianum*	Report concerning *T. viride*, *T. koningii*, and *T. pseudokoningii* not substantiated
Coelomycetes *Colletotrichum*	Colonies fast growing, woolly, tan to gray-brown, occasionally greenish and sometimes with lavender shades, with honey-colored masses of conidia. Brown appressoria usually present; conidiomata (fruit bodies) acervular, conidiogenous cells phialidic. Conidia hyaline, aseptate, straight to curved; also formed in aerial mycelium. Setae and sclerotia may be present.	*C. gloeosporioides* *C. coccodes* *C. dematium* *C. crassipes*	Colonies may be darker with better sporulation on potato carrot agar. Compare *C. dematium* with *Fusarium*.
Phoma	Colonies pale to tan to gray-brown, woolly; conidiomata pycnidial, usually dark, separate or aggregated, ostioles single to several, immersed or semi-immersed, mostly thin walled. Conidiogenous cells phialidic, conidia one celled, small, hyaline, often guttulate.	Several species reported in the literature, but most not well documented	Morphologically similar to *Pleurophoma*. Species-level identification difficult. See chapter 122 for additional coelomycetous genera.

[a]On potato dextrose agar (PDA) after 4 days of incubation at 25°C unless otherwise noted. See references cited in the text for a more detailed description of the features noted in this table. List is not all-inclusive.

[b]Species listed produce their teleomorph (sexual structures) in culture.

CLINICAL SIGNIFICANCE

The spectrum of disease caused by hyaline moulds is diverse, and disease is largely determined by the local and general immunologic and physiological state of the host and may be symptomatic or asymptomatic. In most instances, the portal of entry for fungal propagules is either through a break in the epidermis or by way of the lungs. Exceptions to this include introduction into the body by means of contaminated surgical instruments, intraocular lenses, prosthetic devices, or other contaminated materials or solutions associated with surgery or routine health care. Individuals whose resistance is lowered as a result of a severe debilitating disease or immunosuppressive therapy typically suffer from invasive pulmonary or paranasal sinus infection, but in some instances, the infecting fungus may spread to surrounding tissues or disseminate to virtually any organ. Fungemia is uncommon except in disseminated *Fusarium* infection. Noninvasive forms of infection also have been noted to occur in debilitated individuals as well as in individuals with apparently normal defense mechanisms. In such cases, the fungus colonizes a preexisting cavity in the lungs such as an ectatic bronchus, a tuberculous cavity, or a lung cyst. Other clinical syndromes usually occurring in immunocompetent individuals include chronic sinusitis, onychomycosis, subcutaneous abscess, keratitis, otomycosis, and allergic manifestations, including bronchopulmonary mycosis and sinusitis in atopic patients.

Although the majority of saprobic and plant-pathogenic moulds are not considered pathogenic for humans and other animals and appear unlikely to be able to adapt to or take advantage of risk factors predisposing to opportunistic infection, those capable of growing at or near body temperature must be considered to have latent pathogenic capability. The diversity of fungi known to be capable of colonizing or invading human tissue has increased dramatically in recent years, as reflected by new reports of proven infection. Moreover, certain fungi are isolated often enough to be suspicious for pathogenic potential. Still, there is a need for definitive evidence of infection due to a normally saprobic mould. The laboratory procedure for confirming fungal etiology includes (i) detection in the specimen of hyphal elements which are compatible with the morphology of the isolated mould, (ii) isolation of several colonies of a fungus or isolation of the same fungus from a repeat specimen, (iii) accurate identification of the isolated mould, and (iv) confirmation of the mould's ability to grow at or near body temperature. Species of *Fusarium* or other hyaline moulds isolated from all deep tissue or body fluids must be considered potentially invasive pathogens. No fungal isolate should be discarded as a contaminant without thorough examination of the clinical specimen. Quality control measures to ensure that isolation media are not contaminated and inspection of the slant or plate to evaluate where the fungus is growing relative to where the specimen was placed may also be important in evaluating whether an isolate is involved in disease. Close communication between microbiologists and physicians also is essential, especially for rare or unusual opportunists seen in individuals maintained on long-term immunosuppressive therapy.

COLLECTION, TRANSPORT, AND STORAGE OF SPECIMENS

Clinical specimens from patients with suspected mycosis are to be collected with prudence and transported to the laboratory and processed as soon as possible by using the standard procedures described in chapter 112 of this *Manual*. Because of the diverse clinical manifestations, various sites may need to be examined for fungal elements. Biopsy material, transtracheal aspirates, and sputum samples collected in the early morning all may be useful specimens for the isolation and detection of hyaline moulds, as are infected nails. Swabs taken from mucous membranes and skin lesions are not recommended. Although the reliability in determining whether an isolate is a possible pathogen is increased if cultures of two different specimens yield the same organism, a tissue biopsy sample is more informative, since the significance of culture can be verified by histological examination of the tissue. While blood cultures are generally of limited use for the detection of invasive hyaline moulds with dry conidia, such as *Aspergillus* (56), *Fusarium* and other species with slimy conidia may be reliably detected (170). For optimum recovery, the specimen should be inoculated onto several types of media and incubated at 28 to 30°C. The opportunistic moulds are variably sensitive to cycloheximide, so media containing this selective agent should be used cautiously. Suspicious isolates, especially of uncommon species, should be tested for their ability to grow at 35 to 37°C. Potentially neurotropic species may also grow at 40°C and above (3, 21).

FUSARIUM SPECIES

Taxonomy

Fusarium species are cosmopolitan soil saprobes and facultative plant pathogens that can cause infection or toxicosis in humans and animals (47, 48, 115, 131, 210). They belong to the order Hypocreales, family Hypocreaceae. Clinically significant species are mostly heterothallic, with the anamorphic (asexual) state seen in culture. Teleomorphs occur in *Gibberella*, *Neocosmospora*, and other genera. Characterization at the molecular level has shown that organisms once considered individual species by morphological features are now known to represent several closely related species (4, 67, 72, 134, 145, 151, 210, 211, 237). These phylogenetically related species comprise a species complex (SC). Multilocus phylogenetic studies demonstrated that the most frequently recovered SC, the *Fusarium solani* SC (FSSC) (Fig. 1A), was comprised of over 45 phylogenetically distinct species within three major clades, and that human isolates were restricted to clade 3. Clade 3 was also shown to be associated with four major lineages, designated groups 1 through 4, with many strains clustered in groups 1 and 2 (34, 145, 237). Subsequently, more robust typing studies based on polymorphisms in portions of the internal transcribed spacer (ITS) region and domains D1 plus D2 of the nuclear large-subunit rRNA, the translation elongation factor 1 alpha gene (EF-1α), and the second largest subunit of the RNA polymerase II gene (RPB2) identified 34 species within clade 3 of the FSSC (150). The FSSC currently also includes *Fusarium falciforme* (FSSC groups 3 and 4) (previously *Acremonium falciforme*), *Acremonium lichenicola* (*Cylindrocarpon lichenicola*), and *Neocosmospora vasinfecta* (145, 211). Although the *Fusarium oxysporum* SC (FOSC) is best known as an economically devastating vascular wilt pathogen on a wide range of agriculturally important plant

hosts (51), it is also the second most common *Fusarium* SC associated with human disease (Fig. 1B). The FOSC is also a phylogenetically diverse SC. Multilocus sequence typing and amplified fragment length polymorphism (AFLP) analyses of over 100 isolates of *Fusarium oxysporum* from the environment, hospital bronchoscopy and water sources, and clinical isolates revealed a geographically widespread clonal lineage comprising >70% of isolates genotyped (151). These studies have further supported hospital water distribution systems as a potential source of nosocomial infection (8, 229). Several medically important species are included within the species-rich *Gibberella fujikuroi* species complex (GFSC) as defined by multilocus genotyping (134, 146, 147). These include *Fusarium verticillioides* (Fig. 1C), *Fusarium proliferatum* (Fig. 1D), *Fusarium napiforme*, and *Fusarium nygamai*. The *Fusarium chlamydosporum* species complex (FCSC) is also phyogenetically diverse and represents four species based on multilocus genotyping (149). Similarly, the *Fusarium dimerum* SC (FDSC) (Fig. 1E and F) currently contains seven named and two unnamed species (191). These strains are unlike those in the aforementioned SCs in that they frequently display slower growth, and aerial mycelium is either absent or only sparsely developed, so colonies appear mucoid to slimy (usually some shade of orange). Another morphologically and phylogenetically diverse group of fusaria includes those previously referred to as *Fusarium semitectum* or *Fusarium incarnatum* and now known to reside in the *Fusarium incarnatum-Fusarium equiseti* species complex (FIESC) (148). Multilocus phylogenetic studies have demonstrated that this complex encompasses 28 species (149).

Description of the Agents

As can be seen from the taxonomic discussion, the *Fusarium* species cited as etiologic agents of human and animal disease fall within six SCs. Based upon our current understanding of the genus and recognizing the likelihood of future taxonomic changes, the more common species within these complexes are as follows: FSSC, *F. solani*, *F. falciforme*, *Fusarium lichenicola*, and *Neocosmospora vasinfecta*; FOSC, *F. oxysporum*; GFSC, *F. verticillioides*, *Fusarium thapsinum*, and *F. proliferatum*; FCSC, *F. chlamydosporum*; FDSC, *F. dimerum* and *Fusarium delphinoides*; and FIESC, *F. incarnatum/F. pallidoroseum*, which may be separate species. See also Table 2.

Epidemiology and Transmission

There are numerous toxins and metabolites produced by *Fusarium* species that have been implicated in human disease, especially associated with the consumption of contaminated food products (see chapter 124). Alimentary toxic aleukia was described to occur in individuals who ate grain contaminated with *Fusarium sporotrichioides* or *Fusarium poae* that produce trichothecene mycotoxins (92). Besides orally ingested mycotoxins, systemic effects of exposure to inhaled mycotoxins have also been attributed to *Fusarium*, although these effects have been much less well characterized (109). The more common clinical presentation in human disease is associated with the fusarial conidia gaining access to the host and germinating, and with subsequent tissue invasion by hyphae. The portal of entry, however, is unknown in most cases of invasive infection. Ingestion or access through mucosal membranes may occur in some (24, 137). Disseminated infection may also follow onychomycosis, often associated with cellulitis (69). Hospital water supply and distribution systems have also been implicated

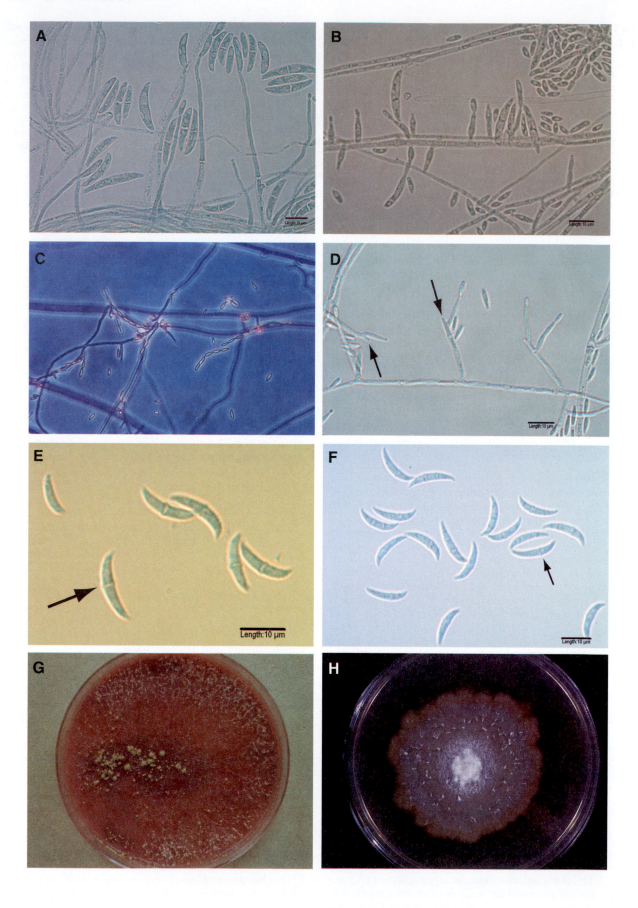

as a source of infection of immunocompromised patients by Anaissie et al. (8) and O'Donnell et al. (151). The most common mode of transmission, however, appears to be inhalation of airborne conidia (169).

Although invasive infection by *Fusarium* is uncommon, an increased incidence of disseminated infection has been seen in neutropenic patients with hematologic cancer, in recipients of solid-organ transplants, and in allogeneic hematopoietic stem cell transplant (HSCT) recipients (12, 19, 70, 75, 116, 131, 135–137, 139–141, 170, 186). The incidence of fusariosis among allogeneic HSCT recipients varied from 4.21 to 5.0 cases per 1,000 in human leukocyte antigen (HLA)-matched related transplant recipients and 20.19 cases per 1,000 in HLA-mismatched transplant recipients (141). Among allogeneic HSCT recipients, a trimodal distribution was observed: a first peak before engraftment, a second peak at a median of 62 days after transplantation, and a third peak >1 year after transplantation. The actuarial survival rate was 13% (median, 13 days), with persistent neutropenia (hazard ratio of 5.43) and use of corticosteroids (hazard ratio of 2.18) being the most important factors associated with poor outcome (136, 141).

Clinical Significance

The spectrum of clinical presentations by *Fusarium* species includes those seen in both the healthy and the immunocompromised host, although these distinctions may be ill defined in some settings. A frequent infection in the healthy host is keratitis resulting from trauma and penetration of the cornea, contamination of soft contact lenses and/or solutions (34, 88, 102, 139, 148, 173), or local immunosuppression by corticosteroid drops (139). The keratitis outbreaks recognized in Hong Kong (173), Singapore (102), the United Kingdom, and the United States (34) in 2005 and 2006 in contact lens wearers using ReNu with MoistureLoc Solution (Bausch & Lomb, Rochester, NY) resulted in the largest investigation and molecular characterization of fusarial keratitis isolates to date and clearly demonstrated that these strains occurred in nearly the full spectrum of clinically significant fusarial SCs. Other presentations in the immunocompetent host include those listed in Table 1. Cutaneous lesions in various stages of evolution (141), fungemia (236), rhinocerebral involvement, pneumonia, endogenous endophthalmitis (175, 221), or combinations of these are common clinical findings in disseminated fusarial disease (131, 136–141, 165, 170, 186). Unlike in invasive cases of aspergillosis, recovery of *Fusarium* species from the blood in disseminated disease approaches 60% (140, 170). Members of the FSSC (typically reported as *Fusarium solani*) are the most frequently cited agents of disease, and most cases involve keratitis (48, 205). Mayayo et al. (121) consider this species to be the most virulent, and it has been suggested that production

of cyclosporine may contribute to its pathogenicity (208). Additional species in the FSSC, including *Neocosmospora vasinfecta*, *F. lichenicola* (*Cylindrocarpon lichenicola*), and *F. falciforme* (*Acremonium falciforme*), are also agents of disease. *Fusarium oxysporum* (FOSC) (151) and *Fusarium verticillioides* (17) in the GFSC appear to be the next most common organisms recovered with a similar spectrum of infection. *Fusarium verticillioides* was the most frequently isolated species in deep-seated infections in Italy (222). Given our current understanding of the genus, it is now difficult to attribute older clinical case reports to the newly defined species. See references 16, 47, 48, 191, and 222 for a more complete list of *Fusarium* species known as etiologic agents in human and animal disease.

Collection, Transport, and Storage of Specimens

Methods of collection, transport, and storage of specimens are detailed in chapter 112. Like invasive aspergillosis, invasive *Fusarium* infections are difficult to diagnose and usually require a combination of clinical, culture, and radiographic findings. However, unlike *Aspergillus*, *Fusarium* is more frequently recovered from blood, nails, and skin lesions of the immunocompromised host (24, 129). The recovery from a normally sterile site and microscopic evidence of invasive growth in tissue provide the most convincing evidence of invasive fusariosis.

Direct Examination

Microscopy

In direct examination, the hyphae of *Fusarium* species resemble those of *Aspergillus*, *Paecilomyces*, or *Scedosporium* species in size (3 to 6 μm in width), septation, branching pattern, and predilection for vascular invasion. The hyphae are irregular in width and may show areas of collapse. Hyphae exhibit both dichotomous branching (i.e., branching at 45°), as is commonly seen in invasive aspergillosis, and branching at right angles (33, 117). Microconidia and, rarely, macroconidia and budding cells, as well as phialides, may be found in blood vessel lumens or in aerated tissues (117). Immunohistological methods may help to distinguish between infections caused by some hyaline moulds, but cross-reactivity is problematic and serological tests are not in common use (98). Definitive diagnosis requires isolation and identification of the fungus, along with demonstration of fungal elements in tissue.

Antigen Detection

There is no commercial system available for detection of genus-specific or species-specific antigens released by *Fusarium* species in human infection. The diagnostic utility of polyclonal fluorescent-antibody reagents to members of the FSSC in tissue sections from patients with invasive

FIGURE 1 (A) A member of the FSSC. Microconidia are borne from long monophialides. Macroconidia borne in the aerial mycelium are also present. (B) *Fusarium oxysporum* in the FOSC. Microconidia are borne from short monophialides. A few macroconidia are also present. (C) Chains of microconidia produced by *Fusarium verticillioides* (formerly *Fusarium moniliforme*) in the GFSC. (D) *Fusarium proliferatum* in the GFSC. Note polyphialides (arrows) with more than one opening not delimited by a septum. Truncate conidia that have been borne in chains as well as false heads are also present. (E) Macroconidia of *Fusarium dimerum* in the FDSC. Note that conidia are two celled and that the septum is in the middle. (F) Macroconidia of *Fusarium delphinoides* in the FDSC. Note that the septum in two-celled conidia is off-center, and three-celled conidia are also present. (G) Colony of *Achaetomium strumarium* showing yellowish surface mycelium and pink pigment on cornmeal agar after 5 weeks. (H) An isolate of *Gymnascella hyalinospora* described in reference 106 was glabrous and sterile when grown on potato dextrose agar for 15 days at 30°C.

fusariosis was evaluated, but extensive cross-staining was observed with sections containing aspergilli, *Paecilomyces lilacinus*, and *Pseudallescheria boydii* (98).

There is one report that suggests that exoantigens from *F. oxysporum* cross-react with the Pastorex *Aspergillus* antigen latex agglutination kit (95), but no significant cross-reactivity with *F. solani* and *F. oxysporum* was found with the Platelia *Aspergillus* assay despite the fact that the two kits employ the same monoclonal antibody (218). There are no reports that indicate that sera from patients with invasive fusariosis show reactivity with these antigen detection kits. Antigens prepared from *F. verticillioides* were found to cause borderline cross-reactivity with the Platelia *Candida* antigen assay (Bio-Rad) (178). This reactivity appeared to be specific for *F. verticillioides*, since extracts prepared from *F. solani* and *F. oxysporum* showed no cross-reactivity in vitro.

Circulating $(1\rightarrow3)$-β-D-glucan can be detected in the blood of patients with *Fusarium* fungemia and pneumonia (143, 154), although the presence of this marker is not specific for *Fusarium* (142). The sensitivity for detection of *Fusarium* infection was found to be 100% at a cutoff value of 60 pg/ml among three patients with invasive fusariosis (154). The clinical experience of $(1\rightarrow3)$-β-D-glucan detection in patients with invasive fusariosis is limited, but the test is of value for patients with suspicion of invasive fungal infection as part of the diagnostic workup. In a mouse model, $(1\rightarrow3)$-β-D-glucan remains high throughout the infection, suggesting that this marker may provide a specific and sensitive diagnostic tool for the detection of invasive fusariosis (100). False-positive reactions of $(1\rightarrow3)$-β-D-glucan are known to occur in some patients. These include subjects who had experienced renal failure and who were undergoing hemodialysis with cellulose membranes (97), subjects treated with certain immunoglobulin products (87), and specimens (or subjects) exposed to glucan-containing gauze or related materials (130). This underscores the need to combine $(1\rightarrow3)$-β-D-glucan monitoring with clinical examination of the patient and other diagnostic procedures, such as high-resolution computed tomography scan, when making a diagnosis.

Nucleic Acid Detection Techniques

Given the difficulty in species level identification of *Fusarium* isolates utilizing microscopic and macroscopic features, and the expertise required, application of molecular tools makes them an attractive alternative method for the early diagnosis of invasive fusariosis. However, within the field of clinical mycology only a very limited number of studies have been published. In one study using PCR, *Fusarium* DNA was detected in tissues in a mouse model of disseminated fusariosis (86). In another study, a panfungal and species-specific *F. solani* PCR was designed based on the 18S rRNA gene sequence and applied to ocular specimens from three patients with suspected bacterial or fungal endophthalmitis. Although *F. solani* was detected in spiked specimens, no clinical samples from patients with endophthalmitis due to *Fusarium* were analyzed (91). PCR-based identification was also applied to *Fusarium* isolates obtained from patients with onychomycosis (133). The *Fusarium* species identified were the same as those known to cause disseminated fusariosis in immunocompromised patients.

Panfungal PCR systems that detect a wide range of fungi, including *Fusarium*, have been developed. In one study the PCR was positive with blood samples from a patient with an invasive fusariosis and blood cultures positive for *F. solani* (227). Luminex microbead hybridization technology using 75 genus-specific hybridization probes has recently been reported to detect a variety of fungal pathogens, including *Fusarium*, from clinical blood and pulmonary samples (111). As with other opportunistic fungi, molecular methods such as PCR appear to have promise for the detection and identification of *Fusarium* infections; however, the value of these tools in the management of patients remains to be investigated.

Isolation Procedures

In general, *Fusarium* species can be recovered easily on routine mycological media, and there are no specific growth requirements. Given the aggressive nature of fusaria in neutropenic, immunocompromised individuals, however, the use of a medium for direct plating of specimens that can aid an early diagnosis by displaying consistent morphological features, such as potato dextrose agar, is highly recommended. See chapter 112 for detailed information on specimen collection and processing.

Identification

Microscopic features of phialide shape, the number of openings on the phialides (i.e., monophialides or polyphialides), the formation of conidia in heads or chains, micro- and macroconidial shape and septation, the presence and arrangement of chlamydospores, colonial features (including growth rates and color of colony obverse and reverse [105]), and color of conidial masses are important characters for species identification. However, considerable proficiency is required to identify *Fusarium* species with certainty, and a reference laboratory should be consulted. Alternatively, molecular tools are being developed to help identify clinical *Fusarium* isolates (133). Although fusaria grow well on most mycological media, the medium can profoundly influence the colonial topography, color, and conidium development. Synthetic nutrient agar, potato dextrose agar, and tap water agar supplemented with either sterilized carnation leaves or potassium chloride are widely employed (131, 132). Use of a rich medium to maintain isolates can result in cultural degeneration.

A recently recommended biosafety level (BSL) classification for fusaria is either BSL 1 or BSL 2, depending upon the species (48). Filamentous clinical isolates should be handled in a biological safety cabinet.

Typing Systems

Typing systems that have been applied to *Aspergillus* have also been used to differentiate strains of *Fusarium* (4, 72, 84, 190), although most experience has been obtained in the field of agricultural research rather than in clinical mycology. Recently the Clinical and Laboratory Standards Institute published a document for identification of bacteria and fungi by DNA target sequencing (41), and a consortium of international experts assembled as an International Society for Human and Animal Mycology working group on fungal identification has provided clinical laboratories with initial recommendations for molecular typing of *Aspergillus*, *Fusarium*, and the Mucorales (20). These single-locus (ITS) guidelines for placing fusaria within an SC are based upon knowledge gained from multilocus sequencing (*ITS-LSU rDNA*, *EF-1α*, β-tubulin [β-*TUB*], calmodulin [*CAM*], and *RPB2*) analyzed by phylogenetic methods (145–151). These guidelines propose that if the ITS sequence yields a >99% identity with a type or reference strain by comparative sequence analysis with GenBank/EMBL/DDBJ, then the isolate can be placed within one of the six SCs. Additional loci mentioned above would be required with less than 99%

identity or for species identification (20). Additional public databases, such as FUSARIUM-ID, are also available (67).

Serologic Tests

Conventional serologic tests have been developed and used to measure exposure of specific patient populations to *Fusarium*, most commonly in the setting of occupational exposure or indoor dampness problems (90, 112, 184). In these populations, immunoglobulin G (IgG) directed against *Fusarium* can be detected. Elevated levels of IgE and IgG antibody directed against *F. oxysporum* were found in a patient with allergic bronchopulmonary mycosis due to this species (185). Anti-*Fusarium* antibodies have not been evaluated as a diagnostic tool for patients with invasive fusariosis.

Antimicrobial Susceptibilities

In vitro studies show relatively high MICs of amphotericin B and itraconazole for members of the FSSC (MIC$_{90}$s, 4 and >8 µg/ml, respectively) and *F. oxysporum* (MIC$_{90}$s, 1.0 and >8 µg/ml, respectively) (59). Higher MICs of these drugs were obtained with the Etest, which showed an agreement of less than 80% for these species with the NCCLS M38-A method (43). In a later study using Etest, 60% of the *Fusarium* isolates had amphotericin B Etest MICs of less than 1 µg/ml; however, all were resistant to itraconazole (168). Voriconazole, posaconazole, itraconazole, and ravuconazole show variable to no in vitro activity against clinical *Fusarium* isolates (161). In one series voriconazole was active against *F. solani*, *F. oxysporum*, *F. proliferatum*, and *F. verticillioides* (reported as *Fusarium moniliforme*) (MIC$_{90}$, 2 µg/ml) but was not fungicidal against most isolates (10, 39). However, in another study both azoles showed no activity (50). The correlation between in vitro activity and clinical outcome remains suboptimal for *Fusarium*, given the clinical responses observed in patients with invasive fusariosis treated with voriconazole (158) and the efficacy of posaconazole in experimental fusariosis (119). The echinocandins show no meaningful activity against *Fusarium* in vitro (11, 160), and the Fks1 gene appears to confer intrinsic resistance in *F. solani* (96). Universal in vitro resistance was found in four clades in the FSSC (15), and testing of *F. solani* by the European Committee on Antimicrobial Susceptibility Testing method indicated a lack of activity by any agent tested (114). In an Italian study, *F. solani* demonstrated high azole MICs, while *F. verticillioides* showed low posaconazole MICs (222). Azor et al. also reported in vitro posaconazole activity against *F. verticillioides*, as well as terbinafine activity gainst both *F. verticillioides* and *F. thapsinum* (17). In vitro testing of less-frequent *Fusarium* species in the GFSC, the FCSC, and the FIESC showed that terbinafine was the most active agent against all species except for *F. incarnatum*, against which amphotericin B was the most active (16, 42). In contrast, terbinafine showed high MIC$_{90}$s against *F. solani* and *F. oxysporum* (65). Synergy studies in a murine model with *F. oxysporum* showed prolonged survival and reduced fungal burden with the combination of amphotericin B and posaconazole (182), and silver nitrate was shown to exhibit in vitro activity against several species of ocular fusaria (234).

Evaluation, Interpretation, and Reporting of Results

The early diagnosis of fusariosis is often key to appropriate management strategies, and the recovery of *Fusarium* isolates should be reported to the clinician long before a final identification is made. Strains identified by phenotypic features or ITS sequence data should be reported as members of one of the SCs.

OTHER OPPORTUNISTIC HYALINE MOULDS

Taxonomy

Other opportunistic hyaline moulds known to cause human or animal disease are located in various taxonomic groupings as seen in Table 3. A few are homothallic ascomycetes and filamentous basidiomycetes; however, the majority are genera that, although connected to ascomycetes, only display their asexual anamorphs in culture. Most are hyaline or only lightly pigmented; however, some, like *Acrophialophora*, become dark centrally. Others, such as *Phialemonium* and *Lecythophora*, have been considered as agents of phaeohyphomycosis but are included here as they are pale in culture. Two coelomycetous genera, *Colletotrichum* and *Phoma*, are also included. Unlike the hyphomycetes, which bear their conidia free, coelomycetes produce their conidia within semi-enclosed or enclosed structures known as acervuli or pycnidia, respectively. Coelomycetes are frequently acquired as a result of some type of implantation of the fungus rather than inhalation (213, 214).

Description of the Agents

Ascomycetes

Homothallic Ascomycetes

Homothallic ascomycetous genera that may be seen in culture include those producing cleistothecia (ascomata without openings or ostioles) such as *Thermoascus*, *Aphanoascus*, and *Cephalotheca*, those displaying perithecia (ascomata with ostioles) such as *Achaetomium* (Fig. 1G), *Chaetomium*, and *Microascus* (Fig. 2C), and those whose ascospores are borne in naked clusters as in *Gymnascella*. *Thermoascus* species are non-ostiolate, thermophilic ascomycetes with growth to 50°C. They produce pale yellow, elliptical, thick-walled ascospores and have anamorphs in the genus *Paecilomyces*. *Aphanoascus* is a keratinolytic ascomycete characterized by yellowish, lens-shaped reticulate ascospores and a *Chrysosporium* anamorph. *Cephalotheca foveolata* is characterized by cleistothecial ascomata covered with yellow to brown hairs, foveolate (delicately pitted or dimpled as seen by electron microscopy) ascospores (Fig. 2D), and a *Phialemonium*-like anamorph (Fig. 2E) (235). *Achaetomium* and *Chaetomium* produce brown lemon-shaped to fusiform ascospores within ascomata that are ornamented with hairs (or setae), especially around the upper part near the opening. Anamorphs are uncommon. *Microascus* species produce yellowish to reddish orange, variously shaped ascospores extruded in a long cirrus (like toothpaste squeezed from a tube) and have anamorphs in the genus *Scopulariopsis*. Species identification in the genus *Microascus* is based primarily on the features of the perithecia such as size and length of necks, as well as the shape of the ascospores. *Gymnascella* species are onygenalean fungi that produce clusters of ascospores surrounded by yellow or orange filaments, but differentiated ascomata are not formed (Fig. 1H and 2A and B). A case isolate and the reference isolate of this species both displayed false-positive results in the Gen-Probe test for *Blastomyces dermatitidis* (89).

Basidiomycetes

Schizophyllum and Other Genera

Filamentous basidiomycetes are uncommon causes of human or animal disease and are still poorly characterized. However, those that have been well documented are included in genera that may remain sterile in culture. A clinical isolate may be confirmed as a basidiomycete by the presence

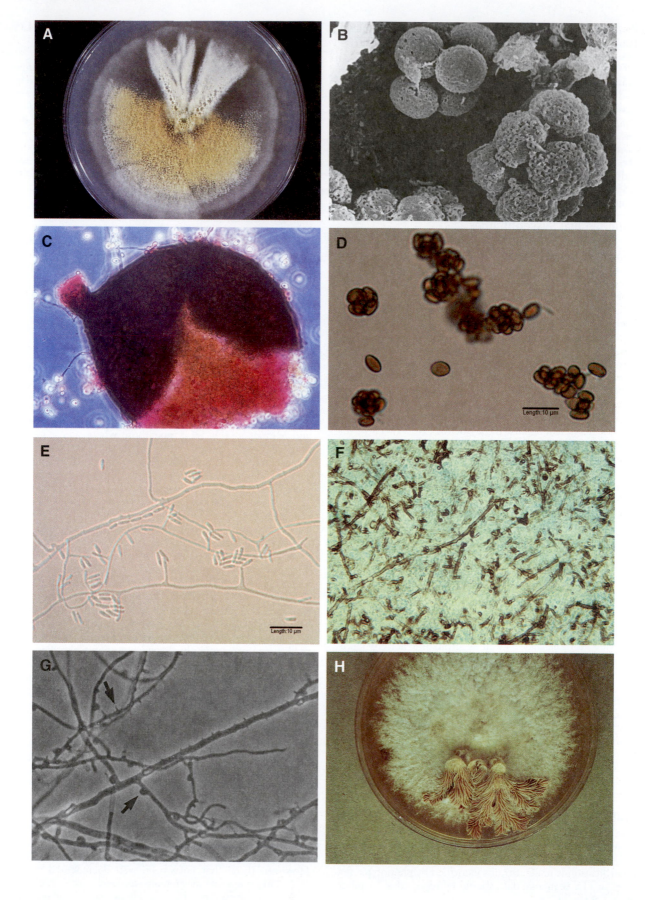

of clamp connections on the hyphae, but these diagnostic structures may be lacking. A nonsporulating hyaline mould may be suspected as a basidiomycete when the isolate is fast growing, displays growth on benomyl agar, grows at 37°C, and fails to grow on medium with cycloheximide (196).

Schizophyllum commune is recognized as a significant cause of allergic sinusitis, allergic bronchopulmonary mycosis, and related allergic disease and as an occasional cause of invasive infection in both immunocompetent and immunosuppressed patients (204). In culture, isolates of *Schizophyllum commune* may be dikaryotic, producing diagnostic spicules and clamp connections on the hyphae (Fig. 2G), as well as basidiocarps (mushrooms) under conditions of light (Fig. 2H). Other isolates are monokaryotic, remaining sterile, lacking clamps and sometimes lacking spicules. When spicules are absent, hyphae of *S. commune* then resemble those of *Aspergillus* species or other moulds both in culture and in tissue (7, 196, 199) (Fig. 2F). Monokaryotic isolates can be difficult to identify, and techniques such as vegetative compatibility tests or sequencing of the ITS region of rRNA may be required to confirm their identification as *S. commune* (198, 199).

Other uncommon basidiomycetes causing disease in humans or animals include *Inonotus tropicalis* (Fig. 3A) (45, 217), *Oxyporus corticola* (25), *Coprinus* species with arthroconidium-forming *Hormographiella* anamorphs (110, 228), and the *Sporothrix*-like organism previously known as *Sporothrix cyanescens* (200), *Cerinosterus cyanescens* (121, 123), and *Fugomyces cyanescens* (195). Phylogenetic studies have placed this species in the family Quambalariaceae as *Quambalaria cyanescens* (46). Another basidiomycete with less convincing pathogenic potential is *Sporotrichum pruinosum*, the anamorph of *Phanerochaete chrysosporium* (101).

Hyphomycetes

Scopulariopsis

The annellidic genus *Scopulariopsis* (Fig. 4F) contains both lightly colored and dark species, some of which have teleomorphs in the genus *Microascus* of the Microascaceae (2, 52, 53, 127) or the genus *Kernia*. Members of the genus *Scopulariopsis* are common soil fungi and agents of deterioration, especially of cellulosic substrates. Of the 30 species known, only a few are reliably reported from human infections.

Acremonium, Lecythophora, and *Phialemonium*

Fungi belonging to the genera *Acremonium*, *Lecythophora*, and *Phialemonium* form single-celled conidia in slimy masses from slender phialides. The genus *Acremonium*, formerly called *Cephalosporium*, includes approximately 100 species associated with soil, insects, sewage, rhizospheres of plants, and other environmental substrates. Teleomorphs, where known, are in the genera *Nectria*, *Emericellopsis*, and *Thielavia*, which are placed in different ascomycete orders. Teleomorph connections and molecular data provide evidence for some restructuring of the genus along phylogenetic lines (47, 71, 76). The genus *Lecythophora* contains two significant species, *L. hoffmannii* and *L. mutabilis*; human etiologic agents in the genus *Phialemonium* include *P. obovatum* and *P. curvatum* (47, 48). Genus recognition of *Acremonium* in culture is usually possible, but identification to the species level is very difficult, and many reports of infection are based on unidentified species (76, 210). Species of *Acremonium* grow well on Sabouraud dextrose agar, and some species can tolerate cycloheximide. The genus *Phaeoacremonium*, including *P. parasiticum* and some other species associated with human infections, is distinguished from *Acremonium* by its brownish pigmented hyphae and conidiophores (see chapter 122). The genera *Lecythophora* and *Phialemonium* differ from *Acremonium* by their formation of short, stumpy phialides without basal septa (called adelophialides) in addition to the more spindle-shaped phialides (64), but these distinctions are not always readily observed. *L. mutabilis* differs from *L. hoffmannii* in forming accessory brown chlamydospores on sporulation media. Three species of *Phialemonium* were distinguished originally by conidial shape and colony color (64), but the PCR-restriction fragment length polymorphism banding patterns showed a close relationship between isolates of *P. curvatum* and *Phialemonium dimorphosporum*, and these two species were synonymized (80).

Arthrographis and *Onychocola*

The genera *Arthrographis* and *Onychocola* are hyaline, arthroconidium-forming fungi. The thermotolerant *Arthrographis kalrae* is a rare opportunist recovered from skin, lung, corneal ulcer, and sinus (36, 159, 195). Because initial growth is often yeastlike, an isolate may not be recognized as a pleomorphic mould and may be subjected to tests commonly used for yeast identification. *Onychocola canadensis* (Fig. 3F and G) is a cycloheximide-tolerant hyphomycete.

Beauveria and *Engyodontium*

Beauveria and *Engyodontium* species have solitary conidia borne sympodially. *Beauveria bassiana* is a well-known insect pathogen with limited virulence for humans. *Engyodontium album* is closely related (47) and was formerly placed in the genus *Beauveria*.

Chrysosporium, Myceliophthora, and *Myriodontium*

Members of the genera *Chrysosporium* (Fig. 3B and C), *Myriodontium*, and *Myceliophthora* (Fig. 3E) produce solitary, usually single-celled conidia which are called aleurioconidia because of their lytic method of conidium dehiscence (94). Members of these genera are related to the dermatophytes and the dimorphic pathogens, sharing with them a tolerance of cycloheximide and having teleomorphs in the ascomycete order *Onygenales* (94, 194).

Metarhizium and *Trichoderma*

Metarhizium anisopliae is an insect pathogen of wide distribution. A taxonomic revision of the genus was made by Driver et al. in 2000 (54). Conidia are produced in chains that adhere together, in contrast to *Trichoderma* species, which form conidia in slimy heads. Morphological criteria for recognition

---

FIGURE 2 (A) The same isolate of *Gymnascella hyalinospora* as in Fig. 1H turned yellow on oatmeal agar, with development of ascospores after 15 days at 30°C. (B) Ascospores of *Gymnascella hyalinospora* observed by scanning electron microscopy. Magnification, ×6,000. (C) Perithecium of a *Microascus* species. (D) Brown ascospores of *Cephalotheca foveolata* that formed after 8 weeks on carnation leaf agar at 25°C. (E) *Phialemonium*-like anamorph of *Cephalotheca foveolata* showing adelophialides (reduced phialides without a septum) and ellipsoidal conidia. (F) Tissue section stained with Gomori methenamine silver stain showing monokaryotic (clampless) hyphae of *Schizophyllum commune* in a pulmonary fungus ball. (G) *Schizophyllum commune* in slide culture preparation showing clamp connections and narrow pegs or spicules (arrows). Magnification, ×580. (H) Dikaryotic culture of *Schizophyllum commune* showing development of gilled fruiting bodies on potato dextrose agar after 7 weeks in the light.

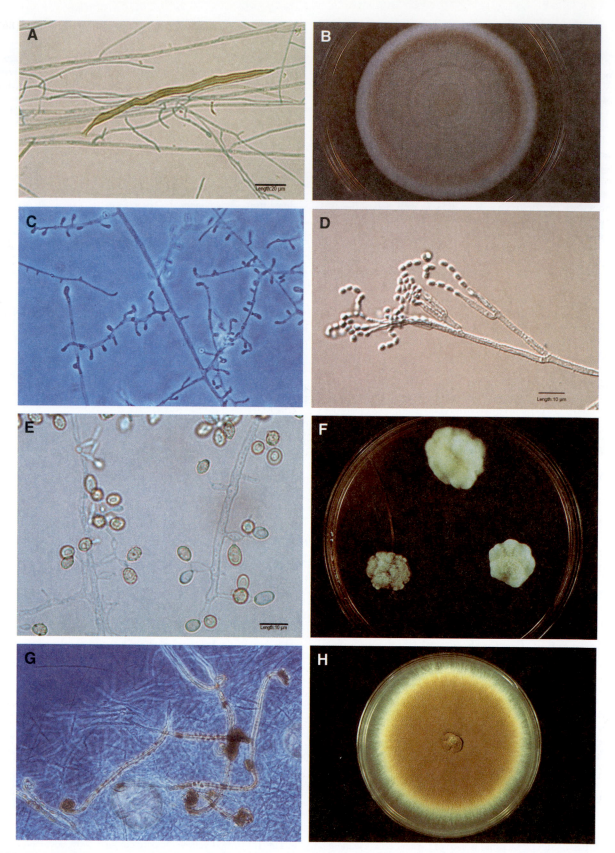

FIGURE 3   (A) Setal hyphae of *Inonotus tropicalis*, slide culture preparation on potato flake agar, 10 days, 25°C. Bar, 20 µm. (B) Colony of *Chrysosporium zonatum* on potato dextrose agar after 14 days at 37°C. (C) Conidia of *Chrysosporium zonatum* formed on short curved stalks. (D) Rough stipe, metulae, and phialides of *Geosmithia argillacea*. Note also that conidia are initially cuneiform (wedge shaped). Bar, 10 µm. (E) Conidia of *Myceliophthora thermophila* in various stages of maturity. Mature conidia are dark and rough. Bar, 10 µm. (F) Culture of three different isolates of *Onychocola canadensis* after 5 weeks on Mycosel agar. (G) Setae (appendages) of *Onychocola canadensis*. (H) Colony of *Paecilomyces variotii* on potato dextrose agar after 7 days.

of the *Trichoderma longibrachiatum* SC include (i) fast-growing yellowish green colonies with a radius greater than 35 mm at 40°C after 3 days of growth on potato dextrose agar; (ii) a strong yellow diffusing pigment present at 30°C but absent at 40°C; (iii) hyphae sparingly branched and forming phialides that are mostly solitary, longer, and more gradually tapered (cylindrical); and (iv) smooth oblong to ellipsoidal conidia (Fig. 4G and H). Intercalary phialides and chlamydospores are common. Some reports concerning *Trichoderma pseudokoningii* may actually refer to *Trichoderma citrinoviride*, a thermotolerant species closely related to *T. longibrachiatum* (47, 108). An oligonucleotide barcode program, *TrichOKEY*, was published in 2006 for sequence-based identification (55).

Paecilomyces, Acrophialophora, Phialosimplex, and Geosmithia

Species of *Paecilomyces* occur worldwide as soil saprophytes, insect parasites, and agents of biodeterioration. The two most important medically significant species are *Paecilomyces lilacinus* and *P. variotii*. Their teleomorphs are unknown, but their affinity is within the ascomycete family *Trichocomaceae*, which also includes *Penicillium* and *Aspergillus* species; some other species have teleomorphs in the genus *Thermoascus* (*Thermoascaceae*). The colonial and morphological features of these two species (Fig. 3H and 4A and B) are described in Table 3. A similar species not confirmed as an agent of infection, *P. marquandii*, displays a yellow diffusing pigment and fails to grow at 37°C (204).

Acrophialophora is a thermotolerant and potentially neurotropic genus widespread in temperate to tropical regions. Colonies are initially pale but darken centrally at maturity. Also described under the name *Paecilomyces fusisporus*, it differs by producing unbranched, erect, brown, echinulate conidiophores that are fertile at the apex and anchored by a foot cell, and basally swollen monophialidic but occasionally polyphialidic conidiogenous cells. Conidia are borne in chains, and distinct spiral bands may be present (6). The organism may superficially resemble *Scedosporium prolificans* (77, 202).

Phialosimplex is a newly described species seen primarily in dogs and also having phylogenetic affinity to the *Trichocomaceae* (203). Colonies are moderately fast-growing and white to gray to yellowish, with *Phialosimplex caninus* distinguished by a yellow diffusible pigment (Fig. 4D). Hyaline subglobose to pyriform to ovoid truncate conidia are borne in long chains or heads from single narrow, mostly monophialidic conidiogenous cells (Fig. 4E). *Sagenomella chlamydospora* (68) and *Sagenomella sclerotialis* (63) were transferred to *Phialosimplex* as *Phialosimplex chlamydosporus* comb. nov. and *Phialosimplex sclerotialis* comb. nov., respectively. Compare with *Acremonium* species that produce conidia in chains and with *Acrophialophora fusispora*.

Geosmithia is a genus that closely resembles *Penicillium*. *G. argillacea* (formerly *Penicillium argillaceum*), teleomorph *Talaromyces eburneus*, was an agent of disseminated disease in a German shepherd dog (74). It is distinguished from *Penicillium* species by roughened stipes, metulae, and phialides, and by cuneiform to ellipsoidal conidia (Fig. 3D).

Coelomycetes

Colletotrichum and *Phoma*

Colletotrichum species are acervular coelomycetes occasionally recovered as agents of disease. They are fast-growing colonies of various shades that are most easily recognized in the laboratory by the production of brown, variably shaped appressoria. Honey-colored masses of conidia may be present in culture as well as setae and sclerotia in some species.

Cano et al. have described the salient features seen in clinical strains (28). Species in the genus *Phoma* are pycnidial coelomycetes that may be pale or darker in culture, and several species are described. They are usually recognized by small dark dots (pycnidia) that form on the surface or are immersed in the agar. Boerema et al. have recently published a *Phoma* identification manual (22); however, species differentiation is best handled in a reference laboratory. See chapter 122 for additional coelomycetous genera.

Epidemiology and Transmission

The methods of transmission and sources of infection for the other opportunistic hyaline moulds are similar to those seen in aspergillosis and fusariosis, and acquisition is typically through inhalation or traumatic implantation. Coelomycetous fungi, although ubiquitous, are mostly reported from cases of keratitis and subcutaneous mycoses in compromised individuals (81) and appear to be acquired primarily through external inoculation (213).

Clinical Significance

Ascomycetes

Homothallic Ascomycetes

Species of *Chaetomium* and *Achaetomium* (Fig. 1G) are neurotropic agents of cerebral infection (3, 9, 21), while *Chaetomium globosum* occurs most commonly as a contaminant or as a rare agent of onychomycosis (195, 201). *Microascus* spp. are also agents of deep infections, including endocarditis (31) and a brain abscess (18) by *Microascus cinereus*, disseminated infections by *Microascus cirrosus*, and a fatal pneumonia by *Microascus trigonosporus* (126). Additional rarely implicated genera include *Gymnascella* (Fig. 1H and 2A and B) and *Cephalotheca* (Fig. 2D and E). Please see references 18, 31, 47, 48, 89, 107, 126, and 226.

Basidiomycetes

Schizophyllum and Other Genera

Filamentous basidiomycetes, as well as species of smuts which may appear yeastlike (*Ustilaginaceae* and *Tilletiaceae*), are commonly isolated from respiratory specimens and sometimes from blood; however, their significance can be difficult to evaluate (181, 196).

Schizophyllum commune is recognized as a significant cause of allergy-related sinusitis and pulmonary disease, including allergic bronchopulmonary mycosis and bronchial mucoid impaction (7, 27, 40, 93, 196, 198, 199) as well as infections of the brain, lungs, and buccal mucosa in both immunocompetent and immunosuppressed patients (93, 177, 179, 195, 196). *Coprinus cinereus* or its anamorph *Hormographiella aspergillata* has been reported from prosthetic valve endocarditis, fatal lung infections in leukemic patients, a lung abscess in a patient with non-Hodgkin's lymphoma, keratomycosis in a dog, and cutaneous lesions (110, 172, 195, 212, 228). *Inonotus tropicalis* was reported as an agent of osteomyelitis in a patient with X-linked chronic granulomatous disease (45, 217) and has also been seen in an additional patient with this disease (D. Sutton, unpublished data).

Hyphomycetes

Scopulariopsis

Scopulariopsis brevicaulis, the most common etiologic agent and contaminant (Fig. 4F), and other species are occasional agents of onychomycosis (2, 94, 194). They are also rarely invasive, causing otomycosis, keratitis, prosthetic

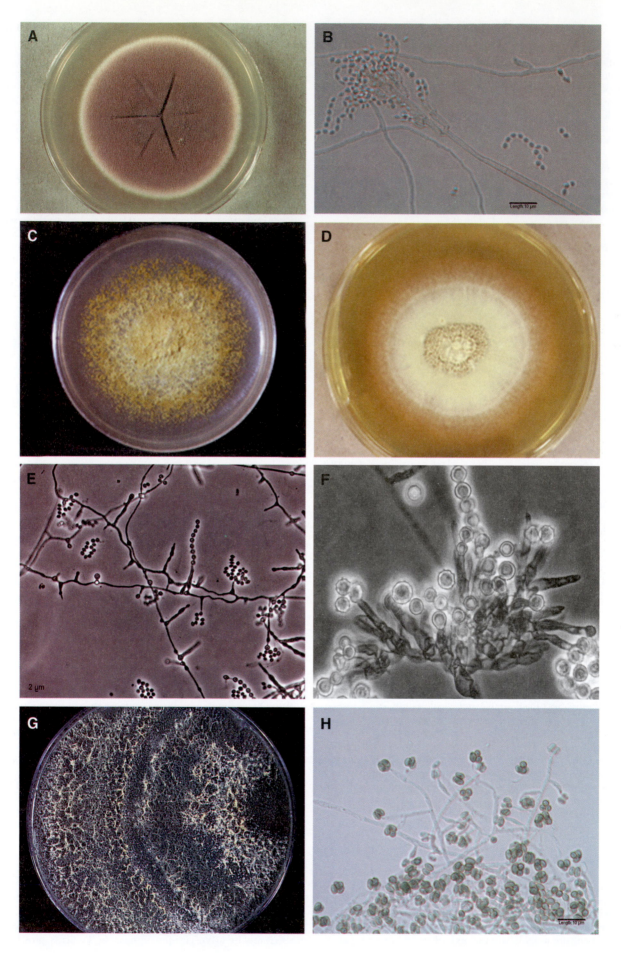

valve endocarditis, sinusitis, pneumonia, brain abscess, and subcutaneous and bone invasion in immunocompetent and immunosuppressed individuals (14, 47, 107, 120, 124, 162, 189). *Scopulariopsis candida* and *Scopulariopsis acremonium* have been reported from invasive sinusitis, but few details concerning the latter species were provided in the report (58, 106). Brain abscess caused by *Scopulariopsis brumptii* and invasive cutaneous infection caused by *M. cirrosus* have been reported to occur in liver transplant and bone marrow recipients, respectively (107, 157). A case of fatal *Scopulariopsis acremonium* was reported to occur in a lung transplant recipient (233).

Acremonium, Lecythophora, and Phialemonium

Many reports concerning *Acremonium* species involve infections of the nail, skin, eye, or mycetoma (see also chapter 123) (47, 94). Localized and disseminated infections occur in patients following valve replacement, dialysis, or transplantation or in patients with hematologic or solid-organ malignancies (47, 76, 188, 201, 210, 230). Fungemia is common. Several cases of invasive *Acremonium strictum* have been reported (61, 99, 125). *Phialemonium obovatum* was an agent of endocarditis (66), while arthritis, fungemia, endovascular infections, and ophthalmitis have been reported for *P. curvatum* (44, 80, 166, 231).

Onychocola

Onychocola canadensis (Fig. 3F and G) causes distal subungual onychomycosis or, less commonly, white superficial onychomycosis and infection of the glabrous skin (82, 94, 194, 197). Although *O. canadensis* is an uncommon cause of onychomycosis, more than 60 isolates from nails have now been recorded from New Zealand, Australia, Europe, and the United States, with two additional cases from Spain (118).

Beauveria and Engyodontium

Beauveria bassiana has caused several cases of fungal keratitis (104, 122). A recent molecular study comparing clinical keratitis isolates with Environmental Protection Agency-registered strains showed that these strains were unrelated (155, 223). An isolate that failed to grow at 35°C also caused disseminated disease in a patient with acute lymphoblastic leukemia (224). *E. album* was a cause of endocarditis (13).

Chrysosporium and Myceliophthora Species

The thermotolerant *Chrysosporium zonatum* is an etiologic agent of human pneumonia and osteomyelitis (180) (Fig. 3B and C), while the *Chrysosporium* anamorph of *Nannizziopsis vriesii*, *Chrysosporium ophiodiicola* (171), *Chyrysosporium guarroi* (1), and other, as-yet-undescribed species are pathogenic for reptiles. The thermophilic species *Myceliophthora thermophila* (Fig. 3E) has been reported to cause fatal aortic vasculitis in two patients, was isolated from the brain of a patient who developed a bacterial cerebral abscess after trauma, and is an agent of severe osteomyelitis following a pitchfork injury (23, 49, 60, 220).

Metarhizium and Trichoderma Species

Metarhizium anisopliae is an insect pathogen of wide distribution documented to cause keratitis, sinusitis, invasive infections, and disseminated skin lesions (26, 32, 153, 174). Species of *Trichoderma* in the section *Longibrachiatum*, which includes *T. longibrachiatum* (Fig. 4G and H) and *T. citrinoviride*, appear to be the most important pathogenic species (37, 128, 176, 192).

Paecilomyces, Acrophialophora, Phialosimplex, and Geosmithia Species

Clinical manifestations of both *P. lilacinus* and *P. variotii* include cutaneous and subcutaneous infections, pulmonary infection, pyelonephritis, sinusitis, cellulitis, endocarditis, and fungemia in both immunocompetent and immunocompromised patients (30, 35, 47, 201, 210, 232). The clinical manifestations, treatment options, and outcomes for *P. lilacinus* infections have recently been reviewed (152, 156). *Acrophialophora fusispora* was the etiologic agent in a brain abscess in a child with leukemia (6) and has been recovered in pulmonary infections (79, 216) and cases of keratitis (79). It also appears to be a frequent colonizer in patients with cystic fibrosis (38, 163). *Phialosimplex caninus* sp. nov., seen primarily in dogs, has also been recovered from pleural fluid and tissue from a human (203).

Coelomycetes

Colletotrichum and Phoma

Colletotrichum species are primarily phytopathogens but occasionally are recovered as agents of keratitis (47, 48). There are also rare reports of subcutaneous infection following trauma (81).

Collection, Transport, and Storage of Specimens

Methods of collection, transport, and storage of specimens are detailed in chapter 112. As with other invasive mycoses, infections are difficult to diagnose and usually require a combination of clinical, culture, and radiographic findings. The recovery from a normally sterile site and microscopic evidence of invasive growth in tissue provide the most convincing evidence of disease.

Direct Examination

Microscopy

Histopathological findings for most opportunistic hyaline moulds are typically indistinguishable from those of species of *Aspergillus*, *Fusarium*, and *Pseudallescheria* (162). Ascospores may occasionally be seen, as was demonstrated with *Gymnascella* (89), and clamp connections may also be seen in tissue sections with *Schizophyllum commune* (177). Budding forms may also rarely be seen (117, 188, 230).

Antigen Detection

Detection of $(1{\rightarrow}3)$-β-D-glucan (142, 143) in patients with invasive hyalohyphomycosis may assist with an early

---

FIGURE 4 (A) Colony of *Paecilomyces lilacinus* on potato dextrose agar after 14 days. (B) Verticillate conidiophores of *Paecilomyces lilacinus* bearing whorls of phialides. Bar, 10 μm. (C) Yellowish colony of *Phialemonium curvatum* on potato flake agar after 14 days at 25°C. (D) Colony of *Phialosimplex caninus* with yellow diffusible pigment on potato dextrose agar after 21 days at 30°C. (E) Conidia of *Phialosimplex caninus* borne in long chains or heads from simple basally inflated phialides. Bar, 2 μm. (F) Rough-walled conidia in chains formed on annellides in *Scopulariopsis brevicaulis*. Note branched conidiogenous apparatus. Magnification, ×580. (G) Colony of *Trichoderma longibrachiatum* on potato dextrose agar after 4 days at 37°C. Note that the plate has been inoculated on one side. (H) Green, oval conidia of *Trichoderma longibrachiatum*. Bar, 10 μm.

diagnosis, but monitoring of this marker needs to be combined with clinical examination of the patient and other diagnostic procedures, such as high-resolution computed tomography scanning.

Nucleic Acid Detection

Luminex microbead hybridization technology using 75 species- and genus-specific hybridization probes has recently been reported to detect a variety of fungal pathogens from clinical blood and pulmonary samples. This method appears to have promise for the early detection and identification of various invasive fungal pathogens (111).

Isolation Procedures

Opportunistic hyaline moulds are usually easily recovered on routine mycological media, and there are no specific growth requirements; however, media with and without cycloheximide should be employed. The fungicide benomyl at a final concentration of 10 μg/ml in the culture medium can be useful to distinguish filamentous basidiomycetes, which are tolerant to benomyl, from isolates of ascomycetous origin, which may be sensitive to benomyl (209). Coelomycetes grow well on most fungal media; however, they are notorious for remaining sterile without extended incubation (up to several weeks for some genera) (213). See chapter 112 for detailed information on appropriate media for initial plating and isolation.

Identification

More detailed descriptions of these hyaline fungi are found in several identification manuals and in the references cited therein (47, 48, 94, 215). Many can be identified to the genus level with little difficulty; however, several require sequencing. See Table 3 for salient phenotypic features of the organisms reviewed.

Typing Systems

Although comparative sequence analysis of clinical isolates is becoming more common in large tertiary-care and research centers, it is far from standardized. Various methods of DNA extraction are available (62), and several different genes or portions thereof may be sequenced (20, 41, 145–151, 167, 191, 237). The use of molecular characterization to identify isolates that remain sterile in culture presents significant problems in that the species identification, when determined by percent identity, cannot be confirmed by phenotypic features. Several nonsporulating moulds were sequenced by Pounder et al. (164), and this practice will likely continue. It should be highlighted, however, that several database entries in public databases are incorrect, making comparative sequence analysis without phenotypic correlation fraught with uncertainty (20). On the other hand, molecular characterization has become the "gold standard" for classification of species for taxonomic categorization and will continue to provide a better understanding of the evolutionary relationships of clinically significant fungi (85, 145–151, 191).

Serologic Tests

Serologic procedures currently have little clinical utility in the diagnosis of uncommon hyaline opportunistic fungi.

Antimicrobial Susceptibilities

Uncommon hyaline moulds display various antifungal susceptibility patterns. Their infrequent isolation makes reference laboratory susceptibility testing of a group of similar isolates useful for empirical antifungal therapy; however, patient isolates should be assessed individually for appropriate patient management. Please see references relating to the genera discussed for published in vitro data. Treatment failures in *Chaetomium* infections have been reported when patients were treated with amphotericin B alone or in combination with itraconazole. Voriconazole and the experimental triazoles ravuconazole and albaconazole showed potent activity in vitro, with MICs of less than 0.5 μg/ml (193). The echinocandin micafungin was not active in vitro. Evaluation of antifungal activitiy in 44 clinical isolates of filamentous basidiomycetous fungi, including *Schizophyllum commune* (n = 5), *Coprinus* species (n = 8), *Bjerkandera adusta* (n = 14), and sterile, uncharacterized basidiomycetes (n = 17), demonstrated low MICs of amphotericin B, itraconazole, voriconazole, and posaconazole, in contrast to those of fluconazole and flucytosine (73). No statistically significant differences among the genera were noted.

Antifungals, including amphotericin B and itraconazole, have limited in vitro activity against *Scopulariopsis* species, and conflicting results have been reported for voriconazole and terbinafine (65, 206). In vitro, promising interaction was observed between terbinafine and fluconazole, itraconazole, and voriconazole against isolates of *S. brevicaulis*, although clinical experience with combination therapy is very limited (183). When *Paecilomyces* species were evaluated by the European Committee on Antimicrobial Susceptibility Testing methodology (113, 114), amphotericin B, itraconazole, and the echinocandins showed poor activity against 27 strains of *P. lilacinus*; however, the newer triazoles voriconazole, ravuconazole, and posaconazole and the allylamine terbinafine showed low MIC₉₀s. In contrast, 31 strains of *P. variotii* demonstrated low MICs of all of the above agents except voriconazole and ravuconazole (29).

Evaluation, Interpretation, and Reporting of Results

As for the fusaria, the early diagnosis of invasive hyalohyphomycosis caused by other hyaline moulds is often key to appropriate management strategies. The identification of uncommon hyaline moulds should always be evaluated in light of the patient's immune status as well as the anatomic site of recovery and frequency of isolation.

We thank Lynne Sigler, University of Alberta Microfungus Collection & Herbarium, Devonian Botanic Garden, Edmonton, Alberta, Canada, and Kerry O'Donnell, Bacterial Foodborne Pathogens and Mycology, NCAUR-ARS-USDA, Peoria, IL, for their helpful comments and review of this chapter.

REFERENCES

1. Abarca, M. L., G. Castellá, J. Martorell, and F. J. Cabanes. 2010. *Chrysosporium guarroi* sp. nov. a new emerging pathogen of pet green iguanas (*Iguana iguana*). Med. Mycol. 48:365–372.
2. Abbott, S. P., and L. Sigler. 2001. Heterothallism in the Microascaceae demonstrated by three species in the *Scopulariopsis brevicaulis* series. Mycologia 93:1211–1220.
3. Abbott, S. P., L. Sigler, R. McAleer, D. A. McGough, M. G. Rinaldi, and G. Mizell. 1995. Fatal cerebral mycoses caused by the ascomycete *Chaetomium strumarium*. J. Clin. Microbiol. 33:2692–2698.
4. Abd-Elsalam, K. A., J. R. Guo, F. Schnieder, A. M. Asran-Amal, and J. A. Verreet. 2004. Comparative assessment of genotyping methods for study of genetic diversity of *Fusarium oxysporum* isolates. Pol. J. Microbiol. 53:167–174.
5. Ajello, L. 1986. Hyalohyphomycosis and phaeohyphomycosis: two global disease entities of public health importance. Eur. J. Epidemiol. 2:243–251.
6. Al-Mohsen, I. Z., D. A. Sutton, L. Sigler, E. Almodovar, N. Mahgoub, H. Frayha, S. Al-Hajjar, M. G. Rinaldi, and

T. J. Walsh. 2000. *Acrophialophora fusispora* brain abscess in a child with acute lymphoblastic leukemia: review of cases and taxonomy. *J. Clin. Microbiol.* **38:**4569–4576.

7. **Amitani, R., K. Nishimura, A. Niimi, H. Kobayashi, R. Nawada, T. Murayama, H. Taguchi, and F. Kuze.** 1996. Bronchial mucoid impaction due to the monokaryotic mycelium of *Schizophyllum commune. Clin. Infect. Dis.* **22:**146–148.

8. **Anaissie, E. J., R. T. Kuchar, J. H. Rex, A. Francesconi, M. Kasai, F.-M. Müller, M. Lozano-Chiu, R. C. Summerbell, M. C. Dignani, S. J. Chanock, and T. J. Walsh.** 2001. Fusariosis associated with pathogenic *Fusarium* species colonization of a hospital water system: a new paradigm for the epidemiology of opportunistic mold infections. *Clin. Infect. Dis.* **33:**1871–1878.

9. **Aribandi, M., C. Bazan, and M. G. Rinaldi.** 2005. Magnetic resonance imaging findings in a fatal primary cerebral infection due to *Chaetomium strumarium. Australas. Radiol.* **49:**166–169.

10. **Arikan, S., M. Lozano-Chiu, V. Paetznick, S. Nangia, and J. H. Rex.** 1999. Microdilution susceptibility testing of amphotericin B, itraconazole, and voriconazole against clinical isolates of *Aspergillus* and *Fusarium* species. *J. Clin. Microbiol.* **37:**3946–3951.

11. **Arikan, S., M. Lozano-Chiu, V. Paetznick, and J. H. Rex.** 2001. In vitro susceptibility testing methods for caspofungin against *Aspergillus* and *Fusarium* isolates. *Antimicrob. Agents Chemother.* **45:**327–330.

12. **Ascioglu, S., J. H. Rex, B. de Pauw, J. E. Bennett, J. Bille, F. Crokaert, et al.** 2002. Invasive Fungal Infections Cooperative Group of the European Organization for Research and Treatment of Cancer; Mycoses Study Group of the National Institute of Allergy and Infectious Diseases. Defining opportunistic invasive fungal infections in immunocompromised patients with cancer and hematopoietic stem cell transplants: an international consensus. *Clin. Infect. Dis.* **34:**7–14.

13. **Augustinsky, J., P. Kammeyer, A. Husain, G. S. de Hoog, and C. R. Libertin.** 1990. *Engyodontium album* endocarditis. *J. Clin. Microbiol.* **28:**1479–1481.

14. **Aznar, C., C. de Bievre, and C. Guiguen.** 1989. Maxillary sinusitis from *Microascus cinereus* and *Aspergillus repens. Mycopathologia* **105:**93–97.

15. **Azor, M., J. Gené, J. Cano, and J. Guarro.** 2007. Universal in vitro antifungal resistance of genetic clades of the *Fusarium solani* species complex. *Antimicrob. Agents Chemother.* **51:**1500–1503.

16. **Azor, M., J. Gené, J. Cano, P. Manikandan, N. Venkatapathy, and J. Guarro.** 2009. Less frequent species of *Fusarium* of clinical interest: correlation between morphological and molecular identification and antifungal susceptibility. *J. Clin. Microbiol.* **47:**1463–1468.

17. **Azor, M., J. Gené, J. Cano, D. A. Sutton, A. W. Fothergill, M. G. Rinaldi, and J. Guarro.** 2008. In vitro antifungal susceptibility and molecular characterization of clinical isolates of *Fusarium verticillioides* (*F. moniliforme*) and *Fusarium thapsinum. Antimicrob. Agents Chemother.* **52:**2228–2231.

18. **Baddley, J. W., S. A. Moser, D. A. Sutton, and P. G. Pappas.** 2000. *Microascus cinereus* (anamorph *Scopulariopsis*) brain abscess in a bone marrow transplant recipient. *J. Clin. Microbiol.* **38:**395–397.

19. **Baddley, J. W., T. P. Stroud, D. Salzman, and P. G. Pappas.** 2001. Invasive mold infections in allogenic bone marrow transplant recipients. *Clin. Infect. Dis.* **32:**1319–1324.

20. **Balajee, S. A., A. M. Borman, M. E. Brandt, J. Cano, M. Cuenca-Estrella, E. Dannaoui, J. Guarro, G. Haase, C. C. Kibler, K. O'Donnell, C. A. Petti, J. L. Rodriguez-Tudela, D. Sutton, A. Velegraki, and B. L. Wickes.** 2009. Sequence-based identification of *Aspergillus*, *Fusarium*, and *Mucorales* species in the clinical mycology laboratory: where are we and where should we go from here? *J. Clin. Microbiol.* **47:**877–884.

21. **Barron, M. A., D. A. Sutton, R. Veve, J. Guarro, M. Rinaldi, E. Thompson, P. J. Cagnoni, K. Moultney, and N. E. Madinger.** 2003. Invasive mycotic infections caused by *Chaetomium perlucidum*, a new agent of cerebral phaeohyphomycosis. *J. Clin. Microbiol.* **41:**5302–5307.

22. **Boerema, G. H., J. de Gruyter, M. E. Noordeloos, and M. E. C. Hamers.** 2004. Phoma *Identification Manual. Differentiation of Specific and Infra-Specific Taxa in Culture.* CABI Publishing, Cambridge, MA.

23. **Bourbeau, P., D. A. McGough, H. Fraser, N. Shah, and M. G. Rinaldi.** 1992. Fatal disseminated infection caused by *Myceliophthora thermophila*, a new agent of mycosis: case history and laboratory characteristics. *J. Clin. Microbiol.* **30:**3019–3023.

24. **Boutati, E. I., and E. J. Anaissie.** 1997. *Fusarium*, a significant emerging pathogen in patients with hematologic malignancy: ten years' experience at a cancer center and implications for management. *Blood* **90:**999–1008.

25. **Brockus, C. W., R. K. Myers, J. M. Crandell, D. A. Sutton, B. L. Wickes, and K. K. Nakasone.** 2009. Disseminated *Oxyporus corticola* infection in a German shepherd dog. *Med. Mycol.* **47:**862–868.

26. **Bugner, D., G. Eagles, M. Burgess, P. Procopis, M. Rogers, D. Muir, R. Pritchard, A. Hocking, and M. Priest.** 1998. Disseminated invasive infection due to *Metarrhizium anisopliae* in an immunocompromised child. *J. Clin. Microbiol.* **36:**1146–1150.

27. **Buzina, W., D. Lang-Loidolt, H. Braun, K. Freudenschuss, and H. Stammberger.** 2001. Development of molecular methods for identification of *Schizophyllum commune* from clinical samples. *J. Clin. Microbiol.* **39:**2391–2396.

28. **Cano, J., J. Guarro, and J. Gené.** 2004. Molecular and morphological identification of *Colletotrichum* species of clinical interest. *J. Clin. Microbiol.* **42:**2450–2454.

29. **Castelli, M. V., A. Alastruey-Izquierdo, I. Cuesta, A. Monzon, E. Mellado, J. L. Rodríguez-Tudela, and M. Cuenca-Estrella.** 2008. Susceptibility testing and molecular classification of *Paecilomyces* spp. *Antimicrob. Agents Chemother.* **52:**2926–2928.

30. **Castro, L. G. M., A. Salebian, and M. N. Sotto.** 1990. Hyalohyphomycosis by *Paecilomyces lilacinus* in a renal transplant patient and a review of human *Paecilomyces* species infections. *J. Med. Vet. Mycol.* **28:**15–26.

31. **Célard, M., E. Dannaoui, M. A. Piens, E. Guého, G. Kirkorian, T. Greenland, F. Vandenesch, and S. Picot.** 1999. Early *Microascus cinereus* endocarditis of a prosthetic valve implanted after *Staphylococcus aureus* endocarditis of the native valve. *Clin. Infect. Dis.* **29:**691–692.

32. **Cepero de Garcia, M. C., M. L. Arboleda, F. Barraquer, and E. Grose.** 1997. Fungal keratitis caused by *Metarrhizium anisopliae. J. Med. Vet. Mycol.* **35:**361–363.

33. **Chandler, F. W., and J. C. Watts.** 1987. *Pathologic Diagnosis of Fungal Infections.* American Society of Clinical Pathologists, Inc., Chicago, IL.

34. **Chang, D. C., G. B. Grant, K. O'Donnell, K. A. Wannemuehler, J. Noble-Wang, C. Y. Rao, L. M. Jacobson, C. S. Crowell, R. S. Sneed, F. M. T. Lewis, J. K. Schaffzin, M. A. Kainer, C. A. Genese, E. C. Alfonso, D. B. Jones, A. Srinivasan, S. K. Fridkin, and B. J. Park for the *Fusarium* Keratitis Investigation Team.** 2006. Multistate outbreak of *Fusarium* keratitis associated with use of a contact lens solution. *JAMA* **296:**953–963.

35. **Chan-Tack, K. M., C. L. Thio, N. S. Miller, C. L. Karp, C. Ho, and W. G. Merz.** 1999. *Paecilomyces lilacinus* fungemia in an adult bone marrow transplant recipient. *Med. Mycol.* **37:**57–60.

36. **Chin-Hong, P. V., D. A. Sutton, M. Roemer, M. A. Jacobson, and J. A. Aberg.** 2001. Invasive fungal sinusitis and meningitis due to *Arthrographis kalrae* in a patient with AIDS. *J. Clin. Microbiol.* **39:**804–807.

37. **Chouaki, T., V. Lavarde, L. Lachaud, C. P. Raccurt, and C. Hennequin.** 2002. Invasive infections due to *Trichoderma* species; report of 2 cases, findings of in vitro susceptibility testing, and review of the literature. *Clin. Infect. Dis.* **35:**1360–1367.

38. **Cimon, B., S. Challier, H. Béguin, J. Carrère, C. Chabasse, and J.-P. Bouchara.** 2005. Airway colonization by *Acrophialophora fusispora* in patients with cystic fibrosis. *J. Clin. Microbiol.* **43:**1484–1487.

39. **Clancy, C. J., and M. H. Nguyen.** 1998. In vitro efficacy and fungicidal activity of voriconazole against *Aspergillus*

and *Fusarium* species. *Eur. J. Clin. Microbiol. Infect. Dis.* **17:**573–575.

40. **Clark, S., C. K. Campbell, A. Sandison, and D. I. Choa.** 1996. *Schizophyllum commune:* an unusual isolate from a patient with allergic fungal sinusitis. *J. Infect.* **32:**147–150.

41. **Clinical and Laboratory Standards Institute.** 2008. *Interpretive Criteria for Identification of Bacteria and Fungi by DNA Target Sequencing: Guideline.* Clinical and Laboratory Standards Institute document MM18-A. Clinical and Laboratory Standards Institute, Wayne, PA.

42. **Clinical and Laboratory Standards Institute.** 2008. *Reference Method for Broth Dilution Antifungal Susceptibility Testing of Filamentous Fungi.* Approved standard, 2nd ed. Clinical and Laboratory Standards Institute document M38-A2. Clinical and Laboratory Standards Institute, Wayne, PA.

43. **Clinical and Laboratory Standards Institute/NCCLS.** 2002. *Reference Method for Broth Dilution Antifungal Susceptibility Testing of Filamentous Fungi.* Approved standard. NCCLS document M38-A. Clinical and Laboratory Standards Institute/NCCLS, Wayne, PA.

44. **Dan, M., O. Yossepowitch, D. Hendel, O. Shwartz, and D. A. Sutton.** 2006. *Phialemonium curvatum* arthritis of the knee following intra-articular injection of a corticosteroid. *Med. Mycol.* **44:**571–574.

45. **Davis, C. M., L. M. Noroski, M. K. Dishop, D. A. Sutton, R. M. Broverman, M. E. Paul, and H. M. Rosenblatt.** 2007. Basidiomycetous fungal *Inonotus tropicalis* sacral osteomyelitis in X-linked chronic granulomatous disease. *Pediatr. Infect. Dis. J.* **26:**655–656.

46. **De Beer, Z. W., D. Begerow, R. Bauer, G. S. Pegg, P. W. Crous, and M. J. Wingfield.** 2006. Phylogeny of the *Quambalariaceae* fam. nov., including important *Eucalyptus* pathogens in South Africa and Australia. *Stud. Mycol.* **55:**289–298.

47. **De Hoog, G. S., J. Guarro, J. Gené, and M. J. Fígueras.** 2000. *Atlas of Clinical Fungi,* 2nd ed. Centraalbureau voor Schimmelcultures, Baarn, The Netherlands.

48. **De Hoog, G. S., J. Guarro, J. Gene, and M. J. Fígueras.** 2009. *Atlas of Clinical Fungi,* pilot version of 3rd ed., CD-ROM. Centraalbureau voor Schimmelcultures, Baarn, The Netherlands.

49. **Destino, L., D. A. Sutton, A. L. Helon, P. L. Havens, J. G. Thometz, R. E. Willoughby, Jr., and M. J. Chusid.** 2006. Severe osteomyelitis caused by *Myceliophthora thermophila* after a pitchfork injury. *Ann. Clin. Microbiol. Antimicrob.* **5:**21.

50. **Diekema, D. J., S. A. Messer, R. J. Hollis, R. N. Jones, and M. A. Pfaller.** 2003. Activities of caspofungin, itraconazole, posaconazole, ravuconazole, voriconazole, and amphotericin B against 448 recent clinical isolates of filamentous fungi. *J. Clin. Microbiol.* **41:**3623–3626.

51. **Di Pietro, A., M. P. Madred, Z. Caracuel, J. Delgado-Jarana, and M. I. G. Roncero.** 2003. *Fusarium oxysporum:* exploring the molecular arsenal of a vascular wilt pathogen. *Mol. Plant Pathol.* **4:**315–325.

52. **Domsch, K. H., W. Gams, and T.-H. Anderson.** 1980. *Compendium of Soil Fungi.* IHW-Verlag, Eching, Germany. [Reprinted in 1993.]

53. **Domsch, K. H., W. Gams, and T.-H. Anderson.** 2007. *Compendium of Soil Fungi,* 2nd ed. IHW-Verlag, Eching, Germany.

54. **Driver, F., R. J. Milner, and J. W. H. Trueman.** 2000. A taxonomic revision of *Metarhizium* based on a phylogenetic analysis of rDNA sequence data. *Mycol. Res.* **104:**134–150.

55. **Druzhinina, I. S., A. G. Kopchinskiy, and C. P. Kubicek.** 2006. The first 100 *Trichoderma* species characterized by molecular data. *Mycoscience* **47:**55–64.

56. **Duthie, R., and D. W. Denning.** 1995. *Aspergillus* fungemia: report of two cases and review. *Clin. Infect. Dis.* **20:**598–605.

57. **Ellis, D., S. Davis, H. Alexiou, R. Handke, and R. Bartley.** 2007. *Descriptions of Medical Fungi.* Nexus Print Solutions, Underdale, South Australia, Australia.

58. **Ellison, M. D., R. T. Hung, K. Harris, and B. H. Campbell.** 1998. Report of the first case of invasive fungal sinusitis caused by *Scopulariopsis acremonium.* *Arch. Otolaryngol. Head Neck Surg.* **124:**1014–1016.

59. **Espinel-Ingroff, A.** 2001. Comparison of the E-test with the NCCLS M38-P method for antifungal susceptibility testing of common and emerging pathogenic filamentous fungi. *J. Clin. Microbiol.* **39:**1360–1367.

60. **Farina, C., A. Gamba, R. Tambini, H. Beguin, and J. L. Trouillet.** 1998. Fatal aortic *Myceliophthora thermophila* infection in a patient affected by cystic medial necrosis. *Med. Mycol.* **36:**113–118.

61. **Foell, J. L., M. Fischer, M. Seibold, M. Borneff-Lipp, A. Wawer, G. Horneff, and S. Burdach.** 2006. Lethal double infection with *Acremonium strictum* and *Aspergillus fumigatus* during induction chemotherapy in a child with ALL. *Pediatr. Blood Cancer* **49:**858–861.

62. **Fredricks, D. N., C. Smith, and A. Meier.** 2005. Comparison of six DNA extraction methods for recovery of fungal DNA as assessed by quantitative PCR. *J. Clin. Microbiol.* **43:**5122–5128.

63. **Gams, W.** 1978. Connected and disconnected chains of phialoconidia and *Sagenomella* gen. nov. segregated from *Acremonium. Persoonia* **10:**97–110.

64. **Gams, W., and M. R. McGinnis.** 1983. *Phialemonium,* a new anamorphic genus intermediate between *Phialophora* and *Acremonium. Mycologia* **75:**977–987.

65. **Garcia-Effron, G., A. Gomez-Lopez, E. Mellado, A. Monzon, J. L. Rodriguez-Tudela, and M. Cuenca-Estrella.** 2004. In vitro activity of terbinafine against medically important non-dermatophyte species of filamentous fungi. *J. Antimicrob. Chemother.* **53:**1086–1089.

66. **Gavin, P. J., D. A. Sutton, and B. Z. Katz.** 2002. Fatal endocarditis caused by the dematiaceous fungus *Phialemonium obovatum:* case report and review of the literature. *J. Clin. Microbiol.* **40:**2207–2212.

67. **Geiser, D. M., M. del Mar Jiménez-Gasco, S. Kang, I. Makalowska, N. Veeraraaghavan, T. J. Ward, N. Zhang, G. A. Kuldau, and K. O'Donnell.** 2004. FUSARIUM-ID v. 1.0: a DNA sequence database for identifying *Fusarium. Eur. J. Plant Pathol.* **110:**473–479.

68. **Gené, J., J. L. Blanco, J. Cano, M. E. García, and J. Guarro.** 2003. New filamentous fungus *Sagenomella chlamydospora* responsible for a disseminated infection in a dog. *J. Clin. Microbiol.* **41:**1722–1725.

69. **Girmenia, C., W. Arcese, A. Micozzi, P. Martino, P. Bianco, and G. Morace.** 1992. Onychomycosis as a possible origin of disseminated *Fusarium solani* infection in a patient with severe aplastic anemia. *Clin. Infect. Dis.* **14:**1167.

70. **Girmenia, C., L. Pagano, L. Corvatta, L. Mele, A. Del Favero, and P. Martino for the Gimena Infection Programme.** 2000. The epidemiology of fusariosis in patients with haematological diseases. *Br. J. Haematol.* **111:**272–276.

71. **Glenn, A. F., C. W. Bacon, R. Price, and R. T. Hanlin.** 1996. Molecular phylogeny of *Acremonium* and its taxonomic implications. *Mycologia* **88:**369–383.

72. **Godoy, P., J. Cano, J. Gene, J. Guarro, A. L. Hofling-Lima, and A. L. Colombo.** 2004. Genotyping of 44 isolates of *Fusarium solani,* the main agent of fungal keratitis in Brazil. *J. Clin. Microbiol.* **42:**4494–4497.

73. **González, G. M., D. A. Sutton, E. Thompson, R. Tijerina, and M. G. Rinaldi.** 2001. In vitro activities of approved and investigational antifungal agents against 44 clinical isolates of basidiomycetous fungi. *Antimicrob. Agents Chemother.* **45:**633–635.

74. **Grant, D. C., D. A. Sutton, C. A. Sandberg, R. D. Tyler, Jr., E. H. Thompson, A. M. Romanelli, and B. L. Wickes.** 2009. Disseminated *Geosmithia argillacea* infection in a German shepherd dog. *Med. Mycol.* **47:**221–226.

75. **Grossi, P., C. Farina, R. Fiocchi, and D. Dalla Gasperina.** 2000. Prevalence and outcome of invasive fungal infections in 1,963 thoracic organ transplant recipients: a multicenter retrospective study. *Transplantation* **70:**112–116.

76. **Guarro, J., W. Gams, I. Pujol, and J. Gene.** 1997. *Acremonium* species: new emerging fungal opportunists—in vitro antifungal susceptibilities and review. *Clin. Infect. Dis.* **25:**1222–1229.

77. **Guarro, J., and J. Gené.** 2002. *Acrophialophora fusispora* misidentified as *Scedosporium prolificans*. *J. Clin. Microbiol.* **40:**3544–3545. (Authors' reply, **40:**3545.)

78. **Guarro, J., J. Gené, and A.M. Stchigel.** 1999. Developments in fungal taxonomy. *Clin. Microbiol. Rev.* **12:**454–500.

79. **Guarro, J., D. K. Mendiratta, H. De Sequeira, V. Rodríguez, D. Thamke, A. M. Gomes, A. K. Shuklal, F. Menezes, P. Narang, J. R. Vieira, and J. Gené.** 2007. *Acrophialophora fusispora*: an emerging agent of human mycoses. A report of 3 new clinical cases. *Diagn. Microbiol. Infect. Dis.* **59:**85–88.

80. **Guarro, J., M. Nucci, T. Akiti, J. Gené, J. Cano, M. Da Gloria, C. Barreiro, and C. Aguilar.** 1999. *Phialemonium* fungemia: two documented nosocomial cases. *J. Clin. Microbiol.* **37:**2493–2497.

81. **Guarro, J., T. E. Svidzinski, L. Zaror, M. H. Forjaz, J. Gené, and O. Fischman.** 1998. Subcutaneous hyalohyphomycosis caused by *Colletotrichum gloeosporioides*. *J. Clin. Microbiol.* **36:**3060–3065.

82. **Gupta, A. K., C. B. Horgan-Bell, and R. C. Summerbell.** 1998. Onychomycosis associated with *Onychocola canadensis*: ten case reports and a review of the literature. *J. Am. Acad. Dermatol.* **39:**410–417.

83. **Hay, R. J.** 2007. *Fusarium* infections of the skin. *Curr. Opin. Infect. Dis.* **20:**115–117.

84. **Healy, M., K. Reece, D. Walton, J. Huong, S. Frye, I. I. Raad, and D. P. Kontoyiannis.** 2005. Use of the DiversiLab System for species and strain differentiation of *Fusarium* species isolates. *J. Clin. Microbiol.* **43:**5278–5280.

85. **Hibbett, D. S., M. Binder, J. F. Bischoff, M. Blackwell, P. F. Cannon, O. E. Eriksson, S. Huhndorf, T. James, P. M. Kirk, R. Lucking, H. Thorsten Lumbsch, F. Lutzoni, P. B. Matheny, D. J. McLaughlin, M. J. Powell, S. Redhead, C. L. Schoch, J. W. Spatafora, A. Stalpers, R. Vilgalys, M. C. Aime, A. Aptroot, R. Bauer, D. Begerow, G. L. Benny, L. A. Castlebury, P. W. Crous, Y. C. Dai, W. Gams, D. M. Geiser, G. W. Griffith, C. Gueidan, D. L. Hawksworth, G. Hestmark, K. Hosaka, R. A. Humber, K. D. Hyde, J. E. Ironside, U. Koljalg, C. P. Kurtzman, K. H. Larsson, R. Lichtwardt, J. Longcore, J. Miadlikowska, A. Miller, J. M. Moncalvo, S. Mozley-Standridge, F. Oberwinkler, E. Parmasto, V. Reeb, J. D. Rogers, C. Roux, L. Ryvarden, J. P. Sampaio, A. Schussler, J. Sugiyama, R. G. Thorn, L. Tibell, W. A. Untereiner, C. Walker, Z. Wang, A. Weir, M. Weiss, M. M. White, K. Winka, Y. J. Yao, and N. Zhang.** 2007. A higher-level phylogenetic classification of the fungi. *Mycol. Res.* **111:**509–547.

86. **Hue, F.-X., M. Huerre, M. A. Rouffault, and C. de Bievre.** 1999. Specific detection of *Fusarium* species in blood and tissues by a PCR technique. *J. Clin. Microbiol.* **37:**2434–2438.

87. **Ikemura, K., K. Ikegami, T. Shimazu, T. Yoshioka, and T. Sugimoto.** 1989. False-positive result in *Limulus* test caused by *Limulus* amebocyte lysate-reactive material in immunoglobulin products. *J. Clin. Microbiol.* **27:**1965–1968.

88. **Imamura, Y., J. Chandra, P. K. Mukherjee, A. A. Lattif, L. B. Szczotka-Flynn, E. Pearlman, J. H. Lass, K. O'Donnell, and M. A. Ghannoum.** 2008. *Fusarium* and *Candida albicans* on soft contact lenses: model development, influence of lens type, and susceptibility to lens care solutions. *Antimicrob. Agents Chemother.* **52:**171–182.

89. **Iwen, P. C., L. Sigler, S. R. Tarantolo, D. A. Sutton, M. G. Rinaldi, R. P. Lackner, D. I. McCarthy, and S. H. Hinrichs.** 2000. Pulmonary infection caused by *Gymnascella hyalinospora* in a patient with acute myelogenous leukemia. *J. Clin. Microbiol.* **38:**375–381.

90. **Jaakkola, M. S., S. Laitinen, R. Piipari, J. Uitti, H. Nordman, A. M. Haapala, and J. J. Jaakkola.** 2002. Immunoglobulin G antibodies against indoor dampness-related microbes and adult onset asthma: a population-based incident case-control study. *Clin. Exp. Immunol.* **129:**107–112.

91. **Jaeger, E. E., N. M. Carroll, S. Choudhury, A. A. Dunlop, H. M. Towler, M. M. Matheson, P. Adamson, N. Okhravi, and S. Lightman.** 2000. Rapid detection and identification of *Candida, Aspergillus,* and *Fusarium* species in ocular samples using nested PCR. *J. Clin. Microbiol.* **38:**2902–2908.

92. **Joffe, A. Z.** 1978. *Fusarium poae* and *F. sporotrichoides* as principal causal agents of alimentary toxic aleukia, p. 27–41. *In* T. Willie and L. Morehouse (ed.), *Mycotoxic Fungi, Mycotoxins, Mycotoxicoses. An Encyclopedic Handbook*. Marcel Dekker, Inc., New York, NY.

93. **Kamai, K., H. Unno, J. Ito, K. Nishimura, and M. Miyakji.** 1999. Analysis of the cases in which *Schizophyllum commune* was isolated. *Jpn. J. Med. Mycol.* **40:**175–181.

94. **Kane, J., R. Summerbell, L. Sigler, S. Krajden, and G. Land.** 1997. *Laboratory Handbook of Dermatophytes*. Star Publishing Co., Belmont, CA.

95. **Kappe, R., and A. Schulze-Berge.** 1993. New cause for false-positive results with the Pastorex *Aspergillus* antigen latex agglutination test. *J. Clin. Microbiol.* **31:**2489–2490.

96. **Katiyar, S. K., and T. D. Edlind.** 2009. Role of Fks1 in the intrinsic echinocandin resistance of *Fusarium solani* as evidenced by hybrid expression in *Saccharomyces cerevisiae*. *Antimicrob. Agents Chemother.* **53:**1772–1778.

97. **Kato, A., T. Takita, M. Furuhashi, T. Takahashi, Y. Maruyama, and A. Hishida.** 2001. Elevation of blood (1,3)-beta-D-glucan concentrations in hemodialysis patients. *Nephron* **89:**159.

98. **Kaufman, L., P. G. Standard, M. Jalbert, and D. Kraft.** 1997. Immunohistologic identification of *Aspergillus* spp. and other hyaline fungi by using polyclonal fluorescent antibodies. *J. Clin. Microbiol.* **35:**2206–2209.

99. **Keynan, Y., H. Sprecher, and G. Weber.** 2007. *Acremonium* vertebral osteomyelitis: molecular diagnosis and response to voriconazole. *Clin. Infect. Dis.* **45:**e5–e6.

100. **Khan, Z. U., S. Ahmad, and A. M. Theyyathel.** 2008. Diagnostic value of DNA and (1→3)-β-D-glucan detection in serum and bronchoalveolar lavage of mice experimentally infected with *Fusarium oxysporum*. *J. Med. Microbiol.* **57**(Pt. 1)**:**36–42.

101. **Khan, Z. U., H. S. Randhawa, T. Kowshik, S. N. Gaur, and G. A. de Vries.** 1988. The pathogenic potential of *Sporotrichum pruinosum* isolated from the human respiratory tract. *J. Med. Vet. Mycol.* **26:**145–151.

102. **Khor, W.-B., T. Aung, S.-M. Saw, T.-Y.Wong, P. A. Tambyah, A.-L.Tan, R. Beuerman, L. Lim, W.-K. Chan, W.-J. Heng, J. Lim, R. S. K. Loh, S.-B. Lee, and D. T. H. Tan.** 2006. An outbreak of *Fusarium* keratitis associated with contact lens wear in Singapore. *JAMA* **295:**2867–2873.

103. **Kirk, P. M., P. G. Cannon, J. C. David, and J. A. Stalpers.** 2001. *Ainsworth & Bisby's Dictionary of the Fungi*, 9th ed. CABI Bioscience, Surrey, United Kingdom.

104. **Kisla, T. A., A. Cu-Unjieng, L. Sigler, and J. Sugar.** 2000. Medical management of *Beauveria bassiana* keratitis. *Cornea* **19:**405–406.

105. **Kornerup, A., and J. H. Wanscher.** 1983. *Methuen Handbook of Colour*. Eyre Methuen Ltd., London, United Kingdom.

106. **Kriesel, J. D., E. E. Adderson, W. M. Gooch III, and A. T. Pavia.** 1994. Invasive sinonasal disease due to *Scopulariopsis candida*: case report and review of *Scopulariopsis*. *Clin. Infect. Dis.* **19:**317–319.

107. **Krisher, K. K., N. B. Holdridge, M. M. Mustafa, M. G. Rinaldi, and D. A. McGough.** 1995. Disseminated *Microascus cirrosus* infection in a pediatric bone marrow transplant patient. *J. Clin. Microbiol.* **33:**735–737.

108. **Kuhls, K., E. Lieckfeldt, T. Börner, and E. Guého.** 1999. Molecular reidentification of human pathogenic *Trichoderma* isolates as *Trichoderma longibrachiatum* and *Trichoderma citrinoviride*. *Med. Mycol.* **37:**25–33.

109. **Kuhn, D. M., and M. A. Ghannoum.** 2003. Indoor mold, toxigenic fungi, and *Stachybotrys chartarum*: infectious disease perspective. *Clin. Microbiol. Rev.* **16:**144–172.

110. **Lagrou, K., C. Massonet, K. Theunissen, W. Meersseman, M. Lontie, E. Verbeken, J. Van Eldere, and J. Maertens.** 2005. Fatal pulmonary infection in a leukaemic patient caused by *Hormographiella aspergillata*. *J. Med. Microbiol.* **54:**685–688.

111. **Landlinger, C., S. Preuner, B. Willinger, B. Haberpursch, Z. Racil, J. Mayer, and T. Lion.** 2009. Species-specific identification of a wide range of clinically relevant fungal

pathogens by use of Luminex xMAP technology. *J. Clin. Microbiol.* **47**:1063–1073.

112. **Lappalainen, S., A. L. Pasanen, M. Reiman, and P. Kalliokoski.** 1998. Serum IgG antibodies against *Wallemia sebi* and *Fusarium* species in Finnish farmers. *Ann. Allergy Asthma Immunol.* **81**:585–592.

113. **Lass-Flörl, C., M. Cuenca-Estrella, D. W. Denning, and J. L. Rodriguez-Tudela.** 2006. Antifungal susceptibility testing in *Aspergillus* spp. according to EUCAST methodology. *Med. Mycol.* **44**(Suppl.):319–325.

114. **Lass-Flörl, C., A. Mayr, S. Perkhofer, G. Hinterberger, J. Hausdorfer, C. Speth, and M. Fille.** 2008. Activities of antifungal agents against yeasts and filamentous fungi: assessment according to the methodology of the European Committee on Antimicrobial susceptibility Testing. *Antimicrob. Agents Chemother.* **52**:3637–3641.

115. **Leslie, J. F., and B. F. Summerell.** 2006. *The* Fusarium *Laboratory Manual.* Blackwell Publishing, Ames, IA.

116. **Lionakis, M. S., and D. P. Kontoyiannis.** 2004. The significance of isolation of saprophytic molds from the lower respiratory tract in patients with cancer. *Cancer* **100**:165–172.

117. **Liu, K., D. N. Howell, J. R. Perfect, and W. A. Schell.** 1998. Morphologic criteria for the preliminary identification of *Fusarium, Paecilomyces,* and *Acremonium* species by histopathology. *Am. J. Clin. Pathol.* **109**:45–54.

118. **Llovo, J., E. Prieto, H. Vazquez, and A. Muñoz.** 2002. Onychomycosis due to *Onychocola canadensis*: report of the first two Spanish cases. *Med. Mycol.* **40**:209–212.

119. **Lozano-Chiu, M., S. Arikan, V. L. Paetznick, E. J. Anaissie, D. Loebenberg, and J. H. Rex.** 1999. Treatment of murine fusariosis with SCH 56592. *Antimicrob. Agents Chemother.* **43**:589–591.

120. **Marques, A. R., K. J. Kwon-Chung, S. M. Holland, M. L. Turner, and J. J. Gallin.** 1995. Suppurative cutaneous granulomata caused by *Microascus cinereus* in a patient with chronic granulomatous disease. *Clin. Infect. Dis.* **20**:110–114.

121. **Mayayo, E., I. Pujol, and J. Guarro.** 1999. Experimental pathogenicity of four opportunistic *Fusarium* species in a murine model. *J. Med. Microbiol.* **48**:363–366.

122. **McDonnell, P. J., T. P. Werblin, L. Sigler, and W. R. Green.** 1985. Mycotic keratitis due to *Beauveria alba*. *Cornea* **3**:213–216.

123. **Middelhoven, W. J., E. Guého, and G. S. de Hoog.** 2000. Phylogenetic position and physiology of *Cerinosterus cyanescens*. *Antonie van Leeuwenhoek* **77**:313–320.

124. **Migrino, R. Q., G. S. Hall, and D. L. Longworth.** 1995. Deep tissue infections caused by *Scopulariopsis brevicaulis*: report of a case of prosthetic valve endocarditis and review. *Clin. Infect. Dis.* **21**:672–674.

125. **Miyakis, S., A. Velegraki, S. Delikou, A. Parcharidou, V. Papadakis, V. Kitra, I. Papadatos, and S. Polychronopoulou.** 2006. Invasive *Acremonium strictum* infection in a bone marrow transplant recipient. *Pediatr. Infect. Dis. J.* **25**:273–275.

126. **Mohammedi, I., M. A. Piens, C. Audigier-Valette, J. C. Gantier, L. Argaud, O. Martin, and D. Robert.** 2004. Fatal *Microascus trigonosporus* (anamorph *Scopulariopsis*) pneumonia in a bone marrow transplant recipient. *Eur. J. Microbiol. Infect. Dis.* **23**:215–217.

127. **Morton, F. J., and G. Smith.** 1963. The genera *Scopulariopsis* Bainier, *Microascus* Zukal, and *Doratomyces* Corda. *Mycol. Pap.* **86**:1–96.

128. **Munoz, F. M., G. J. Demmler, W. R. Travis, A. K. Ogden, S. N. Rossmann, and M. G. Rinaldi.** 1997. *Trichoderma longibrachiatum* infection in a pediatric patient with aplastic anemia. *J. Clin. Microbiol.* **35**:499–503.

129. **Musa, M. O., A. Al Eisa, M. Halim, E. Sahovic, M. Gyger, N. Chaudhri, F. Al Mohareb, P. Seth, M. Aslam, and M. Aljurf.** 2000. The spectrum of *Fusarium* infection in immunocompromised patients with haematological malignances and in non-immunocompromised patients: a single institution experience over 10 years. *Br. J. Haematol.* **108**:544–548.

130. **Nakao, A., M. Yasui, T. Kawagoe, H. Tamura, S. Tanaka, and H. Takagi.** 1997. False-positive endotoxemia derives from gauze glucan after hepatectomy for hepatocellular carcinoma with cirrhosis. *Hepatogastroenterology* **44**:1413–1418.

131. **Nelson, P. E., M. C. Dignani, and E. J. Anaissie.** 1994. Taxonomy, biology and clinical aspects of *Fusarium* species. *Clin. Microbiol. Rev.* **7**:479–504.

132. **Nelson, P. E., T. A. Toussoun, and W. F. O. Marasas.** 1983. Fusarium *Species: an Illustrated Manual of Identification.* Pennsylvania State University Press, State College.

133. **Ninet, B., I. Jan, O. Bontems, B. Lechenne, O. Jousson, D. Lew, J. Schrenzel, R. G. Panizzon, and M. Monod.** 2005. Molecular identification of *Fusarium* species in onychomycoses. *Dermatology* **210**:21–25.

134. **Nirenberg, H. I., and K. O'Donnell.** 1998. New *Fusarium* species and combinations within the *Gibberella fujikuroi* species complex. *Mycologia* **90**:434–458.

135. **Nir-Paz, R., J. Strahilevitz, M. Shapiro, N. Keller, A. Goldschmied-Reouven, O. Yarden, C. Block, and I. Polacheck.** 2004. Clinical and epidemiological aspects of infections caused by *Fusarium* species: a collaborative study from Israel. *J. Clin. Microbiol.* **42**:3456–3461.

136. **Nucci, M.** 2003. Emerging moulds: *Fusarium, Scedosporium* and Zygomycetes in transplant recipients. *Curr. Opin. Infect. Dis.* **16**:607–612.

137. **Nucci, M., and E. Anaissie.** 2006. Emerging fungi. *Infect. Dis. Clin. N. Am.* **20**:563–579.

138. **Nucci, M., and E. Anaissie.** 2007. *Fusarium* infections in immunocompromised patients. *Clin. Microbiol. Rev.* **20**:695–704.

139. **Nucci, M., and E. J. Anaissie.** 2009. Hyalohyphomycosis, p. 309–327. *In* E. J. Anaissie, M. R. McGinnis, and M. A. Pfaller (ed.), *Clinical Mycology,* 2nd ed. Elsevier, London, United Kingdom.

140. **Nucci, M., E. J. Anaissie, F. Queiroz-Telles, C. A. Martins, P. Trabasso, C. Solza, C. Mangini, B. P. Simoes, A. L. Colombo, J. Vaz, C. E. Levy, S. Costa, V. A. Moreira, J. S. Oliveira, N. Paraguay, G. Duboc, J. C. Voltarelli, A. Maiolino, R. Pasquini, and C. A. Souza.** 2003. Outcome predictors of 84 patients with hematologic malignancies and *Fusarium* infection. *Cancer* **98**:315–319.

141. **Nucci, M., K. A. Marr, F. Queiroz-Telles, C. A. Martins, P. Trabasso, S. Costa, J. C. Voltarelli, A. L. Colombo, A. Imhof, R. Pasquini, A. Maiolino, C. A. Souza, and E. Anaissie.** 2004. *Fusarium* infection in hematopoietic stem cell transplant recipients. *Clin. Infect. Dis.* **38**:1237–1242.

142. **Obayashi, T., M. Yoshida, T. Mori, H. Goto, A. Yasuoka, H. Iwasaki, H. Teshima, S. Kohno, A. Horiuchi, A. Ito, H. Yamaguchi, K. Shimada, and T. Kawai.** 1995. Plasma $(1\rightarrow3)$-β-D-glucan measurement in diagnosis of invasive deep mycosis and fungal febrile episodes. *Lancet* **345**:17–20.

143. **Odabasi, Z., G. Mattiuzzi, E. Estey, H. Kantarjian, F. Saeki, R. J. Ridge, P. A. Ketchum, M. A. Finkelman, J. H. Rex, and L. Ostrosky-Zeichner.** 2004. Beta-D-glucan as a diagnostic adjunct for invasive fungal infections: validation, cutoff development, and performance in patients with acute myelogenous leukemia and myelodysplastic syndrome. *Clin. Infect. Dis.* **39**:199–205.

144. **Odds, F., T. Arai, A. F. DiSalvo, E. G. V. Evans, R. J. Hay, H. S. Randhawa, M. G. Rinaldi, and T. J. Walsh.** 1992. Nomenclature of fungal diseases: a report and recommendations from a subcommittee of the International Society for Human and Animal Mycology (ISHAM). *J. Med. Vet. Mycol.* **30**:1–10.

145. **O'Donnell, K.** 2000. Molecular phylogeny of the *Nectria haematococca-Fusarium solani* species complex. *Mycologia* **92**:919–938.

146. **O'Donnell, K., E. Cigelnik, and H. I. Nirenberg.** 1998. Molecular systematic and phylogeography of the *Gibberella fujikuroi* species complex. *Mycologia* **90**:465–493.

147. **O'Donnell, K., H. I. Nirenberg, A. Takayuki, and E. Cigelnik.** 2000. A multigene phylogeny of the *Gibberella fujikuroi* species complex: detection of additional phylogenetically distinct species. *Mycoscience* **41**:61–78.

148. **O'Donnell, K., B. A. J. Sarver, M. Brandt, D. C. Chang, J. Noble-Wang, B. J. Park, D. A. Sutton, L. Benjamin, M. Lindsley, A. Padhye, D. M. Geiser, and T. J. Ward.** 2007. Phylogenetic diversity and microsphere array-based genotyping of human pathogenic fusaria, including isolates from the multistate contact lens-associated U.S. keratitis outbreaks of 2005 and 2006. *J. Clin. Microbiol.* **45:**2235–2248.

149. **O'Donnell, K., D. A. Sutton, M. G. Rinaldi, C. Gueidan, P. W. Crous, and D. M. Geiser.** 2009. Novel multilocus sequence typing scheme reveals high genetic diversity of human pathogenic members of the *Fusarium incarnatum-F. equiseti* and *F. chlamydosporum* species complexes within the United States. *J. Clin. Microbiol.* **47:**3851–3861.

150. **O'Donnell, K., D. A. Sutton, A. Fothergill, D. McCarthy, M. G. Rinaldi, M. E. Brandt, N. Zhang, and D. M. Geiser.** 2008. Molecular phylogenetic diversity, multilocus haplotype nomenclature, and in vitro antifungal resistance within the *Fusarium solani* species complex. *J. Clin. Microbiol.* **46:**2477–2490.

151. **O'Donnell, K., D. A. Sutton, M. G. Rinaldi, K. C. Magnon, P. A. Cox, S. G. Revankar, S. Sanche, D. M. Geiser, J. H. Juba, J. A. van Burik, A. Padhye, E. J. Anaissie, A. Francesconi, T. J. Walsh, and J. S. Robinson.** 2004. Genetic diversity of human pathogenic members of the *Fusarium oxysporum* complex inferred from multilocus DNA sequence data and amplified fragment length polymorphism analyses: evidence for the recent dispersion of a geographically widespread clonal lineage and nosocomial origin. *J. Clin. Microbiol.* **42:**5109–5120.

152. **Okhravi, N., and S. Lightman.** 2007. Clinical manifestations, treatment and outcome of *Paecilomyces lilacinus* infections. *Clin. Microbiol. Infect. Dis.* **13:**553–554.

153. **Osorio, S., R. de la Cámara, M. C. Monteserin, R. Granados, F. Oña, J. L. Rodríguez-Tudela, and M. Cuenca-Estrella.** 2007. Recurrent disseminated skin lesions due to *Metarrhizium anisopliae* in an adult patient with acute myelogenous leukemia. *J. Clin. Microbiol.* **45:**651–655.

154. **Ostrosky-Zeichner, L., B. D. Alexander, D. H. Kett, J. Vazquez, P. G. Pappas, F. Saeki, P. A. Ketchum, J. Wingard, R. Schiff, H. Tamura, M. A. Finkelman, and J. H. Rex.** 2005. Multicenter clinical evaluation of the (1→3) beta-D-glucan assay as an aid to diagnosis of fungal infections in humans. *Clin. Infect. Dis.* **41:**654–659.

155. **Pariseau, B., S. Nehls, G. S. H. Ogawa, D. A. Sutton, B. L. Wickes, and A. M. Romanelli.** 2010. *Beauveria* keratitis and biopesticides: case histories and a random amplification of polymorphic DNA comparison. *Cornea* **29:**152–158.

156. **Pastor, F. J., and J. Guarro.** 2006. Clinical manifestations, treatment and outcome of *Paecilomyces lilacinus* infections. *Clin. Microbiol. Infect. Dis.* **12:**948–960.

157. **Patel, R., C. A. Gustaferro, R. A. F. Krom, R. H. Wiesner, G. D. Roberts, and C. V. Paya.** 1994. Phaeohyphomycosis due to *Scopulariopsis brumptii* in a liver transplant patient. *Clin. Infect. Dis.* **19:**198–200.

158. **Perfect, J. R., K. A. Marr, T. J. Walsh, R. N. Greenberg, B. DuPont, J. de la Torre-Cisneros, G. Just-Nubling, H. T. Schlamm, I. Lutsar, A. Espinel-Ingroff, and E. Johnson.** 2003. Voriconazole treatment for less-common, emerging, or refractory fungal infections. *Clin. Infect. Dis.* **36:**1122–1131.

159. **Perlman, E. M., and L. Binns.** 1997. Intense photophobia caused by *Arthrographis kalrae* in a contact lens wearing patient. *Am. J. Ophthalmol.* **123:**547–549.

160. **Pfaller, M. A., F. Marco, S. A. Messer, and R. N. Jones.** 1998. In vitro activity of two echinocandin derivatives, LY303366 and MK-0991 (L-743,792), against clinical isolates of *Aspergillus, Fusarium, Rhizopus,* and other filamentous fungi. *Diagn. Microbiol. Infect. Dis.* **30:**251–255.

161. **Pfaller, M. A., S. A. Messer, R. J. Hollis, and R. N. Jones, and the SENTRY Participants Group.** 2002. Antifungal activities of posaconazole, ravuconazole, and voriconazole compared to those of itraconazole and amphotericin B against 239 clinical isolates of *Aspergillus* spp. and other filamentous fungi: report from SENTRY Antimicrobial Surveillance Program, 2000. *Antimicrob. Agents Chemother.* **46:**1032–1037.

162. **Phillips, P., W. S. Wood, G. Phillips, and M. G. Rinaldi.** 1989. Invasive hyalohyphomycosis caused by *Scopulariopsis brevicaulis* in a patient undergoing allogeneic bone marrow transplant. *Diagn. Microbiol. Infect. Dis.* **12:**429–432.

163. **Pihet, M., J. Carrère, B. Cimon, D. Chabasse, L. Delhaes, F. Symoens, and J.-P. Bouchara.** 2009. Occurrence and relevance of filamentous fungi in respiratory secretions of patients with cystic fibrosis—a review. *Med. Mycol.* **47**(Special Issue)**:**387–397.

164. **Pounder, J. I., K. E. Simmon, C. A. Barton, S. L. Hohmann, M. E. Brandt, and C. A. Petti.** 2007. Discovering potential pathogens among fungi identified as nonsporulating molds. *J. Clin. Microbiol.* **45:**568–571.

165. **Prins, C., P. Chavez, K. Tamm, and C. Hauser.** 1995. Ecthyma gangrenosum-like lesions: a sign of disseminated *Fusarium* infection in the neutropenic patient. *Clin. Exp. Dermatol.* **20:**428–430.

166. **Proia, L. A., M. K. Hayden, P. L. Kammeyer, J. Ortiz, D. A. Sutton, T. Clark, H.-J. Schroers, and R. C. Summerbell.** 2004. *Phialemonium:* an emerging mold pathogen that caused 4 cases of hemodialysis-associated endovascular infection. *Clin. Infect. Dis.* **39:**373–379.

167. **Pryce, T. M., S. Palladino, I. D. Kay, and G. W. Coombs.** 2003. Rapid identification of fungi by sequencing the ITS1 and ITS2 regions using an automated capillary electrophoresis system. *Med. Mycol.* **41:**369–381.

168. **Qiu, W. Y., Y. F. Yao, Y. F. Zhu, Y. M. Zhang, P. Zhou, Y. Q. Jin, and B. Zhang.** 2005. Fungal spectrum identified by a new slide culture and in vitro drug susceptibility using Etest in fungal keratitis. *Curr. Eye Res.* **30:**1113–1120.

169. **Raad, I., J. Tarrand, H. Hanna, M. Albitar, E. Janssen, M. Boktour, G. Bodey, M. Mardani, R. Hachem, D. Ontoyiannis, E. Whimbey, and K. Rolston.** 2002. Epidemiology, molecular mycology, and environmental sources of *Fusarium* infection in patients with cancer. *Infect. Control Hosp. Epidemiol.* **23:**532–537.

170. **Rabodonirina, M., M. A. Piens, M. F. Monier, E. Gueho, D. Fiere, and M. Mojon.** 1994. *Fusarium* infections in the immunocompromised patients: case reports and literature review. *Eur. J. Clin. Microbiol. Infect. Dis.* **13:**152–161.

171. **Rajeev, S., D. A. Sutton, B. L. Wickes, D. L. Miller, D. Giri, M. Wan Meter, E. H. Thompson, M. G. Rinaldi, A. M. Romanelli, J. F. Cano, and J. Guarro.** 2009. Isolation and characterization of a new fungal species, *Chrysosporium ophiodiicola,* from a mycotic granuloma of a black rat snake (*Elaphe obsoleta obsoleta*). *J. Clin. Microbiol.* **47:**1264–1268.

172. **Rampazzo, A., P. Kuhnert, J. Howard, and V. Bornand.** 2009. *Hormographiella aspergillata* keratomycosis in a dog. *Vet. Ophthalmol.* **12:**43–47.

173. **Rao, S. K., P. T. H. Lam, E. Y. M. Li, H. K. L. Yuen, and D. S. C. Lam.** 2007. A case series of contact lens-associated *Fusarium* keratitis in Hong Kong. *Cornea* **26:**1205–1209.

174. **Revankar, S. G., D. A. Sutton, S. E. Sanche, J. Rao, M. Zervos, F. Dashti, and M. G. Rinaldi.** 1999. *Metarrhizium anisopliae* as a cause of sinusitis in immunocompetent hosts. *J. Clin. Microbiol.* **37:**195–198.

175. **Rezai, K. A., D. Eliott, O. Plous, J. A. Vasquez, and G. W. Abrams.** 2005. Disseminated *Fusarium* infection presenting as bilateral endogenous endophthalmitis in a patient with acute myeloid leukemia. *Arch. Ophthalmol.* **123:**702–703.

176. **Richter, S., M. G. Cormican, M. A. Pfaller, C. K. Lee, R. Gingrich, M. G. Rinaldi, and D. A. Sutton.** 1999. Fatal disseminated *Trichoderma longibrachiatum* infection in an adult bone marrow transplant patient: species identification and review of the literature. *J. Clin. Microbiol.* **37:**1154–1160.

177. **Rihs, J. D., A. A. Padhye, and C. B. Good.** 1996. Brain abscess caused by *Schizophyllum commune:* an emerging basidiomycete pathogen. *J. Clin. Microbiol.* **34:**1628–1632.

178. **Rimek, D., J. Singh, and R. Kappe.** 2003. Cross reactivity of the PLATELIA CANDIDA antigen detection enzyme

immunoassay with fungal antigen extracts. *J. Clin. Microbiol.* **41:**3395–3398.

179. **Roh, M. L., C. U. Tuazon, R. Mandler, K. J. Kwon-Chung, and C. E. Geist.** 2005. Sphenocavernous syndrome associated with *Schizophyllum commune* infection of the sphenoid sinus. *Ophthal. Plast. Reconstr. Surg.* **21:**71–74.

180. **Roilides, E., L. Sigler, E. Bibashi, H. Katsifa, N. Flaris, and C. Panteliadis.** 1999. Disseminated infection due to *Chrysosporium zonatum* in a patient with chronic granulomatous disease and review of non-*Aspergillus* infections in these patients. *J. Clin. Microbiol.* **37:**18–25.

181. **Romanelli, A. M., D. A. Sutton, E. H. Thompson, M. G. Rinaldi, and B. L. Wickes.** 2010. Sequence-based identification of filamentous basidiomycetous fungi from clinical specimens: a cautionary note. *J. Clin. Microbiol.* **48:**741–752.

182. **Ruíz-Cendoya, M., M. Mariné, M. Mar Rodríguez, and J. Guarro.** 2009. Interactions between triazoles and amphotericin B in the treatment of disseminated murine infection by *Fusarium oxysporum*. *Antimicrob. Agents Chemother.* **53:**1705–1708.

183. **Ryder, N. S.** 1999. Activity of terbinafine against serious fungal pathogens. *Mycoses* **42:**115–119.

184. **Rydjord, B., G. Hetland, and H. G. Wiker.** 2005. Immunoglobulin G antibodies against environmental moulds in a Norwegian healthy population show a bimodal distribution for *Aspergillus versicolor*. *Scand. J. Immunol.* **62:**281–288.

185. **Saini, S. K., S. R. Boas, A. Jerath, M. Roberts, and P. A. Greenberger.** 1998. Allergic bronchopulmonary mycosis to *Fusarium vasinfectum* in a child. *Ann. Allergy Asthma Immunol.* **80:**377–380.

186. **Sampathkumar, P., and C. V. Paya.** 2001. *Fusarium* infection after solid-organ transplantation. *Clin. Infect. Dis.* **32:**1237–1240.

187. **Samson, R. A., E. S. Hoekstra, J. Frisvad, and O. Filtenborg.** 2000. *Introduction to Food- and Airborne Fungi*, 6th ed. Centraalbureau voor Schimmelcultures, Utrecht, The Netherlands.

188. **Schell, W. A., and J. R. Perfect.** 1996. Fatal, disseminated *Acremonium strictum* infection in a neutropenic host. *J. Clin. Microbiol.* **34:**1333–1336.

189. **Schinabeck, M. K., and M. A. Ghannoum.** 2003. Human hyalohyphomycoses: a review of human infections due to *Acremonium* spp., *Paecilomyces* spp., *Penicillium* spp., and *Scopulariopsis* spp. *J. Chemother.* **15**(Suppl. 2):5–15.

190. **Schmidt, A. L., and V. Mitter.** 2004. Microsatellite mutation directed by an external stimulus. *Mutat. Res.* **568:**233–243.

191. **Schroers, H.-J., K. O'Donnell, S. C. Lamprecht, P. L. Kammeyer, S. Johnson, D. A. Sutton, M. G. Rinaldi, D. M. Geiser, and R. C. Summerbell.** 2009. Taxonomy and phylogeny of the *Fusarium dimerum* species group. *Mycologia* **101:**44–70.

192. **Seguin, P., B. Degeilh, I. Grulois, A. Gacouin, S. Maugendre, T. Dufour, B. Dupont, and C. Camus.** 1995. Successful treatment of a brain abscess due to *Trichoderma longibrachiatum* after surgical resection. *Eur. J. Clin. Microbiol. Infect. Dis.* **14:**445–448.

193. **Serena, C., M. Ortoneda, J. Capilla, F. J. Pastor, D. A. Sutton, M. G. Rinaldi, and J. Guarro.** 2003. In vitro activities of new antifungal agents against *Chaetomium* spp. and inoculum standardization. *Antimicrob. Agents Chemother.* **47:**3161–3164.

194. **Sigler, L.** 2003. Ascomycetes: the *Onygenaceae* and other fungi from the order *Onygenales*, p. 195–236. *In* D. H. Howard (ed.), *Fungi Pathogenic for Humans and Animals*, 2nd ed. Marcel Dekker, Inc., New York, NY.

195. **Sigler, L.** 2003. Miscellaneous opportunistic fungi: *Microascaceae* and other ascomycetes, hyphomycetes, coelomycetes and basidiomycetes, p. 637–676. *In* D. H. Howard (ed.), *Fungi Pathogenic for Humans and Animals*, 2nd ed. Marcel Dekker, Inc., New York, NY.

196. **Sigler, L., and S. P. Abbott.** 1997. Characterizing and conserving diversity of filamentous basidiomycetes from human sources. *Microbiol. Cult. Collect.* **13:**21–27.

197. **Sigler, L., S. P. Abbott, and A. Woodgyer.** 1994. New records of nail and skin infection due to *Onychocola canadensis* and description of its teleomorph *Arachnomyces nodosetosus* sp. nov. *J. Med. Vet. Mycol.* **32:**275–285.

198. **Sigler, L., J. R. Bartley, D. H. Parr, and A. J. Morris.** 1999. Maxillary sinusitis caused by medusoid form of *Schizophyllum commune*. *J. Clin. Microbiol.* **37:**3395–3398.

199. **Sigler, L., L. De La Maza, G. Tan, K. N. Egger, and R. K. Sherburne.** 1995. Diagnostic difficulties caused by a nonclamped *Schizophyllum commune* isolate in a case of fungus ball of the lung. *J. Clin. Microbiol.* **33:**1979–1983.

200. **Sigler, L., J. L. Harris, D. M. Dixon, A. L. Flis, I. F. Salin, M. Kemna, and R. A. Duncan.** 1990. Microbiology and potential virulence of *Sporothrix cyanescens*, a fungus rarely isolated from blood and skin. *J. Clin. Microbiol.* **28:**1009–1015.

201. **Sigler, L., and M. J. Kennedy.** 1999. *Aspergillus*, *Fusarium*, and other opportunistic moniliaceous fungi, p. 1212–1241. *In* P. R. Murray, E. J. Baron, M. A. Pfaller, F. C. Tenover, and R. H. Yolken (ed.), *Manual of Clinical Microbiology*, 7th ed. American Society for Microbiology, Washington, DC.

202. **Sigler, L., and D. A. Sutton.** 2002. *Acrophialophora fusispora* misidentified as *Scedosporium prolificans*. *J. Clin. Microbiol.* **40:**3544–3545. (Authors' reply, **40:**3545.)

203. **Sigler, L., D. A. Sutton, C. F. C. Gibas, R. C. Summerbell, R. K. Noel, and P. C. Iwen.** 2010. *Phialosimplex*, a new anamorphic genus associated with infections in dogs and having phylogenetic affinity to the Trichocomaceae. *Med. Mycol.* **48:**335–345.

204. **Sigler, L., and P. E. Verweij.** 2003. *Aspergillus*, *Fusarium*, and other opportunistic moniliaceous fungi, p. 1726–1760. *In* P. R. Murray, E. J. Baron, J. H. Jorgensen, M. A. Pfaller, and R. H. Yolken (ed.), *Manual of Clinical Microbiology*, 8th ed. ASM Press, Washington, DC.

205. **Sponsel, W. E., J. R. Graybill, H. L. Nevarez, and D. Dang.** 2002. Ocular and systemic posaconazole (SCH-56592) treatment of invasive *Fusarium solani* keratitis and endophthalmitis. *Br. J. Ophthalmol.* **86:**829–830.

206. **Steinbach, W. J., W. A. Schell, J. L. Miller, J. R. Perfect, and P. L. Martin.** 2004. Fatal *Scopulariopsis brevicaulis* infection in a paediatric stem cell transplant patient treated with voriconazole and caspofungin and a review of *Scopulariopsis* infections in immunocompromised patients. *J. Infect.* **48:**112–116.

207. **St-Germain, G., and R. Summerbell.** 1996. *Identifying Filamentous Fungi*. Star Publishing Co., Belmont, CA.

208. **Sugiura, Y., J. R. Barr, D. B. Barr, J. W. Brock, C. M. Elie, Y. Ueno, D. G. Patterson, M. E. Potter, and E. Reiss.** 1999. Physiological characteristics and mycotoxins of human clinical isolates of *Fusarium* species. *Mycol. Res.* **103:**1462–1468.

209. **Summerbell, R. C.** 1993. The benomyl test as a fundamental diagnostic method for medical mycology. *J. Clin. Microbiol.* **31:**572–577.

210. **Summerbell, R. C.** 2003. *Aspergillus*, *Fusarium*, *Sporothrix*, *Piedraia*, and their relatives, p. 237–498. *In* D. H. Howard (ed.), *Fungi Pathogenic for Humans and Animals*, 2nd ed. Marcel Dekker, Inc., New York, NY.

211. **Summerbell, R. C., and H.-J. Schroers.** 2002. Analysis of phylogenetic relationship of *Cylindrocarpon lichenicola* and *Acremonium falciforme* to the *Fusarium solani* species complex and a review of similarities in the spectrum of opportunistic infections caused by these fungi. *J. Clin. Microbiol.* **40:**2866–2875.

212. **Surmonta, I., F. van Aelst, J. Verbanck, and G. S. de Hoog.** 2002. A pulmonary infection caused by *Coprinus cinereus* (*Hormographiella aspergillata*) diagnosed after a neutropenic episode. *Med. Mycol.* **40:**217–219.

213. **Sutton, D. A.** 1999. Coelomycetous fungi in human disease. A review: clinical entities, pathogenesis, identification and therapy. *Rev. Iberoam. Micol.* **16:**171–179.

214. **Sutton, D. A.** 2008. Rare and emerging agents of hyalohyphomycosis. *Curr. Fungal Infect. Rep.* **2:**134–142.

215. **Sutton, D. A., A. W. Fothergill, and M. G. Rinaldi.** 1998. *Guide to Clinically Significant Fungi*. Williams & Wilkins, Baltimore, MD.

216. Sutton, D. A., L. Sigler, K. G. Kalassian, A. W. Fothergill, and M. G. Rinaldi. 1997. Pulmonary *Acrophialophora fusispora*: case history, literature review and mycology, p. 160. *Abstr. 13th ISHAM Congr.*

217. Sutton, D. A., E. H. Thompson, M. G. Rinaldi, P. C. Iwen, K. K. Nakasone, H. S. Jung, H. M. Rosenblatt, and M. E. Paul. 2005. Identification and first report of *Inonotus (Phellinus) tropicalis* as an etiologic agent in a patient with chronic granulomatous disease. *J. Clin. Microbiol.* **43:**982–987.

218. Swanink, C. M., J. F. Meis, A. J. Rijs, J. P. Donnelly, and P. E. Verweij. 1997. Specificity of a sandwich enzyme-linked immunosorbent assay for detecting *Aspergillus* galactomannan. *J. Clin. Microbiol.* **35:**257–260.

219. Tan, D. H. S., L. Sigler, C. F. C. Gibas, and I. W. Fong. 2008. Disseminated fungal infection in a renal transplant recipient involving *Macrophomina phaseolina* and *Scytalidium dimidiatum*: case report and review of taxonomic changes among medically important members of the Botryosphaeriaceae. *Med. Mycol.* **46:**285–292.

220. Tekkok, I. H., M. J. Higgins, and E. C. Ventureyra. 1996. Posttraumatic gas-containing brain abscess caused by *Clostridium perfringens* with unique simultaneous fungal suppuration by *Myceliophthora thermophila*: case report. *Neurosurgery* **39:**1247–1251.

221. Tiribelli, M., F. Zaja, C. Fili, T. Michelutti, S. Prosdocimo, A. Candoni, and R. Fanin. 2002. Endogenous endophthalmitis following disseminated fungemia due to *Fusarium solani* in a patient with acute myeloid leukemia. *Eur. J. Haematol.* **68:**314–317.

222. Tortorano, A. M., A. Prigitano, G. Dho, M. C. Esposto, C. Gianni, A. Grancini, C. Ossi, and M. A. Viviani. 2008. Species distribution and in vitro antifungal susceptibility patterns of 75 clinical isolates of *Fusarium* spp. from northern Italy. *Antimicrob. Agents Chemother.* **52:**2683–2685.

223. Tu, E., and A. J. Park. 2007. Recalcitrant *Beauveria bassiana* keratitis: confocal microscopy findings and treatment with posaconazole (Noxafil). *Cornea* **26:**1008–1010.

224. Tucker, D. L., C. H. Beresford, L. Sigler, and K. Rogers. 2004. Disseminated *Beauveria bassiana* infection in a patient with acute lymphoblastic leukemia. *J. Clin. Microbiol.* **42:**5412–5414.

225. Ulloa, M., and R. T. Hanlin. 2000. *Illustrated Dictionary of Mycology.* The American Phytopathological Society, St. Paul, MN.

226. Ustun, C., G. Huls, M. Stewart, and K. Marr. 2006. Resistant *Microascus cirrosus* penumonia can be treated with a combination of surgery, multiple anti-fungal agents and a growth factor. *Mycopathologia* **162:**299–302.

227. Van Burik, J.-A., D. Myerson, R. W. Schreckhise, and R. A. Bowden. 1998. Panfungal PCR assay for detection of fungal infection in human blood specimens. *J. Clin. Microbiol.* **36:**1169–1175.

228. Verweij, P. E., M. Van Kasteren, J. Van de Nes, G. S. De Hoog, B. E. de Pauw, and J. F. G. M. Meis. 1997. Fatal pulmonary infection caused by the basidiomycete *Hormographiella aspergillata*. *J. Clin. Microbiol.* **35:**2675–2678.

229. Warris, A., P. Gaustad, J. F. Meis, A. Voss, P. E. Verweij, and T. G. Abrahamsen. 2001. Recovery of filamentous fungi from water in a paediatric bone marrow transplantation unit. *J. Hosp. Infect.* **47:**143–148.

230. Warris, A., F. Wesenberg, P. Gaustad, P. E. Verweij, and T. G. Abrahamsen. 2000. *Acremonium strictum* fungaemia in a paediatric patient with acute leukaemia. *Scand. J. Infect. Dis.* **32:**442–444.

231. Weinberger, M., I. Mahrshak, N. Keller, A. Goldscmied-Reuven, N. Amariglio, M. Kramer, A. Tobar, Z. Samra, S. D. Pitlik, M. G. Rinaldi, E. Thompson, and D. Sutton. 2006. Isolated endogenous endophthalmitis due to a sporodochial-forming *Phialemonium curvatum* acquired through intracavernous autoinjections. *Med. Mycol.* **44:**253–259.

232. Williamson, P. R., K. J. Kwon-Chung, and J. J. Gallin. 1992. Successful treatment of *Paecilomyces variotii* infection in a patient with chronic granulomatous disease and a review of *Paecilomyces* species infections. *Clin. Infect. Dis.* **14:**1023–1026.

233. Wuyts, W. A., H. Molzahn, J. Maertens, E. K. Verbeken, K. Lagrou, L. J. Dupont, and G. M. Verleden. 2005. Fatal *Scopulariopsis* infection in a lung transplant recipient: a case report. *J. Heart Lung Transplant.* **24:**2301–2304.

234. Xu, Y., G. Pang, C. Gao, D. Zhao, L. Zhou, S. Sun, and B. Wang. 2009. In vitro comparison of the efficacies of natamycin and silver nitrate against ocular fungi. *Antimicrob. Agents Chemother.* **53:**1636–1638.

235. Yaguchi, T., A. Sano, K. Yarita, M. K. Suh, K. Nishimura, and S.-I. Udagawa. 2006. A new species of *Cephalotheca* isolated from a Korean patient. *Mycotaxon* **96:**309–322.

236. Yücesoy, M., M. C. Ergon, H. Oren, and Z. Gülay. 2004. Case report: a *Fusarium* fungemia. *Mikrobiyol. Bul.* **38:**265–271.

237. Zhang, N., K. O'Donnell, D. A. Sutton, F. A. Nalim, R. C. Summerbell, A. A. Padhye, and D. M. Geiser. 2006. Members of the *Fusarium solani* species complex that cause infections in both humans and plants are common in the environment. *J. Clin. Microbiol.* **44:**2186–2190.

Agents of Systemic and Subcutaneous Mucormycosis and Entomophthoromycosis

DEA GARCIA-HERMOSO, ERIC DANNAOUI, OLIVIER LORTHOLARY, AND
FRANÇOISE DROMER

119

Mucormycosis and entomophthoromycosis are invasive fungal infections caused by environmental nonseptate filamentous fungi. Mucormycosis is caused by the ubiquitous Mucorales fungi and occurs mostly in immunocompromised patients or those with diabetes mellitus. These fungi are responsible for rhinocerebral, pulmonary, cutaneous, and disseminated infections characterized by angio-invasion and necrosis and have severe outcomes despite current antifungal and surgical therapies. Entomophthoromycosis is caused by the Entomophthorales fungi, found mostly in warm climates. It includes basidiobolomycosis and conidiobolomycosis and occurs mostly in immunocompetent hosts. It presents as a subcutaneous infection, with a favorable outcome after prolonged azole therapy.

TAXONOMY

The classification of the kingdom Fungi has undergone significant changes in recent years (see chapter 111 in this *Manual*). Traditionally, the etiologic agents of mucormycosis (order Mucorales) and entomophthoromycosis (order Entomophthorales) were assigned to the lower fungi, i.e., the phylum Zygomycota. Following a comprehensive phylogenetic study based on multigene sequence analyses, this phylum was abolished due to its polyphyletic nature (51). Taxa have been redistributed among the phylum Glomeromycota and four new subphyla incertae sedis: Mucoromycotina (which includes three orders, namely, the core group of Mucorales, Endogonales, and Mortierellales), the Entomophthoromycotina (with the order Entomophthorales), the Zoopagomycotina (with the order Zoopagales), and finally, the subphylum Kickxellomycotina (which includes the orders Kickxellales, Dimargaritales, Harpellales, and Asellariales). The relationships among clades within the Zygomycota await further phylogenetic resolution.

In recent years, phylogenetic interactions among members of the order Mucorales have been studied (86, 124, 125) and have revealed the polyphyletic nature of families (Thmnidiaceae, Mucoraceae, and Chaetocladiaceae) and genera such as *Absidia* and *Mucor*. Revisions of other genera published in recent years are detailed below (41, 52, 124). Of note, the first analysis of a genome sequence from a member of the Mucorales (*Rhizopus oryzae*) was published recently (77). Table 1 displays the species of Mucorales that have been described as human pathogens or potential human pathogens (98).

The creation of the subphylum Entomophthoromycotina has recently come under question, and it has been proposed that the order remain grouped with the subphylum Mucoromycotina (123). A consensus involving resolution of the different lineages is thus still pending. According to the classification proposed by Hibbet et al. (51), the subphylum Entomophthoromycotina contains the order Entomophthorales, which is subdivided into two families: the Ancylistaceae and Basidiobolaceae, containing the genera *Conidiobolus* and *Basidiobolus*, respectively. There are 27 species in the genus *Conidiobolus*, but only two (*C. coronatus* and *C. incongruus*) have been recovered from clinical specimens, while in the genus *Basidiobolus*, *B. ranarum* is the only species known to cause human disease.

MUCORMYCOSIS

■ Epidemiology and Transmission

Mucorales are ubiquitous molds widely distributed in the environment (soil, plants, and decaying organic material) (98). They are frequent pathogens of plants and contaminants of grains and foods such as fruit or bread. Airborne spores are thought to be the infectious particles responsible for disease, particularly in immunocompromised individuals, and this explains the most frequent body localizations (skin, sinuses, and lungs). These molds are frequently found as laboratory contaminants and may cause nosocomial infections (68; B. Rammaert, F. Lanternier, J. R. Zahar, E. Dannaoui, M. E. Bougnoux, M. Lecuit, and O. Lortholary, *Abstr. 49th Intersci. Conf. Antimicrob. Agents Chemother.*, abstr. K944, 2009). Specific geographic distributions and environmental niches are described for relevant species in the corresponding sections.

Several recent reports have suggested that the incidence of mucormycosis is increasing, based on single-center studies (20, 65, 79, 80, 93). In a retrospective analysis of hospital records in France, we recently provided a population-based estimate of mucormycosis incidence and trends for the country over a 10-year period from 1997 through 2006 (10). The average annual incidence rate of 0.9 case per million was lower than that reported for a population-based study in San Francisco in 1992 and 1993 (1.7 cases per million) (97) but higher than that reported from Spain in 2005 (0.43 case per million) (118). The sex ratio (1.8 versus 1.1) and mean

TABLE 1 Species of Mucorales (subphylum Mucoromycotina Benny, subphylum nova) involved in human mucormycosis[a]

Family	Genus	Species
Lichtheimiaceae	*Lichtheimia*	*L. corymbifera (Mycocladus corymbifer, Absidia corymbifera)*
		L. ramosa (Absidia ramosa)
Mucoraceae	*Absidia*	*A coerulea*[b]
	Apophysomyces	*A. elegans*
	Actinomucor	*A. elegans*
	Mucor	*M. circinelloides*
		M. hiemalis
		M. indicus
		M. racemosus[b]
		M. ramosissimus
	Rhizomucor	*R. pusillus*
		R. variabilis
	Rhizopus	*R. azygosporus*
		R. microsporus
		R. oryzae
		R. schipperae
		R. stolonifer[b]
Thamnidiaceae	*Cokeromyces*	*C. recurvatus*
Cunninghamellaceae	*Cunninghamella*	*C. bertholletiae*
Syncephalastraceae	*Syncephalastrum*	*S. racemosum*
Saksenaeaceae	*Saksenaea*	*S. vasiformis*

[a]Data from references 31 and 51.
[b]Implication in human infection is not confirmed.

age (38.8 versus 57.1 years) in our study differ from those reported in a review of 929 cases published from 1940 to 1999 (10, 101).

Diabetes is a major risk factor for mucormycosis (36% of cases; 20% of cases are in patients with type 1 diabetes) (70, 101), with significant increases in the incidence of diabetes-associated infection recently documented in France (10) and in a tertiary care center in North India (16). In the latter study, 131 of 178 cases (73.6%) were observed in patients with uncontrolled diabetes, and more importantly, mucormycosis led to the diagnosis of diabetes in 56 cases (42.7% of diabetes cases). Diabetes mellitus was found in 15% (type 1 diabetes in 13%) of 157 pediatric cases (130). Diabetes was also an independent risk factor for mucormycosis in patients with leukemia and/or bone marrow transplantation (65) and significantly influenced the occurrence of mucormycosis during solid organ transplantion (SOT) (111).

Among patients with hematological malignancies, patients with acute leukemia (profound neutropenia or relapse) or allogeneic stem cell transplantation are more prone to develop mucormycosis. In that setting, mucormycosis most often occurs later than 3 months after transplantation, in the setting of graft-versus-host disease (19, 65, 67, 79, 80, 84, 89, 90). Mucormycosis now represents 7 to 8% of invasive fungal infections in bone marrow transplant patients (82; D. P. Kontoyiannis, K. A. Marr, K. Wannemuehler, B. J. Park, J. I. Ito, and P. G. Pappas, *Abstr. 47th Intersci. Conf. Antimicrob. Agents Chemother.*, abstr. M-1196, 2007). An increased incidence of mucormycosis has been observed in patients with hematological malignancies and in stem cell transplant recipients in France (10), as noted in one U.S. center in the 1990s (79). In that population, a potential role of prior exposure to antifungal agents that lacked activity against zygomycetes, such as voriconazole and caspofungin, was reported (14, 42, 58, 65, 80, 103, 111).

Mucormycosis represents 2% of invasive fungal infections following SOT, mostly after kidney transplantation (P. G. Pappas, C. Kauffman, B. Alexander, D. Andes, S. Hadley, T. Patterson, R. Walker, V. Morrison, T. Perl, K. Wannemuehler, and T. Chiller, *Abstr. 47th Intersci. Conf. Antimicrob. Agents Chemother.*, abstr. M-1195, 2007). In a recent international study of SOT recipients, renal failure, diabetes mellitus, and prior voriconazole and/or caspofungin use were associated with a higher risk, whereas tacrolimus was associated with a lower risk of mucormycosis (111). Liver transplant recipients were more likely to have disseminated disease and developed infection significantly earlier after transplantation than other SOT recipients.

Mucormycosis can also develop in human immunodeficiency virus-infected patients or intravenous drug abusers. It can affect otherwise healthy individuals following cutaneous injuries with contaminated soil, accounting for almost 20% of cases in some studies. Finally, it may present as a community-acquired or health care-related disease. A review of cases published between 1970 and 2009 revealed a total of 169 individual (including 49 in children) mucormycosis cases associated with health care, of which 72% were published after 1990 (Rammaert et al., *Abstr. 49th Intersci. Conf. Antimicrob. Agents Chemother.*). Outbreaks of mucormycosis are rare but have been related to building construction or use of contaminated adhesive tape, ostomy bags, or wooden tongue depressors.

■ **Clinical Manifestations**

Localized and disseminated forms of disease need to be differentiated (84). The most frequent localized forms are sinusitis and pneumonia, which represented 39% and 24% of clinical sites involved, respectively, in a recent review of the literature (101). Dissemination rates vary from 3% to more than 50% for patients with hematological malignancies (depending to some extent on the underlying diseases and the site of infection) (84, 90, 101).

Sinus involvement (isolated sinusitis, rhinocerebral, and sino-orbital forms) is the most common presentation in diabetes patients and intravenous drug abusers, while pulmonary infection is the second most common presentation; the reverse is true for hematology patients (65, 101). Infection causes necrosis and hemorrhage and may be localized or associated with dissemination. The clinicoradiological presentation is similar to that of invasive aspergillosis in patients with hematological malignancies. In a recent study of 58 SOT patients with mucormycosis, pulmonary localization was present in 31 (53%) of the patients, including 23 with localized infection (114).

Cutaneous lesions are encountered most often in immunocompetent hosts (101) and follow injury with contaminated soil or contamination with airborne spores (2, 122), surgery, or burns. Local and hematogenous dissemination may occur. In contrast, skin lesions resulting from dissemination of infection from other sites are rare.

Cerebral infection can complicate sinusitis or occur independently, especially in intravenous drug abusers. Patients may be lethargic, confused, or obtunded; focal neurological deficits are often present. Gastrointestinal lesions have been described in 7% of cases; they occur in low-birth-weight premature infants and malnourished individuals and after peritoneal dialysis (101). They are responsible for abdominal pain and digestive hemorrhage, and complications include digestive tract perforation, peritonitis, and dissemination to the liver.

■ Treatment

Prophylaxis

There is no benefit of the prophylactic use of azoles such as fluconazole or itraconazole in immunocompromised patients due to a lack of activity against Mucorales (67, 79, 90). The best preventive measure is the reduction of environmental exposure, notably with the use of HEPA-filtered rooms (90). The specific role of posaconazole as a prophylactic agent against mucormycosis has not been demonstrated (23, 121).

Curative Treatment

In a recent review, only 3% of untreated patients survived, compared with 64% of those who received antifungal therapy (101). Combined medical and surgical treatment, in association with correction of the underlying disease wherever possible, offers the best chance of survival (127). Lipid derivatives of amphotericin B given early in the course of the disease are probably more effective and better tolerated than amphotericin B deoxycholate (69). A clinical response was obtained with high doses of lipid-associated amphotericin B in patients who experienced failure with the conventional drug (12, 92). The performance of oral posaconazole, iron chelators, or echinocandins in combination with polyenes is still under evaluation. Other therapeutic measures include optimal control of the underlying risk factor, such as ketoacidosis (18, 67, 84, 90). Global case fatality rates vary from 84% to 47% over time (101), with those for rhinocerebral forms ranging from 20 to 69% (16, 93).

■ Collection, Transport, and Storage of Specimens

Mucormycosis is a rapidly progressive infection, and a timely diagnosis is mandatory for optimal therapeutic management; this remains difficult (34). The clinical and radiological features are not specific and often mimic those of other invasive filamentous fungal infections, particularly invasive aspergillosis. Unfortunately, the therapies of choice for these diseases are different, and delaying treatment has an important impact on outcome (18). Thus, a high index of suspicion is needed for patients with predisposing risk factors and compatible clinical signs. For these patients, specimens should be obtained rapidly for both microbiological and histopathological laboratories, as direct microscopic examination and culture remain the most useful diagnostic techniques. Although recent advances have been made in molecular diagnosis, these methods are not yet standardized or commercially available. Various specimens can be obtained, depending on the clinical form and localization(s) of infection. In all cases, tissue biopsy samples or specimens obtained aseptically from sterile sites are preferred. For cutaneous infection, a skin biopsy should be performed. For the rhinocerebral forms, nasal discharge, scraping of the nasal mucosa, sinus aspirate, or tissue specimens from the affected area should be obtained. For the pulmonary form, broncho-alveolar lavage fluid and fluids obtained by bronchoscopy can be examined, although they are not always positive (43). Sputum culture is insensitive (74). When feasible, biopsy samples of pulmonary lesions (either transbronchial or percutaneous computerized tomography-guided biopsy) are the specimens of choice (43, 83). Blood cultures have no diagnostic value, as they are almost always negative, despite the fact that mucormycosis is an angioinvasive disease. Similarly, in central nervous system infections, the fungus is rarely seen in or cultured from the cerebrospinal fluid. Samples should be collected in sterile receptacles, tissue samples should be kept moist with a few drops of saline, and further samples should be placed in formalin for histopathological analysis. Samples must be transported rapidly and processed in the microbiology laboratory. They should not be refrigerated (32).

■ Direct Examination and Histopathology

Demonstration of hyphae in clinical samples is important for the diagnosis of mucormycosis. This demonstration provides a rapid (within hours) and definitive means of diagnosis. It may be the only means of diagnosis due to the frequent lack of positive cultures from tissue samples. Occasionally, contamination of culture by airborne spores can lead to a false-positive diagnosis of mucormycosis, underlying the importance of direct examination (119).

Microscopy

Wet mounts of clinical samples can be observed directly after adding a few drops of potassium hydroxide. Alternatively, staining with optical brighteners (calcofluor white, Blankophor P, or Uvitex 2B) can increase sensitivity in cases where few hyphal elements are present (102). These fluorescent dyes can also be applied to Gram-stained slides if fresh samples are not available. Hyphae can also be visualized easily by Gomori methenamine-silver (GMS) staining. Giemsa staining is not recommended because the hyphae of mucoraceous molds stain poorly. The specific morphological characteristics suggestive of Mucorales are thin, hyaline, non- or pauciseptate walls and ribbon-like hyphae with a large diameter (between 5 and 25 μm) compared with that of hyaline hyphomycetes. Width is generally irregular, with a twisted or folded appearance. Wide branching angles ($\geq$90°) are suggestive of Mucorales, contrasting with the acute (45°) branching pattern of common hyaline hyphomycetes such as *Aspergillus*. Mucoraceous molds do not sporulate in tissues unless there is an air interface. When hyphae are fragmented and scant, a definite diagnosis of mucormycosis can be difficult based on direct examination only. In these cases, only a culture yielding a Mucorales isolate or molecular identification will allow the diagnosis of mucormycosis as opposed to invasive infection due to a hyaline hyphomycete.

Tissue samples should also be processed in the histopathology laboratory (Fig. 1). Tissue sections can be stained by GMS or periodic acid-Schiff stain. Hyphae are often poorly stained by hematoxylin and eosin compared to those

of other filamentous fungi. The morphology of hyphae is similar to that seen with fresh samples. Nevertheless, cross sections of the hyphae can produce vacuolated or yeast-like images that can be misinterpreted. Necrosis, hemorrhage, and inflammation are common in infected tissues. Areas of acute inflammation filled with neutrophils and, sometimes, granulomatous reactions can be seen. Hyphae typically penetrate the walls of blood vessels, with subsequent invasion of the lumen and tissue infarction. Perineural invasion has been demonstrated in a significant number of cases (37).

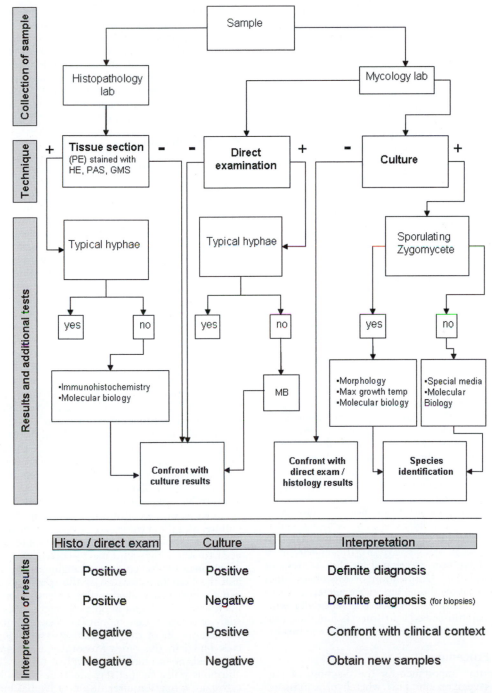

FIGURE 1 Flow diagram following the processing of a sample in the mycology/microbiology laboratory or the histopathology laboratory. PE, paraffin embedded; HE, hematoxylin-eosin stain; PAS, periodic acid-Schiff stain; GMS, Gomori methenamine silver stain.

Immunohistochemistry with commercially available antibodies can be performed to gather additional evidence of the presence of Mucorales in difficult cases (60).

Antigen Detection

There are currently no specific antigen detection methods available for the diagnosis of mucormycosis. Moreover, testing for the presence of β-D-glucan is not helpful.

Detection of Nucleic Acids in Clinical Materials

In a significant number of cases, culture is negative or not performed and the only available samples are formalin-fixed, paraffin-embedded tissue specimens (25). There is currently no consensus on the best technical parameters to use, and there are no commercially available molecular detection techniques. Different approaches have been tried. Both formalin-fixed, paraffin-embedded tissues and fresh or frozen tissues can be used; lower yields have been obtained using the former. Most studies have used PCR-based techniques. Internal transcribed spacer 1 (ITS1) sequencing after PCR with panfungal primers allowed reliable identification to the species level for histopathologically positive tissue samples obtained from mice experimentally infected with Mucorales (E. Dannaoui, P. Schwarz, M. Slany, J. Loeffler, A. T. Jorde, M. Cuenca-Estrella, P. Hauser, P. Warn, M. Huerre, T. Freiberger, P. Gaustad, J. L. Rodriguez-Tudela, J. Bille, D. Denning, S. Bretagne, and O. Lortholary, *Abstr. 47th Intersci. Conf. Antimicrob. Agents Chemother.* abstr. M-567, 2007). However, the sensitivity of the molecular tool was lower than that of conventional histopathology. For patients, a similar approach was used, with positive PCR results obtained for five of nine tissue samples from patients with proven or probable mucormycosis according to culture or histopathology (72). Another technique, using an 18S rRNA-targeted seminested PCR specific for Mucorales, also showed promising results (8, 99). The latter technique was prospectively evaluated, and the yield of PCR was superior to that of culture for histopathologically positive samples (100). More recently, a real-time PCR assay targeting a conserved region of the Mucorales cytochrome *b* gene had a sensitivity and specificity of 56 and 100%, respectively, with formalin-fixed, paraffin-embedded tissue samples (49). Of note, an in situ hybridization technique using Mucorales-specific DNA probes targeting the 18S rRNA subunit also showed promising results (50). Molecular identification of Mucorales can be achieved more readily with fresh or frozen tissue samples, as shown with samples from experimentally infected animals (61, 108) or from patients with positive histopathology or culture (72). In addition, molecular identification using various DNA targets and techniques proved useful in several case reports of infection by Mucorales organisms belonging to different genera and species (59, 63, 71, 73, 78). In summary, new molecular tools have been developed for the diagnosis of mucormycosis and the identification of Mucorales fungi in tissues. Nevertheless, the technical parameters need to be optimized, especially to improve the sensitivity with formalin-fixed, paraffin-embedded tissues, before their routine use can be envisioned in microbiology laboratories.

■ Isolation Procedures

Culture is of prime importance for the diagnosis of mucormycosis, for several reasons. First, when hyphae in tissues are not morphologically typical or are scant, the distinction between Mucorales and hyaline hyphomycetes such as *Aspergillus*, *Fusarium*, or *Scedosporium* spp. can be difficult, keeping in mind that they can induce the same clinical presentation and radiological lesions. Second, even when hyphae are typical, identification to the species or genus level is impossible based on morphology in tissues. Third, culture is required to allow antifungal susceptibility testing. However, cultures are often negative even if their yields have increased noticeably over time (101). Due to the nonseptate nature of the hyphae, tissue grinding may induce a loss of viability and should therefore be avoided. Alternatively, biopsy specimens should be sliced and small pieces of tissues placed on the culture media. Mucorales are not fastidious organisms and can grow on common microbiological agar media, but mycological media such as Sabouraud dextrose agar containing antibiotics are preferred. Cycloheximide-containing media should not be used because this inhibitor of protein synthesis suppresses the growth of several species of Mucorales, even at low concentrations (109). Cultures should be incubated at 37°C for optimal yields (64), but incubation of a second tube at 25 to 30°C is recommended because some species have an optimum temperature of growth below 37°C (107).

■ Identification

Phenotypic Identification

General Description

Routine identification of Mucorales fungi to the species level is based mainly on the examination of their macroscopic and asexual microscopic characteristics, although some other criteria, such as physiological tests (109) or maximum growth temperature, can be used. The formation of zygospores is not useful for routine identification because they are not produced unless the isolate is mated with tester strains of the opposite mating type. The use of media with a high carbohydrate content favors massive formation of mycelia and prevents production of the asexual fruiting bodies required for identification. Therefore, media such as 2% malt, potato dextrose, and cherry decoction (acidic) agars are recommended for subculture of most of the Mucorales, although some of these media are not commercially available. To trigger sporulation in species such as *Apophysomyces* and *Saksenaea*, nutritionally deficient media containing a low percentage of yeast extract solution are advisable (88). Multiple factors, such as light and temperature, also influence the growth, morphology, and sporulation of these fungi. Several species are thermotolerant, being capable of growing at temperatures well over 40°C. Mycelial development of the Mucorales tends to be rapid (24 to 48 h) and extensive. Colony appearance varies according to the species, the age of the culture, and the media used. It is recommended for an accurate morphological study of Mucorales to use subculture at 27 to 30°C. Important macroscopic features include the appearance of the colonies (height, color, and texture) and the branching pattern of the sporangiophores; these can be observed under a 10× objective or a binocular microscope. For microscopic characteristics, a detailed study of adhesive tape mounts or tease mounts is essential for description of the sporulating structures of the species. Fungi in the order Mucorales are characterized by branched, nonseptate, wide hyphae (10 to 20 μm) with chitinous walls. Sexual reproduction occurs by means of zygospore formation after fusion of hyphal branches from the same (homothallic) or sexually differentiated (heterothallic) mycelia (39). The mature zygospore is often thick-walled and undergoes an obligatory dormant period

TABLE 2 Differential characteristics of zygospores in genera involved in mucormycosis

Genus	Type of sexual reproduction	Characteristics of zygospores
Lichtheimia	Heterothallic	Ellipsoidal with equatorial ridges; almost equal suspensors
Rhizopus	Heterothallic	Reddish brown; unequal spherical suspensors
Mucor	Heterothallic	Without appendages on suspensors
Rhizomucor	Heterothallic or homothallic	Spherical with blunt outgrowths
Cokeromyces	Homothallic	Spherical and brown, with sharp projections between opposite suspensors
Cunninghamella	Heterothallic	Spherical and brownish, with broad-ended projections
Syncephalastrum	Heterothallic	Spherical and black, with conical projections between equal suspensors

*a*Data from reference 31.

before germination. Table 2 details the characteristics of the zygospores of the principal genera involved in human disease. Asexual multiplication is by means of nonmotile sporangiospores (endospores) borne in closed sac-like structures named sporangia. They can exist as multispored sporangia or sporangiola (small sporangia) having few (or one) spores. Sporangia are supported by specialized hyphae named sporangiophores. In some species, these arise from a branched system of rhizoids which anchor the sporangiophore to the substratum. The rhizoids are connected by a rooting branch called a stolon. Additional morphological structures are the columella (central axis of the sporangium) and the apophysis (a swelling of the sporangiophore just below the columella). Some species can produce thick-walled and/or thin-walled swollen structures, named chlamydospores and oidia, respectively. The liberation of sporangiospores occurs by breakage or deliquescence of the sporangial wall (Fig. 2). Structures of Mucorales used for routine identification include branching of sporangiophores, type of sporangia (merosporangia or sporangiola), shape, color, and presence or absence of apophyses and columellae, and presence or absence of rhizoids or chlamydospores. Of note, several potentially useful websites are available online (tolweb.org/Zygomycota, www.doctorfungus.org, www.mycology.adelaide.edu.au, and www.cbs.knaw.nl).

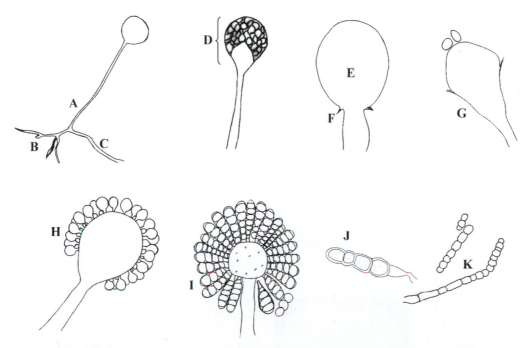

FIGURE 2 Schematic drawings of morphological structures observed in Mucorales. Sporangiophores (A) bear sporangia containing sporangiospores (D), can be anchored to the substrate by rhizoids (B), and expand by the means of stolons (C). The columella (E) is produced at the apex of the sporangiophore, and in some species an apophysis (G) is present. (F) For some species, after liberation of sporangiospores, a thin sporangium membrane may be visible. Sporangia with single or few spores are called sporangiola (H), and sporangia with few spores aligned in rows are called merosporangia (I). Thick-walled chlamydospores (J) and oidia (thin-walled swollen vesicles) (K) can be observed. (Drawings by Dea Garcia-Hermoso.)

Description of Specific Genera and Species

Morphological (macroscopic and microscopic) characteristics frequently implicated in human infections are described below. Only major features from our own experience and from specialized books (31, 35, 68) are mentioned. All colony morphology descriptions are made for subcultures on 2% malt agar at 30°C (unless otherwise specified). Colonies of Mucorales fungi have mostly floccose textures, with colors varying from white (*Saksenaea*) to yellow (*Mucor*), brownish (*Apophysomyces*), or gray (*Lichtheimia* and *Rhizomucor*). *Rhizopus* produces a high aerial mycelium, whereas *Rhizomucor* forms a 2- to 3-μm-high mycelium. The morphology of sporangiophores (height and branching) can vary depending on the genus. They can be branched, as in *Lichtheimia* or *Mucor*; irregularly branched, as in *Rhizomucor*; or mostly unbranched, as in *Rhizopus*. In addition, the site from which the sporangiophore arises (between rhizoids or directly from the stolon) is a supplementary clue for the identification of the different genera (Fig. 3).

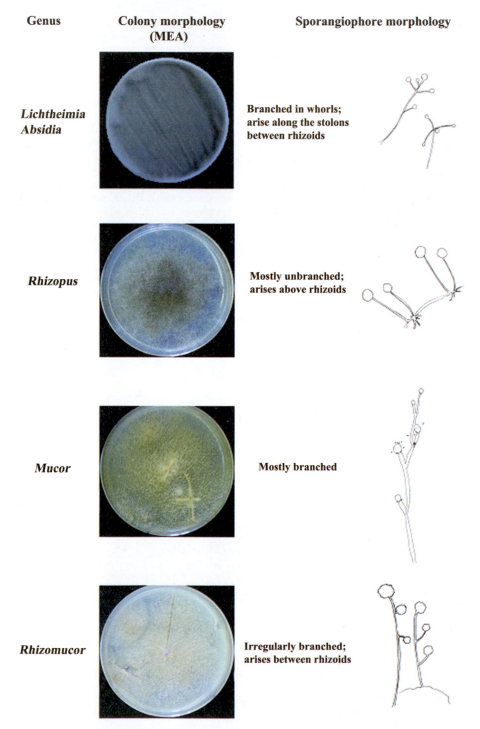

Genus	Colony morphology (MEA)	Sporangiophore morphology
Lichtheimia Absidia		Branched in whorls; arise along the stolons between rhizoids
Rhizopus		Mostly unbranched; arises above rhizoids
Mucor		Mostly branched
Rhizomucor		Irregularly branched; arises between rhizoids

FIGURE 3   Culture variability of some of the genera of Mucorales and their branching development.

Microscopic Characteristics

A morphological key to the principal genera of Mucorales is illustrated in Fig. 4. The combination of asexual fruiting bodies and criteria such as maximum growth temperature is useful for the differentiation of these fungi to the species level.

Family Lichtheimiaceae

Genus *Lichtheimia*. *LICHTHEIMIA CORYMBIFERA (MYCOCLADUS CORYMBIFER, ABSIDIA CORYMBIFERA).* The genus *Absidia* was recently revised on the basis of phylogenetic, physiological, and morphological characteristics (52). The thermotolerant species of *Absidia corymbifera*, *Absidia blakesleeana* and *Absidia hyalospora*, were placed in the new family Mycocladiaceae and the genus *Mycocladus*. More recently, the same authors made a nomenclatural correction, creating the family Lichtheimiaceae (instead of Mycocladiaceae) and reassigning the genus *Lichtheimia* in place of *Mycocladus* (53). Recently, 38 isolates morphologically identified as *L. corymbifera* were studied by a multigene sequence analysis. The results uncovered the presence of a different species (named *Lichtheimia ramosa*), which differed in morphology and sequence content from *L. corymbifera* (41).

Lichtheimia corymbifera has a worldwide distribution and has been isolated from diverse substrates, including seeds, soil, and decaying vegetable debris. It produces white, fast-growing, woolly colonies which become grayish brown with age. The maximum growth temperature is between 46 and 52°C. Microscopically, sporangiophores are usually erect and highly branched and arise singly or in small corymbs from stolons, but not opposite the rhizoids as in *Rhizopus*. Rhizoids are present but are generally indistinguishable. Multispored sporangia are small and spherical to pyriform. Columellae are hemispherical or ellipsoidal, with marked conical apophyses, and sporangiospores are smooth and hyaline (2.73 by 2.24 μm in diameter). Giant cells of irregular shape are frequently present (Fig. 5).

Family Mucoraceae

Genus *Rhizopus*. The genus *Rhizopus* is commonly found in air, soil, and compost and is characterized by the rapid production of white cottony colonies, which turn brownish to black with time due to the presence of pigmented sporangiophores and sporangia. The sporangiophores are unbranched, arising singly or in groups, with well-developed rhizoids at the base, which distinguish the genus *Rhizopus* from the genera *Lichtheimia* and *Rhizomucor*. Differences in the length of sporangiophores, the shape and ornamentation of sporangiospores, and the maximum growth temperature are useful to identify the different species of *Rhizopus*, as shown in Table 3. *Rhizopus oryzae* and *Rhizopus microsporus* are the most common species involved in mucormycosis. Detailed descriptions of these species are provided below. Other species, such as *Rhizopus schipperae* and *Rhizopus azygosporus*, are rarely recovered from clinical specimens.

RHIZOPUS ORYZAE. Microscopic features include single or clustered brown sporangiophores of 1 to 2 mm in height bearing multispored sporangia (150 to 170 μm in diameter).

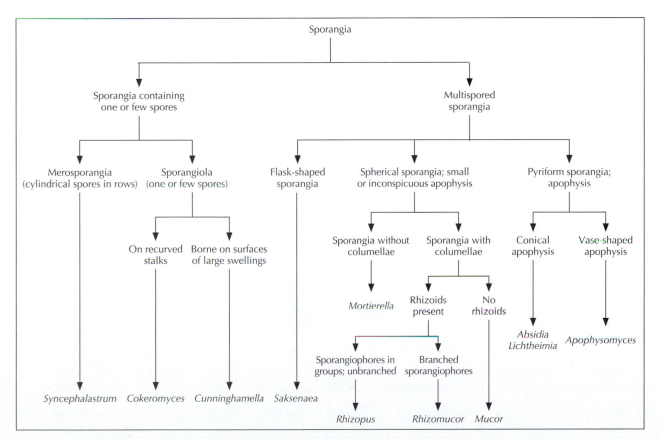

FIGURE 4 Flow diagram for the identification of the different genera of Mucorales. Data from references 31 and 68.

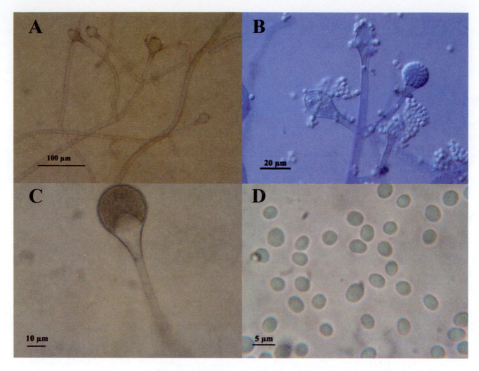

FIGURE 5 *Lichtheimia corymbifera.* (A) Branched sporangiophores; (B) hemispheric columellae and sporangiospores; (C) pyriform multispored sporangium and marked conical apophysis; (D) sporangiospores.

Columellae are ellipsoidal and brown to gray and generally have a truncate base. Rhizoids are well developed and easily observed under a stereomicroscope. Sporangiospores are angular and round to ellipsoidal, with longitudinal ridges measuring 6 to 8 by 4.5 to 5.0 μm. Chlamydospores (10 to 35 μm in diameter) can be present (Fig. 6). This thermotolerant species can grow at 40°C but not at 45°C. *Rhizopus oryzae* differs from the nonpathogenic organism *Rhizopus stolonifer*, which harbors longer sporangiophores (>2 mm) and larger columellae (up to 275 μm in diameter) and does not grow at 40°C (105).

RHIZOPUS MICROSPORUS. According to a recent U.S. review, *Rhizopus microsporus* is the second most frequent agent of mucormycosis (4). It can be isolated from soil or wood products. Colonies are pale brownish gray, with sporangiophores arising from stolons and measuring up to 400 μm in length (106). Sporangia are dark brown (up to 80 μm in diameter), columellae are conical, and sporangiospores are striate and angular to ellipsoidal (Fig. 7). In addition to the typical variety, *Rhizopus microsporus* var. *microsporus,* there are three supplementary varieties: *Rhizopus microsporus* var. *chinensis, Rhizopus microsporus* var. *oligosporus,* and *Rhizopus microsporus* var. *rhizopodiformis.* They can be distinguished on the basis of the morphology of sporangiospores and their temperature tolerance (Table 3). *Rhizopus microsporus* var. *rhizopodiformis,* the predominant variety identified among

TABLE 3 Main characteristics allowing distinction between *Rhizopus* species and *R. microsporus* varieties

Species	Sporangiophore ht (mm)	Sporangiospore shape and ornamentation	Growth at indicated temp (°C)				
			30	37	40	45	50
R. oryzae	Often >1	Angular, round to ellipsoidal, striate	+	+	+	−	−
R. stolonifer	Often >1	Angular, round to ellipsoidal, striate	+	−	−	−	−
R. microsporus var. *microsporus*	Not exceeding 0.8	Angular-ellipsoidal, striate	+	+	+	+	−
R. microsporus var. *oligosporus*	Not exceeding 0.8	Large, round, irregularly ornamented	+	+	+	Limited growth	−
R. microsporus var. *rhizopodiformis*	Not exceeding 0.8	Small, round, spinulose	+	+	+	+	+
R. microsporus var. *chinensis*	Not exceeding 0.8	Angular, homogeneous	+	+	+	+ (immature sporangia)	−
R. schipperae	Not exceeding 0.8	Round to ellipsoidal, striate	+	+	+	Very limited growth	−
R. azygosporus	Not exceeding 0.8	Round, barely striate	+	+	+	+	+

^aData from references 31 and 106.

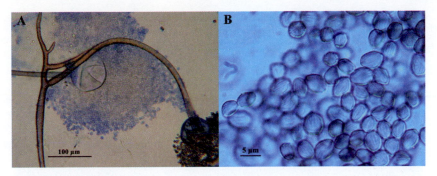

FIGURE 6   Typical microscopic features of *Rhizopus oryzae*. (A) Melanized sporangiophore arising opposite rhizoids; (B) striate angular sporangiospores.

clinical isolates (68), differs from the other varieties by its growth at 50°C and spinulose sporangiospores.

Genus *Rhizomucor*. Species of the genus *Rhizomucor* are frequently isolated from composting or fermenting organic matter (112). Macroscopically, *Rhizomucor* produces rapidly growing gray to brown wooly colonies. Sporangiophores are single or branched and arise from aerial mycelium or from stolons. Rhizoids are present but often difficult to recognize. Sporangia are multispored, apophyses are absent, and the fungus grows at high temperatures (is thermotolerant). The genus *Rhizomucor* differs from the genus *Mucor* by its thermotolerance and the presence of rhizoids and stolons. To distinguish between the three pathogenic—or potentially pathogenic—species of *Rhizomucor* (*Rhizomucor pusillus*, *Rhizomucor miehei*, and *Rhizomucor variabilis*), parameters such as maximal growth temperature, size of sporangia, sucrose assimilation, and the capacity to grow in the presence of thiamine can be used. *R. variabilis* does not grow at temperatures of more than 38°C, while growth is observed at 45°C for *R. pusillus* and *R. miehei*. The latter has smaller spo-

rangia than *R. pusillus* (60 μm versus 100 μm in diameter) and fails to assimilate sucrose, and its growth depends on the presence of thiamine. Due to the uncertain taxonomic position of the species *R. variabilis* (phylogenetic analyses place this species close to *Mucor hiemalis*) (124), only the description of the species *Rhizomucor pusillus* is provided.

RHIZOMUCOR PUSILLUS. Colonies are brown, compact, and short. Apical branches arise from the tops of sporangiophores, supporting globose sporangia of 100 μm in diameter. Simple and branched rhizoids can be observed. Columellae are round to pyriform, without apophyses. Sporangiospores are round, hyaline, and smooth-walled (Fig. 8). Maximum growth temperature is 55°C.

Genus *Mucor*. The most important feature of the species belonging to the genus *Mucor* is the absence of basal rhizoids and stolons, which distinguishes them from *Lichtheimia*, *Rhizopus*, and *Rhizomucor*. Colonies are usually fast-growing and white to yellow, becoming gray with time. The tall sporangiophores (they can reach several centimeters

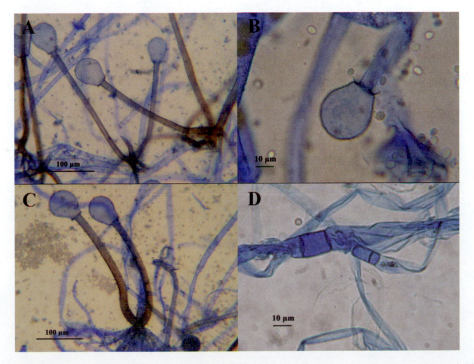

FIGURE 7   Short pigmented sporangiophores arising in pairs in *Rhizopus microsporus*. (A and C) Rhizoids; (B) conical columella; (D) chlamydospores.

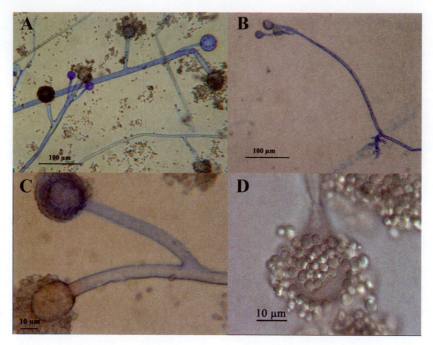

FIGURE 8 *Rhizomucor pusillus.* Sporangiophores with apical branching (A), simple rhizoids (B), and globose sporangia with round and smooth-walled sporangiospores (C and D) are shown.

in height) are simple or branched, supporting multispored sporangia. For some species, residues of the sporangial wall (collarette) can be present, and some species can produce chlamydospores (Fig. 9). Maximum growth temperatures for pathogenic *Mucor* species range from 32°C (*Mucor racemosus*) to 42°C (*Mucor indicus*). *Mucor circinelloides* is a very variable species and comprises four varieties, based mainly on differences in the shapes of columellae and sporangiospores. Major phenotypic differences among the thermotolerant *Mucor* species involved in human infections are summarized in Table 4. The identification of these species can be complicated under unsuitable growth conditions,

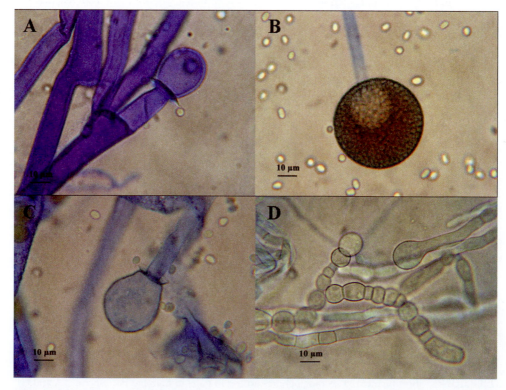

FIGURE 9 Micromorphology of *Mucor circinelloides.* (A) Sporangiophore; (B) sporangia; (B and C) ellipsoidal sporangiospores; (D) oidia.

TABLE 4 Macroscopic and microscopic features of *Mucor* species involved in human infection

Species	Colony morphology	Colony ht (mm)	Sporangium diam (μm)	Columella shape	Sporangiospore shape	Maximum growth temp (°C)	Presence of chlamydospores	Other characteristics
M. *circinelloides*	Light gray to brown	Up to 6	Up to 80	Obovoid to ellipsoidal	Ellipsoidal	36–40	Rare	Assimilation of ethanol
M. *racemosus*	Light gray to brown	Up to 20	Up to 90	Obovoid, ellipsoidal, pyriform with truncate base	Ellipsoidal to subglobose	32	Abundant, mainly in sporangio-phores	
M. *ramosissimus*	Olive gray	Up to 2	Up to 80	Applanate	Subglobose to ellipsoidal	36	Absent	Presence of oidia in substrate mycelium
M. *indicus*	Deep yellow	Up to 10	Up to 75	Subglobose	Subglobose to cylindrical-ellipsoidal	42	Abundant	Light-dependent sporulation

*a*Data from reference 104.

which can induce morphological variations such as sterile sporangia, swelling in sporangiophores, and modifications in the size and shape of sporangia, columellae, and sporangiospores (104).

Genus *Apophysomyces*. *APOPHYSOMYCES ELEGANS.* *Apophysomyces elegans* is a soil fungus with a tropical to subtropical distribution. It produces fast-growing white to gray colonies. Sporangiophores are erect, unbranched, and single, bearing multispored, usually pyriform, sporangia of 20 to 60 μm in diameter. The production of prominent vase-shaped or bell-shaped apophyses is a distinctive feature of this species. These apophyses differ from the conical apophyses produced by *Lichtheimia*. Columellae are hemispheric, and sporangiospores are smooth-walled and cylindrical (Fig. 10). Good growth is observed at 42°C (35). The use of nutrient-poor media (e.g., water-yeast extract medium) can improve

sporulation, which is often lacking on primary isolation media (88).

Family Thamnidiaceae

Genus *Cokeromyces*. *COKEROMYCES RECURVATUS.* *Cokeromyces recurvatus* remains a rare agent of mucormycosis. It has been recovered mostly from soil or from rabbit, rat, or lizard dung in North America (United States and Mexico). Colonies are slow growing (less than 1 mm high) and grayish to brown. Microscopic features include the presence of long, recurved, twisted stalks arising from terminal vesicles of unbranched sporangiophores, globose sporangiola (8 to 11 μm in diameter) borne on those stalks, and smooth-walled spherical sporangiospores of 2 to 4 μm (Fig. 11). A yeast-like form can be obtained by subculture on media such as brain heart infusion agar

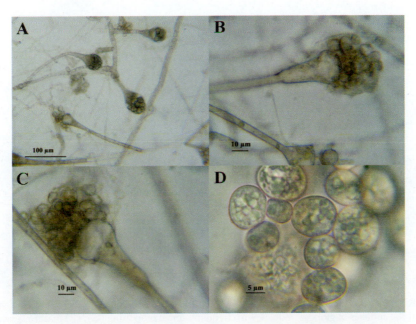

FIGURE 10 *Apophysomyces elegans*. (A) Unbranched sporangiophores bearing multispored sporangia with a vase-shaped apophysis (B and C); (D) cylindrical sporangiospores.

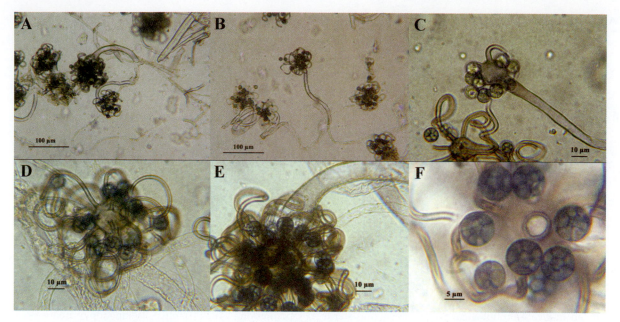

FIGURE 11 *Cokeromyces recurvatus.* (A and B) Mostly unbranched sporangiophores without rhizoids; (C) young sporangiolum; (D to F) recurved stalks arising from terminal vesicles and bearing few spored sporangiola.

or yeast extract-glucose-peptone agar. Yeasts are thin- to thick-walled and spherical, measuring 10 to 100 μm in diameter. Some cells produce single buds on the whole surface (68). The species is homothallic and produces lemon-shaped zygospores.

Family Cunninghamellaceae

Genus Cunninghamella. CUNNINGHAMELLA BERTHOLLETIAE. Although it is a rare agent of human disease, *Cunninghamella bertholletiae* has the capacity to infect immunocompetent individuals. It is traditionally considered the only clinically relevant species of the genus. Another species, *Cunninghamella echinulata*, has also been implicated in a case of human mucormycosis (75). *C. bertholletiae* is a thermotholerant fungus isolated from soil. It produces white to dark gray expanding colonies. Sporangiophores are erect, with lateral branching at the apical zone. Each branch produces a globose vesicle (up to 40 μm in diameter) which bears a one-spored sporangiolum. At maturity, each sporangiolum becomes a finely echinulate spherical sporangiospore (7 to 11 μm in diameter) (Fig. 12). Key features for the

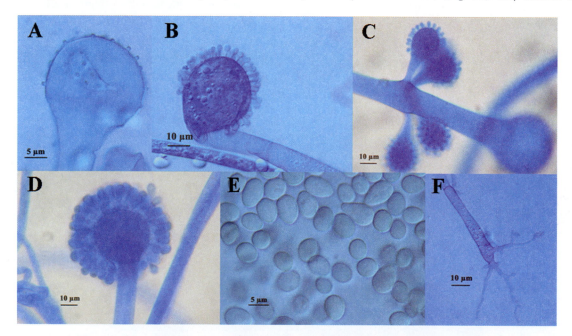

FIGURE 12 *Cunninghamella bertholletiae.* (A, B, and D) Development of single-spored sporangiola on the surfaces of globose vesicles, with frequent apical branching (C); (E) mature sporangiola grow to be single echinulate sporangiospores; (F) rhizoids.

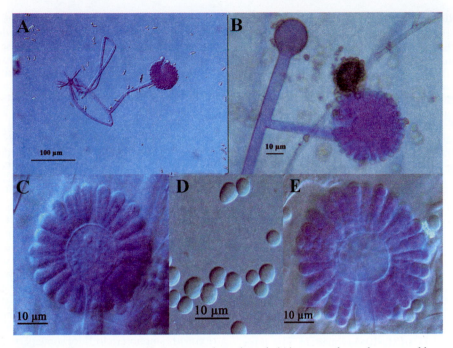

FIGURE 13   Short sporangiophores arising from rhizoids (A), terminal vesicles covered by mero-sporangia (B, C, and E), and merospores (D) characteristic of *Syncephalastrum racemosus*.

identification of C. *bertholletiae* are essentially its growth at 45°C (with a maximum of 50°C) and the presence of monosporic sporangiola borne on terminal vesicles.

Family Syncephalastraceae

Genus *Syncephalastrum*. Species of the genus *Syncephalastrum* have a worldwide distribution and have been isolated from soil, plants, and diverse foodstuffs (98). The only species associated with cases of human infection is *Syncephalastrum racemosum*, described below.

SYNCEPHALASTRUM RACEMOSUM. In culture, S. *racemosum* grows rapidly and produces expanding white to grayish colonies turning darker due to the formation of sporangia and resembling the colonies formed by *Rhizopus* spp. The maximal temperature for growth is 40°C. Sporangiophores are short, erect, and mostly branched, arising from rhizoids and forming terminal globose vesicles. The whole surface of these vesicles is covered with cylindrical

merosporangia containing 3 to 14 smooth-walled, spherical to ovoidal merospores disposed in single rows (Fig. 13). This is a distinctive feature of the genus compared to other members of the Mucorales.

Family Saksenaeaceae

Genus *Saksenaea*. SAKSENAEA VASIFORMIS. *Saksenaea vasiformis* is the only species in the genus *Saksenaea*. It is a saprophytic fungus with a worldwide distribution and was first isolated from forest soil (98). It produces white to grayish expanding colonies, with a maximum growth temperature of 44°C. The use of specific nutrient-poor media (e.g., water-yeast extract medium) can induce sporulation (88). Czapek medium at 30°C or 37°C also induces sporulation. Microscopically, sporangiophores are unbranched, with melanized rhizoids. The formation of distinctive flask-shaped multi-spored sporangia is a key feature for the identification of this species. Sporangiospores are smooth-walled and cylindrical, measuring 11 to 15 μm in diameter, as seen in Fig. 14.

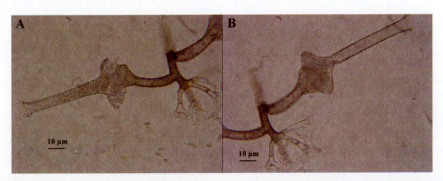

FIGURE 14   *Saksenaea vasiformis.* (A and B) Unbranched sporangiophores with dark rhizoids and typical multispored flask-shaped sporangia.

Molecular Identification

Phenotypic identification of Mucorales to the species level remains difficult because the various species that can be responsible for infection share common morphological characteristics (107). Moreover, some pathogenic species, such as *S. vasiformis* and *A. elegans*, regularly fail to sporulate on standard mycological media (54). In a recent study, Mucorales were erroneously identified by morphology in >20% of cases (65). The correct identification often requires specialized expertise found only in reference laboratories (128). Therefore, sequence-based identification is interesting because it provides rapidly obtainable and easily comparable data (40).

DNA bar coding of Mucorales requires a DNA target shared by all species, with sufficient interspecific variability to allow distinction between the species. The intraspecific variability should be minimal for the purpose of species identification. Besides the choice of the best target and technique, a comprehensive and reliable database is mandatory. It has been shown that a commercially available sequencing kit may incorrectly identify many of the pathogenic Mucorales species (44, 48), probably due to the incomplete associated sequence database. Most studies have focused on ribosomal DNA targets, including 18S (78), 28S (124), and ITS (81, 108) sequences. The intra- and interspecific variabilities of the whole ITS1-5.8S-ITS2 region were evaluated with a large number of isolates of Mucorales, including most of the human-pathogenic species (108). The sequence variability was low (<2%) within a given species, contrasting with large variations between species. Even species belonging to a given genus, such as *R. oryzae* and *R. microsporus*, were easily differentiated based on their ITS sequences (<70% similarity). ITS sequencing has also been used successfully in individual cases (13, 59, 62). Other DNA targets (a fragment of the high-affinity iron permease FTR1 gene [85]) and techniques (real-time PCR assay targeting the cytochrome *b* gene [49]) have also been evaluated.

Based on available data and expert opinions, an international consensus was reached on the best sequence-based identification strategy for Mucorales and other filamentous fungi. ITS sequencing is thus recommended as the first-line choice for identification of Mucorales to the species level (5, 21). The D1/D2 region of the 28S rRNA can be used as an alternative target. Although some issues remain to be addressed to thoroughly standardize these new molecular tools, they already represent considerable advances. These techniques should impact routine procedures in the clinical microbiology laboratory and the current knowledge on the epidemiology of mucormycosis.

■ Typing Systems

Few methods have been evaluated for the typing of clinical isolates of Mucorales (1, 17, 65). The methods used proved to be inefficient due to their low discriminatory power.

■ Serologic Tests

Serologic diagnosis of mucormycosis has been attempted (27, 98), but no commercial assays are available at this time.

■ Antifungal Susceptibilities

Antifungal susceptibility can be evaluated both in vitro and in vivo (in animal models of infection) (24). In vitro antifungal susceptibility can be evaluated by using the reference microdilution broth techniques developed by the Clinical and Laboratory Standards Institute (22) or the European Committee on Antimicrobial Susceptibility Testing (113) or by using the commercially available Etest (bioMérieux, Marcy l'Etoile, France) (36). Although Mucorales fungi share most antifungal susceptibility patterns, there is some specificity depending on genus and even species. Amphotericin B is the most active drug against Mucorales, as shown both in vitro (3, 27, 28, 115, 120) and in animal models of infection (26, 29, 56, 116). Nevertheless, some species, such as *Cunninghamella bertholletiae*, exhibit higher amphotericin B MICs, and experimental data from animals infected with this species suggest a limited in vivo efficacy. Among the new azoles, voriconazole has poor activity, which is highlighted by breakthrough mucormycosis in patients treated with this agent. In contrast, posaconazole has relatively low MICs (3, 28, 115). Furthermore, in vivo efficacy of posaconazole in various animal models has been demonstrated for its use both as a curative treatment and prophylactically (6, 26, 116). Echinocandins have no significant in vitro activity, despite the fact that *Rhizopus oryzae* possesses the target enzyme for this class of compounds. In vivo, caspofungin alone exhibits modest efficacy (57), and it showed promising clinical efficacy in combination with amphotericin B for some patients (96).

■ Evaluation, Interpretation, and Reporting of Results

Culture results should always be interpreted in light of the clinical presentation and along with the results of direct examination and histopathology (Fig. 1). A positive Mucorales culture can occur due to contamination during collection of the sample or processing of the sample in the laboratory. A recent study in Spain showed that fewer than 8% of the Mucorales isolates recovered in the laboratory were from patients with invasive mucormycosis (118, 119). In the revised consensus definitions for the diagnosis of invasive fungal infections developed by the European Organization for Research and Treatment of Cancer and the Mycoses Study Group, proven disease requires that "histopathologic, cytopathologic, or direct microscopic examination of a specimen obtained by needle aspiration or biopsy shows hyphae accompanied by evidence of associated tissue damage" or "the recovery of a mold by culture of a specimen obtained by a sterile procedure from a normally sterile and clinically or radiologically abnormal site consistent with an infectious disease process, excluding bronchoalveolar lavage fluid, a cranial sinus cavity specimen, and urine" (33). However, "the failure to meet the criteria for invasive fungal infection does not mean that there is none, only that there is insufficient evidence to support the diagnosis. This is the most compelling reason for not employing these definitions in daily clinical practice." One may thus have proof of an invasive fungal infection and a high suspicion of mucormycosis without evidence of the latter in the absence of positive culture. As mentioned before, attempts to establish a definite diagnosis are important to offer the best management for the patient.

ENTOMOPHTHOROMYCOSIS

■ Epidemiology and Transmission

The majority of members of the Entomophthorales are pathogens of arthropods and other animals. They are present in soil, decaying vegetables, and dung worldwide but are found more abundantly in warm climates of Africa and Asia (68). Infections due to *Basidiobolus ranarum* have been described in Asia (Indonesia, where the first cases were described, India, and Myanmar) and several African countries (mostly Uganda and Nigeria) and, rarely, in South America. Infections due to *Conidiobolus* spp. have been described in Africa, Madagascar, Mayotte, India, China, and South America (15, 95).

■ Clinical Manifestations

One of the major differences between mucormycosis and entomophthoromycosis is that the former occurs mainly in predisposed individuals and the latter occurs mostly in immunocompetent hosts.

Basidiobolus ranarum is responsible for subcutaneous infections which affect mostly the limbs, buttocks, trunk, and perineum and, less often, the face and neck. The disease presents mostly in male children as a hard, painless nodule that enlarges peripherally without affecting the overlying skin (47). Invasive infections with gastrointestinal involvement (131) have been described as a small cluster in Arizona (76) and sporadically worldwide. Disseminated infections are extremely rare (9).

In contrast to basidiobolomycosis, infections due to *Conidiobolus* spp. affect adults (mostly males) and outdoor workers and are usually limited to the nose and face. The onset of infection is thought to take place in the nasal mucosa after inoculation of spores following a minor trauma. Swelling extends locally to the nose, nasolabial folds, cheeks, eyebrows, upper lip, and even the palate and pharynx, producing characteristic facies in severe forms (46). Conjunctival inoculation of the fungus was documented once in Brazil (11). Rare cases of dissemination have been reported for immunosuppressed individuals (126). Tissue lesions caused by *Conidiobolus coronatus* and *Conidiobolus incongruus* are similar (110).

■ Treatment and Outcome

Therapeutic strategies for basidiobolomycosis and conidiobolomycosis are not standardized because of the lack of trials for these rare infections. Surgical excision, potassium iodide, and prolonged azole therapy have been used successfully for infection due to *Basidiobolus* (15, 93). For infections due to *Conidiobolus* spp., potassium iodide was historically used, with variable results. Prolonged oral azole therapy should now be used and is successful (95).

■ Collection, Transport, and Handling of Specimens

Since several differential diagnoses are possible, confirmation of the fungal etiology should be obtained. The diagnosis relies on classical procedures combining direct examination or histology and culture. Tissue biopsy specimens should be obtained from the affected area. For the gastrointestinal form of basidiobolomycosis, biopsy specimens obtained during endoscopy are the samples of choice. Specimens should be processed immediately and should not be refrigerated (47).

■ Direct Examination

Microscopy

A direct examination can be performed after maceration of the tissue sample in KOH or after staining of the sample

with calcofluor white or Gomori-Grocott stain. Typically, hyphae are broad, thin-walled, and generally more septate than those of the Mucorales. Histopathology shows simultaneous acute and chronic inflammatory reactions. Hyphae can be observed by use of routine staining procedures (hematoxylin and eosin, periodic acid-Schiff, and Gomori-Grocott stains). The presence of the Splendore-Hoeppli phenomenon in tissue sections stained with hematoxylin-eosin is suggestive of entomopthoromycosis. The pink structure corresponds to a sheath of amorphous eosinophilic material around hyphal fragments. Although the Splendore-Hoeppli phenomenon is strongly suggestive of entomophthoromycosis, it can also be observed in various bacterial, fungal, and parasitic infections as well as in cases of noninfectious disease (55). In contrast to the case for mucormycosis, there is typically no necrosis and no invasion of blood vessels.

Antigen Tests

No antigen tests are currently available for the detection of entomophthoromycosis.

Detection of Nucleic Acids in Clinical Materials

Molecular techniques have not been developed for the diagnosis of entomophthoromycosis from tissues.

■ Isolation Procedures

Biopsy specimens should be sliced and inoculated onto Sabouraud agar or potato dextrose agar (PDA). Media containing cycloheximide should be avoided because this drug inhibits the growth of Entomophthorales. Cultures must be incubated at both 37°C and 25 to 30°C because *Basidiobolus* and *Conidiobolus* have different optimum growth temperatures. *Basidiobolus* grows well at 30°C but less rapidly at 37°C, whereas *Conidiobolus* spp. grow rapidly at 37°C (98).

■ Identification

Phenotypic Identification

Members of the Entomophthorales are characterized by the presence of primary and secondary conidia, which are discharged by force at maturity. Primary conidia with papillate bases are produced straight from the thallus, in repetitive cycles (31). They generate a germ tube or can produce smaller secondary conidia (similar in morphology to the primary conidia) in the presence of suitable substrate conditions. Villose conidia (old conidia with hair-like appendages) can also develop. Passive release of microconidia may also occur. In some species, thin sporangiophores bear capilliconidia at the apex. These spores are characterized by an adhesive tip. Zygospores (thick-bilayer-walled spores) are produced after conjugation of undifferentiated gametangia and can have beak-like appendages coming from gametangial remains (31, 35, 68). Sporulation occurs after 3 to 10 days of culture. Colonies are usually waxy or powdery, with radial folds and with colors ranging from cream to gray (68). A key feature of these fungi is their capacity to forcibly discharge conidia. Therefore, placing a cover slide inside a petri dish lid can be helpful for recovery of the papillate conidia. For a detailed description and additional information, see the taxonomic classification study of Ben-Ze'ev and Kenneth (7).

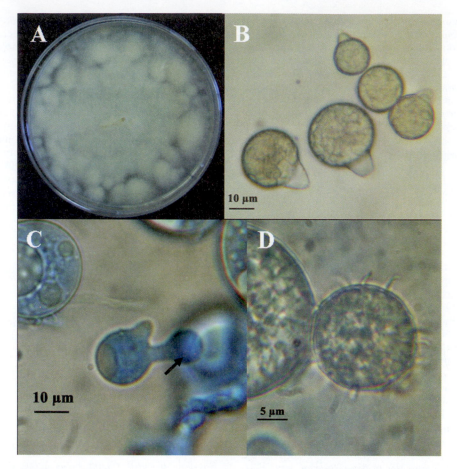

FIGURE 15 *Conidiobolus coronatus.* (A) Ten-day-old powdery colony on PDA medium; (B) primary conidia with papilla; (C) passively released secondary conidium (arrow); (D) villose conidium.

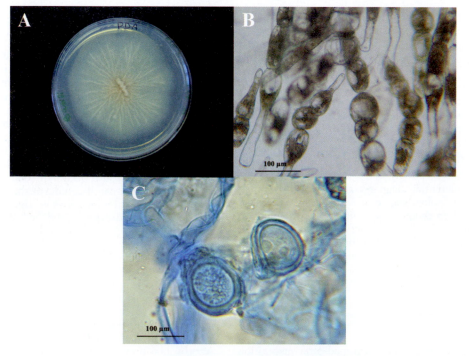

FIGURE 16 *Basidiobolus ranarum.* (A) Ten-day-old wrinkled colony on PDA medium; (B) uninucleated hyphal elements; (C) young zygospores.

Family Ancylistaceae

Genus *Conidiobolus*. *CONIDIOBOLUS CORONATUS*. *C. coronatus* is a fast-growing fungus present in soil and on decaying leaves (35) and is isolated most frequently in tropical forests of Africa (38). *C. coronatus* is an occasional pathogen of insects and has been recovered from diverse animals, such as dolphins, chimpanzees, and horses (98). Colonies are hyaline and radially folded, with an initially waxy appearance becoming powdery when mycelia become visible. The lid of the dish can be covered with conidia forcibly discharged by the conidiophores. These primary conidia are spherical (40 μm in diameter) and possess a prominent papilla. Villose conidia are present in older cultures (Fig. 15). Replicative, passively discharged microconidia are regularly produced (31).

Family Basidiobolaceae

Genus *Basidiobolus*. *BASIDIOBOLUS RANARUM*. *Basidiobolus ranarum* is present in decaying fruit and vegetable matter (35). It can be present as a commensal in the intestinal tracts of amphibians and reptiles (87). Colonies on PDA agar are yellowish and waxy, have radial folds, and do not form an aerial mycelium when they are young. They grow well at 25 to 37°C. Microscopic examination after 7 to 10 days of culture reveals large aseptate hyphae which can break up into free hyphal elements that are basically uninucleated. *B. ranarum* is homothallic. Sexual reproduction occurs by gametangial conjugation, producing thick-walled zygospores with lateral protuberances of gametangial remains (beaks) (Fig. 16). Primary conidiophores with swollen apices forcibly discharge spherical primary conidia. Secondary conidia are pyriform (clavate) and are passively released from the sporophore. These conidia possess a knob-like adhesive tip. Occasionally, elongated cells with a terminal adhesive tip (capilliconidia) are present (31, 38).

Molecular Identification

There is no technique published for the molecular identification of Entomophthorales.

■ Typing Systems

To date, there is no typing method developed for Entomophthorales.

■ Serologic Tests

There are no commercially available diagnostic tests for Entomophthorales.

■ Antimicrobial Susceptibilities

In vitro susceptibility data are scarce, and some technical issues (such as inoculum preparation) remain to be addressed. Potassium iodide shows no in vitro activity, despite in vivo efficacy (129). Amphotericin B exhibits relatively high MICs (45, 117), while itraconazole and ketoconazole have good in vitro activities (45). Overall, *Basidiobolus* spp. are more susceptible than *Conidiobolus* spp. to the different antifungals tested.

■ Evaluation, Interpretation, and Reporting of Results

In areas where entomophthoromycosis is endemic, final diagnosis is based on a direct examination showing broad thin-walled hyphae with the Splendore-Hoeppli phenomenon, without necrosis or invasion of blood vessels. In cases of positive culture, results of antifungal susceptibility testing do not currently influence therapeutic decisions.

REFERENCES

1. **Abe, A., T. Sone, I. N. Sujaya, K. Saito, Y. Oda, K. Asano, and F. Tomita.** 2003. rDNA ITS sequence of *Rhizopus oryzae*: its application to classification and identification of lactic acid producers. *Biosci. Biotechnol. Biochem.* **67:**1725–1731.
2. **Almaslamani, M., S. J. Taj-Aldeen, D. Garcia-Hermoso, E. Dannaoui, H. Alsoub, and A. Alkhal.** 2009. An increasing trend of cutaneous zygomycosis caused by *Mycocladus corymbifer* (formerly *Absidia corymbifera*): report of two cases and review of primary cutaneous *Mycocladus* infections. *Med. Mycol.* **47:**532–538.
3. **Almyroudis, N. G., D. A. Sutton, A. W. Fothergill, M. G. Rinaldi, and S. Kusne.** 2007. In vitro susceptibilities of 217 clinical isolates of zygomycetes to conventional and new antifungal agents. *Antimicrob. Agents Chemother.* **51:**2587–2590.
4. **Alvarez, E., D. A. Sutton, J. Cano, A. W. Fothergill, A. Stchigel, M. G. Rinaldi, and J. Guarro.** 2009. Spectrum of zygomycete species identified in clinically significant specimens in the United States. *J. Clin. Microbiol.* **47:**1650–1656.
5. **Balajee, S. A., A. M. Borman, M. E. Brandt, J. Cano, M. Cuenca-Estrella, E. Dannaoui, J. Guarro, G. Haase, C. C. Kibbler, W. Meyer, K. O'Donnell, C. A. Petti, J. L. Rodriguez-Tudela, D. Sutton, A. Velegraki, and B. L. Wickes.** 2009. Sequence-based identification of *Aspergillus*, *Fusarium*, and *Mucorales* species in the clinical mycology laboratory: where are we and where should we go from here? *J. Clin. Microbiol.* **47:**877–884.
6. **Barchiesi, F., E. Spreghini, A. Santinelli, A. W. Fothergill, E. Pisa, D. Giannini, M. G. Rinaldi, and G. Scalise.** 2007. Posaconazole prophylaxis in experimental systemic zygomycosis. *Antimicrob. Agents Chemother.* **51:**73–77.
7. **Ben-Ze'ev, I., and R. Kenneth.** 1982. Criteria of taxonomic value in the *Entomophthorales*. *Mycotaxon* **14:**393–455.
8. **Bialek, R., F. Konrad, J. Kern, C. Aepinus, L. Cecenas, G. M. Gonzalez, G. Just-Nubling, B. Willinger, E. Presterl, C. Lass-Florl, and V. Rickerts.** 2005. PCR based identification and discrimination of agents of mucormycosis and aspergillosis in paraffin wax embedded tissue. *J. Clin. Pathol.* **58:**1180–1184.
9. **Bigliazzi, C., V. Poletti, D. Dell'Amore, L. Saragoni, and T. V. Colby.** 2004. Disseminated basidiobolomycosis in an immunocompetent woman. *J. Clin. Microbiol.* **42:**1367–1369.
10. **Bitar, D., D. Van Cauteren, F. Lanternier, E. Dannaoui, D. Che, F. Dromer, J. Descenclos, and O. Lortholary.** 2009. Increasing incidence of zygomycosis (mucormycosis), France, 1997–2006. *Emerg. Infect. Dis.* **15:**1395–1401.
11. **Bittencourt, A. L., R. Marback, and L. M. Nossa.** 2006. Mucocutaneous entomophthoramycosis acquired by conjunctival inoculation of the fungus. *Am. J. Trop. Med. Hyg.* **75:**936–938.
12. **Bjorkholm, M., G. Runarsson, F. Celsing, M. Kalin, B. Petrini, and P. Engervall.** 2001. Liposomal amphotericin B and surgery in the successful treatment of invasive pulmonary mucormycosis in a patient with acute T-lymphoblastic leukemia. *Scand. J. Infect. Dis.* **33:**316–319.
13. **Blanchet, D., E. Dannaoui, A. Fior, F. Huber, P. Couppie, N. Salhab, D. Hoinard, and C. Aznar.** 2008. *Saksenaea vasiformis* infection, French Guiana. *Emerg. Infect. Dis.* **14:**342–344.
14. **Blin, N., N. Morineau, F. Gaillard, O. Morin, N. Milpied, J. L. Harousseau, and P. Moreau.** 2004. Disseminated mucormycosis associated with invasive pulmonary aspergillosis in a patient treated for post-transplant high-grade non-Hodgkin's lymphoma. *Leuk. Lymphoma* **45:**2161–2163.
15. **Cameron, H. M.** 1989. Entomophthoromycosis, p. 186–198. *In* E. S. Mahgoub (ed.), *Tropical Mycosis*. Janssen Research Council, Beerse, Belgium.

16. **Chakrabarti, A., A. Das, J. Mandal, M. R. Shivaprakash, V. K. George, B. Tarai, P. Rao, N. Panda, S. C. Verma, and V. Sakhuja.** 2006. The rising trend of invasive zygomycosis in patients with uncontrolled diabetes mellitus. *Med. Mycol.* **44:**335–342.

17. **Chakrabarti, A., A. Ghosh, G. S. Prasad, J. K. David, S. Gupta, A. Das, V. Sakhuja, N. K. Panda, S. K. Singh, S. Das, and T. Chakrabarti.** 2003. *Apophysomyces elegans:* an emerging zygomycete in India. *J. Clin. Microbiol.* **41:**783–788.

18. **Chamilos, G., R. E. Lewis, and D. P. Kontoyiannis.** 2008. Delaying amphotericin B-based frontline therapy significantly increases mortality among patients with hematologic malignancy who have zygomycosis. *Clin. Infect. Dis.* **47:**503–509.

19. **Chamilos, G., E. M. Marom, R. E. Lewis, M. S. Lionakis, and D. P. Kontoyiannis.** 2005. Predictors of pulmonary zygomycosis versus invasive pulmonary aspergillosis in patients with cancer. *Clin. Infect. Dis.* **41:**60–66.

20. **Chayakulkeeree, M., M. A. Ghannoum, and J. R. Perfect.** 2006. Zygomycosis: the re-emerging fungal infection. *Eur. J. Clin. Microbiol. Infect. Dis.* **25:**215–229.

21. **Clinical and Laboratory Standards Institute (CLSI).** 2007. *Interpretive Criteria for Identification of Bacteria and Fungi by DNA Target Sequencing; Approved Guideline MM-18A.* CLSI, Wayne, PA.

22. **Clinical and Laboratory Standards Institute (CLSI).** 2002. *Reference Method for Broth Dilution Antifungal Susceptibility Testing of Filamentous Fungi: Approved Standard.* Document M-38A. CLSI, Wayne, PA.

23. **Cornely, O. A., J. Maertens, D. J. Winston, J. Perfect, A. J. Ullmann, T. J. Walsh, D. Helfgott, J. Holowiecki, D. Stockelberg, Y. T. Goh, M. Petrini, C. Hardalo, R. Suresh, and D. Angulo-Gonzalez.** 2007. Posaconazole vs. fluconazole or itraconazole prophylaxis in patients with neutropenia. *N. Engl. J. Med.* **356:**348–359.

24. **Dannaoui, E.** 2006. Animal models for evaluation of antifungal efficacy against filamentous fungi, p. 115–136. *In* K. Kavanagh (ed.), *Medical Mycology: Cellular and Molecular Techniques.* John Wiley & Sons, Bognor Regis, United Kingdom.

25. **Dannaoui, E.** 2009. Molecular tools for identification of Zygomycetes and diagnosis of zygomycosis. *Clin. Microbiol. Infect.* **15**(Suppl. 5):66–70.

26. **Dannaoui, E., J. F. Meis, D. Loebenberg, and P. E. Verweij.** 2003. Activity of posaconazole in treatment of experimental disseminated zygomycosis. *Antimicrob. Agents Chemother.* **47:**3647–3650.

27. **Dannaoui, E., J. F. Meis, J. W. Mouton, and P. E. Verweij.** 2002. In vitro susceptibilities of Zygomycota to polyenes. *J. Antimicrob. Chemother.* **49:**741–744.

28. **Dannaoui, E., J. Meletiadis, J. W. Mouton, J. F. Meis, and P. E. Verweij.** 2003. In vitro susceptibilities of zygomycetes to conventional and new antifungals. *J. Antimicrob. Chemother.* **51:**45–52.

29. **Dannaoui, E., J. W. Mouton, J. F. Meis, and P. E. Verweij.** 2002. Efficacy of antifungal therapy in a nonneutropenic murine model of zygomycosis. *Antimicrob. Agents Chemother.* **46:**1953–1959.

30. Reference deleted.

31. **de Hoog, G. S., J. Guarro, J. Gené, and M. J. Figueras.** 2009. *Atlas of Clinical Fungi CD-ROM. A Pilot CD-ROM Version of the 3rd Edition.* Centraalbureau voor Schimmelcultures, Utrecht, The Netherlands.

32. **Denning, D. W., C. C. Kibbler, and R. A. Barnes.** 2003. British Society for Medical Mycology proposed standards of care for patients with invasive fungal infections. *Lancet Infect. Dis.* **3:**230–240.

33. **De Pauw, B., T. J. Walsh, J. P. Donnelly, D. A. Stevens, J. E. Edwards, T. Calandra, P. G. Pappas, J. Maertens, O. Lortholary, C. A. Kauffman, D. W. Denning, T. F. Patterson, G. Maschmeyer, J. Bille, W. E. Dismukes, R. Herbrecht, W. W. Hope, C. C. Kibbler, B. J. Kullberg, K. A. Marr, P. Munoz, F. C. Odds, J. R. Perfect, A. Restrepo, M. Ruhnke, B. H. Segal, J. D. Sobel, T. C. Sorrell, C. Viscoli,

J. R. Wingard, T. Zaoutis, and J. E. Bennett.** 2008. Revised definitions of invasive fungal disease from the European Organization for Research and Treatment of Cancer/Invasive Fungal Infections Cooperative Group and the National Institute of Allergy and Infectious Diseases Mycoses Study Group (EORTC/MSG) Consensus Group. *Clin. Infect. Dis.* **46:**1813–1821.

34. **Dromer, F., and M. R. McGinnis.** 2002. Zygomycosis, p. 297–308. *In* E. Anaissie, M. R. McGinnis, and M. A. Pfaller (ed.), *Clinical Mycology.* Churchill Livingstone, New York, NY.

35. **Ellis, D., S. Davis, H. Alexiou, R. Handke, and R. Bartley.** 2007. *Descriptions of Medical Fungi,* 2nd ed. Mycology Unit, Women's and Children's Hospital, Adelaide, Australia.

36. **Espinel-Ingroff, A.** 2006. Comparison of three commercial assays and a modified disk diffusion assay with two broth microdilution reference assays for testing zygomycetes, *Aspergillus* spp., *Candida* spp., and *Cryptococcus neoformans* with posaconazole and amphotericin B. *J. Clin. Microbiol.* **44:**3616–3622.

37. **Frater, J. L., G. S. Hall, and G. W. Procop.** 2001. Histologic features of zygomycosis: emphasis on perineural invasion and fungal morphology. *Arch. Pathol. Lab. Med.* **125:**375–378.

38. **Fromentin, H., and P. Ravisse.** 1977. Tropical entomophthoromycoses. *Acta Trop.* **34:**375–394.

39. **Gams, W., E. Hoekstra, and A. Aptroot.** 1998. *CBS Course of Mycology.* Centraalbureau voor Schimmelcultures, Baarn, The Netherlands.

40. **Garcia-Hermoso, D., and E. Dannaoui.** 2007. The Zygomycetes, p. 159–183. *In* K. Kavanagh (ed.), *New Insights in Medical Mycology.* Springer Science, New York, NY.

41. **Garcia-Hermoso, D., D. Hoinard, J. C. Gantier, F. Grenouillet, F. Dromer, and E. Dannaoui.** 2009. Molecular and phenotypic evaluation of *Lichtheimia corymbifera* (formerly *Absidia corymbifera*) complex isolates associated with human mucormycosis: rehabilitation of *L. ramosa. J. Clin. Microbiol.* **47:**3862–3870.

42. **Girmenia, C., M. L. Moleti, A. Micozzi, A. P. Iori, W. Barberi, R. Foa, and P. Martino.** 2005. Breakthrough *Candida krusei* fungemia during fluconazole prophylaxis followed by breakthrough zygomycosis during caspofungin therapy in a patient with severe aplastic anemia who underwent stem cell transplantation. *J. Clin. Microbiol.* **43:**5395–5396.

43. **Glazer, M., S. Nusair, R. Breuer, J. Lafair, Y. Sherman, and N. Berkman.** 2000. The role of BAL in the diagnosis of pulmonary mucormycosis. *Chest* **117:**279–282.

44. **Greenberg, R. N., L. J. Scott, H. H. Vaughn, and J. A. Ribes.** 2004. Zygomycosis (mucormycosis): emerging clinical importance and new treatments. *Curr. Opin. Infect. Dis.* **17:**517–525.

45. **Guarro, J., C. Aguilar, and I. Pujol.** 1999. In-vitro antifungal susceptibilities of *Basidiobolus* and *Conidiobolus* spp. strains. *J. Antimicrob. Chemother.* **44:**557–560.

46. **Gugnani, H. C.** 1992. Entomophthoromycosis due to *Conidiobolus. Eur. J. Epidemiol.* **8:**391–396.

47. **Gugnani, H. C.** 1999. A review of zygomycosis due to *Basidiobolus ranarum. Eur. J. Epidemiol.* **15:**923–929.

48. **Hall, L., S. Wohlfiel, and G. D. Roberts.** 2004. Experience with the MicroSeq D2 large-subunit ribosomal DNA sequencing kit for identification of filamentous fungi encountered in the clinical laboratory. *J. Clin. Microbiol.* **42:**622–626.

49. **Hata, D. J., S. P. Buckwalter, B. S. Pritt, G. D. Roberts, and N. L. Wengenack.** 2008. Real-time PCR method for detection of zygomycetes. *J. Clin. Microbiol.* **46:**2353–2358.

50. **Hayden, R. T., X. Qian, G. W. Procop, G. D. Roberts, and R. V. Lloyd.** 2002. In situ hybridization for the identification of filamentous fungi in tissue section. *Diagn. Mol. Pathol.* **11:**119–126.

51. **Hibbett, D. S., M. Binder, J. F. Bischoff, M. Blackwell, P. F. Cannon, O. E. Eriksson, S. Huhndorf, T. James, P. M. Kirk, R. Lucking, H. Thorsten Lumbsch, F. Lutzoni, P. B. Matheny, D. J. McLaughlin, M. J. Powell, S. Redhead, C. L. Schoch, J. W. Spatafora, J. A. Stalpers, R. Vilgalys, M. C. Aime, A. Aptroot, R. Bauer, D. Begerow, G. L. Benny, L. A. Castlebury, P. W. Crous, Y. C. Dai, W. Gams, D. M. Geiser, G. W. Griffith, C. Gueidan, D. L. Hawksworth, G. Hestmark, K. Hosaka, R. A. Humber, K. D. Hyde, J. E. Ironside,

U. Koljalg, C. P. Kurtzman, K. H. Larsson, R. Lichtwardt, J. Longcore, J. Miadlikowska, A. Miller, J. M. Moncalvo, S. Mozley-Standridge, F. Oberwinkler, E. Parmasto, V. Reeb, J. D. Rogers, C. Roux, L. Ryvarden, J. P. Sampaio, A. Schussler, J. Sugiyama, R. G. Thorn, L. Tibell, W. A. Untereiner, C. Walker, Z. Wang, A. Weir, M. Weiss, M. M. White, K. Winka, Y. J. Yao, and N. Zhang. 2007. A higher-level phylogenetic classification of the Fungi. *Mycol. Res.* **111:**509–547.

52. Hoffmann, K., S. Discher, and K. Voigt. 2007. Revision of the genus *Absidia* (Mucorales, Zygomycetes) based on physiological, phylogenetic, and morphological characters; thermotolerant *Absidia* spp. form a coherent group, Mycocladiaceae fam. nov. *Mycol. Res.* **111:**1169–1183.

53. Hoffmann, K., G. Walther, and K. Voight. 2009. *Mycocladus* vs. *Lichtheimia*: a correction (*Lichtheimiaceae* fam. nov., Mucorales, Mucoromycotina). *Mycol. Res.* **113:**277–278.

54. Holland, J. 1997. Emerging zygomycoses of humans: *Saksenaea vasiformis* and *Apophysomyces elegans*. *Curr. Top. Med. Mycol.* **8:**27–34.

55. Hussein, M. R. 2008. Mucocutaneous Splendore-Hoeppli phenomenon. *J. Cutan. Pathol.* **35:**979–988.

56. Ibrahim, A. S., V. Avanessian, B. Spellberg, and J. E. Edwards, Jr. 2003. Liposomal amphotericin B, and not amphotericin B deoxycholate, improves survival of diabetic mice infected with *Rhizopus oryzae*. *Antimicrob. Agents Chemother.* **47:**3343–3344.

57. Ibrahim, A. S., J. C. Bowman, V. Avanessian, K. Brown, B. Spellberg, J. E. Edwards, Jr., and C. M. Douglas. 2005. Caspofungin inhibits *Rhizopus oryzae* 1,3-beta-D-glucan synthase, lowers burden in brain measured by quantitative PCR, and improves survival at a low but not a high dose during murine disseminated zygomycosis. *Antimicrob. Agents Chemother.* **49:**721–727.

58. Imhof, A., S. A. Balajee, D. N. Fredricks, J. A. Englund, and K. A. Marr. 2004. Breakthrough fungal infections in stem cell transplant recipients receiving voriconazole. *Clin. Infect. Dis.* **39:**743–746.

59. Iwen, P. C., A. G. Freifeld, L. Sigler, and S. R. Tarantolo. 2005. Molecular identification of *Rhizomucor pusillus* as a cause of sinus-orbital zygomycosis in a patient with acute myelogenous leukemia. *J. Clin. Microbiol.* **43:**5819–5821.

60. Jensen, H. E., J. Salonen, and T. O. Ekfors. 1997. The use of immunohistochemistry to improve sensitivity and specificity in the diagnosis of systemic mycoses in patients with haematological malignancies. *J. Pathol.* **181:**100–105.

61. Kasai, M., S. M. Harrington, A. Francesconi, V. Petraitis, R. Petraitiene, M. G. Beveridge, T. Knudsen, J. Milanovich, M. P. Cotton, J. Hughes, R. L. Schaufele, T. Sein, J. Bacher, P. R. Murray, D. P. Kontoyiannis, and T. J. Walsh. 2008. Detection of a molecular biomarker for zygomycetes by quantitative PCR assays of plasma, bronchoalveolar lavage, and lung tissue in a rabbit model of experimental pulmonary zygomycosis. *J. Clin. Microbiol.* **46:**3690–3702.

62. Khan, Z. U., S. Ahmad, A. Brazda, and R. Chandy. 2009. *Mucor circinelloides* as a cause of invasive maxillofacial zygomycosis: an emerging dimorphic pathogen with reduced susceptibility to posaconazole. *J. Clin. Microbiol.* **47:**1244–1248.

63. Kobayashi, M., K. Togitani, H. Machida, Y. Uemura, Y. Ohtsuki, and H. Taguchi. 2004. Molecular polymerase chain reaction diagnosis of pulmonary mucormycosis caused by *Cunninghamella bertholletiae*. *Respirology* **9:**397–401.

64. Kontoyiannis, D. P., G. Chamilos, S. A. Hassan, R. E. Lewis, N. D. Albert, and J. J. Tarrand. 2007. Increased culture recovery of Zygomycetes under physiologic temperature conditions. *Am. J. Clin. Pathol.* **127:**208–212.

65. Kontoyiannis, D. P., M. S. Lionakis, R. E. Lewis, G. Chamilos, M. Healy, C. Perego, A. Safdar, H. Kantarjian, R. Champlin, T. J. Walsh, and I. I. Raad. 2005. Zygomycosis in a tertiary-care cancer center in the era of *Aspergillus*-active antifungal therapy: a case-control observational study of 27 recent cases. *J. Infect. Dis.* **191:**1350–1360.

66. Reference deleted.

67. Kontoyiannis, D. P., V. C. Wessel, G. P. Bodey, and K. V. Rolston. 2000. Zygomycosis in the 1990s in a tertiary-care cancer center. *Clin. Infect. Dis.* **30:**851–856.

68. Kwon-Chung, K., and J. Bennett. 1982. *Medical Mycology.* Lea & Febiger, Philadelphia, PA.

69. Lanternier, F., and O. Lortholary. 2008. Liposomal amphotericin B: what is its role in 2008? *Clin. Microbiol. Infect.* **14**(Suppl. 4):71–83.

70. Lanternier, F., and O. Lortholary. 2009. Zygomycosis in diabetes. *Clin. Microbiol. Infect.* **15**(Suppl. 5):21–25.

71. Larche, J., M. Machouart, K. Burton, J. Collomb, M. F. Biava, A. Gerard, and B. Fortier. 2005. Diagnosis of cutaneous mucormycosis due to *Rhizopus microsporus* by an innovative PCR-restriction fragment-length polymorphism method. *Clin. Infect. Dis.* **41:**1362–1365.

72. Lau, A., S. Chen, T. Sorrell, D. Carter, R. Malik, P. Martin, and C. Halliday. 2007. Development and clinical application of a panfungal PCR assay to detect and identify fungal DNA in tissue specimens. *J. Clin. Microbiol.* **45:**380–385.

73. Lechevalier, P., D. Garcia Hermoso, A. Carol, S. Bonacorsi, L. Ferkdadji, F. Fitoussi, O. Lortholary, A. Bourrillon, A. Faye, E. Dannaoui, and F. Angoulvant. 2008. Molecular diagnosis of *Saksenaea vasiformis* cutaneous infection after scorpion sting in an immunocompetent adolescent. *J. Clin. Microbiol.* **46:**3169–3172.

74. Lee, F. Y., S. B. Mossad, and K. A. Adal. 1999. Pulmonary mucormycosis: the last 30 years. *Arch. Intern. Med.* **159:**1301–1309.

75. Lemmer, K., H. Losert, V. Rickerts, G. Just-Nubling, A. Sander, M. L. Kerkmann, and K. Tintelnot. 2002. Molecular biological identification of *Cunninghamella* species. *Mycoses* **45**(Suppl. 1):31–36.

76. Lyon, G. M., J. D. Smilack, K. K. Komatsu, T. M. Pasha, J. A. Leighton, J. Guarner, T. V. Colby, M. D. Lindsley, M. Phelan, D. W. Warnock, and R. A. Hajjeh. 2001. Gastrointestinal basidiobolomycosis in Arizona: clinical and epidemiological characteristics and review of the literature. *Clin. Infect. Dis.* **32:**1448–1455.

77. Ma, L. J., A. S. Ibrahim, C. Skory, M. G. Grabherr, G. Burger, M. Butler, M. Elias, A. Idnurm, B. F. Lang, T. Sone, A. Abe, S. E. Calvo, L. M. Corrochano, R. Engels, J. Fu, W. Hansberg, J. M. Kim, C. D. Kodira, M. J. Koehrsen, B. Liu, D. Miranda-Saavedra, S. O'Leary, L. Ortiz-Castellanos, R. Poulter, J. Rodriguez-Romero, J. Ruiz-Herrera, Y. Q. Shen, Q. Zeng, J. Galagan, B. W. Birren, C. A. Cuomo, and B. L. Wickes. 2009. Genomic analysis of the basal lineage fungus *Rhizopus oryzae* reveals a whole-genome duplication. *PLoS Genet.* **5:**e1000549.

78. Machouart, M., J. Larche, K. Burton, J. Collomb, P. Maurer, A. Cintrat, M. F. Biava, S. Greciano, A. F. Kuijpers, N. Contet-Audonneau, G. S. de Hoog, A. Gerard, and B. Fortier. 2006. Genetic identification of the main opportunistic *Mucorales* by PCR-restriction fragment length polymorphism. *J. Clin. Microbiol.* **44:**805–810.

79. Marr, K. A., R. A. Carter, F. Crippa, A. Wald, and L. Corey. 2002. Epidemiology and outcome of mould infections in hematopoietic stem cell transplant recipients. *Clin. Infect. Dis.* **34:**909–917.

80. Marty, F. M., L. A. Cosimi, and L. R. Baden. 2004. Breakthrough zygomycosis after voriconazole treatment in recipients of hematopoietic stem-cell transplants. *N. Engl. J. Med.* **350:**950–952.

81. Nagao, K., T. Ota, A. Tanikawa, Y. Takae, T. Mori, S. Udagawa, and T. Nishikawa. 2005. Genetic identification and detection of human pathogenic *Rhizopus* species, a major mucormycosis agent, by multiplex PCR based on internal transcribed spacer region of rRNA gene. *J. Dermatol. Sci.* **39:**23–31.

82. Neofytos, D., D. Horn, E. Anaissie, W. Steinbach, A. Olyaei, J. Fishman, M. Pfaller, C. Chang, K. Webster, and K. Marr. 2009. Epidemiology and outcome of invasive fungal infection in adult hematopoietic stem cell transplant recipients: analysis of Multicenter Prospective Antifungal Therapy (PATH) Alliance registry. *Clin. Infect. Dis.* **48:**265–273.

83. Nosari, A., M. Anghilieri, G. Carrafiello, C. Guffanti, L. Marbello, M. Montillo, G. Muti, S. Ribera, A. Vanzulli, M. Nichelatti, and E. Morra. 2003. Utility of percutaneous lung biopsy for diagnosing filamentous fungal infections in hematologic malignancies. *Haematologica* **88:**1405–1409.

84. **Nosari, A., P. Oreste, M. Montillo, G. Carrafiello, M. Draisci, G. Muti, A. Molteni, and E. Morra.** 2000. Mucormycosis in hematologic malignancies: an emerging fungal infection. *Haematologica* **85:**1068–1071.

85. **Nyilasi, I., T. Papp, A. Csernetics, K. Krizsan, E. Nagy, and C. Vagvolgyi.** 2008. High-affinity iron permease (FTR1) gene sequence-based molecular identification of clinically important Zygomycetes. *Clin. Microbiol. Infect.* **14:**393–397.

86. **O'Donnell, K., F. Lutzoni, T. J. Ward, and G. L. Benny.** 2001. Evolutionary relationships among mucoralean fungi (Zygomycota): evidence for family polyphyly on a large scale. *Mycologia* **93:**286–296.

87. **Okafor, J. I., D. Testrake, H. R. Mushinsky, and B. G. Yangco.** 1984. A *Basidiobolus* sp. and its association with reptiles and amphibians in southern Florida. *Sabouraudia* **22:**47–51.

88. **Padhye, A. A., and L. Ajello.** 1988. Simple method of inducing sporulation by *Apophysomyces elegans* and *Saksenaea vasiformis. J. Clin. Microbiol.* **26:**1861–1863.

89. **Pagano, L., M. Caira, A. Candoni, M. Offidani, L. Fianchi, B. Martino, D. Pastore, M. Picardi, A. Bonini, A. Chierichini, R. Fanci, C. Caramatti, R. Invernizzi, D. Mattei, M. E. Mitra, L. Melillo, F. Aversa, M. T. Van Lint, P. Falcucci, C. G. Valentini, C. Girmenia, and A. Nosari.** 2006. The epidemiology of fungal infections in patients with hematologic malignancies: the SEIFEM-2004 study. *Haematologica* **91:**1068–1075.

90. **Pagano, L., M. Offidani, L. Fianchi, A. Nosari, A. Candoni, M. Piccardi, L. Corvatta, D. D'Antonio, C. Girmenia, P. Martino, and A. Del Favero.** 2004. Mucormycosis in hematologic patients. *Haematologica* **89:**207–214.

91. Reference deleted.

92. **Parkyn, T., A. W. McNinch, T. Riordan, and M. Mott.** 2000. Zygomycosis in relapsed acute leukaemia. *J. Infect.* **41:**265–268.

93. **Prabhu, R. M., and R. Patel.** 2004. Mucormycosis and entomophthoramycosis: a review of the clinical manifestations, diagnosis and treatment. *Clin. Microbiol. Infect.* **10(Suppl. 1):**31–47.

94. Reference deleted.

95. **Receveur, M. C., C. Roussin, B. Mienniel, O. Gasnier, J. P. Riviere, D. Malvy, and O. Lortholary.** 2005. Rhinofacial entomophthoromycosis. About two new cases in Mayotte. *Bull. Soc. Pathol. Exot.* **98:**350–353. (In French.)

96. **Reed, C., R. Bryant, A. S. Ibrahim, J. Edwards, Jr., S. G. Filler, R. Goldberg, and B. Spellberg.** 2008. Combination polyene-caspofungin treatment of rhino-orbital-cerebral mucormycosis. *Clin. Infect. Dis.* **47:**364–371.

97. **Rees, J. R., R. W. Pinner, R. A. Hajjeh, M. E. Brandt, and A. L. Reingold.** 1998. The epidemiological features of invasive mycotic infections in the San Francisco Bay area, 1992–1993: results of population-based laboratory active surveillance. *Clin. Infect. Dis.* **27:**1138–1147.

98. **Ribes, J. A., C. L. Vanover-Sams, and D. J. Baker.** 2000. Zygomycetes in human disease. *Clin. Microbiol. Rev.* **13:**236–301.

99. **Rickerts, V., G. Just-Nubling, F. Konrad, J. Kern, E. Lambrecht, A. Bohme, V. Jacobi, and R. Bialek.** 2006. Diagnosis of invasive aspergillosis and mucormycosis in immunocompromised patients by seminested PCR assay of tissue samples. *Eur. J. Clin. Microbiol. Infect. Dis.* **25:**8–13.

100. **Rickerts, V., S. Mousset, E. Lambrecht, K. Tintelnot, R. Schwerdtfeger, E. Presterl, V. Jacobi, G. Just-Nubling, and R. Bialek.** 2007. Comparison of histopathological analysis, culture, and polymerase chain reaction assays to detect invasive mold infections from biopsy specimens. *Clin. Infect. Dis.* **44:**1078–1083.

101. **Roden, M. M., T. E. Zaoutis, W. L. Buchanan, T. A. Knudsen, T. A. Sarkisova, R. L. Schaufele, M. Sein, T. Sein, C. C. Chiou, J. H. Chu, D. P. Kontoyiannis, and T. J. Walsh.** 2005. Epidemiology and outcome of zygomycosis: a review of 929 reported cases. *Clin. Infect. Dis.* **41:**634–653.

102. **Ruchel, R., and M. Schaffrinski.** 1999. Versatile fluorescent staining of fungi in clinical specimens by using the optical brightener Blankophor. *J. Clin. Microbiol.* **37:**2694–2696.

103. **Safdar, A., S. O'Brien, and I. F. Kouri.** 2004. Efficacy and feasibility of aerosolized amphotericin B lipid complex therapy in caspofungin breakthrough pulmonary zygomycosis. *Bone Marrow Transplant.* **34:**467–468.

104. **Schipper, M. A. A.** 1976. On *Mucor circinelloides, Mucor racemosus* and related species. *Stud. Mycol.* **12:**1–40.

105. **Schipper, M. A. A.** 1984. A revision of the genus *Rhizopus.* I. The *Rhizopus stolonifer* group and *Rhizopus oryzae. Stud. Mycol.* **25:**1–19.

106. **Schipper, M. A. A., and J. A. Stalpers.** 1984. A revision of the genus *Rhizopus.* II. The *Rhizopus microsporus* group. *Stud. Mycol.* **25:**30–34.

107. **Schipper, M. A. A., and J. A. Stalpers.** 2002. Zygomycetes. The order *Mucorales,* p. 67–125. *In* D. H. Howard (ed.), *Pathogenic Fungi in Humans and Animals,* 2nd ed. Marcel Dekker, New York, NY.

108. **Schwarz, P., S. Bretagne, J. C. Gantier, D. Garcia-Hermoso, O. Lortholary, F. Dromer, and E. Dannaoui.** 2006. Molecular identification of zygomycetes from culture and experimentally infected tissues. *J. Clin. Microbiol.* **44:**340–349.

109. **Schwarz, P., O. Lortholary, F. Dromer, and E. Dannaoui.** 2007. Carbon assimilation profiles as a tool for identification of zygomycetes. *J. Clin. Microbiol.* **45:**1433–1439.

110. **Sharma, N. L., V. K. Mahajan, and P. Singh.** 2003. Orofacial conidiobolomycosis due to *Conidiobolus incongruus. Mycoses* **46:**137–140.

111. **Singh, N., J. M. Aguado, H. Bonatti, G. Forrest, K. L. Gupta, N. Safdar, G. T. John, K. J. Pursell, P. Munoz, R. Patel, J. Fortun, P. Martin-Davila, B. Philippe, F. Philit, A. Tabah, N. Terzi, V. Chatelet, S. Kusne, N. Clark, E. Blumberg, M. B. Julia, A. Humar, S. Houston, C. Lass-Florl, L. Johnson, E. R. Dubberke, M. A. Barron, and O. Lortholary.** 2009. Zygomycosis in solid organ transplant recipients: a prospective, matched case-control study to assess risks for disease and outcome. *J. Infect. Dis.* **200:**1002–1011.

112. **St.-Germain, G., and R. Summerbell.** 1996. *Identifying Filamentous Fungi. A Clinical Laboratory Handbook.* Star Publishing Company, Belmont, CA.

113. **Subcommittee on Antifungal Susceptibility Testing (AFST) of the ESCMID European Committee for Antimicrobial Susceptibility Testing (EUCAST), J. L. Rodriguez-Tudela, J. P. Donnelly, M. C. Arendrup, S. Arikan, F. Barchiesi, J. Bille, E. Chryssanthou, M. Cuenca-Estrella, E. Dannaoui, D. Denning, W. Fegeler, P. Gaustad, C. Lass-Florl, C. Moore, M. Richardson, A. Schmalreck, A. Velegraki, and P. E. Verweij.** 2008. EUCAST technical note on the method for the determination of broth dilution minimum inhibitory concentrations of antifungal agents for conidia-forming moulds. *Clin. Microbiol. Infect.* **14:**982–984.

114. **Sun, H. Y., J. M. Aguado, H. Bonatti, G. Forrest, K. L. Gupta, N. Safdar, G. T. John, K. J. Pursell, P. Munoz, R. Patel, J. Fortun, P. Martin-Davila, B. Philippe, F. Philit, A. Tabah, N. Terzi, V. Chatelet, S. Kusne, N. Clark, E. Blumberg, M. B. Julia, A. Humar, S. Houston, C. Lass-Florl, L. Johnson, E. R. Dubberke, M. A. Barron, O. Lortholary, and N. Singh.** 2009. Pulmonary zygomycosis in solid organ transplant recipients in the current era. *Am. J. Transplant.* **9:**2166–2171.

115. **Sun, Q. N., A. W. Fothergill, D. I. McCarthy, M. G. Rinaldi, and J. R. Graybill.** 2002. In vitro activities of posaconazole, itraconazole, voriconazole, amphotericin B, and fluconazole against 37 clinical isolates of zygomycetes. *Antimicrob. Agents Chemother.* **46:**1581–1582.

116. **Sun, Q. N., L. K. Najvar, R. Bocanegra, D. Loebenberg, and J. R. Graybill.** 2002. In vivo activity of posaconazole against *Mucor* spp. in an immunosuppressed-mouse model. *Antimicrob. Agents Chemother.* **46:**2310–2312.

117. **Taylor, G. D., A. S. Sekhon, D. L. Tyrrell, and G. Goldsand.** 1987. Rhinofacial zygomycosis caused by *Conidiobolus coronatus:* a case report including in vitro sensitivity to antimycotic agents. *Am. J. Trop. Med. Hyg.* **36:**398–401.

118. **Torres-Narbona, M., J. Guinea, J. Martinez-Alarcon, P. Munoz, I. Gadea, and E. Bouza.** 2007. Impact of zygomycosis on microbiology workload: a survey study in Spain. *J. Clin. Microbiol.* **45:**2051–2053.

119. **Torres-Narbona, M., J. Guinea, J. Martinez-Alarcon, P. Munoz, T. Pelaez, and E. Bouza.** 2008. Workload and clinical significance of the isolation of zygomycetes in a tertiary general hospital. *Med. Mycol.* **46:**225–230.

120. **Torres-Narbona, M., J. Guinea, J. Martinez-Alarcon, T. Pelaez, and E. Bouza.** 2007. In vitro activities of amphotericin B, caspofungin, itraconazole, posaconazole, and voriconazole against 45 clinical isolates of zygomycetes: comparison of CLSI M38-A, Sensititre YeastOne, and the Etest. *Antimicrob. Agents Chemother.* **51:**1126–1129.

121. **Ullmann, A. J., J. H. Lipton, D. H. Vesole, P. Chandrasekar, A. Langston, S. R. Tarantolo, H. Greinix, W. Morais de Azevedo, V. Reddy, N. Boparai, L. Pedicone, H. Patino, and S. Durrant.** 2007. Posaconazole or fluconazole for prophylaxis in severe graft-versus-host disease. *N. Engl. J. Med.* **356:**335–347.

122. **Vitrat-Hincky, V., B. Lebeau, E. Bozonnet, D. Falcon, P. Pradel, O. Faure, A. Aubert, C. Piolat, R. Grillot, and H. Pelloux.** 2009. Severe filamentous fungal infections after widespread tissue damage due to traumatic injury: six cases and review of the literature. *Scand. J. Infect. Dis.* **41:**491–500.

123. **Voight, K., E. Hoffman, E. Einax, M. Erckart, T. Papp, C. Vagvolgyi, and L. Olsson.** 2009. Revision of the family structure of the *Mucorales* (*Mucoromycotina*, Zygomycetes) based on multigene-genealogies: phylogenetic analyses suggest a bigeneric *Phycomycetaceae* with *Spinellus* as sister group to *Phycomyces*, p. 313–332. *In* Y. Gherbawy, R. Mach, and M. Rai (ed.), *Current Advances in Molecular Mycology.* Nova Science Publishers, Inc., New York, NY.

124. **Voigt, K., E. Cigelnik, and K. O'Donnell.** 1999. Phylogeny and PCR identification of clinically important zygomycetes based on nuclear ribosomal-DNA sequence data. *J. Clin. Microbiol.* **37:**3957–3964.

125. **Voigt, K., and J. Wostemeyer.** 2001. Phylogeny and origin of 82 zygomycetes from all 54 genera of the *Mucorales* and *Mortierellales* based on combined analysis of actin and translation elongation factor EF-1alpha genes. *Gene* **270:**113–120.

126. **Walker, S. D., R. V. Clark, C. T. King, J. E. Humphries, L. S. Lytle, and D. E. Butkus.** 1992. Fatal disseminated *Conidiobolus coronatus* infection in a renal transplant patient. *Am. J. Clin. Pathol.* **98:**559–564.

127. **Walsh, T. J., and D. P. Kontoyiannis.** 2008. What is the role of combination therapy in management of zygomycosis? *Clin. Infect. Dis.* **47:**372–374.

128. **Weitzman, I., S. Whittier, J. C. McKitrick, and P. Della-Latta.** 1995. Zygospores: the last word in identification of rare or atypical zygomycetes isolated from clinical specimens. *J. Clin. Microbiol.* **33:**781–783.

129. **Yangco, B. G., J. I. Okafor, and D. TeStrake.** 1984. In vitro susceptibilities of human and wild-type isolates of *Basidiobolus* and *Conidiobolus* species. *Antimicrob. Agents Chemother.* **25:**413–416.

130. **Zaoutis, T. E., E. Roilides, C. C. Chiou, W. L. Buchanan, T. A. Knudsen, T. A. Sarkisova, R. L. Schaufele, M. Sein, T. Sein, P. A. Prasad, J. H. Chu, and T. J. Walsh.** 2007. Zygomycosis in children: a systematic review and analysis of reported cases. *Pediatr. Infect. Dis. J.* **26:**723–727.

131. **Zavasky, D. M., W. Samowitz, T. Loftus, H. Segal, and K. Carroll.** 1999. Gastrointestinal zygomycotic infection caused by *Basidiobolus ranarum*: case report and review. *Clin. Infect. Dis.* **28:**1244–1248.

Histoplasma, Blastomyces, Coccidioides, and Other Dimorphic Fungi Causing Systemic Mycoses

MARY E. BRANDT, BEATRIZ L. GOMEZ, AND DAVID W. WARNOCK

120

TAXONOMY

The dimorphic fungi causing systemic disease belong to the class Euascomycetes, order Onygenales. This order contains three families of medical importance, the Onygenaceae (dimorphic pathogens), the Arthrodermataceae (dermatophytes), and the Gymnoascaceae (agents of onychomycosis and dermatomycosis). The Onygenales share several general characteristics: their sexual stages (teleomorphs) form rudimentary asci surrounded by a network of hyphae, which may have complex appendages; and their asexual (anamorph) species generally possess one of two forms, either unicellular aleurioconidia or arthroconidia in chains of alternately viable and nonviable cells.

The family Onygenaceae was originally defined based on morphological characteristics of the teleomorphs and of the conidia of the anamorphs. The teleomorph genus *Ajellomyces* contains three species, *A. dermatitidis*, *A. capsulatus*, and *A. crescens*, the anamorphs of which are placed in the genera *Blastomyces*, *Histoplasma*, and *Emmonsia*, respectively (62). The teleomorphs of *Coccidioides* and *Paracoccidioides* have not been discovered, although genetic data suggest that *Coccidioides* and *Paracoccidioides* are recombining in nature (41, 48).

Molecular phylogenetic studies have indicated that species of the Onygenales are divided into several clades (descendants of a common ancestor). The family name Ajellomycetaceae has recently been proposed for one of these clades (72), which includes *Emmonsia crescens* and *Emmonsia parva*, *Histoplasma capsulatum*, *Paracoccidioides brasiliensis*, *Blastomyces dermatitidis*, and *Lacazia loboi*, the agent of lacaziosis (33, 66). A second clade, which retains the family name Onygenaceae, includes the pathogens *Coccidioides immitis* and *Coccidioides posadasii* with, among others, species of *Aphanoascus*, *Chrysosporium*, *Nannizziopsis*, and *Uncinocarpus* (72). The Onygenaceae and Ajellomycetaceae are well separated from the other families Gymnoascaceae and Arthrodermataceae. In all of these phylogenetic trees, pathogenic organisms are interspersed with nonpathogenic relatives, which suggests that the capacity to infect humans has arisen numerous times during the evolution of the Onygenales.

This chapter covers the dimorphic members of the families Onygenaceae and Ajellomycetaceae, which include *B. dermatitidis*, *H. capsulatum*, *P. brasiliensis*, and *Coccidioides immitis* and *C. posadasii* as well as *Emmonsia* species. Nonpathogenic species of *Chrysosporium*, *Uncinocarpus*, and other related genera are not covered here. It should be noted that because the three species with *Ajellomyces* teleomorphs appear in the same clade, an argument has been made that all of the anamorphs should be placed in the same genus. At the time of this writing, this proposal has not been implemented, in part due to the widespread usage of the anamorph names. The dimorphic fungus *Penicillium marneffei* is covered in chapter 117.

Histoplasma capsulatum

Historically, *H. capsulatum* was divided into three varieties: *H. capsulatum* var. *capsulatum*, a human pathogen found in North and South America; var. *duboisii*, a human pathogen found in Africa; and var. *farciminosum*, a pathogen of horses and mules found in parts of northern Africa and the Middle East. Recent phylogenetic studies have defined at least eight clades within *H. capsulatum*: North American class 1, North American class 2, Latin American group A, Latin American group B, Australian, Netherlands (Indonesian), Eurasian, and African clades (37). Seven of these eight clades comprise genetically and geographically distinct populations that can be regarded as phylogenetic species. The single exception, the Eurasian clade, originated from within the Latin American group A clade. *H. capsulatum* var. *farciminosum* was placed within the Eurasian clade. In addition to the seven phylogenetic species, another seven lineages represented by single isolates from Latin America were identified (37). These may represent additional phylogenetic species.

At this time, the disease African histoplasmosis is considered a distinct entity, but the taxonomic placement of *H. capsulatum* var. *duboisii* has been called into question by the finding of one var. *capsulatum* isolate from South Africa that was placed in the African (var. *duboisii*-containing) clade (37). This extends the results of earlier studies that had shown that var. *duboisii* had mitochondrial DNA restriction patterns identical to those of var. *capsulatum* strains.

Blastomyces dermatitidis

The genus *Blastomyces* is represented by the single species *B. dermatitidis*. Phylogenetic data show that, within the single branch occupied by the anamorphs of the three dimorphic *Ajellomyces* species, *B. dermatitidis* is most closely related to the genus *Emmonsia*. Isolates of *E. parva* are closer to *B. dermatitidis* than they are to *E. crescens*. The recognition of this close relationship between *Blastomyces* and *Emmonsia* has suggested that they be consolidated into one genus. However, this proposal has not been implemented.

Coccidioides Species

Phylogenetic studies have led to the recognition of two species within the genus *Coccidioides*. The species name *C. immitis* is now restricted to isolates from California, while the name *C. posadasii*, in honor of Posadas, the author of the first description of coccidioidomycosis in Argentina in 1892, has been proposed for all other isolates belonging to this genus (25). Zimmerman et al. first divided *C. immitis* into two groups, named group I (non-CA) and group II (CA), after comparing restriction fragment length polymorphisms (RFLPs) within total genomic DNA (80). The genealogies of five nuclear genes were later used to confirm that *C. immitis* consists of two taxa, non-CA (Arizona, Texas, Mexico, and Argentina) and CA. These two taxa did not interbreed, although genetic recombination had occurred between individuals within each of the two groups. Later, a more extensive population sample, including isolates from Venezuela, Mexico, and Brazil, was studied by using a set of nine microsatellite markers (25). This study showed that two major clades could be distinguished. These clades, now named *C. posadasii* and *C. immitis*, respectively, correspond to the previous group I (non-CA) and group II (CA).

Paracoccidioides brasiliensis

Phylogenetic analysis of *P. brasiliensis* has shown that this fungus can be divided into at least three distinct species: S1 (isolates from various locations), PS2 (Brazil and Venezuela), and PS3 (Colombia) (48). These species have not been formally named. A proposal has also been made to name the highly divergent "Pb01-like" group "*Paracoccidioides lutzii*" (71). Comparison of 18S and chitin synthetase sequences has indicated that *P. brasiliensis* is related to the uncultivable pathogen *Lacazia loboi*, the agent of lacaziosis (33). However, these sequences demonstrated sufficient differences that *L. loboi* was kept as an independent genus (33).

Emmonsia Species

The genus *Emmonsia* currently includes three species: *E. crescens*, *E. parva*, and *E. pasteuriana* (66). The last has thus far only been recovered from a single case of disseminated cutaneous infection in a patient with AIDS (31). *E. crescens* is known to form a sexual stage in the genus *Ajellomyces*, but *E. parva* has no known teleomorph.

DESCRIPTION OF THE AGENTS

Histoplasma capsulatum

H. capsulatum is a thermally dimorphic fungus, displaying a filamentous mold form in the environment and in culture at temperatures below 35°C and a yeast phase in tissue and at temperatures above 35°C. The mold phase may contain two types of conidia (Fig. 1). Macroconidia are thick walled with a diameter of 8 to 15 μm and display characteristic tubercles or projections on their surfaces. Microconidia, smooth walled with a diameter of 2 to 4 μm, are the infectious particles (38, 42). The yeast phase develops as small oval budding cells with a diameter of 2 to 4 μm, often within macrophages (Fig. 2 and 3A). The yeast cell found in African histoplasmosis is thick walled and larger, 8 to 15 μm in diameter.

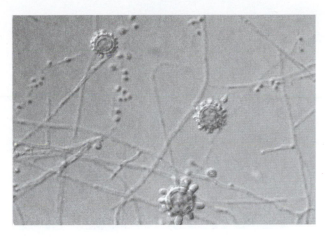

FIGURE 1 Mycelial phase of *H. capsulatum* showing tuberculate macroconidia and microconidia. Lactophenol cotton blue stain. Magnification, ~×245.

H. capsulatum is found in soils throughout the world. It grows best in soils with a high nitrogen content, particularly those enriched with bird or bat guano. Birds do not become colonized or infected with *H. capsulatum* (due to their high body temperatures), and their droppings are primarily a nutrient source. Soil samples from sites where birds have roosted have remained contaminated for at least 10 years after the roost has been cleared (42).

Histoplasmosis is the most common endemic mycosis in North America, but it is also found throughout Central and South America. In the United States, the disease is most prevalent in states surrounding the Mississippi and Ohio Rivers, but foci of endemicity exist throughout the eastern half of the continent. Other endemic regions include parts of Africa, Australia, and eastern Asia, in particular India and Malaysia.

Blastomyces dermatitidis

B. dermatitidis is thermally dimorphic, converting from the mold phase to the yeast phase under appropriate conditions of temperature and nutrition. At room temperature, a floccose white mold can be recovered (Fig. 4). The microconidia are oval or pyriform (pear shaped) with a diameter of 2 to 10 μm; no macroconidia are produced. Large round thick-walled yeast cells, 5 to 15 μm in size, with broad-based budding daughter cells are found in tissue and on

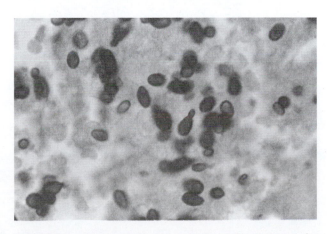

FIGURE 2 GMS stain showing blastoconidia of *H. capsulatum*. Magnification, ~×290.

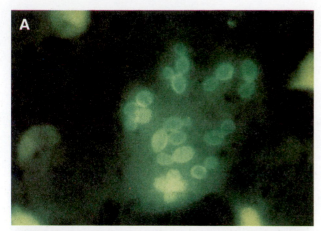

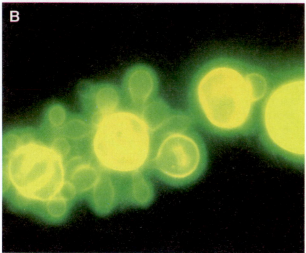

FIGURE 3 (A) Calcofluor white wet mount of sputum showing blastoconidia of *H. capsulatum*. Original magnification, ×475. (Courtesy of the American Society of Clinical Pathology.) (B) Calcofluor white wet mount of sputum showing blastoconidia of *P. brasiliensis*. Magnification, ~×255.

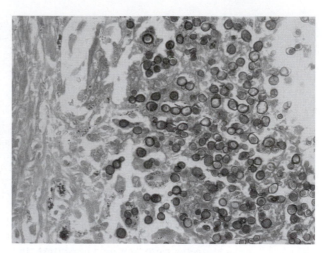

FIGURE 5 Blastoconidia of *B. dermatitidis*. GMS stain. Magnification, ~×290.

appropriate media at 37°C (Fig. 5). Yeast cells may occur inside or outside macrophages.

The natural habitat of *B. dermatitidis* is the soil. It appears to survive best in moist acidic soils that contain a high nitrogen and organic content. Higher soil temperatures and recent rainfall facilitate growth of the fungus.

The largest number of cases of blastomycosis has been reported from North America, but the disease is also endemic in Africa and parts of Central and South America. In the United States, the organism is most commonly found in states surrounding the Mississippi and Ohio Rivers; in Canada, the disease occurs in the provinces that border the Great Lakes.

Coccidioides Species

In the environment and in culture at room temperature, the *Coccidioides* fungus exists as a mold producing septate hyphae and arthroconidia that usually develop in alternate hyphal cells (Fig. 6). As the arthroconidia mature, the alternating disjunctor cells undergo lytic degradation, releasing the barrel-shaped arthroconidia, approximately 2 to 5 μm, which are the infectious particles. Inside the host and on special media,

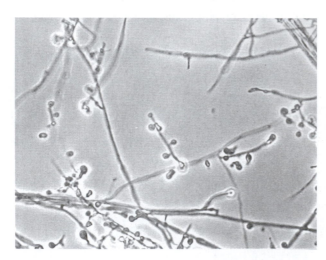

FIGURE 4 Mycelial phase of *B. dermatitidis*. Magnification, ~×240.

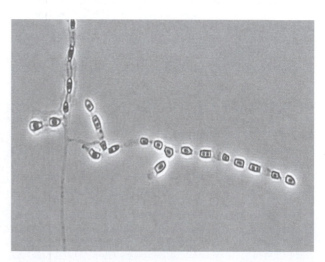

FIGURE 6 Mycelial phase of *Coccidioides immitis* showing alternating arthroconidia. Lactofuchsin stain. Magnification, ~×250.

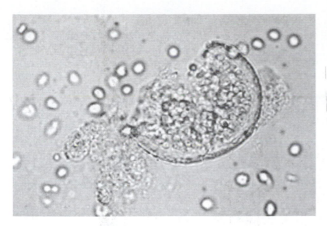

FIGURE 7 KOH preparation of pus from a lesion showing *Coccidioides* spherule and endospores. Magnification, ~×290. (Reprinted from reference 73 with permission).

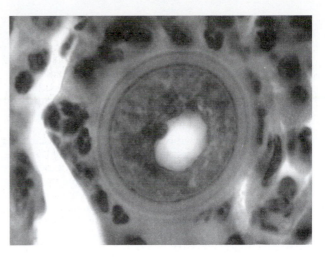

FIGURE 9 *E. parva* adiaspore in mouse tissue. PAS stain. Magnification, ~×280.

the arthroconidia transform into a structure called a spherule. A spherule is a large (up to 120 μm), thick-walled spherical structure containing many internal endospores, each approximately 2 to 4 μm, which can be released if the spherule ruptures (Fig. 7). Each endospore can develop into a spherule as well, continuing the process within the host.

Coccidioides is a soil-inhabiting fungus with a restricted geographical distribution (26). It is confined to regions of the Western Hemisphere that correspond to the lower Sonoran desert life zone. In the United States, the region of endemicity includes central and southern California, southern Arizona, southern New Mexico, part of Utah, and western Texas. The region of endemicity extends southwards into the desert regions of northern Mexico and parts of Central and South America.

Paracoccidioides brasiliensis

P. brasiliensis is a thermally dimorphic fungus. At room temperature, it grows as a mold. Growth requires a lengthy incubation, of up to 30 days. Isolates incubated on rich media produce thin septate hyphae and occasional chlamydospores. Under conditions of nutritional deprivation, some isolates produce conidia, which vary in structure from arthroconidia to microconidia of less than 5 μm. Conidia transform into yeast cells under appropriate nutritional and temperature conditions of approximately 37°C. Yeast cells are mostly oval and characteristically display a mother cell surrounded by multiple buds, a structure thought to resemble a ship's "pilot wheel" (Fig. 3B and 8).

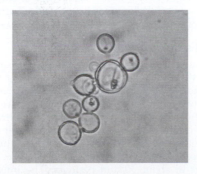

FIGURE 8 Wet mount showing blastoconidia of *P. brasiliensis*. Magnification, ~×290

Although *P. brasiliensis* has been isolated from soil, understanding of its precise environmental habitat remains limited. The region of endemicity extends from Mexico to Argentina, sparing certain countries (Chile, Suriname, the Guyanas, Nicaragua, Belize, and most of the Caribbean islands) within these latitudes. Within countries where the disease is endemic, the mycosis is diagnosed only in areas with relatively well-defined ecologic characteristics (presence of tropical and subtropical forest, abundant watercourses, mild temperatures, high rainfall, and coffee/tobacco crops). The greatest numbers of reported cases have come from Brazil, Colombia, and Venezuela (63).

Emmonsia Species

In the environment and in culture at room temperature, *Emmonsia* species exist as a mold that produces small single-celled conidia (about 4 μm in size) on the sides of the hyphae or on short side branches. Inside the host, the conidia of *E. crescens* and *E. parva* transform into structures termed adiaspores, which resemble the spherules of *Coccidioides* species (Fig. 9). Although adiaspores enlarge to become enormous, thick-walled structures, no endospores are produced and the spores eventually die. Adiaspores can also be generated in vitro in rich media. *E. crescens* and *E. parva* are largely indistinguishable: the former produces large (20- to 140-μm) multinucleate adiaspores at 37°C, while the latter produces smaller (8- to 20-μm) adiaspores at 40°C. *E. pasteuriana* does not produce adiaspores in tissue; rather, at 37°C on rich media it produces structures that resemble budding yeast cells.

The natural habitat of *Emmonsia* species is the soil. Infection has occurred in numerous species of burrowing mammals. Human cases are rare but have been reported from North, Central, and South America, as well as from several European and Asian countries (66).

EPIDEMIOLOGY AND TRANSMISSION

Histoplasmosis

Inhalation of microconidia is the usual mode of *H. capsulatum* infection in humans. The incubation period is 1 to 3 weeks. In cases of reinfection, the incubation period appears to be shorter (4 to 7 days after exposure). Histoplasmosis is not contagious, but there have been occasional reports of transmission from an organ donor to a recipient (15).

The major risk factor for infection is environmental exposure (16). The risk depends on several factors including the nature of the environmental site, the activities performed, and the duration and degree of dust or soil exposure. Longer and more intense exposures usually result in more severe pulmonary disease. Most reported outbreaks have been associated with exposures to sites contaminated with *H. capsulatum* or have followed activities that disturbed accumulations of bird or bat guano (42).

Persons with underlying illnesses are at increased risk for some forms of histoplasmosis. Disseminated infection is more common among individuals with underlying cell-mediated immunological defects, including those with HIV infection, transplant recipients, and individuals receiving tumor necrosis factor alpha inhibitors for rheumatoid arthritis. Immunocompromised persons with histoplasmosis have a higher mortality rate than those who are not immunosuppressed.

Blastomycosis

Inhalation of conidia is the usual mode of infection leading to blastomycosis. The incubation period has been estimated to be 4 to 6 weeks (12). Blastomycosis is not contagious.

Outbreaks have been associated with occupational and recreational activities, often along streams or rivers, and have resulted from exposures to moist soil enriched with decaying vegetation. Apart from outbreaks, blastomycosis is more commonly seen in adults than in children. More men than women are affected. The disease often occurs in individuals with an outdoor occupation or recreational interest.

B. dermatitidis is uncommon as an opportunistic pathogen, but it causes more-aggressive disease in persons with underlying cell-mediated immunological defects, such as those with HIV infection and transplant recipients. Immunocompromised persons with blastomycosis have a higher mortality rate than those who are not immunosuppressed.

Coccidioidomycosis

Inhalation of arthroconidia is the usual mode of infection leading to coccidioidomycosis in humans. The incubation period is 1 to 3 weeks. In contrast to what is observed with histoplasmosis, once individuals have recovered from *Coccidioides* infection, they are usually immune to reinfection. The infection is not contagious, but occasional person-to-person spread has occurred via contaminated fomites (22) or by transmission from an organ donor to a recipient (79).

The major risk factor for infection is environmental exposure. The risk depends on a number of factors including the nature of the environmental site, the activities performed, and the duration and degree of dust or soil exposure. Infection has been associated with ground-disturbing activities, such as building construction, landscaping, farming, archaeological excavation, and numerous recreational pursuits. Natural events that result in the generation of dust clouds, such as earthquakes and windstorms, have been associated with an increased risk of infection and have resulted in large outbreaks.

Disseminated infection is more common among those of black, Asian, or Filipino race and among pregnant women in the third trimester. Individuals with underlying cell-mediated immunological defects, such as those with AIDS and those receiving immunosuppressive medications, are also at increased risk of disease dissemination.

Paracoccidioidomycosis

Inhalation of conidia is the usual mode of infection leading to paracoccidioidomycosis in humans. The incubation period is unknown, but it is clear that the fungus can remain dormant for very long periods in the lymph nodes following asymptomatic primary infection.

Paracoccidioidomycosis predominates in adults, who display 85% to 95% of cases, and in persons in agriculture-related occupations. The disease is more often diagnosed in males than in females (ratio of 15:1). Estrogen-mediated inhibition of the mold-to-yeast transformation could help to account for this (63). Sporadic cases have been reported in individuals with underlying immunosuppressive conditions, including HIV infection.

Adiaspiromycosis

Inhalation of conidia is the usual mode of infection leading to adiaspiromycosis in animals and humans. The incubation period is unknown. No risk factors have been identified.

CLINICAL SIGNIFICANCE

Histoplasmosis

There is a wide spectrum of clinical manifestations of histoplasmosis, ranging from a transient pulmonary infection that subsides without treatment to chronic pulmonary infection or to more widespread disseminated disease (16, 38). Many healthy individuals develop no symptoms when exposed to *H. capsulatum* in a setting of endemicity. Higher levels of exposure result in an acute symptomatic and often severe flu-like illness. The symptoms, which include fever, chills, headache, nonproductive cough, myalgia, pleuritic chest pain, loss of appetite, and fatigue, usually disappear within a few weeks. The most severe and rarest form of this disease is disseminated histoplasmosis. The clinical manifestations range from an acute illness that is fatal within a few weeks if left untreated (often seen in infants, persons with AIDS, and solid-organ transplant recipients) to an indolent, chronic illness that can affect a wide range of sites.

Hepatic infection is common in nonimmunosuppressed individuals with disseminated histoplasmosis, and adrenal gland destruction is a frequent problem. Mucosal ulcers are found in over 60% of these patients. The mouth and throat are often affected, but lesions also occur on the lip, nose, and other sites. Central nervous system disease occurs in 5 to 20% of patients, presenting as chronic meningitis or focal brain lesions. In persons with AIDS, disseminated histoplasmosis is usually associated with low CD4 T-lymphocyte counts and presents with nonspecific symptoms, such as fever and weight loss. Mucosal lesions are uncommon, but multiple cutaneous lesions may be present. Central nervous system involvement occurs in 10 to 20% of cases.

African Histoplasmosis

The clinical manifestations of African histoplasmosis differ from those of classical histoplasmosis. The illness is indolent at onset, and the predominant sites affected are the skin and bones. Individuals with more widespread infection involving the liver, spleen, and other organs have a febrile wasting illness that is fatal within weeks or months if left untreated. Multiple cutaneous lesions often develop on the face and trunk. These lesions often enlarge and ulcerate. Osteomyelitis occurs in about 30% of patients. The infection may spread into contiguous joints causing arthritis, or into adjacent soft tissue, causing a purulent subcutaneous abscess.

Blastomycosis

Blastomycosis encompasses a wide clinical spectrum, ranging from a transient pulmonary infection that subsides without treatment to chronic pulmonary infection or to widespread disseminated disease (12). Acute pulmonary blastomycosis usually presents as a nonspecific influenza-like illness, similar to that seen with histoplasmosis or coccidioidomycosis. Otherwise healthy persons generally recover after 2 to 12 weeks of symptoms, but some infected individuals return months later with infection of other sites. Other patients with acute blastomycosis fail to recover and develop chronic pulmonary disease or disseminated infection.

The skin and bones are the most common sites of extrapulmonary disease. The skin is involved in more than 70% of cases, the lesions presenting either as raised verrucous lesions with irregular borders or as ulcers. The latter can also appear on the mucosa of the nose, mouth, and throat. Osteomyelitis occurs in about 30% of patients with disseminated infection, with the spine, ribs, and long bones being the commonest sites of involvement. Arthritis occurs in about 10% of patients. Meningitis is rare, except in immunocompromised individuals. Other organs, such as the male genitourinary tract, adrenal glands, thyroid, liver, spleen, and gastrointestinal tract are sometimes involved.

Coccidioidomycosis

Coccidioidomycosis includes a wide clinical spectrum, ranging from a transient pulmonary infection that resolves without treatment to chronic pulmonary infection or to widespread disseminated disease (26). About 40% of newly infected persons develop an acute symptomatic and often severe flu-like illness (valley fever). Higher rates of symptomatic infection (50 to 100%) have often been reported during outbreaks. The symptoms include fever, headache, chills, nonproductive cough, myalgia, and pleuritic chest pain. Up to 50% of patients develop a mild, diffuse erythematous or maculopapular rash covering the trunk and limbs within the first few days of the onset of symptoms. More dramatic and persistent is the rash of erythema nodosum or erythema multiforme, which occurs in about 5% of infected persons but is more common in women. Otherwise healthy persons recover without treatment, their symptoms disappearing in a few weeks.

Fewer than 1% of infected individuals develop disseminated coccidioidomycosis. This progressive disease usually develops within 3 to 12 months of the initial infection, although it can occur much later following reactivation of a quiescent infection in an immunosuppressed individual. The clinical manifestations range from a fulminant illness that is fatal within a few weeks if left untreated to an indolent chronic disease that persists for months or years. One or more sites may be involved, but the skin, soft tissue, bones, joints, and meninges are most commonly affected. Cutaneous and subcutaneous lesions are common. Osteomyelitis occurs in about 40% of patients, with the spine, ribs, cranial bones, and ends of the long bones being the most common sites. The disease may spread into contiguous joints causing arthritis, or into adjacent soft tissue, causing subcutaneous abscess formation. Meningitis is the most serious complication of coccidioidomycosis, occurring in 30 to 50% of patients with disseminated disease. Without treatment, it is almost always fatal.

Paracoccidioidomycosis

The lungs are the usual initial site of *P. brasiliensis* infection, but the organism then spreads through the lymphatics to the regional lymph nodes. In most cases the primary infection is asymptomatic. However, children and adolescents sometimes present with an acute disseminated form of infection in which superficial and/or visceral lymph node enlargement is the major manifestation. This presentation is also seen in immunocompromised patients. It has a poor prognosis.

Most adults with paracoccidioidomycosis present with chronic progressive infection involving one or more organs, with the severity of the symptoms varying with the patient (63). In 80% of cases the disease involves the lungs. The disease is slowly progressive and may take months or even years to become established. Ulcerative mucocutaneous lesions of the face, mouth, and nose are the most obvious presenting sign. Other sites of infection include the small or large intestine, liver and spleen, adrenal glands, bones and joints, central nervous system, and male genitourinary tract. In 60 to 80% of cases, active pulmonary involvement and residual fibrotic lesions are observed; these lesions can alter respiratory function and incapacitate the patient.

Adiaspiromycosis

In most cases, adiaspiromycosis is a self-limited, localized pulmonary infection with few or no symptoms. Because the adiaspores enlarge but do not reproduce, symptoms and clinical signs appear to depend upon the number of conidia inhaled. Some patients have presented with nonproductive cough, dyspnea, and fever. A few cases of fatal, multifocal pulmonary disease have been reported (66).

COLLECTION, TRANSPORT, AND STORAGE OF SPECIMENS

Clinical Specimens

Methods of collection, transport, and storage of specimens are detailed in chapter 112. Tissue samples should be obtained when appropriate and should be divided and submitted for microbiological and histopathological examination. If possible, special tissue stains such as the Grocott-Gomori methenamine silver (GMS) and periodic acid-Schiff (PAS) stains should be requested. Since colonization with the dimorphic fungal pathogens does not occur, their microscopic detection and/or isolation in culture is consistent with a firm diagnosis of infection. Blood, urine, and cerebrospinal fluid (CSF) can also be collected as appropriate for antigen and/or antibody testing.

Histoplasma capsulatum

H. capsulatum organisms can be isolated from sputum or bronchoalveolar lavage fluid specimens in 60 to 85% of cases of chronic pulmonary histoplasmosis if multiple specimens are tested (75). In disseminated disease, useful specimens for culture include blood, urine, lymph node, and bone marrow samples. Bone marrow cultures are positive in over 75% of cases. Blood cultures collected with the Isolator lysis-centrifugation system (Wampole Laboratories, Princeton, NJ) or Bactec Mycolytic bottles (BD Diagnostic Systems, Franklin Lakes, NJ) show the greatest sensitivity. Biopsy specimens of oral, cutaneous, and gastrointestinal lesions, adrenal glands, or liver and spleen have also provided a diagnosis. *Histoplasma* meningitis is difficult to diagnose, with CSF cultures being positive in no more than two-thirds of cases. The best results are obtained when large volumes of CSF (10 to 20 ml) are cultured on multiple occasions.

Blastomyces dermatitidis

Sputum samples, bronchoalveolar lavage fluid, or lung biopsy specimens may be submitted. Skin biopsy specimens are useful in the diagnosis of cutaneous disease. Collection of urine after prostatic massage may be helpful in the diagnosis of genitourinary blastomycosis.

Coccidioides Species

In addition to lower respiratory tract samples, material for microscopy and culture can be collected from suppurative cutaneous and soft tissue lesions. Organisms can be recovered only infrequently from CSF, and usually only after culture of large volumes (10 to 20 ml).

Paracoccidioides brasiliensis

In addition to lower respiratory samples, material can be collected from oral or pharyngeal lesions, cutaneous lesions, lymph nodes, adrenal glands, and the gastrointestinal tract.

Emmonsia Species

Sputum and bronchoalveolar lavage fluids are seldom culture positive in patients with disease. The diagnosis is usually based on histopathologic demonstration of adiaspores in lung tissue.

DIRECT EXAMINATION

Microscopy

Direct microscopic examination of clinical materials may provide a rapid presumptive diagnosis of a systemic fungal infection. However, it is important to appreciate that tissue form cells of *H. capsulatum* and *B. dermatitidis* can appear similar to each other as well as to yeast cells of various *Candida* species, *Cryptococcus neoformans,* and *Penicillium marneffei* and to endospores of *Coccidioides* species. It is often helpful to stain fresh, wet preparations of sputum, bronchoalveolar lavage fluid, CSF, urine, pus, or other material with calcofluor white, a fluorescent compound that binds to the fungal cell wall.

Histoplasma capsulatum

Giemsa and Wright's stains can be used to detect yeast cells of *H. capsulatum* in blood or bone marrow smears. These cells can also be seen in tissue sections stained with GMS or PAS but usually not with hematoxylin and eosin (H&E). Detection of the small (2- to 4-μm) oval budding yeasts allows a presumptive diagnosis of histoplasmosis. Organisms can be found within macrophages or free in the tissues. It is unusual to find yeast cells on cytological examination of sputum or other respiratory tract fluids. The thick-walled narrow-based budding yeast cells causing African histoplasmosis, approximately 10 to 15 μm in diameter, are about fourfold larger than those of classical *H. capsulatum* in tissue sections.

Blastomyces dermatitidis

Direct calcofluor white or KOH mounts or Gram stains of sputum, tissues, and exudates often permit the detection of the large round yeast cells of *B. dermatitidis*. The broad-based buds often attain the same size as the parent cells before becoming detached. Histopathologic examination using PAS or GMS stains also can be of value.

Coccidioides Species

Tissue sections should be stained with PAS, GMS, or H&E to permit the detection of the characteristic large, thick-walled spherules of *Coccidioides* species. Microscopic examination of wet preparations of sputum, bronchoalveolar lavage fluid, pus, or other samples treated with KOH is also helpful but is less sensitive. *Prototheca wickerhamii* may resemble small spherules, and *Rhinosporidium seeberi* may simulate larger ones.

Paracoccidioides brasiliensis

The characteristic translucent-walled yeast cells of *P. brasiliensis* with multiple buds can often be found on direct microscopic examination of sputum, bronchoalveolar lavage fluid, pus from draining lymph nodes, or tissue biopsy specimens. Staining of wet preparations with lactophenol cotton blue, methylene blue, Gram stain, or calcofluor white can be helpful. Tissue sections can be stained with PAS, GMS, or H&E.

Emmonsia Species

Tissue sections stained with PAS or GMS are most helpful in demonstrating the characteristic adiaspores of *Emmonsia* species in lung tissue. It is important to appreciate that in the chronic stage the organism may collapse, forming various shapes that may resemble other fungi, helminths, or pollen grains. Adiaspores must also be distinguished from the spherules of *Coccidioides*. Adiaspores do not contain endospores.

Antigen Detection

Histoplasma capsulatum

The *Histoplasma* polysaccharide antigen (HPA) test is a microtiter plate-based double-antibody sandwich enzyme immunoassay (EIA) to detect antigen in urine, serum, or CSF in cases of disseminated histoplasmosis (14). This test is also useful in the early diagnosis of acute pulmonary histoplasmosis and during treatment follow-up (75). This test is performed on a fee-for-service basis by MiraVista Diagnostics (Indianapolis, IN) (www.miravistalabs.com). Similar tests have also been developed for detection of antigenuria (Specialty Laboratories, Valencia, CA; and ImmunoMycologics [IMMY], Norman, OK) (13), although varying results were reported when these tests were compared (51).

Ten milliliters of urine, 5 ml of serum, or 1 ml of CSF is the preferred volume for the HPA test, although a minimum volume of 0.5 ml of any specimen is required for a single test. To obtain maximum test sensitivity, it is recommended that both serum and urine specimens be tested in parallel. Treatment success or failure may be assessed by collecting specimens at least 14 days after starting treatment and testing the newly acquired samples in parallel with the last specimen that was positive before initiation of treatment.

Blastomyces dermatitidis

The *Blastomyces* antigen test is a microtiter plate-based double-antibody sandwich EIA to detect antigenuria and antigenemia in disseminated blastomycosis (20). This test is performed on a fee-for-service basis by MiraVista Diagnostics. The sample requirements are the same as those for the HPA test.

Coccidioides Species

An EIA using antibodies against *Coccidioides* galactomannan has been developed for detecting the more severe forms of coccidioidomycosis (71% sensitivity) (21). This test is performed on a fee-for-service basis by MiraVista Diagnostics. The sample requirements are the same as those for the HPA test.

Paracoccidioides brasiliensis

At present, paracoccidioidomycosis antigen testing is not available as a routine diagnostic test. A 43-kDa glycoprotein and an 87-kDa heat shock protein have been described as useful targets for serum antigen detection (27, 53). Several reports have described the detection of *P. brasiliensis* antigen in urine, CSF, and bronchoalveolar fluid samples (45, 64). Others have noted that antigen levels in serum diminished or even disappeared during successful treatment (28, 46).

Emmonsia Species

No serologic tests exist at this time for the diagnosis of adiaspiromycosis in humans.

Nucleic Acid Detection in Clinical Materials

No commercially available systems exist for detection of fungal nucleic acids in human clinical samples. However, a number of methods are currently under investigation, several of which are highlighted in this section. Conserved regions of rRNA genes have been used as targets in a number of PCR-based detection assays. It is important to appreciate that amplification of conserved genes can result in products derived both from pathogenic fungi and from genetically related nonpathogenic fungal species. The nonspecific nucleic acids could arise from colonization of the original sample with saprophytic organisms, from contamination during sample collection, or from contamination of PCR reagents with fungal DNA. It is very important that the identity of amplicons detected using conserved genes be verified by direct sequencing (56). In more recent studies, genes specific for the fungus of interest have been chosen as PCR targets, thus eliminating this specificity problem.

Histoplasmosis

At the time of this writing (March 2010), more than 10 publications have described the use of PCR to detect *H. capsulatum* DNA in fixed paraffin-embedded tissue samples, blood, bronchial lavage fluids, bone marrow, and ophthalmic samples. Early studies targeted the internal transcribed spacer (ITS) rRNA gene region, but the use of targets unique to *H. capsulatum* has provided better assay specificity. Bialek et al. designed a nested PCR that targeted the gene coding for a unique 100-kDa protein of *H. capsulatum* (3), which was used to detect *H. capsulatum* DNA in clinical samples from patients with histoplasmosis in French Guiana (55). In another study, a portion of the *H. capsulatum* H antigen gene was amplified (8). The original format of nested or seminested PCR has recently been adapted to real-time PCR with promising results (34, 54).

Blastomycosis

A nested-PCR assay targeting the WI-1 gene has been described for the detection of *B. dermatitidis* DNA in paraffin-embedded tissue (4, 6). The PCR amplified DNA from 8 of 13 tissue samples in which yeast cells were detected by microscopy, and all products were homologous to the WI-1 gene on direct sequencing.

Coccidioidomycosis

Single- and nested-PCR assays have been used to amplify DNA from sera of mice infected with *C. posadasii* and from sera of seropositive patients (reviewed in reference 6). The antigen 2/proline-rich antigen (Ag2/PRA) gene was targeted for direct detection of *Coccidioides* DNA in sputum and in three human paraffin-embedded tissue samples that were microscopically positive for spherules (5). A real-time PCR study of 266 respiratory specimens and 66 fresh tissue specimens targeting the ITS-2 region showed excellent sensitivity and specificity when compared with culture (7).

Paracoccidioidomycosis

A nested-PCR assay targeting the immunogenic gp43 gene was evaluated in the detection of *P. brasiliensis* DNA in lung homogenates from infected and uninfected mice (2). Assays targeting gp43 used with clinical samples from infected patients lacked sensitivity when applied to serum but were able to detect 10 yeast cells per ml of sputum. A real-time PCR with a molecular beacon probe targeting the ITS-1 region has also been developed for the detection of *Paracoccidioides brasiliensis* DNA in clinical samples (10).

Adiaspiromycosis

A panfungal PCR targeting the ribosomal ITS-1 and -2 regions identified *Emmonsia crescens* from a bronchoalveolar lavage fluid sample of a patient with confirmed adiaspiromycosis (19).

ISOLATION PROCEDURES

Biosafety

Laboratory-associated infections with *Coccidioides* species, *H. capsulatum*, and *B. dermatitidis* have occurred in healthy immunocompetent individuals after exposure to airborne conidia (69, 74), which can be released from contaminated soil samples as well as from sporulating mold phase cultures of the organisms. Even the mere lifting of a culture plate lid is often sufficient to cause the release of large numbers of conidia into the air. Should a sporulating culture be dropped, millions of conidia may be dispersed. It is also important to note that local infections including granuloma formation have been reported following accidental percutaneous inoculation during injection of laboratory animals, or while performing autopsies of humans with histoplasmosis, coccidioidomycosis, or blastomycosis.

All procedures involving the manipulation of sporulating cultures of *Coccidioides* species, *B. dermatitidis*, and *H. capsulatum* and for processing soil or other environmental materials known or likely to contain these organisms should be performed inside a class II biological safety cabinet under conditions of biosafety level 3 containment. Biosafety level 2 practices and facilities are recommended for handling and processing clinical specimens and animal tissues (78). Hyaline (colorless) molds of unknown identity should always be examined and manipulated inside a class II biosafety cabinet. Such molds should never be handled on an open laboratory bench. In Europe, these organisms are classified as hazard group 3, which means that even clinical samples suspected of containing the organisms should be handled under containment level 3 conditions. Recommendations for handling inadvertent exposure to *Coccidioides* in the laboratory have been published (67).

Biosecurity

In the United States, both species of *Coccidioides* are classified as select agents. The select agent regulations in the Code of Federal Regulations (42 C.F.R. Part 73, 7 C.F.R. Part 331, and 9 C.F.R. Part 121 [www.selectagents.gov]) govern the possession, use, and transfer of these agents. Any entity in the United States that possesses, uses, or transfers isolates that are known to be *Coccidioides* species must have a certificate of registration issued by the Secretary of the Department of Health and Human Services (DHHS). Isolates that are known to be *Coccidioides* may be transferred only between registered laboratories. In addition, individuals may not handle or possess isolates that are known to be *Coccidioides* species unless they have been approved by DHHS based on a security risk assessment from the U.S. Attorney General. Clinical or diagnostic laboratories that possess, use, or transfer an isolate suspected to be *Coccidioides* that is contained in a specimen presented for diagnosis, verification, or confirmation are exempt from these requirements. These exempt laboratories must destroy or transfer the isolate within seven calendar days of identification of the agent. The exempt laboratory, as well as the registered laboratory, must submit a completed APHIS/CDC Form 4 within seven calendar days of identification, specifying the final status of the isolate. Application forms, Form 4, and a copy of the regulations can be found at www.selectagents.gov.

Culture for Mold Phase

In general, the organisms discussed in this chapter can be readily cultivated in the mold phase on general fungal media such as Sabouraud dextrose agar or potato dextrose agar incubated at 25°C. Incubation at 37°C is also helpful to recover the yeast phase of dimorphic organisms. Media containing antibiotics such as chloramphenicol or gentamicin should be used when culturing clinical materials, such as sputum, that may be contaminated with bacteria. Media containing cycloheximide are useful to inhibit saprophytic fungi and to provide a useful differential tool in identification. Many unrelated saprophytic soil fungi fail to grow on media containing cycloheximide, fail to grow altogether at 37°C, or fail to convert to the yeast phase at 37°C. Screw-cap slants are preferable to plates for culturing dimorphic fungi. If plates are used, they should be sealed so that mold spores cannot escape into the ambient air. Seals that are permeable to air such as Shrink Seals (Scientific Device Laboratory, Des Plaines, IL) are useful for this purpose. In general, colonies develop within 3 to 7 days, but some strains of *H. capsulatum* and *P. brasiliensis* may require incubation for as much as 4 to 6 weeks.

Culture for Yeast Phase

H. capsulatum, *B. dermatitidis*, and *P. brasiliensis* can be recovered in the yeast phase by using appropriate media incubated at 37°C. *Coccidioides* species do not have a yeast phase. *E. parva* and *E. crescens* produce adiaspores at elevated temperatures.

Histoplasma capsulatum

The yeast phase of *H. capsulatum* can be recovered in rich media such as brain heart infusion agar (BHI) or BHI with blood (BHIB). Plates or slants should be incubated at 37°C under aerobic conditions for at least 4 weeks.

Blastomyces dermatitidis

The yeast phase of *B. dermatitidis* can be recovered in rich media such as BHI, BHIB, Pine's medium, or Kelley's agar by incubation at 37°C under aerobic conditions. Yeasts are usually visible within 1 week, but media should be held for at least 4 weeks before being discarded.

Paracoccidioides brasiliensis

The yeast phase of *P. brasiliensis* can be recovered in media such as BHI, Pine's medium, or Kelley's agar by incubation at 37°C. The organism grows slowly, and plates or slants should be held for at least 4 weeks.

Emmonsia Species

E. parva and *E. crescens* produce adiaspores in vitro when cultivated on phytone yeast extract agar, BHI, or BHIB at 37°C to 40°C depending on the species. *E. pasteuriana* produces yeast-like cells after culture on BHI at 37°C for approximately 10 days.

IDENTIFICATION

In general, these organisms are identified by their characteristic morphologic features, by conversion to the yeast phase, by DNA probe testing if available, and/or by direct DNA sequencing. Slide cultures should not be performed on suspected dimorphic isolates due to the possibility of laboratory infection from accidental inhalation of infectious conidia.

Histoplasma capsulatum

The mold phase can be recovered after incubation at 25°C. The colony is initially white or buff-brown. Both types may be isolated from the same patient, and eventually the brown type may convert to the white type. The brown type generally produces more of the characteristic tuberculate macroconidia than the white type. On subculture, only about 30% of macroconidia show tubercles. Microconidia are abundant in fresh isolates of *H. capsulatum*. After multiple subcultures, the production of both macroconidia and microconidia may be diminished. The presence of both macroconidia and microconidia is not required for identification of *H. capsulatum*, as authentic *H. capsulatum* isolates that fail to produce either macroconidia or microconidia have been recognized. Macroconidia but no microconidia can also be seen in the saprophytic fungus *Sepedonium* as well as in the related fungus *Renispora flavissima*. Authentic *H. capsulatum* isolates can be recognized by their thermal dimorphism as well as by their growth on inhibitory mold agar.

Once the characteristic morphology has been recognized, mold phase *H. capsulatum* isolates can be confirmed by conversion to the yeast phase. The isolate is transferred to BHI or BHIB agar and incubated at 37°C for at least 7 to 10 days. Hyphal cells may form buds directly or develop enlarged, transitional cells that subsequently begin to bud. The microconidia may also convert to budding yeast cells. Complete conversion rarely is achieved, and multiple transfers to fresh BHI or BHIB medium may be required. The colony develops a white, smooth, yeast-like appearance, and microscopic examination reveals oval, budding yeasts approximately 1 to 3 by 3 to 5 μm. The cells have a narrower base of attachment between the bud and parent cell than do those of *B. dermatitidis*.

The AccuProbe test (GenProbe, San Diego, CA) can also be used to confirm isolates as *H. capsulatum*. This test requires actively growing cultures: mold phase cells not more than 4 weeks of age or yeast cells not older than 1 week. Isolates can be taken from solid media or broth cultures. In this assay, formation of specific DNA-RNA hybrids is quantitated in relative light units by use of a luminometer. Extracts that display relative light unit values of >50,000 are considered positive. The AccuProbe test has largely replaced exoantigen testing for identification of *H. capsulatum*. Several studies have shown that this test is sensitive and specific for identification of *H. capsulatum* (32, 58, 68), although false-positive results can be obtained when isolates that are genetically related to the *Ajellomycetaceae* are tested (9). An exoantigen testing kit to identify the organism is commercially available from IMMY.

African *Histoplasma* isolates display colonial morphology similar to that of non-African isolates and yield positive results in the AccuProbe test for *Histoplasma capsulatum* (58). Histopathologic examination of tissue forms is required to distinguish members of the African clade.

Blastomyces dermatitidis

At 25 to 30°C, isolates of *B. dermatitidis* produce a variety of forms ranging from a fluffy white colony that is visible within 2 to 3 days to a glabrous, tan, nonconidiating colony that grows more slowly. Microscopic examination shows microconidia that are oval or pyriform, usually smooth walled, and formed on short lateral or terminal branches along the hyphae. *B. dermatitidis* also grows readily on inhibitory media containing cycloheximide. Conidia of the hyaline hyphomycete *Scedosporium apiospermum*, of some *Chrysosporium* species, and of the dermatophyte *Trichophyton rubrum* are morphologically similar and can be mistaken for *B. dermatitidis*. These species either fail to grow at 37°C (some *Chrysosporium* species) or grow as molds when incubated at 37°C (*S. apiospermum* and *T. rubrum*).

The identification can be confirmed by conversion to the yeast phase. Generally, isolates of *B. dermatitidis* convert readily to the yeast phase on BHI, BHIB, or Pine's or Kelley's medium incubated at 37°C. Yeast cells are hyaline, smooth walled and thick walled, generally 8 to 15 μm in diameter, with the bud connected to the parent cell by a broad base of up to 4 to 5 μm in diameter. Conversion can be accomplished in 2 to 3 days, although occasional isolates may take several weeks.

Identification can also be confirmed using the AccuProbe test for *B. dermatitidis*. False-positive *Blastomyces dermatitidis* Gen-Probe results were obtained with *P. brasiliensis* (59) and with *Gymnascella hyalinospora*, so care must be taken to distinguish these organisms (reviewed in reference 6). An exoantigen testing kit to identify the organism is commercially available from IMMY.

Coccidioides Species

At 25 to 30°C, isolates of *Coccidioides* species display considerable variation in colonial morphology. Colonies can range from moist, glabrous, and grayish to abundant, floccose, and white. Colonies may become tan and even red with age (69). Microscopic examination shows hyphae that are thin and septate, with fertile (spore-producing) hyphae usually arising at right angles. Arthroconidia are hyaline, one-celled, short, cylindrical to barrel-shaped, moderately thick walled, smooth walled, and 2 to 8 by 3 to 5 μm. Arthroconidia alternate with thin-walled empty disjunctor cells. At maturity, the disjunctor cells undergo lytic degradation, releasing the arthroconidia. After this fragmentation, the arthroconidia may display frill-like remains of the disjunctor cells on each end. Isolates of *Coccidioides* grow well on inhibitory mold agar containing cycloheximide, which helps to distinguish this organism from similar soil saprophytes such as *Malbranchea* species. It is also important to distinguish true alternate arthroconidia from aging mycelia that, due to cytoplasmic shrinkage, display an appearance that can be misinterpreted as arthroconidia. True arthroconidia eventually fragment and disperse; aging mycelia do not. The two species of *Coccidioides* cannot be readily distinguished morphologically.

When incubated at 37°C, no yeast form is produced. The organism can produce spherules in vitro when incubated at 37 to 40°C in appropriate media and increased CO_2 tension, but this procedure is rarely performed on routine clinical isolates.

The AccuProbe for *Coccidioides* may be used for confirmation of unknown isolates as *Coccidioides* species. This test is generally sensitive and specific, although pretreatment of isolates with formaldehyde leads to false-negative results. The test does not distinguish between the two species of *Coccidioides*. An exoantigen testing kit to identify the organism is commercially available from IMMY. A TaqMan real-time PCR assay that distinguishes between the two species has also been described (65).

Paracoccidioides brasiliensis

When incubated at 25 to 30°C, isolates display slow growth and produce a variety of forms ranging from glabrous leathery, brownish, flat colonies with a few tufts of aerial mycelium to wrinkled, folded, floccose colonies to velvety, white-to-beige forms. The colonies are very similar in appearance to those of *B. dermatitidis*. Most strains grow for long periods of time without the production of conidia.

When cultures are transferred to 37°C on rich media such as BHI or Pine's or Kelley's agar, the resulting yeast colonies are generally folded (cerebriform) in appearance. Mycelial elements may be seen mixed with yeast cells. Conversion to the yeast phase also is quite slow. Yeasts are 2 to 30 μm in diameter and are oval or irregular in shape, displaying the characteristic "pilot's wheel" appearance of multiple thin-necked round buds developing around the parent cell. The walls are thinner than those of *B. dermatitidis* yeast cells, and the buds are not broad based.

Identification is usually confirmed by demonstrating thermal dimorphism. There is no commercial DNA probe test for *P. brasiliensis*. The AccuProbe test for *B. dermatitidis* cross-reacts with *P. brasiliensis* (59), so care must be taken when employing this test on isolates that may actually be *P. brasiliensis*. Slow-growing, nonsporulating isolates are more characteristic of *P. brasiliensis* than of *B. dermatitidis*.

Emmonsia Species

At 25°C, *Emmonsia* species organisms grow as glabrous (waxy), colorless colonies, which produce yellowish white aerial mycelia in time. Some strains display pale orange to grayish orange aerial mycelia. The colonies often have areas that alternate between a tufted mycelium and a glabrous consistency. Reverse pigmentation is pale gray to grayish brown. On microscopic examination, the hyphae are septate and branching. Sporulation is enhanced on potato dextrose or Pablum cereal agar. Numerous conidia are produced either directly from the sides of the hyphae or on short stalks that branch at right angles from the hyphae. Each stalk bears a single terminal conidium. Sometimes the swollen end may bear one to three secondary spine-like pegs, which in turn form a secondary conidium in a flower-like arrangement (66). The conidia are round, oval, or pyriform and measure 2 to 4 μm by 3 to 5 μm. The conidial wall is smooth but may roughen with age. *E. parva* and *E. crescens* are indistinguishable in morphology and appearance at 25°C.

E. crescens displays no hyphal growth at 37°C and forms larger adiaspores (20 to 140 μm in diameter) on BHI or phytone yeast extract agar at this temperature. *E. parva* produces hyphae at 37°C and produces smaller adiaspores (8 to 20 μm in diameter) at 40°C. *E. pasteuriana* displays features at 25°C that are similar to those of *E. crescens* and *E. parva*. At 37°C on BHIB, this species produces yeast-like cells that are oval or lemon shaped, budding on a narrow base, and 2 to 4 μm. The colonies are creamy and smooth. This species does not produce adiaspores in vitro or in vivo (31).

TYPING SYSTEMS

In general, typing systems have been used to show geographic differences among isolates and cryptic species. In some genera, diversity can be shown among isolates collected from a single geographic area.

Histoplasma capsulatum

Isolates can be divided into at least eight clades as described earlier (37). This typing system can be used to place an unknown isolate into one of the major worldwide geographic groupings. For further delineation, RFLP typing with the yeast phase-specific nuclear gene yps-3 and/or mitochondrial DNA probes and random amplified polymorphic DNA-based and ITS-based typing methods have been used in several studies (reviewed in reference 70). These studies have shown that considerable polymorphisms can be demonstrated among individual patient isolates from a particular geographic location (70); that animal and soil strains from Brazil display indistinguishable subtypes (17); and that strains from patients in Brazil, where mucocutaneous histoplasmosis is much more common than in the United States, display distinct ITS and yps-3 subtypes not seen in strains from U.S. patients (36).

Blastomyces dermatitidis

In a study using RFLP with several rRNA gene probes to study 55 isolates from the United States, India, and Africa, three major groups were defined. These groups were further divided using random amplified polymorphic DNA fingerprinting into 5, 15, and 12 types, respectively, that correlated with the geographic origin of the isolate (49). Interestingly, these studies showed that soil isolates collected from an outbreak of blastomycosis in Eagle River, WI, were not responsible for the majority of cases of disease in that outbreak. A study exploring polymorphisms in the promoter region upstream of the BAD-1 virulence gene as potential subtyping tools showed that significant size differences in the subtypes were due to large insertions in the promoter region (52).

Coccidioides Species

Two major clades, corresponding to the two species C. immitis and C. posadasii, were defined when an extensive population sample, including isolates from Venezuela, Mexico, and Brazil, was studied by using a set of nine microsatellite markers (25). Typing of isolates to C. immitis (CA) or C. posadasii (non-CA) species can be accomplished by examining any of 17 sites fixed for alternate alleles (40, 65). Microsatellite typing conducted with 121 clinical isolates from Arizona concluded that this disease in Arizona could not be linked to a dominant hypervirulent strain of C. posadasii (35).

Paracoccidioides brasiliensis

Multilocus sequence typing at eight loci demonstrated the existence of at least three distinct species within this organism (48). The gp43 gene encoding a dominant glycoprotein antigen has been studied by several groups as a useful target for subtyping. In an earlier study, microsatellite sequences were compared as markers to discriminate among a set of P. brasiliensis human isolates causing either chronic or acute disease (57). These authors did not observe any clustering of isolates associated with either acute or chronic disease.

Emmonsia Species

Based on ITS sequences, isolates of E. crescens fall into two phylogenetic groups, North American and Eurasian, depending on the continents from which the isolates were obtained (62). Isolates of E. parva separate into two groups as well, one group isolated from the North American prairies and the second group from the desert southwest of the United States or from Italy.

SEROLOGIC TESTS

Histoplasmosis

Serologic tests have an important role in the rapid diagnosis of several forms of H. capsulatum infection but are most useful for persons with chronic pulmonary or disseminated histoplasmosis (44). Of the different methods that have been developed, the immunodiffusion (ID), complement fixation (CF), and latex agglutination (LA) tests are the most popular. The principal antigen used in these tests is histoplasmin, a soluble filtrate of mycelial-phase broth cultures. Histoplasmin contains three antigenic components of particular interest. The H antigen is a β-glucosidase against which antibodies are formed during acute histoplasmosis. The M antigen is a catalase against which antibodies are produced during all phases of the disease. The C antigen is a heat-stable galactomannan polysaccharide that is cross-reactive with B. dermatitidis and C. immitis. The H and M antigens were once thought to be specific proteins for the detection of anti-H. capsulatum antibodies. The M antigen, however, was found to be not specific unless used in a deglycosylated form.

The ID test is a qualitative method that detects precipitins to the H and M glycoprotein antigens of H. capsulatum present in histoplasmin. Both serum and CSF can be used. Patients with negative serum reactions during the acute phase of infection should have additional samples taken 3 to 4 weeks later. ID test kits and reagents are available from Gibson Laboratories (Lexington, KY), IMMY, and Meridian Bioscience (Cincinnati, OH). Commercial kits include mycelial-phase culture filtrates containing H. capsulatum H and M antigens, positive-control sera containing antibodies against both H and M antigens, and ID plates. Positive-control sera must be included each time the test is performed and must react with both the H and M antigens. The ID test is a useful screening procedure or can be used as an adjunct to the CF test. It is more specific but less sensitive than the CF test.

The CF test is a quantitative procedure in which two antigens are employed: histoplasmin and a suspension of intact merthiolate-killed H. capsulatum yeast phase cells. The latter is more sensitive (~80% versus ~20%) but less specific (~90% versus ~99%) than histoplasmin. Serum, peritoneal fluid, or CSF can be used in the CF test. Patients with negative serum reactions during the acute phase of infection should have additional samples taken 3 to 4 weeks later. No commercial kits are available, but antigens, antisera, and other reagents can be purchased from several commercial sources (e.g., IMMY and Meridian). Negative-control serum and positive-control serum from human histoplasmosis cases demonstrating a CF titer of 1:32 or greater with the homologous antigen should be tested each time the CF test is performed.

An LA test using histoplasmin as antigen is commercially available (LA-Histo antibody system; IMMY). This semiquantitative test detects immunoglobulin M (IgM) antibodies and is used primarily for the presumptive diagnosis of acute histoplasmosis. It is less helpful for the detection of chronic infection.

Blastomycosis

The most useful serologic test is ID, but CF and enzyme-linked immunosorbent assay procedures have also been developed and evaluated. Substantial improvement in the performance of these tests has been achieved by the use of two purified surface antigens of *B. dermatitidis*, one termed the A antigen and the other the WI-1 antigen. Both molecules are released from the yeast phase of *B. dermatitidis* by autolysis and can be recovered from culture filtrates. Immunological comparison of the two antigens has shown that they are very similar, but WI-1 is a 120-kDa protein that is not glycosylated while the A antigen is a 135-kDa glycosylated protein.

The ID test is a qualitative method that detects precipitins to the A antigen of *B. dermatitidis*. Patients with negative serum reactions during the acute phase of infection should have additional samples taken 3 to 4 weeks later. ID test kits and reagents are available from Gibson, IMMY, and Meridian. Commercial kits include purified *B. dermatitidis* A antigen, positive-control serum containing antibodies against A antigen, and ID plates. The positive-control serum must be included each time the test is performed and must react with the homologous reference antigen to form the A precipitin line.

Coccidioidomycosis

Despite the fact that sensitive procedures such as EIA have been developed, the ID and CF tests remain the most reliable methods for the serologic diagnosis of coccidioidomycosis (44). The principal antigen used in these tests is coccidioidin, a soluble filtrate of mycelial-phase broth cultures.

The simultaneous use of heated and unheated coccidioidin antigens permits the ID test to be employed to detect either IgM or IgG antibodies on a single plate. The IDTP test utilizes heated coccidioidin as antigen, detects IgM, and gives results comparable to those obtained with the classical tube precipitin test. It is most useful for diagnosing recent infection. The IDCF test utilizes unheated coccidioidin, detects IgG antibodies, and gives results comparable to those obtained by the CF method (see below). It is less sensitive but more specific than the CF test (61). Commercial kits are available (Gibson, IMMY, and Meridian) and include unheated and heat-treated coccidioidin antigens, positive-control sera containing IgM or IgG antibodies, and ID plates. The sensitivity of the IDTP and IDCF tests can be improved by 10-fold concentration of serum prior to testing. Positive-control sera must be included each time the test is performed and must react with the homologous reference antigen to form a precipitin line. The ID test is useful for initial screening of specimens and can be followed by other tests if positive.

The CF test is a sensitive quantitative method in which unheated coccidioidin is used to detect IgG antibodies. The major disadvantage of CF is that it is a laborious and time-consuming procedure that requires experienced personnel for optimum performance. No commercial kits are available, but reagents for in-house use can be obtained from several commercial sources (IMMY and Meridian). Negative-control serum and a positive-control serum from a human case of coccidioidomycosis (with a titer of ≥1:32) should be included each time the test is performed. Anticomplementary activity in serum samples can occur and may be resolved by subsequent ID testing. In addition to serum, the CF test can be performed with CSF, pleural, or joint fluid samples.

A qualitative LA test using heat-treated coccidioidin as antigen is available from several commercial sources (e.g., LA-Cocci antibody system from IMMY and Coccidioides latex agglutination system from Meridian). This test is simple and rapid to perform. It detects IgM antibodies and is more sensitive than the IDTP test in detecting early infection. However, it has a false-positive rate of 5 to 10%, and the results should be confirmed using the IDTP and/or CF methods. It is not recommended for screening CSF specimens because false-positive reactions can occur (60).

The Premier *Coccidioides* EIA (Meridian) is a qualitative test for detection of IgM and IgG antibodies in serum or CSF specimens. The antigen used in this test is a mixture of purified TP and CF antigens. Published evaluations suggest this test has a sensitivity of >95% and a specificity of ~95% (39, 47). However, false-positive reactions have been obtained with sera from some patients with blastomycosis. Positive EIA results should be confirmed by the IDTP and IDCF tests.

Paracoccidioidomycosis

The most popular serologic methods for diagnosis of paracoccidioidomycosis are ID and CF, but other tests, such as enzyme-linked immunosorbent assays, have also been employed. The principal antigens used in these tests are derived from culture filtrates of mycelial-phase or yeast phase broth cultures of *P. brasiliensis*. The major diagnostic antigen found in these preparations is a 43-kDa glycoprotein. Cell wall antigens have proved less useful than culture filtrate antigens, largely because wall antigens are dominated by cross-reactive galactomannan (63).

The ID test is a qualitative method that can be performed on a fee-for-service basis by Cerodex Laboratories, Inc., Washington, OK. Commercial mycelial-form culture filtrate antigen can be obtained for in-house use from IMMY. No commercial kits are available for this test. The CF test is performed with *P. brasiliensis* yeast form culture filtrate antigen. No commercial kits or reagents are available.

Adiaspiromycosis

No serologic tests are available for diagnosis of adiaspiromycosis.

ANTIMICROBIAL SUSCEPTIBILITIES

Established treatment options for *H. capsulatum*, *B. dermatitidis*, *Coccidioides* species, and *P. brasiliensis* include amphotericin B, the azoles voriconazole, posaconazole, itraconazole, ketoconazole, and fluconazole, and the echinocandins, although no comparative trials of these agents have been performed. In vitro antifungal susceptibility testing for dimorphic fungi remains unstandardized, and no susceptibility breakpoints have been determined for these organisms (69). Table 1 lists the in vitro susceptibilities of these organisms to established and investigational antifungal agents as reported in studies that were performed in accordance with CLSI documents M38 (for filamentous fungi) and M27 (for yeast). Fluconazole treatment failures have been reported in some cases of histoplasmosis and coccidioidomycosis, partially attributed to organisms that demonstrated drug MICs of ≥64 µg/ml (69, 77).

EVALUATION, INTERPRETATION, AND REPORTING OF RESULTS

Histoplasmosis

The definitive diagnosis of histoplasmosis can be accomplished by direct microscopic detection of *H. capsulatum*

TABLE 1   In vitro susceptibilities of dimorphic fungi to antifungal agents

Fungus	Antifungal agent	MIC range (μg/ml)	MIC$_{90}$ range (μg/ml)	Reference(s)
B. dermatitidis	Amphotericin B	≤0.03–1	0.5	23, 43, 50
	Fluconazole	1–64	NR[a]	49
	Itraconazole	≤0.03–1	0.125	23, 43, 50
	Posaconazole	≤0.03–0.06	NR	24
	Voriconazole	≤0.03–16	0.25	23, 43, 50
	Anidulafungin	2–8	NR	24
	Caspofungin	0.5–8	NR	24
Coccidioides spp.	Amphotericin B	0.125–2	0.5–1	29, 43, 50
	Fluconazole	2–64	64	29, 50
	Itraconazole	0.125–2	1	43, 50
	Posaconazole	0.25–1	1	30
	Voriconazole	≤0.03–0.5	0.25	43, 50
	Caspofungin	8–64	32	29
H. capsulatum	Amphotericin B	≤0.03–2	0.25	23, 43, 50
	Fluconazole	≤0.125–64	NR	49
	Itraconazole	≤0.03–8	0.06	23, 43, 50
	Posaconazole	≤0.03–0.06	NR	24
	Voriconazole	≤0.03–2	0.25	23, 43, 50
	Anidulafungin	2–4	NR	24
	Caspofungin	0.5–4	NR	24
P. brasiliensis	Amphotericin B	0.125–4	NR	50
	Fluconazole	≤0.125–64	NR	50
	Itraconazole	≤0.03–1	NR	50
	Voriconazole	≤0.03–2	NR	50

[a]NR, not reported.

in clinical specimens or its isolation in culture. However, isolation and identification may take 2 to 4 weeks.

Antigen detection complements other diagnostic methods for histoplasmosis and is particularly useful in immunocompromised patients with more extensive disease, often providing a rapid diagnosis before positive cultures can be identified. HPA has been detected in serum, urine, CSF, and bronchoalveolar lavage fluid specimens obtained from individuals with disseminated histoplasmosis. Antigen levels are higher in urine than in serum. For patients with AIDS and disseminated histoplasmosis, sensitivity is 95% in urine and 86% in serum (75). Specificity is about 98%. Antigen has been detected in the CSF of patients with *Histoplasma* meningitis.

Antigen levels in the urine and serum decline with effective treatment, becoming undetectable in most patients. Failure of antigen concentrations to fall during treatment suggests therapeutic failure. In patients who have responded to treatment and in whom antigen levels have previously fallen, an increase in antigen levels in the urine or serum is suggestive of relapse.

The LA test for *Histoplasma* antibodies is most useful for the diagnosis of acute infection, positive results being obtained within 2 to 3 weeks after exposure. An LA titer of 1:16 is presumptive evidence of infection, and a titer of ≥1:32 is considered strong presumptive evidence of active or recent infection (44). Because false-positive reactions can occur, the results should be confirmed by the ID test. Low-titer results from single specimens should be interpreted with caution. In such cases, the test should be performed on another specimen collected 4 to 6 weeks later.

In the ID test, precipitins to the M antigen of *H. capsulatum* are the first to appear (4 to 8 weeks after exposure) and can be detected in up to 75% of persons with acute histoplasmosis.

However, they can also be found in nearly all individuals with chronic pulmonary infection, as well as in those who have undergone a recent skin test with histoplasmin. Precipitins to the H antigen are specific for active disease but occur in fewer than 20% of cases. They usually disappear within the first 6 months of infection and are seldom, if ever, found in the absence of M precipitins. The presence of precipitins to both H and M antigens is highly suggestive of active histoplasmosis, regardless of other serologic test results.

The CF test is useful in the diagnosis of acute, chronic, disseminated, and meningeal forms of histoplasmosis. In acute infections, antibodies to the yeast antigen are the first to appear (about 4 weeks after exposure) and the last to disappear after resolution of the infection. Antibodies to histoplasmin appear later and reach lower titers than those observed for the yeast antigen. In contrast, histoplasmin titers are usually higher in persons with chronic histoplasmosis. CF test results can be difficult to interpret because cross-reactions can occur with sera from persons with blastomycosis, coccidioidomycosis, and other fungal infections. In such instances, titers usually range between 1:8 and 1:32 and occur mainly against the yeast form antigen. However, many serum samples from culture-confirmed cases of disseminated histoplasmosis yield titers in the same range. CF titers of 1:8 or greater with either antigen are considered presumptive evidence of histoplasmosis. Titers above 1:32 and rising titers in serial samples offer stronger evidence of infection.

Titers of CF antibodies to *H. capsulatum* decrease following resolution of the infection but increase in individuals with chronic progressive disease. However, clinical and microbiological findings should also be considered in assessing the patient's prognosis or making treatment decisions. In some patients, positive CF titers decline slowly and persist long after the disease has been cured. The significance of persistently elevated or fluctuating CF titers is unclear, as is the effect of antifungal treatment on antibody clearance (16).

Serologic tests are particularly useful in patients with *Histoplasma* meningitis (76). The detection of precipitins to H and M antigens in CSF specimens is sufficient to make a diagnosis in the appropriate clinical setting and often is the only positive diagnostic test.

Blastomycosis

Although microscopic examination and culture remain the most sensitive means of establishing the diagnosis of blastomycosis, serologic tests can also provide useful information. A positive reaction in an ID test using the A antigen of *B. dermatitidis* is specific and diagnostic for blastomycosis (44). However, a negative ID test does not rule out the diagnosis because the sensitivity of this method has been reported to range from ~30% for cases of localized infection to ~90% for cases of disseminated blastomycosis. In established cases of the disease, a decline in the number or the disappearance of precipitin lines is evidence of a favorable prognosis.

With urine specimens, the *Blastomyces* antigen test has been reported to have a sensitivity of 89% for disseminated infection and 100% for pulmonary disease (20). However, cross-reactive antigens occurred in urine from all patients with paracoccidioidomycosis and from 96% of patients with histoplasmosis.

Coccidioidomycosis

Although the definitive laboratory diagnosis of coccidioidomycosis depends on microscopic examination and culture, serologic tests are of proven usefulness in diagnosis and management. A positive IDTP test result is indicative of acute coccidioidomycosis. IDTP-reactive IgM antibodies can be detected in up to 75% of cases within 1 week of symptom onset, and ~90% are positive within 3 weeks. Although infrequent, a positive IDTP test result with CSF is indicative of acute meningitis. In cases where the IDTP test is negative but the CF test is positive, patients should be investigated for microbiologic or histopathologic evidence of histoplasmosis or blastomycosis. In addition, sera should be obtained at 3-week intervals and examined by CF and ID tests for coccidioidomycosis, histoplasmosis, and blastomycosis. False-positive IDTP reactions have been reported to occur in 15% of sera obtained from cystic fibrosis patients in the absence of a positive culture (18).

A positive IDCF test result is presumptive evidence of recent or chronic infection. IDCF-reactive IgG antibodies can usually be detected within 2 to 6 weeks after onset of symptoms. Although the IDCF test is generally not performed as a quantitative test, it can be used in this manner after serial dilution of patient serum to obtain an endpoint titer. Titers obtained using the quantitative IDCF are not identical to titers obtained from the CF test, but the observed trends are comparable.

The LA test is more sensitive than the IDTP test in detecting acute infection but is less specific. For this reason, a positive test result with undiluted serum should be confirmed by the ID and/or CF test.

The CF test does not become positive until about 4 to 12 weeks after infection, but CF antibodies persist for long periods in individuals with chronic pulmonary or disseminated coccidioidomycosis. Testing of serial specimens to detect rising or falling titers can reveal the progression or regression of illness and the response to antifungal treatment. A CF titer to coccidioidin at any dilution should be considered presumptive evidence of coccidioidomycosis.

In most instances, the titer is proportional to the extent of the infection, and failure of the CF titer to fall during treatment of disseminated coccidioidomycosis is an ominous sign (61). Titers of 1:2 or 1:4 are usually indicative of early, residual, or meningeal disease; however, similar titers are sometimes found in individuals without coccidioidomycosis. The parallel use of the IDCF and CF tests can help to confirm or refute the diagnosis. CF titers of >1:16 should lead to a careful assessment of the patient for possible spread of the disease beyond the respiratory tract. More than 60% of patients with disseminated coccidioidomycosis have CF titers of >1:32. However, false-negative results can occur in immunocompromised individuals, such as persons with AIDS (1). Patients with clinical presentations consistent with coccidioidomycosis but with negative or low serum CF titers should be retested at 3- to 4-week intervals.

The detection of CF antibodies in the CSF is usually diagnostic of coccidioidal meningitis and remains the single most useful test for diagnosis of that infection. However, ~5% of CSF specimens from patients with coccidioidal meningitis are negative in the CF test.

Paracoccidioidomycosis

The definitive diagnosis of paracoccidioidomycosis depends on microscopic examination and culture. However, isolation and identification of *P. brasiliensis* from clinical specimens may take up to 4 weeks.

Serologic tests are useful for the rapid presumptive diagnosis of paracoccidioidomycosis, particularly in cases of disseminated infection (11, 63). The ID test with yeast form culture filtrate antigen is highly specific and is positive in 65 to 100% of cases of acute or chronic pulmonary infection or disseminated paracoccidioidomycosis. The CF test with yeast form culture filtrate antigen is less specific than the ID test, and cross-reactions can occur with cases of histoplasmosis. However, CF titers of ≥1:8 are considered presumptive evidence of paracoccidioidomycosis. Low CF titers are usually associated with localized infection, while higher titers are found in those with multifocal disease. Falling CF titers are often predictive of successful treatment, and high or fluctuating CF titers are suggestive of a poor prognosis. Some reports, however, have indicated that ID and CF results do not correlate well with the clinical status of the patient (28, 46).

Adiaspiromycosis

The definitive diagnosis of adiaspiromycosis can be accomplished by direct microscopic detection of *Emmonsia* species in clinical specimens or their isolation in culture.

REFERENCES

1. Antoniskis, D., R. A. Larsen, B. Akil, M. U. Rarik, and J. M. Leedom. 1990. Seronegative disseminated coccidioidomycosis in patients with HIV infection. *AIDS* **4:**691–693.
2. Bialek, R., A. Ibricevic, C. Aepinus, L. K. Najvar, A. W. Fothergill, J. Knobloch, and J. R. Graybill. 2000. Detection of *Paracoccidioides brasiliensis* in tissue samples by a nested PCR assay. *J. Clin. Microbiol.* **38:**2940–2942.
3. Bialek, R., A. Feucht, C. Aepinus, G. Just-Nubling, V. J. Robertson, J. Knobloch, and R. Hohle. 2002. Evaluation of two nested PCR assays for detection of *Histoplasma capsulatum* DNA in human tissue. *J. Clin. Microbiol.* **40:**1644–1647.
4. Bialek, R., A. C. Cirera, T. Herrmann, C. Aepinus, V. I. Shearn-Bochsler, and A. M. Legendre. 2003. Nested PCR assays for detection of *Blastomyces dermatitidis* DNA in paraffin-imbedded canine tissue. *J. Clin. Microbiol.* **41:**205–208.

5. **Bialek, R., J. Kern, T. Herrmann, R. Tijerina, L. Cecenas, U. Reischl, and G. M. Gonzalez.** 2004. PCR assays for identification of *Coccidioides posadasii* based on the nucleotide sequence of the antigen 2/proline rich antigen. *J. Clin. Microbiol.* **42:**778–783.

6. **Bialek, R., G. M. Gonzalez, D. Begerow, and U. E. Zelck.** 2005. Coccidioidomycosis and blastomycosis: advances in molecular diagnosis. *FEMS Immunol. Med. Microbiol.* **45:**355–360.

7. **Binnicker, M. J., S. P. Buckwalter, J. J. Eisberner, R. A. Stewart, A. E. McCullough, S. L. Wohlfiel, and N. L. Wegenack.** 2007. Detection of *Coccidioides* species in clinical specimens by real-time PCR. *J. Clin. Microbiol.* **45:**173–178.

8. **Bracca, A., M. E. Tosello, J. E. Girardini, S. L. Amigot, C. Gomez, and E. Serra.** 2003. Molecular detection of *Histoplasma capsulatum* var. *capsulatum* in human clinical samples. *J. Clin. Microbiol.* **41:**1753–1755.

9. **Brandt, M. E., D. Gaunt, N. Iqbal, S. McClinton, S. Hambleton, and L. Sigler.** 2005. False-positive *Histoplasma capsulatum* Gen-Probe chemiluminescent test result caused by a *Chrysosporium* species. *J. Clin. Microbiol.* **43:**1456–1458.

10. **Buitrago, M. J., P. Merino, S. Puente, A. Gomez-Lopez, A. Arribi, R. M. Zancope-Oliveira, M. C. Gutierrez, J. L. Rodriguez-Tudela, and M. Cuenca-Estrella.** 2009. Utility of real-time PCR for the detection of *Paracoccidioides brasiliensis* DNA in the diagnosis of imported paracoccidioidomycosis. *Med. Mycol.* **31:**1–4.

11. **Cano, L. E., and A. Restrepo.** 1987. Predictive value of serologic tests in the diagnosis and follow-up of patients with paracoccidioidomycosis. *Rev. Inst. Med. Trop. Sao Paulo* **29:**276–283.

12. **Chapman, S. W.** 2005. *Blastomyces dermatitidis,* p. 3026–3040. *In* G. L. Mandell, J. E. Bennett, and R. Dolin (ed.), *Principles and Practice of Infectious Diseases,* 6th ed. Elsevier, Philadelphia, PA.

13. **Cloud, J. L., S. K. Bauman, B. P. Neary, K. G. Ludwig, and E. R. Ashwood.** 2007. Performance characteristics of a polyclonal enzyme immunoassay for the quantitation of *Histoplasma* antigen in human urine samples. *Am. J. Clin. Pathol.* **128:**18–22.

14. **Connolly, P. A., M. M. Durkin, A. M. LeMonte, E. J. Hackett, and L. J. Wheat.** 2007. Detection of *Histoplasma* antigen by quantitative enzyme immunoassay. *Clin. Vaccine Immunol.* **14:**1587–1591.

15. **Cuellar Rodriguez, J., R. K. Avery, M. Budey, S. M. Gordon, N. K. Shrestha, D. van Duin, M. Oethinger, and S. D. Mawhorter.** 2009. Histoplasmosis in solid organ transplant recipients: 10 years of experience at a large transplant center in an endemic area. *Clin. Infect. Dis.* **49:**710–716.

16. **Deepe, G. S., Jr.** 2005. *Histoplasma capsulatum,* p. 3012–3026. *In* G. L. Mandell, J. E. Bennett, and R. Dolin (ed.), *Principles and Practice of Infectious Diseases,* 6th ed. Elsevier, Philadelphia, PA.

17. **de Medeiros Muniz, M., C. V. Pizzini, J. M. Peralta, E. Reiss, and R. Zancopé-Oliveira.** 2001. Genetic diversity of *Histoplasma capsulatum* strains isolated from soil, animals, and clinical specimens in Rio de Janeiro State, Brazil, by a PCR-based random amplified polymorphic DNA assay. *J. Clin. Microbiol.* **39:**4487–4494.

18. **Dosanjh, A., J. Theodore, and D. Pappagianis.** 1998. Probable false positive coccidioidal serologic results in patients with cystic fibrosis. *Pediatr. Transplant.* **2:**313–317.

19. **Dot, J. M., A. Debourgogne, J. Champigneulle, Y. Salles, M. Brizion, J. M. Puyhardy, J. Collomb, F. Plénat, and M. Machouart.** 2009. Molecular diagnosis of disseminated adiaspiromycosis due to *Emmonsia crescens.* *J. Clin. Microbiol.* **47:**1269–1273.

20. **Durkin, M., J. Witt, A. LeMonte, B. Wheat, and P. Connolly.** 2004. Antigen assay with the potential to aid in diagnosis of blastomycosis. *J. Clin. Microbiol.* **42:**4873–4875.

21. **Durkin, M., P. Connolly, T. Kuberski, R. Myers, B. M. Kubak, D. Bruckner, D. Pegues, and L. J. Wheat.** 2008. Diagnosis of coccidioidomycosis with use of the *Coccidioides* Antigen Enzyme Immunoassay. *Clin. Infect. Dis.* **47:**69–73.

22. **Eckmann, B. H., G. L. Schaefer, and M. Huppert.** 1964. Bedside interhuman transmission of coccidioidomycosis via growth on fomites. *Am. Rev. Respir. Dis.* **89:**179–185.

23. **Espinel-Ingroff, A.** 1998. In vitro activity of the new triazole voriconazole (UK-109,496) against opportunistic filamentous and dimorphic fungi and common and emerging yeast pathogens. *J. Clin. Microbiol.* **36:**198–202.

24. **Espinel-Ingroff, A.** 1998. Comparison of in vitro activities of the new triazole SCH56592 and the echinocandins MK-0991 (L-743,872) and LY303366 against opportunistic filamentous and dimorphic fungi and yeasts. *J. Clin. Microbiol.* **36:**2950–2956.

25. **Fisher, M. C., G. L. Koenig, T. J. White, and J. W. Taylor.** 2002. Molecular and phenotypic description of *Coccidioides posadasii* sp. nov., previously recognized as the non-California population of *Coccidioides immitis.* *Mycologia* **94:**73–84.

26. **Galgiani, J.** 2005. *Coccidioides* species, p. 3040–3051. *In* G. L. Mandell, J. E. Bennett, and R. Dolin (ed.), *Principles and Practice of Infectious Disease,* 6th ed. Elsevier, Philadelphia, PA.

27. **Gomez, B. L., J. I. Figueroa, A. J. Hamilton, B. Ortiz, M. A. Robledo, R. J. Hay, and A. Restrepo.** 1997. Use of monoclonal antibodies in diagnosis of paracoccidioidomycosis: new strategies for detection of circulating antigens. *J. Clin. Microbiol.* **35:**3278–3283.

28. **Gomez, B. L., J. I. Figueroa, A. J. Hamilton, S. Diez, M. Rojas, A. M. Tobon, R. J. Hay, and A. Restrepo.** 1998. Antigenemia in patients with paracoccidioidomycosis: detection of the 87-kilodalton determinant during and after antifungal therapy. *J. Clin. Microbiol.* **36:**3309–3316.

29. **Gonzalez, G. M., R. Tijerina, L. K. Najvar, R. Bocanegra, M. Luther, M. G. Rinaldi, and J. R. Graybill.** 2001. Correlation between antifungal susceptibilities of *Coccidioides immitis* in vitro and antifungal treatment with caspofungin in a mouse model. *Antimicrob. Agents Chemother.* **45:**1854–1859.

30. **Gonzalez, G. M., R. Tijerina, L. K. Najvar, R. Bocanegra, M. Rinaldi, D. Loebenberg, and J. R. Graybill.** 2002. In vitro and in vivo activities of posaconazole against *Coccidioides immitis.* *Antimicrob. Agents Chemother.* **46:**1352–1356.

31. **Gori, S., E. Drouhet, E. Gueho, M. Huerre, A. Lofaro, M. Parenti, and B. Dupont.** 1998. Cutaneous disseminated mycosis in a patient with AIDS due to a new dimorphic fungus. *J. Mycol. Med.* **8:**57–63.

32. **Hall, G. S., K. Pratt-Rippin, and J. A. Washington.** 1992. Evaluation of a chemiluminescent probe assay for identification of *Histoplasma capsulatum* isolates. *J. Clin. Microbiol.* **30:**3003–3004.

33. **Herr, R. A., E. J. Tarcha, P. R. Taborda, J. W. Taylor, L. Ajello, and L. Mendoza.** 2001. Phylogenetic analysis of *Lacazia loboi* places this previously uncharacterized pathogen within the dimorphic onygenales. *J. Clin. Microbiol.* **39:**309–314.

34. **Imhof, A., C. Schaer, G. Schoedon, D. J. Schaer, R. B. Walter, A. Schaffner, and M. Schneemann.** 2003. Rapid detection of pathogenic fungi from clinical specimens using LightCycler real-time fluorescence PCR. *Eur. J. Clin. Microbiol. Infect. Dis.* **22:**558–560.

35. **Jewell, K., R. Cheshier, and G. D. Cage.** 2008. Genetic diversity among clinical *Coccidioides* spp. isolates in Arizona. *Med. Mycol.* **46:**449–455.

36. **Karimi, K., L. J. Wheat, P. Connolly, G. Cloud, R. Hajjeh, E. Wheat, K. Alves, C. da Silva Lacaz, and E. Keath.** 2002. Differences in histoplasmosis in patients with acquired immunodeficiency syndrome in the United States and Brazil. *J. Infect. Dis.* **186:**1655–1660.

37. **Kasuga, T., T. J. White, G. Koenig, J. McEwen, A. Restrepo, E. Castaneda, C. DaSilva Lacaz, E. M. Heins-Vaccari, R. S. De Freitas, R. M. Zancope-Oliveira, Z. Qin, R. Negroni, D. A. Carter, Y. Mikami, M. Tamura, M. L. Taylor, G. F. Miller, N. Poonwan, and J. W. Taylor.** 2003. Phylogeography of the fungal pathogen *Histoplasma capsulatum.* *Mol. Ecol.* **12:**3383–3401.

38. **Kauffman, C. A.** 2009. Histoplasmosis. *Clin. Chest Med.* **30:**217–225.

39. **Kaufman, L., A. S. Sekhon, N. Moledina, M. Jalbert, and D. Pappagianis.** 1995. Comparative evaluation of commercial Premier EIA and microimmunodiffusion and complement fixation tests for *Coccidioides immitis* antibodies. *J. Clin. Microbiol.* **33:**618–619.

40. **Koufopanou, V., A. Burt, and J. W. Taylor.** 1997. Concordance of gene genealogies reveals reproductive isolation in the pathogenic fungus *Coccidioides immitis*. *Proc. Natl. Acad. Sci. USA* **94:**5478–5482.

41. **Koufopanou, V., A. Burt, T. Szaro, and J. W. Taylor.** 2001. Gene genealogies, cryptic species, and molecular evolution in the human pathogen *Coccidioides immitis* and relatives (Ascomycota, Onygenales). *Mol. Biol. Evol.* **18:**1246–1258.

42. **Lenhart, S. W., M. P. Schafer, M. Singal, and R. A. Hajjeh.** 2004. *Histoplasmosis: Protecting Workers at Risk.* DHHS (NIOSH) publication no. 2005–109. www.cdc.gov/niosh/docs/2005-109.

43. **Li, R. K., M. A. Ciblak, N. Nordoff, L. Pasarell, D. W. Warnock, and M. R. McGinnis.** 2000. In vitro activities of voriconazole, itraconazole, and amphotericin B against *Blastomyces dermatitidis, Coccidioides immitis,* and *Histoplasma capsulatum. Antimicrob. Agents Chemother.* **44:**1734–1736.

44. **Lindsley, M. D., D. W. Warnock, and C. J. Morrison.** 2006. Serological and molecular diagnosis of fungal infection, p. 569–605. *In* N. R. Rose, R. G. Hamilton, and B. Detrick (ed.), *Manual of Molecular and Clinical Laboratory Immunology,* 7th ed. ASM Press, Washington, DC.

45. **Marques da Silva, S. H., A. L. Colombo, M. H. Blotta, J. D. Lopes, F. Queiroz-Telles, and Z. Pires de Camargo.** 2003. Detection of circulating gp43 antigen in serum, cerebrospinal fluid, and bronchoalveolar lavage fluid of patients with paracoccidioidomycosis. *J. Clin. Microbiol.* **41:**3675–3680.

46. **Marques da Silva, S. H., F. Queiroz-Telles, A. L. Colombo, M. H. Blotta, J. D. Lopes, and Z. P. Camargo.** 2004. Monitoring of gp43 antigenemia in paracoccidioidomycosis patients during therapy. *J. Clin. Microbiol.* **42:**2419–2424.

47. **Martins, T. B., T. D. Jaskowski, C. L. Mouritsen, and H. R. Hill.** 1995. Comparison of commercially available enzyme immunoassay with traditional serological tests for detection of antibodies to *Coccidioides immitis. J. Clin. Microbiol.* **33:**940–943.

48. **Matute, D. R., J. G. McEwen, R. Puccia, B. A. Montes, G. San-Blas, E. Bagagli, J. T. Rauscher, A. Restrepo, F. Morais, G. Niño-Vega, and J. W. Taylor.** 2006. Cryptic speciation and recombination in the fungus *Paracoccidioides brasiliensis* as revealed by gene genealogies. *Mol. Biol. Evol.* **23:**65–73.

49. **McCullough, M. J., A. F. DiSalvo, K. V. Clemons, P. Park, and D. A. Stevens.** 2000. Molecular epidemiology of *Blastomyces dermatitidis. Clin. Infect. Dis.* **30:**328–335.

50. **McGinnis, M. R., L. Pasarell, D. A. Sutton, A. W. Fothergill, C. R. Cooper, and M. G. Rinaldi.** 1997. In vitro evaluation of voriconazole against some clinically important fungi. *Antimicrob. Agents Chemother.* **41:**1832–1834.

51. **McKinsey, D. S., J. P. McKinsey, N. Northcutt, and J. C. Sarria.** 2009. Interlaboratory discrepancy of antigenuria results in 2 patients with AIDS and histoplasmosis. *Diagn. Microbiol. Infect. Dis.* **63:**111–114.

52. **Meece, J. K., J. L. Anderson, B. S. Klein, T. D. Sullivan, S. L. Foley, D. J. Baumgardner, C. F. Brummitt, and K. D. Reed.** 2009. Genetic diversity in *Blastomyces dermatitidis:* implications for PCR detection in clinical and environmental samples. *Med. Mycol.* **22:**1–7.

53. **Mendes-Giannini, M. J., J. P. Bueno, M. A. Shikanai-Yasuda, A. W. Ferreira, and A. Masuda.** 1989. Detection of the 43,000-molecular-weight glycoprotein in sera of patients with paracoccidioidomycosis. *J. Clin. Microbiol.* **27:**2842–2845.

54. **Martagon-Villamil, J., N. Shrestha, M. Sholtis, C. M. Isada, G. S. Hall, T. Byrne, B. A. Lodge, L. B. Reller, and G. W. Procop.** 2003. Identification of *Histoplasma capsulatum* from culture extracts by real-time PCR. *J. Clin. Microbiol.* **41:**1295–1298.

55. **Maubon, D., S. Simon, and C. Aznar.** 2007. Histoplasmosis diagnosis using a polymerase chain reaction method.

Application on human samples in French Guiana, South America. *Diagn. Microbiol. Infect. Dis.* **58:**441–444.

56. **Millar, B. C., X. Jiru, M. J. Walker, J. P. Evans, and J. E. Moore.** 2003. False identification of *Coccidioides immitis*: do molecular methods always get it right? *J. Clin. Microbiol.* **41:**5778–5780.

57. **Nascimento, E, R. Martinez, A. R. Lopes, L. A. de Souza Bernardes, C. P. Barco, M. H. S. Goldman, J. W. Taylor, J. G. McEwen, M. P. Nobrega, F. G. Nobrega, and G. H. Goldman.** 2004. Detection and selection of microsatellites in the genome of *Paracocccidioides brasiliensis* as molecular markers for clinical and epidemiological studies. *J. Clin. Microbiol.* **42:**5007–5014.

58. **Padhye, A. A., G. Smith, D. McLaughlin, P. G. Standard, and L. Kaufman.** 1992. Comparative evaluation of a chemiluminescent DNA probe and an exoantigen test for rapid identification of *Histoplasma capsulatum. J. Clin. Microbiol.* **30:**3108–3111.

59. **Padhye, A. A., G. Smith, P. G. Standard, D. McLaughlin, and L. Kaufman.** 1994. Comparative evaluation of chemiluminescent DNA probe assays and exoantigen tests for rapid identification of *Blastomyces dermatitidis* and *Coccidioides immitis. J. Clin. Microbiol.* **32:**867–870.

60. **Pappagianis, D., I. Krasnow, and S. Beall.** 1976. False-positive reactions of cerebrospinal fluid and diluted sera with the coccidioidal latex agglutination test. *Am. J. Clin. Pathol.* **66:**916–921.

61. **Pappagianis, D.** 1996. Serology of coccidioidomycosis, p. 33–35. *In* H. E. Einstein and A. Catanzaro (ed.), *Coccidioidomycosis: Proceedings of the 5th International Conference.* National Foundation for Infectious Diseases, Washington, DC.

62. **Peterson, S. W., and L. Sigler.** 1998. Molecular genetic variation in *Emmonsia crescens* and *Emmonsia parva,* etiologic agents of adiaspiromycosis, and their phylogenetic relationship to *Blastomyces dermatitidis* (*Ajellomyces dermatitidis*) and other systemic fungal pathogens. *J. Clin. Microbiol.* **36:**2918–2925.

63. **Restrepo, A., and A. M. Tobón.** 2005. *Paracoccidioides brasiliensis,* p. 3062–3068. *In* G. L. Mandell, J. E. Bennett, and R. Dollin (ed.), *Principles and Practice of Infectious Diseases,* 6th ed. Elsevier, Philadelphia, PA.

64. **Salina, M. A., M. A. Shikanai-Yasuda, R. P. Mendes, B. Barraviera, and M. J. Mendes Giannini.** 1998. Detection of circulating *Paracoccidioides brasiliensis* antigen in urine of paracoccidioidomycosis patients before and during treatment. *J. Clin. Microbiol.* **36:**1723–1728.

65. **Sheff, K. W., E. R. York, E. M. Driebe, B. M. Barker, S. D. Rounsley, V. G. Waddell, S. M. Beckstrom-Sternberg, J. S. Beckstrom-Sternberg, P. S. Keim, and D. M. Engelthaler.** 2010. Development of a rapid, cost-effective TaqMan real-time PCR assay for identification and differentiation of *Coccidioides immitis* and *Coccidioides posadasii. Med. Mycol.* **48:**466–469.

66. **Sigler, L.** 2005. Adiaspiromycosis and other infections caused by *Emmonsia* species, p. 809–824. *In* R. Hay and W. Merz (ed.), *Medical Mycology, Topley & Wilson's Microbiology and Microbial Infections,* 10th ed. Hodder Arnold, London, United Kingdom.

67. **Stevens, D. A., K. V. Clemons, H. B. Levine, D. Pappagianis, E. J. Baron, J. R. Hamilton, S. C. Deresinski, and N. Johnson.** 2009. Expert opinion: what to do when there is *Coccidioides* exposure in a laboratory. *Clin. Infect. Dis.* **49:**919–923.

68. **Stockman, L., K. A. Clark, J. M. Hunt, and G. D. Roberts.** 1993. Evaluation of commercially available acridinium ester-labeled chemiluminescent DNA probes for culture identification of *Blastomyces dermatitidis, Coccidioides immitis, Cryptococcus neoformans,* and *Histoplasma capsulatum. J. Clin. Microbiol.* **31:**845–850.

69. **Sutton, D. A.** 2007. Diagnosis of coccidioidomycosis by culture: safety considerations, traditional methods, and susceptibility testing. *Ann. N. Y. Acad. Sci.* **1111:**315–325.

70. **Taylor, J. W., D. M. Geiser, A. Burt, and V. Koufopanou.** 1999. The evolutionary biology and population genetics underlying fungal strain typing. *Clin. Microbiol. Rev.* **12:**126–146.

71. **Teixeira, M. M., R. C. Theodoro, M. J. A. deCarvalho, L. Fernandes, H. C. Paes, R. C. Hahn, L. Mendoza, E. Bagagli, G. San-Blas, and M. S. S. Felipe.** 2009. Phylogenetic analysis reveals a high level of speciation in the *Paracoccidioides* genus. *Mol. Phylogenet. Evol.* **52:**273–283.

72. **Untereiner, W. A., J. A. Scott, F. A. Naveau, L. Sigler, J. Bachewich, and A. Angus.** 2004. The Ajellomycetaceae, a new family of vertebrate-associated Onygenales. *Mycologia* **96:**812–821.

73. **Verghese, S., D. Arjundas, K. C. Krishnakumar, P. Padmaja, D. Elizabeth, A. A. Padhye, and D. W. Warnock.** 2002. Coccidioidomycosis in India: report of a second imported case. *Med. Mycol.* **40:**307–309.

74. **Warnock, D. W.** 2000. Mycotic agents of human disease, p. 111–120. *In* D. O. Fleming and D. L. Hunt (ed.), *Biological Safety: Principles and Practices,* 3rd ed. ASM Press, Washington, DC.

75. **Wheat, L. J.** 2006. Improvements in diagnosis of histoplasmosis. *Expert Opin. Biol. Ther.* **6:**1207–1221.

76. **Wheat, J., M. French, B. Batteiger, and R. Kohler.** 1985. Cerebrospinal fluid *Histoplasma* antibodies in central nervous system histoplasmosis. *Arch. Intern. Med.* **145:**1237–1240.

77. **Wheat, L. J., P. Connolly, M. Smedema, E. Brizendine, and R. Hafner.** 2001. Emergence of resistance to fluconazole as a cause of failure during treatment of histoplasmosis in patients with acquired immunodeficiency syndrome. *Clin. Infect. Dis.* **33:**1910–1913.

78. **Wilson, D. E., and C. L. Chosewood.** 2007. *Biosafety in Microbiological and Biomedical Laboratories,* 5th ed. U.S. Government Printing Office, Washington, DC.

79. **Wright, P. W., D. Pappagianis, M. Wilson, A. Louro, S. A. Moser, K. Komatsu, and P. G. Pappas.** 2003. Donor-related coccidioidomycosis in organ transplant recipients. *Clin. Infect. Dis.* **37:**1265–1269.

80. **Zimmerman, C. R., C. J. Snedker, and D. Pappagianis.** 1994. Characterization of *Coccidioides immitis* isolates by restriction fragment length polymorphisms. *J. Clin. Microbiol.* **32:**3040–3042.

Trichophyton, Microsporum, Epidermophyton, and Agents of Superficial Mycoses*

RICHARD C. SUMMERBELL

121

TAXONOMY

The etiologic agents of dermatophytosis are classified, along with some nonpathogenic relatives, in the anamorphic genera *Trichophyton, Microsporum,* and *Epidermophyton.* Those capable of reproducing sexually, i.e., producing ascomata with asci and ascospores, are classified in the teleomorphic genus *Arthroderma* (123), family Arthrodermataceae, order Onygenales (27), and phylum Ascomycota. The recorded connections between the teleomorphic (sexual) and anamorphic (asexual) states of the dermatophytes as well as the dermatophytoids (i.e., the soil-borne *Trichophyton* and *Microsporum* species that are best not called "dermatophytes" [Greek for "skin plants"] because they are not pathogenic [4, 112]) are given in Table 1.

Phylogenetic studies have tended to support the ongoing classification of dermatophytes in the three traditional anamorph genera mentioned above. Some normally nonpathogenic, geophilic dermatophytoids currently placed in *Trichophyton,* e.g., *T. ajelloi* and *T. terrestre,* appear to belong to a distinct clade in most phylogenies based on the ribosomal internal transcribed spacer (ITS) region sequences, but the degree of bootstrap support for this clade does not support its distinction as a separate genus (19, 41, 45).

As part of the ongoing molecular revolution in biology, fungal taxonomy is ever more strongly influenced by our greatly increased understanding of population genetics (21). Dermatophytes show two population genetics patterns differing among species having "population hosts" (53) in different zoological families, orders, or classes (109, 110). (A population host, which is the normal epidemiologic reservoir of the species, is distinguished from "occasional host" species that may acquire infection but do not support ongoing populations; for example, *Microsporum canis* has mostly feline population hosts, and while humans are frequently infected by feline carriers, the species is seldom directly transmitted from human to human, making our species only an occasional host.) Some dermatophyte species, including pathogens with population hosts in the rodent, rabbit, pig, dog, and cat families, are potentially sexual, with sexual reproduction occurring only off the host, i.e., on hair or other keratinous debris in contact with soil. Other species, particularly those with human, ungulate, equine, or avian population hosts, have no access to a soil-based location suitable for sexual reproduction and host reinfection; these species are found on investigation to be asexual and clonal. They consist, in all known cases, of genetically highly uniform isolates (44, 80, 90) sharing, where known, a single mating type factor (109, 115). Most appear to have evolved from a single strain of a sexual ancestral species that was able to make the rare, successful switch to ongoing contagious infection of a new animal host. A few epidemiological and phenotypic characters in the clonal species appear to have undergone accelerated evolution due to strong selection for increased compatibility with the new host. This process has tended to produce differences allowing relatively easy laboratory identification of these species. At the same time, the basic cellular "housekeeping" genes investigated in phylogenetic taxonomic studies have evolved at a normal rate and thus strongly tend to resemble forms seen in ancestral species complexes or in sibling species. This has led to considerable recent confusion about species concepts. Long-recognized dermatophyte species, such as *Trichophyton equinum* and *Microsporum gallinae,* that have distinct epidemiologies and that are easily identified in the routine diagnostic laboratory have nonetheless been suggested not to be distinct species as traditionally conceived (41, 43), since their ITS and some other sequences are strongly similar to those of related species (e.g., *Trichophyton tonsurans* and *Arthroderma grubyi,* respectively, for the examples mentioned). The ITS sequences of the dermatophytes proposed for synonymy, however, generally show a small number of consistent sequence polymorphisms compared with sequences of the species with which synonymy has been proposed. This suggests that further genetic study will tend to support the lineages in question as recently diverged but nonetheless separate at the species level. *Trichophyton equinum,* for example, was reinstated as a recognized distinct species after more detailed genetic study (45, 113). The present chapter retains a relatively cautious approach to the ongoing debates in this area (128), synonymizing traditionally recognized species primarily when there is unequivocal, multigene molecular evidence that they are not supported at the species level. The list of recognized species is in Table 1.

---

*This chapter contains information presented in chapter 124 by Richard C. Summerbell, Irene Weitzman, and Arvind A. Padhye in the ninth edition of this *Manual.*

TABLE 1 Important characteristics of clinically isolated dermatophytes and dermatophytoids

Dermatophyte species and abundance (teleomorph name[s] if formation of sexual state is known)	Growth	Macromorphology	Micromorphology	BCPMSG medium pH results (for 7–10 days)	Urea test (7 days, broth)	Hair perforation	Other comments
Epidermophyton floccosum[a]	Moderately rapid	Flat, slightly granular at first, soon developing white puffs of degeneration; sandy to olive-brown (Fig. 18e); reverse pale to yellowish	Macroconidia abundant, club-shaped with broadly rounded apex, usually with fewer than 6 cells (Fig. 12); no microconidia formed; many chlamydospores in primary isolates	Alkaline	Pos	Neg	Invades skin and nails, rarely hair; no microconidia
Microsporum audouinii[b]	Moderately rapid	Flat to velvety, thin, pale salmon to pale brownish reverse	Rare, deformed macroconidia, often with beak, constricted midregion, and at least trace granulation (Fig. 13); drop-shaped microconidia and aerial arthroconidia may be present; pectinate branching, apiculate terminal chlamydospores often seen	No pH change or alkaline	Neg	Neg	Poor growth and no or brownish pigment on polished rice medium; usually connected with patient or index patient in or recently from Africa; only children typically infected
M. canis[a] (*Arthroderma otae*)	Rapid	Flat to velvety (Fig. 18g), thin, pale to yellow, with yellow (rarely pale) reverse	Macroconidia thick walled, roughened and beaked (Fig. 14); microconidia drop shaped	No pH change; macroconidia often abundant	Pos	Pos	Good growth and yellow pigment on polished rice medium; human infection usually from cat or dog; *M. canis* "distortum" phenotype has macroconidia distorted, bizarrely shaped; "*M. equinum*" phenotype from horses has few, short macroconidia
M. cookei[b] (*A. cajetani*)	Moderately rapid	Granular to velvety; reverse wine red	Macroconidia rough, thick walled with cellular compartments rather than true cross walls (Fig. 15); microconidia drop shaped	No pH change	Pos	Pos	Probably nonpathogenic; existing case reports poorly substantiated
M. ferrugineum[c]	Slow	Flat or folded, waxy to slightly velvety; surface and reverse yellow, rusty, or pale	No conidia, coarse, straight "bamboo" hyphae with prominent septa may be present	No pH change	Neg	Neg	Yellow colony on Lowenstein-Jensen medium (compare *T. soudanense*); geographically restricted to parts of Africa, Asia, and eastern Europe
M. gallinae[c]	Moderately rapid	Flat to velvety; surface white tinged with pink; reverse red; red pigment diffuses into agar	Macroconidia smooth to slightly rough, often bent and with thickest cells near the apex, sometimes slightly rough; microconidia drop shaped	No data	Neg	Neg	Rare; human infection usually from chicken; species may be an asexual phenotype within *A. grubyi* according to Gräser et al. (41)

Species	Growth rate	Colony morphology	Conidia	pH			Comments
M. gypseum complex[a] (A. gypseum, A. incurvatum, A. fulvum)	Rapid	Granular, sandy in color, or occasionally light cinnamon or rosy buff; reverse usually pale to brownish	Macroconidia abundant, thin walled, fusoid (tapered at both ends), roughened, with up to 6 septa (Fig. 16); microconidia drop shaped, mostly formed along sparsely branched hyphae (a feature only noted if M. racemosum is queried)	No pH change	Pos	Pos	Human infection usually from soil contact
M. nanum[b] (A. obtusum)	Moderately rapid	Powdery, sandy in color; reverse often reddish brown	Macroconidia rough, usually only 1–3 cells long, egg shaped to ellipsoidal	No data	Pos	Pos	Human infection usually from pig; now rare
M. persicolor[b] (A. persicolor)	Rapid	Powdery, sandy in color; reverse pale to yellowish, sometimes with rosy tones	Macroconidia fusoid (tapered on both ends), often absent or smooth walled on Sabouraud agar but usually common and rough walled on Sabouraud with added salt (3% or 5% NaCl) (Fig. 17); microconidia formed on pedicels (must be checked within 5 days)	No pH change	Pos	Pos	Usually poor growth at 37°C in vitro; rose to wine red reverse on sugar-free media, e.g., glucose-free Sabouraud agar; human infection usually from soil (fomites from voles)
M. praecox[b]	Rapid	Powdery, sandy in color, reverse yellow	As M. gypseum	No pH change	Pos	Neg	Uncommon
M. racemosum[c] (A. racemosum)	Rapid	Powdery, sandy in color, reverse red	Macroconidia as M. gypseum; microconidia mostly formed in densely branched formations structured like grape clusters (racemes)	No pH change	Pos	Pos	Rare
M. vanbreuseghemii[c] (A. grubyi)	Rapid	Powdery, pinkish or buff; pale to yellow reverse	Macroconidia rough, thick walled, cylindrical, often more than 8 cells long, with cellular compartments rather than true cross walls	No data	Pos	Pos	Rare; anamorph may be conspecific with phenotypically and epidemiologically different M. gallinae according to Gräser et al. (41)
Trichophyton ajelloi[b] (A. uncinatum)	Moderately rapid	Powdery, rich tan to medium orange-brown in color; reverse pale, brownish or with purple-black pigment	Macroconidia smooth, thick walled, cylindrical, often more than 7 cells long, with cellular compartments rather than true cross walls (Fig. 5)	No data	Pos	Pos	Nonpathogenic in humans
T. concentricum[c]	Slow	Folded, honey brown to reddish brown, glabrous or slightly velvety colony	No conidia	No data	Pos or neg	Neg	Only from indigenous Asian Austronesian/Melanesian or indigenous Central and South American people with distinct tinea imbricata infection
T. equinum[b]	Moderately rapid	Flat to velvety colony with cream-colored surface and yellow to red-brown reverse	Macroconidia uncommon, cylindrical to club shaped, smooth; microconidia abundant, on small pedicels (examine before 5 days)	Alkaline	Pos	Usually neg, sometimes pos	Human infection usually from horse; has a nicotinic acid requirement except in autotrophic variant from Australia and New Zealand

(Continued on next page)

TABLE 1 Important characteristics of clinically isolated dermatophytes and dermatophytoids (*Continued*)

Dermatophyte species and abundance (teleomorph name[s] if formation of sexual state is known)	Growth	Macromorphology	Micromorphology	BCPMSG medium pH results (for 7–10 days)	Urea test (7 days, broth)	Hair perforation	Other comments
T. erinacei hedgehog form[b] (*A. benhamiae*)	Rapid	Granular to powdery, yellow-cream to buff surface, yellow reverse	Macroconidia uncommon, club shaped, smooth; microconidia nearly spherical, abundant, mostly produced in dense tufts; spiral appendages present	Alkaline	Neg (European/ New Zealand form); pos (African form)	Pos	Human infection usually from hedgehog or its fomites; therefore, mostly restricted to regions with wild hedgehogs or to pet hedgehog owners
T. megninii[b]	Moderately rapid	Cottony, with white down sometimes suffused with rosy pigment; reverse red to red-brown	Macroconidia seldom seen, pencil shaped; microconidia drop shaped	Alkaline	Pos or weak pos	Neg	Endemic in Portugal and nearby areas; requires histidine; considered a subtype of *T. rubrum* by Gräser et al. (41).
T. mentagrophytes complex (zoophilic)[a] inclusive of *T. mentagrophytes* sensu stricto (= the former *T. mentagrophytes* var. *quinckeanum*) plus animal-adapted forms of *T. interdigitale* and the *Trichophyton* anamorph of *A. benhamiae* (*A. vanbreuseghemii*, *A. benhamiae*)	Rapid	Granular to powdery, yellow-cream to buff surface (Fig. 18b), pale to red-brown reverse	Macroconidia uncommon, club shaped, smooth; microconidia nearly spherical, abundant, mostly produced in dense tufts; spiral appendages present	Alkaline (rarely weak)	Pos	Pos	Human infection usually from rodent or rabbit. Macroconidia induced on SGA + 3% or 5% sodium chloride (Fig. 6).
T. mentagrophytes complex (anthropophilic)[a] inclusive of human-adapted forms of *T. interdigitale* and possibly of the *Trichophyton* anamorph of *A. benhamiae* (*A. vanbreuseghemii*, *A. benhamiae*)	Rapid	Powdery to cottony, yellow-cream to buff or white surface, pale to red-brown reverse	Macroconidia uncommon, club shaped, smooth; microconidia nearly spherical or drop shaped, produced mainly in dense tufts when round and on sparsely branched hyphae when drop shaped; spiral appendages present but rare in very cottony isolates	Alkaline	Pos	Pos	Macroconidia often induced on SGA + 3% or 5% sodium chloride

Species	Growth rate	Colony morphology	Microscopic morphology				Comments
T. mentagrophytes ("nodular" variant[b] formerly called T. krajdenii, now known to be a distinct morph of T. interdigitale)	Moderately slow	Cottony, cream to white surface often with yellow marginal zone (Fig. 18a); intense yellow reverse	Macroconidia rare, microconidia usually drop shaped, sometimes also round; coiled, yellow "nodular bodies" and yellow pigment granules present in submerged mycelium; spiral appendages seldom seen	Alkaline	Pos	Pos	Although usually very different in morphology, this variant so far is not genetically distinguishable from other anthropophilic isolates of T. interdigitale
T. rubrum[a] (cosmopolitan variant)	Moderately slow	Cottony to velvety, white to reddish surface (Fig. 18c), typically wine red reverse (Fig. 18d) but yellow variants occasional; red color poorly formed in presence of common bacterial contamination	Macroconidia seldom seen, pencil shaped (Fig. 8); microconidia drop shaped, abundant, scanty or not formed; lateral hyphal projections often present	No pH change (alkalinity after 14 days)	Neg (rarely weak)	Neg	Melanoid variants secreting brown pigment rarely seen
T. rubrum (Afro-Asiatic variant[b] formerly called T. raubitschekii, T. fluviomuniense, or, when microconidia absent, T. kanei)	Moderately slow	Powdery to low velvety, cream to deep red; reverse wine red	Macroconidia abundant (Fig. 7), club shaped, sometimes with "rat-tail" extension; microconidia drop shaped to round; many chlamydospores in primary isolates	No pH change (alkality after 14 days)	Pos	Neg	Although usually very different in morphology, this variant so far is genetically distinguished from typical T. rubrum only at microsatellite markers; it is often from upper body infection (tinea corporis, tinea cruris)
T. schoenleinii[c]	Slow	Convoluted, slightly velvety whitish colony	No conidia seen; "favic chandeliers" or "nailhead hyphae" present	Alkaline	variable	Neg	Very rare; associated with clinically recognizable "favus" lesions; now extirpated except in rural central Asia, rural Africa
T. simii[b] (A. simii)	Rapid	Granular to powdery, yellow-cream to buff surface, pale to red-brown reverse	Macroconidia abundant, often with some cells swollen as chlamydospores; microconidia drop shaped	Alkaline	Pos	Pos	Endemic to India and Africa; similar to zoophilic T. mentagrophytes, but macroconidial number and shape are atypical; reference distinction is by mating or molecular study

(Continued on next page)

TABLE 1 Important characteristics of clinically isolated dermatophytes and dermatophytoids (*Continued*)

Dermatophyte species and abundance (teleomorph name[s] if formation of sexual state is known)	Growth	Macromorphology	Micromorphology	BCPMSG medium pH results (for 7–10 days)	Urea test (7 days, broth)	Hair perforation	Other comments
T. soudanense[b]	Moderately slow	Flat, bright yellow to (less commonly) wine-red colony with radial striations and star-like margin; uncommonly cottony; reverse yellow to wine red	Macroconidia not seen, microconidia drop shaped, scarce or absent; reflexive hyphal branches in radial striations	Alkaline, with small zone of clearing	Usually neg, occasionally pos	Neg	Endemic to sub-Saharan Africa but widely disseminated in cosmopolitan parts of Europe and Americas; dark colony on Lowenstein-Jensen medium (compare *M. ferrugineum*); may or may not grow on growth factor test media; considered a subtype of *T. rubrum* by Gräser and colleagues (42, 85)
T. terrestre complex[b] (*A. lenticulare*, *A. quadrifidum*, *A. insingulare*)	Moderately rapid	Powdery white to cream or pinkish surface; pale or rarely yellow to red reverse	Macroconidia numerous, mostly small (5 or fewer cells) intergrading with large club-shaped microconidia in a continuous series (Fig. 9), so that 3-, 2-, and 1-celled conidia are present	Alkaline	Pos	Pos	No growth at 37°C in vitro; nonpathogenic
T. tonsurans[a]	Moderately slow	Powdery to velvety, white to yellowish or red-brown surface; reverse chestnut red-brown (Fig. 18f) and/or sulfur yellow, rarely pale yellow	Macroconidia uncommon, small pencil or club shaped; microconidia abundant (Fig. 10), often on broad "matchstick" pedicels; "balloon forms" and "filiform branches" may be seen	Alkaline, sometimes weak	Pos	Usually neg, sometimes pos	Stimulated by thiamine; a form producing only macroconidia has been described
T. vanbreuseghemii[c] (*A. gertleri*)	Moderately slow	Buff colony, leathery, finely grainy; reverse whitish or pale yellow	Abundant macroconidia with cells of uneven length, tending to fragment into single cells; microconidia small, boxy	No data	Pos	Pos	Geophilic; very rare in clinical laboratory
T. verrucosum[a]	Slow	Convoluted, slightly velvety whitish or less commonly tan to ochraceous colony	Macroconidia seldom seen, with "rat-tail extension"; microconidia round to drop shaped; chains of symmetrical chlamydospores seen on milk solids	Alkaline (may be weak) with broad zone of clearing	Neg	Neg	Human infection usually from cattle; growth stimulated at 37°C
T. violaceum[b]	Slow	Glabrous (bald-looking), smooth or convoluted colony; purple-red, sometimes with white sectors; some East African isolates purely whitish	Macroconidia seldom seen; microconidia drop shaped, formed mostly on thiamine medium or on sporulation media; chains of asymmetrical chlamydospores seen on milk solids media at 37° (Fig. 11)	No pH change or weak alkaline with small to broad zone of clearing (always broad after 14 days)	Pos or weak	Neg	Endemic to north Africa and Middle East but widely disseminated in cosmopolitan parts of Europe, Americas, and South Africa

[a]Common.
[b]Uncommon but likely to be seen by large labs in Americas and Europe.
[c]Unlikely to be seen except in region where endemic or proficiency test or soil isolation experiment.

EPIDEMIOLOGY AND TRANSMISSION

Dermatophytes are keratinophilic fungi that are capable of invading the keratinous tissues of living animals. They are grouped into three categories based on host preference and natural habitat (Table 2) (3). Anthropophilic species almost exclusively infect humans; animals are rarely infected. Geophilic species are soil-associated organisms, and soil per se or soil-borne keratinous debris (e.g., shed hairs or molted feathers) is a source of infection for humans as well as other animals. Zoophilic species are essentially pathogens of nonhuman mammals or, rarely, birds; however, animal-to-human transmission is not uncommon. Understanding this ecological classification for case isolates may be helpful in determining the source of infection; e.g., human infections caused by *Microsporum canis* are often the result of contact between susceptible children and newly acquired or stray kittens (73). Clinical species identification of dermatophytes assists in controlling infections that may have a family pet or other domesticated animal as an ongoing source of inoculum.

Some dermatophytes, e.g., *Trichophyton rubrum*, are cosmopolitan, whereas others, e.g., *Trichophyton concentricum*, are geographically limited (94). *T. concentricum* is found only in the Pacific Islands and regions in Southeast Asia and tropical America.

Anthropophilic fungi are usually transmitted either directly through close human contact or indirectly through sharing of clothes, combs, brushes, towels, bedsheets, etc. Tinea capitis (scalp infection) is highly contagious and may spread rapidly within a family, institution, or school. Transmission of tinea cruris (infection of the groin) is associated with shared clothing, towels, and sanitary facilities. The transmission of tinea pedis (athlete's foot) and tinea unguium (nail infection) often involves communal showers, baths, or other aquatic facilities but may depend on both environmental and host factors (98, 125). Acquisition of chronic *T. rubrum* tinea pedis has been suggested to require a dominant autosomal susceptibility gene (131).

Infections with geophilic dermatophytes involve transmission of soil-borne inoculum to humans or other mammals. Outbreaks originating from infected soil with secondary human-to-human transmission have been reported (6). Infections by zoophilic species result from animal-to-human contact (cats, dogs, cattle, laboratory animals, etc.) or from indirect transmission involving fomites. The fungi may then be transmitted among humans to a limited extent, especially in institutions (103).

CLINICAL SIGNIFICANCE

The dermatophytoses (tinea or ringworm) generally manifest as infections of the keratinized tissues (hair, nails, skin, etc.) of humans, other mammals, and birds. Cutaneous infections resembling dermatophytoses may be caused by yeasts or by unrelated filamentous fungi that are normally saprobes or plant pathogens; these infections are referred to as opportunistic dermatomycoses (125).

Dermatophytes are among the few fungal species that cause contagious, directly host-to-host-transmissible diseases of humans and animals. The transmission of these fungi is usually carried out by arthroconidia that have formed in or on infected host tissue. These conidia may be spread by direct skin contact or via fomites containing free arthroconidia, shed skin scales, or hairs. Typical fomites include such materials as hats, shoes, shower room floors, bedding, clothing of nursing staff in chronic care institutes, and farm fence posts used by animals for scratching. Tissue invasion is normally cutaneous; dermatophytes are usually unable to penetrate deeper tissues as a result of nonspecific inhibitory factors in serum (68), inhibition of fungal keratinases (32), a barrier formed of epidermal keratinocytes (69), and other immunological barriers (84, 126). In acute cases, there is a strong Th1 reaction mediated in part by $CD4^+$ lymphocytes (70), while in chronic cases, there is an immediate hypersensitivity-type reaction characterized by high levels of immunoglobulin E and immunoglobulin G4 antibodies and production of Th2 cytokines by mononucleocytes (121). Moreover many dermatophytes grow slowly, or, in rare cases, not at all at 37°C, so are better suited to the temperature of superficial tissues.

Dermatophytes tend to grow in an annular fashion on most affected skin regions, producing a "ringworm" infection form with a more or less raised and erythematous active area at the periphery and a relatively scurfy inactive zone at center of established lesions. The organism can often only be isolated from the active, peripheral ring. Infection may

TABLE 2 Grouping of dermatophytes on the basis of host preference and natural habitat[a]

Anthropophilic	Zoophilic (main animal host groups)	Geophilic
Epidermophyton floccosum	*Microsporum* spp.	*Microsporum* spp.
	M. canis (especially cats, dogs, and horses)	M. gypseum complex
Microsporum spp.	M. gallinae (especially poultry)	M. praecox
M. audouinii	M. nanum (especially pigs)	M. racemosum
M. ferrugineum	M. persicolor (especially rodents and other small mammals)	M. vanbreuseghemii
Trichophyton spp.	*Trichophyton* spp.	*Trichophyton vanbreuseghemii*
T. concentricum	Trichophyton equinum (especially horses)	
T. megninii	T. erinacei (especially hedgehogs)	
T. mentagrophytes complex	T. mentagrophytes complex (granular isolates) (especially	
(velvety and cottony isolates)	rodents, rabbits, and cavies)	
T. rubrum	T. simii (said to be monkeys; not well evidenced)	
T. schoenleinii	T. verrucosum (especially cattle)	
T. soudanense		
T. tonsurans		
T. violaceum		

[a]Normally nonpathogenic, soil-associated dermatophytoids such as *T. terrestre* and *M. cookei* are not included in this table.

range from mild to severe, partly as a consequence of the reaction of the host to the metabolic products of the fungus. Also important in determining the severity of infection are the virulence of the infecting strain, the anatomic location of the infection, the status of the host's immune system, and local environmental factors. Occasionally, especially in immunocompromised patients, subcutaneous tissue may be invaded, e.g., in Majocchi's granuloma, kerion, mycetoma-like processes (12, 127), or, more rarely, a generalized systemic infection (10). A *T. rubrum* infection suggestive of cutaneous blastomycosis has been reported in an immunocompromised patient (105).

In synopsis, the principal current risk factors for common forms of dermatophytosis are age (youth for tinea capitis or advanced age for onychomycosis); family history of chronic dermatophytosis; participation in sports featuring extensive body contact (e.g., wrestling and judo) or foot maceration (e.g., marathon running); barefoot use of communal aquatic facilities (showers and swimming areas); exchange of headgear, footwear or inadequately cleaned bedding; contact with feral domestic animals (especially street kittens) or animals recently supplied by en masse breeding operations (especially cats, guinea pigs, rabbits, laboratory rats, and cattle); inhabitation of rodent-infested dwellings; and, especially for children in developing countries, contact with livestock suffering from untreated dermatophytosis and contact with barbering instruments that have not been effectively disinfected (2, 8, 24, 52, 58, 71, 75, 96, 126, 131).

Anatomic Specificity

Infections caused by dermatophytes are named according to the anatomic location involved, e.g., tinea barbae (beard and moustache), tinea capitis (scalp), tinea facei (face, eyebrows, and eyelashes), tinea corporis (trunk and major limbs), tinea cruris (groin and perineal and perianal areas), tinea pedis (soles and toe webs), tinea manuum (palms), and tinea unguium (nails). Different dermatophyte species may produce clinically identical lesions; conversely, a single species may infect many anatomic sites.

Tinea barbae (infection of the beard area) is usually caused by zoophilic fungi, e.g., *Trichophyton verrucosum* and granular, zoophilic forms of the *T. mentagrophytes* complex. It is typically highly inflamed and may present as acute pustular folliculitis that can progress to suppurative boggy lesions (kerion). A less severe form appears as dry, erythematous, scaly lesions. Tinea capitis may vary from highly erythematous, patchy, scaly areas with dull gray hair stumps to highly inflamed lesions with folliculitis, kerion formation, alopecia, and scarring. *Trichophyton tonsurans* (anthropophilic) and *M. canis* (zoophilic) are the most common agents, and both are highly contagious (94). Favus (tinea favosa), usually caused by *Trichophyton schoenleinii* but also potentially caused by *Trichophyton violaceum* or *Microsporum gypseum*, is a now very rare chronic infection of the scalp and glabrous skin characterized by the formation of cup-shaped crusts (scutula) resembling honeycombs. Tinea corporis, which can be caused by any dermatophyte but is often associated with zoophiles, classically manifests as circular, erythematous lesions with scaly, raised, active, and often vesicular borders. Chronic lesions on the trunk and extremities usually are caused by *T. rubrum*, in particular by Afro-Asiatic forms of this fungus (formerly often called *Trichophyton raubitschekii*, a name now considered to be a synonym of *T. rubrum*). Tinea cruris ("jock itch"), usually caused by *T. rubrum* or *Epidermophyton floccosum*,

typically appears as scaly, erythematous to tawny brown, bilateral and asymmetric lesions extending down to the inner thigh and exhibiting a sharply marginated border frequently studded with small vesicles. Tinea pedis varies in appearance: the most common manifestation is maceration, peeling, itching, and painful fissuring between the fourth and fifth toes, but an acute inflammatory condition with vesicles and pustules can also occur, as can a hyperkeratotic chronic infection of the sole ("moccasin foot"). Members of the *T. mentagrophytes* complex frequently cause the more inflammatory type of infections, whereas *T. rubrum* usually causes the more chronic type. Infection of the sole by human-adapted forms of *Trichophyton interdigitale*, one of the members of the *T. mentagrophytes* complex, can be recognized by the formation of bullous vesicles in the thin skin of the plantar arch and along the sides of the feet and heel adjacent to the thick plantar stratum corneum (130). Tinea unguium, or nail infection by dermatophytes, is a subcategory of the more general phenomenon of onychomycosis, fungal nail infection. It is most often caused by *T. rubrum* and usually appears as thickened, deformed, friable, discolored nails with accumulated subungual debris. This type of presentation results from invasion of the underside of the distal nail and is therefore termed "distal-subungual onychomycosis." A less common infection type usually caused by *T. interdigitale* typically manifests, especially in its earlier stages, as "superficial white onychomycosis," i.e., white patches in the superficial portions of the nail. "Proximal-subungual tinea unguium" may also occur. This infection, in which the nail is subungually infected beginning near its point of origin in the area of the lunula, is usually caused by *T. rubrum* and often signals immunosuppression, e.g., AIDS (28).

COLLECTION, TRANSPORT, AND STORAGE OF SPECIMENS

Preliminary Patient Examination

In areas where tinea capitis caused by *Microsporum canis* is common, patients may be examined with a Wood's lamp (filtered UV light with a wavelength of 365 nm) in a darkened room for the presence of bright green fluorescent hairs. These are ideal for collection as laboratory specimens, though in some cases diagnosis may be done by Wood's light alone. The fluorescent hairs, considered "Wood's light positive," typically show a small-arthroconidial, ectothrix type of hair invasion in direct microscopy. Apart from *M. canis*, *M. audouinii*, and *M. ferrugineum* also cause this type of fluorescent ectothrix infection. Hairs infected with *T. schoenleinii* may show a dull green color (96). The Wood's lamp can also be used to differentiate between dermatophytosis and nonfungal skin conditions that may be similar clinically, e.g., erythrasma. In erythrasma, the skin fluoresces orange to coral red, whereas in the dermatophytosis, the skin is not fluorescent.

Sampling Preparations and Practice

Sufficient clinical material should be collected for both direct microscopic examination and culture. Whenever feasible, aseptic technique is to be used to minimize contamination. The following equipment should be available for the collection and transport of specimens: forceps for epilating hairs, sterile no. 15 scalpel blades or sharp curette, sterile nail clippers, scissors, sterile gauze squares, 70% alcohol for disinfection, sterile water for cleansing painful areas, and clean pill packets or clean paper envelopes to contain and transport the clinical specimens, such as hairs, skin scrapings, or nail clippings. Black photographic paper or strong black paper may be used for collecting and better visualizing scrapings. After collection, the paper is folded, tightly taped in the corners and placed in an envelope for transport. There are several commercial transport package systems available; MycoTrans (Biggar, Lanarkshire, United Kingdom) and Dermapak (Dermaco, Toddington, Bedfordshire, United Kingdom) are two of these. Closed tubes are not recommended for specimens, since they retain moisture, which may result in an overgrowth of bacterial as well as fungal contaminants. Disposable sterilized brushes or disposable, nonpasted toothbrushes have been recommended for collection of specimens from the scalp or from the fur of animals (76). If histopathological processing is done, the nail plate may be placed in a 4% formaldehyde solution (106). Culture media (detailed below) may be inoculated directly on collection.

Hairs from the scalp should be epilated with sterile forceps. If the specimen is Wood's light positive, epilate only fluorescent hairs. Nonfluorescent hairs, especially those infected with endothrix fungi such as *T. tonsurans*, may need to be dug out with the tip of a sterile scalpel blade because the hairs often break off at scalp level and are thus difficult to grasp with a forceps. Rubbing with a sterile moistened swab has been successful with pediatric patients (57). Where possible, skin scrapings from the adjacent area should also be included. In the rare event that favus is seen, the scutulum at the mouth of the hair follicle is suitable for culture and microscopic examination. In lower-body dermatophytoses, lesions with defined borders should be preliminarily disinfected with alcohol or cleansed with sterile water, and then active border areas should be scraped with a blunt scalpel to collect epidermal scales. Where borders are not visible to indicate the area of maximal fungal activity, as in tinea manuum, the preliminarily cleansed infected area can be broadly scraped in order to obtain specimens from a variety of areas that may imperceptibly differ in current fungal activity. In vesicular tinea pedis, the tops of the vesicles can be removed with sterile scissors for direct examination and culture. Culture of the vesicle fluid is not recommended.

Nails should be disinfected with alcohol gauze squares. The most desirable material for culture in typical subungual onychomycosis is the waxy subungual debris, which contains the fungal elements. The highest proportion of viable elements for culturing is often found close to the juncture of the nail bed. In order to remove contaminating saprobic fungi and bacteria, the crumbly debris directly underneath the nail near the tips is removed with the scalpel before material is collected for culture. Some investigators will clip the nail short first and perform this scraping-away of contaminated material on the clipping. If the dorsal nail plate is diseased (superficial white onychomycosis), scrape and discard the outer surface before underlying material is removed for culture. In rare cases with a presentation consistent with *Trichophyton soudanense* endonyx nail infection (118), in which the internal strata of the nail plate are milky white but the upper and lower nail surfaces appear relatively unaffected, clippings may be taken or the milky area may be exposed and scraped.

Any specimen needing to be transported, or for any other reason not processed immediately, should be retained in the paper packets described above. Closed tubes are not recommended for specimens since they may retain moisture, resulting in an overgrowth of contaminants. Dermatophytes in dry specimens of skin, hair, and nails may be stored for years in viable condition, provided the material is not subjected to temperature extremes.

LABORATORY TESTING OF SPECIMENS

Direct Microscopic Examination

Direct microscopic examination of skin, hair, and nails is the most rapid method of determining fungal etiology and is traditionally accomplished by examining the clinical material in 10% potassium hydroxide (KOH) or sodium hydroxide (NaOH) (66, 97). Another common procedure is to use 25% potassium or sodium hydroxide mixed with 5% glycerin to impede desiccation (66). Addition of fluorescent brighteners such as calcofluor white may significantly increase accuracy (93). In nails, histopathology based on staining nail biopsy material with periodic acid-Schiff stain has been shown to have potential for generating results more accurate than those afforded by hydroxide-based direct microscopy (72). The suggestion, however, that biopsy/periodic acid-Schiff can also replace culturing (72) is unsound, in that this technique does not permit reliable distinction of dermatophytes from other nail-invading species (111).

Nail clippings should be aseptically cut into smaller fragments and, where possible, pounded with a heavy object inside their collection packet in order to release friable, flaky material containing the greatest amount of dermatophyte inoculum. Skin or nail scrapings, nail fragments, or hair roots are placed in 1 or 2 drops of one of the above-mentioned KOH or NaOH solutions on a clean glass slide. A coverslip is placed on top, and the preparation is heated gently (short of boiling) by being passed rapidly over a Bunsen burner three or four times and then allowed to sit at room temperature for a few minutes for clearing. The exact time needed will depend on concentration of hydroxide used, thickness of specimen fragments, and exact amount of heat imparted by contact with flame. Clearing is evident to the naked eye as a pronounced decrease in the opacity of the scraping. Alternatively, a slide warmer set at 51 to 54°C may be used to heat the slides for 1 hour (66). Laboratories using a 10% KOH or NaOH solution for skin may find that nail scrapings may require a stronger alkali solution (up to 25% KOH or NaOH). If the specimens are in 20% KOH for 20 to 30 min, the heating step is unnecessary. Demonstration of fungal elements may be facilitated by use of glucan-binding fluorescent brighteners such as calcofluor white (97) or Congo red (66). These require use of a fluorescence microscope set up to visualize the specific fluorescence obtained. Calcofluor white is added directly to the KOH drop on the slide as an approximately equal drop of 0.1% solution (77). Some laboratories presoften nails before the addition of calcofluor; otherwise it does not penetrate the nail tissue well. Moreover, since calcofluor deteriorates in light, it is best to view preparations as soon as possible after adding the dye. One routinely used procedure is to place three drops of 20% KOH into the bottom of a small microcentrifuge tube, place about half a dozen fragments of skin or nail into the tube, and leave it to soften for at least 30 min (it can be left for several hours). After this time, the softened material is removed with a pastette, placed onto a glass slide, covered with a drop of calcofluor, and squashed down under a coverslip to produce a monolayer of epidermal cells before viewing under the microscope. Hairs are placed directly onto slides with the KOH so that there

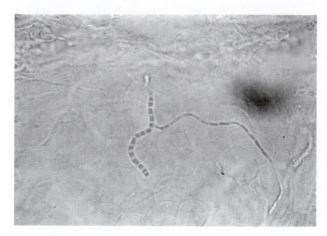

FIGURE 1 Dermatophyte hyphae in skin scraping. NaOH mount. Magnification, ×400.

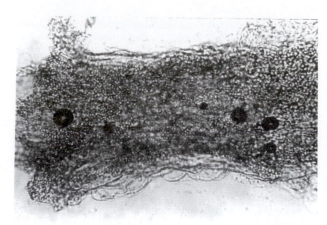

FIGURE 2 *M. audouinii*, ectothrix type of hair invasion. Magnification, ×400.

is minimal disruption of the architecture. All preparations should be examined under low power and confirmed under high power.

Skin and nails infected by dermatophytes may reveal one or more of the following: hyaline hyphal fragments; septate, often branched hyphae; and chains of arthroconidia (Fig. 1).

The appearance of infected hairs depends on the invading dermatophyte species. Hyphae invade the hairs, and arthroconidia are formed by fragmentation of these hyphae. The appearances and locations of the arthroconidia may suggest the infecting genera or species (Table 3), as may the sizes (96). Three main types of colonizations (ectothrix, endothrix, and favic) are observed by direct microscopic examination. The terms "ectothrix" and "endothrix" refer to the location of the arthroconidia in relation to the hair shaft (ecto- and endo- meaning outside and inside, respectively), while favic refers to the distinctive infection caused by *T. schoenleinii*, a fungus that is now extremely rare except in some parts of central Asia and the African Sahel.

In ectothrix colonization, arthroconidia appear as a mosaic sheath around the hair or as chains on the surface of the hair shaft (Fig. 2). In *M. canis*, *M. audouinii*, and *M. ferrugineum* infections, colonized hairs fluoresce green under a Wood's lamp; other ectothrix infections (Table 3) are nonfluorescent. Endothrix hair invasion is observed as chains of arthroconidia filling the insides of shortened hair

stubs (Fig. 3). Hairs are Wood's lamp negative. In favic hairs, hyphae, air bubbles, or tunnels and fat droplets are observed within the hair (Fig. 4). These hairs are dull green under the Wood's lamp. In general, infected hairs from all infection types show hyphae within the hair shaft at some time during the course of infection, usually during the early stages.

Isolation Procedures

Scrapings, hairs, and other materials collected as outlined above for direct examination are plated on selected isolation media and incubated at 32°C for optimal growth; temperatures between 24°C and 32°C are also acceptable if the total incubation time is suitably adjusted to compensate for slower outgrowth expected at lower temperatures. Generally from 5 to 15 skin or nail fragments are planted per plate or tube used for isolation, and these fragments are separated so that antibiotic-resistant mold or bacterial contaminants from one piece cannot overgrow the others. Hairs are also well separated. Cultures on primary isolation medium are routinely incubated at 25 to 30°C and examined weekly for up to 4 weeks.

The most common medium used for the isolation of dermatophytes is Sabouraud glucose agar (SGA) (original

TABLE 3 Hair invasion by dermatophytes on the human host

Ectothrix	Endothrix	Favic
Microsporum audouinii	*Trichophyton soudanense*	*Trichophyton schoenleinii*
M. canis	*T. tonsurans*	
M. ferrugineum	*T. violaceum*	
M. gypseum complex		
M. praecox		
T. megninii		
T. mentagrophytes complex		
T. verrucosum		

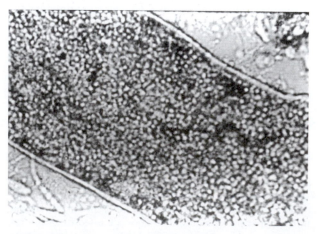

FIGURE 3 *T. tonsurans*, endothrix type of hair invasion. Magnification, ×1,000.

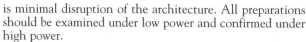

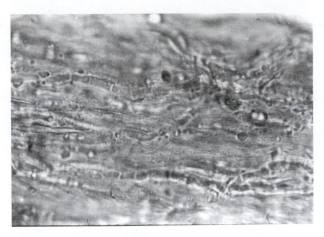

FIGURE 4 Hair infected by *T. schoenleinii* from a patient with favus. Magnification, ×1,000.

formulation with 4% glucose or Emmons' modification with 2% glucose), supplemented with chloramphenicol (0.05 g liter^{-1}) and cycloheximide (0.4 g liter^{-1}) to inhibit bacterial and saprobic fungal contamination. This type of medium is available commercially as, for example, Mycobiotic agar (Acumedia Manufacturers, Lansing, MI; Remel, Lenexa, KS; Delasco, Council Bluffs, IA), Mycosel (BD Diagnostic Systems, Sparks, MD), or Dermasel Selective Supplement (Oxoid, Basingstoke, Hampshire, United Kingdom; note that Remel is currently the U.S. distributor for Oxoid). An alternative medium promoting more rapid conidiation and colony pigmentation development is potato flake agar supplemented with cycloheximide and chloramphenicol (Hardy Diagnostics, Santa Maria, CA). For the isolation of cycloheximide-susceptible fungi that cause clinical infections resembling dermatophytosis, any of the SGA with chloramphenicol (Remel or BD), inhibitory mold agar (BD, Remel, or Hardy), or Littman oxgall agar (BD) may be recommended (97). Inhibitory mold agar and Littman oxgall agar have the advantage of restricting contaminant colony diameters. For all media, the addition of gentamicin is recommended for specimens heavily contaminated by bacteria (116). SGA with cycloheximide, chloramphenicol, and gentamicin is routinely used as an isolation medium in some laboratories (66).

Additional and alternative media may be used in special circumstances. For example, vitamin-free Casamino Acids (BD)-erythritol-albumin agar medium plus cycloheximide, chloramphenicol, and gentamicin may be used for filament-positive skin and nail specimens, especially from body sites where *Candida* overgrowth may be a problem (e.g., groin or fingernails). This medium (currently not commercially available to our knowledge) prevents the common suppression of dermatophyte outgrowth by heavy inoculum of *Candida albicans*, *Candida parapsilosis*, and related biotin-requiring yeasts (35). Dermatophyte species with vitamin requirements (very uncommon in these types of cases) may grow poorly on it, and it is always used in combination with a cycloheximide-containing SGA.

Another primary isolation medium that may be used is dermatophyte test medium (DTM; available commercially from BD, Hardy, and Remel, among others). This selective medium screens for the presence of dermatophytes in heavily contaminated material (nails, etc.). The growth of dermatophytes causes a rise in pH, thus changing the phenol red indicator from yellow to red (117). The use of DTM should be combined with morphological study, since dermatophytoids such as *Trichophyton terrestre*, as well as various *Chrysosporium* species and other nondermatophytic fungi, can grow and turn the medium red (66, 78, 100). Rapid sporulation medium, mentioned above for potato flake agar, contains a pH indicator that works on a similar principle but turns from yellow to blue-green, leaving the red reverse pigment of typical *T. rubrum* visible (7). DTM may uncommonly give false-negative results with some *Microsporum* isolates (81).

Nucleic Acid-Based Direct Detection Techniques

Numerous techniques have been published for directly detecting dermatophyte DNA in tissue, but as yet none is established as a routine diagnostic procedure. This is due mainly to the relatively low cost of traditional procedures. However, in terms of accuracy, traditional procedures are not optimal; in onychomycosis, for example, they disclose at best circa 85% of true-positive cases from the initial patient specimen, and this percentage is much lower in many laboratories (111). This has given strong incentive for development of molecular detection techniques. At present, a large number of primary studies related to rapid PCR of dermatological specimens for dermatophytosis and related mycoses (e.g., nondermatophyte filamentous fungal onychomycosis) have been published. Techniques employed include the PCR-enzyme-linked immunosorbent assay (14), PCR-reverse line blotting (15), PCR coupled with restriction fragment length polymorphism study (17), multiplex PCR (20), nested PCR (37), PCR based in part on a microsatellite locus permitting strain typing of *T. rubrum* (67), and direct PCR with sequencing (119). These techniques require comparative assessment and comprehensive review, which is beyond the scope of this chapter. Also, related techniques, such as real-time PCR (9, 16, 56), have been shown to work well in trial studies but also need to prove themselves as consistently practical and cost-effective in interlaboratory study related to routine diagnosis. In unusual situations, molecular direct-detection methods may be invaluable: for example, in a deep dermatophytosis case in which all conventional tests had given negative results, *Trichophyton rubrum* was identified by means of a nested PCR study directed at amplifying a portion of the ITS region from paraffin-embedded sections (82).

IDENTIFICATION

At present, the great majority of dermatophytes are identified phenotypically. Identification is often based on (i) colony characteristics in pure culture on SGA and (ii) microscopic morphology. These criteria alone, however, may be insufficient, since colonial appearance may vary or be similar for different species. Characteristic pigmentation may fail to appear, and isolates, especially *Trichophyton* spp., may not sporulate. Special media may be required to stimulate pigment production; it may be necessary to use sporulation and physiologic tests in conjunction with morphology to identify the species correctly. Various molecular identification mechanisms have also been described (discussed above) but are seldom practically applicable except in high-level reference laboratories. The majority of isolates are easily identified when visual examination is combined with any needed testing for characteristic growth factor requirements; phenotypic studies thus remain the least expensive option for routine identification.

Colony Characteristics

In observing gross colony morphology, note the color of the surface and the reverse of the colony, texture of the surface (powdery, granular, woolly, cottony, velvety, or glabrous), topography (elevation, folding, margins, etc.), and rate of growth.

Microscopic Morphology

Microscopic morphology, especially the appearance and arrangement of the conidia (macroconidia or microconidia) and other structures, may be determined by teased mounts, sticky tape mounts, or slide culture preparations mounted in lactophenol cotton blue (LCB), in lactophenol aniline blue (phenol, an ingredient of LCB and lactophenol aniline blue, is listed as a hazardous chemical; therefore, solutions containing phenol should be prepared, stored, and used in an approved chemical safety cabinet), in lacto-fuchsin (66), or in more permanent mounting fluids (122). Sometimes a special medium, such as cornmeal or cornmeal-glucose agar, potato-glucose agar, SGA plus 3 to 5% NaCl (63, 65), pablum cereal agar (66), rapid sporulation medium (7), or lactrimel agar (18, 62) may be required to stimulate sporulation.

Physiological Tests

In Vitro Hair Perforation Test

The in vitro hair perforation test distinguishes between atypical isolates of the *T. mentagrophytes* complex and *T. rubrum* (5). It may also be used to assist in making other distinctions such as *M. canis* versus *Microsporum audouinii* and *Microsporum praecox* versus *M. gypseum* (89). Hairs exposed to *T. mentagrophytes* complex members, *M. canis*, and *M. gypseum* show wedge-shaped perforations perpendicular to the hair shaft (a positive test result), whereas *T. rubrum*, *M. audouinii*, and *M. praecox* do not form these perforating structures.

Place short strands of human hair (ideally hair from a child under 18 months old) in petri dishes, and autoclave the dishes at 121°C for 10 min; add 25 ml of sterile distilled water and 2 or 3 drops of 10% sterilized yeast extract. Inoculate these plates with several fragments of the test fungus that has been grown on SGA; incubate the plates at 25°C, and examine them at regular intervals over a period of 21 days. Hairs may be examined microscopically for perforations by removing a few segments and placing them in a drop of LCB mounting fluid. Gently heating the mounts aids in the detection of the fungus. A positive control test should always be run with a known perforating species; *M. canis* is recommended. Some hair samples may prove unsuitable for unknown reasons, e.g., possible prior contact with shampoos containing antifungal inhibitors.

Special Nutritional Requirements

Nutritional tests aid in the routine identification of *Trichophyton* species that seldom produce conidia or that resemble each other morphologically (38). Certain species have distinctive nutritional requirements, whereas others do not. The method employs a Casamino Acids basal medium that is vitamin free (*Trichophyton* agar 1 [T1]) and to which various vitamins are added, i.e., inositol (T2), thiamine plus inositol (T3), thiamine (T4), and nicotinic acid (T5). In addition, the series includes an ammonium nitrate basal medium (T6) to which histidine is added (T7). These media are available commercially in dehydrated form from BD Biosciences and in prepared form from Remel. A small fragment (about the size of the head of a pin) from the culture to be tested is placed on the surface of the basal medium (controls) and the media containing the vitamin and amino acid additives. Care must be taken to avoid transferring agar from the fungal inoculum to the nutritional media. Cultures are incubated at room temperature (or 37°C if *T. verrucosum* is suspected) and read after 7 and 14 days. The amount of growth is graded from 0 to 4+. Commonly observed reactions are summarized in Table 4.

TABLE 4 Dermatophyte nutritional response as elucidated by *Trichophyton* agars[a]

Species	Response in vitamin tests					Response in amino acid tests	
	1	2	3	4	5	6	7
	Vitamin free	Inositol	Thiamine + inositol	Thiamine	Nicotinic acid	Amino acid free	Histidine
M. gallinae						4	4
T. concentricum, 50%	4	4	4	4	4		
T. concentricum, 50%	2	2	4	4	2		
T. equinum var. equinum	0	0	0	0	4		
T. equinum var. autotrophicum-T. megninii	4	4	4	4	4	0	4
T. soudanense	v	v	v	v	v	v	v
T. tonsurans	1	1	4	4	1		
T. verrucosum, 84%	1	2	4	2	1		
T. verrucosum, 16%	1	1	4	4	1		
T. violaceum (typical)	1	1	4	4	1		
T. violaceum (rare "T. yaoundei" form)	4	4	4	4	4		

[a]Only the growth responses for organisms with growth factor requirements and the selected organisms that must be most closely compared with them are included in this table. The numbers in the table body indicate the relative degree of growth according to traditional 1+ to 4+ visually approximated scale: 0, no growth; 1, slight growth, strongly nutrient deprived colony morphology (very sparse, subsurface colonial growth only or colony diameter strongly reduced compared to Sabouraud agar control); 2, partially stimulated growth but still significantly suppressed compared to that of the control; 4, growth comparable to that of the control (the table includes no 3+ reactions); v, variable. Blank spaces in the table indicate growth responses that are not customarily examined but that are insignificantly different from control growth responses on Sabouraud agar.

Urea Hydrolysis

The ability to hydrolyze urea provides additional data to aid in distinguishing the typical, cosmopolitan form of *T. rubrum* (urease negative) from members of the *T. mentagrophytes* complex (typically urease positive), and from the urease-positive Afro-Asiatic or "granular" form of *T. rubrum*, formerly often called *T. raubitschekii* (99, 102). Christensen urea agar and broth may both be used; the broth appears to be the more sensitive of these alternatives (64). After the urea medium is inoculated, it is incubated at 25 to 30°C up to 7 days. The tubes should be examined every 2 or 3 days for the color change from orange or pale pink to purple-red that indicates the presence of urease, a positive test result. Negative and positive controls should always be done on new batches of these media. See Table 1.

Growth on BCPMSG

Bromcresol purple (BCP)-milk solids-glucose (BCPMSG) medium is available commercially as dermatophyte milk agar (Hardy). Type of growth (profuse versus restricted) and a change in the pH indicator (BCP) indicating alkalinity are especially useful for distinguishing *T. rubrum* from the *T. mentagrophytes* complex, and *T. mentagrophytes* from *Microsporum persicolor* (65, 66, 114). *T. rubrum* shows restricted growth and produces no alkaline reaction on BCPMSG, whereas members of the *T. mentagrophytes* complex typically show profuse growth and an alkaline reaction. Although *M. persicolor* shows profuse growth, it does not result in an alkaline reaction. Other tests for distinguishing *T. mentagrophytes* and close relatives from *M. persicolor* are described elsewhere (86).

Cultures to be tested are inoculated onto slants of BCPMSG and examined for pH change and growth characteristics at the end of a 7-day incubation at 25°C. A color change from pale blue to violet purple indicates an alkaline reaction.

Growth on Polished Rice Grains

Unlike most dermatophytes, *M. audouinii* grows poorly on rice grains and produces a brownish discoloration of the rice (23, 66). This test distinguishes this species from *M. canis* and other dermatophytes that grow and sporulate on rice grains. It may be especially useful in areas where *M. audouinii* is still endemic, e.g., sub-Saharan Africa, or where immigrants or travelers from such areas are reintroducing it.

The medium is prepared in 12-ml flasks by mixing 1 part raw unfortified rice grains and 3 parts water (23) or 8.0 g of rice grains and 125 ml of distilled water. Autoclave at 15 lb/in² for 15 min. Inoculate the surface of the rice, and incubate the sample for 2 weeks at 25 to 30°C.

Temperature Tolerance and Temperature Enhancement

Tests for temperature tolerance and enhancement are useful for distinguishing the *T. mentagrophytes* complex from *Trichophyton terrestre* (87), *T. mentagrophytes* from *M. persicolor* (65), *T. verrucosum* from *T. schoenleinii* (96), and *Trichophyton soudanense* from *M. ferrugineum* (124). At 37°C, members of the *T. mentagrophytes* complex show good growth, whereas *T. terrestre* does not grow and *M. persicolor* generally grows poorly or not at all (a single atypical isolate with good growth has been observed); growth of *T. verrucosum* and *T. soudanense* is enhanced, but that of *T. schoenleinii* and *M. ferrugineum* is not.

Inoculate two slants of SGA with an equivalent fragment of the culture. Incubate one slant at room temperature (25 to 30°C) and one at 37°C. Compare the growth at the two temperatures when mature colonies appear at room temperature. Appropriate controls are recommended and should be compared first.

Molecular Identification Techniques

Routine diagnostic sequencing of the ITS region (91) remains the gold standard for molecular identification of dermatophytes. The recommendation of standard DNA barcodes (113) is in progress. Many other nucleic acid-based identification techniques for dermatophytes were published in previous years but have not been adopted widely. Some recent contenders for rapid, state-of-the-art species identification include PCR using a (GACA)$_4$ primer (104) and restriction fragment length polymorphism of the ITS 2 gene region (31).

DESCRIPTION OF THE ETIOLOGIC AGENTS

Characteristic features of dermatophyte species are presented in Table 1. The table also includes data on some similar but rarely or never pathogenic *Microsporum* and *Trichophyton* species that must be distinguished from pathogenic species.

Two types of conidia may be produced on the aerial mycelium of the dermatophytes: large multicellular, smooth or rough, thin- or thick-walled macroconidia and smaller unicellular, smooth-walled microconidia. The three genera are classically grouped according to the presence or absence of these two types of conidia and the appearance of the surface of the macroconidia, i.e., rough versus smooth. In reality, when atypical isolates and species are taken into account, the genera show considerable overlap in morphology (88). For this reason, it is often more convenient to identify isolates directly at the species level than it is to try to identify them at the genus level first. Identification of species is based on the microscopic appearance and arrangement of the conidia (Fig. 5 through 17), colonial morphology on SGA (Fig. 18), and physiological tests (Table 5).

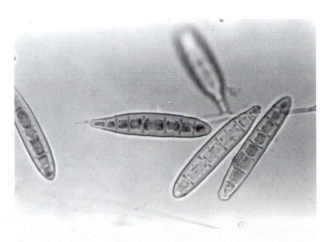

FIGURE 5 Smooth-walled macroconidia of *Trichophyton ajelloi*. Magnification, ×400.

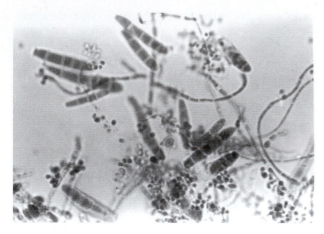

FIGURE 6 Macroconidia and microconidia of *Trichophyton mentagrophytes* complex on SGA with 5% NaCl. Magnification, ×400.

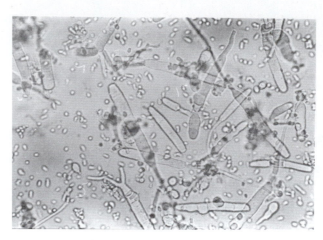

FIGURE 7 Smooth-walled macroconidia of Afro-Asiatic type *Trichophyton rubrum* (*T. raubitschekii*) from primary isolate on SGA. Magnification, ×1,000.

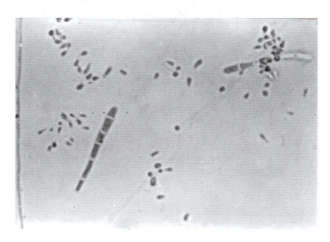

FIGURE 8 Long, narrow macroconidium and clavate to pyriform microconidia of *T. rubrum*. Magnification, ×400.

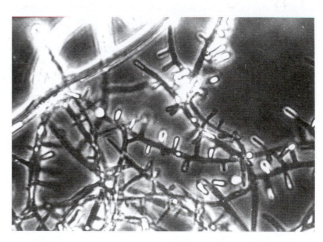

FIGURE 9 Clavate macroconidium, microconidia, and intermediate conidia of *Trichophyton terrestre*. Phase contrast; magnification, ×400.

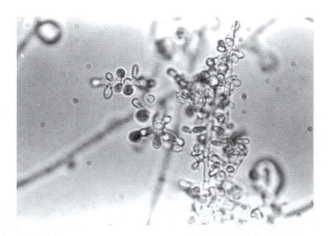

FIGURE 10 Microconidia with typical refractile cytoplasm of *Trichophyton tonsurans*. Magnification, ×400.

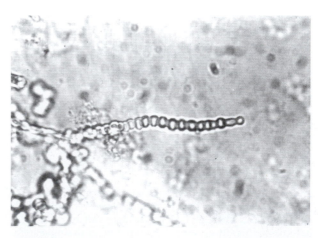

FIGURE 11 Characteristic chlamydospores produced by *Trichophyton verrucosum* or BCP-milk solids-yeast extract agar. Magnification, ×400.

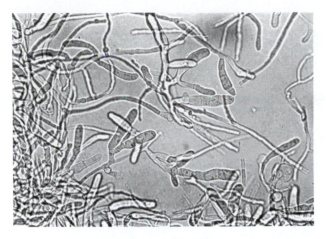

FIGURE 12 Macroconidia of *Epidermophyton floccosum* on SGA. Note the absence of microconidia. Magnification, ×400.

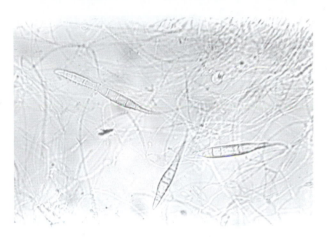

FIGURE 13 Macroconidia of *Microsporum audouinii* on SGA with 3% NaCl. Magnification, ×400.

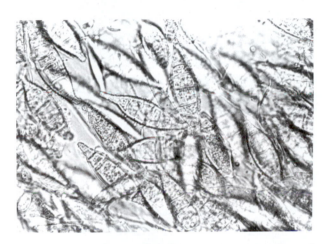

FIGURE 14 Macroconidia of *Microsporum canis* with rough thick walls. Magnification, ×400.

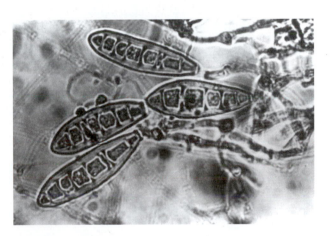

FIGURE 15 Macroconidia of *Microsporum cookei*, showing thick walls and pseudosepta. Magnification, ×400.

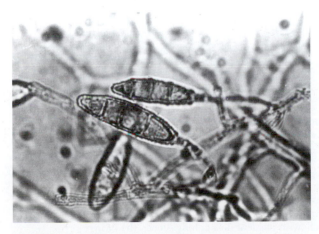

FIGURE 16 Macroconidia of *Microsporum gypseum*. Magnification, ×400.

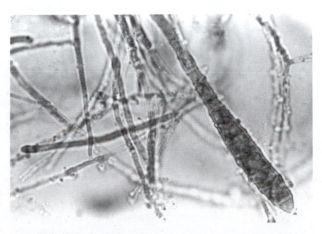

FIGURE 17 Rough-walled macroconidium of *Microsporum persicolor* on SGA with 3% NaCl. Magnification, ×1,000.

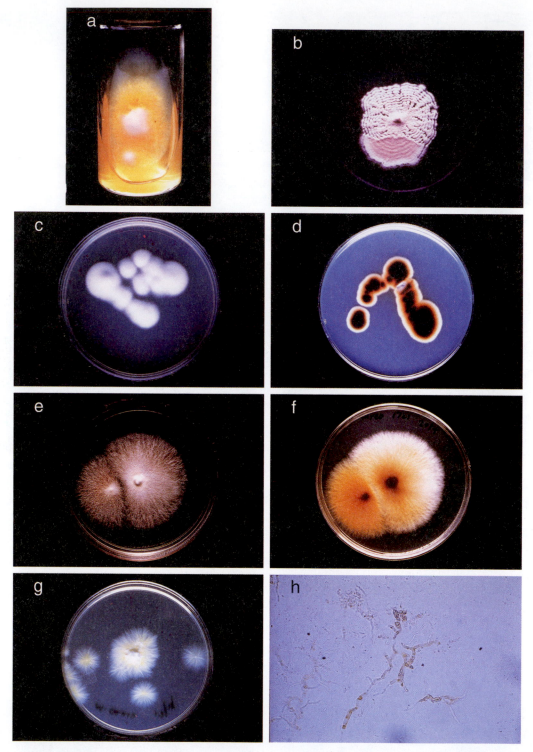

FIGURE 18 (a) *Trichophyton mentagrophytes* complex: "nodular" variant of *Trichophyton interdigitale* (formerly *Trichophyton krajdenii*), SGA, 12 days, showing typical bright yellow pigmentation. (b) *Trichophyton mentagrophytes* complex: granular, zoophilic type *Trichophyton interdigitale* (mating tester strain of *Arthroderma vanbreuseghemii*), 14 days. (c) *Trichophyton rubrum*, SGA, 10 days, surface showing cottony white mycelium. (d) *Trichophyton rubrum*, SGA, 10 days, reverse showing typical red pigment. (e) *Trichophyton tonsurans*, SGA, 14 days, surface showing low velvety texture, mixed white and brownish mycelium. (f) *Trichophyton tonsurans*, SGA, 14 days, reverse showing mixture of mahogany red-brown and sulfur yellow coloration. (g) *Microsporum canis*, SGA, 10 days, relatively flat colony showing pale striate margin and yellowish pigment near colony center. (h) Brown filaments of *Hortaea werneckii* in NaOH mount of scraping from tinea nigra. Magnification, ×400.

TABLE 5 Sequence of procedures for phenotypic identification of dermatophytes in pure culture[a]

1. Examine colony at day 7 and, if necessary, day 14, for colors of surface and reverse, topography, texture, and rate of growth. Proceed to step 2.
2. Prepare tease mounts and search for identifying microscopic morphology, especially presence, appearance, and arrangement, of macroconidia and microconidia (consult Fig. 5 to 18 and Table 1). If the results are inconclusive, proceed to step 3.
3. Prepare slide cultures or transparent tape mounts and examine for characteristic morphology as indicated above if tease mounts do not provide sufficient information. Consider special media if sporulation is absent (potato glucose agar, lactrimel, BCPMSG, SGA with 3–5% NaCl). At the same time, proceed to step 4.
4. Perform as many of the following physiologic and other special tests as necessary for identification.
   a. Urease (ensure culture is bacteria free!)
   b. Nutritional requirements if *Trichophyton* is suspected
   c. Growth on rice grains if an unusual *Microsporum* sp. is suspected
   d. Elevated temperature response (37°C on SGA or, if *T. verrucosum* is suspected, BCPMSG)
   e. Special differentiation media: e.g., BCPMSG to distinguish *T. mentagrophytes* complex from *T. rubrum* and *M. persicolor*; Lowenstein-Jensen or BCPMSG to distinguish *T. soudanense* from *M. ferrugineum*; SGA + 3–5% NaCl to distinguish *T. mentagrophytes* complex from *M. persicolor* and atypical *T. rubrum*; DTM to distinguish nonsporulating dermatophytes from most other nonsporulating hyaline fungi
   f. In vitro hair perforation test
   g. Molecular or mating studies (to be performed in reference laboratories)

[a]It may be necessary to incubate cultures on brain-heart infusion agar or BCPMSG to ensure absence of antibiotic-resistant bacterial contamination before proceeding to step 4. Procedures are adapted from Weitzman and colleagues (125) and Kane et al. (66).

Trichophyton Species

Macroconidia have smooth, thin to thick walls, are variable in shape (clavate, fusiform to cylindrical), vary in number of septa (1 to 12) and in size (8 to 86 by 4 to 14 μm), and are borne singly or in clusters. Microconidia, which are usually present and more numerous than macroconidia, may be globose, pyriform, or clavate and are borne singly along the sides of hyphae or in grapelike clusters. Though species in this genus generally produce microconidia more readily than macroconidia, two lineages producing macroconidia but lacking microconidia have been described: (i) "*Trichophyton kanei*" (108), now known to be a variant of the Afro-Asiatic genotype of *T. rubrum*, and (ii) a variant all-macroconidial form of *T. tonsurans* (88). Fresh isolates of the dermatophytoid *T. ajelloi* may also produce many macroconidia and few or no microconidia. Some species such as *T. schoenleinii* rarely produce conidia of any kind in culture, and nonsporulating isolates of normally conidial species, especially *T. rubrum*, may also be encountered.

Microsporum Species

Microsporum species produce macroconidia and microconidia that may be rare or numerous, depending on the species and the substrate. The distinguishing characteristic is the macroconidium, which is typically rough walled (varying from minutely to strongly roughened). Macroconidia also vary in shape (obovate, fusiform to cylindrofusiform), number of septa (1 to 15), size (6 to 160 by 6 to 25 μm), and width of the cell wall. Microconidia are pyriform or clavate and usually are arranged singly along the sides of the hyphae. *Microsporum* species invade skin, hair, and, rarely, nails. Biological (teleomorphic) species within the *M. gypseum* complex can be provisionally recognized on the basis of colonial and microscopic features on Takashio's medium (33), but these species are best distinguished by mating or molecular testing.

Epidermophyton floccosum

In *E. floccosum*, microconidia are lacking; only smooth-walled, broadly clavate macroconidia are produced. They have one to six septa, are 20 to 40 μm long by 7 to 12 μm wide, and are borne singly or in clusters of two or three. *E. floccosum* is currently the only recognized *Epidermophyton* species; the former *E. stockdaleae* is now considered a synonym of *Trichophyton ajelloi* (41).

STRAIN TYPING SYSTEMS

Dermatophyte strains within anthropophilic species tend to be very closely related, delaying the development of useful techniques for epidemiological analysis, but strains of *T. rubrum* were eventually distinguished by polymorphisms in the numbers of subrepeat elements in the ribosomal nontranscribed spacer region (55, 60, 92, 129). In addition, the Afro-Asiatic lineage of *T. rubrum* was distinguished from the now-cosmopolitan epidemic *T. rubrum* form by means of a microsatellite marker designated T1 (85). More recently, an elegant system involving multiple microsatellite markers has been developed (42). Nontranscribed spacer polymorphisms can also be applied to distinguish *Trichophyton interdigitale* and *T. tonsurans* isolates (36, 55, 79). While it is beyond the scope of this chapter to review all current molecular differentiation techniques for dermatophytes or their applications in outbreaks, the multilocus genotyping system of Abdel-Rahman et al. (1) should be cited as an example of how such methods can foster the development of epidemiological insight.

ANTIMICROBIAL SUSCEPTIBILITIES

Dermatophytes can in principle be tested for susceptibility to antifungal drugs using the Clinical and Laboratory Standards Institute M38-A3 standard procedure for molds (83). A trial has shown that this type of methodology can be applied with good inter- and intralaboratory reproducibility to the commonly used drugs ciclopirox, fluconazole, griseofulvin, itraconazole, posaconazole, terbinafine, and voriconazole (39). Treatment failures in dermatophytoses, however, are almost always due to factors other than drug resistance (54), and potentially burdensome requests for dermatophyte susceptibility testing should be closely screened for scientific and clinical appropriateness.

EVALUATION, INTERPRETATION, AND REPORTING OF LABORATORY RESULTS

For nonimmunocompromised patients, positive direct microscopy compatible with dermatophytosis is conventionally interpreted as presumptively indicating this condition in hair and in skin specimens other than those from nails, soles, and palms. The positive microscopic report itself conveys this information; it should be issued within 2 working days of specimen receipt. With soles and palms, persons who have lived in tropical areas or who are of south Asian heritage may have dermatophytosis-like *Neoscytalidium* (26) (previously called *Scytalidium*, *Nattrassia*, and *Hendersonula toruloidea*) infections, which are similar to dermatophytoses both clinically and in direct microscopy (66); no presumptive diagnosis can be inferred until the culture result is available. The direct microscopic result, however, is still reported immediately. For patients without risk factors for *Neoscytalidium*, qualified physicians may make presumptive diagnoses of dermatophytosis for sole and palm skin as for other skin sites. In onychomycosis, over 35 different mold species may be involved in producing conditions clinically and microscopically resembling tinea unguium (66), particularly in geriatric patients. Microscopic results are still reported promptly, but culture results are of high interest. At the same time, the outgrowth of known onychomycosis-causing nondermatophytes may or may not be significant, excepting the nail-infecting *Neoscytalidium* species, which are always considered significant when grown. The complexities of accurately reporting nondermatophytes from nail specimens are beyond the scope of this chapter but are discussed in light of rigorous validation studies on this topic by Summerbell et al. (111).

Isolation of a dermatophyte culture from lesional skin, hair, or nails is interpreted as diagnostic whether or not fungal elements are seen in the initial direct microscopy examination. Note that dermatophytoids such as *Microsporum cookei* and *Trichophyton terrestre* are presumed to be contaminants until proven otherwise; they are, however, reported along with the comment "normally nonpathogenic" when grown. These fungi have been the subjects of numerous false and questionable case reports in the literature, and there may be some confusion about their status. If such a fungus were to infect human epidermis, the gold standard for scientifically evidencing the case would be three successive, consistent repeat isolations of the fungus from the lesion in specimens collected on different days, plus demonstration of compatible fungal elements in direct microscopy of the affected tissue. No inferential diagnoses from lower quality evidence should be accepted as conclusive, even if the patient is said to have been successfully treated. A common dermatophyte such as *T. rubrum* that failed to grow out in initial culture(s) is very likely to be the actual etiologic agent in such cases (111). In onychomycosis in particular, true causal dermatophytes have only at best a circa 75% chance of being grown from the initial specimen taken from any given patient; another circa 15% will be recovered from a second specimen, while circa 10% can be detected only by doing three or more serial specimens, something very seldom done in practice (111). Cycloheximide-tolerant dermatophytoids that grow (in any quantity whatsoever) from single, otherwise unproductive specimens should not be assumed to be causal simply because they share a genus name with dermatophyte species.

SUPERFICIAL MYCOSES

In the superficial mycoses, the causative fungi colonize the cornified layers of the epidermis or the suprafollicular portion of the hair. There is little tissue damage, and cellular response from the host generally is lacking. The diseases are largely cosmetic in impact, involving charges in the pigmentation of the skin (tinea versicolor or tinea nigra) or formation of nodules along the distal hair shaft (black piedra and white piedra).

In contrast to agents of the dermatophytoses, the etiologic agents are diverse and unrelated.

Tinea Versicolor (Pityriasis Versicolor)

Tinea versicolor is an infection of the stratum corneum caused by a group of closely similar lipophilic yeast species of the *Malassezia furfur* complex. Members of this complex infecting human skin were often treated in former times as a single species but were then shown by molecular, physiological, and serotyping studies to be separate (48, 50). The complex includes *M. furfur* (synonyms: *Pityrosporum furfur* and *Pityrosporum ovale* pro parte), *M. sympodialis*, *M. globosa* (probable synonym *Pityrosporum orbiculare*), *M. restricta*, *M. slooffiae*, *M. obtusa*, *M. dermatis*, *M. japonica*, and *M. yamatoensis* (48, 107). Some additional species have been reported for animals. In routine clinical reporting, referring to these organisms as members of the *M. furfur* complex is normally sufficient. *Malassezia pachydermatis*, which causes animal ear infections and occasional human iatrogenic fungemias, is not considered a member of the *M. furfur* complex and, if reported, is reported under its individual species name. It is easily distinguished from *M. furfur* complex members by its ability to grow on ordinary laboratory media such as Sabouraud agar (see comments on *Malassezia* culture, below). It is insignificant when grown from human skin except where investigations of catheter-related problems are involved.

Tinea versicolor lesions appear as scaly, discrete or concrescent, hypopigmented or hyperpigmented (fawn, yellow-brown, brown, or red) patches chiefly on the neck, torso, and limbs. The infection is largely cosmetic, becoming apparent when the skin fails to tan normally. The disease has a worldwide distribution: in tropical climates 30 to 35% of the population may be affected, while incidence in areas of temperate climate is much lower, with only 1.0 to 4.0% of the population affected. *M. furfur* and related yeasts are found on the normal skin and elicit disease only under conditions, local or systemic, that favor the overgrowth of the organism.

The *M. furfur* complex has been associated with folliculitis (11), obstructive dacryocystitis (95), systemic infections in patients receiving intralipid therapy (29), and seborrheic dermatitis, especially in patients with AIDS (46). Excellent reviews on human infections caused by *Malassezia* spp. and on the characteristics of the genus are available (13, 30, 51, 101). Additional information is also found in chapter 115 of this *Manual*.

Direct Examination

The fungi are observed readily when scrapings are mounted in 10% KOH plus ink (22), 25% NaOH plus 5% glycerin, calcofluor white, or Kane's formulation (glycerol, 10 ml; Tween 80, 10 ml; phenol, 2.5 g; methylene blue, 1.0 g; distilled water, 480 ml). In cases in which skin scrapings from unspecified body sites are examined, Kane's formulation has the advantage of vividly staining both fungi and the differential-diagnostic organisms causing erythrasma and pitted keratolysis. (These two bacterial infections, often confused with superficial mycosis, are mainly from intertriginous sites and foot soles, respectively.) Tinea versicolor is signaled in microscopy by the presence of "spaghetti and meatballs," i.e., short, septate, occasionally branching filaments 2.5 to

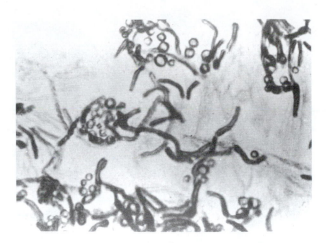

FIGURE 19 *Malassezia furfur* in skin scrapings from a lesion of tinea versicolor (Kane's stain). Magnification, ×1,000.

4 μm in diameter and of variable lengths intermingled with clusters of small, unicellular, oval, or round budding yeast cells (Fig. 19). The yeasts show the presence of a collarette between mother and daughter cells (budding is phialidic and unipolar) and average 4 μm (up to 8 μm) in size.

Isolation and Culture

Culture is not essential for identification unless the findings of direct microscopic examination are atypical or unless full species identification is desired for research purposes. Also, *M. furfur* complex members are part of the normal flora of the skin, and positive culture does not indicate infection. The species require exogenous lipid and do not grow on routine mycology media. If culture is desired, scrapings may be inoculated on Leeming-Notman medium, which uses whole milk as a major lipid source (74), on Dixon agar (25), or on modified Dixon agar, consisting of malt extract (3.6%), mycological peptone (Oxoid) (0.6%), desiccated ox bile (bile salts; Oxoid) (2%), Tween 40 (1%), glycerol (0.2%), oleic acid (0.2%), and agar (1.2%). Growth of the yeasts is slow; colonies are cream colored, glossy or rough, and raised (Fig. 20), later becoming dull, dry, and tan to brownish. Only budding yeast cells generally appear in culture (Fig. 21).

Tinea Nigra

Tinea nigra is characterized by the appearance, primarily on the palms of the hands and less commonly on the dorsa of the feet, of flat, sharply marginated, brownish black, non-scaly macules that may resemble melanoma (101).

The disease, almost always caused by *Hortaea werneckii* (*Phaeoannellomyces werneckii*, *Exophiala werneckii*, or *Cladosporium werneckii*), is most common in tropical areas (95) but has been contracted occasionally in coastal areas in and near the southeastern United States (120, 101). Cases diagnosed outside the area of endemicity have resulted mostly from travel to the American tropics or the Caribbean islands (95). *H. werneckii* is a member of the ascomycetous order Capnodiales (59) (see chapter 122).

Direct Microscopic Examination

Microscopic examination of skin scrapings in KOH or NaOH reveals numerous light brown, frequently branching septate filaments 1.5 to 5 μm in diameter (Fig. 18h); short, sinuous filaments; and budding cells, some septate.

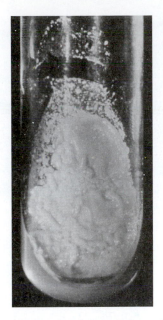

FIGURE 20 Culture of *Malassezia furfur* on Littman oxgall agar overlaid with olive oil.

Isolation

On SGA with or without antibiotics, *H. werneckii* grows slowly and usually appears within 2 to 3 weeks as moist, shiny olive to greenish black yeast-like colonies. The yeast-like cells are usually two-celled when reproductive and, instead of budding, produce new yeast cells from thick (up to 2 μm in diameter) distinctly annelled (multiply ringed as if wearing several bracelets) pegs. After 7 or more days, colonies may develop a fringe of thick, dark, conspicuously septate hyphae that also bear annelled fertile structures. These produce conidia that are indistinguishable from young yeast cells.

Black Piedra

Black piedra is a fungal infection of the scalp hair, less commonly of the beard or moustache, and rarely of axillary or pubic hairs. The disease is characterized by the presence of

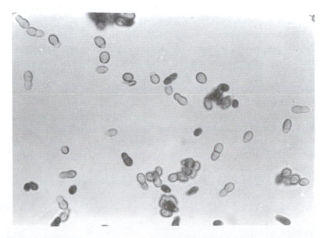

FIGURE 21 Microscopic appearance of *Malassezia furfur* yeast cells on Littman oxgall overlaid with olive oil. Magnification, ×400.

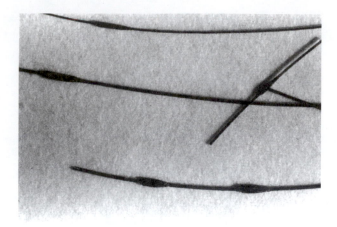

FIGURE 22 Black piedra nodules on scalp hair. NaOH mount. Magnification, ×100.

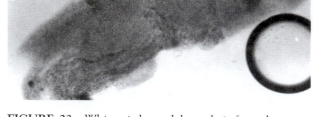

FIGURE 23 White piedra nodule on hair from the groin. Magnification, ×1,000.

discrete, hard, gritty, dark brown to black nodules adhering firmly to the hair shaft (Fig. 22). It is found mostly in tropical regions in Africa, Asia, and Central and South America. Humans as well as other primates are infected (40, 95, 101).

The etiologic agent in humans is *Piedraia hortae*, an ascomycete (order Dothideales) forming nodules that serve as ascostromata containing locules that harbor the asci and ascospores.

Direct Microscopic Examination

Hair fragments containing one or more black nodules are placed in 25% KOH or NaOH with 5% glycerol. The preparation is heated gently and carefully squashed so as not to break the coverslip, as the nodules are very hard. A squashed preparation of a mature nodule should reveal compact masses of dark, septate hyphae and round or oval asci containing 2 to 8 hyaline, aseptate banana-shaped (fusiform) ascospores that bear one or more appendages. The preparation should first be observed under the low-power objective to reveal the dark mass of compacted hyphae around the surface of the hair, and then examined under the high-power objective to observe the asci and ascospores.

Isolation, Culture, and Identification

When ascospores are seen in direct specimen microscopy, culture is unnecessary. Otherwise, SGA with chloramphenicol and SGA with chloramphenicol and cycloheximide may be used for isolation. Some reports have indicated that cycloheximide may be inhibitory; however, others have used this antibiotic successfully. SGA supplemented with chloramphenicol alone may be used for successful isolation.

Colonies are very slow growing, appear dark brown-to-black, are glabrous at first, and later are covered with short dark brown-to-black aerial mycelium. They tend to be heaped in the center with a flat periphery. Some colonies produce a reddish brown diffusible pigment on the agar. Microscopic examination reveals only highly septate dark hyphae and swollen intercalary cells. Conidia and ascospores are usually not found on routine mycological media.

White Piedra

White piedra is a fungal infection of the hair shaft characterized by the presence of soft white, yellowish, beige, or greenish nodules found chiefly on facial, axillary, or genital hairs (Fig. 23) and less commonly on scalp, eyebrows, and eyelashes. Nodules may be discrete or more often coalescent, forming an irregular transparent sheath.

The infection occurs sporadically in North America and Europe and more commonly in South America, Africa, and parts of Asia (95). Although white piedra is uncommon, genital white piedra is occasionally but regularly seen in certain populations (61, 101).

Microscopic examination of hairs containing the adherent nodules mounted in 10% KOH or 25% NaOH–5% glycerin and squashed under a coverslip will reveal intertwined hyaline septate hyphae, hyphae breaking up into oval or rectangular arthroconidia 2 to 4 μm in diameter (Fig. 24), occasional blastoconidia, and bacteria that may surround the nodule as a zooglea.

The isolates were formerly described as *Trichosporon beigelii* or *Trichosporon cutaneum* but are now correctly identified in most cases as *Trichosporon ovoides* (causes scalp hair white piedra), *Trichosporon inkin* (causes most cases of pubic white piedra), and *Trichosporon asahii* (34, 49). As with the M. *furfur* complex, these species form a complex of difficult-to-identify species whose distinction, except in demonstrated cases of piedra, is not known to have strong clinical implications in dermatologic mycology. They are

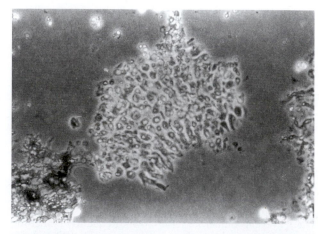

FIGURE 24 Arthroconidia from a crushed nodule of white piedra. Magnification, ×1,000.

also very common skin contaminants. Ordinarily, they may be reported for skin, hair, and nails of nonneutropenic patients simply as members of the genus *Trichosporon*, based on production of budding yeast cells, arthroconidia, and a positive urease test, unless a research-level identification of a proven etiologic agent is attempted. The causal agents of white piedra may be readily isolated on SGA with chloramphenicol or other isolation media containing antibacterial antibiotics. The isolation medium should not contain cycloheximide, since this drug is inhibitory to some of the species. Growth is rapid, yielding white to cream-colored colonies that exhibit a variety of colonial morphologies depending on the species. A description of the genus and characteristics of the species involved in white piedra are given in papers by Guého et al. (47, 49). More information about *Trichosporon* is found in chapter 115 of this *Manual*.

REFERENCES

1. **Abdel-Rahman, S. M., B. Preuett, and A. Gaedigk.** 2007. Multilocus genotyping identifies infections by multiple strains of *Trichophyton tonsurans. J. Clin. Microbiol.* **45:**1949–1953.
2. **Adams, B. B.** 2002. Tinea corporis gladiatorum. *J. Am. Acad. Dermatol.* **47:**286–290.
3. **Ajello, L.** 1960. Geographic distribution and prevalence of the dermatophytes. *Ann. N. Y. Acad. Sci.* **89:**30–38.
4. **Ajello, L.** 1974. Natural history of the dermatophytes and related fungi. *Mycopathol. Mycol. Appl.* **53:**93–110.
5. **Ajello, L. and L. K. Georg.** 1957. In vitro cultures for differentiating between atypical isolates of *Trichophyton mentagrophytes* and *Trichophyton rubrum. Mycopathol. Mycol. Appl.* **8:**3–7.
6. **Alsop, J., and A. P. Prior.** 1961. Ringworm infection in a cucumber greenhouse. *Br. Med. J.* **1:**1081–1083.
7. **Aly, R.** 1994. Culture media for growing dermatophytes. *J. Am. Acad. Dermatol.* **31:**S107–S108.
8. **Aly, R., R. J. Hay, A. Del Palacio, and R. Galimberti.** 2000. Epidemiology of tinea capitis. *Med. Mycol.* **38**(Suppl. 1):183–188.
9. **Arabatzis, M., L. E. Bruijnesteijn van Coppenraet, E. J. Kuijper, G. S. de Hoog, A. P. Lavrijsen, K. Templeton, E. M van der Raaij-Helmer, A. Velegraki, Y. Gräser, and R. C. Summerbell.** 2007. Diagnosis of common dermatophyte infections by a novel multiplex real-time polymerase chain reaction detection/identification scheme. *Br. J. Dermatol.* **157:**681–689.
10. **Araviysky, A. N., R. A. Araviysky, and G. A. Eschkov.** 1975. Deep generalized trichophytosis. *Mycopathologia* **56:**47–65.
11. **Back, O., J. Faergemann, and R. Hornquist.** 1985. *Pityrosporum* folliculitis: a common disease of the young and middle-aged. *J. Am. Acad. Dermatol.* **12:**56–61.
12. **Barson, W. J.** 1985. Granuloma and pseudogranuloma of the skin due to *Microsporum canis. Arch. Dermatol.* **121:**895–897.
13. **Batra, R., T. Boekhout, E. Guého, F. J. Cabanes, T. L. Dawson, Jr., and A. K. Gupta.** 2005. *Malassezia* Baillon, emerging clinical yeasts. *FEMS Yeast Res.* **5:**1101–1113.
14. **Beifuss, B., G. Bezold, P. Gottlöber, C. Borelli, J. Wagener, M. Schaller, and H. C. Korting.** 2011. Direct detection of five common dermatophyte species in clinical samples using a rapid and sensitive 24-h PCR-ELISA technique open to protocol transfer. *Mycoses* **54:**137–145.
15. **Bergmans, A. M., L. M. Schouls, M. van der Ent, A. Klaassen, N. Böhm, and R. G. Wintermans.** 2008. Validation of PCR-reverse line blot, a method for rapid detection and identification of nine dermatophyte species in nail, skin and hair samples. *Clin. Microbiol. Infect.* **14:**778–788.
16. **Bergmans, A. M., M. van der Ent, A. Klaassen, N. Böhm, G. I. Andriesse, and R. G. Wintermans.** 15 July 2009. Evaluation of a single-tube real-time PCR for detection and identification of 11 dermatophyte species in clinical material. *Clin. Microbiol. Infect.* **16:**704–710. [Epub ahead of print.]
17. **Bontems, O., P. M. Hauser, and M. Monod.** 2009. Evaluation of a polymerase chain reaction-restriction fragment length polymorphism assay for dermatophyte and nondermatophyte identification in onychomycosis. *Br. J. Dermatol.* **161:**791–796.
18. **Borelli, D.** 1962. Medios caseros para micologia. *Arch. Venez. Med. Trop. Parasitol. Med.* **4:**301–310.
19. **Brasch, J., and Y. Gräser.** 2005. *Trichophyton eboreum* sp. nov. isolated from human skin. *J. Clin. Microbiol.* **43:**5230–5237.
20. **Brillowska-Dabrowska, A., D. M. Saunte, and M. C. Arendrup.** 2007. Five-hour diagnosis of dermatophyte nail infections with specific detection of *Trichophyton rubrum. J. Clin. Microbiol.* **45:**1200–1204.
21. **Burnett, J.** 2003. *Fungal Populations & Species.* Oxford University Press, Oxford, United Kingdom.
22. **Cohen, M. M.** 1954. A simple procedure for staining tinea versicolor (*M. furfur*) with fountain pen ink. *J. Investig. Dermatol.* **22:**9–10.
23. **Conant, N. F.** 1936. Studies on the genus *Microsporum.* I. Cultural studies. *Arch. Dermatol.* **33:**665–683.
24. **Connole, M. D., H. Yamaguchi, D. Elad, A. Hasegawa, E. Segal, and J. M. Torres-Rodriguez.** 2000. Natural pathogens of laboratory animals and their effects on research. *Med. Mycol.* **38**(Suppl. 1):59–65.
25. **Crespo Erchiga, V., A. Ojeda Martos, A. Vera Casano, A. Crespo Erchiga, and F. Sanchez Fajardo.** 2000. *Malassezia globosa* as the causative agent of pityriasis versicolor. *Br. J. Dermatol.* **143:**799–803.
26. **Crous, P. W., B. Slippers, M. J. Wingfield, J. Rheeder, W. F. Marasas, A. J. Philips, A. Alves, T. Burgess, P. Barber, and J. Z. Groenewald.** 2006. Phylogenetic lineages in the Botryosphaeriaceae. *Stud. Mycol.* **55:**235–253.
27. **Currah, R. S.** 1985. Taxonomy of the Onygenales: Arthrodermataceae, Gymnoascaceae, Myxotrichaceae and Onygenaceae. *Mycotaxon* **24:**1–216.
28. **Daniel, C. R., III, L. A. Norton, and R. K. Scher.** 1992. The spectrum of nail disease in patients with human immunodeficiency virus infection. *J. Am. Acad. Dermatol.* **27:**93–97.
29. **Danker, W. M., S. A. Spector, J. Fierer, and C. E. Davis.** 1987. *Malassezia* fungemia in neonates and adults: complication of hyperalimentation. *Rev. Infect. Dis.* **9:**743–753.
30. **Dawson, T. L., Jr.** 2007. *Malassezia globosa* and *M. restricta*: breakthrough understanding of the etiology and treatment of dandruff and seborrheic dermatitis through whole-genome analysis. *J. Investig. Dermatol. Symp. Proc.* **12:**15–19.
31. **De Baere, T., R. C. Summerbell, B. Theelen, T. Boekhout, and M. Vaneechoutte.** 2010. Evaluation of internal transcribed spacer 2-RFLP analysis for the identification of dermatophytes. *J. Med. Microbiol.* **59:**48–54.
32. **Dei Cas, E., and A. Vernes.** 1986. Parasitic adaptation of pathogenic fungi to mammalian hosts. *Crit. Rev. Microbiol.* **13:**173–218.
33. **Demange, C., N. Contet-Audonneau, M. Kombila, M. Miegeville, M. Berthonneau, C. DeVroey, and G. Percebois.** 1992. *Microsporum gypseum* complex in man and animals. *J. Med. Vet. Mycol.* **30:**301–308.
34. **Douchet, C., M. Therizol-Ferly, M. Kombila, T. H. Duong, M. Gomez de Diaz, A. Barrabes, and D. Richard-Lenoble.** 1994. White piedra and *Trichosporon* species in equatorial Africa. III. Identification of *Trichosporon* species by slide agglutination test. *Mycoses* **37:**261–264.
35. **Fischer, J. B., and J. Kane.** 1974. The laboratory diagnosis of dermatophytosis complicated with *Candida albicans. Can. J. Microbiol.* **20:**167–182.
36. **Gaedigk, A., R. Gaedigk, and S. M. Abdel-Rahman.** 2003. Genetic heterogeneity in the rRNA gene locus of *Trichophyton tonsurans. J. Clin. Microbiol.* **41:**5478–5487.
37. **Garg, J., R. Tilak, S. Singh, A. K. Gulati, A. Garg, P. Prakash, and G. Nath.** 2007. Evaluation of pan-dermatophyte nested PCR in diagnosis of onychomycosis. *J. Clin. Microbiol.* **45:**3443–3445.
38. **Georg, L. K., and L. B. Camp.** 1957. Routine nutritional tests for the identification of dermatophytes. *J. Bacteriol.* **74:**113–121.

39. **Ghannoum, M. A., V. Chaturvedi, A. Espinel-Ingroff, M. A. Pfaller, M. G. Rinaldi, W. Lee-Yang, and D. W. Warnock.** 2004. Intra- and interlaboratory study of a method for testing the antifungal susceptibilities of dermatophytes. *J. Clin. Microbiol.* **42:**2977–2979.

40. **Gip, L.** 1994. Black piedra: the first case treated with terbinafine (Lamisil®). *Br. J. Dermatol.* **130**(Suppl. 43)**:**26–28.

41. **Gräser, Y., G. S. de Hoog, and A. F. A. Kuijpers.** 2000. Recent advances in the molecular taxonomy of dermatophytes, p. 17–21. *In* R. K. S. Kushwaha and J. Guarro (ed.), *Biology of Dermatophytes and Other Keratinophilic Fungi.* Revista Iberoamericana de Micología, Bilbao, Spain.

42. **Gräser, Y., J. Fröhlich, W. Presber, and S. de Hoog.** 2007. Microsatellite markers reveal geographic population differentiation in *Trichophyton rubrum. J. Med. Microbiol.* **56:**1058–1065.

43. **Gräser, Y., A. F. A. Kuijpers, W. Presber, and G. S. de Hoog.** 1999. Molecular taxonomy of *Trichophyton mentagrophytes* and *T. tonsurans. Med. Mycol.* **37:**315–330.

44. **Gräser, Y., A. F. A. Kuijpers, W. Presber, and G. S. de Hoog.** 2000. Molecular taxonomy of the *Trichophyton rubrum* complex. *J. Clin. Microbiol.* **38:**3329–3336.

45. **Gräser, Y., J. Scott, and R. Summerbell.** 2008. The new species concept in dermatophytes—a polyphasic approach. *Mycopathologia* **166:**239–256.

46. **Groisser, D., E. J. Bottone, and M. Lebwohl.** 1989. Association of *Pityrosporum orbiculare* (*Malassezia furfur*) with seborrheic dermatitis in patients with acquired immunodeficiency syndrome (AIDS). *J. Am. Acad. Dermatol.* **20:**770–773.

47. **Guého, E., G. S. de Hoog, and M. T. Smith.** 1992. Neotypification of the genus *Trichosporon. Antonie van Leeuwenhoek* **61:**285–288.

48. **Guého, E., G. Midgley, and J. Guillot.** 1996. The genus *Malassezia* with description of four new species. *Antonie van Leeuwenhoek* **69:**337–355.

49. **Guého, E., M. T. Smith, G. S. de Hoog, G. Billon-Grand, R. Christen, and W. H. Batenburg-van der Vegte.** 1992. Contributions to a revision of the genus *Trichosporon. Antonie van Leeuwenhoek* **61:**289–316.

50. **Guillot, J., S. Hadina, and E. Guého.** 2008. The genus *Malassezia:* old facts and new concepts. *Parassitologia* **50:**77–79.

51. **Gupta, A. K., R. Batra, R. Bluhm, T. Boekhout, and T. L. Dawson, Jr.** 2004. Skin diseases associated with *Malassezia* species. *J. Am. Acad. Dermatol.* **51:**785–798.

52. **Gupta, A. K., and J. Q. De Rosso.** 1999. Management of onychomycosis in children. *Postgrad. Med.* **1999**(Spec. No.)**:**31–37.

53. **Gupta, A. K., Y. Kohli, and R. C. Summerbell.** 2002. Exploratory study of single-copy genes and ribosomal intergenic spacers for distinction of dermatophytes. *Stud. Mycol.* **47:**87–96.

54. **Gupta, A. K., and Y. Kohli.** 2003. Evaluation of *in vitro* resistance in patients with onychomycosis who fail antifungal therapy. *Dermatology* **207:**375–380.

55. **Gupta, A. K., Y. Kohli, and R. C. Summerbell.** 2001. Variation in restriction fragment length polymorphisms among serial isolates from patients with *Trichophyton rubrum* infection. *J. Clin. Microbiol.* **39:**3260–3266.

56. **Gutzmer, R., S. Mommert, U. Küttler, T. Werfel, and A. Kapp.** 2004. Rapid identification and differentiation of fungal DNA in dermatological specimens by LightCycler PCR. *J. Med. Microbiol.* **53:**1207–1214.

57. **Head, E. S., J. C. Henry, and E. M. MacDonald.** 1984. The cotton swab technic for the culture of dermatophyte infections: its efficacy and merit. *J. Am. Acad. Dermatol.* **11:**797–801.

58. **Hirose, N., Y. Shiraki, M. Hiruma, and H. Ogawa.** 2005. An investigation of *Trichophyton tonsurans* infection in university students participating in sports clubs. *Nippon Ishinkin Gakkai Zasshi* (Jpn. J. Med. Mycol.) **46:**119–123.

59. **Holker, U., J. Bend, R. Pracht, L. Tetsch, T. Muller, M. Hofer, and G. S. de Hoog.** 2004. *Hortaea acidophila,* a new acid-tolerant black yeast from lignite. *Antonie Van Leeuwenhoek* **86:**287–294.

60. **Jackson, C. J., R. C. Barton, S. L. Kelly and E. G. V. Evans.** 2000. Strain identification of *Trichophyton rubrum* by specific amplification of subrepeat elements in the ribosomal DNA nontranscribed spacer. *J. Clin. Microbiol.* **38:**4527–4534.

61. **Kalter, D. C., J. A. Tschen, P. L. Cernoch, M. E. McBride, J. Sperber, S. Bruce, and J. E. Wolf, Jr.** 1986. Genital white piedra: epidemiology, microbiology, and therapy. *J. Am. Acad. Dermatol.* **14:**982–993.

62. **Kaminski, G. W.** 1985. The routine use of modified Borelli's lactrimel (MBLA). *Mycopathologia* **91:**57–59.

63. **Kane, J., and J. B. Fischer.** 1975. The effect of sodium chloride on the growth and morphology of dermatophytes and some other keratolytic fungi. *Can. J. Microbiol.* **21:**742–749.

64. **Kane, J., and J. B. Fischer.** 1976. The differentiation of *Trichophyton rubrum* from *T. mentagrophytes* by use of Christensen's urea broth. *Can. J. Microbiol.* **17:**911–913.

65. **Kane, J., L. Sigler, and R. C. Summerbell.** 1987. Improved procedures for differentiating *Microsporum persicolor* from *Trichophyton mentagrophytes. J. Clin. Microbiol.* **25:**2449–2452.

66. **Kane, J., R. C. Summerbell, L. Sigler, S. Krajden, and G. Land.** 1997. *Laboratory Handbook of Dermatophytes and Other Filamentous Fungi from Skin, Hair and Nails.* Star Publishing Co., Belmont, CA.

67. **Kardjeva, V., R. C. Summerbell, T. Kantardjiev, D. Devliotou-Panagiotidou, E. Sotiriou, and Y. Gräser.** 2006. Forty-eight-hour diagnosis of onychomycosis with subtyping of *Trichophyton rubrum* strains. *J. Clin. Microbiol.* **44:**1419–1427.

68. **King, R. D., H. A. Khan, J. C. Foye, J. H. Greenberg, and H. E. Jones.** 1975. Transferrin, iron and dermatophytes. Serum dermatophyte inhibitory component definitively identified as unsaturated transferrin. *J. Lab. Clin. Med.* **86:**204–212.

69. **Koga, T.** 2003. Immune response in dermatophytosis. *Nippon Ishinkin Gakkai Zasshi* (Jpn. J. Med. Mycol.) **44:**273–275.

70. **Koga, T., H. Duan, K. Urabe and M. Furue.** 2001. Immunohistochemical detection of interferon-gamma-producing cells in dermatophytosis. *Eur. J. Dermatol.* **11:**105–107.

71. **Lacroix, C., M. Baspeyras, P. de la Salmonière, M. Benderdouche, B. Couprie, I. Accoceberry, F. X. Weill, F. Derouin, and M. Feuilhade de Chauvin.** 2002. Tinea pedis in European marathon runners. *J. Eur. Acad. Dermatol. Venereol.* **16:**139–142.

72. **Lawry M. A., E. Haneke, K. Strobeck, S. Martin, B. Zimmer and P. S. Romano.** 2000. Methods for diagnosing onychomycosis. *Arch. Dermatol.* **136:**1112–1116.

73. **Lawson, G. T. N., and W. J. McLeod.** 1957. *Microsporum canis*—an intensive outbreak. *Br. Med. J.* **2:**1159–1160.

74. **Leeming, J. and F. Notman.** 1987. Improved methods for isolation and enumeration of *Malassezia furfur* from human skin. *J. Clin. Microbiol.* **25:**2017–2019.

75. **Levy, L. A.** 1997. Epidemiology of onychomycosis in special-risk populations. *J. Am. Podiatr. Med. Assoc.* **87:**546–550.

76. **Mackenzie, D. W. R.** 1963. "Hairbrush diagnosis" in detection and eradication of nonfluorescent scalp ringworm. *Br. Med. J.* **2:**363–365.

77. **McGinnis, M. R., J. H. Rex, S. Arikan, and L. Rodrigues.** Examination of specimens page, Lab procedures section, Doctor Fungus website. http://www.doctorfungus.org/thelabor/sec5.pdf.

78. **Merz, W. G., C. L. Berger, and M. Silva-Hutner.** 1970. Media with pH indicators for the isolation of dermatophytes. *Arch. Dermatol.* **102:**545–547.

79. **Mochizuki, T., H. Ishizaki, R. C. Barton, M. K. Moore, C. J. Jackson, S. L. Kelly, and E. G. Evans.** 2003. Restriction fragment length polymorphism analysis of ribosomal DNA intergenic regions is useful for differentiating strains of *Trichophyton mentagrophytes. J. Clin. Microbiol.* **41:**4583–4588.

80. **Mochizuki, T., S. Watanabe, and M. Uehara.** 1996. Genetic homogeneity of *Trichophyton mentagrophytes* var. *interdigitale* isolated from geographically distant regions. *J. Med. Vet. Mycol.* **34:**139–143.

81. **Moriello, K. A., and D. J. DeBoer.** 1991. Fungal flora of the haircoat of cats with and without dermatophytosis. *J. Med. Vet. Mycol.* **29:**285–292.

82. **Nagao, K., T. Sugita, T. Ouchi, and T. Nishikawa.** 2005. Identification of *Trichophyton rubrum* by nested PCR analysis from paraffin embedded specimen in trichophytia profunda acuta of the glabrous skin. *Nippon Ishinkin Gakkai Zasshi (Jpn. J. Med. Mycol.)* **46:**129–132.

83. **National Committee for Clinical Laboratory Standards.** 2002. *Reference Method for Broth Dilution Antifungal Susceptibility Testing of Filamentous Fungi,* 2nd ed. Approved Standard. Document M38-A2. National Committee for Clinical Laboratory Standards, Wayne, PA.

84. **Ogawa, H., R. C. Summerbell, K. V. Clemons, P. G. Sohnle, T. Koga, R. Tsuboi, A. Rashid, D. A. Stevens, and Y.-P. Ran.** 1998. Dermatophytes and host defense in cutaneous mycoses. *Med. Mycol.* **36**(Suppl. 1)**:**166–173.

85. **Ohst, T., G. S. de Hoog, W. Presber, V. Stavrakieva, and Y. Gräser.** 2004. Origins of microsatellite diversity in the *Trichophyton rubrum-T. violaceum* clade (dermatophytes). *J. Clin. Microbiol.* **42:**4444–4448.

86. **Padhye, A. A., F. Blank, P. J. Koblenzer, S. Spatz, and L. Ajello.** 1973. *Microsporum persicolor* infection in the United States. *Arch. Dermatol.* **108:**561–562.

87. **Padhye, A. A., and J. Carmichael.** 1971. The genus *Arthroderma* Berkeley. *Can. J. Bot.* **49:**1525–1540.

88. **Padhye, A. A., I. Weitzman, and E. Domenech.** 1994. An unusual variant of *Trichophyton tonsurans* var. *sulfureum. J. Med. Vet. Mycol.* **32:**147–150.

89. **Padhye, A. A., C. N. Young, and L. Ajello.** 1980. Hair perforation as a diagnostic criterion in the identification of *Epidermophyton, Microsporum* and *Trichophyton* species, p. 115–120. *In Superficial Cutaneous and Subcutaneous Infections.* Scientific publication no. 396. Pan American Health Organization, Washington, DC.

90. **Probst, S., G. S. de Hoog, and Y. Gräser.** 2002. Development of DNA markers to explore host shifts in dermatophytes. *Stud. Mycol.* **47:**57–74.

91. **Pryce, T. M., S. Palladino, I. D. Kay, and G. W. Coombs.** 2003. Rapid identification of fungi by sequencing the ITS1 and ITS2 regions using an automated capillary electrophoresis system. *Med. Mycol.* **41:**369–381.

92. **Rad, M. M., C. Jackson, R. C. Barton, and E. G. Evans.** 2005. Single strains of *Trichophyton rubrum* in cases of tinea pedis. *J. Med. Microbiol.* **54:**725–726.

93. **Richardson, M. D.** 1990. Diagnosis and pathogenesis of dermatophyte infections. *Br. J. Clin. Pract.* **71**(Suppl.)**:**98–102.

94. **Rippon, J. W.** 1985. The changing epidemiology and emerging patterns of dermatophyte species, p. 209–234. *In* M. R. McGinnis (ed.), *Current Topics in Medical Mycology.* Springer-Verlag, New York, NY.

95. **Rippon, J. W.** 1988. *Medical Mycology: the Pathogenic Fungi and the Pathogenic Actinomycetes,* 3rd ed., p. 154–168. The W. B. Saunders Co., Philadelphia, PA.

96. **Rippon, J. W.** 1988. *Medical Mycology: the Pathogenic Fungi and the Pathogenic Actinomycetes,* 3rd ed., p. 169–275. The W. B. Saunders Co., Philadelphia, PA.

97. **Robinson, B. E., and A. A. Padhye.** 1988. Collection transport and processing of clinical specimens, p. 11–32. *In* B. B. Wentworth (ed.), *Diagnostic Procedures for Mycotic and Parasitic Infections,* 7th ed. American Public Health Association, Inc., Washington, DC.

98. **Rosenthal, S. A.** 1974. The epidemiology of tinea pedis, p. 515–526. *In* H. M. Robinson, Jr. (ed.), *The Diagnosis and Treatment of Fungal Infections.* Charles C Thomas, Springfield, IL.

99. **Rosenthal, S. A., and H. Sokolsky.** 1965. Enzymatic studies with pathogenic fungi. *Dermatol. Int.* **4:**72–79.

100. **Salkin, I. F.** 1973. Dermatophyte test medium: evaluation with nondermatophytic pathogens. *Appl. Microbiol.* **26:**134–137.

101. **Schwartz, R. A.** 2004. Superficial fungal infections. *Lancet* **364:**1173–1182.

102. **Sequeira, H., J. Cabrita, C. DeVroey, and C. Wuytack-Raes.** 1991. Contributions to our knowledge of *Trichophyton megninii. J. Med. Vet. Mycol.* **29:**417–418.

103. **Shah, P. C., S. Krajden, J. Kane, and R. C. Summerbell.** 1988. Tinea corporis caused by *Microsporum canis:* report of a nosocomial outbreak. *Eur. J. Epidemiol.* **4:**33–38.

104. **Shehata, A. S., P. K. Mukherjee, H. N. Aboulatta, A. I. el-Akhras, S. H. Abbadi, and M. A. Ghannoum.** 2008. Single-step PCR using (GACA)4 primer: utility for rapid identification of dermatophyte species and strains. *J. Clin. Microbiol.* **46:**2641–2645.

105. **Squeo, R. F., R. Beer, D. Silvers, I. Weitzman, and M. Grossman.** 1998. Invasive *Trichophyton rubrum* resembling blastomycosis infection in the immunocompromised host. *J. Am. Acad. Dermatol.* **39:**379–380.

106. **Suarez, S. M., D. N. Silvers. R. K. Scher, H. H. Pearlstein, and R. Auerbach.** 1991. Histologic evaluation of nail clippings for diagnosing onychomycosis. *Arch. Dermatol.* **127:**1517–1519.

107. **Sugita, T., M. Tajima, M. Takashima, M. Amaya, M. Saito, R. Tsuboi, and A. Nishikawa.** 2004. A new yeast, *Malassezia yamatoensis,* isolated from a patient with seborrheic dermatitis, and its distribution in patients and healthy subjects. *Microbiol. Immunol.* **48:**579–583.

108. **Summerbell, R. C.** 1987. *Trichophyton kanei,* sp. nov. a new anthropophilic dermatophyte. *Mycotaxon* **28:**509–523.

109. **Summerbell, R. C.** 2000. Form and function in the evolution of dermatophytes, p. 30–43. *In* R. K. S. Kushwaha and J. Guarro (ed.), *Biology of Dermatophytes and Other Keratinophilic Fungi.* Revista Iberoamericana de Micologia, Bilbao, Spain.

110. **Summerbell, R. C.** 2002. What is the evolutionary and taxonomic status of asexual lineages in the dermatophytes? *Stud. Mycol.* **47:**97–101.

111. **Summerbell, R. C., E. Cooper, U. Bunn, F. Jamieson, and A. K. Gupta.** 2005. Onychomycosis: a critical study of techniques and criteria for confirming the etiologic significance of nondermatophytes. *Med. Mycol.* **43:**39–59.

112. **Summerbell, R. C., A. Li, and R. Haugland.** 1997. What constitutes a functional species in the asexual dermatophytes? *Microbiol. Cult. Coll.* **13:**29–37.

113. **Summerbell, R. C., M. K. Moore, M. Starink-Willemse, and A. Van Iperen.** 2007. ITS barcodes for *Trichophyton tonsurans* and *T. equinum. Med. Mycol.* **45:**193–200.

114. **Summerbell, R. C., S. A. Rosenthal, and J. Kane.** 1988. Rapid method for differentiation of *Trichophyton rubrum, Trichophyton mentagrophytes,* and related dermatophyte species. *J. Clin. Microbiol.* **26:**2279–2282.

115. **Summerbell, R. C., I. Weitzman, and A. Padhye.** 2002. The *Trichophyton mentagrophytes* complex: biological species and mating type prevalences of North American isolates, and a review of the worldwide distribution and host associations of species and mating types. *Stud. Mycol.* **47:**75–86.

116. **Taplin, D.** 1965. The use of gentamicin in mycology. *J. Investig. Dermatol.* **45:**549–550.

117. **Taplin, D., N. Zaias, G. Rebell, and H. Blank.** 1969. Isolation and recognition of dermatophytes on a new medium (DTM). *Arch. Dermatol.* **99:**203–209.

118. **Tosti, A., R. Baran, B. M. Piraccini, and P. A. Fanti.** 1999. "Endonyx" onychomycosis: a new modality of nail invasion by dermatophytes. *Acta Derm. Venereol.* **79:**52–53.

119. **Uchida, T., K. Makimura, K. Ishihara, H. Goto, Y. Tajiri, M. Okuma, R. Fujisaki, K. Uchida, S. Abe, and M. Iijima.** 2009. Comparative study of direct polymerase chain reaction, microscopic examination and culture-based morphological methods for detection and identification of dermatophytes in nail and skin samples. *J. Dermatol.* **36:**202–208.

120. **Van Velsor, H., and H. Singletary.** 1964. Tinea nigra palmaris. *Arch. Dermatol.* **90:**59–61.

121. **Vermout, S., J. Tabart, A. Baldo, A. Mathy, B. Losson, and B. Mignon.** 2008. Pathogenesis of dermatophytosis. *Mycopathologia* **166:**267–275.

122. **Weeks, R. J., and A. A. Padhye.** 1982. A mounting medium for permanent preparations of micro-fungi. *Mykosen* **25:**702–704.

123. **Weitzman, I., M. R. McGinnis, A. A. Padhye, and L. Ajello.** 1986. The genus *Arthroderma* and its later synonym *Nannizzia. Mycotaxon* **25:**505–518.

124. **Weitzman, L., and S. A. Rosenthal.** 1984. Studies in the differentiation between *Microsporum ferrugineum* Ota and *Trichophyton soudanense* Joyeaux. *Mycopathologia* **84:**95–101.

125. **Weitzman, I., S. A. Rosenthal, and M. Silva-Hutner.** 1988. Superficial and cutaneous infections caused by molds: dermatomycoses, p. 33–97. *In* B. B. Wentworth (ed.), *Diagnostic Procedures for Mycotic and Parasitic Infections*, 7th ed. American Public Health Association, Inc., Washington, DC.

126. **Weitzman, I., and R. C. Summerbell.** 1995. The dermatophytes. *Clin. Microbiol. Rev.* **8:**240–259.

127. **West, B. C., and K. J. Kwon-Chung.** 1980. Mycetoma caused by *Microsporum audouinii. Am. J. Clin. Pathol.* **73:**447–454.

128. **Woodgyer, A.** 2004. The curious adventures of *Trichophyton equinum* in the realm of molecular biology: a modern fairy tale. *Med. Mycol.* **42:**397–403.

129. **Yazdanparast, A., C. J. Jackson, R. C. Barton, and E. G. Evans.** 2003. Molecular strain typing of *Trichophyton rubrum* indicates multiple strain involvement in onychomycosis. *Br. J. Dermatol.* **148:**51–54.

130. **Zaias, N., and G. Rebell.** 2003. Clinical and mycological status of the *Trichophyton mentagrophytes* (*T. interdigitale*) syndrome of chronic dermatophytosis of the skin and nails. *Int. J. Dermatol.* **42:**779–788.

131. **Zaias, N., A. Tosti, G. Rebell, R. Morelli, F. Bardazzi, H. Bieley, M. Zaiac, B. Glick, B. Paley, M. Allevato, and R. Baran.** 1996. Autosomal dominant pattern of distal subungual onychomycosis caused by *Trichophyton rubrum. J. Am. Acad. Dermatol.* **34:**302–304.

Bipolaris, Exophiala, Scedosporium, Sporothrix, and Other Melanized Fungi*

JOSEP GUARRO AND G. SYBREN DE HOOG

122

This chapter covers most of the agents of phaeohyphomycosis, chromoblastomycosis, and sporotrichosis, as well as a number of agents of superficial and cutaneous disease. Hyaline fungal agents and members of the Sordariales (*Chaetomium* and *Achaetomium*) are discussed in chapter 118. Agents causing mycetoma are covered in chapter 123. The genera discussed in this chapter belong to the ascomycetous orders Botryosphaeriales (*Lasiodiplodia* and *Neoscytalidium*), Chaetothyriales (*Cladophialophora, Exophiala, Fonsecaea, Ochroconis, Phialophora,* and *Rhinocladiella*), Calosphaeriales (*Phaeoacremonium* and *Pleurostomophora*; the genus *Phialemonium* is discussed in chapter 118), Dothideales (*Aureobasidium* and *Hormonema*), Microascales (*Scedosporium*), Ophiostomatales (*Sporothrix*), and Pleosporales (*Alternaria, Bipolaris, Curvularia,* and *Exserohilum*). In this chapter, the genera are treated according to their ordinal relationships (Table 1). Definitions of mycological terms are provided in chapter 111.

The term dematiaceous applies to fungi with black (containing melanin) hyphae in general (57), but it has been recommended in medical mycology to reserve this term for the rapidly growing members of Pleosporales only (38), as these are very different from Chaetothyriales in all respects. Also, the term phaeoid indicates brown hyphae; "phaeohyphomycosis" is an umbrella term for infection caused by moulds that display brownish yeastlike cells, pseudohyphae, or hyphae or a combination of these forms in host tissue. "Black yeasts and relatives" is preferably used to indicate members of Chaetothyriales and Dothideales only (38). The black yeasts are not a formal taxonomic group, but the term is applied to a wide range of unrelated ascomycetous and basidiomycetous fungi that are able to produce budding cells at some stage in their life cycle.

Pleoanamorphism (multiple morphological forms) is particularly striking in members of the black yeasts and in the genus *Scedosporium*. These fungi are frequently seen in the clinical laboratory to produce more than one asexual form of propagation (anamorphs), which may bear separate names. When a single fungus produces more than one anamorph, the term synanamorph is used to designate any of the concurrently existing forms. In addition, some isolates of some species of *Scedosporium* have the ability to produce a sexual form (teleomorph), characterized by the formation of fruiting bodies with meiotic ascospores. In each organism only a single teleomorph can be produced. The fungus involving all its forms of propagation is preferably referred to by its teleomorph name.

TAXONOMY AND DESCRIPTION OF THE AGENTS

Botryosphaeriales

Lasiodiplodia

Lasiodiplodia is a coelomycete genus characterized by spherical fruit bodies filled with asexual conidia. The conidia initially are ellipsoidal and hyaline but gradually become brown and develop a median septum at maturation. *Lasiodiplodia theobromae* (Fig. 1) is the only species involved in human infection.

Neoscytalidium

Neoscytalidium dimidiatum (formerly known as *Scytalidium dimidiatum*) is a plant pathogen that produces arthroconidia in culture, and some isolates also produce pycnidia (flask-shaped structures containing conidiogenous cells) under appropriate growth conditions. The coelomycetous synanamorph has been given the separate name *Nattrassia mangiferae*, previously known as *Hendersonula toruloidea*. However, molecular studies have demonstrated that *N. dimidiatum* and *N. mangiferae* are two different species and that the latter, which is not pathogenic to humans, must be accommodated in the recently described genus *Neofusicoccum* (35).

Inside multilocular fruit bodies hyaline, ellipsoidal conidia develop, which in part become brownish and have one or two septa. In culture, usually only a rapidly growing, jet black, floccose anamorph with dark arthroconidia (*Neoscytalidium dimidiatum* [Fig. 1]) is seen; the pycnidia are only produced after 2 months' growth on a moistened plant leaf. Melaninless mutants (140), which also show reduced conidiation, were until recently referred to as *Scytalidium hyalinum*. The fungus is a common plant pathogen in the tropics.

Calosphaeriales

Recently, some melanized phialidic fungi were segregated from *Phialophora* on molecular grounds; these now constitute small islands of clinical significance in the order Calosphaeriales, which otherwise contains plant-associated

*This chapter contains information presented in chapter 125 by G. Sybren de Hoog and Roxana G. Vitale in the ninth edition of this *Manual*.

TABLE 1 Overview of the clinically most relevant species and their attribution to the ordinal level

Order, genus, and species	Synanamorph	Teleomorph	Obsolete name(s)
Botryosphaeriales			
Lasiodiplodia theobromae		Botryosphaeria theobromae	Botryodiplodia theobromae
Neoscytalidium dimidiatum			Nattrassia mangiferae, Scytalidium hyalinum, Hendersonula toruloidea, Scytalidium dimidiatum
Calosphaeriales			
Phaeoacremonium			
alvesii			
griseobrunneum			
krajdenii			
parasiticum			Phialophora parasitica
rubrigenum			
venezuelense			
Phialemonium			
curvatum			
obovatum			
Pleurostomophora			
repens			Phialophora repens
richardsiae			Phialophora richardsiae
Capnodiales			
Cladosporium			
cladosporioides			
oxysporum			
Hortaea werneckii			Exophiala werneckii, Phaeoannellomyces werneckii
Chaetothyriales			
Cladophialophora			
arxii			
bantiana			Xylohypha bantiana, Cladosporium trichoides
boppii			
carrionii	Unnamed Phialophora		
devriesii			
emmonsii			
modesta			
mycetomatis			
samoënsis			
saturnica			
Coniosporium epidermidis			
Cyphellophora			
laciniata			Pseudomicrodochium suttonii, Pseudomicrodochium fusarioides
pluriseptata			
Exophiala			
attenuata			
bergeri			
dermatitidis	Unnamed Phialophora		Wangiella dermatitidis
jeanselmei			
oligosperma			
phaeomuriformis	Sarcinomyces phaeomuriformis		
spinifera	Unnamed Phialophora		
Fonsecaea			
monophora			
pedrosoi	Unnamed Phialophora		Fonsecaea compacta
Ochroconis gallopava			Dactylaria gallopava, D. constricta var. gallopava
Phialophora			
americana		Capronia semiimmersa	
europaea			
verrucosa			
Rhinocladiella			
mackenziei			Ramichloridium mackenziei
aquaspersa			
similis	Unnamed Exophiala		
Dothideales			
Aureobasidium pullulans		Discosphaerina fulvida	
Hormonema dematioides		Sydowia polyspora	

(Continued on next page)

TABLE 1 (Continued)

Order, genus, and species	Synanamorph	Teleomorph	Obsolete name(s)
Microascales			
Scedosporium			
apiospermum	Unnamed *Graphium*	*Pseudallescheria apiosperma*	
aurantiacum	Unnamed *Graphium*		
boydii	Unnamed *Graphium*	*Pseudallescheria boydii*	
prolificans			*Scedosporium inflatum*
Ophiostomatales			
Sporothrix			
brasiliensis			
globosa			
luriei			
schenckii			
Pleosporales			
Alternaria			
alternata			*Alternaria tenuissima*
infectoria		*Lewia infectoria*	
Bipolaris			
australiensis		*Cochliobolus australiensis*	*Drechslera australiensis*
hawaiiensis		*Cochliobolus hawaiiensis*	*Drechslera hawaiiensis, Dissitimurus exedrus*
spicifera		*Cochliobolus spicifera*	*Drechslera spicifera*
Curvularia			
geniculata		*Cochliobolus geniculatus*	
lunata		*Cochliobolus lunatus*	
Exserohilum rostratum		*Setosphaeria rostrata*	*Exserohilum longirostratum, Exserohilum macginnisii*
Sordariales			
Achaetomium strumarium			*Chaetomium strumarium*
Chaetomium			
globosum			
perlucidum			

moulds. Infections are mostly of traumatic nature and are supposed to originate directly from the woody plant material of the fungal habitat. *Phialemonium* species (see chapter 118) are also found in this order.

Phaeoacremonium

Phaeoacremonium (34) is morphologically characterized by slender, tubular and often tapering or inflated, brown phialides. Hyaline, slimy conidia are produced through inconspicuous collarettes. Six species are known from opportunistic infections in humans (Table 1), *Phaeoacremonium parasiticum* (Fig. 2) being the most common.

Pleurostomophora

Pleurostomophora is a genus of mainly wood-inhabiting fungi. Hyphae are dark and bear pale, tapering phialides that may be single or aggregated in dense brushes; hyaline, slimy conidia are produced through small or large collarettes. *Pleurostomophora repens*, until recently known as *Phialophora repens*, was occasionally reported from subcutaneous infections in humans. The second species of the genus involved also in human infections is *Pleurostomophora richardsiae* (Fig. 2) (syn. *Phialophora richardsiae*), a soft-rot fungus on wood.

Capnodiales

Cladosporium

Species of *Cladosporium*, especially *Cladosporium cladosporioides* (Fig. 3) and *C. oxysporum*, are extremely common contaminants in the clinical laboratory but have also been described as occasional human pathogens.

Hortaea

Members of the genus *Hortaea* have rather wide hyphae which become profusely septate during growth of the fungus, and they have annellidic conidiogenesis from broad scars. The halophilic species *H. werneckii* (Fig. 1) lives in evaporation ponds at the subtropical seashore and causes superficial infections.

Chaetothyriales

The rather small order Chaetothyriales is clinically highly relevant, because about half of the species known to date are able to cause infections in humans.

Cladophialophora

Catenate (in chains), dry conidia and an absence of differentiated conidiophores characterize *Cladophialophora*. This genus contains 10 pathogenic species (Table 1), 7 of which are almost exclusively known from humans and other warm-blooded animals. The most significant species are *Cladophialophora bantiana* and *C. carrionii*. *C. bantiana*, a remarkable neurotropic mould, is recognizable by very long, coherent, poorly branched conidial chains and by an ability to grow at 40°C (Fig. 2; see also Fig. 5). It has a characteristic 558-bp intron at position 1768 of the small-subunit (SSU) ribosomal operon (67). *C. carrionii* is a common agent of chromoblastomycosis, with small conidia in profusely branched chains.

Coniosporium

Although most species of *Coniosporium* have been described from rock and wood, recently *Coniosporium epidermidis* was recovered from human infections (101).

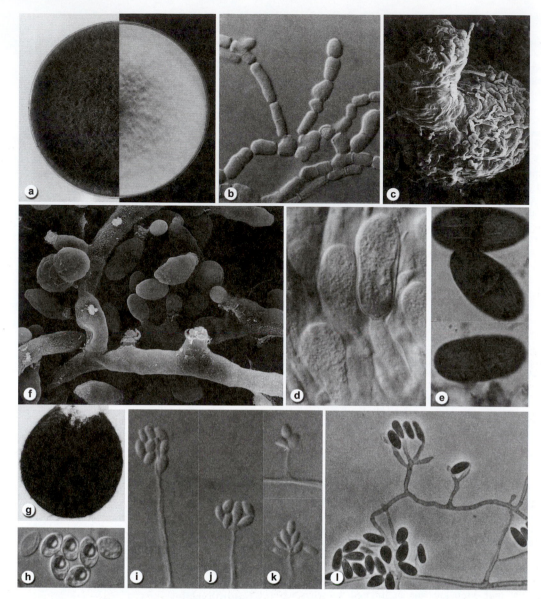

FIGURE 1 (a and b) *Neoscytalidium dimidiatum*; (c to e) *Lasiodiplodia theobromae*; (f) *Hortaea werneckii*; (g and h) *Pseudallescheria boydii*; (i to l) *Scedosporium boydii*. Reproduced from reference 38.

Cyphellophora

Cyphellophora is a rare group of infective agents characterized by slender, curved, mostly 1–3-septate conidia. Cultures are evenly melanized and show limited expansion growth; budding cells are absent. Conidia are produced from poorly developed collarettes alongside the hyphae. *Cyphellophora laciniata*, also known under the generic name *Pseudomicrodochium*, and *C. pluriseptata* (Fig. 2) are rare agents of mycoses.

Exophiala

Exophiala is the main genus of clinically relevant black yeasts. Strains show high degrees of morphological diversity. Most isolates initially grow in a yeast form that is succeeded by a hyphal anamorph. As a result, colonies are moist and slimy at first, becoming velvety to woolly with age. The process of conidium production is annellidic, from narrow, inconspicuous scars or extensions. Occasionally a very slowly growing, meristematic morphology ("*Sarcinomyces*") is preponderant.

Fresh isolates or strains cultivated on nutritionally deficient media frequently produce conidia in chains (43) and may produce scattered or compacted phialides with huge collarettes (44). The most frequently identified species are *Exophiala dermatitidis* (Fig. 2) and *E. jeanselmei*. The latter has recently been subdivided into a number of taxa on molecular grounds (45, 167). *E. oligosperma* is morphologically distinguished from *E. jeanselmei* only by subtle differences such as the presence of short and irregular annellated zones in the former, which are pronounced and tapering in the latter. *E. dermatitidis* is recognizable morphologically by phialides without collarettes, which are wide, scar-like, very short annellated zones. In addition, growth at 40°C and the inability to assimilate nitrate are characteristic (123). The related species *E. phaeomuriformis* differs by having a growth maximum at 38°C (112). The less frequent species *E. spinifera* can be recognized by the presence of large, stiff conidiophores. Recently a similar species with reduced conidiogenous cells, *E. attenuata*, was described (167).

Fonsecaea

The two species known in the genus *Fonsecaea*, characterized by conidia produced in chains of maximally four, are both human pathogens. In culture, *Fonsecaea* species mostly have one morphological form, but they may produce additional phialides with collarettes releasing balls of one-celled conidia. No budding cells are produced on routine media. *Fonsecaea pedrosoi* (Fig. 2; including the mutant *F. compacta*) is one of the etiologic agents of human chromoblastomycosis. The second species, *F. monophora* (37), is morphologically indistinguishable.

Ochroconis

The phylogenetic position of the genus *Ochroconis* is unclear. All species have rust brown to olivaceous colonies and produce 1- to 3-septate conidia from small, open denticles inserted in low numbers on sympodial cells. *O. gallopava* (Fig. 3) has hyaline, clavate conidia and grows well at 40°C.

Phialophora

When phialides are the only form of propagation in chaetothyrialean fungi, the generic name *Phialophora* is applied.

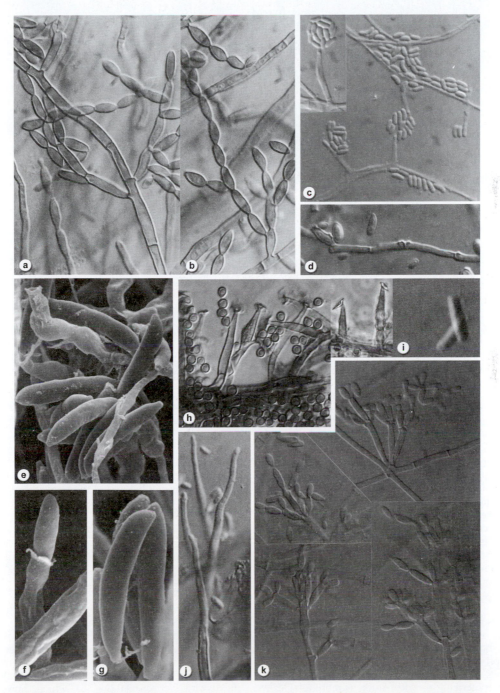

FIGURE 2 (a and b) *Cladophialophora bantiana*; (c) *Phialemonium curvatum*; (d) *Exophiala dermatitidis*; (e to g) *Cyphellophora pluriseptata*; (h and i) *Pleurostomophora richardsiae*; (j) *Phaeoacremonium parasiticum*; (k) various pictures of *Fonsecaea pedrosoi*. Reproduced from reference 38.

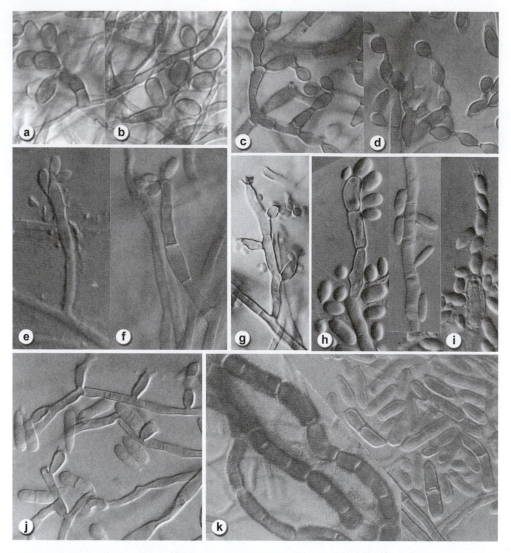

FIGURE 3 (a and b) *Rhinocladiella mackenziei*; (c and d) *Cladosporium cladosporioides*; (e and f) *Rhinocladiella aquaspersa*; (g) *Phialophora verrucosa*; (h and i) *Aureobasidium pullulans*; (j) *Ochroconis gallopava*; (k) *Hormonema dematioides*. Reproduced from reference 38.

Dematiaceous phialidic fungi belonging to other orders are now classified in genera such as *Cadophora*, *Phaeoacremonium*, and *Pleurostomophora* (66). No budding cells are produced in *Phialophora*. *Phialophora verrucosa*, with darkened, funnel-shaped collarettes (Fig. 3), is one of the commonest species of this genus. *P. americana* differs mainly by having vase-shaped collarettes (46). Given the close molecular similarity, there is no consensus as to whether *P. verrucosa* and *P. americana* comprise two species or one (46, 172).

Rhinocladiella

Rhinocladiella is morphologically characterized by pale brown conidiophores bearing noncatenate conidia on denticles and occasionally shows exophiala-like budding cells in culture (6). It comprises three pathogenic species, *Rhinocladiella mackenziei* (Fig. 3), *R. aquaspersa* (Fig. 3), and *R. atrovirens*. *R. mackenziei*, described from leaf litter, is morphologically similar to *Pleurothecium obovoideum* (formerly *Ramichloridium obovoideum*) and for a long time was thought to be conspecific. However, on the basis of ribosomal DNA (rDNA) data

it is distantly related, not even belonging to the same order (the latter species belongs to the Sordariales) (6).

Dothideales

The order Dothideales comprises numerous saprobes which thrive well under conditions of decreased water activity, such as on sugary leaf surfaces, rock, glass, and moist medical devices.

Aureobasidium and *Hormonema*

The genus *Aureobasidium* contains a single, ubiquitous and highly polymorphic species, *A. pullulans* (Fig. 3). Colonies in vitro are often pink due to the preponderance of wide, hyaline, oligokaryotic (having 3 to 10 nuclei) hyphae bearing synchronously produced conidia and containing scattered endoconidia (conidia formed inside a hypha). *Aureobasidium* is often confused with *Hormonema* (Fig. 3), which, however, produces conidia in a basipetal succession with the youngest at the base (47). In addition, the ITS (internal transcribed spacer) rDNA sequences of the two species are clearly different (176).

Microascales

The order Microascales comprises *Scopulariopsis* with its *Microascus* teleomorphs (see chapter 118) but also *Scedosporium*, linked to *Pseudallescheria* and *Petriella* teleomorphs.

Pseudallescheria/Scedosporium

The genus *Pseudallescheria* (anamorph *Scedosporium*) comprises several species of clinical interest (68, 69). This fungus has become one of the most frequently misidentified organisms in medical mycology, largely due to the differential abundance of each of the phenotypes of *Pseudallescheria boydii*. This has led to a large number of new introductions in totally unrelated genera (38). However, it is currently accepted that *P. boydii* and *Scedosporium apiospermum* are two different species, i.e., *P. boydii* (anamorph *Scedosporium boydii*) and *Pseudallescheria apiosperma* (anamorph *Scedosporium apiospermum*) (69). The former species is homothallic, and the teleomorph (Fig. 1) is frequently found in clinical samples. The latter species is heterothallic, and the teleomorph is not present in cultures of clinical samples. The anamorphs of these two species are morphologically difficult to distinguish from each other and are characterized by hyaline, Fontana-Masson-negative hyphae from which slimy, pale brown conidia are produced in basipetal succession from inconspicuous annellides. In addition, some isolates are able to produce a *Graphium* synanamorph. A closely related species with a high incidence in Australia is *S. aurantiacum*, which is characterized by the production of a yellow to orange pigment (48). Another clinically important species that does not belong to the *P. boydii* species complex is *S. prolificans*. However, the latter fungus has flask-shaped conidiogenous cells and is monomorphic (see Fig. 6).

Ophiostomatales

Ophiostomatales is a large order of plant-pathogenic fungi. Most are blue-stain fungi in wood and live in association with bark beetles. Only a few species are human or animal pathogens. The main teleomorph genus is *Ophiostoma*.

Sporothrix

Sporothrix schenckii has colorless hyphae that bear a cluster of thin denticles with hyaline, tear-shaped conidia at their tips. Additional spherical and sessile conidia may or may not be present; this is the only melanized part of the fungus. The mould can be transformed in vitro to a stable yeast at 37°C on enriched media such as chocolate agar or brain heart infusion agar. Occasional isolates are difficult to convert and may require multiple subcultures and extended incubation. Transition is observed in environmental as well as clinical isolates.

Recent molecular studies have demonstrated that *S. schenckii* sensu lato is a complex of numerous phylogenetic species (106–108). The combination of phenotypic (morphology of the sessile pigmented conidia; growth at 30, 35, and 37°C; and assimilation of sucrose, raffinose, and ribitol) and genetic approaches (analysis of the calmodulin gene sequences) allows differentiation of some of these species. Apart from *S. schenckii* sensu stricto, the species *S. brasiliensis*, *S. globosa*, and *S. luriei* are also involved in human infections. The last is a rare species that has only been reported from three cases (107).

Pleosporales

Most members of the order Pleosporales have rapidly expanding, floccose colonies, which show optimal conidium production on media poor in nutrients, such as potato carrot agar. The large conidia are then mostly visible with the aid of a stereomicroscope. Conidia are generally produced on septate, dark brown, erect conidiophores. Conidia consist of several compartments. True septa are found in those conidia where the outer wall and septum are continuous; such conidia are euseptate (in *Alternaria* and *Curvularia*). False septa are observed in those conidia where only the inner wall layers are involved in septation and the outer wall forms a sac-like structure around the individual cells; such conidia are distoseptate (in *Bipolaris* and *Exserohilum*).

Alternaria

Since clinical strains are very likely to belong to only two species of *Alternaria*, *Alternaria infectoria* and *A. alternata*, isolates are easily identified down to the species level. Available criteria comprise characteristics of growth, sporulation, and morphology, and very large differences in the rDNA ITS, which can be displayed by sequencing or by restriction fragment length polymorphisms (39). *Alternaria infectoria* in tissue may present with hyaline yeast cells rather than melanized hyphae. Cultures of *A. infectoria*, in contrast to those of *A. alternata*, frequently exhibit creamish patches and show reduced sporulation. Conidia of *A. infectoria* bear long apical beaks which serve as secondary conidiophores. *A. alternata* displays conidia in chains.

Bipolaris

The preponderant *Bipolaris* species in human infections are *Bipolaris australiensis*, *B. hawaiiensis* (Fig. 4), and *B. spicifera*. They are characterized by large, ellipsoidal, straight or curved conidia.

Curvularia

Most species of the genus *Curvularia* are easily recognizable on the basis of the characteristics of their conidia, which are ellipsoidal, often curved, and with dark and flat scars (57). Saprobic members of *Curvularia*, particularly *Curvularia geniculata* and *C. lunata* (Fig. 4), have been identified as potential agents of human infections.

Exserohilum

Exserohilum (1, 114) is characterized by very long, distoseptate conidia with a distinct, protruding basal hilum. Three species have been recognized as opportunistic agents (*Exserohilum longirostratum*, *E. macginnisii*, and *E. rostratum* [Fig. 4]), but given their close molecular similarities, they may be morphological variants of a single species (38).

Sordariales

Sordariales is a large and diverse order of ascomycetes. *Madurella mycetomatis* was recently proven to be another member of Sordariales (36); this species is treated in chapter 123. The genera *Chaetomium* and *Achaetomium* are treated in chapter 118.

EPIDEMIOLOGY AND TRANSMISSION

Phaeohyphomycoses are usually subcutaneous, but they can also be superficial or even systemic. The fungi more commonly involved in phaeohyphomycosis are *Scedosporium* spp., *Exophiala jeanselmei*, *E. dermatitidis*, and *Bipolaris* spp. *E. jeanselmei*, regarded in the literature as a major agent of cutaneous and subcutaneous infections, was rarely observed in a recent study of a large number of clinical strains of *Exophiala*, identified by molecular methods, from the United States (178).

The route of infection is likely traumatic implantation, with the fungus causing a reaction leading to the formation of an inflammatory cyst. It is unknown why the inoculation of

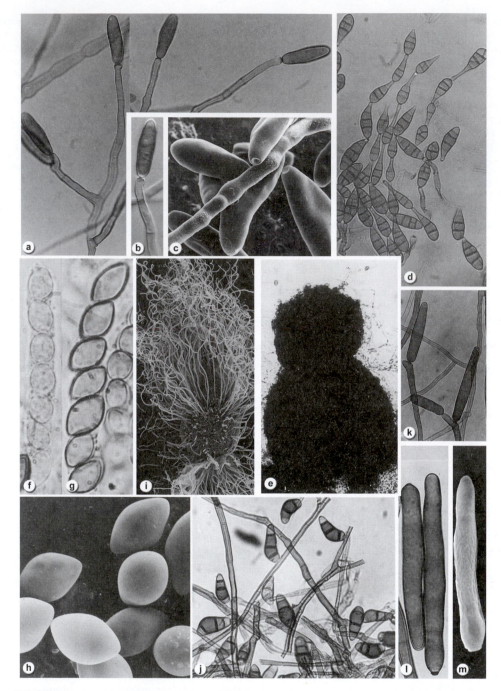

FIGURE 4 (a to c) *Bipolaris hawaiiensis;* (d) *Alternaria alternata;* (e to h) *Achaetomium strumarium;* (i) *Chaetomium globosum;* (j) *Curvularia lunata;* (k to m) *Exserohilum rostratum.* Reproduced from reference 38.

some fungi leads to the development of phaeohyphomycosis and others to chromoblastomycosis, but several fungi can cause both. The species that cause subcutaneous infections are generally uncommon in the environment and occupy hitherto-unrevealed microhabitats. Some thermotolerant species seem to be associated with environmental xenobiotics or occur in animal feces (40); others are found on slightly osmotic surfaces such as fruit (111). Psychrophilic species that cause infections in cold-blooded vertebrates are frequent in water, either ocean water (96, 97), municipal drinking water

(75), or hospital water (132). In the indoor environment *Exophiala* has been found in steam baths (111).

Many members of the Dothideales are tolerant of extreme growth conditions and are found in Antarctic or Mediterranean rock (146, 156) or in hypersaline ponds (177). These species have the ability to transition morphologically to a tolerant, meristematic ecotype consisting of clumps of amorphous, thick-walled, highly melanized cells. *Aureobasidium pullulans* has a yeast phase that colonizes moist surfaces; i.e., it forms isodiametrically expanding cells that become subdivided in all directions and may eventually fall apart into small cell clumps.

Chromoblastomycosis

Chromoblastomycosis is one of the most frequently found subcutaneous mycoses. It occurs usually in the tropical and subtropical regions, with higher prevalences in Africa and Latin America, affecting mainly adult males working in agriculture or related activities. The fact that males are predominantly affected has been related to a possible role of human sex hormones. The fungus usually penetrates the cutaneous barrier through puncture wounds, usually by a thorn or a splinter. The fungal agents causing these infections are saprobic dematiaceous fungi living in soil or rotting wood. Several reports have associated some of these fungi with palm trees and xerophyte plants. Inoculation of cactus plants with *C. carrionii* showed that this fungus is able to persist in cactus tissue, producing muriform cells in the spines morphologically similar to those known as the invasive form in chromoblastomycosis. These cells can be regarded as the extremotolerant survival phase and are likely to play an essential role in the natural life cycle of these organisms (41). The ecology of the fungi causing chromoblastomycosis is clearly differentiated. *F. pedrosoi* is the only species isolated in the evergreen forests of tropical areas and is clearly prevalent in temperate zones, while *C. carrionii* is identified only in spiny desert areas (60).

Sporotrichosis

The species of the *Sporothrix schenckii* complex can be found in soil and thorny plants. Infection is acquired through traumatic inoculation of fungi from contaminated soil or plants. However, transmission from bites or scratches from animals has also been reported. Although this fungus has a worldwide distribution, it is most common in the tropics and warm parts of temperate areas of the globe. Occasional outbreaks occur in different populations, such as gardeners, rural workers, armadillo hunters, and persons in contact with domestic cats. This fungus has been recognized as opportunistic in immunocompromised individuals.

CLINICAL SIGNIFICANCE

Disorders caused by the fungi described in this chapter are mainly localized and occur in otherwise healthy hosts. The infections arise mostly after traumatic inoculation of contaminated material from the environment; less frequently, e.g., in the case of sinusitis, otitis, or growth in the mucous lungs of patients with cystic fibrosis, asymptomatic or mildly symptomatic colonization of cavities is observed. These fungi are typical opportunists, causing infections increasing in severity in individuals with impaired innate immunity and metabolic diseases such as diabetes. Infections also arise in patients with severe immunological disorders, such as neutropenic patients, solid-organ transplantation recipients, or patients undergoing long-term corticosteroid therapy. Some species of Chaetothyriales (such as *C. bantiana*) are able to cause deep or disseminated infections in hosts with no known immune disorder. If untreated, such infections may take a chronic, fatal course after a destructive disease process. The frequency of these infections is relatively to extremely low, but given the potentially severe course of the disease, as well as the sometimes very high degrees of resistance to antifungal drugs, attentiveness to these fungi is mandatory. *Sporothrix* (order Ophiostomatales) is the only agent of infection that increases in severity with defects of acquired cellular immunity, such as AIDS (134).

Among the specific disease entities caused by the melanized fungi are the following.

Phaeohyphomycosis

Superficial

Botryosphaeriales
Neoscytalidium dimidiatum is a common plant pathogen in the tropics and is regularly involved in syndromes very similar to dermatophytosis on skin and nails (56, 102, 115).

Capnodiales
The halophilic species *H. werneckii* can adhere to exceptionally salty human hands (75), causing a syndrome in the dead keratin layers known as tinea nigra (147).

Chaetothyriales
A few species of the order Chaetothyriales can cause occasional superficial infections in humans. Recently described was *Coniosporium epidermidis*, which so far has almost exclusively been found on human skin (101). The species may cause asymptomatic infections, may be found in association with dermatophyte infections, or may cause mild cutaneous infections. *Cyphellophora laciniata* and *C. pluriseptata* are occasionally isolated from human skin and nails (50, 51), but their etiology has not unambiguously been proven. *Phialophora europaea* is fairly commonly involved in mild skin and nail infections, but due to its slow growth, it is frequently overlooked.

Cutaneous and Corneal

Botryosphaeriales
Lasiodiplodia theobromae is occasionally found to cause ocular infections following injury to the cornea (135, 154).

Capnodiales
Species of *Cladosporium*, especially *C. cladosporioides* and *C. oxysporum*, are associated with allergic disease in the indoor environment, with numerous (sub)cutaneous (80, 128, 166) and even deep (94) infections, but there remains some doubt about their pathogenic role.

Chaetothyriales
Cladophialophora emmonsii, *Cladophialophora boppii*, and *Cladophialophora saturnica* are rare agents of mild cutaneous infections (8, 124).

Pleosporales
One of the main recognized clinical entities associated with Pleosporales is cutaneous infection in immunosuppressed patients caused by *Alternaria* and mainly affecting patients on long-term steroid usage, tacrolimus, or other immunosuppressive agents (125, 127). Nearly all cases were caused by *Alternaria infectoria* (17, 120, 142) and *A. alternata* (113, 155), the two main saprobic species of the genus (39). Infections attributed to *A. chlamydospora* (10, 153) probably concerned meristematic segregants of *A. alternata*. Several cutaneous infections have been attributed to *A. tenuissima* (141), which is only doubtfully separate from *A. alternata* (39). *Exserohilum* spp. can occasionally cause infections of the skin and cornea (114).

Subcutaneous

Botryosphaeriales
Rare cases of subcutaneous infection by *Lasiodiplodia theobromae* (158) and *Neoscytalidium dimidiatum* (151) have been reported.

Calosphaeriales

Members of the order Calosphaeriales are typical agents of subcutaneous infections. Most of the six pathogenic species of *Phaeoacremonium* cause this type of infection, *P. parasiticum* being the most common (62, 77, 117, 122). Human infections by *Pleurostomophora richardsiae* mostly involve subcutaneous cysts in which the fungus is encapsulated by a collagen layer (78), occasionally with bone involvement (164). Most patients have some underlying condition such as diabetes (131) or transplantation (137).

Chaetothyriales

Exophiala dermatitidis is the most commonly encountered species in clinical settings, causing infections of cutaneous and subcutaneous tissues (83) in mostly immunocompromised patients. *E. oligosperma* is a common etiologic agent of subcutaneous infections in immunosuppressed, elderly, diabetic, or otherwise debilitated individuals (45, 74, 157).

Microascales

Several species of *Scedosporium* are common causes of subcutaneous infections (33, 76).

Pleosporales

Members of the order Pleosporales (most commonly *Bipolaris*, *Curvularia*, and *Exserohilum*) are able to cause subcutaneous infections, although more commonly they produce allergic sinusitis with occasional cerebral involvement in otherwise healthy individuals (4, 11, 24, 25, 55, 88, 98, 110, 114, 126, 138, 174).

Systemic

Botryosphaeriales

Lasiodiplodia theobromae has been involved in a case of pneumonia (170). *Neoscytalidium dimidiatum* caused deep infections in immunocompromised patients (12, 168).

Calosphaeriales

Phaeoacremonium parasiticum is able to cause disseminated infections in debilitated patients (9).

Chaetothyriales

A disease entity that is largely confined to Chaetothyriales is primary cerebral infection in immunocompromised or immunocompetent individuals, i.e., cerebritis where the first symptoms of disease are of a neurological nature. Hyphal elements that show melanization either directly or after Fontana-Masson staining are observed in abscesses in the brain parenchyma. The portal of entry may be the lung, but frequently symptoms are confined to the brain. Six fungal species account for most nontraumatic brain infections. *Cladophialophora bantiana* has caused about one-third of the cases in otherwise healthy individuals (52, 85, 92, 137). If untreated, the infections are fatal within 1 to 6 months. *Exophiala dermatitidis* is responsible for a striking number of fatal, neurotropic infections in young, healthy individuals, all in Asia (28). The other four species are *Cladophialophora modesta*, *Fonsecaea monophora*, *Ochroconis gallopava*, and *Rhinocladiella mackenziei*. *O. gallopava* is also the cause of epizootic encephalitis in flocks of turkeys and chickens (86) and is able to cause pulmonary infections in immunocompetent individuals (84, 121).

Rhinocladiella mackenziei is a remarkable fungus because it is exclusively known from fatal brain infections in the Middle East or from immigrants from that region (91, 160). Several patients had no known immune disorder; the environmental niche of the species is unknown. *R. atrovirens* has been reported to cause cerebral phaeohyphomycosis in an AIDS patient (49), but as *R. atrovirens* in a modern, molecular circumscription is limited to isolates growing on conifer wood in northern countries, these cases probably concerned the sibling species *R. similis* (45).

Occasionally systemic dissemination is observed in patients with or without proven immune disorder; these infections are fatal if they go untreated. Secondary cutaneous lesions often lead to marked eruptions with high morbidity. The disorder has been observed repeatedly in *Cladophialophora devriesii*, *C. modesta*, *C. arxii*, *Exophiala dermatitidis*, and *E. spinifera* (73, 162). The last two species have capsule-like extracellular polysaccharides around yeast cells (175) and have a high virulence to humans. The rare infections by *E. spinifera* can be localized, but in about one-half of the cases fatal, disseminated mycoses are observed in adolescents (reviewed by de Hoog et al. [42]).

The etiologic agents in cases of phaeohyphomycosis published under the name *F. pedrosoi* (116, 152) should be reconsidered, since it has been observed that the second species of the genus, *F. monophora*, has a more diverse clinical spectrum which includes brain infection (119, 159, 161). Occasionally, opportunistic infections including endocarditis and osteomyelitis caused by *Phialophora verrucosa* have been reported (54, 163). It is possible that some of these infections were attributable to *P. americana*.

Dothideales

Aureobasidium pullulans has been implicated as an agent of catheter-related septicemia, peritonitis, and disseminated infection (21, 30, 82, 89, 90, 143), and *Hormonema dematioides* has been implicated in a case of peritonitis (149).

Microascales

Relatively common deep and disseminated infections caused by *Scedosporium* are noted for immunosuppressed or otherwise debilitated patients. The reported clinical spectrum of *S. apiospermum*/*P. boydii* has changed over time, from prevalently chronic mycetoma in otherwise healthy patients between 1911 and 1980 to systemic opportunistic infection after 1980 (33, 76). Systemic infections after solid-organ transplantation are relatively frequent (103); occasionally infections are noted with the application of invasive devices (148). Osteomyelitis (76) and arthritis (71) are frequent. Fisher et al. (63) were the first to describe the near-drowning syndrome caused by *S. apiospermum*, which characteristically leads to delayed, potentially fatal brain infection after the patient has recovered from the primary effects of aspiration of polluted water. Berenguer et al. stressed the species' neurotropism (13). In severely compromised patients, cerebral dissemination may take place from local foci (87, 93). *P. boydii* shows a high incidence in cystic fibrosis patients (29, 33, 76).

Despite its rather frequent occurrence in clinical settings, the history of *Scedosporium prolificans*, one of the most virulent species of Microascales, is remarkably short (76). Malloch and Salkin described the first clinical cases in 1984 (105). Since then numerous strains have been recovered, mostly from clinical cases with major immunosuppression, and since no older reports of cases in immunocompetent patients are known, the species is a truly emerging opportunist (13, 33, 139). The species has been reported from bone and soft tissue infections (139, 169, 171) as well as from (secondary) cutaneous infection, fungemia, and endocarditis (16, 22). The fungus may disseminate to visceral organs in immunocompromised individuals (13, 118). A nosocomial outbreak has been described (79).

Pleosporales

A wide spectrum of opportunistic infections has been attributed to *Curvularia*, including endocarditis, pulmonary infection, cerebral infection, and peritonitis (18, 55, 61, 130, 138, 173).

Chromoblastomycosis

Chromoblastomycosis occurs in otherwise healthy patients; it is characterized by chronic, cutaneous to subcutaneous lesions and frequently with marked hyperplasia. A primary lesion is represented by a papula at the site of inoculation that slowly enlarges over time, becoming a tumoral (cauliflower-like) lesion that can spread via the lymphatic system, although hematogenous dissemination has also been proposed. Lesions contain the typical and resistant spherical and mostly cruciately septate muriform (sclerotic) bodies, indicative of chromoblastomycosis.

Three fungal species of Chaetothyriales account for virtually all cases of chromoblastomycosis: *Cladophialophora carrionii*, *Fonsecaea pedrosoi*, and *Phialophora verrucosa*. Infections by *C. carrionii* mainly occur in arid climates (59, 100, 133), probably acquired via traumatic inoculation of cactus spines (179). Occasionally *Cladophialophora boppii* (15) and, more recently, the new species *Cladophialophora samoënsis* have also been reported as causes of chromoblastomycosis (8). Infections by *P. verrucosa* mainly occur in tropical climatic zones (65, 165). *Rhinocladiella aquaspersa* is a rare agent of chromoblastomycosis in South America (5, 129, 150).

Sporotrichosis

Sporotrichosis is a cutaneous to subcutaneous chronic infection that can undergo lymphatic spread. Musculoskeletal involvement and disseminated infection are relatively rare, as are the nasal and pulmonary infections that may arise from inhalation of conidia (26, 31, 75). Most infections originate from traumatic implantation of the fungus. Some disseminated cases were observed in AIDS patients (14, 53). In addition, infections have been described as being transmitted by animals (2, 144). Apart from *S. schenckii* sensu stricto, the species *S. brasiliensis*, *S. globosa*, and *S. luriei* are also involved in human infections. The last is a rare species known by only three isolates (107).

COLLECTION, TRANSPORT, AND STORAGE OF SPECIMENS

Collection, transport, and storage of specimens are described in chapter 112. Appropriate collection of specimens is essential for mycological study. There should be sufficient quantity for direct microscopic examination as well as for isolation.

DIRECT EXAMINATION

Microscopy

Melanization of vegetative cells or conidia, which results in colony coloration ranging from olive or gray to black, is caused by the deposition of dihydroxynaphthalene melanin in cell walls. This property occurs commonly among species classified in very different parts of the fungal kingdom. The amount of melanin expressed in host tissue may be very small and difficult to observe using traditional histologic stains. The use of the Fontana-Masson stain (95; see chapter 113) for demonstrating the presence of melanin is therefore recommended as a routine to distinguish fungi with melanized hyphae from those causing "hyalohyphomycosis," e.g., *Aspergillus*. This does not apply for *Sporothrix* and *Scedosporium*, which are not melanized but are able to produce melanized conidia either in vitro or in vivo or both. *Sporothrix* has a characteristic yeast form in tissue; the recognition of *Scedosporium* rests upon methods other than histopathology.

There are numerous procedures for treating the specimen to enhance fungal detection, including treatment with potassium hydroxide or calcofluor white and Giemsa, Wright, or Gram stain (see chapter 113). Histopathology procedures using periodic acid-Schiff (PAS), hematoxylin and eosin, or methenamine silver enhance observation. Fontana-Masson staining is useful to detect melanization in cells that appear hyaline with light microscopy. To summarize, some characteristic features include the following.

Skin Infections

Pigmented hyphal fragments, occasionally melanized yeast-like cells, are visible in infected skin tissue (Fig. 5).

Sinusitis

In sinusitis, the sinuses are occluded by amorphous fungus balls. Histologic examination reveals the presence of dense masses of pigmented, branched, and septate hyphae not invading the mucosa.

Cerebral Infection

In cases of cerebral infection, the hyphae are often poorly colored and scantily branched. In advanced cases, abscesses are formed (Fig. 5).

Disseminated Infection

Pigmented or poorly colored fungal elements such as hyphae or yeast-like cells can be observed in cases of disseminated infection (Fig. 6).

Chromoblastomycosis

The hallmark of chromoblastomycosis is the presence of muriform or sclerotic cells in tissue sections or wet preparations of pus, scrapings, or biopsy samples. Muriform cells are swollen, spherical, dark brown, thick-walled cells which often develop a septum and may finally become divided by intersecting septa in more than one plane (Fig. 6).

Sporotrichosis

In sporotrichosis, hyaline yeast-like cells are occasionally present, bearing slender daughter cells at very narrow bases. They are usually few in number and may easily be missed during microscopy, so Gomori methenamine-silver (GMS) or PAS staining is therefore recommended; Fontana-Masson staining is negative (Fig. 6).

Antigen and Nucleic Acid Detection

There are few data for detection of antigens or nucleic acids in human clinical samples for diagnosis of the mycoses included in this chapter. A panfungal PCR assay has been developed that targets the ITS1 region of the rDNA gene cluster for detecting fungal DNA in fresh and paraffin-embedded tissue specimens. This method was useful for the identifying species of *Scedosporium*, *Exophiala*, and *Exserohilum*. PCR products were sequenced and compared with sequences in the GenBank database (99).

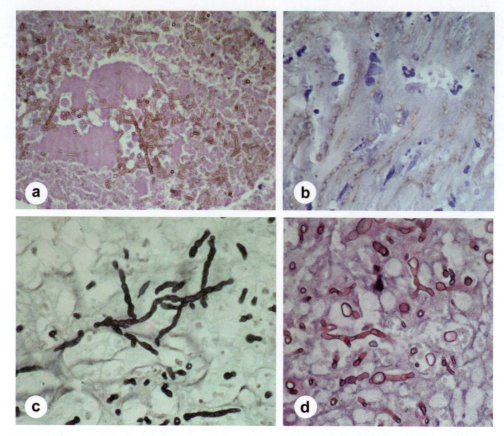

FIGURE 5 (a) Hematoxylin and eosin stain of subcutaneous nodule biopsy sample showing branching hyphae of *Fonseacea monophora;* (b to d) brain tissue showing irregular, branching, and septate hyphae of *Cladophialophora bantiana,* stained with hematoxylin and eosin stain (b), GMS stain (c), and PAS stain (d). Magnifications, ×250 (a) and ×400 (b to d). (Courtesy of E. Mayayo, Universitat Rovira i Virgili.)

ISOLATION PROCEDURES

The use of nutritionally minimal media such as 2% water agar, moistened sterile wooden sticks, or moistened sterile filter paper stimulates the formation of conidia. In the case of infection due to more than one agent, the strain that grows in a more limited manner may pass unnoticed for a long period. Therefore, a loopful of cells suspended in 0.1% Tween and streaked onto a fresh culture plate is useful to select an individual colony for identification.

IDENTIFICATION

For the identification of most of the species included in this chapter, the "gold standard" is to grow the fungi in culture and to examine the relevant morphological characteristics described above. Appropriate culture media are described in chapter 113. Slide culture preparations (114) using potato dextrose agar or cornmeal dextrose agar, to be handled only within a biological safety cabinet, are ideal for determining conidiogenesis. For morphological features of the fungi treated in this chapter, the reader is referred to de Hoog et al. (38).

Molecular identification of most species is currently performed by sequencing of ribosomal genes and comparison with dedicated databases (32). Care should be taken when the GenBank database is used for the purpose of identification in less-known fungal groups, because over 10% of the sequences may be incorrect (39). Sequences should be evaluated not only from a technical point of view but also nomenclaturally, i.e., by comparison with ex-type strains.

When ribosomal genes are used, the phylogenetic position of taxa can be established by sequencing the nuclear SSU (18S) rRNA gene. This gene is mostly invariant between closely related species. In most fungal groups, species diagnostics is possible with ITS sequences. But application of this technique as a gold standard for melanized fungi is still in dispute. In some genera, such as *Alternaria*, the numerous species described on the basis of morphology prove to be invariant in the ITS region. In this case the question as to whether ITS shows insufficient polymorphism or whether simply too many species have been introduced remains. In contrast, ITS-based species distinction with black yeasts provides satisfactory results. In some genera, such as *Sporothrix*, sequencing of the calmodulin gene is necessary to gain resolution of species within the complex (108). In *Scedosporium* (69) and *Phaeoacremonium* (117), β-tubulin gene sequencing is used for this purpose.

TYPING SYSTEMS

A diversity of high-resolution molecular typing systems has been developed in recent years. These have been applied mainly to epidemiological tracking of fungal pathogens in the hospital and the community but also to show geographical differences among isolates and to detect cryptic species.

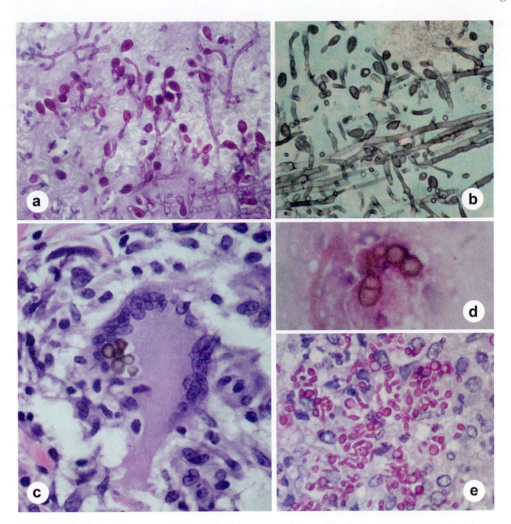

FIGURE 6 (a and b) Lung tissue with numerous conidia and hyphae of *Scedosporium prolificans* stained with PAS (a) and GMS (b); (c) PAS stain of a subcutaneous nodule biopsy sample showing sclerotic cells of *Fonsecaea pedrosoi* within a giant cell; (d) PAS stain of a fine-needle aspirate of a subcutaneous nodule showing sclerotic cells of *Fonsecaea pedrosoi*; (e) PAS stain of a hepatic vessel showing a massive embolization by *Sporothrix schenckii* showing characteristic elongate cells. Magnifications, ×400. (Courtesy of E. Mayayo, Universitat Rovira i Virgili.)

Chaetothyriales

On the basis of a multigene phylogeny, it has been demonstrated that important phenotypic features have evolved independently several times in the order Chaetothyriales, and that most of the species of *Cladophialophora* belong to a monophyletic group comprising two main clades (*carrionii* and *bantiana* clades) (8).

In a study that investigated the molecular diversity of oligotrophic and neurotropic members of the genus *Exophiala* using ITS sequences and M-13 fingerprint and SSU intron data, two main groups could be distinguished within *E. dermatitidis*. The environmental strains were mainly placed in one of these groups, while the clinical strains were in the second one. Interestingly, strains from East Asia that clustered in the clinical group caused severe brain and disseminated infections, and strains of the same group recovered from outside East Asia only caused a relatively mild fungemia (112).

The natural niche of *Fonsecaea*, one of the most common agents causing chromoblastomycosis, remains uncertain. To elucidate where and how patients acquire the infection, probably through traumatic inoculation, numerous isolates with *Fonsecaea*-like morphology from environmental sources were typed using random amplified polymorphic DNA methodology. The results revealed a high degree of strain diversity and showed that most strains isolated from environments to which symptomatic human patients were exposed were found to be more closely related to species of *Cladophialophora* than to *Fonsecaea* (37).

Dothideales

Multilocus typing at four loci demonstrated the existence of at least five different sequence types in isolates of *Neoscytalidium dimidiatum*, from which two were detected exclusively in isolates from plants, two were found only in clinical isolates, and one was observed in isolates from humans and from a mango tree. This has been proposed as the possible source of infection in a case of mycetoma in an agricultural field worker and should be considered as a potential reservoir of pathogenic strains of the fungus (104).

Microascales

In numerous molecular studies there has been a high genetic diversity among isolates of *Scedosporium* from different origins (reviewed in reference 81). However, recent multilocus sequence analysis has shown that such variability could be explained by the existence of numerous cryptic species in the *Pseudallescheria boydii* complex (68, 69). By contrast, in *S. prolificans* genetic variation seems to be low to absent.

Ophiostomatales

With *Sporothrix*, as with *Scedosporium*, numerous molecular studies (reviewed in reference 108) have proved the existence of a high level of intraspecific variability, with isolates mainly grouped according to their geographical origin. But recent multilocus studies have demonstrated that *S. schenckii* sensu lato comprises several phylogenetic species and morphospecies (106, 107) with a marked geographical distribution; i.e., *S. brasiliensis* isolates are mainly found in Brazil, and all the isolates from India tested molecularly belong to *S. globosa*. This likely correlates with the genetic and morphological diversity shown within *S. schenckii* by many authors.

SEROLOGIC TESTS

A latex agglutination test is commercially available (Immuno-Mycologics Inc., Norman, OK) for detecting antibodies against *S. schenckii*, particularly in disseminated cases, but despite a study (19) reporting a sensitivity of 90 to 94% and a specificity of 95 to 100%, the test has not been used widely. However, the detection of antibodies was demonstrated to be useful in the diagnosis of central nervous system sporotrichosis in several patients when culture-based diagnosis had failed (145).

ANTIFUNGAL SUSCEPTIBILITIES

The available in vitro data for dematiaceous fungi are increasing every day, and in general the antifungal susceptibility of the most clinically relevant species is known. However, interpretive breakpoints have not been defined, and clinical correlation data are practically nonexistent.

Azole antifungal drugs in general have demonstrated the most consistent in vitro activity against dematiaceous fungi, except *S. prolificans*, which is resistant to all the azoles (23). Itraconazole has shown good activity against numerous dematiaceous fungi (64), although some instances of azole resistance have been observed in sequential isolates of *F. pedrosoi* from patients on long-term itraconazole treatment (3). The newer triazoles posaconazole and voriconazole have a broad spectrum of activity against most of the fungi included in this chapter. The activities of these triazoles were similar against agents of chromoblastomycosis (72) and *Pseudallescheria boydii* complex (70). Posaconazole activity is higher than voriconazole activity against *Alternaria* spp. (7), *Exophiala* spp. (64), and *Sporothrix* spp. (109), although against the last the activity of both drugs was very poor. Other azoles have a much more limited role in the therapy of these infections.

Amphotericin B generally has good in vitro activity against most clinically important dematiaceous fungi, such as *Exophiala* (64) and *Alternaria* (7). However, some species have been consistently resistant in vitro, including all the species of *Scedosporium* tested (23, 70). Other species have occasionally found to be resistant, including *Curvularia* spp., *Exophiala* spp., and *R. mackenziei* (27). Flucytosine has shown some activity against a variety of dematiaceous

fungi, including agents of chromoblastomycosis and phaeohyphomycosis (20, 136). However, in other studies this drug was inactive (27). Terbinafine showed a clear in vitro fungicidal activity against filamentous fungi. Studies of in vitro activity against dematiaceous fungi are emerging and fairly broad-spectrum activity is seen, including against *Alternaria*, *Curvularia*, and *Bipolaris* (136). Echinocandins appear to have variable and species-dependent fungistatic activity for the dematiaceous fungi (58).

EVALUATION, INTERPRETATION, AND REPORTING OF RESULTS

More than 100 species of melanized fungi have caused infection in humans and animals, and many of these are relatively rare as etiologic agents. As a result, few clinicians are familiar with these fungi and they are frequently overlooked. Infections caused by dematiaceous fungi are being diagnosed increasingly among healthy as well as compromised patients. Concurrently, the expanding diversity of etiology within this group of fungi is becoming apparent.

Determining whether a particular dematiaceous fungus is involved in a disease process can be difficult because most of these fungi are occasionally recovered as contaminants from clinical specimens. Repeated recovery of a suspected etiologic agent is significant, while DNA sequence identity of clinical material and the isolate is highly supportive. Isolation of a dematiaceous fungus from a normally sterile body site should not be dismissed as contamination, particularly if colonies are numerous or more than one culture plate shows growth. If isolated from a nonsterile pulmonary specimen such as skin, sputum, or bronchial lavage fluid, well-documented opportunists from genera such as *Cladophialophora*, *Fonsecaea*, *Ochroconis*, or *Scedosporium*, which are not seen as contaminants, also are highly indicative. Correlation between culture and histopathology results should also be determined.

Failure to order fungus culture when tissues are collected during surgical procedures is an increasing problem in the management of these infections, and clinicians should order fungus culture whenever warranted. In the future, direct identification of fungal genera from tissue blocks using immunohistochemistry, in situ DNA hybridization, or DNA sequencing will be a promising approach to rapid detection and identification of these agents.

REFERENCES

1. **Alcorn, J. L.** 1983. Generic concepts in *Drechslera*, *Bipolaris* and *Exserohilum*. Mycotaxon **17:**1–86.
2. **Amaya Tapia, A., E. Uribe Jimenez, R. Diaz Perez, M. A. Covarrubias Velasco, D. Diaz Santana Bustamante, G. Aguirre Avalos, and A. Rodriguez Toledo.** 1996. Esporotricosis cutanea transmitida por mordedura de tejon. Med. Cutanea Ibero-Lat.-Am. **24:**87–89.
3. **Andrade, T. S., L. G. Castro, R. S. Nunes, V. M. Gimenes, and A. E. Cury.** 2004. Susceptibility of sequential *Fonsecaea pedrosoi* isolates from chromoblastomycosis patients to antifungal agents. Mycoses **47:**216–221.
4. **Aquino, V. M., J. M. Norvell, K. Krisher, and M. M. Mustafa.** 1995. Fatal disseminated infection due to *Exserohilum rostratum* in a patient with aplastic anemia: case report and review. Clin. Infect. Dis. **20:**176–178.
5. **Arango, M., C. Jaramillo, A. Cortes, and A. Restrepo.** 1998. Auricular chromoblastomycosis caused by *Rhinocladiella aquaspersa*. Med. Mycol. **36:**43–45.
6. **Arzanlou, M., J. Z. Groenewald, W. Gams, U. Braun, H. D. Shin, and P. W. Crous.** 2007. Phylogenetic and morphotaxonomic revision of *Ramichloridium* and allied genera. Stud. Mycol. **58:**57–93.

7. Badali, H., G. S. de Hoog, I. Curfs-Breuker, B. Andersen, and J. F. Meis. 2009. *In vitro* activities of eight antifungal drugs against 70 clinical and environmental isolates of *Alternaria* species. *J. Antimicrob. Chemother.* doi:10.1093/jac/dkp109.

8. Badali, H., C. Gueidan, M. J. Najafzadeh, A. Bonifaz, A. H. G. Gerrits van den Ende, and G. S. de Hoog. 2008. Biodiversity of the genus *Cladophialophora*. *Stud. Mycol.* 61:175–191.

9. Baddley, J. W., L. Mostert, R. C. Summerbell, and S. A. Moser. 2006. *Phaeoacremonium parasiticum* infections confirmed by beta-tubulin sequence analysis of case isolates. *J. Clin. Microbiol.* 44:2207–2211.

10. Bartolome, B., R. Valks, J. Fraga, V. Buendia, J. Fernandez-Herrera, and A. Garcia-Diez. 1999. Cutaneous alternariosis due to *Alternaria chlamydospora* after bone marrow transplantation. *Acta Dermato-Venereol.* 79:244.

11. Bartynski, J. M., T. V. McCaffrey, and E. Frigas. 1990. Allergic fungal sinusitis secondary to dematiaceous fungi—*Curvularia lunata* and *Alternaria*. *Otolaryngology* 103:32–39.

12. Benne, C. A., C. Neeleman, M. Bruin, G. S. de Hoog, and A. Fleer. 1993. Disseminating infection with *Scytalidium dimidiatum* in a granulocytopenic child. *Eur. J. Clin. Microbiol. Infect. Dis.* 12:118–121.

13. Berenguer, J., J. L. Rodriguez-Tudela, C. Richard, M. Alvarez, M. A. Sanz, L. Gaztelurrutia, J. Ayats, and J. V. Martinez-Suarez. 1997. Deep infections caused by *Scedosporium prolificans*. A report on 16 cases in Spain and a review of the literature. *Medicine* 76:256–265.

14. Bolao, F., D. Podzamczer, M. Ventin, and F. Gudiol. 1994. Efficacy of acute phase and maintenance therapy with itraconazole in an AIDS patient with sporotrichosis. *Eur. J. Clin. Microbiol. Infect. Dis.* 13:609–612.

15. Borelli, D. 1983. *Taeniolella boppii*, nova species, agente de cromomicosis. *Med. Cutanea Ibero-Lat.-Am.* 11:227–232.

16. Bouza, E., P. Munoz, L. Vega, M. Rodriguez-Creixems, J. Berenguer, and A. Escudero. 1996. Clinical resolution of *Scedosporium prolificans* fungemia associated with reversal of neutropenia following administration of granulocyte colony-stimulating factor. *Clin. Infect. Dis.* 23:192–193.

17. Brasch, J., J. O. Busch, and G. S. de Hoog. 2008. Cutaneous phaeohyphomycosis caused by *Alternaria infectoria*. *Acta Dermato.-Venereol.* 88:160–161.

18. Bryan, C. S., C. W. Smith, D. E. Berg, and R. B. Karp. 1993. *Curvularia lunata* endocarditis treated with terbinafine: case report. *Clin. Infect. Dis.* 16:30–32.

19. Bulmer, S. O., L. Kaufman, W. Kaplan, D. W. McLaughlin, and D. E. Kraft. 1973. Comparative evaluation of five serological methods for the diagnosis of sporotrichosis. *Appl. Microbiol.* 26:4–8.

20. Caligiorne, R. B., M. A. Resende, P. H. C. Melillo, C. P. Peluso, F. H. S. Carmo, and V. Acevedo. 1999. In vitro susceptibility of chromoblastomycosis and phaeohyphomycosis agents to antifungal drugs. *Med. Mycol.* 37:405–409.

21. Caporale, N. E., L. Calegari, D. Perez, and E. Gezuele. 1996. Peritoneal catheter colonization and peritonitis with *Aureobasidium pullulans*. *Perit. Dial. Int.* 16:97–98.

22. Carreter de Granda, M. E., C. Richard, E. Conde, A. Iriondo, F. Marco de Lucas, R. Salesa, and A. Zubizarreta. 2001. Endocarditis caused by *Scedosporium prolificans* after autologous peripheral blood stem cell transplantation. *Eur. J. Clin. Microbiol. Infect. Dis.* 20:215–217.

23. Carrillo, A. J., and J. Guarro. 2001. In vitro activities of four novel triazoles against *Scedosporium* spp. *Antimicrob. Agents Chemother.* 45:2151–2153.

24. Carter, E., and C. Boudreaux. 2004. Fatal cerebral phaeohyphomycosis due to *Curvularia lunata* in an immunocompetent patient. *J. Clin. Microbiol.* 42:5419–5423.

25. Castelnuovo, P., F. De Bernardi, C. Cavanna, F. Pagella, P. Bossolesi, P. Marone, and C. Farina. 2004. Invasive fungal sinusitis due to *Bipolaris hawaiiensis*. *Mycoses* 47:76–81.

26. Castrejon, O. V., M. Robles, and O. E. Zubieta Arroyo. 1995. Fatal fungaemia due to *Sporothrix schenckii*. *Mycoses* 38:373–376.

27. Cermeño-Vivas, J. R., and J. M. Torres-Rodriguez. 2001. In vitro susceptibility of dematiaceous fungi to ten antifungal drugs using an agar diffusion test. *Rev. Iberoam. Micol.* 18:113–117. (In Spanish.)

28. Chang, C. L., D.-S. Kim, D. J. Park, H. J. Kim, C. H. Lee, and J. H. Shin. 2000. Acute cerebral phaeohyphomycosis due to *Wangiella dermatitidis* accompanied by cerebrospinal fluid eosinophilia. *J. Clin. Microbiol.* 38:1965–1966.

29. Cimon, B., J. Carrere, J. F. Vinatier, J. P. Chazalette, D. Chabasse, and J. P. Bouchara. 2000. Clinical significance of *Scedosporium apiospermum* in patients with cystic fibrosis. *Eur. J. Clin. Microbiol. Infect. Dis.* 19:53–56.

30. Clark, E. C., S. M. Silver, G. E. Hollick, and M. G. Rinaldi. 1995. Continuous ambulatory peritoneal dialysis complicated by *Aureobasidium pullulans* peritonitis. *Am. J. Nephrol.* 15:353–355.

31. Clay, B. M., and V. K. Anand. 1996. Sporotrichosis: a nasal obstruction in an infant. *Am. J. Otolaryngol.* 17:75–77.

32. Clinical and Laboratory Standards Institute. 2008. *Interpretive Criteria for Identification of Bacteria and Fungi by DNA Sequencing; Approved Guideline.* CLSI document MM18-A. Clinical and Laboratory Standards Institute, Wayne, PA.

33. Cortez, K. J., E. Roilides, F. Queiroz-Telles, J. Meletiadis, C. Antachopoulos, T. Knudsen, W. Buchanan, J. Milanovich, D. A. Sutton, A. Fothergill, M. G. Rinaldi, Y. R. Shea, T. Zaoutis, S. Kottilil, and T. J. Walsh. 2008. Infections caused by *Scedosporium* spp. *Clin. Microbiol. Rev.* 21:157–197.

34. Crous, P. W., W. Gams, M. J. Wingfield, and P. S. van Wyk. 1996. *Phaeoacremonium* gen. nov. associated with wilt and decline disease of woody hosts and human infections. *Mycologia* 88:786–796.

35. Crous, P. W., B. Slippers, M. J. Wingfield, J. Rheeder, W. F. Marasas, A. J. Philips, A. Alves, T. Burgess, P. Barber, and J. Z. Groenewald. 2006. Phylogenetic lineages in the Botryosphaeriaceae. *Stud. Mycol.* 55:235–253.

36. de Hoog, G. S., D. Adelmann, A. O. A. Ahmed, and A. van Belkum. 2004. Phylogeny and typification of *Madurella mycetomatis*, with a comparison of other agents of eumycetoma. *Mycoses* 47:121–130.

37. de Hoog, G. S., D. Attili-Angelis, V. A. Vicente, and F. Queiroz-Telles. 2004. Molecular ecology and pathogenic potential of *Fonsecaea* species. *Med. Mycol.* 42:405–416.

38. de Hoog, G. S., J. Guarro, J. Gené, and M. J. Figueras. 2000. *Atlas of Clinical Fungi*, 2nd ed. Centraalbureau voor Schimmelcultures, Utrecht, The Netherlands, and Universitat Rovira i Virgili, Reus, Spain.

39. de Hoog, G. S., and R. Horré. 2002. Molecular taxonomy of the *Alternaria* and *Ulocladium* species described from humans and their identification in the routine laboratory. *Mycoses* 45:259–276.

40. de Hoog, G. S., T. Matos, M. Sudhadham, K. F. Luijsterburg, and G. Haase. 2005. Intestinal prevalence of the neurotropic black yeast *Exophiala* (*Wangiella*) *dermatitidis* in healthy and impaired individuals. *Mycoses* 48:142–145.

41. De Hoog, G. S., A. S. Nishikaku, G. Fernandez-Zeppenfeldt, C. Padín-González, E. Burger, H. Badali, N. Richard-Yegres, and A. H. van den Ende. 2007. Molecular analysis and pathogenicity of the *Cladophialophora carrionii* complex, with the description of a novel species. *Stud. Mycol.* 58:219–234.

42. de Hoog, G. S., N. Poonwan, and A. H. G. Gerrits van den Ende. 1999. Taxonomy of *Exophiala spinifera* and its relationship to *E. jeanselmei*. *Stud. Mycol.* 43:133–142.

43. de Hoog, G. S., K. Takeo, E. Göttlich, K. Nishimura, and M. Miyaji. 1995. A human isolate of *Exophiala* (*Wangiella*) *dermatitidis* forming a catenate synanamorph that links the genera *Exophiala* and *Cladophialophora*. *J. Med. Vet. Mycol.* 33:355–358.

44. de Hoog, G. S., K. Takeo, S. Yoshida, E. Göttlich, K. Nishimura, and M. Miyaji. 1994. Pleoanamorphic life cycle of *Exophiala* (*Wangiella*) *dermatitidis*. *Antonie van Leeuwenhoek* 65:143–153.

45. de Hoog, G. S., V. Vicente, R. B. Caligiorne, S. Kantarcioglu, K. Tintelnot, A. H. G. Gerrits van den Ende, and G. Haase. 2003. Species diversity and polymorphism in the *Exophiala spinifera* clade containing opportunistic black yeast-like fungi. *J. Clin. Microbiol.* 41:4767–4778.

46. de Hoog, G. S., X. O. Weenink, and A. H. G. Gerrits van den Ende. 1999. Taxonomy of the *Phialophora verrucosa* complex with the description of four new species. *Stud. Mycol.* **43:**107–142.

47. de Hoog, G. S., and N. A. Yurlova. 1994. Conidiogenesis, nutritional physiology and taxonomy of *Aureobasidium* and *Hormonema. Antonie van Leeuwenhoek* **65:**41–54.

48. Delhaes, L., A. Harun, S. C. A. Chen, O. Nguyen, M. Slavin, C. H. Heath, K. Maszewska, C. Halliday, V. Robert, T. C. Sorrell, W. Meyer, and the Australian Scedosporium (AUSCEDO) Study Group. 2008. Molecular typing of Australian *Scedosporium* isolates showing genetic variability and numerous *S. aurantiacum. Emerg. Infect. Dis.* **14:**282–290.

49. del Palacio-Hernanz, A., M. K. Moore, C. K. Campbell, A. del Palacio-Perez-Medel, and R. del Castillo-Cantero. 1989. Infection of the central nervous system by *Rhinocladiella atrovirens* in a patient with acquired immunodeficiency syndrome. *J. Med. Vet. Mycol.* **27:**127–130.

50. de Vries, G. A. 1962. *Cyphellophora laciniata* nov. gen., nov. sp. and *Dactylium fusarioides* Fragoso et Ciferri. *Mycopathol. Mycol. Appl.* **16:**47–54.

51. de Vries, G. A., M. C. C. Elders, and M. H. F. Luykx. 1986. Description of *Cyphellophora pluriseptata* sp. nov. *Antonie van Leeuwenhoek* **52:**141–143.

52. Dixon, D. M., and T. J. Walsh. 1989. Infections due to *Xylohypha bantiana* (*Cladosporium trichoides*). *Rev. Infect. Dis.* **11:**515–525.

53. Donabedian, H., E. O'Donnell, C. Olszewski, R. D. MacArthur, and N. Budd. 1994. Disseminated cutaneous and meningeal sporotrichosis in an AIDS patient. *Diagn. Microbiol. Infect. Dis.* **18:**111–115.

54. Duggan, J. M., M. D. Wolf, and C. A. Kauffman. 1995. *Phialophora verrucosa* infection in an AIDS patient. *Mycoses* **38:**215–218.

55. Ebright, J. R., P. H. Chandrasekar, S. Marks, M. R. Fairfax, A. Aneziokoro, and M. R. McGinnis. 1999. Invasive sinusitis and cerebritis due to *Curvularia clavata* in an immunocompetent adult. *Clin. Infect. Dis.* **28:**687–689.

56. Elewski, B. E. 1996. Onychomycosis caused by *Scytalidium dimidiatum. J. Am. Acad. Dermatol.* **35:**336–338.

57. Ellis, M. B. 1971. *Dematiaceous Hyphomycetes.* Commonwealth Mycological Institute, Kew, United Kingdom.

58. Espinel-Ingroff, A. 2003. In vitro antifungal activities of anidulafungin and micafungin, licensed agents and the investigational triazole posaconazole as determined by NCCLS methods for 12,052 fungal isolates: review of the literature. *Rev. Iberoam. Micol.* **20:**121–136.

59. Esterre, P., A. Andriantsimahavandy, E. R. Ramarcel, and J.-L. Pecarrere. 1996. Forty years of chromoblastomycosis in Madagascar: a review. *Am. J. Trop. Med. Hyg.* **55:**45–47.

60. Esterre, P., and F. Queiroz-Telles. 2006. Management of chromoblastomycosis: novel perspectives. *Curr. Opin. Infect. Dis.* **19:**148–152.

61. Fernandez, M., D. E. Noyola, S. N. Rosemann, and M. S. Edwards. 1999. Cutaneous phaeohyphomycosis caused by *Curvularia lunata* and a review of *Curvularia* infections in pediatrics. *Pediatr. Infect. Dis. J.* **18:**727–731.

62. Fincher, R. M. E., J. F. Fisher, A. A. Padhye, L. Ajello, and J. C. H. Steele, Jr. 1988. Subcutaneous phaeohyphomycotic abscess caused by *Phialophora parasitica* in a renal allograft recipient. *J. Med. Vet. Mycol.* **26:**311–314.

63. Fisher, J. F., S. Shadomy, J. R. Teabeaut, J. Woodward, G. E. Michaels, M. A. Newman, E. White, P. Cook, A. Seagraves, F. Yaghmai, and J. P. Rissing. 1982. Near-drowning complicated by brain abscess due to *Petriellidium boydii. Arch. Neurol.* **39:**511–513.

64. Fothergill, A. W., M. G. Rinaldi, and D. A. Sutton. 2009. Antifungal susceptibility testing of *Exophiala* spp.: a head-to-head comparison of amphotericin B, itraconazole, posaconazole and voriconazole. *Med. Mycol.* **47:**41–43.

65. Fukushiro, R. 1983. Chromomycosis in Japan. *Int. J. Dermatol.* **22:**221–229.

66. Gams, W. 2000. *Phialophora* and some similar morphologically little-differentiated anamorphs of divergent ascomycetes. *Stud. Mycol.* **45:**187–199.

67. Gerrits van den Ende, A. H. G., and G. S. de Hoog. 1999. Variability and molecular diagnostics of the neurotropic species *Cladophialophora bantiana. Stud. Mycol.* **43:**151–162.

68. Gilgado, F., J. Cano, J. Gené, and J. Guarro. 2005. Molecular phylogeny of the *Pseudallescheria boydii* complex. Proposal of two new species. *J. Clin. Microbiol.* **43:**4930–4942.

69. Gilgado, F., J. Cano, J. Gené, D. A. Sutton, and J. Guarro. 2008. Molecular and phenotypic data supporting distinct species statuses for *Scedosporium apiospermum* and *Pseudallescheria boydii* and the proposed new species *Scedosporium dehoogii. J. Clin. Microbiol.* **46:**766–771.

70. Gilgado, F., C., Serena, J. Cano, J. Gené, and J. Guarro. 2006. Antifungal susceptibilities of the species of the *Pseudallescheria boydii* complex. *Antimicrob. Agents Chemother.* **50:**4211–4213.

71. Ginter, G., G. S. de Hoog, A. Pschaid, M. Fellinger, A. Bogiatzis, C. Berghold, E. M. Reich, and F. C. Odds. 1995. Arthritis without grains caused by *Pseudallescheria boydii. Mycoses* **38:**369–371.

72. González, G. M., A. W. Fothergill, D. A. Sutton, M. G. Rinaldi, and D. Loebenberg. 2005. In vitro activities of new and established triazoles against opportunistic filamentous and dimorphic fungi. *Med. Mycol.* **43:**281–284.

73. Gonzalez, M. S., B. Alfonso, D. Seckinger, A. A. Padhye, and L. Ajello. 1984. Subcutaneous phaeohyphomycosis caused by *Cladosporium devriesii. Sabouraudia* **22:**427–432.

74. González-López, M. A., R. Salesa, M. C. González-Vela, H. Fernández-Llaca, J. F. Val-Bernal, and J. Cano. 2007. Subcutaneous phaeohyphomycosis caused by *Exophiala oligosperma* in a renal transplant recipient. *Br. J. Dermatol.* **156:**762–764.

75. Göttlich, E., W. van der Lubbe, B. Lange, S. Fiedler, I. Melchert, M. Reifenrath, H.-C. Flemming, and G. S. de Hoog. 2002. Fungal flora in groundwater-derived public drinking water. *Int. J. Hyg. Environ. Health* **205:**269–279.

76. Guarro, J., A. S. Kantarcioglu, R. Horré, J. L. Rodriguez-Tudela, M. Cuenca, J. Berenguer, and G. S. de Hoog. 2006. *Scedosporium* infection, an emerging fungal disease entity. *Med. Mycol.* **44:**295–327.

77. Guarro, J., A. M. Silvestre, Jr., G. Verkley, J. Cano, O. F. Gompertz, J. Gené, M. M. Ogawa, J. Tomimori-Yamashita, S. P. Teixeira, and F. A. de Almeida. 2006. Limitations of DNA sequencing for diagnosis of a mixed infection by two fungi, *Phaeoacremonium venezuelense* and a *Plectophomella* sp., in a transplant recipient. *J. Clin. Microbiol.* **44:**4279–4282.

78. Guého, E., A. Bonnefoy, J. Luboinski, J.-C. Petit, and G. S. de Hoog. 1989. Subcutaneous granuloma caused by *Phialophora richardsiae*: case report and review of the literature. *Mycoses* **32:**219–223.

79. Guerrero, A., P. Torres, M. T. Duran, B. Ruiz-Diez, M. Rosales, and J. L. Rodriguez-Tudela. 2001. Airborne outbreak of nosocomial *Scedosporium prolificans* infection. *Lancet* **357:**1267–1268.

80. Gugnani, H. C., V. Ramesh, N. Sood, J. Guarro, Moin-Ul-Haq, A. Paliwal-Joshi, and B. Singh. 2006. Cutaneous phaeohyphomycosis caused by *Cladosporium oxysporum* and its treatment with potassium iodide. *Med. Mycol.* **44:**285–288.

81. Harun, A., H. Perdomo, F. Gilgado, S. C. A. Chen, J. Cano, J. Guarro, and W. Meyer. 2009. Genotyping of *Scedosporium* species: a review of molecular approaches. *Med. Mycol.* **47:**406–414.

82. Hirsch, B. E., B. F. Farber, J. F. Shapiro, and S. Kennelly. 1996. Successful treatment of *Aureobasidium pullulans* prosthetic hip infection. *Infect. Dis. Clin. Pract.* **5:**205–207.

83. Hohl, P. E., H. P. Holley, E. Prevost, L. Ajello, and A. A. Padhye. 1983. Infections due to *Wangiella dermatitidis* in humans: report of the first documented case from the United States and a review of the literature. *Rev. Infect. Dis.* **5:**854–864.

84. Hollingsworth, J. W., S. Shofer, and A. Zaas. 2007. Successful treatment of *Ochroconis gallopavum* infection in an immunocompetent host. *Infection* **35:**367–369.

85. Horré, R., and G. S. de Hoog. 1999. Primary cerebral infections by melanized fungi: a review. *Stud. Mycol.* **43:**176–193.

86. Horré, R., G. S. de Hoog, C. Kluczny, G. Marklein, and K. P. Schaal. 1999. rDNA diversity of *Ochroconis* and *Scolecobasidium* species isolated from humans and animals. *Stud. Mycol.* **43:**194–205.

87. Horré, R., E. Feil, A. P. Stangel, H. Zhou, S. Gilges, A. Wohrmann, G. S. de Hoog, J. F. Meis, G. Marklein, and K. P. Schaal. 2000. Scedosporiosis of the brain with fatal outcome after traumatization of the foot. *Mycoses* **43:**33–36.

88. Hsu, M. M., and Y.-Y. Lee. 1993. Cutaneous and subcutaneous phaeohyphomycosis caused by *Exserohilum rostratum*. *J. Am. Acad. Dermatol.* **28:**340–344.

89. Huang, Y. T., S. J. Liaw, C. H. Liao, J. L. Yang, D. M. Lai, Y. C. Lee, and P. R. Hsueh. 2008. Catheter-related septicemia due to *Aureobasidium pullulans*. *Int. J. Infect. Dis.* **12:**137–139.

90. Ibanez Perez, R., J. Chacon, A. Fidalgo, J. Martin, V. Paraiso, and J. L. Munoz-Bellido. 1997. Peritonitis by *Aureobasidium pullulans* in continuous ambulatory peritoneal dialysis. *Nephrol. Dial. Transplant.* **12:**1544–1545.

91. Kanj, S. S., S. S. Amr, and G. D. Roberts. 2001. *Ramichloridium mackenziei* brain abscess: report of two cases and review of the literature. *Med. Mycol.* **39:**97–102.

92. Kantarcioglu, A. S., and G. S. de Hoog. 2004. Infections of the central nervous system by melanized fungi: a review of cases presented between 1999 and 2004. *Mycoses* **47:**4–13.

93. Kantarcioglu, A. S., J. Guarro, and G. S. de Hoog. 2008. Central nervous system infections by members of the *Pseudallescheria boydii* species complex in healthy and immunocompromised hosts: epidemiology, clinical characteristics and outcome. *Mycoses* **51:**275–290.

94. Kantarcioglu, A. S., A. Yücel, and G. S. de Hoog. 2002. Isolation of *Cladosporium cladosporioides* from cerebrospinal fluid. *Mycoses* **45:**500–503.

95. Kimura, M., and M. R. McGinnis. 1998. Fontana-Masson stained tissue from culture-proven mycoses. *Arch. Pathol. Lab. Med.* **122:**1107–1111.

96. Langdon, J. S., and W. L. McDonald. 1987. Cranial *Exophiala pisciphila* infection in *Salmo salar* in Australia. *Bull. Eur. Assoc. Fish Pathol.* **7:**35–37.

97. Langvad, F., O. Pedersen, and K. Engjom. 1985. A fungal disease caused by *Exophiala* sp. nova in farmed Atlantic salmon in Western Norway, p. 323–328. *In* A. E. Ellis (ed.), *Fish and Shellfish Pathology.* Academic, London, United Kingdom.

98. Latham, R. H. 2000. *Bipolaris spicifera* meningitis complicating a neurosurgical procedure. *Scand. J. Infect. Dis.* **32:**102–103.

99. Lau, A., S. Chen, T. Sorrell, D. Carter, R. Malik, P. Martin, and C. Halliday. 2007. Development and clinical application of a panfungal PCR assay to detect and identify fungal DNA in tissue specimens. *J. Clin. Microbiol.* **45:**380–385.

100. Lavelle, P. 1980. Chromoblastomycosis in Mexico. *PAHO Sci. Publ.* **396:**235–247.

101. Li, D. M., G. S. de Hoog, D. M. Lindhardt Saunte, A. H. G. Gerrits van den Ende, and X. R. Chen. 2008. *Coniosporium epidermidis* sp. nov., a new species from human skin. *Stud. Mycol.* **61:**131–136.

102. Little, M. G., and M. L. Hammond. 1995. *Scytalidium dimidiatum* in Australia. *Australas. J. Dermatol.* **36:**204–205.

103. Lopez, F. A., R. S. Crowley, L. Wastila, H. A. Valantine, and J. S. Remington. 1999. *Scedosporium apiospermum* (*Pseudallescheria boydii*) infection in a heart transplant recipient: a case of mistaken identity. *J. Heart Lung Transplant.* **17:**321–324.

104. Madrid, H., M. Ruíz-Cendoya, J. Cano, A. Stchigel, R. Orofino, and J. Guarro. 2009. Genotyping and in vitro antifungal susceptibility of *Neoscytalidium dimidiatum* isolates from different origins. *Int. J. Antimicrob. Agents* **34:**351–354.

105. Malloch, D., and I. F. Salkin. 1984. A new species of *Scedosporium* associated with osteomyelitis in humans. *Mycotaxon* **21:**247–255.

106. Marimon, R., J. Cano, J. Gené, D. A. Sutton, M. Kawasaki, and J. Guarro. 2007. *Sporothrix brasiliensis*, *S. globosa*, and *S. mexicana*, three new *Sporothrix* species of clinical interest. *J. Clin. Microbiol.* **45:**3198–3206.

107. Marimon, R., J. Gene, J. Cano, and J. Guarro. 2008. *Sporothrix luriei*: a rare fungus from clinical origin. *Med. Mycol.* **10:**1–5.

108. Marimon, R., J. Gené, J. Cano, L. Trilles, M. D. S. Lazera, and J. Guarro. 2006. Molecular phylogeny of *Sporothrix schenckii*. *J. Clin. Microbiol.* **44:**3251–3256.

109. Marimon, R., C. Serena, J. Gené, J. Cano, and J. Guarro. 2008. In vitro antifungal susceptibilities of five species of *Sporothrix*. *Antimicrob. Agents Chemother.* **52:**732–734.

110. Mathews, M. S., and S. V. Maharajan. 1999. *Exserohilum rostratum* causing keratitis in India. *Med. Mycol.* **37:**131–132.

111. Matos, T., G. S. de Hoog, A. G. de Boer, I. de Crom, and G. Haase. 2002. High prevalence of the neurotrope *Exophiala dermatitidis* and related oligotrophic black yeasts in sauna facilities. *Mycoses* **45:**373–377.

112. Matos, T., G. Haase, A. H. G. Gerrits van den Ende, and G. S. de Hoog. 2003. Molecular diversity of oligotrophic and neurotropic members of the black yeast genus *Exophiala*, with accent on *E. dermatitidis*. *Antonie van Leeuwenhoek* **83:**293–303.

113. Mayser, P., M. Nilles, and G. S. de Hoog. 2002. Cutaneous phaeohyphomycosis due to *Alternaria alternata*. *Mycoses* **45:**338–340.

114. McGinnis, M. R., M. G. Rinaldi, and R. E. Winn. 1986. Emerging agents of phaeohyphomycosis: pathogenic species of *Bipolaris* and *Exserohilum*. *J. Clin. Microbiol.* **24:**250–259.

115. Moore, M. K. 1986. *Hendersonula toruloidea* and *Scytalidium hyalinum* infections in London, England. *J. Med. Vet. Mycol.* **24:**219–230.

116. Morris, A., W. A. Schell, D. McDonagh, S. Chafee, and J. R. Perfect. 1995. *Fonsecaea pedrosoi* pneumonia and *Emericella nidulans* cerebral abscesses in a bone marrow transplant patient. *Clin. Infect. Dis.* **21:**1346–1348.

117. Mostert, L., J. Z. Groenewald, R. C. Summerbell, V. Robert, D. A. Sutton, A. A. Padhye, and P. W. Crous. 2005. Species of *Phaeoacremonium* associated with infections in humans and environmental reservoirs in infected woody plants. *J. Clin. Microbiol.* **43:**1752–1767.

118. Nenoff, P., U. Gutz, K. Tintelnot, A. Bosse-Henck, M. Mierzwa, J. Hofmann, L. C. Horn, and U. F. Haustein. 1996. Disseminated mycosis due to *Scedosporium prolificans* in an AIDS patient with Burkitt lymphoma. *Mycoses* **39:**461–465.

119. Nobrega, J. P., S. Rosemberg, A. M. Adami, E. M. Heins-Vaccari, C. S. Lacaz, and T. de Brito. 2003. *Fonsecaea pedrosoi* cerebral phaeohyphomycosis ("chromoblastomycosis"): first human culture-proven case reported in Brazil. *Rev. Inst. Med. Trop. São Paulo* **45:**217–220.

120. Nulens, E., E. De Laere, H. Vandevelde, L. B. Hilbrands, A. J. Rijs, W. J. Melchers, and P. E. Verweij. 2006. *Alternaria infectoria* phaeohyphomycosis in a renal transplant patient. *Med. Mycol.* **44:**379–382.

121. Odell, J. A., S. Alvarez, D. G. Cvitkovich, D. A. Cortese, and B. L. McComb. 2000. Multiple lung abscesses due to *Ochroconis gallopavum*, a dematiaceous fungus, in a nonimmunocompromised wood pulp worker. *Chest* **118:**1503–1505.

122. Padhye, A. A., D. Davis, P. N. Baer, A. Reddick, K. K. Sinha, and J. Ott. 1998. Phaeohyphomycosis caused by *Phaeoacremonium inflatipes*. *J. Clin. Microbiol.* **36:**2763–2765.

123. Padhye, A. A., M. R. McGinnis, and L. Ajello. 1978. Thermotolerance of *Wangiella dermatitidis*. *J. Clin. Microbiol.* **8:**424–426.

124. Padhye, A. A., M. R. McGinnis, L. Ajello, and F. W. Chandler. 1988. *Xylohypha emmonsii* sp. nov., a new agent of phaeohyphomycosis. *J. Clin. Microbiol.* **26:**702–708.

125. Pastor, F. J., and J. Guarro. 2008. *Alternaria* infections: laboratory diagnosis and relevant clinical features. *Clin. Microbiol. Infect.* **14:**734–746.

126. Pauzner, R., A. Goldschmied-Reouven, I. Hay, Z. Vared, Z. Ziskind, N. Hassin, and Z. Farfel. 1997. Phaeohyphomycosis following cardiac surgery: case report and review of serious infection due to *Bipolaris* and *Exserohilum* species. *Clin. Infect. Dis.* **25:**921–923.

127. Pereiro, M., M. F. Pereiro, G. S. de Hoog, and J. Toribio. 2004. Cutaneous infection caused by *Alternaria* in patients receiving tacrolimus. *Med. Mycol.* **42:**277–282.

128. Pereiro, M., Jr., J. Jo-Chu, and J. Toribio. 1998. Phaeohyphomycotic cyst due to *Cladosporium cladosporioides*. *Dermatology* **197:**90–92.

129. Perez-Blanco, M., G. Fernandez-Zeppenfeldt, V. R. Hernandez, F. Yegres, and D. Borelli. 1998. Cromomicosis por *Rhinocladiella aquaspersa*: descripción del primer caso en Venezuela. *Revta Iberoam. Micol.* **15**:51–54.

130. Pimentel, J. D., K. Mahadevan, A. Woodgyer, L. Sigler, C. Gibas, O. C. Harris, M. Lupino, and E. Athan. 2005. Peritonitis due to *Curvularia inaequalis* in an elderly patient undergoing peritoneal dialysis and a review of six cases of peritonitis associated with other *Curvularia* spp. *J. Clin. Microbiol.* **43**:4288–4292.

131. Pitrak, D. L., E. W. Koneman, R. C. Estupinan, and J. Jackson. 1988. *Phialophora richardsiae* in humans. *Rev. Infect. Dis.* **10**:1195–1203.

132. Porteous, N. B., A. M. Grooters, S. W. Redding, E. H. Thompson, M. G. Rinaldi, G. S. de Hoog, and D. A. Sutton. 2003. *Exophiala mesophila* in dental unit waterlines. *J. Clin. Microbiol.* **41**:3885–3889.

133. Queiroz-Telles, F., P. Esterre, M. Pérez-Blanco, R. G. Vitale, C. Guedes Salgado, and A. Bonifaz. 2009. Chromoblastomycosis: an overview of clinical manifestations, diagnosis and treatment. *Med. Mycol.* **47**:3–15.

134. Ramos-e-Silva, M., C. Vasconcelos, S. Carneiro, and T. Cestari. 2007. Sporotrichosis. *Clin. Dermatol.* **25**:181–187.

135. Rebell, G., and R. K. Forster. 1976. *Lasiodiplodia theobromae* as a cause of keratomycoses. *Sabouraudia* **14**:155–170.

136. Revankar, S. G. 2007. Dematiaceous fungi. *Mycoses* **50**: 91–101.

137. Revankar, S. G., D. A. Sutton, and M. G. Rinaldi. 2004. Primary central nervous system phaeohyphomycosis: a review of 101 cases. *Clin. Infect. Dis.* **38**:206–216.

138. Rinaldi, M. G., P. Phillips, J. G. Schwartz, R. E. Winn, G. R. Holt, F. W. Shagets, J. Elrod, G. Nishioka, and T. B. Aufdemorte. 1987. Human *Curvularia* infections. Report of five cases and review of the literature. *Diagn. Microbiol. Infect. Dis.* **6**:27–39.

139. Rodriguez-Tudela, J. L., J. Berenguer, J. Guarro, A. S. Kantarcioglu, R. Horre, G. S. de Hoog, and M. Cuenca-Estrella. 2009. Epidemiology and outcome of *Scedosporium prolificans* infection, a review of 162 cases. *Med. Mycol.* **47**:359–370.

140. Roeijmans, H. J., G. S. de Hoog, C. S. Tan, and M. J. Figge. 1997. Molecular taxonomy and GC/MS of metabolites of *Scytalidium hyalinum* and *Nattrassia mangiferae* (*Hendersonula toruloidea*). *J. Med. Vet. Mycol.* **35**:181–188.

141. Romano, C., M. Fimiani, M. Pellegrino, L. Valenti, L. Casini, C. Miracco, and E. Faggi. 1996. Cutaneous phaeohyphomycosis due to *Alternaria tenuissima*. *Mycoses* **39**:211–215.

142. Roosje, P. J., G. S. de Hoog, J. P. Koeman, and T. Willemse. 1993. Phaeohyphomycosis in a cat caused by *Alternaria infectoria* Simmons. *Mycoses* **36**:451–454.

143. Salkin, I. F., J. A. Martinez, and M. E. Kemna. 1986. Opportunistic infection of the spleen caused by *Aureobasidium pullulans*. *J. Clin. Microbiol.* **23**:828–831.

144. Saravanakumar, P. S., P. Eslami, and F. A. Zar. 1996. Lymphocutaneous sporotrichosis associated with a squirrel bite: case report and review. *Clin. Infect. Dis.* **23**:647–648.

145. Scott, E. N., and H. G. Muchmore. 1989. Immunoblot analysis of antibody responses to *Sporothrix schenckii*. *J. Clin. Microbiol.* **27**:300–304.

146. Selbmann, L., G. S. de Hoog, A. Mazzaglia, E. I. Friedmann, and S. Onofri. 2005. Fungi at the edge of life: cryptoendolithic black fungi from Antarctic deserts. *Stud. Mycol.* **51**:1–26.

147. Severo, L. C., M. C. Bassanesi, and A. T. Londero. 1994. Tinea nigra: report of four cases observed in Rio Grande do Sul (Brazil) and a review of Brazilian literature. *Mycopathologia* **126**:157–162.

148. Severo, L. C., F. de M. Oliveira, C. D. Garcia, A. Uhlmann, and A. T. Londero. 1999. Peritonitis by *Scedosporium apiospermum* in a patient undergoing continuous ambulatory peritoneal dialysis. *Rev. Inst. Med. Trop. São Paulo* **41**:263–264.

149. Shin, J. H., S. K. Lee, S. P. Suh, D. W. Ryang, N. H. Kim, M. G. Rinaldi, and D. A. Sutton. 1998. Fatal *Hormonema dematioides* peritonitis in a patient on continuous ambulatory peritoneal dialysis: criteria for organism identification

150. Sidrim, J. J. C., R. H. O. Menezes, G. C. Paixao, M. F. G. Rocha, R. S. N. Brilhante, A. M. A. Oliveria, and M. J. N. Diogenes. 1999. *Rhinocladiella aquaspersa*: limite imprecise entre chromoblastomycose et phaeohyphomycose? *J. Mycol. Med.* **9**:114–118.

151. Sigler, L., R. C. Summerbell, L. Poole, M. Wieden, D. A. Sutton, M. G. Rinaldi, M. Aguirre, G. W. Estes, and J. N. Galgiani. 1997. Invasive *Nattrassia mangiferae* infections: case report, literature review, and therapeutic and taxonomic appraisal. *J. Clin. Microbiol.* **35**:433–440.

152. Singh, N., R. Agarwal, D. Gupta, M. R. Shivaprakash, and A. Chakrabarti. 2006. An unusual case of mediastinal mass due to *Fonsecaea pedrosoi*. *Eur. Respir. J.* **28**:662–664.

153. Singh, S. M., J. Naidu, and M. Pouranik. 1990. Ungual and cutaneous phaeohyphomycosis caused by *Alternaria alternata* and *Alternaria chlamydospora*. *J. Med. Vet. Mycol.* **28**:275–282.

154. Slomovic, A. R., R. K. Forster, and H. Gelender. 1985. *Lasiodiplodia theobromae* panophthalmitis. *Can. J. Ophthalmol.* **20**:225–228.

155. Sood, N., H. C. Gugnani, J. Guarro, A. Paliwal-Joshi, and V. K. Vijayan. 2007. Subcutaneous phaeohyphomycosis caused by *Alternaria alternata* in an immunocompetent patient. *Int. J. Dermatol.* **46**:412–413.

156. Sterflinger, K., G. S. de Hoog, and G. Haase. 1999. Phylogeny and ecology of meristematic ascomycetes. *Stud. Mycol.* **43**:5–22.

157. Sudduth, E. J., A. J. Crumbley, and W. E. Farrar. 1992. Phaeohyphomycosis due to *Exophiala* species: clinical spectrum of disease in humans. *Clin. Infect. Dis.* **15**:639–644.

158. Summerbell, R. C., S. Krajden, R. Levine, and M. Fuksa. 2004. Subcutaneous phaeohyphomycosis caused by *Lasiodiplodia theobromae* and successfully treated surgically. *Med. Mycol.* **42**:543–547.

159. Surash, S., A. Tyagi, G. S. de Hoog, J.-S. Zeng, R. C. Barton, and R. P. Hobson. 2005. Cerebral phaeohyphomycosis caused by *Fonsecaea monophora*. *Med. Mycol.* **43**:465–472.

160. Sutton, D. A., M. Slifkin, R. Yakulis, and M. G. Rinaldi. 1998. U.S. case report of cerebral phaeohyphomycosis caused by *Ramichloridium obovoideum* (*R. mackenziei*): criteria for identification, therapy, and review of other known dematiaceous neurotropic taxa. *J. Clin. Microbiol.* **36**:708–715.

161. Takei, H., J. C. Goodman, and S. Z. Powell. 2007. Cerebral phaeohyphomycosis caused by *Cladophialophora bantiana* and *Fonsecaea monophora*: report of three cases. *Clin. Neuropathol.* **26**:21–27.

162. Tintelnot, K., P. von Hunnius, G. S. de Hoog, A. Polak-Wyss, E. Guého, and F. Masclaux. 1995. Systemic mycosis caused by a new *Cladophialophora* species. *J. Med. Vet. Mycol.* **33**:349–354.

163. Turiansky, G. W., P. M. Benson, L. C. Sperling, P. Sau, I. F. Salkin, M. R. McGinnis, and W. D. James. 1995. *Phialophora verrucosa*: a new cause of mycetoma. *J. Am. Acad. Dermatol.* **32**:311–315.

164. Uberti-Foppa, C., L. Fumagalli, N. Gianotti, A. M. Viviani, R. Vaiani, and E. Guého. 1995. First case of osteomyelitis due to *Phialophora richardsiae* in a patient with HIV infection. *AIDS* **9**:975–976.

165. Velazquez, L. F., A. Restrepo, and G. Calle. 1976. Cromomicosis: experiencia de doce años. *Acta Med. Colomb.* **1**:165–171.

166. Vieira, M. R., A. Milheiro, and F. A. Pacheco. 2001. Phaeohyphomycosis due to *Cladosporium cladosporioides*. *Med. Mycol.* **39**:135–137.

167. Vitale, R. G., and G. S. de Hoog. 2002. Molecular diversity, new species and antifungal susceptibilities in the *Exophiala spinifera* clade. *Med. Mycol.* **40**:545–556.

168. Willinger, B., G. Kopetzky, F. Harm, P. Apfalter, A. Makristathis, A. Berer, A. Bankier, and S. Winkler. 2004. Disseminated infection with *Nattrassia mangiferae* in an immunosuppressed patient. *J. Clin. Microbiol.* **42**:478–480.

169. Wilson, C. M., E. J. O'Rourke, M. R. McGinnis, and I. F. Salkin. 1990. *Scedosporium inflatum*: clinical spectrum of a newly recognized pathogen. *J. Infect. Dis.* **161**:102–107.

170. **Woo, P. C., S. K. Lau, A. H. Ngan, H. Tse, E. T. Tung, and K. Y. Yuen.** 2008. *Lasiodiplodia theobromae* pneumonia in a liver transplant recipient. *J. Clin. Microbiol.* **46:**380–384.

171. **Wood, G. M., J. G. McCormack, and D. B. Muir.** 1992. Clinical features of human infection with *Scedosporium inflatum. Clin. Infect. Dis.* **14:**1027.

172. **Yamagishi, Y., K. Kawasaki, and H. Ishizaki.** 1997. Mitochondrial DNA analysis of *Phialophora verrucosa. Mycoses* **40:**329–334.

173. **Yau, Y. C., J. de Nanassy, R. C. Summerbell, A. G. Matlow, and S. E. Richardson.** 1994. Fungal sternal wound infection due to *Curvularia lunata* in a neonate with congenital heart disease: case report and review. *Clin. Infect. Dis.* **19:**735–740.

174. **Young, C. N., J. G. Swart, D. Ackerman, and K. Davidge-Pitts.** 1978. Nasal obstruction and bone erosion caused by *Drechslera hawaiiensis. J. Laryngol. Otol.* **92:**137–143.

175. **Yurlova, N. A., and G. S. de Hoog.** 2002. Exopolysaccharides and capsules in human pathogenic *Exophiala* species. *Mycoses* **45:**443–448.

176. **Yurlova, N. A., G. S. de Hoog, and A. H. G. Gerrits van den Ende.** 1999. Taxonomy of *Aureobasidium* and allied genera. *Stud. Mycol.* **43:**63–69.

177. **Zalar, P., G. S. de Hoog, and N. Gunde-Cimerman.** 1999. Ecology of halotolerant dothideaceous black yeasts. *Stud. Mycol.* **43:**38–48.

178. **Zeng, J. S., D. A. Sutton, A. W. Fothergill, M. G. Rinaldi, M. J. Harrak, and G. S. de Hoog.** 2007. Spectrum of clinically relevant *Exophiala* species in the United States. *J. Clin. Microbiol.* **45:**3713–3720.

179. **Zeppenfeldt, G., N. Richard-Yegres, F. Yegres, and R. Hernández.** 1994. *Cladosporium carrionii:* hongo dimorfo en cactáceas de la zona endémica para la cromomicosis en Venezuela. *Rev. Iberoam. Micol.* **11:**61–63.

Fungi Causing Eumycotic Mycetoma*

ABDALLA O. A. AHMED AND G. SYBREN DE HOOG

123

Eumycetoma is a chronic, granulomatous, progressive subcutaneous fungal disease characterized by the production of large masses of fungal organisms called grains, which are discharged through sinus tracts. Eumycetoma is seen more frequently in tropical and subtropical regions and less frequently in temperate countries. Several hyaline and dematiaceous fungi can cause eumycetoma, and their distributions are greatly affected by climate, especially rainfall.

TAXONOMY

All fungi known to cause eumycetoma probably belong to the phylum Ascomycota, although for many species no ascus-producing state is known (26). Ordinal relationships are hypothesized on the basis of ribosomal small subunit (24) and internal transcribed spacer (ITS) DNA sequences (28) (Table 1; see also listing by order below). The etiologic agents described in this chapter are species that are isolated most commonly from human or lower-animal mycetoma.

Order Pleosporales

Curvularia Species
Numerous species of Curvularia are known, mostly occurring in decaying vegetations. Curvularia is a hyphomycete dematiaceous mold, with some known teleomorphs belonging to the class Euascomycetes in the phylum Ascomycota (26).

Leptosphaeria senegalensis
L. senegalensis is a dematiaceous filamentous fungus with a known teleomorph belonging to the class Euascomycetes in the phylum Ascomycota (26).

Madurella grisea
Molecular phylogeny and diagnostics of members of the genus Madurella based on the ribosomal operon showed that this genus encompasses a hidden diversity beyond the two currently recognized species (24). An rRNA restriction fragment length polymorphism was used for species distinction by Ahmed et al. (3, 4), and a specific ITS PCR was used by Ahmed et al. (4).

Pyrenochaeta romeroi
Pyrenochaeta is a coelomycete anamorphic fungus. The genus Pyrenochaeta contains three species: Pyrenochaeta mackinnonii, Pyrenochaeta unguis-hominis, and Pyrenochaeta romeroi. Pyrenochaeta mackinnonii and Pyrenochaeta romeroi might be misidentified as Madurella grisea when cultures are lacking pycnidia (asexual fruiting bodies containing conidia) (26). Pyrenochaeta romeroi is indistinguishable from Phoma leveillei (coelomycete), and it should be classified in the genus Phoma rather than in Pyrenochaeta (26).

Order Chaetothyriales

Exophiala jeanselmei
E. jeanselmei is one of the black yeasts, which belong to the ascomycete order Chaetothyriales. Members of this order are frequently involved in black grain mycetoma in the tropics (8, 26).

Order Sordariales

Madurella mycetomatis
Phylogenetic studies suggest that M. mycetomatis and M. grisea are distantly related. M. mycetomatis is probably a member of the order Sordariales, while M. grisea clusters with known members of the Pleosporales (24).

Neotestudina rosatii
Neotestudina rosatii is classified in the class Ascomycetes, order Dothideales (24, 26). This species has been isolated from human mycetoma and soil from tropical countries (24, 26).

Order Microascales

Phaeoacremonium Species
Phaeoacremonium is the anamorph filamentous fungus of the teleomorph genus Togninia, which belongs to the order Diaporthales in the class Ascomycetes (66). Phaeoacremonium contains many species associated with plants and human infections (66).

---

*Some of the material in this chapter was presented in chapter 126 by G. Sybren de Hoog, Abdalla O. A. Ahmed, Michael R. McGinnis, and Arvind A. Padhye in the ninth edition of this Manual.

TABLE 1 Overview of main species causing eumycotic mycetoma

Order	Species	Geographic distribution	Color of grains	Size of grains (mm)
Pleosporales	*Curvularia geniculata*	Worldwide	Black	0.5–1.0
Pleosporales	*Curvularia lunata*	Worldwide	Black	0.5–1.0
Chaetothyriales	*Exophiala jeanselmei*	Worldwide	Black	0.5–1.0
Hypocreales	*Fusarium falciforme*	Worldwide	Whitish	0.2–0.5
Pleosporales	*Leptosphaeria senegalensis*	West Africa, India	Black	0.5–2.0
Pleosporales	*Madurella grisea*	South America, India	Black	0.3–0.6
Sordariales	*Madurella mycetomatis*	East Africa, Middle East	Black	Up to 5.0 or more
Sordariales	*Neotestudina rosatii*	Central Africa	Whitish	0.5–1.0
Diaporthales	*Phaeoacremonium* spp.	South America, India	White or black	0.5–2.0
Microascales	*Pseudallescheria boydii*	North and South America	Whitish	0.2–2.0
Pleosporales	*Pyrenochaeta mackinnonii*	Central and South America	Black	0.3–1.0
Pleosporales	*Pyrenochaeta romeroi*	Arid subtropics	Black	0.3–1.0

Order Hypocreales

Fusarium falciforme

F. falciforme is the filamentous fungus previously known as *Acremonium falciforme* (86). The genus *Fusarium* is classified in the order Hypocreales in the class Ascomycetes.

Order Microascales

Pseudallescheria Species

The genus *Pseudallescheria* comprises a larger number of species than supposed originally (36, 37, 75). Recently, *Pseudallescheria boydii* and *Scedosporium apiospermum* have been separated from each other as different species. In addition, new species have been proposed in the two genera, namely *P. minutispora*, *S. aurantiacum*, and *S. dehoogii* (36, 37). Therefore, previously reported mycetoma cases attributed to *P. boydii* might actually have been caused by a different species.

DESCRIPTION OF THE AGENTS

Order Pleosporales

Curvularia geniculata

The common saprobe *Curvularia geniculata* has occasionally been reported as an etiologic agent of mycetoma in dogs in the United States (16).

Curvularia lunata

The ubiquitous saprobe *Curvularia lunata* (Fig. 1 and 2) has been described as an etiologic agent of mycetoma in humans in Senegal and Sudan (56, 84).

Leptosphaeria senegalensis

L. senegalensis and the related species *L. tompkinsii* cause mycetomata in the northern tropical portion of Africa, especially in Senegal and Mauritania, and in India (29, 31).

Madurella grisea

M. grisea occurs as an etiologic agent of black grain mycetoma in South America, India, Africa, and North and Central America (17, 55, 56, 65). As the fungus is strictly sterile, molecular confirmation is overdue for all these cases.

Pyrenochaeta romeroi

Mycetomata caused by *P. romeroi* (Fig. 3) have been reported from Somalia, India, and South America (13, 49, 58).

The close resemblance of the granules produced by the coelomycete *P. romeroi* and the gray cultures of that species suggests that *Madurella grisea* may be a nonsporulating counterpart of *P. romeroi*. Molecular rRNA ITS data (24) show that all these species are very different from one another.

Order Chaetothyriales

Exophiala jeanselmei

E. jeanselmei (Fig. 4) has been reported as an agent of eumycetoma in India (87, 88), Malaysia, Thailand (74), Argentina (63), and the United States (70), but only a few cases (51, 68) have been confirmed by molecular data (27a).

The related fungus *Cladophialophora bantiana*, a species that in humans is mainly linked with brain infections (47), was recently reported to cause mycetoma in humans (10, 97) and dogs (39).

Order Sordariales

Madurella mycetomatis

Madurella mycetomatis is common in the arid climatic zone of Africa (Sudan, Mali, and Djibouti) and is occasionally encountered in the Middle East and India.

Neotestudina rosatii

Mycetomata caused by *N. rosatii* have been described in Australia, Cameroon, Guinea, Senegal, and Somalia (58, 82).

Order Diaporthales

Phaeoacremonium Species

Members of the genus *Phaeoacremonium* are occasionally reported as agents of mycetoma. de Albornoz (22) described a case of infection caused by *Phaeoacremonium inflatipes*, Rowland and Farrar (79) and Hemashettar et al. (45) described cases of infection by *Phaeoacremonium krajdenii*, and Hood et al. (46) described a case of infection by *Phaeoacremonium parasiticum*.

Order Hypocreales

Fusarium falciforme

F. falciforme (86) (Fig. 5) is occasionally found as a cause of mycetoma in the United States and Argentina (42, 64, 69). It was also reported as the cause of an opportunistic mycetoma infection in a renal transplant recipient (94).

Order Microascales

Pseudallescheria boydii (Anamorph: *Scedosporium boydii*)

P. boydii is the most common agent of mycetoma in humans as well as lower animals in temperate climates (19), occurring mostly in the limbs (95). Subcutaneous infections frequently lack the formation of grains when the patients' immunity is impaired (73). In addition, arthritis is frequently observed, due to the predilection of this species for cartilaginous tissues (38, 44, 53, 71).

EPIDEMIOLOGY AND TRANSMISSION

The number of species involved in mycetoma is increasing, but little is known about the epidemiology and mode of transmission of these species. Case reports are indicative of the presence of certain species in particular geographical locations but do not provide a clear understanding of the environmental distribution of species and the possible ecological niches.

The causal agents of eumycetoma are largely saprobes that live on hard plant materials, such as various types of thorns and spines, associated with soil (5, 9, 33, 54). Segretain and coworkers (82, 84), using specific isolation media and techniques, showed that *L. senegalensis* and *L. tompkinsii* could be recovered from about 50% of the dry thorns of *Acacia* trees that they examined, particularly those that had been stained by mud during the rainy season. *N. rosatii* was reportedly isolated from sandy ground (58), and *M. mycetomatis* was isolated from soil and anthills (81, 90). It should be noted, however, that the identity of these fungi has not been verified with molecular methods; the possibility that environmental strains do not always belong to the same species as the clinical strains cannot be excluded. Using ITS sequencing, Badali et al. (8) reidentified a collection of *E. jeanselmei* clinical and environmental strains. *E. jeanselmei* identification was confirmed in all mycetoma or mycetoma-like infections, while other environmental strains were found to belong to other *Exophiala* species, suggesting some predilection for human invasion with particular species. Another example of possible human predilection is *M. mycetomatis*, which is a common agent of black grain mycetoma in the arid climate zones of East Africa. The direct isolation of this species from the environment is difficult (1).

Borelli (11) isolated another sterile fungus, reported as *Madurella grisea*, from soil in Venezuela; the ecological niche and clinical potential of this rare species have not yet been determined. *P. boydii* is associated with manure and polluted environments (27, 35) and has been known as an agent of human mycetoma in temperate climates since the 1920s (85).

Mycetoma may infect all people living in areas of endemicity but develops more commonly among persons who are in contact with contaminated materials, such as field workers, farmers, and fishermen. Areas of endemicity are particularly located in tropical climate zones. *M. mycetomatis* is limited to semiarid to arid climates, while *Leptosphaeria* species are found in the rain forest. Locally acquired mycetomata in temperate climates invariably are caused by *P. boydii*. Cases observed in the United States and Europe caused by species other than *P. boydii* are imported by immigrants from tropical countries. For example, de Hoog et al. (25) reported cases in The Netherlands originating from Indonesia and Suriname, and Ahmed et al. (3) reported *M. mycetomatis* mycetoma cases seen in France but originating in Mali.

Climate has a definite influence on the prevalence and distribution of mycetoma. Rivers that flood each year during the wet season in many countries of Africa and Asia influence the distribution of the causal agents. Rainfall also aids the spread of the etiologic agents on organic matter (30).

CLINICAL SIGNIFICANCE

A mycetoma (plural, mycetomata) (62) is a localized, chronic, noncontiguous, granulomatous infection involving cutaneous and subcutaneous tissues and eventually, in some cases, bones. Mycetomata are generally confined to either the feet or the hands but occasionally affect sites such as the back, shoulders, buttocks, and, rarely, the scalp. The characteristic triad of a painless subcutaneous mass, sinuses, and discharge containing grains (masses of fungal organisms) is characteristic of mycetoma; however, a similar condition (actinomycetoma) may be caused by aerobic actinomycete bacteria.

The disease is more commonly seen in humans than in lower animals. Only a few cases of mycetoma involving such animals as cats, dogs, horses, and goats have been described in the literature (16, 48, 50, 52, 56; L. Ajello, presented at the Primer Simposio Internacional de Micetomas, Barquisimeto, Venezuela, 1978). Most cases occur in otherwise healthy patients. The development of mycetoma after an accidental implantation of the etiologic agent following surgery (72) and in a renal transplant recipient (94) has been reported.

A mycetoma develops after a traumatic injury by microbe-contaminated thorns, splinters, fish scales or fins, snake bites, insect bites, farm implements, and knives. The initial lesion is often characterized by a feeling of discomfort and pain at the point of inoculation. Weeks or months later, the subcutaneous tissue at the site of inoculation becomes indurated, abscesses develop, and fistulae may drain to the surface. Mycetomata are characterized by swelling, granulomas, abscesses, and sinuses from which serosanguinous fluid containing fungal grains are discharged. Grains can vary from approximately 0.2 to over 5 mm in diameter. The size, color, shape, and internal architecture of the grains vary depending on the species of the etiologic agent. Some of the host material, especially at the periphery of the grain, provides a protective barrier for the fungus against antifungal agents and humoral immune responses such as antibodies.

A mycetoma develops slowly beneath thick fibrosclerous tissue. The subsequent phase of proliferation involves the invasion of muscles and intramuscular layers by portions of the sclerotium that break free from their parent structure. The granulomatous lesions can extend as deep as bone, where severe bone destruction, formation of small cavities, and complete remodeling may occur. Early osteolytic damage includes loss of the cortical margin and external erosion of the bone. As the infection progresses, blood, lymphatic vessels, and nerves may be damaged. Frequently, secondary bacterial infections and osteomyelitis producing total bone destruction occur. Pain is often associated with the development of multiple fistulas.

Fungus balls in preexisting lung cavities are sometimes inappropriately called mycetomata (34, 40). In the absence of well-organized grains, they should be referred to as aspergillomas, or simply as fungus balls, depending on the etiologic agent (59). Similarly, mycelial aggregates formed by dermatophytes in cutaneous or subcutaneous tissues differ from grains of mycetomata by lacking granule ontogeny, a distinct Splendore-Hoeppli reaction (see "Microscopy" below) surrounding the mycelial aggregates, and the entry of the fungus from the hair follicles into deeper tissue following the rupture of the follicular epithelium. Such infections caused by dermatophytes have been referred to as pseudomycetomata (6).

COLLECTION, TRANSPORT, AND STORAGE OF SPECIMENS

Methods of collection, transport, and storage of specimens are described in detail in chapter 112. Different specimens can be obtained from patients with eumycetoma, but direct examination and culture of fungi causing mycetoma always require surgical tissue biopsies and/or bone curettage. Tissue materials should be divided and submitted for both microbiology and histopathology examination. It should be noted that tissue biopsy specimens without visible grains usually result in negative cultures. The best specimen for fungal cultures is usually collected during surgery as excisional or incisional biopsy. Grains are not always present in tissue specimens obtained by a cutaneous biopsy procedure with local anesthesia. However, incisional biopsy specimens obtained under local anesthesia, when containing grains, can also result in positive cultures. Grains collected with cotton swabs from the sinus tracts are not recommended, because such grains can be contaminated or dead.

Several grains are usually needed for direct examination and culture, and therefore, as much tissue as possible should be obtained. Tissue should be collected in sterile dry leakproof containers and transported to the laboratory as soon as possible at room temperature. If transport is delayed for more than 2 h, specimens can be refrigerated. Small biopsy samples can be covered with 2 to 3 ml of sterile saline to prevent drying during transportation to the laboratory.

DIRECT EXAMINATION

Microscopy

The grains of eumycetomata are composed of septate mycelial filaments at least 2 to 5 μm in diameter. The mycelium may be distorted and unusual in form and size, and the cell walls of the fungi, especially toward the periphery of the grains, are thickened. Vesicles are frequently present, especially at the periphery of the grain. The mycelium of the grains may be embedded in a cementlike substance, depending on the species involved. Wethered et al. (98) described the cement surrounding grains of M. *mycetomatis* as being an amorphous, electron-dense material with areas containing different-sized membrane-bound vesicular inclusions. Often the sclerotia elicit an immune response, known as the Splendore-Hoeppli reaction (6, 62), seen histologically in the form of an eosinophilic deposit of amorphous material around the grain. A similar tissue reaction in experimental eumycetoma in mice has been described (4a).

Grains are white or yellow-brown ("white grain mycetoma") when the agent is producing mostly hyaline mycelia, and black ("black grain mycetoma") in the case of melanized fungi. Melanin is a high-molecular-weight compound that is anchored to extracellular proteins. A precursor for production of melanin in ascomycetous fungi is 1,8-dihydroxynaphthalene (DHN-melanin) (61, 62). In *Madurella mycetomatis*, melanin was shown to be produced through the DHN pathway and offers the fungus protection against strong oxidants and antifungal drugs (91). Reports

of hyaline fungi such as *Acremonium kiliense* and *Fusarium solani* var. *coeruleum* forming black grains (89) are probably erroneous. Etiologic agents with melanized hyphae or conidia such as *P. inflatipes* and *P. boydii* produce whitish grains in tissue (21, 22, 54, 63). Melanin production in *Phaeoacremonium* species is facultative, while in *P. boydii* dark pigmentation is limited to the conidia.

Curvularia geniculata

C. *geniculata* grains are black to dark brown, firm, and 0.5 to 1.0 mm or more in size. In tissue sections, grains are spherical, ovoid, or irregularly shaped and are often surrounded by a zone of epithelioid cells. The periphery of the grain is a dense, interwoven mass of dematiaceous mycelium and thick-walled, chlamydospore-like cells embedded in a cement-like substance. The interior of the grains is vacuolar and consists of a loose network of septate, hyphal filaments.

Curvularia lunata

The grains of C. *lunata* resemble those of C. *geniculata* in their morphologic characteristics.

Leptosphaeria Species

The grains of the two *Leptosphaeria* species are indistinguishable from each other. They are black, 0.5 to 2 mm in size, and firm to hard. In tissue sections, the grains are round to polylobulated, with large vesicles. At the periphery, the mycelium is embedded in a black, cementlike substance. The central portion of each grain consists of a loose network of hyphae.

M. grisea

Grains of M. *grisea* are black, 0.3 to 0.6 mm in diameter, and soft to firm. In tissue sections, the grains are oval, lobulated, or reniform (kidney-shaped), and sometimes vermiform (worm-shaped). They are composed of a dense network of hyphae weakly pigmented in the center and brown to blackish brown in the peripheral region as the result of the presence of a brown, cementlike interstitial material.

P. romeroi

P. *romeroi* produces soft to firm black sclerotia that are oval, lobulated, sometimes vermiform and about 1.0 mm in diameter. They resemble those of M. *grisea* (83).

E. jeanselmei

In host tissue, E. *jeanselmei* produces dark sclerotia that are brown to black, irregular in shape, and fragile. Detached portions or fragments of the sclerotia often are found within giant cells. When extruded through fistulae, the grains often look like worms (vermiform) because of their elongated shapes and irregular surfaces. In tissue sections, grains appear as hollow structures or as sinuous bands that are vermiform. The external surface is composed of brown, thick-walled hyphae and thick-walled chlamydosporelike cells. The grains are cement free. Within the hollow grains, smaller, degenerated hyphal fragments with leukocytes and giant cells may be seen.

M. mycetomatis

The grains produced by M. *mycetomatis* are reddish brown to black. They may reach 5 mm or more in diameter and are firm to hard. In tissue sections, the sclerotia are compact, variable in size and shape, and frequently multilobulated. They are composed of hyphae 1.2 to 5 μm in diameter that terminate in enlarged hyphal cells at the periphery of the grains, which measure 12 to 15 μm in diameter. The cell wall pigment is minimal, but hyphal cells contain brown particles. The hyphae are embedded in a conspicuous brown matrix that is characteristic of M. mycetomatis. Some grains are vesicular and more regular in size and shape. The vesicles are predominantly visible in the peripheral zone in a dense, brown, cementlike matrix.

N. rosatii

The sclerotia of N. rosatii are white to brownish white, 0.5 to 1.0 mm in diameter, and soft. In tissue sections, the sclerotia appear to be polyhedral to subregular and consist of hyphae, which are embedded in the peripheral cementing material. The sclerotia demonstrate an eosinophilic border. The central portion of each sclerotium consists of more or less disintegrated mycelium and chlamydospores.

Phaeoacremonium Species

Although Phaeoacremonium is a dematiaceous fungus and the well-known agent of phaeohyphomycosis, it seems that melanin production is facultative in eumycetoma. White grain mycetoma caused by P. krajdenii has been reported by Hemashettar et al. (45).

F. falciforme

The grains of F. falciforme are white to pale yellow, soft, and 0.2 to 0.5 mm in diameter. They are composed of slender, polymorphic, septate hyphae 1.5 to 2.0 μm in diameter with irregular bulbous swellings and peripheral cementing material.

Pseudallescheria Species

Grains of Pseudallescheria species in tissue are white to yellowish white and soft to firm; they vary from globose to subglobose or lobulated and are 0.2 to 2.0 mm in diameter. They are composed of hyaline hyphae 1.5 to 5.0 μm in diameter that radiate from the center into terminal thick-walled cells 15 to 20 μm in diameter at the peripheries. The central portion of each grain consists of loosely interwoven hyaline mycelium.

Antigen Detection

There are no commercially available assays for detection of antigen from these agents.

Nucleic Acid Detection Techniques

Molecular diagnostics have been developed for selected agents. PCR-based assays for rapid diagnosis of Scedosporium apiospermum infections from infected tissue are useful (41, 57). Willinger et al. (99) used molecular techniques for detection of S. apiospermum and similar organisms from fungus balls in the maxillary sinus.

ISOLATION PROCEDURES

To maximize the chances of obtaining pure cultures of the etiologic agents, grains from the eumycotic mycetomata should be washed several times with saline containing antibacterial antibiotics such as penicillin and streptomycin. The grains are then cultured on Sabouraud dextrose agar (SDA) containing chloramphenicol (50 mg/liter) and SDA containing chloramphenicol and cycloheximide (500 mg/liter) in petri dishes. Plates should be incubated at 25 and 37°C. Because many of the fungi that cause mycetoma grow slowly, culture plates should be incubated for 4 weeks before being discarded as negative. Identification of the isolated fungus is based on gross morphology of fruit bodies and conidia, if present.

Certain species (M. grisea, M. mycetomatis, N. rosatii, P. mackinnonii, and P. romeroi) do not sporulate readily but can be recognized by molecular techniques (4, 96). Borman and his coworkers developed a rapid protocol for identifying agents of black grain mycetoma by sequence data of the rRNA ITS (15). The black yeast E. jeanselmei (3) and agents of the genus Phaeoacremonium can be identified by using the same marker (66, 67). Wedde et al. (96) also developed specific primers based on rRNA ITS sequences for the identification of Pseudallescheria and Scedosporium species. Given the large infraspecific variability of the species, a less variable region, such as the 26S rRNA operon (80), might also provide successful detection of S. apiospermum-like genotypes.

IDENTIFICATION

C. geniculata

In culture, C. geniculata develops a rapidly growing, floccose to downy, olive gray to black colony. Microscopically, the melanized, septate hyphae bear solitary, geniculate (bent like a knee) conidiogenous cells. The conidia are without protruding hila. They are smooth walled, predominantly five celled, curved, with the swollen median cell pale to dark brown, in contrast to the lighter end cells.

C. lunata

In culture, C. lunata produces geniculate conidiophores that are sympodial in their development. Conidia are without protruding hila. They are smooth and predominantly four celled, with the penultimate cell being pale to dark brown.

Leptosphaeria Species

In culture, L. senegalensis and L. tompkinsii grow rapidly and produce gray-brown colonies. On cornmeal agar, both species produce ascostromata that are nonostiolate (without natural opening), scattered, immersed or superficial, globose to subglobose, black, and covered with brown, smoothly bent hyphae. The asci, produced after prolonged incubation on plant stems, are eight spored, clavate to cylindrical, and double walled. The major difference between the two species is found in the ascospores, which differ in size, shape, septation, and the nature of the gelatinous sheath that surrounds them (31, 32).

M. grisea

In culture, M. grisea forms slow-growing, velvety colonies that are cerebriform, radially furrowed or smooth, and dark gray to olive brown to black. The reverses of the colonies are black. Microscopically, the hyphae are septate, light to dark brown, 1 to 3 μm in diameter, and nonsporulating. Chlamydospores are rare. Large moniliform hyphae, 3 to 5 μm in diameter, are often present. Some isolates of M. grisea have been described as producing abortive or fertile pycnidia (60, 83). Such isolates are morphologically indistinguishable from Pyrenochaeta mackinnonii (12, 78), but rRNA ITS sequence data (24) show large differences between these species.

P. romeroi

In culture, colonies of P. romeroi are fast growing and floccose to velvety, with a gray surface and whitish margin. The reverse of the colony is black, with no diffusible pigment. On nutritionally deficient media such as oatmeal agar under near-UV light, pycnidia develop after 3 to 4 weeks.

The conidiomata (asexual fruiting bodies) are subglobose, 80 to 160 μm in diameter, and dark brick to fawn, later becoming dark brown with short necks. They are ostiolate (with natural opening), and setae around ostioles are septate and roughened and measure 80 to 100 by 3 μm. The conidiophores inside the conidiomata are sparse and have lateral branches. Conidiogenous cells are hyaline and are borne on branches or arise directly from cells lining the conidiomatal cavity, which produce hyaline to yellowish, shortly cylindrical conidia measuring 1 to 2 by 1.0 μm.

E. jeanselmei

Initially, the colonies of E. jeanselmei may be yeastlike and black, gradually spreading, becoming raised or dome shaped, with limited expansion growth. After 2 weeks on SDA, the colonies are covered with short aerial hyphae and appear olive gray with an olive black reverse. Microscopically, annellidic, rocket-shaped conidiogenous cells are inserted at right angles on undifferentiated hyphae. The septate mycelium is sometimes toruloid, branched, and pale brown. The conidia, which aggregate in masses at the tips of annellides, tend to slide down the conidiophore or along the hyphae. The smooth conidia are exogenous, nonseptate, subspherical, and ellipsoidal to cylindrical, measuring 1.5 to 2.8 μm.

M. mycetomatis

In culture, M. mycetomatis shows wide variation. Colonies are slow growing and white at first, becoming olivaceous, yellow, or brown; flat or dome shaped; and velvety to glabrous, often with a rust brown diffusible pigment. On nutritionally deficient media, sclerotial bodies 750 μm in diameter develop. These are black and consist of undifferentiated polygonal cells. On SDA, the mycelium is sterile. On nutritionally poor media, such as soil extract or hay infusion agar, about 50% of the isolates produce round to pyriform conidia 3 to 4 μm in diameter at the tips of phialides. The phialides are tapering, ranging from 3 to 15 μm in length, often with an inconspicuous collarette (Fig. 6).

M. mycetomatis grows better at 37 than at 30°C, with a maximum of 40°C, whereas M. grisea grows better at 30 than at 37°C. M. mycetomatis is slowly proteolytic and utilizes glucose, maltose, and galactose but not sucrose. It utilizes potassium nitrate, ammonium sulfate, asparagine, and urea, and it hydrolyzes starch. M. grisea, on the other hand, is weakly proteolytic and assimilates glucose, maltose, and sucrose but not lactose.

N. rosatii

In culture, colonies of N. rosatii are slow growing, attaining diameters of 25 to 28 mm in 2 weeks, and have an aerial mycelium that is grayish black to brownish black. On potato-carrot or cornmeal agar incubated at 30°C, most of the ascomata are submerged. The ascostromal walls are smooth and are surrounded by interwoven brown to hyaline hyphae. The eight-spored asci, 12 to 35 by 10 to 25 μm, are scattered in the central part of the ascostroma (Fig. 7) and are globose to subglobose, thick walled, and bitunicate, becoming evanescent as the ascospores mature. The ascospores vary in size (9 to 12.5 by 4.5 to 8.0 μm) and shape, ranging from ellipsoidal to rhomboidal, asymmetrical, or slightly curved; are constricted at the median transverse septum; and have brown smooth walls.

Phaeoacremonium Species

Members of the genus Phaeoacremonium are morphologically characterized by slender, gradually tapering, melanized conidiophores with narrow phialide openings producing ellipsoidal to reniform conidia.

F. falciforme

Colonies of F. falciforme on SDA are slow growing, reaching 60 to 65 mm in diameter in 2 weeks. They are downy and gray-brown, becoming gray-violet. The reverse of the colony develops a violet-purple pigment. The hyphae are hyaline, septate, smooth, branched, and 1.5 to 2.5 μm in diameter. They bear erect, undifferentiated, unbranched, repeatedly septate conidiophores. The conidia are borne at the tip of phialidic conidiogenous cells, where they accumulate in mucoid clusters. The conidia are allantoid (sausage shaped), slightly curved, and nonseptate to monoseptate and measure 7 to 8.5 by 2.7 to 3.2 μm. The intercalary or, rarely, terminal chlamydospores are smooth, thick walled, and 5 to 8 μm in diameter.

P. boydii

Colonies grow rapidly and are floccose and white at first, becoming gray as conidia are produced. With age, the colonies become dark grayish brown. Submerged ascocarps (cleistothecia) (Fig. 8) may be produced when isolates are grown on cornmeal agar and are visible macroscopically as small black dots. They are globose, nonostiolate, 140 to 200 μm in diameter, and often covered with brown, thick-walled, septate hyphae 2 to 3 μm wide. They have a wall 4 to 6 μm thick that is composed of two or three layers of interwoven, flattened, dark brown cells, each 2 to 6 μm wide. The cleistothecia open at maturity by an irregular rupture of the wall. The eight-spored asci are ellipsoidal to nearly spherical and 12 to 18 by 9 to 13 μm. The ascospores are ellipsoidal to oblate, symmetrical or slightly flattened, measure 6 to 7 by 3.5 to 4.0 μm, are straw colored, and have two germ pores.

The anamorph, Scedosporium boydii (Fig. 9), produces conidia that are oval to clavate, truncate, and subhyaline, becoming pale gray to pale brown in mass. Conidia are produced singly. They remain attached at the tips of annellides. Annellations can be detected at the tips of conidiogenous cells as swollen rings. Some isolates also produce a Graphium synanamorph (Fig. 10), which is characterized by ropelike bundles of hyphae with annellidic conidiogenesis. The hyphae are fused into long stalks known as synnemata. The conidia produced are hyaline, cylindric to clavate, and truncate at the base. A fungus consisting of elongate, multicellular conidia and described as Polycytella hominis (18) was recently proven to be a degenerate anamorph of P. boydii (14).

TYPING SYSTEMS

Over the years, many molecular typing techniques have been established for a number of fungal species, including those causing mycetoma. Such techniques are useful not only in genotyping, but also in accurate species identification (4). Genotyping enables differentiation of environmental and clinical isolates, and therefore it is an important tool in understanding the environmental distribution of species and source of infection. Harun et al. (43) provided a comprehensive review of the methods used in the genotyping of Scedosporium species. van de Sande et al. (92) in an amplified fragment length polymorphism study revealed clones of Madurella species differing in virulence and geographic distribution. Subspecific typing of S. apiospermum at the population level is unproblematic because of

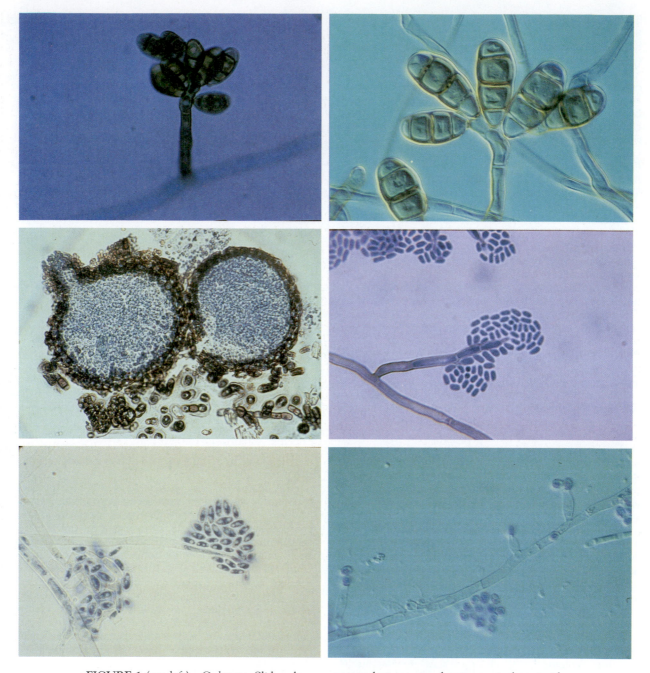

FIGURE 1 (top left) *C. lunata.* Slide culture on potato dextrose agar showing geniculate conidiogenous cell and septate, curved conidia. Magnification, ×160.

FIGURE 2 (top right) *C. lunata.* Geniculate conidiogenous cell bearing smooth, predominantly four-celled conidia. Magnification, ×160.

FIGURE 3 (middle left) *P. romeroi.* Ostiolate conidiomata (pycnidia) containing numerous cylindric conidia. Magnification, ×250.

FIGURE 4 (middle right) *E. jeanselmei.* Lateral, septate conidiophore bearing closely annellated conidiogenous cell producing smooth, nonseptate, ellipsoidal to cylindric conidia. Magnification, ×160.

FIGURE 5 (bottom left) *F. falciforme.* Slide culture on SDA showing erect, septate conidiophore, phialidic conidiogenous cell, and slightly curved conidia. Magnification, ×160.

FIGURE 6 (bottom right) *M. mycetomatis.* Slide culture on soil extract agar showing lateral phialides and globose conidia. Magnification, ×250.

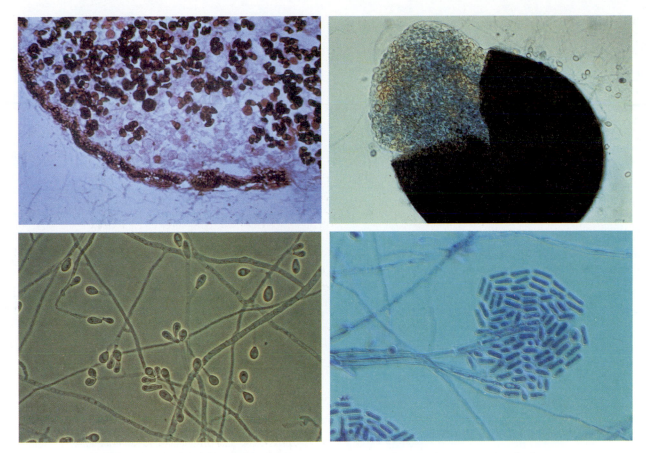

FIGURE 7 (top left) *N. rosatii*. Cross section of an ascocarp showing the ascomatal wall of interwoven hyphae and containing dark asci and ascospores. Magnification, ×250.
FIGURE 8 (top right) *P. boydii*. Globose, nonostiolate, ruptured cleistothecium containing ellipsoid to oblate ascospores. Magnification, ×160.
FIGURE 9 (bottom left) *S. boydii*. Slide culture on potato dextrose agar showing lateral, single, egg-shaped to clavate, truncate conidia. Magnification, ×160.
FIGURE 10 (bottom right) *Graphium* synanamorph of *P. boydii*. Slide culture on potato dextrose agar showing ropelike bundles of hyphae producing cylindric, smooth conidia. Magnification, ×160.

the large degree of heterogeneity. Rainer et al. (76) found with M-13 fingerprinting that nearly all strains analyzed belonged to different genotypes; several genotypes could be recovered from a single sampling site. The high degree of polymorphism enabled Zouhair et al. (100) to monitor the dissemination of a strain colonizing the lungs of a patient with cystic fibrosis to cutaneous locations by using multilocus enzyme electrophoresis and randomly amplified polymorphic DNA. In a longitudinal study, Defontaine et al. (23) analyzed nine patients with cystic fibrosis, none of which were found to harbor strains that shared the same genotype.

SEROLOGIC TESTS

There are no commercially available serologic tests for these agents.

ANTIMICROBIAL SUSCEPTIBILITIES

With the exception of *P. boydii* and *Fusarium* species, most fungi causing eumycotic mycetoma are susceptible in vitro to ketoconazole, itraconazole, voriconazole, and posaconazole. However, it should be noted that in vitro activities and clinical responses to these agents are variable (2, 7, 8, 20, 93). Ketoconazole and itraconazole are the common agents used for the treatment of mycetoma, but their clinical response is poor (2, 7). The newer triazoles, such as voriconazole and posaconazole, have the highest in vitro and in vivo efficacy (7). For instance, *Madurella* species have low MICs to ketoconazole, itraconazole, and voriconazole. Most *M. mycetomatis* strains (MIC$_{90}$) are inhibited by concentrations ranging from 0.064 to 0.125 μg/ml. The only systemic azole with a high MIC against *M. mycetomatis* is fluconazole, whose MIC$_{90}$ reaches 16 μg/ml (93).

Itraconazole and posaconazole have the highest in vitro antifungal activity against *E. jeanselmei*, but their clinical effects need to be determined (8). However, Cerar et al. showed that *P. romeroi* strains had an itraconazole MIC of >32 μg/ml, while the MICs of voriconazole and posaconazole were as low as 0.25 μg/ml (20).

Most fungi causing eumycotic mycetoma have a similar susceptibility to amphotericin B with mean MICs ranging from 0.016 to 2 or 4 μg/ml, with the exception of *P. boydii*, for which the MIC may reach 16 μg/ml or even more (26).

M. mycetomatis has amphotericin B MICs ranging from <0.016 to 4 μg/ml, but flucytosine does not inhibit the growth of this species (93).

EVALUATION, INTERPRETATION, AND REPORTING OF RESULTS

Because agents of eumycotic mycetoma are soil or plant saprobes, their etiologic role in mycetoma must be carefully established. A definitive diagnosis is based on the demonstration of grains in tissue, which are expelled through draining sinuses. Grains may become entangled on gauze bandages placed over fistulae. Pus, exudate, or biopsy material should be examined for the presence of grains that are detectable with the naked eye. Their color, internal architecture, size, and shape give a fair indication of the identity of the possible etiologic agents.

Actinomycotic mycetomata are differentiated from eumycotic mycetomata by the examination of crushed, Gram-stained grains. Actinomycotic grains, as well as coccoid and bacillary forms, are composed of gram-positive, interwoven, thin filaments, 0.5 to 1.0 μm in diameter. Grains of the eumycotic agents, on the other hand, are composed of broader, interwoven, septate hyphae, 2 to 5 μm in diameter, with many unusually shaped, swollen cells up to 15 μm in diameter, especially at the periphery of the grains. In many species, the grains are embedded in cementlike material.

Although the gross and microscopic characteristics of the grains provide insight into the identity of the etiologic agent or a particular group to which it belongs (77), definitive identification of the etiologic agent should be based on isolation of the same fungus from several grains. Clinical microbiology laboratories should avoid reporting patients' specimens as "black grain mycetoma" or "pale grain mycetoma," and isolation and identification of species involved should be attempted. Careful evaluation of culture results is important, especially when new or uncommon fast-growing species are reported, since some of these species might represent contamination during collection of specimens or isolation. On the other hand, physicians should avoid planning a patient's therapy based on grain morphology in clinical materials alone; rather, results of laboratory diagnosis with species identification should be awaited.

REFERENCES

1. **Ahmed, A., D. Adelmann, A. Fahal, H. Verbrugh, A. van Belkum, and S. de Hoog.** 2002. Environmental occurrence of *Madurella mycetomatis*, the major agent of human eumycetoma in Sudan. *J. Clin. Microbiol.* **40:**1031–1036.
2. **Ahmed, A. A., W. W. van de Sande, A. Fahal, I. Bakker-Woudenberg, H. Verbrugh, and A. van Belkum.** 2007. Management of mycetoma: major challenge in tropical mycoses with limited international recognition. *Curr. Opin. Infect. Dis.* **20:**146–151.
3. **Ahmed, A. O., N. Desplaces, P. Leonard, F. Goldstein, S. De Hoog, H. Verbrugh, and A. van Belkum.** 2003. Molecular detection and identification of agents of eumycetoma: detailed report of two cases. *J. Clin. Microbiol.* **41:**5813–5816.
4. **Ahmed, A. O., M. M. Mukhtar, M. Kools-Sijmons, A. H. Fahal, S. de Hoog, B. G. van den Ende, E. E. Zijlstra, H. Verbrugh, E. S. Abugroun, A. M. Elhassan, and A. van Belkum.** 1999. Development of a species-specific PCR-restriction fragment length polymorphism analysis procedure for identification of *Madurella mycetomatis*. *J. Clin. Microbiol.* **37:**3175–3178.
4a. **Ahmed, A. O., W. van Vianen, M. T. ten Kate, W. W. Van de Sande, A. Van Belkum, A. H. Fahal, H. A. Verbrugh, and I. A. Bakker-Woudenberg.** 2003. A murine model of *Madurella mycetomatis* eumycetoma. *FEMS Immunol. Med. Microbiol.* **37:**29–36.
5. **Ajello, L.** 1962. Epidemiology of human fungus infections, p. 69–83. *In* G. Dalldorf (ed.), *Fungi and Fungous Diseases.* Charles C Thomas, Springfield, IL.
6. **Ajello, L., W. Kaplan, and F. W. Chandler.** 1980. *Superficial, Cutaneous and Subcutaneous Infections,* p. 135–140. Scientific Publication no. 396. Pan American Health Organization, Washington, DC.
7. **Ameen, M., and R. Arenas.** 2009. Developments in the management of mycetomas. *Clin. Exp. Dermatol.* **34:**1–7.
8. **Badali, H., M. J. Najafzadeh, M. Van Esbroeck, E. van den Enden, B. Tarazooie, J. F. Meis, and G. S. de Hoog.** 29 July 2009. The clinical spectrum of *Exophiala jeanselmei*, with a case report and in vitro antifungal susceptibility of the species. *Med. Mycol.* July 29:1–10. [Epub ahead of print.]
9. **Baylet, R., R. Camain, and M. Rey.** 1961. Champignons de mycétomes isolés des épineux au Sénégal. *Bull. Soc. Med. Afr. Noire Lang. Fr.* **6:**317–319.
10. **Bonifaz, A., S. De Hoog, M. R. McGinnis, A. Saul, O. Rodriguez-Cortes, J. Araiza, M. Cruz, and P. Mercadillo.** 2009. Eumycetoma caused by *Cladophialophora bantiana* successfully treated with itraconazole. *Med. Mycol.* **47:**111–114.
11. **Borelli, D.** 1962. *Madurella mycetomi* y *Madurella grisea. Arch. Venez. Med. Trop. Parasitol. Med.* **4:**195–211.
12. **Borelli, D.** 1976. *Pyrenochaeta mackinnonii* nova species agente de micetoma. *Castellania* **4:**227–234.
13. **Borelli, D.** 1959. *Pyrenochaeta romeroi* n. sp. *Rev. Dermatol. Venez.* **1:**325–327.
14. **Borman, A. M., C. K. Campbell, C. J. Linton, P. D. Bridge, and E. M. Johnson.** 2006. *Polycytella hominis* is a mutated form of *Scedosporium apiospermum. Med. Mycol.* **44:**33–39.
15. **Borman, A. M., C. J. Linton, S. J. Miles, and E. M. Johnson.** 2008. Molecular identification of pathogenic fungi. *J. Antimicrob. Chemother.* **61**(Suppl. 1):i7–i12.
16. **Brodey, R. S., H. F. Schryver, M. J. Deubler, W. Kaplan, and L. Ajello.** 1967. Mycetoma in a dog. *J. Am. Vet. Med. Assoc.* **151:**442–451.
17. **Butz, W. C., and L. Ajello.** 1971. Black grain mycetoma. A case due to *Madurella grisea. Arch. Dermatol.* **104:**197–201.
18. **Campbell, C. K.** 1987. *Polycytella hominis* gen. et sp. nov., a cause of human pale grain mycetoma. *J. Med. Vet. Mycol.* **25:**301–305.
19. **Castro, L. G., W. Belda Junior, A. Salebian, and L. C. Cuce.** 1993. Mycetoma: a retrospective study of 41 cases seen in Sao Paulo, Brazil, from 1978 to 1989. *Mycoses* **36:**89–95.
20. **Cerar, D., Y. M. Malallah, S. J. Howard, P. Bowyer, and D. W. Denning.** 2009. Isolation, identification and susceptibility of *Pyrenochaeta romeroi* in a case of eumycetoma of the foot in the UK. *Int. J. Antimicrob. Agents* **34:**613–614.
21. **Crous, P. W., W. Gams, M. J. Wingfield, and P. S. van Wyk.** 1996. *Phaeoacremonium* gen. nov. associated with wilt and decline diseases of woody hosts and human infections. *Mycologia* **88:**786–796.
22. **de Albornoz, M. B.** 1974. *Cephalosporium serrae*, an etiologic agent of mycetoma. *Mycopathol. Mycol. Appl.* **54:**485–498.
23. **Defontaine, A., R. Zouhair, B. Cimon, J. Carrere, E. Bailly, F. Symoens, M. Diouri, J. N. Hallet, and J. P. Bouchara.** 2002. Genotyping study of *Scedosporium apiospermum* isolates from patients with cystic fibrosis. *J. Clin. Microbiol.* **40:**2108–2114.
24. **de Hoog, G. S., D. Adelmann, A. O. Ahmed, and A. van Belkum.** 2004. Phylogeny and typification of *Madurella mycetomatis*, with a comparison of other agents of eumycetoma. *Mycoses* **47:**121–130.
25. **de Hoog, G. S., A. Buiting, C. S. Tan, A. B. Stroebel, C. Ketterings, E. J. de Boer, B. Naafs, R. Brimicombe, M. K. Nohlmans-Paulssen, G. T. Fabius, et al.** 1993. Diagnostic problems with imported cases of mycetoma in The Netherlands. *Mycoses* **36:**81–87.
26. **de Hoog, G. S., J. Guarro, J. Gene, and M. J. Figueras.** 2000. *Atlas of Clinical Fungi*, 2nd ed. Centraalbureau voor Schimmelcultures/Universitat Rovira i Virgili, Utrecht/Reus, The Netherlands.

27. de Hoog, G. S., F. D. Marvin-Sikkema, G. A. Lahpoor, J. C. Gottschall, R. A. Prins, and E. Gueho. 1994. Ecology and physiology of the emerging opportunistic fungi *Pseudallescheria boydii* and *Scedosporium prolificans*. *Mycoses* **37:**71–78.

27a. de Hoog, G. S., V. Vicente, R. B. Caligiorne, S. Kantarcioglu, K. Tintelnot, A. H. G. Gerrits van den Ende, and G. Haase. 2003. Species diversity and polymorphism in the *Exophiala spinifera* clade containing opportunistic black yeast-like fungi. *J. Clin. Microbiol.* **41:**4767–4778.

28. Desnos-Ollivier, M., S. Bretagne, F. Dromer, O. Lortholary, and E. Dannaoui. 2006. Molecular identification of black-grain mycetoma agents. *J. Clin. Microbiol.* **44:**3517–3523.

29. Destombes, P., F. Mariat, L. Rosati, and G. Segretain. 1977. Mycetoma in Somalia—results of a survey done from 1959 to 1964. *Acta Trop.* **34:**355–373.

30. Destombes, P., P. Ravisse, and O. Nazimoff. 1970. Summary of deep mycoses established in 20 years of histopathology in the Institut Pasteur de Brazzaville. *Bull. Soc. Pathol. Exot. Filiales* **63:**315–324.

31. El-Ani, A. S. 1966. A new species of *Leptosphaeria*, an etiologic agent of mycetoma. *Mycologia* **58:**406–411.

32. El-Ani, A. S., and M. A. Gordon. 1965. The ascospore sheath and taxonomy of *Leptosphaeria senegalensis*. *Mycologia* **57:**275–278.

33. Emmons, C. W. 1962. Soil reservoirs of pathogenic fungi. *J. Wash. Acad. Sci.* **52:**3–9.

34. Fahey, P. J., M. J. Utell, and R. W. Hyde. 1981. Spontaneous lysis of mycetomas after acute cavitating lung disease. *Am. Rev. Respir. Dis.* **123:**336–339.

35. Fisher, J. F., S. Shadomy, J. R. Teabeaut, J. Woodward, G. E. Michaels, M. A. Newman, E. White, P. Cook, A. Seagraves, F. Yaghmai, and J. P. Rissing. 1982. Near-drowning complicated by brain abscess due to *Petriellidium boydii*. *Arch. Neurol.* **39:**511–513.

36. Gilgado, F., J. Cano, J. Gene, and J. Guarro. 2005. Molecular phylogeny of the *Pseudallescheria boydii* species complex: proposal of two new species. *J. Clin. Microbiol.* **43:**4930–4942.

37. Gilgado, F., J. Cano, J. Gene, D. A. Sutton, and J. Guarro. 2008. Molecular and phenotypic data supporting distinct species statuses for *Scedosporium apiospermum* and *Pseudallescheria boydii* and the proposed new species *Scedosporium dehoogii*. *J. Clin. Microbiol.* **46:**766–771.

38. Ginter, G., G. S. de Hoog, A. Pschaid, M. Fellinger, A. Bogiatzis, C. Berghold, E. M. Reich, and F. C. Odds. 1995. Arthritis without grains caused by *Pseudallescheria boydii*. *Mycoses* **38:**369–371.

39. Guillot, J., D. Garcia-Hermoso, F. Degorce, M. Deville, C. Calvie, G. Dickele, F. Delisle, and R. Chermette. 2004. Eumycetoma caused by *Cladophialophora bantiana* in a dog. *J. Clin. Microbiol.* **42:**4901–4903.

40. Hadjiliadis, D., T. A. Sporn, J. R. Perfect, V. F. Tapson, R. D. Davis, and S. M. Palmer. 2002. Outcome of lung transplantation in patients with mycetomas. *Chest* **121:**128–134.

41. Hagari, Y., S. Ishioka, F. Ohyama, and M. Mihara. 2002. Cutaneous infection showing sporotrichoid spread caused by *Pseudallescheria boydii* (*Scedosporium apiospermum*): successful detection of fungal DNA in formalin-fixed, paraffin-embedded sections by seminested PCR. *Arch. Dermatol.* **138:**271–272.

42. Halde, C., A. A. Padhye, L. D. Haley, M. G. Rinaldi, D. Kay, and R. Leeper. 1976. *Acremonium falciforme* as a cause of mycetoma in California. *Sabouraudia* **14:**319–326.

43. Harun, A., H. Perdomo, F. Gilgado, S. C. Chen, J. Cano, J. Guarro, and W. Meyer. 2009. Genotyping of *Scedosporium* species: a review of molecular approaches. *Med. Mycol.* **47:**406–414.

44. Hayden, G., C. Lapp, and F. Loda. 1977. Arthritis caused by *Monosporium apiospermum* treated with intraarticular amphotericin B. *Am. J. Dis. Child.* **131:**927.

45. Hemashettar, B. M., B. Siddaramappa, B. S. Munjunathaswamy, A. S. Pangi, J. Pattan, A. T. Andrade, A. A. Padhye, L. Mostert, and R. C. Summerbell. 2006. *Phaeoacremonium krajdenii*, a cause of white grain eumycetoma. *J. Clin. Microbiol.* **44:**4619–4622.

46. Hood, S. V., C. B. Moore, J. S. Cheesbrough, A. Mene, and D. W. Denning. 1997. Atypical eumycetoma caused by *Phialophora parasitica* successfully treated with itraconazole and flucytosine. *Br. J. Dermatol.* **136:**953–956.

47. Horré, R., and G. S. de Hoog. 1999. Primary cerebral infections by melanized fungi: a review. *Stud. Mycol.* **43:**176–193.

48. Kano, R., K. Edamura, H. Yumikura, H. Maruyama, K. Asano, S. Tanaka, and A. Hasegawa. 2009. Confirmed case of feline mycetoma due to *Microsporum canis*. *Mycoses* **52:**80–83.

49. Klokke, A. H., G. Swamidasan, R. Anguli, and A. Verghese. 1968. The causal agents of mycetoma in South India. *Trans. R. Soc. Trop. Med. Hyg.* **62:**509–516.

50. Lambrechts, N., M. G. Collett, and M. Henton. 1991. Black grain eumycetoma (*Madurella mycetomatis*) in the abdominal cavity of a dog. *J. Med. Vet. Mycol.* **29:**211–214.

51. Langeron, M. 1928. Mycétome à *Torula jeanselmei* Langeron, 1928. Nouveau type de mycétome à grains noirs. *Ann. Parasitol. Hum. Comp.* **6:**385–403.

52. Lopez, M. J., S. O. Robinson, A. J. Cooley, M. A. Prichard, and M. R. McGinnis. 2007. Molecular identification of *Phialophora oxyspora* as the cause of mycetoma in a horse. *J. Am. Vet. Med. Assoc.* **230:**84–88.

53. Lutwick, L. I., M. W. Rytel, J. P. Yanez, J. N. Galgiani, and D. A. Stevens. 1979. Deep infections from *Petriellidium boydii* treated with miconazole. *JAMA* **241:**272–273.

54. Mackinnon, J. E., I. A. Conti-Diaz, E. Gezuele, and E. Civila. 1971. Datos sobre ecologia de *Allescheria boydii*, Shear. *Rev. Urug. Pathol. Clin. Microbiol.* **9:**37–43.

55. Mackinnon, J. E., L. V. Ferrada, and L. Montemayor. 1949. *Madurella grisea* n. sp., a new species of fungus producing black variety of maduromycosis in South America. *Mycopathol. Mycol. Appl.* **4:**385–392.

56. Mahgoub, E. S. 1973. Mycetomas caused by *Curvularia lunata*, *Madurella grisea*, *Aspergillus nidulans*, and *Nocardia brasiliensis* in Sudan. *Sabouraudia* **11:**179–182.

57. Mancini, N., C. M. Ossi, M. Perotti, S. Carletti, C. Gianni, G. Paganoni, S. Matusuka, M. Guglielminetti, A. Cavallero, R. Burioni, P. Rama, and M. Clementi. 2005. Direct sequencing of *Scedosporium apiospermum* DNA in the diagnosis of a case of keratitis. *J. Med. Microbiol.* **54:**897–900.

58. Mariat, F., P. Destombes, and G. Segretain. 1977. The mycetomas: clinical features, pathology, etiology and epidemiology. *Contrib. Microbiol. Immunol.* **4:**1–39.

59. Matsumoto, T., and L. Ajello. 1986. No granules, no mycetomas. *Chest* **90:**151–152.

60. Mayorga, R., and J. E. Close de Leon. 1966. On a limb from which spore bearing *Madurella grisea* was isolated from a black grained mycetoma in a Guatemalan. *Sabouraudia* **4:**210–214.

61. McGinnis, M. 1992. Black fungi: a model for understanding tropical mycosis, p. 129–149. *In* D. H. Walker (ed.), *Global Infectious Diseases: Prevention, Control, and Eradication*. Springer Verlag, New York, NY.

62. McGinnis, M. R. 1996. Mycetoma. *Dermatol. Clin.* **14:**97–104.

63. McGinnis, M. R., A. A. Padhye, and L. Ajello. 1982. *Pseudallescheria boydii* Negroni et Fischer, 1943, and its later synonym *Petriellidium* Malloch, 1970. *Mycotaxon* **14:**94–102.

64. Milburn, P. B., D. M. Papayanopulos, and B. M. Pomerantz. 1988. Mycetoma due to *Acremonium falciforme*. *Int. J. Dermatol.* **27:**408–410.

65. Montes, L. F., R. G. Freeman, and W. McClarin. 1969. Maduromycosis due to *Madurella grisea*. *Arch. Dermatol.* **99:**74–79.

66. Mostert, L., J. Z. Groenewald, R. C. Summerbell, W. Gams, and P. W. Crous. 2006. Taxonomy and pathology of *Togninia* (Diaporthales) and its *Phaeoacremonium* anamorphs. *Stud. Mycol.* **54:**1–113.

67. Mostert, L., J. Z. Groenewald, R. C. Summerbell, V. Robert, D. A. Sutton, A. A. Padhye, and P. W. Crous. 2005. Species of *Phaeoacremonium* associated with infections in humans and environmental reservoirs in infected woody plants. *J. Clin. Microbiol.* **43:**1752–1767.

68. Murray, I. G., G. E. Dunkerley, and K. E. Hughes. 1964. A case of Madura foot caused by *Phialophora jeanselmei*. *Sabouraudia* **3:**175–177.

69. **Negroni, R., G. Lopez Daneri, A. Arechavala, M. H. Bianchi, and A. M. Robles.** 2006. Clinical and microbiological study of mycetomas at the Muniz hospital of Buenos Aires between 1989 and 2004. *Rev. Argent. Microbiol.* **38:**13–18.

70. **Neilsen, H. S., Jr., N. F. Conant, T. Weinberg, and J. F. Reback.** 1968. Report of a mycetoma due to *Phialophoria jeanselmei* and undescribed characteristics of the fungus. *Sabouraudia* **6:**330–333.

71. **Ochiai, N., C. Shimazaki, R. Uchida, S. Fuchida, A. Okano, E. Ashihara, T. Inaba, N. Fujita, and M. Nakagawa.** 2003. Disseminated infection due to *Scedosporium apiospermum* in a patient with acute myelogenous leukemia. *Leuk. Lymphoma* **44:**369–372.

72. **Pankovich, A. M., B. J. Auerbach, W. I. Metzger, and T. Barreta.** 1981. Development of maduromycosis *(Madurella mycetomi)* after nailing of a closed tibial fracture: a case report. *Clin. Orthop. Relat. Res.* **January-February:**220–222.

73. **Posteraro, P., C. Frances, B. Didona, R. Dorent, B. Posteraro, and G. Fadda.** 2003. Persistent subcutaneous *Scedosporium apiospermum* infection. *Eur. J. Dermatol.* **13:**603–605.

74. **Pupaibul, K., W. Sindhuphak, and A. Chindamporn.** 1982. Mycetoma of the hand caused by *Phialophora jeanselmei*. *Mykosen* **25:**321–330.

75. **Rainer, J., and G. S. De Hoog.** 2006. Molecular taxonomy and ecology of *Pseudallescheria, Petriella* and *Scedosporium prolificans* (Microascaceae) containing opportunistic agents on humans. *Mycol. Res.* **110:**151–160.

76. **Rainer, J., G. S. de Hoog, M. Wedde, Y. Graser, and S. Gilges.** 2000. Molecular variability of *Pseudallescheria boydii*, a neurotropic opportunist. *J. Clin. Microbiol.* **38:**3267–3273.

77. **Rippon, J. W.** 1988. *Medical Mycology: the Pathogenic Fungi and the Pathogenic Actinomycetes*, 3rd ed. W. B. Saunders Company, Philadelphia, PA.

78. **Romero, H., and D. W. Mackenzie.** 1989. Studies on antigens from agents causing black grain eumycetoma. *J. Med. Vet. Mycol.* **27:**303–311.

79. **Rowland, M. D., and W. E. Farrar.** 1987. Case report: thorn-induced *Phialophora parasitica* arthritis treated successfully with synovectomy and ketoconazole. *Am. J. Med. Sci.* **30:**393–395.

80. **Sandhu, G. S., B. C. Kline, L. Stockman, and G. D. Roberts.** 1995. Molecular probes for diagnosis of fungal infections. *J. Clin. Microbiol.* **33:**2913–2919.

81. **Segretain, G.** 1972. Recherches sur l'écologie de *Madurella mycetomi* au Sénégal. *Bull. Soc. Fr. Mycol. Med.* **14:**121–124.

82. **Segretain, G., and P. Destombes.** 1961. Description d'un nouvel agent de maduromycose *Neotestudina rosatii*, n. gen., n. sp. isolé en Afrique. *C. R. Hebd. Seances Acad. Sci.* **253:**2577–2579.

83. **Segretain, G., and P. Destombes.** 1969. Recherches sur mycetomes à *Madurella grisea* et *Pyrenochaeta romeroi*. *Sabouraudia* **7:**51–61.

84. **Segretain, G., and F. Mariat.** 1968. Recherches sur la présence d'agents de mycétomes dans le sol et sur les épineux du Sénégal et de la Mauritanie. *Bull. Soc. Pathol. Exot. Filiales* **61:**194–202.

85. **Shear, C. L.** 1922. Life history of an undescribed ascomycete isolated from a granular mycetoma of man. *Mycologia* **14:**239–243.

86. **Summerbell, R. C., and H. J. Schroers.** 2002. Analysis of phylogenetic relationship of *Cylindrocarpon lichenicola* and *Acremonium falciforme* to the *Fusarium solani* species complex and a review of similarities in the spectrum of opportunistic infections caused by these fungi. *J. Clin. Microbiol.* **40:**2866–2875.

87. **Talwar, P., and S. C. Sehgal.** 1979. Mycetomas in North India. *Sabouraudia* **17:**287–291.

88. **Thammayya, A., and M. Sanyal.** 1980. *Exophiala jeanselmei* causing mycetoma pedis in India. *Sabouraudia* **18:**91–95.

89. **Thianprasit, M., and A. Sivayathorn.** 1984. Black dot mycetoma. *Mykosen* **27:**219–226.

90. **Thirumalachar, M. J., and A. A. Padhye.** 1968. Isolation of *Madurella mycetomi* from soil in India. *Hindustan Antibiot. Bull.* **10:**314–318.

91. **van de Sande, W. W., J. de Kat, J. Coppens, A. O. Ahmed, A. Fahal, H. Verbrugh, and A. van Belkum.** 2007. Melanin biosynthesis in *Madurella mycetomatis* and its effect on susceptibility to itraconazole and ketoconazole. *Microbes Infect.* **9:**1114–1123.

92. **van de Sande, W. W., R. Gorkink, G. Simons, A. Ott, A. O. Ahmed, H. Verbrugh, and A. van Belkum.** 2005. Genotyping of *Madurella mycetomatis* by selective amplification of restriction fragments (amplified fragment length polymorphism) and subtype correlation with geographical origin and lesion size. *J. Clin. Microbiol.* **43:**4349–4356.

93. **van de Sande, W. W., A. Luijendijk, A. O. Ahmed, I. A. Bakker-Woudenberg, and A. van Belkum.** 2005. Testing of the in vitro susceptibilities of *Madurella mycetomatis* to six antifungal agents by using the Sensititre system in comparison with a viability-based 2,3-bis(2-methoxy-4-nitro-5-sulfophenyl)-5- [(phenylamino)carbonyl]-2H-tetrazolium hydroxide (XTT) assay and a modified NCCLS method. *Antimicrob. Agents Chemother.* **49:**1364–1368.

94. **Van Etta, L. L., L. R. Peterson, and D. N. Gerding.** 1983. *Acremonium falciforme (Cephalosporium falciforme)* mycetoma in a renal transplant patient. *Arch. Dermatol.* **119:**707–708.

95. **Venugopal, P. V., and T. V. Venugopal.** 1995. Pale grain eumycetomas in Madras. *Australas. J. Dermatol.* **36:**149–151.

96. **Wedde, M., D. Muller, K. Tintelnot, G. S. De Hoog, and U. Stahl.** 1998. PCR-based identification of clinically relevant *Pseudallescheria/Scedosporium* strains. *Med. Mycol.* **36:**61–67.

97. **Werlinger, K. D., and A. Yen Moore.** 2005. Eumycotic mycetoma caused by *Cladophialophora bantiana* in a patient with systemic lupus erythematosus. *J. Am. Acad. Dermatol.* **52:**S114–S117.

98. **Wethered, D. B., M. A. Markey, R. J. Hay, E. S. Mahgoub, and S. A. Gumaa.** 1987. Ultrastructural and immunogenic changes in the formation of mycetoma grains. *J. Med. Vet. Mycol.* **25:**39–46.

99. **Willinger, B., A. Obradovic, B. Selitsch, J. Beck-Mannagetta, W. Buzina, H. Braun, P. Apfalter, A. M. Hirschl, A. Makristathis, and M. Rotter.** 2003. Detection and identification of fungi from fungus balls of the maxillary sinus by molecular techniques. *J. Clin. Microbiol.* **41:**581–585.

100. **Zouhair, R., A. Defontaine, C. Ollivier, B. Cimon, F. Symoens, J. N. Halle, J. Deunff, and J. P. Bouchara.** 2001. Typing of *Scedosporium apiospermum* by multilocus enzyme electrophoresis and random amplification of polymorphic DNA. *J. Med. Microbiol.* **50:**925–932.

Mycotoxins

NANCY C. ISHAM, WILLIAM J. HALSALL, AND MAHMOUD A. GHANNOUM

124

Mycotoxins are nonvolatile secondary metabolites produced by many different species of ubiquitous fungi having adverse effects on humans and animals. Recently, two events brought interest in mycotoxins to the forefront: (i) the report of black mold as the possible cause of acute idiopathic pulmonary hemosiderosis in newborn infants in Cleveland, OH, which suggested that the presence of fungi in buildings (termed sick building syndrome [SBS]) could have deleterious health effects, and (ii) the flooding of New Orleans, LA, and the Gulf Coast as a result of Hurricane Katrina, which led to extensive fungal proliferation in homes and businesses. In this chapter we review various mycotoxins and their relevance to SBS, veterinary problems, bioterrorism, and food safety. We do not describe the health effects of mycotoxins, as this topic has been reviewed extensively elsewhere (35, 38, 43, 49, 66). The reader is also referred to an excellent review on mycotoxins by Bennett and Klich (7).

MAJOR CATEGORIES OF MYCOTOXINS

Not all toxic compounds produced by fungi are classified as mycotoxins; for example, compounds mainly toxic to bacteria are termed antibiotics, while those toxic to plants are called phytotoxins (7). There are some 300 to 400 compounds, toxic to vertebrates in low concentrations, which are currently recognized as mycotoxins. Table 1 provides a listing of some of the most commonly encountered mycotoxin-producing fungi, many of which produce more than one mycotoxin class.

Aflatoxins

The aflatoxin class of mycotoxins is one of the first to be discovered and studied. Some of the most common aflatoxins (Fig. 1) (7) are aflatoxins B_1, B_2, G_1, and G_2 (based on their blue or green fluorescence under UV light) (82), with aflatoxin B_1 being the most potent natural carcinogen known (73).

Aflatoxins are produced by several species of *Aspergillus*, in particular *Aspergillus flavus* and *A. parasiticus*. *A. flavus* is a common contaminant of agricultural products, among which are cereals, rice, figs, nuts, and tobacco (19, 21). Contamination of crops can occur in the fields before harvest, especially in times of drought (21, 41), or during storage, depending upon the moisture content of the substrate and the relative humidity of the storage conditions (19, 79).

Aflatoxin contamination can be the cause of a variety of economic and health problems. For instance, the presence of aflatoxin in grain significantly lowers the grain's value as feed or an export commodity because of the toxin's link to increased mortality in farm animals (72). Further, ingestion of aflatoxin by dairy cows can lead to the presence of aflatoxin M_1 (a hydroxylated form of B_1) in their milk (77).

There are substantial differences in the susceptibilities of different vertebrate species to aflatoxin exposure. One of the first indications of the effects of aflatoxins was observed in 1960, when more than 100,000 turkey poults died from aflatoxin-contaminated feed, an outbreak named "turkey X disease" (1, 8). Other outbreaks have occurred in ducklings and chickens (4), swine (31, 50), and calves (51), due mostly to contaminated Brazilian peanut meal used as feed. The most recent and notable outbreak of acute aflatoxicosis occurred in Kenya in 2004 in humans (5, 10, 48). This outbreak illustrates the need for a regulatory body to monitor the amount of mycotoxins present in foods meant for human consumption, a luxury not normally available to developing countries.

Citrinin

Citrinin (Fig. 2) (7) is a simple, low-molecular-weight compound that crystallizes as lemon-colored needles. It had been tested for use as an antibiotic (46, 47, 84) and as a treatment for ulcers (46) before its mycotoxic effects were discovered.

The most common organisms producing citrinin are *Penicillium citrinum*, *Penicillium expansum*, *Penicillium viridicatum*, *Penicillium camemberti* (used to produce cheese), *Aspergillus niveus*, *Aspergillus oryzae* (used to produce sake and soy sauce), *Aspergillus terreus*, and *Monascus* spp. (used to produce red food dyes) (11).

Citrinin, first isolated from *P. citrinum*, has been associated with Japanese yellow rice disease (71). It has also been found in various other grains, peanuts, and fruits, and there is limited evidence of its surviving unchanged in cereal food products (7). Citrinin has demonstrated nephrotoxic effects on all animal species tested (9) and was shown to inhibit dehydrogenase activity in rats' kidneys, liver, and brain (33). However, there have been no reported outbreaks of human citrinin poisoning, and its relevance to human health is unknown.

TABLE 1 Simplified taxonomy of mycotoxin-producing fungi

Mycotoxin class	Genera	Representative species
Aflatoxin	Aspergillus, Penicillium	A. fumigatus, A. flavus, A. parasiticus, P. puberulum
Citrinin	Penicillium	P. citrinin, P. expansum
Ergot alkaloid	Aspergillus, Balansia, Claviceps, Epichloë, Neotyphodium	A. fumigatus, C. purpurea
Fumonisin	Fusarium	F. verticillioides (syn. F. moniliforme), F. proliferatum
Ochratoxin	Aspergillus, Penicillium	A. ochraceus, P. verrucosum
Patulin	Aspergillus, Byssochlamys, Penicillium	A. clavatus, B. fulva, B. nivea, P. griseofulvium, P. expansum
Trichothecene	Stachybotrys	S. chartarum
Zearalenone	Fusarium	F. crookwellense, F. culmorum, F. graminearum, F. semitectum

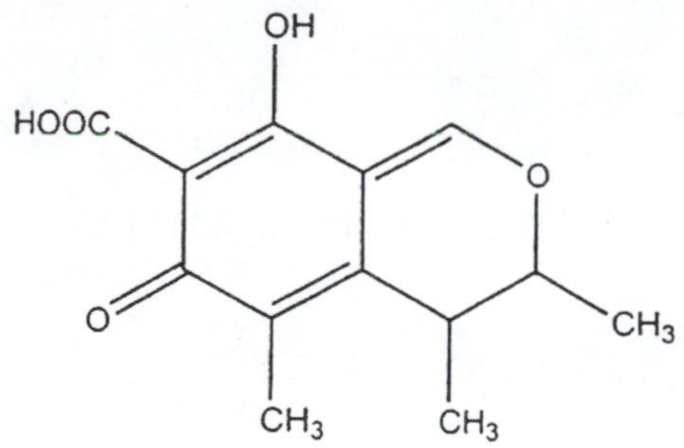

Ergot Alkaloids

Ergot alkaloids, produced by the ergot fungus *Claviceps purpurea*, are the causative agent of ergotism (also called St. Anthony's fire), which can manifest in either a gangrenous or convulsive condition following ingestion of contaminated grains (especially rye) (6). Two main classes of ergot alkaloids exist: lysergic acid derivatives and clavines. Both are indole alkaloids derived from a tetracyclic ergoline ring system. Lysergic acid, a component common to all ergot alkaloids, often forms amide, amino acid, or peptide derivatives (e.g., ergine, ergonovine, lysergic acid diethylamide [LSD], and ergovaline). The clavines contain the ergoline structure but do not have amino acid or peptide components (e.g., pergolide and lisuride) (6). A representative chemical structure, that of ergotamine, is shown in Fig. 3 (7).

Semisynthetic ergot alkaloids have been developed through decades of research, which began with the series of lysergic acid derivatives that included the infamous hallucinogen LSD (25). Most recently, ergot alkaloids have been investigated for their anticancer potential (26), as well

FIGURE 2 Citrinin. (Reprinted from reference 7 with permission of the publisher.)

as their effect on serotonin and serotonin receptors (67, 81). However, definition of the mechanisms of action for the myriad of ergot alkaloids is beyond the scope of this chapter.

Aspergillus, Balansia, Claviceps, Epichloë, and *Neotyphodium* spp. have been found to produce ergot alkaloids. *Aspergillus fumigatus* has been shown to produce fumigaclavines A, B, and C and festuclavine (first described for *C. purpurea* and later for *Neotyphodium* spp.) (15, 65).

Modern methods of cleaning grains have all but eliminated the threat to the human food chain. However, ergotism remains an important veterinary concern, as symptoms of gangrene, convulsions, and abortion in cattle, sheep, pigs, and chickens mimic those in humans (52).

Fumonisins

Fumonisins (Fig. 4) (7) are among the most recently discovered mycotoxins. In 1988, Gelderblom et al. (30) determined that fumonisins produced by *Fusarium verticillioides* (then called *Fusarium moniliforme*) were the causative agent of leukoencephalomalacia in horses (55) and hepatocarcinoma in rats (40, 56). As of 2002, there were 28 known fumonisin analogs, separated into four main groups: A, B, C, and P (68).

Fusarium proliferatum, Fusarium nygamai, Alternaria alternata, and *Gibberella fujikuroi,* the teleomorph (sexual form) of *F. verticillioides,* also produce these mycotoxins (18). See reference 68 by Rheeder et al. for a review of the taxonomy of fumonisin-producing fungi.

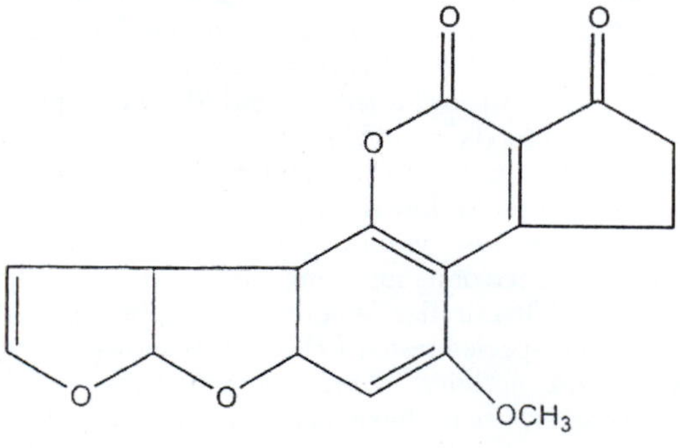

FIGURE 1 Aflatoxin B₁. (Reprinted from reference 7 with permission of the publisher.)

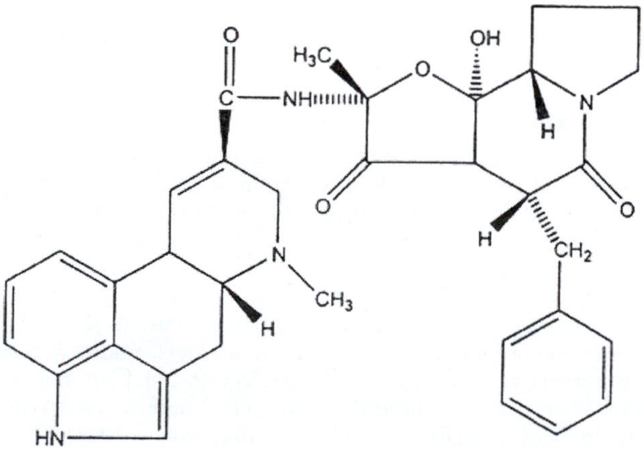

FIGURE 3 Ergotamine. (Reprinted from reference 7 with permission of the publisher.)

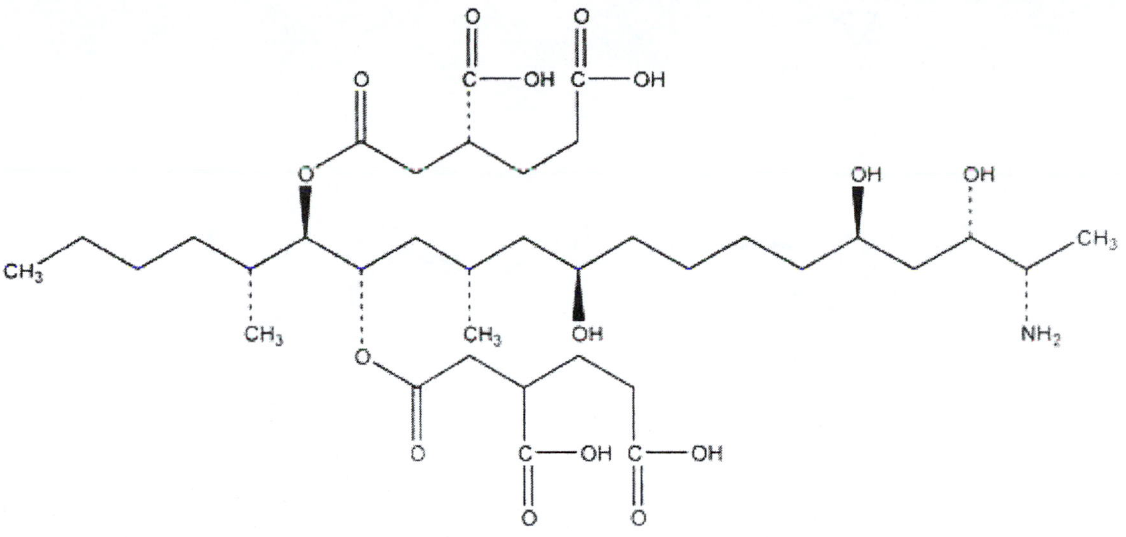

FIGURE 4 Fumonisin B$_1$. (Reprinted from reference 7 with permission of the publisher.)

Besides the syndromes mentioned above, fumonisins have also been shown to cause pulmonary edema and hydrothorax in swine (32). *F. verticillioides*, the major producer of fumonisins, can have an important economic effect on the supply of corn, as it can cause a variety of blights and rots depending on environmental conditions (62).

Ochratoxins

Ochratoxins A and B (Fig. 5) (7) are produced by *Penicillium verrucosum* and many species of *Aspergillus*, especially *A. ochraceus*. These toxins can be carcinogenic, immunosuppressive, and nephrotoxic (44, 72). Ochratoxin A, first discovered to be toxic to animals in 1965 (78), is more common than ochratoxin B and can be metabolized after ingestion by cytochrome P450 liver enzymes (86).

Ochratoxins are found most often in contaminated barley but may also be present in oats, rye, wheat, and coffee beans (7, 78). They are of particular concern because of their ability to be carried through the food chain, especially in milk and in the tissues of pork (24, 57). Scandinavian countries (Denmark in particular) have had a high incidence of porcine nephropathy and high levels of ochratoxin A contamination (42).

Patulin

Patulin (Fig. 6) (7) was first isolated in the 1940s from *Penicillium griseofulvum*, and efforts were made to mass-produce this mycotoxin for its antibiotic effects (63). However, patulin was reclassified as a mycotoxin in the 1960s, following the discovery of its toxicity to plants and animals (7).

One of the most common occurrences of patulin is in unfermented juices made from fruit contaminated with *P. expansum* (76). Patulin is toxic at high concentrations in vitro, but natural poisoning in humans has yet to be proven (7).

Trichothecenes

Trichothecene mycotoxins are secondary metabolites of a variety of *Fusarium* spp., but also of *Myrothecium*, *Phomopsis*, *Stachybotrys*, *Trichoderma*, and *Trichothecium*, among others. Some of the most common and well-studied *Fusarium* trichothecenes (Fig. 7) (7) are T-2 toxin, HT-2 toxin, diacetoxyscirpenol, nivalenol, and deoxynivalenol (also called DON or vomitoxin). DON is one of the most common mycotoxins found in grain, including barley, oats, rye, and wheat. When ingested in large quantities by agricultural animals, it can cause nausea, vomiting, and diarrhea; ingestion of smaller quantities results in weight loss and feed refusal (70). DON can also suppress bovine and porcine neutrophil function in vitro (75).

Stachybotrys chartarum produces several macrocyclic trichothecenes, including verrucarins B and J; roridin E; satratoxins F, G, and H; and isosatratoxins F, G, and H (37, 39). *Stachybotrys*-contaminated straw was first described

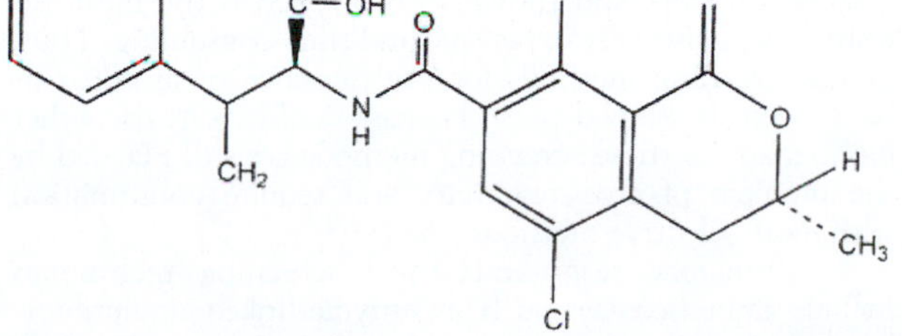

FIGURE 5 Ochratoxin A. (Reprinted from reference 7 with permission of the publisher.)

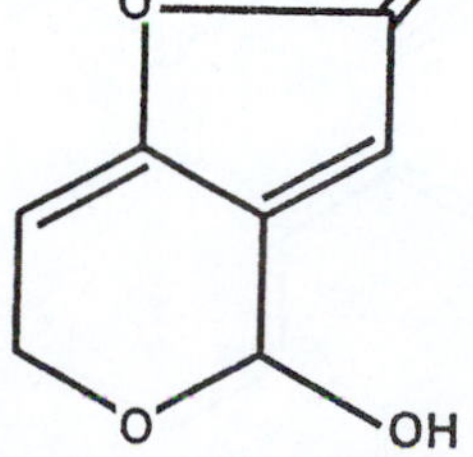

FIGURE 6 Patulin. (Reprinted from reference 7 with permission of the publisher.)

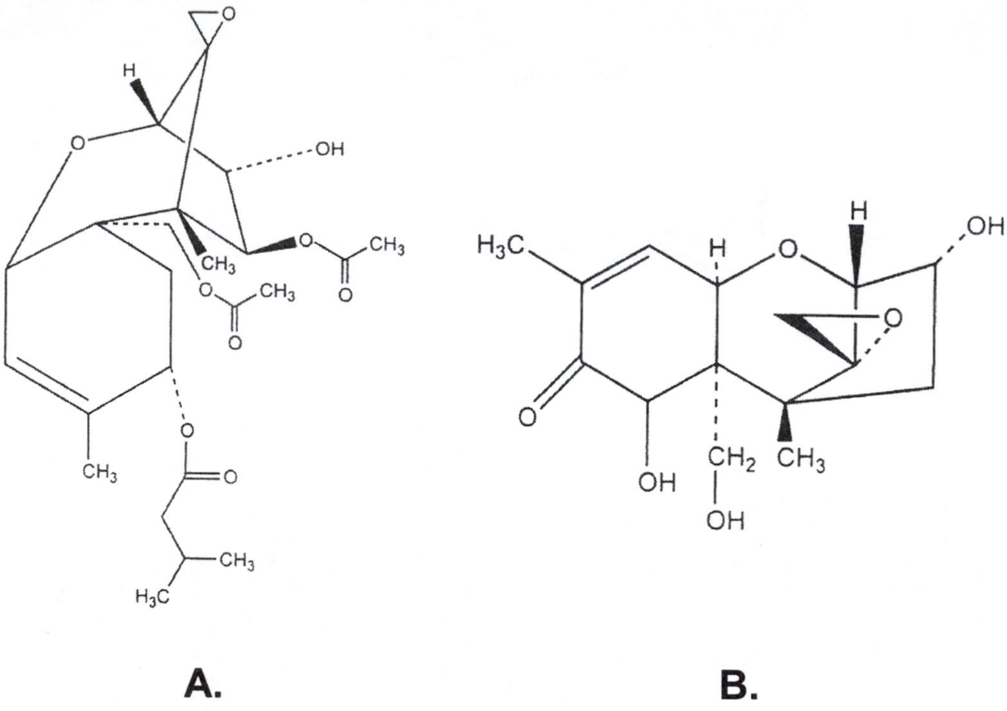

FIGURE 7 (A) T-2 toxin; (B) deoxynivalenol. (Modified and reprinted from reference 7 with permission of the publisher.)

as causing a highly fatal equine disease (28) and has since become better known as a factor in SBS, discussed below.

Zearalenone

Zearalenone (Fig. 8) (7) is a nonsteroidal estrogen or phytoestrogen produced by various species of *Fusarium*, including *F. roseum* and *F. tricinctum* (23). Zearalenone is a common contaminant of cereal crops worldwide and has been implicated in the hyperestrogenism of farm animals as a result of digestion of moldy corn and grains (34, 60). Some of the symptoms of hyperestrogenism are enlargement of the uterus and nipples, vaginal prolapse, and infertility (61).

FOOD SAFETY

Consumption of moldy food products is the leading cause of mycotoxicoses in agricultural animals and humans alike.

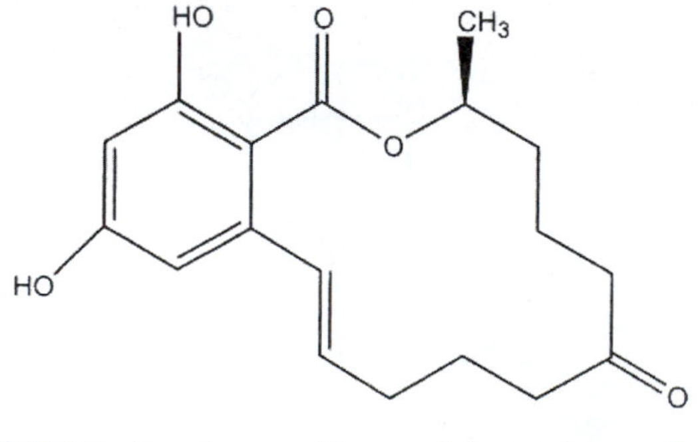

FIGURE 8 Zearalenone. (Reprinted from reference 7 with permission of the publisher.)

Contamination can occur at any point, ranging from the crop in the field through storage and shipping. The economic consequences of mycotoxin contamination are immense, and mycotoxins pose a higher chronic dietary risk than synthetic contaminants, plant toxins, food additives, or pesticide residues (45). Tables 2 and 3 list the mycotoxins discussed within this chapter, their common food substrates, and the agricultural animals most commonly affected.

Recent Advances in Detection

Since it would be impossible to prevent all mycotoxin contamination, methods of monitoring food intended for human and animal consumption must be established. The regulatory guidelines for the limits of mycotoxins in food and feed differ from country to country, but they have been summarized in a series of compendia published by the Food and Agriculture Organization of the United Nations (27). The chemical diversity of the mycotoxin group requires that each be separated from its substrate and studied by a unique assay. The mycotoxins are comprised of a large variety of chemical structures, which are often present in smaller amounts than other interfering substances. Generally, sample preparation consists of an extraction step followed by a purification step, and though this method is the most definitive, it is also very expensive and time-consuming. Thus, newer screening methods for the presence of mycotoxins have been developed over the past decade. On the other hand, many of these screening methods are still plagued by the problem of cross-reactivity and require confirmation with more selective methods.

Confirmatory tests and novel screening techniques include immunoassays such as enzyme-linked immunosorbent assay, fluorescence polarization immunoassay, surface-plasmon resonance, and other conductometric measurements (12, 14). High-performance liquid chromatography (HPLC)

TABLE 2 Mycotoxins and their common food substrates

Mycotoxin class	Barley	Coffee beans	Corn	Fruits	Oats	Peanuts	Rice	Rye	Wheat
Aflatoxin			X			X	X		X
Citrinin	X		X		X		X	X	X
Ergot alkaloid	X				X			X	X
Fumonisin			X						
Ochratoxin	X	X			X			X	X
Patulin				X					
Trichothecene			X						
Zearalenone			X						

and gas chromatography are widely used, and since the introduction of atmospheric pressure ionization, liquid chromatography-mass spectrometry has become a routine technique for detecting the presence of mycotoxins, including tricothecenes, ochratoxins, zearalenone, fumonisins, and aflatoxins (87). The latest official methods, validated by the Association of Official Analytical Chemists International, are based on immunoaffinity column cleanup of conventional extracts, followed by fluorescently labeled HPLC (72). The reader is referred to the article by Cigic and Prosen for a comprehensive review of recent developments in analytical protocols (14).

Effects of Climate Change

It is estimated that one-quarter of the world's crops are contaminated to some extent with mycotoxins (54); this proportion varies from year to year based on environmental factors. There is much evidence of the influence of environmental factors, mainly temperature, relative humidity, drought, insect attack, and other plant stressors, on the ability of molds to produce mycotoxins. Further, the pathogenicity of different molds may be partially additive, and the advantage of one mold species over another may be temperature dependent (61). Each species and its ability to produce mycotoxins must be evaluated independently within its own optimum growth conditions. For wheat species, infection of the cereal ears by *Fusarium* spp. (particularly *F. graminearum*, which is a predominant producer of DON) is enhanced by prolonged periods of warm, humid weather (59). At the other extreme, production of fumonisins and aflatoxins is more abundant under drought conditions. Warmer temperatures and fewer frost days result in more insect and other plant pathogens being capable of surviving the winter and thus causing plants to be more susceptible to mycotoxin-producing mold infestation. In summary, climate changes in any particular geographical region may result in radical changes in the amount and type of crop damage and mycotoxin contamination.

The Future of Prevention and Amelioration of Mycotoxin Contamination

Several different approaches are currently being developed in order to protect the food supply from mycotoxin contamination, including measures taken before, during, and after cultivation of crops. One of the most promising control measures is the development of transgenic strains of cereal crops. A trichothecene resistance gene, *TR1101*, has recently been identified, and expression of these genes in cereal crops has the potential to reduce levels of *Fusarium* head blight and resultant mycotoxin contamination (17). Though most breeding successes have been reported for wheat and barley strains, it is also essential to breed for resistance in other crops, such as corn and oats, in order to reduce soilborne sources of fungal inocula (29).

During the planting process, it has been demonstrated that removal of debris from the previous crop, wet planting of seed, and lower levels of nitrogen fertilizer significantly reduce the risk of fumonisin contamination in corn (3). Other biological controls are being studied to reduce mycotoxins during the growing cycle. These include the use of insecticides to control insect pests such as *Lobesia botrana* (grape berry moth) larvae that encourage the growth of *Aspergillus* and resultant accumulation of ochratoxin A (16). Another biological control is the application of mycoviruses, which are typically easily spread through asexual fungal spores. Though many mycoviruses have minimal effects on their host fungi, they have the potential to be used as gene vectors for the transmission of resistant genes. This approach may expand rapidly with the increasing availability of virus-specific molecular detection methods (66). Additionally, a recent study has shown that the application of nontoxigenic strains of A. *flavus* to corn plant whorls prior to tasseling was able to significantly reduce

TABLE 3 Mycotoxins and animal outbreaks

Mycotoxin class	Cattle	Poultry	Swine	Horses	Sheep
Aflatoxin	X	X	X		
Citrinin					
Ergot alkaloid					
Fumonisin		X			
Ochratoxin		X	X		
Patulin					
Trichothecene	X		X		
Zearalenone	X			X	X

the aflatoxin accumulation in the crop, presumably through competition with toxin-producing strains (22).

Finally, several recent studies have concentrated on degradation of mycotoxins following crop harvest. Many microorganisms such as soil and water bacteria, fungi, protozoa, and specific enzymes isolated from microbial systems have been shown to degrade mycotoxins (specifically aflatoxins) (83). The addition of sodium carbonate and other feed additives has demonstrated success in lowering mortality and reducing adverse effects of mycotoxin-contaminated feed in livestock (20, 68).

BIOTERRORISM

In response to a concern about the possible use of mycotoxins in bioterrorism, the Committee on Protection from Mycotoxins was formed by the National Research Council in 1982 (17). Following years of research, Ciegler proposed the use of mycotoxins as a new class of chemical weapons in 1986 (13). However, the choice of aflatoxin as a weapon of mass destruction is odd at best, since the effects (liver cancer) of aflatoxicosis are too long-term to be effective during war.

Trichothecenes are much more suited for warfare than aflatoxins because they act immediately upon contact, and several milligrams can be lethal. Of historical note is the "yellow rain" incident of 1981 (69). The United States accused the Soviet Union of using nivalenol, DON, and T-2 toxin as biological weapons against Hmong tribesmen in Cambodia and Laos. However, it was later concluded that this "yellow rain" was not a weapon but simply the excreta of swarms of wild Asian honeybees (64).

The use of mycotoxins in bioterrorism has been assessed by several investigators in recent years (7, 36, 53, 74, 85). Aflatoxins and trichothecenes have been recently tested for combined toxicity and were found to have additive effects in most cases. The combination of these two mycotoxins resulted in a synergistic effect in a human bronchial epithelial cell line (58). Interestingly, it has been shown that chlorine dioxide may be effective in the detoxification of trichothecenes, roridin A, and verrucarin A (80) in the case of widespread exposure. In general, it is accepted that while the presence of mycotoxin weapons may cause terror, the actual use of such weapons would not be effective or reliable in a time of war.

SICK BUILDING SYNDROME

SBS is a loosely defined condition that applies to indoor environments suspected of causing a variety of health complaints for occupants. The buildings usually have many problems, including water damage; improper heating, ventilation, and air conditioning systems; poor construction; and bacterial, fungal, and/or insect infestations. Symptoms may include eye, nose, and throat irritation; fatigue; headache; lack of concentration; frequent respiratory tract infections; shortness of breath; dizziness; and nausea (2).

Mycotoxins are just one of the many factors considered as possible contributors to SBS. Several mycotoxin-producing fungi have been implicated, including *Alternaria*, *Aspergillus*, *Cladosporium*, *Chaetomium*, and *Penicillium* spp. One of the most widely investigated species is *S. chartarum* (for a comprehensive review, see the work of Kuhn and Ghannoum) (43).

However, it has not been definitively proven that occupants develop illnesses either from these "sick" buildings or from the molds present inside them. Several recent reviews of SBS conclude that (i) there is no evidence that mold presents an imminent threat to life for healthy members of the general population in typical exposures; (ii) indoor airborne microorganisms are only weakly correlated with human disease, and a definite causal relationship has not been established; and (iii) the concentration of mold contamination required to create infective doses is improbable and inconsistent with the reported spore concentrations in buildings (2, 43).

A further argument against mycotoxins as the cause of SBS symptoms is the fact that mycotoxins are not volatile, and therefore, widespread exposure is unlikely. Moreover, the conditions conducive for mold growth are not necessarily the same as for mycotoxin production, and fungi differ in their abilities to produce mycotoxins. To conclude that the presence of mold found within a sick building is indeed associated with symptoms suffered by occupants, the following must be established: (i) existence of the mold presenting a potential health risk in the indoor environment, (ii) mode of transmission (the source colony must be in direct contact or close proximity for contact with spores and related by-products), and (iii) portal of entry (the mold must be absorbed into the body through inhalation, ingestion, or skin absorption). The mere presence of a fungus in an indoor environment is not sufficient evidence to establish a cause-effect relationship and does not necessarily prove that mycotoxin is also present.

CONCLUSIONS

There are several classes of mycotoxins, produced by a wide range of fungal species, which have been linked to various environmental issues such as SBS, veterinary problems, bioterrorism, and food safety. Over the past decade, there have been many developments in the processes for identifying mycotoxin contamination, as well as advances in methods to control its production. Much research is yet needed to reduce the threat of mycotoxin-producing fungal species to the health of human, livestock, and plant populations and its resultant effects on the international economy.

REFERENCES

1. **Allcroft, R., and R. B. A. Carnaghan.** 1963. Toxic products in groundnuts: biological effects. *Chem. Ind.* (London) **1963:**50–53.
2. **Anonymous.** 2002. *Adverse Human Health Effects Associated with Molds in the Indoor Environment.* American College of Occupational and Environmental Medicine, Arlington Heights, IL. http://www.acoem.org/guidelines/pdf/Mold-10-27-02.pdf.
3. **Arino, A., M. Herrera, T. Juan, G. Estopanan, J. J. Carraminana, C. Rota, and A. Herrera.** 2009. Influence of agricultural practices on the contamination of maize by fumonisin mycotoxins. *J. Food Prot.* **72:**898–902.
4. **Asplin, F. D., and R. B. A. Carnaghan.** 1961. The toxicity of certain groundnut meals for poultry with special reference to their effect on ducklings and chickens. *Vet. Rec.* **73:**1215–1219.
5. **Azziz-Baumgartner, E., K. Lindblade, K. Gieseker, H. S. Rogers, S. Kieszak, H. Njapau, R. Schleicher, L. F. McCoy, A. Misore, K. DeCock, C. Rubin, L. Slutsker, and the Aflatoxin Investigative Group.** 2005. Case-control study of an acute aflatoxicosis outbreak, Kenya, 2004. *Environ. Health Perspect.* **113:**1779–1783.
6. **Bennett, J. W., and R. Bentley.** 1999. Pride and prejudice: the story of ergot. *Perspect. Biol. Med.* **42:**333–355.
7. **Bennett, J. W., and M. Klich.** 2003. Mycotoxins. *Clin. Microbiol. Rev.* **16:**497–516.
8. **Blount, W. P.** 1961. Turkey "X" disease. *Turkeys* **9:**52, 55–58, 61, 77.
9. **Carlton, W. W., and J. Tuite.** 1977. Metabolites of *P. viridicatum* toxicology, p. 525–555. *In* J. V. Rodricks, C. W. Hesseltine, and M. A. Mehlman (ed.), *Mycotoxins in Human and Animal Health.* Pathotox Publications, Inc., Park Forest South, IL.

10. **Centers for Disease Control and Prevention.** 2004. Outbreak of aflatoxin poisoning—eastern and central provinces, Kenya, January–July 2004. *MMWR Morb. Mortal. Wkly. Rep.* **53:**790–793.

11. **Chu, F. S.** 1991. Current immunochemical methods for mycotoxin analysis, p. 140–157. *In* M. Vanderlaan, L. H. Stanker, B. E. Watkins, and D. W. Roberts (ed.), *Immunoassays for Trace Chemical Analysis: Monitoring Toxic Chemicals in Humans, Food, and the Environment.* American Chemical Society, Washington, DC.

12. **Chun, H. S., E. H. Choi, H. J. Chang, S. W. Choi, and S. A. Eremin.** 2009. A fluorescence polarization immunoassay for the detection of zearalenone in corn. *Anal. Chim. Acta* **639:**83–89.

13. **Ciegler, A.** 1986. Mycotoxins: a new class of chemical weapons. *NBC Defense Technol. Int.* **1**(April):52–57.

14. **Cigic, I. K., and H. Prosen.** 2009. An overview of conventional and emerging analytical methods for the determination of mycotoxins. *Int. J. Mol. Sci.* **10:**62–115.

15. **Cole, P.** 1977. Drug-induced lung disease. *Drugs* **13:**422–444.

16. **Cozzi, G., M. Haidukowski, G. Perrone, A. Visconti, and A. Logrieco.** 2009. Influence of Lobesia botrana field control on black aspergilli rot and ochratoxin A contamination in grapes. *J. Food Prot.* **72:**894–897.

17. **Desjardins, A. E.** 2009. From yellow rain to green wheat: 25 years of tricothecene biosynthesis research. *J. Agric. Food Chem.* **57:**4478–4484.

18. **Desjardins, A. E., R. D. Plattner, T. C. Nelsen, and J. F. Leslie.** 1995. Genetic analysis of fumonisin production and virulence of *Gibberella fujikuroi* mating population A (*Fusarium moniliforme*) on maize (*Zea mays*) seedlings. *Appl. Environ. Microbiol.* **61:**79–86.

19. **Detroy, R. W., E. B. Lillehoj, and A. Ciegler.** 1971. Aflatoxin and related compounds, p. 3–178. *In* A. Ciegler, S. Kadis, and S. J. Ajl (ed.), *Microbial Toxins,* vol. VI. *Fungal Toxins.* Academic Press, New York, NY.

20. **Diaz, G. J., A. Cortes, and L. Botero.** 2009. Evaluation of the ability of a feed additive to ameliorate the adverse effects of aflatoxins in turkey poults. *Br. Poult. Sci.* **50:**240–250.

21. **Diener, U. L., R. J. Cole, T. H. Sanders, G. A. Payne, L. S. Lee, and M. A. Klich.** 1987. Epidemiology of aflatoxin formation by *Aspergillus flavus. Annu. Rev. Phytopathol.* **25:**249–270.

22. **Dorner, J. W.** 2009. Biological control of aflatoxin contamination in corn using a nontoxigenic strain of *Aspergillus flavus. J. Food Prot.* **72:**801–804.

23. **El-Nezami, H., N. Polychronaki, S. Salminen, and H. Mykkänen.** 2002. Binding rather than metabolism may explain the interaction of two food-grade *Lactobacillus* strains with zearalenone and its derivative α-zearalenol. *Appl. Environ. Microbiol.* **68:**3545–3549.

24. **Fink-Gremmels, J.** 1999. Mycotoxins: their implications for human and animal health. *Vet. Q.* **21:**115–120.

25. **Floss, H. G.** 1976. Recent advances in the chemistry and biosynthesis of ergot alkaloids. *Cesk. Farm.* **25:**409–419.

26. **Floss, H. G.** 2006. From ergot to ansamycins—45 years in biosynthesis. *J. Nat. Prod.* **69:**158–169.

27. **Food and Agriculture Organization.** 1997. *Worldwide Regulations for Mycotoxins: a Compendium.* Food and Agriculture Organization of the United Nations Food and Nutrition Paper 64. Food and Agriculture Organization, Rome, Italy.

28. **Forgacs, J.** 1972. Stachybotryotoxicosis, p. 95–128. *In* S. Kadis, A. Ciegler, and S. J. Ajl (ed.), *Microbial Toxins,* vol. VI. *Fungal Toxins.* Academic Press, New York, NY.

29. **Foroud, N. A., and F. Eudes.** 2009. Tricothecenes in cereal grains. *Int. J. Mol. Sci.* **10:**147–173.

30. **Gelderblom, W. C., K. Jaskiewicz, W. F. Marasas, P. G. Thiel, R. M. Horak, R. Vleggaar, and N. P. Kriek.** 1988. Fumonisins—novel mycotoxins with cancer-promoting activity produced by *Fusarium moniliforme. Appl. Environ. Microbiol.* **54:**1806–1811.

31. **Harding, J. D. J., J. T. Done, G. Lewis, and R. Allcroft.** 1963. Experimental groundnut poisoning in pigs. *Res. Vet. Sci.* **4:**217–229.

32. **Harrison, L. R., B. M. Colvin, J. T. Greene, L. E. Newman, and J. R. Cole, Jr.** 1990. Pulmonary edema and hydrothorax in swine produced by fumonisin B₁, a toxic metabolite of *Fusarium moniliforme. J. Vet. Diagn. Investig.* **2:**217–221.

33. **Hashimoto, K., and Y. Morita.** 1957. Inhibitory effect of citrinin (C13H1405) on the dehydrogenase system of rat's kidney, liver and brain tissue, specially concerning the mechanism of polyuria observed in the poisoned animal. *Jpn. J. Pharmacol.* **7:**48–54.

34. **Hawkins, M. B., J. W. Thornton, D. Crews, et al.** 2000. Identification of a third distinct estrogen receptor and reclassification of estrogen receptors in teleosts. *Proc. Natl. Acad. Sci. USA* **97:**10751–10756.

35. **Hayes, R. B., J. P. van Nienwenhuise, J. W. Raatgever, and F. J. W. Ten Kate.** 1984. Aflatoxin exposure in the industrial setting: an epidemiological study of mortality. *Food Chem. Toxicol.* **22:**39–43.

36. **Henghold, W. B.** 2004. Other biologic toxin bioweapons: ricin, staphylococcal enterotoxin B, and trichothecene mycotoxins. *Dermatol. Clin.* **22:**257–262.

37. **Hinkley, S. F., E. P. Mazzola, J. C. Fettinger, Y. F. Lam, and B. B. Jarvis.** 2000. Atranones A–G, from the toxigenic mold *Stachybotrys chartarum. Phytochemistry* **55:**663–673.

38. **Hsieh, D.** 1988. Potential human health hazards of mycotoxins, p. 69–80. *In* S. Natori, K. Hashimoto, and Y. Ueno (ed.), *Mycotoxins and Phytotoxins.* Third Joint Food and Agriculture Organization/W.H.O./United Nations Program International Conference of Mycotoxins. Elsevier, Amsterdam, The Netherlands.

39. **Jarvis, B. B., W. G. Sorenson, E. Hintikka, M. Nikulin, Y. Zhou, J. Jiang, S. Wang, S. Hinkley, R. A. Etzel, and D. Dearborn.** 1998. Study of toxin production by isolates of *Stachybotrys chartarum* and *Memnoniella echinata* isolated during a study of pulmonary hemosiderosis in infants. *Appl. Environ. Microbiol.* **64:**3620–3625.

40. **Jaskiewicz, K., S. J. van Rensburg, W. F. O. Marasas, and W. C. A. Gelderblom.** 1987. Carcinogenicity of *Fusarium moniliforme* culture material in rats. *JNCI* **78:**321–325.

41. **Klich, M. A.** 1987. Relation of plant water potential at flowering to subsequent cottonseed infection by *Aspergillus flavus. Phytopathology* **77:**739–741.

42. **Krogh, P.** 1987. Ochratoxins in food, p. 97–121. *In* P. Krogh (ed.), *Mycotoxins in Food.* Academic Press, London, United Kingdom.

43. **Kuhn, D. M., and M. A. Ghannoum.** 2003. Indoor mold, toxigenic fungi, and *Stachybotrys chartarum:* infectious disease perspective. *Clin. Microbiol. Rev.* **16:**144–172.

44. **Kuiper-Goodman, T.** 1990. Uncertainties in the risk assessment of three mycotoxins: aflatoxin, ochratoxin, and zearalenone. *Can. J. Physiol. Pharmacol.* **68:**1017–1024.

45. **Kuiper-Goodman, T.** 1998. Food safety: mycotoxins and phycotoxins in perspective, p. 25–48. *In* M. Miraglia, H. van Edmond, C. Brera, and J. Gilbert (ed.), *Mycotoxins and Phycotoxins—Developments in Chemistry, Toxicology and Food Safety.* Alaken Inc., Fort Collins, CO.

46. **LeJeune, P.** 1957. Use of a new antibiotic, citrinin, in treatment of tropical ulcer. *Ann. Soc. Belg. Med. Trop.* **37:**139–146.

47. **Leusch, L.** 1952. Notes on the trial therapeutic use of citrinin. *J. Pharm. Belg.* **7:**77–79.

48. **Lewis, L., M. Onsongo, H. Njapau, H. Schurz-Rogers, G. Luber, S. Kieszak, J. Nyamongo, L. Backer, A. M. Dahiye, A. Misore, K. DeCock, C. Rubin, and the Kenya Aflatoxicosis Investigation Group.** 2005. Aflatoxin contamination of commercial maize products during an outbreak of acute aflatoxicosis in eastern and central Kenya. *Environ. Health Perspect.* **113:**1763–1767.

49. **Li, F. Q., T. Yoshizawa, S. Kawamura, S. Y. Luo, and Y. W. Li.** 2001. Aflatoxins and fumonisins in corn from the high-incidence area for human hepatocellular carcinoma in Guangxi, China. *J. Agric. Food Chem.* **49:**4122–4126.

50. **Loosemore, R. M., and J. D. J. Harding.** 1961. A toxic factor in Brazilian groundnut causing liver damage in pigs. *Vet. Rec.* **73:**1362–1364.

51. **Loosemore, R. M., and L. M. Markson.** 1961. Poisoning of cattle by Brazilian groundnut meal. *Vet. Rec.* **73:**813–814.

52. **Lorenz, K.** 1979. Ergot on cereal grains. *Crit. Rev. Food Sci. Nutr.* **11:**311–354.

53. **Madsen, J. M.** 2001. Toxins as weapons of mass destruction. A comparison and contrast with biological-warfare and chemical-warfare agents. *Clin. Lab. Med.* **21:**593–605.

54. **Mannon, J., and E. Johnson.** 1985. Fungi down on the farm. *New Sci.* **105:**12–16.

55. **Marasas, W. F. O., T. S. Kellerman, J. G. Pienaar, and T. W. Naudé.** 1976. Leukoencephalomalacia: a mycotoxicosis of Equidae caused by *Fusarium moniliforme. J. Vet. Res.* **43:**113–122.

56. **Marasas, W. F. O., N. P. J. Kriek, J. E. Fincham, and S. J. van Rensburg.** 1984. Primary liver cancer and oesophageal basal cell hyperplasia in rats caused by *Fusarium moniliforme. Int. J. Cancer* **34:**383–387.

57. **Marquardt, R. R., and A. A. Frohlich.** 1992. A review of recent advances in understanding ochratoxicosis. *J. Anim. Sci.* **70:**3968–3988.

58. **McKean, C. M., L. Tang, M. Billam, M. Tang, C. W. Theodorakis, R. J. Kendall, and J. S. Wang.** 2006. Comparative acute and combinative toxicity of aflatoxin B$_1$ and T-2 toxin in animals and immortalized human cell lines. *J. Appl. Toxicol.* **26:**139–147.

59. **Mirocha, C. J., C. M. Christensen, and G. H. Nelson.** 1971. F-2 (zearalenone) estrogenic mycotoxin from *Fusarium*, p. 107–138. *In* S. Kadis, A. Ciegler, and S. J. Ajl (ed.), *Microbial Toxins*, vol. VII. *Algal and Fungal Toxins*. Academic Press, New York, NY.

60. **Mirocha, C. J., S. V. Pathre, and C. M. Christensen.** 1977. Zearalenone, p. 345–364. *In* J. V. Rodricks, C. W. Hesseltine, and M. A. Mehlman (ed.), *Mycotoxins in Human and Animal Health*. Pathotox Publishers Inc., Park Forest South, IL.

61. **Mirocha, C. J., B. Schauerhamer, and S.V. Pathre.** 1974. Isolation, detection, and quantitation of zearalenone in maize and barley. *J. Assoc. Off. Anal. Chem.* **57:**1104–1110.

62. **Nelson, P. E., A. E. Desjardins, and R. D. Plattner.** 1993. Fumonisins, mycotoxins produced by *Fusarium* species: biology, chemistry and significance. *Annu. Rev. Phytopathol.* **31:**233–252.

63. **Norstadt, F. A., and T. M. McCalla.** 1969. Patulin production by *Penicillium urticae* Bainier in batch culture. *Appl. Microbiol.* **17:**193–196.

64. **Nowicke, J. W., and M. Meselson.** 2000. Yellow rain—a palynological analysis. *Nature* **309:**205–206.

65. **Panaccione, D. G., and C. M. Coyle.** 2005. Abundant respirable ergot alkaloids from the common airborne fungus *Aspergillus fumigatus. Appl. Environ. Microbiol.* **71:**3106–3111.

66. **Pitt, J. I.** 2000. Toxigenic fungi: which are important? *Med. Mycol.* **38:**17–22.

67. **Reissig, J. E., and A. M. Rybarczyk.** 2005. Pharmacologic treatment of opioid-induced sedation in chronic pain. *Ann. Pharmacother.* **39:**727–731.

68. **Rheeder, J. P., W. F. O. Marasas, and H. F. Vismer.** 2002. Production of fumonisin analogs by *Fusarium* species. *Appl. Environ. Microbiol.* **68:**2101–2105.

69. **Rosen, R. T., and J. D. Rosen.** 1982. Presence of four *Fusarium* mycotoxins and synthetic material in 'yellow rain'. Evidence for the use of chemical weapons in Laos. *Biomed. Mass. Spectrom.* **9:**443–450.

70. **Rotter, B. A., D. B. Prelusky, and J. J. Pestka.** 1996. Toxicology of deoxynivalenol (vomitoxin). *J. Toxicol. Environ. Health* **48:**1–34.

71. **Saito, M., M. Enomoto, and T. Tatsuno.** 1971. Yellowed rice toxins: luteroskyrin and related compounds, chlorine-containing compounds and citrinin, p. 299–380. *In* A. Ciegler, S. Kadis, and S. J. Ajl (ed.), *Microbial Toxins*, vol. VI. *Fungal Toxins*. Academic Press, New York, NY.

72. **Smith, J. E., and M. O. Moss.** 1985. *Mycotoxins. Formation, Analyses and Significance.* John Wiley and Sons, Chichester, United Kingdom.

73. **Squire, R. A.** 1981. Ranking animal carcinogens: a proposed regulatory approach. *Science* **214:**877–880.

74. **Stark, A. A.** 2005. Threat assessment of mycotoxins as weapons: molecular mechanisms of acute toxicity. *J. Food Prot.* **68:**1285–1293.

75. **Takayama, H., N. Shimada, O. Mikami, and H. Murata.** 2005. Suppressive effect of deoxynivalenol, a *Fusarium* mycotoxin, on bovine and porcine neutrophil chemiluminescence: an in vitro study. *J. Vet. Med. Sci.* **67:**531–533.

76. **Trucksess, M. W., and Y. Tang.** 2001. Solid phase extraction method for patulin in apple juice and unfiltered apple juice, p. 205–213. *In* M. W. Trucksess and A. F. Pohland (ed.), *Mycotoxin Protocols*. Humana Press, Totowa, NJ.

77. **Van Egmond, H. P.** 1989. Aflatoxin M$_1$: occurrence, toxicity, regulation, p. 11–55. *In* H. P. Van Egmond (ed.), *Mycotoxins in Dairy Products*. Elsevier Applied Science, London, United Kingdom.

78. **Van Egmond, H. P., and G. J. A. Speijers.** 1994. Survey of data on the incidence and levels of ochratoxin A in food and animal feed worldwide. *Nat. Toxins* **3:**125–144.

79. **Wilson, D. M., and G. A. Payne.** 1994. Factors affecting *Aspergillus flavus* group infection and aflatoxin contamination of crops, p. 309–325. *In* D. L. Eaton and J. D. Groopman (ed.), *The Toxicology of Aflatoxins. Human Health, Veterinary and Agricultural Significance*. Academic Press, San Diego, CA.

80. **Wilson, S. C., T. L. Brasel, J. M. Martin, C. Wu, L. Andriychuk, D. R. Douglas, L. Cobos, and D. C. Straus.** 2005. Efficacy of chlorine dioxide as a gas and in solution in the inactivation of two trichothecene mycotoxins. *Int. J. Toxicol.* **24:**181–186.

81. **Winter, J. C., K. Kiers, M. D. Zimmerman, C. J. Reissig, J. R. Eckler, T. Ullrich, K. C. Rice, A. Rabin, and J. B. Richards.** 2005. The stimulus properties of LSD in C57BL/6 mice. *Pharmacol. Biochem. Behav.* **81:**830–837.

82. **Wogan, G. N.** 1966. Chemical nature and biological effects of the aflatoxins. *Bacteriol. Rev.* **30:**460–470.

83. **Wu, Q., A. Jezkova, Z. Yuan, L. Pavlikova, V. Dohnal, and K. Kuca.** 2009. Biological degradation of aflatoxins. *Drug Metab. Rev.* **41:**1–7.

84. **Yu, S. J., C. S. Kiang, S. V. Denn, H. T. Tsai, and Y. Wang.** 1951. A preliminary report on the topical use of citrinin. *Chin. Med. J.* **69:**199–203.

85. **Zapor, M., and J. T. Fishbain.** 2004. Aerosolized biologic toxins as agents of warfare and terrorism. *Respir. Care Clin. N. Am.* **10:**111–122.

86. **Zepnik, H., A. Pähler, U. Schauer, and W. Dekant.** 2001. Ochratoxin A-induced tumor formation: is there a role of reactive ochratoxin A metabolites? *Toxicol. Sci.* **59:**59–67.

87. **Zollner, P., and B. Mayer-Helm.** 2006. Trace mycotoxin analysis in complex biological and food matrices by liquid chromatography-atmospheric pressure ionisation mass spectrometry. *J. Chromatogr. A* **1136:**123–169.

Lacazia, Pythium, and *Rhinosporidium*

LEONEL MENDOZA AND RAQUEL VILELA

125

In the past 100 years the microbial pathogens described in this chapter have been classified as fungal and/or parafungal protistan pathogens (1, 2, 13, 22). Based on their apparent epidemiological connection with water, they were at one point also placed in a new category of hydrophilic infectious agents (1). However, based on taxonomic and other morphological characteristics, these three anomalous species were not well understood (1, 22). This frustrating situation fueled a strong controversy that has only recently been resolved with the advent of molecular methodologies (26, 27). Despite the recent finding that both *Pythium insidiosum* and *Rhinosporidium seeberi* are protistan pathogens, they are still studied by medical mycologists, continuing a historical tradition. Table 1 summarizes the most prominent features of the pathogens covered in this chapter.

LACAZIA LOBOI

Taxonomy

Jorge de Oliveira Lobo first described lacaziosis occurring in a patient from the state of Pernambuco, Brazil (23). He stated that the new pathogen was phenotypically similar to the parasitic stages of the genera *Blastomyces* and *Paracoccidioides*. The earliest attempts to isolate this pathogen in culture met with failure, and soon it became clear that this pathogen cannot be cultured (22, 52). This fact led to great controversy regarding its epidemiological and taxonomic affinities, reflected by the numerous names under which this pathogen has been known. Taborda et al. in 1999 (44) suggested the binomial *Lacazia loboi* to end more than 70 years of taxonomic ambiguity. Because the epithet lobomycosis was derived from the obsolete genus *Lobomyces* (22), Vilela et al. (53) suggested the name lacaziosis as a better term. Their suggestion was based on the proposal of Taborda et al. (44) and the placement of *L. loboi* as a separate taxon from the genus *Paracoccidioides* (18). Initial phylogenetic studies placed *L. loboi* near *P. brasiliensis* (18, 26), but besides the long branches described in phylogenetic analysis between these pathogens, there were not sufficient DNA sequences to support this claim. Vilela et al. (51), using at least five different loci and 20 *L. loboi* human strains, presented a strong argument for the phylogenetic placement of this pathogen as an independent taxon. This proposal was supported by another study indicating that an ancestor of both pathogens gave rise to two *Paracoccidioides* species

(*P. brasiliensis* and *Paracoccidioides lutzii*) and to *L. loboi* (45). Thus, *L. loboi* should be classified within the Ascomycota in the order Onygenales, family Ajellomycetaceae. Whether the teleomorphic stages of *Paracoccidioides* and *Lacazia* are located within the genus *Ajellomyces* together with *Ajellomyces capsulatus* and *Ajellomyces dermatitidis* is at this point unclear.

Description of the Agent

Because *L. loboi* cannot be cultured, our knowledge of this pathogen is based on the morphological features observed in its parasitic stage. Its in vivo phenotype is characterized by the development of unicellular, thick-walled yeastlike cells that can be found forming one, two, or more branches in chains of three or more cells characteristically connected by short tubules (Fig. 1). The yeastlike cells of *L. loboi* measure 5 to 12 μm in diameter and can be easily observed with most stains. Interestingly, the in vivo phenotype of *L. loboi* is very similar to the parasitic stage of *P. brasiliensis*, which led Lacaz et al. (22) to classify this pathogen in the genus *Paracoccidioides*. Electron microscopic analysis of *L. loboi* showed thick chitinous yeastlike cell walls and an amorphous cytoplasmic content. Approximately 60% of the yeastlike cells observed lacked a defined cytoplasmic region, a finding in agreement with results of viability studies.

Epidemiology and Transmission

Lacaziosis (lobomycosis or Jorge Lobo's disease) is known to occur only in patients inhabiting the tropical areas of the Americas (23). In addition to the many human cases, reports of the disease in species of dolphins around the coasts of South America, Florida, and the Gulf of Mexico have also been found (31). Although the majority of patients with lacaziosis have been from Brazil, cases from Mexico, Central America, Colombia, Surinam, Venezuela, and other nearby countries have also been reported (22). Two European patients apparently acquired the infection after contact with an infected bottle-nosed dolphin in an aquarium. In addition, American and Canadian patients were recently reported with the infection after visiting or working in areas of endemicity (8, 14).

It is believed that the infection is acquired through small traumatic skin lesions after contact with the pathogen in aquatic ecological niches in nature. The report of dolphins with lacaziosis tends to support this idea. However, the real ecological niche of this pathogen is unknown. The disease

TABLE 1 Taxonomical, epidemiological, clinical, and mycological features of the hydrophilic microbes *Lacazia loboi*, *Pythium insidiosum*, and *Rhinosporidium seeberi*

Pathogen	Taxonomy/phylogeny	Epidemiology	Clinical/in vivo form	In vitro form
Lacazia loboi	Ascomycete fungus located within the dimorphic Onygenales	Restricted to South America; cases of infection occur in dolphins; acquired by trauma; hydrophilic	Parakeloidal skin lesions; yeast-like cells in chains connected by small tubules	Uncultivated
Pythium insidiosum	Kingdom Stramenopila (Protista), class Oomycetes (Peronosporomycetes); better known as the "aquatic fungi"	Found in tropical, subtropical, and temperate areas; acquired in aquatic or terrestrial environments by trauma; hydrophilic	Cutaneous, intestinal, and vascular infection disseminated by metastasis/coenocytic hyphae exhibiting Splendore-Hoeppli phenomenon	Flat colonies without aerial mycelia; coenocytic hyphae without fruiting bodies; biflagellate zoospores in water cultures
Rhinosporidium seeberi	Kingdom Protista, class Mesomycetozoea; located at the animal-fungal divergence	Found on all continents except Australia; infection is endemic in India and Sri Lanka; acquired by trauma; hydrophilic	Polypoidal mucosal and skin lesions/spherical sporangia, with or without endospores at different stages of development	Uncultivated

seems to occur in apparently healthy hosts. It is quite possible that *L. loboi* cells possess hyphae with propagules (perhaps conidia) similar to those in *Paracoccidioides brasiliensis* that may make contact with hosts through trauma, thus causing lacaziosis. Transmission of the disease from one patient to another is rare, but some cases of autoinoculation and accidental infection by physicians in contact with infected patients (22, 36) or with infected dolphins (43) have been reported. In addition, the disease can be experimentally reproduced in mice (5).

Clinical Significance

Infections caused by *L. loboi* are rarely observed in the tropical areas of the Americas where the organism is endemic. Recent reports estimate that some 500 human cases, mostly in males with cutaneous lesions, have been diagnosed so far in the areas of endemicity, but the real number could be higher. The disease occurs in apparently healthy patients inhabiting such. A genetic-predisposition theory was abandoned after the finding that the number of cases in a Brazilian tribe with a high occurrence of the disease dramatically decreased when the tribe was moved to a new location. One common problem in the areas of endemicity is that patients with the disease do not seek

medical attention until years later, when the lesions have increased in size and spread to other skin areas. One explanation may be that the affected population is usually poor, with no access to health care, and that the lesions are rarely painful.

Frequently affected areas are the arms, ears, back, chest, face, and lower limbs. Some investigators believe that the distribution of lesions on cooler areas of skin in humans and in dolphins may indicate that the pathogen does not tolerate well a temperature of 37°C. Initially, a single small (0.5 to 1.0 cm in diameter), smooth, parakeloidal skin lesion develops. Some patients complain of slight pruritus at this stage. The infection is not life threatening and usually evolves very slowly, sometimes over 20 or more years. Usually, when patients seek medical attention they have already developed more than one lesion. In the chronic phase, the lesions are polymorphic. At least five clinical manifestations are recognized, including the typical parakeloidal type and the infiltrative, gummatous, ulcerated, and verrucous forms. However, Lacaz et al. (22) pointed out that two or more forms, including a macular type, could be found in a single patient. The differential diagnosis includes chromoblastomycosis, leprosy, neoplasia, paracoccidioidomycosis, and similar skin conditions.

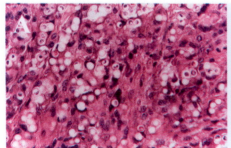 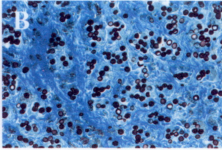 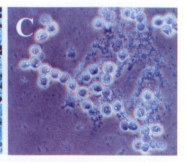

FIGURE 1 *L. loboi*. Histological sections stained with H&E (A) and silver stain (B) show the typical morphological features found in patients with cutaneous lacaziosis. (A) The yeastlike cells of *L. loboi* are poorly stained with H&E and are observed as empty round structures surrounded by an area of granulomatous reaction. (B) The presence of abundant yeastlike cells in chains is the main feature in silver-stained sections. (C) Numerous yeastlike cells of *L. loboi* in chains connected with slender tubules and containing small dancing bodies in their cytoplasm. Magnification for all panels, ×40. Panels A and B are courtesy of P. S. Rosa.

Collection, Transport, and Storage of Specimens

The guidelines for the collection, processing, storage, and examination of specimens are provided in chapter 112. Clinical specimens collected in cases of lacaziosis are mostly biopsy tissues from the infected sites. Since *L. loboi* cannot be cultured, clinical specimens from the infected areas are usually fixed in formaldehyde for later histopathological evaluation.

Direct Examination

Microscopy

In contrast to the systemic spread of *P. brasiliensis* infections, *L. loboi* is typically confined to cutaneous and subcutaneous tissues. The lesions are characterized by fibrosis and granulomatous reaction, with numerous histiocytes and giant cells containing many yeastlike cells of *L. loboi*. Areas of necrosis and the presence of other inflammatory cells have been reported. When tissue is stained with hematoxylin and eosin (H&E), the yeastlike cells arranged in linear chains are not well stained and appear as empty spaces with thick cell walls (Fig. 1A). Special fungal stains such as Gomori methenamine silver (GMS) and periodic acid-Schiff (PAS) stains should be used for the histopathological diagnosis of lacaziosis. With GMS, *L. loboi* yeastlike cells are dark or have the appearance of empty cells (Fig. 1B). The yeastlike cells are in chains of two or more cells and form branches, similar to the yeast cells observed in the infected tissue of patients with paracoccidioidomycosis. The cells are typically connected with small tubules, a feature also observed using other fungal stains such as PAS stain.

For the diagnosis of lacaziosis using direct microscopy, biopsy specimens should be cut into pieces 2 to 5 mm in diameter. One or more pieces are then placed with 1 or 2 drops of 10% KOH on a glass slide with a coverslip. The slide should be heated without boiling and then held for about 15 min at room temperature before microscopic evaluation. In 10% KOH, *L. loboi* yeastlike cells appear in great quantities (Fig. 1C). Cells 2 to 12 μm in diameter and uniform in size can be found as single yeast cells or as chains connected by short tubules of three or more cells. Moving protoplasmic granules can also be detected within some of the yeastlike cells (Fig. 1C).

Nucleic Acid Detection Techniques

At present, there are no commercially available nucleic acid probes for the detection of this pathogen in clinical samples.

Isolation Procedures, Identification, and Typing Systems

Claims that *L. loboi* has been isolated in pure culture have not yet been validated. Most of the recovered organisms were fungal contaminants or *P. brasiliensis* (22, 52). The identification of the etiologic agent is based on the clinical features and the phenotypic characteristics on wet-mount preparations and/or histopathological analyses of the infected tissues. No typing systems for this organism exist at this time.

Serologic Tests

One major obstacle to developing serologic assays for lacaziosis has been the lack of cultures. Thus, most of the serologic approaches have been carried out using parasitic forms in infected tissues as antigen or using cultures of closely related pathogens (22). These tests showed that *L. loboi* possesses cross-reactive antigens in common with fungal pathogens such as *Blastomyces dermatitidis, Histoplasma capsulatum,* and *P. brasiliensis* (22). Mendoza et al. (24), using antigenic proteins derived from the yeastlike cells of *L. loboi* from experimentally infected mice, found that the antibodies in the sera of humans, dolphins, and mice with lacaziosis detected a 193-kDa *L. loboi* immunodominant protein. Although antibodies in these sera did react with a *P. brasiliensis* purified gp43 antigen (24), they did not detect the corresponding gp43 antigen of the *L. loboi* parasitic stage. This finding suggests that the 193-kDa protein of *L. loboi* may have epitopes in common with gp43 of *P. brasiliensis*. It also implies that the 193-kDa antigen expressed during lacaziosis infection, although it cross-reacts with the antibodies against gp43 of *P. brasiliensis*, might be an entirely different antigenic protein. The role of this *L. loboi* antigenic protein in the pathogenesis of lacaziosis is under investigation. The use of *L. loboi* antigens in serologic surveys to study the epidemiology of lacaziosis has been suggested (24). Although serology is not commercially available, Biomedical Laboratory Diagnostics, Michigan State University, has developed a Western blot assay that can be requested at http://bld.msu.edu/.

Antimicrobial Susceptibilities

Although fungal therapy has cured some cases of lacaziosis, *L. loboi* is well known for its resistance to antimicrobial drugs, including most antifungals (22). This fact has left clinicians with only one choice: surgery. Due to the intractability of this organism to culture, susceptibility testing is not possible.

Evaluation, Interpretation, and Reporting of Results

Clinical samples from patients suspected of having lacaziosis submitted to the laboratory comprise deep-skin scrapings and tissue biopsy samples. The samples have to be processed as described above (see "Microscopy") and evaluated for the presence of uniform yeastlike cells connected by small tubules forming short chains. Because *P. brasiliensis* in the parasitic phase could also form yeast cells connected by tubules, the significant variation in size could be used to separate *L. loboi* from *P. brasiliensis*. The latter pathogen tends to develop large and small yeast cells in the infected tissues, whereas *L. loboi* yeastlike cells have uniform size. In addition, the lack of fungal growth in culture could also be used as an aid in the diagnosis of this uncultivated pathogen. After laboratory evaluation of the clinical material, the presence of uniform yeastlike cells that yielded no fungal growth in culture is used to confirm lacaziosis. This is particularly important for patients who have visited the areas where the disease is endemic. The report of the results should include the finding of uniform yeastlike cells connected by tubules, the lack of fungal growth in culture, and the histopathological results of the evaluated tissue samples.

PYTHIUM INSIDIOSUM

Taxonomy

P. insidiosum was first reported more than 150 years ago to occur in Indonesian equines (13), but successful isolation of this organism in pure culture was not possible until the beginning of the 20th century. Later a similar organism was isolated again from horses and the name *Hyphomyces destruens* was introduced. The finding that a strain from New Guinea (3) developed zoospores suggested that this pathogen was an organism in the genus *Pythium*. deCock et al. (13) introduced the binomial *P. insidiosum*, placing this pathogen within the protist kingdom Stramenopila and phylum Oomycota. Molecular studies (35, 39) showed that strains of *P. insidiosum* cluster phylogenetically according to their geographic origin. Thus, it is likely that *P. insidiosum* could be a phylogenetic complex of closely related species, or perhaps a complex of different strains belonging to one single species, *P. insidiosum*, including *Lagenidium*-like strains recovered from dogs (15, 24).

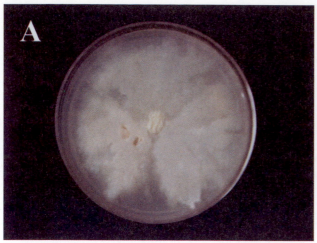
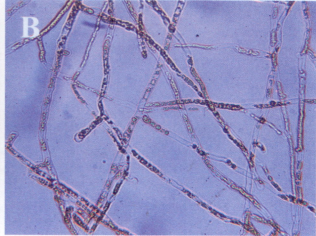

FIGURE 2 *P. insidiosum.* (A) Colony of *P. insidiosum* on Sabouraud dextrose agar. *P. insidiosum* produces cream to white submerged colonies at 25 and 37°C. (B) Sparsely septate hyphae are found on agar plates. No fruiting bodies can be found on dry cultures. Panel B magnification, ×40.

Description of the Agent

Unlike the other organisms described in this chapter, *P. insidiosum* can be readily isolated on most mycological media (13). This pathogen develops white submerged colonies with a characteristic radiate pattern and few to no aerial hyphae (Fig. 2A). The hyphae have perpendicular lateral branches measuring 4 to 10 μm in diameter and possess few cross septa. Zoosporogenesis (generation of zoospores) is only possible in water cultures containing various ions, including Ca^{2+} (11, 13, 28). The structures in which the zoospores develop are termed sporangia.

The zoospores form by progressive cleavage and mature inside large sporangia (20 to 60 μm in diameter). Once fully formed, the biflagellate zoospores mechanically break the sporangial wall, swim, and then encyst. It has been proposed that the zoospores may be the infectious units due to their motility. Zoospores are kidney-like in shape, and two unequal flagella arise from inside a lateral groove. Upon encystment the zoospores lose their flagella and become spherical. Under the right conditions the encysted zoospores develop a germ tube and form long filaments (29). *P. insidiosum* oogonia (teleomorphic stage) have been rarely observed and are believed to represent a resistant stage in nature.

Epidemiology and Transmission

Infections caused by this hydrophilic pathogen have been recorded in tropical, subtropical, and some temperate areas of the world. In the Americas, pythiosis is common in tropical Central, North, and South America, with most cases reported in Brazil, Colombia, Costa Rica, the United States, and Venezuela (13, 29). In the United States, infections are more prevalent in animals and humans inhabiting southern states such as Alabama, Georgia, Florida, Louisiana, Mississippi, North Carolina, South Carolina, and Texas. However, cases of the disease have been also reported in more northern states, including California, Illinois, Indiana, Kansas, New Jersey, Missouri, Tennessee, and Virginia; cases as far north as Wisconsin and New York have also been recorded. In Asia, pythiosis has been reported in Japan, India, Indonesia, the Pacific Islands, South Korea, and Thailand; it has also been reported in nearby areas such as Australia, New Guinea, and New Zealand. Tropical Africa is ideal for pythiosis; however, only one case in a dog with the cutaneous form was reported in the northwest African country of Mali. This might

suggest that the disease has most likely been misdiagnosed in this geographic region (35).

Until recently, infections caused by *P. insidiosum* were considered exotic. The disease was believed to be restricted to animals in tropical regions, with few or no occurrences in other geographic areas. Interestingly, in the last 10 years the number of pythiosis cases has increased on all continents (13, 46). The finding that humans (37, 46, 50, 55), dogs (17, 48), and other animals can be infected indicates that previously pythiosis was erroneously diagnosed as a fungal infection. Most cases of pythiosis occur in apparently healthy humans and animals. In Thailand, however, the disease in humans is associated with thalassemia or similar blood disorders (37). No such association has been reported so far in other areas.

The infection is acquired after *P. insidiosum* propagules enter the skin or the intestinal tract through traumatic lesions (29, 48). The infection is believed to be acquired from wet environments. Supabandhu et al. (42) cultured and identified *P. insidiosum* from environmental samples, confirming the presence of this oomycete in wet agricultural environments in Thailand. In addition, cases of pythiosis in the absence of water suggest that *P. insidiosum* can cause infection after contact with resting spores from terrestrial environments. The transmission of *P. insidiosum* from one individual to another (human to animal or vice versa) has not been yet recorded. Only rabbits seem to be susceptible to experimental inoculation (32).

Clinical Significance

The clinical manifestations of pythiosis vary according to the infection site. Most patients with the disease state that they had a skin injury prior to the infection. The lesions caused by *P. insidiosum* in humans can be classified into superficial infections (keratitis); cutaneous and subcutaneous forms, including orbital pythiosis; and vascular forms that usually lead to systemic infection and death. Keratitis caused by *P. insidiosum* is similar to that caused by fungi and other etiologic agents (4, 33, 54). It begins with trauma to the superficial layers of the eye, followed by the development of conjunctivitis, photophobia, corneal ulcers, and hypopyon (pus in the interior chamber of the eye). Cutaneous and subcutaneous infections are characterized by the formation of granulomatous plaques and/or ulcerated swellings that remain localized. Once the pathogen has reached the subcutaneous tissues, itchy papules may develop. The orbital form of subcutaneous pythiosis is rare and has been observed mainly in children in Australia and the United States (49). Vascular pythiosis starts with a traumatic lesion, usually on the lower limbs, followed by dissemination of the pathogen to the nearby arteries (37, 46). Initially the infected skin shows signs of dry gangrene, and for some patients the formation of painful necrotic ulcers has also been reported (46). Clinical symptoms are claudication (limping) of the affected limb, local ischemia, swelling, pain, and the absence of the dorsalis pedis pulse. As the infection progresses, an ascending arteritis with the formation of thrombi and aneurysms of the large arteries is the main feature. If not treated, *P. insidiosum* may spread through the arteries and reach the iliac and renal arteries and abdominal aorta, causing disseminated pythiosis. This form of pythiosis is more common in Thailand among patients with thalassemia, and it is usually life threatening (46, 50, 55). Human pythiosis should be differentiated from subcutaneous tuberculosis, cutaneous leishmaniasis, arteriosclerosis, diabetes mellitus, mycotic keratitis, subcutaneous zygomycosis, and other mycoses associated with filamentous fungi.

Collection, Transport, and Storage of Specimens

The clinical specimens required for diagnosis of pythiosis vary according to the infected host and the clinical form (29, 46). For patients with keratitis, swabs or scrapings of the affected eyes should be collected. Dryness of clinical specimens from keratitis patients could prevent the microscopic detection of the hyphal elements and subsequent culture of *P. insidiosum.*

Swabs must be immediately transported at room temperature in tubes with high humidity (or containing small quantities of sterile distilled water) to the laboratory and should be processed upon arrival. The collected eye scrapings should be placed in small aseptic petri dishes and immediately transported at room temperature to the laboratory. Biopsy or necropsy samples are usually collected in sterile distilled water and transported at room temperature to the laboratory. Specimens collected from patients with cutaneous, subcutaneous, vascular, and disseminated pythiosis can be also placed in tubes containing sterile distilled water plus 100 U of penicillin/ml and 0.25 mg of streptomycin or 0.4 mg of chloramphenicol/ml. If these antibiotics are not available, the use of sterile distilled water is encouraged. Although some studies indicate that transportation or storage at 4°C of specimens from patients suspected of having pythiosis did not interfere with the isolation of the pathogen in the laboratory, others report a considerable reduction in the number of positive cultures from samples stored at 4°C (29).

Direct Examination

Microscopy

Clinical specimens of *P. insidiosum* in 10% KOH characteristically show the presence of long (4.0 to 9.0 μm in diameter), hyaline, sparsely septated hyphal structures (Fig. 3D). Some hyphal elements may reach more than 15 μm and develop lateral branches at a 90° angle, a typical feature of

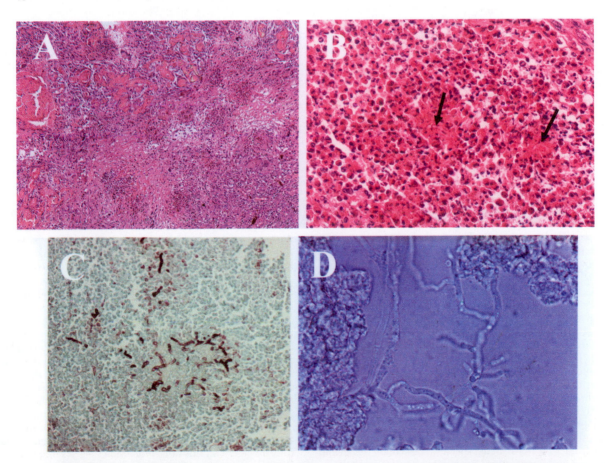

FIGURE 3 *P. insidiosum.* (A) Low magnification (×10) tissue section showing several eosinophilic microabscesses. (B) Numerous eosinophils around the unstained hyphal elements of *P. insidiosum* (Splendore-Hoeppli phenomenon [arrows]), a typical feature of pythiosis. Magnification, ×40. (C) Silver stain showing the typical hyphal features of *P. insidiosum.* Magnification, ×40. Panel courtesy of M. G. Rinaldi. (D) 10% KOH wet-mount preparation. Note sparsely septate slender hyaline hyphae with branches at 90° angles. Magnification, ×40.

this oomycete. In histopathological preparations stained with H&E, *P. insidiosum* appears as short or long hyaline coenocytic (without septa) hyphae 6 to 10 μm in diameter. The fact that in vivo structures of *P. insidiosum* are detectable in H&E has been used to differentiate this oomycete from the hyphal elements developed by members of the order Enthomophthorales (genera *Basidiobolus* and *Conidiobolus*). In infected tissues *P. insidiosum* triggers an eosinophilic granuloma with giant cells, mast cells, and other inflammatory cells (Fig. 3A and B). The hyphal elements of *P. insidiosum* are found in the center of microabscesses with numerous eosinophils that usually degranulate over the organism's hyphae (Splendore-Hoeppli phenomenon) (Fig. 3B). The activation of an eosinophilic inflammatory response with the Splendore-Hoeppli phenomenon is a feature in common with the order Entomophthorales, from which it must be differentiated. Although most experts in the diagnosis of pythiosis agree that it is difficult to distinguish between the hyphal structures of *P. insidiosum* and those of the Entomophthorales, features of the Entomophthorales such as the poor staining capabilities in H&E, the ribbon-type morphology, and the bigger size of their hyphal filaments sometimes help to distinguish these fungi from *P. insidiosum*. *P. insidiosum*'s hyphal elements are well stained by GMS and appear as short or long, sparsely septate, tubular dark structures (Fig. 3C). Transversely sectioned poorly stained (with GMS or PAS stain) hyphae can be also found as ring-shaped bodies.

The most important immunohistological tests for the specific identification of the hyphal elements of *P. insidiosum* in infected tissues have been the peroxidase and the immunofluorescence tests (6). Because the hyphal structures of *P. insidiosum* are difficult to differentiate from those in the fungi, especially the mucormycetes and Entomophthorales (formerly zygomycetes), these assays have been of paramount importance for the accurate identification of this oomycete in the absence of culture. Most of these assays are available through reference laboratories for pythiosis in the United States at Michigan State University (http://bld.msu.edu) and Pan American Veterinary Laboratories (http://www.pavlab.com) and in other countries such as Brazil and Thailand.

Nucleic Acid Detection Techniques

The first molecular approach for the diagnosis of *P. insidiosum* from clinical specimens was carried out with a patient with keratitis (4). The hyphal elements present in the specimen were identified by sequencing part of the 18S ribosomal DNA region using the NS1 and NS2 and internal transcribed spacer (ITS) universal primers. This approach has been successful with clinical specimens (4, 50). Grooters and Gee (16) introduced a PCR technique for the identification of *P. insidiosum* from cultures and from clinical specimens. A set of primers (PI-1 and PI-2) that amplified 105 bp of the ITS-1 region of *P. insidiosum* were tested. These primers have been used by several laboratories (50) and were entirely specific when tested against several filamentous fungi. Schurko et al. (38) introduced a dot blot hybridization technique by constructing a 530-bp species-specific DNA probe for the detection of *P. insidiosum*. This DNA probe specifically binds to intergenetic spacer 1 of this pathogen, and it did not hybridize with the genomic DNA from 23 other *Pythium* species, *Lagenidium giganteum*, or several pathogenic fungi, including the entomophthoromycetes *Conidiobolus coronatus* and *Basidiobolus ranarum*. This probe may be ideal for the detection of *P. insidiosum* from environmental samples and for the specific diagnosis of pythiosis from clinical specimens from susceptible hosts.

Isolation Procedures, Identification, and Typing Systems

In contrast with the other hydrophilic pathogens covered in this chapter, *P. insidiosum* can be cultured on various media. The most common media used for the isolation of *P. insidiosum* are 2% Sabouraud dextrose agar or broth with or without antibiotics (see "Collection, Transport, and Storage of Specimens" above), blood agar, cornmeal agar (Difco), potato dextrose agar, and nutritive agar (Difco). Biopsy or necropsy tissues from humans and animals and kunkers (stony hard masses found only in horses with pythiosis) from horses suspected of pythiosis are usually cut into fragments 2 to 5 mm in diameter, placed into tubes containing sterile distilled water, and vigorously washed two or three times before plating. The small fragments are then physically pushed into the agar, and the plates are incubated at 25 and 37°C for 2 or more days. The relative humidity of the incubator should be enhanced by placing a beaker of water inside the chamber. Specimens that have been transported for more than 24 h can also be inoculated into tubes containing broth and then incubated at 37°C. Usually, cottony colonies surrounding the clinical specimens are detectable after 24 to 48 h of incubation. On solid media *P. insidiosum* develops only sparsely septate hyphae (Fig. 2B). The appearance of *P. insidiosum* on solid media is described above.

P. insidiosum can be identified definitively only if the isolate develops the characteristic oogonia (teleomorphic stage) on culture plates. The formation of oogonia, however, is extremely rare, which further complicates the final identification of this pathogen in the clinical setting. Based on the fact that *P. insidiosum* is the only pathogen that develops zoospores in water, some laboratories have been using this characteristic for identification (50). This approach, however, does not guarantee that the species involved in that particular case is indeed *P. insidiosum*. The identification of this pathogen using molecular methods as described above is recommended. A drawback to this approach is that only a few laboratories possess these capabilities.

Currently, there are no typing systems available for *P. insidiosum*.

Serologic Tests

Early serologic tests showed that anti-*P. insidiosum* antibodies could be detected in the sera of infected hosts and thus could be used for the diagnosis of pythiosis. The most common assays for pythiosis are agglutination, enzyme-linked immunosorbent assay (ELISA), immunodiffusion, and Western blotting. Immunodiffusion has proven to be a very specific test, with several precipitin bands, but it is too insensitive and yields many false negatives, especially when performed with sera from humans and dogs with pythiosis (21). To overcome this drawback, an ELISA and a Western blot assay were later introduced (17, 21, 28, 30, 50). These assays are extremely sensitive and specific in detecting anti-*P. insidiosum* immunoglobulin G. Recently, an agglutination test was used for the rapid diagnosis of pythiosis. Although it proved to be a good screening test, it had a high rate of false positives and false negatives. The finding that antibodies in the sera of different hosts recognize different antigenic proteins when evaluated with several geographically divergent strains of *P. insidiosum* suggests frequent subclinical infections with multiple *P. insidiosum* strains (12).

Antimicrobial Susceptibility

Pythium insidiosum, like the other oomycetes, does not possess ergosterol in its cytoplasmic membrane. Despite this obvious contraindication, amphotericin B and other antifungal drugs that target ergosterol have been used, with mixed results. For instance, two children with orbital pythiosis were successfully treated with amphotericin B in Australia (49). However, this antifungal did not have effects in humans from Thailand with the disease (37, 55). Recently, susceptibility testing on a strain isolated from a child in Tennessee with orbital pythiosis showed the strain to have low mean inhibitory concentrations to terbinafine and itraconazole (40). Although this combination of drugs was successfully used in this case, the same combination was less effective when tested in other humans and animals. The inconsistent results obtained with most antifungal drugs for the treatment of pythiosis in humans and animals have led to the use of unconventional treatments such as immunotherapy (55). Immunotherapy has been found effective in 55% of the humans and dogs and in 70% of the equines with the disease (25). In addition, some investigators have evaluated in vitro combinations of several antifungals against *P. insidiosum,* with promising results (7, 9, 10). These studies indicate that terbinafine plus fluconazole or ketoconazole (9), or terbinafine plus amphotericin B (10), substantially reduced the in vitro growth of *P. insidiosum.* However, these combinations of antifungal drugs have yet to be tested in clinical cases.

Evaluation, Interpretation, and Reporting of Results

Culture is the "gold standard" test for pythiosis. Because *P. insidiosum* morphological features in infected tissues are identical to those displayed by the fungal entomophthoromycetes *Conidiobolus* and *Basidiobolus,* wet mounts, histopathological examination of tissue sections, serologic assays, and culture have to be evaluated as a whole for a proper interpretation and identification of this pathogen in the laboratory. For instance, the finding of sparsely septate hyaline hyphae in a wet-mount preparation must be confirmed by culture. Moreover, serologic assays such as ELISA and Western blotting identifying anti-*P. insidiosum* antibodies in hosts with a putative clinical diagnosis of pythiosis should be interpreted with caution. *P. insidiosum* can cause subclinical infections in humans and animals inhabiting the areas of endemicity. Thus, false positives have been found for apparently healthy individuals (25). When culture is not possible, the use of molecular approaches and/or peroxidase and immunofluorescence tests could be of help. The presence of hyaline hyphae in wet-mount preparations and in histopathology should be reported as suggestive of pythiosis, whereas positive results in culture (development of zoospores in water cultures) or positive reactions in molecular assays and/or in immunostaining tests are reported as confirmatory tests for the disease. In such cases the report of results should include the following: pythiosis caused by *P. insidiosum* confirmed by culture and supported by serologic and molecular assays.

RHINOSPORIDIUM SEEBERI

Taxonomy

The first two cases of rhinosporidiosis were reported in 1900 by Guillermo Rodolfo Seeber in his M.D. thesis in Argentina (1, 2). He stated that in 1896 he had found two patients with nasal polyps containing an organism similar to that reported by Posadas in 1892 (coccidioidomycosis). He also mentioned that in 1892, Malbran had studied a case of a nasal polyp showing a spherical microbe with identical

morphological features. A nasal case of rhinosporidiosis observed by O'Kinealy in 1903 in India was studied in detail by Minchin and Fanthan in 1905 (2). These investigators suggested the binomial *Rhinosporidium kinealyi* to identify this strain. Seeber in 1912 introduced the name *Rhinosporidium seeberi* and called attention to its priority over *R. kinealyi.* Ashworth in 1923 stated that the genus *Rhinosporidium* proposed by Minchin and Fanthan should be adopted and that, based on the description of Seeber (2) and the name *Coccidioides seeberia* reintroduced by Belou, the binomial *R. seeberi* has priority.

The fact that this pathogen has not been cultured led some investigators to extreme hypotheses. The suggestion that *R. seeberi* is a cyanobacterium in the genus *Microcystis* is the most recent in a long list of similar views. The placement of *R. seeberi* within the Mezomycetozoea came as a surprise. This group comprises orphan aquatic fish and amphibian parasites with spherical forms and endospores strikingly similar to those of *R. seeberi* (26, 27). Using the ribosomal DNA ITS, it was recently found that *R. seeberi* may include several species-specific strains that could represent new species (41).

Description of the Agent

This anomalous pathogen has resisted culture; thus, its morphological features are only known through in vivo microscopic and ultramicroscopic studies (1, 2). In infected tissues, *R. seeberi* has a complex parasitic cell cycle. It appears as multiple spherical structures known as sporangia (cysts in most mesomycetozoans) in different stages of development (Fig. 4A and B). Its in vivo cell cycle starts with the release of hundreds of oval or spherical endospores, 7 to 15 μm in diameter, from a pore developed only in mature sporangia. The endospores increase in size and progressively develop from juvenile (10 to 100 μm) to intermediate (100 to 150 μm) and then to mature (150 to more than 450 μm) size. The endospores are released from the mature sporangia, and then its in vivo cycle is somehow reinitiated (Fig. 4C). Although the diameter of the sporangium has been used to identify its in vivo stages, the mature sporangium differs from other stages by the presence of well-developed endospores.

Epidemiology and Transmission

Rhinosporidiosis usually occurs in most tropical and subtropical areas of the world except Australia (1). Although the infection was first recognized in Argentina, India and Sri Lanka show the highest occurrence of the disease (47). Rhinosporidiosis occurs sporadically in other geographic areas such as the Americas, Africa, Europe, and Asian countries, including in the Middle East. Because some cases of rhinosporidiosis occur in dry areas, especially after sand storms, the hydrophilic nature of this pathogen has long been questioned (1, 2, 47). Based on accounts from patients with the disease, it is believed that rhinosporidiosis is acquired through contact with aquatic environments contaminated with *R. seeberi,* but the precise mechanism of infection from natural sources is unknown.

The finding linking *R. seeberi* to aquatic pathogens of fish and amphibians (19, 26, 27) tends to confirm its hydrophilic nature. Most probably, this pathogen evolved from an aquatic niche, in which it still can be found, to terrestrial environments by the development of resistant spores. This is a very likely scenario since the formation of zoospores, as in the other members of the Dermocystida among which *R. seeberi* is phylogenetically located, has not been established

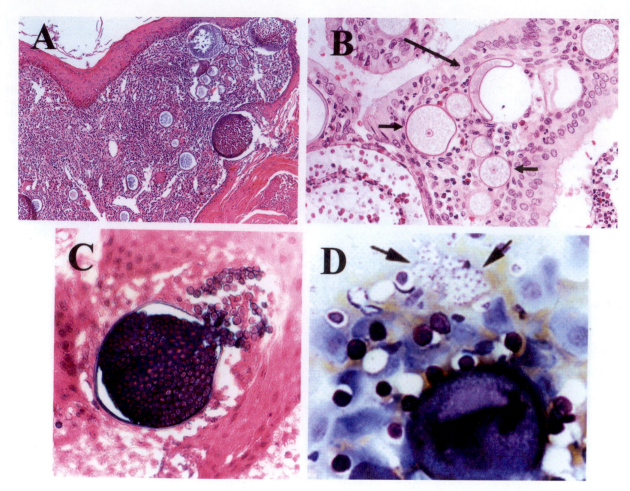

FIGURE 4 *R. seeberi.* (A) H&E-stained mature sporangia with endospores and numerous juvenile sporangia of different sizes. Magnification, ×10. (B) A collapsed sporangium in U shape and juvenile sporangia with prominent nuclei and nucleoli (long and short arrows, respectively). Magnification, ×30. (C) Mature sporangia releasing endospores through a cell wall pore. Magnification, ×30. (D) Wright-Giemsa impression smears from a dog with nasal rhinosporidiosis. An immature collapsed sporangium is shown in the lower section. Numerous endospores surrounded by a clear halo are shown in the upper section. Magnification, ×70. Panel D is courtesy of W. A. Meier.

(1, 2, 26, 47). The disease tends to occur as single cases, but two outbreaks of rhinosporidiosis in humans in Serbia (34) and in swans from Florida (20) have also been recorded. The resistant spores present in water and soil may gain entry through small cutaneous or mucocutaneous wounds and establish infection. Although the disease occurs in apparently healthy hosts, some investigators have suggested associations with particular occupational and social conditions (1, 47). Little is known about the predisposing factors leading to the disease. The disease has not been induced in experimental animals, and transmission from one host to another has yet to be reported.

Clinical Significance

In addition to humans, rhinosporidiosis around the facial areas has been reported to occur in several animal species, including cattle, cats, dogs, goats, horses, river dolphins, and birds (1, 27). In humans the most common clinical manifestation is the formation of painless polyps usually located on mucosal areas of the nose, eyes, larynx, genitalia, and rectum. Multicentric skin lesions have also been

recorded (47). The disease is not life threatening, but it can cause breathing difficulties when the polyps obstruct the nose or laryngeal passages. Rhinorrhea and bleeding are common with polyps located in the nose. The slow-growing polypoidal masses are usually found as single or multiple, pedunculate (attached to the skin), sessile red lesions that bleed easily. Pruritus of the affected areas is also common. The differential diagnosis includes bacterial and fungal infection, neoplasia, and other similar mucosal and skin conditions.

Collection, Transport, and Storage of Specimens

Guidelines for the collection, processing, storage, and examination of specimens are provided in chapter 112. Clinical specimens collected in cases of rhinosporidiosis are usually biopsy tissues from infected sites. Since *R. seeberi* cannot be cultured, clinical specimens are usually fixed in formaldehyde upon collection to be histopathologically evaluated later. Nonetheless, fresh samples should also be examined in the laboratory to rule out other etiologic agents and to confirm the histopathological findings. In these cases, biopsy specimens should be aseptically collected and transported immediately to the laboratory. For samples collected far from the laboratory, cooling (−80 to 4°C) of collected specimens for shipping or storage purposes may be necessary.

Direct Examination

Microscopy

Wet-mount preparations from clinical specimens from cases of rhinosporidiosis usually show the presence of mature and immature spherical sporangia and numerous endospores. Mature sporangia with endospores have thin cell walls and measure more than 400 μm in diameter. Juvenile and intermediate sporangia are smaller and may have thicker cell walls. For fresh specimens treated only with water, the release of endospores from mature sporangia has been reported (27). A purification system to study *R. seeberi* phenotypes was recently proposed (1). The presence of *R. seeberi* sporangia and endospores can also be found on smears stained with Giemsa or Gram stain (Fig. 4D). The spherical unstained elements of *R. seeberi* develop autofluorescence when viewed with a fluorescence microscope.

The parasitic spherical structures of this mesomycetozoan pathogen stain very well with H&E, but they also stain with GMS and PAS stains, a feature used by many in the past to suggest a link with the members of the kingdom Fungi. Biopsy tissue from polypoidal lesions stained with H&E is characterized by the presence of numerous sporangia at different stages of development (Fig. 4A and B). Hyperplasia of the mucous membranes and/or skin with fibrovascular and fibromyxomatous connective tissue containing numerous sporangia is the main feature of the infection. Inflammatory infiltrates of lymphocytes, neutrophils, plasma cells, and, more rarely, giant cells and eosinophils are usually observed in cases of nasal, ocular, and skin infections. Juvenile and intermediary sporangia possess a central nucleus with a prominent nucleolus (Fig. 4B). The collapse of immature sporangia may cause the formation of U-shaped structures. Mature sporangia possessing several thousand endospores are usually found near the mucosal epithelium, where they are transported from the internal infected areas by a transepidermal elimination phenomenon (Fig. 4A and C) (47). The cell walls of the mature sporangia are usually thin, and the enclosed endospores contain clusters of eosinophilic spherical structures. Endospores have a mucoid capsule that does not stain in H&E preparations. The presence of a pore on the sporangial wall is also observed depending on the plane of the sectioned tissue (Fig. 4C).

Nucleic Acid Detection in Clinical Materials

Currently there are no available DNA-based techniques for the diagnosis of *R. seeberi*.

Isolation Procedures, Identification, and Typing Systems

Despite numerous reports claiming that *R. seeberi* has been isolated in pure culture, such claims have not yet been validated. Most of the organisms recovered from cases of rhinosporidiosis have proven to be fungal or bacterial contaminants (1, 47). Because *R. seeberi* has not yet been cultured, the identification of this pathogen is based on its phenotypic characteristics on wet-mount preparations and/or histopathological analyses. The morphological characteristics of *R. seeberi* in infected tissues are almost pathognomonic. Nonetheless, the organism's epidemiological features and

the clinical signs of disease should be taken into consideration when making a final diagnosis. Morphologically, the parasitic (spherule) stages of *Coccidioides immitis* and *C. posadasii* mimic the *R. seeberi* sporangia with endospores. However, the epidemiological, clinical, and phylogenetic features of coccidioidomycosis and the fact that *Coccidioides* species can be readily cultured categorically separate this pathogen from *R. seeberi*.

Serologic Tests

Although early investigators did not find *R. seeberi* antibodies in the sera of infected hosts by using endospores or sporangia as antigens, others suggest that the reason for the failure was the use of insensitive assays such as immunodiffusion. Herr et al., using an immunoelectron microscopic approach, showed for the first time that anti-*R. seeberi* antibodies against a specific antigen, detected only in mature sporangia, are present in the sera of patients with rhinosporidiosis (19). Despite these efforts, there are no available serologic diagnostic assays for rhinosporidiosis in the clinical setting.

Antimicrobial Susceptibility

R. seeberi is resistant to most antifungal drugs (1, 38). However, the use of dapsone was found to be helpful to control some cases (1). Because this pathogen cannot be isolated in culture, susceptibility testing is not possible. Treatment consists of surgical removal of the infected tissues.

Evaluation, Interpretation, and Reporting of Results

The finding of spherical structures at different stages of development, some of them containing numerous endospores on histopathology, in cytological samples stained with Giemsa and Gram stains and in wet-mount preparations is suggestive of rhinosporidiosis. Since the *R. seeberi* spherical structures with endospores mimic the parasitic stage of *Coccidioides* species, a differential diagnosis is required, especially in the areas where coccidioidomycosis is endemic. The finding of >300-μm spherical sporangia with endospores and negative cultures is confirmatory of rhinosporidiosis. The report of the results should contain the finding of typical spherical structures that resisted culture.

REFERENCES

1. **Arseculeratne, S. N., and L. Mendoza.** 2005. Rhinosporidiosis, p. 436–475. *In* W. G. Merz and R. J. Hay (ed.), *Topley and Wilson's Microbiology and Microbial Infections,* 10th ed., vol. 5. *Medical Mycology.* Arnold, London, England.
2. **Ashworth, J. H.** 1923. On *Rhinosporidium seeberi* (Wernicke, 1903) with special reference to its sporulation and affinities. *Trans. R. Soc. Edinb.* **53:**301–342.
3. **Austwick, P. K.C., and J. W. Copland.** 1974. Swamp cancer. *Nature* (London) **250:**84.
4. **Badenoch, P. R., and D. J. Coster.** 2001 *Pythium insidiosum* keratitis confirmed by DNA sequence analysis. *Br. J. Ophthalmol.* **85:**502–503.
5. **Belone, A. F. F., S. Madeira, P. S. Rosa, and D. V. A. Opromolla.** 2002. Experimental reproduction of the Jorge Lobo's disease in BALB/c mice inoculated with *Lacazia loboi* obtained from a previously infected mouse. *Mycopathologia* **155:**191–194.
6. **Brown, C. C., J. J. McClure, P. Triche, and C. Crowder.** 1988. Use of immunohistochemical methods for diagnosis of equine pythiosis. *Am. J. Vet. Res.* **49:**1866–1868.
7. **Brown, T. A., A. M. Grooters, and G. L. Hosgood.** 2008. In vitro susceptibility of *Pythium insidiosum* and a *Lagenidium* sp. to itraconazole, posaconazole, voriconazole, terbinafine, caspofungin and mefenoxam. *Am. J. Vet. Res.* **69:**1463–1468.

8. **Burns, R. A., J. S. Roy, C. Woods, A. A. Padhye, and D. W. Warnock.** 2000. Report of the first case of lobomycosis in the United States. *J. Clin. Microbiol.* **38:**1283–1285.

9. **Cavalheiro, A. S., G. Maboni, M. I. de Azevedo, J. S. Argenta, D. I. Pereira, T. B. Spader, S. H. Spader, S. H. Alves, and J. M. Santurio.** 2009. In vitro activity of terbinafine combined with caspofungin and azoles against *Pythium insidiosum. Antimicrob. Agents Chemother.* **53:**2136–2138.

10. **Cavalheiro, A. S., R. A. Zanette, T. B. Spader, L. Lovato, M. I. Azevedo, S. Botton, S. H. Alves, and J. M. Santurio.** 2009. In vitro activity of terbinafine associated to anphotericin B, fluvastatin, rifampicin, metronidazole, and ibuprofen against *Pythium insidiosum. Vet. Microbiol.* **137:**408–411.

11. **Chaiprasert, A., K. Samerpitak, W. Wanachiwanawin, and P. Thasnakorn.** 1990. Induction of zoospores formation in Thai isolates of *Pythium insidiosum. Mycoses* **33:**317–323.

12. **Chindamporn, A., R. Vilela, K. A. Hoag, and L. Mendoza.** 2009. Antibodies in the sera of host species with pythiosis recognized a variety of unique immunogens in geographically divergent *Pythium insidiosum* strains. *Clin. Vaccine Immunol.* **16:**330–336.

13. **deCock, A. W., L. Mendoza, A. A. Padhye, L. Ajello, and L. Kaufman.** 1987. *Pythium insidiosum* sp. nov., the etiologic agent of pythiosis. *J. Clin. Microbiol.* **25:**344–349.

14. **Elsayed, S., S. M. Kuhn, D. Barber, D. L. Church, S. Adams, and R. Kasper.** 2004. Human case of lobomycosis. *Emerg. Infect. Dis.* **10:**715–718.

15. **Grooters, A. M.** 2003. Pythiosis, lagenidiosis, and zygomycosis in small animals. *Vet. Clin. Small Anim.* **33:**695–720.

16. **Grooters, A. M., and M. K. Gee.** 2002. Development of nested polymerase chain reaction for the detection and identification of *Pythium insidiosum. J. Vet. Intern. Med.* **16:**147–152.

17. **Grooters, A. M., B. S. Leise, M. K. Lopez, M. K. Gee, and K. L. O'Reilly.** 2002. Development and evaluation of an enzyme-linked immunosorbent assay for the diagnosis of pythiosis in dogs. *J. Vet. Intern. Med.* **16:**142–146.

18. **Herr, R. A., E. J. Tarcha, P. R. Taborda, J. W. Taylor, L. Ajello, and L. Mendoza.** 2001. Phylogenetic analysis of *Lacazia loboi* places this previously uncharacterized pathogen within the dimorphic Onygenales. *J. Clin. Microbiol.* **39:**309–314.

19. **Herr, R. A., L. Ajello, J. W. Taylor, S. N. Arseculeratne, and L. Mendoza.** 1999. Phylogenetic analysis of *Rhinosporidium seeberi*'s 18S small-subunit ribosomal DNA groups this pathogen among members of the protoctistan Mesomycetozoa clade. *J. Clin. Microbiol.* **37:**2750–2754.

20. **Kennedy, F. A., R. R. Buggage, and L. Ajello.** Rhinosporidiosis: a description of an unprecedented outbreak in captive swans (*Cygnus* spp.) and a proposal for revision of the ontogenic nomenclature of *Rhinosporidium seeberi. J. Med. Vet. Mycol.* **33:**157–165.

21. **Krajaejun, T., M. Kunakorn, S. Niemhom, P. Chogtrakool, and R. Pracharktam.** 2002. Development and evaluation of an in-house enzyme-linked immunosorbent assay for early diagnosis and monitoring of human pythiosis. *Clin. Diagn. Lab. Immunol.* **9:**378–382.

22. **Lacaz, C. S., R. G. Baruzzi, and M. C. B. Rosa.** 1986. *Doenca de Jorge Lôbo*, p. 92. Editora da Universidade de São Paulo, Brazil. IPIS Gráfica e Editora, São Paulo, Brazil.

23. **Lobo, J. O.** 1930. Nova especie de blastomycose. *Brasil. Med.* **44:**1227.

24. **Mendoza, L., A. F. Belone, R. Vilela, M. Rehtanz, G. D. Bossart, J. S. Reif, P. A. Fair, W. N. Durden, J. St. Leger, L. R. Travassos, and P. S. Rosa.** 2008. Use of sera from humans and dolphins with lacaziosis and sera from experimentally infected mice for Western blot analyses of *Lacazia loboi* antigens. *Clin. Vaccine Immunol.* **15:**164–167.

25. **Mendoza, L., and J. C. Newton.** 2005. Immunology and immunotherapy of the infections caused by *Pythium insidiosum. Med. Mycol.* **43:**477–486.

26. **Mendoza, L., and V. Silva.** 2004. The use of phylogenetic analysis to investigate uncultivated microbes in medical mycology,

p 275–298. *In* G. San-Blas and R. A. Calderone (ed.), *Pathogenic Fungi: Structural Biology, and Taxonomy.* Caister Academic Press, Norfolk, England.

27. **Mendoza, L., J. W. Taylor, and L. Ajello.** 2002. The class Mesomycetozoea: a heterogeneous group of microorganisms at the animal-fungal boundary. *Annu. Rev. Microbiol.* **56:**315–344.

28. **Mendoza, L., L. Kaufman, W. Mandy, and R. Glass.** 1997. Serodiagnosis of human and animal pythiosis using an enzyme-linked immunosorbent assay. *Clin. Diagn. Lab. Immunol.* **4:**715–718.

29. **Mendoza, L., F. Hernandez, and L. Ajello.** 1993. Life cycle of the human and animal Oomycete pathogen *Pythium insidiosum. J. Clin. Microbiol.* **31:**2967–2973.

30. **Mendoza, L., V. Nicholson, and J. F. Prescott.** 1992. Immunoblot analysis of the humoral immune response to *Pythium insidiosum* in horses with pythiosis. *J. Clin. Microbiol.* **30:**2980–2983.

31. **Migaki, G., M. G. Valerio, B. Irvine, and F. M. Gradner.** 1971. Lobo's disease in an Atlantic bottle-nosed dolphin. *J. Am. Vet. Med. Assoc.* **159:**578–582.

32. **Miller, R. I., and R. S. Campbell.** 1983. Experimental pythiosis in rabbits. *Sabouraudia* **21:**331–334.

33. **Murdoch, D., and D. Parr.** 1997. *Pythium insidiosum* keratitis. *Aust. N. Z. J. Ophthalmol.* **25:**177–179.

34. **Radovanovic, Z., Z. Vukovic, and S. Jankovic.** 1997. Attitude of involved epidemiologists toward the first European outbreak of rhinosporidiosis. *Eur. J. Epidemiol.* **13:**157–160.

35. **Rivierre, C., C. Laprie, O. Guiard-Marigny, P. Bergeaud, M. Berthelemy, and J. Guillot.** 2005. Pythiosis in Africa. *Emerg. Infect. Dis.* **11:**479–481.

36. **Rosa, S. M., C. T. Soares, A. F. F. Belone, R. Vilela, S. Ura, M. C. Filho, and L. Mendoza.** 2009. Accidental Jorge Lobo's disease in a worker dealing with *Lacazia loboi* infected mice: a case report. *J. Med. Case Rep.* **3:**67–71.

37. **Sathapatayavongs, B., P. Leelachaikul, R. Prachaktam, V. Atichartakarn, S. Sriphojanart, P. Trairatvorakul, S. Jirasiritham, S. Nontasut, C. Eurvilaichit, and T. Flegel.** 1989. Human pythiosis associated with thalassemia hemoglobinopathy syndrome. *J. Infect. Dis.* **159:**274–280.

38. **Schurko, A. M., L. Mendoza, A. W. A. M. deCock, J. E. J. Bedard, and G. R. Klassen.** 2004. Development of species-specific probe for *Pythium insidiosum* and the diagnosis of pythiosis. *J. Clin. Microbiol.* **42:**2411–2418.

39. **Schurko, A. M., L. Mendoza, C. A. Lévesque, N. L. Désaulniers, A. W. A. M. deCock, and G. R. Klassen.** 2003. A molecular phylogeny of *Pythium insidiosum. Mycol. Res.* **107:**537–544.

40. **Shenep, J. L., B. K. English, L. Kaufman, T. A. Pearson, J. W. Thompson, R. A. Kaufman, G. Frisch, and M. G. Rinaldi.** 1998. Successful medical therapy for deeply invasive facial infection due to *Pythium insidiosum* in a child. *Clin. Infect. Dis.* **27:**1388–1393.

41. **Silva, V., C. N. Pereira, L. Ajello, and L. Mendoza.** 2005. Molecular evidence for multiple host-specific strains in the genus *Rhinosporidium. J. Clin. Microbiol.* **43:**1865–1868.

42. **Supabandhu, J., M. C. Fisher, L. Mendoza, and N. Vanittanakom.** 2008. Isolation and identification of the human pathogen *Pythium insidiosum* from environmental samples collected in Thai agricultural areas. *Med. Mycol.* **46:**41–52.

43. **Symmers, W. S.** 1983. A possible case of Lobo's disease acquired in Europe from a bottle-nose dolphin (*Tursiops truncatus*). *Bull. Soc. Pathol. Exot. Filiales* **76:**777–784.

44. **Taborda, P. R., V. A. Taborda, and M. R. McGinnis.** 1999. *Lacazia loboi* gen. nov., the etiologic agent of lobomycosis. *J. Clin. Microbiol.* **37:**139–145.

45. **Teixeira, M. M., R. C. Theodoro, M. J. de Carvalho, L. Fernades, H. C. Paes, R. C. Hahn, L. Mendoza, E. Bagali, G. San-Blas, and M. S. Felipe.** 2009. Phylogenetic analysis reveals a high level of speciation in the *Paracoccidioides* genus. *Mol. Phylogenet. Evol.* **52:**273–283.

46. **Thianprasit, M., A. Chaiprasert, and P. Imwidthaya.** 1996. Human pythiosis. *Curr. Top. Med. Mycol.* **7:**43–54.

47. **Thianprasit, M., and K. Thagerngpol.** 1989. Rhinosporidiosis. *Curr. Top. Med. Mycol.* **3:**61–85.

48. **Thomas, R. C., and D. T. Lewis.** 1998. Pythiosis in dogs and cats. *Compend. Contin. Educ. Pract. Vet.* **20:**63–75.
49. **Triscott, J. A., D. Weedon, and E. Cabana.** 1993. Human subcutaneous pythiosis. *J. Cutan. Pathol.* **20:**267–271.
50. **Vanittanakom, N., J. Supabandhu, C. Khamwan, J. Praparattanapan, S. Thirach, N. Prasertwitayakij, W. Louthrenoo, S. Cheiwchanvit, and N. Tananuvat.** 2004. Identification of emerging human-pathogenic *Pythium insidiosum* by serological and molecular assay-based methods. *J. Clin. Microbiol.* **42:**3970–3974.
51. **Vilela, R., P. S. Rosa, A. F. Belone, J. W. Taylor, S. M. Dório, and L. Mendoza.** 2009. Molecular phylogeny of animal pathogen *Lacazia loboi* inferred from rDNA and DNA coding sequences. *Mycol. Res.* **113:**851–857.
52. **Vilela, R., J. E. Martins, C. N. Pereira, N. Melo, and L. Mendoza.** 2007. Molecular study of archival fungal strains isolated from cases of lacaziosis (Jorge Lobo's disease). *Mycoses* **50:**470–474.
53. **Vilela, R., L. Mendoza, P. S. Rosa, A. F. F. Belone, S. Madeira, D. V. A. Opromolla, and M. A. de Resende.** 2005. Molecular model for studying the uncultivated fungal pathogen *Lacazia loboi. J. Clin. Microbiol.* **43:**3657–3661.
54. **Virgil, R., H. D. Perry, B. Pardanani, K. Szabo, E. K. Rahn, J. Stone, I. Salkin, and D. M. Dixon.** 1993. Human infectious corneal ulcer caused by *Pythium insidiosum. Cornea* **12:**81–83.
55. **Wanachiwanawin, W., L. Mendoza, S. Visuthisakchi, P. Mutsikapan, B. Sathapatayavongs, A. Chaiprasert, P. Suwanagool, W. Manuskiatti, C. Ruangsetakit, and L. Ajello.** 2004. Efficacy of immunotherapy using antigens of *Pythium insidiosum* in the treatment of vascular pythiosis in humans. *Vaccine* **22:**3613–3621.

section VII ANTIFUNGAL AGENTS AND SUSCEPTIBILITY TEST METHODS

VOLUME EDITORS: JAMES H. JORGENSEN AND DAVID W. WARNOCK

SECTION EDITORS: MARY E. BRANDT AND ELIZABETH M. JOHNSON

Antifungal Agents*

DAVID W. WARNOCK

126

After a long period of slow development, the last decade has seen the introduction of an important new class of antifungal agents (the echinocandins), expansion of the spectrum of an established class of agents through chemical modification (the triazoles), and the development of novel methods for delivering established agents (lipid-based formulations of amphotericin B). These developments have changed the standards of care for the treatment of many invasive fungal infections, particularly aspergillosis and candidiasis. This chapter reviews the four major families of antifungal drugs that are currently available for systemic administration: the allylamines, the azoles, the echinocandins, and the polyenes. The comparative activities of the major systemic antifungal agents against important groups of fungi are summarized in Table 1. This chapter also discusses the characteristics of several other agents that can be used for the oral or parenteral treatment of superficial, subcutaneous, or systemic fungal infections. Novel agents that are currently in clinical trials are briefly reviewed.

ALLYLAMINES

The allylamines are a group of synthetic antifungal compounds effective in the topical and oral treatment of dermatophytoses. Two drugs, terbinafine and naftifine, are licensed for clinical use. Naftifine is available as a topical preparation only.

Mechanism of Action

The allylamines inhibit squalene epoxidase, a critical enzyme in the formation of ergosterol, the principal sterol in the membrane of susceptible fungal cells. The consequent accumulation of squalene leads to membrane disruption and cell death (122).

Terbinafine

Terbinafine (Lamisil; Novartis Pharmaceuticals) is a lipophilic drug that is available for oral or topical administration. It is widely used for the treatment of superficial fungal infections caused by dermatophytes.

Spectrum of Activity

Terbinafine is effective against several groups of pathogenic fungi, including dermatophytes (*Epidermophyton*, *Microsporum*, and *Trichophyton* spp.) (40, 41, 99) and dematiaceous fungi (81). It also has some activity against *Aspergillus* spp. (85), *Candida* spp. (123), *Blastomyces dermatitidis* and *Histoplasma capsulatum* (128), *Paracoccidioides brasiliensis* (52), *Penicillium marneffei* (80), and *Sporothrix schenckii* (142).

Acquired Resistance

There have been no reports of development of resistance to terbinafine among dermatophytes even after prolonged exposure.

Pharmacokinetics

Terbinafine is well absorbed after oral administration and is then rapidly and extensively distributed to body tissues (69). It reaches the stratum corneum as a result of diffusion through the dermis and epidermis and secretion in sebum. Diffusion from the nail bed is the major factor in its rapid penetration of nails. Terbinafine has been found to persist in nail for long periods after cessation of treatment. It is extensively metabolized by the human hepatic cytochrome P-450 enzyme system, and the inactive metabolites are mostly excreted in the urine (149).

Clinical Use

Terbinafine is the drug of choice for dermatophyte infections of the skin and nails in cases where topical treatment is considered inappropriate or has failed (32, 79). It is not as effective as itraconazole for treatment of fungal nail infections (onychomycosis) involving nondermatophytes. Terbinafine has also proven effective in some patients with aspergillosis, chromoblastomycosis, and sporotrichosis (118), but it is not licensed for these indications. Anecdotal evidence suggests that the use of terbinafine in combination with voriconazole may be beneficial in the treatment of infections with *Scedosporium prolificans*.

Drug Interactions

Although terbinafine is metabolized by the human hepatic cytochrome P-450 enzyme system, it does not inhibit most CYP enzymes at clinically relevant concentrations (149).

---

*This chapter contains information presented in chapter 129 by Sevtap Arikan and John H. Rex in the ninth edition of this *Manual*.

TABLE 1 Spectrums and extents of activity of commonly used systemic antifungal agents[a]

Organism	Activity[b] of antifungal agent							
	Amphotericin	Fluconazole	Itraconazole	Posaconazole	Voriconazole	Anidulafungin	Caspofungin	Micafungin
Aspergillus spp.	+++	−	++	+++	+++	++	++	++
B. dermatitidis	+++	+	+++	+++	+++	−	−	−
Candida spp.								
C. *albicans*	+++	+++	+++	+++	+++	+++	+++	+++
C. *glabrata*	++	++	++	++	++	+++	+++	+++
C. *krusei*	++	−	+++	+++	+++	+++	+++	+++
C. *lusitaniae*	++	+++	+++	+++	+++	+++	+++	+++
C. *parapsilosis*	+++	+++	+++	+++	+++	++	++	++
C. *tropicalis*	+++	+++	+++	+++	+++	+++	+++	+++
Coccidioides spp.	+++	+++	+++	+++	+++	−	−	−
Cryptococcus spp.	+++	+++	++	+++	+++	−	−	−
Fusarium spp.	++	−	+	++	++	−	−	−
H. capsulatum	+++	++	+++	+++	+++	−	−	−
Mucoraceous molds	+++	−	−	++	−	−	−	−
P. brasiliensis	+++	++	+++	+++	+++	−	−	−

[a]This table is a general overview for comparison of the activities of some systemic drugs against various fungi. Readers are recommended to refer to the text for more detailed information.

[b]−, no meaningful activity; +, occasional activity; ++, moderate activity but resistance is noted; +++, reliable activity with occasional resistance.

Concentrations of terbinafine in blood are reduced when it is given together with drugs, such as rifampin, that induce the hepatic cytochrome P-450 system.

Toxicity and Adverse Effects
Terbinafine produces few adverse reactions. These include abdominal discomfort, nausea, diarrhea, impairment of taste, and transient skin rashes (53). Rare but serious side effects include Stevens-Johnson syndrome and hepatotoxic reactions including cholestasis and hepatitis.

AZOLES
The azoles constitute a large group of synthetic agents containing many compounds that are effective in the topical treatment of dermatophyte infections and superficial forms of candidiasis; a number are suitable for systemic administration. Members of this group have in common an imidazole or triazole ring with *N*-carbon substitution.

Mechanism of Action
Azole compounds inhibit a fungal cytochrome P-450-dependent enzyme, lanosterol 14 α-demethylase, which is responsible for the conversion of lanosterol to ergosterol, the principal sterol in the membrane of susceptible fungal cells (144). This results in the accumulation of various methylated sterols and the depletion of ergosterol with subsequent disruption of membrane structure and function. The activity is essentially fungistatic, although some of the newer triazoles can exert fungicidal effects against some mold species at the concentrations achieved with recommended dosages (77).

Several mechanisms of resistance have been described (see chapter 127). These include upregulation of multidrug efflux transporter genes; upregulation of the *ERG11* gene that encodes the target enzyme, lanosterol 14 α-demethylase; and decreased affinity of this enzyme for azole agents due to amino acid substitutions (126). Changes in other enzymes involved in the ergosterol biosynthesis pathway, such as loss of $\Delta^{5,6}$-sterol desaturase activity, may also contribute to azole resistance (126).

Pharmacokinetics
With the exception of fluconazole, food has a significant effect on the absorption of azole antifungals (34). Administration with food improves the absorption of ketoconazole, posaconazole, and the capsule formulation of itraconazole (22, 29, 39, 57). In contrast, absorption of voriconazole and the oral solution formulation of itraconazole is reduced when the drug is given with a high-fat meal (6, 115).

Peak concentrations of azoles in blood are typically reached within 2 to 3 h after oral administration. With fluconazole and posaconazole, blood levels increase in proportion to dosage (21, 34). In contrast, increases in itraconazole and ketoconazole dosage produce disproportionate changes in peak blood concentrations due to saturable first-pass metabolism in the liver (28, 33). In adults, there is a disproportionate increase in blood levels of voriconazole with increasing oral and parenteral dosage (114). In children, however, increases in dosage produce proportional changes in drug levels, and clearance of the drug is more rapid (153).

Due to its low protein binding (about 12%), fluconazole attains high concentrations in most tissues and body fluids. Levels of the drug in cerebrospinal fluid (CSF) usually exceed 50% of the simultaneous concentration in blood (34). Likewise, voriconazole is extensively distributed into tissues (140), with CSF levels that are around 30 to 60% of the simultaneous concentration in blood (76). Voriconazole concentrations in vitreous and aqueous fluids are around 40 to 50% of the simultaneous level in blood (55). Levels of itraconazole and ketoconazole in the CSF are minimal (23, 57).

Levels of itraconazole in tissues such as lung, liver, brain, and bone are two to three times higher than in serum. High concentrations are also found in the stratum corneum as a result of drug secretion in sebum (17). Itraconazole has been found to persist in the skin and nails for weeks to months after the end of a course of treatment, thereby allowing intermittent pulse regimens for dermatophyte infections and onychomycosis (17, 156).

With the exception of fluconazole and posaconazole, the azoles are extensively metabolized by the human hepatic cytochrome P-450 enzyme system and are eliminated as inactive metabolites in the bile or urine. More than 90% of a dose of fluconazole is eliminated in the urine, predominantly as unchanged drug (13). More than 75% of a dose of posaconazole is eliminated in the feces, predominantly as unchanged drug, with the remainder being excreted as glucuronidated derivatives in the urine (70). Itraconazole is unusual because its major metabolite, hydroxyitraconazole, is bioactive and has a spectrum of activity similar to that of the parent compound (89). This metabolite is found at concentrations in serum about twofold higher than those of the parent drug (57).

Voriconazole is metabolized by several different hepatic cytochrome P-450 enzymes, primarily CYP-2C19, with more than 80% of a dose being eliminated as inactive metabolites in the urine (61, 121). However, as a result of a point mutation in the gene encoding this enzyme, some persons are poor metabolizers while others are extensive metabolizers. About 3 to 5% of Caucasians and 15 to 20% of non-Indian Asians are poor metabolizers (140). Voriconazole concentrations in blood are as much as fourfold lower in individuals who metabolize the drug more extensively.

Drug Interactions

Most azole antifungal agents are extensively metabolized by the human hepatic cytochrome P-450 enzyme system and are potent inhibitors of CYP-3A4; some also inhibit CYP-2C9 and CYP-2C19. Their coadministration with other drugs that are metabolized by these enzymes can result in increased concentrations of the azole, the interacting drug, or both, in blood (147). When an azole agent is discontinued, the change in metabolism that occurs may necessitate upward or downward adjustment of the dosage of the other drugs. Administration of azoles with drugs that are potent inducers of the human cytochrome P-450 enzyme system, such as rifampin, results in a marked reduction in concentrations in blood, especially with itraconazole and ketoconazole (147).

Fluconazole

Fluconazole (Diflucan; Pfizer) is a water-soluble bis-triazole and is available in both oral and parenteral formulations. It is extensively used, particularly in the treatment of candidiasis and cryptococcosis.

Spectrum of Activity

Fluconazole possesses the narrowest spectrum of all the azole antifungals currently available for systemic use. It is active against most *Candida* spp. and *Cryptococcus neoformans* (105, 110). However, *Candida krusei* appears to be intrinsically resistant (91). The spectrum of activity also includes several dimorphic fungi (*B. dermatitidis*, *Coccidioides* spp., and *H. capsulatum*) (48). Fluconazole has no activity against *Aspergillus* spp., *Fusarium* spp. (95), or mucoraceous molds (1).

Acquired Resistance

There have been few reports of resistance developing in *Candida albicans* during short-term fluconazole treatment in patients with mucosal or deep-seated forms of candidiasis (126). In contrast, many strains of *Candida glabrata* rapidly become resistant to fluconazole during treatment (11). In persons with AIDS, resistant strains of *C. albicans* have appeared following repeated courses of low-dose fluconazole treatment for oral or esophageal infection (120). However, with the widespread use of highly active antiretroviral treatment for HIV infection, resistant strains are now rarely encountered (78, 119). There are a few reports of resistant strains of *C. neoformans* from AIDS patients with relapsed infection following long-term maintenance treatment with fluconazole (14).

Clinical Use

Fluconazole is widely used in the treatment of mucosal and systemic candidiasis (96), coccidioidomycosis (42), and cryptococcosis (100). It is also widely used for the prevention of candidiasis in neutropenic patients (96), as well as for the prevention of relapse of cryptococcal meningitis in persons with AIDS (100). Fluconazole is an alternative for the treatment of histoplasmosis and sporotrichosis but is less effective than itraconazole (66, 154).

Therapeutic Drug Monitoring

Concentrations of fluconazole in serum are predictable from dosing and organ function, and routine monitoring of drug levels is not required (2, 49, 59).

Toxicity and Adverse Effects

Fluconazole is one of the least-toxic and best-tolerated azole drugs, and side effects during treatment are rare. The most common patient complaints include headache, hair loss, and loss of appetite (135). Transient abnormalities of liver enzymes and rare serious skin reactions, including Stevens-Johnson syndrome, have been reported.

Itraconazole

Itraconazole (Sporanox; Ortho-McNeil-Janssen Pharmaceuticals) is a lipophilic triazole drug available for oral or parenteral administration. It is extensively used, particularly in the treatment of superficial fungal infections, as well as in a range of subcutaneous and systemic infections.

Spectrum of Activity

Itraconazole has good activity against a broad spectrum of pathogenic fungi, including *Aspergillus* spp. (25, 31, 35, 102, 111), *Candida* spp. (25, 102, 110), many dematiaceous molds (63, 81), dermatophytes (40, 41, 99), and dimorphic fungi (*B. dermatitidis*, *Coccidioides* spp., *H. capsulatum*, *P. brasiliensis*, *P. marneffei*, and *S. schenckii*) (19, 48, 52, 74, 80, 124, 142). Itraconazole has modest activity against *C. neoformans* (102, 110) but is ineffective against *Pseudallescheria boydii* (46) and most mucoraceous molds (1, 30).

Acquired Resistance

Acquired resistance is rare, but ketoconazole-resistant *C. albicans* strains from patients with chronic mucocutaneous candidiasis have been found to be cross-resistant to itraconazole (132), as have many fluconazole-resistant *C. albicans* strains from AIDS patients with chronic relapsing oropharyngeal candidiasis (5). Itraconazole-resistant strains of *A. fumigatus* have been reported following treatment, but azole resistance remains an uncommon problem among *Aspergillus* spp. (82, 109).

Clinical Use

Itraconazole has been widely used to treat various superficial fungal infections, including the dermatophytoses, onychomycosis, pityriasis versicolor, and mucosal and cutaneous forms of candidiasis (especially in patients who have experienced treatment failure with fluconazole) (16). It is also effective in patients with paracoccidioidomycosis, chromoblastomycosis, sporotrichosis, and certain forms of phaeohyphomycosis (15, 66, 131). Despite its limitations, itraconazole continues to be a drug of choice in the management of mild to moderate forms of blastomycosis and histoplasmosis (18, 154). It was the first orally active drug for aspergillosis, but its use in seriously ill patients with life-threatening forms of this disease is not recommended (152). Itraconazole is the drug of choice for long-term maintenance treatment to prevent relapse in AIDS patients with histoplasmosis (154), but it is less effective than fluconazole as maintenance treatment in AIDS patients with cryptococcosis (100).

Therapeutic Drug Monitoring

Absorption of the capsule formulation of itraconazole after oral administration shows marked variation between individuals. Because low concentrations in serum are often predictive of treatment failure, measurement of blood levels is advisable in situations where the drug is used to treat or prevent serious invasive fungal infections (2, 49, 59). For prophylaxis, a target trough concentration of >0.5 μg/ml has been proposed; for treatment, a trough of >1 to 2 μg/ml has been recommended (2).

Toxicity and Adverse Effects

Most side effects associated with itraconazole are mild and reversible. The most frequently reported adverse events are headache, loss of appetite, nausea, abdominal discomfort, diarrhea, skin rashes, and transient elevations of liver enzymes (54). Gastrointestinal intolerance is more common with itraconazole oral solution and is sometimes severe enough to necessitate discontinuation of treatment (51, 145). Rare, but serious, side effects include Stevens-Johnson syndrome, hepatitis, and congestive heart failure.

Ketoconazole

Ketoconazole (Nizoral; Ortho-McNeil-Janssen Pharmaceuticals) is a lipophilic drug formulated for oral or topical use. It is the only antifungal imidazole still available for systemic administration, but its main use is now as a topical agent.

Spectrum of Activity

Ketoconazole has useful activity against dermatophytes (40, 41, 99) and dimorphic fungi (B. dermatitidis, Coccidioides spp., H. capsulatum, P. brasiliensis, and S. schenckii) (19, 129, 142). It is also active against Candida spp. and C. neoformans, although it is less effective than the newer triazoles. It has no activity against P. boydii or mucoraceous molds (1, 46).

Acquired Resistance

Acquired resistance is rare, but several instances were documented in the 1980s among patients given long-term treatment for chronic mucocutaneous candidiasis due to C. albicans (132). In the 1990s, many fluconazole-resistant isolates of C. albicans from AIDS patients with relapsing oropharyngeal or esophageal candidiasis were cross-resistant to ketoconazole (64).

Clinical Use

Due to the availability of less toxic, more efficacious alternatives, ketoconazole is now little used, except in resource-limited environments. It is a second-line agent for mild or moderate forms of blastomycosis, histoplasmosis, and paracoccidioidomycosis (75). However, prolonged administration of high dosage is often required and later relapse is a common problem. Ketoconazole remains a useful topical agent for dermatophytosis, cutaneous candidiasis, pityriasis versicolor, and seborrheic dermatitis.

Toxicity and Adverse Effects

Unwanted effects include loss of appetite, abdominal pain, nausea, and vomiting. Transient elevations of liver enzymes are common with oral ketoconazole, and fatal hepatitis is a rare but well-recognized adverse event (72). High doses of ketoconazole inhibit human adrenal and testicular steroid synthesis, with clinical consequences such as alopecia, gynecomastia, and impotence (113).

Posaconazole

Posaconazole (Noxafil; Schering) is a broad-spectrum triazole compound that is currently available only as an oral suspension. An intravenous formulation is in a phase I clinical trial. Posaconazole is highly lipophilic and has a chemical structure similar to that of itraconazole.

Spectrum of Activity

Posaconazole is highly active against most Aspergillus spp. (25, 35, 111), as well as Candida spp., C. neoformans, and Trichosporon spp. (25, 94, 110, 124). It has potent activity against a number of dimorphic fungi, including B. dermatitidis, Coccidioides spp., H. capsulatum, P. marneffei, and S. schenckii (48, 124). It is less active against Fusarium spp. and P. boydii but appears to be effective against dematiaceous fungi (46, 48, 95, 124). Unlike other azole antifungals, posaconazole has significant activity against some mucoraceous molds (1, 25, 30, 124).

Acquired Resistance

Acquired resistance to posaconazole has not been reported. Posaconazole sometimes has activity against strains of Aspergillus and Candida spp. that show resistance to itraconazole, fluconazole, and/or voriconazole (82, 124).

Clinical Use

The lack of an intravenous formulation of posaconazole is a major disadvantage in the treatment of seriously ill patients. In the United States, the drug has been approved for the treatment of oropharyngeal candidiasis (including infections refractory to itraconazole and/or fluconazole), as well as for prophylaxis of invasive aspergillosis and candidiasis in high-risk patients, such as hematopoietic stem cell transplant (HSCT) recipients with graft-versus-host disease and neutropenic cancer patients. In the European Union, posaconazole has been licensed for similar indications, as well as for salvage treatment of invasive aspergillosis, coccidioidomycosis, chromoblastomycosis, Fusarium infections, and mycetoma. Other indications for which posaconazole has proved effective but is not currently licensed include histoplasmosis (117) and infections caused by mucoraceous molds (143).

Therapeutic Drug Monitoring

Similar to itraconazole and voriconazole, there appears to be a relationship between posaconazole trough concentrations in serum and clinical response, and measurement of drug levels may therefore be useful. For prophylaxis, a target trough concentration of >0.5 μg/ml has been proposed; for treatment, a trough of >0.5 to 1.5 μg/ml has been suggested (2).

Toxicity and Adverse Effects

Posaconazole is well tolerated, even among patients receiving the drug for longer than 6 months (116). The most frequently reported side effects have been gastrointestinal symptoms and headache. Transient transaminase abnormalities have also been reported. Rare cases of cholestasis or hepatic failure have occurred during treatment with posaconazole.

Voriconazole

Voriconazole (Vfend; Pfizer) is a broad-spectrum triazole compound available for oral or intravenous administration. Its chemical structure is similar to that of fluconazole.

Spectrum of Activity

Voriconazole is highly active against most *Aspergillus* spp., *Fusarium* spp., and *P. boydii* (25, 35, 46, 63, 95, 111), as well as *Candida* spp., *C. neoformans*, and *Trichosporon* spp. (25, 94, 124). Voriconazole has potent activity against a number of dimorphic fungi, including *B. dermatitidis*, *Coccidioides* spp., *H. capsulatum*, and *P. marneffei* (48, 74), as well as dematiaceous moulds (63). Voriconazole is ineffective against mucoraceous molds (1, 30, 63, 124).

Acquired Resistance

Acquired resistance to voriconazole has not been reported. However, some fluconazole-resistant strains of *Candida* spp. show reduced susceptibility to voriconazole, as do some itraconazole-resistant strains of *Aspergillus* spp. (82, 124).

Clinical Use

The availability of both an intravenous formulation and a well-absorbed oral formulation of voriconazole is a distinct advantage when treating seriously ill patients. In the United States, the drug has been approved for the treatment of invasive aspergillosis and has become the drug of choice for these infections (152). It is also licensed for the treatment of candidemia in nonneutropenic patients, for disseminated infections caused by *Candida* spp., and for esophageal candidiasis, as well as for salvage treatment of *Fusarium* and *Scedosporium* infections. In the European Union, voriconazole has been approved for similar indications. Voriconazole has no activity against mucoraceous molds, and its use in immunocompromised patients has sometimes been associated with breakthrough infections caused by these organisms (68).

Therapeutic Drug Monitoring

Voriconazole concentrations in serum are highly variable, largely due to differences in the rate of metabolism between individuals, and it may be beneficial to monitor drug levels (2, 49, 59). For prophylaxis, a target trough concentration of >0.5 μg/ml has been proposed; for treatment, a trough of >1 to 2 μg/ml has been recommended (2). To avoid toxicity, trough concentrations of 6 μg/ml of voriconazole should not be exceeded.

Toxicity and Adverse Effects

Voriconazole is generally well tolerated. About 30% of patients experience transient visual disturbances, usually during the first week of treatment (140). Other side effects include skin rashes and transient abnormalities of liver enzymes. Rare, but serious, adverse effects include Stevens-Johnson syndrome, hepatic failure, and cardiovascular events.

ECHINOCANDINS

The echinocandins are a new class of semisynthetic lipopeptide antifungal agents that target the fungal cell wall. Three echinocandins have been approved for the treatment of serious fungal infections: anidulafungin, caspofungin, and micafungin. Due to their high molecular weight and low oral bioavailability, these drugs are available as intravenous preparations only. They are now widely used, particularly in the treatment of candidiasis.

Mechanism of Action

The echinocandins disrupt fungal cell wall synthesis by inhibiting the enzyme 1,3-β-D-glucan synthase. This results in inhibition of the formation of 1,3-β-D-glucan, an essential polysaccharide component of the cell wall of susceptible fungi (71). Inhibition leads to osmotic lysis of the cell and eventual cell death. Echinocandin drugs bind to FKSp, the major subunit of 1,3-β-D-glucan synthase, which is encoded by three FKS genes in *Candida* spp. (97). The echinocandins are fungicidal for *Candida* spp. but fungistatic for *Aspergillus* spp. (8, 139), where they block the growth of the apical tips of the hyphae (12).

Although rare at present, resistance to echinocandin drugs among clinical isolates has been associated with mutations in the *C. albicans FKS1* gene that lead to amino acid substitutions in the FKS1p subunit of 1,3-β-D-glucan synthase (36, 97, 101). These changes result in altered drug binding and confer cross-resistance to all echinocandin drugs. Mutations in the *FKS1* and *FKS2* genes are responsible for reduced susceptibility to caspofungin and micafungin in *C. glabrata* (45).

Spectrum of Activity

The echinocandins have a limited spectrum of activity. They are highly active against a broad range of *Candida* spp., including fluconazole-resistant strains (83, 84, 103, 104, 108, 139). However, *Candida parapsilosis*, *Candida lusitaniae*, and *Candida guilliermondii* appear to be less susceptible (84, 103, 104, 139). The echinocandins are also active against *Aspergillus* spp., including those that are intrinsically resistant to amphotericin B (35, 84, 87, 139).

The echinocandins are ineffective against fungi that lack a significant amount of 1,3-β-D-glucan in their cell wall, including *C. neoformans* and *Trichosporon* spp. as well as *Fusarium* spp. and the mucoraceous molds (1, 25, 35, 84, 87, 88, 139). Micafungin has been reported to be active against the mycelial forms of several dimorphic fungi, including *B. dermatitidis* and *H. capsulatum* but is ineffective against the tissue forms of these pathogens (86).

Acquired Resistance

Acquired resistance to echinocandins is rare at present, but resistant strains of several *Candida* spp. have been recovered from patients failing caspofungin treatment (20, 44, 65, 141), and a resistant strain of *C. albicans* was recovered from a patient failing micafungin treatment (73). These strains were cross-resistant to anidulafungin. Resistance has been associated with acquisition of mutations in the *FKS1* and/ or *FKS2* genes that led to amino acid substitutions within the FKS1p and FKS2p subunits of 1,3-β-D-glucan synthase (20, 44, 45, 65, 73, 141).

Pharmacokinetics

Concentrations of all three echinocandins in blood increase in proportion to dosage (37, 56, 58, 136). These drugs are extensively distributed to body tissues, but levels in the CSF are negligible. The predominant differences among these agents lie in their metabolism and half-life. Caspofungin and micafungin are metabolized by the liver and eliminated as inactive metabolites in the feces and urine (4, 24, 125, 137). Anidulafungin is not eliminated by hepatic metabolism but undergoes slow nonenzymatic degradation in the blood to an inactive open-ring peptide (27). Less than 1 to 3% of an echinocandin dose is excreted unchanged in the urine (24, 27, 37, 137). In adults, the half-life of caspofungin is about 9 to 10 h (136), while that of micafungin is 13 h (24) and that of anidulafungin is 18 to 27 h (27, 37). The three echinocandins have a shorter half-life in children (10, 127, 151).

Drug Interactions

The echinocandins do not interact with the human hepatic cytochrome P-450 system, and their use has been associated with very few significant drug interactions.

Therapeutic Drug Monitoring

At this time, there is no established relationship between efficacy or toxicity of the echinocandins and concentrations in serum (49). Routine monitoring of serum levels during treatment with these drugs is not required.

Toxicity and Adverse Effects

As a class, the echinocandins are well tolerated, and their use is associated with very few significant adverse effects (10, 24, 127, 146). The most common side effects are gastrointestinal in nature but occur in only around 5% of patients. Occasional cases of infusion-related pain and phlebitis have been noted with anidulafungin and micafungin, but these are less common than with caspofungin. Transient elevations of liver enzymes have been reported in a few patients.

Anidulafungin

Anidulafungin (Ecalta or Eraxis; Pfizer) was the first echinocandin to go into development and the most recent to be licensed for clinical use. It differs from caspofungin and micafungin in that it is insoluble in water. Anidulafungin is derived from a fermentation product of *Aspergillus nidulans* and is formulated for intravenous infusion.

Clinical Use

In the United States, anidulafungin is currently approved for the treatment of esophageal candidiasis, candidemia, and two invasive forms of candidiasis (abdominal abscesses and peritonitis). In the European Union, anidulafungin is approved for the treatment of invasive candidiasis in nonneutropenic patients. Anidulafungin has not been evaluated in sufficient numbers of neutropenic patients to determine its effectiveness in that group.

Caspofungin

Caspofungin (Cancidas; Merck) is a water-soluble lipopeptide, derived from a fermentation product of *Glarea lozoyensis*. It is formulated for intravenous infusion.

Clinical Use

In the United States, caspofungin is currently approved for the treatment of esophageal candidiasis, candidemia, and certain invasive forms of candidiasis, including abdominal abscesses, peritonitis, and pleural space infections. Caspofungin is also licensed for the salvage treatment of invasive aspergillosis in patients who have failed to respond to, or are intolerant of, other antifungal agents. Caspofungin is approved for the empiric treatment of presumed fungal infections in febrile neutropenic patients. It has simi-

lar indications in the European Union with a license for the treatment of invasive candidiasis in adult and pediatric patients, salvage treatment of aspergillosis, and empiric treatment of febrile neutropenia in adult or pediatric patients.

Micafungin

Micafungin (Mycamine; Astellas Pharma) is a water-soluble antifungal agent, derived from a fermentation product of *Coleophoma empetri*. It is formulated for intravenous administration.

Clinical Use

In the United States, micafungin is currently approved in adults for the treatment of esophageal candidiasis, candidemia, and several invasive forms of candidiasis, including abdominal abscesses and peritonitis. In the European Union, the drug is approved for the treatment of esophageal candidiasis in adults and for invasive candidiasis in adults and children, including neonates. In addition, micafungin is licensed as prophylactic treatment to prevent *Candida* infections in HSCT recipients in the United States and the European Union.

POLYENES

Around 100 polyene antibiotics have been described, but few have been developed for clinical use. Amphotericin B and its lipid formulations are used for the treatment of systemic fungal infections. Nystatin, natamycin, and mepartricin are topical polyene agents used in the treatment of oral, vaginal, and ocular fungal infections. A liposomal formulation of nystatin entered clinical trials, but its development has ceased. The polyenes are large molecules that consist of a closed macrolide lactone ring. One side of the ring is composed of a rigid lipophilic chain with a variable number of conjugated double bonds, and on the opposite side there are a similar number of hydroxyl groups. Thus, the molecule is amphipathic, and this feature of its structure is believed to be important in its mechanism of action.

Mechanism of Action

The polyenes bind to sterols, principally ergosterol, in the membranes of susceptible fungal cells causing impairment of membrane barrier function, leakage of cell constituents, metabolic disruption, and cell death (67). In addition to its membrane-permeabilizing effects, amphotericin B can cause oxidative damage to fungal cells through a cascade of oxidative reactions linked to lipoperoxidation of the cell membrane (133). More recently, however, an antioxidant effect of amphotericin B has been observed, and the relevance of pro-oxidant effects thus remains unclear (92).

Amphotericin B

Amphotericin B (Fungizone; Apothecon) is a fermentation product of *Streptomyces nodosus* available for intravenous infusion. The conventional micellar suspension formulation of this drug (amphotericin B deoxycholate) is often associated with serious toxic side effects, particularly renal damage. During the 1990s, three new lipid-associated formulations of amphotericin B were developed in an effort to alleviate the toxicity of the agent. These are liposomal amphotericin B (AmBisome; Astellas Pharma), in which the drug is encapsulated in phospholipid-containing liposomes; amphotericin B lipid complex (ABLC) (Abelcet; Enzon Pharmaceuticals), in which the drug is complexed with phospholipids to produce ribbon-like structures; and amphotericin B colloidal dispersion (ABCD) (Amphotec; Three Rivers Pharmaceuticals), in which the drug is packaged into small lipid disks containing cholesterol sulfate. These formulations possess the same broad spectrum of activity as the micellar suspension but are less nephrotoxic.

Spectrum of Activity

Amphotericin B is active against a broad spectrum of pathogenic fungi including most *Aspergillus* spp., *Candida* spp., *C. neoformans*, and the mucoraceous molds (1, 25, 30, 31, 35, 84, 111, 124). However, most isolates of *Aspergillus terreus* are resistant to amphotericin B (31, 35, 111, 138), as are isolates of *Aspergillus lentulus*, a new sibling species of *Aspergillus fumigatus* (3). *Candida krusei* also demonstrates reduced susceptibility to amphotericin B (106). Amphotericin B is effective against dimorphic fungi (*B. dermatitidis*, *Coccidioides* spp., *H. capsulatum*, and *P. brasiliensis)* and many dematiaceous fungi (63, 74, 124). Strains of *P. boydii*, *Fusarium* spp., and *Trichosporon* spp. are often intrinsically resistant to amphotericin B (46, 94, 95, 124).

Acquired Resistance

Acquired resistance is rare, but amphotericin-B-resistant strains of *C. albicans*, *C. glabrata*, *C. guilliermondii*, *C. lusitaniae*, *C. tropicalis*, and *C. neoformans* with alterations in the cell membrane, including reduced amounts of ergosterol, have been reported following prolonged treatment (134).

Pharmacokinetics

Amphotericin B is poorly absorbed after oral administration and must be administered as a slow intravenous infusion. The drug is widely distributed to many tissues, with the highest concentrations being found in the liver, spleen, and kidneys. Levels in the CSF are less than 5% of the simultaneous concentration in blood. Amphotericin B is mostly excreted as unchanged drug in the urine (21%) and feces (42%) (9). No metabolites have been identified. The drug is cleared very slowly, with the conventional deoxycholate formulation having a terminal half-life of around 127 h.

The pharmacokinetics of lipid-based formulations of amphotericin B are quite diverse. Maximal concentrations of the liposomal formulation in serum are much higher than those of the deoxycholate formulation, while levels of ABCD and ABLC are lower due to more rapid distribution of the drug to tissue (62). Administration of lipid-associated formulations of amphotericin B results in higher drug concentrations in the liver and spleen than are achieved with the conventional formulation (150). Renal concentrations of the drug are lower, and the nephrotoxic side effects are greatly reduced.

Clinical Use

Although other agents have subsequently been introduced, amphotericin B remains the treatment of choice for many serious fungal infections, including blastomycosis, coccidioidomycosis, histoplasmosis, sporotrichosis, and mucormycosis (18, 42, 66, 154). However, with the advent of voriconazole and the echinocandins, amphotericin B is no longer regarded as the drug of first choice for many cases of aspergillosis or candidiasis (96, 152). The three lipid-based formulations of amphotericin B are currently licensed for treatment of invasive fungal infections in patients who are refractory to, or intolerant of, conventional amphotericin B. In addition, liposomal amphotericin B is licensed for the treatment of cryptococcal meningitis in persons with AIDS, as well as for the empirical treatment of presumed fungal infection in febrile neutropenic patients. Clinical experience with these preparations has demonstrated that they are safer and no less active than the conventional formulation and, for some infections, they are more effective (93).

Drug Interactions

Amphotericin B can augment the nephrotoxicity of many other agents, including aminoglycoside antibiotics and cyclosporine (43).

Therapeutic Drug Monitoring

Concentrations of amphotericin B in serum and tissue show marked variation with formulation, especially among the lipid-based products, and there are few data relating either efficacy or toxicity to blood levels. Therefore, there is no need to monitor concentrations of amphotericin B in serum during therapy.

Toxicity and Adverse Effects

Amphotericin B deoxycholate causes infusion-related reactions, including hypotension, fever, rigors, and chills, in approximately 70% of patients (50). The major adverse effect of the drug is nephrotoxicity. This is dose related and may occur in more than 80% of patients receiving treatment (43). The lipid-associated formulations all lower the risk of amphotericin B-induced renal failure (157). However, infusion-related side effects, such as hypoxia and chills, are more common in patients treated with ABCD (155). In contrast, infusion-related reactions are uncommon in patients receiving liposomal amphotericin B or ABLC (7).

OTHER MISCELLANEOUS AGENTS

Flucytosine

Flucytosine (5-fluorocytosine; Ancobon; Valeant Pharmaceuticals) is a synthetic fluorinated analogue of cytosine and the only available antifungal agent acting as an antimetabolite. In the United States, flucytosine is available as oral tablets; elsewhere it is also available as an infusion for parenteral administration.

Mechanism of action

Flucytosine disrupts pyrimidine metabolism and thus the synthesis of DNA, RNA, and proteins within susceptible fungal cells (112). Flucytosine is transported into these cells by the enzyme cytosine permease and is there converted by cytosine deaminase to 5-fluorouracil (5-FU). Two mechanisms then account for the antifungal activity. The first involves the conversion of 5-FU into 5-fluorouridine triphosphate, which is incorporated into fungal RNA in place of uridylic acid, with resulting inhibition of protein synthesis. The second mechanism involves the conversion of 5-FU to 5-fluorodeoxyuridine monophosphate, which blocks the enzyme thymidylate synthetase, causing inhibition of fungal DNA synthesis. Fungi lacking cytosine deaminase are intrinsically resistant to flucytosine.

Spectrum of Activity

Flucytosine has a narrow spectrum of activity. It includes *Candida* spp., *C. neoformans*, and some dematiaceous fungi causing chromoblastomycosis (25, 84). Primary resistance to flucytosine is very uncommon among *Candida* spp., occurring in around 2 to 3% of isolates (84, 107).

Acquired Resistance

Monotherapy with flucytosine often leads to the induction of resistance among *Candida* spp. and *C. neoformans* (60).

Pharmacokinetics

Flucytosine is rapidly and almost completely absorbed after oral administration (26). The drug is widely distributed, with levels in most body tissues and fluids usually exceeding 50% of the simultaneous blood concentration (148). Flucytosine is primarily eliminated by renal excretion of unchanged drug. The serum half-life is between 3 and 6 h but may be greatly extended in renal failure, necessitating modification of the dosage regimen.

Clinical Use

Due to the risk of resistance, flucytosine is rarely administered as a single agent. It is most commonly used in combination with amphotericin B in the treatment of candidiasis and cryptococcosis (96, 100). Combination treatment with fluconazole has also been shown to be effective in AIDS-associated cryptococcal meningitis (100).

Drug Interactions

The antifungal activity of flucytosine is competitively inhibited by cytarabine (cytosine arabinoside), and the two drugs should not be administered together (148). Nephrotoxic drugs, such as amphotericin B, decrease the elimination of flucytosine, and concentrations of the latter in serum should be monitored when these agents are administered together. Flucytosine is myelosuppressive (see below) and should be used with caution in patients receiving other drugs, such as zidovudine, that could enhance its immunosuppressive side effects.

Therapeutic Drug Monitoring

Regular monitoring of drug concentrations of flucytosine in serum is advisable to reduce the risk of hepatotoxicity and hematological toxicity; this is essential when there is renal impairment. To avoid toxicity, a peak concentration of 100 μg/ml of flucytosine should not be exceeded (49). In contrast to toxicity, there are few data relating efficacy to blood levels for flucytosine. A reasonable goal is to maintain a trough concentration of >20 to 25 μg/ml (2, 49).

Toxicity and Adverse Effects

The most common, and least harmful, side effects of flucytosine are gastrointestinal and include nausea, diarrhea, vomiting, and abdominal pain. The most severe adverse effects include bone marrow depression and hepatotoxicity (148). These complications are more likely to occur if excessively high concentrations in blood are maintained.

Griseofulvin

Griseofulvin is an antifungal antibiotic derived from a number of *Penicillium* species, including *Penicillium griseofulvum*. Introduced in 1958, oral griseofulvin transformed the treatment of dermatophytosis.

Mechanism of Action

Griseofulvin is a fungistatic drug that binds to microtubular proteins and inhibits fungal cell mitosis (67).

Spectrum of Activity

The spectrum of useful activity is restricted to dermatophytes causing skin, nail, and hair infections (*Epidermophyton*, *Microsporum*, and *Trichophyton* spp.) (40, 99). Resistance has rarely been reported.

Pharmacokinetics

Absorption of griseofulvin from the gastrointestinal tract differs between individuals but is improved if the drug is given with a high-fat meal (90). Griseofulvin appears in the stratum corneum within a few hours of ingestion, as a result of secretion in perspiration (38, 130). However, levels begin to fall soon after the drug is discontinued, and within 48 to 72 h it can no longer be detected. Griseofulvin is metabolized by the liver to 6-desmethyl griseofulvin, which is excreted in the urine.

Clinical Use

Newer oral agents such as terbinafine or itraconazole are often preferred for nail infections, but griseofulvin remains a useful second-line agent for moderate to severe dermatophytoses of the skin and scalp hair, where topical treatment is considered inappropriate or has failed.

Drug Interactions

Absorption of griseofulvin is reduced in persons receiving concomitant treatment with barbiturates. Griseofulvin may decrease the effectiveness of oral anticoagulants, oral contraceptives, and cyclosporine.

Toxicity and Adverse Effects

In most cases, prolonged courses and high doses are well tolerated. Adverse effects occur in around 15% of patients and include headache, nausea, vomiting, abdominal discomfort, and rashes.

NOVEL ANTIFUNGAL AGENTS IN DEVELOPMENT

Two promising broad-spectrum triazole compounds, isavuconazole and albaconazole, were undergoing clinical trials at the time of writing (March 2010) (47, 98). Isavuconazole (Basilea Pharmaceutica and Astellas Pharma) is a water-soluble compound that can be administered orally or intravenously. The drug has predictable and dose-proportional pharmacokinetics and was in phase III clinical trials for the treatment of invasive candidiasis and candidemia, treatment of invasive aspergillosis, and treatment of rare mold infections. Albaconazole (Stiefel) is an oral agent that has demonstrated high levels of bioavailability and antifungal activity. It was evaluated in a phase I trial for tinea pedis and was at the time of writing in a phase II trial for the treatment of toenail onychomycosis.

CONCLUSION

The recent surge in development of new antifungal agents has greatly increased the number of drugs available to combat the growing number of serious fungal infections. There are now few life-threatening conditions for which there is no effective treatment, and there are many for which there are several therapeutic options. With judicious use of the available agents, antifungal drug resistance should continue to be a minor clinical problem. As more compounds have become licensed, the number of novel antifungal drugs entering preclinical development appears to have diminished. It remains to be seen which, if any, of these will reach the marketplace.

REFERENCES

1. **Almyroudis, N. G., D. A. Sutton, A. W. Fothergill, M. G. Rinaldi, and S. Kusne.** 2007. In vitro susceptibilities of 217 clinical isolates of zygomycetes to conventional and new antifungal agents. *Antimicrob. Agents Chemother.* **51:**2587–2590.
2. **Andes, D., A. Pascual, and O. Marchetti.** 2009. Antifungal therapeutic drug monitoring: established and emerging indications. *Antimicrob. Agents Chemother.* **53:**24–34.

3. Balajee, S. A., J. L. Gribskov, E. Hanley, D. Nickle, and K. A. Marr. 2005. *Aspergillus lentulus*, sp. nov., a new sibling species of *A. fumigatus*. *Eukaryot. Cell* **4:**625–632.

4. Balani, S. K., X. Xu, B. H. Arison, M. V. Silva, A. Gries, F. A. DeLuna, D. Cui, P. H. Kari, T. Ly, C. E. Hop, R. Singh, M. A. Wallace, D. C. Dean, J. H. Lin, P. G. Pearson, and T. A. Baillie. 2000. Metabolites of caspofungin acetate, a potent antifungal agent, in human plasma and urine. *Drug Metab. Dispos.* **28:**1274–1278.

5. Barchiesi, F., A. L. Colombo, D. A. McGough, A. W. Fothergill, and M. G. Rinaldi. 1994. In vitro activity of itraconazole against fluconazole-susceptible and -resistant *Candida albicans* isolates from oral cavities of patients infected with human immunodeficiency virus. *Antimicrob. Agents Chemother.* **38:**1530–1533.

6. Barone, J. A., B. L. Moskovitz, J. Guarnieri, A. E. Hassell, J. L. Colaizzi, R. H. Bierman, and L. Jessen. 1998. Enhanced bioavailability of itraconazole in hydroxypropyl-β-cyclodextrin solution versus capsules in healthy volunteers. *Antimicrob. Agents Chemother.* **42:**1862–1865.

7. Barrett, J. P., K. A. Vardulaki, C. Conlon, J. Cooke, P. Daza-Ramirez, E. G. Evans, P. M. Hawkey, R. Herbrecht, D. I. Marks, J. M. Moraleda, G. R. Park, S. J. Sen, and C. Viscoli. 2003. A systematic review of the antifungal effectiveness and tolerability of amphotericin B formulations. *Clin. Ther.* **25:**1295–1320.

8. Bartizal, K., C. J. Gill, G. K. Abruzzo, A. M. Flattery, L. Kong, P. M. Scott, J. G. Smith, C. E. Leighton, A. Bouffard, J. F. Dropinski, and J. Balkovec. 1997. In vitro preclinical evaluation studies with the echinocandin antifungal MK-0991 (L-743,872). *Antimicrob. Agents Chemother.* **41:**2326–2332.

9. Bekersky, I., R. N. Fielding, D. E. Dressler, J. W. Lee, D. N. Buell, and T. J. Walsh. 2002. Pharmacokinetics, excretion, and mass balance of liposomal amphotericin B (AmBisome) and amphotericin B deoxycholate in humans. *Antimicrob. Agents Chemother.* **46:**828–833.

10. Benjamin, D. K., T. Driscoll, N. L. Seibel, C. E. Gonzalez, M. M. Roden, R. Kilaru, K. Clark, J. A. Dowell, J. Schranz, and T. J. Walsh. 2006. Safety and pharmacokinetics of intravenous anidulafungin in children with neutropenia at high risk for invasive fungal infection. *Antimicrob. Agents Chemother.* **50:**632–638.

11. Borst, A., M. T. Raimer, D. W. Warnock, C. J. Morrison, and B. A. Arthington-Skaggs. 2005. Rapid acquisition of stable azole resistance by *Candida glabrata* isolates obtained before the clinical introduction of fluconazole. *Antimicrob. Agents Chemother.* **49:**783–787.

12. Bowman, J. C., P. S. Hicks, M. B. Kurtz, H. Rosen, D. M. Schmatz, P. A. Liberator, and C. M. Douglas. 2002. The antifungal echinocandin caspofungin acetate kills growing cells of *Aspergillus fumigatus* in vitro. *Antimicrob. Agents Chemother.* **46:**3001–3012.

13. Brammer, K. W., A. J. Coakley, S. G. Jezequel, and M. H. Tarbit. 1991. The disposition and metabolism of [14C] fluconazole in humans. *Drug Metab. Dispos.* **19:**764–767.

14. Brandt, M. E., M. A. Pfaller, R. A. Hajjeh, R. J. Hamill, P. G. Pappas, A. L. Reingold, D. Rimland, and D. W. Warnock. 2001. Trends in antifungal drug susceptibility of *Cryptococcus neoformans* isolates in the United States: 1992 to 1994 and 1996 to 1998. *Antimicrob. Agents Chemother.* **45:**3065–3069.

15. Brandt, M. E., and D. W. Warnock. 2003. Epidemiology, clinical manifestations, and therapy of infections caused by dematiaceous fungi. *J. Chemother.* **15**(Suppl. 2):36–47.

16. Caputo, R. 2003. Itraconazole (Sporanox) in superficial and systemic fungal infections. *Expert Rev. Anti-Infect. Ther.* **1:**531–542.

17. Cauwenbergh, G., H. Degreed, J. Heykants, R. Woestenborghs, P. Van Rooy, and K. Haeverans. 1988. Pharmacokinetic profile of orally administered itraconazole in human skin. *J. Am. Acad. Dermatol.* **18:**263–268.

18. Chapman, S. W., W. E. Dismukes, L. A. Proia, R. W. Bradsher, P. G. Pappas, M. G. Threlkeld, and C. A. Kauffman.

2008. Clinical practice guidelines for the management of blastomycosis: 2008 update by the Infectious Diseases Society of America. *Clin. Infect. Dis.* **46:**1801–1812.

19. Chapman, S. W., P. D. Rogers, M. G. Rinaldi, and D. C. Sullivan. 1998. Suceptibilities of clinical and laboratory isolates of *Blastomyces dermatitidis* to ketoconazole, itraconazole, and fluconazole. *Antimicrob. Agents Chemother.* **42:**978–980.

20. Cleary, J. D., G. Garcia-Effron, S. W. Chapman, and D. S. Perlin. 2008. Reduced *Candida glabrata* susceptibility secondary to an *FKS1* mutation developed during candidemia treatment. *Antimicrob. Agents Chemother.* **52:**2263–2265.

21. Courtney, R., S. Pai, M. Laughlin, J. Lim, and V. Batra. 2003. Pharmacokinetics, safety and tolerability of oral posaconazole administered in single and multiple doses in healthy adults. *Antimicrob. Agents Chemother.* **47:**2788–2795.

22. Courtney, R., E. Radwanski, J. Lim, and M. Laughlin. 2004. Pharmacokinetics of posaconazole coadministered with antacid in fasting or nonfasting healthy men. *Antimicrob. Agents Chemother.* **48:**804–808.

23. Craven, P. C., J. R. Graybill, J. H. Jorgensen, W. E. Dismukes, and B. E. Levine. 1983. High-dose ketoconazole for treatment of fungal infections of the central nervous system. *Ann. Intern. Med.* **98:**160–167.

24. Cross, S. A., and L. J. Scott. 2008. Micafungin: a review of its use in adults for the treatment of invasive and oesophageal candidiasis, and as prophylaxis against *Candida* infections. *Drugs* **68:**2225–2255.

25. Cuenca-Estrella, M., A. Gomez-Lopez, E. Mellado, M. J. Buitrago, A. Monzon, and J. L. Rodriguez-Tudela. 2006. Head-to-head comparison of the activities of currently available antifungal agents against 3,378 Spanish clinical isolates of yeasts and filamentous fungi. *Antimicrob. Agents Chemother.* **50:**917–921.

26. Cutler, R. E., A. D. Blair, and M. R. Kelly. 1978. Flucytosine kinetics in subjects with normal and impaired renal function. *Clin. Pharmacol. Ther.* **24:**333–342.

27. Damle, B. D., J. A. Dowell, R. L. Walsky, G. L. Weber, M. Stogniew, and P. B. Inskeep. 2009. In vitro and in vivo studies to characterize the clearance mechanism and potential cytochrome P450 interactions of anidulafungin. *Antimicrob. Agents Chemother.* **53:**1149–1156.

28. Daneshmend, T. K., D. W. Warnock, M. D. Ene, E. M. Johnson, G. Parker, M. D. Richardson, and C. J. Roberts. 1983. Multiple-dose pharmacokinetics of ketoconazole and their effects on antipyrine kinetics in man. *J. Antimicrob. Chemother.* **12:**185–188.

29. Daneshmend, T. K., D. W. Warnock, M. D. Ene, E. M. Johnson, M. R. Potten, M. D. Richardson, and P. J. Williamson. 1984. Influence of food on the pharmacokinetics of ketoconazole. *Antimicrob. Agents Chemother.* **25:**1–3.

30. Dannaoui, E., J. Meletiadis, J. W. Mouton, J. F. Meis, and P. E. Verweij. 2003. In vitro susceptibilities of zygomycetes to conventional and new antifungals. *J. Antimicrob. Chemother.* **51:**45–52.

31. Dannaoui, E., F. Persat, M. F. Monier, E. Borel, M. A. Piens, and S. Picot. 1999. In-vitro susceptibility of *Aspergillus* spp. isolates to amphotericin B and itraconazole. *J. Antimicrob. Chemother.* **44:**553–555.

32. Darkes, M. J., L. J. Scott, and K. L. Goa. 2003. Terbinafine: a review of its use in onychomycosis in adults. *Am. J. Clin. Dermatol.* **4:**39–65.

33. DeBeule, K., and J. Van Gestel. 2001. Pharmacology of itraconazole. *Drugs* **61**(Suppl. 1):27–37.

34. Debruyne, D., and J. P. Ryckelynck. 1993. Clinical pharmacokinetics of fluconazole. *Clin. Pharmacokinet.* **24:**10–27.

35. Diekema, D. J., S. A. Messer, R. J. Hollis, R. N. Jones, and M. A. Pfaller. 2003. Activities of caspofungin, itraconazole, posaconazole, ravuconazole, voriconazole, and amphotericin B against 448 recent clinical isolates of filamentous fungi. *J. Clin. Microbiol.* **41:**3623–3626.

36. Douglas, C. M., J. A. D'Ippolito, G. J. Shei, M. Meinz, J. Onishi, J. A. Marrinan, W. Li, G. K. Abruzzo, A. Flattery, K. Bartizal, A. Mitchell, and M. B. Kurtz. 1997.

Identification of the *FSK1* gene of *Candida albicans* as the essential target of 1,3-β-D-glucan synthase inhibitors. *Antimicrob. Agents Chemother.* **41**:2471–2479.

37. **Dowell, J. A., W. Knebel, T. Ludden, M. Stogniew, D. Krause, and T. Henkel.** 2004. Population pharmacokinetic analysis of anidulafungin, an echinocandin antifungal. *J. Clin. Pharmacol.* **44**:590–598.

38. **Epstein, W. L., V. P. Shah, and S. Riegelman.** 1972. Griseofulvin levels in stratum corneum: study after oral administration. *Arch. Dermatol.* **106**:344–348.

39. **Ezzet, F., D. Wexler, R. Courtney, G. Krishna, J. Lim, and M. Laughlin.** 2005. Oral bioavailability of posaconazole in fasted healthy subjects: comparison between three regimens and basis for clinical dosage recommendations. *Clin. Pharmacokinet.* **44**:211–220.

40. **Favre, B., B. Hofbauer, K. S. Hildering, and N. S. Ryder.** 2003. Comparison of in vitro activities of 17 antifungal drugs against a panel of 20 dermatophytes by using a microdilution assay. *J. Clin. Microbiol.* **41**:4817–4819.

41. **Fernandez-Torres, B., A. J. Carrillo, E. Martin, A. del Palacio, M. K. Moore, A. Valverde, M. Serrano, and J. Guarro.** 2001. In vitro activities of 10 antifungal drugs against 508 dermatophyte strains. *Antimicrob. Agents Chemother.* **45**:2524–2528.

42. **Galgiani, J. N., N. M. Ampel, J. E. Blair, A. Catanzaro, R. H. Johnson, D. A. Stevens, and P. L. Williams.** 2005. Coccidioidomycosis. *Clin. Infect. Dis.* **41**:1217–1223.

43. **Gallis, H. A., R. H. Drew, and W. W. Pickard.** 1990. Amphotericin B: 30 years of clinical experience. *Rev. Infect. Dis.* **12**:308–329.

44. **Garcia-Effron, G., D. P. Kontoyiannis, R. E. Lewis, and D. S. Perlin.** 2008. Caspofungin–resistant *Candida tropicalis* strains causing breakthrough fungemia in patients at high risk for hematologic malignancies. *Antimicrob. Agents Chemother.* **52**:4181–4183.

45. **Garcia-Effron, G., S. Lee, S. Park, J. D. Cleary, and D. S. Perlin.** 2009. Effect of *Candida glabrata FKS1* and *FKS2* mutations on echinocandin sensitivity and kinetics of 1,3-β-D-glucan synthase: implication for the existing susceptibility breakpoint. *Antimicrob. Agents Chemother.* **53**:3690–3699.

46. **Gilgado, F., C. Serena, J. Cano, J. Gene, and J. Guarro.** 2006. Antifungal susceptibilities of the species of the *Pseudallescheria boydii* complex. *Antimicrob. Agents Chemother.* **50**:4211–4213.

47. **Girmenia, C.** 2009. New generation azole antifungals in clinical investigation. *Expert Opin. Investig. Drugs* **18**:1279–1295.

48. **Gonzalez, G. M., A. W. Fothergill, D. A. Sutton, M. G. Rinaldi, and D. Loebenberg.** 2005. In vitro activities of new and established triazoles against opportunistic filamentous and dimorphic fungi. *Med. Mycol.* **43**:281–284.

49. **Goodwin, M. L., and R. H. Drew.** 2008. Antifungal serum concentration monitoring: an update. *J. Antimicrob. Chemother.* **61**:17–25.

50. **Goodwin, S. D., J. D. Cleary, C. A. Walawander, J. W. Taylor, and T. H. Grasela.** 1995. Pretreatment regimens for adverse events related to infusion of amphotericin B. *Clin. Infect. Dis.* **20**:755–761.

51. **Groll, A. H., L. Wood, M. Roden, D. Mickiene, C. C. Chiou, E. Townley, L. Dad, S. C. Piscitelli, and T. J. Walsh.** 2002. Safety, pharmacokinetics, and pharmacodynamics of cyclodextrin itraconazole in pediatric patients with oropharyngeal candidiasis. *Antimicrob. Agents Chemother.* **46**:2554–2563.

52. **Hahn, R. C., C. J. Fontes, R. D. Batista, and J. S. Hamdan.** 2002. In vitro comparison of activities of terbinafine and itraconazole against *Paracoccidioides brasiliensis*. *J. Clin. Microbiol.* **40**:2828–2831.

53. **Hall, M., C. Monka, P. Krupp, and D. O'Sullivan.** 1997. Safety of oral terbinafine: results of a postmarketing surveillance study in 25,884 patients. *Arch. Dermatol.* **133**:1213–1219.

54. **Haria, M., H. M. Bryson, and K. L. Goa.** 1996. Itraconazole: a reappraisal of its pharmacological properties and therapeutic use in the management of superficial fungal infections. *Drugs* **51**:585–620.

55. **Hariprasad, S. M., W. F. Mieler, E. R. Holz, H. Gao, J. E. Kim, J. Chi, and R. A. Prince.** 2004. Determination of vitreous, aqueous, and plasma concentration of orally administered voriconazole in humans. *Arch. Ophthalmol.* **122**:42–47.

56. **Hebert, M. F., H. E. Smith, T. C. Marbury, S. K. Swan, W. B. Smith, R. W. Townsend, D. Buell, J. Keirns, and I. Bekersky.** 2005. Pharmacokinetics of micafungin in healthy volunteers, volunteers with moderate liver disease, and volunteers with renal dysfunction. *J. Clin. Pharmacol.* **45**:1145–1152.

57. **Heykants, J., A. Van Peer, V. Van de Velde, P. Van Rooy, W. Meuldermans, K. Lavrijsen, R. Woestenborghs, J. Van Cutsem, and G. Cauwenbergh.** 1989. The clinical pharmacokinetics of itraconazole: an overview. *Mycoses* **32**(Suppl. 1):67–87.

58. **Hiemenz, J., P. Cagnoli, D. Simpson, S. Devine, N. Chao, J. Keirns, W. Lau, D. Facklam, and D. Buell.** 2005. Pharmacokinetics and maximum tolerated dose study of micafungin in combination with fluconazole versus fluconazole alone for prophylaxis of fungal infections in adult patients undergoing a bone marrow or peripheral stem cell transplant. *Antimicrob. Agents Chemother.* **49**:1331–1336.

59. **Hope, W. W., E. M. Billaud, J. Lestner, and D. W. Denning.** 2008. Therapeutic drug monitoring for triazoles. *Curr. Opin. Infect. Dis.* **21**:580–586.

60. **Hospenthal, D. R., and J. E. Bennett.** 1998. Flucytosine monotherapy for cryptococcosis. *Clin. Infect. Dis.* **27**:260–264.

61. **Hyland, R., B. C. Jones, and D. A. Smith.** 2003. Identification of the cytochrome P450 enzymes involved in the N-oxidation of voriconazole. *Drug Metab. Dispos.* **31**:540–547.

62. **Janknegt, R., S. De Marie, I. A. Bakker-Woudenberg, and D. J. Crommelin.** 1992. Liposomal and lipid formulations of amphotericin B: clinical pharmacokinetics. *Clin. Pharmacokinet.* **23**:279–291.

63. **Johnson, E. M., A. Szekely, and D. W. Warnock.** 1998. In-vitro activity of voriconazole, itraconazole and amphotericin B against filamentous fungi. *J. Antimicrob. Chemother.* **42**:741–745.

64. **Johnson, E. M., D. W. Warnock, J. Luker, S. R. Porter, and C. Scully.** 1995. Emergence of azole drug resistance in *Candida* species from HIV-infected patients receiving prolonged azole therapy for oral candidosis. *J. Antimicrob. Chemother.* **35**:103–114.

65. **Kahn, J. N., G. Garcia-Effron, M. J. Hsu, S. Park, K. A. Marr, and D. S. Perlin.** 2007. Acquired echinocandin resistance in a *Candida krusei* isolate due to modification of glucan synthase. *Antimicrob. Agents Chemother.* **51**:1876–1878.

66. **Kauffman, C. A., B. Bustamante, S. W. Chapman, and P. G. Pappas.** 2007. Clinical practice guidelines for the management of sporotrichosis: 2007 update by the Infectious Diseases Society of America. *Clin. Infect. Dis.* **45**:1255–1265.

67. **Kerridge, D.** 1986. Mode of action of clinically important antifungal drugs. *Adv. Microb. Physiol.* **27**:1–72.

68. **Kontoyiannis, D. P., M. S. Lionakis, R. E. Lewis, G. Chamilos, M. Healy, C. Perego, A. Safdar, H. Kantarjian, R. Champlin, T. J. Walsh, and I. I. Raad.** 2005. Zygomycosis in a tertiary-care cancer center in the era of *Aspergillus*-active antifungal therapy: a case-control observational study of 27 recent cases. *J. Infect. Dis.* **191**:1350–1360.

69. **Kovarik, J. M., E. G. Mueller, H. Zehender, J. Denouel, H. Caplain, and L. Millerioux.** 1995. Multiple-dose pharmacokinetics and distribution in tissue of terbinafine and metabolites. *Antimicrob. Agents Chemother.* **39**:2738–2741.

70. **Krieter, P., B. Flannery, T. Musick, M. Gohdes, M. Martinho, and R. Courtney.** 2004. Disposition of posaconazole following single-dose oral administration in healthy subjects. *Antimicrob. Agents Chemother.* **48**:3543–3551.

71. **Kurtz, M. B., and C. M. Douglas.** 1997. Lipopeptide inhibitors of fungal glucan synthase. *J. Med. Vet. Mycol.* **35**:79–86.

72. **Lake-Bakaar, G., P. J. Scheuer, and S. Sherlock.** 1987. Hepatic reactions associated with ketoconazole in the United Kingdom. *Br. Med. J.* **294**:419–422.

73. **Laverdiere, M., R. G. Lalonde, J. G. Baril, D. C. Sheppard, S. Park, and D. S. Perlin.** 2006. Progressive loss of echinocandin activity following prolonged use for treatment of *Candida albicans* oesophagitis. *J. Antimicrob. Chemother.* **57:**705–708.

74. **Li, R. K., M. A. Ciblak, N. Nordoff, L. Pasarell, D. W. Warnock, and M. R. McGinnis.** 2000. In vitro activities of voriconazole, itraconazole, and amphotericin B against *Blastomyces dermatitidis*, *Coccidioides immitis*, and *Histoplasma capsulatum*. *Antimicrob. Agents Chemother.* **44:**1734–1736.

75. **Lortholary, O., D. W. Denning, and B. Dupont.** 1999. Endemic mycoses: a treatment update. *J. Antimicrob. Chemother.* **43:**321–331.

76. **Lutsar, I., S. Roffey, and P. Troke.** 2003. Voriconazole concentrations in the cerebrospinal fluid and brain tissue of guinea pigs and immunocompromised patients. *Clin. Infect. Dis.* **37:**728–732.

77. **Manavathu, E. K., J. L. Cutwright, and P. H. Chandrasekar.** 1998. Organism-dependent fungicidal activities of azoles. *Antimicrob. Agents Chemother.* **42:**3018–3021.

78. **Martins, M. D., M. Lozano-Chiu, and J. H. Rex.** 1998. Declining rates of oropharyngeal candidiasis and carriage of *Candida albicans* associated with trends towards reduced rates of carriage of fluconazole-resistant C. *albicans* in human immunodeficiency virus-infected patients. *Clin. Infect. Dis.* **27:**1291–1294.

79. **McClellan, K. J., L. R. Wiseman, and A. Markham.** 1999. Terbinafine: an update of its use in superficial mycoses. *Drugs* **58:**179–202.

80. **McGinnis, M. R., N. G. Nordoff, N. S. Ryder, and G. B. Nunn.** 2000. In vitro comparison of terbinafine and itraconazole against *Penicillium marneffei*. *Antimicrob. Agents Chemother.* **44:**1407–1408.

81. **McGinnis, M. R., and L. Pasarell.** 1998. In vitro evaluation of terbinafine and itraconazole against dematiaceous fungi. *Med. Mycol.* **36:**243–246.

82. **Mellado, E., G. Garcia-Effron, L. Alcazar-Fuoli, W. J. Melchers, P. E. Verweij, M. Cuenca-Estrella, and J. L. Rodriguez-Tudela.** 2007. A new *Aspergillus fumigatus* resistance mechanism conferring in vitro cross-resistance to azole antifungals involves a combination of cyp51A alterations. *Antimicrob. Agents Chemother.* **51:**1897–1904.

83. **Messer, S. A., D. J. Diekema, L. Boyken, S. Tendolkar, R. J. Hollis, and M. A. Pfaller.** 2006. Activities of micafungin against 315 invasive clinical isolates of fluconazole-resistant *Candida* spp. *J. Clin. Microbiol.* **44:**324–326.

84. **Messer, S. A., G. J. Moet, J. T. Kirby, and R. N. Jones.** 2009. Activity of contemporary antifungal agents, including the novel echinocandin anidulafungin, tested against *Candida* spp., *Cryptococcus* spp., and *Aspergillus* spp.: report from the SENTRY antimicrobial surveillance program (2006 to 2007). *J. Clin. Microbiol.* **47:**1942–1946.

85. **Moore, C. B., C. M. Walls, and D. W. Denning.** 2001. In vitro activities of terbinafine against *Aspergillus* species in comparison with those of itraconazole and amphotericin B. *Antimicrob. Agents Chemother.* **45:**1882–1885.

86. **Nakai, T., J. Uno, F. Ikeda, S. Tawara, K. Nishimura, and M. Miyaji.** 2003. In vitro antifungal activity of micafungin (FK463) against dimorphic fungi: comparison of yeast-like and mycelia forms. *Antimicrob. Agents Chemother.* **47:**1376–1381.

87. **Nakai, T., J. Uno, K. Otomo, F. Ikeda, S. Tawara, T. Goto, K. Nishimura, and M. Miyaji.** 2002. In vitro activity of FK463, a novel lipopeptide antifungal agent, against a variety of clinically important molds. *Chemotherapy* **48:**78–81.

88. **Odabasi, Z., V. L. Paetznick, J. R. Rodriguez, E. Chen, and L. Ostrosky-Zeichner.** 2004. In vitro activity of anidulafungin against selected clinically important mold isolates. *Antimicrob. Agents Chemother.* **48:**1912–1915.

89. **Odds, F. C., and H. Vanden Bossche.** 2000. Antifungal activity of itraconazole compared with hydroxyl-itraconazole in vitro. *J. Antimicrob. Chemother.* **45:**371–373.

90. **Ogunbona, F. A., I. F. Smith, and O. S. Olawoye.** 1985. Fat contents of meals and bioavailability of griseofulvin in man. *J. Pharm. Pharmacol.* **37:**283–284.

91. **Orozco, A. S., L. M. Higginbotham, C. A. Hitchcock, T. Parkinson, D. Falconer, A. S. Ibrahim, M. A. Ghannoum, and S. G. Filler.** 1998. Mechanism of fluconazole resistance in *Candida krusei*. *Antimicrob. Agents Chemother.* **42:**2645–2649.

92. **Osaka, K., V. B. Ritov, J. F. Bernardo, R. A. Branch, and V. E. Kagan.** 1997. Amphotericin B protects cis-parinaric acid against perosyl radical-induced oxidation: amphotericin B as an antioxidant. *Antimicrob. Agents Chemother.* **41:**743–747.

93. **Ostrosky-Zeichner, L., K. A. Marr, J. H. Rex, and S. H. Cohen.** 2003. Amphotericin B: time for a new "gold standard." *Clin. Infect. Dis.* **37:**415–425.

94. **Paphitou, N. I., L. Ostrosky-Zeitner, V. L. Paetznick, J. R. Rodriguez, E. Chen, and J. H. Rex.** 2002. In vitro antifungal susceptibilities of *Trichosporon* species. *Antimicrob. Agents Chemother.* **46:**1144–1146.

95. **Paphitou, N. I., L. Ostrosky-Zeitner, V. L. Paetznick, J. R. Rodriguez, E. Chen, and J. H. Rex.** 2002. In vitro activities of investigational triazoles against *Fusarium* species: effects of inoculum size and incubation time on broth microdilution susceptibility test results. *Antimicrob. Agents Chemother.* **46:**3298–3300.

96. **Pappas, P. G., C. A. Kauffman, D. Andes, D. K. Benjamin, T. F. Calandra, J. E. Edwards, S. G. Filler, J. F. Fisher, B. J. Kullberg, L. Ostrosky-Zeichner, A. C. Reboli, J. H. Rex, T. J. Walsh, and J. D. Sobel.** 2009. Clinical practice guidelines for the management of candidiasis: 2009 update by the Infectious Diseases Society of America. *Clin. Infect. Dis.* **48:**503–535.

97. **Park, S., R. Kelly, J. N. Kahn, J. Robles, M. J. Hsu, E. Register, W. Li, V. Vyas, H. Fan, G. Abruzzo, A. Flattery, C. Gill, G. Chrebet, S. A. Parent, M. Kurtz, H. Teppler, C. M. Douglas, and D. S. Perlin.** 2005. Specific substitutions in the echinocandin target Fks1p account for reduced susceptibility of rare laboratory and clinical *Candida* sp. isolates. *Antimicrob. Agents Chemother.* **49:**3264–3273.

98. **Pasqualotto, A. C., K. O. Thiele, and L. Z. Goldani.** 2010. Novel triazole antifungal drugs: focus on isavuconazole, ravuconazole and albaconazole. *Curr. Opin. Investig. Drugs* **11:**165–174.

99. **Perea, S., A. W. Fothergill, D. A. Sutton, and M. G. Rinaldi.** 2001. Comparison of in vitro activities of voriconazole and five established antifungal agents against different species of dermatophytes using a broth macrodilution method. *J. Clin. Microbiol.* **39:**385–388.

100. **Perfect, J. R., W. E. Dismukes, F. Dromer, D. L. Goldman, J. R. Graybill, R. J. Hamill, T. S. Harrison, R. A. Larsen, O. Lortholary, M. H. Nguyen, P. G. Pappas, W. G. Powderly, N. Singh, J. D. Sobel, and T. C. Sorrell.** 2010. Clinical practice guidelines for the management of cryptococcal disease: 2010 update by the Infectious Diseases Society of America. *Clin. Infect. Dis.* **50:**291–322.

101. **Perlin, D. S.** 2007. Resistance to echinocandin-class antifungal drugs. *Drug Resist. Updat.* **10:**121–130.

102. **Pfaller, M. A., L. Boyken, R. J. Hollis, S. A. Messer, S. Tendolkar, and D. J. Diekema.** 2005. In vitro susceptibilities of clinical isolates of *Candida* species, *Cryptococcus neoformans*, and *Aspergillus* species to itraconazole: global survey of 9,359 isolates tested by Clinical and Laboratory Standards Institute broth microdilution methods. *J. Clin. Microbiol.* **43:**3807–3810.

103. **Pfaller, M. A., L. Boyken, R. J. Hollis, S. A. Messer, S. Tendolkar, and D. J. Diekema.** 2005. In vitro activities of anidulafungin against more than 2,500 clinical isolates of *Candida* spp., including 315 isolates resistant to fluconazole. *J. Clin. Microbiol.* **43:**5425–5427.

104. **Pfaller, M. A., L. Boyken, R. J. Hollis, S. A. Messer, S. Tendolkar, and D. J. Diekema.** 2006. In vitro susceptibilities of *Candida* spp. to caspofungin: four years of global surveillance. *J. Clin. Microbiol.* **44:**760–763.

105. **Pfaller, M. A., and D. J. Diekema.** 2004. Twelve years of fluconazole in clinical practice: global trends in species distribution and fluconazole susceptibility of bloodstream isolates of *Candida*. *Clin. Microbiol. Infect.* **10**(Suppl. 1):11–23.

106. **Pfaller M. A., S. A. Messer, and A. Bolmstrom.** 1998. Evaluation of Etest for determining in vitro susceptibility of yeast isolates to amphotericin B. *Diagn. Microbiol. Infect. Dis.* **32:**223–227.

107. **Pfaller, M. A., S. A. Messer, L. Boyken, H. Huynh, R. J. Hollis, and D. J. Diekema.** 2002. In vitro activities of 5-fluorocytosine against 8,803 clinical isolates of *Candida* spp.: global assessment of primary resistance using National Committee for Clinical Laboratory Standards susceptibility testing methods. *Antimicrob. Agents Chemother.* **46:**3518–3521.

108. **Pfaller, M. A., S. A. Messer, L. Boyken, C. Rice, S. Tendolkar, R. J. Hollis, and D. J. Diekema.** 2003. Caspofungin activity against clinical isolates of fluconazole-resistant *Candida*. *J. Clin. Microbiol.* **41:**5729–5731.

109. **Pfaller, M. A., S. A. Messer, L. Boyken, C. Rice, S. Tendolkar, R. J. Hollis, and D. J. Diekema.** 2008. In vitro survey of triazole cross-resistance among more than 700 clinical isolates of *Aspergillus* species. *J. Clin. Microbiol.* **46:**2568–2572.

110. **Pfaller, M. A., S. A. Messer, R. J. Hollis, and R. N. Jones.** 2001. In vitro activities of posaconazole (Sch 56592) compared with those of itraconazole and fluconazole against 3,685 clinical isolates of *Candida* spp. and *Cryptococcus neoformans*. *Antimicrob. Agents Chemother.* **45:**2862–2864.

111. **Pfaller, M. A., S. A. Messer, R. J. Hollis, and R. N. Jones.** 2002. Antifungal activities of posaconazole, ravuconazole, and voriconazole compared to those of itraconazole and amphotericin B against 239 clinical isolates of *Aspergillus* spp. and other filamentous fungi: report from SENTRY Antimicrobial Surveillance Program, 2000. *Antimicrob. Agents Chemother.* **46:**1032–1037.

112. **Polak, A., and H. J. Scholer.** 1975. Mode of action of 5-fluorocytosine and mechanisms of resistance. *Chemotherapy* **21:**113–130.

113. **Pont, A., J. R. Graybill, P. C. Craven, J. N. Galgiani, W. E. Dismukes, R. E. Reitz, and D. A. Stevens.** 1984. High-dose ketoconazole therapy and adrenal and testicular function in humans. *Arch. Intern. Med.* **144:**2150–2153.

114. **Purkins, L., N. Wood, K. Greenhalgh, M. J. Allen, and S. D. Oliver.** 2003. Voriconazole, a novel wide-spectrum triazole: oral pharmacokinetics and safety. *Br. J. Clin. Pharmacol.* **56**(Suppl. 1):10–16.

115. **Purkins, L., N. Wood, D. Kleinermans, K. Greenhalgh, and D. Nichols.** 2003. Effect of food on the pharmacokinetics of multiple-dose oral voriconazole. *Br. J. Clin. Pharmacol.* **56**(Suppl. 1):17–23.

116. **Raad, I. I., J. R. Graybill, A. B. Bustamante, O. A. Cornely, V. Gaona-Flores, C. Afif, D. R. Graham, R. N. Greenberg, S. Hadley, A. Langston, R. Negroni, J. R. Perfect, P. Pitisuttithum, A. Restrepo, G. Schiller, L. Pedicone, and A. J. Ullmann.** 2006. Safety of long-term oral posaconazole use in the treatment of refractory invasive fungal infections. *Clin. Infect. Dis.* **42:**1726–1734.

117. **Restrepo, A., A. Tobon, B. Clark, D. R. Graham, G. Corcoran, R. W. Bradsher, M. Goldman, G. Pankey, T. Moore, R. Negroni, and J. R. Graybill.** 2007. Salvage treatment of histoplasmosis with posaconazole. *J. Infect.* **54:**319–327.

118. **Revankar, S. G., M. D. Nailor, and J. D. Sobel.** 2008. Use of terbinafine in rare and refractory mycoses. *Future Microbiol.* **3:**9–17.

119. **Revankar, S. G., S. E. Sanche, O. P. Dib, M. Caceres, and T. F. Patterson.** 1998. Effect of highly active antiretroviral therapy on recurrent oropharyngeal candidiasis in HIV-infected patients. *AIDS* **12:**2511–2513.

120. **Rex, J. H., M. G. Rinaldi, and M. A. Pfaller.** 1995. Resistance of *Candida* species to fluconazole. *Antimicrob. Agents Chemother.* **39:**1–8.

121. **Roffey, S. J., S. Cole, P. Comby, D. Gibson, S. G. Jezequel, A. N. Nedderman, D. A. Smith, D. K. Walker, and N. Wood.** 2003. The disposition of voriconazole in mouse, rat, rabbit, guinea pig, dog, and human. *Drug Metab. Dispos.* **31:**731–741.

122. **Ryder, N. S.** 1991. Squalene epoxidase as a target for the allylamines. *Biochem. Soc. Trans.* **19:**774–777.

123. **Ryder, N. S., S. Wagner, and I. Leitner.** 1998. In vitro activities of terbinafine against cutaneous isolates of *Candida albicans* and other pathogenic yeasts. *Antimicrob. Agents Chemother.* **42:**1057–1061.

124. **Sabatelli, F., R. Patel, P. A. Mann, C. A. Mendrick, C. C. Norris, R. Hare, D. Loebenberg, T. A. Black, and P. M. McNicholas.** 2006. In vitro activities of posaconazole, fluconazole, itraconazole, voriconazole, and amphotericin B against a large collection of clinically important molds and yeasts. *Antimicrob. Agents Chemother.* **50:**2009–2015.

125. **Sandhu, P., W. Lee, X. Xu, B. F. Leake, M. Yamazaki, J. A. Stone, J. H. Lin, P. G. Pearson, and R. B. Kim.** 2005. Hepatic uptake of the novel antifungal agent caspofungin. *Drug Metab. Dispos.* **33:**676–682.

126. **Sanglard, D., and F. C. Odds.** 2002. Resistance of *Candida* species to antifungal agents: molecular mechanisms and clinical consequences. *Lancet Infect. Dis.* **2:**73–85.

127. **Seibel, N. L., C. Schwartz, A. Arrieta, P. Flynn, A. Shad, E. Albano, J. Keirns, W. M. Lau, D. P. Facklam, D. N. Buell, and T. J. Walsh.** 2005. Safety, tolerability, and pharmacokinetics of micafungin (FK463) in febrile neutropenic pediatric patients. *Antimicrob. Agents Chemother.* **49:**3317–3324.

128. **Shadomy, S., A. Espinel-Ingroff, and R. J. Gebhart.** 1985. In-vitro studies with SF 86-327, a new orally active allylamine derivative. *Sabouraudia* **23:**125–132.

129. **Shadomy, S., S. C. White, H. P. Yu, and W. E. Dismukes.** 1985. Treatment of systemic mycoses with ketoconazole: in vitro susceptibilities of clinical isolates of systemic and pathogenic fungi to ketoconazole. *J. Infect. Dis.* **152:**1249–1256.

130. **Shah, V. P., W. L. Epstein, and S. Riegelman.** 1974. Role of sweat in accumulation of orally administered griseofulvin in skin. *J. Clin. Investig.* **53:**1673–1678.

131. **Shikanai-Yasuda, M. A., G. Benard, Y. Higaki, G. M. Del Negro, S. Hoo, E. H. Vaccari, R. C. Gryschek, A. A. Segurado, A. A. Barone, and D. R. Andrade.** 2002. Randomized trial with itraconazole, ketoconazole and sulfadiazine in paracoccidioidomycosis. *Med. Mycol.* **40:**411–417.

132. **Smith, K. J., D. W. Warnock, C. T. Kennedy, E. M. Johnson, V. Hopwood, J. Van Cutsem, and H. Vanden Bossche.** 1986. Azole resistance in *Candida albicans*. *J. Med. Vet. Mycol.* **24:**133–144.

133. **Sokol-Anderson, M. L., J. Brajtburg, and G. Medoff.** 1986. Amphotericin B-induced oxidative damage and killing of *Candida albicans*. *J. Infect. Dis.* **154:**76–83.

134. **Sterling, T. R., and W. G. Merz.** 1998. Resistance to amphotericin B: emerging clinical and microbiological patterns. *Drug Resist. Updat.* **1:**161–165.

135. **Stevens, D. A., M. Diaz, R. Negroni, F. Montero-Gei, L. G. Castro, S. A. Sampaio, D. Borelli, A. Restrepo, L. Franco, J. L. Bran, E. G. Arathoon, et al.** 1997. Safety evaluation of chronic fluconazole therapy. *Chemotherapy* **43:**371–377.

136. **Stone, J. A., S. D. Holland, P. J. Wickersham, A. Sterrett, M. Schwartz, C. Bonfiglio, M. Hesney, G. A. Winchell, P. J. Deutsch, H. Greenberg, T. L. Hunt, and S. A. Waldman.** 2002. Single- and multiple-dose pharmacokinetics of caspofungin in healthy men. *Antimicrob. Agents Chemother.* **46:**739–745.

137. **Stone, J. A., X. Xu, G. A. Winchell, P. J. Deutsch, P. G. Pearson, E. M. Migoya, G. C. Mistry, L. Xi, A. Miller, P. Sandhu, R. Singh, F. deLuna, S. C. Dilzer, and K. C. Lasseter.** 2004. Disposition of caspofungin: role of distribution in determining pharmacokinetics in plasma. *Antimicrob. Agents Chemother.* **48:**815–823.

138. **Sutton, D. A., S. E. Sanche, S. G. Revankar, A. W. Fothergill, and M. G. Rinaldi.** 1999. In vitro amphotericin B resistance in clinical isolates of *Aspergillus terreus*, with a head-to-head comparison to voriconazole. *J. Clin. Microbiol.* **37:**2343–2345.

139. **Tawara, S., F. Ikeda, K. Maki, Y. Morishita, K. Otomo, N. Teratani, T. Goto, M. Tomashima, H. Ohki, A. Yamada, K. Kawabata, H. Takasugi, K. Sakane, H. Tanaka, F.**

Matsumoto, and S. Kuwahara. 2000. In vitro activities of a new lipopeptide antifungal agent, FK463, against a variety of clinically important fungi. *Antimicrob. Agents Chemother.* **44:**57–62.

140. **Theuretzbacher, U., F. Ihle, and H. Derendorf.** 2006. Pharmacokinetic/pharmacodynamic profile of voriconazole. *Clin. Pharmacokinet.* **45:**649–663.

141. **Thompson, G. R., N. P. Wiederhold, A. C. Vallor, N. C. Villareal, J. S. Lewis, and T. F. Patterson.** 2008. Development of caspofungin resistance following prolonged therapy for invasive candidiasis secondary to *Candida glabrata* infection. *Antimicrob. Agents Chemother.* **52:**3783–3785.

142. **Trilles, L., B. Fernandez-Torres, M. dos Santos Lazera, B. Wanke, A. de Oliveira Schubach, R. de Almeida Paes, I. Inza, and J. Guarro.** 2005. In vitro antifungal susceptibilities of *Sporothrix schenckii* in two growth phases. *Antimicrob. Agents Chemother.* **49:**3952–3954.

143. **Van Burik, J. A., R. S. Hare, H. P. Solomon, M. L. Corrado, and D. P. Kontoyiannis.** 2006. Posaconazole is effective as salvage therapy in zygomycosis: a retrospective summary of 91 cases. *Clin. Infect. Dis.* **42:**e61–e65.

144. **Vanden Bossche, H.** 1985. Biochemical targets for antifungal azole derivatives: hypothesis on the mode of action. *Curr. Top. Med. Mycol.* **1:**313–351.

145. **Vandewoude, K., D. Vogelaers, J. Decruyenaere, P. Jaqmin, K. De Beule, A. Van Peer, R. Woestenborghs, K. Groen, and F. Colardyn.** 1997. Concentrations in plasma and safety of 7 days of intravenous itraconazole followed by 2 weeks of oral itraconazole solution in patients in intensive care units. *Antimicrob. Agents Chemother.* **41:**2714–2718.

146. **Vazquez, J.** 2006. The safety of anidulafungin. *Expert Opin. Drug Saf.* **5:**751–758.

147. **Venkatakrishnan, K., L. L. von Moltke, and D. J. Greenblatt.** 2000. Effects of the antifungal agents on oxidative drug metabolism. *Clin. Pharmacokinet.* **38:**111–180.

148. **Vermes, A., H. J. Guchelaar, and J. Dankert.** 2000. Flucytosine: a review of its pharmacology, clinical indications, pharmacokinetics, toxicity and drug interactions. *J. Antimicrob. Chemother.* **46:**171–179.

149. **Vickers, A. E., J. R. Sinclair, M. Zollinger, F. Heitz, U. Glanzel, L. Johanson, and V. Fischer.** 1999. Multiple cytochrome P-450s involved in the metabolism of terbinafine suggest a limited potential for drug-drug interactions. *Drug Metab. Dispos.* **27:**1029–1038.

150. **Vogelsinger, H., S. Weller, A. Djanani, J. Kountchev, R. Bellmann-Weiler, C. J. Wiedermann, and R. Bellmann.** 2006. Amphotericin B tissue distribution in autopsy material after treatment with liposomal amphotericin B and amphotericin B colloidal dispersion. *J. Antimicrob. Chemother.* **57:**1153–1160.

151. **Walsh, T. J., P. C. Adamson, N. L. Seibel, P. M. Flynn, M. N. Neely, C. Schwartz, A. Shad, S. L. Kaplan, M. M. Roden, J. A. Stone, A. Miller, S. K. Bradshaw, S. X. Li, C. A. Sable, and N. A. Kartsonis.** 2005. Pharmacokinetics, safety, and tolerability of caspofungin in children and adolescents. *Antimicrob. Agents Chemother.* **49:**4536–4545.

152. **Walsh, T. J., E. J. Anaissie, D. W. Denning, R. Herbrecht, D. K. Kontoyiannis, K. A. Marr, V. A. Morrison, B. H. Segal, W. J. Steinbach, D. A. Stevens, J. A. van Burik, J. R. Wingard, and T. F. Patterson.** 2008. Treatment of aspergillosis: clinical practice guidelines of the Infectious Diseases Society of America. *Clin. Infect. Dis.* **46:**327–360.

153. **Walsh, T. J., M. O. Karlsson, T. Driscoll, A. G. Arguedas, P. Adamson, X. Saez-Llorens, A. J. Vora, A. C. Arrieta, J. Blumer, I. Lutsar, P. Milligan, and N. Wood.** 2004. Pharmacokinetics and safety of intravenous voriconazole in children after single- or multiple-dose administration. *Antimicrob. Agents Chemother.* **48:**2166–2172.

154. **Wheat, L. J., A. G. Freifeld, M. B. Kleiman, J. W. Baddley, D. S. McKinsey, J. E. Loyd, and C. A. Kauffman.** 2007. Clinical practice guidelines for the management of patients with histoplasmosis: 2007 update by the Infectious Diseases Society of America. *Clin. Infect. Dis.* **45:**807–825.

155. **White, M. H., R. A. Bowden, E. S. Sandler, M. L. Graham, G. A. Noskin, J. R. Wingard, M. Goldman, J. A. Van Burik, A. McCabe, J. S. Lin, M. Gurwith, and C. B. Miller.** 1998. Randomized, double-blind clinical trial of amphotericin B colloidal dispersion vs. amphotericin B in the empirical treatment of fever and neutropenia. *Clin. Infect. Dis.* **27:**296–302.

156. **Willemsen, M., P. De Doncker, J. Willems, R. Woestenborghs, V. Van de Velde, J. Heykants, J. Van Cutsem, G. Cauwenbergh, and D. Roseeuw.** 1992. Post-treatment itraconazole levels in the nail: new implications for treatment in onychomycosis. *J. Am. Acad. Dermatol.* **26:**731–735.

157. **Wong-Beringer, A., R. A. Jacobs, and B. J. Guglielmo.** 1998. Lipid formulations of amphotericin B: clinical efficacy and toxicities. *Clin. Infect. Dis.* **27:**603–618.

Mechanisms of Resistance to Antifungal Agents

THEODORE C. WHITE AND SAMANTHA J. HOOT

127

The significant rise in incidence of fungal infections during the last 20 years is the result of several factors usually associated with immune dysfunction. The number of patients with immune dysfunction has grown dramatically because of the AIDS epidemic, increased bone marrow transplants (BMTs) and solid organ transplants, and aggressive cancer chemotherapy. Hospital-acquired fungal infections are also emerging as significant problems. With the increase in fungal infections, there has been a dramatic rise in the use of antifungals for the treatment of both systemic and localized fungal infections. The currently available antifungal agents and new drugs under development are summarized in chapter 126. It is not surprising that the expanded use of antifungal drugs has accelerated the development of resistance to these compounds. This chapter is an updated version of the chapter in the previous edition of this *Manual* (39). Detailed reviews of the background of antifungal drug resistance have been presented previously (20, 32, 40, 41) and should be consulted for background. Primary references published before 2006 can be found in these reviews.

Classes of antifungal drugs include polyenes, azoles, allylamines, flucytosine, and echinocandins. The mechanisms of action for these antifungal drugs are summarized in chapter 126. The azoles, such as fluconazole, and the allylamines, such as terbinafine, target ergosterol biosynthesis and are termed ergosterol biosynthesis inhibitors. Ergosterol is the major sterol in fungal plasma membrane, similar to cholesterol in mammalian cells. The polyenes, such as amphotericin B, bind to ergosterol in the plasma membrane. Flucytosine (5-fluorocytosine) inhibits pyrimidine metabolism and DNA synthesis. The echinocandins, including caspofungin, anidulafungin, and micafungin, target glucan synthetase in the plasma membrane and inhibit cell wall synthesis and stability.

CLINICAL COMPONENTS OF ANTIFUNGAL DRUG RESISTANCE

Clinically, infections that are recalcitrant to treatment with these classes of antifungal drugs are considered resistant. A recalcitrant infection can be the result of a variety of factors associated with the host, the drug, and the fungus (summarized in Table 1).

Host Factors

The single factor that is most important in the resolution of a fungal infection is the immune status of the host. The antifungal drugs and the host immune system work together in controlling the infection. Infections in patients with nonfunctional immune systems are more recalcitrant to treatment, as the drug must combat the infection without the additive effect of the immune system. The site of the infection (systemic or localized to skin, oral mucosa, vaginal mucosa, eye, brain, etc.) contributes to clinical resistance, since the site may be protected or inaccessible to drug therapy. Thus, early diagnosis, when fungal levels are low, is key to effective therapies. The presence of foreign objects, such as catheters, artificial heart valves, and other surgical devices, can also contribute to a recalcitrant infection, as the fungus can attach to and invade these objects, creating a source of constant inoculation and protection from drug therapy. Finally, the patient's adherence to prescribed therapy regimens is extremely important for effective treatment. Poor adherence to a drug regimen reduces the effectiveness of the drug and fails to resolve the infection. Poor adherence also contributes substantially to the development of antifungal drug resistance, as intermittent or low-dose therapies commonly allow organisms that are incrementally more resistant to persist and become the dominant strain.

Drug Characteristics

The characteristics of the antifungal drug are also factors in the treatment of a recalcitrant infection. Fungistatic drugs, such as the azoles, do not kill the cells and are thus more likely to allow cells to develop resistance than fungicidal drugs, such as amphotericin B or the echinocandins. As discussed above, the dosing of the antifungal drug, including the quantity, frequency, schedule, and cumulative dose, can also contribute to resolution of a fungal infection. The absorption, distribution, and metabolism of the drug within the host also contribute to the overall efficacy at the site of infection. Finally, other drug therapies administered to the patient can alter the efficacy of antifungal drugs.

Fungal Factors

Several factors of the fungus affect the treatment of the infection. First and foremost, the species and strain will clearly determine which drugs are effective. Secondly, the cell type can alter drug efficacy. Fungi exist in a variety of cell types or

TABLE 1 Factors that contribute to clinical antifungal drug resistance

Host factors	Drug factors	Fungal factors
Immune status	Fungistatic nature of drug	Species and strain
Site of infection	Dosing	Cell type
Severity of infection	Frequency	Morphology
Presence of foreign materials	Quantity	Cell states
Poor adherence to drug regimen	Cumulative dose	Serotypes
	Pharmacokinetics	Biofilms
	Absorption	Genomic stability of strain
	Distribution	Size of population
	Metabolism	Population "bottlenecks"
	Drug-drug interactions	Strain MIC

morphologies, including yeasts (blastospores), hyphae, chlamydospores, conidia, and mycelia, each of which can have a specific susceptibility to antifungal drugs. For example, *Candida albicans* exists in yeast and hyphal forms; azole drugs interfere with hyphal production at subinhibitory concentrations of the drug in susceptible strains. However, resistant strains form hyphae in the presence of high concentrations of azole drugs. In addition to morphology, several fungi including *C. albicans* exist in different switch phenotypes or cell states. These cell states vary in susceptibility to antifungal drugs. An important cell state that has received considerable attention in recent years is fungal biofilms, in which cells grow as a plaque or mat on a surface. Fungal biofilms are known to have altered antifungal susceptibilities. Recent evidence suggests that the extracellular matrix material in the biofilm can act as a sponge and absorb antifungal drugs, so that the cell surface is not exposed to high drug concentrations (22).

The genome stability of the fungus can also affect antifungal susceptibility. The best example is the development of resistance in *Candida* with different ploidy (copies of the genome). The development of resistance is a common occurrence in haploid *Candida glabrata* but infrequent in diploid *C. albicans*, where mutations in both copies may be needed to have an effect.

The severity of the infection can also contribute to clinical resistance, as higher concentrations of fungal cells will require higher concentrations of drug and/or longer treatments. The population size can also have an effect on resistance. Large numbers of organisms in a severe infection can increase the chance of a random mutation in the population, which could result in a resistant fungal cell in the infection. In large populations, population bottlenecks may dramatically alter the susceptibility pattern of the cells in an infection. For example, an infected catheter is removed and replaced with a new catheter in a patient with a systemic infection who is receiving antifungal drugs. The remaining fungal cells in the bloodstream could colonize the new catheter, and those cells may be more resistant due to exposure to antifungal drugs. Such a shift in the population structure is known as a population bottleneck, and it can clearly have effects on the development of resistance.

The final fungal factor that has an effect on a recalcitrant infection is the level of susceptibility of the fungal isolate to antifungal drugs, usually measured as the MIC using standardized Clinical and Laboratory Standards Institute (CLSI) protocols as described in chapter 128. CLSI protocols include M27–A3, which employs broth dilutions for yeasts; M38–A2, which employs broth dilutions for filamentous fungi, such as *Aspergillus*; and M44–A, which employs disk diffusion for yeasts. Other protocols with comparable results include

the European Committee on Antimicrobial Susceptibility Testing (EUCAST) methodology and commercially available test systems such as Etest, Sensititre, and VITEK 2. The specifics of the susceptibility testing protocols and other factors associated with the standardized methods are discussed in chapter 128. The standardized CLSI methodology has been used to demonstrate the existence of true, clinically relevant fungal resistance and the extent of the resistance in various patient populations.

COMPLICATIONS OF SUSCEPTIBILITY TESTING

Clinical Breakpoints

The CLSI and EUCAST protocols determine levels of susceptibility in vitro. These MICs can then be used to predict resistance in vivo by defining clinical breakpoints, the MIC values above which a strain is clinically resistant to drug treatment (Table 2). For both itraconazole and fluconazole, the CLSI M27-A3 protocol defines MICs for *C. albicans* that predict treatment outcomes and can guide patient treatment (31). While breakpoints for other azoles have not been determined for *C. albicans*, it is likely that those breakpoints are similar to the 1.0-μg/ml breakpoint used for itraconazole (Table 2), as the MIC values for clinical isolates to most azoles have the same relative distributions (29). Clinical breakpoints for the echinocandins have also been suggested (28) (Table 2).

The difference between MIC and clinical breakpoints has created some confusion. A clinical breakpoint is defined as the MIC at which a strain behaves as a resistant strain. The clinical breakpoint must be set for every drug and fungal species. The problem with clinical interpretations is that strains with MICs to itraconazole or other azoles above 1.0 μg/ml are frequently and incorrectly regarded as susceptible, since their MIC is below the 64-μg/ml value that is the clinical breakpoint for the more common azole fluconazole. It is important to remember that MICs are numbers determined in vitro, and clinical significance can be determined only by using clinical breakpoints to correctly interpret these numerical results. In addition, it is vitally important that antifungal pharmacokinetics and pharmacodynamics be taken into account when dealing with clinical resistance.

Some studies have correlated the distribution of in vitro MICs for wild-type clinical isolates with the treatment outcome to determine breakpoints for prediction of clinical outcome. This type of work was recently addressed for *Aspergillus fumigatus* with three triazoles, and wild-type

TABLE 2 Clinical breakpoints for *Candida albicans*[a]

Drug	Clinical breakpoint (μg/ml) for strains that are:			
	Susceptible	Susceptible dose dependent or intermediate	Resistant	Reference
Fluconazole	≤8.0	16–32	≥64	31
Itraconazole	≤0.125	0.25–0.5	≥1.0	31
Voriconazole	≤1.0	2	≥4.0	29
Echinocandins[b]	≤2.0		≥4.0	28
Flucytosine	≤4.0	8.0–16	≥32	31

[a]For a more complete list of clinical breakpoints in other species, refer to chapter 128.
[b]Includes caspofungin, anidulafungin, and micafungin.

distributions and data on clinical outcome were used to assign epidemiological cutoff values or breakpoints for *A. fumigatus* (27).

The 90–60 Rule

A very important consideration for MIC interpretation is the 90–60 rule (30). Essentially, this rule states that infections respond to therapy about 90% of the time if the infectious agent is judged to be susceptible in vitro, while infections respond to therapy about 60% of the time if the infectious agent is judged to be resistant in vitro, even with the correct interpretation of clinical breakpoints. This rule appears to be applicable to most, if not all, microbial infections: fungal, bacterial, and parasitic infections. It implies that patients with susceptible strains will respond 90% of the time, and patients with a fluconazole-resistant strain of *C. albicans* will respond to fluconazole 60% of the time. The most likely reasons for successful treatment of a resistant strain, or failure to treat a susceptible strain, are found in Table 1. The 90–60 rule is important when drug therapies are compared. Case reports or studies of salvage therapy do not necessarily imply that one drug is effective against a strain that is resistant to another drug; the successful treatment may be part of the 60% success rate that is true even for drugs to which the strain is resistant in vitro.

The factors that contribute to a recalcitrant or resistant clinical infection have been described above and are summarized in Table 1. The rest of this chapter focuses on the resistance of fungal isolates, as determined by their MIC.

INTRINSIC AND ACQUIRED RESISTANCE

There are two types of resistance: intrinsic resistance, which is an inherited characteristic of a species or strain, and acquired resistance, which occurs when a previously susceptible isolate develops a resistant phenotype, usually as a result of prolonged treatment with antifungals. The ideal antifungal drug would be effective against all fungi, both yeasts and molds. However, with each of the current antifungal drugs, there are genera and species that are intrinsically resistant. Fungal genera and species that are intrinsically resistant to antifungal drugs are summarized in chapter 126. In certain genera, some species are susceptible and other species are resistant to specific antifungals. These unique species are briefly discussed below.

Intrinsic Azole Resistance

Candida krusei is intrinsically resistant to azoles. In addition, many strains of *C. glabrata* are intrinsically resistant or susceptible dose-dependent. Other strains can quickly acquire resistance during therapy. *C. krusei* and *C. glabrata*

are increasing in frequency in oral and systemic candidiasis in patient populations that use azole drugs for treatment or prophylaxis (26). In addition, the frequency of vaginitis caused by these azole-resistant *Candida* species is increasing, although these strains continue to respond to azole therapy for vaginitis.

Intrinsic Amphotericin B and Flucytosine Resistance

Resistance to amphotericin B has been seen with the yeasts *C. krusei* and *Candida lusitaniae* and the molds *Aspergillus terreus* and *Scedosporium* spp. These fungal infections are not common, and there is no indication that the frequency of these species has increased in patient populations exposed to long-term treatment with or large doses of amphotericin B. Intrinsic or, more commonly, acquired resistance to flucytosine is relatively frequent in many fungi, and flucytosine monotherapy is rarely used to treat fungal infections.

Acquired Azole Resistance

Acquired azole resistance was rare in the 1980s, when long-term azole therapy was used primarily to treat patients with chronic mucocutaneous candidiasis; some isolates of *C. albicans* became resistant following prolonged treatment. However, in the 1990s azole resistance became a significant problem in *C. albicans* isolates from AIDS patients. Oral candidiasis was a common opportunistic infection in human immunodeficiency virus (HIV)-infected patients, occurring in over 90% of all patients with low CD4 counts. Azole drugs were commonly prescribed at relatively low doses for long-term suppressive therapy that was administered intermittently. Not surprisingly, azole resistance in oral candidiasis became a significant problem. Resistant strains of *C. albicans* were found in 20 to 33% of symptomatic oral candidiasis patients with HIV and up to 14% of asymptomatic patients with HIV. In recent years, most HIV-infected patients in developed countries have received highly active antiretroviral therapy, which reduces the frequency of most opportunistic infections, including oral candidiasis; this reduces the need for azole prophylaxis and reduces issues of azole resistance. At this time, the frequency of antifungal resistance in strains from patients receiving highly active antiretroviral therapy is not known. Children with HIV infection are particularly susceptible to oral candidiasis, and many receive substantial clotrimazole prophylaxis. A survey demonstrated that up to 10% of oral isolates from these children are resistant to clotrimazole and cross resistant to other azoles and require amphotericin B for treatment. Unlike oral isolates, vaginal isolates of *C. albicans* do not increase their resistance to azoles, even after long-term exposure. In addition to *C. albicans*, *Candida dubliniensis* is a recently described closely related species that is very difficult to distinguish from C. *albicans* but which also has the ability to develop resistance to azole drugs.

Acquired resistance has best been described in several matched sets of azole-susceptible and azole-resistant isolates from the same strain of C. *albicans*, usually obtained from oral candidiasis in AIDS patients or systemic infections in BMT patients. Azole resistance in a patient can be the result of (i) a commensal strain that was already intrinsically resistant, (ii) a commensal strain that developed resistance during therapy, or (iii) a resistant strain that was acquired from another individual by nosocomial transmission or intimate contact.

In addition to *Candida*, acquired resistance to azoles has also developed in isolates of *Cryptococcus neoformans* from AIDS patients who have been on maintenance azole therapy to prevent recurrence of cryptococcal meningitis and in isolates of A. *fumigatus* from patients who have received repeated treatment with itraconazole or voriconazole. Resistance mechanisms in these fungi are similar to mechanisms seen in *Candida* species and include efflux pump overexpression and alteration of the azole target enzyme.

Azoles are commonly used in surgical wards to prevent systemic candidiasis; as nonprescription drugs to treat fungal infections of the skin, including athlete's foot; and in agriculture. Epidemiological studies of azole resistance in these settings are not extensive, although some data suggest a link between agricultural azole use and resistance in A. *fumigatus*. The use of azoles as fungal pesticides in Europe is thought to have led to the emergence of resistance-conferring *cyp51A* mutations (37). In A. *fumigatus*, a specific G138C *cyp51* mutation was identified, and cross-resistance to multiple azoles was demonstrated (15).

Acquired Polyene Resistance

Acquired resistance to fungicidal amphotericin B is rare; it occurs mostly in yeasts from cancer patients who have received repeated doses of the drug to treat recalcitrant or recurring systemic fungal infections. The MICs of amphotericin B for yeasts from cancer patients are higher than the MICs of colonizing isolates from controls. Case reports about acquired resistance to amphotericin B may be increasing. Intrinsic amphotericin B resistance in C. *lusitaniae* may be related to cell switching between two cell states.

Change to a More Resistant Species or Strain

Clear differences have been documented in the patterns of antifungal resistance of different species, and between strains within a species, due to randomly occurring genetic differences. These small differences in strain susceptibility result in a distribution of MICs for strains within a species. Intrinsically resistant species and strains may be present in individuals by chance as commensal colonizers. If infection or disease develops, the infectious agent will already be resistant to treatment with antifungal therapy.

Resistant species and strains may also be acquired by nosocomial transmission or intimate contact. The frequency with which fungal strains move from person to person has been investigated to some extent with C. *albicans*, where replacement rates are usually under 50%, although the sensitivity of the techniques used to differentiate strains can have a significant impact on determining if strains are indistinguishable, similar, or unrelated. Transmission of a resistant strain either orally or sexually between patients has been documented.

MOLECULAR MECHANISMS OF AZOLE DRUG RESISTANCE

Molecular analyses of antifungal drug resistance have focused on C. *albicans*, but studies have been done on C. *glabrata* and C. *krusei*, as well as C. *neoformans* and A. *fumigatus*. This section concentrates on the mechanisms identified in C. *albicans*, with discussion of mechanisms identified in other fungi when applicable.

Matched Sets

The molecular analysis of antifungal drug resistance in C. *albicans* is complicated by the clonal nature of this diploid yeast. C. *albicans* grows vegetatively with limited sexual reproduction. However, C. *albicans* does have mating loci similar to *Saccharomyces cerevisiae*, and "mating" of two diploid cells into a tetraploid cell can be detected under controlled circumstances. Still, mating in C. *albicans* is limited, and most strains have diverged by acquiring mutations asexually, resulting in strains with considerable differences in their genomes. Genetic or expression differences identified between unmatched susceptible and resistant isolates could be the cause(s) of resistance or could simply be the result of strain divergence. Thus, it is important to determine the relatedness of a susceptible isolate and resistant isolate before comparing them by molecular analyses.

Strain differences can be detected by several molecular techniques, including restriction fragment length polymorphisms, chromosome karyotyping, and random amplification of polymorphic DNA. Perhaps the most appropriate method for strain typing is multilocus sequence typing, which has been used to sort C. *albicans* into 17 distinct clades and to detect even minor strain differences between clinical isolates (23). Given the genetic diversity and clonal nature of clinical isolates from many fungal species, including C. *albicans* and C. *neoformans*, it is important to compare matched sets of susceptible and resistant isolates when determining the molecular mechanisms of resistance.

Alterations in Ergosterol Biosynthesis

The target enzyme of the azole antifungals is lanosterol demethylase, the product of the *ERG11* gene (Erg11p) and part of the biosynthetic pathway leading to ergosterol. A defective Erg11p does not remove methyl groups at the 14α carbon of ergosterol precursors, resulting in an accumulation of 14α-methyl sterols, including a diol, 14α-methyl-ergosta-8,24(28)-dien-3β,6α-diol. The 14α-methyl sterols alter the fluidity and function of the fungal plasma membrane, and the resulting cells are more susceptible to oxygen-dependent microbicidal systems of the host. The diol also accumulates in these cells. This diol is fungicidal in S. *cerevisiae*, though its effect in C. *albicans* is not clear. Frequently, fungal cells escape the effects of 14α-methyl sterols and the diol with a mutation in the sterol desaturase, the product of the *ERG3* gene.

Alterations in *ERG11*

Several alterations in *ERG11* have been associated with resistance in C. *albicans*, including (i) point mutations in the coding regions, (ii) overexpression of the gene, (iii) gene amplification (which leads to overexpression), and (iv) gene conversion or mitotic recombination.

There are point mutations within the coding region of *ERG11* that are present in a resistant isolate and which are not present in the susceptible isolate of the same strain. *ERG11* mutations include 29 catalogued amino acid substitutions occurring a total of 98 times in 53 sequences. The 29 substitutions are distributed throughout the sequence and cluster in three regions of the gene, suggesting three hot spots of mutation. These mutations are predicted to result in proteins in which the substitution interferes with several protein regions, including the active site, the channel leading to the active site, and the flexible helix that interacts with and covers the channel. Of these 29 substitutions, six mutations—Y132H, D278E, S405F, F449L, G464S, and R467K (letters represent amino acids; the wild-type amino acid precedes the numerical position in the protein sequence, and the mutant amino acid follows)—have been experimentally linked to resistance either directly in *C. albicans* or by heterologous expression in *S. cerevisiae*.

Point mutations in *ERG11* have also been reported in other fungi, including *C. neoformans* and *A. fumigatus* (8). In *Aspergillus* species, the most common *cyp51A* (*ERG11*) mutations are G54W, L98H, and multiple different substitutions at M220. The point mutation L98H is always seen in combination with duplication of a portion of promoter sequence leading to overexpression of the mutated *cyp51A* (36). Similar to the situation with *C. albicans*, it is thought that *cyp51A* mutations in *A. fumigatus* are often found in combination with alteration of efflux pumps. Similarly, *C. neoformans* can develop azole resistance due to mutations in *ERG11*, most commonly a mutation that results in a G484S amino acid substitution (7).

Overexpression of *ERG11* contributes to resistance, as increased amounts of protein require increased amounts of drug. *ERG11* overexpression has been identified in several clinical isolates, although the level of overexpression has usually been less than fivefold. The effect of overexpression alone has not been determined, as these clinical isolates usually have additional alterations, such as point mutations within the *ERG11* gene.

Overexpression can be the result of localized gene amplification. In *C. albicans*, gene amplification has been shown to occur by the creation of an isochromosome of the left arm of chromosome 5, which includes the *ERG11* gene, as well as the *MTL* mating locus and *TAC1*, a transcription factor that regulates efflux pump expression (see below). The mechanism by which these isochromosomes are created is not known in detail, but it has been suggested that they are created by recombination at an inverted repeat in the centrosome region of the chromosome (3, 34, 35).

Gene amplification has also been identified in an azole-resistant clinical isolate of *C. glabrata*, although this isolate demonstrated other resistance mechanisms as well. The gene amplification was due to a chromosome duplication that was lost when the strain was grown in the absence of drug, although partial resistance was maintained.

Two groups have documented changes in *ERG11* allelic sequences as strains develop resistance (10a, 38a). In both cases, it appears that a mutation initially occurred in one allele of *ERG11*, which resulted in a strain that was heterozygous at *ERG11*. Random gene conversion or mitotic recombination then appears to have copied the mutation into the other allele, so that both alleles of the *ERG11* gene contained the mutation, a process known as loss of heterozygosity. These homozygous strains may then have been selected under drug pressure, as the cells express only a resistant Erg11p.

Resistant clinical isolates usually contain mutated but functional *ERG11* genes. In *C. albicans* and *C. glabrata*, deletions of the *ERG11* genes have been shown to cause increased azole resistance but also an increased susceptibility to oxidative killing by the host. Therefore, it is unlikely that clinical isolates would have a nonfunctional *ERG11* gene.

The *ERG11* gene appears to be important for the intrinsic resistance of *C. krusei*. *C. krusei* cell extracts with Erg11p enzyme activity are 24- to 46-fold less susceptible to fluconazole than extracts from *C. albicans*. The intrinsic resistance of *C. krusei* is likely to be due to both reduced Erg11p enzyme susceptibility and reduced drug accumulation associated with drug efflux (see below).

Additional Alterations in Ergosterol Synthesis

Several other genes in the ergosterol pathway (*ERG* genes) have been analyzed for their effects on drug susceptibility. In clinical isolates, changes have been observed in the profile of sterols from the cells that suggest mutation in *ERG* genes. However, only rarely are mutations identified in *ERG* genes to explain the altered sterol profiles.

In *C. neoformans*, the azoles appear to inhibit other gene products in the ergosterol pathway in addition to Erg11p. The drugs appear to act directly or indirectly to inhibit the C-4 sterol demethylase complex (Erg25p, Erg26p, and Erg27p). Inhibition of this complex reduces the production of the growth-arresting diol without alterations in Erg3p. Itraconazole appears to have an additional inhibitory effect on Erg24p, at least in *C. neoformans* and *Histoplasma capsulatum*, where itraconazole has an increased effectiveness compared to other azoles.

Drug Accumulation

Drug accumulation within a fungal cell is the result of a balance between drug import, drug efflux, and drug metabolism. Azole drug accumulation has been studied primarily in *C. albicans*, where radioactively labeled azoles and the fluorescent dye rhodamine-123 have been used to show drug accumulation within the cells. Drug accumulation has also been observed in *C. glabrata*, *C. krusei*, *C. dubliniensis*, *C. neoformans*, and *A. fumigatus*. This accumulation was saturable, suggesting an import or efflux mechanism other than diffusion. This azole accumulation is dependent on energy, cell viability, pH, and temperature. Drug accumulation is also dependent on the sterol composition of the cell membrane, as modified membranes lacking ergosterol are less fluid and have altered permeability and reduced azole accumulation. Intracellular drug levels are reduced in resistant clinical isolates compared to matched susceptible controls, and several studies have shown that this reduced accumulation is energy dependent.

Drug Import

It was commonly assumed that azole drugs enter the cell by passive diffusion, although this has not been documented clearly. Recently, azole import has been studied in detail (18). Import of radiolabeled fluconazole was shown to be saturable in de-energized cells, suggesting that azole import is facilitated by diffusion involving a surface protein. Other azoles were shown to specifically compete with fluconazole import. Fluconazole import was demonstrated for *C. albicans*, *C. krusei*, *C. neoformans*, and *S. cerevisiae*. Some resistant clinical isolates were shown to have significant reductions in azole import, which suggests that altered import may be a mechanism of resistance.

Drug Metabolism

To date, studies on azole modification, activation, or degradation have not been reported. It has been suggested but not published that azoles are not metabolized in susceptible isolates of *C. albicans*, although it is not clear if this has been studied in resistant isolates of *C. albicans* or in other species.

Drug Efflux

Two classes of efflux pumps, the ATP binding cassette transporters (ABCTs) and the major facilitators (MFs), are involved in movement of small molecules across the plasma membrane of cells in both directions. Specific members of each class of pump have been associated with drug resistance in one or more systems. The ABCT pumps are associated with active efflux of small molecules that are toxic to the cells. These small molecules tend to be hydrophobic or lipophilic, as are the azole drugs. The MF pumps are also associated with relatively hydrophobic molecules, such as tetracycline.

ABCT Pumps

The ABCT pumps consist of two membrane-spanning domains that assemble into a channel in the plasma membrane and two nucleotide binding domains that bind and use ATP as an energy source for the pump. The nucleotide binding domains contain an ATP binding cassette (ABC; hence the name), which is a conserved motif among proteins that use ATP as an energy source. In *C. albicans*, azole drug resistance is associated with the ABCT genes *CDR1* and *CDR2*, members of the *Candida* drug resistance (CDR) gene family, which is homologous to the pleiotrophic drug resistance (PDR) gene family of *S. cerevisiae*.

Deletion of the *CDR1* gene of *C. albicans*, like its *S. cerevisiae* homolog *PDR5*, causes cells to be hypersusceptible to azoles, terbinafine, amorolfine (another ergosterol biosynthesis inhibitor), several metabolic inhibitors, and other compounds, although there is no change in susceptibility to amphotericin B or flucytosine. Overexpression of *CDR1* has been demonstrated in a variety of resistant and susceptible clinical isolates from oral and systemic disease.

Deletion of the *CDR2* gene, which is closely related to *CDR1*, does not alter drug susceptibilities, although the double gene disruption of *CDR1* and *CDR2* causes hypersusceptibility compared to the single *CDR1* gene disruption. Increased mRNA levels of *CDR2* have been detected in several resistant clinical isolates; most of these isolates also have increased mRNA levels of *CDR1*. The coregulation of *CDR1* and *CDR2* suggests that the genes are both transcriptionally regulated by the same or similar factors and that those factors are involved in clinical resistance (see below).

PDR16 is another ABCT gene that is overexpressed in some *C. albicans* clinical isolates. Deletion of *PDR16* results in hypersusceptibility to azole drugs, and overexpression results in increased azole resistance in vitro. *PDR16* is coexpressed with *CDR1* and *CDR2*.

ABCT pumps associated with azole resistance have been identified in *C. krusei*, *C. glabrata*, *Candida tropicalis*, *C. dubliniensis*, *C. neoformans*, *A. fumigatus*, *Aspergillus nidulans*, and *Aspergillus flavus*. In *C. glabrata*, strains with disruptions of pump genes are hypersusceptible to azoles, and overexpression of pump genes is associated with the development of resistance at a high frequency. In *A. fumigatus*, overexpression of both ABCT and MF pumps has been associated with decreased intracellular levels of azole drugs, resulting in reduced susceptibility (10). The *C. neoformans* ABCT pump encoded by *AFR1* was overexpressed following in vitro azole exposure and resulted in reduced azole susceptibility. Deletion of this ABCT pump resulted in azole sensitivity, which confirms its role in azole resistance (6).

MF Pumps

The MF pumps also consist of two membrane-spanning domains that assemble into a channel, but the MF pumps do not have nucleotide binding domains. Instead, these pumps use the proton gradient of the membrane as an energy source. The MF pumps commonly transport molecules by antiport: protons enter the cell and small molecules are removed from the cell.

Disruption of the *MDR1* gene in *C. albicans* increased susceptibilities to azoles and several other stress-inducing drugs and reduced virulence in an animal model of systemic candidiasis. Increased mRNA levels of the *MDR1* gene have been correlated with azole resistance in several clinical isolates of *C. albicans*. The *MDR1* gene has been disrupted in azole-resistant clinical isolates overexpressing *MDR1*. The resulting disruptants had an increased susceptibility to azole drugs, demonstrating that *MDR1* is in fact a cause of azole resistance (13). In *C. neoformans*, *MDR1* is present and appears to be functionally homologous to *MDR1* from other fungi, but it has not been definitively shown to lead to azole resistance (7).

Transcriptional Regulation of Resistance Genes

Increased mRNA levels of resistance genes, including *ERG11*, *CDR1*, *CDR2*, *PDR16*, and *MDR1*, are commonly the result of increased expression, which is usually the result of altered transcriptional regulation.

The *ERG11* gene appears to be coordinately regulated with other genes in the *ERG* pathway by a transcription factor encoded by *UPC2* (Table 3). Upc2p is one member of a large family of fungus-specific transcription regulators containing a Zn_2Cys_6 binding motif. Upc2p contains a transcription activation domain at the N terminus and a transmembrane segment at the C terminus. Activation may occur by cleavage of the protein, which releases the N terminus from the endoplasmic reticulum membrane and allows the transcription activation domain to enter the nucleus and activate genes (19). This mechanism is similar to the sterol response element binding protein transcription factor that regulates cholesterol in mammalian cells. Deletion of *UPC2* in *C. albicans* results in cells that are hypersusceptible to all drugs associated with the ergosterol pathway as well as drugs associated with cell wall stability. The deletion also affects other aspects of sterol metabolism and is important for azole regulation of the ergosterol pathway, which suggests that *UPC2* is a master regulator of sterols. Upc2p is known to interact with the promoters of over 200 genes, including many *ERG* genes, and the efflux pump genes *CDR1* and *MDR1* (42). The *ERG* genes are induced in the presence of ergosterol biosynthesis inhibitors, including the azoles; and the induction is dependent on *UPC2* (25). Most importantly, a mutation in *UPC2* that results in overexpression of the *ERG* genes has been identified in a clinical isolate (9).

To date, the efflux genes *CDR1* and *CDR2* appear to be regulated together, although there are a small number of clinical isolates that overexpress only one or the other gene, which suggests that these isolates may contain promoter mutations. Regions of the *CDR1* and *CDR2* promoters that are important for regulation have been identified, including the drug response element, which is important for overexpression of the pumps in clinical isolates. Two other elements, steroid response element 1 and steroid response element 2, are responsible for steroid induction of the pump genes but not induction by other drugs. A negative response element which binds to an as yet unidentified 55-kDa protein has also been identified.

Several transcription factors that regulate expression of *CDR1* and *CDR2* have been identified. The factor that recognizes the drug response elements is known as *TAC1*,

TABLE 3 Transcriptional regulation of resistance

Overexpressed gene(s)	Inducible by azoles	Other inducers	Transcription factor gene(s)	Mutation in clinical isolates
ERG11	Yes	Ergosterol biosynthesis inhibitors	*UPC2*	Yes
CDR1, CDR2	No	Fluphenazine	*TAC1*	Yes
			NDT80	None reported
			FCR1, FCR3	None reported
MDR1	No	Stress inducers, oxidizing agents	*MRR1*	Yes
			CAP1	None reported
			MCM1	None reported

another member of the Zn_2Cys_6 transcription factor family (Table 3). Gain-of-function mutations in *TAC1* have been identified in many clinical isolates in which *CDR1*, *CDR2*, and/or *PDR16* are overexpressed (3, 4). *TAC1* appears to act as a recessive allele; it causes efflux pump overexpression only when a mutation is present in both alleles of *TAC1*.

Additional factors that are known to regulate expression of *CDR1* and *CDR2* include *NDT80*, *FCR1*, and *FCR3*. *NDT80* is a unique transcription factor, *FCR1* encodes another Zn_2Cys_6 transcription factor, and *FCR3* encodes a member of the bZip transcription factor family. To date, no mutations in these genes have been associated with resistance.

The *C. albicans MDR1* gene is transcriptionally regulated by three transcription factors, *MRR1*, *CAP1*, and *MCM1* (Table 3). The Zn_2Cys_6 transcription factor gene *MRR1* has recently been identified as the transcription factor that is mutated in clinical isolates; its mutation results in overexpression of *MDR1* (8, 21, 33). The unrelated transcription factors *CAP1* and *MCM1* regulate the response of fungal cells to oxidative stress and other stress conditions, in part by inducing MF pump genes including *MDR1* (12), but they have not been linked to azole resistance in clinical isolates.

While mutations in *UPC2*, *TAC1*, and *MRR1* have all been linked to overexpression of their respective resistance genes in clinical isolates, only the *UPC2* transcription factor that controls *ERG* genes responds to azole drugs (14, 25). The efflux pumps *CDR1*, *CDR2*, *PDR16*, and *MDR1* do not respond to azole drugs, but they do respond to steroids, fluphenazine, stress inducers, and oxidizing agents (Table 3).

mRNA Stability

In addition to transcriptional regulation by transcription factors, recent studies have demonstrated increased mRNA stability and increased transcriptional initiation for the *CDR1* gene in resistant isolates, which is possibly the result of altered sequences in the 3' untranslated region of the mRNA (17).

Identification of Additional Genes

Transcription profiling using microarrays has been used to identify other genes associated with resistance. Many of the identified genes are upregulated either with *CDR1* and *CDR2* or with *MDR1*. This suggests that some of these additional genes might be coregulated by the transcription factors described above. In each of these analyses, the genes are correlated with resistance, but their role in resistance is yet to be demonstrated.

Genetic screens have also been used in both *C. albicans* and *C. glabrata* to identify additional genes associated with

resistance. A genetic screen identified the *C. albicans CKA2* gene, encoding casein kinase II, which suggests a role for kinase signaling in resistance (2). A screen in *C. glabrata* identified genes encoding efflux pumps and transporters, as expected from the molecular mechanisms described above, and Ca^{2+} channel regulators and genes involved in mitochondrial function, as expected from the phenotypes described below.

Summary of Molecular Mechanisms

The resistance mechanisms described to date are summarized in Fig. 1. In a susceptible cell, azole drugs enter the cell by facilitated diffusion and target lanosterol demethylase, Erg11p, which is part of the ergosterol biosynthesis pathway.

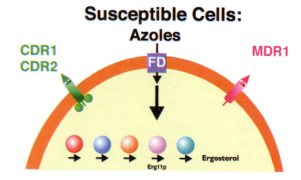

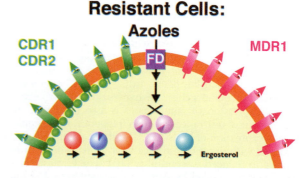

FIGURE 1 Molecular mechanisms of azole resistance. See text for details. Gene products shown in the figure include Erg11p (pink sphere), the *CDR* efflux pumps (green tubes) with ATP binding cassette domains (green spheres), the *MDR* efflux pump (red tubes), and other ergosterol biosynthetic enzymes (spheres of assorted colors). Point mutations are shown as dark slices in pink and blue spheres. Reprinted with modification from reference 41 with permission of the publisher.

The *CDR* pumps and the *MDR1* pump are expressed at low levels in susceptible cells. The drug enters resistant cells by facilitated diffusion, which may be altered in these cells. The interaction between the azoles and Erg11p can be altered by mutation or overexpression of the *ERG11* gene. Alterations in other enzymes in ergosterol biosynthesis can also affect azole susceptibility. Both the *CDR* gene family and the *MDR1* pump can be overexpressed, reducing the amount of drug within the cell.

Resistance Is a Composite

Resistance in *C. albicans* clinical isolates is not usually the result of a single alteration. Instead, several alterations usually contribute to the generation of a resistant cell. Each alteration allows the corresponding isolate to outgrow the other cells in the population, becoming fixed as the major strain. Subsequent alterations, each of which increases the resistance of the cell only slightly, allow the strain to gradually develop a highly resistant phenotype. This has been well documented in a series of 17 sequential isolates from a single patient (41). In this series, all of the isolates were indistinguishable from each other, although early in the series, a substrain appears to have become the major strain. After substrain selection, the *MDR1* gene was overexpressed, correlating with a significant increase in resistance. Later in the series, isolates acquired an R467K mutation in *ERG11*, so that the Erg11p enzyme became more resistant to azole and the cells had an increased azole resistance. At the same time, the *ERG11* gene was overexpressed and allelic differences were eliminated, which suggests that a gene conversion or mitotic recombination copied the R467K mutation to both alleles. Even later in the infection, the *CDR1* and *CDR2* genes were overexpressed, again correlating with a significant rise in azole resistance. The timing and the order in which each of these changes occurred is unlikely to have been critical to the development of resistance, but the sum of each of these alterations results in a resistant phenotype.

Unidentified Mechanisms

While significant progress has been made in the characterization of molecular mechanisms associated with azole resistance, most of the resistant isolates characterized are oral isolates from AIDS patients with oral candidiasis. When a series of systemic isolates was characterized, some isolates were identified with the same molecular mechanisms of resistance. However, a significant number of azole-resistant systemic isolates showed no alterations in the target enzyme or efflux pumps. It is likely that these strains have alterations in drug metabolism or other, as yet unidentified mechanisms.

Resistance in Perspective

Several generalizations concerning resistance can be made based on the work from the last 15 years. First, the predominant molecular mechanism of azole drug resistance in oral isolates is overexpression of efflux pumps, especially *CDR1* and *CDR2*. Second, unlike resistance in parasite and mammalian systems, drug resistance in the fungi is not normally associated with gene amplification. Fungi in general have elaborate systems for the regulation of gene transcription, and thus gene amplification is not necessary to alter gene expression. Third, unlike studies with prokaryotes, studies with fungi have not yet identified any plasmids or other episomes containing resistance markers. Finally, there is no documented situation in which the resistance markers from one isolate were transferred to another isolate.

PHENOTYPES ASSOCIATED WITH AZOLE RESISTANCE

MIC susceptibility testing is important in determining a strain's basic response to antifungal drugs. However, in the last several years, additional phenotypes associated with resistance (Table 4) which do not fit simply into the standard susceptible versus resistant definitions of MIC testing and which do not appear to be directly the result of the molecular mechanisms described above have been identified. Understanding of these phenotypes will give additional insight into how a fungal cell responds to antifungal drugs.

Mating Type

As mentioned above, *C. albicans* has two mating types, a and α, defined by the gene set at the *MTL* (mnemonic for mating-type-like) locus. Most strains are diploid a/α. However, strains that are homozygous at the *MTL* locus do exist (a/a and α/α). These homozygous strains are able to undergo phenotypic switching between two cell states, white and opaque. Opaque cells are the mating-competent forms of *C. albicans* that can undergo fusion to form tetraploids. A correlation has been identified between homozygosity at the *MTL* locus and azole resistance. All *MTL* homozygotes are not resistant, and all azole-resistant isolates are not homozygous at the *MTL* locus, but there is an increased frequency of *MTL* homozygotes in azole-resistant strains. This correlation between azole resistance and *MTL* homozygosity has several possible explanations. The transcription factor *TAC1*, which regulates expression of the *CDR1* and *CDR2* efflux pump genes, is genetically linked to the *MTL* locus (5). It is also possible that a mating reaction creates genetic variation, and drug pressure may then select for strains with new genetic compositions. As 50% of the progeny of a mating reaction should be *MTL* homozygotes, then the correlation between azole resistance and *MTL* homozygosity may be the link to mating and genetic variability. Finally, it is possible that isochromosome formation associated with azole resistance leads to *MTL* homozygosity.

Trailing

Standard susceptibility testing monitors growth at 24 or 48 h, and the MIC is defined as the concentration of drug that inhibits growth by 50% or 80% compared to the control. Some fungal isolates appear susceptible at 24 h of growth but resistant at 48 h of growth. This difference between the 24- and 48-h growth is known as trailing. Trailing growth at 48 h is usually the result of growth inhibition near the 50% or 80% cutoff, while growth of true resistant

TABLE 4 Cellular phenotypes associated with resistance

Cellular phenotype	Characterization by MIC[a]
Homozygosity at *MTL* locus	Associated with resistant MIC
Trailing	Resistant MIC
Calcineurin effects	No change in standard MIC
Heterogeneous resistance	Susceptible MIC
High-frequency azole resistance	Susceptible → resistant MIC
Inducible resistance	Susceptible → resistant MIC
Transient resistance	Resistant → susceptible MIC
Stable resistance	Consistently resistant MIC
Cross-resistance	Resistant MIC for many drugs
Altered fitness	No change in standard MIC

[a]Standard MIC_{80} at 48 h.

strains is usually similar to the no-drug control. Trailing is a result of residual growth, which is growth of cells with drug concentrations above the MIC, because the azole drugs are fungistatic rather than fungicidal. Clinically, infections with these trailing isolates are usually treatable with azole drugs at standard drug concentrations. Consistent with this, trailing isolates behave as susceptible isolates in animal models of candidiasis. It has been observed that trailing can be reduced in acidic media. This may have consequences in treatment of vaginal isolates, because the vaginal pH is more acidic than that of blood. Under those conditions, trailing would be reduced, which is consistent with the observation that resistance has not been observed in vaginal yeast infections.

Tolerance

Strains that show significant residual growth, or trailing, show drug tolerance, which is associated with fungistatic drugs. Azole drug tolerance is lost in the presence of cyclosporine, which inhibits fungal calcineurin, an important factor in Ca^{2+} regulation. Cyclosporine eliminates trailing and drug tolerance, essentially making a fungistatic drug fungicidal. However, cyclosporine does not alter the MIC of the isolate, just its residual growth above the MIC. The use of cyclosporine with azole drugs decreases the fungal load in animal models, suggesting that the drug combination may have important clinical significance.

Recently, it has been shown that the heat shock protein Hsp90p is important for drug tolerance and resistance (6). Hsp90p is involved in folding of proteins, and one of its clients is calcineurin. Hsp90p and calcineurin are both involved in mediating the fungal stress response, which allows cells to persist during drug treatments. The subsequent persistence would then allow time for stable drug-resistant mutants to arise.

Heterogeneous Antifungal Resistance

Heterogeneous resistance is an unusual phenomenon in which a small percentage of the cells in a population are resistant. Only 1 to 5% of isolates in a collection exhibit heterogeneous resistance. When a strain capable of heterogeneous resistance is spread on an agar plate containing drug, colonies form at a low frequency (1 in 10 to 1 in 100,000). The important observation is that these colonies are not 100% resistant; they contain only a small percentage of resistant cells. If the colony is respread on another plate, the same low proportion of resistant cells is observed. The resistant phenotype is not genetically fixed, but the ability of a small percentage to be resistant is fixed in these strains. This phenomenon of heterogeneous resistance has been observed in bacteria, including *Staphylococcus* and *Enterococcus*. Heterogeneous resistance has been observed for azoles in *C. albicans* and *C. neoformans*. The genetic mechanisms of heterogeneous resistance have not been identified in any organism. This heterogeneous resistance is a significant problem, since the strains that show heterogeneous resistance test as susceptible by the standard methods for determining MICs yet can behave as resistant in vivo.

High-Frequency Azole Resistance

A resistance phenotype that resembles heterogeneous resistance is known as high-frequency azole resistance (HFAR). HFAR isolates are able to form colonies at low frequencies (1 in 10 to 1 in 10,000) on agar containing azole drugs. However, unlike heterogeneous resistant colonies, these HFAR colonies retain their resistance even when grown in the absence of drug. HFAR colonies selected for fluconazole resistance are cross resistant to all azoles and hypersusceptible to amphotericin B. HFAR has been observed in *C. albicans*, *C. glabrata*, and even *S. cerevisiae*. HFAR in *C. glabrata* has been associated with loss of mitochondrial function. This is consistent with the observation that *C. glabrata* petites (cells lacking mitochondrial DNA) are azole resistant and with the observation that genes with mitochondrial function are identified in a screen for azole resistance (16, 24). It is unlikely that fungal cells without mitochondrial function would survive in an animal model of infection, but these observations provide information on the mechanism behind HFAR.

Inducible Azole Resistance

Most susceptible strains of *C. albicans* cannot be induced in vitro to form resistance, perhaps because *C. albicans* is diploid and point mutations have no effect unless they are dominant or codominant mutations. However, there is a small number of strains in which resistance can be induced. It is possible that these strains have preexisting alterations in genes associated with drug resistance, although the mechanisms allowing the induction of resistance have not been studied. In one set of induced strains, the induction of resistance is associated with an increased expression of the efflux pumps *CDR1* and *CDR2*.

Transient Resistance

Resistance mutations are usually genetically stable and persist in cells in the absence of drug pressure. However, there are reversible mechanisms by which cells can be induced to be resistant in the presence of drug, including gene activation and repression. If resistance is the result of a reversible cell state, then resistance will persist in the presence of drug and the cells will revert to a susceptible phenotype in the absence of drug. Such inducible resistance has been documented in vitro and in vivo.

Clinical isolates of *C. albicans* from BMT patients have been shown to have transient azole resistance, and some strains are predisposed to induction. When characterized, this transient resistance is associated with increased expression of the *CDR* efflux pumps, while the loss of resistance is associated with reduced expression of the same pumps.

Stable Resistance

Mutations occur randomly in a strain, including alterations that render the strain resistant. Such mutations might include point mutations in *ERG11*, in the promoters of efflux pumps, or in the transcription factors that regulate those pumps. When these resistance mutations occur during an infection, the mutation would allow those cells to selectively outgrow the other cells in the population under drug pressure. Genetically fixed mutations should render the cell stably resistant to drugs. When these strains are grown in the absence of drugs, the resistant phenotype will persist if the isolates are relatively fit compared to a susceptible version of the strain. In general, stable and fit resistant isolates are obtained from patients who have received long-term antifungal treatment, such as AIDS patients.

Cross-Resistance

Based on the molecular mechanisms outlined above, it is expected that clinical isolates that are resistant to one azole, such as fluconazole, should be cross resistant to other azoles, although the *MDR1* efflux pump has an effect on fluconazole and to some extent voriconazole but does not have an effect on other drugs. Point mutations in the target enzyme Erg11p may alter the active site or another part of the enzyme such that one or more azoles are unable to inhibit the enzyme. This is consistent with MIC testing for azole-resistant clinical isolates. The CDR pumps alter susceptibility to fluconazole, voriconazole, itraconazole, and ketoconazole, as well as nystatin, terbinafine, and amorolfine. They do not have an effect on amphotericin B or flucytosine or two other antifungals, nikkomycin and griseofulvin.

Fitness

Alterations in the drug resistance genes described above may affect the overall fitness of a strain, such that the strain might be less fit in the absence of drug than its susceptible counterparts. Lack of fitness may compromise the virulence of a strain. Fitness has been assessed in vivo by testing the virulence of matched susceptible and resistant isolates, with no obvious correlation. In vitro, when an inducible susceptible isolate was grown in the presence of drug, it developed resistance. The developing resistant population was initially less fit than the susceptible parent when grown in the absence of drug. However, fitness improved under continued drug pressure until the resistant strain was as fit as the parent susceptible strain in the absence of drug. This fitness appears to be independent of the molecular mechanisms of resistance.

Phenotypes and MIC

In this section, several phenotypes associated with resistance have been described. These phenotypes are not usually detected with standard MIC susceptibility testing (Table 4). Even trailing will not be detected unless the investigator measures growth at both 24 and 48 h. Strains can exhibit one or more of these phenotypes. The molecular basis has not been determined for most of these phenotypes. Understanding these phenotypes is important, in addition to MIC characterizations, to determine how a strain will behave in a patient.

MOLECULAR MECHANISMS OF NONAZOLE DRUG RESISTANCE

Resistance to Flucytosine

Up to 10% of C. albicans clinical isolates have intrinsic resistance to flucytosine, and 30% of the susceptible isolates develop acquired resistance during drug therapy. Resistance can be associated with mutations in any of the following: cytosine deaminase, which converts flucytosine to 5-fluorouracil; uracil phosphoribosyl transferase, which is important for nucleic acid synthesis; or either of two purine-cytosine permeases. Mutations in one of the purine-cytosine permeases of C. lusitaniae were shown to result in cross-resistance to flucytosine and fluconazole.

C. albicans can be divided into five clades, or groupings, based on molecular markers such as multilocus sequence typing (see above). Recently, flucytosine resistance in C. albicans has been shown to be specific to clade 1 and linked to mutations in the uracil phosphoribosyl transferase gene FUR1. In haploid C. neoformans, flucytosine resistance can result from a single mutation at either of two specific gene loci, FCY1 or FCY2.

Polyene Resistance

Amphotericin B-resistant clinical isolates of C. tropicalis have been identified, and amphotericin B-resistant isolates of C. albicans, C. neoformans, A. nidulans, and Aspergillus fennelliae

have been constructed either by mutagenesis or serial passage in the presence of increasing amounts of drug. Most isolates have greatly reduced levels of ergosterol in their plasma membranes, which decreases the binding ability of amphotericin B. Sterol analysis suggests that these isolates are defective in ERG2 or ERG3, although definitive molecular analyses have not been performed. Alterations in the structure of the membrane or the sterol/phospholipid ratio may also be associated with amphotericin B resistance. Acquired resistance has also been described when environmental isolates of C. neoformans were passaged in a mouse model of cryptococcosis. The passaged isolates become more resistant to amphotericin B in the absence of drug, suggesting that resistance levels can be altered by interactions with the host.

Echinocandin Resistance

The echinocandins have not been in clinical use for as long as the other agents, so echinocandin-resistant clinical isolates are limited in number. In vitro, resistance is usually generated by mutation in genes encoding one of three subunits of the target enzyme glucan synthetase (11). There is some indication that both C. albicans and A. fumigatus strains that overexpress CDR2 may have increased resistance to caspofungin, although this change in susceptibility is not detected by standard MIC analyses. Some C. albicans isolates show growth at high concentrations of echinocandins, above the MIC. This is called paradoxical growth or Eagle's effect, and it may be mediated by the fungal stress response, which includes increased synthesis of chitin, a component of the cell wall (38). Susceptibility testing of Candida isolates against all three clinically available echinocandins (caspofungin, anidulafungin, and micafungin) has been done using a variety of accepted methods. In general, the testing methods can distinguish between resistant and susceptible isolates for the echinocandins (1).

CLINICAL IMPLICATIONS AND FUTURE DIRECTIONS

Dosing

There have been no clinical studies to determine the optimal dosing of antifungal drugs to prevent resistance. In general, azole drugs should not be used prophylactically in the prevention of oral or vaginal candidiasis. However, the azoles are clearly important in the prevention of systemic infections and in the prevention of recurrent cryptococcal meningitis infections. Based on drug resistance in a variety of organisms, continuous treatment with a large and safe dose of drug for the minimum period required to cure the infection will have the least risk for the development of resistance.

Detection

The CLSI and EUCAST susceptibility test methods are satisfactory for determining the MICs of most yeasts and filamentous fungi. Given the multiple molecular mechanisms of resistance presented in Fig. 1 and the real possibility that there exist other mechanisms of resistance which have not been identified, a simple molecular test for resistance would be difficult to develop.

Drug Development

There is always a need for new antifungal agents that are effective against strains and species that show resistance to current therapies. New azole drugs, such as posaconazole, need to be carefully monitored for their effect on strains that are resistant to fluconazole.

The multiple efflux pumps in fungal genomes and the broad substrate specificity of each of these pumps suggest that strains or species with high levels of efflux may be resistant to many classes of drug. Strategies to interfere with the pumps or inhibit pump activity are currently the focus of drug development in several industry and biotechnology settings.

Drug combinations are likely to become more important in future antifungal drug strategies. Amphotericin B is currently used in combination with flucytosine and with azole drugs. The use of azoles in combination with flucytosine or with terbinafine has been discussed and tested. With the development of new antifungal drugs, such as the echinocandins, the possible drug combinations increase dramatically.

The best way to improve treatment success in a patient is to improve their immune status. Strategies using cytokines have been tested in the treatment of fungal disease, but further work is clearly required before such strategies become clinically applicable.

An increased understanding of antifungal drug resistance should allow for the development of new diagnostic strategies to identify resistant clinical isolates in a patient, new treatment strategies to treat these resistant infections, and new prevention strategies that would forestall the development of antifungal drug resistance in these patient populations. One fact is clear: as strategies emerge to treat resistant fungal infections, the fungal cells will continue to evolve new mechanisms of antifungal drug resistance.

REFERENCES

1. **Arendrup, M. C., G. Garcia-Effron, C. Lass-Flörl, A. G. Lopez, J.-L. Rodriguez-Tudela, M. Cuenca-Estrella, and D. S. Perlin.** 2010. Echinocandin susceptibility testing of *Candida* species: comparison of EUCAST EDef 7.1, CLSI M27-A3, Etest, disk diffusion, and agar dilution methods with RPMI and isosensitest media. *Antimicrob. Agents Chemother.* **54:**426–439.
2. **Bruno, V. M., and A. P. Mitchell.** 2005. Regulation of azole drug susceptibility by *Candida albicans* protein kinase CK2. *Mol. Microbiol.* **56:**559–573.
3. **Coste, A., A. Selmecki, A. Forche, D. Diogo, M.-E. Bougnoux, C. d'Enfert, J. Berman, and D. Sanglard.** 2007. Genotypic evolution of azole resistance mechanisms in sequential *Candida albicans* isolates. *Eukaryot. Cell* **6:**1889–1904.
4. **Coste, A., V. Turner, F. Ischer, J. Morschhauser, A. Forche, A. Selmecki, J. Berman, J. Bille, and D. Sanglard.** 2006. A mutation in Tac1p, a transcription factor regulating CDR1 and CDR2, is coupled with loss of heterozygosity at chromosome 5 to mediate antifungal resistance in *Candida albicans*. *Genetics* **172:**2139–2156.
5. **Coste, A. T., M. Karababa, F. Ischer, J. Bille, and D. Sanglard.** 2004. TAC1, transcriptional activator of CDR genes, is a new transcription factor involved in the regulation of *Candida albicans* ABC transporters CDR1 and CDR2. *Eukaryot. Cell* **3:**1639–1652.
6. **Cowen, L. E.** 2008. The evolution of fungal drug resistance: modulating the trajectory from genotype to phenotype. *Nat. Rev. Microbiol.* **6:**187–198.
7. **Cowen, L. E., and W. J. Steinbach.** 2008. Stress, drugs, and evolution: the role of cellular signaling in fungal drug resistance. *Eukaryot. Cell* **7:**747–764.
8. **Dunkel, N., J. Blass, P. D. Rogers, and J. Morschhauser.** 2008. Mutations in the multi-drug resistance regulator MRR1, followed by loss of heterozygosity, are the main cause of MDR1 overexpression in fluconazole-resistant *Candida albicans* strains. *Mol. Microbiol.* **69:**827–840.
9. **Dunkel, N., T. T. Liu, K. S. Barker, R. Homayouni, J. Morschhäuser, and P. D. Rogers.** 2008. A gain-of-function mutation in the transcription factor Upc2p causes upregulation of ergosterol biosynthesis genes and increased fluconazole resistance in a clinical *Candida albicans* isolate. *Eukaryot. Cell* **7:**1180–1190.
10. **Ferreira, M. E., A. L. Colombo, I. Paulsen, Q. Ren, J. Wortman, J. Huang, M. H. Goldman, and G. H. Goldman.** 2005. The ergosterol biosynthesis pathway, transporter genes, and azole resistance in *Aspergillus fumigatus*. *Med. Mycol.* **43**(Suppl 1):S313–S319.
10a. **Franz, R., S. L. Kelly, D. C. Lamb, D. E. Kelly, M. Ruhnke, and J. Morschhäuser.** 1998. Multiple molecular mechanisms contribute to a stepwise development of fluconazole resistance in clinical *Candida albicans* strains. *Antimicrob. Agents Chemother.* **42:**3065–3072.
11. **Garcia-Effron, G., S. Lee, S. Park, J. D. Cleary, and D. S. Perlin.** 2009. Effect of *Candida glabrata* FKS1 and FKS2 mutations on echinocandin sensitivity and kinetics of 1,3-β-D-glucan synthase: implication for the existing susceptibility breakpoint. *Antimicrob. Agents Chemother.* **53:**3690–3699.
12. **Harry, J. B., B. G. Oliver, J. L. Song, P. M. Silver, J. T. Little, J. Choiniere, and T. C. White.** 2005. Drug-induced regulation of the MDR1 promoter in *Candida albicans*. *Antimicrob. Agents Chemother.* **49:**2785–2792.
13. **Hiller, D., D. Sanglard, and J. Morschhäuser.** 2006. Overexpression of the MDR1 gene is sufficient to confer increased resistance to toxic compounds in *Candida albicans*. *Antimicrob. Agents Chemother.* **50:**1365–1371.
14. **Hoot, S. J., B. G. Oliver, and T. C. White.** 2008. *Candida albicans* UPC2 is transcriptionally induced in response to antifungal drugs and anaerobicity through Upc2p-dependent and -independent mechanisms. *Microbiology* **154:**2748–2756.
15. **Howard, S. J., I. Webster, C. B. Moore, R. E. Gardiner, S. Park, D. S. Perlin, and D. W. Denning.** 2006. Multi-azole resistance in *Aspergillus fumigatus*. *Int. J. Antimicrob. Agents* **28:**450–453.
16. **Kaur, R., I. Castano, and B. P. Cormack.** 2004. Functional genomic analysis of fluconazole susceptibility in the pathogenic yeast *Candida glabrata*: roles of calcium signaling and mitochondria. *Antimicrob. Agents Chemother.* **48:**1600–1613.
17. **Manoharlal, R., N. A. Gaur, S. L. Panwar, J. Morschhäuser, and R. Prasad.** 2008. Transcriptional activation and increased mRNA stability contribute to overexpression of CDR1 in azole-resistant *Candida albicans*. *Antimicrob. Agents Chemother.* **52:**1481–1492.
18. **Mansfield, B. E., H. N. Oltean, B. G. Oliver, S. E. Leyde, L. Hedstrom, and T. C. White.** 2010. Azole drug import requires a transporter in *Candida albicans* and other pathogenic fungi. Presented at the 10th ASM Conference on Candida and Candidiasis, Miami, Florida, March 23–26, 2010.
19. **Marie, C., S. Leyde, and T. C. White.** 2008. Cytoplasmic localization of sterol transcription factors Upc2p and Ecm22p in *S. cerevisiae*. *Fungal Genet. Biol.* **45:**1430–1438.
20. **Marie, C., and T. C. White.** 2009. Genetic basis of antifungal drug resistance. *Curr. Fungal Infect. Rep.* **3:**163–169.
21. **Morschhauser, J., K. S. Barker, T. T. Liu, B. W. J. Bla, R. Homayouni, and P. D. Rogers.** 2007. The transcription factor Mrr1p controls expression of the MDR1 efflux pump and mediates multidrug resistance in Candida albicans. *PLoS Pathog.* **3:**e164.
22. **Nett, J., L. Lincoln, K. Marchillo, R. Massey, K. Holoyda, B. Hoff, M. VanHandel, and D. Andes.** 2007. Putative role of β-1,3 glucans in *Candida albicans* biofilm resistance. *Antimicrob. Agents Chemother.* **51:**510–520.
23. **Odds, F. C., M. E. Bougnoux, D. J. Shaw, J. M. Bain, A. D. Davidson, D. Diogo, M. D. Jacobsen, M. Lecomte, S. Y. Li, A. Tavanti, M. C. Maiden, N. A. Gow, and C. d'Enfert.** 2007. Molecular phylogenetics of *Candida albicans*. *Eukaryot. Cell* **6:**1041–1052.
24. **Oliver, B. G., P. M. Silver, C. Marie, S. J. Hoot, S. E. Leyde, and T. C. White.** 2008. Tetracycline alters drug susceptibility in *Candida albicans* and other pathogenic fungi. *Microbiology* **154:**960–970.

25. **Oliver, B. G., J. L. Song, J. H. Choiniere, and T. C. White.** 2007. *cis*-acting elements within the *Candida albicans ERG11* promoter mediate the azole response through transcription factor Upc2p. *Eukaryot. Cell* **6:**2231–2239.

26. **Pfaller, M. A., and D. J. Diekema.** 2004. Rare and emerging opportunistic fungal pathogens: concern for resistance beyond *Candida albicans* and *Aspergillus fumigatus. J. Clin. Microbiol.* **42:**4419–4431.

27. **Pfaller, M. A., D. J. Diekema, M. A. Ghannoum, J. H. Rex, B. D. Alexander, D. Andes, S. D. Brown, V. Chaturvedi, A. Espinel-Ingroff, C. L. Fowler, E. M. Johnson, C. C. Knapp, M. R. Motyl, L. Ostrosky-Zeichner, D. J. Sheehan, and T. J. Walsh.** 2009. Wild-type MIC distribution and epidemiological cutoff values for *Aspergillus fumigatus* and three triazoles as determined by the Clinical and Laboratory Standards Institute broth microdilution methods. *J. Clin. Microbiol.* **47:**3142–3146.

28. **Pfaller, M. A., D. J. Diekema, L. Ostrosky-Zeichner, J. H. Rex, B. D. Alexander, D. Andes, S. D. Brown, V. Chaturvedi, M. A. Ghannoum, C. C. Knapp, D. J. Sheehan, and T. J. Walsh.** 2008. Correlation of MIC with outcome for *Candida* species tested against caspofungin, anidulafungin, and micafungin: analysis and proposal for interpretive MIC breakpoints. *J. Clin. Microbiol.* **46:**2620–2629.

29. **Pfaller, M. A., D. J. Diekema, J. H. Rex, A. Espinel-Ingroff, E. M. Johnson, D. Andes, V. Chaturvedi, M. A. Ghannoum, F. C. Odds, M. G. Rinaldi, D. J. Sheehan, P. Troke, T. J. Walsh, and D. W. Warnock.** 2006. Correlation of MIC with outcome for *Candida* species tested against voriconazole: analysis and proposal for interpretive breakpoints. *J. Clin. Microbiol.* **44:**819–826.

30. **Rex, J. H., and M. A. Pfaller.** 2002. Has antifungal susceptibility testing come of age? *Clin. Infect. Dis.* **35:**982–989.

31. **Rex, J. H., M. A. Pfaller, J. N. Galgiani, M. S. Bartlett, A. Espinel-Ingroff, M. A. Ghannoum, M. Lancaster, F. C. Odds, M. G. Rinaldi, T. J. Walsh, and A. L. Barry.** 1997. Development of interpretive breakpoints for antifungal susceptibility testing: conceptual framework and analysis of *in vitro*-*in vivo* correlation data for fluconazole, itraconazole, and *Candida* infections. *Clin. Infect. Dis.* **24:**235–247.

32. **Sanglard, D., and J. Bille.** 2002. Current understanding of the mode of action and of resistance mechanisms to conventional and emerging antifungal agents for treatment of *Candida* infections, p. 349–383. *In* R. Calderone (ed.), *Candida and Candidiasis.* ASM Press, Washington, DC.

33. **Schubert, S., P. D. Rogers, and J. Morschhäuser.** 2008. Gain-of-function mutations in the transcription factor *MRR1* are responsible for overexpression of the *MDR1* efflux pump in fluconazole-resistant *Candida dubliniensis* strains. *Antimicrob. Agents Chemother.* **52:**4274–4280.

34. **Selmecki, A., A. Forche, and J. Berman.** 2006. Aneuploidy and isochromosome formation in drug-resistant *Candida albicans. Science* **313:**367–370.

35. **Selmecki, A., M. Gerami-Nejad, C. Paulson, A. Forche, and J. Berman.** 2008. An isochromosome confers drug resistance in vivo by amplification of two genes, ERG11 and TAC1. *Mol. Microbiol.* **68:**624–641.

36. **Verweij, P. E., S. J. Howard, W. J. Melchers, and D. W. Denning.** 2009. Azole-resistance in *Aspergillus*: proposed nomenclature and breakpoints. *Drug Resist. Updates* **12:**141–147.

37. **Verweij, P. E., E. Snelders, G. H. Kema, E. Mellado, and W. J. Melchers.** 2009. Azole resistance in *Aspergillus fumigatus*: a side-effect of environmental fungicide use? *Lancet Infect. Dis.* **9:**789–795.

38. **Walker, L. A., C. A. Munro, I. de Bruijn, M. D. Lenardon, A. McKinnon, and N. A. Gow.** 2008. Stimulation of chitin synthesis rescues *Candida albicans* from echinocandins. *PLoS Pathog.* **4:**e1000040.

38a. **White, T. C.** 1997. The presence of an R467K amino acid substitution and loss of allelic variation correlate with an azole-resistance 14α demethylase in *Candida albicans. Antimicrob. Agents Chemother.* **41:**1488–1494.

39. **White, T. C.** 2007. Mechanisms of resistance to antifungal agents, p. 1961–1971. *In* P. R. Murray, E. J. Baron, J. H. Jorgensen, M. L. Landry, and M. A. Pfaller (ed.), *Manual of Clinical Microbiology,* 9th ed., vol. 2. ASM Press, Washington, DC.

40. **White, T. C., J. B. Harry, and B. G. Oliver.** 2004. Antifungal drug resistance: pumps and permutations, p. 319–338. *In* J. W. Domer and G. S. Koybayashi (ed.), *Human Fungal Pathogens,* vol. XII. Springer, Berlin.

41. **White, T. C., K. A. Marr, and R. A. Bowden.** 1998. Clinical, cellular, and molecular factors that contribute to antifungal drug resistance. *Clin. Microbiol. Rev.* **11:**382–402.

42. **Znaidi, S., S. Weber, O. Z. Al-Abdin, P. Bomme, S. Saidane, S. Drouin, S. Lemieux, X. De Deken, F. Robert, and M. Raymond.** 2008. Genomewide location analysis of *Candida albicans* Upc2p, a regulator of sterol metabolism and azole drug resistance. *Eukaryot. Cell* **7:**836–847.

Susceptibility Test Methods: Yeasts and Filamentous Fungi

ELIZABETH M. JOHNSON, ANA V. ESPINEL-INGROFF, AND MICHAEL A. PFALLER

128

The introduction of modern patient management technologies and therapies has resulted in a rapidly expanding number of chemically induced immunosuppressed patients who are highly susceptible to severe fungal infections. Fungi are also important nosocomial pathogens causing severe morbidity and mortality in hospitalized patients with a combination of a variety of risk factors and immunosuppression (44, 82, 83, 100, 105). Systemic infections caused by *Candida* spp. other than *C. albicans*, *Aspergillus* spp., and other filamentous fungi (molds) are being reported more frequently (82). As fungal infections became an important public health problem and resistance to established antifungal agents began to emerge (22, 23, 53, 61, 82, 117), pharmaceutical companies developed new agents with either a broader spectrum or different targets of activity.

Thirteen agents have been approved for the treatment of systemic fungal diseases: the polyene macrolide antibiotics conventional amphotericin B (Fungizone; Apothecon) and its three lipid formulations; flucytosine (5-fluorocytosine) (Ancobon; Valeant Pharmaceuticals), a synthetic pyrimidine; the azoles ketoconazole (Nizoral; Ortho-McNeil-Janssen Pharmaceuticals), fluconazole (Diflucan; Pfizer), itraconazole (Sporanox; Ortho-McNeil-Janssen Pharmaceuticals), voriconazole (Vfend; Pfizer), and posaconazole (Noxafil; Schering-Plough); and the echinocandins caspofungin (Cancidas; Merck), micafungin (Mycamine; Astellas Pharma Fujisawa Healthcare), and anidulafungin (Eraxis in the United States, Ecalta in Europe; Pfizer).

The mechanisms of resistance to antifungal agents and more detailed information on new and established agents are found elsewhere (chapters 126 and 127).

ANTIFUNGAL SUSCEPTIBILITY TESTING

Rationale

Ideally, in vitro susceptibility tests (i) provide a reliable measure of the relative activities of two or more antifungal agents, (ii) correlate with in vivo activity and predict the likely outcome of therapy, (iii) provide a means with which to monitor the development of resistance among a normally susceptible population of organisms, and (iv) predict the therapeutic potential of newly discovered investigational agents (44). The development of the Clinical and Laboratory Standards Institute (CLSI; formerly the National Committee for Clinical Laboratory Standards [NCCLS]) reference method M27-A3 (14) has improved the reproducibility of in vitro antifungal susceptibility data and facilitated the establishment of interpretive breakpoints for the triazoles fluconazole, itraconazole, and voriconazole (14, 15, 89, 104) and the echinocandins (85). Based on historical data and the pharmacokinetics of flucytosine, interpretive breakpoints for flucytosine and *Candida* spp. also have been established (15). Some correlation has been suggested between amphotericin B MIC results obtained by nonstandardized methods and clinical outcome. Unfortunately, most M27-A amphotericin B MICs for yeasts are within a very narrow range (0.25 to 1 μg/ml) (14), precluding a clear discrimination between susceptible and potentially resistant isolates. Although the use of Etest or an alternative medium in broth-based tests has been suggested, data are not available for the evaluation of an optimal procedure for the detection of amphotericin B resistance (121).

With the use of both established and investigational agents has come the recognition of resistance to one or more antifungal agents in selected isolates. As a result, clinical laboratories are now being asked to assume a greater role in the selection and monitoring of antifungal chemotherapy. New developments in the standardization of susceptibility testing procedures for both yeast and mold mean that susceptibility testing has become a useful aid in selecting the most appropriate antifungal agent (29, 37, 56, 76). The methods that have been more frequently applied to antifungal susceptibility testing are listed in Table 1. The CLSI Subcommittee on Antifungal Susceptibility Testing has developed reference methods for broth macro- and microdilution susceptibility testing of yeasts (CLSI M27-A3 document) and molds (CLSI M38-A2 document) and more recently a disk diffusion method for yeasts (CLSI M44-A2 document) and a proposed disk diffusion method for molds (M51-P) (Tables 2 to 8) (13–17). The European Committee on Antifungal Susceptibility Testing (EUCAST) has developed a modified broth microdilution method for yeast and has developed breakpoints for itraconazole and fluconazole to be applied to this method (19, 112).

In vitro antifungal susceptibility testing is influenced by a number of technical variables, including inoculum size and preparation, medium formulation and pH, duration and temperature of incubation, and the criterion used for MIC endpoint determination. In addition, antifungal

TABLE 1 Methods used for antifungal susceptibility testing

Test method	Means of endpoint determination
Broth macrodilution (yeasts)	Visual comparison of turbidity (≥50% inhibition) with that of growth control (M27-A3 document)
Broth microdilution (yeasts)	Visual comparison of turbidity (≥50% inhibition) with that of growth control (M27-A3 document)
Colorimetric microdilution (yeasts [YeastOne] and molds)	Visual observation of color change
Spectrophotometric microdilution (yeasts)	Turbidimetric MIC determination by spectrophotometer (EUCAST)
Macro- and microdilution (filamentous fungi)	Visual comparison of growth (50% inhibition or more [nondermatophytes] or 80% or more [dermatophytes] or MEC) with that of growth control (M38-A2 document)
Agar macrodilution (yeasts and molds, standard dishes)	Visual
Agar diffusion (yeasts and molds)	
Disk	Zone diameter (visual)
Antifungal strip (Etest)	Ellipse of inhibition (visual)

TABLE 2 CLSI M27-A3 document broth dilution guidelines for antifungal susceptibility testing of yeasts[a]

Parameter	Description
Broth medium	RPMI 1640 broth buffered with MOPS buffer (0.165 M) and 0.2% dextrose to a pH of 7.0 at 25°C
Medium modifications	(i) Yeast nitrogen base broth (pH 7.0) with MOPS provides better growth for C. neoformans and (ii) RPMI 1640 with 2% dextrose
Inoculum preparation	Five colonies from 24-h (Candida spp.) or 48-h (C. neoformans) cultures on Sabouraud dextrose agar or potato dextrose agar
Stock inoculum suspension	Adjusted by spectrophotometer at 530 nm to match the turbidity of a 0.5 McFarland standard (1×10^6 to 5×10^6 CFU/ml)
Test inoculum	1:2,000 (macrodilution) or 1:1,000 (microdilution) dilutions with medium of the stock inoculum suspension; inoculum size after inoculation, 0.5×10^3 to 2.5×10^3 CFU/ml (both methods)
Drug dilutions	Additive 10× (macrodilution) or 2× (microdilution) twofold drug dilutions with medium (fluconazole, caspofungin, micafungin, and flucytosine) or 100× with solvent (amphotericin B, other azoles, and anidulafungin)
Drug dilution ranges	
Flucytosine and fluconazole	0.12–64 μg/ml
Other drugs	0.03–16 μg/ml
Methods	
Macrodilution	0.9 ml of diluted test inoculum plus 0.1 ml of 10× drug concn
Microdilution	100 μl of diluted test inoculum plus 100 μl of 2× drug concn
Growth control(s)	
Macrodilution	0.9 ml of diluted inoculum plus 0.1 ml of drug-free medium (or plus 2% of solvent)
Microdilution	100 μl of diluted inoculum plus 100 μl of drug-free medium (or plus 2% of solvent)
Time of reading	Amphotericin B, 24 or 48 h; fluconazole, 24 or 48 h; echinocandins, 24 h only; 5-FC and other azoles, 48 h
MIC by visual examination	
Amphotericin B, macro- and microdilution	Lowest drug concn that prevents any discernible growth (100% inhibition)
Flucytosine, azoles, caspofungin, and other echinocandins	Lowest drug concn that shows prominent (~50%) decrease in turbidity

[a]Data from reference 14.

TABLE 3 MIC ranges for QC and reference isolates for CLSI broth macrodilution and microdilution methods[a]

QC or reference isolate	Antifungal agent	MIC range (μg/ml)		
		48 h, macrodilution	24 h, microdilution	48 h, microdilution
QC isolates				
Candida parapsilosis	Amphotericin B	0.25–1.0	0.25–2.0	0.5–4.0
ATCC 22019	Anidulafungin	NA	0.25–2.0	0.5–2.0
	Caspofungin	NA	0.25–1.0	0.5–4.0
	Flucytosine (5FC)	0.12–0.5	0.06–0.25	0.12–0.5
	Fluconazole	2.0–8.0	0.5–4.0	1.0–4.0
	Itraconazole	0.06–0.25	0.12–0.5	0.12–0.5
	Ketoconazole	0.06–0.25	0.03–0.25	0.06–0.5
	Micafungin	NA	0.5–2.0	0.5–4.0
	Posaconazole	NA	0.06–0.25	0.06–0.25
	Ravuconazole	NA	0.016–0.12	0.03–0.25
	Voriconazole	NA	0.016–0.12	0.03–0.25
Candida krusei	Amphotericin B	0.25–2.0	0.5–2.0	1.0–4.0
ATCC 6258	Anidulafungin	NA	0.03–0.12	0.03–0.12
	Caspofungin	NA	0.12–1.0	0.25–1.0
	Flucytosine (5FC)	4.0–16	4.0–16	8.0–32
	Fluconazole	16–64	8.0–64	16–128
	Itraconazole	0.12–0.5	0.12–0.5	0.25–1.0
	Micafungin	NA	0.12–0.5	0.12–0.5
	Ketoconazole	0.12–0.5	0.12–1.0	0.25–1.0
	Posaconazole	NA	0.06–0.5	0.12–1.0
	Ravuconazole	NA	0.06–0.5	0.25–1.0
	Voriconazole	NA	0.06–0.5	0.12–1.0
Paecilomyces variotii	Amphotericin B	NA	NA	1.0–4.0
ATCC MYA-3630	Anidulafungin (MEC)	NA	≤0.015	NA
	Itraconazole	NA	NA	0.06–0.5
	Posaconazole	NA	NA	0.03–0.25
	Voriconazole	NA	NA	0.015–0.12
Reference isolates				
Aspergillus flavus	Amphotericin B	NA	NA	0.5–4.0
ATCC 204304	Itraconazole	NA	NA	0.25–0.5
	Posaconazole	NA	NA	0.06–0.5
	Ravuconazole	NA	NA	0.5–4.0
	Voriconazole	NA	NA	0.5–4.0
Aspergillus flavus	Amphotericin B	NA	NA	1.0–8.0
ATCC MYA-3631	Posaconazole	NA	NA	0.12–1.0
	Voriconazole	NA	NA	0.5–2.0
Aspergillus fumigatus	Amphotericin B	NA	NA	0.5–4.0
ATCC MYA-3626	Anidulafungin (MEC)	NA	≤0.015	NA
	Posaconazole	NA	NA	0.25–2.0
	Voriconazole	NA	NA	0.25–1.0
Aspergillus fumigatus	Amphotericin B	NA	NA	0.5–4.0
ATCC MYA-3627	Itraconazole	NA	NA	≥16
	Voriconazole	NA	NA	0.25–1.0
Aspergillus terreus	Amphotericin B	NA	NA	2.0–8.0
ATCC MYA-3633	Anidulafungin (MEC)	NA	≤0.015	NA
	Voriconazole	NA	NA	0.25–1.0
Fusarium moniliforme	Amphotericin B	NA	NA	2.0–8.0
ATCC MYA-3629	Anidulafungin (MIC)	NA	NA	≥8.0
	Itraconazole	NA	NA	>16
	Posaconazole	NA	NA	0.5–2.0
	Voriconazole	NA	NA	1.0–4.0

(Continued on next page)

TABLE 3 *(Continued)*

QC or reference isolate	Antifungal agent	MIC range (μg/ml)		
		48 h, macrodilution	24 h, microdilution	48 h, microdilution
Fusarium solani ATCC 3636	Anidulafungin (MIC)	NA	NA	≥8.0
Scedosporium apiospermum ATCC MYA-3635	Amphotericin B	NA	NA	4.0–16[c]
	Posaconazole	NA	NA	1.0–4.0[c]
	Voriconazole	NA	NA	0.5–2.0[c]
Scedosporium apiospermum ATCC MYA-3634	Anidulafungin (MEC)	NA	NA	1.0–4.0
Trichophyton mentagrophytes MRL 1957 (ATCC MYA-4439)	Ciclopirox	NA	NA	0.5–2.0[b]
	Griseofulvin	NA	NA	0.12–0.5[b]
	Itraconazole	NA	NA	0.03–0.25[b]
	Posaconazole	NA	NA	0.03–0.25[b]
	Terbinafine	NA	NA	0.002–0.008[b]
	Voriconazole	NA	NA	0.03–0.25[b]
Trichophyton rubrum MRL 666 (ATCC MYA-4438)	Ciclopirox	NA	NA	0.5–2.0[b]
	Fluconazole	NA	NA	0.5–4.0[b]
	Voriconazole	NA	NA	0.008–0.06[b]

[a]Data from CLSI documents M27-S3 (15) and M38-A2 (16). NA, not available (for yeasts) or not applicable (for molds).
[b]After 4 days of incubation.
[c]After 72 h of incubation.

TABLE 4 Zone diameters for QC isolates for CLSI disk diffusion method[a]

Antifungal agent	Disk content (μg)	Zone diameter (mm)			
		C. albicans ATCC 90028	*C. parapsilosis* ATCC 22019	*C. tropicalis* ATCC 750	*C. krusei* ATCC 6258
Caspofungin	5	18–27	14–23	20–27	19–26
Fluconazole	25	28–39	22–33	26–37	—[b]
Posaconazole	5	24–34	25–36	23–33	23–31
Voriconazole	1	31–42	28–37	—[b]	16–25

[a]Data from CLSI document M44-S3 (13).
[b]—, zone diameters not established due to lack of interlaboratory reproducibility.

TABLE 5 CLSI M44-A2 document guidelines for antifungal disk diffusion susceptibility testing of *Candida* spp.[a]

Parameter	Description
Agar medium	Mueller-Hinton agar + 2% dextrose and 0.5 μg of methylene blue dye/ml
Inoculum preparation	From 24-h cultures on Sabouraud dextrose agar as described in Table 2 for broth micro- and macrodilution methods
Test inoculum	Stock inoculum suspension, adjusted by spectrophotometer at 530 nm to match the turbidity of a 0.5 McFarland standard: 1×10^6 to 5×10^6 CFU/ml
Disk contents	Caspofungin, 5 μg; fluconazole, 25 μg; posaconazole, 5 μg; voriconazole, 1 μg
Incubation conditions	20–24 h at 35°C
Reading zone diameter	To the nearest whole millimeter at the point at which there is prominent reduction in growth. Pinpoint microcolonies at the zone edge or large colonies within the zone should be ignored.

[a]Data from CLSI M44-A2 (17).

TABLE 6 Interpretive MIC breakpoints and corresponding zone diameters for in vitro susceptibility testing of *Candida* species with CLSI-recommended methods[a]

Antifungal agent	MIC breakpoint, in μg/ml[b] (zone diameter, in mm[c])				
	Susceptible	Susceptible (dose dependent)	Intermediate	Resistant	Nonsusceptible
Fluconazole[d]	≤8 (≥19)	16–32 (15–18)		≥64 (≤14)	
Voriconazole	≤1 (≥17)	2 (14–16)		≥4 (≤13)	
Itraconazole	≤0.125 (NA)	0.25–0.5 (NA)		≥1 (NA)	
Flucytosine	≤4 (NA)		8–16 (NA)	≥32 (NA)	
Anidulafungin[e]	≤2				>2
Caspofungin[e]	≤2.0 (≥11)				>2 (≤11)
Micafungin[e]	≤2				>2

[a]Subject to modification. Consult the latest CLSI supplements for currently validated breakpoints.
[b]Method performed as described in CLSI document M27-A3 (14).
[c]Method performed as described in CLSI document M44-A2 (17); NA, not available.
[d]Fluconazole breakpoints apply to both 24- and 48-h readings. Isolates of *Candida krusei* are assumed to be intrinsically resistant to fluconazole. The results of fluconazole susceptibility testing of this species (zone diameter and MIC) should not be interpreted using this scale.
[e]There is no Resistant category assigned to the echinocandins; isolates with MICs higher than 2.0 μg/ml may be described as nonsusceptible.

TABLE 7 Optical density ranges for filamentous fungi[a]

Fungus	OD range at 530 nm	Approx mean inoculum size (10^6 CFU/ml)
Alternaria spp.	0.25–0.3	
Aspergillus spp.	0.09–0.13	1.6
Bipolaris spp.	0.25–0.3	0.6
Cladophialophora bantiana	0.15–0.17	1.1
Exophiala dermatitidis	0.09–0.13	
Fusarium spp.	0.15–0.17	3.0
Ochroconis gallopava	0.15–0.17	1.1
Paecilomyces lilacinus	0.09–0.13	2.1
Paecilomyces variotii	0.09–0.13	
Rhizopus arrhizus and other mucoraceous molds	0.15–0.17	1.3
Scedosporium apiospermum	0.15–0.17	1.0
Sporothrix schenckii	0.09–0.13	2.0

[a]Data from CLSI document M38-A2 (16). Suspensions are diluted 1:50 in the standard medium to produce an inoculum density twice that of the final required density (0.4×10^4 to 5×10^4 CFU/ml).

TABLE 8 CLSI M38-A2 document guidelines for broth dilution antifungal susceptibility testing of filamentous fungi[a]

Parameter	Description
Medium for conidial growth	Potato dextrose, 35°C (7 days); *Fusarium* spp. may need 25–28°C incubation for the last 4 days
Inoculum morphology	Conidia or sporangiospores
Recommended OD ranges (see Table 7)	For *Aspergillus* and for *R. arrhizus*, 0.09–0.13; for *Fusarium* and *S. apiospermum*, 0.15–0.17; stock inoculum suspensions, 0.4×10^6–5×10^6 CFU/ml
Inoculum concn (final)	0.4×10^4 to 5×10^4 CFU/ml or 1:50 dilution of stock suspension (*S. apiospermum*, 2:50)
Test medium	RPMI 1640 as for the yeasts (pH, 7.0 ± 0.1)
Format	Microdilution assay; total volume/well, 200 μl
Drug concn	Amphotericin B, ketoconazole, itraconazole, posaconazole, ravuconazole, and voriconazole, 0.0313–16.0 μg/ml; flucytosine and fluconazole, 0.125–64.0 μg/ml; anidulafungin, caspofungin, and micafungin, 0.015–8.0 μg/ml. Different ranges should be used for testing dermatophytes: ciclopirox, 0.06–32 μg/ml; fluconazole and griseofulvin, 0.125–64 μg/ml; itraconazole, voriconazole, and terbinafine, 0.001–0.5 μg/ml; posaconazole, 0.004–8.0 μg/ml.
Incubation duration at 35°C without agitation	For *R. arrhizus* and other mucoraceous molds, 21–26 h; for *Scedosporium* spp., 70–74 h; for most other opportunistic filamentous fungi, 46–50 h. Echinocandin MECs should be read at 21–26 h or at 46–72 h for *Scedosporium* spp.
Endpoint determination, visual	Growth relative to that for positive growth control read with a reading mirror. The MIC is read as the lowest drug concn that substantially inhibits growth (100% for amphotericin B and most azoles, 50% or more for other drugs, 80% or more for dermatophytes). For echinocandins an MEC is determined as the lowest concentration that leads to the growth of small, rounded, compact hyphal forms as compared to the hyphal growth seen in the control well.
Colorimetric (Alamar Blue)	For amphotericin B, first blue well or without color change; for azoles, first blue well or slightly purple well

[a]Data from reference 16.

susceptibility testing is complicated by problems unique to fungi, such as slow growth rates (relative to bacteria) and the ability of certain fungi (dimorphic) to grow either as a unicellular yeast form that produces blastoconidia or as a hyphal or filamentous fungal form that may have the ability to produce conidia or sporangiospores. Finally, the basic properties of the antifungal agents themselves, such as solubility, chemical stability, modes of action, and the tendency to produce partial inhibition of growth over a wide range of concentrations above the MIC, must be taken into account.

SUSCEPTIBILITY TESTING METHODS FOR YEASTS

Standardized Broth Dilution Methods for Yeasts

As a result of several collaborative studies (8, 43, 47, 80), the M27-A3 document (approved standard, 3rd ed.) is available for testing yeasts such as *Candida* spp. and *Cryptococcus neoformans* by both macrodilution and microdilution broth formats (14); breakpoints for fluconazole, itraconazole, voriconazole, anidulafungin, caspofungin, micafungin, and flucytosine versus *Candida* spp. have been established (Table 6), although these may be subject to revision (76a). Other relationships between results obtained with the reference method and patient response have not been established, e.g., among others, for *C. neoformans* and other yeast genera and yeast-like organisms or other agents. The main differences between the previous version (M27-A2/S2) and M27-A3/S3 are the inclusion of quality control (QC) parameters for several new agents, additional breakpoint recommendations, and the reading of amphotericin B and fluconazole MICs after 24 hours of incubation. There are warnings about the applicability of fluconazole breakpoints with *Candida glabrata* isolates and the suggestion that if the MIC is ≤32 μg/ml with this species, patients should receive a maximum-dosage regimen of fluconazole.

Microdilution

The broth microdilution test (Table 2) has become the most widely used technique for antifungal susceptibility testing; this approach is described in the M27-A3 document (14) and also below. Although the antifungal broth macrodilution test was the first method proposed by the CLSI Subcommittee, this test is cumbersome for use in the clinical laboratory. The microdilution test provides consistent MIC results, and interlaboratory agreement of the microdilution MICs can be higher than that of the macrodilution MICs for some drugs (43).

Standard Medium

The test medium recommended by the Subcommittee is the RPMI 1640 broth medium with L-glutamine and a pH indicator and without sodium bicarbonate (04-525Y from BioWhittaker, Walkersville, MD, and American Bioganics, Inc., Niagara Falls, NY; and R-6504 from Sigma Chemical Co., St. Louis, MO). The medium should be buffered to a pH of 7.0 at 25°C with MOPS (morpholinepropanesulfonic acid) (final molarity at pH 7.0, 0.165). The RPMI medium is suitable for testing most fungi (14, 16, 34, 43, 47), but it may not be adequate to support the growth of some strains of *C. neoformans* or to determine amphotericin B MICs. RPMI medium containing 2% dextrose (14, 19) and yeast nitrogen base broth (1, 110) may enhance the growth of yeasts, facilitating the determination of MICs. However, 2% dextrose does not have a significant impact

on the growth density at 24 h and it could falsely elevate the MICs at 48 h (70) and produce lower MICs at 24 h. The EUCAST method includes the use of this modified RPMI medium (19, 112).

Drug Stock Solutions

Antifungal standards can be obtained directly from the drug manufacturers or from the U.S. Pharmacopeia (Rockville, MD). Clinical intravenous or oral preparations should not be used (14, 16). Antifungal stock solutions should be prepared at concentrations at least 10 times the highest concentration to be tested (e.g., 1,280 μg/ml for fluconazole and flucytosine). Solutions of standard powders of flucytosine, fluconazole, caspofungin, or any other water-soluble agent are prepared in distilled water. For testing non-water-soluble agents, sufficient drug standard should be weighed to prepare a solution of 1,600 μg/ml. Commonly used solvents include dimethyl sulfoxide, ethyl alcohol, polyethylene glycol, and carboxymethyl cellulose. The actual amount to be weighed must be adjusted according to the specific biological activity of each standard. Amphotericin B solutions must be protected from light, and drug stock solutions prepared with solvents should be allowed to stand for 30 min before use.

The sterile stock solutions may be stored in small volumes in sterile polypropylene or polyethylene vials carefully sealed at −60°C (preferably) or below for 6 months or more without significant loss of activity but should never be stored at a temperature higher than −20°C. Vials should be removed as needed and used on the same day. Any unused drug should be discarded at the end of the day. The use of QC strains (8, 14, 15, 40, 58), such as those listed in Table 3, will help in evaluating drug activity.

Preparation of Inocula

Inocula should be prepared by the spectrophotometric method (14, 80) as outlined in Table 2. The yeasts are grown on plates of Sabouraud agar (Emmons 11589 Sabouraud dextrose agar from BBL or modified 0747 Sabouraud agar from Difco) or potato dextrose agar at 35°C and subcultured at least twice to ensure purity and viability. The inoculum suspension is prepared by picking five colonies, each at least 1 mm in diameter, from 24-h-old cultures of *Candida* spp. or 48-h-old cultures of *C. neoformans* and suspending the material in 5 ml of sterile 0.85% NaCl. The turbidity of the cell suspension measured at 530 nm is adjusted with sterile saline to match the transmittance produced by a 0.5 McFarland barium sulfate standard. This procedure produces a cell suspension containing 1×10^6 to 5×10^6 CFU/ml, which is then diluted 1:1,000 with RPMI medium to provide the 2× test inoculum (1×10^3 to 5×10^3 CFU/ml). The 2× inoculum is diluted 1:1 when the wells are inoculated to achieve the desired final inoculum size (0.5×10^3 to 2.5×10^3 CFU/ml).

Drug Dilutions and Performance of Microdilution Test for Yeasts

For drugs dissolved in solvents other than water (e.g., the polyenes, itraconazole, posaconazole, voriconazole, and anidulafungin), intermediate test drug dilutions are prepared from stock solutions to be 100 times the strength of the final drug concentration, with 100% solvent (e.g., dimethyl sulfoxide) used as a diluent according to the standard additive twofold drug dilution schema (14) (e.g., 1,600 to 3 μg/ml for amphotericin B, anidulafungin, aminocandin, and all azoles except fluconazole). This procedure prevents precipitation of agents with low solubility in aqueous media. Despite this procedure, itraconazole and some other agents do not remain completely solubilized upon dilution into aqueous media. Thus, at high concentrations, a certain amount of turbidity is encountered and may interfere with the interpretation of MIC endpoints. For water-soluble drugs (e.g., fluconazole and caspofungin), drug dilutions are prepared from the stock to be 10 times the final test drug concentrations directly in RPMI medium according to the additive, twofold drug dilution schema (14) (e.g., 640 to 1.2 µg/ml for fluconazole and flucytosine). The 10× and 100× drug concentrations should be diluted 1:5 and 1:50, respectively, with RPMI to achieve the 2× drug concentrations needed for the microdilution test; after the inoculation step the drug concentrations are 16 to 0.03 µg/ml for amphotericin B, echinocandins, and triazoles and 64 to 0.12 µg/ml for fluconazole and flucytosine.

The broth microdilution test is performed by using sterile, disposable, multiwell microdilution plates (96 U-shaped wells) (e.g., Dynatech Laboratories, Inc., Alexandria, VA). A multichannel pipette (or a large dispensing instrument for 96-well trays) is used to dispense the 2× drug concentrations in 100-µl volumes into the wells of rows 1 to 10 of the microdilution plates. Row 1 contains the highest drug concentration (either 64 or 16 µg/ml), and row 10 contains the lowest drug concentration (either 0.12 or 0.03 µg/ml). Microdilution trays can be stored at −60°C for 3 to 6 months. Each well is inoculated on the day of the test with 100 µl of the corresponding 2× inoculum, which brings the drug dilutions and inoculum densities to the final test concentrations (final volume in each well, 200 µl). The growth control wells contain 100 µl of sterile drug-free medium (for water-soluble agents) or 100 µl of sterile drug-free medium with 2% solvent (for non-water-soluble agents) and are inoculated with 100 µl of the corresponding 2× inoculum. The QC yeasts are tested in the same manner as the other isolates and are included each time an isolate is tested. Row 11 of the microdilution plate can be used for the sterility control (drug-free medium only).

Incubation and Determination of Microdilution MICs for Yeasts

The microdilution plates are incubated at 35°C for 24 to 48 h (*Candida*) and 70 to 74 h (*C. neoformans*) in ambient air. The determination of MIC endpoints is a critical step in antifungal susceptibility testing, especially with the azoles (for yeasts) and echinocandins (for yeasts and molds). The growth in each well is compared with that in the growth control (drug-free) well with the aid of a reading mirror (e.g., Cooke Engineering Co., Alexandria, VA). The MIC for amphotericin B is defined as the lowest concentration at which complete absence of growth (optically clear) is observed.

The partial inhibition or trailing that is observed with flucytosine, the azoles, and most of the new and investigational agents precludes the determination of well-defined endpoints and creates a great deal of variability in interpretation. Therefore, the MIC of flucytosine and the azoles is defined as the lowest concentration at which prominent growth inhibition is observed (~50% or less of the growth in the growth control well) (Table 2). Agitation of the microdilution trays (2) (see below) is highly recommended prior to MIC determination; this step facilitates the visual estimate of prominent growth inhibition. In most instances when testing *Candida* spp., azole MICs may be read following incubation for 24 h. The shorter incubation time minimizes much of the difficulty with trailing and may improve

the clinical correlation slightly (32, 103). Another means to overcome the presence of trailing is the cumbersome measurement of ergosterol production in cells exposed to selected concentrations of fluconazole (6). Heavily trailing endpoints are seen with about 5% of isolates when reading fluconazole MICs, but studies of the in vivo response of such isolates in animal models of infection and in patients with oropharyngeal candidiasis suggest that they respond in the same way to low-dose fluconazole therapy as do fully susceptible strains (6, 103).

Trailing growth is also a problem when reading MICs of the echinocandins for some *Candida* spp. It appears that a 50% inhibition endpoint after 24 h of incubation may be the best approach for the echinocandins when testing yeasts (14, 71).

Macrodilution

Broth macrodilution tests are adequate for the testing of all antifungal agents and are suitable for small laboratories in which the volume of these tests is low. Only the steps and testing conditions that are relevant to the macrodilution test are discussed in detail here (Table 2). Each intermediate drug concentration solution is further diluted (1:10) in RPMI medium to obtain 10 times the final strength (e.g., 160 to 0.3 µg/ml). This step reduces the final solvent concentration to 10%. The 10× drug dilutions are dispensed in 0.1-ml volumes into round-bottom, snap-cap, sterile polystyrene tubes (12 by 75 mm; e.g., Falcon 2054; Becton Dickinson Labware, Lincoln Park, NJ); these tubes can be stored at −60°C for 3 to 6 months. On the day of the test, each tube is inoculated with a 0.9-ml volume of the corresponding diluted yeast inoculum suspension. This step brings the drug dilutions to the final test drug concentrations mentioned above and the corresponding solvent to 1% in each MIC tube. The stock inoculum suspensions are prepared and adjusted as described above for the microdilution test and are then diluted 1:2,000 with RPMI to provide an inoculum of 0.5×10^3 to 2.5×10^3 CFU/ml. The growth control tube(s) is inoculated with a 0.9-ml volume(s) of the inoculum suspension(s) and a 0.1-ml volume(s) of drug-free medium with 1% of the corresponding solvent. The QC yeasts (Table 3) are tested in the same manner as the other isolates and are included each time an isolate is tested. In addition, 1 ml of uninoculated drug-free medium (for water-soluble agents) or drug-free medium with 1% of the corresponding solvent is included as a sterility control.

Incubation and Determination of Macrodilution MICs for Yeasts

The MIC tubes are incubated at 35°C without agitation for 24 to 48 h (*Candida*) and 70 to 74 h (*C. neoformans*) in ambient air; the turbidity or growth in each tube is visually graded. For amphotericin B, the MIC is read as the lowest concentration that prevents any discernible growth. For azoles and flucytosine, the MIC is defined as the lowest drug concentration that causes a prominent decrease in turbidity to about 50% relative to that of the growth control (Table 2) (14).

Quality Control for Yeast Testing

QC of MIC tests is essential to good laboratory practice. *Candida parapsilosis* ATCC 22019 and *Candida krusei* ATCC 6258 have been selected as the QC strains according to the CLSI guidelines for such selection. Table 3 summarizes the expected MIC ranges of 11 antifungal agents for these two QC isolates in both macrodilution (48-h ranges only) and microdilution (both 24- and 48-h ranges) testing

(CLSI M27-S3) (15). Each new batch of medium and lot of macrodilution tubes and microdilution trays should be checked with one of the two QC strains to determine if the MICs are within these ranges (8, 15, 58). In addition, the overall performance of the test system should be monitored by testing either or both QC isolates each day on which a test is performed for each drug. Details regarding corrective measures when the MICs for the QC isolates are not within the expected ranges are found in the M27-A3 document (14). A selection of potentially useful reference strains has been deposited with the American Type Culture Collection (ATCC) (Table 3).

Expected Results

About 95% of clinical yeast isolates are inhibited by ≤8.0 μg of flucytosine/ml (83, 95, 99), although *Candida krusei* isolates tend to have higher levels of resistance (28%) (95). However, isolates of *C. neoformans* for which MICs are ≥16 may be recovered from patients during treatment with flucytosine. *Candida* isolates for which flucytosine MICs are ≥32 μg/ml and ≤4 μg/ml are considered resistant and susceptible, respectively (Table 6) (15). Amphotericin B MICs determined by the microdilution M27-A method are clustered between 0.25 and 1.0 μg/ml for 94% of clinical yeast isolates and >2 μg/ml for the other 6% (14). An amphotericin B MIC of 2.0 μg/ml (or greater) suggests probable clinical resistance, since this MIC only approximates the concentrations achievable in serum at high doses of amphotericin B (1 mg/kg of body weight per day) and exceeds that achievable in cerebrospinal fluid. The difference in amphotericin B MICs for susceptible and potentially resistant isolates is probably very small, so caution should be exercised in the interpretation of results. Although it has been suggested that antibiotic medium 3 provides reliable detection of resistant isolates, lot-to-lot variability has been documented (63). In addition, this medium did not improve the detection of potentially amphotericin B-resistant isolates recovered from patients with candidemia who had failed amphotericin B therapy (microbiologic failure) (69). The application of Etest methodology may more readily detect amphotericin B resistance in vitro (121).

Ketoconazole is fungistatic for most yeast isolates, with MICs of 0.03 to 16 μg/ml by the M27-A3 microdilution method. Fluconazole inhibits the majority (~90%) of *Candida* spp. and *C. neoformans* at concentrations of ≤8 μg/ml; however, MICs for *Candida glabrata* and *C. krusei* generally are 4 to 16 μg/ml and 16 to ≥64 μg/ml, respectively (96). Itraconazole is generally quite active in vitro, with MICs of 0.01 to 1.0 μg/ml or less for most yeast isolates, except for *C. glabrata* (0.06 to 8 μg/ml) and *C. krusei* (0.5 to 2 μg/ml). Overall, ≥99% of isolates of *Candida* spp. and *C. neoformans* are inhibited by ≤1 μg of posaconazole, ravuconazole, or voriconazole per ml, but high voriconazole MICs have been reported for *Sporobolomyces salmonicolor, Rhodotorula rubra,* and for some *Candida albicans* and *C. glabrata* isolates (24, 48, 96). MICs of the echinocandins are usually ≤2 μg/ml for most *Candida* isolates, except for *Candida guilliermondii* and some *C. parapsilosis* and *C. lusitaniae* isolates (24, 28, 68, 97); trailing is observed with these species. Pfaller and Diekema have reported caspofungin susceptibility results on thousands of *Candida* isolates undertaken as part of a global surveillance program to examine geographical and temporal trends (83). Results indicate that >99% of isolates tested in each year since the introduction of caspofungin (2001 to 2004) have MICs of ≤1.0 mg/liter, which mirrors the susceptibility profiles encountered in the years prior to its introduction, suggesting that there is little problem with innate or emerging resistance in this genus.

Broth-Based Alternative Approaches for Yeasts

Although the CLSI methods for in vitro susceptibility testing were essential for standardization and for improving interlaboratory reproducibility, they may not be the best methods for testing all organisms or for routine use in clinical laboratories. Modifications of reference methods offer promise as alternative approaches that may better serve clinical laboratory needs; some of these methods are described below.

Spectrophotometric Methods

Microdilution methods allow the determination of endpoints with automated plate reading and yield MIC values that are more accurate and objective than those by other tests. Agitation of microtiter plates (2) at 50 rpm for at least 5 min by use of a microdilution tray shaker before spectrophotometric MIC determination is essential to obtain homogeneous cell suspensions in the wells and hence a more precise MIC determination. However, the inability to obtain homogeneous cell suspensions with some yeasts demands manual mixing of the cells in each well by using a micropipette tip. The spectrophotometric method allows the determination of different levels (percentages) of growth inhibition (GI), e.g., a GI_{50} corresponds to the first well that shows a 50% decrease in optical density (OD) relative to the OD in the drug-free growth control well. Turbidimetric growth inhibition levels of 50% (GI_{50}) with the azoles and flucytosine and of 90% (GI_{90}) with amphotericin B (530- to 550-nm wavelength) have provided the most accurate values (24, 44, 70, 110).

EUCAST Method

A method similar to the CLSI M27-A3 method for broth microdilution testing of yeasts has been developed under the auspices of the Subcommittee on Antifungal Susceptibility Testing of the EUCAST (19, 112, 114). Although similar to the M27-A3 method (Table 2), this method employs flat-bottom microtiter plates, a higher inoculum (10^5 cells/ml), and RPMI medium supplemented with additional glucose (2%) in order to encourage rapid yeast growth and facilitate early reading (24 h) of endpoints. Moreover, to reduce variation due to observer subjectivity in determination of MIC endpoints, spectrophotometric readings are performed after incubation at 35 to 37°C for 24 h. Although good intralaboratory reproducibility of the EUCAST method as well as good agreement between EUCAST and CLSI microdilution methods has been documented (108), CLSI breakpoints should not be used to interpret EUCAST MICs; the latter MICs are consistently lower than reference values, and falsely susceptible results could be reported (31). EUCAST has reported data on MIC distributions and epidemiological cutoffs for amphotericin B, flucytosine, fluconazole, itraconazole, and voriconazole for *Candida* species and has introduced QC strains (18, 107). With the change in incubation time of the CLSI method to 24 h the two methods are moving closer together. Global collaboration in standardization of an antimicrobial susceptibility testing method is rare but is being encouraged by the International Organization for Standardization, which marks a very positive step in the improvement of antifungal susceptibility testing worldwide.

Colorimetric Methods

Colorimetric indicators or fluorescent dyes can facilitate determination of MIC endpoints. Commercial (Sensititre YeastOne and Fungitest) and noncommercial (tetrazolium salt methods and substrate uptake indicators) procedures have been adapted for antifungal susceptibility testing (21, 44, 45, 77, 90). The Sensititre YeastOne (TREK Diagnostic Systems, Inc., Cleveland, OH) panel follows the same microdilution format as the CLSI reference method and has been approved by the U.S. Food and Drug Administration (FDA) for the testing of fluconazole, itraconazole, and flucytosine. Other systemic antifungal agents including amphotericin B, the extended-spectrum triazoles, and the echinocandins are also available on prepared trays for nondiagnostic use. Reading of endpoints is enhanced by the inclusion of Alamar Blue as the oxidation-reduction colorimetric indicator. If wells remain blue, there is no growth; pink wells indicate growth, and purple wells indicate partial inhibition. Agreement to within two doubling dilutions with reference broth microdilution MICs has been excellent with posaconazole, ravuconazole, and voriconazole (95.4%) and with anidulafungin, caspofungin, and micafungin (100%) all read after 24-h incubation (81, 90). This method minimizes the trailing effect of azoles.

Vitek 2 Yeast Susceptibility Testing

In an effort to automate yeast susceptibility testing, bioMérieux (Hazelwood, MO) has developed the Vitek 2 yeast susceptibility test, a commercial test system based on spectrophotometric analysis. This was shown to produce reproducible, rapid, and accurate results consistent with those produced by the CLSI broth microdilution method for amphotericin B, flucytosine, fluconazole, and voriconazole with several hundred isolates of Candida spp. (86, 87). A recent study has investigated the potential of the Vitek 2 system to specifically detect resistance to fluconazole and voriconazole in 36 isolates of C. albicans and 86 isolates of C. glabrata with well-characterized resistance mechanisms (102). The Vitek 2 system exhibited excellent agreement with the reference broth microdilution method for detecting resistance with overall categorical agreement of 97.5% for both fluconazole and voriconazole. Inclusion of the most recently licensed antifungal agents, posaconazole and the echinocandins, would be a major step in producing rapid, quantitative antifungal susceptibility data to assist in optimizing therapy of invasive candidal infection when resistance to one or more of the established agents is detected. To date, the FDA has only cleared this system for testing fluconazole as part of patient care.

Flow Cytometry

Flow cytometric methods also have been adapted for antifungal susceptibility testing by introducing DNA-binding vital dyes into the culture to detect fungal cell damage after exposure to an antifungal agent (11, 44, 122). MICs determined by this approach have been comparable to those obtained by the M27-A3 methods (11, 122). Although these methods produce faster results (in 4 to 6 h), the need for a flow cytometer for MIC determination would preclude their use in small laboratories; moreover, they are not FDA approved.

Standardized Disk Diffusion Method for Yeasts

Worldwide, the most commonly used technique for antibacterial susceptibility testing is the disk diffusion test, which yields a quantitative result (zones of inhibition) and a qualitative interpretive category (e.g., susceptible or resistant). Agar disk diffusion testing is a simple, flexible, and cost-effective alternative to broth dilution testing. Disk diffusion testing of antifungal agents has been slow to develop despite the fact that early studies with fluconazole disks showed promise for testing Candida spp. The CLSI Subcommittee on Antifungal Susceptibility Testing has developed a disk diffusion method (Table 5) for testing Candida spp. with caspofungin, fluconazole, posaconazole, and voriconazole, although interpretive criteria are available only for caspofungin, fluconazole, and voriconazole and as yet there are no commercially available FDA-approved disks (M44-A2 document) (13, 17). One significant advantage of the M44-A2 disk diffusion method is that results can be obtained after 20 to 24 h of incubation. Early multicenter testing was very positive; a comparison of results of fluconazole disk diffusion testing from 54 laboratories (2,949 isolates of Candida spp.) with results from a central reference laboratory showed an overall categorical agreement of 90.4% with only 0.4% very major (false-susceptible) errors (91). Since then, it has undergone extensive worldwide testing with fluconazole and voriconazole as part of a global survey and performed very well (84). It has also demonstrated good performance with caspofungin (64). The M44 disk test method has also been shown to be a useful approach for determining the susceptibility of C. neoformans and other genera of yeasts (84, 98).

Zone interpretive criteria (Table 6) have been approved for fluconazole, voriconazole, and caspofungin (CLSI M44-S3) (13, 17).

Standard Medium

The CLSI M44-A2 method uses Mueller-Hinton agar supplemented with 2% glucose and 0.5 μg of methylene blue/ml (17). The increased glucose and the methylene blue supplementation improve yeast growth and provide sharper zones surrounding the fluconazole, posaconazole, and voriconazole disks (17); in addition, this medium is readily available and has shown acceptable batch-to-batch reproducibility. The pH of the medium should be 7.2 to 7.4 at room temperature after gelling, and the surface of the agar should be moist, but moisture droplets on the agar surface or on the petri dish cover should not be present (17). The medium can be prepared and poured with the two supplements, or the supplements can be added to commercially prepared Mueller-Hinton agar plates; the latter method enables the use of the routine agar plates from the bacteriology laboratory. A detailed instruction for the preparation of the agar plates is found in the M44-A2 document (17).

Preparation of Inocula

The M44-A2 method employs an inoculum suspension adjusted to the turbidity of a 0.5 McFarland standard by the spectrophotometer, as described above for broth dilution standard methods (Tables 2 and 5) (14, 17).

Performance of Disk Diffusion Method for Yeasts

The agar plates are inoculated within 15 min of adjusting the inoculum suspension as follows (Table 5). Briefly, a sterile cotton swab is dipped into the undiluted inoculum suspension, rotated several times, and pressed firmly against the inside wall of the tube above the fluid level to remove excess fluid. The entire dried agar surface is evenly streaked in three different directions, swabbing the rim of the plate as the final step. The lid of the plate should be left ajar to allow the agar surface to dry for no more than 15 min. Fluconazole (25 μg), posaconazole

(5 μg), voriconazole (1 μg), and caspofungin (5 μg) disks are dispensed onto the inoculated agar surface. Disks must be pressed down to ensure complete contact with the agar and distributed evenly so they are not closer than 24 mm from center to center. After the disks are placed, they cannot be moved because drug diffusion is almost instantaneous. Plates should be incubated within 15 min after disks have been placed (17).

Incubation and Determination of Disk Diffusion Zone Diameters for Yeasts

After 20 to 24 h of incubation at 35°C, the resulting inhibition zones should be uniformly circular and a confluent lawn of growth should be present. The plates are read above a black, nonreflecting background illuminated with reflected light (17). The zone diameters surrounding the 25-μg fluconazole disks, 5-μg posaconazole disks, 1-μg voriconazole disks, and 5-μg caspofungin disks are measured to the nearest whole millimeter at the point at which there is prominent reduction in growth. Pinpoint microcolonies at the zone edge or large colonies within a zone are encountered frequently and should be ignored. If growth is insufficient, the plates should be read at 48 h (Table 5) (17).

Quality Control for Antifungal Susceptibility Disk Testing of Yeasts

QC zone diameter limits have been defined for fluconazole, posaconazole, voriconazole, and caspofungin when testing *Candida* spp. (Table 4) (7, 13, 17, 78).

Agar-Based Alternative Approaches for Yeasts

NeoSensitabs Tablets

A commercial agar diffusion test, Neo-Sensitabs tablets, from Rosco Diagnostica (Rosco Laboratory, Taastrup, Denmark; distributor, Key Scientific Products, Stamford, TX) is available for antifungal susceptibility testing of yeasts. Tablets of established and some of the new antifungal agents (e.g., voriconazole, caspofungin, and posaconazole) are available. Preliminary comparisons with both M27-A2 and M44-A methods have provided promising results (36).

Etest

The Etest (bioMérieux, Marcy l'Etoile, France, and Durham, NC) is based on the diffusion of a stable concentration gradient of an antimicrobial agent from a plastic strip onto an agar medium. Etest strips for amphotericin B, fluconazole, flucytosine, ketoconazole, itraconazole, posaconazole, voriconazole, caspofungin, micafungin, and anidulafungin are commercially available. However, for clinical use FDA has approved only fluconazole, itraconazole, and flucytosine strips. Agreement of Etest and reference MICs has been species and medium dependent; low agreement has been reported for *C. glabrata*, *C. tropicalis*, and *C. neoformans* (44). The medium that provides the best performance for Etest MICs is solidified RPMI medium supplemented with 2% glucose, and reading requires expertise and close adherence to the manufacturer's instructions. If a clear zone is seen, the MIC can easily be read where the zone of inhibition intersects the strip, and false susceptibility has not been reported. Problems can arise when inexperienced readers incorrectly interpret faint background growth of small colonies within the zone as resistance. This is most often seen with fluconazole, and if an isolate is unexpectedly found to be fluconazole resistant by Etest, it should be

retested by a reference method. The Etest may be useful in testing yeasts suspected of being potentially resistant to amphotericin B (74, 79, 121). Amphotericin B MICs of ≥0.38 μg/ml determined by Etest for *Candida* spp. have been associated with therapeutic failure in patients treated with amphotericin B for candidemia (12). However, there are conflicting reports suggesting that even when isolates are tested by this methodology, susceptibility data for *Candida* spp. do not appear to correlate with treatment failure or success, suggesting that factors other than MIC may have a greater impact on the outcome of invasive candidiasis (72). This method has also been evaluated for testing the susceptibilities of *Candida* spp. to triazoles and echinocandins (93, 94).

Fungicidal Activity

Standard testing parameters are not available for the evaluation of the fungicidal activity of antifungal agents. The determination of minimum fungicidal concentrations (MFCs) requires the subculturing onto an agar medium of fixed volumes from each MIC tube or well that shows complete inhibition of growth. The criteria for MFC determination vary in different publications, and the MFC has been described as the lowest drug concentration resulting in either no growth or three to five colonies (9, 101). It has been reported that amphotericin B MFCs can be better predictors of microbiological failure than MICs in candidemia (69) and trichosporonosis (119). The clinical relevance and the development of standard guidelines for MFC determination need to be addressed.

Molecular Methods

There are multiple mechanisms that lead to reduced susceptibility or overt resistance to azole antifungal drugs in *Candida* species; these include changes in cell wall composition leading to reduced uptake, increased efflux, and mutation in the target enzymes (see chapter 127). One or more of these may be present in a cell, and stepwise acquisition appears to be common. Thus, any method for molecular determination of resistance must be a multiplex system and must also be capable of determining not just presence but upregulation of housekeeping genes. For this reason such methods are currently the province of research laboratories. Resistance to echinocandins usually centers around two hot spot mutations of the *FKS* genes, although other mutations have been induced in the laboratory setting. These are easier to detect by simple sequencing (73).

SUSCEPTIBILITY METHODS FOR FILAMENTOUS FUNGI

Standardized Broth Dilution Methods for Molds

Although the number of serious infections caused by the filamentous fungi is lower than the number of yeast infections, antifungal susceptibility testing of these opportunistic pathogens may be important in guiding the selection of antifungal agents for the treatment of invasive disease. On the basis of results from multicenter studies (33, 34, 38, 39, 41), the CLSI Subcommittee has developed both broth micro- and macrodilution methods for testing molds that are more frequently associated with invasive infections (16). These optimal testing conditions are described below (Tables 3, 7, and 8). The other steps are similar to the ones described for broth dilution methods for yeasts (see above).

Microdilution

Standard Medium

The test medium is the same MOPS-buffered standard RPMI recommended for yeast testing (14, 16).

Drug Stock Solutions

Drug stock solutions are prepared as described above for yeast testing (14) and in the CLSI M38-A2 document (16).

Preparation of Inocula

Since nongerminated conidia are easier to prepare and standardize, this is the method of inoculum preparation described in the M38-A2 document (16). A comparison of germinated versus nongerminated conidial suspensions has demonstrated that MICs and MFCs of amphotericin B, itraconazole, posaconazole, and voriconazole for *Aspergillus* spp. are similar or within 2 dilutions with both types of inocula (44).

The inoculum for each isolate is prepared by first growing the mold on potato dextrose agar slants (Remel, Lenexa, KS) for 7 days at 35°C. A conidial suspension is prepared by flooding each slant with approximately 1 ml of sterile 0.85% NaCl. The resulting mixture is withdrawn, and the heavy particles are allowed to settle for 3 to 5 min. The upper homogeneous suspension, containing the mixture of nongerminated conidia or sporangiospores and hyphal fragments, is mixed for 15 s with a vortex. The turbidity of the mixed suspension is measured by using a spectrophotometer at 530 nm and adjusted to a specific final OD range (Table 7) for each species tested (16, 38, 39). Stock inoculum suspensions are diluted 1:50 in medium to obtain 2× the strength needed for the test.

Drug Dilutions and Performance of Microdilution Test for Molds

Drug dilutions are prepared and dispensed in sterile, disposable, multiwell microdilution trays, as described above for yeast testing. On the day of the test, each well is inoculated with 100-μl volumes of the 1:50 conidial or sporangiospore suspensions.

Incubation and Determination of Broth Microdilution MICs for Molds

All microdilution trays are incubated at 35°C, and MICs are determined as described in the M38-A2 document (16) and as recommended for some uncommon molds (38): (i) after 21 to 26 h for *Rhizopus* spp.; (ii) after 46 to 50 h for most other opportunistic filamentous fungi such as *Aspergillus* spp., *Exophiala* spp., *Fusarium* spp., *Paecilomyces* spp., and *Sporothrix schenckii*; and (iii) after 70 to 74 h for *Scedosporium* spp. The MIC endpoint criterion for molds is the lowest drug concentration that shows complete growth inhibition when testing amphotericin B, itraconazole, voriconazole, and posaconazole (16). Experience with both established and investigational agents has demonstrated that MICs for other opportunistic and slower-growing filamentous fungi can be determined (sufficient or heavy growth present in the growth control) after 48 to 96 h of incubation. Testing of the dimorphic fungi may require 5 to 7 days of incubation (24, 44). Endpoint determination with the echinocandin agents is difficult to assess and requires evaluation of the minimum effective concentration (MEC) (see below). For most molds this is read at 21 to 26 h, and for *Scedosporium* spp. it is read at 46 to 72 h.

Macrodilution

Good agreement between results obtained by both micro- and macrodilution methods for molds has been documented (39). Some laboratories would rather perform broth macrodilution testing because of safety concerns and low testing volume. Macrodilution testing conditions are described in the CLSI M38-A2 document (16). Briefly, inoculum stock suspensions and drug dilutions are prepared as for the microdilution test. The 100-fold drug dilutions should be diluted 1:10 with RPMI medium to achieve 10 times the strength needed for the macrodilution test. The stock inoculum suspensions are diluted 1:100 with medium to obtain 0.4×10^4 to 5×10^4 CFU/ml. The 10× drug concentrations are dispensed into 12- by 75-mm sterile tubes in 0.1-ml volumes. Each tube is inoculated on the day of the test with 0.9 ml of the corresponding suspension.

Incubation and Determination of Broth Macrodilution MICs for Molds

Tubes are incubated at 35°C without agitation and observed for the presence or absence of visible growth. The MICs are determined as described above for the microdilution method for molds.

Quality Control for Mold Testing

Either one of the QC yeast organisms or the QC *Paecilomyces variotii* ATCC MYA-3630 isolate may be tested in the same manner as the other mold isolates or as described above for yeasts and should be included each time an isolate is evaluated with any antifungal agent. In addition, other molds have been selected as reference isolates (Table 3) (40).

Expected Results

Amphotericin B MICs determined by the M38-A2 microdilution method are ≤1.0 μg/ml for most mold species. High amphotericin B MICs (>2 μg/ml) have been reported for *Paecilomyces lilacinus*, most *Scedosporium apiospermum* isolates, *Scedosporium prolificans*, and some isolates of *Alternaria* spp., *Aspergillus* spp. (especially *A. terreus*), *Fusarium* spp., *Penicillium marneffei*, *Phialophora* spp., and *S. schenckii* (25, 29, 42, 44). MICs of itraconazole are also usually ≤2.0 μg/ml; the exceptions are its high MICs for *Aspergillus ustus/calidoustus* (some isolates), *Fusarium solani*, *Fusarium oxysporum*, *P. lilacinus*, *S. schenckii*, *S. prolificans*, *Trichoderma longibrachiatum*, and some isolates of *Rhizopus arrhizus* (25, 29, 42, 44). Similar results are obtained with the other triazoles, but in addition good in vitro activity against the mucoraceous molds has been reported with posaconazole (20, 115).

Publications have cited resistance to itraconazole and some cross-resistance to voriconazole in *Aspergillus fumigatus* from certain chronic clinical conditions necessitating long-term use of these agents (22, 55). More recently there has been a report from The Netherlands of azole resistance in 6 to 12.8% of recent clinical isolates (118). However, a recent publication of more than 700 clinical isolates of *Aspergillus* spp. showed that only 2.2% had itraconazole MIC of ≥4 μg/ml (resistant) although a further 9.6% had a MIC of 2.0 μg/ml (intermediate) (106). A group of 43 isolates with itraconazole MICs higher than the normal epidemiological cutoff levels was examined for cross-resistance to other triazoles. Cross-resistance to posaconazole was encountered in 53.5% of the isolates, whereas only 7% of the isolates appeared to be cross-resistant to voriconazole (88).

EUCAST Method for Molds

EUCAST has developed a method for the susceptibility testing of filamentous fungi in which test parameters are similar to the CLSI method M38-A2 but, as with the yeast method, differ in the addition of 2% glucose to the RPMI broth and a higher inoculum concentration (2×10^5 to 5×10^5 CFU/ml) (113). Under these test conditions EUCAST has proposed epidemiological cutoffs of ≤ 1 μg/ml for itraconazole, ravuconazole, and voriconazole with *A. fumigatus* and a lower cutoff of ≤ 0.25 μg/ml for posaconazole (106). Identical epidemiological cutoffs have been proposed for the CLSI method with *A. fumigatus* (88).

Broth Microdilution Method for Dermatophytes

Susceptibility testing of dermatophytes has lagged behind that of other molds, but the M38-A2 broth microdilution method has been successfully adapted, with minor modifications, to the testing of dermatophytes (51, 52). These modifications include the use of oatmeal agar for inoculum preparation when testing *Trichophyton rubrum* in order to induce conidium formation and 4 to 5 days of incubation at 35°C for MIC determination (80% growth inhibition endpoints). Two isolates of *Trichophyton* spp. have been validated as reference strains (Table 3).

Broth-Based Alternative Approaches for Molds

Evaluation of Morphologic Changes

Trailing growth is not a problem when testing investigational or established azoles against most molds. However, when testing the echinocandins, most *Aspergillus* isolates show trailing growth and conventional MIC determination could categorize these trailing isolates as resistant to caspofungin. A more careful examination of the microdilution wells reveals the presence of compact, round microcolonies. Under microscopic examination, these microcolonies correspond to significant morphologic alterations. The hyphae grow abnormally as short, highly branched filaments with swollen germ tubes. Kurtz et al. (59) defined the concentration of drug producing these morphologic changes as the minimum effective concentration (MEC) to distinguish it from conventional MICs. A multicenter study has demonstrated that caspofungin MECs were reliable endpoints in 14 of 17 laboratories (71), and in another study, 8 of these laboratories evaluating anidulafungin MECs against a variety of mold species provided reliable endpoints (41). However, because conflicting results were reported from three laboratories, caution and further refinement of this testing approach are needed.

MICs/MECs of the echinocandins are usually <1.0 μg/ml for *Aspergillus* spp. but higher for other molds (MICs > 8 μg/ml). However, MICs of <1.0 μg/ml have been reported for some isolates of the dimorphic fungi, *Phialophora* spp., and *S. apiospermum* (28).

Colorimetric Methods

The YeastOne method has also been evaluated for molds, and it appears to be applicable for such testing (10, 62, 65). The measurement of metabolic activity by reading the Alamar Blue color change (OD) produced when tetrazolium salts (yellow) are cleaved to their formazan derivative (purple), using a microtiter plate spectrophotometer, has also been evaluated for molds (54, 66). Again, further evaluations, including interlaboratory studies, are needed with more isolates and species.

Agar-Based Alternative Approaches for Filamentous Fungi

As for yeasts, agar-based methods have been applied to susceptibility testing of molds, including agar dilution, disk diffusion, and Etest methods and semisolid agar (60).

Agar Dilution Methods

Agar dilution methods involve the preparation of 10× double dilutions of the agent, which are incorporated into molten agar. Drug-containing plates are inoculated with suspensions of the organism being tested. Since standard methods are not available, the size of the inoculum varies among the different studies.

Disk Diffusion Method

Disk diffusion methodology has been evaluated for amphotericin B, caspofungin, itraconazole, posaconazole, and voriconazole against a wide range of opportunistic pathogenic molds (5, 30, 35, 111). The CLSI Subcommittee is developing a proposed method for testing caspofungin, amphotericin B, and the triazoles (M51-P). It is similar to that for yeasts (M44-A2) but employs Mueller-Hinton agar not supplemented with methylene blue or increased dextrose, as in a collaborative multicenter study these conditions were found to be unsuitable for many molds (30). The inoculum concentration is prepared as for CLSI M38-A2, and plates are inoculated in the same way as in the yeast disk diffusion methodology. After incubation at 35°C for 16 to 24 h for mucoraceous molds, 24 h for *Aspergillus* spp., and 48 h for other molds, there should be a confluent lawn of growth surrounding a circular inhibition zone, which is measured to the nearest whole millimeter. Microcolonies near the zone edge or large isolated colonies within a zone should be ignored for all drugs except amphotericin B (30). Good levels of overall categorical agreement were found in comparisons to CLSI M38 results when testing large numbers of isolates from many mold species. However, there were reservations about using amphotericin B disks except with mucoraceous molds, and the itraconazole disks should not currently be used to test mucoraceous molds but are suitable for other genera (30).

Neo-Sensitabs Diffusion Method for Molds

The Neo-Sensitabs diffusion method, a commercial agar diffusion test, is available in Europe for antifungal susceptibility testing of yeasts, but early studies have proved disappointing for some drug-organism combinations when testing molds (35). The reliability and clinical utility of this method for mold testing need to be assessed in multicenter studies (37).

Etest

The Etest is a convenient method that has also been adapted in several studies for testing mold pathogens (25, 27, 46, 65, 75, 92, 111, 116). Since the trailing effect is not a major problem for azole testing against most molds, Etest inhibition ellipses are usually sharp and MICs are easily interpreted. Overall, comparisons of Etest and M38-A methods have demonstrated better agreement when testing the triazoles (>90%) than amphotericin B (>80%). Amphotericin B Etest MICs for *A. flavus*, *S. apiospermum*, and *S. prolificans* are usually higher than reference values, especially after 48 h of incubation (25). The reliability of the Etest method and the clinical relevance of its MICs for molds should be addressed. Although Etest strips for amphotericin B, anidulafungin, ketoconazole, posaconazole, voriconazole, and caspofungin are commercially available, the FDA has not to date approved any antifungal strip for clinical use in susceptibility testing of molds.

Molecular Tests

The application of molecular methods to the detection of resistance in isolates of filamentous fungi has proven easier in mold isolates than in yeasts as resistance mechanisms appear to be fewer. A multiplex-PCR assay to detect specific *A. fumigatus cyp51A* gene mutations leading to triazole resistance and cross-resistance has been developed (49). Moreover, echinocandin resistance has been detected in clinical isolates by sequencing of the *FKS1* gene (50). Gene expression profiling by Northern blotting and real-time PCR has revealed overexpression of the *FKS1* gene leading to reduced susceptibility in an isolate of *A. fumigatus* from a patient for whom caspofungin therapy had failed (4). Caspofungin resistance of this isolate had not been detected by CLSI or EUCAST broth microdilution MEC tests, but the Etest endpoint and testing in an animal model suggested reduced susceptibility. This suggests that further studies are needed to determine the ideal parameters for the detection of echinocandin resistance.

Fungicidal Activity

A CLSI study has demonstrated that laboratories may reliably perform MFC testing (38) and time-kill curves. In contrast to what is observed with yeasts, the azoles appear to have a certain degree of fungicidal activity as mentioned above for a variety of common and rare opportunistic mold pathogens. MFCs of 0.2 to 4 μg/ml have been reported with the triazoles for various mold species (26, 38). However, standardization of this procedure is needed to reliably assess the potential value of the MFC endpoint in patient management. These standardization efforts should include the correlation of in vitro results with the clearing of target organs of the infecting organism in animal models and the further clinical relevance of MFC data. Recent studies incorporating an indicator of metabolic activity [2,3-bis(2-methoxy-4-nitro-5-sulfophenyl)-2H-tetrazolium-5-carboxanilide] in microdilution broth-based formats have examined fungicidal activity of amphotericin B and voriconazole and have revealed a concentration-dependent sigmoid pattern of fungicidal effects (67). Such developments will need careful evaluation and standardization.

CLINICAL RELEVANCE

In order to be useful clinically, in vitro susceptibility testing should reliably predict the in vivo response to therapy in human infections. However, factors related to the drug, the host immune response and/or the status of the current underlying disease, proper patient management, the infecting organism, and the interactions of the organism with both the host and the therapeutic agent appear to have more value than the MIC as predictors of clinical outcome (104). As so many factors can influence the process of antifungal therapy for an infection caused by a presumably susceptible isolate, a low MIC does not necessarily predict clinical success. However, in vitro resistance may be able to identify, among a population of susceptible strains, those isolates that are less likely to respond to a specific antifungal regimen. In order to appreciate the clinical value of the in vitro antifungal testing result, one must understand that the predictive value of in vitro susceptibility in bacterial infections has been accurately summarized as the "90-60 rule" (105). Infections due to susceptible isolates respond to therapy ~90% of the time, whereas infections due to resistant isolates respond ~60% of the time. There is now a considerable body of data indicating that standardized antifungal susceptibility testing (CLSI M27-A3) for *Candida* spp. and some triazoles provides results that have a predictive utility consistent with the 90-60 rule.

Interpretive MIC breakpoints (Table 6) have been established for fluconazole, itraconazole, and voriconazole following correlation with clinical data (oropharyngeal candidiasis [fluconazole and itraconazole], candidemia in nonneutropenic patients [fluconazole and voriconazole], and other infections [voriconazole]) (13, 14, 104). Isolates inhibited by ≥64 μg of fluconazole per ml and ≥1 μg of itraconazole per ml are considered resistant to these agents, whereas isolates inhibited by ≤8 μg of fluconazole per ml and ≤0.12 g of itraconazole per ml are considered susceptible. In addition, fluconazole MICs of 16 to 32 μg/ml and itraconazole MICs of 0.25 to 0.5 μg/ml have been designated susceptible-dose dependent (S-DD). For fluconazole, this novel designation encompasses isolates in which susceptibility is dependent on achievable peak levels in serum of 40 to 60 μg/ml at fluconazole dosages of 800 mg/day versus the expected peak levels of ≤30 μg/ml at lower dosages. The pharmacodynamic parameter that predicts efficacy for fluconazole is ~25 (area under the concentration-time curve [AUC]/MIC ratio). However, a recent publication highlights the need for a reevalution and the introduction of species-specific breakpoints (76a). For itraconazole, an MIC within the S-DD range indicates the need for serum concentrations of >0.5 μg/ml for an optimal response. However, host factors, rather than azole resistance, can be responsible for clinical failure. Recently, a susceptible breakpoint of ≤1 μg/ml, S-DD of 2 μg/ml, and a resistant breakpoint of ≥4 μg/ml were established for voriconazole and *Candida* spp. (15) (Table 6). Isolates for which the voriconazole MIC is ≥4 μg/ml (resistant endpoint) are mostly *C. glabrata* (>93%) and represent a concentration of voriconazole that cannot be maintained with the currently recommended doses (200 to 300 mg administered orally or an intravenous dose of 4 mg/kg every 12 h); as a consequence, patients infected with these isolates are less likely to respond clinically to voriconazole therapy (<60% response). Therefore, the 60% clinical response rate at the voriconazole-resistant breakpoint is consistent with the 90-60 rule. In support of the susceptible breakpoint of ≤1 μg/ml, concentrations of ≥1 μg/ml in plasma are determined throughout the dosing interval with the recommended doses; the 1-μg/ml MIC encompasses 99% of all clinical isolates of *Candida*. Pharmacokinetics and pharmacodynamic parameters indicate that a 24-h free-drug AUC/MIC ratio of 20 is predictive of efficacy and recommended doses would produce free-drug AUCs of ~20 μg · h/ml (3). Therefore, it can be predicted that current recommended dosing regimens could be used successfully to treat patients infected with isolates for which voriconazole MICs are ≤1 μg/ml as determined by the reference method.

Lack of response to fluconazole therapy has been documented in a few cases of fluconazole resistance in invasive candidal infections (23). In cryptococcal infections, fluconazole MICs of >16 μg/ml have correlated with clinical failure to fluconazole maintenance therapy (1).

For the echinocandins, a susceptible breakpoint of ≤2.0 μg/ml has been proposed for *Candida* spp. based on pharmacokinetic and pharmacodynamic parameters as well as limited correlation with clinical outcome data (M38-A). To date, there have been few reports of clinical failure due to emergent resistance to this class of agents (109), and Kartsonis and colleagues (57) failed to establish any relationship between baseline caspofungin MIC and clinical outcome with isolates from esophageal and invasive *Candida* infections; however, their data set only included three isolates with reduced susceptibility to caspofungin (MIC, $\geq$4.0 mg/liter). For this reason the CLSI Antifungal Subcommittee proposed a "susceptible only" breakpoint MIC of $\leq$2.0 mg/liter for caspofungin, anidulafungin, and micafungin; isolates with MICs of >2.0 mg/liter should be classified as nonsusceptible (85).

Very few correlations of in vitro results with in vivo response have been reported for mold infections (37). Clinical failure with amphotericin B has been associated with MICs of >8.0 μg/ml for *Aspergillus fumigatus* and *Acremonium strictum* and >2 μg/ml for *Scedosporium boydii* infections (37); both primary resistance and acquired resistance have been demonstrated. Clinical failures of itraconazole and amphotericin B in the treatment of aspergillosis have been correlated with MICs of >8 μg/ml and >2 μg/ml, respectively (22, 61). Two recent publications have agreed on epidemiological breakpoints for *A. fumigatus* based on 637 isolates tested by the CLSI method (88) and 393 isolates tested by the EUCAST method (106). The consensus epidemiological cutoff results were $\leq$1.0 μg/ml for itraconazole, ravuconazole, and voriconazole and $\leq$0.25 μg/ml for posaconazole. The agreement between the two methods for testing of *A. fumigatus* and the establishment of wild-type distributions and epidemiological cutoffs is an important development that will enhance surveillance of resistance and facilitate the development of clinical breakpoints for this important mold pathogen.

SUMMARY AND CONCLUSIONS

A great deal of progress has been achieved in the field of antifungal susceptibility testing with both yeasts and filamentous fungi since testing began in earnest in the early 1980s. Standardized broth macrodilution and microdilution methods are available for testing molds and yeasts, as are the 24-h disk diffusion methodology to test caspofungin, fluconazole, posaconazole, and voriconazole against *Candida* spp. and a proposed method for mold disk diffusion. Progress is also being made in establishing the relationship between test results and patient responses to therapy in varied clinical settings and with many of the currently available antifungal agents. However, particularly with filamentous fungi, tests are currently most useful for detecting resistance or outliers based on either assigned in vitro breakpoints or epidemiological cutoffs. Moreover, some commercial methods have been approved for the antifungal susceptibility testing of *Candida* spp. and there is a move towards consensus in the standardized methodology employed in the United States and Europe. This should help to improve surveillance of resistance patterns worldwide and help in the development of universal clinically relevant breakpoints.

REFERENCES

1. Aller, A. I., E. Martin-Mazuelos, F. Lozano, J. Gomez-Mateos, L. Steele-Moore, W. J. Holloway, M. J. Gutiérrez, F. J. Recio, and A. Espinel-Ingroff. 2000. Correlation of fluconazole MICs with clinical outcome in cryptococcal infection. *Antimicrob. Agents Chemother.* 44:1544–1548.
2. Anaissie, E. J., V. L. Paetznick, L. G. Ensign, A. Espinel-Ingroff, J. N. Galgiani, C. A. Hitchcock, M. LaRocco, T. Patterson, M. A. Pfaller, J. H. Rex, and M. G. Rinaldi. 1996. Microdilution antifungal susceptibility testing of *Candida albicans* and *Cryptococcus neoformans* with and without agitation: an eight-center collaborative study. *Antimicrob. Agents Chemother.* 40:2387–2391.
3. Andes, D., K. Marchillo, T. Stamstad, and R. Conklin. 2003. In vivo pharmacokinetics and pharmacodynamics of a new triazole, voriconazole, in a murine candidiasis model. *Antimicrob. Agents Chemother.* 47:3165–3169.
4. Arendrup, M. C., S. Perkhofer, S. J. Howard, G. Garcia-Effron, A. Vishukumar, D. Perlin, and C. Lass-Flörl. 2008. Establishing in vitro-in vivo correlations for *Aspergillus fumigatus*: the challenge of azoles versus echinocandins. *Antimicrob. Agents Chemother.* 52:3504–3511.
5. Arikan, S., V. Paetznick, and J. H. Rex. 2002. Comparative evaluation of disk diffusion with microdilution assay in susceptibility testing of caspofungin against *Aspergillus* and *Fusarium* isolates. *Antimicrob. Agents Chemother.* 46:3084–3087.
6. Arthington-Skaggs, B. A., H. Jradi, T. Desai, and C. J. Morrison. 1999. Quantitation of ergosterol content: novel method for determination of fluconazole susceptibility of *Candida albicans. J. Clin. Microbiol.* 37:3332–3337.
7. Barry, A., J. Bille, S. Brown, D. Ellis, J. Meis, M. Pfaller, R. Rennie, M. Rinaldi, T. Rogers, and M. Traczewski. 2003. Quality control limits for fluconazole disk susceptibility tests on Mueller-Hinton agar with glucose and methylene blue. *J. Clin. Microbiol.* 41:3410–3412.
8. Barry, A. L., M. A. Pfaller, S. D. Brown, A. Espinel-Ingroff, M. A. Ghannoum, C. Knapp, R. P. Rennie, J. H. Rex, and M. G. Rinaldi. 2000. Quality control limits for broth microdilution susceptibility tests of ten antifungal agents. *J. Clin. Microbiol.* 38:3457–3459.
9. Cantón, E., J. Peman, A. Viudes, G. Quindós, M. Gobernado, and A. Espinel-Ingroff. 2003. Minimum fungicidal concentrations of amphotericin B for bloodstream *Candida* species. *Diagn. Microbiol. Infect. Dis.* 45:203–206.
10. Castro, C., M. C. Serrano, B. Flores, A. Espinel-Ingroff, and E. Martin-Mazuelos. 2004. Comparison of the Sensititre YeastOne colorimetric antifungal panel with a modified NC-CLS M38-A method to determine the activity of voriconazole against clinical isolates of *Aspergillus* spp. *J. Clin. Microbiol.* 42:4358–4360.
11. Chaturvedi, V., R. Ramani, and M. A. Pfaller. 2004. Collaborative study of the NCCLS and flow cytometry methods for antifungal susceptibility testing of *Candida albicans*: a two-center collaborative study. *J. Clin. Microbiol.* 42:2249–2251.
12. Clancy, C. J., and M. H. Nguyen. 1999. Correlation between in vitro susceptibility determined by E test and response to therapy with amphotericin B: results from a multicenter prospective study of candidemia. *Antimicrob. Agents Chemother.* 43:1289–1290.
13. Clinical and Laboratory Standards Institute. 2009. *Zone Diameter Interpretive Standards and Corresponding Minimal Inhibitory Concentration (MIC) Interpretive Breakpoints. Supplement M44-S3.* Clinical and Laboratory Standards Institute, Wayne, PA.
14. Clinical and Laboratory Standards Institute. 2008. *Reference Method for Broth Dilution Susceptibility Testing of Yeasts, 3rd ed. Approved Standard. Document M27-A3.* Clinical and Laboratory Standards Institute, Wayne, PA.
15. Clinical and Laboratory Standards Institute. 2008. *Reference Method for Broth Dilution Antifungal Susceptibility Testing of Yeasts; Third Informational Supplement. Supplement M27-S3.* Clinical and Laboratory Standards Institute, Wayne, PA.
16. Clinical and Laboratory Standards Institute. 2008. *Reference Method for Broth Dilution Antifungal Susceptibility Testing of Filamentous Fungi, 2nd ed. Approved Standard. Document M38-A2.* Clinical and Laboratory Standards Institute, Wayne, PA.
17. Clinical and Laboratory Standards Institute. 2009. *Method for Antifungal Disk Diffusion Susceptibility Testing of Yeasts. Approved Guideline, 2nd ed. Document M44-A2.* Clinical and Laboratory Standards Institute, Wayne, PA.
18. Cuenca-Estrella, M., M. C. Arenderup, E. Chrysanthou, E. Danaoui, C. Lass-Florl, P. Sandven, A. Velagraki, and J. L. Rodriguez-Tudela. 2007. Multicenter determination of quality control strains and quality control ranges for antifungal susceptibility testing of yeasts and filamentous fungi using the methods of the Antifungal Susceptibility Testing Subcommittee on Antimicrobial Susceptibility Testing (AFST-EUCAST). *Clin. Microbiol. Infect.* 13:1018–1022.
19. Cuenca-Estrella, M., C. B. Moore, F. Barchiesi, J. Bille, E. Chryssanthou, D. W. Denning, J. P. Donnelly, F. Dromer,

B. Dupont, J. H. Rex, M. D. Richardson, B. Sancak, P. E. Verweij, L. L. Rodriguez-Tudela, and the AFST Subcommittee of the European Committee on Antimicrobial Susceptibility Testing. 2003. Multicenter evaluation of the reproducibility of the proposed antifungal susceptibility testing method for fermentative yeasts of the Antifungal Susceptibility Testing Subcommittee of the European Committee on Antimicrobial Susceptibility Testing (AFST-EUCAST). *Clin. Microbiol. Infect.* **9:**467–474.

20. Dannaoui, E., J. Meletiadis, J. W. Mouton, J. F. G. M. Meis, P. E. Verweij, and the Eurofong Network. 2003. In vitro susceptibilities of zygomycetes to conventional and new antifungals. *J. Antimicrob. Chemother.* **51:**45–52.

21. Davey, K. G., A. D. Holmes, E. M. Johnson, A. Szekely, and D. W. Warnock. 1998. Comparative evaluation of FUNGITEST and broth microdilution methods for antifungal drug susceptibility testing of *Candida* species and *Cryptococcus neoformans.* *J. Clin. Microbiol.* **36:**926–930.

22. Denning, D. W., S. A. Radford, K. L. Oakley, L. Hall, E. M. Johnson, and D. W. Warnock. 1997. Correlation between in-vitro susceptibility testing to itraconazole and in-vivo outcome of *Aspergillus fumigatus* infection. *J. Antimicrob. Chemother.* **40:**401–414.

23. Espinel-Ingroff, A. 1997. Clinical relevance of antifungal resistance. *Infect. Dis. Clin. N. Am.* **11:**929–944.

24. Espinel-Ingroff, A. 1998. Comparison of in vitro activities of the new triazole SCH56592 and the echinocandins MK-0991 (L-743,872) and LY303366 against opportunistic filamentous and dimorphic fungi and yeasts. *J. Clin. Microbiol.* **36:**2950–2956.

25. Espinel-Ingroff, A. 2001. Comparison of the E-test with the NCCLS M38-P method for antifungal susceptibility testing of common and emerging pathogenic filamentous fungi. *J. Clin. Microbiol.* **39:**1360–1367.

26. Espinel-Ingroff, A. 2001. In vitro fungicidal activities of voriconazole, itraconazole, and amphotericin B against opportunistic moniliaceous and dematiaceous fungi. *J. Clin. Microbiol.* **39:**954–958.

27. Espinel-Ingroff, A. 2003. Evaluation of broth microdilution testing parameters and agar diffusion Etest procedure for testing susceptibilities of *Aspergillus* spp. to caspofungin acetate (MK-0991). *J. Clin. Microbiol.* **41:**403–409.

28. Espinel-Ingroff, A. 2003. In vitro antifungal activities of anidulafungin and micafungin, licensed agents and the investigational triazole posaconazole as determined by NCCLS methods for 12,052 fungal isolates: review of the literature. *Rev. Iberoam. Micol.* **20:**121–136.

29. Espinel-Ingroff, A. 2008. In vitro susceptibility testing: when, where and what to use. *J. Invasive Fungal Infect.* **2:**52–61.

30. Espinel-Ingroff, A., B. Arthington-Skaggs, N. Iqbal, D. Ellis, M. A. Pfaller, S. Messer, M. Rinaldi, A. Fothergill, D. L. Gibbs, and A. Wang. 2007. Multicenter evaluation of a new disk agar diffusion method for susceptibility testing of filamentous fungi with voriconazole, posaconazole, itraconazole, amphotericin B, and caspofungin. *J. Clin. Microbiol.* **45:**1811–1820.

31. Espinel-Ingroff, A., F. Barchiesi, M. Cuenca-Estrella, M. A. Pfaller, M. Rinaldi, J. L. Rodríguez-Tudela, and P. E. Verweij. 2005. International and multicenter comparison of EUCAST 7.1 and CLSI M27-A2 broth microdilution methods for testing susceptibilities of *Candida* spp. to fluconazole, itraconazole, posaconazole, and voriconazole. *J. Clin. Microbiol.* **43:**3884–3889.

32. Espinel-Ingroff, A., F. Barchiesi, M. Cuenca-Estrella, A. Fothergill, M. A. Pfaller, M. Rinaldi, J. L. Rodríguez-Tudela, and P. E. Verweij. 2005. Comparison of visual 24-hour and spectrophotometric 48-hour MICs to CLSI microdilution MICs of fluconazole, itraconazole, posaconazole, and voriconazole for *Candida* spp.: a collaborative study. *J. Clin. Microbiol.* **43:**4535–4540.

33. Espinel-Ingroff, A., M. Bartlett, R. Bowden, N. X. Chin, C. Cooper, Jr., A. Fothergill, M. R. McGinnis, P. Menezes, S. A. Messer, P. W. Nelson, F. C. Odds, L. Pasarell, J. Peter, M. A. Pfaller, J. H. Rex, M. G. Rinaldi, G. S. Shankland, T. Walsh, and I. Weitzman. 1997. Multicenter evaluation of proposed standardized procedure for antifungal susceptibility testing of filamentous fungi. *J. Clin. Microbiol.* **35:**139–143.

34. Espinel-Ingroff, A., M. Bartlett, V. Chaturvedi, M. Ghannoum, K. C. Hazen, M. A. Pfaller, M. Rinaldi, and T. J. Walsh. 2001. Optimal susceptibility testing conditions for detection of azole resistance in *Aspergillus* spp.: NCCLS collaborative evaluation. *Antimicrob. Agents Chemother.* **45:**1828–1835.

35. Espinel-Ingroff, A., and E. Canton. 2008. Comparison of Neo-Sensitabs tablet diffusion assay with CLSI broth microdilution M38-A and disk diffusion methods for testing susceptibility of filamentous fungi with amphotericin B, caspofungin, itraconazole, posaconazole, and voriconazole. *J. Clin. Microbiol.* **46:**1793–1803.

36. Espinel-Ingroff, A., E. Canton, D. Gibbs, and A. Wang. 2007. Comparison of Neo-Sensitabs tablet diffusion assay results on three different agar media with CLSI broth microdilution M27-A2 and disk diffusion M44-A results for testing susceptibility of *Candida* spp. and *Cryptococcus neoformans* to amphotericin B, caspofungin, itraconazole, and voriconazole. *J. Clin. Microbiol.* **45:**858–864.

37. Espinel-Ingroff, A., E. Canton, and J. Peman. 2009. Updates in antifungal susceptibility testing of filamentous fungi. *Curr. Fungal Infect. Rep.* **3:**133–141.

38. Espinel-Ingroff, A., V. Chaturvedi, A. Fothergill, and M. G. Rinaldi. 2002. Optimal testing conditions for determining MICs and minimum fungicidal concentrations of new and established antifungal agents for uncommon molds: NCCLS collaborative study. *J. Clin. Microbiol.* **40:**3776–3781.

39. Espinel-Ingroff, A., K. Dawson, M. Pfaller, E. Anaissie, B. Breslin, D. Dixon, A. Fothergill, V. Paetznick, J. Peter, M. Rinaldi, and T. Walsh. 1995. Comparative and collaborative evaluation of standardization of antifungal susceptibility testing for filamentous fungi. *Antimicrob. Agents Chemother.* **39:**314–319.

40. Espinel-Ingroff, A., A. Fothergill, M. Ghannoum, E. Manavathu, L. Ostrosky-Zeichner, M. Pfaller, M. Rinaldi, W. Schell, and T. Walsh. 2005. Quality control and reference guidelines for CLSI broth microdilution susceptibility method (M38-A document) of amphotericin B, itraconazole, posaconazole, and voriconazole. *J. Clin. Microbiol.* **43:**5243–5246.

41. Espinel-Ingroff, A., A. Fothergill, M. Ghannoum, E. Manavathu, L. Ostrosky-Zeichner, M. Pfaller, M. Rinaldi, W. Schell, and T. Walsh. 2007. Quality control and reference guidelines for CLSI broth microdilution method (M38-A) document for susceptibility testing of anidulafungin against moulds. *J. Clin. Microbiol.* **45:**2180–2182.

42. Espinel-Ingroff, A., E. Johnson, H. Hockey, and P. F. Troke. 2008. Activities of voriconazole, itraconazole and amphotericin B in vitro against 590 moulds from 323 patients in voriconazole phase III clinical studies. *J. Antimicrobial. Chemother.* **61:**616–620.

43. Espinel-Ingroff, A., C. W. Kish, Jr., T. M. Kerkering, R. A. Fromtling, K. Bartizal, J. N. Galgiani, K. Villareal, M. A. Pfaller, T. Gerarden, M. G. Rinaldi, and A. Fothergill. 1992. Collaborative comparison of broth macrodilution and microdilution antifungal susceptibility tests. *J. Clin. Microbiol.* **30:**3138–3145.

44. Espinel-Ingroff, A., and M. Pfaller. 2003. Susceptibility test methods: yeasts and filamentous fungi, p. 1972–1986. *In* P. R. Murray, E. J. Baron, J. H. Jorgensen, M. A. Pfaller, and R. H. Yolken (ed.), *Manual of Clinical Microbiology*, 9th ed. ASM Press, Washington, DC.

45. Espinel-Ingroff, A., M. A. Pfaller, S. A. Messer, C. C. Knapp, N. Holliday, and S. B. Killian. 2004. Multicenter comparison of the Sensititre YeastOne colorimetric antifungal panel with the NCCLS M27-A2 reference method for testing new antifungal agents against clinical isolates of *Candida* spp. *J. Clin. Microbiol.* **42:**718–721.

46. Espinel-Ingroff, A., and A. Rezusta. 2002. E-test method for testing susceptibilities of *Aspergillus* spp. to the new triazoles voriconazole and posaconazole and to established antifungal agents: comparison with NCCLS broth microdilution method. *J. Clin. Microbiol.* **40:**2101–2107.

47. Fromtling, R. A., J. N. Galgiani, M. A. Pfaller, A. Espinel-Ingroff, K. F. Bartizal, M. S. Bartlett, B. A. Body, C. Frey, G. Hall, G. D. Roberts, F. B. Nolte, F. C. Odds, M. G. Rinaldi, A. M. Sugar, and K. Villareal. 1993. Multicenter evaluation of a macrobroth antifungal susceptibility test for yeasts. *Antimicrob. Agents Chemother.* **37:**39–45.

48. Fung-Tomc, J. C., E. Huczko, B. Minassian, and D. P. Bonner. 1998. In vitro activity of a new oral triazole, BMS-207147 (ER-30346). *Antimicrob. Agents Chemother.* **42:**313–318.

49. Garci-Effron, G., A. Dilger, L. Alcazar-Fuoli, S. Park, E. Mellado, and D. S. Perlin. 2008. Rapid detection of triazole antifungal resistance in *Aspergillus fumigatus*. *J. Clin. Microbiol.* **46:**1200–1206.

50. Gardiner, R. E., P. Souteropoulis, S. Park, and D. S. Perlin. 2005. Characterization of *Aspergillus fumigatus* mutants with reduced susceptibility to caspofungin. *Med. Mycol.* **43**(Suppl. 1):S299–S305.

51. Ghannoum, M. A., V. Chaturvedi, A. Espinel-Ingroff, M. A. Pfaller, M. G. Rinaldi, W. Lee-Yang, and D. W. Warnock. 2004. Intra- and interlaboratory study of a method for testing the antifungal susceptibilities of dermatophytes. *J. Clin. Microbiol.* **42:**2977–2979.

52. Ghannoum, M. A., N. C. Isham, and D. V. Chand. 2009. Susceptibility testing of dermatophytes. *Curr. Fungal Infect. Rep.* **32:**142–146.

53. Hadfield, T. L., M. B. Smith, R. E. Winn, M. G. Rinaldi, and C. Guerra. 1987. Mycoses caused by *Candida lusitaniae*. *Rev. Infect. Dis.* **9:**1006–1012.

54. Hawser, S. P., C. Jessup, J. Vitullo, and M. A. Ghannoum. 2001. Utility of 2,3-bis(2-methoxy-4-nitro-5-sulfophenyl)-5-[(phenylamino)carbonyl]-2H-tetrazolium hydroxide (XTT) and minimum effective concentration assays in the determination of antifungal susceptibility of *Aspergillus fumigatus* to the lipopeptide class of compounds. *J. Clin. Microbiol.* **39:**2738–2741.

55. Howard, S. J., I. Webster, C. B. Moore, R. E. Gardiner, S. Park, D. S. Perlin, and D. W. Denning. 2006. Multi-azole drug resistance in *Aspergillus fumigatus*. *Int. J. Antimicrob. Agents* **28:**450–453.

56. Johnson, E. M. 2008. Issues in antifungal susceptibility testing. *J. Antimicrob. Chemother.* **61**(Suppl. 1):13–18.

57. Kartsonis, N., J. Killar, L. Mixson, C.-M. Hoe, C. Sable, K. Bartizal, and M. Motyl. 2005. Caspofungin susceptibility testing of isolates from patients with esophageal candidiasis or invasive candidiasis: relationship of MIC to treatment outcome. *Antimicrob. Agents Chemother.* **49:**3616–3623.

58. Krisher, K., S. D. Brown, and M. M. Traczewski. 2004. Quality control parameters for broth microdilution tests of anidulafungin. *J. Clin. Microbiol.* **42:**490.

59. Kurtz, M. B., I. B. Heath, J. Marrinan, S. Dreikom, J. Onishi, and C. Douglas. 1994. Morphological effects of lipopeptides against *Aspergillus fumigatus* correlate with activities against (1,3)-beta-D-glucan synthase. *Antimicrob. Agents Chemother.* **38:**1480–1489.

60. Kuzucu, C., B. Rapino, L. McDermott, and S. Hadley. 2004. Comparison of the semisolid agar antifungal susceptibility test with the NCCLS M38-P broth microdilution test for screening of filamentous fungi. *J. Clin. Microbiol.* **42:**1224–1227.

61. Lass-Flörl, C., G. Kofler, G. Kropshofer, J. Hermans, A. Kreczy, M. P. Dierich, and D. Niederwieser. 1998. In vitro testing of susceptibility to amphotericin B is a reliable predictor of clinical outcome in invasive aspergillosis. *J. Antimicrob. Chemother.* **42:**497–502.

62. Linares, M. J., G. Charriel, F. Solis, F. Rodriguez, A. Ibarra, and M. Casal. 2005. Susceptibility of filamentous fungi to voriconazole tested by two microdilution methods. *J. Clin. Microbiol.* **43:**250–253.

63. Lozano-Chiu, M., P. W. Nelson, M. Lancaster, M. A. Pfaller, and J. H. Rex. 1997. Lot-to-lot variability of antibiotic medium 3 used for testing susceptibility of *Candida* isolates to amphotericin B. *J. Clin. Microbiol.* **35:**270–272.

64. Lozano-Chiu, M., P. W. Nelson, V. L. Paetznick, and J. H. Rex. 1999. Disk diffusion method for determining susceptibilities of *Candida* spp. to MK-0991. *J. Clin. Microbiol.* **37:**1625–1627.

65. Martin-Mazuelos, E., J. Peman, A. Valverde, M. Chaves, M. C. Serrano, and E. Canton. 2003. Comparison of the Sensititre YeastOne colorimetric antifungal panel and Etest with the NCCLS M38-A method to determine the activity of amphotericin B and itraconazole against clinical isolates of *Aspergillus* spp. *J. Antimicrob. Chemother.* **52:**365–370.

66. Meletiadis, J., J. F. G. M. Meis, J. W. Mouton, J. P. Donnelly, and P. E. Verweij. 2000. Comparison of NCCLS and 3-(4,5-dimethyl-2-thiazyl)-2,5-diphenyl-2H-tetrazolium bromide (MTT) methods of in vitro susceptibility testing of filamentous fungi and development of a new simplified method. *J. Clin. Microbiol.* **38:**2949–2954.

67. Meletiadis, J., C. Antachopoulos, T. Stergiopoulos, S. Pournaras, E. Roilides, and T. J. Walsh. 2007. Differential fungicidal activities of amphotericin B and voriconazole against *Aspergillus* species by microbroth methodology. *Antimicrob. Agents Chemother.* **51:**3329–3337.

68. Messer, S. A., J. T. Kirby, H. S. Sader, T. R. Fritsche, and R. N. Jones. 2004. Initial results from a longitudinal international surveillance programme for anidulafungin. *J. Antimicrob. Chemother.* **54:**1051–1056.

69. Nguyen, M. H., C. J. Clancy, V. L. Yu, Y. C. Yu, A. J. Morris, D. R. Snydman, D. A. Sutton, and M. G. Rinaldi. 1998. Do in vitro susceptibility data predict the microbiologic response to amphotericin B? Results of a prospective study of patients with *Candida* fungemia. *J. Infect. Dis.* **177:**425–430.

70. Nguyen, M. H., and C. Y. Yu. 1999. Influence of incubation time, inoculum size, and glucose concentrations on spectrophotometric endpoint determinations for amphotericin B, fluconazole, and itraconazole. *J. Clin. Microbiol.* **37:**141–145.

71. Odds, F. C., M. Motyl, R. Andrade, J. Bille, E. Canton, M. Cuenca-Estrella, A. Davidson, C. Durussel, D. Ellis, E. Foraker, A. W. Fothergill, M. A. Ghannoum, R. A. Giacobbe, M. Gobernado, R. Handke, M. Laverdiere, W. Lee-Yang, W. G. Merz, L. Ostrosky-Zeichner, J. Peman, S. Perea, J. R. Perfect, M. A. Pfaller, L. Proia, J. H. Rex, M. G. Rinaldi, J. Rodriguez-Tuleda, W. A. Schell, C. Shields, D. A. Sutton, P. E. Verweij, and D. W. Warnock. 2004. Interlaboratory comparison of results of susceptibility testing with caspofungin against *Candida* and *Aspergillus* species: an interlaboratory comparison. *J. Clin. Microbiol.* **42:**3475–3482.

72. Park, B. J., B. A. Arthington-Skaggs, R. A. Hajjeh, N. Iqbal, M. A. Ciblak, W. Lee-Yang, M. D. Hairston, M. Phelan, B. D. Plikaytis, A. N. Sofair, L. H. Harrison, S. K. Fridkin, and D. W. Warnock. 2006. Evaluation of amphotericin B interpretive breakpoints for *Candida* bloodstream isolates by correlation with therapeutic outcome. *Antimicrob. Agents Chemother.* **50:**1287–1292.

73. Perlin, D. S. 2007. Resistance to echinocandin-class antifungal drugs. *Drug Resist. Update* **10:**121–130.

74. Peyron, F., A. Favel, A. Michel-Nguyen, M. Gilly, P. Regli, and A. Bolmström. 2001. Improved detection of amphotericin B-resistant isolates of *Candida lusitaniae* by Etest. *J. Clin. Microbiol.* **39:**339–342.

75. Pfaller, J. B., S. A. Messer, R. J. Hollis, D. J. Diekema, and M. A. Pfaller. 2003. In vitro susceptibility testing of *Aspergillus* spp.: comparison of Etest and reference microdilution methods for determining voriconazole and itraconazole MICs. *J. Clin. Microbiol.* **41:**1126–1129.

76. Pfaller, M. A. 2008. New developments in the antifungal susceptibility testing of *Candida*. *Curr. Fungal Infect. Rep.* **2:**125–133.

76a. Pfaller, M. A., D. Andes, D. J. Diekema, A. Espinel-Ingroff, D. Sheehan, and the CLSI Subcommittee for Antifungal Susceptibility Testing. 2010. Wild-type MIC distributions, epidemiological cutoff values, and species-specific clinical breakpoints for fluconazole and *Candida*: time for harmonization of CLSI and EUCAST broth microdilution methods. *Drug Resist. Updates* **13:**180–195.

77. Pfaller, M. A., S. Arikan, M. Lozano-Chiu, Y.-S. Chen, S. Coffman, S. A. Messer, R. Rennie, C. Sand, T. Heffner, J. H. Rex, J. Wang, and N. Yamane. 1998. Clinical evaluation of the ASTY colorimetric microdilution panel for antifungal susceptibility testing. *J. Clin. Microbiol.* **36:**2609–2612.

78. **Pfaller, M. A., A. Barry, J. Bille, S. Brown, D. Ellis, J. F. Meis, R. Rennie, M. Rinaldi, T. Rogers, and M. Traczewski.** 2004. Quality control limits for voriconazole disk susceptibility tests on Mueller-Hinton agar with glucose and methylene blue. *J. Clin. Microbiol.* **42:**1716–1718.

79. **Pfaller, M. A., L. Boyken, S. A. Messer, S. Tendolkar, R. J. Hollis, and D. J. Diekema.** 2004. Evaluation of the Etest method using Mueller-Hinton agar with glucose and methylene blue for determining amphotericin B MICs for 4,936 clinical isolates of *Candida* species. *J. Clin. Microbiol.* **42:**4977–4979.

80. **Pfaller, M. A., L. Burmeister, M. S. Bartlett, and M. G. Rinaldi.** 1988. Multicenter evaluation of four methods of yeast inoculum preparation. *J. Clin. Microbiol.* **26:**1437–1441.

81. **Pfaller, M. A., V. Chateurvedi, D. J. Diekema, M. A. Ghannoum, N. M. Holliday, S. B. Killian, C. C. Knapp, S. A. Messer, A. Miskov, and R. Ramani.** 2008. Clinical evaluation of the Sensititre YeastOne colorimetric antifungal plate for antifungal susceptibility testing of the echinocandins anidulafungin, caspofungin, and micafungin. *J. Clin. Microbiol.* **46:**2155–2159.

82. **Pfaller, M. A., and D. J. Diekema.** 2004. Rare and emerging opportunistic fungal pathogens: concern for resistance beyond *Candida albicans* and *Aspergillus fumigatus.* *J. Clin. Microbiol.* **42:**4419–4431.

83. **Pfaller, M. A., and D. J. Diekema.** 2007. The epidemiology of invasive candidiasis: a persistent public health problem. *Clin. Microbiol. Rev.* **20:**133–163.

84. **Pfaller, M. A., D. J. Diekema, D. L. Gibbs, V. A. Newell, J. F. Meis, I. M. Gould, W. Fu, A. L. Colombo, E. Rodriguez-Noviega, and the Global Antifungal Surveillance Group.** 2007. Results from the ARTEMIS DISK Global Antifungal Surveillance Study, 1997 to 2005: an 8.5 year analysis of susceptibility of *Candida* species and other yeast species to fluconazole and voriconazole determined by CLSI standardized disk diffusion testing. *J. Clin. Microbiol.* **45:**1735–1745.

85. **Pfaller, M. A., D. J. Diekema, L. Ostrosky-Zeichner, J. H. Rex, B. D. Alexander, D. Andes, S. D. Brown, V. Chateurvedi, M. A. Ghannoum, C. C. Knapp, D. J. Sheenan, and T. J. Walsh.** 2008. Correlation of MIC with outcome for *Candida* species tested against caspofungin, anidulafungin, and micafungin: analysis and proposal for interpretive MIC breakpoints. *J. Clin. Microbiol.* **46:**2020–2029.

86. **Pfaller, M. A., D. J. Diekema, G. W. Procop, and M. G. Rinaldi.** 2007. Multicenter comparison of the VITEK 2 yeast susceptibility test with the CLSI broth microdilution reference method for testing fluconazole against *Candida* spp. *J. Clin. Microbiol.* **45:**796–802.

87. **Pfaller, M. A., D. J. Diekema, G. W. Procop, and M. G. Rinaldi.** 2007. Multicenter comparison of the VITEK 2 antifungal susceptibility test with the CLSI broth microdilution reference method for testing amphotericin B, flucytosine, and voriconazole against *Candida* spp. *J. Clin. Microbiol.* **45:**3522–3528.

88. **Pfaller, M. A., D. J. Diekema, M. A. Ghannoum, J. H. Rex, B. D. Alexander, D. Andes, S. D. Brown, V. Chateurvedi, A. Espinel-Ingroff, C. L. Fowler, E. M. Johnson, C. C. Knapp, M. R. Motyl, L. Ostrosky-Zeichner, D. J. Sheenan, T. J. Walsh, and the Clinical and Laboratory Standards Institute Antifungal Testing Subcommittee.** 2009. Wild-type MIC distribution and epidemiological cutoff values for *Aspergillus fumigatus* and three triazoles as determined by the Clinical and Laboratory Standards Institute broth microdilution methods. *J. Clin. Microbiol.* **47:**3142–3146.

89. **Pfaller, M. A., D. J. Diekema, J. H. Rex, A. Espinel-Ingroff, E. M. Johnson, D. Andes, V. Chaturvedi, M. A. Ghannoum, F. C. Odds, M. G. Rinaldi, D. J. Sheehan, P. Troke, T. J. Walsh, and D. W. Warnock.** 2006. Correlation of MIC with outcome for *Candida* species tested against voriconazole: analysis and proposal for interpretive MIC breakpoints. *J. Clin. Microbiol.* **44:**819–826.

90. **Pfaller, M. A., A. Espinel-Ingroff, and R. N. Jones.** 2004. Clinical evaluation of the Sensititre YeastOne colorimetric antifungal plate for antifungal susceptibility testing of the new triazoles voriconazole, posaconazole, and ravuconazole. *J. Clin. Microbiol.* **42:**4577–4580.

91. **Pfaller, M. A., K. C. Hazen, S. A. Messer, L. Boyken, S. Tendolkar, R. J. Hollis, and D. J. Diekema.** 2004. Comparison of fluconazole disk diffusion testing for *Candida* species with results from a central reference laboratory in the ARTEMIS Global Antifungal Surveillance Program. *J. Clin. Microbiol.* **42:**3607–3612.

92. **Pfaller, M. A., S. A. Messer, K. Mills, and A. Bolmström.** 2000. In vitro susceptibility testing of filamentous fungi: comparison of Etest and reference microdilution methods for determining itraconazole MICs. *J. Clin. Microbiol.* **38:**3359–3361.

93. **Pfaller, M. A., S. A. Messer, K. Mills, A. Bolmström, and R. N. Jones.** 2001. Evaluation of Etest method for determining caspofungin (MK-0991) susceptibilities of 726 clinical isolates of *Candida* species. *J. Clin. Microbiol.* **39:**4387–4389.

94. **Pfaller, M. A., S. A. Messer, K. Mills, A. Bolmström, and R. N. Jones.** 2001. Evaluation of Etest method for determining posaconazole MICs for 314 clinical isolates of *Candida* species. *J. Clin. Microbiol.* **39:**3952–3954.

95. **Pfaller, M. A., S. A. Messer, L. Boyken, H. Huynh, R. J. Hollis, and D. J. Diekema.** 2002. In vitro activities of 5-fluorocytosine against 8,803 clinical isolates of *Candida* spp.: global assessment of primary resistance using National Committee for Clinical Laboratory Standards susceptibility testing methods. *Antimicrob. Agents Chemother.* **46:**3518–3521.

96. **Pfaller, M. A., S. A. Messer, L. Boyken, R. J. Hollis, C. Rice, S. Tendolkar, and D. J. Diekema.** 2004. In vitro activities of voriconazole, posaconazole, and fluconazole against 4,169 clinical isolates of *Candida* spp. and *Cryptococcus neoformans* collected during 2001 and 2002 in the ARTEMIS global antifungal surveillance program. *Diagn. Microbiol. Infect. Dis.* **48:**201–205.

97. **Pfaller, M. A., S. A. Messer, L. Boyken, C. Rice, S. Tendolkar, R. J. Hollis, and D. J. Diekema.** 2004. Further standardization of broth microdilution methodology for in vitro susceptibility testing of capsofungin against *Candida* species by use of an international collection of more than 3,000 clinical isolates. *J. Clin. Microbiol.* **42:**3117–3119.

98. **Pfaller, M. A., S. A. Messer, L. Boyken, C. Rice, S. Tendolkar, R. J. Hollis, and D. J. Diekema.** 2004. Evaluation of the NCCLS M44-P disk diffusion method for determining fluconazole susceptibility of 276 clinical isolates of *Cryptococcus neoformans.* *J. Clin. Microbiol.* **42:**380–383.

99. **Pfaller, M. A., S. A. Messer, L. Boyken, C. Rice, S. Tendolkar, R. J. Hollis, G. V. Doern, and D. J. Diekema.** 2005. Global trends in the antifungal susceptibility of *Cryptococcus neoformans:* 1990 to 2004. *J. Clin. Microbiol.* **43:**2163–2167.

100. **Pfaller, M. A., J. H. Rex, and M. G. Rinaldi.** 1997. Antifungal testing: technical advances and potential clinical applications. *Clin. Infect. Dis.* **24:**776–784.

101. **Pfaller, M. A., D. J. Sheehan, and J. H. Rex.** 2004. Determination of fungicidal activity against yeasts and molds: lessons learned from bactericidal testing and the need for standardization. *Clin. Microbiol. Rev.* **17:**268–280.

102. **Posteraro, B., R. Martucci, M. La Sorda, B. Fiori, D. Sanglard, E. De Carolis, A. R. Florio, G. Fadda, and M. Sanguinetti.** 2009. Reliability of the Vitek 2 yeast susceptibility test for the detection of in vitro resistance to fluconazole and voriconazole in clinical isolates of *Candida albicans* and *Candida glabrata.* *J. Clin. Microbiol.* **47:**1927–1930.

103. **Revanker, S. G., W. R. Kirkpatrick, R. K. McAtec, A. W. Fothergill, S. W. Redding, M. G. Rinaldi, and T. F. Patterson.** 1998. Interpretation of trailing endpoints in antifungal susceptibility testing by the National Committee for Clinical Laboratory Standard method. *J. Clin. Microbiol.* **36:**153–156.

104. **Rex, J. H., M. A. Pfaller, J. N. Galgiani, M. S. Bartlett, A. Espinel-Ingroff, M. A. Ghannoum, M. Lancaster, F. C. Odds, M. G. Rinaldi, T. J. Walsh, and A. L. Barry for the Subcommittee on Antifungal Susceptibility Testing of the National Committee for Clinical Laboratory Standards.** 1997. Development of interpretive breakpoints for antifungal susceptibility testing: conceptual framework and analysis of in vitro-in vivo correlation data for fluconazole, itraconazole, and *Candida* infections. *Clin. Infect. Dis.* **24:**235–247.

105. **Rex, J. H., and M. A. Pfaller.** 2002. Has antifungal susceptibility testing come of age? *Clin. Infect. Dis.* **35:**982–989.
106. **Rodriguez-Tudela, J. L., L. Alcazar-Fuoli, E. Mellado, A.
Alastruey-Izquierdo, A. Monzon, and M. Cuenca-Estrella.**
2008. Epidemiological cutoffs and cross-resistance to azole
drugs in *Aspergillus fumigatus. Antimicrob. Agents Chemother.*
52:2468–2472.
107. **Rodriguez-Tudela, J. L., M. Arenderup, E. Chryssanthou,
E. Dannaoui, D. W. Denning, J. P. Donnelly, A.
Schmalrek, P. E. Verweij, and M. Cuenca-Estrella.** 2008.
Minimal inhibitory concentration distributions and epidemiological cut-offs of amphotericin B, flucytosine, fluconazole, itraconazole and voriconazole for *Candida* species
using the EUCAST methodology for susceptibility testing.
Clin. Microbiol. Infect. **14:**982–984.
108. **Rodriguez-Tudela, J. L., J. P. Donnelly, M. A. Pfaller, E.
Chryssanthou, P. Warn, D. W. Denning, A. Espinel-Ingroff,
F. Barchiesi, and M. Cuenca-Estrella.** 2007. Statistical analysis of correlation between fluconazole MICs for *Candida* spp.
assessed by standard methods set forth by the European Committee on Antimicrobial Susceptibility Testing (E.Dis.7.1)
and CLSI (M27-A2). *J. Clin. Microbiol.* **45:**109–111.
109. **Rogers, T. R., E. M. Johnson, and C. E. Munro.** 2007. Echinocandin drug resistance. *J. Invasive Fungal Infect.* **1:**99–105.
110. **Sanati, H., S. A. Messer, M. Pfaller, M. Witt, R. Larsen,
A. Espinel-Ingroff, and M. Ghannoum.** 1996. Multicenter
evaluation of broth microdilution for susceptibility testing of
Cryptococcus neoformans against fluconazole. *J. Clin. Microbiol.* **34:**1280–1282.
111. **Serrano, M. C., M. Ramirez, D. Morilla, A. Valverde, M.
Chavez, A. Espinel-Ingroff, R. Claro, A. Fernandex, C.
Almeida, and E. Martin-Mazuelos.** 2004. A comparative
study of the disc diffusion method with the broth microdilution and Etest methods for voriconazole susceptibility testing
of *Aspergillus* spp. *J. Antimicrob. Chemother.* **53:**739–742.
112. **Subcommittee on Antifungal Susceptibility Testing
(AFST) of the ESCMID European Committee for Antimicrobial Susceptibility Testing (EUCAST).** 2008. EUCAST
definitive document EDef 7.1: method for the determination
of broth dilution MICs of antifungal agents for fermentative
yeasts. *Clin. Microbiol. Infect.* **14:**398–405.
113. **Subcommittee on Antifungal Susceptibility Testing (AFST)
of the ESCMID European Committee for Antimicrobial
Susceptibility Testing (EUCAST).** 2008. EUCAST technical
note on the method for the determination of broth dilution

114. **Subcommittee on Antifungal Susceptibility Testing (AFST)
of the ESCMID European Committee for Antimicrobial
Susceptibility Testing (EUCAST).** 2008. EUCAST technical note on voriconazole. *Clin. Microbiol. Infect.* **14:**985–987.
115. **Sun, Q. N., A. W. Fothergill, D. I. McCarthy, M. G.
Rinaldi, and J. R. Graybill.** 2002. In vitro activities of
posaconazole, itraconazole, voriconazole, amphotericin B,
and fluconazole against 37 clinical isolates of zygomycetes.
Antimicrob. Agents Chemother. **46:**1581–1582.
116. **Szekely, A., E. M. Johnson, and D. W. Warnock.** 1999.
Comparison of E-test and broth microdilution methods
for antifungal drug susceptibility testing of molds. *J. Clin.
Microbiol.* **37:**1480–1483.
117. **Troke, P., K. Aguirrebengoa, C. Arteaga, D. Ellis, C. H.
Heath, I. Lustsar, M. Rovira, Q. Nguyen, M. Slavin, and
S. C. A. Chen on behalf of the Global Scedosporium Study
Group.** 2008. Treatment of scedosporiosis with voriconazole:
clinical experience with 107 patients. *Antimicrob. Agents
Chemother.* **52:**1743–1750.
118. **Verweij, P. E., E. Snelders, G. H. J. Kema, E. Mullado,
and W. J. G. Melchers.** 2009. Azole resistance in *Aspergillus fumigatus:* a side-effect of environmental fungicide use?
Lancet Infect. Dis. **9:**789–795.
119. **Walsh, T. J., G. P. Melcher, M. G. Rinaldi, J. Lecciones, D.
A. McGough, P. Kelly, J. Lee, D. Callender, M. Rubin, and
P. A. Pizzo.** 1990. *Trichosporon beigelii,* an emerging pathogen
resistant to amphotericin B. *J. Clin. Microbiol.* **28:**1616–1622.
120. **Walsh, T. J., H. Teppler, G. R. Donowitz, J. A. Maertens, L. R. Baden, A. Dmoszynska, O. A. Cornely, M. R.
Bourque, R. J. Lupinacci, C. A. Sable, and B. E. dePaw.**
2004. Caspofungin versus liposomal amphotericin B for
empirical antifungal therapy in patients with persistent fever
and neutropenia. *N. Engl. J. Med.* **351:**1391–1402.
121. **Wanger, A., K. Mills, P. W. Nelson, and J. H. Rex.** 1995.
Comparison of Etest and National Committee for Clinical
Laboratory Standards broth macrodilution method for antifungal susceptibility testing: enhanced ability to detect amphotericin B-resistant *Candida* isolates. *Antimicrob. Agents
Chemother.* **39:**2520–2522.
122. **Wenisch, C., C. B. Moore, R. Krause, E. Presterl, P.
Pichna, and D. W. Denning.** 2001. Antifungal susceptibility testing of fluconazole by flow cytometry correlates with
clinical outcome. *J. Clin. Microbiol.* **39:**2458–2462.

PARASITOLOGY

VOLUME EDITOR: DAVID W. WARNOCK

SECTION EDITORS: LYNNE S. GARCIA AND GARY W. PROCOP

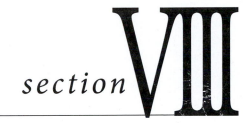

section VIII

Taxonomy and Classification of Human Parasitic Protozoa and Helminths

FRANCIS E. G. COX

129

The term parasite is traditionally applied to several disparate groups of eukaryotic organisms, mainly protozoa and helminths (embracing nematode, cestode, trematode, and acanthocephalan worms) but also some arthropods, annelids, and molluscs. Medical parasitology is concerned with the 200 or so species of helminth worms and about 80 species of protozoa that infect humans. Many of these are rare and accidental parasites, but about 100 species of protozoa and helminths are commonly found in humans, of which a small number are responsible for a disproportionate number of important diseases, particularly in the poorer parts of the world, and these inevitably require and receive the most attention. This chapter is concerned with the classification of the parasitic protozoa and helminths that are commonly encountered in humans together with a number that are only occasionally encountered.

Taxonomy is the science of establishing and defining systematic groups of organisms in a hierarchical manner that reflects the evolutionary past and present relationships among the groups. The basic unit is the species, a grouping in which, among higher organisms, all members are morphologically similar and able to interbreed successfully. The taxonomic groups of higher organisms are largely defined on morphological criteria. The classification of the multicellular helminth worms, which have well-defined morphological characters, clear affinities with free-living species, and characteristic life cycles involving sexual reproduction, is therefore based on sound taxonomic principles. The single-celled protozoa are more difficult to classify and have always constituted an enigmatic group, a subject that is discussed further below.

Over the past 30 years, the five traditionally accepted kingdoms of living organisms, Prokaryota (bacteria), Animalia (animals), Plantae (plants), Fungi (fungi), and Protista, an unnatural assemblage of single-celled eukaryotic organisms including animals, plants, and fungi (19), have been subjects of controversy and have undergone a number of modifications, often on a somewhat arbitrary basis. With the advent of molecular and biochemical techniques, a new consensus has emerged that has made it possible to arrange the so-called "lower organisms" within groups based on evolutionary distances but not necessarily in a hierarchical way. The identification of certain organelles found in eukaryotic cells with their prokaryote origins has now also made it possible to organize all living organisms within a realistic and evolutionarily sound overall scheme (3), and this is the basis of the one adopted here. The most important aspect of this classification is that the major elements in it are compatible with more traditional classifications. Essentially six kingdoms are recognized, the five classical groups, Bacteria, Protozoa, Animalia, Fungi, and Plantae, plus the Stramenopila (formerly Chromista). This classification regards the Protozoa as the basal eukaryotic kingdom and reestablishes the validity of the kingdom Protozoa, thus bringing the protozoa and helminths under the same rules whereby all species are named according to the guidelines set out in the International Code of Zoological Nomenclature (http://www.iczn.org). From a practical point of view, this confers stability in the naming of species and ensures priority for the name originally given while permitting corrections or amendments when necessary. It must be remembered, however, that the International Code is not a panacea for solving all taxonomic problems.

The concept of species as the basic unit that underlies the logical classification of all eukaryotes is scientifically sound but does not necessarily meet the needs of those whose interests are in the diseases caused by parasites and not the parasites themselves. This subject is discussed in some detail by Tibayrenc (25), who points out that there have been some 24 concepts of species and that "Biological researchers need more-pragmatic approaches that can be understood by non-specialists. Decision makers need precise answers for cost-effective and efficient control measures against transmissible diseases." It is worth bearing this in mind when considering the classification adopted here, which is intended to serve simply as a framework within which researchers and "decision-makers" can communicate with one another.

This revised classification has necessitated the redistribution of some taxa, including some parasites of humans, and in this chapter some of the generic and specific names are different from those in the previous edition of this *Manual*, but all such changes can be justified on grounds of new discoveries and interpretations.

CLASSIFICATION OF THE PROTOZOA

There are estimated to be over 200,000 named species of single-celled eukaryotic organisms (8), of which only about 10,000, some 5%, are parasitic; thus, any system of classification must primarily satisfy zoologists and protozoologists working with free-living protozoa. Traditionally, the phylum Protozoa embraced four great groups of single-celled organisms, recognized on the basis of their mode of locomotion: Rhizopoda or Sarcodina (amoebae, moving by pseudopodia), Mastigophora (flagellates, moving by flagella), Ciliophora or Ciliata (ciliates, moving by cilia) and Sporozoa (sporozoans, spore-forming protozoans without any obvious means of locomotion). Rapid developments in our understanding of the protozoa during the 1960s and 1970s necessitated a new classification, and in 1980, the Society of Protozoologists published a classification (18) which recognized seven phyla: Sarcomastigophora (amoebae and flagellates), Apicomplexa (essentially equivalent to the Sporozoa), Ciliophora (ciliates), Microspora, Myxozoa, Ascetospora, and Labyrinthomorpha. However, by the beginning of the 1990s a number of protozoologists (9, 23) had reverted to what was essentially the traditional four "groups": the flagellated protozoa, the amoeboid protozoa, the ciliated protozoa, and the sporozoans (including the microsporidians and myxosporidians). This approach had the merit of simplicity and maintained clear links with the traditional classification but was merely a classification of convenience and did not stand up to rigorous analysis at either the evolutionary or molecular level. Further attempts to resolve this problem resulted in an "interim user friendly" classification (8) that served its purpose well until more rational and natural classifications emerged.

Over the past decade or so, developments in molecular biology have given us a clearer understanding of phylogenetic relationships involving particular groups of single-celled eukaryotic organisms, but unfortunately, this has once again resulted in a plethora of classifications. In 2005, a quarter of a century after the publication of the Society of Protozoologists' classification, another attempt was made by the then International Society of Protozoologists to produce an updated and comprehensive classification of the single-celled eukaryotes, or protists (1). The authors of this classification abandoned the traditional higher taxa in favor of a series of groups and ranks, but the classification is so complex that it is unlikely to be of use to any scientists except specialist protozoologists working with free-living organisms. It now seems unlikely that protozoologists, particularly those working with free-living organisms, will ever come up with a scheme of classification acceptable to everyone. These apparent vacillations have confused parasitologists, (most of whom are concerned with fewer than 0.05% of all species), who simply require a stable framework within which to classify parasites, particularly those

of medical and veterinary importance. As a consequence, the now-outdated 1980 classification continues to appear in recently published and well-respected textbooks (16, 21). This classification has a number of drawbacks that are discussed below. Table 1 summarizes the differences among the traditional, 1980, and current classifications.

The classification in Table 2 is based on that developed over many years by Cavalier-Smith (3–6) and embraces traditional and novel elements, meets the requirements of parasitologists, and bridges the gap between those working with free-living and those working with parasitic protozoa. There are several major and important differences between the traditional (1980) classification and the one outlined below.

1. The myxosporidians, formerly classified among the sporozoans (but which do not affect humans), are now clearly recognized as metazoans and placed in the kingdom Animalia.

2. Microsporidians, some of which do infect humans (mainly immunocompromised individuals), have traditionally been classified with the protozoa sensu strictu but are now known to be more closely related to other fungi than to protozoa and should be classified with the Fungi (15). However, some parasitologists have been reluctant to part with this group, so it seems sensible, at least for time being, to retain the microsporidians alongside the Protozoa while acknowledging that they are, in fact, fungi.

3. The taxonomic position of *Blastocystis* has always been enigmatic, and this genus has been shuffled between the Fungi and Protozoa but is now placed in the kingdom Stramenopila (formerly Chromista) (26).

With the removal of these groups, the Protozoa becomes a kingdom containing between 11 and 13 phyla, depending on which classification is used, of which 7 contain parasites that infect humans. The phylum Amoebozoa, containing the amoebae, is equivalent to the old Rhizopoda (Sarcodina), the flagellates belonging to the former Mastigophora are now distributed among three phyla: Metamonada, Percolozoa, and Euglenozoa. Two phyla remain unchanged, the Ciliophora, containing the ciliates, and the Apicomplexa (Sporozoa). The status of the phylum Apicomplexa requires some explanation. Sporozoa is the traditional name applied to a large group of sexually reproducing, spore-forming protozoans with recognizably similar morphology at the electron microscope level and comparable life cycles. In the 1970s, a new parasite genus, *Perkinsus*, was allocated to this group; this genus, containing parasites of marine molluscs, was quite different from any of the other sporozoans.

TABLE 1 Comparison of the "traditional," "1980," and current classifications of the Protozoa

Common name	Traditional classification	1980 classification	Current classification
Protozoa	Phylum Protozoa	Subkingdom Protozoa	Kingdom Protozoa
Flagellates	Class Mastigophora	Phylum Sarcomastigophora (subphylum Mastigophora)	Phylum Metamonada
			Phylum Parabasalia
			Phylum Percolozoa
			Phylum Euglenozoa
Amoebae	Class Rhizopoda	Phylum Sarcomastigophora (subphylum Sarcodina)	Phylum Amoebozoa
Sporozoans	Class Sporozoa	Phylum Apicomplexa	Phylum Sporozoa
Ciliates	Class Ciliata	Ciliophora	Phylum Ciliophora
Cnidosporidians	Class Cnidosporidia	Phylum Microspora	Now kingdom Fungi
		Phylum Myxozoa	Now kingdom Animalia

TABLE 2 Outline classification of parasitic protozoa and helminths that infect humans[a]

KINGDOM PROTOZOA
  Group 1 (flagellates)
    Phylum Metamonada (flagellates)
      Class Trepomonadea (intestinal flagellates)
        Order Diplomonadida: **Giardia duodenalis,**[b] *Enteromonas hominis*
      Class Retortamonadea (intestinal flagellates)
        Order Retortamonadida: *Chilomastix mesnili, Retortamonas intestinalis*
      Class Trichomonadea (intestinal and related flagellates)
        Order Trichomonadida: **Dientamoeba fragilis, Trichomonas vaginalis,** *T. tenax, Pentatrichomonas hominis*
    Phylum Percolozoa (flagellates and amoebae)
      Class Heterolobosea (free-living and opportunistic flagellated amoebae and amoebae)
        Order Schizopyrenida: **Naegleria fowleri**
    Phylum Euglenozoa (flagellates)
      Class Kinetoplastidea (blood- and tissue-inhabiting flagellates)
        Order Trypanosomatida: **Leishmania donovani, L. infantum, L. major,** *L. tropica, L. braziliensis, L. mexicana,*
          L. aethiopica, L. amazonensis,* L. colombiensis, L. garnhami, L. guyanensis, L. lainsoni,* L. naiffi,* L. panamensis,
          L. peruviana, L. pifanoi, L. shawi,* Leishmania sp. (Thailand), **Trypanosoma cruzi, T. brucei gambiense,**[c] **T. brucei**
          rhodesiense,[c] *T. rangeli*
  Group 2 (amoebae)
    Phylum Amoebozoa (amoebae)
      Class Amoebaea (amoebae, free-living and opportunistic parasites)
        Order Acanthopodida: **Acanthamoeba castellanii,** *A. culbertsoni,* A. hatchetti,* A. polyphaga,** **Balamuthia mandrillaris**
      Class Archamoebae (intestinal amoebae)
        Order: Euamoebida: **Entamoeba histolytica, E. coli, E. dispar, E. hartmanni,** *E. gingivalis, E. moshkovskii,* E. chattoni,**
          E. polecki,* Endolimax nana, Iodamoeba bütschlii
  Group 3 (sporozoans)
    Phylum Apicomplexa (sporozoans and dinoflagellates)
      Subphylum Sporozoa
      Class Coccidea (sporozoan parasites)
        Order Eimeriida: **Cryptosporidium parvum,** *C. baileyi,* C. canis,* C. felis,* C. hominis, C. meleagridis,** **Toxoplasma**
          gondii, Cyclospora cayetanensis, *Isospora belli,* Sarcocystis hominis, S. lindemanni,* S. suihominis*
        Order Piroplasmida: *Babesia duncani,* **B. microti,** *B. divergens,* B. gibsoni,* Babesia* spp.[d]
        Order Haemosporida: **Plasmodium knowlesi,**[e] **P. falciparum, P. malariae, P. ovale, P. vivax**
  Group 4 (ciliates)
    Phylum Ciliophora (ciliates)
      Class Litostomatea (free-living and parasitic ciliates)
        Order Vestibulifera: *Balantidium coli*

KINGDOM STRAMENOPILA (FORMERLY CHROMISTA)
  Subkingdom Chromobiota
    Phylum Bigyra
      Class Blastocystea: **Blastocystis hominis**[f]

KINGDOM FUNGI
  Phylum Microsporidia (microsporidians)[g]: **Encephalitozoon cuniculi,*** *E. hellem,** **E. intestinalis,* Enterocytozoon bieneusi,**
    Nosema ocularum,* Anncaliia (Brachiola) algerae,* A. connori,* A. vesicularum,* Microsporidium ceylonensis,* M. africanum,*
    Pleistophora ronneafiei,* Trachipleistophora hominis,* T. anthropophthera,* Vittaforma corneae

KINGDOM ANIMALIA
  Subkingdom 1, Radiata (no parasites of humans)
  Subkingdom 2, Myxozoa (no parasites of humans)
  Subkingdom 3, Bilateria
    Infrakingdom 1, Ecdysozoa
      Phylum Nemathelminthes (Nematoda, roundworms)
        Class Adenophorea (Aphasmidia)
          Superfamily Trichinelloidea
            Family Trichinellidae: **Trichinella spiralis,** *T. britovi,* T. murrelli,* T. nativa,* T. nelsoni,* T. papuae,**
             T. pseudospiralis,* T. zimbabwensis*
           Family Trichuridae: **Trichuris trichiura,** *T. suis,* T. vulpis,* Capillaria philippinensis (Paracapillaria philippinensis),*
             Capillaria spp.[h]

(Continued on next page)

TABLE 2 Outline classification of parasitic protozoa and helminths that infect humans (*Continued*)

Class Secernentea (Phasmidea)
 Superfamily Ancylostomatoidea
  Family Ancylostomatidae: **Ancylostoma duodenale,** *A. braziliense,*[+] *A. caninum,*[+] *A. ceylanicum, Necator americanus*
 Superfamily Ascaridoidea
  Family Ascarididae: **Ascaris lumbricoides,** *A. suum,*[*] *Toxocara canis,*[+] *T. cati,*[+] *Parascaris equorum,*[+] *Lagochilascaris minor,*[+] *Baylisascaris procyonis*[+]
  Family Anisakidae: *Anisakis physeteris,*[+] *A. simplex,*[+] *Phocanema decipiens*[+]
 Superfamily Dracunculoidea
  Family Dracunculidae: **Dracunculus medinensis**
 Superfamily Filarioidea
  Family Onchocercidae: **Brugia malayi,** *B. timori, B. beaveri,*[*] *B. guyanensis,*[*] **Loa loa, Wuchereria bancrofti, Onchocerca volvulus,** *Dipetalonema* spp.,[*] *Dirofilaria immitis, D. repens, D. striata,*[*] *D. tenuis,*[*] *D. ursi,*[*] *Mansonella ozzardi, M. perstans, M. streptocerca, M. semiclarum, M. rodhaini*[+]
 Superfamily Gnathostomatoidea
  Family Gnathostomatidae: **Gnathostoma spinigerum,**[+] *G. binucleatum,*[+] *Gnathostoma* sp.[+]
 Superfamily Metastrongyloidea
  Family Metastrongylidae: *Metastrongylus elongatus*[*]
  Family Angiostrongylidae: *Parastrongylus cantonensis, P. costaricensis*
 Superfamily Oxyuroidea
  Family Oxyuridae: **Enterobius vermicularis,** *E. gregorii*
 Superfamily Physalopteroidea
  Family Physalopteridae: *Physaloptera caucasica*[*]
 Superfamily Rhabditoidea
  Family Strongyloididae: **Strongyloides fuelleborni, S. stercoralis,** *Strongyloides* spp.[+]
 Superfamily Spiruroidea
  Family Gongylonematidae: *Gongylonema pulchrum*[*]
 Superfamily Strongyloidea
  Family Chabertiidae: *Oesophagostomum bifurcum, Oesophagostomum* spp.,[*] *Ternidens deminutus*
  Family Sygamidae: *Mammomonogamus laryngeus*[*]
 Superfamily Thelazioidea
  Family Thelaziidae: *Thelazia californiensis,*[*] *T. callipaeda*[*]
 Superfamily Trichostrongyloidea
  Family Trichostrongylidae: *Trichostrongylus axei,*[*] *T. brevis,*[*] *T. capricola, T. colubriformis, T. orientalis, T. probolurus, T. skrjabini, T. vitrinus, Trichostrongylus* spp.,[*] *Haemonchus contortus*[*]
  Family Dioctophymatidae: *Dioctophyma renale*
Infrakingdom 2, Platyzoa
 Phylum 1, Acanthognatha (thorny- or spiny-headed worms)
  Class Archiacanthocephala
   Order Moniliformida
    Family Moniliformidae: *Moniliformis moniliformis*[*]
   Order Oligacanthorhynchida
    Family Oligacanthorhynchidae: *Macracanthorhynchus hirudinaceus,*[*] *M. ingens*[*]
 Phylum 2, Platyhelminthes
  Class Trematoda, subclass Digenea (flukes)
   Order Strigeida
    Superfamily Diplostomoidea
     Family Diplostomidae: *Alaria alata,*[+] *A. americana,*[+] *Diplostomum spathaceum,*[+] *Neodiplostomum seoulense*[*]
    Superfamily Gymnophalloidea
     Family Gymnophallidae: *Gymnophalloides*
    Superfamily Schistosomatoidea
     Family Schistosomatidae: **Schistosoma haematobium, S. japonicum, S. mansoni, S. mekongi, S. intercalatum,** *S. bovis,*[+] *S. malayensis,*[+] *S. mattheei, Schistosoma* spp.,[+] *Austrobilharzia terrigalensis,*[+] *Bilharziella polonica,*[+] *Gigantobilharzia sturniae,*[+] *G. huttoni,*[+] *Heterobilharzia americana, Microbilharzia variglandis,*[+] *Orientobilharzia turkestanica,*[+] *Trichobilharzia* spp.[+]
     Family Clinostomidae: *Clinostomum complanatum*[+]
   Order Echinostomida
    Superfamily Echinostomatoidea
     Family: Echinostomatidae *Acanthoparyphium kurogamo,*[*] *A. tyosenense,*[+] *Artyfechinostomum malayanum,*[*] *Echinostoma echinatum, E. hortense,*[*] *E. ilocanum,*[*] *Echinostoma* spp.,[*] *Echinoparyphium recurvatum,*[*] *Echinochasmus* spp.,[*] *Hypoderaeum conoideum*
     Family Fasciolidae: **Fasciola hepatica, Fasciolopsis buski,** *Fasciola gigantica*
    Superfamily Paramphistomoidea
     Family Zygocotylidae: **Gastrodiscoides hominis,** *Watsonius watsoni*[*]

(*Continued on next page*)

TABLE 2 *(Continued)*

          Order Plagiorchiida
             Superfamily Opisthorchioidae
                Family Heterophyidae: *Apophallus donicus,* Heterophyes heterophyes, Heterophyes* spp.,* *Haplorchis* spp.,* *Metagonimus yokogawai, M. takahashi,* M. miyatai, Centrocestus cuspidatus,* C. formosana,* Stellantchasmus falcatus,* Stichodora* spp.,* *Cryptocotyle lingua**
                Family Opisthorchiidae: **Clonorchis sinensis, Opisthorchis felineus, O. viverrini,** *O. guayaquilensis,* Metorchis* spp.,* *Prosthodendrium molenkampi*
             Superfamily Dicrocoelioidea
                Family Dicrocoeliidae: **Dicrocoelium dendriticum,** *Eurytrema pancreaticum**
             Superfamily Plagiorchioidea
                Family Lecithodendriidae: *Phaneropsolus bonnei*
                Family Paragonimidae: **Paragonimus westermani,** *P. africanus, P. heterotremus, P. mexicanus,* P. miyazakii, P. ohirai,* P. pulmonalis, P. skrjabini, P. uterobilateralis, Paragonimus* spp.*
                Family Plagiorchiidae: *Plagiorchis* spp.*
                Family Troglotrematidae: *Nanophyetus salmincola**
                Family Achillurbainiidae: *Achillurbainia* spp.*

        Class Cestoidea (Cestoda, tapeworms)
          Order Pseudophyllidea
             Family Diphyllobothriidae: **Diphyllobothrium latum,** *D. dalliae, D. klebanovskii, D. pacificum, Diphylobothrium* spp.,* *Diplogonoporus grandis, Diplogonoporus* spp.,* *Ligula intestinalis,* Schistocephalus solidus,* Spirometra* spp.*
          Order Cyclophyllidea
             Family Anoplocephalidae: *Bertiella mucronata,* B. studeri,* Inermicapsifer cubensis, I. madagascariensis, Mathevotaenia symmetrica**
            Family Davaineidae: *Buginetta alouattae,* Raillietina celebensis,* R. demerariensis**
            Family Dipylidiidae: *Dipylidium caninum*
             Family Hymenolepididae: **Hymenolepis nana,**[i] *Hymenolepis diminuta*
            Family Mesocestoidae: *Mesocestoides* spp.*
            Family Taeniidae: **Taenia saginata, T. solium,** *Taenia* spp.,* **Echinococcus granulosus,** *E. multilocularis, Echinococcus* spp.,* *Multiceps* spp.*
Subkingdom 4, Mesozoa (no parasites of humans)

---

[a]Parasites in bold type are the most important species. Symbols: *, rare or very rare parasites of humans; +, accidental infections with larval forms and in which the parasite fails to develop to its adult stage.

[z]This organism is also known as *Giardia lamblia* or *G. intestinalis.* Molecular and epidemiological evidence now suggests that at least two assemblages of *Giardia* infect humans, one of which is *Giardia duodenalis* and the other possibly a new species, *G. enterica* (20).

[c]*Trypanosoma brucei gambiense* and *T. brucei rhodesiense* are subspecies but are often referred to as species, *T. gambiense* and *T. rhodesiense.*

[d]Molecular phylogenetic studies of *Babesia* species indicate that humans also harbor a small number of *Babesia* parasites that cannot be identified as *B. divergens, B. microti,* or *B. duncani,* for example, forms from Korea that resemble ovine babesias, a *B. divergens*-like parasite from the United States, two as-yet-unclassified forms from Japan, and others from Brazil, Mexico, China, Taiwan, Egypt, and South Africa (4).

[e]*Plasmodium knowlesi,* a malaria parasite of macaque monkeys in Southeast Asia that occasionally infected humans in the past, has now been established as a naturally transmitted parasite of humans in Malaysia and other parts of Southeast Asia, where it has now caused a number of deaths (11). *Plasmodium knowlesi* now brings the number of human malaria parasites to five.

[f]The designation *Blastocystis hominis* is commonly used in the scientific literature, but it is now clear that this organism exists as a number of serotypes, and it has been recommended that all isolates from birds and mammals, including humans, should be in future designated as *Blastocystis* sp. serotypes ST1 to ST10 plus ST Unknown. Of these, all except ST5 and ST10 have been identified in humans, and all of these except ST9 are found in other hosts (24).

[g]The classification of the microsporidians is in a state of flux pending agreement as to how they should be classified within the fungi, so they are not assigned to any class or order in this classification.

[h]Some zoologists have assigned certain *Capillaria* species, including those found in humans, to other genera (*Calodium, Eucoleus, Pearsonema, Paracapillaria,* and *Crossicapillaria*), but these genera have been largely ignored by medical parasitologists and, in order to avoid confusion, are not listed here.

[i]Zoologists have assigned this worm commonly known as *Hymenolepis nana* to the genus *Rodentolepis* (12), but this change has not been widely accepted by parasitologists working with human parasites.

The phylum Sporozoa was downgraded to a class and the name of the phylum was changed to Apicomplexa in order to incorporate two classes, Sporozoea and Perkinsea (18). Not all parasitologists liked this change, but the word Apicomplexa has gradually crept into the literature and is now widely used. It is now clear that *Perkinsus* spp. do not belong with the sporozoans and should be classified close to, or with, the dinoflagellates (22). Since its original description, the taxon Apicomplexa has also acquired a number of nonparasitic flagellated species belonging to the order Colpodellida; therefore, Apicomplexa now embraces both the traditional sporozoans and a number of nonparasitic species. Unfortunately, Apicomplexa has now become largely synonymous with Sporozoa, and the two names are often used interchangeably. Nevertheless, the compact group of species of most interest to parasitologists, the sporozoans sensu stricto, are members of the class Coccidea in the subphylum Sporozoa, a taxon that has been included in Table 2. Therefore, when considering these important parasitic protozoans, reference should be made to the subphylum Sporozoa and sporozoans rather than to the phylum Apicomplexa and apicomplexans.

OUTLINE CLASSIFICATION OF EUKARYOTIC PARASITES

Table 2 shows an outline classification of parasites, and its sole purpose is to provide a taxonomically sound and convenient set of pigeon holes to which the various parasitic organisms can be assigned. Elsewhere there are full annotated lists of the parasitic protozoa, helminths and arthropods (2), and parasitic helminths (7) of humans and more explanatory classifications of the parasitic protozoa (10) and parasitic helminth worms (12). There are also comprehensive classifications of all the trematode worms, including those found in humans (13, 17).

The levels of the taxa used differ between the protozoa and helminths, and this is deliberate. In the classification of the Protozoa, the higher taxa, subkingdoms and infrakingdoms, have been omitted for simplicity and protozoans are classified as far as orders, as this is the lowest taxonomic level normally used by parasitologists. The groups have been included in the table to enable parasitologists to cross-refer to familiar categories but have no taxonomic significance. Helminth worms are usually classified as far as superfamilies and families, taxa rarely used by protozoologists. For simplicity and clarity, orders are omitted in the lists of nematodes. As well as the formal taxa, common names such as flagellates and flukes widely used by parasitologists are included for convenience. The most important parasites, either because of their capacity to cause disease or because they are very common, and therefore likely to feature in textbooks, are given in bold.

I thank Tom Cavalier-Smith, Department of Zoology, University of Oxford, for his helpful discussions while I was writing this and previous versions of this chapter.

REFERENCES

1. **Adl, S. M., A. G. B. Simpson, M. A. Farmer, R. A. Andersen, O. R. Anderson, J. R. Barta, S. S. Bowser, G. Brugerolle, R. A. Fensome, S. Fredericq, T. Y. James, S. Karpov, P. Kugrens, J. Krug, C. E. Lane, L. A. Lewis, J. Lodge, D. H. Lynn, D. G. Mann, R. M. McCourt, L. Mendoza, Ø. Moestrup, S. E. Mozley-Standridge, T. A. Nerad, C. A. Shearer, A. V. Smirnov, F. W. Spiegel, and M. F. J. R. Taylor.** 2005. The new higher level classification of eukaryotes with emphasis on the taxonomy of protists. *Eukaryot. Microbiol.* **52:**399–451.
2. **Ashford, R. W., and W. Crewe.** 2003. *The Parasites of Homo sapiens,* 2nd ed. Taylor and Francis, London, United Kingdom.
3. **Cavalier-Smith, T.** 1998. A revised six-kingdom system of life. *Biol. Rev.* **73:**203–267.
4. **Cavalier-Smith, T.** 1999. Principles of protein and lipid targeting in secondary symbiogenesis: eugelenoid, dinoflagellate, and sporozoan plastid origins and the eukaryote family tree. *J. Eukaryot. Microbiol.* **46:**347–366.
5. **Cavalier-Smith, T.** 2003. Protist phylogeny and the high-level classification of Protozoa. *Eur. J. Protistol.* **39:**338–348.
6. **Cavalier-Smith, T., and E. E. Chao.** 2004. Protalveolate phylogeny and systematics and the origins of Sporozoa and dinoflagellates (phylum Myzozoa nom. nov.). *Eur. J. Protistol.* **40:**185–212.
7. **Coombs, I., and D. W. T. Crompton.** 1991. *A Guide to Human Helminths.* Taylor and Francis, London, United Kingdom.
8. **Corliss, J. O.** 1994. An interim utilitarian ('user-friendly') hierarchical classification and characterization of the protists. *Acta Protozool.* **3:**31–51.
9. **Cox, F. E. G.** 1991. Systematics of parasitic protozoa, p. 55–80. *In* J. P. Kreier and J. R. Baker (ed.), *Parasitic Protozoa,* 2nd ed., vol. 1. Academic Press Inc., San Diego, CA.
10. **Cox, F. E. G.** 2005. Classification of the parasitic protozoa, p. 186–199. *In* F. E. G. Cox, D. D. Despommier, S. Gillespie, and D. Wakelin (ed.), *Topley and Wilson's Microbiology and Microbial Infections,* 10th ed., part 6. *Parasitology.* Arnold, London, United Kingdom.
11. **Cox-Singh, J., and B. Singh.** 2008. Knowlesi malaria: newly emergent and of public health importance? *Trends Parasitol.* **24:**406–410.
12. **Gibson, D. I.** 2005. Nature and classification of parasitic helminths, p. 573–599. *In* F. E. G. Cox, D. D. Despommier, S. Gillespie, and D. Wakelin (ed.), *Topley and Wilson's Microbiology and Microbial Infections,* 10th ed., part 6. *Parasitology.* Arnold, London, United Kingdom.
13. **Gibson, D. I., A. Jones, and R. A. Bray.** 2002. *Keys to the Trematoda,* vol. 1. CABI Publishing, Wallingford, United Kingdom.
14. **Gray, J. S., and L. M.Weiss.** 2008. *Babesia microti,* p. 303–349. *In* N. A. Khan (ed.), *Emerging Protozoan Pathogens.* Taylor and Francis, New York, NY.
15. **Hirt, R. P., J. M. Logsdon, B. Healey, M. W. Dorey, W. F. Doolittle, and T. M. Embley.** 1999. Microsporidia are related to Fungi: evidence from the largest subunit of RNA polymerase II and other proteins. *Proc. Natl. Acad. Sci. USA* **96:**580–585.
16. **John, D. I., and W. Petri.** 2006. *Markell and Voge's Medical Parasitology,* 9th ed. Elsevier, Amsterdam, The Netherlands.
17. **Jones, A., R. A. Bray, and D. I. Gibson.** 2005. *Keys to the Trematoda,* vol. 2. CABI Publishing, Wallingford, United Kingdom.
18. **Levine, N. D., J. O. Corliss, F. E. G. Cox, G. Deroux, J. Grain, B. M. Honigberg, G. F. Leedale, A. R. Loeblich, J. Lom, D. Flynn, G. Merinfield, F. C. Page, G. Plojansky, V. Sprague, J. Vavra, and F. G. Wallace.** 1980. A newly revised classification of the protozoa. *J. Protozool.* **27:**37–59.
19. **Margulis, L.** 1974. Five-kingdom classification and the origin and evolution of cells. *Evol. Biol.* **7:**45–78.
20. **Monis, P. T., S. M. Caccio, and R. C. A. Thompson.** 2009. Variation in *Giardia:* towards a taxonomic revision of the genus. *Trends Parasitol.* **25:**93–100.
21. **Peters, W., and G. Pasvol.** 2007. *Atlas of Tropical Medicine and Parasitology,* 6th ed. Elsevier, Amsterdam, The Netherlands.
22. **Siddall, M. E., K. S. Reece, J. E. Graves, and E. M. Burreson.** 1997. 'Total evidence' refutes the inclusion of *Perkinsus* species in the phylum Apicomplexa. *Parasitology* **115:**165–176.
23. **Sleigh, M. A.** 1991. The nature of protozoa, p. 1–53. *In* J. P. Kreier and J. R. Baker (ed.), *Parasitic Protozoa,* 2nd ed., vol. 1. Academic Press, San Diego, CA.
24. **Tan, K. S.** 2008. New insights on classification, identification and clinical relevance of *Blastocystis* spp. *Clin. Microbiol. Rev.* **21:**639–665.
25. **Tibayrenc, M.** 2006. The species concept in parasites and other pathogens: a pragmatic approach. *Trends Parasitol.* **22:**66–70.
26. **Webster, J., and R. W. S. Weber.** 2007. *Introduction to Fungi,* 3rd ed. Cambridge University Press, Cambridge, United Kingdom.

Specimen Collection, Transport, and Processing: Parasitology

ROBYN Y. SHIMIZU, FELIX GRIMM, LYNNE S. GARCIA, AND PETER DEPLAZES

130

Routine diagnostic parasitology generally includes laboratory procedures that are designed to detect organisms within clinical specimens by using morphological criteria rather than culture, biochemical tools, and/or physical growth characteristics (Table 1). Parasite identification is frequently based on light microscopic analysis of concentrated and/or stained preparations. Small organisms often require high magnification such as with oil immersion ($\times$1,000) (from 1.5 μm [microsporidia] upwards). Electron microscopy for species characterization of organisms has been replaced in recent years mainly by molecular methods (PCR and sequence analyses of selected genes). Furthermore, new commercial test kits designed especially for detection of antigens (e.g., coproantigens of *Giardia*, *Cryptosporidium*, and *Entamoeba histolytica* [Table 2] or circulating *Plasmodium* antigens [Table 3]) have expanded the methodological repertoire. In addition to those methods for direct parasite detection (morphology, antigens, and DNA), methods for indirect detection of parasite infections demonstrating specific antibodies directed to a variety of native or recombinant parasite antigens have been developed and made commercially available (Table 4). Diagnostic techniques are available to detect a large range of protozoan and helminth species in different clinical specimens. An important precondition for reliable diagnostic results is the proper collection, processing, and examination of clinical specimens. Based on the biology of the parasites and the procedural features of the tests, multiple specimens must often be submitted and examined before the suspected organism(s) is found and its identity is confirmed or a suspected infection can be excluded.

SPECIMEN COLLECTION AND TRANSPORT

Various collection methods are available for specimens suspected of containing parasites or parasitic elements (Tables 5, 6, 7, and 8) (3, 8, 9, 17, 20, 24, 32). When collection methods are selected, the decision should be based on a thorough understanding of the value and limitations of each. The final laboratory results are based on parasite recovery and identification and depend on the initial handling of the specimen. Unless the appropriate specimens are properly collected and processed, these infections may not be detected. Therefore, specimen rejection criteria have become much more important for all diagnostic microbiology procedures.

Diagnostic laboratory results based on improperly collected specimens may require inappropriate expenditures of time and supplies and may also mislead the physician. As a part of any continuous quality improvement program for the laboratory, the generation of test results must begin with stringent criteria for specimen acceptance or rejection. Additionally, diagnostic laboratories should provide clear information on preanalytical requirements to the physicians.

All fresh specimens should be handled carefully, since each specimen represents a potential source of infectious material. Safety precautions should include proper labeling of fixatives; specific areas designated for specimen handling (biological safety cabinets may be necessary under certain circumstances, such as parasite cultures); proper containers for centrifugation; acceptable discard policies; appropriate policies of no eating, drinking, or smoking within the work areas; and, if applicable, correct techniques for organism culture and/or animal inoculation. Precautions must be followed when applicable, particularly when blood and other body fluids are being handled (28, 31).

Collection of Fresh Stool

Collection of stool for parasite detection should always be performed before barium is used for radiological examination. Stool specimens containing the opaque, chalky sulfate suspension of barium are unacceptable for examination, and intestinal protozoa may be undetectable for 5 to 10 days after barium is given to the patient. Certain substances and medications also interfere with the detection of intestinal protozoa; these include mineral oil, bismuth, antibiotics (metronidazole and tetracyclines), antimalarial agents, and nonabsorbable antidiarrheal preparations. After administration of any of these compounds, parasites may not be recovered for a week to several weeks. Therefore, specimen collection should be delayed for 5 to 10 days or at least 2 weeks after barium or antibiotics, respectively, are administered (8, 9, 19, 23). Some laboratories add the following comment to their negative reports: "Certain antibiotics such as metronidazole or tetracycline may interfere with the recovery of intestinal parasites, particularly the protozoa."

Fecal specimens should be collected in clean, wide-mouthed containers; often a waxed cardboard or plastic container with a tight-fitting lid is selected for this purpose. The specimens should not be contaminated with water or urine because water may contain free-living organisms

TABLE 1 Body sites and possible parasites recovered[a]

Site	Parasites
Blood	
RBCs	*Plasmodium* spp., *Babesia* spp.
Leukocytes	*Leishmania* spp., *Toxoplasma gondii*
Whole blood/plasma	*Trypanosoma* spp., microfilariae
Bone marrow	*Leishmania* spp., *Trypanosoma cruzi*, *Plasmodium* spp.
Central nervous system	*Taenia solium* (cysticerci), *Echinococcus* spp., *Naegleria fowleri*, *Acanthamoeba* spp., *Balamuthia mandrillaris*, *Toxoplasma gondii*, microsporidia, *Trypanosoma* spp.
Cutaneous ulcers	*Leishmania* spp., *Acanthamoeba* spp.
Intestinal tract	*Entamoeba histolytica*, *Entamoeba dispar*, *Entamoeba coli*, *Entamoeba hartmanni*, *Endolimax nana*, *Iodamoeba bütschlii*, *Blastocystis hominis*, *Giardia lamblia* (*intestinalis*), *Chilomastix mesnili*, *Dientamoeba fragilis*, *Pentatrichomonas hominis*, *Balantidium coli*, *Cryptosporidium* spp., *Cyclospora cayetanensis*, *Isospora belli*, *Enterocytozoon bieneusi*, *Encephalitozoon* spp., *Ascaris lumbricoides*, *Enterobius vermicularis*, hookworm, *Strongyloides stercoralis*, *Trichuris trichiura*, *Hymenolepis nana*, *Hymenolepis diminuta*, *Taenia saginata*, *Taenia solium*, *Diphyllobothrium latum*, *Clonorchis sinensis* (*Opisthorchis*), *Paragonimus* spp., *Schistosoma* spp., *Fasciolopsis buski*, *Fasciola hepatica*, *Metagonimus yokogawai*, *Heterophyes heterophyes*
Liver, spleen	*Echinococcus* spp., *Entamoeba histolytica*, *Leishmania* spp., microsporidia, *Capillaria hepatica*, *Clonorchis sinensis* (*Opisthorchis*)
Lungs	*Cryptosporidium* spp.,[b] *Echinococcus* spp., *Paragonimus* spp., *Toxoplasma gondii*, helminth larvae
Muscle	*Trichinella* spp., *Taenia solium* (cysticerci), *Onchocerca volvulus* (nodules), *Trypanosoma cruzi*, microsporidia
Skin	*Leishmania* spp., *Onchocerca volvulus*, microfilariae
Urogenital system	*Trichomonas vaginalis*, *Schistosoma* spp., microsporidia, microfilariae
Eyes	*Acanthamoeba* spp., *Toxoplasma gondii*, *Loa loa*, microsporidia, *Thelazia* spp.

[a]Parasites include trophozoites, cysts, oocysts, spores, adults, larvae, eggs, and amastigote and trypomastigote stages. This table does not include every possible parasite that could be found in a particular body site. However, the most likely organisms have been listed.

[b]Disseminated in severely immunosuppressed individuals.

that can be mistaken for human parasites and urine may destroy motile organisms. Stool specimen containers should be placed in plastic bags when transported to the laboratory for testing. If postal delivery services are used, any diagnostic specimens must be packed according to national or international rules (e.g., labeling with UN code 3373; three-container approach). Specimens should be identified with the following information: patient's name and identification number, physician's name, and the date and time the specimen was collected. The specimen must also be accompanied by a request form indicating which laboratory procedures should be performed. The presumptive diagnosis or relevant travel history information is helpful and should accompany the test request. In some situations, it may be necessary to contact the physician for additional patient history.

In the past, it has been recommended that a normal examination for stool parasites before therapy include three specimens. Three specimens, collected as outlined above, have also been recommended for posttherapy examinations. However, a patient who has received treatment for a protozoan infection should be checked 3 to 4 weeks after therapy, and those treated for *Taenia* infections should be checked 5 to 6 weeks after therapy. In many cases, the posttherapy specimens are not collected, often as a cost containment measure; if the patient becomes symptomatic again, additional specimens can be submitted (17, 20).

Although some recommend collection of only one or two specimens, there are differences of opinion regarding this approach. It has also been suggested that three specimens be pooled and examined as a single specimen; again, this approach is somewhat controversial. However, physicians should be aware that the probability of detecting clinically relevant parasites in a single stool specimen may be as low as 50 to 60% but is >95% if three samples are examined (20).

If a series of three specimens is collected, they should be submitted on separate days. If possible, the specimens should be submitted every other day; otherwise, the series of three specimens should be submitted within no more than 10 days. If a series of six specimens is requested, the specimens should also be collected on separate days or within no more than 14 days. Many organisms, particularly the intestinal protozoa, do not appear in the stool in consistent numbers on a daily basis, and the series of three specimens is considered the minimum for an adequate examination. Multiple specimens from the same patient should not be submitted on the same day. One possible exception would be a patient who has severe, watery diarrhea, in whom any organisms present might be missed because of a tremendous dilution factor related to fluid loss. These specimens should be accepted only after consultation with the physician. It is also not recommended that the three specimens be submitted one each day for three consecutive days; however, use of this collection time frame would not be cause enough to reject the specimens.

To evaluate patients who are at risk for giardiasis, the negative predictive value of some of the immunoassays on a single stool specimen is not sufficiently high to exclude the possibility of a *Giardia lamblia* infection. In cases where the clinical suspicion for *G. lamblia* infection is moderate or high and the first assay yields a negative result, testing of a second specimen may be recommended (16).

Fresh specimens are mandatory for the recovery of motile trophozoites (amebae, flagellates, or ciliates). The protozoan trophozoite stage is normally found in cases

TABLE 2 Commercially available kits for immunodetection of parasitic organisms or antigens in stool samples

Organism and kit name[a]	Manufacturer and/or distributor	Type of test[b]	Comment(s)[c]
Cryptosporidium spp.			The tests detect *C. hominis*, different *C. parvum* genotypes, and other species depending on intensity of the infection.
ProSpecT Cryptosporidium Microplate Assay	Remel	EIA	Can be used with fresh, frozen, or formalin-preserved stool; http://www.remel.com
Xpect *Cryptosporidium* Kit	Remel	Cartridge, IC	
PARA-TECT *Cryptosporidium*	Medical Chemical Corp.	EIA	Contact manufacturer; http://www.med-chem.com
Crypto-CELISA	Cellabs	EIA	Can be used with fresh, frozen, or formalin-preserved stool; http://www.cellabs.com
Crypto Cel	Cellabs	DFA	
Cryptosporidium II Test	TechLab	EIA	http://www.techlabinc.com
Cryptosporidium Test	Inverness Medical	EIA	http://www.invernessmedicalpd.com
Cryptosporidium	IVD Research	EIA	http://www.ivdresearch.com
Entamoeba histolytica			These tests differentiate between *E. histolytica* and *E. dispar*.
Entamoeba histolytica II Test	TechLab	EIA	Requires fresh or frozen stool
Entamoeba CELISA Path	Cellabs	EIA	
Entamoeba histolytica/*E. dispar* group			These tests *do not* differentiate *E. histolytica* from *E. dispar*.
ProSpecT *Entamoeba histolytica*	Remel	EIA	
Giardia lamblia			
ProSpecT *Giardia*	Remel	EIA	Different EIA formats; contact manufacturer
PARA-TECT *Giardia*	Medical Chemical	EIA	
Giardia-CELISA	Cellabs	EIA	
Giardia-Cel	Cellabs	DFA	
Xpect *Giardia*	Remel	Cartridge IC	Can be used with fresh, frozen, or formalin-preserved stool
Giardia II	TechLab	EIA	
Giardia lamblia II	Inverness Medical	EIA	
Giardia	IVD Research	EIA	
Combination tests: *Cryptosporidium* and *Giardia*			
ProSpecT *Giardia*/*Cryptosporidium*	Remel	EIA	Can be used with fresh, frozen, or formalin-preserved stool
MERIFLUOR *Cryptosporidium*/*Giardia*	Meridian Bioscience	DFA	http://www.meridianbioscience.com
PARA-TECT *Cryptosporidium*/*Giardia* DFA	Medical Chemical	DFA	
Crypto/Giardia-Cel	Cellabs	DFA	
ImmunoCard STAT! *Cryptosporidium*/*Giardia*	Meridian Bioscience	Cartridge IC	Can be used with fresh, frozen, or formalin-preserved stool
Xpect Giardia/Cryptosporidium	Remel	Cartridge IC	Can be used with fresh, frozen, or formalin-preserved stool
Giardia/*Cryptosporidium* Chek	TechLab	EIA	
Cryptosporidium/*Giardia*	IVD Research	DFA	
Combination tests: *Cryptosporidium*, *Giardia*, and *Entamoeba*			
Triage Parasite Panel	Biosite Diagnostics, Inc.	Cartridge, IC	Requires fresh or frozen stool; combination test with *Giardia* and *E. histolytica*/*E. dispar* group; does not differentiate between *E. histolytica* and *E. dispar*; http://www.biosite.com

[a]A number of the kits are manufactured by a single manufacturer but labeled under different company names; consequently, some of the data for sensitivity and specificity may be identical to those of kits produced under another name or by another company.
[b]EIA, enzyme immunoassay; DFA, direct fluorescent antibody; IC, immunochromatography.
[c]URLs are given only the first time the company name appears in the table.

TABLE 3 Commercially available test kits for immunodetection or molecular detection of parasitic organisms or antigens in serum, plasma, blood, or vaginal discharge

Disease or organism and manufacturer	Test	Company website	Usable specimen(s)
Malaria			
ACON Laboratories	Malaria P.f. Rapid Test	http://www.aconlabs.com	Whole blood
AmeriTek, Inc.	One Step Malaria Test	http://www.ameritek.org	Whole blood
Binax	NOW Malaria P.f./P.v.	http://www.binax.com	Whole blood
Core Diagnostics Ltd.	CORE Malaria (Pf, Pf/Pv, Pan Pf)	http://www.corediag.com	Whole blood
Cortez Diagnostics, Inc.	OneStep RapiCard InstaTest	http://www.rapidtest.com	Whole blood
DiaMed SA	OptiMAL Rapid Malaria Test, OptiMAL-IT Rapid Malaria Test	http://diamed.com	Whole blood
Genix Technology	Malaria (P. fal.) Ag	http://www.genixtech.com	Whole blood
International Immuno-Diagnostics	One-Step Malaria (PF/PV)	http://www.intlimmunodiagnostics.com	Whole blood
Mega Diagnostics, Inc.	MegaKwik Malaria (Pf) Card Test	http://www.mega-dx.com	Whole blood
Orchid Biomedical Systems	Paracheck Pf	http://www.tulipgroup.com/Orchid	Plasma, whole blood
Premier Medical Corporation	First Response Malaria P.f/P.v Antigen Strips	http://www.premiermedcorp.com	Whole blood
	First Response Malaria Ag pLDH Card Test		
	First Response Antigen (HRP2) Detection Card Test		
Princeton BioMeditech Corporation	BioSign Malaria Pf, Pf/Pv	http://www.pbmc.com	Whole blood
SPAN Diagnostics	ParaHIT f Parahit-Total	http://www.span.co.in	Whole blood
Standard Diagnostics Inc.	Malaria P.f/P.v Antigen Test	http://www.standardia.com	Whole blood, serum
Filariasis			
Cellabs Pty Ltd.	Filariasis-CELISA	http://www.cellabs.com.au	Whole blood, serum
Binax Inc.	NOW Filariasis Test	http://www.binax.com	Whole blood, plasma, serum
Trichomonas vaginalis			
Genzyme Diagnostics	OSOM Trichomonas Rapid Test	http://www.genzymediagnostics.com	Genital swab
Kalon Biological Limited	Kalon Tvaginalis latex kit	http://www.kalonbio.co.uk	Genital swab
Millipore	Light Diagnostics *T. vaginalis* DFA Kit	http://www.millipore.com	Genital swab
Becton-Dickinson "RNA Probe"	BD Affirm VP III	http://www.bd.com	Genital swab

of diarrhea; the intestinal tract contents move through the system too rapidly for cyst formation to occur. Once the stool specimen is passed from the body, trophozoites do not encyst but may disintegrate if not examined or preserved within a short time after passage. However, most helminth eggs and larvae, coccidian oocysts, and microsporidian spores survive for extended periods. Liquid specimens should be examined within 30 min of passage, not 30 min from the time they reach the laboratory. If this general time recommendation of 30 min is not possible, the specimen should be placed in one of the available fixatives (8). Soft (semiformed) specimens may have a mixture of protozoan trophozoites and cysts and should be examined within 1 h of passage; again, if this time frame is not possible, preservatives should be used. Immediate examination of formed specimens is not as critical; in fact, if the specimen is examined any time within 24 h after passage, the protozoan cysts should still be intact.

Preservation of Stool

If there are delays from the time of specimen passage until examination in the laboratory, the use of stool preservatives should be considered. To preserve protozoan morphology and to prevent the continued development of some helminth eggs and larvae, the stool specimens can be placed in preservative either immediately after passage (by the patient using a collection kit) or once the specimen is received by the laboratory. There are several fixatives available; these include formalin, sodium acetate-acetic acid-formalin (SAF), Schaudinn's fluid, and polyvinyl alcohol (PVA) (Table 8). Regardless of the fixative selected, adequate mixing of the specimen and preservative is mandatory. Specimens preserved in stool fixatives should be stored at room temperature. It is also important to use the correct ratio of stool and fixative to ensure proper fixation. If commercial vials are used, they are marked with a "fill-to" line for the addition of stool to the container.

TABLE 4 Commercially available kits or antigens for immunodetection of specific serum antibodies

Disease (organism)	Manufacturer and/or distributor[a]	Type of test[b]	Comment(s)
Protozoa			
Toxoplasmosis (*Toxoplasma gondii*)			See chapter 135 for serologic tests
Amebiasis (*Entamoeba histolytica*)	Millipore	EIA	Early extraintestinal infections may be missed
	IVD Research	EIA	(follow-ups recommended); infections with
	NovaTec	EIA	*E. dispar* do not induce detectable antibodies.
Chagas' disease (*Trypanosoma cruzi*)	IVD Research	EIA	
	Millipore	EIA	
	Hemagen	EIA	
	Diagnostics	EIA	
	InBios	Rapid	
	NovaTec	EIA	
Leishmaniasis	Bordier Affinity Products	EIA	
	NovaTec	EIA	
Helminths			
Ascariasis	IVD Research	EIA	
	NovaTec	EIA	
Cysticercosis (*Taenia solium*)	IVD Research	EIA	Cross-reactions in cases of other helminthic
	Millipore	EIA	infections (especially echinococcosis) may occur.
	NovaTec	EIA	
Schistosomiasis (*Schistosoma* spp.)	IVD Research	EIA	
	Bordier Affinity Products	EIA	
	NovaTec	EIA	
Cystic echinococcosis (*Echinococcus granulosus*)	IVD Research	EIA	Not species specific. Cases of alveolar echinococcosis
	Bordier Affinity Products	EIA	cross-react. False-positive reactions may occur for patients suffering from other helminth infections.
Alveolar echinococcosis (*E. multilocularis*)	Bordier Affinity Products	EIA	Screening test for alveolar echinococcosis; cases of cystic echinococcosis may cross-react.
Strongyloidiasis (*Strongyloides stercoralis*)	IVD Research	EIA	Cross-reactions in patients with other helminth
	Bordier Affinity Products	EIA	infections may occur.
Toxocariasis (*Toxocara canis*)	IVD Research	EIA	
	Bordier Affinity Products	EIA	
	NovaTec	EIA	
Trichinellosis (*Trichinella spiralis*)	IVD Research	EIA	Numerous cross-reactions with other helminth infections may occur.
Filariasis	Bordier Affinity Products	EIA	
	NovaTec	EIA	

[a]Bordier Affinity Products, Chatanerie 2, CH-1023 Crissier, Switzerland (http://www.bordier.ch); Hemagen, 34–40 Bear Hill Rd., Waltham, MA 02154 (http://www.hemagen.com); Immunetics, 380 Green St., Cambridge, MA 02139 (http://www.immunetics.com); InBios, 562 1st Ave. South, Suite 600, Seattle, WA 98104 (http://www.inbios.com); IVD Research, 5909 Sea Lion Place, Suite D, Carlsbad, CA 92008 (http://ivd@ivdresearch.com), bioMérieux SA, F-69280 Marcy l'Etoile, France (http://bioMerieux-diagnostics.com); Millipore Coporation, 290 Concord Rd., Billerica, MA (http://millipore.com); NovaTec, Immunodiagnostica GmbH, Waldstrasse 23 a6, 63128 Dietzenbach, Germany (http://www.novatec-id.com).
[b]Abbreviations: EIA, enzyme immunoassay; Rapid, rapid immunochromatographic (some are dipstick, cartridge, or other rapid test formats).

When selecting an appropriate fixative, keep in mind that a permanent stained smear is mandatory for a complete examination for parasites (8, 9, 19, 23, 26). You may also want to use some of the newer immunoassay procedures or molecular diagnostic methods (PCR); make sure that the fixative you are using is compatible with the kit or the method you have selected. It is also important to remember that disposal regulations for compounds containing mercury are becoming stricter; each laboratory must check applicable regulations to help determine fixative options.

Formalin

Formalin is an all-purpose fixative that is appropriate for helminth eggs and larvae and for protozoan cysts. Two concentrations are commonly used: 5%, which is recommended for preservation of protozoan cysts, and 10%, which is recommended for helminth eggs and larvae. Although 5% is often recommended for all-purpose use, most commercial manufacturers provide 10%, which is more likely to kill all helminth eggs. To help maintain organism morphology, the formalin can be buffered with sodium phosphate buffers, i.e., neutral formalin. Selection of specific formalin formulations is at the user's discretion. Aqueous formalin permits the examination of the specimen as a wet mount only, a technique much less accurate than a stained smear for the identification of intestinal protozoa.

Protozoan cysts (not trophozoites), coccidian oocysts, helminth eggs, and larvae are well preserved for long periods in 10% aqueous formalin. Hot (60°C) formalin can be used for specimens containing helminth eggs, since in cold formalin some thick-shelled eggs may continue to develop, become infective, and remain viable for long periods. Several

TABLE 5 Specimen preparation and procedures, recommended stain(s) and relevant parasites, and additional information

Body site	Procedures[a] and specimens	Recommended methods and relevant parasites[a]	Additional information
Blood	Microscopy[b]: thin and thick blood films. Fresh blood (preferred) or EDTA-blood (fill EDTA tube completely with blood and then mix).	Giemsa stain (all blood parasites); hematoxylin-based stain (sheathed microfilariae) Malaria: thick and thin blood films are definitely recommended and should be prepared within 30 to 60 min of blood collection via venipuncture (other tests may be used complementarily)	Most drawings and descriptions of blood parasites are based on Giemsa-stained blood films. Although Wright's stain (or Wright-Giemsa combination stain) works, stippling in malaria may not be visible and the organisms' colors do not match the descriptions. However, with other stains (those listed above, in addition to some of the "quick" blood stains), the organisms should be detectable on the blood films.
	Concentration methods: EDTA-blood	Buffy coat, fresh blood films for detection of moving microfilariae or trypanosomes QBC, a screening method for blood parasites (hematocrit tube contains acridine orange), has been used for malaria, *Babesia*, trypanosomes, and microfilariae. It is usually impossible to identify malaria organisms to the species level; requires high levels of training.	The use of blood collected with anticoagulant (rather than fresh) has direct relevance to the morphology of malaria organisms seen in peripheral blood films. If the blood smears are prepared after more than 1 h, stippling may not be visible, even if the correct pH buffers are used. Also, if blood is kept at room temperature (with the stopper removed), the male microgametocyte may exflagellate and fertilize the female macrogametocyte, and development continues within the tube of blood (as it would in the mosquito host). The ookinete may actually resemble *Plasmodium falciparum* gametocytes.
	Antigen detection: EDTA-blood for malaria, serum or plasma for circulating antigens (hemolyzed blood can interact in some tests)	Commercial immunoassay test kits for malaria and some microfilariae. Sensitivity is not higher than for thick films for *Plasmodium* spp., much more sensitive for *Leishmania* (peripheral blood is used from immunodeficient patients only).	
	PCR[c]: EDTA-blood, ethanol fixed or unfixed thin and thick blood films, coagulated blood, possibly with hemolyzed or frozen blood samples	Sequencing of PCR product is often used for species or genotype identification	PCR: so far no commercial tests are available; high laboratory standards are needed (may work with frozen, coagulated, or hemolyzed blood samples).
	Specific antibody detection: serum or plasma, anticoagulated or coagulated blood (hemolyzed blood can cause problems in some tests)	Most commonly used are EIA (many test kits commercially available), EITB (commercially available for some parasites), and IFA	Many laboratories use in-house tests; only a few fully defined antigens are available; sensitivities and specificities of the tests should be documented by the laboratory.
Bone marrow	Biopsy samples or aspirates Microscopy: thin and thick films with aspirate collected in EDTA	Giemsa stain (all blood parasites)	*Leishmania* amastigotes are recovered in cells of the reticuloendothelial system; if films are not prepared directly after sample collection, infected cells may disintegrate. Sensitivity of microscopy is low; use only in combination with other methods.
	Cultures: sterile material in EDTA or culture medium	Culture for *Leishmania* (or *Trypanosoma cruzi*)	
	PCR: aspirate in EDTA	PCR for blood parasites, including *Leishmania* and *Toxoplasma* and rare other parasites	
Central nervous system	Microscopy: spinal fluid and CSF (wet examination, stained smears), brain biopsy (touch or squash preparations, stained)	Stains: Giemsa (trypanosomes, *Toxoplasma*); Giemsa, trichrome, or calcofluor (amebae [*Naegleria*-PAM, *Acanthamoeba*- or *Balamuthia*-GAE]); Giemsa, acid-fast, PAS, modified trichrome, silver methenamine (microsporidia) (tissue Gram stains also recommended for microsporidia in routine histologic preparations); H&E, routine histology (larval cestodes, *Taenia solium* [cysticerci], *Echinococcus* spp.)	If CSF is received (with no suspect organism suggested), Giemsa would be the best choice; however, modified trichrome or calcofluor is also recommended as a second stain (amebic cysts, microsporidia). If brain biopsy material is received (particularly from an immunocompromised patient), PCR is recommended for diagnosis and for identification to the species or genotype level.
	Culture: sterile aspirate or biopsy material (in physiological saline)	Free-living amebae (exception: *Balamuthia* does not grow in the routine agar/bacterial overlay method). *Toxoplasma* can be cultured in tissue culture media.	A small amount of the sample should always be stored frozen for PCR analyses in case the results of the other methods are inconclusive.

(Continued on next page)

TABLE 5 *(Continued)*

Body site	Procedures[a] and specimens	Recommended methods and relevant parasites[a]	Additional information
	PCR: aspirate or biopsy material, native, frozen, or fixed in ethanol	Protozoa and helminths; species and genotype characterization	
Cutaneous ulcers	Microscopy: aspirate, biopsy material (smears, touch or squash preparations, histologic sections)	Giemsa (*Leishmania*); H&E, routine histology (*Acanthamoeba* spp., *Entamoeba histolytica*)	Most likely causative parasites would be *Leishmania*, which would stain with Giemsa. PAS could be used to differentiate *Histoplasma capsulatum* from *Leishmania* in tissue. Sensitivity of microscopy may be low.
	Cultures (less common)	*Leishmania*, free-living amebae (often bacterial contaminations)	In immunocompromised patients, skin ulcers have been documented with amebae as causative agents.
	PCR: aspirate, biopsy material, native, frozen, or fixed in ethanol	*Leishmania* (species identification), free-living amebae	Cultures of material from cutaneous ulcers may be contaminated with bacteria; PCR would be the method of choice.
Eye	Microscopy: biopsy material (smears, touch or squash preparations), scrapings, contact lens, sediment of lens solution	Calcofluor (*Acanthamoeba* cyst only); Giemsa (trophozoites, cysts [amebae]; modified trichrome (preferred) or silver methenamine stain, PAS, acid-fast (microsporidial spores); H&E, routine histology (cysticerci, *Loa loa*, *Toxoplasma*)	Some free-living amebae (most commonly *Acanthamoeba*) have been implicated as a cause of keratitis. Although calcofluor stains the cyst walls, it does not stain the trophozoites. Therefore, in suspected cases of amebic keratitis, both stains should be used. H&E (routine histology) can be used to detect and confirm cysticercosis. The adult worm of *Loa loa*, when removed from the eye, can be stained with a hematoxylin-based stain (Delafield's) or can be stained and examined by routine histology.
	Culture: native material (see above) in PBS supplemented with antibiotics if possible to avoid bacterial growth	Cultures: free-living amebae and *Toxoplasma*	
	PCR: native material in physiological NaCl or PBS, ethanol or frozen	Free-living amebae, *Toxoplasma*, microsporidial species and genotype identification	Microsporidial confirmation to the species or genotype level is done by PCR and sequence analyses; however, the spores could be found by routine light microscopy with modified trichrome and/or calcofluor stain. Sensitivity of microscopic methods may be low.
Intestinal tract	Stool and other intestinal material		Stool fixation with formalin or formalin-containing fixatives preserves trophozoite morphology, allows prolonged storage (room temperature) and long transportation, and prevents hatching of *Schistosoma* eggs but makes *Strongyloides* larval concentration impossible and impedes further PCR analyses.
	Microscopy: stool, sigmoidoscopy material, duodenal contents (all fresh or preserved (see Table 4), direct wet smear, concentration methods	Concentration methods: formalin-ethyl acetate sedimentation of formalin or SAF-fixed stool samples (most protozoa); flotation or combined sedimentation flotation methods (helminth ova); agar or Baermann concentration (larvae of *Strongyloides* spp.; unpreserved stool required)	Taeniid eggs cannot be identified to the species level.
		Direct wet smear (direct examination of unpreserved fresh material is also used (motile protozoan trophozoites; helminth eggs and protozoan cysts may also be detected)	Microsporidia: confirmation to the species or genotype level requires PCR; however, modified trichrome and/or calcofluor stain can be used to confirm the presence of spores.
		Stains: trichrome or iron hematoxylin (intestinal protozoa); modified trichrome (microsporidia); modified acid-fast (*Cryptosporidium*, *Cyclospora*, *Isospora*)	
	Anal impression smear	Adhesive cellulose tape, no stain (*Enterobius vermicularis*)	Four to six consecutive negative tapes are required to rule out infection with pinworm (*Enterobius vermicularis*).
	Adult worms or tapeworm segments (proglottids)	Carmine stains (rarely used for adult worms or cestode segments). Proglottids can usually be identified to the genus level (*Taenia*, *Diphyllobothrium*, *Hymenolepis*) without using tissue stains	Worm segments can be stained with special stains. However, after dehydration through alcohols and xylenes (or xylene substitutes), the sexual organs and the branched uterine structure will be visible, allowing identification of the proglottid to the species level.

(Continued on next page)

TABLE 5 Specimen preparation and procedures, recommended stain(s) and relevant parasites, and additional information (*Continued*)

Body site	Procedures[a] and specimens	Recommended methods and relevant parasites[a]	Additional information
	Antigen detection: fresh native or frozen material; suitability of fixation is test dependent	Commercial immunoassays: (Table 2, e.g., EIA, FA, cartridge formats (*Entamoeba histolytica*, the *Entamoeba histolytica/E. dispar* group, *Giardia*, and, *Cryptosporidium*). In-house tests for *Taenia solium* and *Taenia saginata*.	Coproantigens can be detected in the pre-patent period and independently from egg excretion.
	PCR: native material, fresh, frozen or ethanol-fixed	No commercial tests available. Primers for genus or species identification of most helminths and protozoa are published.	Due to potential inhibition after DNA extraction from stool samples, concentration or isolation methods may be required prior to DNA extraction. However, new DNA isolation kits facilitate isolation of high-quality DNA from stool. Sequence analyses may be required for species or genotype identification.
	Biopsy material Microscopy: fixed for histology or touch or squash preparations for staining PCR: see above	H&E, routine histology (*Entamoeba histolytica*, *Cryptosporidium*, *Cyclospora*, *Isospora belli*, *Giardia*, microsporidia); less common findings include *Schistosoma* spp., hookworm, or *Trichuris*	Special stains may be helpful for the identification of microsporidia (tissue Gram stains, silver stains, PAS, and Giemsa) or coccidia (modified acid-fast stain).
Liver and spleen	Biopsy samples or aspirates Microscopy: unfixed material in physiological NaCl; fixed for histology	Examination of wet smears for *Entamoeba histolytica* (trophozoites), protoscolices of *Echinococcus* spp. or eggs of *Capillaria hepatica*. Giemsa stain (*Leishmania*, other protozoa and microsporidia); H&E (routine histology).	There are definite risks associated with punctures (aspirates and/or biopsy) of spleen or liver lesions (*Echinococcus*). Always keep a small amount of material frozen for PCR.
	Culture: sterile preparation of native material	For *Leishmania* (not common)	
	Animal inoculation: sterile preparation of native material	Intraperitoneal inoculation of *E. multilocularis* cyst material for viability test after long-term chemotherapy	
	PCR: native material, frozen or ethanol fixed	Species or genotype identification (e.g., *Echinococcus* spp.)	
Respiratory tract	Sputum, induced sputum, nasal and sinus discharge, bronchoalveolar lavage fluid, transbronchial aspirate, tracheobronchial aspirate, brush biopsy sample, open-lung biopsy sample	Helminth larvae (*Ascaris*, *Strongyloides*), eggs (*Paragonimus*, *Capillaria*), or hooklets (*Echinococcus*) can be recovered in unstained respiratory specimens Stains: Giemsa for many protozoa, including *Toxoplasma* tachyzoites, modified acid-fast stains (*Cryptosporidium*); modified trichrome (microsporidia)	There are immunoassay reagents (FA) available for the diagnosis of pulmonary cryptosporidiosis. Routine histologic procedures allow the identification of any of the helminths or helminth eggs present in the lung. Disseminated toxoplasmosis and microsporidiosis are well documented, with organisms being found in many different respiratory specimens.
	Microscopy: unfixed material, treated for smear preparation PCR: unfixed native material, frozen or fixed in ethanol	Routine histology (H&E; silver methenamine stain, PAS, acid-fast, tissue Gram stains for helminths, protozoa, and microsporidia)	
Muscle	Biopsy material Microscopy: unfixed, touch and squash preparations or fixed for histology and EM	Larvae of *Trichinella* spp. can be identified unstained (species identification with single larvae by PCR). H&E, routine histology (*Trichinella* spp., cysticerci); silver methenamine stain, PAS, acid-fast, tissue Gram stains, EM (rare microsporidia).	If *Trypanosoma cruzi* organisms are present in the striated muscle, they could be identified in routine histology preparations. Modified trichrome and/or calcofluor stain can be used to confirm the presence of microsporidial spores.
	PCR: unfixed or native, frozen or ethanol fixed	Microsporidial identification to the species level requires subsequent sequencing	Larvae of *Trichinella* may be detected in heavy infections only. Biopsies are not recommended as standard procedures.
Skin	Aspirates, skin snips, scrapings, biopsy samples	See Cutaneous ulcer (above)	Any of the potential parasites present can be identified by routine histology procedures, but the sensitivities of these methods may be low.

(Continued on next page)

TABLE 5 *(Continued)*

Body site	Procedures[a] and specimens	Recommended methods and relevant parasites[a]	Additional information
	Microscopy: wet examination, stained smear (or fixed for histology or EM)	Wet preparations (microfilariae), Giemsa-stained smears or H&E, routine histology (*Onchocerca volvulus*, *Dipetalonema streptocerca*, *Dirofilaria repens*, other larvae causing cutaneous larva migrans [zoonotic *Strongyloides* spp., hookworms], *Leishmania*, *Acanthamoeba* spp., *Entamoeba histolytica*, microsporidia, and arthropods [*Sarcoptes* and other mites]	
	PCR: unfixed native, frozen or fixed in ethanol	Primers for most parasite species available	
Amniotic fluid	PCR (and/or culture): native material Animal inoculation (*Toxoplasma*)	PCR based on the detection of highly repetitive gene sequences is the method of choice	Only applicable to confirm suspected prenatal *Toxoplasma* infections
Urogenital system	Vaginal discharge, saline swab, transport swab (no charcoal), air-dried smear for FA, urethral discharge, prostatic secretions, urine (single unpreserved, 24-h unpreserved, or early-morning specimen).	Giemsa, immunoassay reagents (*Trichomonas vaginalis*); Delafield's hematoxylin (microfilariae); modified trichrome (microsporidia); H&E, routine histology, PAS, acid-fast, tissue Gram stains (microsporidia). Direct examination of urine sediment for *Schistosoma haematobium* eggs or microfilariae.	Although *T. vaginalis* is probably the most common parasite identified, there are others to consider, the most recently implicated organisms being in the microsporidial group. Microfilariae could also be recovered and stained. Fixation of urine with formalin prevents hatching of *Schistosoma* eggs.
	Microscopy: wet smears, smears of urine sediment, stained smears Cultivation: vaginal or urethral discharge or swab preparations PCR: native material, frozen or fixed in ethanol	Identification and propagation of *T. vaginalis* (commercial plastic envelope culture systems available); moving trophozoites can be detected microscopically (or in Giemsa-stained smears)	Material must be put into culture medium immediately after collection; do not cool or freeze.

[a]CSF, cerebrospinal fluid; EIA, enzyme immunoassay; EITB, enzyme-linked immunoelectrotransfer blot (Western blot); EM, electron microscopy; FA, fluorescent antibody; GAE, granulomatous amebic encephalitis; GI, gastrointestinal; H&E, hematoxylin and eosin; IFA, indirect immunofluorescence assay; PAM, primary amebic encephalitis; PAS, periodic acid-Schiff stain; PBS, phosphate-buffered saline; QBC, quantitative buffy coat.

[b]Many parasites or parasite stages may be detected in standard histologic sections of tissue material. However, species identification is difficult and additional examinations may be required. Usually, these techniques are not considered first-line methods. Additional methods like EM are carried out only by specialized laboratories and are not available for standard diagnostic purposes. EM examination for species identification has largely been replaced by PCR.

[c]Material/specimens suitable for PCR: native (unfixed), in saline, PBS (ethanol), or frozen; avoid formalin.

grams of fecal material should be thoroughly mixed in 5 or 10% formalin (ratio, 1:10).

Formaldehyde vapor concentrations must be monitored and maintained at concentrations below the 8-h time-weighted average. In the United States, these limits are 0.75 ppm and the 15-min short-term exposure limit, i.e., 2.0 ppm (8). However, these limits may vary from country to country. Generally, the amount of formaldehyde used in microbiology is quite small; laboratory monitoring values are usually well below the required maximum concentrations. Initial monitoring must be repeated any time there is a change in production, equipment, process, personnel, or control measures which may result in new or additional exposure to formaldehyde. Stool fixatives that contain formaldehyde indicate that fact on the label. A number of single-vial fixative collection systems are now available; although they may not contain formaldehyde, the actual formulas are proprietary.

Sodium Acetate-Acetic Acid-Formalin

Both the concentration and the permanent stained smear can be performed with specimens preserved in SAF, which does not contain mercuric chloride, which is found in Schaudinn's fluid and PVA. It is a liquid fixative, much like the 10% formalin described above. The sediment is used to prepare the permanent smear, and it is frequently recommended that the stool material be placed on an albumin-coated slide to improve adherence to the glass (29, 34).

SAF is considered to be a "softer" fixative than mercuric chloride. The organism morphology is not quite as sharp after staining as that of organisms originally fixed in solutions containing mercuric chloride. The pairing of SAF-fixed material with iron hematoxylin staining provides better organism morphology than does staining of SAF-fixed material with trichrome (personal observation). Although SAF has a long shelf life and is easy to prepare, the smear preparation technique may be a bit more difficult for less experienced personnel who are not familiar with fecal

TABLE 6 Fecal specimens for parasites: options for collection and processing[a]

Options	Pros	Cons
Although physicians can order stools for parasitology when deemed appropriate, many laboratories include in their protocols the rejection of stools from inpatients who have been in-house for >3 days.	Patients may become symptomatic with diarrhea after they have been inpatients for a few days; symptoms are usually not attributed to parasitic infections but are generally due to other causes.	There is always a chance that the problem is related to a nosocomial parasitic infection (rare), but *Cryptosporidium, Giardia,* and microsporidia may be possible considerations.
Examination of a single stool (O&P examination)	If parasites are diagnosed in the first sample or if the patient becomes asymptomatic after collection of the first stool, subsequent specimens may not be necessary. However, with some intestinal parasitic infections, patients may alternate with constipation and diarrhea.	Diagnosis from examination of a single stool specimen depends on the parasite load in the specimen. Of organisms present, 40 to 50% are found with only a single stool exam; two O&P examinations are acceptable, but three specimens are more sensitive; any patient remaining symptomatic would require additional testing. In a series of three stool specimens, frequently not all three specimens are positive and/or may be positive for different organisms (may be a cost-effective approach).
Examination a second stool specimen only after the first one is negative and the patient is still symptomatic	With additional examinations, yield of protozoa increases (*E. histolytica,* 22.7%; *G. lamblia,* 11.3%; and *D. fragilis,* 31.1%).	Assumes that the second (or third) stool specimen is collected within the recommended 10-day time frame for a series of stools; protozoa are shed periodically. May be inconvenient for the patient, and the correct diagnosis might be delayed.
Examination of a single stool and a *Giardia* immunoassay	If the examinations are negative and the patient's symptoms subside, then probably no further testing is required.	Patients may exhibit symptoms (off and on), so it may be difficult to rule out parasitic infections with only a single stool and immunoassay. If the patient remains symptomatic, then even if the *Giardia* immunoassay is negative, other protozoa may be missed (*Cryptosporidium, E. histolytica/E. dispar,* and *D. fragilis*).
Pooling of three specimens for examination; one concentration and one permanent stain are performed. The laboratory will pool the specimens.	Three specimens are collected over 7–10 days, which may save time and expense.	Procedure not recommended. Decreases strongly the sensitivity of the procedure; organisms present in low numbers may be missed due to the dilution factor.
Permanent stained smears are performed, one from each of the three specimens; subsequently, three specimens are pooled for a single concentration on the pooled specimen.	Three specimens are collected over 7–10 days; would maximize recovery of protozoa in areas of the United States where these organisms are most common	Might miss light helminth infection (eggs and larvae) due to the pooling procedure.
Three stool specimens are collected, but samples of stool from all three are put into a single vial (patient is given a single vial only).	Pooling of the specimens would require only a single vial.	Absolutely not recommended. Lack of sensitivity; proper mixing of specimen and fixative complicates patient collection and depends on patient compliance.
Immunoassays are performed only for selected patients[b] (children <5 yr old, children from day care centers, patients with immunodeficiencies, and patients from diarrheal outbreaks) for intestinal protozoa.	Would be more cost-effective than performing immunoassay procedures on all specimens	The competence and the information needed to group patients are often not available in the laboratory. Ordering guidelines for clients are highly recommended (see Table 7).

[a]See key references 25 and 30.

[b]It is difficult to recognize an early outbreak situation where screening of all specimens for either *Giardia lamblia, Cryptosporidium* spp., or both may be relevant. If it appears that an outbreak is in the early stages, then performing the immunoassays on request can be changed to screening all stools.

specimen techniques. Laboratories that have considered using only a single preservative have selected this option. Helminth eggs and larvae, protozoan trophozoites and cysts, coccidian oocysts, and microsporidian spores are preserved using this method.

Schaudinn's Fluid
Schaudinn's fluid (contains mercuric chloride) is used with fresh stool specimens or samples from the intestinal mucosal surface. Many laboratories that receive specimens from in-house patients (no problem with delivery times) often select this approach. Permanent stained smears are then prepared from fixed material. A concentration technique using Schaudinn's fluid-preserved material is also available but is not widely used (3, 8, 19, 23).

Polyvinyl Alcohol
PVA is a plastic resin that is normally incorporated into Schaudinn's fixative. The PVA powder serves as an adhesive for the stool material; i.e., when the stool-PVA mixture is

TABLE 7 Approaches to stool parasitology: test ordering[a]

Patient and/or situation	Test ordered	Follow-up test ordered
Immunocompromised patients with diarrhea Potential waterborne outbreak from (municipal) water supply	*Cryptosporidium* or *Giardia/Cryptosporidium* immunoassay[b,c] (see Table 2)	If immunoassays are negative and symptoms continue, special tests for microsporidia (modified trichrome stain) and coccidia (modified acid-fast stain) and O&P examination should be performed.
Patient with diarrhea (from a nursery school or day care center or a camper or backpacker) Patient with diarrhea and potential waterborne outbreak (resort setting) Patient from area within the United States where *Giardia* is the most common organism found	*Giardia* or *Giardia/Cryptosporidium* immunoassay[b,c]	If immunoassays are negative and symptoms continue, special tests for microsporidia and coccidia (see above) and O&P examination should be performed.
Patient with diarrhea and relevant travel history Patient with diarrhea who is a past or present resident of a developing country Patient in area of the United States where parasites other than *Giardia* are found (e.g., in large metropolitan area)	O&P examination, the *Entamoeba histolytica/E. dispar* group immunoassay, confirmation for *E. histolytica*, *Cryptosporidium* or *Giardia/Cryptosporidium* immunoassay[b,c]	If examinations are negative and symptoms continue, special tests for coccidia and microsporidia should be performed.
Patient with unexplained eosinophilia (may be low or high); may or may not have diarrhea; may be immunocompromised, often due to receipt of steroids; patient may actually present with hyperinfection and severe diarrhea (symptoms may also include pneumonia and/or episodes of sepsis and/or meningitis)	O&P examination with emphasis on helminths (unfixed stool, for sedimentation/flotation techniques); it is very important to make sure that an infection with *Strongyloides stercoralis* has been ruled out—particularly if the patient is immunosuppressed or may become immunosuppressed from therapy, etc. (unfixed stool, Baermann concentration or agar plate culture)	If the O&P examinations are negative, agar plate cultures for *S. stercoralis* are recommended, particularly if the history is suggestive for this infection. The serological detection of specific antibody is an additional diagnostic option.
Patient with diarrhea (suspected foodborne outbreak)	Test for *Cyclospora cayetanensis* (modified acid-fast stain)	If test is negative and symptoms continue, special procedures for microsporidia and other coccidia and O&P examination should be performed.

[a]Modified from reference 9.

[b]Depending on the particular immunoassay kit used, various single or multiple organisms may be included. Selection of a particular kit depends on many variables: clinical relevance, cost, ease of performance, training, personnel availability, number of test orders, training of physician clients, sensitivity, specificity, equipment, time to result, etc. Very few laboratories handle this type of testing in exactly the same way. Many options are clinically relevant and acceptable for patient care.

[c]Two stool specimens should be tested using an immunoassay in order to rule out an infection with *Giardia*; fecal immunoassays may also be negative in cases with a low parasite load.

spread onto the glass slide, it adheres because of the PVA component. Fixation is still accomplished by Schaudinn's fluid itself. Perhaps the greatest advantage in the use of PVA is that a permanent stained smear can be prepared. Like SAF, PVA fixative solution is recommended as a means of preserving cysts and trophozoites for later examination and permits specimens to be shipped (by regular mail service) from any location in the world to a laboratory for subsequent examination. PVA is particularly useful for liquid specimens and should be used in the ratio of 3 parts PVA to 1 part fecal specimen (5).

Modified Polyvinyl Alcohol

Although preservatives that do not contain mercury compounds have been developed, substitute compounds have not provided the quality of preservation necessary for good protozoan morphology on the permanent stained smear. Copper sulfate has been tried but does not provide results equal to those seen with mercuric chloride (18). Zinc sulfate has proven to be an acceptable mercury substitute and is used with trichrome stain. Although zinc substitutes have become widely available, each manufacturer has a proprietary formula for the fixative (13, 15).

Single-Vial Collection Systems

Several manufacturers now have available single-vial stool collection systems, similar to SAF or modified PVA methods. From the single vial, both the concentration and permanent stained smear can be prepared. It is also possible to perform immunoassays from some of these vials. Ask the manufacturer about all diagnostic capabilities (concentrate, permanent stained smear, immunoassay procedures, and molecular analyses) and for specific information indicating that there are no formula components that would interfere with any of the methods. Like the zinc substitutes, these formulas are proprietary (15). The ability to perform immunoassays using fixed specimens varies depending on the fixative and specific immunoassay being used.

New-Formulation Single-Vial Collection Systems

New formulations continue to be developed, and some of them appear to adhere to the slide without the use of albumin or PVA. These formulations can be used to perform concentrations and some of the immunoassays and to prepare permanent stained smears.

TABLE 8 Fecal preservatives: pros and cons

Stool preservative	Pros	Cons
Formalin	Good overall fixative for stool concentration. Easy to prepare; long shelf life. Concentrated sediment can be used with different stains[a] but not with all immunoassays (Table 5).	Does not preserve trophozoites well. Does not adequately preserve organism morphology for a good permanent stained smear; not optimal for all immunoassays; not appropriate for molecular diagnosis (PCR).
SAF	Can be used for concentration and permanent stained smears. Contains no mercury compounds. Easy to prepare; long shelf life. Concentrated sediment can be used with most of the new immunoassay methods and special stains.	Poor adhesive properties; albumin-coated slides recommended. Protozoan morphology better if iron hematoxylin stain is used for permanent stained smears (trichrome is not quite as good). May be a bit more difficult to use; however, this is really not a limiting factor. Not appropriate for molecular diagnosis (PCR).
Schaudinn's fixative	Fixative for smears prepared from fresh fecal specimens or samples from the intestinal mucosal surfaces. Provides excellent preservation of protozoan trophozoites and cysts.	Not generally recommended for concentration procedures. Contains mercuric chloride; creates disposal problems. Poor adhesive qualities with liquid or mucoid specimens.
PVA	Can prepare permanent stained smears and perform concentration techniques (less common). Provides excellent preservation of protozoan trophozoites and cysts. Specimens can be shipped to the laboratory for subsequent examination; organism morphology excellent after processing. Suitable for PCR analysis.	*Trichuris trichiura* eggs and *Giardia lamblia* cysts are not concentrated as easily as from formalin-based fixatives. *Strongyloides stercoralis* larval morphology is poor (better from formalin-based preservation). *Isospora belli* oocysts may not be visible from PVA-preserved material (better from formalin-based preservation). Contains mercury compounds (Schaudinn's fluid). May turn white and gelatinous when it begins to dehydrate or when refrigerated. Difficult to prepare in the laboratory. Specimens containing PVA cannot be used with the immunoassay methods.
Modified PVA	Can prepare permanent stained smears and perform concentration techniques (less common). Many workers prefer the zinc substitutes over those prepared with copper sulfate. Does not contain mercury compounds.	Overall protozoan morphology of trophozoites and cysts is poor when they are preserved in the copper-sulfate-based fixative, particularly compared with organisms preserved in mercuric chloride-based fixatives. Zinc-based fixatives appear to be some of the better alternatives. Staining characteristics of protozoa are not consistent; some are good, and some are poor. Organism identification may be difficult, particularly with small protozoan cysts (*Endolimax nana*).
Single-vial systems	Can prepare permanent stained smears and perform concentration techniques. Can perform immunoassays—"universal fixative" currently now available. Do not contain formalin or mercury compounds. Unless organism numbers are rare, acceptable organism recovery and identification are possible; additional training may be required to recognize the organisms because the overall morphology is not comparable to that seen with mercury-based fixatives.	Overall protozoan morphology of trophozoites and cysts is not as good as that of organisms preserved with mercuric chloride-based fixatives; similar to modified PVA options. Staining characteristics of protozoa are not consistent; some are good, and some are poor. Identification of *Endolimax nana* cysts may be difficult. Not all immunoassays can be performed from stool specimens preserved in these fixatives. However, in spite of the cons, single-vial systems are becoming more widely used for concentrations, permanent stained smears, and fecal immunoassays.

[a]Modified acid-fast and modified trichrome stains.

Collection of Blood

Depending on the life cycle, there are a number of parasites that may be recovered in a blood specimen, either whole blood, buffy coat preparations, or various types of concentrations (9, 19, 23). These parasites include *Plasmodium, Babesia, Trypanosoma, Leishmania, Toxoplasma,* and microfilariae. Although some organisms may be motile in fresh, whole blood, species identification is normally accomplished from the examination of permanent stained blood thin and/or thick films. Blood films can be prepared from fresh, whole blood collected with no anticoagulants, anticoagulated blood, or sediment from the various concentration procedures.

Unless it is certain that well-prepared slides will be available, it is necessary to request a tube of fresh blood (EDTA anticoagulant is preferred) and prepare the smears. The tube should be filled with blood to provide the proper blood/anticoagulant ratio. For detection of stippling, the smears should be prepared within 1 h after the specimen is drawn. After that time, stippling may not be visible on stained films; however, the overall organism morphology will still be excellent. Most laboratories routinely use commercially available blood collection tubes; preparation of EDTA collection tubes in-house is neither necessary nor cost-effective.

The time the specimen was drawn should be clearly indicated on the tube of blood and also on the result report. The physician will then be able to correlate the results with any fever pattern or other symptoms that the patient may have. There should also be some comments on the test result report that is sent back to the physician, stating that one negative specimen does not rule out the possibility of a parasitic infection (8, 27).

Collection of Specimens from Other Body Sites

Although clinical specimens for examination can be obtained from many other body sites, these specimens and appropriate diagnostic methods are not as commonly performed as those used for the routine stool specimen or for blood specimens. The majority of specimens from other body sites (Table 1) would be submitted as fresh specimens for further testing.

DIRECT DETECTION BY ROUTINE METHODS

Intestinal Tract Specimens

The most common specimen submitted to the diagnostic laboratory is the stool specimen, and the most commonly performed procedure in parasitology is the ova and parasite (O&P) examination, which is composed of three separate protocols: the direct wet mount, the concentration, and the permanent stained smear. The direct wet mount requires fresh stool, is designed to allow the detection of motile protozoan trophozoites, and is examined microscopically at low and high dry magnifications (×100, entire 22- by 22-mm coverslip [larvae, larger helminth eggs]; ×400, one-third to one-half of a 22- by 22-mm coverslip [protozoan cysts and/or trophozoites, smaller helminth eggs]). However, due to potential problems with the lag time between specimen passage and receipt in the laboratory, the direct wet examination has been eliminated from the routine O&P examination in favor of receipt of specimens collected in stool preservatives; if specimens are received in the laboratory in stool collection preservatives, the direct wet preparation is not performed.

The second part of the O&P examination is the concentration, which is designed to facilitate the recovery of protozoan cysts, coccidian oocysts, microsporidial spores, and helminth eggs and larvae. Both flotation (zinc sulfate, zinc chloride, and others) and sedimentation methods are available, the most common procedure being the formalin-ethyl acetate sedimentation method (formerly called the formalin-ether method). The concentrated specimen is examined as a wet preparation, with or without iodine, using low and high dry magnifications (×100 and ×400) as indicated for the direct wet smear examination. It is important to remember that large, heavy helminth eggs (unfertilized *Ascaris* eggs) or eggs that are operculated (trematode and some cestode eggs) do not float optimally when flotation fluids with densities of <1.35 are used; both the surface film and sediment must be examined by this method. It is also important to note that the flotation media with high densities may change the morphological characteristics of some parasites.

The third part of the O&P examination is the permanent stained smear, which is designed to facilitate the identification of intestinal protozoa. Several staining methods are available, the two most common being the Wheatley modification of the Gomori tissue trichrome and the iron hematoxylin stains. This part of the O&P examination is critical for the confirmation of suspicious objects seen in the wet examination and identification of protozoa that might not have been seen in the wet preparation. The permanent stained smears are examined using oil immersion objectives (×600 for screening and ×1,000 for final review of ≥300 oil immersion fields).

Other specimens from the intestinal tract such as duodenal aspirates or drainage, mucus from the Entero-Test Capsule technique (HDC Corp., San Jose, CA), and sigmoidoscopy material can also be examined as wet preparations and as permanent stained smears after processing with either trichrome or iron hematoxylin staining. Although not all laboratories examine these types of specimens, they are included to give some idea of the possibilities for diagnostic testing.

Amniotic Fluid

Methods for the diagnosis of congenital *Toxoplasma* infection are summarized in chapter 135. Amniotic fluid collected under sterile conditions allows both mouse or tissue culture inoculation and molecular diagnosis by PCR. PCR is the recommended test of choice for the detection of *Toxoplasma* in amniotic fluid.

Urogenital Tract Specimens

The identification of *Trichomonas vaginalis* is usually based on the examination of wet preparations of vaginal and urethral discharges and prostatic secretions or urine sediment. Multiple specimens may have to be examined before the organisms are detected. These specimens are diluted with a drop of saline and examined under low power (×100) and reduced illumination for the presence of motile organisms; as the jerky motility begins to diminish, it may be possible to observe the undulating membrane, particularly under high dry power (×400). Culture systems (InPouch TV; BioMed Diagnostics, San Jose, CA, and Empyrean Diagnostics, Inc., Mountain View, CA) that allow direct inoculation, transport, culture, and microscopic examination are available commercially (2, 8). Rapid tests that allow detection of *T. vaginalis* antigens are also commercially available (Table 3).

Stained smears such as Papanicolaou- or Giemsa-stained smears can be used, but they are usually not necessary for the identification of this organism and can be difficult to interpret. If a dry smear is received by the laboratory, it can be fixed with absolute methanol and stained with Giemsa stain; this approach is not optimal, but the smear can be examined and may confirm a positive infection. The number of false-positive and false-negative results reported on the basis of stained smears strongly suggests the value of confirmation by observation of motile organisms from the direct mount, from appropriate culture media, or from direct detection by more sensitive immunological or molecular methods (Table 3) (6).

Examination of urinary sediment may be indicated in certain filarial infections. Administration of the drug diethylcarbamazine (Hetrazan) has been reported to enhance the recovery of microfilariae from urine. The triple-concentration technique is recommended for the recovery of microfilariae (8). The membrane filtration technique can also be used with urine for the recovery of microfilariae (8). *Schistosoma haematobium* eggs can be concentrated by centrifugation of urine specimens; a membrane filter technique for the egg recovery has also been useful (8). Fresh samples or fixed samples in formalin should be used to prevent hatching of eggs.

Microsporidial spores of *Encephalitozoon intestinalis* can also be recovered from urine sediment. This organism primarily infects the intestinal tract but can also disseminate to the kidneys in immunocompromised individuals.

Sputum

Although not one of the more common specimens, expectorated sputum may be submitted for examination for parasites. Organisms in sputum that may be detected and may cause pneumonia, pneumonitis, or Loeffler's syndrome include the migrating larval stages of *Ascaris lumbricoides*, *Strongyloides stercoralis*, and hookworm; the eggs of *Paragonimus* spp.; *Echinococcus granulosus* hooklets; and *Entamoeba histolytica*, *Entamoeba gingivalis*, *Trichomonas tenax*, *Cryptosporidium* spp., and possibly the microsporidia. In a *Paragonimus* infection, the sputum may be viscous and tinged with brownish flecks, which are clusters of eggs ("iron filings"), and may be streaked with blood. Sputum is usually examined as a wet mount (saline or iodine), using low and high dry power ($\times 100$ and $\times 400$). The specimen is not concentrated before preparation of the wet mount. If the sputum is thick, an equal amount of 3% sodium hydroxide (NaOH) (or undiluted chlorine bleach) can be added; the specimen is thoroughly mixed and then centrifuged at $500 \times g$ for 5 min. NaOH should not be used if one is looking for *Entamoeba* spp. or *T. tenax*. After centrifugation, the supernatant fluid is discarded and the sediment can be examined as a wet mount with saline or iodine. If examination has to be delayed for any reason, the sputum should be fixed in 5 or 10% formalin to preserve helminth eggs or larvae or in PVA fixative to be stained later for protozoa.

Aspirates

The examination of aspirated material for the diagnosis of parasitic infections may be extremely valuable, particularly when routine testing methods have failed to demonstrate the organisms. These specimens should be transported to the laboratory immediately after collection. Aspirates include liquid specimens collected from a variety of sites where organisms might be found. The aspirates most commonly processed in the parasitology laboratory include fine-needle and duodenal aspirates. Fluid specimens collected by bronchoscopy include bronchoalveolar lavage fluid and bronchial washings (22).

Fine-needle aspirates may be submitted for slide preparation, culture, and/or molecular analyses. Aspirates of cysts and abscesses for amebae may require concentration by centrifugation, digestion, microscopic examination for motile organisms in direct preparations, and cultures and microscopic evaluation of stained preparations. Antigen detection and PCR are other possibilities, depending on individual laboratory testing options.

Bone marrow aspirates for *Leishmania* sp. amastigotes, *Trypanosoma cruzi* amastigotes, or *Plasmodium* spp. require Giemsa staining. Examination of these specimens may confirm an infection that has been missed by examination of routine blood films. In certain situations, culture, immunoassays for antigen detection, or PCR also provide more sensitive results (21).

Biopsy Specimens

Biopsy specimens are recommended for the detection of tissue parasites (Table 5). The following procedures may be used for this purpose in addition to standard histologic preparations: impression smears and teased and squash preparations of biopsy tissue from skin, muscle, cornea, intestine, liver, lung, and brain. Tissue to be examined by permanent sections or electron microscopy should be fixed as specified by the laboratories that will process the tissue. In certain cases, a biopsy may be the only means of confirming a suspected parasitic infection. Specimens that are going to be examined as fresh material rather than as tissue sections should be kept moist in saline and submitted to the laboratory immediately.

Detection of parasites in tissue depends in part on specimen collection and on having sufficient material to perform the recommended diagnostic procedures. Biopsy specimens are usually quite small and may not be representative of the diseased tissue. Multiple tissue samples often improve diagnostic results. To optimize the yield from any tissue specimen, all areas should be examined by as many procedures as possible. Tissues are obtained by invasive procedures, many of which are very expensive and lengthy; consequently, these specimens deserve the most comprehensive procedures possible.

Tissue submitted in a sterile container in sterile saline or on a sterile sponge dampened with saline may be used for cultures or molecular analyses of protozoa after mounts for direct examination or impression smears for staining have been prepared. Bacteriological transport media should be avoided. If cultures for parasites are to be made, sterile slides should be used for smear and mount preparation.

Blood

Depending on the life cycle, a number of parasites may be recovered in a blood specimen, either whole blood, buffy coat preparations, or various types of concentrations (8, 27). Although some organisms may be motile in fresh whole blood, species identification is normally accomplished from the examination of permanent stained blood films, both thick and thin films. Blood films can be prepared from fresh whole blood collected with no anticoagulants, anticoagulated blood, or sediment from the various concentration procedures. The recommended stain of choice is Giemsa stain; however, the parasites can also be seen on blood films stained with Wright's stain. Delafield's hematoxylin stain is often used to stain the microfilarial sheath; in some cases, Giemsa stain does not provide sufficient stain quality to allow differentiation of the microfilariae.

Thin Blood Films

In any examination of thin blood films for parasitic organisms, the initial screen should be carried out with the low-power objective ($10 \times$) of a microscope. Microfilariae may be missed if the entire thin film is not examined. Microfilariae are rarely present in large numbers, and frequently only a few organisms are present in each thin film preparation. Microfilariae are commonly found at the edges of the thin film or at the feathered end of the film because they are carried to these sites during spreading of the blood. The feathered end of the film, where the erythrocytes (RBCs) are drawn out into one single, distinctive layer of cells, should be examined for the presence of malaria parasites and trypanosomes. In these areas, the morphology and size of the infected RBCs are most clearly seen.

Depending on the training and experience of the microscopist, examination of the thin film usually takes 15 to 20 min (≥ 300 oil immersion fields) for the thin film at a magnification of $\times 1,000$. Although some people use a $50 \times$ or $60 \times$ oil immersion objective to screen stained blood films, there is some concern that small parasites such as plasmodia, *Babesia* spp., or *Leishmania* spp. may be missed at this lower total magnification ($\times 500$ or $\times 600$) compared with the $\times 1,000$ total magnification obtained using the more traditional $100 \times$ oil immersion objective. Because people tend to scan blood films at different rates, it is important to examine a minimum number of fields. If something suspicious has been seen in the thick film, the number of fields examined on the thin film is often considerably greater than 300. The request for blood film examination should always be considered a STAT procedure, with all reports (negative as well as positive) being relayed by telephone to the physician as soon as possible. If positive, notification of appropriate governmental agencies (local, state, and federal) should be done within a reasonable time frame in accordance with guidelines and laws. Most county or state public health laboratories require reporting of *Plasmodium*- and *Babesia*-positive cases; the local public health facility should be consulted for a list of reportable parasitic diseases relevant for your location.

Both malaria and *Babesia* infections have been missed with automated differential instruments, and therapy was delayed. Although these instruments are not designed to detect intracellular blood parasites, the inability of the automated systems to discriminate between uninfected RBCs and those infected with parasites may pose serious diagnostic problems (14).

Thick Blood Films

In the preparation of a thick blood film, the highest concentration of blood cells is in the center of the film. The examination should be performed at low magnification to detect microfilariae more readily. Examination of a thick film usually requires 5 to 10 min (approximately 100 oil immersion fields). The search for malarial organisms and trypanosomes is best done under oil immersion (total magnification, × 1,000). Intact RBCs are frequently seen at the very periphery of the thick film; such cells, if infected, may prove useful in malaria diagnosis, since they may demonstrate the characteristic morphology necessary to identify the organisms to the species level.

Blood Stains

For accurate identification of blood parasites, a laboratory should develop proficiency in the use of at least one good staining method. It is better to select one method that will provide reproducible results than to use several on a hit-or-miss basis. Blood films should be stained as soon as possible, since prolonged storage may result in stain retention. Failure to stain positive malarial smears within a month may result in failure to demonstrate typical staining characteristics for individual species.

The most common stains are of two types. Wright's stain has the fixative in combination with the staining solution, so that both fixation and staining occur at the same time; therefore, the thick film must be laked before staining. In Giemsa stain, the fixative and stain are separate; therefore, the thin film must be fixed with absolute methanol before staining.

Buffy Coat Films

Trypanosomes, occasionally *Histoplasma capsulatum* (a fungus which manifests as small oval yeast cells resembling those of *Leishmania* amastigote stages), and, in immunocompromised patients, potentially *Leishmania* spp. (*L. infantum, L. chagasi,* and *L. donovani*) are detected in the peripheral blood. The parasite or fungus is found in the large mononuclear cells in the buffy coat (a layer of leukocytes resulting from centrifugation of whole anticoagulated blood). The nuclear material stains dark red-purple, and the cytoplasm stains light blue (*Leishmania* spp.). *H. capsulatum* appears as a large dot of nuclear material (dark red-purple) surrounded by a clear halo area. Trypanosomes in the peripheral blood also concentrate with the buffy coat cells.

Screening Methods

Microhematocrit centrifugation with use of the QBC malaria tube, a glass capillary tube and closely fitting plastic insert (QBC malaria blood tubes; Becton Dickinson, Tropical Disease Diagnostics, Sparks, MD), has been used for the detection of blood parasites. At the end of centrifugation of 50 to 60 μl of capillary or venous blood (5 min in a QBC centrifuge, 14,387 × g), parasites or RBCs containing parasites are concentrated into a 1- to 2-mm region near the top of the RBC column and are held close to the wall of the tube by the plastic float, making them readily visible by microscopy. Tubes precoated with acridine orange provide a stain which induces fluorescence in the parasites. This method automatically prepares a concentrated smear, which represents the distance between the float and the walls of the tube. Once the tube is placed into the plastic holder (Para-viewer) and immersion oil is applied to the top of the hematocrit tube (no coverslip is necessary), the tube is examined with a 40× to 60× oil immersion objective (which must have a working distance of 0.3 mm or greater) (8).

Antigen and DNA Detection for Blood Parasites

Several antigen detection tests are available. Many among them are designed for rapid and individual diagnoses (Table 3; see also below). Most of the kits are not available in the United States but have proven to be very useful in other countries. Rapid tests are available to diagnose specifically *Plasmodium falciparum* or, on a genus level, *Plasmodium* sp. infections (Table 3). These tests are simple to perform and can be applied during the more time-consuming microscopic identification of the thin and thick blood smears. However, one has to be aware that false-positive and false-negative reactions do occur (4, 7, 33). The general recommendation is to use these tests only in addition to the microscopic examination of thick and thin blood smears. There are various PCR-based methods have been described in the scientific literature. Although the methods are more sensitive than standard microscopic examinations of blood films, they are not routinely used for malaria diagnosis.

Knott Concentration

The Knott concentration procedure is used primarily to detect the presence of microfilariae in the blood, especially when a light infection is suspected. The disadvantage of the procedure is that the microfilariae are killed by the formalin and are therefore not seen as motile organisms.

Membrane Filtration Technique

The membrane filtration technique using Nuclepore filters (25-mm Nuclepore filter [5-μm porosity]) has proved highly efficient in demonstrating filarial infections when microfilaremias are of low density. It has also been successfully used in field surveys (8).

Culture Methods

Very few clinical laboratories offer specific culture techniques for parasites. The methods for in vitro culture are often complex, while quality control is difficult and not really feasible for the routine diagnostic laboratory. In certain institutions, some techniques may be available, particularly where consultative services are provided and for research purposes.

Few parasites can be routinely cultured, and the only procedures that are in general use are for *Entamoeba histolytica, Naegleria fowleri, Acanthamoeba* spp., *Trichomonas vaginalis, Toxoplasma gondii, Trypanosoma cruzi, Encephalitozoon* spp., and the leishmanias. These procedures are usually available only after consultation with the laboratory and on special request. Commercial tests are available only for *T. vaginalis* (InPouch TV; BioMed Diagnostics).

Animal Inoculation and Xenodiagnosis

Most routine clinical laboratories do not have the animal care facilities necessary to provide animal inoculation capabilities for the diagnosis of parasitic infections. Host specificity for many animal parasite species is well known and limits the types of animals available for these procedures. In certain suspect infections animal inoculation may be requested and can be very helpful in making the diagnosis, although animal inoculation certainly does not take the place of other, more routine procedures. Mouse inoculation with amniotic fluid has been used in the past for diagnosis of congenital toxoplasmosis; this method, however, has mostly been replaced by PCR. Intraperitoneal inoculation of *Echinococcus multilocularis* metacestode material from surgical resection or from biopsy samples from mice or gerbils is still the most reliable procedure available for viability testing after long-term chemotherapy.

Xenodiagnosis is a technique that uses the arthropod host as an indicator of infection. Uninfected reduviid bugs are allowed to feed on the blood of a patient who is suspected of having Chagas' disease (*T. cruzi* infection). After 30 to 60 days, feces from the bugs are examined over a 3-month time frame for the presence of developmental stages of the parasite, which are found in the hindgut of the vector. This type of procedure is used primarily in South America for fieldwork, and the appropriate bugs are raised in various laboratories specifically for this purpose.

Antigen Detection

The detection of parasite-specific antigen is indicative of current infection. Immunoassays are generally simple to perform. Some formats allow the processing of large numbers of tests at one time, thereby reducing overall costs; others are specially designed for rapid individual diagnoses (immunochromatographic formats) (Tables 2 and 3). A major disadvantage of antigen detection is that in most cases the method can detect only a single pathogen at one time. Therefore, additional parasitological examinations must be performed to detect other parasitic pathogens. The current commercially available immunoassays for the detection of intestinal protozoa have excellent sensitivity and specificity compared to routine microscopy (1, 10–12). Specific ordering approaches using both immunoassays and routine O&P examinations are listed in Table 7. Rapid tests for the diagnosis of malaria should be used only in parallel to the examination of thick and thin blood smears.

Parasite DNA Detection

Nucleic acid-based diagnostic tests (particularly PCR, with its inherent potential for highly efficient and specific amplification of DNA) have been developed for almost all species of parasites. However, only a few are routinely used in diagnostic settings. The main reason for this minor role of diagnostic PCR in parasitology is the fact that many parasite stages can be adequately diagnosed using established, more traditional techniques (microscopy, detection of antigens and antibodies, or in vitro cultivation) that are generally less expensive than PCR and technically less demanding. Therefore, diagnosis by PCR is of great value in cases where these techniques are insufficient, i.e., in cases where (i) the immune response is not informative (e.g., acute infections, short-term follow-up after therapy, and congenital infections); (ii) high sensitivity is needed because of low parasite levels (e.g., cutaneous leishmaniasis); or (iii) morphologically indistinguishable organisms need to be identified (e.g., *Entamoeaba histolytica*/*Entabmoeba dispar* and eggs of taeniid tapeworms).

Diagnostic PCR may become more widespread when simple, fully standardized (commercial) test kits are available and costs are reduced through the implementation of pre- and post-PCR automated techniques. Furthermore, the possibilities to not only detect and identify but also quantify organisms and determine their genotypes by analyzing the diagnostic PCR product extend the diagnostic power of PCR. Indeed, PCR coupled with genetic characterization is already widely being used in parasitology to address questions such as parasite host range and host specificity, ways of transmission, and molecular epidemiology. Such genotyping applications should increase in the future with increasing knowledge of the relationship between genetic variation in parasites and features such as virulence or drug resistance. An important limitation of PCR-based diagnosis is the fact that sensitivity dramatically decreases with material stored for more than 1 day in formalin due to the fragmentation (fragment length of a few hundred base pairs) of the DNA. However, by selecting primers that produce PCR products as short as possible, which is recommended for real-time PCR, sensitivity might be reasonably high. Such tests, however, are not yet widely available in parasitology. Therefore, it seems to be the best choice to avoid formalin fixation if PCR analyses have to be considered.

APPENDIX

Parasite images

Parasites and parasitological resources

University of Delaware
http://www.udel.edu/medtech/dlehman/medt372/index.html

Parasite image library
http://www.dpd.cdc.gov/DPDx/HTML/Image_Library.htm

Protozoan images
http://www.medicine.cmu.ac.th

University of Georgia College of Agricultural and Environmental Sciences
http://sacs.cpes.peachnet.edu/nemabc/slideset1.htm

Parasitology information

Centers for Disease Control and Prevention
http://www.dpd.cdc.gov/DPDx/

World Health Organization
http://www.who.int

Medical Chemical Corporation
http://www.med-chem.com

Additional parasitology websites

Department of Parasitology, Faculty of Medicine, Chiang Mai University, Chiang Mai, Thailand
http://www.med.cmu.ac.th/dept/parasite/Default.htm

Biosystematics & the United States, National Parasite Collection Unit
http://www.lpsi.barc.usda.gov/bnpcu/

Medical parasitology links
http://www.hanmat.org/links.htm

Oklahoma State University
http://www.cvm.okstate.edu/instruction/kocan/vpar5333/vpar5333.Htm

University of California, Davis, Department of Nematology
http://ucdnema.ucdavis.edu/imagemap/nemmap/ENT156H-TML/E156charac

University of Edinburgh
http://www.ed.ac.uk/cpb/websites/htm

Literature

NCBI National Library of Medicine (PubMed)
http://www.ncbi.nim.nih.gov/entrez/query.fcgi

REFERENCES

1. **Aldeen, W. E., K. Carroll, A. Robison, M. Morrison, and D. Hale.** 1998. Comparison of nine commercially available enzyme-linked immunosorbent assays for detection of *Giardia lamblia* in fecal specimens. *J. Clin. Microbiol.* **36:**1338–1340.

2. **Beal, C., R. Goldsmith, M. Kotby, M. Sherif, A. El-Tagi, A. Farid, S. Zakaria, and J. Eapen.** 1992. The plastic envelope method, a simplified technique for culture diagnosis of trichomoniasis. *J. Clin. Microbiol.* **30:**2265–2268.

3. **Beaver, P. C., R. C. Jung, and E. W. Cupp.** 1984. *Clinical Parasitology*, 9th ed. Lea & Febiger, Philadelphia, PA.

4. **Bell, D., R. Go, C. Miguel, J. Walker, L. Cacal, and A. Saul.** 2001. Diagnosis of malaria in a remote area of the Philippines: comparison of techniques and their acceptance by health workers and the community. *Bull. W. H. O.* **79:**933–941.

5. **Brooke, M. M., and M. Goldman.** 1949. Polyvinyl alcohol-fixative as a preservative and adhesive for protozoa in dysenteric stools and other liquid material. *J. Lab. Clin. Med.* **34:**1554–1560.

6. **Chernesky, M., S. Morse, and J. Schachter.** 1999. Newly available and future laboratory tests for sexually transmitted diseases (STDs) other than HIV. *Sex. Transm. Dis.* **26:**8–11.

7. **Craig, M. H., B. L. Bredenkamp, C. H. Williams, E. J. Rossouw, V. J. Kelly, I. Kleinschmidt, A. Martineau, and G. F. Henry.** 2002. Field and laboratory comparative evaluation of ten rapid malaria diagnostic tests. *Trans. R. Soc. Trop. Med. Hyg.* **96:**258–265.

8. **Garcia, L. S.** 2007. *Diagnostic Medical Parasitology*, 5th ed. ASM Press, Washington, DC.

9. **Garcia, L. S.** 2009. *Practical Guide to Diagnostic Parasitology*, 2nd ed. ASM Press, Washington, DC.

10. **Garcia, L. S., and R. Y. Shimizu.** 1997. Evaluation of nine immunoassay kits (enzyme immunoassay and direct fluorescence) for detection of *Giardia lamblia* and *Cryptosporidium parvum* in human fecal specimens. *J. Clin. Microbiol.* **35:**1526–1529.

11. **Garcia, L. S., and R. Y. Shimizu.** 2000. Detection of *Giardia lamblia* and *Cryptosporidium parvum* antigens in human fecal specimens using the ColorPAC combination rapid solid-phase qualitative immunochromatographic assay. *J. Clin. Microbiol.* **38:**1267–1268.

12. **Garcia, L. S., R. Y. Shimizu, and C. N. Bernard.** 2000. Detection of *Giardia lamblia, Entamoeba histolytica/Entamoeba dispar*, and *Cryptosporidium parvum* antigens in human fecal specimens using the Triage parasite panel enzyme immunoassay. *J. Clin. Microbiol.* **38:**3337–3340.

13. **Garcia, L. S., R. Y. Shimizu, T. C. Brewer, and D. A. Bruckner.** 1983. Evaluation of intestinal parasite morphology in polyvinyl alcohol preservative: comparison of copper sulfate and mercuric chloride base for use in Schaudinn's fixative. *J. Clin. Microbiol.* **17:**1092–1095.

14. **Garcia, L. S., R. Y. Shimizu, and D. A. Bruckner.** 1986. Blood parasites: problems in diagnosis using automated differential instrumentation. *Diagn. Microbiol. Infect. Dis.* **4:**173–176.

15. **Garcia, L. S., R. Y. Shimizu, A. Shum, and D. A. Bruckner.** 1993. Evaluation of intestinal protozoan morphology in polyvinyl alcohol preservative: comparison of zinc sulfate- and mercuric chloride-based compounds for use in Schaudinn's fixative. *J. Clin. Microbiol.* **31:**307–310.

16. **Hanson, K. L., and C. P. Cartwright.** 2001. Use of an enzyme immunoassay does not eliminate the need to analyze multiple stool specimens for sensitive detection of *Giardia lamblia. J. Clin. Microbiol.* **39:**474–477.

17. **Hiatt, R. A., E. K. Markell, and E. Ng.** 1995. How many stool examinations are necessary to detect pathogenic intestinal protozoa? *Am. J. Trop. Med. Hyg.* **53:**36–39.

18. **Horen, W. P.** 1981. Modification of Schaudinn fixative. *J. Clin. Microbiol.* **13:**204–205.

19. **Markell, E. K., D. T. John, and W. A. Krotoski.** 1999. *Medical Parasitology*, 8th ed. The W. B. Saunders Co., Philadelphia, PA.

20. **Marti, H., and J. C. Koella.** 1993. Multiple stool examinations for ova and parasites and rate of false-negative results. *J. Clin. Microbiol.* **31:**3044–3045.

21. **Mathis, A., and P. Deplazes.** 1995. PCR and in vitro cultivation for detection of *Leishmania* spp. in diagnostic samples from humans and dogs. *J. Clin. Microbiol.* **33:**1145–1149.

22. **Mathis, A., R. Weber, H. Kuster, and R. Speich.** 1997. Simplified sample processing combined with a sensitive one-tube nested PCR assay for detection of *Pneumocystis carinii* in respiratory specimens. *J. Clin. Microbiol.* **35:**1691–1695.

23. **Melvin, D. M., and M. M. Brooke.** 1982. *Laboratory Procedures for the Diagnosis of Intestinal Parasites*, 3rd ed. U.S. Department of Health, Education, and Welfare publication (CDC) 82-8282. U.S. Government Printing Office, Washington, DC.

24. **Morgan, U., R. Weber, L. Xiao, I. Sulaiman, R. C. A. Thompson, W. Ndiritu, A. Lal, A. Moore, and P. Deplazes.** 2000. Molecular characterization of *Cryptosporidium* isolates obtained from human immunodeficiency virus-infected individuals living in Switzerland, Kenya, and the United States. *J. Clin. Microbiol.* **38:**1180–1183.

25. **Morris, A. J., M. L. Wilson, and L. B. Reller.** 1992. Application of rejection criteria for stool ovum and parasite examinations. *J. Clin. Microbiol.* **30:**3213–3216.

26. **National Committee for Clinical Laboratory Standards/ Clinical and Laboratory Standards Institute.** 2005. *Procedures for the Recovery and Identification of Parasites from the Intestinal Tract*. Approved standard M28-A2. Clinical and Laboratory Standards Institute, Wayne, PA.

27. **National Committee for Clinical Laboratory Standards/ Clinical and Laboratory Standards Institute.** 2000. *Use of Blood Film Examination for Parasites*. Approved standard M15-A. National Committee for Clinical Laboratory Standards, Wayne, PA.

28. **Occupational Safety and Health Administration.** 1991. Occupational exposure to bloodborne pathogens. 29 CFR 1910.1030. *Fed. Regist.* **56:**64175–64182.

29. **Scholten, T. H., and J. Yang.** 1974. Evaluation of unpreserved and preserved stools for the detection and identification of intestinal parasites. *Am. J. Clin. Pathol.* **62:**563–567.

30. **Siegel, D. L., P. H. Edelstein, and I. Nachamkin.** 1990. Inappropriate testing for diarrheal diseases in the hospital. *JAMA* **263:**979–982.

31. **U.S. Department of Health and Human Services.** 2007. *Biosafety in Microbiological and Biomedical Laboratories*, 5th ed. U.S. Government Printing Office, Washington, DC.

32. **Weber, R., D. A. Schwartz, and P. Deplazes.** 1999. Laboratory diagnosis of microsporidiosis, p. 315–361. *In* M. I. Wittner and L. M. Weiss (ed.), *The Microsporidia and Microsporidiosis.* ASM Press, Washington, DC.

33. **Wongsrichanalai, C.** 2001. Rapid diagnostic techniques for malaria control. *Trends Parasitol.* **17:**307–309.

34. **Yang, J., and T. Scholten.** 1977. A fixative for intestinal parasites permitting the use of concentration and permanent staining procedures. *Am. J. Clin. Pathol.* **67:**300–304.

Reagents, Stains, and Media: Parasitology

ANDREA J. LINSCOTT AND SUSAN E. SHARP

131

The evaluation of clinical specimens for ova and parasites in the clinical laboratory can involve the use of direct macroscopic examination of the specimen and microscopic examination of fresh and preserved specimens, as well as culture for some parasitic organisms. These examinations necessitate the use of a variety of stains, reagents, and media, the most common of which are discussed in this chapter.

As many parasitic organisms cannot be cultured, microscopic examination is the mainstay of diagnostic parasitology. Examination after proficient staining of fresh and unconcentrated specimens, as well as preserved and/or concentrated specimens with permanent stained preparations, most often provides for a rapid and accurate diagnosis. A variety of reagents and stains are available for these purposes, and each laboratory must decide which ones to use to best serve its patient population. In addition, as most specimens are submitted in fixatives and preservatives, the reader should note the specific interference of polyvinyl alcohol (PVA) and mercury reagents with immunoassays that are commonly used for parasitic diagnosis.

Caution should be taken when using reagents in the parasitology laboratory. Many routinely used compounds can be dangerous if not handled appropriately. For example, formalin and formaldehyde solutions can cause severe skin irritation and if swallowed can cause violent vomiting and diarrhea; mercury compounds are local irritants and systemic poisons that can be absorbed through the skin; phenol is a skin irritant and can affect the central nervous system if one is exposed to large amounts; and xylene can cause serious skin irritation, with extended exposure causing gastrointestinal, neurologic, and tissue damage (5).

REAGENTS

All of the following reagents listed are preservatives and/or fixatives. Table 1 lists several types of preservatives along with their content, specific permanent stained smears that can be performed, and immunoassays for which they can be used, as well as additional comments concerning the fixative.

Formalin Preparations

■ Formalin

Formalin has always been used in parasitology as an all-purpose preservative and in concentration procedures.

Formalin alone cannot be used for concentration techniques or permanent stained smears. It is easy to prepare and has a long shelf life. It is most routinely used as a preservative for stool and duodenal aspirate specimens. Formalin works well to preserve the morphologies of helminth ova and larvae and those of protozoan cysts, oocysts, and spores, although it does not preserve protozoan trophozoites well. Although both 5 and 10% solutions of formalin are currently used (5% for the best preservation of protozoan stages and 10% for ova and larvae), the 10% formulation is most widely used in clinical parasitology today. Formalin (10%) is prepared as indicated below:

Formaldehyde (37 to 40% HCHO solution)	100 ml
Saline (0.85% NaCl) OR distilled water...........	900 ml

Buffered formalin

Formalin buffered with sodium and potassium phosphates can be used to help maintain the morphology of parasites for long-term storage. To make buffered formalin, mix the following dry ingredients together and store in a tightly closed container. Add 0.8 g of this mixture to 1 liter of 10% (or 5%) formalin.

Sodium phosphate, dibasic (Na_2HPO_4)...........	6.1 g
Potassium phosphate, monobasic (KH_2PO_4)....	0.15 g

■ Merthiolate-iodine-formalin (MIF)

Protozoa and helminth ova and larvae can be distinguished on direct wet mount after stool and duodenal aspirate specimens are fixed in MIF. MIF allows not only for fixation but also for staining of the organisms, although organism morphology is not as good as when other permanent staining compounds are used. This method requires that two stock solutions, listed below, be combined into a fresh working solution immediately prior to use. In addition, after mixing of specimens with MIF, the mixture must be left undisturbed for 24 h prior to preparation of smears from the bottom two layers of the three layers that will form. Parasitological examination of specimens placed in MIF can be performed for several weeks after preservation, making it very useful for field surveys. MIF is also readily available commercially.

TABLE 1 Preservatives used in diagnostic parasitology (intestinal tract specimens)

Preservative	Preservative can be used for:		
	Concentrated examination	Permanent stained smear	Immunoassays[f]
5 or 10% formalin	Yes	No	Yes (EIA, FA, rapid)
5 or 10% buffered formalin	Yes	No	Yes (EIA, FA, rapid)
MIF	Yes	Polychrome IV stain[e]	No There are no published data for immunoassay systems
SAF	Yes	Iron hematoxylin, trichrome (not as good)	Yes (EIA, FA, rapid)
Hg-PVA[a]	Yes	Trichrome or iron hematoxylin	No PVA plastic powder interferes with immunoassays
Cu-PVA[b]	Yes	Trichrome or iron hematoxylin	No PVA plastic powder interferes with immunoassays
Zn-PVA[c]	Yes	Trichrome or iron hematoxylin	Some, but not all PVA plastic powder interferes with immunoassays
Single-vial systems[d]	Yes	Trichrome or iron hematoxylin	Some, but not all If no PVA or mercury, may be compatible with fecal immunoassays
Schaudinn's (without PVA)[a]	No	Trichrome or iron hematoxylin	No Mercury interferes with immunoassays

[a]PVA (plastic powder used as "glue" to attach stool onto the glass slide/no fixation properties per se) and Schaudinn's fixative (mercuric chloride base) are still considered to be the "gold standard" against which all other fixatives are evaluated for organism morphology after permanent staining. Additional fixatives prepared with nonmercuric chloride-based compounds are continuing to be developed and tested.

[b]This modification uses a copper sulfate base rather than mercuric chloride.

[c]This modification uses a zinc base rather than mercuric chloride and apparently works well with both trichrome and iron hematoxylin stains.

[d]These modifications use a combination of ingredients (including zinc) but are prepared from proprietary formulas. The aim is to provide a fixative that can be used for the fecal concentration, permanent stained smear, and available immunoassays for G. lamblia and Cryptosporidium spp. Some of these fixatives are now available commercially (check suppliers such as Medical Chemical Corp. and Meridian Bioscience). Testing for E. histolytica and/or the E. histolytica/E. dispar group still require fresh or frozen specimens.

[e]This stain can be used in place of trichrome for staining fecal smears preserved with MIF, PVA, or SAF methods. It is available commercially.

[f]EIA, enzyme immunoassay; FA, fluorescent antibody; rapid, cartridge (membrane flow/immunochromatographic method).

Solution I (store in brown bottle)

Distilled water	50 ml
Formaldehyde (USP)	5 ml
Thimerosal (tincture of merthiolate, 1:1,000)	40 ml
Glycerol	1 ml

Solution II (Lugol's solution) (good for several weeks in a tightly stopped brown bottle)

Distilled water	100 ml
Potassium iodide crystals (KI)	10 g
Iodine crystals (add after KI dissolves)	5 g

Combine 9.4 ml of solution I with 0.6 ml of solution II just before use.

PVA-Containing Preservatives and Fixatives

PVA acts as an adhesive for stool material, allowing the stool to adhere to glass slides. Several modifications are commercially available. The accompanying compound with the PVA, specifically, mercuric chloride, zinc sulfate, or cupric sulfate, acts as the preservative and allows fixation of protozoan cysts and trophozoites for use with trichrome or iron hematoxylin stains for permanent smears. All PVA-containing preservatives interfere with immunoassays.

■ Hg-PVA

The Hg-PVA fixative uses mercuric chloride as the pre-servative. Protozoan morphology is best preserved with PVA incorporating mercury compounds. However, due to the toxic nature of mercury compounds and the difficulty in preparation, most laboratories no longer prepare Hg-PVA.

■ Zn-PVA

The Zn-PVA fixative uses zinc sulfate in place of mercury as a preservative and fixative for protozoans. Specimens treated with Zn-PVA may also be stained with trichrome or iron hematoxylin stains for permanent smears.

■ Cu-PVA

The Cu-PVA fixative uses cupric sulfate in place of mercury as a preservative and fixative for protozoans. Specimens treated with Cu-PVA may also be stained with trichrome or iron hematoxylin stains for permanent smears.

Studies have shown that zinc sulfate provides a satisfactory, but not equal, substitute for mercury in the permanent staining procedures and that copper sulfate does not preserve morphology equal to that seen with mercuric chloride (7, 8).

■ Schaudinn's fixative/solution

Schaudinn's solution is a fixative made of mercuric chloride, distilled water, and 95% ethyl alcohol that gives excellent morphological preservation of protozoan organisms. It is used primarily in the preparation of permanent stained smears for parasitological examination from fresh, nonpreserved specimens. Specimens fixed in Schaudinn's solution can be used with either trichrome or iron hematoxylin stains. As with Hg-PVA, due to the toxic nature of mercuric compounds and the difficulty in preparation of this fixative, Schaudinn's solution is not routinely made in the clinical microbiology laboratory. In addition, Schaudinn's fixative is becoming increasingly more difficult to purchase commercially.

■ Sodium acetate-acetic acid-formalin (SAF)

SAF is very similar to formalin in that it is a liquid fixative and contains no mercury. However, unlike formalin, SAF can be used for both concentration techniques and permanent stained smears. The sediment from the concentration procedure is used for both the wet preparation and the permanent stain. Albumin-coated slides allow for better adhesion of the concentrated material to the slide and are recommended for use with SAF. SAF is an acceptable substitute for PVA or Schaudinn's solution for permanent smears stained with either trichrome or iron hematoxylin. SAF is available commercially and has a long shelf life, but it can also readily be made in the laboratory by mixing the reagents listed below:

Sodium acetate	1.5 g
Glacial acetic acid...	2.0 ml
Formaldehyde (37 to 40% HCHO solution)..........	4.0 ml
Distilled water	92.0 ml

■ Nonmercury, nonformalin fixatives: single-vial systems

There are several nonmercury, nonformalin proprietary fixatives commercially available that can be used for concentration of stool specimens, preparations of permanently stained smears, and fecal immunoassays (check with manufacturers for specific uses). Special stains are also available for use with some of these fixatives. Several of these all-purpose fixatives are currently available (Medical Chemical Corporation, Torrance, CA; Meridian Bioscience, Cincinnati, OH).

STAINS

Table 2 lists the stains that are most commonly used to detect and aid in the identification of parasitic organisms. The description and procedures for stains used in parasitology are listed below.

■ Iodine (Lugol's or D'Antoni's)

A solution of iodine can be used when preparing direct or concentrated wet mounts for parasitological examination. These nonspecific dyes allow the differentiation of parasitic cysts from leukocytes, the former of which retain the iodine and appear light brown. Iodine stains can be purchased commercially for use in routine parasitology. These solutions should be stored in dark containers in a dark environment. D'Antoni's iodine preparation has the advantage of use without further dilution, whereas Lugol's iodine must first be diluted into a working solution (1:5 dilution in distilled water) prior to use. Working solutions of both iodine preparations fade with time and should be discarded and replaced when their dark tea color lightens.

Basic procedure

Place 1 drop of iodine on a slide; add to this a small amount of fecal specimen and mix until homogeneous. The iodine stains fecal material immediately, and the timing of this step is not important. Place a coverslip on top of the

TABLE 2 Stains used for parasitic identification

Organism	Stain(s) used for detection
Cryptosporidium spp., *Isospora belli*, *Cyclospora cayetanensis*	Modified acid-fast stain
Naegleria spp., *Acanthamoeba* spp., *Balamuthia* spp.	Calcofluor white stain using fluorescent microscopy, trichrome stain
Isospora and *Cyclospora* oocysts, *Sarcocystis* sporocysts	Autofluorescence with no stain using fluorescent microscopy
Acanthamoeba	Modified Field's stain, trichrome stain
Cyclospora	Modified safranin stain
Microsporidia	Modified trichrome stain
Blood parasites (agents of malaria, microfilariae, and *Leishmania*, *Babesia*, and *Trypanosoma* spp.)	Giemsa or Wright's stain (rapid blood stains are also acceptable)
Microfilariae (specifically for sheaths and nuclei)	Delafield's hematoxylin stain; Giemsa stain also acceptable except for *Wuchereria bancrofti*
Parasitic helminth eggs/larvae and protozoan cysts	Iodine
Intestinal protozoan parasites	Iron hematoxylin stain, trichrome stain

suspension and view under ×100 magnification. Examine any suspicious material under ×400 magnification.

Acid-Fast Stains (Modified)

■ Modified Kinyoun stain (cold method)

■ Modified Ziehl-Neelsen stain (hot method)

Cryptosporidium, *Isospora belli*, and *Cyclospora cayetanensis* are parasites that can cause diarrheal disease in humans. All three of these organisms require special staining for detection, and modifications of the classic acid-fast staining techniques used for the detection of mycobacteria are used. The modifications include the use of decolorizing agents less harsh than those used for staining of mycobacteria (see chapter 17). In the modified acid-fast staining procedures, a 1% solution of sulfuric acid (1 ml of sulfuric acid in 99 ml of water) is used, as opposed to the 3% solution that is used in the acid-fast bacillus Kinyoun staining procedure, and a 5% sulfuric acid solution (5 ml of concentrated sulfuric acid in 95 ml of distilled water) is used, as opposed to the 3% HCl solution in 95% ethanol that is used in the acid-fast bacillus Ziehl-Neelsen staining procedure. Application of heat in the modified Ziehl-Neelsen staining procedure facilitates the entry of the carbol fuchsin dye into the organisms to stain them pink or red, whereas phenol replaces heat in the modified Kinyoun staining procedure. Staining reagents for mycobacteria are readily available commercially, and the only preparation that is required for these stains is for the modification of the decolorizing agents. See "Modified safranin stain" in "Other Stains" at the end of this section.

Basic procedure (modified Kinyoun stain)

Specimen (1 or 2 drops) is applied to a slide, allowed to air dry, and fixed with absolute methanol for 1 min. Carbol fuchsin is applied to the slide for 5 min, and then the slide is rinsed with 50% ethanol, followed by a water rinse. Sulfuric acid (1%) decolorizer is added for 2 min, and the slide is rinsed again with water. Methylene blue is added for 1 min, and then the slide is rinsed again with water. The slide is then air dried and examined at ×100 to ×1,000 magnification.

Blood Film Stains

■ Giemsa and Wright's stains

Examination of blood films for parasites includes the use of two common stains, the Giemsa stain and Wright's stain, both derivatives of the original Romanowsky stain. These stains are very similar, differing primarily in that no fixative is included in the Giemsa stain and the blood film must be fixed with absolute methanol prior to staining. Erythrocytic stippling, seen in some malaria infections, can be seen only using the Giemsa stain (4). Although stock solutions of these stains can be prepared in the laboratory, the procedure is very cumbersome and involves grinding of powdered stain with methanol and/or glycerol with a mortar and pestle, days to weeks of storage with shaking, and removal of supernatant or filtering prior to use. In addition, it is recommended that the Giemsa stain be prepared fresh each day of use by diluting the stain stock solution with phosphate-buffered water (9). Alternatively, Giemsa, Wright's, and Wright-Giemsa stains are readily available from commercial suppliers in liquid form and may need only dilution in a buffer solution. Blood films may be stained manually, but many laboratories rely on automated hematologic instruments for staining of thin (not thick) blood films, with acceptable results. These stains allow the detection of blood parasites, including the agent of malaria, microfilariae, and *Leishmania*, *Babesia*, and *Trypanosoma* species. Although for many years, Giemsa stain has been the stain of choice, the parasites can also be seen on blood films stained with Wright's stain, a Wright-Giemsa combination stain, or one of the more rapid stains such as Diff-Quik (American Scientific Products, McGaw Park, IL), Wright's Dip Stat Stain (Medical Chemical Corp.), or Field's stain. It is more appropriate to use a stain with which you are familiar, rather than Giemsa, which is somewhat more complicated to use. Polymorphonuclear leukocytes can serve as the quality control organism for any of the blood stains. Any parasites present will stain like the polymorphonuclear leukocytes, regardless of the stain used. Also, the College of American Pathologists checklist does not mandate the use of Giemsa stain.

Basic procedure

Cover the surface of a thin blood film with stain for 1 to 3 min. Add an equal volume of buffered water to the slide, and mix by gently blowing on the surface of the slide. Wait 4 to 8 min and flood the slide with buffered water. Allow the slide to dry and examine it under ×1,000 magnification. Thick films must be laked in distilled water or treated with saponin prior to performance of the staining procedure described above (9, 10). Satisfactorily stained smears show the following characteristics for the Giemsa and Wright's stains: erythrocytes, pale red and light tan, reddish, or buff, respectively; nuclei of leukocytes, purple with pale purple cytoplasm and bright blue with contrasting light cytoplasm, respectively; eosinophilic granules, bright purple-red and bright red, respectively; and neutrophilic granules, deep pink-purple and pink or light purple, respectively.

Hematoxylin Stains

■ Delafield's hematoxylin stain

Delafield's hematoxylin stain is used for thin and concentrated blood films for the detection of microfilariae and may show greater detail of the nuclei and sheaths than that shown with Giemsa and Wright's stains. Although the stain is not procedurally difficult to prepare, it does involve aging processes of 1 week followed by 1 month before it can be used. Delafield's hematoxylin stain is not readily available commercially and is used only in special circumstances. Preparation of the stain involves dissolving 180 g of aluminum ammonium sulfate in 1 liter of distilled water, heating until dissolved, and cooling (ammonium alum). Hematoxylin crystals (4 g) are dissolved in 25 ml of 95% ethyl alcohol, and the solution is then added to 400 ml of the ammonium alum. The solution is then covered with a cotton plug and exposed to sunlight and air for 1 week, after which it is filtered. To this solution, 100 ml each of glycerol and 95% ethyl alcohol is added. This solution is placed in sunlight for at least 1 month (6).

Basic procedure

Allow the specimen on a slide to air dry. Lake blood films with distilled water for 15 min and fix in absolute methanol for 5 min, followed by air drying. Stain for 10 to 15 min and rinse in water. Air dry, add a coverslip with mounting fluid, and examine the slide under ×1,000 magnification.

■ Iron hematoxylin stain

Iron hematoxylin stains are used for the detection, identification, and enumeration of intestinal protozoan parasites. There are many derivations of the iron hematoxylin stain, all of which can be used with fresh fecal specimens, fixed specimens containing PVA, specimens preserved in Schaudinn's solution, or specimens preserved in SAF to make permanent stained smears. Solutions of hematoxylin-ethanol and ferrous ammonium sulfate-hydrochloric acid are combined in equal parts to make working iron hematoxylin stain, and both solutions are available commercially.

Basic procedure

Place prepared slides in 70% ethanol for 5 min. Place the slide in 70% ethanol with iodine for 5 min if mercury-based fixatives are being used and then again in 70% ethanol for 5 min more (these last two steps are not necessary for non-mercury-based fixatives). Wash the slide in running tap water for 10 min, followed by placement in iron hematoxylin working solution for 5 min. After this staining step, wash again in running tap water for 10 min and then place the slide in the following reagents for 5 min each: 70% ethanol, 95% ethanol, 100% ethanol (twice), and xylene (or a substitute) (twice). Add Permount, and add a coverslip. Examine under ×1,000 magnification.

■ Trichrome stain (Wheatley trichrome stain)

The Wheatley trichrome stain, a modification of the Gomori tissue stain, is used for the detection, identification, and enumeration of intestinal protozoan parasites (24). This stain uses chromotrope 2R and light green SF stains to visually distinguish internal elements of protozoan parasitic cysts and trophozoites. Trichrome staining is usually performed on fixed fecal specimens containing PVA or Schaudinn's solution-preserved specimens. MIF- or SAF-preserved specimens may also be stained with the trichrome stain, as well as specimens preserved with single-vial systems. In addition, some proprietary stains are also available that may work better with these and other fixatives to make permanent stained preparations. Trichrome stain can be easily prepared in the laboratory or purchased from a commercial supplier.

Basic procedure
Place a prepared slide in 70% ethanol for 5 min. For mercury-based fixatives only, place the slide in 70% ethanol with iodine for 1 min (fresh specimens) or up to 10 min (for PVA-fixed air-dried specimens). Then place again in 70% ethanol for 5 min (twice). Place in trichrome stain for 10 min, followed by a 1- to 3-s rinse in 90% ethanol with acetic acid. Dip the slide several times in 100% ethanol, and then place it in 100% ethanol for 3 min (twice), followed by xylene for 5 to 10 min (twice). Add Permount, and add a coverslip. Dry overnight or for 1 h at 37°C. Examine under ×1,000 magnification. If 95% alcohol is substituted for 100% ethanol and xylene substitutes are used, it is important to increase the dehydration times for both the alcohol and xylene substitute by at least 5 to 10 min.

Modified Trichrome Stains for Microsporidia

■ Weber green

■ Ryan blue
Modifications of the trichrome stain have been successfully developed for the detection of microsporidia and are commercially available. Smears prepared from fresh or preserved fecal material can be used in this staining procedure. These stains are based on the standard trichrome technique, but a much more concentrated trichrome reagent is used and a longer staining time is incorporated. These changes are necessary because the microsporidia are not easily stained due to the difficulty in penetrating their outer spores. The Weber stain (23) stains the organisms pink with a green background, while the Ryan stain (16) also stains the organisms pink but gives a blue background. Staining at a temperature of 50°C for 10 min (13) or at 37°C for 30 min (3) may provide more intensely staining organisms and a cleaner background.

Basic procedure
Place a prepared smear in absolute methanol for 5 min and air dry prior to placement in trichrome stain for 90 min. Rinse in acid-alcohol (995.5 ml of 90% ethyl alcohol plus 4.5 ml of glacial acetic acid) for 10 s, dip several times in 95% alcohol, and place in 95% alcohol for 5 min. Prior to mounting, the slide is placed in 100% alcohol for 10 min. Examine at ×1,000 magnification. A study evaluating modifications to this procedure can be found in the reference by Kokoskin and colleagues (13).

■ Acid-fast trichrome stain
The acid-fast trichrome staining technique allows the detection of acid-fast organisms (*Cryptosporidium* spp., *I. belli*, and *C. cayetanensis*) and microsporidia from the same smear (12). Smears prepared from fresh or preserved fecal material can be used in this staining procedure. This procedure stains the microsporidial organisms pink and the acid-fast organisms pink to violet on a blue background.

Basic procedure
Place a prepared, air-dried slide in absolute methanol for 5 to 10 min and then again allow it to air dry. Place in carbol fuchsin solution for 10 min before rinsing in tap water. Decolorize with 0.5% acid-alcohol and rinse in tap water. Place in trichrome stain for 30 min at 37°C. Rinse in acid-alcohol for 10 s and then dip the slides several times in 95% alcohol for 10 s. Place the slide in 95% alcohol for 30 s and then allow it to air dry. Examine at ×1,000 magnification.

Other Stains

■ Modified Field's stain
Modified Field's stain facilitates the identification of *Acanthamoeba* species. This stain was evaluated and shown to give very good contrast compared with other stains, such as Wright's, Giemsa, Ziehl-Neelsen, and trichrome stains. For information on preparation and use of modified Field's stain, the reader is referred to the article by Pirehma and colleagues (15).

■ Modified safranin stain
Modified safranin stain allows for the detection of *Cyclospora* oocysts in formalin-fixed specimens and fecal concentrates. The stain most commonly used in the past for these organisms was the modified acid-fast stain; however, tremendous variations in staining properties can be seen with this stain. The modified safranin stain reportedly uniformly stains oocysts of *Cyclospora*. It has also been shown to be fast, reliable, and easy to perform (22).

Basic procedure
Place a prepared, thin smear of stool on a 60°C slide warmer until dried. Cover smear with a 1% safranin solution and heat in a microwave oven at full power (650 W) for 30 to 60 s. Rinse the smear with tap water for 30 s, counterstain with 1% aqueous methylene blue for 1 min, rinse with tap water, and air dry. Examine at ×1,000 magnification.

■ Calcofluor white stain
Calcofluor white, one of a number of optical brighteners, binds to cellulose and chitin and fluoresces best when exposed to long-wavelength UV light. These properties allow for its use in detecting fungi, *Pneumocystis jirovecii*, and free-living amebae like *Naegleria*, *Acanthamoeba*, and *Balamuthia* species, as well as the larvae of *Dirofilaria* species (its cuticle contains chitin). Calcofluor white is available through several commercial suppliers and is also easily made in the laboratory by following the manufacturer's recommendations.

Basic procedure
Place the specimen on a slide and allow it to air dry. Fix the slide in methanol for 1 to 2 min, rinse with distilled water, and allow it to air dry. Add 1 or 2 drops of 10% KOH, place 1 or 2 drops of calcofluor white solution on the specimen for 3 min, and view the slide with a fluorescent microscope and barrier filter (300 to 412 nm) at ×100 to ×400 magnification.

MEDIA
Cultures can be performed for only a few parasitic organisms, including *Acanthamoeba* species, *Naegleria fowleri*, *Plasmodium* species, intestinal amebae (like *Entamoeba histolytica*), *Trichomonas vaginalis*, *Leishmania* species, and *Trypanosoma* species (6). However, most clinical diagnostic microbiology laboratories do not provide parasite cultures. Cultures of these organisms are done only at large reference laboratories or research facilities. The exception is *Trichomonas vaginalis*, for which commercial products have been adapted for the routine laboratory. Many of the media listed in Table 3 are not commercially available but are listed for reference. Additional information regarding these media is available in the literature (1, 2, 11, 17–21).

TABLE 3 Media used for cultivation of parasites

Medium	Organism(s)	Comment(s)
Acanthamoeba monoxenic culture	*Acanthamoeba* and *Naegleria* species	Acanthamoeba medium plus nonnutrient agar overlaid with *Escherichia coli* or *Enterobacter aerogenes* Used for cerebrospinal fluid, tissue, or soil samples
Balamuth's aqueous egg yolk infusion medium	Intestinal amebae	Cannot grow *Balamuthia* *Balamuthia* grows only in cell culture lines
Boeck and Drbohlav's Locke-egg-serum (LES) medium	Intestinal amebae	Inspissated egg base slant with serum and rice powder
Buffered charcoal-yeast extract (BCYE) agar	*Acanthamoeba* species	Some manufacturers' media support growth better than others Some of these media support growth of trophozoites and/ or cysts
Cysteine-peptone-liver-maltose (CPLM) medium	*Trichomonas vaginalis*	Methylene blue dye is added to aid visualization of the organisms
Defined medium (14, 17) for pathogenic *Naegleria* species	*Naegleria fowleri*	Defined medium (14, 17)
DGM-21A medium	*Acanthamoeba* species	Defined medium
Diamond's Trypticase-yeast extract-maltose (TYM) complete medium, Diamond's complete medium, modified by Klass	*Trichomonas vaginalis*	TYM contains no antibiotics; a nonselective medium Klass modification contains penicillin G, streptomycin sulfate, and amphotericin B to inhibit bacterial overgrowth
Evans' modified Tobie's medium	*Leishmania* species and *Trypanosoma cruzi*	Uses beef extract, defibrinated horse blood, and phenol red as a pH indicator
InPouch TV (Biomed Diagnostics, Inc.)	*Trichomonas vaginalis*	Commercially available
Lash's casein hydrolysate-serum medium	*Trichomonas vaginalis*	Contains beef blood serum, which is absent from other media for *T. vaginalis*
LYI-S-2 medium	*Entamoeba histolytica*	Similar to TYI-S-33
M-11 medium	*Acanthamoeba culbertsoni*	Defined medium containing 11 amino acids
Modified Columbia agar	*Trichomonas vaginalis*	Solid agar medium; *T. vaginalis* colonies change pH and appearance of the agar plates
Nelson's medium	*Naegleria fowleri*	Contains fetal calf serum, which is necessary for growth of *N. fowleri*
NIH medium	*Leishmania* and *Trypanosoma* species	Similar to Evans' modified Tobie's medium
Novy-MacNeal-Nicolle (NNN) medium	*Leishmania* and *Trypanosoma* species	NaCl base agar medium
NNN medium with Offutt's modifications	*Leishmania* species	Contains blood in base medium, differentiating it from NNN medium
4 N (NNNN) medium	*Leishmania* and *Trypanosoma* species	Uses a sugar base Uses NIH medium overlay
Nonnutrient agar with live or dead bacteria	*Acanthamoeba* species	Some manufacturers' media support growth better than others
Proteose peptone-yeast extract-glucose (PPYG) medium	*Acanthamoeba* species	Basic medium to support growth of *Acanthamoeba* species
Peptone-yeast extract-glucose (PYG) medium	*Acanthamoeba* species	Similar to PPYG medium
SCGYEM medium (17)	*Naegleria fowleri*	Undefined medium
Schneider's *Drosophila* medium with 30% fetal calf serum	*Leishmania* and *Trypanosoma* species	Liquid medium; less costly than blood-based agars
Trichomonas culture system	*Trichomonas vaginalis*	Commercially available
Trypticase soy agar with 5% sheep, rabbit, or horse blood	*Acanthamoeba* species	Some manufacturers' media support growth better than others
TYI-S-33 medium	*Entamoeba histolytica*	Contains no antibiotics; a nonselective medium
TYSGM-9 medium	*Entamoeba histolytica*	Contains penicillin G and streptomycin sulfate to inhibit bacterial overgrowth
U.S. Army Medical Research Unit (USAMRU)	*Leishmania* species	Particularly useful in isolation of *Leishmania brasiliensis* complex
Yeager's LIT (liver infusion tryptose) medium	*Trypanosoma cruzi*	Hemin and antibiotics are added to isolate *T. cruzi* from triatoma gut specimens
YI-S medium	*Entamoeba histolytica*	Similar to TYI-S-33 medium

REFERENCES

1. **Byers, T. J., R. A. Akins, B. J. Maynard, R. A. Lefken, and S. M. Martin.** 1980. Rapid growth of *Acanthamoeba* in defined media; induction of encystment by glucose-acetate starvation. *J. Protozool.* **27:**216–219.
2. **Clark, C. G., and L. S. Diamond.** 2002. Methods for cultivation of luminal parasitic protists of clinical importance. *Clin. Microbiol. Rev.* **15:**329–341.
3. **Didier, E. S., J. M. Orenstein, A. Aldra, D. Bertucci, L. B. Rogers, and F. A. Janney.** 1995. Comparison of three staining methods for detecting microsporidia in fluids. *J. Clin. Microbiol.* **33:**3138–3145.
4. **Fritsche, T. R., and R. Selvarangan.** 2007. Medical parasitology, p. 1121–1168. *In* J. B. Henry (ed.), *Clinical Diagnosis and Management by Laboratory Methods.* The W. B. Saunders Company, Philadelphia, PA.
5. **Garcia, L. S.** 2007. *Diagnostic Medical Parasitology,* 5th ed., p. 978. ASM Press, Washington, DC.
6. **Garcia, L. S.** 2007. *Diagnostic Medical Parasitology,* 5th ed., p. 881–909. ASM Press, Washington, DC.
7. **Garcia, L. S., R. Y. Shimizu, A. Shum, and D. A. Bruckner.** 1993. Evaluation of intestinal protozoan morphology in polyvinyl alcohol preservative: comparison of zinc sulfate and mercuric chloride-based compounds for use in Schaudinn's fixative. *J. Clin. Microbiol.* **31:**307–310.
8. **Garcia, L. S., R. Y. Shimizu, T. C. Brewer, and D. A. Bruckner.** 1983. Evaluation of intestinal parasite morphology in polyvinyl alcohol preservative: comparison of copper sulfate and mercuric chloride base for use in Schaudinn's fixative. *J. Clin. Microbiol.* **17:**1092–1095.
9. **Garcia, L. S., S. P. Johnston, A. J. Linscott, and R. Y. Shimizu.** 2008. *Cumitech 46: Laboratory Procedures for Diagnosis of Blood-Borne Parasitic Diseases.* Coordinating ed., L. S. Garcia. ASM Press, Washington, DC.
10. **Gleeson, R. M.** 1990. An improved method for thick film preparation using saponin as a lysing agent. *Clin. Lab. Haematol.* **19:**249–251.
11. **Govinda, S., and L. S. Garcia.** 2002. Culture of protozoan parasites. *Clin. Microbiol. Rev.* **15:**327–328.
12. **Ignatius, R., M. Lehmann, K. Miksits, T. Regnath, M. Arvand, E. Engelmann, H. Hahn, and J. Wagner.** 1997. A new acid-fast trichrome stain for simultaneous detection of *Cryptosporidium parvum* and microsporidial species in stool specimens. *J. Clin. Microbiol.* **35:**446–449.
13. **Kokoskin, E., T. W. Gyorkos, A. Camus, L. Cedilotte, T. Purtill, and B. Ward.** 1994. Modified technique for efficient detection of microsporidia. *J. Clin. Microbiol.* **32:**1074–1075.
14. **Nerad, T. A., G. Visvesvara, and P. M. Daggett.** 1983. Chemically defined media for the cultivation of Naegleria: pathogenic and high temperature species. *J. Protozool.* **30:**383–387.
15. **Pirehma, M., K. Suresh, S. Sivanandam, A. K. Anuar, K. Ramakrishnan, and G. S. Kumar.** 1999. Field's stain—a rapid staining method for *Acanthamoeba* spp. *Parasitol. Res.* **10:**791–793.
16. **Ryan, N. J., G. Sutherland, K. Coughlan, M. Globan, J. Doultree, J. Marshall, R. W. Baird, J. Pedersen, and B. Dwyer.** 1993. A new trichrome-blue stain for detection of microsporidial species in urine, stool, and nasopharyngeal specimens. *J. Clin. Microbiol.* **31:**3264–3269.
17. **Schuster, F. L.** 2002. Cultivation of pathogenic and opportunistic free-living amebas. *Clin. Microbiol. Rev.* **15:**342–354.
18. **Schuster, F. L.** 2002. Cultivation of *Babesia* and *Babesia*-like blood parasites: agents of an emerging zoonotic disease. *Clin. Microbiol. Rev.* **15:**365–373.
19. **Schuster, F. L.** 2002. Cultivation of *Plasmodium* species. *Clin. Microbiol. Rev.* **15:**355–364.
20. **Schuster, F. L., and J. L. Sullivan.** 2002. Cultivation of clinically significant hemoflagellates. *Clin. Microbiol. Rev.* **15:**374–389.
21. **Stary, A., A. Kuchinka-Koch, and L. Teodorowicz.** 2002. Detection of *Trichomonas vaginalis* on modified Columbia agar in the routine laboratory. *J. Clin. Microbiol.* **40:**3277–3280.
22. **Visvesvara, G. S., H. Moura, E. Kovacs-Nace, S. Wallace, and M. L. Eberhard.** 1997. Uniform staining of *Cyclospora* oocysts in fecal smears by a modified safranin technique with microwave heating. *J. Clin. Microbiol.* **35:**730–733.
23. **Weber, R., R. T. Bryan, R. L. Owen, C. M. Wilcox, L. Gorelkin, G. S. Visvesvara, and the Enteric Opportunistic Infections Working Group.** 1992. Improved light-microscopical detection of microsporidia spores in stool and duodenal aspirates. *N. Engl. J. Med.* **326:**161–166.
24. **Wheatley, W. B.** 1951. A rapid staining procedure for intestinal amoebae and flagellates. *Am. J. Clin. Pathol.* **21:**990–991.

General Approaches for Detection and Identification of Parasites

LYNNE S. GARCIA, ROBYN Y. SHIMIZU, AND GRAEME P. PALTRIDGE

132

This chapter discusses various approaches and diagnostic methods currently in use for the diagnosis of parasitic infections. Assuming that clinical specimens have been properly collected and processed according to specific specimen rejection and acceptance criteria, the examination of prepared wet mounts, concentrated specimens, permanent stained smears, blood films, and various culture materials can provide critical information leading to organism identification and confirmation of the suspected cause of clinical disease (4, 6, 13, 14, 16). With the exception of relatively few immunoassay diagnostic kits, the majority of this diagnostic work depends on the knowledge and microscopy skills of the microbiologist. The field of diagnostic parasitology has taken on greater importance during the past few years for a number of reasons. Expanded world travel has increased the potential levels of exposure to a number of infectious agents. It is important to be aware of those organisms commonly found within certain areas of the world and the makeup of the patient population being serviced at your institution, particularly if immunocompromised patients are frequently seen as a part of your routine patient population. It is also important for the physician and microbiologist to recognize and understand the efficacy of any diagnostic method for parasite recovery and identification. Specific information on specimen collection and processing can be found in chapter 130.

STOOL SPECIMENS

For review, see the list of options for the collection of fecal specimens in chapter 130, Tables 3 and 6. Algorithms for the processing of stool specimens are presented in Fig. 1 to 3. The procedures that normally comprise the ova and parasite (O&P) examination are provided below and include the direct wet mount in saline, the concentration, and the permanent stained smear (1, 2, 4, 5, 7, 10–12, 14, 17).

Direct Wet Mount in Saline

The purpose of a direct wet mount is to confirm the possibility of infection with certain protozoa and helminths, to assess the worm burden of the patient, and to look for organism motility (Table 1) (4, 7, 12). Any fresh stool specimens that have not been refrigerated and that have been delivered to the laboratory within specified time frames are acceptable for testing; however, it is much more important to examine liquid or soft stools, rather than formed stools. Liquid and soft stools are much more likely to contain motile protozoan trophozoites rather than cysts, which do not demonstrate motility. Low-power examination (magnification, ×100) of the entire coverslip preparation (22 mm by 22 mm) and high dry power examination (magnification, ×400) of at least one-third of the coverslip area are recommended before the preparation is considered negative. Often, results from the direct smear examination should be considered presumptive; however, some organisms (*Giardia lamblia* cysts and trophozoites, *Entamoeba coli* cysts, *Iodamoeba bütschlii* cysts, helminth eggs and larvae, and *Isospora belli* oocysts) can be definitively identified. Reports of results obtained by this method should be considered preliminary, with the final report available after the results of the concentration wet mount and permanent stained smear are available.

If iodine is added to the preparation for increased contrast, the organisms will be killed and motility will be lost. Specimens that arrive in the laboratory in stool preservatives do not require a direct smear examination; proceed to the concentration and permanent stained smear.

Concentration Wet Mount

The purpose of the concentration method is to separate parasites from fecal debris and to concentrate any parasites present through either sedimentation or flotation (4, 7, 12). The concentration is specifically designed to allow recovery of protozoan cysts, coccidian oocysts, microsporidian spores, and helminth eggs and larvae (Table 2). Any stool specimen that is fresh or preserved is acceptable for testing. Wet mounts prepared from concentrated stool are examined in the same manner as that used for the direct wet mount method. The addition of too much iodine may obscure helminth eggs (the eggs may resemble debris). Often, results from the concentration examination should be considered presumptive; however, some organisms (*G. lamblia* cysts, *E. coli* cysts, *I. bütschlii* cysts, helminth eggs and larvae, and *I. belli* oocysts) can be definitively identified. Reports of results obtained by this method should be considered preliminary, with the final report available after the results of the permanent stained smear are available.

The formalin-ethyl acetate sedimentation concentration procedure is the most commonly used procedure, and the recommended centrifugation speed and time are $500 \times g$ and 10 min, respectively. In this procedure, the use of ether has

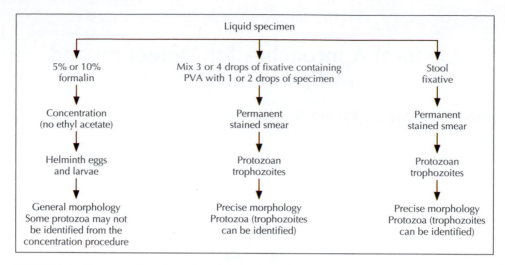

FIGURE 1 Processing liquid stool for O&P examination. Either PVA or Schaudinn's fixative can be used for the preparation of the permanent stained smear. Organism motility is seen when saline is used; iodine kills the organisms, so motility will no longer be visible. The use of ethyl acetate may remove the entire specimen and pull it into the layer of debris that will be discarded (liquid specimen normally contains mucus); centrifuge at 500 × g for 10 min (normal centrifugation time), but do not use ethyl acetate in the procedure. In general, laboratories have switched to nonmercury substitutes; the original Schaudinn's fixative contains mercuric chloride. However, in some instances the term "Schaudinn's fixative" is still used to describe not the original fixative but a formulation that is prepared with a copper or zinc base or other proprietary compounds. When fixatives are selected, it is important to know the contents in order to comply with disposal regulations. Reprinted from reference 5.

been replaced with ethyl acetate. However, it is important to remember that ethyl acetate should not be used for liquid specimens or those containing a great deal of mucus. The ethyl acetate may pull the liquid/mucus specimen contents into the debris layer, which will be discarded. Although the recovery of parasites from a liquid specimen or one containing a lot of mucus may not be successful, this simple centrifugation approach is still recommended. The standard zinc sulfate flotation procedure does not detect operculated or heavy eggs; when using this method, both the surface film and sediment should be examined before a negative result is reported.

Permanent Stained Smears

Trichrome, Iron-Hematoxylin, or Iron-Hematoxylin/ Carbol Fuchsin

The permanent stained smear provides contrasting colors for both the background debris and the parasites present (Tables 3 to 5) (4, 7, 12). Permanent stained stool smears are designed to allow examination and recognition of detailed organism morphology under oil immersion magnification (magnification, ×1,000). This method is primarily designed to allow the recovery and identification of the more common intestinal protozoan trophozoites and cysts, excluding the coccidia (unless the iron-hematoxylin/carbol fuchsin method is used) and microsporidia. Oil immersion examination of a minimum of 300 oil immersion fields is recommended; additional fields may be required if suspect organisms have been seen in the wet mounts. Although review of 300 fields seems like a time-consuming procedure, it takes less time than one would assume. This is particularly true for a trained microscopist in microbiology. Based on their expertise, patient population, and percentage of positive specimens, different laboratories may approach the examination of permanent stained smears by using different guidelines. Some laboratories may use a 60× oil immersion objective for screening purposes (magnification, ×600); however, it is important to examine a sufficient number of fields at a total magnification of ×1,000 before reporting the specimen as negative (no parasites seen).

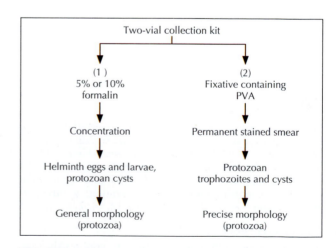

FIGURE 2 Processing preserved stool for O&P examination (two-vial collection kit). The formalin can be buffered or nonbuffered, depending on the laboratory protocol in use. PVA fixative prepared with mercuric chloride provides the best organism preservation. Alternatives are available, including zinc-based PVA, copper sulfate-based PVA, and SAF. Reprinted from reference 5.

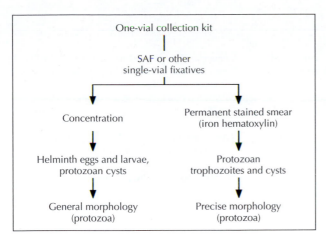

FIGURE 3 Processing preserved stool for O&P examination (one-vial collection kit). There are single-vial collection systems for which the formulas are proprietary; however, many contain zinc sulfate as one of the key ingredients. With the exception of SAF, compatibility of these fixatives with immunoassay reagents is not always possible. Other good options include Unifix, TOTAL FIX, or Z-PVA (Medical Chemical Corp.) with trichrome stain, as well as Ecofix with Ecostain (Meridian Biosciences, Cincinnati, OH). If the iron hematoxylin method containing the carbol fuchsin step is used, the coccidian oocysts will stain pink (*Cryptosporidium* spp., *Cyclospora cayetanensis*, or *Isospora belli*). Also, when using SAF, some recommend the use of an adhesive such as egg albumin to "glue" the fecal material onto the slide prior to staining. It is highly recommended that special stains be performed for the detection and identification of the coccidia (modified acid-fast stains) and the microsporidia (modified trichrome stains) from concentrated sediment to enhance organism recovery. Coccidian oocysts of *Isospora belli* can easily be detected in the concentration sediment wet mount; however, unless a very heavy infection is present, *Cryptosporidium* sp. oocysts may not be seen without special modified acid-fast stains. The small size of the microsporidian spores prevents identification without the use of special modified trichrome stains and microscopic examination with a 100× oil immersion objective. Reprinted from reference 5.

Modified Acid-Fast Staining

The modified acid-fast staining method is used to provide contrasting colors for the background debris and the parasites present and to allow examination and recognition of the acid-fast characteristic of the organisms under high dry magnification (magnification, ×400) (4, 17). Organisms that can be identified with this stain are the coccidia *Cryptosporidium* spp., *Cyclospora cayetanensis*, and *I. belli*. It is important to remember that *C. cayetanensis* stains much more acid-fast variable than *Cryptosporidium* spp. However,

occasionally one can see acid-fast variability with *Cryptosporidium*, particularly if the decolorizer is too strong (18). Although some microsporidian spores are acid-fast positive, their small size makes recognition very difficult; modified trichrome stains are recommended for the detection of microsporidian spores. Oil immersion examination of a minimum of 300 oil immersion fields is recommended.

Both hot and cold modified Ziehl-Neelsen and Kinyoun acid-fast staining methods are excellent for staining coccidian oocysts. Limitations of the procedure are generally related to specimen handling, including proper collection and centrifugation speed and time.

Modified Trichrome

Modified trichrome stains were primarily designed to allow recovery and identification of microsporidial spores from centrifuged stool specimens; internal morphology (horizontal and diagonal stripes of the polar tubule) may be seen in some spores under oil immersion (magnification, ×1,000). Any stool specimen that is submitted fresh or preserved in formalin or sodium acetate-acetic acid-formalin (SAF) is acceptable. Oil immersion examination of a minimum of 300 oil immersion fields is recommended. The identification of microsporidial spores may be possible; however, their small size makes recognition difficult, particularly in infections with few organisms in the clinical specimen. Identification to the species level requires electron microscopy or molecular methods such as PCR.

Immunoassay Methods

Immunoassay reagents are available commercially for several of the protozoan parasites, including *G. lamblia*, *Cryptosporidium* spp., the *Entamoeba histolytica*-*Entamoeba dispar* group, and *Entamoeba histolytica* (Table 6). These methods (enzyme immunoassay [EIA], fluorescent-antibody assay, and immunochromatographic assay [cartridge]) are designed to detect the antigens of select organisms; a negative result does not rule out the possibility that these organisms are present in low numbers or that other intestinal parasites are etiologic agents causing disease, including *Dientamoeba fragilis*, the microsporidia, and helminth parasites (4, 8, 9, 20). Immunoassay reagents are currently under development and trial for *D. fragilis* and the microsporidia.

ADDITIONAL TECHNIQUES FOR STOOL EXAMINATION

Although the routine O&P examination consisting of the direct wet mount, the concentration, and the permanent stained smear is an excellent procedure recommended for the detection of most intestinal parasites, several other diagnostic techniques are available for the recovery and identification of specific parasitic organisms (4, 7). Most laboratories do not routinely offer all of these techniques, but

---

TABLE 1 Diagnostic characteristics of organisms in wet mounts

Specimen	Protozoa	Helminths
Stool, other specimens from gastrointestinal tract, urogenital system	Size, shape, stage (trophozoite, precyst, cyst, oocyst), motility (fresh specimens only), refractility, cytoplasm inclusions (chromatoidal bars, glycogen vacuoles, axonemes, axostyles, median bodies, sporozoites)	Egg, larvae, or adult; size; internal structure: Egg: embryonated, opercular shoulders, abopercular thickenings or projections, hooklets, polar filaments, spines Larvae: head and tail morphology, digestive tract Adult: nematode, cestode, or trematode

TABLE 2 Identification of helminth eggs[a]

1. Eggs small (~25–40 μm)
   A. Operculate, generally oval shoulders (egg <35 μm); *Clonorchis*, operculated shoulders, bile stained, may be an abopercular knob, miracidium present, but difficult to see
      Clonorchis (Opisthorchis) spp. (Chinese liver fluke) or intestinal flukes: (*Heterophyes heterophyes* or *Metagonimus yokogawai*)
   B. Thick, radially striated shell (six-hooked oncosphere, individual eggs resemble those of *Taenia* spp.; eggs passed in egg packets containing 6–10 eggs; each egg is 25–40 μm)
      Dipylidium caninum (dog, cat tapeworm); note: egg packets could measure >150 μm
   C. Thick, radially striated shell (six-hooked oncosphere may not be visible in every egg from formalinized fecal specimens) (eggs cannot be identified to species level without special stains) (each egg is 30–47 μm)
      Taenia spp. (*T. saginata*, beef tapeworm; *T. solium*, pork tapeworm)
   D. Thin eggshell, clear space between developing shell and embryo, spherical or subspherical, containing a six-hooked oncosphere; polar filaments (filamentous strands) present between thin egg shell and embryo (each egg is 31–43 μm)
      Hymenolepis nana (dwarf tapeworm)

2. Eggs medium (~40–100 μm)
   A. Egg barrel-shaped, with clear polar plugs (each egg is 50–54 by 20–23 μm)
      Trichuris trichiura (whipworm)
   B. Egg flattened on one side, may contain larva (each egg is 70–85 by 60–80 μm)
      Enterobius vermicularis (pinworm)
   C. Egg with thick, tuberculated (bumpy) capsule (in decorticate eggs, capsule may be missing) (each egg is 45–75 by 35–50 μm)
      Ascaris lumbricoides (large roundworm), fertilized eggs
   D. Egg bluntly rounded at ends, thin shell (contains developing embryo at 8–16 ball stage of development) (each egg is 56–75 by 36–40 μm)
      Hookworm
   E. Operculate, operculum break in shell sometimes hard to see, smooth transition from shell to operculum; small "bump" may be seen at abopercular end (each egg is 58–75 by 40–50 μm)
      Diphyllobothrium latum (broad fish tapeworm)
   F. Thin eggshell, clear space between developing shell and embryo, spherical or subspherical, containing a six-hooked oncosphere; *no* polar filaments (filamentous strands) present between thin eggshell and embryo (each egg is 70–85 by 60–80 μm)
      Hymenolepis diminuta (rat tapeworm)

3. Eggs large (~100–180 μm)
   A. Egg with opercular shoulders into which the operculum fits (looks like teapot lid and flange into which lid fits), abopercular end somewhat thickened—not always visible (each egg is 80–120 by 48–60 μm); egg has been described as "urn-shaped."
      Paragonimus spp. (lung fluke)
   B. Egg tapered at one or both ends; long thin shell containing developing embryo (each egg is 73–95 by 40–50 μm)
      Trichostrongylus spp.
   C. Egg with thick, tuberculated (bumpy) capsule (in decorticate eggs, capsule may be missing) (each egg is 85–95 by 43–47 μm)
      Ascaris lumbricoides (large roundworm); unfertilized eggs
   D. Egg spined, ciliated miracidium larva may be seen, lateral spine very short (each egg is 70–100 by 55–65 μm)
      Schistosoma japonicum (blood fluke, stool)
      Schistosoma mekongi (rounder and smaller than *S. japonicum*); measure 50–65 by 30–55 μm
   E. Egg spined, ciliated miracidium larva may be seen, spine terminal (each egg is 112–170 by 40–70 μm)
      Schistosoma haematobium (blood fluke, urine)
   F. Egg spined, ciliated miracidium larva may be seen, spine terminal (each egg is 140–240 by 50–85 μm)
      Schistosoma intercalatum (blood fluke, stool)
   G. Egg spined, ciliated miracidium larva may be seen, large lateral spine (each egg is 114–180 by 45–70 μm)
      Schistosoma mansoni (blood fluke, stool)
   H. Egg >85 μm, operculum break in shell sometimes hard to see; smooth transition from shell to operculum; egg passed in undeveloped stage (each egg is 130–140 by 80–85 μm)
      Fasciolopsis buski (giant intestinal fluke) or *Fasciola hepatica* (sheep liver fluke) or *Echinostoma* spp.

[a]This table does not include every possible helminth that could be found as a human parasite; however, the most likely helminth infections are included.

TABLE 3 Diagnostic characteristics of organisms in permanent stained smears

Specimen	Protozoa	Helminths
Stool, other specimens from gastrointestinal tract, urogenital system	Size, shape, stage (trophozoite, precyst, cyst, oocyst, spore) Nuclear arrangement, cytoplasm inclusions (chromatoidal bars, vacuoles, axonemes, axostyles, median bodies, sporozoites, polar tubules)	Egg, larvae, and/or adults may not be identified because of excess stain retention or distortion

TABLE 4 Key to identification of intestinal amebae (permanent stained smear)

1. Trophozoites present 2
   Cysts present 7
2. Trophozoites measure >12 μm 3
   Trophozoites measure <12 μm 4
3. Karyosome central, compact; peripheral nuclear chromatin evenly arranged; "clean" cytoplasm .... *Entamoeba histolytica*[a]
   Karyosome eccentric, spread out; peripheral nuclear chromatin unevenly arranged; "dirty" cytoplasm .... *Entamoeba coli*
4. Peripheral nuclear chromatin 5
   Other than above 6
5. Karyosome central, compact; peripheral nuclear chromatin evenly arranged; "clean" cytoplasm .... *Entamoeba hartmanni*
   Karyosome large, blot-like; extensive nuclear variation .... *Endolimax nana*
6. No peripheral chromatin, karyosome large, junky cytoplasm .... *Iodamoeba bütschlii*
   No peripheral chromatin, karyosome variable, clean cytoplasm .... *Endolimax nana*
7. Cysts measure >10 μm (including any shrinkage "halo") 8
   Cysts measure <10 μm (including any shrinkage "halo") 10
8. Single *Entamoeba*-like nucleus with large inclusion mass .... *Entamoeba polecki*[b]
   Multiple nuclei 9
9. Four *Entamoeba*-like nuclei, chromatoidal bars have smooth, rounded ends .... *Entamoeba histolytica*[a]
   Five or more *Entamoeba*-like nuclei, chromatoidal bars have sharp, pointed ends .... *Entamoeba coli*
10. Single nucleus (may be "basket" nucleus), large glycogen vacuole .... *Iodamoeba bütschlii*[c]
    Multiple nuclei 11
11. Four *Entamoeba*-like nuclei, chromatoidal bars have smooth, rounded ends (nuclei may also number only two) ..... *Entamoeba hartmanni*
    Four karyosomes, no peripheral chromatin, round to oval shape .... *Endolimax nana*

[a]*Entamoeba histolytica* refers to the *Entamoeba histolytica/Entamoeba dispar* group. *E. histolytica* (pathogenic) can be determined by finding red blood cells in the cytoplasm of the trophozoites. Otherwise, on the basis of morphological grounds *E. histolytica* (pathogen) and *E. dispar* (nonpathogen) cannot be differentiated.
[b]It is very difficult to differentiate *Entamoeba polecki* trophozoites from those of the *E. histolytica/E. dispar* group or *E. coli*.
[c]Although some *I. bütschlii* cysts are larger than 10 μm, the majority of cysts measure 9–10 μm and the typical glycogen vacuole ensures the proper identification.

many can be performed relatively simply and inexpensively. Occasionally, it is necessary to examine stool specimens for the presence of scolices and proglottids of cestodes and adult nematodes and trematodes to confirm the diagnosis and/or for species identification (Table 7). A method for the recovery of these stages is also described in this chapter.

Culture of Larval-Stage Nematodes

Nematode infections giving rise to larval stages that hatch in soil or in tissues may be diagnosed by using fecal culture methods to concentrate the larvae (1, 4, 7, 17). *Strongyloides*

TABLE 5 Key to identification of intestinal flagellates

1. Trophozoites present 2
   Cysts present 7
2. Pear shaped 3
   Shape other 6
3. Two nuclei, sucking disk present .... *Giardia lamblia*
   One nucleus present 4
4. Costa length of body .... *Pentatrichomonas hominis*
   No costa 5
5. Cytostome present, >10 μm .... *Chilomastix mesnili*
   Cytostome present, <10 μm .... *Retortamonas intestinalis*
                                                            or *Enteromonas hominis*
6. Ameba shaped, one or two
   fragmented nuclei .... *Dientamoeba fragilis*
   Oval, one nucleus .... *Enteromonas hominis*
7. Oval or round cyst 8
   Lemon-shaped cyst 9
8. Four nuclei, median bodies,
   axoneme, >10 μm .... *Giardia lamblia*
   Two nuclei, no fibrils, <10 μm .... *Enteromonas hominis*
9. One nucleus, (shepherd's) crook fibril .... *Chilomastix mesnili*
   One nucleus, bird's beak fibril .... *Retortamonas intestinalis*

stercoralis larvae are the most common larvae found in stool specimens. Depending on the fecal transit time through the intestine and the patient's condition, rhabditiform and filariform larvae may be present. Caution must be exercised when handling larval cultures because infective filariform larvae may be present. If there is a delay in the preservation of the stool specimen, then embryonated ova as well as larvae of hookworm may be present. Culture of feces for larvae is useful for (i) revealing their presence when they are too scanty to be detected by concentration methods; (ii) distinguishing whether the infection is due to *S. stercoralis* or hookworm on the basis of rhabditiform larval morphology by allowing hookworm egg hatching to occur, releasing first-stage larvae; and (iii) allowing the development of larvae into the filariform stage for further differentiation.

Fecal culture methods are especially helpful for the detection of light infections with hookworm, *S. stercoralis*, and *Trichostrongylus* spp. and for the specific identification of parasites. Also, such techniques are useful for obtaining a large number of infective-stage larvae for research purposes. One enhanced recovery method, the agar plate culture for *Strongyloides*, and several culture techniques are described in this chapter. Since these procedures are less common, brief descriptions are included.

Agar Plate Culture for *S. stercoralis*

Agar plate cultures are recommended for the recovery of *S. stercoralis* larvae and tend to be more sensitive than some of the other diagnostic methods (4, 7). Approximately 2 grams of stool (about 1 inch in diameter) is placed in the center of the agar plate, and the plate is sealed to prevent accidental infections and held for 2 days at room temperature. As the larvae crawl over the agar, they carry bacteria with them, thus creating visible tracks over the agar. The plates are examined under the microscope for confirmation of the presence of larvae, the surface of the agar is then

TABLE 6 Commercially available immunoassays for detection of intestinal parasites

Fresh stool		Preserved in 5–10% formalin, SAF, or other single-vial system[a]	
No concentration	Concentration	No concentration	Concentration
EIA	DFA[b]	EIA	DFA[b]
Cryptosporidium spp.	*Cryptosporidium* spp.	*Cryptosporidium* spp.	*Cryptosporidium* spp.
G. lamblia	*G. lamblia*	*G. lamblia*	*G. lamblia*
E. histolytica		Immunochromatographic assay	
E. histolytica/E. dispar group		(cartridge format)	
Immunochromatographic assay		*Cryptosporidium* spp.	
(cartridge format)		*G. lamblia*	
Cryptosporidium spp.			
G. lamblia			
E. histolytica/E. dispar group			

[a]Some single-vial collection systems may use fixatives that are compatible with immunoassay testing; please consult specific manufacturer.
[b]DFA, direct fluorescent-antibody assay.

washed with 10% formalin, and final confirmation of larval identification is made via wet examination of the sediment from the formalin washings. Although specific agar formulations are often provided, any agar plate where the bacterial colonies are easily seen can be used for this purpose.

Baermann Technique

Another method of examining a stool specimen suspected of having small numbers of *Strongyloides* larvae is the use of a modified Baermann apparatus. The Baermann technique uses a funnel apparatus and relies on the principle that active larvae migrate from a fresh fecal specimen that has been placed on a wire mesh with several layers of gauze, which are in contact with tap water (4). Larvae migrate through the gauze into the water and settle to the bottom of the funnel, where they can be collected and examined. The main difference between this method and the Harada-Mori and petri dish methods is the greater amount of fresh stool used, possibly providing a better chance of larval recovery in a light infection. Besides being used for patient fecal specimens, this technique can be used to examine soil specimens for the presence of larvae.

However, the agar plate method is considered to be a more sensitive method for the recovery of *S. stercoralis* larvae.

Harada-Mori Filter Paper Strip Culture

To detect light infections with hookworm, *S. stercoralis*, and *Trichostrongylus* spp., as well as to facilitate specific identification, the Harada-Mori filter paper strip culture technique is very useful (1, 4, 7). The technique requires filter paper (strip cut to fit into a 15-ml test tube) to which fresh fecal material (about the size of a raisin to a small grape) is added to the middle of the filter paper and a test tube into which the filter paper is inserted. Moisture is provided by adding water to the tube (within a half-inch of the stool, but not covering the stool), which continuously soaks the filter paper by capillary action. Incubation under suitable conditions favors hatching of ova and/or development of larvae. Fecal specimens to be cultured should not be refrigerated, since some parasites are susceptible to cold and may fail to develop after refrigeration. Also, caution must be exercised in handling the filter paper strip itself, since infective *Strongyloides* larvae may migrate upward as well as downward on the paper strip.

TABLE 7 Additional helminth recovery and identification techniques (other than O&P examination)

Organism	Specimen	Procedure
Nematodes		
S. stercoralis	Fresh stool, not refrigerated (all organisms	Harada-Mori filter paper strip
Hookworm	can be recovered by any of the procedures	Filter paper/slant culture
Trichostrongylus spp.	indicated in the column to the right)	Charcoal culture
		Baermann test
		Agar plate culture (primarily for *S. stercoralis*)
Hookworm	Fresh stool, refrigeration acceptable	Direct smear (Beaver)
Ascaris lumbricoides		Dilution egg count (Stoll)
Trichuris trichiura		Either method acceptable for estimation of worm burden
Enterobius vermicularis	Scotch tape preparations, paddles, anal swab,	Direct microscopic examination
	other collection devices	
Trematodes		
Schistosoma spp.	Fresh stool, not refrigerated	Egg hatching test
	Fresh urine (24-h and single collection)	Egg viability test
Cestodes		
Tapeworms	Proglottids (gravid in alcohol)	India ink injection
	Stool in 5–10% formalin	Scolex search

Filter Paper/Slant Culture Technique (Petri Dish)

An alternative technique for culturing *Strongyloides* larvae is a filter paper/slant culture on a microscope slide placed in a glass or plastic petri dish (4). As with the techniques described above, sufficient moisture is provided by continuous soaking of filter paper in water. Fresh stool material is placed on filter paper, which is cut to fit the dimensions of a standard (1- by 3-in.) microscope slide. The filter paper is then placed on a slanted glass slide in a glass or plastic petri dish containing water. This technique allows direct examination of the culture system with a dissecting microscope to look for nematode larvae and free-living stages of *S. stercoralis* in the fecal mass or the surrounding water without having to sample the preparation.

Egg Studies and Scolex Search

Estimation of Worm Burdens

The only human parasites for which it is reasonably possible to correlate egg production with adult worm burdens are *Ascaris lumbricoides*, *Trichuris trichiura*, and the hookworms (*Necator americanus* and *Ancylostoma duodenale*). The specific instances in which information on approximate worm burdens is useful are when one is determining the intensity of infection, deciding on possible chemotherapy, and evaluating the efficacies of the drugs administered. With current therapy, the need for the monitoring of therapy through egg counts is no longer as relevant. Remember that egg counts are estimates; you will obtain count variations regardless of how carefully you follow the procedure. If two or more fecal specimens are being compared, it is best to have the same individual perform the technique with both samples and to do multiple counts. A number of methods have been described (1, 4, 7, 10, 12, 14).

Hatching of Schistosome Eggs

When schistosome eggs are recovered from either urine or stool, they should be carefully examined to determine viability. The presence of living miracidia within the eggs indicates an active infection that may require therapy. The viability of the miracidia can be determined in two ways: (i) the cilia of the flame cells (primitive excretory cells) may be seen on a wet smear by using high dry power and are usually actively moving, and (ii) the miracidia may be released from the eggs by the use of a hatching procedure (4). The eggs usually hatch within several hours when placed in 10 volumes of dechlorinated or spring water (hatching may begin soon after contact with the water). The eggs that are recovered in the urine (24-h specimen collected with no preservatives) are easily obtained from the sediment and can be examined under the microscope to determine viability. A sidearm flask has been recommended, but an Erlenmeyer flask is an acceptable substitute.

Both urine and stool specimens must be collected without preservatives and should not be refrigerated prior to processing. Hatching does not occur until the saline is removed and nonchlorinated water is added. If a stool concentration is performed, use saline throughout the procedure to prevent premature hatching. Make sure that the light is not too close to the side arm or top layer of water in the Erlenmeyer flask. Excess heat kills the miracidia. The lamp light mimics the sun shining on a water source, and the hatched larvae tend to swim toward the light. The absence of live miracidia does not rule out the presence of schistosome eggs. Nonviable eggs or eggs that failed to hatch are not detected by this method. Microscopic examination of direct or concentrated specimens should be used to demonstrate the presence or absence of eggs. Egg viability can be determined by placing some stool or urine sediment (the same material used for the hatching flask) on a microscope slide. Low-power magnification (×100) can be used to locate the eggs. Individual eggs can be examined with high dry magnification (×400); moving cilia on the flame cells (primitive excretory system) confirm egg viability.

Search for Tapeworm Scolices

Since therapy for the elimination of tapeworms is usually very effective, a search for the tapeworm scolex is rarely requested and is no longer clinically relevant. However, stool specimens may have to be examined for the presence of scolices and gravid proglottids of cestodes for proper species identification. This procedure requires mixing a small amount of feces with water and straining the mixture through a series of wire screens (graduated from coarse to fine mesh) to look for scolices and proglottids. Remember to use standard precautions and to wear gloves when performing this procedure. The appearance of scolices after therapy is an indication of successful treatment. If the scolex has not been passed, it may still be attached to the mucosa; the parasite is capable of producing more segments from the neck region of the scolex, and the infection continues.

EXAMINATION OF OTHER SPECIMENS FROM THE INTESTINAL TRACT

Examination for Pinworm

A roundworm parasite that has a worldwide distribution and that is commonly found in children is *Enterobius vermicularis*, known as pinworm or seatworm. The adult female worm migrates out of the anus, usually at night, and deposits her eggs on the perianal area. The adult female (8 to 13 mm long) may occasionally be found on the surface of a stool specimen or on the perianal skin. Since the eggs are usually deposited around the anus, they are not commonly found in feces and must be detected by other diagnostic techniques. Diagnosis of pinworm infection is usually based on the recovery of typical eggs, which are described as thick-shelled, football-shaped eggs with one slightly flattened side. Often each egg contains a fully developed embryo and becomes infective within a few hours after being deposited. Commercial collection devices are available and can be used for specimen collection, similar to the approach with cellulose tape indicated below (4). Many clinicians may treat patients on the basis of clinical symptoms without confirmation of the suspected diagnosis of pinworm infection.

Cellulose Tape Preparations

The most widely used procedure for the diagnosis of pinworm infection is the cellulose tape (adhesive cellophane tape) method (2, 4, 10, 11). Specimens should be obtained in the morning, before the patient bathes or goes to the bathroom. The tape is applied to the anal folds and is then placed sticky side down on a microscope slide for examination. At least four to six consecutive negative slides should be observed before the patient is considered free of infection.

Anal Swabs

The anal swab technique (4) is also available for the detection of pinworm infections; however, most laboratories use the cellulose tape method because it eliminates the necessity of preparing and storing swabs. At least four con-secutive negative preparations should be observed before the patient is considered negative; some recommend six consecutive negative preparations.

A paraffin-coated swab should be gently rubbed over the perianal surface and into the folds. Place the swab into the anal opening about 1/4 in. and then replace the swab in the tube. The tube containing the swab is half filled with xylene substitute and is allowed to stand for a few minutes. After centrifugation, the sediment is examined microscopi-cally for the presence of eggs.

Sigmoidoscopy Material

Material obtained from sigmoidoscopy can be helpful in the diagnosis of amebiasis that has not been detected by routine fecal examinations, and the procedure is recommended for this purpose. However, usually a series of at least three routine stool examinations for parasites should be performed for each patient before a sigmoidoscopy examination is done (4).

Material from the mucosal surface should be aspirated or scraped and must not be obtained with cotton-tipped swabs. At least six representative areas of the mucosa should be sampled and examined (six samples, six slides). Usually, the amount of material is limited and should be processed im-mediately to ensure the best examination possible (Table 8). Three methods of examination can be performed. All three are acceptable; however, depending on the availability of trained personnel, the availability of proper fixation fluids, or the amount of specimen obtained, one or two procedures are recommended. If the amount of material limits the ex-amination to one procedure, the use of polyvinyl alcohol (PVA) fixative is highly recommended for the subsequent preparation of permanent stains.

Although the fecal immunoassays are currently not approved for this purpose and are not the tests of choice, if the material is going to be examined by using any of the fluorescent-antibody assay, EIA, or immunochromato-graphic immunoassay detection kits (*Cryptosporidium* spp. or *G. lamblia*), then 5 or 10% formalin or SAF fixative is

TABLE 8 Recovery of parasites from other intestinal tract specimens

Source	Organism	Procedure
Sigmoidoscopy specimens		
Unpreserved	Ameba trophozoites (motility)	Direct wet mount, immunoassay tests[a]
Air-dried smears	Coccidia	Modified acid-fast stain
	Microsporidia	Modified trichrome, optical brighteners, immunoassay tests[b]
Preserved 5–10% formalin or SAF	Helminth eggs and larvae (rare), ameba and flagellate cysts,[c] and trophozoites (SAF only)	Concentration wet mount, immunoassay tests
	Coccidia	Modified acid-fast smear, immunoassay tests
	Microsporidia	Modified trichrome, optical brighteners, immunoassay tests[b]
PVA	Helminth eggs and larvae (rare), ameba and flagellate cysts[c]	Wet mount
	Ameba and flagellate cysts[c] and trophozoites	Permanent stained smear
Schaudinn's fixative	Ameba and flagellate cysts[c] and trophozoites	Permanent stained smear
Duodenal specimens[d]		
Unpreserved	Helminth eggs and larvae, flagellate trophozoites (motility)	Direct wet mount
Entero-Test capsule		
Preserved 5–10% formalin or SAF	Helminth eggs and larvae, flagellate trophozoites	Concentration wet mount, immunoassay tests Permanent stained smear
Entero-Test capsule	Coccidia	Modified acid-fast smear, immunoassay tests
	Microsporidia	Modified trichrome, optical brighteners, immunoassay tests[b]
PVA	Flagellate trophozoites	Permanent stained smear
Anal impression smear	Pinworm adult and eggs	No stain, cellulose tape preparation and other collection devices
Adult worm or segments	Helminth adult worms or proglottids	Carmine stain (rarely used), India ink
Tissue biopsy specimen	Helminth eggs, larvae, and adults; protozoan cysts; trophozoites; oocysts; sporozoites; and spores	Touch preparations, squash preparations, permanent stains, histology

[a]Immunoassay tests for the *Entamoeba histolytica/E. dispar* group or *Entamoeba histolytica* require fresh or frozen stool; preserved stool specimens are not acceptable for testing. Immunoassays for *Cryptosporidium* spp. and *Giardia lamblia* are approved for use on stool; immunoassay use for other intestinal tract specimens may or may not be appropriate, depending on specimen source, consistency, and volume.
[b]Some genus-specific immunoassay reagents for the microsporidia are available commercially but are not FDA approved.
[c]Although cysts may be present in stool, sigmoidoscopy specimens are often obtained from patients with severe diarrhea or dysentery. In such cases, the cyst forms are usually absent; trophozoites would be the most likely stage seen, particularly in the case of *Entamoeba histolytica*.
[d]Duodenal specimens are often submitted as aspirates; in such cases the volume may be sufficient to perform concentrations. However, if small amounts of duodenal mucus and/or biopsy material are obtained, squash preparations preserved with Schaudinn's fixative are preferred. This approach may require the use of slides precoated with albumin to facilitate adhesion. Mucus obtained from the Entero-Test capsule string may be treated as a fresh specimen; the string can also be immediately placed in preservative after retrieval, and the mucus can be processed as a permanent stained smear.

recommended. However, immunoassays for the detection of the *Entamoeba histolytica/E. dispar* group or confirmation of the pathogen *Entamoeba histolytica* require fresh or frozen stool for testing; preserved stool is not acceptable.

Physicians performing sigmoidoscopy procedures may not realize the importance of selecting the proper fixative for material to be examined for parasites when using the concentration and permanent stained smear methods. It is recommended that a parasitology specimen tray (containing Schaudinn's fixative, PVA, and 5 or 10% formalin) be provided or that a trained technologist be available at the time of sigmoidoscopy to prepare the slides.

Direct Saline Mount

If there is no lag time after collection and a microscope is available in the immediate vicinity, some of the material should be examined as a direct saline mount for the presence of motile trophozoites (4). A drop of material is mixed with a drop of 0.85% sodium chloride and is examined under low light intensity for the characteristic movement of amebae. It may take time for the organisms to become acclimated to this type of preparation; thus, motility may not be obvious for several minutes. There will be epithelial cells, macrophages, and possibly polymorphonuclear leukocytes (PMNs) and erythrocytes, which will require a careful examination to reveal amebae.

Since specific identification of protozoan organisms can be difficult when only the direct saline mount is used, this technique should be used only when there is sufficient material left to prepare permanent stained smears.

Permanent Stained Smear

Most of the material obtained at sigmoidoscopy can be smeared (gently) onto a slide and immediately immersed in Schaudinn's fixative (4). These slides can then be stained with trichrome or iron hematoxylin stain and examined for specific cell morphology, either protozoan or otherwise. The procedure and staining times are identical to those for routine fecal smears.

If the material is bloody, contains a lot of mucus, or is a "wet" specimen, a few (no more than 2 or 3) drops of PVA can be mixed with 1 or 2 drops of material directly on the slide, which is allowed to air dry (a 37°C incubator can be used) for at least 2 h before staining. If time permits, the PVA smears should be allowed to dry overnight; they can be routinely stained with trichrome stain and examined as a permanent mount.

Material from sigmoidoscopy can be placed in small amounts of SAF. After fixation for 30 min, the specimen can be centrifuged at 500 × g for 10 min, and smears from the small amount of sediment can be prepared for permanent staining with iron hematoxylin (trichrome stain would be the second choice). The most relevant organism for consideration when sigmoidoscopy is performed is *E. histolytica*, the morphology of which is normally seen from the permanent stained smear. However, if fresh stool or aspirated material is obtained, then both the permanent stained smear and an antigen detection reagent kit for the detection of the *Entamoeba histolytica/E. dispar* group or confirmation of the pathogen *Entamoeba histolytica* can be used. If enough material is present for only a single procedure, then the permanent stained smear is recommended, particularly if the iron hematoxylin stain (incorporating the carbol fuchsin step) is used (4). This method would enhance the detection of the coccidia, which are modified acid-fast positive. However, this approach is less commonly

used for the detection of *Cryptosporidium* spp. or *G. lamblia*, which can be confirmed by using special stains and/or fecal immunoassays performed on routine stool specimens rather than sigmoidoscopy material.

Duodenal Contents

Duodenal Drainage

In infections with *G. lamblia* or *S. stercoralis*, routine stool examinations may not reveal the organisms. Duodenal drainage material can be submitted for examination (Table 8).

A fresh, unpreserved specimen should be submitted to the laboratory; the amount may vary from <0.5 ml to several milliliters of fluid. The specimen may be centrifuged (at 500 × g for 10 min) and should be examined immediately as a wet mount for motile organisms (iodine may be added later to facilitate identification of any organisms present). If the specimen cannot be completely examined within 2 h after it is taken, any remaining material should be preserved in 5 to 10% formalin.

If the duodenal fluid contains mucus, this is where the organisms tend to be found. Therefore, centrifugation of the specimen is important, and the sedimented mucus should be examined. *Giardia* trophozoites may be caught in mucus strands, and the movement of the flagella on the trophozoites may be the only subtle motility seen for these flagellates. *Strongyloides* larvae are usually very motile. Immunoassay methods for *Cryptosporidium* spp. and *G. lamblia* can also be used with fresh or formalinized material; however, duodenal fluid is not included in many of the package inserts as an acceptable specimen.

If the amount of duodenal material submitted is very small, rather than using any of the specimen for a wet smear examination, permanent stains can be prepared. This approach provides a more permanent record, and the potential problems with unstained organisms, very minimal motility, and a lower-power examination can be avoided by using oil immersion examination of the stained specimen at ×1,000 magnification.

Duodenal Capsule Technique (Entero-Test)

A method of sampling duodenal contents that eliminates the need for intestinal intubation has been devised and consists of the use of a length of nylon yarn coiled inside a gelatin capsule (4, 7). The yarn protrudes through one end of the capsule, and this end of the line is taped to the side of the patient's face. The capsule is then swallowed, the gelatin dissolves in the stomach, and the weighted string is carried by peristalsis into the duodenum. The weight is released and passes out in the stool when the line is retrieved after a period of 4 h. Bile-stained mucus clinging to the yarn is then scraped off with gloved fingers and is collected in a small petri dish. Usually 4 or 5 drops of material are obtained.

The specimen should be examined immediately as a wet mount for motile organisms. Organism motility is similar to that described above for duodenal drainage. If the specimen cannot be completely examined within an hour after the yarn has been removed, the material should be preserved in 5 to 10% formalin or PVA-mucus smears should be prepared.

The pH of the terminal end of the yarn should be checked to ensure adequate passage into the duodenum (a very low pH means that it never left the stomach). Also, since the bile duct drains into the intestine at this point, the terminal end of the yarn should be a yellow-green color.

UROGENITAL SPECIMENS

Several parasites may be recovered and identified from urogenital specimens. Although the most common pathogens are probably *Trichomonas vaginalis* and *Schistosoma haematobium*, other organisms such as the microsporidia are becoming much more important (Table 9). Also, the Knott concentration for the recovery of microfilariae can be performed from blood, as can the membrane filtration approach from urine.

Direct Wet Mount

The identification of *T. vaginalis* is usually based on the examination of a wet preparation of vaginal and urethral discharges and prostatic secretions or urine sediment and may require the testing of multiple specimens to confirm the diagnosis. These specimens are diluted with a drop of saline and are examined under low power and reduced illumination for the presence of actively motile organisms. As the jerky motility begins to diminish, it may be possible to observe the undulating membrane, particularly under high dry power (magnification, ×400).

While the membrane filtration technique can be used for the recovery of microfilariae, examination of urinary sediment may be indicated in certain filarial infections. The occurrence of microfilariae in urine has been reported with increasing frequency in *Onchocerca volvulus* infections in Africa.

Urine is collected in a bottle, this volume is recorded, and thimerosal (1 ml/100 ml of urine) is added. The specimen is placed in a funnel fitted with tubing and a clamp; this preparation is allowed to settle overnight. On the following day, 10 to 20 ml of urine is withdrawn and centrifuged. The supernatant is discarded, and the sediment is resuspended in 0.85% NaCl. This preparation is again centrifuged, and 0.5 to 1.0 ml of the sediment is examined under the microscope for the presence of nonmotile microfilariae. The membrane filtration technique can also be used with urine for the recovery of *Schistosoma haematobium* eggs (4). This approach uses a 25-mm Nuclepore filter (5-μm porosity) (4, 7).

The use of stained smears is usually not necessary for the identification of *T. vaginalis*. Many times the number of false-positive and false-negative results reported on the basis of stained smears strongly suggests the value of confirmation by observation of motile organisms from the direct mount, from appropriate culture media (4, 7, 14), or from direct detection with immunoassay reagents (4).

Stained smears may be prepared from material obtained from the membrane filtration techniques used for the recovery of microfilariae; Delafield's hematoxylin or Giemsa stain may be used. It is important to remember that Giemsa stain may not adequately stain the sheath, and correct identification of the organisms may require staining with a hematoxylin-based stain.

Some microsporidial infections can also be diagnosed from the examination of urine sediment that has been stained by one of the modified trichrome methods or by using optical brightening agents such as calcofluor white (4). Multiple methods are recommended for confirmation of the diagnosis.

Culture

Specimens from women for culture (for *T. vaginalis*) may consist of vaginal exudate collected from the posterior fornix on cotton-tipped applicator sticks or genital secretions collected on polyester sponges. Specimens from men can include semen, urethral samples collected with a polyester sponge, or urine. Urine samples collected from the patient should be the specimen first voided in the morning. It is critical that clinical specimens be inoculated into culture medium as soon as possible after collection (4, 11, 14). Although collection swabs can be used, there are often problems with specimens drying prior to culture; immediate processing is mandatory for maximum organism recovery. Another approach would be to use the plastic envelope methods (*Trichomonas* Culture System [Empyrean Diagnostics, Mountain View, CA] or InPouch TV [BioMed Diagnostics, San Jose, CA]), which are simplified techniques for transport and culture (4). The following control strain should be available when using these cultures for clinical specimens: *T. vaginalis* ATCC 30001. Many media for the isolation of *T. vaginalis* are available, and some of these can be purchased commercially and have relatively long shelf lives, particularly the plastic envelope methods.

If no trophozoites are seen after 4 days of incubation, then discard the tubes and report the culture as negative. Results for patient specimens should not be reported as positive unless control cultures are positive. Since culture may take as long as 3 to 4 days and the clinical specimens may contain nonviable organisms, it is recommended that microscopic examination of wet smears be performed as well (possible dead organisms may be present, although they will be difficult to see).

Antigen Detection *(Trichomonas vaginalis)*

The culture method is considered to be the most sensitive for the diagnosis of trichomoniasis; however, due to the time and effort involved, some laboratories have decided to use some of the new immunoassay detection kits (4). The Osom Trichomonas Rapid Test (Genzyme Diagnostics, Cambridge, MA) is an immunochromatographic method for antigen detection using the dipstick format. Results are available within 10 min, and according to the manufacturer, there is a 95% agreement with the reference standard (culture and wet mount).

TABLE 9 Detection of urogenital parasites

Organism	Procedure
Trichomonas vaginalis	Wet mount (motility)
	Culture
	Giemsa stain
	Direct fluorescent antibody
	DNA probe
	Latex agglutination
	Enzyme-linked immunoassay
	Rapid immunochromatographic assay (dipstick)
Schistosoma haematobium	Wet mount (urine sediment)
	Membrane filtration
	Tissue section
Microfilariae	Knott concentration
	Membrane filtration (Nuclepore filter)
	Giemsa stain
	Delafield's hematoxylin stain
Microsporidia	Modified trichrome stain[a]
	Optical brighteners (calcofluor white)[a]
	Immunoassay tests[a,b]
	Routine histology
	Electron microscopy

[a]Staining procedures and fluorescent antibody tests for organism detection performed on centrifuged sediment (500 × g for 10 min).
[b]Immunoassays are available commercially but are not yet FDA approved.

SPECIMENS FROM OTHER BODY SITES

When routine testing methods have failed to demonstrate the organisms, the examination of aspirated material for the diagnosis of parasitic infections may be extremely valuable (Table 10). Specimens should be transported to the laboratory immediately after collection. Aspirates include liquid specimens collected from a variety of sites as well as fine-needle aspirates and duodenal aspirates. Fine-needle aspirates are often collected by the cytopathology staff who process the specimens, or they may be collected and sent to the laboratory directly for slide preparation and/or culture. Fluid specimens collected by bronchoscopy include bronchoalveolar lavage and bronchial washing fluids.

Procedural details for processing sigmoidoscopic aspirates and scrapings for the recovery of *E. histolytica* and techniques for preparation of duodenal aspirate material have been presented earlier in this chapter.

Biopsy specimens are recommended for use in the diagnosis of parasitic infections in tissues (Table 10). In addition to standard histologic preparations, the following can be used: impression smears and teased and squash preparations of biopsy tissue from skin, muscle, cornea, intestine, liver, lung, and brain. Tissue to be examined as permanent sections or by electron microscopy should be fixed as specified by the laboratories that will process the tissue, and in certain cases, testing of a biopsy specimen may be the only means of confirming a suspected parasitic problem. Specimens that are going to be examined as fresh material rather than as tissue sections should be kept moist in saline and submitted to the laboratory immediately.

Detection of parasites in tissue depends on specimen collection and the retrieval of sufficient material for examination. Biopsy specimens are usually quite small and may not be representative of the diseased tissue. Multiple tissue samples often improve diagnostic results. To optimize the yield from any tissue specimen, examine all areas and use as many procedures as possible. Tissues are obtained from invasive procedures, many of which are very expensive and lengthy; consequently, these specimens deserve the most comprehensive procedures possible.

Tissue submitted in a sterile container on a sterile sponge dampened with saline may be used for cultures of protozoa after mounts for direct examination or impression smears for staining have been prepared. If cultures for parasites will be made, use sterile slides for smear and mount preparation or inoculate cultures prior to smear preparation.

Bone Marrow

Bone marrow aspirates to be evaluated for *Leishmania* amastigotes, *Trypanosoma cruzi* amastigotes (African trypanosomiasis organisms are not relevant), *Plasmodium* spp., or *Toxoplasma gondii* (bone marrow is a less common site for this organism) require Giemsa staining. However, if stained with a hematoxylin/Giemsa combination stain, the organisms will be visible as well. If specimens are to be processed for culture, it is important to maintain sterility of the specimen prior to inoculation of media for parasitology cultures. After inoculation of appropriate media, the remaining specimen can be processed for smear preparation and staining.

Brain

Generally, when cerebrospinal fluid or brain aspirates or biopsy specimens are received, the most likely parasites would include the free-living amebae, *Acanthamoeba* spp., *Balamuthia mandrillaris*, or *Naegleria fowleri*. The use of nonnutrient agar (with bacterial overlays) cultures is recommended for *Acanthamoeba* spp. and *N. fowleri*; quality control cultures with known positive organisms are recommended as a basis for acceptable interpretation of patient culture results. If free-living ameba cultures are ordered for central nervous system specimens, the agar plates should be incubated at 37°C (room air, no CO_2) (4, 7). Unfortunately, cultures for *B. mandrillaris* are difficult to perform; consultation with CDC is recommended if this infection is suspected. The remaining specimen can then be processed for smear preparation and staining. Although *T. gondii* would also be seen in stained smears, one could also use immunospecific reagents, cell line culture, or PCR. Spinal fluid should not be diluted before examination. Impression smears from tissues should be prepared and stained with Giemsa stain. The material is pressed between two slides, with the smear resulting when the slides are pulled apart (one across the other). The smears are allowed to air dry and are then processed like a thin blood film (fixed in absolute methanol and stained with Giemsa stain).

Patients with primary amebic meningoencephalitis are rare, but the examination of spinal fluid may reveal the amebae, usually *Naegleria fowleri*. Unspun sedimented spinal fluid should be placed on a slide, under a coverslip, and observed for motile amebae; smears can also be stained with trichrome, Wright's, or Giemsa stain. Spinal fluid, exudate, or tissue fragments can be examined by light microscopy or phase-contrast microscopy. Care must be taken not to confuse leukocytes with actual organisms and vice versa. The spinal fluid may appear cloudy or purulent (with or without erythrocytes), with a cell count of from a few hundred to more than 20,000 leukocytes (primarily neutrophils) per ml. Failure to find bacteria in this type of spinal fluid should alert one to the possibility of primary amebic meningoencephalitis; however, false-positive bacterial Gram stains have been reported due to the excess debris. Isolation of these organisms from tissues can be done by using special media. When spinal fluid is placed in a counting chamber, organisms that settle to the bottom of the chamber tend to round up and look very much like leukocytes. For this reason, it is better to examine the spinal fluid on a slide directly under a coverslip, not in a counting chamber.

Possible infection with microsporidia (the most likely organism would be *Encephalitozoon* spp.; less common would be *Trachipleistophora antropophtera*) should also be considered. Specific methods would include modified trichrome, acid-fast, and Giemsa stains; a nonspecific optical brightening agent (calcofluor white); routine histology (methenamine silver, PAS, and tissue Gram stains); and electron microscopy. Electron microscopy or immunospecific reagents would be required to identify the microsporidia to the genus and species levels.

Helminth parasite stages such as *Taenia solium* cysticerci and hydatid cysts of *Echinococcus* spp. would generally be identified through examination of routine histologic slides; however, confirmation of hydatid disease could also be made from the hooklets seen in the hydatid cyst fluid contents.

Eyes

Eye specimens could include those from the cornea, conjunctiva, contact lens, or contact lens solutions. Although eye specimens are preferred, *Acanthamoeba* spp. have been cultured from patient contact lenses and lens solution. These specimens would be acceptable; however, due to risk management issues, the laboratory should not accept unopened commercial lens care solutions. These solutions could be referred to laboratories or agencies such as the FDA that handle testing and approval of commercial products. Also,

TABLE 10 Specimen, possible parasite recovered, and appropriate tests (other than intestinal tract)[a]

Body site	Specimen	Possible parasites	Tests
Bone marrow	Aspirate	*Leishmania* spp., *Trypanosoma cruzi*, *Plasmodium* spp., *Toxoplasma gondii*	Giemsa, culture
Brain	Tissue biopsy specimen, cerebrospinal fluid	*Naegleria* spp., *Acanthamoeba* spp.	Giemsa, trichrome, culture
		Balamuthia mandrillaris, Entamoeba histolytica	Giemsa, trichrome
		Toxoplasma gondii	Giemsa, immunospecific reagent, culture, PCR
		Microsporidia (*Encephalitozoon* spp., *Trachipleistophora anthropophthera*)	Modified trichrome, acid-fast stain, Giemsa, optical brightening agent (calcofluor white), histology[b] (methenamine silver, PAS,[c] tissue Gram stains), electron microscopy
		Taenia solium (cysticerci), *Echinococcus* spp.	Routine histology[b]
Eye	Cornea, conjunctiva, contact lens, lens solutions[d]	Microsporidia (*Encephalitozoon* spp., *Trachipleistophora* spp., *Nosema* spp., *Microsporidium* spp.)	Acid-fast stain, Giemsa, modified trichrome, methenamine silver, optical brightening agent calcofluor white), histology[b] (methenamine silver, PAS,[c] tissue Gram stains), electron microscopy
		Acanthamoeba spp.	Giemsa, trichrome, culture, calcofluor white (cysts only)
		Toxoplasma gondii	Giemsa, immunospecific reagent, culture
	Larval or adult worms	*Loa loa, Dipetalonema, Thalezia, Dirofilaria immitis, Gnathostoma* spp., *Toxocara canis, Taenia solium* (cysticerci), *Echinococcus* spp.	Direct examination, routine histology[b]
	Fly larvae, adult lice	Myiasis, lice infestation	Direct examination
Kidney, bladder	Biopsy specimens	Microsporidia (*Encephalitozoon* spp., *Enterocytozoon bieneusi*)	Modified trichrome, acid-fast stain, Giemsa, optical brightening agent (calcofluor white), histology[b] (methenamine silver, PAS,[c] tissue Gram stains), electron microscopy
		Schistosoma haematobium	Direct examination
	Adult worm, eggs	*Dioctyphyma renale*	Direct examination
Liver, spleen	Aspirates, biopsy specimens	*Echinococcus* spp.	Wet mount, routine histology[b]
		Clonorchis spp., *Opisthorchis* spp.	Routine histology[b]
		Capillaria hepatica, Toxocara canis, T. cati, Toxoplasma gondii, Leishmania donovani	Giemsa, culture
		Cryptosporidium spp.	Modified acid-fast stain, immunospecific reagents
		Microsporidia (*Encephalitozoon* spp., *Enterocytozoon bieneusi*)	Modified trichrome, acid-fast stain, Giemsa, optical brightening agent (calcofluor white), histology[b] (methenamine silver, PAS,[c] tissue Gram stains), electron microscopy
		Entamoeba histolytica[e]	Wet mount, trichrome
Lymph node, lymphatics	Aspirates, biopsy specimens	*Toxoplasma gondii, Trypanosoma cruzi, Trypanosoma brucei rhodesiense, T. brucei gambiense*	Direct examination, routine histology,[b] Giemsa, culture
		Microsporidia	Modified trichrome, acid-fast stain, Giemsa, optical brightening agent (calcofluor white), histology[b] (methenamine silver, PAS,[c] tissue Gram stains), electron microscopy
		Wuchereria bancrofti, Brugia malayi, Brugia spp.	Thick blood films, concentration, membrane filtration
Lung	Sputum (expectorated or induced), bronchoalveolar lavage fluid, transbronchial aspirates, brush biopsy specimens, open lung biopsy specimens	*Ascaris lumbricoides, Strongyloides stercoralis*, hookworm, *Paragonimus* spp., *Echinococcus granulosus*	Wet mount, routine histology[b]
		Microsporidia (*Encephalitozoon* spp., *Enterocytozoon bieneusi*)	Modified trichrome, acid-fast stain, Giemsa, optical brightening agent (calcofluor white), histology[b] (methenamine silver, PAS,[c] tissue Gram stains), electron microscopy
		Toxoplasma gondii	Giemsa, immunospecific reagent, culture
		Cryptosporidium spp.	Modified acid-fast stain, immunospecific reagent
	Saliva	*Entamoeba gingivalis, Trichomonas tenax*	Trichrome

(Continued on next page)

TABLE 10 Specimen, possible parasite recovered, and appropriate tests (other than intestinal tract) *(Continued)*

Body site	Specimen	Possible parasites	Tests
Muscle	Biopsy specimen	*Trichinella* spp.	Wet examination, squash preparation, routine histology[b]
		Microsporidia (*Pleistophora* spp., *Nosema* spp., *Trachipleistophora hominis*)	Modified trichrome, acid-fast stain, Giemsa, optical brightening agent (calcofluor white), histology[b] (methenamine silver, PAS,[c] tissue Gram stains), electron microscopy
		Sarcocystis spp., *Baylisascaris procyonis*, *Ancylostoma* spp., *Taenia solium* (cysticerci), *Multiceps* (coenurus), *Echinococcus* spp., *Spirometra* (spargana), *Onchocerca volvulus* (nodules), *Gnathostoma* spp., *Trypanosoma cruzi*	Routine histology[b]
Nasopharynx, sinus cavities	Scraping, biopsy specimens, aspirates	Microsporidia (*Encephalitozoon* spp., *Enterocytozoon bieneusi*, *Trachipleistophora hominis*)	Modified trichrome, acid-fast stain, Giemsa, optical brightening agent (calcofluor white), histology[b] (methenamine silver, PAS,[c] tissue Gram stains), electron microscopy
		Acanthamoeba spp.	Giemsa, trichrome, culture, calcofluor white (cysts only)
		Naegleria spp.	Giemsa, trichrome, culture
		Leishmania spp.	Giemsa, culture
Rectal tissue	Scraping, aspirate, biopsy specimens	*Schistosoma mansoni*, *S. japonicum*	Direct examination
Skin	Skin snips	*Onchocerca volvulus*, *Mansonella streptocerca*	Giemsa, routine histology[b]
	Scraping, aspirates, biopsy specimen	*Leishmania* spp.	Giemsa, culture, routine histology[b]
		Acanthamoeba spp.	Giemsa, trichrome, culture, calcofluor (cysts only)
		Entamoeba histolytica, *Schistosoma* spp.	Routine histology[b]

[a]This table does not include every possible parasite that could be found in a particular body site. Parasite stages include trophozoites, cysts, oocysts, spores, adults, larvae, eggs, hooklets, amastigotes, and trypomastigotes. Although PCR methods have been used in the research setting for most of the organisms listed in the table, reagents are generally not commercially available.

[b]Routine histology can be used for the detection and identification of many parasites. In some cases, it may be the only means of diagnosis.

[c]PAS, periodic acid-Schiff stain.

[d]Although eye specimens are much preferred, free-living amebae have been cultured from patient contact lenses and lens solutions; we would not reject these specimens. An exception would be *unopened* commercial lens care solutions; these solutions would be rejected.

[e]The examination of abscess aspirates for the presence of *Entamoeba histolytica* trophozoites is an uncommon procedure and not always reliable in diagnosing extraintestinal amebiasis; serologic tests would be preferred.

the presence of *Acanthamoeba* in a lens solution does not automatically equate to *Acanthamoeba* keratitis; it is only suggestive at best. A corneal scraping is recommended. After appropriate media have been inoculated, smears from acceptable specimens should be prepared and stained using Giemsa or trichrome stains. Although *T. gondii* could be seen in stained smears, one could also use an immunospecific reagent or PCR for confirmation. Most individuals who are infected with *T. gondii* do not develop ocular disease; however, two populations are at risk, the immunocompromised patient with HIV and neonates who have been exposed transplacentally to the mother's acute infection.

Also, microsporidia are highly suspect from this body site, and specific methods would include modified trichrome, acid-fast, and Giemsa stains; a nonspecific optical brightening agent (calcofluor white); routine histology (methenamine silver, PAS, and tissue Gram stains); and electron microscopy. Electron microscopy or immunospecific reagents would be required to identify the microsporidia to the genus and species levels, which could include *Encephalitozoon* spp., *Trachipleistophora* spp., *Nosema* spp., *Vittaforma* spp., *Anncaliia* spp., and *Microsporidium* spp.

Ocular disease caused by nematodes includes onchocerciasis, loiasis, dirofilariasis, gnathostomiasis, theileriasis, and toxocariasis. Diagnosis of onchocerciasis can be accomplished by confirming the presence of microfilariae in a corneal biopsy or from the microscopic examination of multiple skin snips. The diagnosis of loiasis can be confirmed from the detection of circulating microfilariae of *Loa loa* in the blood or direct eye examination for the presence of the adult worm. Ocular disease can occur with the migration of *Dirofilaria immitis* larvae through periorbital or palpebral tissue; however, laboratory diagnosis of this infection is rare. Diagnosis of infections with *Gnathostoma* spp. and *Toxocara canis* is difficult but should be considered in patients with marked eosinophilia and elevated immunoglobulin E. In the case of visceral and ocular larva migrans, serology for toxocariasis may be very helpful.

Eye disease can also be caused by cestodes, including *T. solium* (cysticercosis) and *Echinococcus* spp. (hydatid disease). These infections would generally be identified through direct ophthalmoscopic demonstration of the larval *T. solium*, computed tomography scans for hydatid cysts, or examination of routine histologic slides.

Ocular myiasis and infestations with lice are also possible; laboratory personnel may be asked to identify various fly larvae (*Dermatobia, Gasterophilus, Oestrus, Cordylobia, Chrysomia, Wohlfahrtia, Cochliomyia,* and *Hypoderma*) and/or lice (*Pediculus humanus corporis* or *P. humanus capitis* [documented, but rare] or *Pthirus pubis* [more common]).

Kidneys and Bladder

The kidneys serve as the primary site for the adult worm *Dioctyphyma renale*. These worms generally live in the pelvis of the right kidney or in body cavities. Although these infections have been isolated from dogs in many areas of the world, they tend to be uncommon in humans. Infections can be confirmed at autopsy, by the migration of worms from the urethra, by discharge of worms from the skin over an abscessed kidney, or by recovery of eggs in the urine. Possible infection with microsporidia (the most likely organism would be *Encephalitozoon* spp.; less common would be *Enterocytozoon bieneusi*) should also be considered. Specific methods would include modified trichrome, acid-fast, and Giemsa stains; a nonspecific optical brightening agent (calcofluor white); routine histology (methenamine silver, PAS, and tissue Gram stains); and electron microscopy. Electron microscopy or immunospecific reagents would be required to identify the microsporidia to the genus and species levels.

Mucosa from the bladder wall may reveal eggs of *Schistosoma haematobium* (tissue squash preparation) when they are not being recovered in the urine. The eggs in the bladder wall should be checked for viability by either a hatching technique or microscopic observation of the functioning flame cells within the miracidium larva (4).

Liver and Spleen

Although the liver and spleen can serve as sites for a number of organisms as the secondary site, specific organisms that need to be considered for these organs as primary sites include the following: *Leishmania donovani, Toxoplasma gondii, Echinococcus* spp., *Toxocara canis, Toxocara cati, Capillaria hepatica, Clonorchis* spp., *Opisthorchis* spp., *Cryptosporidium* spp., *Entamoeba histolytica, Encephalitozoon* spp., and *Encephalitozoon intestinalis* (liver). Typical methods for diagnosis would include wet mounts, routine histology, Giemsa stain, culture, modified acid-fast stains, immunospecific reagents, and trichrome stains (routine and modified).

Examination of aspirates from lung or liver abscesses may reveal trophozoites of *E. histolytica;* however, demonstration of the organisms may be difficult (4). Liver aspirate material should be taken from the margin of the abscess rather than the necrotic center. The organisms are often trapped in the viscous pus or debris and do not exhibit typical motility. A minimum of two separate portions of exudate should be removed (more than two are recommended). The first portion of the aspirate, usually yellowish white, rarely contains organisms. The last portion of the aspirated abscess material is reddish and is more likely to contain amebae. The best material to be examined is that obtained from the actual wall of the abscess. The Amoebiasis Research Unit, Durban, South Africa, has recommended the use of proteolytic enzymes to free the organisms from the aspirate material.

After the addition of the enzyme streptodornase to the thick pus (10 U/ml of pus), the mixture is incubated at 37°C for 30 min and shaken repeatedly. After centrifugation (500 × g for 5 min), the sediment may be examined microscopically as wet mounts or may be used to inoculate culture media. Some of the aspirate can be mixed directly with PVA on a slide and examined as a permanent stained smear (4).

In a suspect case of extraintestinal amebiasis, many laboratories prefer to use a serologic diagnostic approach.

Aspiration of cyst material for the diagnosis of hydatid disease is a dangerous procedure and is usually performed only when open surgical techniques are used for cyst removal. Aspirated fluid usually contains hydatid sand (intact and degenerating scolices, hooklets, and calcareous corpuscles). Some older cysts contain material that resembles curded cottage cheese, and the hooklets may be very difficult to see. Some of this material can be diluted with saline or 10% KOH; usually, scolices or daughter cysts will have disintegrated. However, the diagnosis can be made from seeing the hooklets under high dry power (magnification, ×400). The absence of scolices or hooklets does not rule out the possibility of hydatid disease, since some cysts are sterile and contain no scolices and/or daughter cysts. Histologic examination of the cyst wall should be able to confirm the diagnosis.

Lungs

Expectorated Sputum and Induced Sputum

Although it is not one of the more common specimens, expectorated sputum may be submitted for examination for parasites (Table 10). Organisms in sputum that may be detected and that may cause pneumonia, pneumonitis, or Loeffler's syndrome include the migrating larval stages of *Ascaris lumbricoides, S. stercoralis,* and hookworm; the eggs of *Paragonimus* spp.; *Echinococcus granulosus* hooklets; the protozoa *E. histolytica* and *Cryptosporidium* spp.; and possibly the microsporidia (4). In a *Paragonimus* infection, the sputum may be viscous and tinged with brownish flecks ("iron filings"), which are clusters of eggs, and may be streaked with blood. Although *Entamoeba gingivalis* and *Trichomonas tenax* may be found in sputum, they are generally indicators of poor oral hygiene and/or periodontal disease, not pulmonary disease.

A sputum specimen should be collected properly so that the laboratory receives a "deep sputum" from the lower respiratory tract for examination rather than a specimen that is primarily saliva from the mouth. If the sputum is not induced, then the patient should receive specific instructions regarding collection.

Care should be taken not to confuse *E. gingivalis,* which may be found in the mouth and saliva, with *E. histolytica,* which could result in an incorrect suspicion of pulmonary abscess. *E. gingivalis* usually contains ingested PMNs, while *E. histolytica* may contain ingested erythrocytes but not PMNs. *T. tenax* would also be found in saliva from the mouth and thus would be an incidental finding and normally not an indication of pulmonary problems.

Direct Wet Mount

Sputum is usually examined as a wet mount (saline or iodine), using low and high dry power (magnifications, ×100 and ×400, respectively). The specimen is not concentrated before preparation of the wet mount. If the sputum is thick, an equal amount of 3% sodium hydroxide (or undiluted chlorine bleach) can be added; the specimen is thoroughly mixed and then centrifuged. However, NaOH destroys any protozoan trophozoites that might be present. After centrifugation, the supernatant fluid is discarded, and the sediment can be examined as a wet mount with saline or iodine. If examination must be delayed for any reason, the sputum should be fixed in 5 or 10% formalin to preserve helminth eggs or larvae or in PVA fixative to be stained later for protozoa.

Permanent Stained Smears

If *Cryptosporidium* spp. are suspected (which is rare), then acid-fast or immunoassay techniques normally used for stool specimens can be used (4). Trichrome or iron hematoxylin stains of material may aid in differentiating *E. histolytica* from *E. gingivalis*, and Giemsa stain may better define larvae and juvenile worms.

Bronchoscopy Aspirates

Fluid specimens collected by bronchoscopy may be lavage or washing fluids, with bronchoalveolar lavage fluids preferred. Specimens are usually concentrated by centrifugation prior to microscopic examination of stained preparations. Organisms that may be detected in such specimens are *Paragonimus* spp., *S. stercoralis*, *T. gondii*, *Cryptosporidium* spp., and the microsporidia.

If *T. gondii* is suspected, Giemsa stain, immunospecific reagents, and/or culture (tissue culture) can be used to confirm the diagnosis. A number of cell lines have been used (human foreskin fibroblast is one example), and most routine cell lines work well for the growth and isolation of this organism.

Lymph Nodes and Lymphatics

Material from lymph nodes and lymphatics confirms parasitic infections (toxoplasmosis, Chagas' disease, trypanosomiasis, microsporidiosis, or filariasis) and should be processed as follows. Fluid material can be examined under low power (magnification, ×100) and high dry power (magnification, ×400) as a wet mount (diluted with saline) for the presence of motile organisms.

Material obtained from lymph nodes should be processed for tissue sectioning and as impression smears that should be processed as thin blood films and stained with Giemsa stain. Appropriate culture media can also be inoculated, again making sure that the specimen has been collected under sterile conditions.

If microsporidia are suspected, modified trichrome stains can be used; calcofluor white and immunoassay methods (currently under development) are also excellent options (4). If *T. gondii* is suspected, Giemsa stain, immunospecific reagents, and/or culture (tissue culture) can be used to confirm the diagnosis.

Specific filarial infections generally are caused by *Wuchereria bancrofti*, *Brugia malayi*, and *Brugia* spp. In most cases, the microfilariae can be recovered and identified through examination of thick blood films, specific concentration sediment, and/or membrane filtration methods (4).

Muscle

Muscle is considered the primary site for the following organisms: *Sarcocystis* spp., microsporidia (*Pleistophora* spp. and *Nosema* spp.), *Gnathostoma* spp., *Trichinella* spp. larvae, and cestode larval forms (coenurus [*Taenia* spp.], cysticercosis [*T. solium*], and sparganum). As a secondary site, *T. cruzi* amastigotes can also be found in muscle; *Baylisascaris procyonis* and *Ancylostoma* spp. are also possibilities, as are hydatid cysts (*Echinococcus* spp.). In most cases, biopsy specimens processed by routine histologic methods provide the most appropriate specimens for examination and confirmation of the causative agent.

The presumptive diagnosis of trichinosis is often based on patient history: ingestion of raw or rare pork, walrus meat, or bear meat; diarrhea followed by edema and muscle pain; and the presence of eosinophilia. Generally, the suspected food is not available for examination. The diagnosis

may be confirmed by finding larval *Trichinella spiralis* in a muscle biopsy specimen. The encapsulated larvae can be seen in fresh muscle if small pieces are pressed between two slides and examined under the microscope (4). Larvae are usually most abundant in the diaphragm, masseter muscle, or tongue and may be recovered from these muscles at necropsy. Routine histologic sections can also be prepared.

Human infection with any of the larval cestodes may present diagnostic problems, and frequently, the larvae are referred for identification after surgical removal. In addition to *E. granulosus* (hydatid disease) and the larval stage of *Taenia solium* (cysticercosis), other larval cestodes occasionally cause human disease. The larval stage of tapeworms of the genus *Multiceps*, a parasite of dogs and wild canids, is called a coenurus and may cause human coenurosis. The coenurus resembles a cysticercus but is larger and has multiple scolices developing from the germinal membrane surrounding the fluid-filled bladder. These larvae occur in extraintestinal locations, including the eye, central nervous system, and muscle.

Human sparganosis is caused by the larval stages of tapeworms of the genus *Spirometra*, which are parasites of various canine and feline hosts; these tapeworms are closely related to the genus *Diphyllobothrium*. Sparganum larvae are elongated, ribbon-like larvae without a bladder and with a slightly expanded anterior end lacking suckers. These larvae are usually found in superficial tissues or nodules, although they may cause ocular sparganosis, a more serious disease.

Finding prominent calcareous corpuscles in the tapeworm tissue frequently supports the diagnosis of larval cestodes; specific identification usually depends on referral to specialists.

Nasopharynx and Sinus Cavities

Organisms that might be found in these body sites include the microsporidia, *Acanthamoeba* spp., and *Naegleria*. Specimens submitted for examination could include scrapings, aspirates, and/or biopsy specimens. A number of the special stains would include modified trichrome, acid-fast, and tissue Gram stains. Giemsa, calcofluor white, and regular trichrome stains would also be appropriate. If *Naegleria* or *Acanthamoeba* spp. are suspected, culture is highly recommended. In certain cases of mucocutaneous leishmaniasis, *Leishmania* spp. could also be found from these body sites; Giemsa stain would be recommended for confirmation in both aspirates and biopsy specimens; cultures would also be an option (4).

Rectal Tissue

Often when a patient has an old, chronic infection or a light infection with *Schistosoma mansoni* or *Schistosoma japonicum*, the eggs may not be found in the stool and an examination of the rectal mucosa may reveal the presence of eggs. The fresh tissue should be compressed between two microscope slides and examined under the low power of the microscope (low-intensity light) (4). Critical examination of these eggs should be made to determine whether living miracidia are still found within the egg. Treatment may depend on the viability of the eggs; for this reason, the condition of the eggs should be reported to the physician.

Skin

The use of skin snips is the method of choice for the diagnosis of human filarial infections with *O. volvulus* and *Mansonella streptocerca* (1, 4). Microfilariae of both species occur chiefly in the skin, although *O. volvulus* microfilariae may rarely be found in the blood and occasionally in the urine. Skin snip specimens should be thick enough to include the outer part of the dermal papillae. With a surgical blade, a small slice may be cut from a skin fold held between the thumb and forefinger, or a slice may be taken from a small "cone" of skin pulled up with a needle. Significant bleeding should not occur, and there should be just a slight oozing of fluid. Corneal-scleral punches (either Holth or Walser type) have been found to be successful in taking skin snips of uniform size and depth and an average weight of 0.8 mg (range, 0.4 to 1.2 mg); this procedure is easy to perform and is painless. It has been demonstrated that in African onchocerciasis, it is preferable to take skin snips from the buttock region (above the iliac crest); in Central American onchocerciasis, the preferred skin snip sites are from the shoulders (over the scapula).

Skin snips are placed immediately in a drop of normal saline or distilled water and are covered so that they will not dry; teasing of the specimen with dissecting needles is not necessary but may facilitate release of the microfilariae. Microfilariae tend to emerge more rapidly in saline; however, in either solution, the microfilariae usually emerge within 30 min to 1 h and can be examined with low-intensity light and the 10× objective of the microscope. To see definitive morphological details of the microfilariae, allow the snip preparation to dry, fix it in absolute methyl alcohol, and stain it with Giemsa stain.

Skin biopsy specimens used for the diagnosis of cutaneous amebiasis (*Entamoeba histolytica* or *Acanthamoeba* spp.) and cutaneous leishmaniasis should be processed for tissue sectioning and subsequently stained by the hematoxylin and eosin technique (19).

Although cutaneous disease is an unusual presentation for schistosomiasis, it does occur with skin lesions as the only manifestation. Based on routine histologic examination of skin biopsies, eggs can be found in the cellular infiltrate from within the lesion. When evaluating patients with unusual skin lesions, a complete history may reveal travel to an area where schistosomiasis is endemic.

Material containing intracellular *Leishmania* organisms can be aspirated from below the ulcer bed through the uninvolved skin, not from the surface of the ulcer. The surface of the ulcer must be thoroughly cleaned before specimens are taken; any contamination of the material with bacteria or fungi may prevent recovery of the organism from culture. Aspirated material is placed on a slide and stained with Giemsa stain.

Some prefer to perform a punch biopsy through the active margin of the lesion (after cleaning the lesion); good results have also been seen with the use of dermal scrapings from the bottoms of the ulcers. When microscopic examinations of dermal scrapings of both the ulcer bottom and active margins are combined, the sensitivity of diagnosis may increase to 94% (19). Aspirate culture has been shown to be the most sensitive method for the diagnosis of patients with chronic ulcers. However, any successful culture depends on the prevention of contamination with bacteria and/or fungi; sampling of the ulcer must be done correctly in order to prevent false-negative culture results.

BLOOD

Depending on the life cycle, a number of parasites may be recovered in a blood specimen, either whole blood or buffy coat preparations, or following concentration by various types of procedures. These parasites include *Plasmodium*, *Babesia*, and *Trypanosoma* species, *Leishmania donovani*, and microfilariae. Although some organisms may be motile in fresh, whole blood, species identification is usually accomplished from the examination of permanent stained thick and thin blood films. Blood films can be prepared from fresh, whole blood collected with no anticoagulants, anticoagulated blood (EDTA is recommended; heparin is acceptable, but organism morphology is not as good; other anticoagulants are not recommended), or sediment from the various concentration procedures. Although for many years Giemsa stain has been the stain of choice, the parasites can also be seen on blood films stained with Wright's stain, a Wright/Giemsa combination stain, or one of the more rapid stains such as Diff-Quik (American Scientific Products, McGaw Park, IL), Wright's Dip Stat stain (Medical Chemical Corp., Torrance, CA), or Field's stain. It is more appropriate for personnel to use a stain with which they are familiar than having to use Giemsa stain, which is somewhat more complicated to use. PMNs serve as the quality control cell for any of the blood stains. Any parasites present stain like the PMN nuclear and cytoplasmic material, regardless of the stain used. Delafield's hematoxylin stain is often used to stain the microfilarial sheath; in some cases, Giemsa stain does not provide sufficient stain quality to allow differentiation of the microfilariae (Table 11). When handling blood, as well as other clinical specimens, standard precautions should be observed (3, 4, 14, 15).

Preparation of Thick and Thin Blood Films

Microfilariae and trypanosomes can be detected in fresh blood by their characteristic shape and motility; however, specific identification of the organisms requires a permanent stain. Two types of blood films are recommended. Thick films allow a larger amount of blood to be examined, which increases the possibility of detecting light infections (4, 11, 15). However, only experienced workers can usually make species identification with a thick film, particularly in the case of malaria, and the morphological characteristics of blood parasites are best seen in thin films.

The accurate examination of thick and thin blood films and identification of parasites depend on the use of absolutely clean, grease-free slides for preparation of all blood films. Old (unscratched) slides should be cleaned first in detergent and then with 70% ethyl alcohol; new slides should also be cleaned with alcohol and allowed to dry before use.

Blood films should be prepared when the patient is admitted or seen in the emergency room or clinic; typical fever patterns are frequently absent, and the patient may not be suspected of having malaria. If malaria remains a possible diagnosis, after the first set of negative smears, samples should be taken at intervals of 6 to 8 h for at least 3 successive days. Often, after a day or two, other etiologic agents may be suspected and no additional blood specimens will be received. Another option is to collect blood immediately on admission; if the initial blood films are negative, collect daily specimens for two additional days (ideally between paroxysms if present). Using either collection option, quality patient care depends on the fact that both the physician and laboratory staff know that one negative set of blood films does not eliminate *Plasmodium* spp. as possible etiologic agents.

After a finger stick, the blood should flow freely; blood that has to be "milked" from the finger is diluted with tissue fluids, which decrease the number of parasites per field. An alternative approach to the fingerstick is collection of fresh blood containing anticoagulant (preferably EDTA) for the preparation of blood films. Ideally, the smears should be

TABLE 11 Techniques for the recovery and identification of blood parasites (EDTA or heparin)[a]

Organism	Procedure	Stain
Malaria parasites	Thick and thin films	Giemsa, Wright's, Field's, rapid stains
	QBC[b]	Stain not relevant (centrifugation, acridine orange, microscopy)
	ParaSight F[c]	Stain not relevant (HRP-2 immunochromatographic assay)
	Binax Now Malaria[d]	Stain not relevant (HRP-2 and aldolase immunochromatographic assay)
	PATH IC Falciparum malaria IC[e]	Stain not relevant (HRP-2 immunochromatographic assay)
	Malaria Ag-CELISA[f]	Stain not relevant (HRP-2 immunochromatographic assay)
	Rapimal Dipstick[f]	Stain not relevant (HRP-2 immunochromatographic assay)
	Rapimal Cassette[f]	Stain not relevant (HRP-2 immunochromatographic assay)
	OptiMAL[g]	Stain not relevant (pLDH immunochromatographic assay)
Babesia spp.	Thick and thin films	Giemsa, Wright's, Field's, rapid stains
Microfilariae	Thick and thin films, Knott concentration, membrane filtration, gradient centrifugation	Giemsa, Wright's, or Delafield's hematoxylin
	QBC[b]	Stain not relevant
	NOW ICT Filariasis[d]	Rapid, tends to be dipstick format
	Filariasis Ag-CELISA[f]	EIA
	TropBio[h]	Rapid, tends to be dipstick format
Trypanosomes	Thick and thin films, buffy coat smears, triple centrifugation, culture	Giemsa, Wright's, Field's, rapid stains
	QBC[b]	Stain not relevant
Leishmaniae	Thick and thin films, buffy coat smears, culture	Giemsa, Wright's, Field's, rapid stains

[a]Molecular techniques are still experimental and are not always available; it is always important to verify FDA approval within the United States (contact the manufacturer).

[b]QBC-Blood Parasite Detection Method (Becton-Dickinson Tropical Disease Diagnostics, Sparks, MD).

[c]ParaSight F-Rapid Test for *P. falciparum* malaria (Becton-Dickinson Tropical Disease Diagnostics, Sparks, MD). This test is not licensed for diagnostic use in the United States. This test is a dipstick format.

[d]Binax Now malaria (all four *Plasmodium* species), Binax Now ICT Filariasis (*Wuchereria bancrofti*) (Binax, Inc., Portland, ME). These tests are in a dipstick format.

[e]PATH IC Falciparum malaria IC test (PATH, Seattle, WA). This test is in a dipstick format.

[f]Filariasis Ag-CELISA (*Wuchereria bancrofti*), Malaria Ag-CELISA (*P. falciparum*). Rapimal Dipstick (*P. falciparum*), Rapimal Cassette (*P. falciparum*) (Cellabs, Sydney, New South Wales, Australia).

[g]OptiMAL (differentiates between *P. falciparum* and *P. vivax*) (Flow, Inc., Portland, OR). This test is in a dipstick format.

[h]TropBio (James Cook University, Townsville, Queensland, Australia).

prepared within 1 h after the specimen is drawn. After that time, stippling may not be visible on stained films; however, the overall organism morphology may still be acceptable.

The time that the specimen was drawn should be clearly indicated on the tube of blood and also on the result report. The physician will then be able to correlate the results with any symptoms that the patient may have. There should also be some indication on the slip that is sent back to the physician that one negative specimen does not rule out the possibility of a parasitic infection.

Thick Blood Films

To prepare the thick film, place 2 or 3 small drops of capillary blood directly from the fingerstick (no anticoagulant) on an alcohol-cleaned slide. With the corner of another slide and using a circular motion, mix the drops and spread them over an area 2 cm in diameter. Continue stirring for 30 s to prevent the formation of fibrin strands that may obscure the parasites after staining. If blood containing an anticoagulant is used, 1 or 2 drops may be spread over an area about 2 cm in diameter; it is not necessary to continue stirring for 30 s, since there will be no formation of fibrin strands. If too much blood is used or any grease remains on the slide, the blood may flake off during staining. Allow the film to air dry (room temperature) in a dust-free area. Never apply heat to a thick film, since heat fixes the blood, causing the erythrocytes to

remain intact during staining; the result is stain retention and an inability to identify the parasites. However, the thick films can be placed in a 37°C incubator for 10 to 15 minutes to dry; this seems to work quite well. Remember, do not make the films too thick; one should be able to see newsprint through the wet film prior to drying. After the thick films are thoroughly dry, they can be laked to remove the hemoglobin. To lake the films, place them in buffer solution before staining for 10 min or directly into a dilute, buffered aqueous Giemsa stain. If thick films are to be stained at a later time, they should be laked before storage (4).

Thin Blood Films

The thin blood film is routinely used for specific parasite identification, although the number of organisms per field is much reduced compared with the number in the thick film. The thin film is prepared exactly as one used for a differential count, and a well-prepared film is thick at one end and thin at the other (one layer of evenly distributed erythrocytes with no cell overlap). The thin, feathered end should be at least 2 cm long, and the film should occupy the central area of the slide, with free margins on both sides. Holes in the film indicate the presence of grease on the slide. After the film has air dried (do not apply heat), it may be stained. The necessity for fixation before staining depends on the stain selected.

Staining Blood Films

For accurate identification of blood parasites, a laboratory should develop proficiency in the use of at least one good staining method (2, 4, 10). Since prolonged storage may result in stain retention, blood films should be stained on the same day or within a few days of collection. If thick blood films are not prepared or received, it is possible to stain one of the thin blood films as a thick film and examine the thick portion of the thin film. During staining the red blood cells are laked, thus leaving the white blood cells, platelets, and any parasites present.

Wright's stain has the fixative in combination with the staining solution, so that both fixation and staining occur at the same time; therefore, the thick film must be laked before staining. In aqueous Giemsa stain, the fixative and stain are separate; thus, the thin film must be fixed with absolute methanol before staining.

When slides are removed from either type of staining solution, they should be dried in a vertical position. After being air dried, they may be examined under oil immersion by placing the oil directly on the uncovered blood film. If slides are going to be stored for a considerable length of time for teaching or legal purposes, they should be protected with a coverglass by being mounted in a medium such as Permount. Blood films that have been stained with any of the Romanowsky stains and that have been mounted with Permount or other resinous mounting media are susceptible to fading of the basophilic elements and generalized loss of stain intensity. One can add an antioxidant such as 1% (by volume) 2,6-di-*t*-butyl-*p*-cresol (butylated hydroxytoluene; Sigma-Aldrich) to the mounting medium. Without the addition of this antioxidant, mounted stained blood films eventually become pink; stained films protected with this compound generally remain unchanged in color for many years.

Giemsa Stain

Each new lot number of Giemsa stain should be tested for optimal staining times before being used on patient specimens. If the blood cells appear to be adequately stained, the timing and stain dilution should be appropriate to demonstrate the presence of malaria and other parasites. The use of prepared liquid stain or stain prepared from the powder depends on personal preference; there is apparently little difference between the two preparations.

The commercial liquid stain or the stock solution prepared from powder should be diluted approximately the same amount to prepare the working stain solution (4, 15). Stock Giemsa liquid stain is diluted 1:10 with buffer for both thick and thin blood films, with dilutions ranging from 1:10 up to 1:50. Staining times usually match the dilution factor (e.g., 1:20 for 20 min or 1:50 for 50 min). Some people prefer to use the longer method with more dilute stain for both thick and thin films. The phosphate buffer used to dilute the stock stain should be neutral or slightly alkaline (pH 7.0 to 7.2). Phosphate buffer solution may be used to obtain the right pH. In some laboratories, the pH of tap water may be satisfactory and may be used for the entire staining procedure and the final rinse. Some workers recommend the use of pH 6.8 to emphasize Schüffner's dots.

Giemsa stain colors the blood components as follows: erythrocytes, pale red; nuclei of leukocytes, purple with pale purple cytoplasm; eosinophilic granules, bright purple-red; and neutrophilic granules, deep pink-purple. In malaria parasites, the cytoplasm stains blue and the nuclear material stains red to purple-red. Schüffner's dots and other inclusions

in the erythrocytes stain red. The nuclear and cytoplasmic staining characteristics of the other blood parasites such as *Babesia* spp., trypanosomes, and leishmaniae are like those of the malaria parasites. While the sheath of microfilariae may not always stain with Giemsa, the nuclei within the microfilaria itself stain blue to purple.

Wright's Stain

Wright's stain is available in liquid form and also as a powder, which must be dissolved in anhydrous, acetone-free methyl alcohol before use. Since Wright's stain contains alcohol, the thin blood films do not require fixation before staining. Thick films stained with Wright's stain are usually inferior to those stained with Giemsa solution. Great care should also be taken to avoid excess stain precipitate on the slide during the final rinse. Before staining, thick films must be laked in distilled water (to rupture and remove erythrocytes) and air dried. The staining procedure is the same as that for thin films, but the staining time is usually somewhat longer and must be determined for each batch of stain. Wright's stain colors blood components as follows: erythrocytes, light tan, reddish, or buff; nuclei of leukocytes, bright blue with contrasting light cytoplasm; eosinophilic granules, bright red; and neutrophilic granules, pink or light purple.

In malaria parasites, the cytoplasm stains pale blue and the nuclear material stains red. Schüffner's dots and other inclusions in the erythrocytes usually do not stain or stain very pale with Wright's stain. Nuclear and cytoplasmic staining characteristics of the other blood parasites such as *Babesia* spp., trypanosomes, and leishmaniae are like those seen in the malaria parasites. While the sheath of microfilariae may not always stain with Wright's stain, the nuclei within the microfilaria itself stain pale to dark blue.

Other Stains for Blood

Although Giemsa and Wright's stains are excellent options, the parasites can also be seen on blood films stained with a Wright/Giemsa combination stain or one of the more rapid stains such as Diff-Quik (American Scientific Products), Wright's Dip Stat stain (Medical Chemical Corp.), or Field's stain. PMNs serve as the quality control organism for any of the blood stains. Any parasites present stain like the PMNs, regardless of the stain used. Remember, when using any of the blood stains, that color variations are common.

Proper Examination of Thin and Thick Blood Films

In cases where malaria parasites have not been indicated as the suspect organism, the initial screen of the thin blood film should be carried out with the low-power objective of a microscope because microfilariae may be missed if the entire thin film is not examined. Microfilariae are rarely present in large numbers, and frequently, only a few organisms occur in each thin film preparation. Microfilariae are commonly found at the edges of the thin film or at the feathered end of the film because they are carried to these sites during the process of spreading the blood. This approach to thin film examination is particularly important in cases where a suspect organism has not been indicated. The feathered end of the film where the erythrocytes are drawn out into one single, distinctive layer of cells should be examined for the presence of malaria parasites and trypanosomes. In these areas, the morphology and size of the infected erythrocytes are most clearly seen.

In the case of a suspect malaria diagnosis, the request for blood film examination should always be considered a STAT procedure, with all reports (negative as well as positive) being reported by telephone to the physician as soon as possible (4, 15). Examination of the thin film should include viewing of 200 to 300 oil immersion fields at a magnification of ×1,000. Although some people use a 50× or 60× oil immersion objective to screen stained blood films, there is some concern that small parasites such as *Plasmodium* spp., *Babesia* spp., or *Leishmania donovani* may be missed at this smaller total magnification (×500 or ×600), although they are usually detected at the total magnification of ×1,000 obtained with the more traditional 100× oil immersion objective. Because people tend to scan blood films at different rates, it is important to examine a minimum number of fields, regardless of the time that it takes to perform this procedure. If something suspicious has been seen in the thick film, often the number of fields examined on the thin film may be considerably greater than 200 to 300.

Diagnostic problems with the use of automated differential instruments have been reported (4). Both malaria and *Babesia* infections can be missed with these instruments, and therapy is therefore delayed. Because these instruments are not designed to detect intracellular blood parasites, any reliance on the automated systems for discrimination between uninfected erythrocytes and those infected with parasites may pose serious diagnostic problems.

In the preparation of a thick blood film, the greatest concentration of blood cells is in the center of the film. A search for parasitic organisms should be carried out initially at low magnification to detect microfilariae more readily. Examination of a thick film usually requires 5 to 10 min (approximately 100 oil immersion fields). The search for malarial organisms and trypanosomes is best done under oil immersion (total magnification, ×1,000). Close examination of the very periphery of the thick film may reveal intact erythrocytes; such cells, if infected, may prove useful in malaria diagnosis since the characteristic morphology necessary to identify the organisms to the species level is more easily seen.

Immunochromatographic Tests for Malaria

Immunochromatography relies on the migration of liquid across the surface of a nitrocellulose membrane. Using monoclonal antibodies prepared against a malaria antigen target that has been incorporated onto the strip of nitrocellulose, these tests are based on the capture of parasite antigen from peripheral blood. Currently, the malaria antigens used for these rapid diagnostic tests are histidine-rich protein 2 (HRP-2), parasite lactate dehydrogenase (pLDH), and *Plasmodium* aldolase (Table 11). These dipsticks offer the possibility of more-rapid, nonmicroscopic methods for malaria diagnosis. The tests are easy to perform and interpret; however, there are a number of questions that remain concerning the relevant uses for this type of testing, especially considering the fact that the Binax Now Malaria Test is now FDA approved. A positive-control specimen is also available.

Sensitivity remains a problem, particularly for nonimmune populations. Parasite densities of >100 parasites/µl (0.002% parasitemia) should be detected and are reasonable targets to expect from dipsticks for *Plasmodium falciparum* diagnosis. However, this level of sensitivity is at the lower end of the capability of most devices using capture methods for HRP-2 or pLDH. This level of sensitivity is probably as good as clinical laboratory staff in nonspecialized laboratories with limited exposure to malaria cases could expect to provide using microscopy diagnosis. One of the potential benefits would be for inexperienced evening staff personnel for whom the dipstick identification of a life-threatening parasitemia with *P. falciparum* could prevent a missed infection. However, a negative test could not be accepted and would require confirmation by microscopic examination of both thick and thin blood films for the detection of parasitemia below the present threshold of detection by these rapid tests. Also, there are rare false positives for patients with certain rheumatologic disorders; this is noted in the package insert and has been confirmed by users in this patient population. The U.S. military has conducted FDA-approved trials because of possible use of the devices in the field.

Concentration Procedures

Buffy Coat Films

L. donovani, trypanosomes, and *Histoplasma capsulatum* (a fungus with intracellular elements resembling those of *L. donovani*) may occasionally be detected in the peripheral blood. The parasite or fungus is found in the large mononuclear cells that are found in the buffy coat (a layer of leukocytes resulting from centrifugation of whole citrated blood). The nuclear material stains dark red-purple, and the cytoplasm is light blue (*L. donovani*). *H. capsulatum* appears as a dot of nuclear material (dark red-purple) surrounded by a clear halo area. Trypanosomes in the peripheral blood also concentrate with the buffy coat cells.

Use alcohol-cleaned slides for preparation of the blood films. A microhematocrit tube can also be used; the tube is carefully scored and snapped at the buffy coat interface, and the leukocytes are prepared as a thin film. The tube can also be examined prior to removal of the buffy coat under low and high dry powers of the microscope. If trypanosomes are present, the motility may be observed in the buffy coat. Microfilaria motility would also be visible.

QBC Microhematocrit Centrifugation Method

Microhematocrit centrifugation with use of the QBC malaria tube, a glass capillary tube and closely fitting plastic insert (QBC malaria blood tubes; Becton Dickinson, Tropical Disease Diagnostics, Sparks, MD), has been used for the detection of blood parasites (4). At the end of centrifugation of 50 to 60 µl of capillary or venous blood (5 min in a QBC centrifuge, 14,387 × *g*), parasites or erythrocytes containing parasites are concentrated into a small, 1- to 2-mm region near the top of the erythrocyte column and are held close to the wall of the tube by the plastic float, thereby making them readily visible by microscopy. Tubes precoated with acridine orange provide a stain that induces fluorescence in the parasites. This method automatically prepares a concentrated smear that represents the distance between the float and the walls of the tube. Once the tube is placed into the plastic holder (Paraviewer) and immersion oil is applied onto the top of the hematocrit tube (no coverslip is necessary), the tube is examined with a 40× to 60× oil immersion objective (it must have a working distance of 0.3 mm or greater).

Although a malaria infection could be detected by this method (which is much more sensitive than the thick or the thin blood smear), appropriate thick and thin blood films need to be examined to accurately identify the species of the organism causing the infection.

Knott Concentration

The Knott concentration procedure is used primarily to detect the presence of microfilariae in the blood, especially when a light infection is suspected (4, 11). The disadvantage of the procedure is that the microfilariae are killed by the formalin and are therefore not seen as motile organisms.

Membrane Filtration Technique

The membrane filtration technique is highly efficient in demonstrating filarial infections when microfilaremias are of low density. This method is unsatisfactory for the isolation of *Mansonella perstans* microfilariae because of their small size. A 3-μm-pore-size filter could be used for recovery of this organism. Other filters with similar pore sizes are not as satisfactory as the Nuclepore filter (4).

Delafield's Hematoxylin

Some of the material that is obtained from the concentration procedures can be allowed to dry as thick and thin films and then stained with Delafield's hematoxylin, which demonstrates greater nuclear detail as well as the microfilarial sheath, if present. In addition, fresh thick films of blood containing microfilariae can be stained by this hematoxylin technique (4).

Triple-Centrifugation Method for Trypanosomes

The triple-centrifugation procedure may be valuable in demonstrating the presence of trypanosomes in the peripheral blood when the parasitemia is light (4). After repeated centrifugation of the supernatant, the sediment is examined as a wet preparation or is stained as a thin blood film.

SUMMARY

This chapter covers various approaches and diagnostic methods currently in use for the diagnosis of parasitic infections. If clinical specimens have been properly collected and processed according to specific specimen rejection and acceptance criteria, the examination of prepared wet mounts, concentrated specimens, permanent stained smears, blood films, and various culture materials provides detailed information leading to parasite identification and confirmation of the suspected etiologic agent (4, 6, 14). Although other tests such as immunoassay diagnostic kits continue to become available commercially, the majority of medical parasitology diagnostic work depends on the knowledge and microscopy skills of the microbiologist.

REFERENCES

1. **Ash, L. R., and T. C. Orihel.** 1991. *Parasites: a Guide to Laboratory Procedures and Identification.* ASCP Press, Chicago, IL.
2. **Beaver, P. C., R. C. Jung, and E. W. Cupp.** 1984. *Clinical Parasitology,* 9th ed. Lea & Febiger, Philadelphia, PA.
3. **Code of Federal Regulations.** 1991. Occupational exposure to bloodborne pathogens. *Fed. Regist.* 29CFR1910.1030.
4. **Garcia, L. S.** 2007. *Diagnostic Medical Parasitology,* 5th ed. ASM Press, Washington, DC.
5. **Garcia, L. S.** 2009. *Practical Guide to Diagnostic Parasitology,* 2nd ed. ASM Press, Washington, DC.
6. **Hiatt, R. A., E. K. Markell, and E. Ng.** 1995. How many stool examinations are necessary to detect pathogenic intestinal protozoa? *Am. J. Trop. Med. Hyg.* **53:**36–39.
7. **Isenberg, H. D. (ed.).** 2004. *Clinical Microbiology Procedures Handbook,* 2nd ed. ASM Press, Washington, DC.
8. **Katanik, M. T., S. K. Schneider, J. E. Rosenblatt, G. S. Hall, and G. W. Procop.** 2001. Evaluation of ColorPAC *Giardia/Cryptosporidium* rapid assay and ProSpecT *Giardia/Cryptosporidium* microplate assay for detection of *Giardia* and *Cryptosporidium* in fecal specimens. *J. Clin. Microbiol.* **39:**4523–4525.
9. **Kehl, K. S. C.** 1996. Screening stools for *Giardia* and *Cryptosporidium:* are antigen tests enough? *Clin. Microbiol. Newsl.* **18:**133–135.
10. **Koneman, E. W., S. D. Allen, W. M. Janda, P. C. Schreckenberger, and W. C. Winn, Jr.** 1997. *Color Atlas and Textbook of Diagnostic Microbiology,* 5th ed. J. B. Lippincott Co., Philadelphia, PA.
11. **Markell, E., D. T. John, and W. A. Krotoski.** 1999. *Medical Parasitology,* 8th ed. The W. B. Saunders Co., Philadelphia, PA.
12. **Melvin, D. M., and M. M. Brooke.** 1982. *Laboratory Procedures for the Diagnosis of Intestinal Parasites,* 3rd ed. U.S. Department of Health, Education, and Welfare publication no. (CDC) 82-8282. Government Printing Office, Washington, DC.
13. **Morris, A. J., M. L. Wilson, and L. B. Reller.** 1992. Application of rejection criteria for stool ovum and parasite examinations. *J. Clin. Microbiol.* **30:**3213–3216.
14. **Murray, P. R., E. J. Baron, J. H. Jorgensen, M. L. Landry, and M. A. Pfaller (ed.).** 2007. *Manual of Clinical Microbiology,* 9th ed. ASM Press, Washington, DC.
15. **National Committee for Clinical Laboratory Standards.** 2000. *Laboratory Diagnosis of Blood-Borne Parasitic Diseases. Approved Guideline M15-A.* National Committee for Clinical Laboratory Standards, Villanova, PA.
16. **National Committee for Clinical Laboratory Standards.** 1997. *Protection of Laboratory Workers from Instrument Biohazards and Infectious Disease Transmitted by Blood, Body Fluids, and Tissue. Approved Guideline M29-A.* National Committee for Clinical Laboratory Standards, Villanova, PA.
17. **National Committee for Clinical Laboratory Standards.** 1997. *Procedures for the Recovery and Identification of Parasites from the Intestinal Tract. Approved Guideline M28-A.* National Committee for Clinical Laboratory Standards, Villanova, PA.
18. **Nielsen, C. K., and L. A. Ward.** 1999. Enhanced detection of *Cryptosporidium parvum* in the acid-fast stain. *J. Vet. Diagn. Investig.* **11:**567–569.
19. **Ramirez, J. R., S. Agudelo, C. Muskus, J. F. Alzate, C. Berberich, D. Barker, and I. D. Velez.** 2000. Diagnosis of cutaneous leishmaniasis in Colombia: the sampling site within lesions influences the sensitivity of parasitologic diagnosis. *J. Clin. Microbiol.* **38:**3768–3773.
20. **Sharp, S. E., C. A. Suarez, Y. Duran, and R. J. Poppiti.** 2001. Evaluation of the Triage Micro Parasite Panel for detection of *Giardia lamblia, Entamoeba histolytica/Entamoeba dispar,* and *Cryptosporidium parvum* in patient stool specimens. *J. Clin. Microbiol.* **39:**332–334.

Plasmodium and *Babesia*

WILLIAM O. ROGERS

133

TAXONOMY

The agents of malaria and babesiosis are members of the phylum Apicomplexa, which includes protozoa characterized by the presence of an apical complex consisting of polar rings, conoid, micronemes, rhoptries, subpellicular microtubules, and a small plastid, related to a red algal chloroplast, the apicoplast. The phylum Apicomplexa is classified within the superphylum Alveolata, which includes apicomplexans, ciliates, and dinoflagellates. Although the exact evolutionary pathway is controversial, there is good evidence that the Alveolata acquired chloroplasts by secondary endosymbiosis of a red alga (27). While some dinoflagellates retain functional chloroplasts and are photosynthetic, in apicomplexans the apicoplast does not photosynthesize but is involved in lipid, heme, and isoprenoid synthesis (28, 102). All members of the phylum Apicomplexa are parasitic. The agents of malaria and babesiosis are classified within the orders Haemospororida and Piroplasmorida, respectively.

PLASMODIUM

The genus *Plasmodium* includes at least 172 named species of intraerythrocytic parasites infecting a wide range of mammals, birds, reptiles, and amphibians (59). Four species, *P. falciparum*, *P. vivax*, *P. ovale*, and *P. malariae*, have long been known to infect humans. Recently, it has become clear that a fifth species, *P. knowlesi*, which normally infects long-tailed macaques (*Macaca fascicularis*) and pig-tailed macaques (*Macaca nemestrina*), is a significant cause of human malaria in Southeast Asia. *P. knowlesi* was found to account for more than a quarter of malaria cases in hospitals in Malaysian Borneo (18), and human cases have also been reported from Thailand (79), Singapore (69), and the Philippines (62) and in Western travelers returning from Southeast Asia (9, 15).

Life Cycle

The *Plasmodium* life cycle (Fig. 1) begins with the injection of sporozoites by the bite of an infected mosquito. Sporozoites move rapidly to the liver, where they invade hepatocytes and undergo exoerythrocytic development for 7 to 10 days, leading to the formation of liver schizonts. Rupture of each liver schizont releases thousands of free merozoites into the peripheral blood, where they invade erythrocytes. In the erythrocyte, the early trophozoites (rings) develop into mature trophozoites with an enlarged cytoplasm and an accumulation of hemozoin pigment. Nuclear and cytoplasmic division lead to production of the mature schizont, which ruptures, releasing merozoites and completing the erythrocytic cycle. A fraction of the merozoites undergo sexual differentiation into gametocytes, which undergo fertilization and zygote formation following ingestion with a mosquito blood meal. Fertilized gametes develop into ookinetes, which penetrate the intestinal lining and develop into oocysts on the extraluminal wall of the intestine. Oocysts rupture, releasing sporozoites, which migrate to the salivary glands to complete the life cycle.

There are important species-specific variations in the life cycle. The time required to complete a single erythrocytic stage cycle is 72 hours in *P. malariae*; 48 hours in *P. falciparum*, *P. vivax*, and *P. ovale*; and 24 hours in *P. knowlesi*. The late trophozoites and schizonts of *P. falciparum* insert an antigenically variable, high-molecular-weight protein in the erythrocyte membrane, which causes the infected erythrocyte to adhere to the vascular endothelium (6). Thus, these stages of the life cycle do not circulate in the peripheral blood. *P. vivax* and *P. ovale* may be associated with relapse from the liver months to years after clearance of initial blood stage parasitemia. Sporozoites of these species may enter hepatocytes and complete exoerythrocytic stage development normally, or they may arrest development in the liver as hypnozoites, which subsequently develop into mature liver schizonts, leading to relapse of parasitemia months to a few years later.

Epidemiology and Transmission

Malaria imposes an enormous burden of illness and substantial mortality on the tropical world and in many subtropical regions. There are an estimated 515 (95% confidence interval, 330 to 660) million clinical episodes of malaria due to *Plasmodium falciparum*, the most common cause of malaria (91), and 1.5 million to 2.7 million deaths due to malaria each year (108). Transmission depends on the presence and abundance of an effective anopheline mosquito vector and a reservoir of infected humans, or in the case of *P. knowlesi*, a reservoir of infected macaques. Transmission cannot occur at temperatures outside the range from 16 to 33°C or above 2,000 meters of altitude because development in the mosquito cannot take place. *P. knowlesi* infections have, to date, only been acquired in areas where long-tailed or

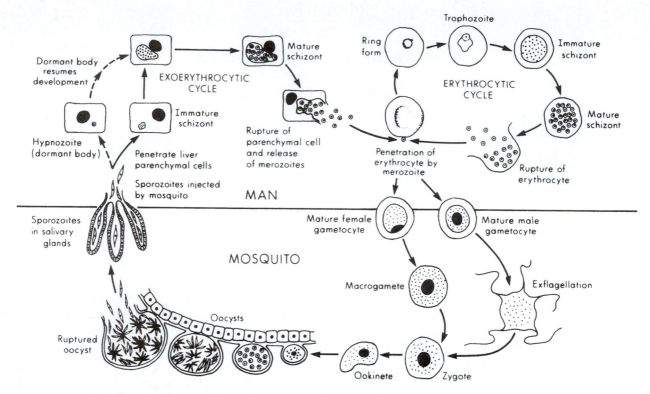

FIGURE 1 Life cycle of the malaria parasite. (Reproduced with permission from reference 54a.)

pig-tailed macaques are present. The intensity of transmission in any location depends on temperature, rainfall, the abundance and behavior of the local anopheline vector, and the existence of a reservoir of infection. The level of endemicity of malaria is classified based on the percentage of children aged 2 to 9 years with splenomegaly or patent parasitemia: hypoendemic, 0 to 10%; mesoendemic, 10 to 50%; hyperendemic, 50 to 75%; holoendemic, >75%. In areas where malaria is holoendemic, such as much of sub-Saharan Africa, the most severe morbidity and mortality occur in early childhood and the majority of deaths are due to severe anemia. Individuals surviving through early childhood develop partial clinical immunity and are less likely to die from malaria. In areas of lesser endemicity, particularly where transmission is seasonal or unstable, development of clinical immunity is less effective, symptomatic and severe malaria occur at all ages, and cerebral malaria is a common manifestation of severe infection.

Although malaria was eradicated from North America by the mid-20th century, competent vector species of anopheline mosquito are widely present, and small, focal outbreaks of malaria can occur when a gametocytemic immigrant or traveler serves as a reservoir of infection (12–14, 56, 63, 95).

Clinical Significance

The classic clinical manifestation of malaria is the febrile paroxysm, which begins with a chill and rigors, leading to an abrupt fever lasting 1 to 2 hours, and finally resolves with profuse sweating and a return to normal temperature. The typical periodicity of these paroxysms, approximately 48 hours in *P. falciparum*, *P. vivax*, and *P. ovale*, 72 hours in *P. malariae*, and 24 hours in *P. knowlesi*, is not always seen, particularly in nonimmune individuals. The fever is frequently accompanied or preceded by headache, myalgias, and malaise. Splenomegaly and anemia are common. Gastrointestinal complaints, nausea, vomiting, and diarrhea, which may be bloody, are also not uncommon and should not distract the clinician from the diagnosis of malaria. Infection with *P. falciparum* may be complicated by various forms of severe malaria. Table 1 shows the World Health Organization criteria for severe malaria (107). Severe malaria due to *P. falciparum* may develop rapidly in a patient who initially presents with mild symptoms and a low parasitemia. It is therefore critical to make the diagnosis of *P. falciparum* quickly. *P. knowlesi* has a short erythrocytic cycle time, 24 hours, may therefore reach high parasite densities rapidly, and may also cause severe malaria (18).

P. vivax and *P. ovale* preferentially invade reticulocytes and therefore only very rarely cause parasitemias greater than 2%. They may relapse from the liver following successful therapy of blood stage infection and must therefore be treated with primaquine to eradicate hypnozoites in the liver. *P. malariae* preferentially infects older erythrocytes and may cause chronic, asymptomatic parasitemia lasting for many years. Proteinuria is a common finding in *P. malariae* infection and may progress to the nephrotic syndrome in children.

Diagnosis

Specimen Collection and Patient History

Because *P. falciparum* can progress rapidly to severe malaria, the diagnosis of malaria is an urgent matter, and all requests for malaria diagnosis should be handled on a STAT basis. Although it is important that thick smears dry completely before staining, drying can be accomplished at 37°C in 15 to 30 minutes; laboratory protocols should not specify

TABLE 1 Classification of severe malaria

Category	Criteria
Cerebral malaria	Unrousable coma or Blantyre coma score of 3 or less
	Coma persists for more than 30 min after any seizures have passed
	Normal cerebrospinal fluid findings
	No other pathological process accounts for coma
Generalized convulsions	Generalized convulsions lasting more than 30 min
	Generalized convulsions more than twice in 24 h in spite of cooling
Severe anemia	Hemoglobin < 5 mg/dl
Respiratory distress	Presence of any of the following: alar flaring, intercostal retractions, use of accessory muscles of respiration, or Kussmaul's respiration
Hypoglycemia	Blood glucose < 40 mg/dl
Circulatory collapse	Systolic blood pressure < 80 mm Hg (adults) or < 50 mm Hg (children)
Renal failure	Urine output < 12 ml/kg/24 h or serum creatinine > 3.0 mg/dl
Malarial hemoglobinuria	Hemoglobinuria by urine dipstick in patient with malaria
Other	Hyperparasitemia (>100,000 parasites/μl)
	Jaundice (serum bilirubin ≥ 3.0 mg/dl)
	Hyperpyrexia (rectal temp ≥ 40°C)
	Impaired consciousness (rousable)

long periods for drying at room temperature (e.g., 4 hours to overnight), as this may unduly delay diagnosis. Ideally, blood for preparation of peripheral smears may be collected by finger prick. If other tests are to be performed, blood may be collected by venipuncture, using EDTA as the anticoagulant. Use of heparin as an anticoagulant may lead to some morphological distortion. Smears should be prepared and stained within an hour of drawing the specimen. Otherwise, confusing alterations in morphology may occur. For example, *P. falciparum* may continue to develop within the stored blood to the mature trophozoite stage, which is normally not seen in peripheral smears, leading to misidentification of the species. Diagnostic malaria smears should always be prepared, stained, and read on a STAT basis. However, if a laboratory is to prepare large numbers of slides from a single patient for later teaching purposes, it is acceptable to prepare the smears immediately but to delay staining for up to a few days. Unstained slides cannot be stored indefinitely, however, as the morphology will degrade over time. It is therefore not possible to maintain a supply of unstained, malaria-positive slides to use for quality control of the Giemsa stain; adequate staining of the normal blood elements in the smear is a sufficient quality control marker. Blood containing malaria parasites is infectious, and universal precautions should be strictly followed.

Requests for malaria smears should include several important pieces of historical information. If the following historical information is not submitted with the request for malaria smears, the laboratory must be proactive in obtaining the history. (i) The patient's travel history and date of return or arrival in the United States can suggest the likelihood of infection and the possible species involved. The interval between exposure to an infective bite and development of symptoms is typically 9 to 14 days for *P. falciparum, P. vivax, P. ovale,* and *P. knowlesi* and up to 40 days for *P. malariae.* Because there may be no primary attack in *P. vivax* or *P. ovale,* if all sporozoites that invaded hepatocytes transformed into hypnozoites, the first symptoms may occur months to as many as 3 years after exposure. There have been extremely rare reports of *P. falciparum* malaria first being detected up to 24 months after exposure (55), but in general, malaria appearing more than 1 month after return from an area of endemic-

ity is relatively unlikely to be due to *P. falciparum,* unless the patient has received antimalarial agents which might have suppressed parasitemia. (ii) A history of prophylaxis or treatment for malaria may result in low parasitemia. Since currently available prophylactic regimens are difficult to comply with and since drug resistance is common in *P. falciparum,* a history of prophylaxis should never be used to exclude malaria from the differential diagnosis. (iii) A history of transfusions or shared needles may suggest direct person-to-person transmission, although cases of transfusion-related malaria are extremely rare in the United States (66). (iv) A history of malaria in the patient suggests the possibility of relapse or recrudescence. (v) Knowledge of the periodicity of the fever pattern and the time in relation to a paroxysm when the specimen was obtained is helpful because, in a regularly periodic *P. falciparum* infection, the circulating parasitemia can be very low and difficult to detect between paroxysms. Regardless of the presence or absence of a fever pattern, blood should be taken immediately for an initial malaria smear when the patient presents.

Blood Film Examination

Detection and identification of the organisms are performed by examination of Giemsa-stained thick and thin blood films. Examination of thick films is the gold standard for detection of organisms because of the relatively large volume of blood (10 μl) that can be examined directly. Hyposmotic lysis of the erythrocytes during staining with Giemsa stain deposits the free parasites onto a background of red cell ghosts, white cell nuclei, and platelets. Approximately 20-fold more blood is examined in each high-power (1,000×) field examined than in a thin film. Although substantial training and practice are required to develop proficiency at distinguishing the free parasites from platelets, leukocyte granules, and other debris present in thick films, thick-film examination is substantially more sensitive than thin-film examination. Early in infection, or following relapse or partial treatment, patients may be symptomatic with parasitemias low enough that they require thick smear examination for detection. While it is often possible to identify parasites to the species level in thick films, thin films are the gold standard for species identification. Although fewer parasites are present in thin films, methanol fixation prior to staining preserves erythrocyte morphology, allowing evaluation of infected erythrocyte size and the position of organisms within the erythrocytes. In difficult cases, therefore, examination of thin films may be necessary to make a specific identification. Morphology is best preserved in thin areas of the smear near the feathered edge; scanning of the thicker areas of the slide may facilitate detection of rare gametocytes or schizonts but must not replace careful examination of the thick film. Smears should be examined at length under oil immersion; a negative report should not be rendered until 200 oil immersion fields of a thick film have been examined. A single set of negative smears does not exclude malaria. Additional specimens should be examined at 12-hour intervals for the subsequent 36 hours.

The morphology of the five species of *Plasmodium* that infect humans in thick and thin blood films is reviewed in references 32 and 57, shown in Fig. 2 to 10, and summarized in Table 2. When abundant organisms encompassing several life cycle stages are present for examination, species identification is not difficult. A high parasitemia consisting only of ring forms suggests *P. falciparum*, even if, as is commonly the case, no gametocytes are found. In samples

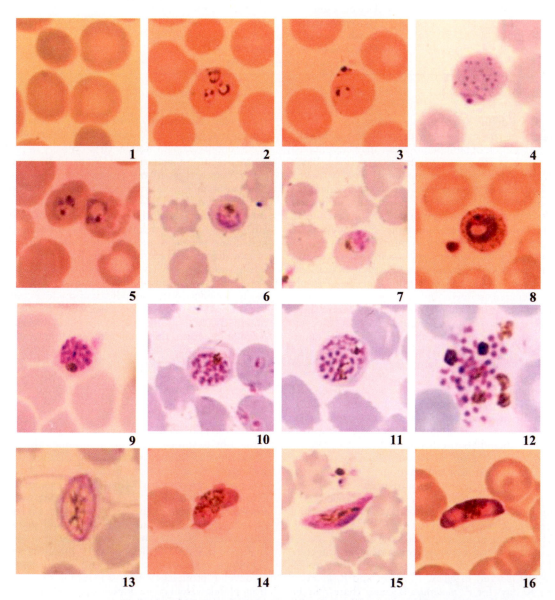

FIGURE 2 *P. falciparum:* morphology of successive developmental stages in Giemsa-stained thin blood smears. Rings and gametocytes will be found in peripheral blood smears; other stages occur in infected erythrocytes but are sequestered in the capillaries and venules of the internal organs and are rarely found in the periphery. Films: 1, normal erythrocyte; 2, young rings; 3, rings with appliqué form; 4, appliqué ring with Maurer's dots; 5, late ring; 6 and 7, mature trophozoites; 8, late trophozoite; 9, young schizont; 10 and 11, mature schizonts; 12, gravid schizont; 13, immature gametocyte; 14, mature microgametocyte; 15 and 16, mature macrogametocytes.

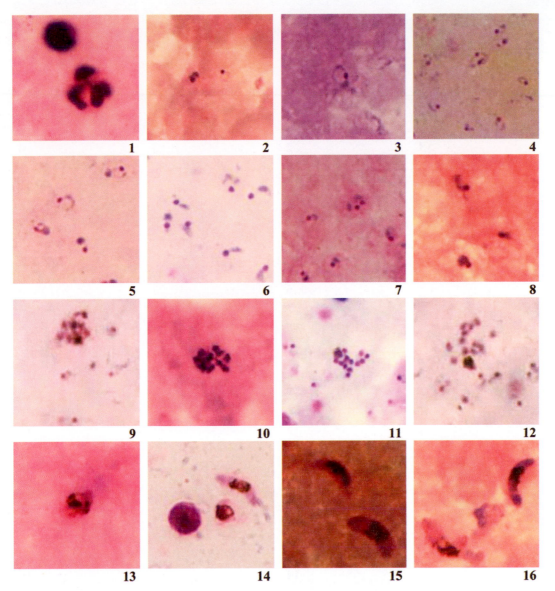

FIGURE 3 *P. falciparum:* morphology of successive developmental stages in Giemsa-stained thick blood smears. Films: 1, leukocyte nuclei and erythrocyte stroma, no parasites; 2 to 4, rings; 5 to 7, trophozoites; 8, mature trophozoite; 9, young schizont; 10 and 11, mature schizonts; 12, gravid schizont; 13, immature gametocyte; 14, immature and mature gametocytes; 15 and 16, mature macrogametocytes (above) and microgametocytes (below).

containing only rare early trophozoites, a species identification may not be possible. Ring morphology is quite variable; early trophozoites of *P. falciparum* may mimic early "band" forms of *P. malariae* or early ameboid trophozoites of *P. vivax*. It is important not to exclude *P. falciparum* solely on the basis of ring morphology. Finally, the possibility of mixed infections should be borne in mind; examination of the smear should not be ended prematurely simply because one species of *Plasmodium* has been identified. *P. knowlesi* infections in humans have frequently been misdiagnosed as *P. malariae*, although there are morphological differences between the species (Table 1). Such misdiagnosis may be dangerous, as *P. knowlesi*, unlike *P. malariae*, can progress to severe malaria. Therefore, patients with a microscopic diagnosis of *P. malariae* and a recent travel history to Southeast Asia should be considered to have *P. knowlesi* infection.

Although many North American clinicians treat all malaria patients with regimens designed to cover drug-resistant *P. falciparum*, species-specific identification of *Plasmodium* spp. is clinically important for several reasons. *P. falciparum* should be identified because it is both more clinically aggressive and more likely to be multiply drug resistant than the other species. *P. vivax* and *P. ovale* should be identified because radical cure of these infections requires supplemental treatment with primaquine to eliminate dormant hypnozoites in the liver. Primaquine may cause hemolytic anemia in some patients with G6PD deficiency; correct species identification prevents its unnecessary use in *P. falciparum* or *P. malariae* infection.

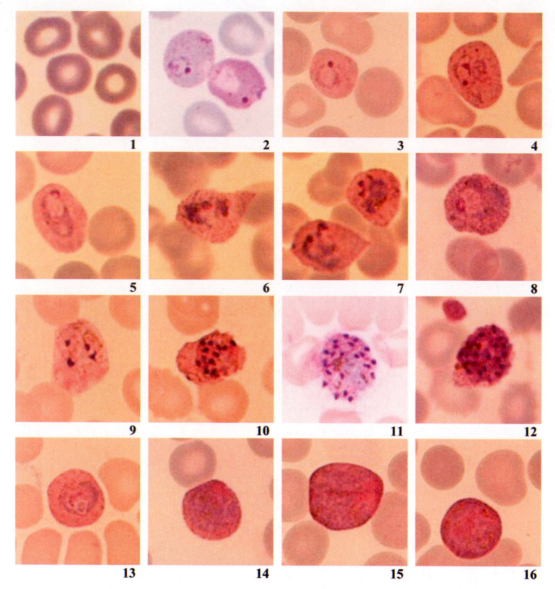

FIGURE 4 *P. vivax:* morphology of successive developmental stages in Giemsa-stained thin blood smears. Films: 1, normal erythrocytes; 2 to 4, rings; 5 to 7, growing trophozoites; 8, mature trophozoite; 9 and 10, immature schizonts; 11 and 12, mature schizonts; 13, immature gametocyte; 14, mature microgametocyte; 15, mature macrogametocyte; 16, mature microgametocyte.

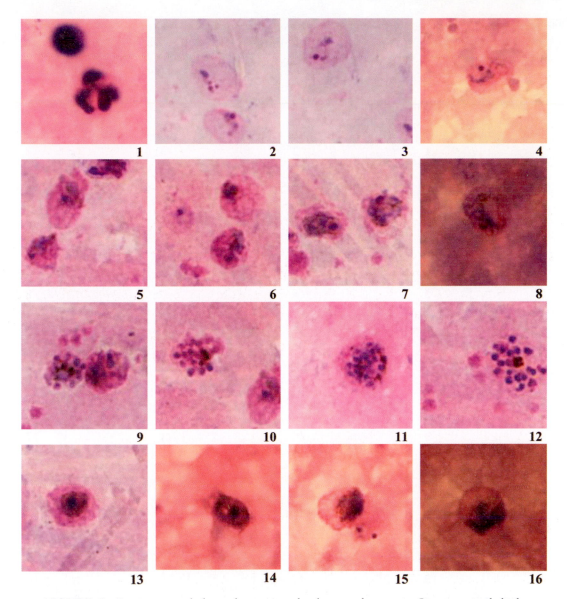

FIGURE 5 *P. vivax:* morphology of successive developmental stages in Giemsa-stained thick blood smears. Films: 1, leukocyte nuclei and erythrocyte stroma, no parasites; 2 to 4, rings; 5 to 7, growing trophozoites; 8, mature trophozoite; 9 and 10, immature schizonts; 11, mature schizont; 12, gravid schizont; 13, immature gametocyte; 14, mature gametocyte, sex undetermined; 15, mature microgametocyte; 16, mature macrogametocyte.

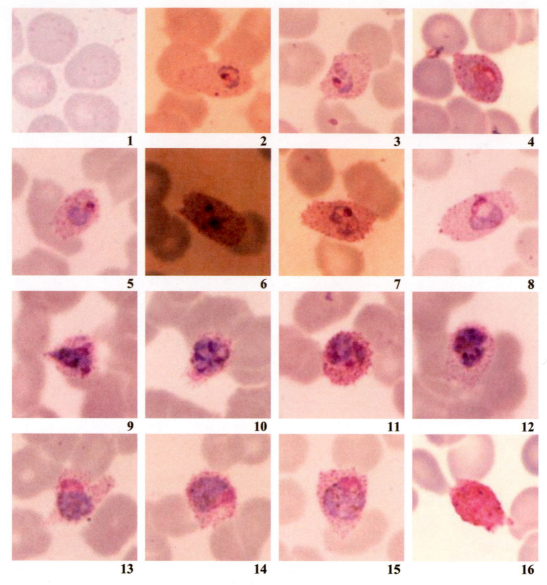

FIGURE 6 *P. ovale:* morphology of successive developmental stages in Giemsa-stained thin blood smears. Films: 1, normal erythrocytes; 2 to 4, rings; 5, young trophozoite; 6 and 7, trophozoites; 8, mature trophozoite; 9 and 10, immature schizonts; 11 and 12, mature schizonts; 13, immature gametocyte; 14 and 15, mature microgametocytes; 16, mature macrogametocyte.

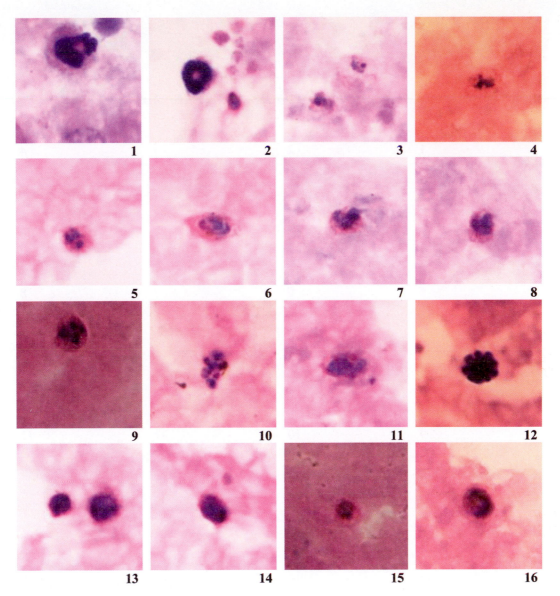

FIGURE 7 *P. ovale:* morphology of successive developmental stages in Giemsa-stained thick blood smears. Films: 1, leukocyte nuclei and erythrocyte stroma, no parasites; 2 to 4, rings; 5 to 7, growing trophozoites; 8, mature trophozoite; 9 and 10, immature schizonts; 11, mature schizont; 12, gravid schizont; 13 and 14, immature gametocytes; 15, mature macrogametocyte; 16, mature microgametocyte.

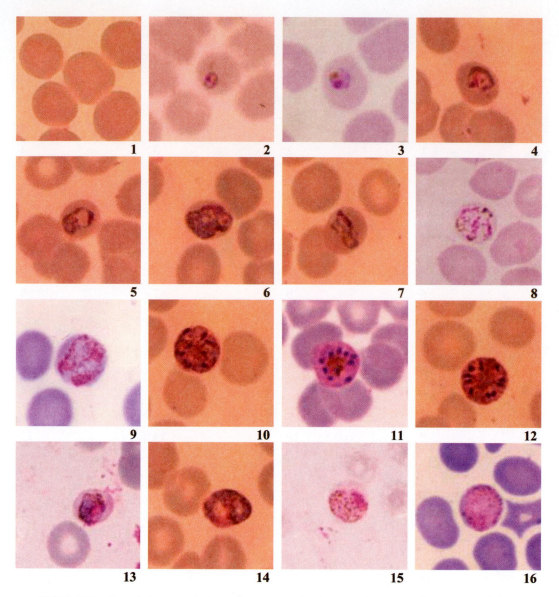

FIGURE 8 *P. malariae:* morphology of successive developmental stages in Giemsa-stained thin blood smears. Films: 1, normal erythrocyte; 2 and 3, rings; 4 and 5, growing trophozoites; 6, mature trophozoite; 7, band form trophozoite; 8 and 9, immature schizonts; 10, schizont; 11 and 12, "daisy head" schizonts; 13, immature gametocyte; 14 and 15, mature macrogametocytes; 16, mature microgametocyte.

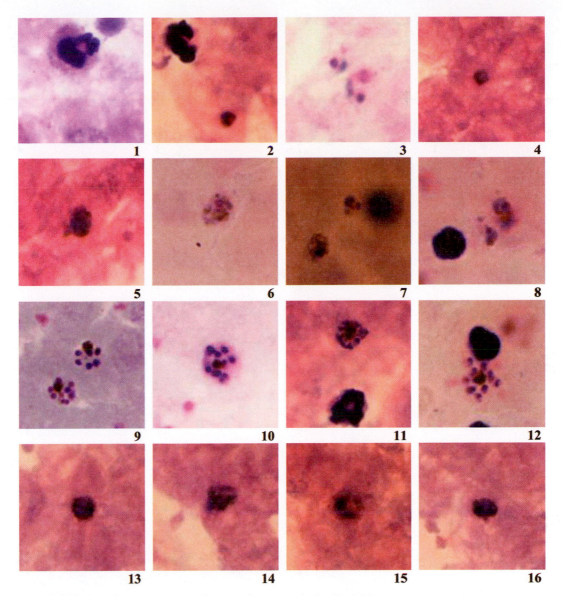

FIGURE 9 *P. malariae:* morphology of successive developmental stages in Giemsa-stained thick blood smears. Films: 1, leukocyte nucleus and erythrocyte stroma, no parasites; 2 to 4, rings; 5 to 8, trophozoites; 9, young schizonts; 10, schizont; 11, "daisy head" schizont; 12, gravid schizont; 13, immature gametocyte; 14, mature gametocyte, sex undetermined; 15, mature microgametocyte; 16, mature macrogametocyte.

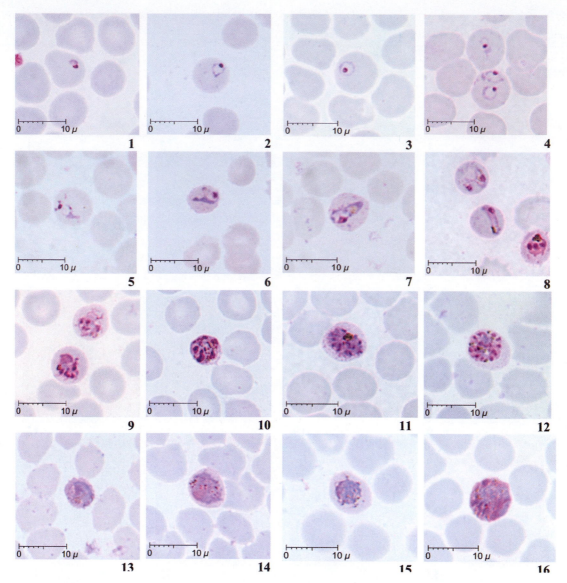

FIGURE 10 *P. knowlesi:* morphology of successive developmental stages in Giemsa-stained thin blood smears. Films: 1 to 4, rings; 5 to 7, growing trophozoites; 8, mature trophozoite; 9 and 10, immature schizonts; 11, mature schizont; 12, mature schizont containing 16 merozoites; 13, immature gametocyte; 14, mature microgametocyte; 15, mature macrogametocyte; 16, mature microgametocyte. (Images reproduced from figures in reference 57 with permission.)

Alternative Diagnostic Methods

A number of new approaches to detection of malaria parasites have been described, including staining with acridine orange (AO) (81), PCR (3), loop-mediated isothermal amplification (42, 70), and antigen detection (19, 89). These and other alternative approaches have been recently reviewed (24) and are summarized in Table 3.

Thin or thick blood films can be stained with AO in place of Giemsa stain. AO is a fluorescent dye that binds to DNA; since mature erythrocytes do not contain DNA, the brightly staining parasite nuclei stand out clearly against a background of uninfected erythrocytes. Nonetheless, particularly in thick films stained with AO, it may be difficult to detect parasite nuclei in the presence of leukocyte nuclei and erythrocytes containing Howell-Jolly bodies. In addition, since it may be difficult to evaluate erythrocyte morphology, species identification can be difficult. The method can be performed on a fluorescence microscope or on a standard microscope with an excitation filter (470 to 490 nm) mounted in the transmitted light path and a separate filter (590 nm) mounted in the ocular. A number of comparisons of AO staining to standard malaria microscopy have been recently reviewed (53, 71); sensitivity and specificity were adequate in most studies. The most frequently cited advantage of AO staining was the speed with which slides could be prepared and read. An alternative version of the AO technique, designated quantitative buffy coat is available in which whole blood is stained with AO and spun in a microcentrifuge tube; the resulting buffy coat is examined directly within the microcentrifuge tube by using a fluorescence microscope fitted with a specialized long-focal-length objective.

TABLE 2 Comparative morphology of *Plasmodium* spp. in Giemsa-stained thin smears

Characteristic	P. falciparum	P. vivax	P. ovale	P. malariae	P. knowlesi
Size and shape of infected erythrocytes	Normal size and shape	Enlarged up to 2-fold; may be oval	Normal to enlarged, frequently oval, may be fimbriated	Small to normal size, normal shape	Normal size and shape
Stippling (best seen with Giemsa stain, pH 7.0–7.2)	Occasional Maurer's dots, less numerous than Schüffner's	Schüffner's dots usually present, except in rings	James' stippling, darker than Schüffner's present in all stages, including rings	Ziemann's dots, rarely seen; requires deliberate overstaining	Irregular stippling in late trophozoites and schizonts
Stages seen in peripheral blood	Rings and gametocytes	All	All	All	All
Multiply infected erythrocytes	Common	Occasional	Occasional	Rare	Common
Early trophozoites	Delicate ring, frequently with two small chromatin dots; often at edge of erythrocyte (appliqué form)	Ring up to 1/3 diam of erythrocyte; larger chromatin dot than P. falciparum	Similar to P. vivax	Smaller than P. vivax; otherwise similar	Double chromatin dots common; infrequent appliqué forms
Mature trophozoites	Not seen in peripheral blood	Ameboid shape, fine golden-brown pigment	Similar to P. vivax except less ameboid, pigment darker brown	Compact cytoplasm, oval, round, or band-shaped, dark brown pigment	Slightly ameboid cytoplasm; band forms common; scattered grains or clumps of golden to brown pigment
Schizonts	Not seen in peripheral blood	12–24 merozoites	8–12 merozoites	6–12 merozoites often radially arranged around central pigment ("daisy head" schizont)	10–16 merozoites
Gametocytes	Crescent- or banana-shaped	Round to slightly oval	Round to slightly oval	Round to slightly oval	Round to slightly oval
Most characteristic findings	Absence of mature trophozoites and schizonts; normal size of infected erythrocytes; multiple infections; appliqué forms; banana-shaped gametocytes	Enlarged infected erythrocytes; Schüffner's dots frequently present; ameboid trophozoite; 12–24 merozoites in each schizont	Normal to enlarged, oval or fimbriated infected erythrocytes; James' stippling may be seen in rings; schizonts with 8–12 merozoites	Normal size of infected erythrocytes; no stippling; "band" trophozoite; "daisy head" schizont with 6–12 merozoites	Rings resemble P. falciparum; trophozoites, schizonts, and gametocytes resemble P. malariae, except that schizonts may contain up to 16 merozoites

The immunochromatographic rapid dipstick antigen detection assays are potentially very useful, both in areas of malaria endemicity where trained laboratory personnel are scarce and in the developed world where they may be inexperienced in malaria diagnosis (67). Rapid immunochromatographic methods for malaria diagnosis have been developed based on several *Plasmodium* antigens. Histidine-rich protein 2 (HRP-2) is a *P. falciparum* protein with roles in heme polymerization and actin binding and is localized in the infected erythrocyte cytoplasm. Dipsticks for diagnosis of *P. falciparum* based on antigen detection of HRP-2 have been widely tested and found to have sensitivity and specificity close to that of expert microscopy (5, 58, 97, 98, 105) and probably superior to that of routine microscopy. These HRP-2-based tests are not appropriate for monitoring therapy, as they may remain positive for up to 28 days after successful therapy (48, 89). HRP-2 is unique to *P. falciparum*; immunochromatographic tests based on HRP-2 cannot detect infection due to the other *Plasmodium* spp. Aldolase is an enzyme within the glycolytic pathway and is found in all species of *Plasmodium*. Monoclonal antibodies raised against *Plasmodium* aldolase recognize aldolase from all *Plasmodium* species which infect humans. Recently, dipsticks combining antibodies

TABLE 3 Alternative methods for diagnosis of malaria

Principle	Method	Comments	Advantages	Disadvantages	Reference(s)
Giemsa stain	Thick film	Gold standard for detection	Screens large volume of blood	Species identification sometimes difficult	22
	Thin film	Traditional method for species identification	Preserves morphology of parasite in erythrocyte	Less sensitive than thick-film examination	32
Fluorescent DNA/RNA stains	AO-stained films	Requires fluorescent microscope	Sensitivity good	May be difficult to read	34, 61
	Centrifugation/AO (QBC)[a]	Requires fluorescent microscope	Rapid	Species identification difficult	60, 81, 92
	Flow cytometry		Automated	Poor sensitivity	99
Hemozoin detection	Dark-field microscopy	Abundant pigment in macrophages suggests poor prognosis		Poor sensitivity	51
	Automated blood analyzers	Detection in unsuspected cases	Automated	Poor sensitivity	43
Nucleic acid detection	DNA/RNA hybridization	First nucleic acid-based method		Poor sensitivity, technically difficult	4, 29
	PCR	Care required to prevent contamination/ false-positive results	Sensitivity comparable to or better than thick film; species identification; best approach to detect mixed infections	Expensive, lengthy procedure	90, 96, 103
	Loop-mediated isothermal amplification	Genus and species specific; performed on whole blood without DNA extraction	Sensitivity and specificity comparable to PCR; less expensive than PCR	Early in development; few field data available	42, 70
Antigen detection	Detection of HRP-2 (Parasight-F, ICT Malaria Pf, PATH Falciparum Malaria IC test)	Immunochromatographic dipstick, *P. falciparum* only	Convenient, rapid, minimal training required	Expensive, cannot be used to monitor therapy, detects only *P. falciparum*	5, 58, 97, 98, 105
	Detection of HRP-2 and aldolase (ICT Pf/Pv, Binax Now ICT Malaria test)	Immunochromatographic dipstick, *P. falciparum* and non-*P. falciparum*	Convenient, rapid, minimal training required	Expensive, cannot be used to monitor therapy	25, 98, 106
	Detection of parasite LDH (OptiMAL)	Immunochromatographic dipstick, *P. falciparum* and non-*P. falciparum*	Convenient, rapid, minimal training required	Expensive	31, 50, 73, 78

[a]QBC, quantitative buffy coat technique.

against HRP-2 and aldolase have been devised which allow detection of *P. falciparum* and non-*P. falciparum* infections (26, 98). An alternative dipstick test uses monoclonal antibodies to capture parasite lactate dehydrogenase (LDH) (78). *P. falciparum* species-specific and *Plasmodium* genus-specific anti-LDH antibodies distinguish between *P. falciparum* and non-*P. falciparum* infection. Preliminary studies suggest that the LDH-based assay may have useful sensitivity and specificity (31, 50, 73, 99). Both HRP-2- and LDH-based assays lose sensitivity when parasitemias are low (<50 to $100/mm^3$). While such assays will not soon replace microscopy, they may shortly become an important adjunct in malaria diagnosis.

Recently, an immunochromatographic test based on HRP-2 and aldolase, the BinaxNOW Malaria (Binax, Inc., Inverness Medical Professional Diagnostics, Scarborough, ME) was approved by the FDA for use in the evaluation of symptomatic patients in laboratories which can both (i) acquire blood samples known to contain *P. falciparum* for use as a positive control and (ii) perform thick- and thin-film examination to confirm negative results in the immunochromatographic test.

It should be pointed out that automated hematology instrumentation will not reliably detect malaria parasites. Finally, it is important that negative results using the alternative diagnostic methods be confirmed by repeated thick-film examination. As of 2010, thick-film examination remains the gold standard for malaria diagnosis.

Serology

Indirect fluorescent antibody tests using antigens prepared from the four species of *Plasmodium* that infect humans have been described previously (94). However, serologic testing is not a reliable method for identifying the infecting species, because of cross-reactions among the four species, and is not useful in clinical diagnosis of malaria because antibodies may be absent in an acute attack and because their presence may reflect past rather than current infection. It has a role in the investigation of transfusion malaria, where it may be used to determine which of a number of potential donors may have been the source of a transfusion-associated case of malaria, and in epidemiological studies, to determine the prevalence of exposure to malaria in a population. Assistance in serological evaluation of suspected transfusion malaria can be obtained from the Malaria Branch, Division of Parasitic Diseases, Centers for Disease Control and Prevention [phone, (770) 488-7788].

Interpretation and Reporting of Results

A positive finding of malaria parasites is a critical result which must be reported immediately to the clinician. The report should include the species identification, if possible. When identification to this level is not possible, an explicit statement that *P. falciparum* cannot be excluded is advisable. If the microscopic diagnosis is *P. malariae* but the patient has traveled to Southeast Asia, the clinician should be informed that *P. knowlesi* cannot be excluded. Because patients with high parasitemias (>3 to 5%) require intensive therapy, quantification of parasitemia is useful. This is typically performed after species identification and may be variously expressed as percent parasitemia (parasites/100 erythrocytes), number of parasites per 200 leukocytes, or number of parasites/mm^3. At high parasitemias, the direct counting of parasites and erythrocytes in a thin film will provide an accurate parasitemia. In low parasitemias and, of course, in thick smears, it is necessary to count parasites/200 leukocytes and to calculate the percent parasitemia or the parasite density based on the patient's complete blood count. A negative report may be accompanied by a reminder that a single negative set of smears does not exclude the diagnosis of malaria. Serial malaria smears may be performed to monitor therapy. Parasitemia normally resolves within 2 to 3 days following initiation of treatment with a drug to which the patient's strain is susceptible. Continued parasitemia at day 3 or failure of the parasitemia to decrease by 75% within the first 48 hours following treatment is an indication of drug resistance. However, gametocytes may continue to circulate for up to 2 weeks after successful cure, and their presence is not an indication that treatment has failed.

Special Considerations in Areas Where Malaria Is Endemic

In travelers returning to areas without malaria transmission, careful parasitological diagnostic testing for malaria is the norm. In areas where malaria is endemic, the appropriate diagnostic strategy depends on the intensity of transmission, the cost of first-line therapy, and the available resources.

In areas of intense transmission, such as much of sub-Saharan Africa or some areas in Southeast Asia, diagnosis of clinical malaria on the basis of a positive peripheral smear is difficult. In such areas, both nonmalarial fevers and asymptomatic parasitemia are common; indeed, the large majority of individuals may harbor *P. falciparum*. Therefore, fever due to nonmalarial causes may frequently coincide with parasitemia. At a population level, it is possible to estimate the fraction of fevers attributable to malaria (39), but this does not help in individual diagnosis. Since high parasitemias are more likely to be associated with fever than low parasitemias, it is tempting to create definitions of clinical malaria based on fever and parasitemia above a specified cutoff. Unfortunately, in many areas of endemicity, no cutoff is satisfactory. For example, in northern Ghana the pretest probability that a child with fever has clinical malaria is 60%. Finding a positive malaria smear raises that probability only to 70%. To obtain a posttest probability of 80% that the fever is due to malaria requires a parasitemia threshold of 20,000 parasites/μl and leads to a sensitivity in the clinical definition of only 55% (83). In such situations, it may be entirely reasonable not to perform a malaria smear and to treat all fevers as malaria empirically.

On the other hand, in areas of lower transmission intensity, empiric therapy not guided by specific diagnosis may lead to substantial overtreatment and to failure to diagnose treatable, nonmalarious causes of fever (74). Whether or not it is cost-effective to attempt to make a laboratory diagnosis of malaria in a given area of endemicity depends on a complex interaction between the local attributable fraction of fevers due to malaria, the cost and side effect profile of recommended first-line antimalarial agents, and the cost and accuracy of available diagnostic methods. As the emergence of drug resistance has forced a shift from older inexpensive drugs such as chloroquine and sulfadoxine-pyrimethamine (Fansidar) to more expensive artemisinin combination therapies (ACT), the importance of accurate diagnosis in areas of low to moderate transmission has increased.

Finally, highly sensitive diagnostic methods are required for use in malaria elimination campaigns. It has become clear that in areas of endemicity, submicroscopic *Plasmodium* infections, detectable by PCR, are common (7) and, in some cases, more common than microscopically detectable ones (23). Individuals carrying submicroscopic gametocytemia may serve as a source of transmission (87). Large-scale screening and treatment programs which used only microscopic diagnosis might leave a substantial reservoir of *Plasmodium* in place (93).

Treatment, Prevention, and Drug Resistance

Prophylaxis and therapy of malaria have been recently reviewed (20, 30, 40). *P. falciparum* resistant to chloroquine is present in all areas of endemicity, with the exception of Central America and the Caribbean. In addition, resistance to other drugs, including sulfadoxine-pyrimethamine and mefloquine is present in many areas and is expanding rapidly. In the face of emerging drug resistance, many countries in areas of endemicity have adopted a policy of first-line treatment of *P. falciparum* with ACT, including artesunate-mefloquine, artemether-lumefantrine (Coartem), and artesunate-amodiaquine. Unfortunately, resistance to artesunate-mefloquine has already appeared in Southeast Asia (84); widespread resistance to ACT would pose a serious problem to malaria control. A formulation of artemether-lumefantrine was recently approved by the U.S. FDA for use in treatment of uncomplicated *P. falciparum* malaria. Distribution of drug resistance in *P. falciparum* as of July 2009 is summarized in Table 4. Current information on the distribution of drug-resistant *P. falciparum* may be obtained from the Centers for Disease Control and Prevention malaria hotline in Atlanta, GA [phone, (770) 488-7788]. In vitro susceptibility testing of *P. falciparum* has been described previously (82) but is not available for clinical use. The combinations of quinine or quinidine and doxycycline or of atovaquone and proguanil remain effective against most strains of *P. falciparum*. Therapy of chloroquine-resistant *P. falciparum* is a complex and rapidly evolving field, and consultation with an infectious disease specialist is essential. Current treatment guidelines from the U.S. CDC are available at http://www.cdc.gov/malaria/pdf/clinicalguidance.pdf. Chloroquine-resistant *P. vivax* emerged in a few areas in the 1990s (2, 68, 77, 88) and has continued to spread (1). More detailed information on specific antimalarial agents and on specialized in vitro susceptibility test methods may be found in chapters 147 and 149, respectively.

Drug and Vaccine Development

In the face of rapidly developing drug resistance, development of new antimalarial drugs and, ultimately, an effective malaria vaccine are high priorities. The sequencing of the *P. falciparum* genome (33), subsequent characterization of the transcriptome and proteome (41), and sequencing of the genomes of *P. vivax* (10), *P. yoelii* (11), and *P. knowlesi* (72) have helped identify a number of potential new drug targets. Even before completion of the *P. falciparum* genome sequence, data mining of the unassembled sequence data led to identification of inhibitors of an isoprenoid biosynthesis pathway with in vitro and in vivo activity against *Plasmodium* (52). These and other advances in antimalarial drug development have been recently reviewed (35, 86).

There remain many difficult obstacles to overcome in malaria vaccine development. Nonetheless, two lines of evidence suggest that a malaria vaccine may be attainable. First, residents of areas where malaria is endemic who do not succumb to malaria in early childhood develop a limited, clinical immunity that greatly reduces their risk of severe disease and death when they become infected (85). Second, human volunteers immunized with radiation-attenuated sporozoites develop solid sterile immunity to sporozoite challenge (17, 21). A wide variety of approaches have been used to develop vaccines targeting the preerythrocytic (65) or erythrocytic (36) stage of the parasite, including synthetic peptides, recombinant viral particles, DNA vaccines, heterologous prime-boost combinations of DNA and recombinant viral vaccines, and attenuated whole-organism vaccines. The current state of clinical testing of malaria vaccines has been recently reviewed (101). No vaccine is yet available for clinical use.

BABESIA

The genus *Babesia* includes approximately 100 species that are transmitted by ticks of the genus *Ixodes* and infect a variety of wild and domestic animals (47). The *Babesia* species are grouped loosely into small *Babesia* (trophozoites measuring 1.0 to 2.5 μm), including *B. microti* and *B. gibsoni*, and the large *Babesia* (trophozoites measuring 2.5 to 5.0 μm), including *B. bovis* and *B. canis*. This morphological division is generally supported by molecular phylogenetic analysis, except that *B. divergens*, which has small trophozoites, groups with the large babesias (47). The taxonomy and phylogeny of *Babesia* are developing rapidly and have been recently reviewed (49). In the United States, *B. microti* and the recently described species *B. duncani* and MO1 (44), a strain closely related to *B. divergens* (38), infect humans. In Europe, the bovine parasites, *B. bovis* and *B. divergens*, have been isolated from human patients. These geographic ranges are not strict. Recently, infection by *B. microti* has been reported from both Europe (45, 64) and Japan (104), and infection with a *B. divergens*-like organism was reported in the northwest United States (46).

Life Cycle

While the life cycle of *Babesia* is roughly similar to that of *Plasmodium*, there are a number of important differences (Fig. 11). First, no exoerythrocytic stage has been described for *Babesia* species; sporozoites injected by the bite of an infected tick invade erythrocytes directly. Within the erythrocyte, the trophozoites reproduce by binary fission rather than schizogony. While gametocytes presumably exist, they have not been morphologically distinguished from trophozoites. As in *Plasmodium* species, fertilization of gametes occurs in the insect intestine within the blood meal and the zygotes pass through the intestinal epithelium to the hemolymph. In *Plasmodium* species, sporogony takes place in oocysts attached to

TABLE 4 Distribution of drug-resistant *P. falciparum*[a]

Region	Chloroquine resistance	Resistance to second-line antimalarials
Caribbean, Central America	No	No
South America	Yes	Sulfadoxine/pyrimethamine (Amazon Basin), mefloquine (Amazon Basin)
West Africa	Yes	Sulfadoxine/pyrimethamine, mefloquine
East Africa	Yes	Sulfadoxine/pyrimethamine
Central Asia	Yes	Sulfadoxine/pyrimethamine
Southeast Asia	Yes	Sulfadoxine/pyrimethamine, mefloquine, halofantrine, mefloquine-artesunate, quinine

[a]Based on information from the World Health Organization Roll Back Malaria Department (http://apps.who.int/malaria/resistancefalciparum.html) as of 10 July 2009.

Events inside the tick:

In the tick gut:

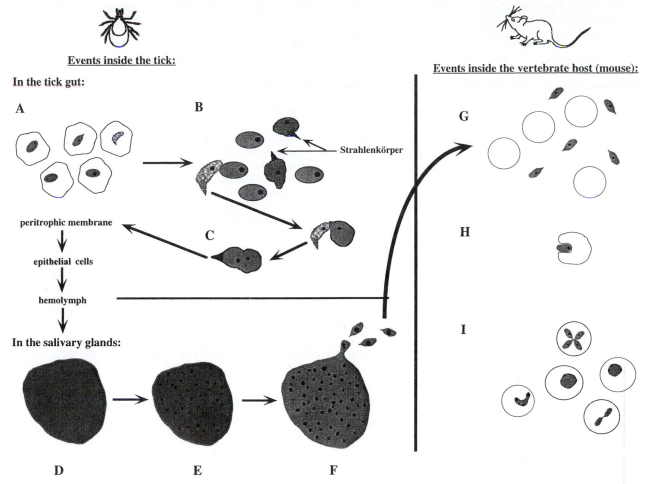

In the salivary glands:

Events inside the vertebrate host (mouse):

FIGURE 11 Life cycle of *Babesia*. Events in the tick begin with the parasites still visible in consumed erythrocytes. Some are beginning to develop Strahlenkörper forms (specialized apical organelles) (A). The released gametes begin to fuse (B). The zygote then goes on to infect and move through other tissues within the tick (C) to the salivary glands. Once a parasite has infected the salivary acini, a multinucleate but undifferentiated sporoblast is formed (D). After the tick begins to feed, the specialized organelles of the future sporozoites form (E). Finally, mature sporozoites bud off the sporoblast (F). As the tick feeds on its vertebrate host, these sporozoites are inoculated into the host (G). Sporozoites (or merozoites) contact a host erythrocyte and begin the process of infection by invagination (H). The parasites become trophozoites and can divide by binary fission within the host erythrocyte, creating the various ring forms and crosses seen on stained blood smears (I). Illustrations are not to scale. (Reproduced with permission from reference 21.)

the transluminal aspect of the intestine and sporozoites released from oocysts migrate to the salivary glands; in *Babesia* species, fertilized gametes migrate through the intestinal wall, through the hemolymph and on to the salivary glands, where they develop into sporoblasts. The final production of sporozoites from sporoblasts only occurs when the tick begins to take a blood meal; the resulting sporozoites are injected into the host during the final hours of attachment and feeding.

Epidemiology and Transmission

Babesiosis is transmitted by the bite of infected *Ixodes scapularis* ticks, and outbreaks of human infection have been described in the Northeast, Midwest, and West Coast of the United States; in Europe; and recently,

in Japan (104). Relatively few cases of babesiosis have been reported in the United States: 10 to 12 cases per year in New York and Nantucket, MA, over the past 30 years (47). However, because babesiosis is a mild and self-limiting infection in most persons, the number of unreported infections may be much higher. Indeed, serological surveys of blood donors have shown a seroprevalence of 3 to 8% for antibodies to *B. microti* (47). With the exception of a few cases attributed to newly described *Babesia* spp. (44, 46, 75, 80), babesiosis in the United States results from infection with *B. microti*. In Europe, a growing number of cases of babesiosis have been reported (49), principally infections of splenectomized individuals with *B. divergens*; however, these infections are clinically serious, with a mortality rate of

42% (37). A handful of cases of transfusion-associated babesiosis, usually involving transmission of *B. microti* from an asymptomatic donor, have been reported from the United States.

The host ranges of *B. microti* and *B. divergens* are wide, and virtually any mammal that serves as a host for *I. scapularis* ticks can be a reservoir of infection. *Babesia* spp. share both vectors and animal reservoirs, i.e., *Ixodes* ticks and white-footed mice, with several other tick-borne pathogens, including the agents of Lyme disease and human granulocytic ehrlichiosis. Not surprisingly, there have been reports of coinfection with *B. microti* and *Borrelia burgdorferi*, and approximately 10% of Lyme disease patients in areas of babesia endemicity may be infected with *B. microti*. Lyme disease patients coinfected with *B. microti* experienced more severe symptoms than those infected with either agent alone (54).

Clinical Significance

There is a wide range of clinical presentations of babesiosis from mild or asymptomatic infection through a fulminant illness clinically similar to malaria and characterized by high fever, myalgias, malaise, fatigue, hepatosplenomegaly, and anemia. In general, infection with *B. microti* in the United States tends to occur in nonsplenectomized individuals and to be relatively mild. Infection with the more recently described babesias from the United States and with *B. divergens* in Europe tends to occur in splenectomized or immunocompromised individuals and to be clinically more severe. Overall, mortality among clinically apparent cases of *B. microti* infection in the United States is 5%, while that in *B. divergens* infection in Europe is 40%. In both the United States and Europe, risk factors for severe disease include increasing age, splenectomy, and immune compromise.

Diagnosis

The diagnosis of babesiosis should be considered for a patient with the appropriate clinical symptoms and a history of travel to areas where the disease is endemic, exposure to ticks, or recent blood transfusion. Examination of Giemsa-stained thin blood smears is the most direct approach to diagnosis. The appearance of *Babesia* in thin films is shown in Fig. 12. Although the trophozoites of *Babesia* can be confused with *Plasmodium* rings, particularly the small-ring trophozoites of *P. falciparum*, *Babesia* can be distinguished from *P. falciparum* by several criteria. *Babesia* trophozoites are quite variable in size (1 to 5 μm), and the smallest are smaller than *P. falciparum* rings. Extracellular trophozoites and multiply infected erythrocytes are more common in *Babesia*. The cytoplasm of the larger *Babesia* trophozoites frequently contains a clear vacuole, which is rare or absent in *P. falciparum*. Finally, diagnostic tetrads, the Maltese cross, though rare in clinical specimens, may be present in *Babesia*. Parasitemias may be very low, particularly in chronic infections in nonsplenectomized patients; in such cases, diagnosis may require serologic testing (16), hamster inoculation (8), or PCR amplification (76).

Treatment and Prevention

Mild cases of infection with *B. microti* usually resolve spontaneously. In more serious cases, treatment with clindamycin and quinine or atovaquone and azithromycin is standard. In very severe cases of *B. microti* infection and in *B. divergens* infection in splenectomized or immunosuppressed patients, antimicrobial therapy may be supplemented with exchange

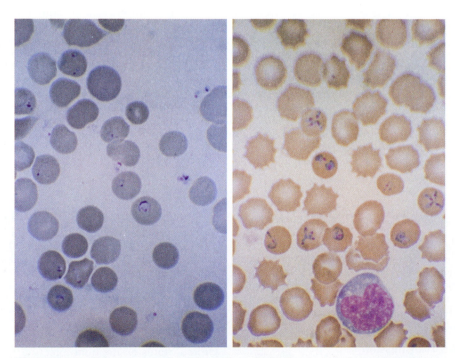

FIGURE 12 *Babesia* spp. in thin blood films. (Left) *B. microti* in human blood: parasites in erythrocytes and extracellular parasites; (right) *Babesia* sp. in classic Maltese cross (tetrad) configuration, a form diagnostic for babesiosis but rare in slides from humans infected with *B. microti*.

transfusion. Appropriate personal protective measures, including use of long pants, long-sleeved shirts, and insect repellant, may reduce the risk of infection when outdoors in areas of endemicity.

REFERENCES

1. **Baird, J. K.** 2004. Chloroquine resistance in *Plasmodium vivax*. *Antimicrob. Agents Chemother.* **48:**4075–4083.
2. **Baird, J. K., H. Basri, Purnomo, M. J. Bangs, B. Subianto, L. C. Patchen, and S. L. Hoffman.** 1991. Resistance to chloroquine by Plasmodium vivax in Irian Jaya, Indonesia. *Am. J. Trop. Med. Hyg.* **44:**547–552.
3. **Barker, R. H., T. Banchongaksorn, J. M. Courval, W. Suwonkerd, K. Rimwungtragoon, and D. F. Wirth.** 1992. A simple method to detect *Plasmodium falciparum* directly from blood using the polymerase chain reaction. *Am. J. Trop. Med. Hyg.* **46:**416–426.
4. **Barker, R. H., Jr., L. Suebsaeng, W. Rooney, G. C. Alecrim, H. V. Dourado, and D. F. Wirth.** 1986. Specific DNA probe for the diagnosis of Plasmodium falciparum malaria. *Science* **231:**1434–1436.
5. **Beadle, C., G. W. Long, W. R. Weiss, P. D. McElroy, S. M. Maret, A. J. Oloo, and S. L. Hoffman.** 1994. Diagnosis of malaria by detection of Plasmodium falciparum HRP-2 antigen with a rapid dipstick antigen-capture assay. *Lancet* **343:**564–568.
6. **Borst, P., W. Bitter, R. McCulloch, F. Van Leeuwen, and G. Rudenko.** 1995. Antigenic variation in malaria. *Cell* **82:**1–4.
7. **Bottius, E., A. Guanzirolli, J. F. Trape, C. Rogier, L. Konate, and P. Druilhe.** 1996. Malaria: even more chronic in nature than previously thought; evidence for subpatent parasitaemia detectable by the polymerase chain reaction. *Trans. R. Soc. Trop. Med. Hyg.* **90:**15–19.
8. **Brandt, F., G. R. Healy, and M. Welch.** 1977. Human babesiosis: the isolation of Babesia microti in golden hamsters. *J. Parasitol.* **63:**934–937.
9. **Bronner, U., P. C. Divis, A. Farnert, and B. Singh.** 2009. Swedish traveller with Plasmodium knowlesi malaria after visiting Malaysian Borneo. *Malar. J.* **8:**15.
10. **Carlton, J. M., J. H. Adams, J. C. Silva, S. L. Bidwell, H. Lorenzi, E. Caler, J. Crabtree, S. V. Angiuoli, E. F. Merino, P. Amedeo, Q. Cheng, R. M. Coulson, B. S. Crabb, H. A. del Portillo, K. Essien, T. V. Feldblyum, C. Fernandez-Becerra, P. R. Gilson, A. H. Gueye, X. Guo, S. Kang'a, T. W. Kooij, M. Korsinczky, E. V. Meyer, V. Nene, I. Paulsen, O. White, S. A. Ralph, Q. Ren, T. J. Sargeant, S. L. Salzberg, C. J. Stoeckert, S. A. Sullivan, M. M. Yamamoto, S. L. Hoffman, J. R. Wortman, M. J. Gardner, M. R. Galinski, J. W. Barnwell, and C. M. Fraser-Liggett.** 2008. Comparative genomics of the neglected human malaria parasite Plasmodium vivax. *Nature* **455:**757–763.
11. **Carlton, J. M., S. V. Angiuoli, B. B. Suh, T. W. Kooij, M. Pertea, J. C. Silva, M. D. Ermolaeva, J. E. Allen, J. D. Selengut, H. L. Koo, J. D. Peterson, M. Pop, D. S. Kosack, M. F. Shumway, S. L. Bidwell, S. J. Shallom, S. E. van Aken, S. B. Riedmuller, T. V. Feldblyum, J. K. Cho, J. Quackenbush, M. Sedegah, A. Shoaibi, L. M. Cummings, L. Florens, J. R. Yates, J. D. Raine, R. E. Sinden, M. A. Harris, D. A. Cunningham, P. R. Preiser, L. W. Bergman, A. B. Vaidya, L. H. van Lin, C. J. Janse, A. P. Waters, H. O. Smith, O. R. White, S. L. Salzberg, J. C. Venter, C. M. Fraser, S. L. Hoffman, M. J. Gardner, and D. J. Carucci.** 2002. Genome sequence and comparative analysis of the model rodent malaria parasite Plasmodium yoelii yoelii. *Nature* **419:**512–519.
12. **Centers for Disease Control and Prevention.** 1995. Local transmission of Plasmodium vivax malaria—Houston, Texas, 1994. *MMWR Morb. Mortal. Wkly. Rep.* **44:**295, 301–303.
13. **Centers for Disease Control and Prevention.** 2002. Local transmission of Plasmodium vivax malaria—Virginia, 2002. *MMWR Morb. Mortal. Wkly. Rep.* **51:**921–923.
14. **Centers for Disease Control and Prevention.** 2003. Local transmission of Plasmodium vivax malaria—Palm Beach County, Florida, 2003. *MMWR Morb. Mortal. Wkly. Rep.* **52:**908–911.
15. **Centers for Disease Control and Prevention.** 2009. Simian malaria in a U.S. traveler—New York, 2008. *MMWR Morb. Mortal. Wkly. Rep.* **58:**229–232.
16. **Chisholm, E. S., T. K. Ruebush, A. J. Sulzer, and G. R. Healy.** 1978. Babesia microti infection in man: evaluation of an indirect immunofluorescent antibody test. *Am. J. Trop. Med. Hyg.* **27:**14–19.
17. **Clyde, D. F.** 1990. Immunity to falciparum and vivax malaria induced by irradiated sporozoites: a review of the University of Maryland studies, 1971–75. *Bull. W. H. O.* **68**(Suppl.):9–12.
18. **Cox-Singh, J., T. M. Davis, K. S. Lee, S. S. Shamsul, A. Matusop, S. Ratnam, H. A. Rahman, D. J. Conway, and B. Singh.** 2008. Plasmodium knowlesi malaria in humans is widely distributed and potentially life threatening. *Clin. Infect. Dis.* **46:**165–171.
19. **Craig, M. H., and B. L. Sharp.** 1997. Comparative evaluation of four techniques for the diagnosis of *Plasmodium falciparum* infections. *Trans. R. Soc. Trop. Med. Hyg.* **91:**279–282.
20. **Deen, J. L., L. von Seidlein, and A. Dondorp.** 2008. Therapy of uncomplicated malaria in children: a review of treatment principles, essential drugs and current recommendations. *Trop. Med. Int. Health* **13:**1111–1130.
21. **Doolan, D. L., and S. L. Hoffman.** 2000. The complexity of protective immunity against liver-stage malaria. *J. Immunol.* **165:**1453–1462.
22. **Earle, W. S., and M. Perez.** 1932. Enumeration of parasites in the blood of malarial patients. *J. Lab. Clin. Med.* **17:**1124.
23. **El Sayed, B., S. E. El Zaki, H. Babiker, N. Gadalla, T. Ageep, F. Mansour, O. Baraka, P. Milligan, and A. Babiker.** 2007. A randomized open-label trial of artesunate-sulfadoxine-pyrimethamine with or without primaquine for elimination of sub-microscopic P. falciparum parasitaemia and gametocyte carriage in eastern Sudan. *PLoS One* **2:**e1311.
24. **Erdman, L. K., and K. C. Kain.** 2008. Molecular diagnostic and surveillance tools for global malaria control. *Travel Med. Infect. Dis.* **6:**82–99.
25. **Farcas, G. A., K. J. Zhong, F. E. Lovegrove, C. M. Graham, and K. C. Kain.** 2003. Evaluation of the Binax NOW ICT test versus polymerase chain reaction and microscopy for the detection of malaria in returned travelers. *Am. J. Trop. Med. Hyg.* **69:**589–592.
26. **Farcas, G. A., K. J. Zhong, T. Mazzulli, and K. C. Kain.** 2004. Evaluation of the RealArt malaria LC real-time PCR assay for malaria diagnosis. *J. Clin. Microbiol.* **42:**636–638.
27. **Fast, N. M., J. C. Kissinger, D. S. Roos, and P. J. Keeling.** 2001. Nuclear-encoded, plastid-targeted genes suggest a single common origin for apicomplexan and dinoflagellate plastids. *Mol. Biol. Evol.* **18:**418–426.
28. **Foth, B. J., and G. I. McFadden.** 2003. The apicoplast: a plastid in Plasmodium falciparum and other Apicomplexan parasites. *Int. Rev. Cytol.* **224:**57–110.
29. **Franzen, L., G. Westin, R. Shabo, L. Aslund, H. Perlmann, T. Persson, H. Wigzell, and U. Pettersson.** 1984. Analysis of clinical specimens by hybridisation with probe containing repetitive DNA from Plasmodium falciparum. A novel approach to malaria diagnosis. *Lancet* **i:**525–528.
30. **Freedman, D. O.** 2008. Clinical practice. Malaria prevention in short-term travelers. *N. Engl. J. Med.* **359:**603–612.
31. **Fryauff, D. J., Purnomo, M. A. Sutamihardja, I. R. Elyazar, I. Susanti, Krisin, B. Subianto, and H. Marwoto.** 2000. Performance of the OptiMAL assay for detection and identification of malaria infections in asymptomatic residents of Irian Jaya, Indonesia. *Am. J. Trop. Med. Hyg.* **63:**139–145.
32. **Garcia, L. S.** 2001. *Diagnostic Medical Parasitology.* ASM Press, Washington, DC.
33. **Gardner, M. J., N. Hall, E. Fung, O. White, M. Berriman, R. W. Hyman, J. M. Carlton, A. Pain, K. E. Nelson, S. Bowman, I. T. Paulsen, K. James, J. A. Eisen, K. Rutherford, S. L. Salzberg, A. Craig, S. Kyes, M. S. Chan, V. Nene, S. J. Shallom, B. Suh, J. Peterson, S. Angiuoli, M. Pertea, J. Allen, J. Selengut, D. Haft, M. W. Mather, A. B. Vaidya, D. M. Martin, A. H. Fairlamb, M. J. Fraunholz, D. S. Roos, S. A. Ralph, G. I. McFadden, L. M. Cummings, G. M. Subramanian, C. Mungall, J. C. Venter, D. J. Carucci,**

S. L. Hoffman, C. Newbold, R. W. Davis, C. M. Fraser, and B. Barrell. 2002. Genome sequence of the human malaria parasite Plasmodium falciparum. *Nature* **419**:498–511.

34. Gay, F., B. Traore, J. Zanoni, M. Danis, and A. Fribourg-Blanc. 1996. Direct acridine orange fluorescence examination of blood slides compared to current techniques for malaria diagnosis. *Trans. R. Soc. Trop. Med. Hyg.* **90**:516–518.

35. Gelb, M. H. 2007. Drug discovery for malaria: a very challenging and timely endeavor. *Curr. Opin. Chem. Biol.* **11**:440–445.

36. Genton, B., and Z. H. Reed. 2007. Asexual blood-stage malaria vaccine development: facing the challenges. *Curr. Opin. Infect. Dis.* **20**:467–475.

37. Gorenflot, A., K. Moubri, E. Precigout, B. Carcy, and T. P. Schetters. 1998. Human babesiosis. *Ann. Trop. Med. Parasitol.* **92**:489–501.

38. Gray, J. S. 2006. Identity of the causal agents of human babesiosis in Europe. *Int. J. Med. Microbiol.* **296**(Suppl. 40):131–136.

39. Greenwood, B. M., A. K. Bradley, A. M. Greenwood, P. Byass, K. Jammeh, K. Marsh, S. Tulloch, F. S. J. Oldfield, and R. Hayes. 1987. Mortality and morbidity from malaria among children in a rural area of The Gambia, West Africa. *Trans. R. Soc. Trop. Med. Hyg.* **81**:478–486.

40. Griffith, K. S., L. S. Lewis, S. Mali, and M. E. Parise. 2007. Treatment of malaria in the United States: a systematic review. *JAMA* **297**:2264–2277.

41. Hall, N., M. Karras, J. D. Raine, J. M. Carlton, T. W. Kooij, M. Berriman, L. Florens, C. S. Janssen, A. Pain, G. K. Christophides, K. James, K. Rutherford, B. Harris, D. Harris, C. Churcher, M. A. Quail, D. Ormond, J. Doggett, H. E. Trueman, J. Mendoza, S. L. Bidwell, M. A. Rajandream, D. J. Carucci, J. R. Yates III, F. C. Kafatos, C. J. Janse, B. Barrell, C. M. Turner, A. P. Waters, and R. E. Sinden. 2005. A comprehensive survey of the Plasmodium life cycle by genomic, transcriptomic, and proteomic analyses. *Science* **307**:82–86.

42. Han, E. T., R. Watanabe, J. Sattabongkot, B. Khuntirat, J. Sirichaisinthop, H. Iriko, L. Jin, S. Takeo, and T. Tsuboi. 2007. Detection of four *Plasmodium* species by genus- and species-specific loop-mediated isothermal amplification for clinical diagnosis. *J. Clin. Microbiol.* **45**:2521–2528.

43. Hanscheid, T., E. Valadas, and M. P. Grobusch. 2000. Automated malaria diagnosis using pigment detection. *Parasitol. Today* **16**:549–551.

44. Herwaldt, B., D. H. Persing, E. A. Precigout, W. L. Goff, D. A. Mathiesen, P. W. Taylor, M. L. Eberhard, and A. F. Gorenflot. 1996. A fatal case of babesiosis in Missouri: identification of another piroplasm that infects humans. *Ann. Intern. Med.* **124**:643–650.

45. Herwaldt, B. L., S. Caccio, F. Gherlinzoni, H. Aspock, S. B. Slemenda, P. Piccaluga, G. Martinelli, R. Edelhofer, U. Hollenstein, G. Poletti, S. Pampiglione, K. Loschenberger, S. Tura, and N. J. Pieniazek. 2003. Molecular characterization of a non-Babesia divergens organism causing zoonotic babesiosis in Europe. *Emerg. Infect. Dis.* **9**:942–948.

46. Herwaldt, B. L., G. de Bruyn, N. J. Pieniazek, M. Homer, K. H. Lofy, S. B. Slemenda, T. R. Fritsche, D. H. Persing, and A. P. Limaye. 2004. Babesia divergens-like infection, Washington State. *Emerg. Infect. Dis.* **10**:622–629.

47. Homer, M. J., I. Aguilar-Delfin, S. R. Telford III, P. J. Krause, and D. H. Persing. 2000. Babesiosis. *Clin. Microbiol. Rev.* **13**:451–469.

48. Humar, A., C. Ohrt, M. A. Harrington, D. Pillai, and K. C. Kain. 1997. Parasight F test compared with the polymerase chain reaction and microscopy for the diagnosis of Plasmodium falciparum malaria in travelers. *Am. J. Trop. Med. Hyg.* **56**:44–48.

49. Hunfeld, K. P., A. Hildebrandt, and J. S. Gray. 2008. Babesiosis: recent insights into an ancient disease. *Int. J. Parasitol.* **38**:1219–1237.

50. Iqbal, J., P. R. Hira, A. Sher, and A. A. Al Enezi. 2001. Diagnosis of imported malaria by Plasmodium lactate dehydrogenase (pLDH) and histidine-rich protein 2 (PfHRP-2)-based immunocapture assays. *Am. J. Trop. Med. Hyg.* **64**:20–23.

51. Jamjoom, G. A. 1983. Dark-field microscopy for detection of malaria in unstained blood films. *J. Clin. Microbiol.* **17**:717–721.

52. Jomaa, H., J. Wiesner, S. Sanderbrand, B. Altincicek, C. Weidemeyer, M. Hintz, I. Turbachova, M. Eberl, J. Zeidler, H. K. Lichtenthaler, D. Soldati, and E. Beck. 1999. Inhibitors of the nonmevalonate pathway of isoprenoid biosynthesis as antimalarial drugs. *Science* **285**:1573–1576.

53. Keiser, J., J. Utzinger, Z. Premji, Y. Yamagata, and B. H. Singer. 2002. Acridine orange for malaria diagnosis: its diagnostic performance, its promotion and implementation in Tanzania, and the implications for malaria control. *Ann. Trop. Med. Parasitol.* **96**:643–654.

54. Krause, P. J., S. R. Telford III, A. Spielman, V. Sikand, R. Ryan, D. Christianson, G. Burke, P. Brassard, R. Pollack, J. Peck, and D. H. Persing. 1996. Concurrent Lyme disease and babesiosis. Evidence for increased severity and duration of illness. *JAMA* **275**:1657–1660.

54a. Krogstad, D. J., and M. A. Pfaller. 1983. Prophylaxis and treatment of malaria. *Curr. Clin. Top. Infect. Dis.* **3**:56–73.

55. Kyronseppa, H., E. Tiula, H. Repo, and J. Lahdevirta. 1989. Diagnosis of falciparum malaria delayed by long incubation period and misleading presenting symptoms: life-saving role of manual leucocyte differential count. *Scand. J. Infect. Dis.* **21**:117–118.

56. Layton, M., M. E. Parise, C. C. Campbell, R. Advani, J. D. Sexton, E. M. Bosler, and J. R. Zucker. 1995. Mosquito-transmitted malaria in New York City, 1993. *Lancet* **346**:729–731.

57. Lee, K. S., J. Cox-Singh, and B. Singh. 2009. Morphological features and differential counts of Plasmodium knowlesi parasites in naturally acquired human infections. *Malar. J.* **8**:73.

58. Lema, O. E., J. Y. Carter, N. Nagelkerke, M. W. Wangai, P. Kitenge, S. M. Gikunda, P. A. Arube, C. G. Munafu, S. F. Materu, C. A. Adhiambo, and H. K. Mukunza. 1999. Comparison of five methods of malaria detection in the outpatient setting. *Am. J. Trop. Med. Hyg.* **60**:177–182.

59. Levine, N. D. 1988. Progress in taxonomy of the Apicomplexan protozoa. *J. Protozool.* **35**:518–520.

60. Long, G. W., T. R. Jones, J. L. Rickman, R. Trimmer, and S. L. Hoffman. 1991. Acridine orange detection of Plasmodium falciparum malaria: relationship between sensitivity and optical configuration. *Am. J. Trop. Med. Hyg.* **44**:402–405.

61. Lowe, B. S., N. K. Jeffa, L. New, C. Pedersen, K. Engbaek, and K. Marsh. 1996. Acridine orange fluorescence techniques as alternatives to traditional Giemsa staining for the diagnosis of malaria in developing countries. *Trans. R. Soc. Trop. Med. Hyg.* **90**:34–36.

62. Luchavez, J., F. Espino, P. Curameng, R. Espina, D. Bell, P. Chiodini, D. Nolder, C. Sutherland, K. S. Lee, and B. Singh. 2008. Human infections with Plasmodium knowlesi, the Philippines. *Emerg. Infect. Dis.* **14**:811–813.

63. Maldonado, Y. A., B. L. Nahlen, R. R. Roberto, M. Ginsberg, E. Orellana, M. Mizrahi, K. McBarron, H. O. Lobel, and C. C. Campbell. 1990. Transmission of Plasmodium vivax malaria in San Diego County, California, 1986. *Am. J. Trop. Med. Hyg.* **42**:3–9.

64. Meer-Scherrer, L., M. Adelson, E. Mordechai, B. Lottaz, and R. Tilton. 2004. Babesia microti infection in Europe. *Curr. Microbiol.* **48**:435–437.

65. Mikolajczak, S. A., A. S. Aly, and S. H. Kappe. 2007. Preerythrocytic malaria vaccine development. *Curr. Opin. Infect. Dis.* **20**:461–466.

66. Mungai, M., G. Tegtmeier, M. Chamberland, and M. Parise. 2001. Transfusion-transmitted malaria in the United States from 1963 through 1999. *N. Engl. J. Med.* **344**:1973–1978.

67. Murray, C. K., R. A. Gasser, Jr., A. J. Magill, and R. S. Miller. 2008. Update on rapid diagnostic testing for malaria. *Clin. Microbiol. Rev.* **21**:97–110.

68. Myat-Phone-Kyaw, Myint-Oo, Myint-Lwin, Thaw-Zin, Kyin-Hla-Aye, and Nwe-Nwe-Yin. 1993. Emergence of chloroquine-resistant *Plasmodium vivax* in Myanmar (Burma). *Trans. R. Soc. Trop. Med. Hyg.* **87**:687.

69. Ng, O. T., E. E. Ooi, C. C. Lee, P. J. Lee, L. C. Ng, S. W. Pei, T. M. Tu, J. P. Loh, and Y. S. Leo. 2008. Naturally acquired human Plasmodium knowlesi infection, Singapore. *Emerg. Infect. Dis.* **14:**814–816.

70. Notomi, T., H. Okayama, H. Masubuchi, T. Yonekawa, K. Watanabe, N. Amino, and T. Hase. 2000. Loop-mediated isothermal amplification of DNA. *Nucleic Acids Res.* **28:**E63.

71. Ochola, L. B., P. Vounatsou, T. Smith, M. L. Mabaso, and C. R. Newton. 2006. The reliability of diagnostic techniques in the diagnosis and management of malaria in the absence of a gold standard. *Lancet Infect. Dis.* **6:**582–588.

72. Pain, A., U. Bohme, A. E. Berry, K. Mungall, R. D. Finn, A. P. Jackson, T. Mourier, J. Mistry, E. M. Pasini, M. A. Aslett, S. Balasubramaniam, K. Borgwardt, K. Brooks, C. Carret, T. J. Carver, I. Cherevach, T. Chillingworth, T. G. Clark, M. R. Galinski, N. Hall, D. Harper, D. Harris, H. Hauser, A. Ivens, C. S. Janssen, T. Keane, N. Larke, S. Lapp, M. Marti, S. Moule, I. M. Meyer, D. Ormond, N. Peters, M. Sanders, S. Sanders, T. J. Sargeant, M. Simmonds, F. Smith, R. Squares, S. Thurston, A. R. Tivey, D. Walker, B. White, E. Zuiderwijk, C. Churcher, M. A. Quail, A. F. Cowman, C. M. Turner, M. A. Rajandream, C. H. Kocken, A. W. Thomas, C. I. Newbold, B. G. Barrell, and M. Berriman. 2008. The genome of the simian and human malaria parasite Plasmodium knowlesi. *Nature* **455:**799–803.

73. Palmer, C. J., L. Validum, J. Lindo, A. Campa, C. Validum, M. Makler, R. R. Cuadrado, and A. Ager. 1999. Field evaluation of the OptiMAL rapid malaria diagnostic test during anti-malarial therapy in Guyana. *Trans. R. Soc. Trop. Med. Hyg.* **93:**517–518.

74. Perkins, M. D., and D. R. Bell. 2008. Working without a blindfold: the critical role of diagnostics in malaria control. *Malar. J.* **7**(Suppl. 1)**:**S5.

75. Persing, D. H., B. L. Herwaldt, C. Glaser, R. S. Lane, J. W. Thomford, D. Mathiesen, P. J. Krause, D. F. Phillip, and P. A. Conrad. 1995. Infection with a Babesia-like organism in northern California. *N. Engl. J. Med.* **332:**298–303.

76. Persing, D. H., D. Mathiesen, W. F. Marshall, S. R. Telford, A. Spielman, J. W. Thomford, and P. A. Conrad. 1992. Detection of Babesia microti by polymerase chain reaction. *J. Clin. Microbiol.* **30:**2097–2103.

77. Phillips, E. J., J. S. Keystone, and K. C. Kain. 1996. Failure of combined chloroquine and high-dose primaquine therapy for Plasmodium vivax malaria acquired in Guyana, South America. *Clin. Infect. Dis.* **23:**1171–1173.

78. Piper, R., J. Lebras, L. Wentworth, A. Hunt-Cooke, S. Houze, P. Chiodini, and M. Makler. 1999. Immunocapture diagnostic assays for malaria using Plasmodium lactate dehydrogenase (pLDH). *Am. J. Trop. Med. Hyg.* **60:**109–118.

79. Putaporntip, C., T. Hongsrimuang, S. Seethamchai, T. Kobasa, K. Limkittikul, L. Cui, and S. Jongwutiwes. 2009. Differential prevalence of Plasmodium infections and cryptic Plasmodium knowlesi malaria in humans in Thailand. *J. Infect. Dis.* **199:**1143–1150.

80. Quick, R. E., B. L. Herwaldt, J. W. Thomford, M. E. Garnett, M. L. Eberhard, M. Wilson, D. H. Spach, J. W. Dickerson, S. R. Telford III, K. R. Steingart, R. Pollock, D. H. Persing, J. M. Kobayashi, D. D. Juranek, and P. A. Conrad. 1993. Babesiosis in Washington State: a new species of Babesia? *Ann. Intern. Med.* **119:**284–290.

81. Rickman, L. S., G. W. Long, R. Oberst, A. Cabanban, R. Sangalang, J. I. Smith, J. D. Chulay, and S. L. Hoffman. 1989. Rapid diagnosis of malaria by acridine orange staining of centrifuged parasites. *Lancet* **i:**68–71.

82. Rieckmann, K. H., G. H. Campbell, L. J. Sax, and J. Mrema. 1978. Drug sensitivity of Plasmodium falciparum: an in vitro microtechnique. *Lancet* **i:**22–23.

83. Rogers, W. O., F. Atuguba, A. R. Oduro, A. Hodgson, and K. A. Koram. 2006. Clinical case definitions and malaria vaccine efficacy. *J. Infect. Dis.* **193:**467–473.

84. Rogers, W. O., R. Sem, T. Thong, C. Phektra, P. Lim, S. Muth, S. Duong, F. Ariey, and C. Wongsrichanalai. 2009. Failure of artesunate-mefloquine combination therapy for uncomplicated P. falciparum malaria in southern Cambodia. *Malar. J.* **8:**10–18.

85. Sabchareon, A., T. Burnouf, D. Ouattara, P. Attanah, H. Bouharoun-Tayooun, P. Chantavanich, C. Foucault, T. Chongsuphajaisiddhi, and P. Druilhe. 1991. Parasitologic and clinical human response to immunoglobulin administration in Falciparum malaria. *Am. J. Trop. Med. Hyg.* **45:**297–308.

86. Sahu, N. K., S. Sahu, and D. V. Kohli. 2008. Novel molecular targets for antimalarial drug development. *Chem. Biol. Drug Des.* **71:**287–297.

87. Schneider, P., J. T. Bousema, L. C. Gouagna, S. Otieno, M. van de Vegte-Bolmer, S. A. Omar, and R. W. Sauerwein. 2007. Submicroscopic Plasmodium falciparum gametocyte densities frequently result in mosquito infection. *Am. J. Trop. Med. Hyg.* **76:**470–474.

88. Schuurkamp, G. J., P. E. Spicer, R. K. Kereu, P. K. Bulungol, and K. H. Rieckmann. 1992. Chloroquine-resistant Plasmodium vivax in Papua New Guinea. *Trans. R. Soc. Trop. Med. Hyg.* **86:**121–122.

89. Shiff, C. J., Z. Premji, and J. N. Minjas. 1993. The rapid manual ParaSight-F test. A new diagnostic tool for Plasmodium falciparum infection. *Trans. R. Soc. Trop. Med. Hyg.* **87:**646–648.

90. Snounou, G. 1996. Detection and identification of the four malaria parasite species infecting humans by PCR amplification. *Methods Mol. Biol.* **50:**263–291.

91. Snow, R. W., C. A. Guerra, A. M. Noor, H. Y. Myint, and S. I. Hay. 2005. The global distribution of clinical episodes of Plasmodium falciparum malaria. *Nature* **434:**214–217.

92. Spielman, A., J. B. Perrone, A. Teklehaimanot, F. Balcha, S. C. Wardlaw, and R. A. Levine. 1988. Malaria diagnosis by direct observation of centrifuged samples of blood. *Am. J. Trop. Med. Hyg.* **39:**337–342.

93. Steenkeste, N., S. Incardona, S. Chy, L. Duval, M. T. Ekala, P. Lim, S. Hewitt, T. Sochantha, D. Socheat, C. Rogier, O. Mercereau-Puijalon, T. Fandeur, and F. Ariey. 2009. Towards high-throughput molecular detection of Plasmodium: new approaches and molecular markers. *Malar. J.* **8:**86.

94. Sulzer, A. J., and M. Wilson. 1971. The indirect fluorescent antibody test for the detection of occult malaria in blood donors. *Bull. W. H. O.* **45:**375–379.

95. Sunstrum, J., L. J. Elliott, L. M. Barat, E. D. Walker, and J. R. Zucker. 2001. Probable autochthonous Plasmodium vivax malaria transmission in Michigan: case report and epidemiological investigation. *Am. J. Trop. Med. Hyg.* **65:**949–953.

96. Tham, J. M., S. H. Lee, T. M. Tan, R. C. Ting, and U. A. Kara. 1999. Detection and species determination of malaria parasites by PCR: comparison with microscopy and with ParaSight-F and ICT malaria Pf tests in a clinical environment. *J. Clin. Microbiol.* **37:**1269–1273.

97. Thepsamarn, P., N. Prayoollawongsa, P. Puksupa, P. Puttoom, P. Thaidumrong, S. Wongchai, J. Doddara, J. Tantayarak, K. Buchachart, P. Wilairatana, and S. Looareesuwan. 1997. The ICT Malaria Pf: a simple, rapid dipstick test for the diagnosis of Plasmodium falciparum malaria at the Thai-Myanmar border. *Southeast Asian J. Trop. Med. Public Health* **28:**723–726.

98. Tjitra, E., S. Suprianto, M. Dyer, B. J. Currie, and N. M. Anstey. 1999. Field evaluation of the ICT malaria P.f/P.v immunochromatographic test for detection of Plasmodium falciparum and Plasmodium vivax in patients with a presumptive clinical diagnosis of malaria in eastern Indonesia. *J. Clin. Microbiol.* **37:**2412–2417.

99. van den Broek, I., O. Hill, F. Gordillo, B. Angarita, P. Hamade, H. Counihan, and J. P. Guthmann. 2006. Evaluation of three rapid tests for diagnosis of P. falciparum and P. vivax malaria in Colombia. *Am. J. Trop. Med. Hyg.* **75:**1209–1215.

100. Van Vianen, P. H., A. van Engen, S. Thaithong, M. van der Keur, H. J. Tanke, H. J. Van der Kaay, B. Mons, and C. J. Janse. 1993. Flow cytometric screening of blood samples for malaria parasites. *Cytometry* **14:**276–280.

101. Vekemans, J., and W. R. Ballou. 2008. Plasmodium falciparum malaria vaccines in development. *Expert Rev. Vaccines* **7:**223–240.

102. **Waller, R. F., and G. I. McFadden.** 2005. The apicoplast: a review of the derived plastid of apicomplexan parasites. *Curr. Issues Mol. Biol.* **7:**57–79.

103. **Warhurst, D. C., F. M. Awad el Kariem, and M. A. Miles.** 1991. Simplified preparation of malarial blood samples for polymerase chain reaction. *Lancet* **337:**303–304.

104. **Wei, Q., M. Tsuji, A. Zamoto, M. Kohsaki, T. Matsui, T. Shiota, S. R. Telford III, and C. Ishihara.** 2001. Human babesiosis in Japan: isolation of *Babesia microti*-like parasites from an asymptomatic transfusion donor and from a rodent from an area where babesiosis is endemic. *J. Clin. Microbiol.* **39:**2178–2183.

105. **Wolday, D., F. Balcha, G. Fessehaye, Y. Birku, and A. Shepherd.** 2001. Field trial of the RTM dipstick method for the rapid diagnosis of malaria based on the detection of *Plasmodium falciparum* HRP-2 antigen in whole blood. *Trop. Doct.* **31:**19–21.

106. **Wongsrichanalai, C., I. Arevalo, A. Laoboonchai, K. Yingyuen, R. S. Miller, A. J. Magill, J. R. Forney, and R. A. Gasser, Jr.** 2003. Rapid diagnostic devices for malaria: field evaluation of a new prototype immunochromatographic assay for the detection of Plasmodium falciparum and non-falciparum Plasmodium. *Am. J. Trop. Med. Hyg.* **69:**26–30.

107. **World Health Organization.** 1990. Severe and complicated malaria. *Trans. R. Soc. Trop. Med. Hyg.* **84**(Suppl. 2)**:**1–65.

108. **World Health Organization.** 1994. World malaria situation in 1992. *Wkly. Epidemiol. Rec.* **69:**309–314.

Leishmania and *Trypanosoma*

DAVID A. BRUCKNER AND JAIME A. LABARCA

134

Leishmania spp. and *Trypanosoma* spp. are protozoa belonging to the family *Trypanosomatidae*. Leishmaniasis is principally a zoonosis, and the organisms are obligate intracellular parasites transmitted to humans by bites from an infected female sand fly. For *Leishmania* in the Old World, there is only one subgenus, *Leishmania*; however, in the New World, the genus has been split into subgenera (*Leishmania* and *Viannia*) according to the development of the organism in the digestive tract (peripylarian or suprapylarian) of the sand fly (38). Depending on the geographic area, many different species can infect humans, producing a variety of diseases (cutaneous, diffuse cutaneous, mucocutaneous, and visceral diseases) (Table 1). The spectrum of clinical presentation is dependent on the host's cell-mediated immune response (89).

Trypanosoma spp. are hemoflagellate protozoa that live in the blood and tissue of the human host. American trypanosomiasis (Chagas' disease) is produced by *Trypanosoma cruzi*, which belongs to the subgenus *Schizotrypanum* and is confined to the American continent. *Trypanosoma rangeli* produces an asymptomatic infection and is also present only on the American continent. African trypanosomiasis (sleeping sickness) is caused by *T. brucei gambiense* and *T. brucei rhodesiense* belonging to the subgenus *Trypanozoon* and is confined to the central belt of Africa. African trypanosomes and *T. rangeli* are transmitted directly into the bite wound by salivary secretions from the insect vector, whereas *T. cruzi* is transmitted through contamination of the bite wound with the feces from the reduviid bug (Table 2). The first documented case of human trypanosomiasis caused by *T. evansi* was detected in India (103).

LEISHMANIA SPP.

Recent estimates suggest that there are approximately 350 million people at risk of acquiring leishmaniasis, with 112 million currently infected. More than 400,000 new cases are reported annually (41). New species of *Leishmania*, particularly in the New World, are being detected frequently. The taxonomy of leishmaniasis is controversial and in a state of dynamic flux. Species differentiation is currently based on molecular techniques rather than geographical distribution and clinical presentation (23, 31, 64).

Life Cycle and Morphology

The parasite has two distinct phases in its life cycle (amastigote and promastigote) (Fig. 1). The amastigote stage (Leishman-Donovan body) is found in reticuloendothelial cells of the mammalian host. The amastigote form is small, is round or oval, measures 3 to 5 μm, and contains a large nucleus and small kinetoplast (Fig. 1 and 2). This stage undergoes multiplication within the reticuloendothelial cells of the host.

Upon ingestion during a blood meal by the insect vector (sand fly), the amastigote transforms into the promastigote stage (Fig. 3). Promastigotes multiply in the gut of the insect, transform to metacyclic promastigotes, and migrate to the hypostome of the sand fly, where they are released when the next blood meal is taken. The complete life cycle in the sand fly is 4 to 18 days. Upon inoculation into the bite site, the promastigote changes to the amastigote form after being engulfed by tissue macrophages. This form change helps to defeat the host's immune response. Changes in the parasite's surface molecules play an important role in macrophage attachment and evading the host's immune response, including manipulating the macrophage's signaling pathways (75, 89, 102).

The life cycles of *Leishmania* organisms are similar for cutaneous, mucocutaneous, and visceral leishmaniasis, except that infected reticuloendothelial cells can be found throughout the body in visceral leishmaniasis.

Epidemiology and Transmission

All adult female sand flies transmitting leishmaniasis belong to the genus *Phlebotomus* in the Old World and *Lutzomyia* in the New World. There are >30 species of sand flies that can transmit leishmaniasis. The disease is considered primarily a zoonosis, with natural reservoirs including rodents, opossums, anteaters, sloths, and dogs. In certain areas of the world where the disease is endemic, the infection can be transmitted by a human-vector-human cycle. The infection may also be transmitted by direct contact with an infected lesion or mechanically through bites by stable or dog flies. Greater than 90% of cutaneous leishmaniasis cases occur in Afghanistan, Algeria, Brazil, Iran, Iraq, Peru, Saudi Arabia, and Syria. There has been an increase in the number of cases among military personnel deployed in Afghanistan, Iraq, and Kuwait (24). Autochthonous human infections

TABLE 1 Features of human leishmanial infections

Species	Disease type[a]	Recommended specimen(s)	Geographic distribution
L. (L.) donovani	VL	Bone marrow, spleen	Africa and Asia
	MCL, CL, DL	Skin or mucosal macrophage	
L. (L.) infantum[b]	VL	Bone marrow, spleen	Africa, Europe, Mediterranean area, Southeast Asia, Central and South America
L. (L.) killicki	CL	Skin macrophage	Algeria, Tunisia
L. (L.) tropica	CL	Skin macrophage	Afghanistan, India, Turkey, former USSR
L. (L.) major	CL	Skin macrophage	Afghanistan, Africa, Middle East, former USSR
L. (L.) aethiopica	CL, DCL, MCL	Skin or mucosal macrophage	Ethiopia, Kenya, former USSR, Yemen
L. (L.) mexicana	CL, DCL, MCL	Skin macrophage	Belize, Guatemala, Mexico, Texas
L. (V.) braziliensis	CL, MCL	Skin or mucosal macrophage	Central and South America
L. (V.) peruviana	CL	Skin macrophage	Colombia, Costa Rica, Panama
L. (L.) garnhami	CL	Skin macrophage	Venezuela
L. (V.) colombiensis	CL	Skin macrophage	Colombia, Panama
L. (V.) panamensis	CL	Skin macrophage	Colombia, Costa Rica, Panama
L. (V.) guyanesis	CL, MCL	Skin or mucosal macrophage	Brazil, Columbia, French Guiana, Peru
L. (V.) venezuelensis	CL	Skin macrophage	Venezuela
L. (V.) lainsoni	CL	Skin macrophage	Brazil
L. (V.) shawii	CL	Skin macrophage	Brazil
L. (L.) amazonensis	CL, DCL	Skin or mucosal macrophage	Brazil, Venezuela
L. (V.) naffi	CL	Skin macrophage	Brazil, Caribbean Islands
L. (L.) pifanoi	CL, DCL	Skin or mucosal macrophage	Brazil, Venezuela

[a]CL, cutaneous leishmaniasis; DCL, diffuse cutaneous leishmaniasis; DL, diffuse leishmaniasis; MCL, mucocutaneous leishmaniasis; VL, visceral leishmaniasis.
[b]L. (L.) infantum in the Old World = L. (L.) chagasi in the New World.

have been described in Texas (104). Most of the diagnosed cases of mucocutaneous leishmaniasis are from Bolivia, Brazil, and Peru.

Visceral leishmaniasis may exist as an endemic, epidemic, and sporadic disease. The disease is a zoonosis except in India, where kala-azar is an anthroponosis. Natural reservoirs are wild Canidae and various rodents for *L. donovani*; dogs, other Canidae, and rats for *L. infantum*; and Canidae and cats for *L. infantum* (*L. chagasi*) in the Americas. Individuals with post-kala-azar dermal leishmaniasis may be very important reservoirs for maintaining the infection during interendemic cycles. More than 90% of the cases of visceral leishmaniasis are found in Bangladesh, Brazil, India, Nepal, and Sudan.

Clinical Significance

Depending on the species involved, infection with *Leishmania* spp. can result in cutaneous, diffuse cutaneous, mucocutaneous, or visceral disease (Table 1) (61). A large number of disease variations have been described, which makes classical

disease categories confusing (23). In areas of endemicity, *Leishmania* coinfection with human immunodeficiency virus (HIV)-positive patients is common. If coinfected patients remain severely immunocompromised, approximately one-quarter will die within the first month of being diagnosed with leishmaniasis. The leishmanial infection will manifest itself like an opportunistic infection, and parasites will be detected in atypical sites (50). The use of highly active antiretroviral therapy has significantly improved the prognosis of patients infected with HIV and visceral leishmaniasis (96).

The first sign of cutaneous disease is the appearance of a firm, painless papule at or near the insect bite site. The incubation period may be as short as 2 weeks (*L. major*) or as long as several months to 3 years (*L. tropica* and *L. aethiopica*). Papules may be intensely pruritic and will grow to 2 cm or more in diameter. Lesions may progress from a simple papule or erythematous macule to a nodule and ulcerate within days to weeks. In simple cutaneous leishmaniasis, the infection remains localized at the insect bite site where a definite self-limiting granulomatous response

TABLE 2 Characteristics of trypanosomiasis

Characteristic	*T. brucei rhodesiense*	*T. brucei gambiense*	*T. cruzi*	*T. rangeli*
Vector	Tsetse fly (*Glossina*)	Tsetse fly (*Glossina*)	Reduviid bug (*Panstrongylus, Rhodnius, Triatoma*)	Reduviid bug (*Rhodnius*)
Primary reservoir	Animals	Humans	Animals	Animals
Illness	Acute, <9 mo	Chronic, months to years	Acute, chronic	Asymptomatic
Epidemiology	Anthropozoonosis[a]	Anthroponosis[b]	Anthropozoonosis	Anthropozoonosis
Diagnostic stage	Trypomastigote	Trypomastigote	Trypomastigote, amastigote	Trypomastigote
Recommended specimen(s)	Blood, CSF, chancre, and lymph node aspirate	Blood, CSF, chancre, and lymph node aspirate	Blood, chagoma, and lymph node aspirate	Blood

[a]Anthropozoonosis: transmission involving human-animal-human cycle.
[b]Anthroponosis: transmission involving a human-human cycle.

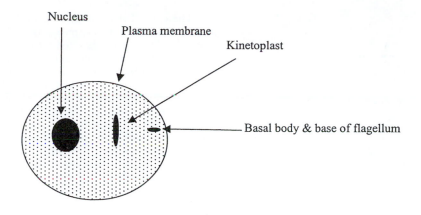

Amastigote

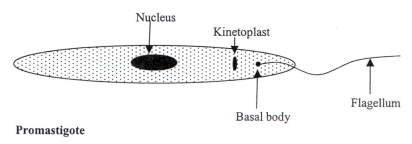

Promastigote

FIGURE 1 Life cycle stages of *Leishmania* spp.

develops. Lesions have been mistaken for basal cell carcinoma, tropical pyoderma, sporotrichosis, or cutaneous mycobacterial infections.

Mucocutaneous leishmaniasis is produced most often by the *L. braziliensis* complex. The primary lesions are similar to those found in other infections of cutaneous leishmaniasis. Untreated primary lesions may develop into the mucocutaneous form in up to 80% of the cases. Metastatic spread to the nasal or oral mucosa may occur in the presence of the active primary lesion or many years later after the primary lesion has healed. Mucosal lesions do not heal spontaneously, and secondary bacterial infections are frequent and may be fatal. A small number of mucocutaneous leishmaniasis cases have been reported with *L. donovani* and *L. aethiopica*. Differential diagnosis has included lymphoma, midline granuloma, Wegener's granulomatosis, paracoccidioidomycosis, histoplasmosis, cutaneous mycobacterial infection, syphilis, and leprosy.

Clinical features of the visceral disease vary from asymptomatic, self-resolving infections to frank visceral leishmaniasis. The incubation period may be as short as 10 days and as long as 2 years; usually it is within 2 to 4 months. Common symptoms include fever, anorexia, malaise, weight loss, and frequently, diarrhea. Individuals coinfected with HIV may not elicit common symptoms seen in immunocompetent individuals, whereas the leukopenia is unusually severe (50). Common clinical signs include nontender hepatomegaly and splenomegaly, lymphadenopathy, and occasional acute abdominal pain; darkening of facial, hand, foot, and abdominal skin (kala-azar) is often seen in light-skinned persons in India. Anemia, cachexia, and

marked enlargement of liver and spleen are noted as the disease progresses. Death may ensue after a few weeks or after 2 to 3 years in chronic cases. The majority of infected individuals are asymptomatic or have very few or minor symptoms that resolve without therapy. There has been a significant increase in leishmaniasis in organ transplant recipients since 1990. Most of the reported cases in organ transplant recipients have been visceral leishmaniasis, with a much smaller number of mucocutaneous leishmaniasis cases and, rarely, cutaneous leishmaniasis cases (3, 74). Differential diagnosis in the acute stage includes amebic liver abscess, Chagas' disease, malaria, typhoid, typhus, and schistosomiasis. Subacute or chronic disease has been confused with malnutrition, bacteremia, brucellosis, histoplasmosis, leukemia, lymphoma, malaria, mononucleosis, and schistosomiasis.

Postdermal leishmaniasis or post-kala-azar dermal leishmaniasis is a condition seen in India and the Sudan in some patients unsuccessfully treated for visceral leishmaniasis. This syndrome is rarely seen in Latin America but has been reported to occur in patients coinfected with HIV. The macular or hypopigmented dermal lesions are associated with few parasites, whereas erythematous and nodular lesions are associated with abundant parasites. This condition must be differentiated from leprosy, syphilis, and yaws.

Diagnosis

In areas where the disease is endemic, the diagnosis may be made on clinical grounds. Prolonged fever, progressive weight loss, anemia, leukopenia, hypergammaglobulinemia, and pronounced hepatomegaly and splenomegaly are highly

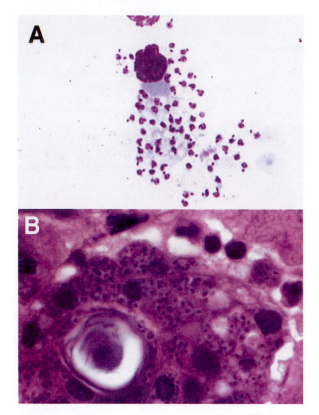

FIGURE 2 (A) *Leishmania donovani* amastigotes from splenic press preparation (Giemsa stain); (B) *Leishmania donovani* amastigotes in liver (hematoxylin and eosin stain).

suggestive of visceral leishmaniasis. The development of one or more chronic skin lesions with a history of exposure in an area of endemicity is suggestive of cutaneous leishmaniasis. In many areas of the world where the disease is endemic, laboratory testing (microscopy, culture, PCR, antigen tests, and serology) is almost impossible to obtain. Definitive diagnosis depends on detecting either the amastigotes in clinical specimens or the promastigotes in culture.

Collection of Specimens

All cutaneous lesions should be thoroughly cleaned with 70% alcohol, and extraneous debris, the eschar and exudates, should be removed. After debridement, with precautions being taken to prevent bleeding, the base of the ulcer can be scraped with a scalpel blade to obtain an exudate for slide preparation, culture, or PCR. Specimens can be collected from the margin of the lesion by aspiration, scraping, or punch biopsy or by making a slit with a scalpel blade. Material scraped from the wall of the slit should be smeared onto a number of slides. PCR-based methods for the diagnosis of leishmaniasis have used a variety of specimens, including urine. PCR has been shown to be more sensitive than direct microscopy, histology, and culture, but availability is limited mainly to large hospitals or clinics. The PCR-based methods have not been standardized, and multicentered studies to validate these tests have not been done (47, 63, 68, 81). Laboratorians may want to contact their state public health laboratory or the Centers for Disease Control and Prevention (CDC) for diagnostic information and help in specimen selection and available tests.

The core of tissue from a punch biopsy can be used to make imprints or touch preparations on a slide. A tissue core should also be submitted for histological examination. Recognition of amastigotes in tissues is more difficult than in smears or imprints because the organisms tend to be crowded within the cells, appear smaller, and are cut at various angles. Fine-needle aspiration can also be performed by using a sterile syringe containing sterile preservative-free buffered saline (0.1 ml) and a 26-gauge needle. The needle is inserted under the outer border of the lesion, the needle is rotated several times, and tissue fluid is aspirated into the needle. Tissue obtained by splenic puncture yields the highest rate of positive specimens; however, this procedure carries significant risk to patients, particularly those with coagulation disorders. Other specimens for the detection of visceral leishmaniasis include lymph node aspirates, liver biopsy specimens, sternal aspirates, iliac crest bone marrow specimens, and buffy coat preparations of venous blood. Amastigotes with reticuloendothelial cells have been detected in bronchoalveolar lavage fluid, pleural effusions, and biopsy specimens collected from the gastrointestinal tract and oropharynx of HIV-positive patients (50). Individuals with post-kala-azar dermal leishmaniasis have large numbers of parasites in the skin, particularly those with erythematous and nodular lesions (51).

Direct Examination

Microscopic and PCR Detection

Amastigote stages are found within macrophages or close to disrupted cells (Fig. 2). This stage can be recognized by its shape, size, staining characteristics, and especially, the presence of an intracytoplasmic kinetoplast. The cytoplasm stains light blue, and the nucleus and kinetoplast stain red or purple with Giemsa stain. Amastigotes can be differentiated from fungal organisms because they do not stain positive with periodic acid-Schiff, mucicarmine, or silver stain. Molecular techniques (none are FDA approved) for the detection of leishmanial DNA or RNA have been used for diagnosis, prognosis, and species identification. These methods are considered more sensitive than slide examination or culture, particularly for the detection of mucocutaneous leishmaniasis (4, 38, 41, 43, 45, 62, 73, 77, 82, 92, 99, 105). Generally, organisms in mucocutaneous lesions are scant and difficult to detect microscopically. Because infections caused by *Leishmania* subgenus *Viannia* are considered more aggressive and are more likely to result in treatment failure, molecular techniques to identify the organism to the species level can be very important (6, 49, 52, 100).

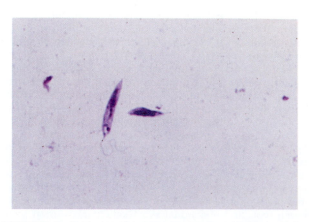

FIGURE 3 *Leishmania donovani* promastigotes (Giemsa stain).

Culture

If material is to be cultured, it must be collected aseptically. Tissues should be minced prior to culture. Culture media successfully employed to recover organisms include Novy, MacNeal, and Nicolle's medium (NNN) and Schneider's *Drosophila* medium supplemented with 30% fetal bovine serum. Cultures, incubated at 25°C, should be examined twice weekly for the first 2 weeks and once a week thereafter for up to 4 weeks before the culture is declared negative. Promastigote stages can be detected microscopically in wet mounts and then stained with Giemsa stain to observe their morphology.

Animal Inoculation and Culture

Animals such as the golden hamster can be inoculated with patient material. Animals are inoculated intranasally for cutaneous and mucocutaneous leishmaniasis and intraperitoneally for visceral leishmaniasis. It may take 2 to 3 months before an animal becomes positive. A combination of tissue smears, culture, and animal inoculation may be needed to optimize the laboratory diagnosis of the infection. PCR testing, if available, can be used as a supplemental diagnostic procedure (82, 85).

Skin Testing

The leishmanin (Montenegro) test (not available in Canada or the United States), a delayed-type hypersensitivity reaction, is useful for epidemiological surveys of a population to identify groups at risk of infection. Positive reactions are usually seen in cutaneous and mucocutaneous leishmaniasis; however, patients with active visceral and diffuse cutaneous leishmaniasis exhibit negative reactions. Post-kala-azar patients may also exhibit a negative reaction. This test is of no value for the diagnosis of visceral leishmaniasis.

Serologic Tests

Serologic tests (none are FDA approved) are available for research or epidemiologic purposes; however, they are not very useful for the diagnosis of mucocutaneous and visceral leishmaniasis. In kala-azar, there is a large increase in gamma globulins, both immunoglobulin G (IgG) and IgM. This is the basis for the aldehyde or formol-gel test, which has been used as a screening test in areas of endemicity (70). The addition of 1 drop of formalin to 1 ml of serum promotes the precipitation of immunoglobulins. A number of serologies including indirect fluorescent antibody (IFA), enzyme linked immunoassay (ELISA), and immunoblot tests have been developed for diagnostic purposes; however, they are not widely available except in areas of endemicity (13, 17, 84). An ELISA, dipstick test, and rapid immunochromatographic strip using *L. infantum/L chagasi* recombinant k39 antigen has good sensitivity and specificity in diagnosing visceral leishmaniasis in immunocompetent people (16, 95, 101). Visceral leishmaniasis patients coinfected with HIV may have no detectable antileishmania antibodies (15, 50, 54). Serologic testing is available at some referral laboratories and the CDC. The detection of urinary antigens has been used for the diagnosis of visceral leishmaniasis (7).

Treatment and Prevention

Lesions in simple cutaneous leishmaniasis generally heal spontaneously. Treatment options have included cryotherapy, heat, photodynamic therapy, surgical excision of lesions, and chemotherapy (98). Treatment is advocated to reduce scarring in cosmetic areas and to prevent dissemination and/or relapse of the infection. Although the optimal treatment for cutaneous leishmaniasis is unknown, standard therapy consists of injections of antimonial compounds. Response to therapy varies depending on the species of *Leishmania* and the type of disease (91, 97); therefore, it is important to identify the species of *Leishmania* causing the infection (78, 88, 105). The risk of relapse is quite high within the first 6 to 12 months posttherapy (57, 69). Patients clinically cured of *L. (V.) braziliensis* infection, which is noted for its chronicity, latency, and metastasis with mucosal membrane involvement, have been found to be PCR positive up to 11 years posttherapy (65). To ensure that treatment has been effective, follow-up smears and cultures should be done 1 to 2 weeks posttherapy. PCR testing has been used to monitor the progress of therapy (65, 80).

In areas where leishmaniasis is endemic, vaccination is still a major goal for eliminating leishmaniasis. Inoculating the serous exudate from naturally acquired lesions of cutaneous leishmaniasis into an inconspicuous area of the body of a nonimmune person has been effective; however, vaccines against other forms of leishmaniasis have not worked. Other possible prevention methods include spraying dwellings with insecticides, applying insect repellents to the skin, and use of fine-mesh bed netting. Reservoir control has been unsuccessful in most areas, although in areas where canines may be a reservoir host, pyrethroid-impregnated collars are being used to prevent infections. Individuals with lesions should be warned to protect the lesion from insect bites, and patients should be educated about the possibility of autoinoculation or infection.

AMERICAN TRYPANOSOMIASIS

■ *Trypanosoma cruzi*

American trypanosomiasis (Chagas' disease) is a zoonosis caused by *Trypanosoma cruzi*. There are 100 million persons at risk of infection in 18 Latin American countries, and 16 to 18 million persons are actually infected (50). Patients can present with either acute or chronic disease. Chagas' disease was considered a disease of rural areas; however, it is now ubiquitous due to social pattern changes of rural to urban migration. A very serious problem is disease acquisition through blood transfusion and organ transplantation (56, 63). A large number of patients with positive serology can remain asymptomatic (30).

Life Cycle and Morphology

Trypomastigotes (Fig. 4 and 5) are ingested by the reduviid bug (triatomids, kissing bugs, or conenose bugs) as it obtains a blood meal. The trypomastigotes transform into epimastigotes (Fig. 4 and 6) that multiply in the posterior portion of the midgut. After 8 to 10 days, metacyclic trypomastigotes develop from the epimastigotes. These metacyclic trypomastigotes are passed in the feces.

Humans contract Chagas' disease when the reduviid bug defecates while taking a blood meal and metacyclic trypomastigotes in the feces are rubbed or scratched into the bite wound or onto mucosal surfaces. In humans, *T. cruzi* can be found in two forms, as amastigotes and trypomastigotes (Fig. 4, 6, and 7). The trypomastigote form is present in the blood and infects the host cells. The amastigote form multiplies within the cell, eventually destroying the cell, and both amastigotes and trypomastigotes are released into the blood.

The trypomastigote is spindle shaped and approximately 20 μm long and characteristically assumes a C or U shape in stained blood films (Fig. 6). Trypomastigotes occur in

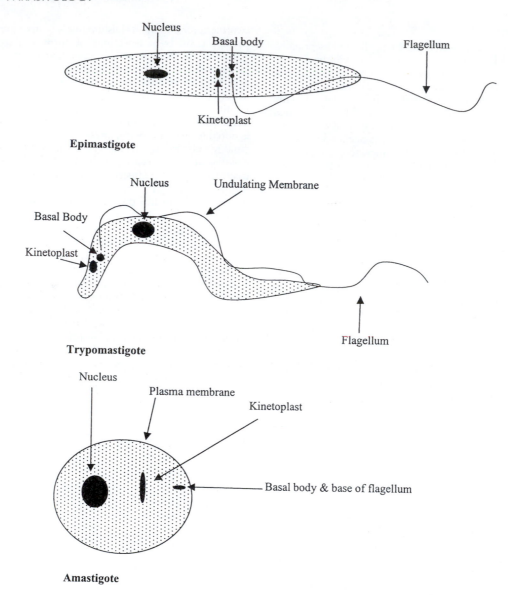

Nucleus

Basal body

Flagellum

Kinetoplast

Epimastigote

Nucleus

Undulating Membrane

Basal Body

Kinetoplast

Flagellum

Trypomastigote

Nucleus

Plasma membrane

Kinetoplast

Basal body & base of flagellum

Amastigote

FIGURE 4 Life cycle stages of trypanosomes.

the blood in two forms, a long, slender form and a short, stubby one. The nucleus is situated in the center of the body, with a large, oval kinetoplast located at the posterior end. A flagellum arises from the basal body and extends along the outer edge of an undulating membrane until it reaches the anterior end of the body, where it projects as a free flagellum. When the trypomastigotes are stained with Giemsa stain, the cytoplasm stains blue and the nucleus, kinetoplast, and flagellum stain red or violet.

The amastigote (2 to 6 μm in diameter) is indistinguishable from those found in leishmanial infections. It contains a large nucleus and a rod-shaped kinetoplast that stains red or violet with Giemsa stain, and the cytoplasm stains blue (Fig. 2 and 7).

Epidemiology and Transmission

Chagas' disease is a zoonosis occurring throughout the American continent, including Central and South America, California, Louisiana, and Texas (66, 71). It involves reduviid bugs living in close association with reservoirs (dogs, cats, armadillos, opossums, raccoons, and rodents). Human infections occur mainly in rural areas where poor sanitary and socioeconomic conditions and poor housing provide excellent breeding places for reduviid bugs (79). Chagas' disease is found in 18 countries in Central and South America. There have been 6 autochthonous cases identified in the United States (66). The disease distribution has been broken into two ecological zones: the southern cone, where the reduviid vector lives inside the human home, and the northern South America, Central America, and Mexico zone, where the reduviid lives inside and outside the home. Strains of *T. cruzi* have large differences in infectivity of potential vectors, antigenicity, histotropism, pathogenicity, and response to therapy (5, 9, 10, 20). Based on molecular epidemiology, *T. cruzi* has been broken into two main genotypes or lineages (*T. cruzi* I and *T. cruzi* II). *T. cruzi* II has been further subdivided in sublineages or subdivisions a to e. *T. cruzi* I is most commonly found in sylvatic cycles, whereas *T. cruzi* II is commonly detected in domestic cycles in the

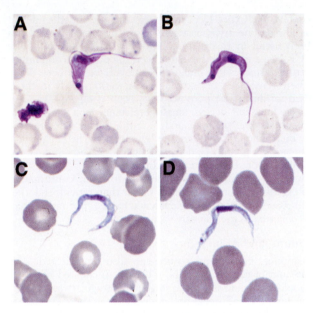

FIGURE 5 (A and B) *Trypanosoma cruzi* trypomastigotes; (C and D) *Trypanosoma brucei gambiense* trypomastigotes.

southern cone. Most human infections are due to *T. cruzi* II in the southern cone, whereas in the northern cone, *T. cruzi* I predominates (36, 42). Transmission by blood or blood product transfusion is a serious concern in areas of endemicity, and serologic screening of blood donors can be used, whereas in areas where the disease is not endemic, questionnaires may be used to defer prospective donors from areas of endemicity (83, 94).

Clinical Significance

In addition to contracting *T. cruzi* infections through the insect's bite wound or exposed mucous membranes, one can be infected by blood transfusion, placental transfer, organ transplant, and accidental ingestion of parasitized reduviid bugs or their feces (83, 94). A localized inflammatory reaction may ensue at the infection site with development of a chagoma (erythematous subcutaneous nodule) or Romaña's sign (edema of the eyelids and conjunctivitis).

Acute systemic signs occur around the second to third week of infection and are characterized by high fevers,

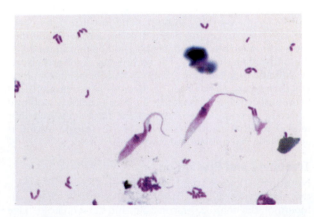

FIGURE 6 *Trypanosoma cruzi* epimastigotes (Giemsa stain).

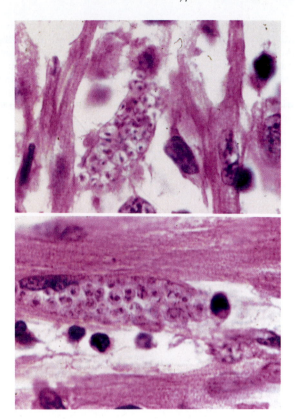

FIGURE 7 *Trypanosoma cruzi* amastigotes in heart muscle (hematoxylin and eosin stain).

hepatosplenomegaly, myalgia, erythematous rash, acute myocarditis, lymphadenopathy, and subcutaneous edema of face, legs, and feet. The acute phase of Chagas' disease in immunosuppressive patients is manifested as acute myocarditis or acute encephalitis with a high mortality rate. Most acute cases resolve over a period of 2 to 3 months into an asymptomatic chronic stage (indeterminate phase or clinical latency period). Approximately 70% of the individuals with chronic Chagas' disease remain asymptomatic (indeterminate phase); however, they are still capable of transmitting the infection. The remaining 30% of these individuals with chronic Chagas' disease develop myocarditis or symptoms associated with denervation of the digestive tract (14). Chronic Chagas' disease may develop years or decades after undetected infection or after the diagnosis of acute disease. The most frequent clinical sign of chronic Chagas' disease is cardiomyopathy manifested by cardiomegaly and conduction changes. Some patients are more likely to develop megaesophagus or megacolon. The "mega" condition has been associated with the destruction of ganglion cells, resulting in dysmotility and causing dysphagia, aspiration, and regurgitation in patients with megaesophagus and severe constipation in patients with megacolon. In chronic Chagas' disease, autoimmunity may also be responsible for tissue destruction in addition to the tissue destruction caused by the parasite. Reactivation of Chagas' disease in HIV-positive patients usually leads to very high parasitemia (32). Central nervous system (CNS) involvement is seldom observed, but in HIV-coinfected individuals, CNS involvement is frequently noted and acute fatal meningoencephalitis and granulomatous encephalitis have been described for these patients (50). Congenital transmission from mother to fetus can occur in both acute and chronic phases of the disease. Congenital infections can cause abortion, prematurity, neurological sequelae, and mental deficiency (30). Infants of seropositive mothers should be monitored for up to a year after birth to rule out infection. Transmission of the infection during transplantation of solid organs and other tissues from seropositive donors has become a significant problem (56). Although transplantation of any organ or tissue from a seropositive donor should be regarded as infectious, the risk of transmission of the infection is dependent on other factors. Some recipients do not develop infections; however, all should be serially monitored for signs of infection.

Diagnosis

Health care personnel working with specimens from patients suspected of having Chagas' disease should follow the blood-borne pathogen guidelines using universal precautions. Trypomastigotes are highly infectious.

Collection of Specimens

The definitive diagnosis depends on demonstration of trypomastigotes in the blood, amastigote stages in tissues, or positive PCR and serologic tests (Table 3). Aspirates from chagomas and enlarged lymph nodes can be examined for amastigotes and trypomastigotes. Histological examination of biopsy specimens may also be done. Trypomastigotes may be easily detected in the blood in acute disease; however, in chronic disease, this stage is rare or absent, except during febrile episodes. Trypomastigotes appear in the blood about 10 days after infection and persist through the acute phase. Laboratorians may want to contact their state public health laboratory or the CDC for diagnostic information and help in specimen selection and available tests.

Direct Examination

Microscopic and PCR Detection

Trypomastigotes may be detected in blood by using thin and thick blood films or the buffy coat concentration technique (93). The stain of choice is Giemsa for both amastigote and trypomastigote stages. Amastigotes can be differentiated from fungal organisms because they do not stain positive with periodic acid-Schiff, mucicarmine, or silver stain. Although not routinely available except in specialized

TABLE 3 Diagnostic methods to detect Chagas' infections

Method[a]	Infection stage		
	Acute	Indeterminate	Chronic
Direct			
Direct microscopy	+	−	−
Thick and thin blood films	+	−	−
PCR	+	+	+
Blood culture	+	−	−
Xenodiagnosis	+	+	+
Indirect			
IFA (IgM and IgG)	+	+	+
EIA	−	+	+
IHA	−	+	+
RIPA/WB	−	+	+

[a]EIA, enzyme immunoassay; IHA, indirect hemagglutinin assay; RIPA, radioimmunoprecipitation assay; WB, Western blot.

centers, PCR (not FDA approved) has been used to detect as few as one trypomastigote in 20 ml of blood and has been useful in treatment follow-up (18, 27, 40, 63). The PCR-based methods have not been standardized, and multicentered studies to validate these tests have not been done. There have been few studies where various PCR methods used for diagnostic purposes have been compared. In areas where kala-azar occurs, amastigote stages look similar, and infections of *L. donovani* and *T. cruzi* must be differentiated by PCR, immunoassay, culture (epimastigote in *T. cruzi* versus promastigote in *L. donovani*), serologic tests, animal inoculation, or xenodiagnosis techniques (27). Patient history, including geographic and/or travel history, and confirmation of organisms in striated muscle rather than reticuloendothelial tissues are very strong evidence for *T. cruzi* rather than *L. donovani* as the causative agent.

Culture and Animal Inoculation

Aspirates, blood, and tissues can also be cultured. The medium of choice is NNN. Cultures, incubated at 25°C, should be examined for epimastigote stages twice weekly during the first 2 weeks and once per week thereafter for up to 4 weeks before they are considered negative. If available, laboratory animals (rats or mice) can be inoculated and the blood can be observed for trypomastigotes.

Xenodiagnosis

Although xenodiagnosis is used less frequently for clinical diagnosis in areas of endemicity, trypanosome-free reduviid bugs are allowed to feed on individuals suspected of having Chagas' disease. The feces, hemolymph, hindgut, and salivary glands can be examined microscopically for flagellated forms over a period of 3 months, or PCR methods can be used to detect infected bugs and provide a rapid diagnosis (106). Xenodiagnosis is positive in less than 50% of the seropositive patients. Some patients may develop a severe anaphylactic reaction to the reduviid bug's salivary secretion.

Serologic Tests

Serologic tests using blood and saliva for the diagnosis of Chagas' disease include complement fixation (Guerreiro-Machado test), chemiluminescence, IFA, indirect hemagglutination, and ELISA (21). Most of these tests use an epimastigote antigen, and cross-reactions have been noted for patients infected with *Trypanosoma rangeli*, *Leishmania* spp., *Toxoplasma gondii*, and hepatitis (29, 41). The use of synthetic peptides and recombinant proteins has improved the sensitivity and specificity of the serodiagnostic techniques (1, 19, 35, 37, 46, 83). The sensitivity and specificity of serologic tests for screening blood donors has improved so that single-assay screening may be justified rather than the two-assay screening method previously recommended (76). Follow-up blood specimens should be reexamined 1 to 2 months after therapy by the techniques described above. A difficult problem using serology has been determining whether a patient has been reinfected or if treatment has been unsuccessful. Changes in *T. cruzi*-specific T cell and antibody response were determined to be an excellent marker for therapeutic response (57). Serologic testing is available at referral laboratories and the CDC.

Treatment and Prevention

Nifurtimox (Lampit) and benznidazole (Radamil) reduce the severity of acute Chagas' disease. Other drugs, allopurinol, fluconazole, itraconazole, and ketoconazole, have been used to treat a limited number of patients. Response to therapy can be monitored by measuring the reduction in antibody response or the reduction in parasite load by PCR (20, 40, 72). Surgery has been successfully used to treat cases of chagasic heart disease, megaesophagus, and megacolon.

Until recently, control of Chagas' disease has been mainly through the use of insecticides to eliminate the reduviid vector. Construction of reduviid-proof dwellings and health education are essential for effective control programs. Bed nets are also effective in preventing infections. Serologic screening of blood products for transfusion from areas in which the disease is endemic is highly recommended (21, 25, 58). An alternative approach to serologic testing for blood donors is the use of questionnaires to defer prospective donors from areas of endemicity.

■ *Trypanosoma rangeli*

T. rangeli infects humans and other vertebrates in both Central and South America, and it is often found in areas where *T. cruzi* is also present (33, 48). Human infections are asymptomatic, and trypomastigotes have been noted to persist in the blood for longer than a year. *T. rangeli* and *T. cruzi* can use the same triatomid vector to transmit infections. *T. rangeli* infections can be transmitted by inoculation of triatomid saliva during feeding or by the vector's feces (25). In some areas, *T. rangeli* infections are five to six times more frequent than infections with *T. cruzi*. Trypomastigotes can be detected from the blood of infected patients by using thin and thick blood smears and buffy coat concentration techniques. The parasites can be stained with Giemsa or Wright stain. Microscopically, the trypomastigote cannot be differentiated from African trypanosomes, which do not occur in the Americas. PCR methods have been used to detect infections in humans and vectors (28, 34). Infections can also be detected by xenodiagnosis. In addition, blood can be cultured (Tobies medium or NNN) or injected into laboratory animals (mice) and examined for epimastigotes and trypomastigotes, respectively. Although there are no serologic tests to detect *T. rangeli* infections, serologic cross-reactions have been noted to occur with tests for *T. cruzi* (2). There are no treatment recommendations for *T. rangeli* infections.

AFRICAN TRYPANOSOMIASIS

African trypanosomiasis is limited to the tsetse fly belt of Central Africa, where there are over 60 million people at risk for African trypanosomiasis (20). The West African (Gambian) form of sleeping sickness, noted for its chronicity and responsible for 99% of the sleeping sickness cases, is caused by *T. brucei gambiense*, whereas the East African (Rhodesian) form, noted for its acute morbidity and mortality within months of infection, is caused by *T. brucei rhodesiense* (87). *T. brucei gambiense* infections can last for months to years with slow CNS involvement. In some areas of endemicity, civil strife has disrupted both the health care infrastructure and vector control, which has led to a resurgence of this disease.

Life Cycle and Morphology

T. brucei rhodesiense and *T. brucei gambiense* are closely related and morphologically indistinguishable. In the past, differentiation was based on clinical signs and geographic area; however, differentiation can now be accomplished using isoenzyme characteristics and DNA and RNA methods.

The trypomastigote forms (Fig. 4 and 6) in the blood range from long, slender-bodied organisms with a long flagellum to short, fat, stumpy forms without a free flagellum (14 to 33 μm long and 1.5 to 3.5 μm wide). The short, stumpy forms are the infective stage for the tsetse fly.

Using Giemsa or Wright stain, the granular cytoplasm stains pale blue and contains dark blue granules and possibly vacuoles. The centrally located nucleus stains reddish. The kinetoplast is located at the organism's posterior end and stains reddish; the remaining intracytoplasmic flagellum (axoneme) may not be visible. The flagellum arises from the kinetoplast, as does the undulating membrane. The flagellum runs along the edge of the undulating membrane until the undulating membrane merges with the trypanosome body at the organism's anterior end. At this point, the flagellum becomes free to extend beyond the body. Trypanosomal forms are ingested by the tsetse fly when a blood meal is taken and transform to epimastigotes (Fig. 4). The organisms multiply in the gut of the fly, and after approximately 2 weeks, the organisms migrate back to the salivary glands. Human are infected when metacyclic forms from the salivary glands are introduced into the bite site as the blood meal is taken by the tsetse fly. The trypomastigote has the ability to change the surface coat of the outer membrane, helping the organism evade the host's humoral immune response (39).

Epidemiology and Transmission

The development cycle in the tsetse fly varies from 12 to 30 days and averages 20 days. Fewer than 10% of the tsetse flies become infective after obtaining blood from infected patients. Both female and male tsetse flies can transmit the infection.

Although there is no evidence of animal-to-human transmission of *T. brucei gambiense*, trypanosomal strains isolated from hartebeest, kob, chickens, dogs, cows, and domestic pigs in West Africa are identical to those isolated from humans in the same area. Evidence suggests that transmission may be entirely interhuman. The tsetse fly vectors of Rhodesian trypanosomiasis are game feeders (including cattle) that may transmit the disease from human to human or from animal to human.

There is molecular evidence of multistrain introduction of the infection with parasites of the *T. brucei* complex that can have epidemiological implications as to virulence, pathogenicity, and response to therapy (8). This phenomenon has not received much attention.

Clinical Significance

After a bite by an infected tsetse fly, a local inflammatory reaction that resolves spontaneously within 1 to 2 weeks can be detected at the bite site. The bite site chancre can be painful, presenting as an erythematous indurated nodule that may ulcerate. The trypomastigotes gain entrance to the bloodstream, causing a symptom-free low-grade parasitemia that may continue for many months. The infection may self-cure during this period without development of symptoms or lymph node invasion. Chancres may be confused with insect bites and bacterial skin infections, with resolution occurring within a few weeks.

The clinical course and disease progression are more acute with *T. brucei rhodesiense* than with *T. brucei gambiense* infections. Diagnostic symptoms include irregular fever, lymph node enlargement (particularly those of the posterior triangle of the neck, known as Winterbottom's sign, which is prominent in *T. brucei gambiense* infections), delayed sensation to pain (Kerandel's sign), and erythematous skin rashes. In addition to lymph node involvement, the spleen and liver become enlarged. With Gambian trypanosomiasis, the blood lymphatic stage (stage I) may last for years before the sleeping sickness syndrome occurs (CNS involvement, meningoencephalitis stage, stage II).

Laboratory findings include anemia, granulocytopenia, increased sedimentation rate, and marked increases in serum IgM. The sustained high IgM levels are a result of the parasite producing variable antigen types to evade the patient's defense system (39). In an immunocompetent host, the lack of elevated serum IgM rules out African trypanosomiasis. Diagnostic differential may include brucellosis, malaria, relapsing fever, and typhoid.

Upon trypomastigote invasion of the CNS, the sleeping sickness stage of the infection is initiated (stage II). Gambian trypanosomiasis is characterized by steady, progressive meningoencephalitis, behavioral changes, apathy, confusion, coordination loss, and somnolence. *T. brucei rhodesiense* produces a more rapid, fulminating disease, and death may occur before there is extensive CNS involvement. In the terminal phase of the disease, the patient becomes emaciated, leading to profound coma and death, usually from secondary infections. Cerebrospinal fluid (CSF) findings include increased protein and IgM levels, lymphocytosis, and morular cells of Mott. Morular (mulberry) cells are altered plasma cells whose cytoplasm is filled with proteinaceous droplets. Morular cells are not seen in all patients; however, they are characteristic of African trypanosomiasis. The diagnostic differential may include cryptococcosis, HIV, meningitis, Parkinson's disease, psychiatric disorders, and space-occupying lesions.

Diagnosis

Definitive diagnosis depends upon demonstration of trypomastigotes in blood, lymph node aspirate, sternum bone marrow, and CSF. Trypomastigotes can be more readily detected in body fluids in infections due to *T. brucei rhodesiense* than in those due to *T. brucei gambiense* because of higher parasitemias. Due to periodicity, parasite numbers in the blood vary, and a number of techniques must be used to detect the trypomastigotes. Laboratorians may want to contact their state public health laboratory or the CDC for diagnostic information and help with specimen selection and available tests.

Collection of Specimens

Trypomastigotes are highly infectious, and health care personnel must be cautious and adhere to blood-borne pathogen guidelines using universal precautions when handling blood, CSF, or aspirates. Blood can be collected from either finger stick or venipuncture. Venous blood should be collected in a tube containing EDTA. Multiple blood exams should be performed before trypanosomiasis is ruled out. Parasites are found in high numbers in the blood during the febrile period and in low numbers in the afebrile periods. If CSF is examined, a volume greater than 1 ml, preferably 5 ml or more, should be collected. In cases in which trypomastigotes are in undetectable numbers in the blood, they may be seen in aspirates of inflamed lymph nodes; however, attempts to demonstrate them in tissue are not practical. Blood and CSF specimens should be examined during therapy to evaluate the clinical response and up to 2 years after therapy.

Direct Examination

Microscopic and PCR Detection

In addition to thin and thick blood films, a buffy coat concentration method is recommended to detect the parasites. Parasites can be detected on thick blood smears when numbers are greater than 2,000/ml, with hematocrit capillary tube concentration when numbers are greater than 100/ml, and on an anion-exchange column when numbers are greater than 4/ml. Unfortunately, anion exchange is not easily adapted to clinical laboratories or field studies (26). In suspected and confirmed cases of trypanosomiasis, a lumbar puncture is mandatory to rule out CNS involvement (stage II). CSF examination must be conducted by using centrifuged sediments (22). The CSF should be examined immediately because the trypomastigotes begin to autolyze within 10 min. Detection of trypomastigotes in the CSF allows immediate classification of stage II illness (CNS involvement). Referral laboratories have used molecular methods (PCR, not FDA approved) to detect infections and differentiate species, but these methods are not routinely used in the field (12, 26). The PCR-based methods have not been standardized and multicentered institutional studies to validate these tests have not been done. There have been few studies where the various PCR methods used for diagnostic purposes have been compared.

Culture and Animal Inoculation

Small laboratory animals (rats and guinea pigs) have been used to detect infections. *T. brucei rhodesiense* is more adaptable to cultivation and animal infection than *T. brucei gambiense*; however, cultivation is not practical for most diagnostic laboratories.

Serologic Tests

Serologic techniques (not FDA approved) that have been used for epidemiologic screening include IFA, ELISA, indirect hemagglutination assay, the card agglutination trypanosomiasis test (CATT), and LATEX/*T. b. gambiense*. CATT is effective in screening the population for suspected cases of *T. brucei gambiense* but not *T. brucei rhodesiense*. Major serodiagnostic problems with CATT include false-positive results due to malarial infections and the fact that many in the population have elevated antibody levels due to exposure to animal trypanosomes that are noninfectious to humans. CATT does not differentiate between current and past infections (26, 44, 90). Both CATT and LATEX/*T. b. gambiense* have good negative predictive values (20). Markedly elevated serum and CSF IgM concentrations are of diagnostic value. CSF antibody titers should be interpreted with caution because of the lack of reference values and the possibility of CSF containing serum due to a traumatic tap. Intrathecal production of immunoglobulins can be found in a number of neuroinflammatory diseases. LATEX/IgM has been developed for field use to measure CSF concentrations of IgM (26).

Antibodies to galactocerebrosides and neurofilaments as well as elevated concentrations of interleukin-10 and CSF protein levels may be markers for CNS involvement, all of which have been used to monitor CNS infections (26, 59, 60). ELISA has been used to detect antigen in serum and CSF. This method could also be used for clinical staging of the disease to determine whether there was CNS infection and as a follow-up to therapy.

Treatment and Prevention

Suramin (Bayer 205; Naphuride or Antrypol) is the drug of choice for treating the early blood or lymphatic stage of *T. brucei rhodesiense* infections, whereas pentamidine isethionate (Lomidine) is the drug of choice for treating the early stages of *T. brucei gambiense* infections (11, 53, 87). Melarsoprol (mel B or Arsobal) is the drug of choice when CNS involvement is suspected (53, 87).

Difluoromethyomithine (DFMO; Eflomithine or Ornidyl) is a cytostatic drug effective against the acute and late stages of *T. brucei gambiense* infections (50). The effectiveness of therapy can be judged microscopically by the absence of trypomastigotes in the blood, lymph fluid, or CSF and by a decrease in CSF white blood cells (67). CSF antibodies (IgM) decrease, as do levels of interleukin-10, after successful therapy (59). Any individual treated for African trypanosomiasis should be monitored for 2 years after completion of therapy (60).

Population-screening programs have been used to control *T. brucei gambiense* infections. The use of vector control measures has met with limited success (10). The most effective control measures include an integrated approach to reduce the human reservoir of infection and the use of insecticide and fly traps. Persons visiting areas in which the infection is endemic should wear protective clothing (long-sleeved shirts and long trousers). Vaccines are not available.

OTHER TRYPANOSOMES INFECTING HUMANS

Trypanosoma evansi

The first human case of *T. evansi* was diagnosed in India (103). This organism is normally considered a parasite of animals (buffalo, camels, cattle, horses, and rats) and has a very wide geographic distribution (Africa, Asia, and Central and South America). The infection is transmitted mechanically by blood-sucking insects such as stable flies or horseflies. In animals, the incubation period is 5 to 60 days and the severity of the disease varies from no symptoms to weakness, weight loss, anemia, abortions, and death. In the above-mentioned human case, the patient complained of transient fevers and sensory disorders. Fever peaks were noted every 7 to 10 days, and large numbers of parasites were detected in the blood at the time of fevers. No parasites were observed in the CSF. The patient was treated with suramin. Laboratory diagnosis is usually done by examination of blood and lymph node aspirates or biopsy specimens. *T. evansi* cannot be differentiated from *T. brucei gambiense*, *T. brucei rhodesiense*, or *T. rangeli* microscopically.

Trypanosoma lewisi

Human cases of *T. lewisi* infections have been described in India and Thailand in pediatric patients (55, 86). Trypomastigotes were detected in the blood of these patients. In both cases, the patients fully recovered from the infection. The kinetoplast is subterminal to the posterior end of the trypomastigote, and the nucleus is found at the anterior end, terminating where the flagellum is free of the trypomastigote body. *T. lewisi* is a natural infection of wild rats and is considered nonpathogenic. The intermediate host is the flea, where the parasite multiplies in the gut and gives rise to epimastigotes that are found in the rectum and feces. The infection is passed to susceptible rats by ingestion of fleas or their feces. Human infections are thought to be transmitted in a similar fashion.

REFERENCES

1. **Almeida, I. C., D. T. Covas, L. M. Soussumi, and L. R. Travassos.** 1997. A highly sensitive and specific chemiluminescent enzyme-linked immunosorbent assay for diagnosis of active *Trypanosoma cruzi* infection. *Transfusion* **37:**850–857.
2. **Anthony, R. L., T. S. Cody, and N. T. Constantin.** 1981. Antigenic differentiation of Trypanosoma C7–2i and *Trypanosoma rangeli* by means of monoclonal–hybridoma antibodies. *Am. J. Trop. Med. Hyg.* **30:**1191–1197.
3. **Antinori, S., A. Cascio, C. Parravicini, R. Bianchi, and M. Corbellino.** 2008. Leishmaniasis among organ transplant recipients. *Lancet Infect. Dis.* **8:**191–199.
4. **Antinori, S., E. Gianelli, S. Calatini, E. Longhi, M. Gramiccia, and M. Corbellino.** 2004. Cutaneous leishmaniasis: an increasing threat for travelers. *Clin. Microbiol. Infect.* **11:**343–346.
5. **Aparicio, I. M., J. Scharfstein, and A. P. C. A. Lima.** 2004. A new cruzipain-mediated pathway of human cell invasion by *Trypanosoma cruzi* requires trypomastigote membranes. *Infect. Immun.* **72:**5892–5902.
6. **Arora, S. K., S. Gupta, S. Bhardwaj, N. Sachdeva, and N. L. Sharma.** 2008. An epitope-specific PCR test for diagnosis of *Leishmania donovani* infections. *Trans. R. Soc. Trop. Med. Hyg.* **102:**41–45.
7. **Attar, Z. J., M. L. Chance, S. el-Safi, J. Carney, A. Azazy, M. El-Hadi, C. Dourado, and M. Hommel.** 2001. Latex agglutination test for the detection of urinary antigens in visceral leishmaniasis. *Acta Trop.* **78:**11–16.
8. **Balmer, O., and A. Caccone.** 2008. Multiple-strain infections of *Trypanosoma brucei* across Africa. *Acta Trop.* **107:**275–279.
9. **Barnabe, C., R. Yaegar, O. Pung, and M. Tibayrenc.** 2001. *Trypanosoma cruzi:* a considerable phylogenic divergence indicates that the agent of Chagas disease is indigenous to the native fauna of the United States. *Exp. Parasitol.* **99:**73–79.
10. **Barrett, M. P., R. J. S. Burchmore, A. Stich, J. O. Lazzari, A. C. Frasch, J. J. Cazzulo, and S. Krishna.** 2003. The trypanosomiasis. *Lancet* **362:**1469–1480.
11. **Barrett, S. V., and M. P. Barrett.** 2000. Anti-sleeping sickness drugs and cancer chemotherapy. *Parasitol. Today* **16:**7–9.
12. **Becker, S., J. R. Franco, P. P. Simarro, A. Stich, P. M. Abel, and D. Steverding.** 2004. Real-time PCR for detection of *Trypanosoma brucei* in human blood samples. *Diagn. Microbiol. Infect. Dis.* **50:**193–199.
13. **Bern, C., S. Jha, A. B. Joshi, G. D. Thakur, and M. B. Bista.** 2000. Use of the recombinant K39 dipstick test and the direct agglutination test in a setting endemic for visceral leishmaniasis in Nepal. *Am. J. Trop. Med. Hyg.* **63:**153–157.
14. **Blum, J. A., M. J. Zellweger, C. Burri, and C. Hatz.** 2008. Cardiac involvement in African and American trypanosomiasis. *Lancet Infect. Dis.* **8:**631–641.
15. **Boarino, A., A. Scalone, L. Gradoni, E. Ferroglio, E. Vitale, R. Zanatta, M. G. Giuffrida, and S. Rosati.** 2005. Development of recombinant chimeric antigen expressing immunodominant B epitopes of *Leishmania infantum* for serodiagnosis of visceral leishmaniasis. *Clin. Diagn. Lab. Immunol.* **12:**647–653.
16. **Braz, R. E. S., E. T. Nascimento, D. R. A. Martins, M. E. Wilson, R. D. Pearson, S. G. Reed, and S. M. B. Jeronimo.** 2002. The sensitivity and specificity of *Leishmania chagasi* recombinant K39 antigen in the diagnosis of American visceral leishmaniasis and in differentiating active from subclinical infection. *Am. J. Trop. Med. Hyg.* **67:**344–348.
17. **Brito, M. E. F, M. G. Mendonca, Y. M. Gomes, M. L. Jardim, and F. G. C. Abath.** 2000. Identification of potentially diagnostic *Leishmania braziliensis* antigens in human cutaneous leishmaniasis by immunoblot analysis. *Clin. Diagn. Lab. Immunol.* **7:**318–321.
18. **Britto, C., M. A. Cardoso, C. M. M. Vanni, A. Hasslocher-Moreno, S. S. Xavier, W. Oelemann, A. Santoro, C. Pirmez, C. M. Morel, and P. Wincker.** 1995. Polymerase chain reaction detection of *Trypanosoma cruzi* in human blood samples as tool for diagnosis and treatment evaluation. *Parasitology* **110:**241–247.
19. **Buchovsky, A. S., O. Campetella, G. Russomando, L. Franco, R. Oddone, N. Candia, A. Luquetti, S. M. G. Cappa, and M. S. Leguizamon.** 2001. *trans*-Sialidase inhibition assay, a highly sensitive and specific diagnostic test for Chagas' disease. *Clin. Diagn. Lab. Immunol.* **8:**187–189.
20. **Campos, R. F., M. L. S. Guerreiro, K. D. S. C. Sobral, R. D. C. P. C. Lima, and S. G. Andrade.** 2005. Response to chemotherapy with benznidazole of clones isolated from the 21SF strain of *Trypanosoma cruzi* (biodeme type II, *Trypanosoma cruzi* II). *Rev. Soc. Bras. Med. Trop.* **38:**142–146.

21. **Castro, E.** 2009. Chagas' disease: lessons from routine donation testing. *Transfusion Med.* **19:**16–23.

22. **Cattand, P., B. T. Miezan, and P. de Rasdt.** 1988. Human African trypanosomiasis: use of double centrifugation of cerebrospinal fluid to detect trypanosomes. *Bull. W. H. O.* **66:**83–86.

23. **Centers for Disease Control.** 1992. Viscerotropic leishmaniasis in persons returning from Operation Desert Storm 1990–1991. *MMWR Morb. Mortal. Wkly. Rep.* **41:**131–134.

24. **Centers for Disease Control and Prevention.** 2003. Cutaneous leishmaniasis in U.S. military personnel—Southwest/Central Asia, 2002–2003. *MMWR Morb. Mortal. Wkly. Rep.* **52:**1009–1012.

25. **Centers for Disease Control and Prevention.** 2007. Blood donor screening for Chagas' disease—United States, 2006–2007. *MMWR Morb. Mortal. Wkly. Rep.* **56:**141–143.

26. **Chappuis, F., L. Loutan, P. Simarro, V. Lejon, and P. Buscher.** 2005. Options for field diagnosis of human African trypanosomiasis. *Clin. Microbiol. Rev.* **18:**133–146.

27. **Chiaramonte, M. G., F. M. Frank, G. M. Furer, N. J. Taranto, R. A. Margni, and E. L. Malchiodi.** 1999. Polymerase chain reaction reveals *Trypanosoma cruzi* infection suspected by serology in cutaneous and mucocutaneous leishmaniasis patients. *Acta Trop.* **72:**295–308.

28. **Chiurillo, M. A., G. Crisante, A. Rojas, A. Peralta, M. Dias, P. Guevara, N. Anez, and J. L. Ramirez.** 2003. Detection of *Trypanosoma cruzi* and *Trypanosoma rangeli* infection by duplex PCR assay based on telomeric sequences. *Clin. Diagn. Lab. Immunol.* **10:**775–779.

29. **Cordeiro, F. D., O. A. Martins-Filho, M. O. C. Rocha, S. J. Adad, R. Correa-Oliveira, and A. J. Romanha.** 2001. Anti-*Trypanosoma cruzi* immunoglobulin G1 can be a useful tool for diagnosis and prognosis of human Chagas' disease. *Clin. Diagn. Lab. Immunol.* **8:**112–118.

30. **Coura, J. R.** 2007. Chagas' disease: what is known and what is needed–a background article. *Mem. Inst. Oswaldo Cruz* **102:**113–122.

31. **Cupolillo, E., E. Medina-Acosta, H. Noyes, H. Momen, and G. Grimaldi, Jr.** 2000. A revised classification for *Leishmania* and *Endotrypanum. Parasitol. Today* **16:**142–144.

32. **Da-Cruz, A. M., R. P. Igreja, W. Dantas, A. C. V. Junqueira, R. S. Pacheco, A. J. Silva-Goncalves, and C. Pirmez.** 2004. Long-term follow-up of co-infected HIV and *Trypanosoma cruzi* Brazilian patients. *Trans. R. Soc. Trop. Med. Hyg.* **98:**728–733.

33. **Da Silva, F. M., H. Noyes, M. Campaner, A. C. V. Junqueira, J. R. Coura, N. Anez, J. J. Shaw, J. R. Stevens, and M. M. G. Teixeira.** 2004. Phylogeny, taxonomy and grouping of *Trypanosoma rangeli* isolates from man, triatomines and sylvatic mammals from widespread geographical origin based on SSU and ITS ribosomal sequences. *Parasitology* **129:**549–561.

34. **Da Silva, F. M., A. C. Rodrigues, M. Campaner, C. S. A. Takata, M. C. Brigido, A. C. V. Junqueira, J. R. Coura, G. F Takeda, J. J. Shaw, and M. M. G. Teixeira.** 2004. Randomly amplified polymorphic DNA analysis of *Trypanosoma rangeli* and allied species from human, monkeys and other sylvatic mammals of the Brazilian Amazon disclosed a new group and a species-specific market. *Parasitology* **128:**283–294.

35. **Da Silveira, J. L., E. S. Umezawa, and A. O. Luquetti.** 2001. Chagas' disease: recombinant *Trypanosoma cruzi* antigens for serological diagnosis. *Trends Parasitol.* **17:**286–291.

36. **D'Avila, D. A., A. M. Macedo, H. M. S. Valadares, E. D. Gontijo, A. M. de Castro, C. R. Machado, E. Chiari, and L. M. C. Galvao.** 2009. Probing population dynamics of *Trypanosoma cruzi* during progression of the chronic phase in chagasic patients. *J. Clin. Microbiol.* **47:**1718–1725.

37. **Di Pentima, M. C., and M. S. Edwards.** 1999. Enzyme linked immunosorbent assay for IgA antibodies to *Trypanosoma cruzi* in congenital infections. *Am. J. Trop. Med. Hyg.* **60:**211–214.

38. **Disch, J., M. J. Pedras, M. Orsini, C. Pirmez, M. C. de Oliveria, M. Castro, and A. Rabello.** 2005. *Leishmania* (*Viannia*) subgenus kDNA amplification for the diagnosis of mucosal leishmaniasis. *Diagn. Microbiol. Infect. Dis.* **51:**185–190.

39. **Dubois, M. E., K. P. Demick, and J. M. Mansfield.** 2005. Trypanosomes expressing a mosaic variant surface glycoprotein coat escape early detection by the immune system. *Infect. Immun.* **73:**2690–2697.

40. **Duffy, T., M. Bisio, J. Altcheh, J. M. Burgos, M. Diez, M. J. Levin, R. R. Favaloro, H. Freilij, A. B. Schijman.** 2009. Accurate real-time PCR strategy for monitoring bloodstream parasitic loads in Chagas disease patients. *PLoS Negl. Trop. Dis.* **3:**e419.

41. **Faber, W. R., L. Oskam, T. van Gool, N. C. M. Kroon, K. J. Knegt-Junk, H. Hofwegen, A. C. van der Wal, and P. A. Kager.** 2003. Value of diagnostic techniques for cutaneous leishmaniasis. *J. Am. Acad. Dermatol.* **49:**70–74.

42. **Freitas, J. M., E. Lages-Silva, E. Crema, S. D. J. Pena, and M. M. Macedo.** 2005. Real time PCR strategy for the identification of major lineages of *Trypanosoma cruzi* directly in chronically infected human tissues. *Int. J. Parasitol.* **35:**411–417.

43. **Gangneux, J., J. Menotti, E. Lorenzo, C. Sarfati, H. Blanche, H. Bui, E. Pratlong, Y. Garin, and F. Derouin.** 2003. Prospective value of PCR amplification and sequencing for diagnosis and typing of Old World *Leishmania* infections in an area of nonendemicity. *J. Clin. Microbiol.* **41:**1419–1422.

44. **Garcia, A., V. Jamonneau, E. Magnus, C. Laveissere, V. Lejon, P. N'Guessan, L. N'Dri, N. van Meirvenne, and P. Buscher.** 2000. Follow-up of card agglutination trypanosomiasis test (CATT) positive but apparently aparasitaemic individuals in Cote d'Ivoire: evidence for a complex and heterogeneous population. *Trop. Med. Int. Health* **5:**786–793.

45. **Garcia, A. L., A. Kindt, K. W. Quispe-Tintaya, H. Bermudez, A. Llanos, J. Arevalo, A. L. Banuls, S. De Doncker, D. Le Ray, and J. C. Dujardin.** 2005. American tegumentary leishmaniasis: antigen-gene polymorphism, taxonomy and clinical pleomorphism. *Infect. Genet. Evol.* **5:**109–116.

46. **Garcia, L. S.** 2007. *Diagnostic Medical Parasitology*, 5th ed. ASM Press, Washington, DC.

47. **Gomes, A. H. S., I. M. Armelin, S. Z. Menon, and V. L. Pereira-Chioccola.** 2008. *Leishmania* (*V.*) *braziliensis*: detection by PCR in biopsies from patients with cutaneous leishmaniasis. *Exp. Parasitol.* **119:**319–324.

48. **Guhl, F., and G. A. Vallejo.** 2003. *Trypanosoma* (*Herpetosoma*) *rangeli* Tejera, 1920–an updated review. *Mem. Inst. Oswaldo Cruz* **98:**435–442.

49. **Haouas, N., N. Chargui, E. Chaker, H. Babba, S. Belhadj, K. Kallel, E. Pratlong, J. P. Dedet, H. Mezhoud, and R. Azaiez.** 2005. Anthroponotic cutaneous leishmaniasis in Tunisia: presence of *Leishmania killicki* outside its original focus of Tataouine. *Trans. R. Soc. Trop. Med. Hyg.* **99:**499–501.

50. **Harms, G., and H. Feldmeier.** 2005. The impact of HIV infection on tropical diseases. *Infect. Dis. Clin. N. Am.* **19:**121–135.

51. **Ismail, A., A. Kharazrni, H. Permin, and A. M. El Hassam.** 1997. Detection and characterization of *Leishmania* in tissues of patients with post kala-azar dermal leishmaniasis using a specific monoclonal antibody. *Trans. R. Soc. Trop. Med. Hyg.* **91:**283–285.

52. **Jamjoom, M. B., R. W. Ashford, P. A. Bates, M. L. Chance, S. J. Kemp, P. C. Watts, and H. A. Noyes.** 2004. *Leishmania donovani* is the only cause of visceral leishmaniasis in East Africa; previous descriptions of *L. infantum* and "*L. archibaldi*" from this region are a consequence of convergent evolution in the isoenzyme data. *Parasitology* **129:**399–409.

53. **Jannin, J., and P. Cattand.** 2004. Treatment and control of human African trypanosomiasis. *Curr. Opin. Infect. Dis.* **17:**565–570.

54. **Karp, C. L., and P. G. Auwaerter.** 2007. Coinfection with HIV and tropical infectious diseases. I. Protozoal pathogens. *Clin. Infect. Dis.* **45:**1208–1213.

55. **Kaur, R., V. K. Gupta, A. C. Dhariwai, D. C. Jain, and L. Shiv.** 2007. A rare case of trypanosomiasis in a two month old infant in Mumbai. *J. Commun. Dis.* **39:**71–74.

56. **Kun, H. A., A. Moore, L. Mascola, F. Steurer, G. Lawrence, B. Kubak, S. Radhakrishna, D. Leiby, R. Herron, T. Mone, R. Hunter, M. Kuehnert, et al.** 2009. Transmission of *Trypanosoma cruzi* by heart transplantation. *Clin. Infect. Dis.* **48:**1534–1540.

57. **Kyambadde, J. W., J. C. K. Enyaru, E. Matovu, M. Odit, and J. F. Carasco.** 2000. Detection of trypanosomes in suspected sleeping sickness patients in Uganda using the polymerase chain reaction. *Bull. W. H. O.* **78:**119–124.

58. **Leiby, D. A., R. M. Herron, Jr., G. Garratty, and B. L. Herwaldt.** 2008. *Trypanosoma cruzi* parasitemia in U.S. blood donors with serologic evidence of infection. *J. Infect. Dis.* **198:**609–613.

59. **Lejon, V., and P. Büscher.** 2005. Cerebrospinal fluid in human African trypanosomiasis: a key to diagnosis, therapeutic decision and post-treatment follow-up. *Trop. Med. Int. Health* **10:**395–403.

60. **Lejon, V., I. Roger, D. M. Ngoyi, J. Menten, J. Robays, F. X. N'Siesi, S. Bisser, M. Boelaert, and P. Buscher.** 2008. Novel markers for treatment outcome in late-stage *Trypanosoma brucei gambiense* trypanosomiasis. *Clin. Infect. Dis.* **47:**15–22.

61. **Magill, A. J.** 2005. Cutaneous leishmaniasis in the returning traveler. *Infect. Dis. Clin. N. Am.* **19:**241–266.

62. **Mahdi, M., E. M. Elamim, S. E. Melville, A. M. Musa, J. M. Blackwell, M. M. Mukhtar, A. M. Elhassan, and M. E. Ibrahim.** 2005. Sudanese mucosal leishmaniasis: isolation of a parasite within the *Leishmania donovani* complex that differs genotypically from *L. donovani* causing classical visceral leishmaniasis. *Infect. Genet. Evol.* **5:**29–33.

63. **Maldonado, C., S. Albino, L. Vettorazzi, O. Salomone, J. C. Zlocowski, C. Abiega, M. Amuchastegui, R. Cordoba, and T. Alvarellos.** 2004. Using polymerase chain reaction in early diagnosis of re-activated *Trypanosoma cruzi* infection after heart transplantation. *J. Heart Lung Transplant.* **23:**1345–1348.

64. **Mauricio, I. L., J. R. Stothard, and M. A. Miles.** 2000. A strange case of *Leishmania chagasi. Parasitol. Today* **16:**188–189.

65. **Mendonca, M. G., M. E. F. deBrito, E. H. G. Rodrigues, V. Bandeira, M. L. Jardim, and F. G. C. Abath.** 2004. Persistence of *Leishmania* parasites in scars after clinical cure of American cutaneous leishmaniasis: is there a sterile cure? *J. Infect. Dis.* **189:**1018–1023.

66. **Milei, J., R. A. Guerri-Guttenberg, D. A. Grana, and R. Storino.** 2009. Prognostic impact of Chagas disease in the United States. *Am. Heart J.* **157:**22–29.

67. **Moore, A. C.** 2005. Prospects for improving African trypanosomiasis chemotherapy. *J. Infect. Dis.* **191:**1793–1795.

68. **Motazedian, M., M. Fakhar, M. H. Motazedian, G. Hatam, and F. Mikaeili.** 2008. A urine-based polymerase chain reaction method for the diagnosis of visceral leishmaniasis in immunocompetent patients. *Diagn. Microbiol. Infect. Dis.* **60:**151–154.

69. **Murray, H. W.** 2005. Prevention of relapse after chemotherapy in a chronic intracellular infection: mechanisms in experimental visceral leishmaniasis. *J. Immunol.* **174:**4916–4923.

70. **Napier, L.** 1922. A new serum test for kala-azar. *Indian J. Med. Res.* **9:**830–846.

71. **Navrn, T. R., R. R. Roberto, D. D. Juranek, K. Limpakarnjanarat, E. W. Mortenson, J. R. Clover, R. E. Yescott, C. Taclindo, F. Stuerer, and D. Allain.** 1985. Human and sylvatic *Trypanosoma cruzi* infection in California. *Am. J. Public Health* **75:**366–369.

72. **Negrette, O. S., F. J. S. Valdez, C. D. Lacunza, M. F. G. Bustos, M. C. Mora, A. D. Uncos, and M. A. Basombrio.** 2008. Serological evaluation of specific-antibody levels in patients treated for chronic Chagas' disease. *Clin. Vaccine Immunol.* **15:**297–302.

73. **Oliveira, J. G. S., F. O. Novais, C. I. de Oliveira, A. C. da Cruz, Jr., L. F. Campos, A. V. da Rocha, V. Boaventura, A. Noronha, J. M. L. Costa, and A. Barral.** 2005. Polymerase chain reaction (PCR) is highly sensitive for diagnosis of mucosal leishmaniasis. *Acta Trop.* **94:**55–59.

74. **Oliveira, R. A., L. S. V. Silva, V. P. Carvalho, A. F. Coutinho, F. G. Pinheiro, C. G. Lima, J. E. Leandro, Jr., G. B. Silva, Jr., and E. F. Daher.** 2008. Visceral leishmaniasis after renal transplantation: report of 4 cases in Northeastern Brazil. *Transpl. Infect. Dis.* **10:**364–368.

75. **Olivier, M., D. J. Gregory, and G. Forget.** 2005. Subversion mechanisms by which *Leishmania* parasites can escape the host immune response: a signaling point of view. *Clin. Microbiol. Rev.* **18:**293–305.

76. **Otani, M. M., E. Vinelli, L. V. Kirchhoff, A. del Pozo, A. Sands, G. Vercauteren, and E. C. Sabino.** 2009. WHO comparative evaluation of serologic assays for Chagas disease. *Transfusion* **49:**1076–1082.

77. **Paiva, B. R., L. N. Passos, A. Falqueto, R. S. Malfronte, and H. F. de Andrade, Jr.** 2004. Single step polymerase chain reaction (PCR) for the diagnosis of the *Leishmania* (Viannia) subgenus. *Rev. Inst. Med. Trop. Sao Paulo* **46:**335–338.

78. **Palumbo, E.** 2008. Oral miltefosine treatment in children with visceral leishmaniasis: a brief review. *Braz. J. Infect. Dis.* **12:**2–4.

79. **Pereira, K. S., F. L. Schmidt, A. M. Guaraldo, R. M. Franco, V. L. Dias, and L. A. Passos.** 2009. Chagas' disease as a foodborne illness. *J. Food Prot.* **72:**441–446.

80. **Pizzuto, M., M. Piazza, D. Senese, C. Scalamogna, S. Calattini, L. Corsico, T. Persico, B. Adriani, C. Magni, G. Guaraldi, G. Gaiera, A. Ludovisi, M. Gramiccia, M. Galli, M. Moroni, M. Corbellino, and S. Antinori.** 2001. Role of PCR in diagnosis and prognosis of visceral leishmaniasis in patients coinfected with human immunodeficiency virus type 1. *J. Clin. Microbiol.* **39:**357–361.

81. **Reithinger, R., and J. Dujardin.** 2007. Molecular diagnosis of leishmaniasis: current status and future applications. *J. Clin. Microbiol.* **45:**21–25.

82. **Romero, G. A. S., M. V. F. Guerra, M. G. Paes, E. Cupolillo, C. B. Toaldo, V. O. Macedo, and O. Fernandes.** 2001. Sensitivity of the polymerase chain reaction for the diagnosis of cutaneous leishmaniasis due to *Leishmania* (Viannia) *guyanensis. Acta Trop.* **79:**225–229.

83. **Saez-Alquezar, A., E. C. Sabino, N. Salles, D. F. Chamone, F. Hulstaert, H. Pottel, E. Stoops, and M. Zrein.** 2000. Serological confirmation of Chagas' disease by a recombinant and peptide antigen line immunoassay: INNO-LIA Chagas. *J. Clin. Microbiol.* **38:**851–854.

84. **Saha, S., T. Mazumdar, K. Anam, R. Ravindran, B. Bairagi, B. Saba, R. Goswami, N. Pramanik, S. K. Guha, S. Kar, D. Banerjee, and N. Ali.** 2005. *Leishmania* promastigote membrane antigen-based enzyme-linked immunosorbent assay and immunoblotting for differential diagnosis of Indian post-kala-azar dermal leishmaniasis. *J. Clin. Microbiol.* **43:**1269–1277.

85. **Salotra, P., G. Sreenivas, G. P. Pogue, N. Lee, H. L. Nakhasi, V. Ramesh, and N. S. Negi.** 2001. Development of a species-specific PCR assay for detection of *Leishmania donovani* in clinical samples from patients with kala-azar and post-kala-azar dermal leishmaniasis. *J. Clin. Microbiol.* **39:**849–854.

86. **Sarataphan, N., M. Vongpakorn, B. Nuansrichay, N. Autarkool, T. Keowkarnkah, P. Rodtian, R. W. Stich, and S. Jittapalpong.** 2007. Diagnosis of a *Trypanosoma lewisi*-like (*Herpetosoma*) infection in a sick infant from Thailand. *J. Med. Microbiol.* **56:**1118–1121.

87. **Schmid, C., M. Richer, C. M. M. Bilenge, T. Josenando, F. Chappuis, C. R. Manthelot, A. Nangouma, F. Doua, P. N. Asumu, P. P. Simarro, and C. Burri.** 2005. Effectiveness of a 10-day melarsoprol schedule for the treatment of late-stage human African trypanosomiasis: confirmation from a multinational study (IMPAMEL II). *J. Infect. Dis.* **191:**1922–1931.

88. **Schraner, C., B. Hasse, U. Hasse, D. Baumann, A. Faeh, G. Burg, F. Grimm, A. Mathis, R. Weber, and H. F. Gunthard.** 2005. Successful treatment with miltefosine of disseminated cutaneous leishmaniasis in a severely immunocompromised patient infected with HIV-1. *Clin. Infect. Dis.* **40:**120–124.

89. **Silveira, F. T., R. Lainson, and C. E. P. Corbett.** 2004. Clinical and immunopathological spectrum of American cutaneous leishmaniasis with special reference to the disease in Amazonian Brazil: a review. *Mem. Inst. Oswaldo Cruz* **99:**239–251.

90. **Simarro, P. P., J. A. Ruiz, J. R. Franco, and T. Josenando.** 1999. Attitude towards CATT-positive individuals without parasitological confirmation in the African trypanosomiasis (*T. b. gambiense*) focus of Quicama (Angola). *Trop. Med. Int. Health* **4:**858–861.

91. **Soto, J., J. Toledo, J. Vega, and J. Berman.** 2005. Short report: efficacy of pentavalent antimony for treatment of Colombian cutaneous leishmaniasis. *Am. J. Trop. Med. Hyg.* **72:**421–422.

92. **Sreenivas, G., B. V. S. Raju, R. Singh, A. Selvapandiyan, R. Duncan, D. Sarkar, H. L. Nakhasi, and P. Salotra.** 2004. DNA polymorphism assay distinguishes isolates of *Leishmania donovani* that cause kala-azar from those that cause post-kala-azar dermal leishmaniasis in humans. *J. Clin. Microbiol.* **42:**1739–1741.

93. **Strout, R. G.** 1962. A method for concentrating haemoflagellates. *J. Parasitol.* **48:**100.

94. **Theis, J. H.** 1990. Latin American immigrants-blood donation and *Trypanosoma cruzi* transmission. *Am. Heart J.* **120:**1483–1484.

95. **Toz, S. O., K. P. Chang, Y. Ozbel, and M. Z. Alkan.** 2004. Diagnostic value of RK39 dipstick in zoonotic visceral leishmaniasis in Turkey. *J. Parasitol.* **90:**1484–1486.

96. **Trudel, N., R. Garg, N. Messier, S. Sundar, M. Quellette, and M. J. Tremblay.** 2008. Intracellular survival of *Leishmania* spp. that cause visceral leishmaniasis is significantly reduced by HIV-1 protease inhibitors. *J. Infect. Dis.* **198:**1292–1298.

97. **Unger, A., S. O'Neal, P. R. L. Machado, L. H. Guimaraes, D. J. Morgan, A. Schriefer, O. Bacellar, M. J. Glesby, and E. M. Carvalho.** 2009. Association of treatment of American cutaneous leishmaniasis prior to ulcer development with high rate of failure in Northeastern Brazil. *Am. J. Trop. Med Hyg.* **80:**574–579.

98. **van der Snoek, E. M., D. J. Robinson, J. J. van Hellemond, and H. A. M. Neumann.** 2008. A review of photodynamic therapy in cutaneous leishmaniasis. *J. Eur. Acad. Dermatol. Venereol.* **22:**918–922.

99. **Vergel, C., J. Walker, and N. G. Saravia.** 2005. Amplification of human DNA by primers targeted to *Leishmania* kinetoplast DNA and post-genome considerations in the detection of parasites by a polymerase chain reaction. *Am. J. Trop. Med. Hyg.* **72:**423–429.

100. **Volpini, A. C., V. M. A. Passos, G. C. Oliveira, and A. J. Romanha.** 2004. PCR-RFLP to identify *Leishmania* (*Viannia*) *brasiliensis* and *L.* (*Leishmania*) *amazonensis* causing American cutaneous leishmaniasis. *Acta Trop.* **90:**31–37.

101. **Welch, R. J., B. L. Anderson, and C. M. Litwin.** 2008. Rapid immunochromatographic strip test for detection of anti-K39 immunoglobulin G antibodies for diagnosis of visceral leishmaniasis. *Clin. Vaccine Immunol.* **15:**1483–1484.

102. **Wilson, M. E., S. M. B. Jeronimo, and R. D. Pearson.** 2005. Immunopathogensis of infection with the visceralizing *Leishmania* species. *Microb. Pathog.* **38:**147–160.

103. **World Health Organization.** 2005. A new form of human trypanosomiasis in India. *Wkly. Epidemiol. Rec.* **80:**62–63.

104. **Wright, N. A., L. E. Davis, K. S. Aftergut, C. A. Parrish, and C. J. Cockerell.** 2008. Cutaneous leishmaniasis in Texas: a northern spread of endemic areas. *J. Am. Acad. Dermatol.* **58:**650–652.

105. **Zelazny, A. M., D. P. Fedorko, L. Li, E. A. Neva, and S. H. Fischer.** 2005. Evaluation of 7SL RNA gene sequences for the identification of *Leishmania* spp. *Am. J. Trop. Med. Hyg.* **72:**415–420.

106. **Zulantay, I., W. Apt, L. C. Gil, C. Rocha, K. Mundaca, A. Solari, G. Sanchez, C. Rodriguez, G. Martinez, L. M. de Pablos, L. Sandoval, J. Rodriguez, S. Vilchez, and A. Osuna.** 2007. The PCR-based detection of *Trypanosoma cruzi* in the faeces of *Triatoma infestans* fed on patients with chronic American trypanosomiasis gives higher sensitivity and a quicker result than routine xenodiagnosis. *Ann. Trop. Med. Parasitol.* **101:**673–679.

Toxoplasma*

JAMES B. McAULEY, JEFFREY L. JONES, AND KAMALJIT SINGH

135

Toxoplasma gondii is a protozoan parasite that infects most species of warm-blooded animals, including humans. Members of the cat family, Felidae, are the only known definitive hosts for the sexual stages of *T. gondii* and thus are the main reservoirs of infection. The three stages of this obligate intracellular parasite are: (i) tachyzoites (trophozoites), which rapidly proliferate and destroy infected cells during acute infection; (ii) bradyzoites, which slowly multiply in tissue cysts; and (iii) sporozoites in oocysts (Fig. 1). Tachyzoites and bradyzoites occur in body tissues; oocysts are excreted in cat feces. Cats become infected with *T. gondii* by carnivorism or by ingestion of oocysts. Cats that are allowed to roam outside are much more likely to become infected than domestic cats that are confined indoors. After tissue cysts or oocysts are ingested by the cat, viable organisms are released and invade epithelial cells of the small intestine where they undergo an asexual cycle followed by a sexual cycle and then form oocysts, which are then excreted. The unsporulated (i.e., uninfective) oocyst takes 1 to 5 days after excretion to become sporulated (infective). Although cats shed oocysts for only 1 to 2 weeks, large numbers may be shed, often exceeding 100,000 per g of feces. Oocysts can survive in the environment for several months to more than a year and are remarkably resistant to disinfectants, freezing, and drying but are killed by heating to 70°C for 10 min (84).

TAXONOMY

Toxoplasma gondii is included in the phylum Apicomplexa, class Conoidasida, subclass Coccidiasina, order Eucoccidiorida, suborder Eimeriorina, family Sarcocystidae (*Sarcocystis*), subfamily Toxoplasmatinae, genus *Toxoplasma*.

EPIDEMIOLOGY AND TRANSMISSION

Serologic prevalence data indicate that toxoplasmosis is one of the most common infections of humans throughout the world. Because *T. gondii* organisms are rarely detected in humans with toxoplasmosis, serologic examination is used to indicate the presence of the infection by detecting *Toxoplasma*-specific antibodies. The prevalence of positive serologic titers increases with age. In many areas of the world, infection is more common in warm climates and at lower altitudes than in cold climates and mountainous regions. This distribution is probably related to conditions favoring the sporulation and survival of oocysts. Variations in the prevalence of infection between geographic areas and between population groups within the same locale are also probably due to differences in exposure. A high prevalence of infection in France (50 to 85%) has been related to a preference for eating raw or undercooked meat. However, a high prevalence in Central America has been related to the frequency of stray cats in a climate favoring the survival of oocysts. In U.S. military recruits in 1962, seroprevalence rates of up to 30% were found in people living along the sea coast, with rates of less than 1% in the Rocky Mountains and the desert Southwest. More recent data comparing antibody prevalence in U.S. military recruits in 1962 and 1989 indicated a one-third decrease in seropositivity (100). The overall seroprevalence in the United States as determined with specimens collected by the Third National Health and Nutritional Assessment Survey between 1988 and 1994 among persons 12 or more years of age was found to be 22.5%, and the seroprevalence among women of childbearing age (15 to 44 years) was 15% (52). More recently, in analysis of National Health and Nutritional Assessment Survey data, *T. gondii* seroprevalence was shown to decline in U.S.-born persons 12 to 49 years old from 14.1% in 1988 to 1994 to 9.0% in 1999 to 2004 (51).

Human infection may be acquired in several ways: (i) ingestion of undercooked contaminated meat containing *T. gondii* cysts; (ii) ingestion of oocysts from food, soil, or water contaminated with cat feces; (iii) organ transplantation or blood transfusion; (iv) transplacental transmission; and (v) accidental inoculation of tachyzoites. The two major routes of transmission of *Toxoplasma* to humans are oral and congenital. In humans, ingesting either the tissue cyst or the oocyst results in the rupture of the cyst wall, which releases organisms that invade the intestinal epithelium, disseminate throughout the body, and multiply intracellularly. The host cell dies and releases tachyzoites, which invade adjacent cells and continue the process. The tachyzoites are pressured by the host's immune response to transform into bradyzoites and form tissue cysts, most commonly in skeletal muscle, myocardium, and brain; these cysts may remain throughout the life of the host.

*We acknowledge the contribution of Marianna Wilson to the *Toxoplasma* chapter in previous editions of this *Manual*; much of it has been retained in the current chapter.

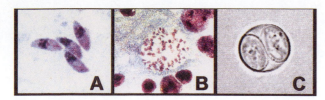

FIGURE 1 Three life stages of *T. gondii*. (A) Tachyzoites, Giemsa stain; (B) cyst with bradyzoites in brain tissue, Giemsa stain; (C) sporulated oocysts, unstained. (Photographs courtesy of J. P. Dubey, U.S. Department of Agriculture, Beltsville, MD.)

Recrudescence of clinical disease may occur if the host becomes immunosuppressed and the cysts rupture, releasing the parasites.

Prevention

Risk factors for *T. gondii* infection identified in epidemiologic studies include eating raw or undercooked pork, mutton, lamb, beef, minced meat products, oysters, clams, mussels, and wild game meat; kitten ownership; cleaning the cat litter box; contact with soil (gardening and yard work); and eating raw or unwashed vegetables or fruits (2, 50, 52, 53). Recommendations for prevention of toxoplasmosis in pregnant women were discussed at a conference at the Centers for Disease Control and Prevention and published (8). These recommendations included the following: (i) food should be cooked to safe temperatures (beef, lamb, and veal roasts and steaks to at least 145°F; pork, ground meat, and wild game to 160°F; poultry to 180°F); (ii) fruits and vegetables should be peeled or washed thoroughly before eating; (iii) cutting boards, dishes, counters, utensils, and hands should always be washed with hot soapy water after they have contacted raw meat, poultry, seafood, or unwashed fruits or vegetables; (iv) pregnant women should wear gloves when gardening and during any contact with soil or sand because cat waste might be in soil or sand and should wash their hands afterwards; (v) pregnant women should avoid changing cat litter if possible. If no one else is available to change the cat litter, pregnant women should use gloves and then wash their hands thoroughly. The litter box should be changed daily because *T. gondii* oocysts require more than 1 day to become infectious. Pregnant women should be encouraged to keep their cats inside and not adopt or handle stray cats. Cats should be fed only canned or dried commercial food or well-cooked table food, not raw or undercooked meats.

CLINICAL SIGNIFICANCE

Toxoplasmosis can be categorized into four groups: (i) acquired in the immunocompetent patient; (ii) acquired or reactivated in the immunodeficient patient; (iii) congenital; and (iv) ocular. Methods of diagnosis and their interpretations may differ for each clinical category.

Acquired infection with *Toxoplasma* in immunocompetent individuals is generally an asymptomatic infection. However, 10 to 20% of patients with acute infection may develop cervical lymphadenopathy and/or a flu-like illness. The clinical course is benign and self-limited; symptoms usually resolve within weeks to months.

Immunodeficient patients often have central nervous system (CNS) disease but may have myocarditis or pneumonitis. In patients with AIDS, toxoplasmic encephalitis is the most common cause of intracerebral mass lesions and is thought to be due to reactivation of chronic infection. Toxoplasmosis in patients being treated with immunosuppressive drugs may be due to either newly acquired or reactivated latent infection (98).

Congenital toxoplasmosis results from an acute primary infection acquired by the mother during pregnancy. The incidence and severity of congenital toxoplasmosis vary with the trimester during which infection was acquired. Because treatment of the mother may reduce the severity of symptoms in the infant due to congenital infection, prompt and accurate diagnosis is extremely important. Many infants with subclinical infection at birth will subsequently develop signs or symptoms of congenital toxoplasmosis; however, treatment may help prevent subsequent symptoms.

Ocular toxoplasmosis, an important cause of chorioretinitis in the United States, may be the result of congenital or acquired infection. Acquired infection is now thought to be more common than congenital infection. Congenitally infected patients are often asymptomatic until the second or third decade of life, when lesions develop in the eye, presumably due to cyst rupture and subsequent release of tachyzoites and bradyzoites. Chorioretinitis is characteristically bilateral in patients with congenital infection but is often unilateral in individuals with acute acquired *T. gondii* infection.

In general, physicians treat *T. gondii* infection in four circumstances: (i) pregnant women with acute infection to prevent fetal infection (14, 30, 35); (ii) congenitally infected infants (38, 63); (iii) immune-suppressed persons, usually with reactivated disease (7, 9, 98, 101); and (iv) acute and recurrent ocular disease (45, 46). Drugs are also prescribed for preventive or suppressive treatment in human immunodeficiency virus (HIV)-infected persons (7, 9). The currently recommended drugs work primarily against the actively dividing tachyzoite form of *T. gondii* and do not eradicate encysted organisms (bradyzoites).

COLLECTION, TRANSPORT, AND STORAGE OF SPECIMENS

Serum, plasma, cerebrospinal fluid (CSF), ocular fluid, and amniotic fluid may be tested for antibodies and/or parasite DNA.

Collection for Determination of Parasite DNA

Blood samples should be collected with an anticoagulant; CSF, ocular fluid, and amniotic fluids do not need an anticoagulant. All samples should be shipped and stored at 4°C prior to testing.

Collection for Antibody Determination

Blood specimens to be tested for the presence of antibodies should be allowed to clot and centrifuged, and the serum should be removed and shipped to a reference laboratory. Hemolysis does not seem to interfere with the antibody reaction in most tests. Serum and CSF specimens may be stored for several days at 4°C or frozen for longer storage. Specimens may be shipped at ambient temperature unless they will be in transit for more than 1 week or will be subjected to temperatures above 30°C. To avoid evaporation of small volumes, ocular fluids should be stored and shipped frozen. CSF and ocular fluid should be tested in parallel with a serum sample drawn on the same date. Long-term storage should take place at −20°C or below.

If the determination of immune status is the reason for testing, a single serum specimen is satisfactory; acute- and convalescent-phase specimens are not necessary. In situations in which determining the time of infection is important, specimens drawn at least 3 weeks apart may or may not be useful. In most cases, detection of an increasing immunoglobulin G (IgG) or IgM titer is not possible because the titers have already reached a plateau by the time the initial sample is drawn. If two specimens are to be compared, they should be tested together. Results from tests done at different times, in different laboratories, or with different procedures should not be compared quantitatively, only qualitatively, as positive or negative.

For tests other than serology, contact a reference laboratory for instructions *before* collecting specimens to ensure proper collection and handling.

DIRECT EXAMINATION

Microscopy
Only very rarely can the diagnosis of toxoplasmosis be documented by the observation of parasites in patient specimens (31, 77). Secretions, excretions, body fluids, and tissues are potential specimens for direct observation of parasites but are generally unrewarding. Fluid specimens such as heparinized blood or CSF should be centrifuged, and the sediment should be smeared on a microscope slide. The slides should be air dried, fixed in methanol, and stained with Giemsa for microscopic examination. Tachyzoites may be observed as free organisms or within host cells such as leukocytes. Well-preserved tachyzoites are crescent shaped and stain well, but degenerating organisms may be oval and stain poorly. Tissue imprints stained with Giemsa may reveal *T. gondii* cysts.

Antigen Detection
Immunologic techniques have been used to identify parasites in tissue sections or tissue cultures; fluorescein isothiocyanate- or peroxidase-labeled antisera may be useful in detecting tachyzoites in tissue sections. Enzyme immunoassay (EIA) antigen detection techniques lack sensitivity for human samples and are not recommended.

Nucleic Acid Detection
PCR technology for *Toxoplasma* has been used to detect congenital infections, toxoplasmic encephalitis in AIDS patients, and ocular disease with various degrees of success (1, 20, 23, 25, 48). The most important use of PCR appears to be in the prenatal diagnosis of congenital toxoplasmosis using amniotic fluid. When maternal serological results indicate potential infection during pregnancy, PCR of amniotic fluid has been shown to be more sensitive for the confirmation of fetal infection than the conventional methods of inoculation of mice and tissue culture cells and fetal blood testing for IgM (29, 43). PCR technology for *Toxoplasma* is offered at the Toxoplasma Serology Laboratory, Palo Alto Medical Foundation, Palo Alto, CA [phone, (650) 853-4828; http://www.pamf.org/serology/], and by a few commercial laboratories. Commercial kits are not yet available. The most common PCR targets include 18S ribosomal DNA and the B1 and AF146257 genes. The requestor should be aware that the reliability of PCR tests may vary widely (1, 39, 66, 67, 68). PCR testing by low-density microarrays has recently been used successfully in the evaluation of granulomatous lymphadenitis (75).

Cell-Mediated Immune Responses
T-cell response has been studied in newborns with congenital toxoplasmosis. A recent study has suggested that measurement of gamma interferon production by T cells in response to stimulation by specific *Toxoplasma* antigens may add to the diagnosis of congenital infection (11), but an assay is not yet commercially available.

ISOLATION AND IDENTIFICATION
Parasites can be isolated with limited success by inoculating patient tissue or body fluids into either mice or tissue culture cells. Fresh tissue samples are ground in saline with a mortar and pestle and inoculated intraperitoneally into mice or directly into tissue culture flasks. The mice should be monitored for 4 to 6 weeks; if the organism is virulent for mice, the parasites can often be demonstrated in the peritoneal fluid after 5 to 10 days. However, if the organism is relatively avirulent for mice, as is usually the case, the mice may not be killed by the infection. If they survive for 6 weeks, serum samples should be obtained for serologic testing. If antibodies are present, the mouse brain should be examined for the presence of *T. gondii* cysts. If cysts are not observed, the murine host may not have been the ideal host. Inoculate additional mice with brain homogenate from the initially inoculated mice and observe and recheck after 6 weeks. *T. gondii* grows in a variety of tissue culture cells. A cytopathic effect may be detected on direct examination after 24 to 96 h in culture. Giemsa staining may reveal parasite structure, but parasitized cells may be difficult to detect. Immunofluorescence allows more sensitive detection of the organisms. The following procedure has been used with some success for parasite isolation from amniotic fluid (19). Centrifuge a 10-ml sample of amniotic fluid at $1,000 \times g$. Resuspend the sediment in 8 ml of minimum essential medium. Inoculate 1 ml into coverslip cultures of human embryonic fibroblast cell line MRC5 in 24-well plates. Incubate the cultures for 96 h with one change of medium at 24 h; fix the cultures with cold acetone. Examine the coverslips by indirect immunofluorescence for the presence of *T. gondii*. The use of tissue culture cells for isolation permits a more rapid diagnosis than mouse inoculation; both methods can be useful for diagnosing congenital toxoplasmosis.

SEROLOGIC TESTS
Serologic testing for *T. gondii*-specific antibodies is the most commonly used method for diagnosis of toxoplasmosis. Many tests for the detection of antibodies to *Toxoplasma* have been used since Sabin and Feldman developed the methylene blue dye test (DT) (68, 84). Commercial kits for agglutination tests, indirect fluorescent antibody (IFA) tests, and EIAs are available worldwide. Because of difficulties in obtaining specimens from patients with clinically documented toxoplasmosis, commercial kit sensitivity and specificity may not be based on documented case specimens but rather on a comparison of results obtained with another kit. Consequently, the true sensitivity and specificity of a kit are generally not known or determined. The rates stated by the manufacturer or published in articles may vary depending upon the samples chosen for testing. Sensitivity and specificity rates determined in prospective studies, when random samples are tested as received for *Toxoplasma* testing, will usually differ from those determined in retrospective studies, when the samples have been chosen as potential problem samples to increase the probability of detecting false-positive or false-negative reactions.

When laboratory personnel decide to initiate *Toxoplasma*-specific antibody testing or when they decide to switch to a different antibody detection kit, the user must carefully review the manufacturer's package insert and published literature for information on the sensitivity and specificity rates. The user should perform an in-laboratory comparison of kits by using positive and negative samples confirmed by a toxoplasmosis reference laboratory. Tables 1 and 2 list commercial kits currently available in the United States and references to published evaluations. However, the test kit industry is in a great deal of flux; company and kit names may change.

In the United States, initial testing for the presence of IgG antibodies in most laboratories is usually performed with an EIA or IFA commercial kit. Results may be stated in international units (based on the WHO international standard reference serum for *Toxoplasma* [62, 68, 86] distributed by the Health Protection Agency, Toxoplasma Reference Laboratory, Singleton Hospital, Swansea SA2 8QA, Wales, United Kingdom; http://www.hpa.org.uk/ProductsServices/InfectiousDiseases/LaboratoriesAndReferenceFacilities/ToxplasmaReferenceLaboratory/), as an index (specific to each kit), as an optical density value (specific to each kit), or as a geometric mean titer. Numerical results are not comparable from kit to kit; comparison may be made only qualitatively as negative (nonreactive or not infected) or positive (reactive or infected). Although elevated *Toxoplasma*-specific IgG levels have been suggested as an indicator of recent infection, high levels may last for many years after primary infection and should not be relied upon for this purpose.

To more definitely distinguish acute and chronic infections, detection of *Toxoplasma*-specific IgM antibodies has been used. The most important use of IgM test results is that a negative reaction essentially excludes recent infection. A guide to the general interpretation of *Toxoplasma* IgG and IgM serology results is presented in Table 3. IFA IgM titers generally increase within 1 week of the onset of symptoms and revert to negative within 6 to 9 months of infection. False-positive reactions caused by rheumatoid factor and false-negative reactions caused by blockage by *Toxoplasma*-specific IgG may occur in IFA IgM and indirect EIA for IgM when whole-serum samples are tested. To decrease the effects of these interfering factors, specimens should be treated to obtain only the IgM fraction for testing.

The IgM capture EIA eliminates potential interference by IgG and other isotypes by binding only IgM antibodies; unbound antibodies are removed by washing, thus eliminating the need for serum fractionation. The most important advantage of the IgM capture EIA compared to IFA is the increased detection of congenital infections: the IgM ELISA was positive for 73% of serum samples from newborn infants with proven congenital toxoplasmosis, whereas only 25% of the same serum samples were found positive by an IFA IgM test (74). Although the capture EIA system is more efficient at detecting acute infections, some persons may have undetectable or low level IgM

TABLE 1 *Toxoplasma* IgG kits available commercially in the United States

Type of test and manufacturer[a]	Kit	Reference(s)
IFA		
GenBio	ImmunoFA Toxoplasma IgG	
Hemagen	Virgo Toxo IgG	
Inverness	Toxoplasma IgG	
Meridian	Toxoplasma IgG	
EIA		
Abbott Laboratories	IMx Toxo IgG	17, 32, 40, 42, 57, 83
	AxSYM Toxo IgG	22, 36, 79, 95
Bayer Diagnostics	Immuno1	83
	Advia Centaur	76
Beckman Coulter	Access Toxo G	17
bioMérieux Vitek	Vidas Toxo IgG	32, 36, 42, 79, 95, 104
Bio-Rad	Platelia Toxo G	42, 79
Biotecx	OptiCoat Toxo IgG ELISA	
Biotest Diagnostics	Toxo IgG	
Diagnostic Products Corp.	Immulite Toxoplasma IgG	22, 27, 104
Diamedix	Toxoplasma IgG	
DiaSorin	Toxoplasma IgG	
	Liaison	99
GenBio	ImmunoDOT TORCH	
Hemagen	Toxoplasma IgG	
Inverness	Toxo IgG II	
Roche Diagnostics	Elecsys Toxo IgG	
Trinity Biotech	Captia Toxoplasma gondii IgG	
Latex		
Biokit	Toxogen	

[a] Abbott Laboratories, Diagnostics Division, North Chicago, IL 60064; Bayer Diagnostics, 511 Benedict Ave., Tarrytown, NY 10591; Beckman Coulter, 4300 N. Harbor Blvd., Fullerton, CA 92834; Biokit USA, 113 Hartwell Ave., Lexington, MA 02173; bioMérieux, 595 Anglum Dr., Hazlewood, MO 63042; Bio-Rad, 4000 Alfred Nobel Dr., Hercules, CA 94547; Biotecx Laboratories, 6023 S. Loop East, Houston, TX 77033; Biotest Diagnostics Corp., 66 Ford Rd., Suite 131, Denville, NJ 07834; Diagnostic Products Corp., 5700 W. 96th St., Los Angeles, CA 90045; Diamedix Corp., 2140 N. Miami Ave., Miami, FL 33127; DiaSorin, P.O. Box 285, Stillwater, MN 55082; GenBio, 15222 A Avenue of Science, San Diego, CA 92128; Hemagen Diagnostics, 34–40 Bear Hill Rd., Waltham, MA 02154; Inverness Medical Professional Diagnostics, 2 Research Way, Princeton, NJ 08540; Meridian Bioscience, 3471 River Hills Dr., Cincinnati, OH 45244; Roche Diagnostics Corp., 9115 Hague Rd., Indianapolis, IN 46250.

TABLE 2 *Toxoplasma* IgM kits available commercially in the United States

Type of test and manufacturer[a]	Kit	Reference(s)
IFA		
GenBio	ImmunoFA Toxoplasma IgM	
Hemagen	VIRGO Toxo IgM	
Inverness	Toxoplasma gondii IgM	
Meridian	Toxoplasma IgM	
EIA		
Abbott Laboratories	IMx Toxo IgM	18, 42, 57, 61, 106
	AxSYM Toxo IgM	17, 36, 79
Bayer Diagnostics	Immuno1	
	Advia Centaur	76
Beckman Coulter	Access Toxo M	17, 18, 26, 59
bioMérieux Vitek	Vidas Toxo IgM	5, 17, 36, 42, 79, 106
Bio-Rad	Platelia Toxo IgM	18, 42, 58, 79, 106
Biotecx	OptiCoat Toxo IgM	
Biotest Diagnostics	Toxo IgM	
Diagnostic Products Corp.	Immulite	27, 104
Diamedix	Toxoplasma IgM	99
DiaSorin	Toxoplasma IgM	
	Liaison	79
Hemagen	Toxoplasma IgM	
Trinity Biotech	Captia Toxoplasma gondii IgM	
Inverness	Toxo IgM	

[a]For company addresses, see Table 1, footnote *a*.

antibodies, and some persons may have detectable IgM antibodies beyond 2 years postinfection (37). Therefore, determining the relative time of infection is not possible with this system alone. Many commercial companies market an EIA kit for IgM: some use the indirect EIA format with a serum pretreatment step, while others use the IgM capture format. False-positive IgM reactions due to unknown factors may be a problem with commercially available kits (106).

The *Toxoplasma* IgG avidity test is an additional tool to help discriminate between past and recently acquired infection (4, 11, 48, 68, 71, 80, 85). The test is based on the observation that, during acute infection, IgG antibodies bind antigen weakly or have low avidity, while patients with chronic infection have more strongly binding (high-avidity) antibodies. Depending on the method used, a high avidity result indicates infection acquired more than 3 to 5 months before. However, a low avidity result does not indicate a recently acquired infection because low-avidity antibodies may be detectable for a year postinfection. Commercial kits are not available in the United States but are available in other countries from Ani Labsystems (3), bioMérieux (48, 69), and DiaSorin (79). Additional refinements to the avidity testing have been recently reported using specific recombinant antigens rather than whole-organism IgG; however, these are not yet commercially available (44, 80).

Other tests may be of assistance in determining current infection. Assays for *Toxoplasma*-specific IgA antibodies

TABLE 3 Guide to general interpretation of *Toxoplasma* serology results obtained with IgG and IgM commercial assays

IgG result	IgM result	Report or interpretation for humans except infants
Negative	Negative	No serological evidence of infection with *Toxoplasma*
Negative	Equivocal	Possible early acute infection or false-positive IgM reaction. Obtain a new specimen for IgG and IgM testing. If results for the second specimen remain the same, the patient is probably not infected with *Toxoplasma*.
Negative	Positive	Possible acute infection or false-positive IgM result. Obtain a new specimen for IgG and IgM testing. If results for the second specimen remain the same, the IgM reaction is probably a false positive.
Equivocal	Negative	Indeterminate: obtain a new specimen for testing or retest this specimen for IgG in a different assay
Equivocal	Equivocal	Indeterminate: obtain a new specimen for both IgG and IgM testing
Equivocal	Positive	Possible acute infection with *Toxoplasma*. Obtain a new specimen for IgG and IgM testing. If results for the second specimen remain the same or if the IgG becomes positive, both specimens should be sent to a reference laboratory with experience in the diagnosis of toxoplasmosis for further testing.
Positive	Negative	Infected with *Toxoplasma* for more than 1 year
Positive	Equivocal	Infected with *Toxoplasma* for probably more than 1 year or false-positive IgM reaction. Obtain a new specimen for IgM testing. If results with the second specimen remain the same, both specimens should be sent to a reference laboratory with experience in the diagnosis of toxoplasmosis for further testing.
Positive	Positive	Possible recent infection within the last 12 months or false-positive IgM reaction. Send the specimen to a reference laboratory with experience in the diagnosis of toxoplasmosis for further testing.

should always be performed in addition to IgM assays for newborns with suspected congenital infection (6, 16, 105). Results of IgA testing in adults have been less consistent (96). The presence of *Toxoplasma*-specific IgE antibodies may also contribute to the determination of acute infections, although reports of the utility of IgE antibody detection have been mixed (28, 55). Immunoblot assays may be useful in determining congenital infections (81) and ocular infections (87). These and other assays (66, 68, 70) are available in the United States at the Toxoplasma Serology Laboratory (see "Nucleic Acid Detection" above) and at many of the *Toxoplasma* reference laboratories in Europe.

A guideline for the clinical use and interpretation of serologic tests for *Toxoplasma gondii* was published (12) by the Clinical and Laboratory Standards Institute and is available for purchase on its website at http://www.clsi.org.

CLINICAL USE OF IMMUNODIAGNOSTIC TESTS

There are four groups of patients for whom diagnosis of toxoplasmosis is critical: pregnant women with infection during gestation, congenitally infected newborns, patients with chorioretinitis, and immunosuppressed individuals.

Determination of Immune Status

An algorithm for serological testing for immune status and acute acquired infection is shown in Fig. 2. Three situations in which baseline information about an individual's immune status would be useful include the following: (i) before

conception, (ii) before receiving immunosuppressive therapy, and (iii) after the initial determination of positive HIV type 1 status. Screening one serum specimen with a sensitive test for IgG antibodies, such as DT, IFA, or EIA, is sufficient. A negative test result indicates that the patient has not been infected. A positive result of any degree indicates infection with *T. gondii* at some undetermined time.

Diagnosis of Acute Acquired Infections

If an acute acquired infection is suspected, the patient's serum specimen should be tested for the presence of *Toxoplasma*-specific antibodies (Fig. 2). A negative result in DT, IgG IFA test, or IgG EIA essentially excludes the diagnosis of acute *Toxoplasma* infection in an immunocompetent person. Demonstration of seroconversion from a negative titer to a positive titer or of more than a fourfold increase in titer confirms the diagnosis of recent infection when specimens drawn several weeks apart are tested in parallel with the same test. However, such situations are rare because specimens are usually drawn after titers have peaked, too late to observe titer changes after initial infection. The presence of typical lymphadenopathy suggestive of acute toxoplasmosis, the presence of a high DT or IgG IFA titer (≥300 IU/ml or ≥1:1,000), and the presence of specific IgM are indicative of acute infection (65, 69, 72). If the patient has clinical illness compatible with toxoplasmosis but the IgG titer is low, a follow-up test 3 weeks later should show an increase in the antibody titer if the illness is due to acute toxoplasmosis and the host is not severely immunosuppressed.

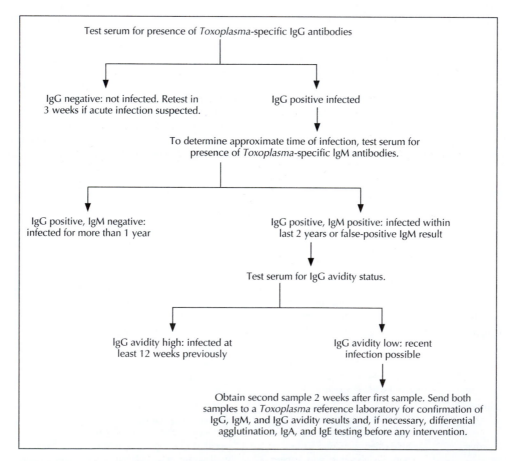

FIGURE 2 Algorithm for the serodiagnosis of toxoplasmosis in people greater than 1 year of age.

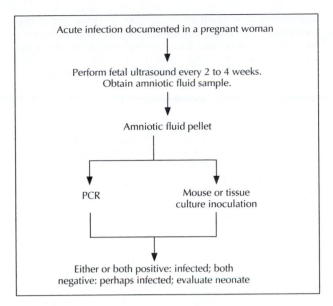

Acute infection documented in a pregnant woman

↓

Perform fetal ultrasound every 2 to 4 weeks.
Obtain amniotic fluid sample.

↓

Amniotic fluid pellet

PCR   Mouse or tissue
             culture inoculation

↓

Either or both positive: infected; both
negative: perhaps infected; evaluate neonate

FIGURE 3 Algorithm for the antenatal diagnosis of congenital toxoplasmosis.

Results of an EIA for IgM and an IgG avidity assay can provide additional evidence for or against acute infection when IgG antibodies are present (68, 71, 90). A negative IgM test essentially rules out infection in the previous 6 months. A positive IgM titer combined with a positive IgG titer may be suggestive of acute infection, due to persistent IgM antibodies, or may be a false-positive reaction.

Diagnosis during Pregnancy

Congenital toxoplasmosis occurs when a woman passes the infection to her fetus after acquiring a primary infection during pregnancy or, more rarely, when a pregnant woman is immunocompromised and a previously acquired infection is reactivated (84). The rate of transmission of infection to the fetus ranges from 11% in the first trimester to 90% in the late third trimester, with an overall transmission rate of approximately 40 to 50%. In France and Austria, the prevention, diagnosis, and treatment of congenital toxoplasmosis begin with mandatory serologic testing of all women before or soon after conception. Although the cost-effectiveness of adopting this approach for all pregnant women in the United States has not been established, this approach does serve as a model for managing individual pregnant patients (14, 41, 43, 82).

Immunocompetent women who have IgG antibody before conception are considered immune and so at very little risk for transmission of infection to the fetus. Women who are seronegative are considered at risk for infection and in France are tested monthly during pregnancy for IgG antibody. If a woman is first tested after conception and has *Toxoplasma*-specific IgG antibodies, IgM and IgG avidity testing should be done to determine if acute infection has occurred during pregnancy (90) (Fig. 2). A high-avidity result in the first 12 weeks of pregnancy essentially rules out an infection acquired during gestation. A low IgG avidity result cannot be used as an indicator of recent infection, because some individuals have persistent low IgG avidity for many months after infection. Immunodiagnosis of acute infection in a pregnant woman should be confirmed by a toxoplasmosis reference laboratory prior to intervention (54, 56, 66, 68).

When the diagnosis of acute toxoplasmosis has been made in a pregnant woman, she can be treated and the fetus can be tested for evidence of infection. The strategy used by Daffos et al. (14) involved initiating treatment with spiramycin once acute maternal infection was indicated and then obtaining amniotic fluid and fetal blood samples between 20 and 26 weeks of gestation for testing (Fig. 3). Amniotic fluid PCR (at 18 weeks gestation or later) is the recommended test of choice to establish the intrauterine diagnosis of congenital toxoplasmosis (66, 91, 92, 103). In addition, fetal ultrasound examinations were performed every 2 to 4 weeks until delivery to search for several nonspecific signs of infection: cerebral or hepatic calcifications, hydrocephalus, hepatomegaly, or ascites.

If collected, fetal blood should be tested for *Toxoplasma*-specific IgG, IgM, and IgA antibodies. Clotted blood should be inoculated into mice or tissue culture cells to demonstrate parasitemia. Nonspecific markers of infection should be tested for; these include leukocytes, eosinophils, platelets, total IgM, gamma-glutamyltransferase, and lactate dehydrogenase. Most infected fetuses have one or more abnormal nonspecific tests, most commonly an elevated total IgM level or an elevated gamma-glutamyltransferase level (14, 41, 81, 82). Demonstrating *Toxoplasma*-specific IgM or IgA antibodies in fetal serum or isolating the parasite from fetal leukocytes is a definitive diagnosis of fetal infection.

Diagnosis in the Newborn

Diagnosis of *Toxoplasma* infection in the newborn is made through a combination of serologic testing, parasite isolation, and nonspecific findings (63, 73, 81, 82, 89). An attempt should be made to isolate *T. gondii* from the placenta, amniotic fluid, and cord blood if the diagnosis has not already been established (Fig. 4). *T. gondii* has been isolated from 95% of the placentas of congenitally infected newborns when the mother has not been treated and from approximately 81% when the mother has been treated. However, *T. gondii* can be isolated from the placentas of uninfected newborns as well. The child's serum should be tested for total IgG and IgM antibody levels and *Toxoplasma*-specific IgG, IgM, and IgA antibodies. CSF should be analyzed for cells, glucose, protein, total IgG antibody, and *Toxoplasma*-specific IgG and IgM antibodies and directly examined for *T. gondii* tachyzoites. A child suspected of having congenital toxoplasmosis should have a thorough general, neurologic, and ophthalmologic examination and a computed tomographic scan of the head (magnetic resonance imaging does not demonstrate calcifications). Because the diagnosis can

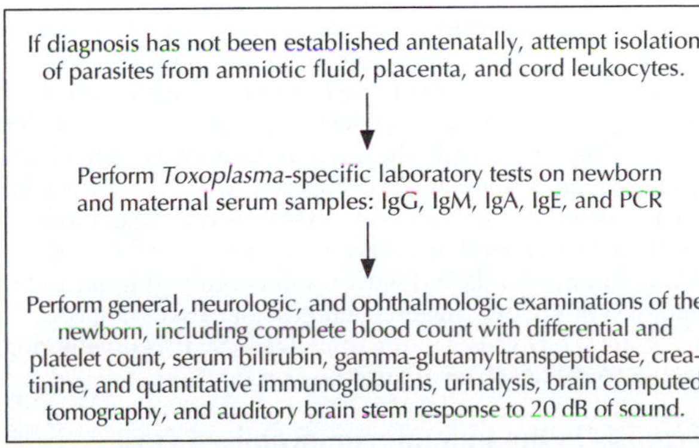

If diagnosis has not been established antenatally, attempt isolation of parasites from amniotic fluid, placenta, and cord leukocytes.

↓

Perform *Toxoplasma*-specific laboratory tests on newborn and maternal serum samples: IgG, IgM, IgA, IgE, and PCR

↓

Perform general, neurologic, and ophthalmologic examinations of the newborn, including complete blood count with differential and platelet count, serum bilirubin, gamma-glutamyltranspeptidase, creatinine, and quantitative immunoglobulins, urinalysis, brain computed tomography, and auditory brain stem response to 20 dB of sound.

FIGURE 4 Algorithm for the diagnosis of neonatal toxoplasmosis.

take several months to confirm, clinicians may have to treat patients based upon early signs, symptoms, and serology while awaiting definitive confirmation. Although the complexity of diagnosing congenital infection necessitates the use of multiple costly laboratory tests, the benefit of early diagnosis and treatment and the cost of unnecessary treatment justify establishing the correct diagnosis.

Persistent or increasing IgG antibody levels in the infant compared with the mother as measured by the DT or IFA test, and/or positive result for Toxoplasma-specific IgM or IgA are diagnostic of congenital infection. Demonstration by IgG and IgM Western blots in the newborn of serum antibodies that are directed against unique Toxoplasma epitopes not found in the mother's serum is also evidence of congenital infection (67, 68, 84, 85, 88).

Placental leak can occasionally lead to false-positive IgM or IgA measurements in the newborn. Positive tests for these antibodies usually must be confirmed by repeat testing of IgM at 2 to 4 days of life and repeat testing for IgA at 10 days of life. Passively transferred maternal IgG has a half-life of approximately 1 month. Maternal antibodies can be detected for several months and have been reported up to 1 year of age. The untreated congenitally infected newborn will begin to produce Toxoplasma-specific IgG antibody within approximately 3 months. Treatment of the infected child may delay antibody production until 9 months of age and, on rare occasion, may prevent production altogether. Persistence of a positive IgG result at 12 months of life in the child confirms infection. Demonstration of a decrease in antibody load (Toxoplasma-specific IgG antibody divided by total IgG) can be helpful in differentiating maternal antibody from fetal antibody.

Although rarely performed, demonstration of IgM antibody or local Toxoplasma-specific IgG antibody production in CSF not contaminated with peripheral blood can help confirm the diagnosis of congenital toxoplasmosis. The calculation is made by dividing the Toxoplasma-specific antibody titer in the body fluid by the Toxoplasma-specific antibody titer in the serum and multiplying the result by the concentration of gamma globulin in serum divided by the concentration of gamma globulin in the body fluid. A result of four or greater corresponds to significant antibody production.

A long-term prospective study is under way in the United States to define optimal therapeutic regimens for the treatment of congenital toxoplasmosis (2, 63). Clinicians should contact Rima McLeod, University of Chicago Hospitals, Chicago, IL [phone, (773) 834-4152] regarding the treatment of infected children.

Diagnosis of Ocular Infection

Toxoplasma chorioretinitis results from both acute infection and congenital infection (45, 46). In addition to demonstrating IgG antibody to Toxoplasma in the serum of a person with compatible eye lesions, demonstration of the local production of antibody and detection of parasite DNA in the aqueous humor have been used to document active ocular toxoplasmosis (25, 33, 102). When the formula described in the section above is used to calculate results obtained in eye fluids and with results obtained in serum, a value of 8 or greater suggests acute ocular toxoplasmosis. If the serum DT titer is greater than 1:1,000, it is usually not possible to calculate local antibody production.

Diagnosis in the Immunocompromised Host

A wide variety of immunosuppressed hosts, including patients with lymphoma, leukemia, multiple myeloma, carcinoma, neuroblastoma, thymoma, systemic lupus erythematosus, scleroderma, autoimmune hemolytic anemia, and kidney, liver, and heart transplants, have been described as having severe, often fatal, toxoplasmosis. The disease is most often related to reactivation of latent infection and commonly involves the CNS, although a wide spectrum of clinical manifestations have been reported. Diagnosis can be very difficult for these patients, as IgM antibody is usually not detectable and the presence of IgG antibody only confirms chronic infection. In the absence of serologic evidence of acute infection, diagnosis can be confirmed by demonstration of the organism histologically or cytologically as replicating within tissue or by isolation or identification of its nucleic acids in a site such as amniotic fluid, CSF, bronchoalveolar fluid, or placenta, in which the encysted organism would not be present as part of a latent infection.

Persons undergoing organ or bone marrow transplantation can benefit from pretransplant testing for Toxoplasma-specific IgG antibodies to determine immune status because they are at risk for either acute acquired infection if they are seronegative before transplantation or reactivation if they are seropositive before transplantation (97). Serial measurement of Toxoplasma DNA in peripheral blood by PCR has been advocated by some as a means of monitoring for development of toxoplasmosis in bone marrow transplant patients (20, 23). Those with acute acquired infection will usually develop detectable Toxoplasma-specific IgG and IgM antibodies, while those with reactivation will not have a detectable Toxoplasma-specific IgM response. Seronegative transplant recipients of hearts from seropositive donors can develop toxoplasmic myocarditis that mimics organ rejection.

Toxoplasmic encephalitis is the most frequent CNS opportunistic infection of AIDS patients and is uniformly fatal if untreated. Among people who died with AIDS from 1992 through 1997 in the United States, 7.2% developed toxoplasmic encephalitis during the course of their AIDS (41). It is recommended that all HIV-infected persons be tested for Toxoplasma-specific IgG antibodies soon after the diagnosis of HIV infection to detect latent infection (4). If Toxoplasma-seropositive, adult/adolescent patients who have a CD4$^+$ T-lymphocyte count of $<100/\mu$l should be administered prophylaxis against toxoplasmic encephalitis with trimethoprim-sulfamethoxazole. Most AIDS patients with toxoplasmic encephalitis have demonstrable IgG antibodies to T. gondii (13, 64). However, approximately 3% of AIDS patients with toxoplasmic encephalitis do not have Toxoplasma-specific antibody in their serum. Local production of Toxoplasma-specific IgG antibody in CSF has been demonstrated for persons with AIDS and with toxoplasmic encephalitis (11). When the formula described above for toxoplasmosis in the newborn is used, a result of greater than 1 corresponds to significant antibody production.

TREATMENT

In general, physicians treat T. gondii infection in four circumstances: (i) pregnant women with acute infection to prevent fetal infection (14, 21, 43); (ii) congenitally infected infants (38, 63); (iii) immunosuppressed persons, usually with reactivated disease (7, 9, 20, 23, 49, 60, 67); and (iv) acute and recurrent ocular disease (24, 46, 93, 94). Drugs are also prescribed for preventive or suppressive treatment in HIV-infected persons (7, 9). The currently recommended drugs work primarily against the actively dividing tachyzoite form of T. gondii and do not eradicate encysted organisms (bradyzoites).

The most common drug combination used to treat congenital toxoplasmosis consists of pyrimethamine and a sulfonamide (sulfadiazine is recommended in the United States), plus folinic acid in the form of leucovorin calcium to protect the bone marrow from the toxic effects of pyrimethamine. Spiramycin [available through the FDA; phone, (301) 796-1600] is recommended for pregnant women with acute toxoplasmosis when fetal infection has not been confirmed in an attempt to prevent transmission of *T. gondii* from the mother to the fetus (70, 84). Randomized prospective studies of treatment during acute infection in pregnant women have not been performed. Some researchers have questioned, or been unable to demonstrate, the effectiveness of treatment during pregnancy in preventing congenital infection (35, 105) or sequelae in infants (34). Nevertheless, a multicenter observational study found that the treatment of acute *T. gondii* infection in pregnancy was associated with a reduction of sequelae in infants but not a reduction in maternal-fetal transmission (30). Pyrimethamine and sulfadiazine (plus leucovorin) are the drugs generally used to treat infants with congenital toxoplasmosis and have led to improved outcomes compared with historic controls (63, 84).

In immunosuppressed persons with toxoplasmosis, a regimen of pyrimethamine and sulfadiazine plus leucovorin is the preferred treatment (7, 9, 67, 70). Clindamycin is a second alternative for use in combination with pyrimethamine and leucovorin in those who cannot tolerate sulfonamides (7, 9, 15, 60, 70). Atovaquone in combination with either pyrimethamine or sulfadiazine has sufficient activity to be considered for treatment in some less severely affected adult patients (10, 70).

The role of other drugs in the treatment of systemic toxoplasmosis has not been defined by controlled trials. There are currently no defined instances of antimicrobial resistance in *T. gondii*, and there are no available standardized assays for testing resistance. In general, alternative drugs such as azithromycin, clarithromycin, and dapsone should be used in combination with another drug, preferably pyrimethamine for patients intolerant of first-line therapy (67).

Because relapse often occurs after toxoplasmosis in HIV-infected patients, maintenance therapy (secondary prophylaxis) with pyrimethamine plus sulfadiazine (first choice) or pyrimethamine plus clindamycin (alternative) is recommended for the patient (7, 9). For prophylaxis to prevent an initial episode of *T. gondii* in *Toxoplasma*-seropositive persons with CD4$^+$ T-lymphocyte counts of less than 100 cells/μl, trimethoprim-sulfamethoxazole is recommended as the first choice, with alternatives consisting of dapsone plus pyrimethamine or atovaquone with or without pyrimethamine. Leucovorin is given with all regimens, including pyrimethamine (7, 9).

Pyrimethamine and sulfadiazine are often used for persons with ocular disease (46). Clindamycin, in combination with other antiparasitic medications is also frequently prescribed for ocular disease (24). A variety of newer agents have been tried in the treatment of ocular toxoplasmosis, including atovaquone (78), rifabutin, trovafloxacin, azithromycin, and clarithromycin (47). In addition to antiparasitic drugs, physicians may add corticosteroids to reduce ocular inflammation. However, the optimal treatment for ocular toxoplasmosis remains to be defined by controlled trials.

EVALUATION, INTERPRETATION, AND REPORTING OF RESULTS

Toxoplasma gondii infection is one of the most common parasitic infections worldwide and, in most instances, is of little clinical significance. The settings in which the laboratory will be required to offer additional evaluation and interpretation include acute primary infection in pregnant women and active disease in hosts who are unable to mount the typical immune response, such as fetuses, neonates, or immunosuppressed individuals. Thus, rarely is the mere presence or absence of *Toxoplasma* IgG sufficient to guide the clinician. The laboratory will need to use additional testing (avidity, IgM, or IgA) in an attempt to define the timing of infection in the case of pregnant women or the presence of actively replicating parasites (PCR or tachyzoites) in the case of the fetus, neonate, or immunosuppressed host.

REFERENCES

1. **Bastien, P., E. Jumas-Bilak, E. Varlet-Marie, and P. Marty.** 2007. Three years of multi-laboratory external quality control for the molecular detection of *Toxoplasma gondii* in amniotic fluid in France. *Clin. Microbiol. Infect.* **13**:430–433.
2. **Boyer, K. M., E. Holfels, N. Roizen, C. Swisher, D. Mack, J. Remington, S. Withers, P. Meier, and R. McLeod.** 2005. Risk factors for *Toxoplasma gondii* infection in mothers of infants with congenital toxoplasmosis: implications for prenatal management and screening. *Am. J. Obstet. Gynecol.* **192**:564–571.
3. **Buffolano, W., M. Lappalainen, L. Hedman, F. Ciccimarra, M. Del Pezzo, R. Rescaldani, N. Gargano, and K. Hedman.** 2004. Delayed maturation of IgG avidity in congenital toxoplasmosis. *Eur. J. Clin. Microbiol. Infect. Dis.* **23**:825–830.
4. **Calderaro, A., S. Peruzzi, G. Piccolo, C. Gorrini, S. Montecchini, S. Rossi, C. Chezzi, and G. Dettori.** 2009. Laboratory diagnosis of *Toxoplasma gondii* infection. *Int. J. Med. Sci.* **6**:135–136.
5. **Candolfi, E., R. Ramirez, M. P. Hadju, C. Shubert, and J. S. Remington.** 1994. The Vitek immunodiagnostic assay for detection of immunoglobulin M toxoplasma antibodies. *Clin. Diagn. Lab. Immunol.* **1**:401–405.
6. **Carvalho, F., D. A. O. Silva, J. Cunha-Junior, M. Souza, T. Oliveira, S. Bela, G. Faria, C. Lopes, and J. Mineo.** 2008. Reverse enzyme-linked immunosorbent assay using monoclonal antibodies against SAG1-related sequence, SAG2A, and p97 antigens from *Toxoplasma gondii* to detect specific immunoglobulin G (IgG), IgM, and IgA antibodies in human sera. *Clin. Vaccine Immunol.* **15**:1265–1271.
7. **Centers for Disease Control and Prevention.** 2009. Guidelines for prevention and treatment of opportunistic infections among HIV-infected adults and adolescents. *MMWR Recommend. Rep.* **58**(RR-04):1–216.
8. **Centers for Disease Control and Prevention.** 2000. Preventing congenital toxoplasmosis. *MMWR Recommend. Rep.* **49**(RR-2):57–75.
9. **Centers for Disease Control and Prevention.** 2009. Guidelines for prevention and treatment of opportunistic infections among HIV-exposed and infected children. *MMWR Recommend. Rep.* **58**(RR-11):1–176.
10. **Chirgwin, K., R. Hafner, C. Leport, J. Remington, J. Andersen, E. M. Bosler, C. Roque, N. Rajicic, V. McAuliffe, P. Morlat, D. T. Jayaweera, J. L. Vilde, and B. J. Luft.** 2002. Randomized phase II trial of atovaquone with pyrimethamine or sulfadiazine for treatment of toxoplasmic encephalitis in patients with acquired immunodeficiency syndrome: ACTG 237/ANRS 039 Study. *Clin. Infect. Dis.* **34**:1243–1250.
11. **Ciardelli, L., V. Meroni, M. A. Avanzini, L. Bollani, C. Tinelli, F. Garofoli, A. Gasparoni, and M. Stronati.** 2008. Early and accurate diagnosis of congenital toxoplasmosis. *Pediatr. Infect. Dis. J.* **27**:125–129.
12. **Clinical and Laboratory Standards Institute/NCCLS.** 2004. *Clinical Use and Interpretation of Serologic Tests for* Toxoplasma gondii; *Approved Guideline.* Clinical and Laboratory Standards Institute, Wayne, PA.
13. **Colombo, F. A., J. E. Vidal, A. C. Penalva de Oliveira, A. V. Hernandez, F. Bonasser-Filho, R. S. Nogueira, R. Focaccia, and V. L. Pereira-Chioccola.** 2005. Diagnosis of

cerebral toxoplasmosis in AIDS patients in Brazil: importance of molecular and immunological methods using peripheral blood samples. *J. Clin. Microbiol.* **43**:5044–5047.

14. **Daffos, F., F. Forestier, M. Capella-Pavlovsky, P. Thulliez, C. Aufrant, D. Valenti, and W. L. Cox.** 1988. Prenatal management of 746 pregnancies at risk for congenital toxoplasmosis. *N. Engl. J. Med.* **318**:271–275.

15. **Dannemann, B., J. A. McCutchan, D. Israelski, D. Antoniskis, C. Leport, B. Luft, J. Nussbaum, N. Clumeck, P. Morlat, J. Chiu, J.-L. Vilde, M. Orellana, D. Feigal, A. Bartok, P. Heseltine, J. Leedom, J. Remington, and The California Collaborative Treatment Group.** 1992. Treatment of toxoplasmic encephalitis in patients with AIDS. A randomized trial comparing pyrimethamine plus clindamycin to pyrimethamine plus sulfadiazine. *Ann. Intern. Med.* **116**:33–43.

16. **Decoster, A., F. Darcy, A. Caron, D. Vinatier, D. Houze de L'Aulnoit, G. Vittu, G. Niel, F. Heyer, B. Lecolier, M. Delcroix, J. C. Monnier, M. Duhamel, and A. Capron.** 1992. Anti-P30 IgA antibodies as prenatal markers of congenital toxoplasma infection. *Clin. Exp. Immunol.* **87**:310–315.

17. **Decoster, A., N. Lambert, C. Germaneau, and C. Masson.** 2000. Serodiagnostic de la toxoplasmose: comparaison de la trousse Access Toxo IgM II aux trousses Axsym Toxo IgM et Vidas Toxo IgM. *Ann. Biol. Clin.* (Paris) **58**:721–727.

18. **Decoster, A., and B. Lecolier.** 1996. Bicentric evaluation of Access Toxo immunoglobulin M (IgM) and IgG assays and IMx toxo IgM and IgG assays and comparison with Platelia Toxo IgM and IgG assays. *J. Clin. Microbiol.* **34**:1606–1609.

19. **Derouin, F., P. Thulliez, E. Candolfi, F. Daffos, and F. Forestier.** 1988. Early prenatal diagnosis of congenital toxoplasmosis using amniotic fluid samples and tissue culture. *Eur. J. Clin. Microbiol. Infect. Dis.* **7**:423–425.

20. **Derouin, F., and H. Pelloux, on behalf of the ESCMID Study Group on Clinical Parasitology.** 2008. Prevention of toxoplasmosis in transplant patients. *Clin. Microbiol. Infect.* **14**:1089–1101.

21. **Desmonts, G., Y. Naot, and J. S. Remington.** 1981. Immunoglobulin M-immunosorbent agglutination assay for diagnosis of infectious diseases: diagnosis of acute congenital and acquired *Toxoplasma* infections. *J. Clin. Microbiol.* **14**:486–491.

22. **Diepersloot, R. J., H. Dunnewold-Hoekstra, J. Kruit-Den Hollander, and F. Vlaspolder.** 2001. Antenatal screening for hepatitis B and antibodies to *Toxoplasma gondii* and rubella virus: evaluation of two commercial immunoassay systems. *Clin. Diagn. Lab. Immunol.* **8**:785–787.

23. **Edvinsson, B., J. Lundquist, P. Ljungman, O. Ringden, and B. Evengard.** 2008. Prevention of toxoplasmosis in transplant patients. *APMIS* **116**:1965–1967.

24. **Engstrom, R. E., Jr., G. N. Holland, R. B. Nussenblatt, and D. A. Jabs.** 1991. Current practices in the management of ocular toxoplasmosis. *Am. J. Ophthalmol.* **111**:601–610.

25. **Fekkar, A., B. Bodaghi, F. Touafek, P. Le Hoang, D. Mazier, and L. Paris.** 2008. Comparison of immunoblotting, calculation of the Goldmann-Witmer coefficient, and real-time PCR using aqueous humor samples for diagnosis of ocular toxoplasmosis. *J. Clin. Microbiol.* **46**:1965–1967.

26. **Flori, P., J. Hafid, H. Raberin, H. Patural, M. N. Varlet, and R. Tran Manh Sung.** 2002. Interet du nouveau test Access Toxo IgM (II) dans l'interpretation serologique de la toxoplasmose au cours de la grossesse. *Ann. Biol. Clin.* (Paris) **60**:65–72.

27. **Fortier, B., A. Dao, C. Coignard-Chatain, and M. F. Biava.** 1997. Application de la chemiluminescence au diagnostic serologique des toxoplasmoses humaines. *Pathol. Biol.* **45**:721–728.

28. **Foudrinier, F., I. Villena, R. Jaussaud, D. Aubert, C. Chemla, F. Martinot, and J. M. Pinon.** 2003. Clinical value of specific immunoglobulin E detection by enzyme-linked immunosorbent assay in cases of acquired and congenital toxoplasmosis. *J. Clin. Microbiol.* **41**:1681–1686.

29. **Foulon, W., J. M. Pinon, B. Stray-Pedersen, A. Pollak, M. Lappalainen, A. Decoster, I. Villena, P. A. Jenum, M. Hayde, and A. Naessens.** 1999. Prenatal diagnosis of congenital toxoplasmosis: a multicenter evaluation of different diagnostic parameters. *Am. J. Obstet. Gynecol.* **181**:843–847.

30. **Foulon, W., I. Villena, B. Stray-Pedersen, A. Decoster, M. Lappalainen, J. M. Pinon, P. A. Jenum, K. Hedman, and A. Naessens.** 1999. Treatment of toxoplasmosis during pregnancy: a multicenter study of impact on fetal transmission and children's sequelae at age 1 year. *Am. J. Obstet. Gynecol.* **180**:410–415.

31. **Fricker-Hidalgo, H., M. P. Brenier-Pinchart, J. P. Schaal, V. Equy, C. Bost-Bru, and H. Pelloux.** 2007. Value of *Toxoplasma gondii* detection in one hundred thirty-three placentas for toxoplasmosis. *Pediatr. Infect. Dis. J.* **26**:845–846.

32. **Galanti, L. M., J. Dell'Omo, B. Wanet, J. L. Guarin, J. Jamart, M. G. Garrino, P. L. Masson, and C. L. Cambiaso.** 1997. Particle counting assay for anti-toxoplasma IgG antibodies. Comparison with four automated commercial enzyme-linked immunoassays. *J. Immunol. Methods* **207**:195–201.

33. **Garweg, J. G.** 2005. Determinants of immunodiagnostic success in human ocular toxoplasmosis. *Parasite Immunol.* **27**:61–68.

34. **Gilbert, R., D. Dunn, M. Wallon, M. Hayde, A. Prusa, M. Lebech, T. Kortbeek, F. Peyron, A. Pollak, and E. Petersen.** 2001. Ecological comparison of the risks of mother-to-child transmission and clinical manifestations of congenital toxoplasmosis according to prenatal treatment protocol. *Epidemiol. Infect.* **127**:113–120.

35. **Gilbert, R., and L. Gras.** 2003. Effect of timing and type of treatment on the risk of mother to child transmission of Toxoplasma gondii. *Br. J. Obstet. Gynaecol.* **110**:112–120.

36. **Goubet, S., H. Pelloux, H. Fricker-Hidalgo, A. Goullier-Fleuret, and P. Ambroise-Thomas.** 1999. Serodiagnostic de la toxoplasmose: comparaison de la trousse Elisa Axsym (Abbott) avec la trousse Vidas (bioMerieux), l'immunofluorence indirecte et l'Isaga. *Ann. Biol. Clin.* (Paris) **57**:481–484.

37. **Gras, L., R. E. Gilbert, M. Wallon, F. Peyron, and M. Cortina-Borja.** 2004. Duration of the IgM response in women acquiring *Toxoplasma gondii* during pregnancy: implications for clinical practice and cross-sectional incidence studies. *Epidemiol. Infect.* **132**:541–548.

38. **Guerina, N. G., H. W. Hsu, H. C. Meissner, J. H. Maguire, R. Lynfield, B. Stechenberg, I. Abroms, M. S. Pasternack, R. Hoff, R. B. Eaton, et al.** 1994. Neonatal serologic screening and early treatment for congenital Toxoplasma gondii infection. *N. Engl. J. Med.* **330**:1858–1863.

39. **Guy, E. C., H. Pelloux, M. Lappalainen, H. Aspock, A. Hassl, K. K. Melby, M. Holberg-Pettersen, E. Petersen, J. Simon, and P. Ambroise-Thomas.** 1996. Interlaboratory comparison of polymerase chain reaction for the detection of *Toxoplasma gondii* DNA added to samples of amniotic fluid. *Eur. J. Clin. Microbiol. Infect. Dis.* **15**:836–839.

40. **Hayde, M., H. R. Salzer, G. Gittler, H. Aspock, and A. Pollak.** 1995. Microparticle enzyme immunoassay (MEIA) for toxoplasma specific immunoglobulin G in comparison to the Sabin-Feldman dye test. A pilot study. *Wien. Klin. Wochenschr.* **107**:133–136.

41. **Hezard, N., C. Marx-Chemla, F. Foudrinier, I. Villena, C. Quereux, B. Leroux, D. Dupouy, M. Talmud, and J. M. Pinon.** 1997. Prenatal diagnosis of congenital toxoplasmosis in 261 pregnancies. *Prenat. Diagn.* **17**:1047–1054.

42. **Hofgartner, W. T., S. R. Swanzy, R. M. Bacina, J. Condon, M. Gupta, P. E. Matlock, D. L. Bergeron, J. J. Plorde, and T. R. Fritsche.** 1997. Detection of immunoglobulin G (IgG) and IgM antibodies to *Toxoplasma gondii*: evaluation of four commercial immunoassay systems. *J. Clin. Microbiol.* **35**:3313–3315.

43. **Hohlfeld, P., F. Daffos, J. M. Costa, P. Thulliez, F. Forestier, and M. Vidaud.** 1994. Prenatal diagnosis of congenital toxoplasmosis with a polymerase-chain-reaction test on amniotic fluid. *N. Engl. J. Med.* **331**:695–699.

44. **Holec-Gasior, L., J. Kur, and E. Hiszczynska-Sawicka.** 2009. GRA2 and ROP1 recombinant antigens as potential markers for detection of *Toxoplasma gondii* specific immunoglobulin G in humans with acute toxoplasmosis. *Clin. Vaccine Immunol.* **16**:510–514.

45. **Holland, G. N.** 2003. Ocular toxoplasmosis: a global reassessment. Part I: epidemiology and course of disease. *Am. J. Ophthalmol.* **136**:973–988.

46. **Holland, G. N.** 2004. Ocular toxoplasmosis: a global reassessment. Part II: disease manifestations and management. *Am. J. Ophthalmol.* **137:**1–17.

47. **Holland, G. N.** 2000. Ocular toxoplasmosis: new directions for clinical investigation. *Ocul. Immunol. Inflamm.* **8:**1–7.

48. **Iqbal, J., and N. Khalid.** 2007. Detection of acute *Toxoplasma gondii* infection in early pregnancy by IgG avidity and PCR analysis. *J. Clin. Microbiol.* **56:**1495–1499.

49. **Israelski, D. M., and J. S. Remington.** 1993. Toxoplasmosis in the non-AIDS immunocompromised host. *Curr. Clin. Top. Infect. Dis.* **13:**322–356.

50. **Jones, J. L., V. Dargelas, J. Roberts, C. Press, J. S. Remington, and J. G. Montoya.** 2009. Risk factors for *Toxoplasma gondii* infection in the United States. *Clin. Infect. Dis.* **49:**878–884.

51. **Jones, J. L., D. Kruszon-Moran, K. Sanders-Lewis, and M. Wilson.** 2007. *Toxoplasma gondii* infection in the United States, 1999–2004, decline from the prior decade. *Am. J. Trop. Med. Hyg.* **77:**405–410.

52. **Jones, J. L., D. Kruszon-Moran, M. Wilson, G. McQuillan, T. Navin, and J. B. McAuley.** 2001. *Toxoplasma gondii* infection in the United States: seroprevalence and risk factors. *Am. J. Epidemiol.* **154:**357–365.

53. **Jones, J. L., A. Lopez, M. Wilson, J. Schulkin, and R. Gibbs.** 2001. Congenital toxoplasmosis: a review. *Obstet. Gynecol. Surv.* **56:**296–305.

54. **Kasper, D. C., A. Prusa, M. Hayde, N. Gerstl, A. Pollak, K. Herkner, and R. Reiter-Reisacher.** 2009. Evaluation of the vitros ECiQ immunodiagnostic system for detection of anti-*Toxoplasma* immunoglobulin G and immunoglobulin M antibodies for confirmatory testing for acute *Toxoplasma gondii* infection in pregnant women. *J. Clin. Microbiol.* **47:**164–167.

55. **Kodym, P., L. Machala, H. Rohacova, B. Sirocka, and M. Maly.** 2007. Evaluation of commercial IgE ELISA in comparison with IgA and IgM ELISAs, IgG avidity assay and complement fixation for the diagnosis of acute toxoplasmosis. *Clin. Microbiol. Infect.* **13:**40–47.

56. **Liesenfeld, O., J. G. Montoya, N. J. Tathineni, M. Davis, B. W. Brown, Jr., K. L. Cobb, J. Parsonnet, and J. S. Remington.** 2001. Confirmatory serologic testing for acute toxoplasmosis and rate of induced abortions among women reported to have positive *Toxoplasma* immunoglobulin M antibody titers. *Am. J. Obstet. Gynecol.* **184:**140–145.

57. **Liesenfeld, O., C. Press, R. Flanders, R. Ramirez, and J. S. Remington.** 1996. Study of Abbott Toxo IMx system for detection of immunoglobulin G and immunoglobulin M toxoplasma antibodies: value of confirmatory testing for diagnosis of acute toxoplasmosis. *J. Clin. Microbiol.* **34:**2526–2530.

58. **Liesenfeld, O., C. Press, J. G. Montoya, R. Gill, J. L. Isaac-Renton, K. Hedman, and J. S. Remington.** 1997. False-positive results in immunoglobulin M (IgM) *Toxoplasma* antibody tests and importance of confirmatory testing: the Platelia Toxo IgM test. *J. Clin. Microbiol.* **35:**174–178.

59. **Liu, X., B. P. Turner, C. E. Peyton, B. S. Reisner, A. O. Okorodudu, A. A. Mohammad, G. D. Hankins, A. S. Weissfeld, and J. R. Petersen.** 2000. Prospective study of IgM to *Toxoplasma gondii* on Beckman Coulter's Access(TM) immunoassay system and comparison with Zeus ELISA and gull IFA assays. *Diagn. Microbiol. Infect. Dis.* **36:**237–239.

60. **Luft, B. J., R. Hafner, A. H. Korzun, C. Leport, D. Antoniskis, E. M. Bosler, D. D. Bourland III, R. Uttamchandani, J. Fuhrer, J. Jacobson, et al.** 1993. Toxoplasmic encephalitis in patients with the acquired immunodeficiency syndrome. *N. Engl. J. Med.* **329:**995–1000.

61. **Luyasu, V., A. R. Robert, L. Schaefer, J. Macioszek, et al.** 1995. Multicenter evaluation of a new commercial assay for detection of immunoglobulin M antibodies to *Toxoplasma gondii*. *Eur. J. Clin. Microbiol. Infect. Dis.* **14:**787–793.

62. **Maudry, A., G. Chene, R. Chatelain, H. Patural, B. Bellete, B. Tisseur, J. Hafid, H. Raberin, S. Beretta, R. T. M. Sung, G. Belot, and P. Flori.** 2009. Bicentric evaluation of six anti-*Toxoplasma* immunoglobulin G (IgG) automated immunoassays and comparison to the Toxo II IgG Western blot. *Clin. Vaccine Immunol.* **16:**1322–1326.

63. **McAuley, J., K. M. Boyer, D. Patel, M. Mets, C. Swisher, N. Roizen, C. Wolters, L. Stein, M. Stein, W. Schey, et al.** 1994. Early and longitudinal evaluations of treated infants and children and untreated historical patients with congenital toxoplasmosis: the Chicago Collaborative Treatment Trial. *Clin. Infect. Dis.* **18:**38–72.

64. **Meira, C. S., T. Costa-Silva, J. Vidal, I. Ferreira, R. Hiramoto, and V. Pereira-Choccola.** 2008. Use of the serum reactivity against *Toxoplasma gondii* excreted-secreted antigens in cerebral toxoplasmosis diagnosis in human immunodeficiency virus-infected patients. *J. Med. Microbiol.* **57:**845–850.

65. **Montoya, J. F., A. Berry, F. Rosso, and J. S. Remington.** 2007. The differential agglutination test as a diagnostic aid in cases of toxoplasmic lymphadenitis. *J. Clin. Microbiol.* **45:**1463–1468.

66. **Montoya, J. F., and J. S. Remington.** 2008. Management of Toxoplasma gondii infection during pregnancy. *Clin. Infect. Dis.* **47:**554–566.

67. **Montoya, J. F., and J. S. Remington.** 2009. *Toxoplasma gondii*, p. 3495–3526. *In* G. L. Mandell, J. E. Bennett, and R. Dolin (ed.), *Principles and Practice of Infectious Diseases*, 7th ed. Churchill Livingstone, Inc., New York, NY.

68. **Montoya, J. G.** 2002. Laboratory diagnosis of *Toxoplasma gondii* infection and toxoplasmosis. *J. Infect. Dis.* **185**(Suppl. 1)**:**S73–S82.

69. **Montoya, J. G., H. B. Huffman, and J. S. Remington.** 2004. Evaluation of the immunoglobulin G avidity test for diagnosis of toxoplasmic lymphadenopathy. *J. Clin. Microbiol.* **42:**4627–4631.

70. **Montoya, J. G., and O. Liesenfeld.** 2004. Toxoplasmosis. *Lancet* **363:**1965–1976.

71. **Montoya, J. G., O. Liesenfeld, S. Kinney, C. Press, and J. S. Remington.** 2002. VIDAS test for avidity of *Toxoplasma*-specific immunoglobulin G for confirmatory testing of pregnant women. *J. Clin. Microbiol.* **40:**2504–2508.

72. **Montoya, J. G., and J. S. Remington.** 1995. Studies on the serodiagnosis of toxoplasmic lymphadenitis. *Clin. Infect. Dis.* **20:**781–789.

73. **Naessens, A., P. A. Jenum, A. Pollak, A. Decoster, M. Lappalainen, I. Villena, M. Lebech, B. Stray-Pedersen, M. Hayde, J. M. Pinon, E. Petersen, and W. Foulon.** 1999. Diagnosis of congenital toxoplasmosis in the neonatal period: a multicenter evaluation. *J. Pediatr.* **135:**714–719.

74. **Naot, Y., G. Desmonts, and J. S. Remington.** 1981. IgM enzyme-linked immunosorbent assay test for the diagnosis of congenital Toxoplasma infection. *J. Pediatr.* **98:**32–36.

75. **Odenthal, M., S. Koenig, P. Farbrother, U. Drebber, Y. Bury, H. P. Dienes, and L. Eichinger.** 2007. Detection of opportunistic infections by low-density microarrays a diagnostic approach for granulomatous lymphadenitis. *Diagn. Mol. Pathol.* **16:**18–26.

76. **Okrongly, D.** 2004. The ADVIA Centaur immunoassay system—designed for infectious disease testing. *J. Clin. Virol.* **30**(Suppl. 1)**:**S19–S22.

77. **Palm, C., H. Tumani, T. Pietzcker, and D. Bengel.** 2008. Diagnosis of cerebral toxoplasmosis by detection of *Toxoplasma gondii* tachyzoites in cerebrospinal fluid. *J. Neurol.* **255:**939–941.

78. **Pearson, P. A., A. R. Piracha, H. A. Sen, and G. J. Jaffe.** 1999. Atovaquone for the treatment of toxoplasma retinochoroiditis in immunocompetent patients. *Ophthalmology* **106:**148–153.

79. **Petersen, E., M. V. Borobio, E. Guy, O. Liesenfeld, V. Meroni, A. Naessens, E. Spranzi, and P. Thulliez.** 2005. European multicenter study of the LIAISON automated diagnostic system for determination of Toxoplasma gondii-specific immunoglobulin G (IgG) and IgM and the IgG avidity index. *J. Clin. Microbiol.* **43:**1570–1574.

80. **Pietkiewicz, H., E. Hiszczynska-Sawicka, J. Kur, E. Petersen, H. V. Nielsen, M. Paul, M. Stankiewicz, and P. Myjak.** 2007. Usefulness of *Toxoplasma gondii* recombinant antigens (GRA1, GRA7, SAG1) in an immunoglobulin G avidity test for the serodiagnosis of toxoplasmosis. *Parasitol. Res.* **100:**333–337.

81. **Pinon, J. M., H. Dumon, C. Chemla, J. Franck, E. Petersen, M. Lebech, J. Zufferey, M. H. Bessieres, P. Marty, R.**

Holliman, J. Johnson, V. Luyasu, B. Lecolier, E. Guy, D. H. Joynson, A. Decoster, G. Enders, H. Pelloux, and E. Candolfi. 2001. Strategy for diagnosis of congenital toxoplasmosis: evaluation of methods comparing mothers and newborns and standard methods for postnatal detection of immunoglobulin G, M, and A antibodies. *J. Clin. Microbiol.* **39:**2267–2271.

82. **Pratlong, F., P. Boulot, I. Villena, E. Issert, I. Tamby, J. Cazenave, and J. P. Dedet.** 1996. Antenatal diagnosis of congenital toxoplasmosis: evaluation of the biological parameters in a cohort of 286 patients. *Br. J. Obstet. Gynaecol.* **103:**552–557.

83. **Rao, L. V., O. A. James, L. M. Mann, A. A. Mohammad, A. O. Okorodudu, M. G. Bissell, and J. R. Petersen.** 1997. Evaluation of Immuno-1 *Toxoplasma* IgG assay in the prenatal screening of toxoplasmosis. *Diagn. Microbiol. Infect. Dis.* **27:**13–15.

84. **Remington, J. S., R. McLeod, P. Thulliez, and G. Desmonts.** 2006. Toxoplasmosis, p. 947–1092. *In* J. S. Remington and J. O. Klein (ed.), *Infectious Diseases of the Fetus and Newborn Infant*, 6th ed. The W. B. Saunders Co., Philadelphia, PA.

85. **Remington, J. S., P. Thulliez, and J. G. Montoya.** 2004. Recent developments for diagnosis of toxoplasmosis. *J. Clin. Microbiol.* **42:**941–945.

86. **Rigsby, P., S. Rijpkema, E. C. Guy, J. Francis, and R. G. Das.** 2004. Evaluation of a candidate international standard preparation for human anti-*Toxoplasma* immunoglobulin G. *J. Clin. Microbiol.* **42:**5133–5138.

87. **Robert-Gangneux, F., P. Binisti, D. Antonetti, A. Brezin, H. Yera, and J. Dupouy-Camet.** 2004. Usefulness of immunoblotting and Goldmann-Witmer coefficient for biological diagnosis of toxoplasmic retinochoroiditis. *Eur. J. Clin. Microbiol. Infect. Dis.* **23:**34–38.

88. **Robert-Gangneux, F., V. Commerce, C. Tourte-Schaefer, and J. Dupouy-Camet.** 1999. Performance of a Western blot assay to compare mother and newborn anti-*Toxoplasma* antibodies for the early neonatal diagnosis of congenital toxoplasmosis. *Eur. J. Clin. Microbiol. Infect. Dis.* **18:**648–654.

89. **Robert-Gangneux, F., M. F. Gavinet, T. Ancelle, J. Raymond, C. Tourte-Schaefer, and J. Dupouy-Camet.** 1999. Value of prenatal diagnosis and early postnatal diagnosis of congenital toxoplasmosis: retrospective study of 110 cases. *J. Clin. Microbiol.* **37:**2893–2898.

90. **Roberts, A., K. Hedman, V. Luyasu, J. Zufferey, M. H. Bessieres, R. M. Blatz, E. Candolfi, A. Decoster, G. Enders, U. Gross, E. Guy, M. Hayde, D. Ho-Yen, J. Johnson, B. Lecolier, A. Naessens, H. Pelloux, P. Thulliez, and E. Petersen.** 2001. Multicenter evaluation of strategies for serodiagnosis of primary infection with Toxoplasma gondii. *Eur. J. Clin. Microbiol. Infect. Dis.* **20:**467–474.

91. **Romand, S., M. Chosson, J. Franck, M. Wallon, F. Kieffer, K. Kaiser, H. Dumon, F. Peyron, P. Thulliez, and S. Picot.** 2004. Usefulness of quantitative polymerase chain reaction in amniotic fluid as early prognostic marker of fetal infection with Toxoplasma gondii. *Am. J. Obstet. Gynecol.* **190:**797–802.

92. **Romand, S., M. Wallon, J. Franck, P. Thulliez, F. Peyron, and H. Dumon.** 2001. Prenatal diagnosis using polymerase chain reaction on amniotic fluid for congenital toxoplasmosis. *Obstet. Gynecol.* **97:**296–300.

93. **Rothova, A.** 1993. Ocular involvement in toxoplasmosis. *Br. J. Ophthalmol.* **77:**371–377.

94. **Rothova, A., C. Meenken, H. J. Buitenhuis, C. J. Brinkman, G. S. Baarsma, T. N. Boen-Tan, P. T. de Jong, N. Klaassen-Broekema, C. M. Schweitzer, Z. Timmerman, J. de Vries, M. J. Zaal, and A. Kijlstra.** 1993. Therapy for ocular toxoplasmosis. *Am. J. Ophthalmol.* **115:**517–523.

95. **Roux-Buisson, N., H. Fricker-Hidalgo, A. Foussadier, D. Rolland, A. S. Suchel-Jambon, M. P. Brenier-Pinchart, and H. Pelloux.** 2005. Comparative analysis of the VIDAS Toxo IgG IV assay in the detection of antibodies to Toxoplasma gondii. *Diagn. Microbiol. Infect. Dis.* **53:**79–81.

96. **Santos Nascimento, F., L. A. Suzuki, and C. L. Rossi.** 2008. Assessment of the value of detecting specific IgA antibodies for the diagnosis of a recently acquired primary *Toxoplasma* infection. *Prenat. Diagn.* **28:**749–752.

97. **Schaffner, A.** 2001. Pretransplant evaluation for infections in donors and recipients of solid organs. *Clin. Infect. Dis.* **33**(Suppl. 1)**:**S9–S14.

98. **Schmidt-Hieber, M., J. Zweigner, L. Uharek, I. W. Blau, and E. Thiel.** 2009. Central nervous system infections in immunocompromised patients - update on diagnosis and therapy. *Leuk. Lymphoma* **50:**24–36.

99. **Singh, S., N. Singh, and S. N. Dwivedi.** 1997. Evaluation of seven commercially available ELISA kits for serodiagnosis of acute toxoplasmosis. *Indian J. Med. Res.* **105:**103–107.

100. **Smith, K. L., M. Wilson, A. W. Hightower, P. W. Kelley, J. P. Struewing, D. D. Juranek, and J. B. McAuley.** 1996. Prevalence of Toxoplasma gondii antibodies in US military recruits in 1989: comparison with data published in 1965. *Clin. Infect. Dis.* **23:**1182–1183.

101. **Soave, R.** 2001. Prophylaxis strategies for solid-organ transplantation. *Clin. Infect. Dis.* **33**(Suppl. 1)**:**S26–S31.

102. **Talabani, H., M. Asseraf, H. Yera, E. Delair, T. Ancelle, P. Thulliez, A. P. Brezin, and J. Dupouy-Camet.** 2009. Contributions of immunoblotting, real-time PCR, and the Goldmann-Witmer coefficient to diagnosis of atypical toxoplasmic retinochoroiditis. *J. Clin. Microbiol.* **47:**2131–2135.

103. **Thalib, L., L. Gras, S. Romand, A. Prusa, M. H. Bessieres, E. Petersen, and R. E. Gilbert.** 2005. Prediction of congenital toxoplasmosis by polymerase chain reaction analysis of amniotic fluid. *Br. J. Obstet. Gynaecol.* **112:**567–574.

104. **Vlaspolder, F., P. Singer, A. Smit, and R. J. Diepersloot.** 2001. Comparison of Immulite with Vidas for detection of infection in a low-prevalence population of pregnant women in The Netherlands. *Clin. Diagn. Lab. Immunol.* **8:**552–555.

105. **Wallon, M., D. Dunn, D. Slimani, V. Girault, F. Gay-Andrieu, and F. Peyron.** 1999. Diagnosis of congenital toxoplasmosis at birth: what is the value of testing for IgM and IgA? *Eur. J. Pediatr.* **158:**645–649.

106. **Wilson, M., J. S. Remington, C. Clavet, G. Varney, C. Press, D. Ware, et al.** 1997. Evaluation of six commercial kits for detection of human immunoglobulin M antibodies to *Toxoplasma gondii*. *J. Clin. Microbiol.* **35:**3112–3115.

Pathogenic and Opportunistic Free-Living Amebae

GOVINDA S. VISVESVARA

136

Small, free-living amebae belonging to the genera *Naegleria*, *Acanthamoeba*, and *Balamuthia* have been identified as agents of central nervous system (CNS) infections of humans and other animals (6, 8, 10, 13, 17, 20, 24, 25, 27–32, 37, 39, 47, 58, 60, 65). Only one species of *Naegleria* (*Naegleria fowleri*), several species of *Acanthamoeba* (e.g., *Acanthamoeba castellanii*, *A. culbertsoni*, *A. hatchetti*, *A. healyi*, *A. polyphaga*, *A. rhysodes*, *A. astronyxis*, and *A. divionensis*), and the only known species of *Balamuthia*, *Balamuthia mandrillaris*, are known to cause disease. *Acanthamoeba* spp. also cause infection of the human cornea, *Acanthamoeba* keratitis (4, 11, 19, 22, 36, 52, 53, 55, 60, 63). Further, both *Acanthamoeba* spp. and *B. mandrillaris* have been identified as agents of cutaneous infections in humans (5, 33, 49, 50). *Sappinia diploidea*, a free-living ameba normally found in soil contaminated with the feces of elk and buffalo, was identified in an excised brain lesion from a 38-year-old immunocompetent man who developed a bifrontal headache, blurry vision, and loss of consciousness following a sinus infection (15). This ameba was recently identified as *Sappinia pedata* based on a real-time PCR assay (38). Additionally, *Paravahlkampfia francinae*, a new species of the free-living ameba genus *Paravahlkampfia*, was recently isolated from the cerebrospinal fluid (CSF) of a patient with a headache, sore throat, and vomiting, symptoms typical of primary amebic meningoencephalitis (PAM) caused by *Naegleria fowleri*. The patient recovered within a few days, indicating that some of the previously reported cases of PAM that survived may have been due to *P. francinae* (61). These findings clearly indicate that there are probably other small amebae that may also cause encephalitis in humans.

The concept that these small, free-living amebae may occur as human pathogens was proposed by Culbertson and colleagues, who isolated *Acanthamoeba* sp. strain A-1 (now designated *A. culbertsoni*) from tissue culture medium thought to contain an unknown virus (7). They also demonstrated the presence of amebae in brain lesions of mice and monkeys that died within a week after intracerebral inoculation with *A. culbertsoni*. Culbertson hypothesized that similar infections might exist in nature in humans. In 1965, Fowler and Carter were the first to describe a fatal infection due to free-living amebae in the brain of an Australian patient (6). The infection is now believed to have been due to *N. fowleri* (6).

TAXONOMY

Until recently, the classical taxonomic classification was based largely on morphologic, ecologic, and physiologic criteria. According to this system, *Acanthamoeba* and *Balamuthia*, along with a heterogeneous group of amebae that include both free-living (e.g., *Hartmannella*, *Vahlkampfia*, and *Vannella*) and parasitic (e.g., *Entamoeba histolytica*) amebae, were classified under the phylum Protozoa, subphylum Sarcodina, superclass Rhizopodea, class Lobosea, and order Amoebida. *Naegleria* was classified under the class Heterolobosea, order Schizopyrenida, and family Vahlkampfiidae. *Sappinia* was classified under the class Lobosea, order Euamoebida, and family Thecamoebidae. Recent information based on modern morphological approaches, biochemical pathways, and molecular phylogenetics has led to the abandonment of the older hierarchical systems consisting of the traditional "kingdom," "phylum," "class," "subclass," "superorder," and "order" and replacement with a new classification system. According to this new schema, the eukaryotes have been classified into six clusters or "supergroups," namely, Amoebozoa, Opisthokonta, Rhizaria, Archaeplastida, Chromalveolata, and Excavata. *Acanthamoeba* and *Balamuthia* are included under the supergroup Amoebozoa: Acanthamoebidae; *Sappinia* is included under the supergroup Flabellinea: Thecamoebidae; and *Naegleria fowleri* is included under the supergroup Excavata: Heterolobosea: Vahlkampfiidae (60).

DESCRIPTION OF THE AGENTS

The genus *Acanthamoeba* contains as many as 24 species in three groups, with groupings based largely on morphologic characteristics. In group I are included those species that have large trophozoites and cysts that measure more than 18 μm. Group II is the largest group, and its members are the most widespread; the endocysts are usually stellate, polygonal, triangular, and oval and measure less than 18 μm. Group III includes those species with cysts that measure less than 18 μm, and the endocysts are either round or oval. Because such morphological characters may change with environmental pressures and culture conditions, efforts were made to utilize nonmorphologic characters for use in taxonomic classification. Therefore, the 18S rRNA gene was considered a good target for the classification and diagnosis of *Acanthamoeba* infection since it has multiple copies and is evolutionarily stable. In the case of *Acanthamoeba*, a substantial sequence variation was seen not only between the species but also within the same species, identified based on morphological features. *Acanthamoeba* is therefore divided into 15 sequence types known as the T1 to T15 genotypes. *Acanthamoeba* genotypes have been identified in corneal tissue, tear fluid, and brain and lung tissue, as well as in the environment. For the detection of *Acanthamoeba*, Booton et al. used nuclear single-subunit rDNA sequences and the genus-specific primers JDP1 (5'-GGCCCAGATCGTTTACCGTGAA-3') and JDP2 (5'-TCTCACAAGCTGCTAGGGGAGTCA-3'), which amplify a region of the single-subunit rDNA that permits genotypic identification of an *Acanthamoeba* isolate following sequence analysis (3). In the case of *N. fowleri*, however, different isolates show similar nuclear 18S rRNA sequences, but variation in the internal transcribed spacer (ITS) sequences has been used to identify six different

genotypes (I, II, III, IV, V, VI) (65). However, in the case of *Balamuthia*, all isolates analyzed so far seem to be largely similar on the basis of their 18S rRNA gene sequences. Mitochondrial 16S rRNA gene sequences show variability of about 1.8%, in contrast to those of *Acanthamoeba* (2).

N. fowleri in its trophic form is a small, slug-like ameba measuring 10 to 35 μm long that exhibits an eruptive locomotion by producing smooth hemispherical bulges. The posterior end, termed the uroid, appears to be sticky and often has several trailing filaments. During its life cycle, this ameba produces a transient pear-shaped biflagellate stage, resulting from altered environmental conditions, and smooth-walled cysts (Fig. 1 to 4). The flagellates do not have cytostomes (mouths). Cysts are usually spherical and measure 7 to 15 μm, and the cyst wall may have one or more pores plugged with a mucoid material (35).

An *Acanthamoeba* organism is a slightly larger ameba (15 to 45 μm) that produces from the surface of its body fine,

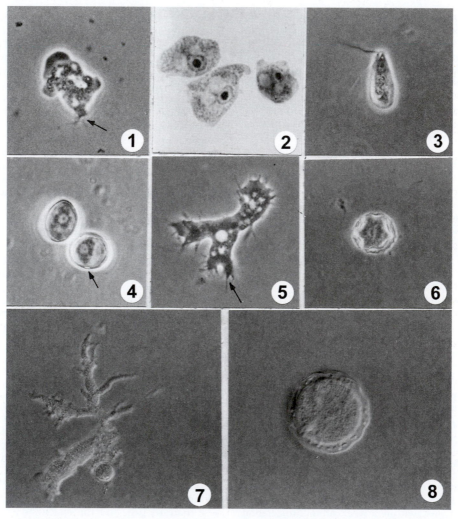

FIGURES 1 through 4 *N. fowleri*. (1) Trophozoite, phase contrast (note the uroid and filaments at arrow); (2) trophozoite, trichrome stain; (3) biflagellate, phase contrast; (4) smooth-walled cyst, phase contrast (note the pore at the arrow). All magnifications, ~×835.
FIGURES 5 and 6 *A. castellanii*. (5) Trophozoite, phase contrast (note the acanthopodia at the arrow); (6) double-walled cyst, phase contrast. Both magnifications, ~×835.
FIGURES 7 and 8 *B. mandrillaris*. (7) Trophozoite, phase contrast; (8) cyst, phase contrast. Both magnifications, ~×1,140.

tapering, hyaline projections called acanthopodia (Fig. 5). It has no flagellate stage but produces a double-walled cyst (10 to 25 μm) (Fig. 6) with a wrinkled outer wall (the ectocyst) and a stellate, polygonal, or even round inner wall (the endocyst) (35). Cysts are resistant to many physical and chemical environmental pressures, including desiccation (51).

Balamuthia trophozoites are in general irregular in shape; a few, however, may be slug-like. Actively feeding amebae may be 12 to 60 μm long, with a mean length of 30 μm (Fig. 7). The trophic forms, while feeding on tissue culture cells, produce broad pseudopodia without any clearly discernible movement. However, when tissue culture cells are destroyed, the trophozoites resort to a spider-like walking movement by producing finger-like determinate pseudopodia (59). Like *Acanthamoeba*, *Balamuthia* does not have a flagellate stage. Cysts are generally spherical and measure 6 to 30 μm in diameter (Fig. 8). Under a light microscope, each cyst appears to have an irregular and slightly wavy outer wall and a round inner wall. A layer of refractile granules immediately below the inner cyst wall is often seen in mature cysts. Under an electron microscope, the cyst wall can be seen to consist of three walls: a thin, irregular outer ectocyst; a thick, electron-dense inner endocyst; and a middle amorphous layer, the mesocyst (58, 59).

Acanthamoeba, *Balamuthia*, and *Naegleria* are predominantly uninucleate, although binucleate forms are occasionally seen. The nucleus is characterized by a large, dense, centrally located nucleolus. *Naegleria* amebae exhibit a promitotic pattern of cell division wherein the nucleolus and the nuclear membrane persist during nuclear division. *Acanthamoeba* spp., however, divide by conventional mitosis, in which the nucleolus and the nuclear membrane disappear during cell division. The pattern of nuclear division in *Balamuthia* is termed metamitosis; the nuclear membrane breaks down, and the nucleolus eventually disappears (59).

EPIDEMIOLOGY

Infection with *N. fowleri* was first described in 1965 from Australia and has now been identified from virtually all over the world. In the United States, PAM has been reported from 1931 to 2008 and is known to affect primarily young males who frequently dive and jump into warm freshwater in the summer, when the temperature of the water in lakes and ponds, especially in the southern tier of the United States, is expected to be high. It has been postulated that higher temperature due to climate change might be responsible for increases in ambient water temperatures and, therefore, increases in the chances of contracting *N. fowleri* infections in areas that had been free of this infection (60, 65). Both *Acanthamoeba* and *Balamuthia* infections have been identified from many parts of the world. However, they are not associated with a particular time of the year. *Acanthamoeba* infections are found mostly in people with immunosuppression, whereas infections with *Balamuthia* are found in both immunocompromised and immunocompetent individuals.

N. fowleri and *Acanthamoeba* spp. are commonly found in soil, freshwater, sewage, and sludge and even on dust in the air. Several species of *Acanthamoeba* have also been isolated from brackish water and seawater and from ear discharges, pulmonary secretions, nasopharyngeal mucosa samples, maxillary sinus samples, mandibular autografts, and stool samples (9, 17, 25, 28, 29, 41, 46, 48, 60). These amebae normally feed on bacteria and multiply in their environmental niche as free-living organisms. *Acanthamoeba* spp. have also been known to harbor *Legionella* spp., *Mycobacterium avium*, and other

bacterial pathogens such as *Listeria monocytogenes*, *Burkholderia pseudomallei*, *Vibrio cholerae*, and *Escherichia coli* serotype O157, which signifies a potential expansion of the public health importance of these organisms (14, 17, 25, 60). Additionally, pure cultures of *A. polyphaga* have been used to isolate *Legionella pneumophila* (40), *Legionella anisa* (23), and, recently, *Mycobacterium massiliense* (1) from human clinical specimens such as sputa, liver and lung abscess specimens, and even human feces. Obligate intracellular pathogens such as *Chlamydia*, *Chlamydophila*, and *Chlamydia*-like bacteria have been found in ~5% of *Acanthamoeba* isolates, and *Chlamydophila pneumophila*, a respiratory pathogen, can survive and grow within *Acanthamoeba* (14). Whether endosymbiont-bearing *Acanthamoeba* strains serve as reservoirs for these bacteria, some of which are potential pathogens for humans, is unknown.

Although *B. mandrillaris* has recently been isolated from soil (12, 42), not much is known about the environmental niche of *B. mandrillaris* and its feeding habits. It is, however, believed that its habitat is similar to those of *Acanthamoeba* and *Naegleria*. Excellent reviews (17, 25, 29, 46, 60) and books (28, 48) have been published on the biology, disease potential, pathology, pathogenicity, and epidemiology of these amebae.

CLINICAL SIGNIFICANCE

Naegleria Meningoencephalitis

In 1966, Butt (5a) described the first case of CNS infection caused by *N. fowleri* in the United States and coined the term "primary amebic meningoencephalitis" (PAM). PAM is an acute fulminating disease with an abrupt onset that occurs generally in previously healthy children and young adults who had contact with freshwater about 7 to 10 days before the onset of symptoms. It is characterized by a severe headache, spiking fever, a stiff neck, photophobia, and a coma, leading to death within 3 to 10 days after the onset of symptoms (6, 28, 29, 47). The portal of entry of the *N. fowleri* amebae is the nasal passages. When people swim in lakes and other bodies of freshwater that harbor these amebae, the amebae may enter the nostrils of the swimmers, make their way into the olfactory lobes via the cribriform plate, and cause acute hemorrhagic necrosis, leading to destruction of the olfactory bulbs and the cerebral cortex. Only a few patients have survived. Upon autopsy, large numbers of amebic trophozoites, many with ingested erythrocytes and brain tissue, are usually seen interspersed with brain tissue (Fig. 9). It is believed that *N. fowleri* directly ingests brain tissue by producing food cups, or amebostomes, as well as by exerting contact-dependent cytolysis, possibly mediated by a multicomponent system consisting of a heat-stable hemolytic protein, a heat-labile cytolysin, and/or phospholipase enzymes (17, 26, 28). Cysts of *N. fowleri* are not usually seen in brain tissue. It was believed until recently that *N. fowleri* infects only humans. In March 1997, however, a report of the first case of PAM in a South American tapir was published, indicating that PAM can occur in animals other than humans (24). A recent report of PAM in Holstein cattle, associated with drinking of surface waters, indicates that this disease is probably more common than is currently appreciated (57).

Acanthamoeba Encephalitis

Several species of *Acanthamoeba* (*A. culbertsoni*, *A. castellanii*, *A. polyphaga*, *A. astronyxis*, *A. healyi*, and *A. divionensis*) have been known to cause a chronic granulomatous amebic encephalitis (GAE), primarily in immunosuppressed

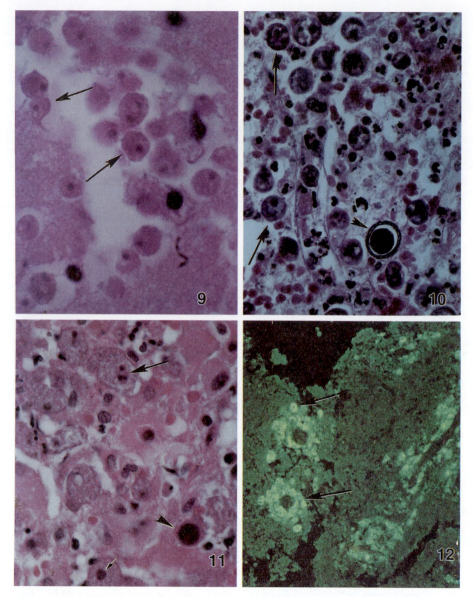

FIGURE 9 Large numbers of *N. fowleri* trophozoites (arrows) in a section of CNS tissue, showing extensive necrosis and destruction of brain tissue. Magnification, ~×564.

FIGURE 10 *A. culbertsoni* trophozoites (arrows) and a cyst (arrowhead) around a blood vessel in a section of CNS tissue from a GAE patient. Magnification, ~×489.

FIGURE 11 *B. mandrillaris* trophozoites and a cyst (arrowhead) in a brain section from a GAE patient. Note the double (small arrow) and triple (large arrow) nucleolar elements within the nuclei of the trophozoites. Magnification. ~×413.

FIGURE 12 Immunofluorescence localization of *B. mandrillaris* in a brain section from a GAE patient. Note the fluorescent amebae (arrows) around blood vessels. Magnification, ~×188.

(either because of iatrogenic suppression or because of human immunodeficiency virus infection or AIDS), chronically ill, or otherwise debilitated persons with no previous history of exposure to recreational freshwater (25, 28, 29, 32, 60). GAE has an insidious onset and is usually chronic, lasting for more than a week and sometimes even for months (10, 25, 27–29, 31, 46, 62). It is characterized by a headache, confusion, dizziness, drowsiness, seizures, and sometimes hemiparesis. Cerebral hemispheres are usually the most heavily affected CNS tissue. They are often edematous, with extensive hemorrhagic necrosis involving the temporal, parietal, and occipital lobes. Amebic trophozoites and cysts are usually scattered throughout the tissue. Many blood vessels are thrombotic and exhibit fibrinoid necrosis; they are also surrounded by polymorphonuclear leukocytes, amebic trophozoites, and cysts (Fig. 10). Multinucleated giant cells forming granulomas may be seen in immunocompetent patients. Some patients, especially those with human immunodeficiency virus infection or AIDS, develop chronic ulcerative skin lesions, abscesses, or erythematous nodules (27–29, 31, 33, 49, 50, 62). It is believed that the route of invasion of and penetration into the CNS is hematogenous, probably from a primary focus in the lower respiratory tract or the skin (27–29). *Acanthamoeba* spp. also cause infections of the CNSs of animals besides humans. Such infections have been recorded in gorillas, monkeys, dogs, ovines, bovines, horses, and kangaroos (29, 39, 60).

Because of the confusion that existed in the earlier literature with regard to the nomenclature of *Acanthamoeba* and *Hartmannella* spp., some workers in the field referred to these amebae as members of the *Hartmannella-Acanthamoeba* group or simply as "*H-A* amebae." Since no true *Hartmannella* species has been found to be pathogenic to humans, all references in the literature to *Hartmannella* in human tissues should be corrected to read *Acanthamoeba* or *Balamuthia*.

Balamuthia (Leptomyxid) Encephalitis

It was believed that all cases of GAE were caused by *Acanthamoeba* spp. Although a number of these cases were confirmed by serologic techniques as being caused by *Acanthamoeba* spp., the causative organisms in a few cases could not be definitively identified. Since cysts were found in the brain tissues of the patients, it was believed that the infections were caused by some other species of *Acanthamoeba* that did not cross-react with the anti-*Acanthamoeba* sera used in the serologic test (29, 60). *B. mandrillaris* (leptomyxid ameba) was definitively identified by an indirect immunofluorescence test as the causal agent in these cases (5, 8, 13, 20, 29, 39, 58, 59). The rabbit anti-*B. mandrillaris* serum used in the indirect immunofluorescence test was made by using culture-derived *Balamuthia* organisms that had been isolated from the CNS tissue of a baboon (58). It is now known that a number of primates, including gorillas, gibbons, baboons, orangutans, and monkeys, as well as dogs, sheep, and horses, have died of CNS infections caused by *B. mandrillaris* (13, 29, 30, 39, 58). According to a recent report, Hispanic Americans have a high incidence of *B. mandrillaris* infection. It is not clearly known whether this is due to environmental factors, genetic predisposition, limited access to medical care, or other socioeconomic factors and pressures (43).

The pathology and pathogenesis of *B. mandrillaris*-induced GAE are similar to those of *Acanthamoeba*-induced GAE. Both trophozoites and cysts are found in CNS tissue (Fig. 11), and their sizes overlap those of *Acanthamoeba* trophozoites and cysts (13, 29, 30, 39, 58, 59). Hence, it is difficult to differentiate *Balamuthia* from *Acanthamoeba* spp. in tissue sections under a light microscope. In some cases, *Balamuthia* trophozoites in tissue sections appear to have more than one nucleolus in the nucleus (Fig. 11). In such cases, it may be possible to distinguish *Balamuthia* amebae from *Acanthamoeba* organisms on the basis of nuclear morphology, since *Acanthamoeba* trophozoites have only one nucleolus. In most cases, electron microscopy, immunohistochemical techniques, or both are necessary to identify *Balamuthia* organisms. Ultrastructurally, the cysts are characterized by three layers in the cyst wall: an outer wrinkled ectocyst, a middle structureless mesocyst, and an inner thin endocyst (58, 59). *Balamuthia* amebae are antigenically distinct from *Acanthamoeba* organisms; they can easily be distinguished by immunofluorescence or other immunochemical assays (Fig. 12) (8, 13, 20, 29, 30, 39, 58, 59).

Acanthamoeba Keratitis

Acanthamoeba spp. also cause a painful vision-threatening disease of the human cornea, *Acanthamoeba* keratitis. If the infection is not treated promptly, it may lead to ulceration of the cornea, loss of visual acuity, and eventually blindness and enucleation (4, 11, 19, 25, 36, 52, 53, 63). The first case of *Acanthamoeba* keratitis in the United States was reported in 1973 in a south Texas rancher with a history of trauma

to his right eye (19). Both trophozoite and cyst stages of *A. polyphaga* were demonstrated to be present in corneal sections and were repeatedly cultured from corneal scrapings and biopsy specimens. Between 1973 and July 1986, 208 cases were diagnosed and reported to the Centers for Disease Control (CDC) (52, 53, 60). The numbers of cases increased gradually between 1973 and 1984, and a dramatic increase began in 1985. An in-depth epidemiologic and case control study (52, 53) revealed that a major risk factor was the use of contact lenses, predominantly daily-wear or extended-wear soft lenses, and that patients with *Acanthamoeba* keratitis were significantly more likely than controls to use home-made saline solution instead of commercially prepared saline (78 and 30%, respectively), to disinfect their lenses less frequently than recommended by the lens manufacturers (72 and 32%), and to wear their lenses while swimming (63 and 30%). Based on a case control study conducted by the CDC to investigate a recent increase in the *Acanthamoeba* keratitis cases during 2004 to 2007, it was revealed that a national increase in the number of such cases was associated with the use of Advanced Medical Optics Complete MoisturePlus multipurpose contact lens solution (54). Further, another study revealed that most contact lens solutions marketed in the United States do not have sufficient disinfection activity against *Acanthamoeba* spp. (18).

Acanthamoeba keratitis is characterized by severe ocular pain, a 360° or partial paracentral stromal ring infiltrate, recurrent corneal epithelial breakdown, and a corneal lesion refractory to the commonly used ophthalmic antibacterial medications. *Acanthamoeba* keratitis in the early stages is frequently misdiagnosed as herpes simplex virus keratitis because of the irregular epithelial lesions, stromal infiltrative keratitis, and edema that are commonly seen in herpes simplex virus keratitis (19, 63). A nonhealing corneal ulcer is often the first clue that *Acanthamoeba* keratitis may be the problem. It is estimated that as of August 2005, more than 4,000 cases of *Acanthamoeba* keratitis have occurred in the United States. Since the diseases caused by *Acanthamoeba* are not required to be reported in the United States, the actual number may be much higher.

COLLECTION, HANDLING, AND STORAGE OF SPECIMENS

For isolation of the etiologic agent, CSF, small pieces of tissue (brain, lung, skin, or corneal biopsy material), or corneal scrapings from the affected area must be obtained aseptically. The specimens should be kept at room temperature (24 to 28°C) and should never be frozen. The specimens may be kept at 4°C for short periods but never for more than 24 h. Personnel handling the specimens must take appropriate precautions, such as wearing surgical masks and gloves and working in a biological safety cabinet. Remaining tissues must be preserved in 10% neutral buffered Formalin so that they can be examined histologically for amebae (55).

CLINICAL AND LABORATORY DIAGNOSIS

Methods of Examination

Direct Examination

Since no distinctive clinical features differentiate PAM from pyogenic or bacterial meningitis, direct examination of the sample as a wet mount preparation is of paramount importance in the diagnosis of PAM and other diseases caused by these amebae. In PAM, the CSF is usually pleocytotic, with a preponderance of polymorphonuclear leukocytes and no bacteria. The CSF pressure may be elevated. The CSF glucose level may be normal or slightly reduced, but the CSF protein level is increased, ranging from 1 to 10 mg/ml. Microscopic detection of amebic organisms in the CSF is the only means of diagnosing PAM. CSF should be examined in situ microscopically for the presence of *N. fowleri* amebae with directional movement. Since the amebae tend to attach to the surface of the container, the container should be shaken gently; then, a small drop of fluid should be placed on a clean microscope slide and covered with a no. 1 coverslip. The CSF may have to be centrifuged at 500 × *g* for 5 min to concentrate the amebae. After the specimen has been centrifuged, most of the supernatant is carefully aspirated and the sediment is gently suspended in the remaining fluid. A drop of this suspension is prepared as described above for microscopic observation. Giemsa or trichrome staining should be performed on CSF smears to visualize the nuclear morphology of the amebae. The slide preparation should be examined under a compound microscope with 10× and 40× lens objectives. Phase-contrast optics is preferable. If regular bright-field illumination is used, the slide should be examined under diminished light. The slide may be warmed to 35°C (to promote amebic movement), and amebae, especially *N. fowleri*, if present, can easily be detected by their active directional movements. Rarely, flagellates with two flagella may be seen. Currently, this is the most sensitive method available for the diagnosis of PAM.

Permanently Stained Preparations

A small drop of the sedimented CSF or other sample is placed in the middle of a slide, which is allowed to stand in a moist chamber for 5 to 10 min at 37°C. This will allow any amebae to attach to the surface of the slide. Several drops of warm (37°C) Schaudinn's fixative are dropped directly onto the sample, which is allowed to stand for 1 min. The slide is then transferred for 1 h to a Coplin jar containing the fixative. It may be stained with Wheatley's trichrome or Heidenhain's iron hematoxylin stain. Corneal scrapings smeared onto microscope slides may be fixed with methanol and stained with Hemacolor stain (Harleco, a division of EM Industries, Inc.) (29, 60). Gram staining is not useful in the detection of amebae. Further, a false-positive Gram stain may lead to inaccurate diagnosis and hence to inappropriate therapy, which will result in death. A recent report describing the transplantation of kidneys and a liver from a donor infected with *N. fowleri* (21) underscores the importance of a correct and timely diagnosis.

Antigen Detection

Pathogenic *N. fowleri* is morphologically indistinguishable from nonpathogenic *Naegleria* at the trophic stage. Differences between these amebae, however, have been demonstrated antigenically by the gel diffusion, immunoelectrophoretic, and immunofluorescence techniques as well as isoenzyme patterns, and these techniques have been utilized to identify the amebae isolated in culture (17, 26, 29, 46, 60). Similarly, antigenic differences have also been shown among various species of *Acanthamoeba* (17, 25, 29, 60). Additionally, *N. fowleri*, *Acanthamoeba* spp., and *B. mandrillaris* have been identified in tissue sections by histochemical methods (5, 8, 10, 20, 24, 29, 31, 33, 39, 46, 58–60).

Nucleic Acid Detection in Clinical Materials

Sequencing of the 5.8S rRNA gene and ITS1 and ITS2 of *N. fowleri* not only can differentiate *N. fowleri* from other *Naegleria* spp. but also can be used in the genotypic analysis of

N. fowleri strains (17, 29, 46, 60, 66). However, this methodology has not been used routinely to identify *N. fowleri* infections in clinical cases until recently. A number of studies have analyzed the mitochondrial DNA and 18S rRNA gene to understand the inter- and intraspecies diversity and phylogeny of *Acanthamoeba* (3, 25, 46, 54). However, only a few studies have used this technique to identify *Acanthamoeba* keratitis or *Acanthamoeba* GAE by using patient specimens (3, 37, 54). Similarly, a PCR assay for the detection of *B. mandrillaris* has been described previously (2). Recently, a PCR assay to detect *B. mandrillaris* in Formalin-fixed archival tissue specimens has also been described (2, 13, 64). A recently developed real-time PCR test simultaneously identifies *Acanthamoeba*, *Balamuthia*, and *N. fowleri* in CSF specimens (37). This real-time PCR assay is better than and has many advantages over conventional PCR. Apart from identifying simultaneously the DNA of all three amebae, it is fast, requiring ~5 h or less. This test is being used routinely at the CDC to identify *Acanthamoeba*, *Balamuthia*, and *N. fowleri* with great success.

ISOLATION

The recommended procedure for isolating free-living pathogenic amebae from biological specimens is as follows.

Materials

1. Page's ameba saline (17, 35). Physiological saline or phosphate-buffered saline solutions that are normally available in the clinical laboratories are not suitable, as the sodium chloride concentrations in these solutions will prevent the growth of amebae, especially *N. fowleri*.

2. Petri dishes containing 1.5% Difco agar made with Page's ameba saline (nonnutrient agar plate) (56). These plates can be stored at 4°C for up to 3 months. Chocolate agar with blood, Trypticase soy agar, and Lowenstein-Jensen agar have been used sometimes. These are not suitable because bacteria that coat the plates or bacteria from the clinical sample may overgrow and either prevent the growth of amebae, especially when they are in small numbers, or obscure their presence.

3. 18- to 24-h-old cultures of *E. coli* or *Enterobacter aerogenes*.

Preparation of Agar Plates

1. Remove plates from the refrigerator and place them in a 37°C incubator for 30 min.

2. Add 0.5 ml of ameba saline to a slant culture of *E. coli* or *Enterobacter aerogenes*. Gently scrape the surface of the slant with a sterile bacteriologic loop (do not break the agar surface). Using a sterile Pasteur pipette, gently and uniformly suspend the bacteria. Add 2 or 3 drops of this suspension to the middle of a warmed (37°C) agar plate, and spread the bacteria over the surface of the agar with a bacteriologic loop. The plate is then ready for inoculation.

Inoculation of Plates with Specimens

1. For CSF samples, centrifuge the CSF at 500 × *g* for 5 to 8 min. With a sterile serologic pipette, carefully transfer all but 0.5 ml of the supernatant to a sterile tube, and store the tube at 4°C for possible future use. Mix the sediment with the remaining fluid. With a sterile Pasteur pipette, place 2 or 3 drops in the center of the agar plate precoated with bacteria, and incubate in room air at 37°C.

2. For tissue samples, gently grind a small piece of the tissue in a small amount of ameba saline. With a sterile Pasteur pipette, place 2 or 3 drops of the mixture in the center of the agar plate. Incubate the plate in room air at

37°C for CNS and lung tissues and at 30°C for tissues from other sites (e.g., skin and cornea).

3. Handle water and soil samples in the same manner as CSF and tissue specimens, respectively.

4. Control cultures are recommended for comparative purposes, although care should be exercised to prevent cross-contamination of patient cultures.

Examination of Plates

1. Using the low-power (10×) lens objective of a microscope, observe the plates daily for 7 days for amebae.

2. If you see amebae anywhere, circle that area with a wax pencil. With the fine spatula, cut a small piece of agar from the circled area and place it face down on the surface of a fresh agar plate precoated with bacteria; incubate as described above. Both *N. fowleri* and *Acanthamoeba* spp. can easily be cultivated in this way and, with periodic transfers, maintained indefinitely. When the plate is examined under a microscope, the amebae will look like small blotches, and if they are observed carefully, their movement can be discerned. After 2 to 3 days of incubation, the amebae will start to encyst. If a plate is examined after 4 to 5 days of incubation, trophozoites as well as cysts will be visible. *B. mandrillaris*, however, will not grow on agar plates seeded with bacteria. While *B. mandrillaris* can be grown on monkey kidney or lung fibroblast cell lines, on human brain microvascular endothelial cells, and axenically in a complex medium (12, 16, 42, 46, 58, 59), such techniques are not routinely available.

Identification and Culture

Identification of living organisms to the genus level is based on characteristic patterns of locomotion, morphologic features of the trophozoite and cyst forms, and results of enflagellation experiments. Immunofluorescence or immunoperoxidase tests using monoclonal or polyclonal antibodies (available at the Centers for Disease Control and Prevention) will be helpful in differentiating *Acanthamoeba* spp. from *B. mandrillaris* in fixed tissue and in identifying the species, especially *Acanthamoeba* spp., in fixed tissue (8, 13, 20, 29, 39, 58, 59).

Enflagellation Experiment

1. Mix 1 drop of the sedimented CSF containing amebae with about 1 ml of sterile distilled water in a sterile tube, or with a bacteriologic loop, scrape the surface of a plate that is positive for amebae, transferring a loopful of scraping to a sterile tube that contains approximately 1 ml of distilled water.

2. Gently shake the tube and transfer a drop of this suspension to the center of a coverslip whose edges have been coated thinly with petroleum jelly. Place a microscope slide over the coverslip and invert the slide. Seal the edges of the coverslip with Vaspar. Place the slide in a moist chamber and incubate as before for 2 to 3 h. In addition, incubate the tube as described above.

3. Periodically examine the tube and the slide preparation microscopically for free-swimming flagellates. *N. fowleri* has a flagellate stage; *Acanthamoeba* spp. and *B. mandrillaris* do not. If the sample contains *N. fowleri*, about 30 to 50% of the amebae will have undergone transformation into pear-shaped biflagellate organisms (Fig. 3).

Other Culture Methods

Axenic Culture

Acanthamoeba spp. can easily be cultivated axenically, without the addition of serum or host tissue, in many different types of nutrient media, e.g., proteose peptone-yeast extract-glucose medium, Trypticase soy broth medium, and chemically defined medium (56). *N. fowleri*, however, requires media containing fetal calf serum or brain extract, e.g., Nelson's medium. A chemically defined medium has only recently been developed for *N. fowleri* (34). *B. mandrillaris* cannot be cultivated on agar plates with bacteria. It can, however, be cultivated on mammalian cell lines (12, 16, 42, 58, 59) or a complex axenic medium (45).

Axenic cultures of *Acanthamoeba* spp. and *N. fowleri* can be established as follows. An actively growing 24- to 36-h-old ameba culture is scraped from the surface of the plate, suspended in 50 ml of ameba saline, and centrifuged at 500 × *g* for 5 min. The supernatant is aspirated, and the sediment is inoculated into proteose peptone-yeast extract-glucose medium or Nelson's medium, depending on the ameba isolate, and incubated at 37°C. Gentamicin, to a final concentration of 50 μg/ml, is added aseptically to the medium before the amebae are inoculated. Three subcultures into the antibiotic-containing medium at weekly intervals are usually sufficient to eliminate the associated bacteria (*E. coli* or *Enterobacter aerogenes*).

Cell Culture

Acanthamoeba spp., *B. mandrillaris*, and *N. fowleri* can also be inoculated onto many types of mammalian cell cultures. Shell vial cultures normally used in the isolation of viruses are suitable for the isolation of the amebae provided that antifungal agents (amphotericin B) are not included in the antibiotic mix. The amebae grow vigorously in these cell cultures and produce cytopathic effects somewhat similar to those caused by viruses (17, 46, 58, 59). Because of such cytopathic effects, *Acanthamoeba* organisms were mistaken for transformed cell types presumed to contain viruses and were erroneously termed lipovirus and Ryan virus (28, 60).

Animal Inoculation

Two-week-old Swiss Webster mice weighing 12 to 15 g each can be infected with these amebae. The mice are anesthetized with ether, and a drop of ameba suspension is instilled into their nostrils. Mice infected with *N. fowleri* die within 5 to 7 days after developing characteristic signs, such as ruffled fur, aimless wandering, partial paralysis, and finally coma and death. Mice infected with *Acanthamoeba* spp. and *B. mandrillaris* may die of acute disease within 5 to 7 days or may die of chronic disease after several weeks. In all cases, the presence of amebae in the mouse brain can be demonstrated either by culture or by histologic examination.

Serology

The serologic techniques discussed here have been developed as research tools and are not routinely available to clinical laboratories. Antibodies (detected by complement fixation, precipitin, etc.) to *Acanthamoeba* spp. have been shown to be present in the sera of patients with upper respiratory tract distress and those with optic neuritis and macular disease and keratitis (17, 19, 25, 29, 46, 60).

An antibody response to *N. fowleri*, however, has not yet been defined. Most of the patients with *Naegleria* PAM died very shortly after infection (5 to 10 days), before they had time to produce detectable levels of antibody. In one case, however, in which the patient survived PAM caused by *N. fowleri*, an antibody response was detected by 10 days after hospitalization, ultimately reaching a titer of 1:4,096 (26, 29, 46, 47, 60).

Since the recognition of *Balamuthia* GAE is relatively new, not much information is available on the serologic responses of patients infected with *Balamuthia*. According to a recent report, four patients with confirmed *Balamuthia* GAE infection had high titers of antibody to *Balamuthia*, whereas six sera from patients with encephalitis of unknown causes (10% of the sera) had titers of 64 and above and none of the control sera had titers of 64 or above. It is therefore possible that patients with *Balamuthia* GAE may be diagnosed premortem by using this serologic test (46, 60).

TREATMENT

There is no single drug that is effective against systemic acanthamebiasis. A number of antimicrobials have shown efficacy against amebae in vitro, but there is no assurance that these same drugs will be effective clinically. An important consideration in corneal infections is using drugs that are not only amebicidal but also cysticidal. As long as cysts remain viable, the infection can recur. Jones et al. (19) found that paromomycin, clotrimazole, and hydroxystilbamidine isethionate were active against *A. polyphaga* in vitro. In a recent study, azithromycin and several phenothiazine compounds protected rat glioma cells from destruction by *Acanthamoeba* (45). Culbertson and others found sulfadiazine to be active against experimental *Acanthamoeba* infections in mice (4, 17, 22, 29, 46, 60). In vitro studies indicate that chlorhexidine gluconate and polyhexamethyl biguanide have excellent amebicidal and cysticidal properties, and they have been used topically in the treatment of *Acanthamoeba* keratitis with success. Several patients with *Acanthamoeba* keratitis have been successfully treated with different drug combinations administered over a long period. For example, in one study, treatment with 0.1% propamidine isethionate (Brolene) eye drops and 0.15% dibromopropamidine ointment together with topical neomycin sulfate was successful in the management of *Acanthamoeba* keratitis (11, 63). Although a few patients with *Acanthamoeba* sp. GAE have survived, most have died in spite of treatment with several drug combinations. The prognoses of patients without CNS infection but with disseminated cutaneous ulcers due to *Acanthamoeba* spp. are good. For example, a patient with Down's syndrome and an immunoglobulin A deficiency who also had undergone cadaveric renal transplantation developed a biopsy specimen-confirmed *Acanthamoeba* skin ulcer. The patient was successfully cured of the infection after prolonged (more than 8 months) therapy with a regimen that included topical as well as systemic administration of a combination of drugs, including topical application of chlorhexidine gluconate solution followed by 2% ketoconazole cream. He also received pentamidine isethionate intravenously for 1 month and thereafter was given oral itraconazole therapy for 8 months; this regimen resulted in complete healing of the cutaneous ulcers (50).

Pathogenic *N. fowleri* is exquisitely susceptible to amphotericin B in vitro, and the minimum amebicidal concentrations were determined to be 0.02 to 0.078 µg/ml for three different clinical isolates of *N. fowleri* (6, 17, 28, 29, 46, 47). Although many patients with PAM have been treated with amphotericin B, only two patients have recovered after receiving intrathecal and intravenous injections of amphotericin B alone or in combination with miconazole (17, 29, 46, 47).

In vitro studies indicate that *B. mandrillaris* is susceptible in vitro to pentamidine isethiocyanate and that patients with *B. mandrillaris* infection may benefit from treatment with this drug (45). Although most patients with *B. mandrillaris* GAE have died of this disease, several patients have survived after treatment initially with pentamidine isethionate and subsequently with a combination of sulfadiazine, clarithromycin, and fluconazole.

Recently, the anticancer drug miltefosine and the antifungal drug voriconazole were tested in vitro against *Balamuthia mandrillaris*, *Acanthamoeba* spp., and *Naegleria fowleri*. *Balamuthia* organisms exposed to <40 mM concentrations of miltefosine survived, while concentrations of ≥40 mM were amebicidal. *Acanthamoeba* spp. recovered from exposure to 40 mM but not 80 mM miltefosine. The inhibitory and amebicidal concentrations for *N. fowleri* were 40 and 55 mM, respectively. Voriconazole had little or no inhibitory effect on *Balamuthia* at concentrations up to 40 mg/ml but had a strong inhibitory effect upon *Acanthamoeba* spp. and *N. fowleri* at all drug concentrations through 40 mg/ml. The ability of miltefosine and voriconazole to penetrate into brain tissue and CSF and their low toxicity make them attractive possibilities in the treatment of the amebic encephalitides. In combination with other antimicrobials, these two drugs may form the basis of an optimal therapy for treatment of *Acanthamoeba*, *Balamuthia*, and *Naegleria* infections (44).

EVALUATION, INTERPRETATION, AND REPORTING OF RESULTS

Most clinical laboratories rely on the agar plate technique for the isolation and identification of these small, free-living, and pathogenic amebae, as other techniques, like PCR, are not available and sometimes not even feasible. The laboratories usually send the specimens to an outside laboratory like the CDC for identification and interpretation. Also, antimicrobial testing is currently not available in most clinical laboratories. Further, it is well known, at least for these free-living amebae, that what works in vitro may not always work in vivo. For example, fluconazole has no activity in vitro against *Balamuthia* but is one of the drugs of choice for treatment. Several patients have survived after receiving fluconazole given along with other drugs; this approach may represent synergistic activities.

Use of trade names is for identification only and does not imply endorsement by the Public Health Service or by the U.S. Department of Health and Human Services.

REFERENCES

1. **Adékambi, T., M. Reynaud-Gaubert, G. Greub, M.-J. Gevaudan, B. La Scola, D. Raoult, and M. Drancourt.** 2004. Amoebal coculture of "*Mycobacterium massiliense*" sp. nov. from the sputum of a patient with hemoptoic pneumonia. *J. Clin. Microbiol.* **42:**5493–5501.
2. **Booton, G. C., J. R. Carmichael, G. S. Visvesvara, T. J. Byers, and P. A. Fuerst.** 2003. Identification of *Balamuthia mandrillaris* by PCR assay using the mitochondrial 16S rRNA gene as a target. *J. Clin. Microbiol.* **41:**453–455.
3. **Booton, G. C., G. S. Visvesvara, T. J. Byers, D. J. Kelly, and P. A. Fuerst.** 2005. Identification and distribution of *Acanthamoeba* species genotypes associated with nonkeratitis infections. *J. Clin. Microbiol.* **43:**1689–1693.
4. **Brasseur, G., L. Favennec, D. Perrine, J. P. Chenu, and P. Brasseur.** 1994. Successful treatment of *Acanthamoeba* keratitis by hexamidine. *Cornea* **13:**459–462.
5. **Bravo, F. G., J. Cabrera, E. Gottuzo, and G. S. Visvesvara.** 2005. Cutaneous manifestations of infection by free-living amebas, p. 49–55. *In* S. K. Tyring, O. Lupi, and U. R. Hengge (ed.), *Tropical Dermatology.* Elsevier Churchill Livingstone, Philadelphia, PA.

5a. **Butt, C. G.** 1966. Primary amebic meningoencephalitis. *N. Engl. J. Med.* **274:**1473–1476.

6. **Carter, R. F.** 1972. Primary amoebic meningoencephalitis. An appraisal of present knowledge. *Trans. R. Soc. Trop. Med. Hyg.* **66:**193–208.

7. **Culbertson, C. G., J. W. Smith, and J. R. Minner.** 1958. *Acanthamoeba:* observations on animal pathogenicity. *Science* **127:**1506.

8. **Deetz, T. R., M. H. Sawyer, G. Billman, F. L. Schuster, and G. S. Visvesvara.** 2003. Successful treatment of *Balamuthia* amebic encephalitis: presentation of two cases. *Clin. Infect. Dis.* **37:**1304–1312.

9. **De Jonckheere, J. F.** 1987. Epidemiology, p. 127–147. *In* E. G. Rondanelli (ed.), *Amphizoic Amoebae Human Pathology.* Piccin Nuova Libraria, Padua, Italy.

10. **Di Gregorio, C., F. Rivasi, N. Mongiardo, B. De Rienzo, and G. S. Visvesvara.** 1991. *Acanthamoeba* meningoencephalitis in an AIDS patient: first report from Europe. *Arch. Pathol. Lab. Med.* **116:**1363–1365.

11. **Driebe, W. T., G. A. Stern, R. J. Epstein, G. S. Visvesvara, M. Adi, and T. Komadina.** 1988. *Acanthamoeba* keratitis: potential role for topical clotrimazole in combination chemotherapy. *Arch. Ophthalmol.* **106:**1196–1201.

12. **Dunnebacke, T. H., F. L. Schuster, S. Yagi, and G. C. Booton.** 2004. *Balamuthia mandrillaris* from soil samples. *Microbiology* **150:**2837–2842.

13. **Foreman, O., J. Sykes, L. Ball, N. Yang, and H. De Cock.** 2004. Disseminated infection with *Balamuthia mandrillaris* in a dog. *Vet. Pathol.* **41:**506–510.

14. **Fritsche, T. R., M. Horn, M. Wagner, R. P. Herwig, K. H. Schleifer, and R. K. Gautom.** 2000. Phylogenetic diversity among geographically dispersed *Chlamydiales* endosymbionts from clinical and environmental isolates of *Acanthamoeba* spp. *Appl. Environ. Microbiol.* **66:**2613–2619.

15. **Gelman, B. B., S. J. Rauf, R. Nader, V. Popov, J. Borkowski, G. Chaljub, H. W. Nauta, and G. S. Visvesvara.** 2001. Amoebic encephalitis due to *Sappinia diploidea*. *JAMA* **285:**2450–2451.

16. **Jayasekera, S., J. Sissons, J. Tucker, C. Rogers, D. Nolder, D. Warhurst, S. Alsam, J. M. L. White, E. M. Higgins, and N. A. Khan.** 2004. Post-mortem culture of *Balamuthia mandrillaris* from the brain and cerebrospinal fluid of a case of granulomatous amoebic meningoencephalitis, using human brain microvascular endothelial cells. *J. Med. Microbiol.* **53:**1007–1012.

17. **John, D. T.** 1993. Opportunistically pathogenic free-living amebae, p. 143–246. *In* J. P. Kreier and J. R. Baker (ed.), *Parasitic Protozoa,* vol. 3. Academic Press, Inc., New York, NY.

18. **Johnston, S. P., R. Sriram, Y. Qvarnstrom, S. Roy, J. Verani, J. Yoder, S. Lorick, J. Roberts, M. J. Beach, and G. S. Visvesvara.** 2009. Resistance of *Acanthamoeba* cysts to disinfection in multiple contact lens solutions. *J. Clin. Microbiol.* **47:**2040–2045.

19. **Jones, D. B., G. S. Visvesvara, and N. M. Robinson.** 1975. *Acanthamoeba polyphaga* keratitis and *Acanthamoeba* uveitis associated with fatal meningoencephalitis. *Trans. Ophthalmol. Soc. U. K.* **95:**221–232.

20. **Jung, S., R. L. Schelper, G. S. Visvesvara, and H. T. Chang.** 2004. *Balamuthia mandrillaris* meningoencephalitis in an immunocompetent patient: a case of unusual clinical course and successful outcome. *Arch. Pathol. Lab. Med.* **128:**466–468.

21. **Kramer, M. H., C. J. Lerner, and G. S. Visvesvara.** 1997. Kidney and liver transplants from a donor infected with *Naegleria fowleri*. *J. Clin. Microbiol.* **35:**1032–1033.

22. **Larkin, D. F. P., S. Kilvington, and J. K. G. Dart.** 1992. Treatment of *Acanthamoeba* keratitis with polyhexamethylene biguanide. *Ophthalmology* **99:**185–191.

23. **La Scola, B., L. Mezi, P. J. Weiller, and D. Raoult.** 2001. Isolation of *Legionella anisa* using an amoebic coculture procedure. *J. Clin. Microbiol.* **39:**365–366.

24. **Lozano-Alarcon, F., G. A. Bradley, B. S. Houser, and G. S. Visvesvara.** 1997. Primary amebic meningoencephalitis due to *Naegleria fowleri* in a South American tapir. *Vet. Pathol.* **34:**239–243.

25. **Marciano-Cabral, F., and G. Cabral.** 2003. The importance of *Acanthamoeba* spp. as agents of disease in humans. *Clin. Microbiol. Rev.* **16:**273–307.

26. **Marciano-Cabral, F., and G. Cabral.** 2007. The immune response to *Naegleria fowleri* amebae and pathogenesis of infection. *FEMS Immunol. Med. Microbiol.* **51:**243–259.

27. **Martinez, A. J.** 1982. Acanthamoebiasis and immunosuppression. Case report. *J. Neuropathol. Exp. Neurol.* **41:**548–557.

28. **Martinez, A. J.** 1985. *Free-Living Amebas: Natural History, Prevention, Diagnosis, Pathology, and Treatment of the Disease.* CRC Press, Inc., Boca Raton, FL.

29. **Martinez, A. J., and G. S. Visvesvara.** 1997. Free-living, amphizoic and opportunistic amebas. *Brain Pathol.* **7:**583–589.

30. **Martinez, A. J., and G. S. Visvesvara.** 2001. *Balamuthia mandrillaris* infection. *J. Med. Microbiol.* **50:**205–207.

31. **Martinez, S. M., G. Gonzales-Madiero, P. Santiago, A. R. DeLope, J. Diz, C. Conde, and G. S. Visvesvara.** 2000. Granulomatous amebic encephalitis in a patient with AIDS: isolation of *Acanthamoeba* sp. group II from brain tissue and successful treatment with sulfadiazine and fluconazole. *J. Clin. Microbiol.* **38:**3892–3895.

32. **Moura, H., S. Wallace, and G. S. Visvesvara.** 1992. *Acanthamoeba healyi* n. sp. and the isoenzyme and immunoblot profiles of *Acanthamoeba* spp., groups 1 and 3. *J. Protozool.* **39:**573–583.

33. **Murakawa, G. J., T. McCalmont, J. Altman, G. H. Telang, M. D. Hoffman, G. R. Kantor, and T. G. Berger.** 1995. Disseminated acanthamoebiasis in patients with AIDS. A report of five cases and a review of the literature. *Arch. Dermatol.* **131:**1291–1296.

34. **Nerad, T. A., G. S. Visvesvara, and P.-M. Daggett.** 1983. Chemically defined media for the cultivation of *Naegleria*: pathogenic and high temperature tolerant species. *J. Protozool.* **30:**383–387.

35. **Page, F. C.** 1985. *A New Key to Fresh Water and Soil Gymnamoebae.* Freshwater Biological Association, Ambleside, Cumbria, England.

36. **Pfister, D. R., J. D. Cameron, J. H. Krachmer, and E. J. Holland.** 1996. Confocal microscopy findings of *Acanthamoeba* keratitis. *Am. J. Ophthalmol.* **121:**119–128.

37. **Qvarnstrom, Y., G. S. Visvesvara, R. Sriram, and A. J. da Silva.** 2006. Multiplex real-time PCR assay for simultaneous detection of *Acanthamoeba* spp., *Balamuthia mandrillaris*, and *Naegleria fowleri*. *J. Clin. Microbiol.* **44:**3589–3595.

38. **Qvarnstrom, Y., A. J. Da Silva, F. L. Schuster, B. B. Gelman, and G. S. Visvesvara.** 2009. Molecular confirmation of *Sappinia pedata* as causative agent of amebic encephalitis. *J. Infect. Dis.* **199:**1139–1142.

39. **Rideout, B. A., C. H. Gardiner, I. H. Stalis, J. R. Zuba, T. Hadfield, and G. S. Visvesvara.** 1997. Fatal infections with *Balamuthia mandrillaris* (a free-living amoeba) in gorillas and other Old World primates. *Vet. Pathol.* **34:**15–22.

40. **Rowbotham, T. J.** 1998. Isolation of *Legionella pneumophila* serogroup 1 from human feces with use of amebic cultures. *Clin. Infect. Dis.* **26:**502–503.

41. **Sawyer, T. K., G. S. Visvesvara, and B. A. Harke.** 1976. Pathogenic amebas from brackish and ocean sediments with a description of *Acanthamoeba hatchetti*, n. sp. *Science* **196:**1324–1325.

42. **Schuster, F. L., T. H. Dunnebacke, G. C. Booton, S. Yagi, C. K. Kohlmeier, C. Glaser, D. Vugia, A. Bakardjiev, P. Azimi, M. Maddux-Gonzalez, A. J. Martinez, and G. S. Visvesvara.** 2003. Environmental isolation of *Balamuthia mandrillaris* associated with a case of amebic encephalitis. *J. Clin. Microbiol.* **41:**3175–3180.

43. **Schuster, F. L., C. Glaser, S. Honarmand, J. H. Maguire, and G. S. Visvesvara.** 2004. *Balamuthia* amebic encephalitis risk, Hispanic Americans. *Emerg. Infect. Dis.* **10:**1510–1512.

44. **Schuster, F. L., J. B. Guglielmo, and G. S. Visvesvara.** 2006. In-vitro activity of miltefosine and voriconazole on clinical isolates of free-living amebas: *Balamuthia mandrillaris*, *Acanthamoeba* spp., and *Naegleria fowleri*. *J. Eukaryot. Microbiol.* **53:**121–126.

45. **Schuster, F. L., and G. S. Visvesvara.** 1996. Axenic growth and drug sensitivity studies of *Balamuthia mandrillaris*, an agent

of amebic meningoencephalitis in humans and other animals. *J. Clin. Microbiol.* **34:**385–388.

46. **Schuster, F. L., and G. S. Visvesvara.** 2004. Free-living amoebae as opportunistic and non-opportunistic pathogens of humans and animals. *Int. J. Parasitol.* **34:**1001–1027.

47. **Seidel, J. S., P. Harmatz, G. S. Visvesvara, A. Cohen, J. Edwards, and J. Turner.** 1982. Successful treatment of primary amebic meningoencephalitis. *N. Engl. J. Med.* **306:**346–348.

48. **Singh, B. N.** 1975. *Pathogenic and Non-Pathogenic Amebae.* John Wiley & Sons, Inc., New York, NY.

49. **Sisson, J. P., C. A. Kemper, M. Loveless, D. McShane, G. S. Visvesvara, and S. C. Deresinski.** 1995. Disseminated *Acanthamoeba* infection in patients with AIDS: case reports and review. *Clin. Infect. Dis.* **20:**1207–1216.

50. **Slater, C. A., J. Z. Sickel, G. S. Visvesvara, R. C. Pabico, and A. A. Gaspari.** 1994. Successful treatment of disseminated *Acanthamoeba* infection in an immunocompromised patient. *N. Engl. J. Med.* **331:**85–87.

51. **Sriram, R., M. Shoff, G. C. Booton, P. A. Fuerst, and G. S. Visvesvara.** 2008. Survival of *Acanthamoeba* cysts after desiccation for more than 20 years. *J. Clin. Microbiol.* **46:**4045–4048.

52. **Stehr-Green, J. K., T. M. Bailey, and G. S. Visvesvara.** 1990. The epidemiology of *Acanthamoeba* keratitis in the United States. *Am. J. Ophthalmol.* **107:**331–336.

53. **Stehr-Green, J. K., T. M. Bailey, F. H. Brandt, J. H. Carr, W. W. Bond, and G. S. Visvesvara.** 1987. *Acanthamoeba* keratitis in soft contact lens wearers: a case-control study. *JAMA* **258:**57–60.

54. **Stothard, D. R., J. M. Schroeder-Diedrich, M. H. Awwad, R. J. Gast, D. R. Ledee, D. S. Rodriguez-Zaragoza, C. L. Dean, P. A. Fuerst, and T. J. Byers.** 1998. The evolutionary history of the genus *Acanthamoeba* and the identification of eight new 18S rRNA gene sequence types. *J. Eukaryot. Microbiol.* **45:**45–54.

55. **Verani, J. R., S. A., Lorick, J. S. Yoder, M. J. Beach, C. R. Braden, J. M. Roberts, C. S. Conover, S. Chen, K. A. McConnell, D. C. Chang, B. J. Park, D. B. Jones, G. S. Visvesvara, and S. L. Roy.** 2009. National outbreak of *Acanthamoeba* keratitis associated with use of contact lens solution, United States. *Emerg. Infect. Dis.* **15:**1236–1242.

56. **Visvesvara, G. S.** 1992. Parasite culture: *Acanthamoeba* and *Naegleria* spp., p. 7.9.2.1–7.9.2.8. *In* H. D. Isenberg (ed.), *Clinical Microbiology Procedures Handbook,* vol. 2. ASM Press, Washington, DC.

57. **Visvesvara, G. S., J. F. De Jonckheere, R. Sriram, and B. Daft.** 2005. Isolation and molecular typing of *Naegleria fowleri* from the brain of a cow that died of primary amebic meningoencephalitis. *J. Clin. Microbiol.* **43:**4203–4204.

58. **Visvesvara, G. S., A. J. Martinez, F. L. Schuster, G. J. Leitch, S. Wallace, T. K. Sawyer, and M. Anderson.** 1990. Leptomyxid ameba, a new agent of amebic meningoencephalitis in humans and animals. *J. Clin. Microbiol.* **28:**2750–2756.

59. **Visvesvara, G. S., F. L. Schuster, and A. J. Martinez.** 1993. *Balamuthia mandrillaris,* new genus, new species, agent of amebic meningoencephalitis in humans and animals. *J. Eukaryot. Microbiol.* **40:**504–514.

60. **Visvesvara, G. S., H. Moura, and F. L. Schuster.** 2007. Pathogenic and opportunistic free-living amoebae: *Acanthamoeba* spp., *Balamuthia mandrillaris,* *Naegleria fowleri,* and *Sappinia diploidea.* *FEMS Immunol. Micribiol.* **50:**1–26.

61. **Visvesvara, G. S., R. Sriram R, Y. Qvarnstrom, K. Bandyopadhyay, A. J. Da Silva, N. J. Pieniazek, and G. A. Cabral.** 2009. *Paravahlkampfia francinae* n. sp. masquerading as an agent of primary amoebic meningoencephalitis. *J. Eukaryot. Microbiol.* **56:**357–366.

62. **Wiley, C. A., R. E. Safrin, C. E. Davis, P. W. Lampert, A. J. Braude, A. J. Martinez, and G. S. Visvesvara.** 1987. *Acanthamoeba* meningoencephalitis in a patient with AIDS. *J. Infect. Dis.* **155:**130–133.

63. **Wright, P., D. Warhurst, and B. R. Jones.** 1985. *Acanthamoeba* keratitis successfully treated medically. *Br. J. Ophthalmol.* **69:**778–782.

64. **Yagi, S., G. C. Booton, G. S. Visvesvara, and F. L. Schuster.** 2005. Detection of mitochondrial 16S ribosomal DNA in clinical specimens by PCR. *J. Clin. Microbiol.* **43:**3192–3197.

65. **Yoder, J. S., B. A. Eddy, G. S. Visvesvara, I. Capwell, and M. J. Beach.** 2010. The epidemiology of primary amoebic meningoencephalitis, 1962–2008. *Epidemiol Infect.* **138:**968–975. doi:10.1017/S0950268809991014.

66. **Zhou, L., R. Sriram, G. S. Visvesvara, and L. Xiao.** 2003. Genetic variations in the internal transcribed spacer and mitochondrial small subunit rRNA gene of *Naegleria* spp. *J. Eukaryot. Microbiol.* **50:**522–526.

Intestinal and Urogenital Amebae, Flagellates, and Ciliates

AMY L. LEBER AND SUSAN NOVAK-WEEKLEY

137

Giardia lamblia and *Entamoeba histolytica* infections are two of the most common protozoal infections seen worldwide and are of serious concern on a global scale due to their prevalence and the pathogenicity of their causative agents. Most of the other protozoa described in this chapter are nonpathogenic organisms. Nevertheless, they need to be detected and differentiated from true pathogens in clinical specimens because they are indicators of exposure to fecal contamination and examination of additional specimens may reveal pathogenic protozoa. The pathogenic and nonpathogenic organisms are categorized as indicated in Table 1; however, reports of disease in patients infected with nonpathogenic species are found in the literature.

Microscopic examination of stool specimens continues to be one of the main tools used in the laboratory diagnosis of intestinal amebic, flagellate, and ciliate infections. The goal of microscopy is to identify pathogenic protozoa, differentiate between these and nonpathogenic species, and properly discriminate among various artifacts that may be present. Other methods for detection include antigen detection assays such as enzyme immunoassays (EIAs), immunochromatographic assays, and direct fluorescent-antibody (DFA) assays for the detection of pathogens such as the *E. histolytica/Entamoeba dispar* group, *E. histolytica*, and *G. lamblia*. Culture for the intestinal ameba is generally not feasible, readily available, or clinically relevant except in certain limited situations. Nucleic acid-based techniques have been developed but are not yet widely available. They are, however, useful particularly to diagnose diseases like amebiasis, where microscopy does not allow differentiation of pathogenic and nonpathogenic *Entamoeba* species. All of these methods may not be available or necessary in every instance. See the sections below and refer to chapters 4, 5, and 132 for additional information.

AMEBAE

Taxonomy

The amebae that parasitize the intestinal tracts of humans belong to four genera: *Entamoeba*, *Endolimax*, *Iodamoeba*, and *Blastocystis*. They all belong to the phylum Amoebozoa, subphylum Conosa, which contains organisms that move by means of cytoplasmic protrusions called pseudopodia (see chapter 129 of this *Manual*). It is noteworthy that *Dientamoeba fragilis*, once classified as an ameba, is now grouped with the flagellates. Even though this reclassification has occurred, *D. fragilis* is still identified on the basis of morphologic comparison to amebae.

Description of the Agents

Of the seven species of intestinal amebae, *E. dispar*, *Entamoeba hartmanni*, *Entamoeba coli*, *Endolimax nana*, and *Iodamoeba bütschlii* are nonpathogenic for humans. *E. histolytica* is pathogenic for humans, causing invasive intestinal and extraintestinal amebiasis. The pathogenicity of *Blastocystis hominis* is still controversial.

Epidemiology, Transmission, and Prevention

All amebae have a common and relatively simple life cycle. The cyst is the infectious form and is acquired by ingestion of contaminated material such as water and food or by direct fecal-oral transmission. Once the cyst arrives in the intestinal tract, excystation occurs, releasing trophozoites. Encystment occurs in the colon, presumably when conditions become unfavorable for the trophozoites. Cysts are passed in the feces and remain viable in the environment for days to weeks in water and soil if protected from desiccation. Improvements in sanitary conditions are necessary to prevent infections in areas where the organisms are endemic. Research to develop a vaccine against *E. histolytica* is ongoing, but none is currently available.

Collection, Transport, and Storage of Specimens

For detection of the amebae, laboratories predominantly receive stool specimens for examination. Both fresh and preserved specimens are useful for the diagnosis of infection, depending on the methodology employed and the circumstances of the laboratory. If fresh specimens are received for the detection of organism motility, they must be examined quickly; wet mounts for the detection of motility cannot be performed on preserved specimens. Other sample types, such as aspirates and tissue samples, may be received and are appropriate for testing depending on the organism suspected. For a more detailed description of collection, refer to chapter 130 of this *Manual*.

Direct Examination

Microscopy

All diagnostic stages of the amebae (trophozoite and cyst) can be detected in fecal specimens, the most common specimen

TABLE 1 Intestinal and urogenital amebae, flagellates, and ciliates of humans

Parasite	Pathogenic	Nonpathogenic
Amebae	Entamoeba histolytica[a]	Entamoeba dispar[b]
	Blastocystis hominis	Entamoeba hartmanni
		Entamoeba coli
		Entamoeba polecki
		Entamoeba gingivalis[c]
		Endolimax nana
		Iodamoeba bütschlii
Flagellates	Giardia lamblia	Chilomastix mesnili
	Trichomonas vaginalis	Pentatrichomonas (Trichomonas) hominis
	Dientamoeba fragilis	Trichomonas tenax[c]
		Enteromonas hominis
		Retortamonas intestinalis
Ciliates	Balantidium coli	

[a]A distinction between *E. histolytica* and *E. dispar* cannot be made on the basis of morphology unless ingested RBCs are seen in the cytoplasm of the trophozoite.

[b]In rare instances, *Entamoeba moshkovskii* may be found in human stool specimens. A free-living ameba, it is nonpathogenic and morphologically identical to *E. histolytica*/*E. dispar* (151).

[c]*E. gingivalis* and *T. tenax* are found in the oral cavity and related specimens.

submitted to the laboratory. The key morphologic features of amebae must be used to differentiate among the various species and to distinguish between somatic cells and other material. Trophozoites must be distinguished from epithelial cells and macrophages. Cysts must be distinguished from polymorphonuclear cells. Also, yeast, pollen, molds, food particles, and other debris present in feces may cause confusion (Table 2; Fig. 1 and 2).

Morphologic examination of fecal specimens can be accomplished with fresh wet mount preparations, wet mounts of concentrated material, and permanent-stained smears. Each of these three types of preparations may be useful for visualizing certain key characteristics. Stained and unstained wet mounts of concentrated material can also be useful for identification, particularly for certain cysts such as those of *Entamoeba coli* and *I. bütschlii*. Iodine will provide color and contrast, both of which may aid in the identification of organisms in wet preparations. However, morphologic examination with permanent-stained smears by oil immersion microscopy (magnification, ×1,000) is the most useful procedure (25).

Trophozoite motility is visible only in saline wet mounts of fresh feces and is often difficult to detect. The arrangement, size, and pattern of nuclear chromatin help differentiate species within the genus *Entamoeba* from other intestinal amebae. The size and position of the nuclear karyosome are also important morphologic features. A ring of nuclear chromatin surrounding the karyosome, resembling a bull's eye, is characteristic of *Entamoeba*. *Endolimax*, *Iodamoeba*, and the flagellate *Dientamoeba* lack peripheral chromatin. The cytoplasm of the trophozoites may contain granules and ingested material such as red blood cells (RBCs), bacteria, yeasts, and molds.

The characteristics of cysts are less variable than those of trophozoites. To aid in differentiation among the genera, the cytoplasm should be examined for the presence of chromatoidal bodies and vacuoles, particularly the large glycogen vacuole seen in *I. bütschlii*.

Evaluation, Interpretation, and Reporting of Results

It is important to remember that identification may not be possible on the basis of one morphologic feature or the characteristics of a single organism in the preparation. Nuclear and cytoplasmic features can vary within species and may overlap between species, making identification challenging. Mixed infections are not uncommon and can be missed in a cursory examination. A complete, overall assessment of the slide is necessary for correct identification. It is important to use an accurate micrometer to measure life cycle stages. Size is reliable only for the differentiation of *E. histolytica*/*E. dispar* from *E. hartmanni*. Also, on permanent-stained smears, shrinkage may occur, affecting the apparent size of the organism. Results of microscopy should clearly indicate the full taxonomic name of the organisms detected along with the forms of the organisms seen (trophozoites versus cysts). Except for *Blastocystis*, quantitation of the amebae on the final report is not appropriate.

E. histolytica

Taxonomy

E. histolytica and the other *Entamoeba* spp. are classified as belonging to the phylum Amoebozoa, subphylum Conosa, class Archamoebea, order Euamoebida (see chapter 129 of this *Manual*).

Description of the Agent

The development of axenic culture methods was a key step in confirming the existence of two species among organisms that had been identified as *E. histolytica* based solely on microscopic findings. Using organisms obtained by such cultures, Sargeaunt and Williams (125) performed isoenzyme analysis of several glycolytic enzymes and identified electrophoretic banding patterns, or zymodemes. Two groups were identified on the basis of these patterns: pathogenic zymodemes (invasive isolates) and nonpathogenic zymodemes (noninvasive isolates). The zymodeme patterns represent stable genetic differences and do not interconvert (107). Additional genetic, biochemical, and immunologic evidence has supported the existence of two distinct species. Diamond and Clark (30) redescribed the two species as *E. histolytica* Schaudinn 1903, which is the invasive human pathogen, and *E. dispar* Brumpt 1925, which is noninvasive and does not cause disease.

A third species of *Entamoeba*, *E. moshkovskii*, has been recognized and is generally considered a free-living amoeba that may be rarely detected in human stool specimens. It is morphologically indistinguishable from *E. histolytica*/*E. dispar*. The prevalence and epidemiology of *E. moshkovskii* is not

TABLE 2 Key features of trophozoites and cysts of common intestinal amebae[a]

Organism	Trophozoites	Cysts
E. histolytica/E. dispar	Size[b]: 12–60 μm; invasive forms, >20 μm Motility: Progressive, directional, rapid Nucleus[c]: 1; peripheral chromatin evenly distributed; karyosome small, compact, centrally located; may resemble E. coli Cytoplasm: Finely granular, like "ground glass"; may contain bacteria Note: RBCs in cytoplasm diagnostic for E. histolytica infection	Size: 10–20 μm; spherical, centrally located Cytoplasm: Chromatoidal bodies may be present; elongate with blunt rounded edges; may be round or oval
E. hartmanni	Size: 5–12 μm Motility: Nonprogressive Nucleus: 1; peripheral chromatin like E. histolytica/E. dispar, may appear as solid ring; karyosome small, compact, centrally located or eccentric Cytoplasm: Finely granular, bacteria, no RBCs Note: Accurate measurement essential for differentiation from E. histolytica/E. dispar	Size: 5–10 μm; spherical Nucleus: Mature cyst, 4; immature cyst, 1 or 2 (very common); peripheral chromatin fine, evenly distributed, may be difficult to see; karyosome small, compact, centrally located Cytoplasm: Chromatoidal bodies usually present, like in E. histolytica/E. dispar
E. coli	Size: 15–50 μm Motility: Sluggish, nondirectional Nucleus: 1; peripheral chromatin clumped and uneven, may be solid ring; karyosome large, not compact, diffuse, eccentric Cytoplasm: Granular, usually vacuolated; contains bacteria, yeast, no RBCs Note: Can resemble E. histolytica/E. dispar; coinfection seen; stained smear essential	Size: 10–35 μm; spherical, rarely oval or triangular Nucleus: Mature cyst, 8; occasionally ≥16; immature cyst, ≥2; peripheral chromatin coarsely granular, unevenly arranged; may resemble E. histolytica/E. dispar; karyosome small, usually eccentric but may be central Cytoplasm: Chromatoidal bodies less frequent than in E. histolytica/E. dispar; splintered, with rough, pointed ends Note: May be distorted on permanent-stained smear due to poor penetration of fixative
E. nana	Size: 6–12 μm Motility: Sluggish, nonprogressive Nucleus: 1; no peripheral chromatin; karyosome large, "blot like" Cytoplasm: Granular, vacuolated; may contain bacteria Note: May be tremendous nuclear variation; can mimic E. hartmanni and D. fragilis	Size: 5–10 μm; oval, may be round Nucleus: Mature cyst, 4; immature cyst, 2; no peripheral chromatin; karyosome smaller than those in trophozoites but larger than those in Entamoeba spp. Cytoplasm: Chromatoidal bodies rare; small granules occasionally seen
I. bütschlii	Size: 8–20 μm Motility: Sluggish, nonprogressive Nucleus: 1; no peripheral chromatin; karyosome large, may have "basket nucleus" Cytoplasm: Coarsely granular, may be highly vacuolated; bacteria, yeast, and debris may be seen Note: Stained smear essential; nucleus may appear to have a halo with chromatin granules fanning around karyosome	Size: 5–20 μm; oval to round Nucleus: Mature cyst, 1; no peripheral chromatin; karyosome large, usually eccentric Cytoplasm: No chromatoidal bodies; small granules occasionally present Note: Glycogen present, large, compact, well-defined mass; cysts may collapse owing to large glycogen vacuole space
B. hominis[d]	Very difficult to identify; rarely seen	Size: 2–200 μm; generally round Description: Usually characterized by a large, central body (looks like a large vacuole) surrounded by small, multiple nuclei; central body area can stain various colors (trichrome) or remain clear

[a]Adapted from reference 37.
[b]Size ranges are based on wet preparations (with permanent stains, organisms usually measure 1 to 2 μm less).
[c]Nuclear and cytoplasmic descriptions are based on permanent-stained smears.
[d]Description of central body form.

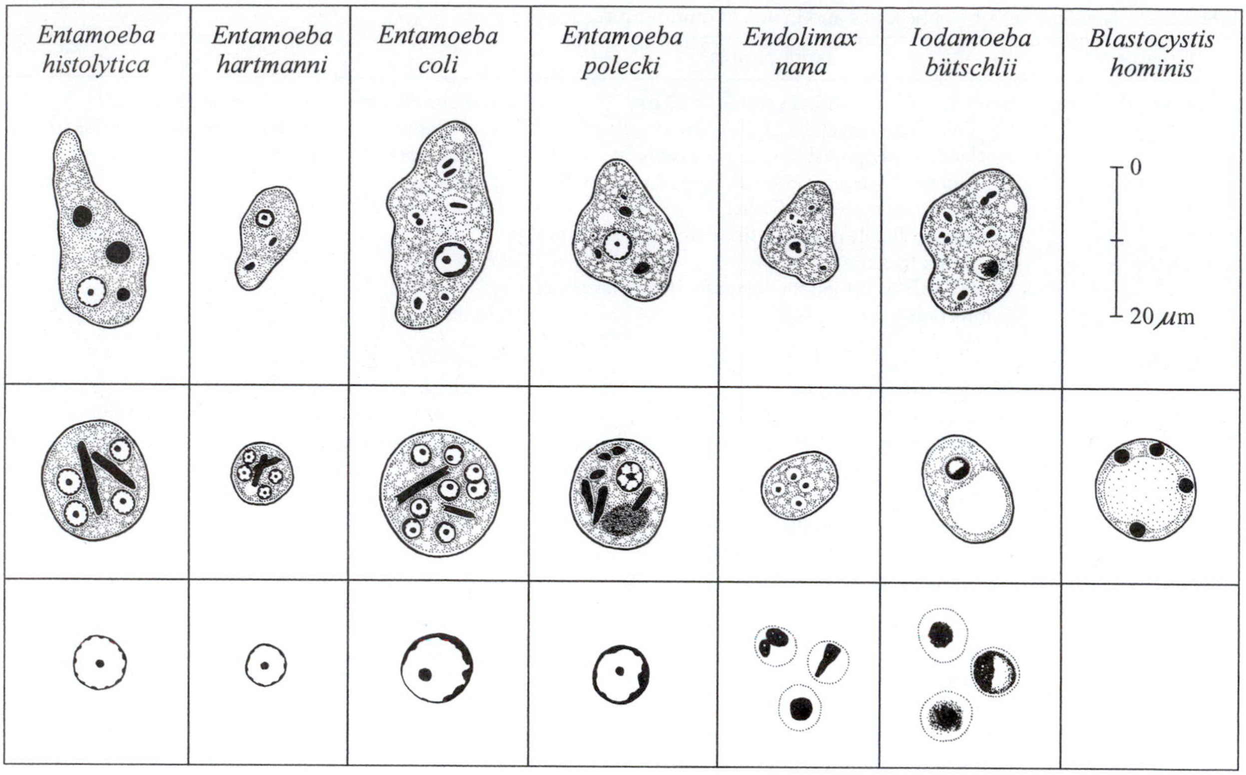

FIGURE 1 Intestinal amebae of humans. (Top row) Trophozoites. *E. histolytica* is shown with ingested RBCs. This is the only microscopic finding that allows differentiation of the pathogenic species *E. histolytica* from the nonpathogenic species *E. dispar*. An ameboid form of *B. hominis* is rarely seen and is difficult to identify. (Middle row) Cysts. For *B. hominis* the central body form is depicted. (Bottom row) Trophozoite nuclei, shown in relative proportion.

well understood. It has been reported as an agent of gastrointestinal disease in some publications (24, 49). More research is needed to understand the role of this organism in human disease and the importance of laboratory diagnosis (35).

Epidemiology, Transmission, and Prevention

E. histolytica can be found worldwide but is more prevalent in tropical and subtropical regions. In areas where the organism is endemic, up to 50% of people may be infected. In temperate climates with poor sanitation, infection rates can approach those seen in tropical regions. Humans are the primary reservoir; infection occurs by ingestion of cysts from fecally contaminated material such as water and food. Sexual transmission also occurs.

Asymptomatic *E. histolytica* infection is equally distributed between the genders, while invasive amebiasis affects men predominantly. In the United States, groups with a higher incidence of amebiasis include immigrants from South and Central America and Southeast Asia. Also, residents of the southern United States and institutionalized individuals are more likely than others to be infected. In one study, short-term travelers to areas where *E. histolytica* and *E. dispar* are endemic were found to be at higher risk of infection with the pathogenic species, *E. histolytica*, than were residents, who were more likely to harbor the nonpathogenic species, *E. dispar* (159). In homosexual males, the infection is often transmitted by sexual behavior, with up to 30% found to be infected in certain studies. These infections are most often asymptomatic. Among human immunodeficiency virus

(HIV)-infected patients in the United States, the incidence of diagnosed *E. histolytica* disease is low (13.5 cases per 10,000 person-years) (88). HIV-infected individuals in non-Western countries, such as Taiwan and Korea, do have a higher risk of invasive amebiasis, in contrast to findings from the United States (61, 104). These differing rates of invasive disease may be attributed to the higher endemicity of *E. histolytica* in the Asia-Pacific regions (62).

Clinical Significance

Among the estimated 500 million people infected each year with *E. histolytica*, there are approximately 50 million cases of colitis and liver abscess and 100,000 deaths (164). The discrepancy between the number of people infected with *E. histolytica* and the morbidity and mortality rates is explained by the existence of two morphologically similar yet distinct species: one capable of producing disease (*E. histolytica*) and the other not (*E. dispar*). *E. dispar* appears to be at least 10 times more common than *E. histolytica* (35).

Infection with *E. histolytica/E. dispar* can result in different clinical presentations: asymptomatic infection, symptomatic infection without tissue invasion, and symptomatic infection with tissue invasion. The majority of infections with *E. histolytica/E. dispar* are asymptomatic. Individuals with such infections will have a negative or weak serologic response and will primarily pass cysts in their stools. Zymodeme analysis shows that most asymptomatic individuals are infected with the noninvasive species *E. dispar* (163, 164). However, it appears that infection with both *E. histolytica*

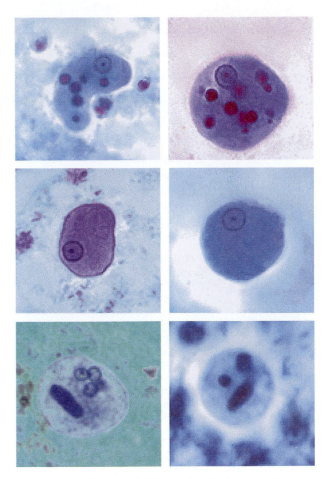

FIGURE 2 (Top row) *Entamoeba histolytica* trophozoites. Note the ingested RBCs in the cytoplasm. (Middle row) *E. histolytica/E. dispar* trophozoites. Note the absence of RBCs in the cytoplasm. (Bottom row) *E. histolytica/E. dispar* cysts. These cysts cannot be identified to the species level on the basis of morphology. Organisms are stained with Wheatley's trichrome stain. (Courtesy of L. Garcia.)

and *E. dispar* can be asymptomatic, with cyst stages being passed in the stool (13). Asymptomatic *E. histolytica* infection may be due to the existence of genetically distinct invasive and noninvasive strains of *E. histolytica* (170).

Intestinal disease results from the penetration of the amebic trophozoites into the intestinal tissues. Approximately 10% of infected individuals will have clinical symptoms, presenting as dysentery, colitis, or rarely, ameboma. The incubation period varies from a few days to several months. Various molecules such as adhesins, amebapores, and proteases have been associated with lysis of the colonic mucosa in intestinal amebiasis (32). The 260-kDa galactose- or *N*-acetylgalactosamine-specific lectin of *E. histolytica* is an important virulence factor, mediating the attachment of the ameba to the intestinal epithelium and contact-dependent cytolysis (115). Symptoms of amebic dysentery include diarrhea with cramping, lower abdominal pain, low-grade fever, and the presence of blood and mucus in stool. The ulcers produced by intestinal invasion by trophozoites start as superficial localized lesions that deepen into the classic flask-shaped ulcers of amebic colitis. The ulcers are separated by segments of normal tissue but can coalesce. Amebae can be

found at the advancing edges of the ulcer but usually not in the necrotic areas. Abdominal perforation and peritonitis are rare but serious complications. A more chronic presentation occurs with amebic colitis. It is characterized by intermittent diarrhea over a long period and can be misdiagnosed as ulcerative colitis or irritable bowel syndrome. Ameboma, a localized tumor-like lesion, results from chronic ulceration and may be mistaken for malignancy. Histologically, it consists of granulomatous tissue.

Extraintestinal disease occurs with the hematogenous spread of the organism. It can occur with or without previous symptomatic intestinal infection. The liver is the most common site of extraintestinal disease, followed by the lungs, pericardium, brain, and other organs. Symptoms can be acute or gradual and may include low-grade fever, right-upper-quadrant pain, and weight loss. Up to 5% of individuals with intestinal symptoms develop liver abscess. However, up to 50% of individuals with liver abscess have no history of gastrointestinal disease.

Direct Examination

The laboratory diagnosis of amebiasis can be made by the examination of feces, material obtained from sigmoidoscopy, tissue biopsy specimens, and abscess aspirates. Serologic testing is also useful for the diagnosis of extraintestinal amebiasis. The choice of methods used by each laboratory is dependent on the available resources, funding, and clinical need. A summary of the laboratory techniques and their performance characteristics is presented in Table 3.

Microscopy

As discussed above, the most important part of the standard microscopic examination of stool and other specimens is the permanent-stained smear. Direct wet preparations and concentration procedures may also be useful (Fig. 1 and Table 2; see also chapter 132). Detection of trophozoites and cysts does not, however, allow differentiation of the pathogenic species, *E. histolytica*, from the nonpathogenic species, *E. dispar* (Fig. 1 and 2). The presence of ingested RBCs in the cytoplasm of the trophozoites is commonly regarded as diagnostic of *E. histolytica* infection. However, the majority of patient samples do not contain trophozoites with ingested RBCs (35). In addition to concerns about sensitivity, Haque et al. (52) found that 16% of *E. dispar* isolates had ingested RBCs; thus, this distinction between the two species is not absolute and may affect specificity (151, 152). In tissue specimens, only the trophozoite is found, and its presence is considered diagnostic of invasive *E. histolytica* disease.

Antigen Detection

For a more definitive differentiation of *E. histolytica* and *E. dispar*, methods other than microscopy are necessary. Zymodeme analysis can accomplish this differentiation, but it requires culture of the organisms from the specimen and is too expensive and complex for routine laboratory use. More recently, antigen detection methods for the detection and differentiation of *E. histolytica* and *E. dispar* have become commercially available in the United States. A listing of commercially available parasite antigen detection kits is given in chapter 130 and has been recently reviewed (35).

The antigen detection assays are designed for use with fresh, fresh-frozen, or unfixed human fecal specimens. Depending on the kit used, the group *E. histolytica/E. dispar* or the individual species can be detected in the feces. Only TechLab (Blacksburg, VA) offers an *E. histolytica*-specific kit, *E. Histolytica II*, which detects the Gal- or GalNAc-

TABLE 3 Sensitivity and specificity of diagnostic tests for amebiasis[a]

Test and specimen type	Colitis		Liver abscess, sensitivity (%)
	Sensitivity (%)	Specificity (%)	
Microscopy			
Stool	>60	10–50	<10
Abscess fluid	NA[b]	NA	<25
Culture with isoenzyme analysis	Lower than antigen or PCR tests	Gold standard	<25
Stool antigen detection (ELISA)[c]	>95	>95	Usually negative
Serum	65 (early)	>90	~75 (late); ~100 (first 3 days)
Abscess fluid	NA	NA	~100 (before treatment)
Saliva	Not done	Not done	70
PCR, stool	>70	>90	Not done
Serum antibody detection (ELISA)	>90	>85	70–80 (acute stage); >90 (convalescent stage)

[a]Reprinted from reference 151 with permission.
[b]NA, not available.
[c]ELISA, enzyme-linked immunosorbent assay.

binding lectin specific to the pathogenic species (52, 114). A rapid, point-of-care test for *E. histolytica* antigen has been reported and would be useful particularly in the developing world; this test is not yet available commercially (86). All the antigen detection methods are relatively simple and are more sensitive and specific than microscopy (Table 3) (41, 52, 106). In comparison to amplified methods such as PCR, antigen detection using stool specimens may be less sensitive and specific for detection of *E. histolytica*/*E. dispar*, depending on the population studied (124, 143). To date, none of the available products can be used with preserved stool, as the fixative appears to denature the antigens. Although some reports of the use of preserved stool have appeared (166), more work is needed to identify additional antigens that withstand fixation before it would be practical to offer antigen tests in laboratories that receive only preserved stool specimens. Antigen assays have been used to test a number of other sample types such as serum, pus, and saliva (1, 51); the detection of antigen in serum may prove to be a sensitive means of diagnosing amebic liver abscess and intestinal disease (51, 151). Because fewer than 10% of patients with amebic liver abscesses have concurrent intestinal disease with amebae detectable in the stool, methods such as routine ova and parasite examination are not useful. Microscopic examination or culture of pus from liver abscesses likewise lacks sensitivity. In a study by Haque et al. (51), serum antigen detection by using the TechLab *E. Histolytica II* kit was a sensitive method for diagnosis with samples collected prior to treatment with metronidazole. Serum antigenemia appears to clear after treatment, suggesting possible utility to monitor therapy; however, this use is still experimental (51, 151).

Nucleic Acid Detection Techniques
Nucleic acid amplification techniques, such as PCR, have been developed for the detection and differentiation of *E. histolytica* and *E. dispar*. The most common genomic targets include the rRNA- or species-specific episomal repeats. Conventional PCR has been applied to specimens such as stool, liver, or brain aspirates, and cerebrospinal fluid and can detect both trophozoite and cyst DNA (34, 118, 122, 136, 171). Several researchers have reported

multiplex PCR methods for detection and differentiation of *E. histolytica*, *E. dispar*, and *E moshkovskii* (35, 75). Use of such a multiplex assay would permit a more accurate diagnosis than microscopy and allow targeted therapy for only true *E. histolytica* infections. More recently, real-time PCR has been used for the detection of *E. histolytica* and *E. dispar* (8, 124) and for the simultaneous detection of *E. histolytica*, *G. lamblia*, and *Cryptosporidium parvum* (157) in clinical specimens. Different extraction techniques, some of which are relatively simple, and the use of fresh and preserved material have been reported (108, 153, 158). Stool can present challenges due to the presence of PCR inhibitors (98), so the inclusion of an amplification control is useful (157).

PCR has proven to be more sensitive and specific than microscopy and at least as sensitive as antigen detection, depending on the study (Table 3) (48, 124, 151). For routine use in clinical laboratories, a PCR method would ideally involve a relatively simple sample preparation procedure and allow the use of preserved material. Because PCR and antigen detection may be approximately equal in sensitivities, an antigen detection test may be preferable due to technical ease of use and shorter time required.

Serologic Tests
Serologic testing is a valuable aid, in conjunction with antigen detection or PCR, for the diagnosis of symptomatic, invasive disease. Multiple serologic methods have been used, including indirect hemagglutination, complement fixation, latex agglutination, and EIA (35, 151). These methods are most useful in populations where *E. histolytica* is not endemic. Of patients with biopsy-proven intestinal amebiasis, 85% have serum antibodies. For patients with extraintestinal disease, serologic tests have a sensitivity approaching 99%. For asymptomatic intestinal diseases, serology is generally not useful unless the patient has invasive infection. Persons infected with *E. dispar* do not produce detectable antibodies. After cure of invasive amebiasis, serum antibodies may persist for up to 10 years; this can complicate diagnosis in areas where infection is endemic (69).

EIAs for the detection of immunoglobulin M (IgM) and IgG are widely used, and most are based on the detection of antilectin antibodies, which appear over 1 week after symptoms of *E. histolytica* infection (151). Indirect hemagglutination is useful and highly specific but may lack sensitivity compared to EIAs (151). Several investigators have reported the utility of IgA antibody testing and a link to partial immunity in individuals with detectable antilectin IgA (50, 51, 140). There are several commercially available serologic kits for diagnosis of amebiasis, some of which are available in the United States. For a recent review of serologic testing see the article by Fotedar et al. (35) and also refer to chapter 5 in this *Manual*.

Treatment

On the basis of the 1997 World Health Organization conference, treatment is not recommended for *E. dispar* infections; if *E. histolytica*/*E. dispar* is detected (no differentiation of species) in symptomatic patients, the physician must evaluate the total clinical presentation to decide whether treatment is indicated. The detection of *E. histolytica* requires treatment of the patient regardless of the symptoms. The use of diagnostics that are species specific (i.e., antigen detection or PCR) allows for targeted chemotherapy.

The drugs used for the treatment of amebiasis are of two classes: luminal amebicides for cysts (paromomycin, iodoquinol, and diloxanide furoate) and tissue amebicides for trophozoites (metronidazole, tinidazole, and dehydroemetine) (2). Invasive disease should be treated with a tissue amebicide followed by a luminal amebicide. Tissue amebicides are not appropriate for treatment of asymptomatic infections (cysts). No high-level resistance to amebicides has been detected to date. Follow-up stool examination is always necessary because of potential treatment failures. Chemoprophylaxis is never appropriate because it may lead to drug resistance and limit the utility of drugs such as metronidazole (155, 164).

Evaluation, Interpretation, and Reporting of Results

Laboratory reporting of *Entamoeba* infection must account for the ability of a particular methodology to detect and differentiate pathogenic and nonpathogenic species. This is based on the report of a World Health Organization panel of experts which made recommendations concerning the reporting and treatment of amebiasis (164). If a microscopic diagnosis is made on the basis of the detection of trophozoites and/or cysts and no method is used to differentiate the two species, the report should indicate "*E. histolytica*/*E. dispar* detected." Laboratory reports must indicate whether trophozoites and/or cysts are present, due to differences in therapy.

Antigen detection methods may or may not allow species differentiation, and the laboratory report should accurately reflect these facts. Reporting of PCR results which are specific for *E. histolytica* or *E. dispar* should state that nucleic acid was detected or not detected. Due to the ability of amplified methods to detect nonviable organisms, the use of PCR for determination of treatment failure should be interpreted cautiously. Neither antigen detection nor PCR allows for determination of the parasite forms present.

B. hominis

Taxonomy

Since its first description in 1912, the taxonomic classification of *Blastocystis hominis* has changed and is still somewhat unclear (19, 134). Current classification of *Blastocystis* is as follows: class Blastocystea, subkingdom Chromobiota, and kingdom Stramenopila (formerly Chromista) (see chapter 129). Molecular studies indicate that *Blastocystis* is closely related to *Proteromonas lacertae* (7, 58, 150). Though *P. lacertae* is a flagellate, interestingly, *B. hominis* does not possess a flagellum and is nonmotile. Genetic, biochemical, and immunologic analyses have revealed that great diversity exists within the species (23, 89, 102). Recent studies have shown that that *Blastocystis* spp. in humans and animals can be divided into 12 or more species (102).

Description of the Agent

The life cycle of *B. hominis* includes vacuolar and fecal cyst forms, granular forms, and ameboid forms with pseudopod-like cytoplasmic extensions. The exact nature of the life cycle of this organism and the infective form has yet to be confirmed experimentally. The cyst form can be varied depending on whether the cyst is observed in fresh stool or in culture (150). *B. hominis* produces pseudopods and reproduces by binary fission or sporulation. It is strictly anaerobic and is capable of ingesting bacteria and other debris. The membrane-bound central body occupies up to 90% of the cell and may function in reproduction. Both thin- and thick-walled cysts have been observed.

Epidemiology, Transmission, and Prevention

B. hominis is a common intestinal parasite of humans and animals, with a worldwide distribution (150). Depending on the geographic location, it may be detected in 1 to 40% of fecal specimens. Human-to-human, animal-to-human, and waterborne modes of transmission have been proposed (84, 102, 150, 168). The organism is polymorphic, consisting of four major forms. The thick-walled cysts are thought to be responsible for external transmission via the fecal-oral route; the thin-walled cysts are thought to cause autoinfection (96). The cyst form is the most recently described form of the life cycle stages. The cysts can vary in shape but are mostly ovoid or spherical. The central vacuole form (also referred to as the central body form) is the most common form found in clinical stool samples. The large central vacuole can occupy the majority of the cellular volume. The ameboid form is rarely reported, and the granular form can be seen when culturing the parasite.

Clinical Significance

The role of *B. hominis* in human disease is still controversial, and studies supporting and refuting its pathogenicity have been published (91, 132, 172). Most recent epidemiological studies point to the fact that *B. hominis* is a pathogen. Since many genotypes appear to exist, there is strong evidence that there are pathogenic and nonpathogenic species (150). Regardless of the number of publications on each side of this debate, clinicians may decide to treat patients with *B. hominis* infection. When *B. hominis* is present in large numbers in the absence of other pathogens, it may be the cause of gastrointestinal disease. The most common symptoms cited include recurrent diarrhea without fever, vomiting, and abdominal pain. The symptoms may be more pronounced and prolonged in patients with underlying conditions such as HIV infection, neoplasia, and abnormal intestinal tract function (60, 154). Other studies suggest that symptomatic patients receiving treatment for *B. hominis* infection may improve due to the elimination of another, undetected pathogen (91). In a study of HIV-infected individuals, Albrecht et al. (5) concluded that, even in patients with severe underlying immunodeficiencies, *B. hominis* is not pathogenic and its detection does not justify treatment.

Direct Examination

Microscopy

Diagnosis of infection is made by detection of the organism, typically the central body form, by routine microscopic stool examination (Table 2; Fig. 1 and 3). The size of the central body form can vary tremendously, from 2 to 200 µm. Extensive size variation exists within and between isolates. The vacuolar form contains a large central vacuole that occupies approximately 90% of the cell (119, 150). Examination of permanent-stained smears is the procedure of choice. Exposure to water before fixation (for the concentration method) will lyse the trophozoites and central body forms, yielding false-negative results. Some type of quantitation (few, moderate, or many) should be included in the laboratory report. Direct wet mounts using iodine as a stain are not recommended, as trichrome staining is more sensitive (150).

Other Diagnostic Methods

Culture of the organism from stool is possible and has been reported to be more sensitive than microscopy but is not routinely available (85). A serologic response to *B. hominis* has been detected using techniques such as EIA and fluorescent-antibody testing (36, 150, 173). It is suggested that this antibody response supports the role of *B. hominis* as a human pathogen but is not useful for diagnosis and should be limited to epidemiological and serologic studies. In asymptomatic individuals, a serologic response may require exposure of up to 2 years before it is detectable (70). A review by Tan describes in detail molecular approaches to the diagnosis and characterization of *B. hominis* (150). Molecular approaches to organism detection might be more sensitive based on some studies but are still not routinely available in the clinical laboratory setting (144–146).

Treatment

Until the role of *B. hominis* as an intestinal pathogen is clearly established, treatment decisions must be based on the overall clinical presentation. Current recommendations for treatment include the use of metronidazole, iodoquinol, or trimethoprim-sulfamethoxazole (2). Metronidazole appears to be the most appropriate choice at present. In vitro data on the susceptibility of *B. hominis* to various drugs are limited (172), but resistance to metronidazole has been reported (55). A failure to clear organisms from the stool has been demonstrated in patients treated with metronidazole and trimethoprim-sulfamethoxazole.

Evaluation, Interpretation, and Reporting of Results

For most laboratories, testing and reporting for *B. hominis* will be limited to detection of the organism by microscopic means. There can be confusion in identifying *Blastocystis* correctly, since the organism can be confused with yeast, fat globules, and even *Cyclospora* spp. It is not necessary to state the form of the organism present (i.e., central body form). This is the sole intestinal parasite that should be routinely reported with quantitation to aid clinicians in determining its clinical significance. Additional commentary may be added to the laboratory report explaining the role of *B. hominis* in disease and the need to exclude other causes for the clinical condition.

NONPATHOGENIC AMEBAE

The other species of intestinal amebae are considered nonpathogenic; except for *Entamoeba polecki*, they have a worldwide distribution and are more prevalent in warmer climates. They must, however, be differentiated from the pathogenic species, *E. histolytica*. A permanently stained smear is often essential to accomplish this goal (Table 2; Fig. 1).

E. hartmanni is a separate species that is morphologically similar to *E. histolytica/E. dispar* (Fig. 4). Size is the key differentiating characteristic. *Entamoeba coli* trophozoites may be difficult to differentiate from *E. histolytica/E. dispar* trophozoites on wet preparations. The mature cyst of *Entamoeba coli* may be refractory to fixation, making it less visible in permanent-stained smears but still detectable by the wet mount method (Fig. 5). It has been reported as the most common ameba isolated from human stool specimens. *E. polecki* is associated with pigs, and in certain areas of the world, such as Papua New Guinea, it is the most common human intestinal parasite. The trophozoite shares characteristics with both *E. histolytica/E. dispar* and *Entamoeba coli*; the cyst normally has one nucleus. *Entamoeba gingivalis* was the first parasitic ameba of humans to be described. It is found in the soft tartar between teeth and can be recovered from sputum. In the trophozoite, the cytoplasm often contains ingested leukocytes. A cyst form has not been observed.

E. nana, like *E. hartmanni*, is one of the smaller intestinal amebae. It is seen in most populations as frequently as *Entamoeba coli*. There is a great deal of nuclear variation, and it can mimic *D. fragilis* and *E. hartmanni* (Fig. 6). The cysts of *E. nana* are usually oval, and both the trophozoites and the cysts are commonly present in fecal material. *I. bütschlii* has the same distribution as other nonpathogenic amebae but is less common than *Entamoeba coli* and *E. nana*. The

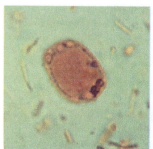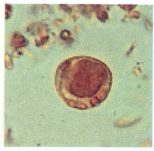

FIGURE 3 *Blastocystis hominis* on an iodine wet mount preparation. Note the peripheral nuclei and the central body form. (Courtesy of L. Garcia.)

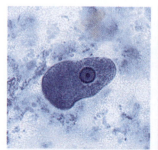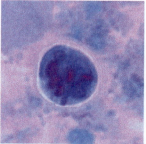

FIGURE 4 *Entamoeba hartmanni* trophozoite (left) and cyst (right). Note the "bull's eye" nucleus in the trophozoite and the numerous chromatoidal bars within the cyst. Organisms are stained with Wheatley's trichrome stain. (Courtesy of L. Garcia.)

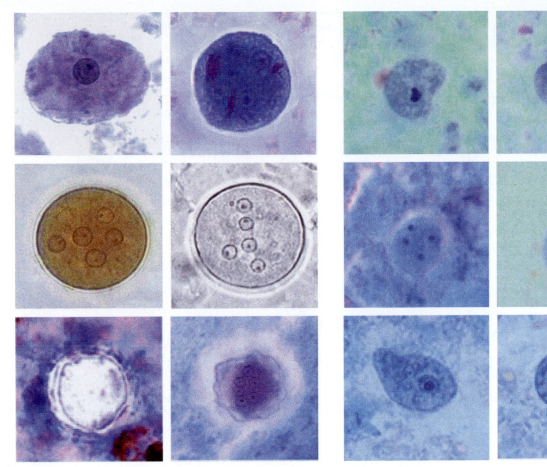

FIGURE 5 (Top row) *Entamoeba coli* trophozoite (left) and cyst (right). Note the large eccentric karyosome in the trophozoite and the chromatoidal bars with sharp pointed ends in the cyst. (Middle row) *Entamoeba coli* cyst in iodine (left) and in saline (right). The nuclei are visible; the presence of five or more nuclei is confirmatory for *Entamoeba coli*. (Bottom row) *Entamoeba coli* cyst (left; trichrome) and cyst (right; trichrome). Both cysts are very distorted and shrunken, although the nuclei can be seen in the cyst on the right. This type of shrinkage is typical of *Entamoeba coli* cysts on permanent-stained smears. (Courtesy of L. Garcia.)

FIGURE 6 (Top row) *Endolimax nana* trophozoites. Note the typical nucleus on the left and the nuclear variation on the right. (Middle row) *E. nana* cysts. Note the typical four nuclei, none of which have peripheral chromatin. (Bottom row) *I. bütschlii* trophozoite (left) and cyst (right). Note the "basket nucleus" in the cyst, along with the large glycogen vacuole. Organisms are stained with Wheatley's trichrome stain. (Courtesy of L. Garcia.)

trophozoite of *I. bütschlii* may be similar to that of *E. nana*, and differentiation between them is difficult. The cyst is very characteristic; it is round to oval and may contain a large glycogen vacuole (Fig. 6).

Treatment is not recommended for infections with any of the nonpathogenic amebae. Methods of prevention of infection with all these amebae include improved personal hygiene and improved sanitary conditions.

FLAGELLATES

Taxonomy

There are six genera of flagellates that parasitize the intestinal tracts of humans; they belong to phylum Metamonada, class Trichomonada, (*Dientamoeba* and *Trichomona*), class Trepomonadea (*Giardia* and *Enteromonas*), and class Retortamonadea (*Chilomastix* and *Retortamonas*) (Fig. 7; see chapter 129).

Description of the Agents

Some flagellates are commensals that reside in the intestinal tract and are harmless to the individual. The flagellates that are pathogenic to humans include *G. lamblia*, *D. fragilis*, and *Trichomonas vaginalis*. The nonpathogenic organisms are *Chilomastix mesnili*, *Enteromonas hominis*, *Retortamonas intestinalis*, and *Pentatrichomonas* (*Trichomonas*) *hominis*. As mentioned above, *D. fragilis* has been reclassified as a flagellate and appears to be closely related to the trichomonads.

Epidemiology, Transmission, and Prevention

Transmission of flagellates, with the exception of *T. vaginalis*, is initiated via the ingestion of contaminated food or water. Of the members of the six genera, all except *D. fragilis* and *Trichomonas* spp. are transmitted in a cyst form. To date, only a trophozoite form has been observed for *D. fragilis* and *Trichomonas* spp. Once in the intestine, the organism excysts, releasing trophozoites that attach to the intestinal epithelium. Completion of the life cycle in humans culminates in the release of viable cysts into the environment via the feces. Infection with any of the flagellates

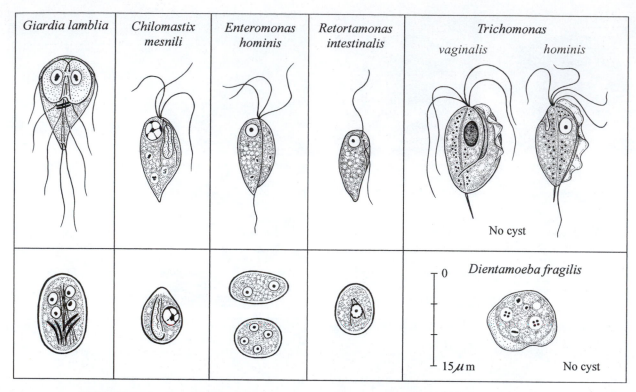

FIGURE 7 Intestinal and urogenital flagellates of humans. (Top row) Trophozoites. *T. vaginalis* is found in urogenital sites; all other flagellates are intestinal. (Bottom row) Cysts. *D. fragilis* trophozoite is shown; no cyst stage.

indicates exposure to feces regardless of the pathogenicity of the organism; preventing this exposure is the key. Measures to improve sanitary conditions are necessary to prevent the spread of infection. As yet, there are no human flagellate vaccines available.

Collection, Transport, and Storage of Specimens

For the detection of flagellates and ciliates, laboratories predominantly receive stool specimens for microscopic examination. String test samples can be submitted for *Giardia* as well. Fresh or preserved specimens can be submitted, but preserved stool is the specimen of choice for most routine clinical laboratories. If fresh specimens are submitted and observed for motility, they must be examined within a specific time period depending on the consistency of the stool. Stool specimens for immunoassay or DFA assay can be fixed in formalin, which can also be used for an ova and parasite exam if immunoassays are negative for *G. lamblia*. Additional information on specimen collection and transport can be found in chapter 130 of this *Manual*.

Direct Examination

Microscopy

In the clinical laboratory, wet preparations and permanent-stained smears of fecal material are still the predominant specimens used to diagnose infections with flagellates. The flagellates have greater morphologic diversity relative to one another than do the amebae (described above), making determination of the genus easier (Table 4; Fig. 7). To aid in the identification of the trophozoite, key features to be noted are the shape, size, number, and position of flagella;

the number of nuclei; and the presence of a spiral groove, cytostome, and characteristic features such as a sucking disk or undulating membrane. Typically, the size, shape, and number of nuclei are diagnostic characteristics used to identify cysts. Examination of permanent-stained smears is always recommended for diagnosis of infection because the wet mount may not be reflective of all organisms and stages present in the specimen.

Other Diagnostic Methods

Antigen-based tests for organisms such as *G. lamblia* are increasing in popularity due to the ease of use and increased throughput compared to microscopy. In addition, nucleic acid amplification methods have been developed to detect *T. vaginalis* in clinical samples and *G. lamblia* in water and clinical samples but are not yet routinely available in the clinical laboratory. Both antigen and amplification tests for the flagellates will be discussed in more detail below. Serologic assays are available for the diagnosis of *G. lamblia* infection but are not routinely used in the clinical setting.

Evaluation, Interpretation, and Reporting of Results

It is important that a representative portion of the slide, either a wet mount or a permanent smear, be scanned before a final opinion on a specimen is given. It is also important to use an accurate micrometer to measure life cycle stages. Reports of microscopy results should clearly indicate the full taxonomic names of the organisms detected along with the forms of the organisms seen (trophozoites versus cysts). Quantitation of the number of organisms seen is not appropriate for the flagellates.

TABLE 4 Key features of trophozoites and cysts of common intestinal and urogenital flagellates[a]

Organism	Trophozoites	Cysts
D. fragilis	Size[b]: 5–15 μm; shaped like amebae Motility: Nonprogressive; pseudopodia are angular Flagella: None Nucleus[c]: 1 (40%) or 2 (60%); no peripheral chromatin; karyosome clusters of 4–8 granules Note: Trophozoites not visible in unstained preparation; variation in size between trophozoites can exist on the same smear; cytoplasm is finely granular, and vacuoles may be present	No cyst stage
G. lamblia	Size: 10–20 μm long, 5–15 μm wide; pear shaped Motility: Falling leaf Flagella: 4 lateral, 2 ventral, 2 caudal Nucleus: 2; not visible in unstained preparation; small central karyosomes present Note: Sucking disk is prominent on ventral side of trophozoite; organism is spoon shaped from side view	Size: 8–19 μm long, 7–10 μm wide; oval, ellipsoidal, or round Nucleus: 4 nuclei usually located on one end; not distinct in unstained preparation; no peripheral chromatin; karyosomes smaller than those in trophozoite Cytoplasm: Staining can cause shrinkage where cytoplasm pulls away from the cyst wall; 4 median bodies present Note: Poorly defined longitudinal fibers may be present
C. mesnili	Size: 6–24 μm long, 4–8 μm wide; pear shaped Motility: Stiff, rotary Flagella: 3 anterior, 1 in cytostome Nucleus: 1; not visible in unstained preparation Cytoplasm: Prominent cytostome extends over 1/3 to 1/2 of body; spiral groove across ventral surface can be hard to see; vacuoles present	Size: 6–10 μm long, 4–6 μm wide; lemon shaped with anterior hyaline knob Nucleus: Same as trophozoite; difficult to see in unstained preparation; indistinct central karyosome present Cytoplasm: Curved fibril alongside cytostome known as "shepherd's crook"
P. hominis	Size: 5–15 μm long, 7–10 μm wide; pear shaped Motility: Jerky, rapid Flagella: 3–5 anterior, 1 posterior (extends beyond end of body) Nucleus: 1; not visible in unstained preparation Cytoplasm: Central longitudinal axostyle; undulating membrane runs the entire length of body Note: May have tremendous nuclear variation; can mimic *E. hartmanni* and *D. fragilis*	No cyst stage
T. vaginalis	Size: 7–23 μm long, 5–15 μm wide Motility: Jerky, rapid Flagella: 3–5 anterior, 1 posterior Nucleus: 1; not visible in unstained preparation Note: Undulating membrane extends 1/2 the length of body; no free posterior flagella	No cyst stage
E. hominis	Size: 4–10 μm long, 5–6 μm wide; oval Motility: Jerky Flagella: 3 anterior, 1 posterior Nucleus: 1; not visible in unstained preparation Note: One side of the body is flat; posterior flagellum extends free posteriorly or laterally	Size: 4–10 μm long, 4–6 μm wide; elongate or oval in shape Nucleus: 1–4; not visible in stained preparation Note: Resemble *E. nana* cysts; fibrils or flagella usually not seen
R. intestinalis	Size: 4–9 μm long, 3–4 μm wide; pear shaped or oval Motility: Jerky Flagella: 1 anterior, 1 posterior Nucleus: 1; not visible in unstained preparation Note: Very difficult to identify; rarely seen; prominent cytostome which extends half the length of body	Size: 4–9 μm long, 5 μm wide; pear or lemon shaped Nucleus: 1; not visible in unstained preparation Note: Resemble *Chilomastix* cysts; bird beak fibril arrangement; shadow outline of cytostome with supporting fibrils extends above nucleus

[a]Adapted from reference 37.
[b]Size ranges are based on wet preparations (with permanent stains, organisms usually measure 1 to 2 μm less).
[c]Nuclear and cytoplasmic descriptions are based on permanent-stained smears.

G. lamblia

Taxonomy

G. lamblia and the other *Giardia* spp. are classified as belonging to the phylum Metamonada (flagellates), subphylum Conosa, class Trepomonadea (intestinal flagellates), order Diplomonadida (see chapter 129 of this *Manual*).

Description of the Agent and Taxonomy

G. lamblia is an intestinal flagellate that infects both humans and animals and is the most common cause of intestinal parasitosis in humans worldwide. Because the literature refers to this organism as G. *lamblia*, *Giardia intestinalis*, and *Giardia duodenalis*, it is evident that there is still debate about the classification and nomenclature of this flagellate. Previous work, based primarily on structural variations of the parasite, resulted in the proposal of three species, *Giardia muris* (mice), *Giardia agilis* (amphibians), and *Giardia duodenalis* (the intestinalis group) (3, 37). Further studies support the existence of additional species, *Giardia ardeae* (herons), *Giardia psittaci* (parakeets), and *Giardia microti* (voles and muskrats). Also, it appears that G. *lamblia* (*intestinalis*) is a species complex that should contain the species G. *microti* as well (97). Further studies are needed to elucidate species designations and groupings. Although these species have been proposed, G. *lamblia* is the name predominantly used in the United States and will continue to be used throughout this chapter.

It is now accepted that there is considerable genetic diversity within G. *lamblia*. Based on molecular biology, the genus *Giardia* is subdivided into major genotypes containing subgenotypes. The major genotypes of G. *lamblia* that are associated with human infections are assemblages A and B. Assemblage A is associated with a mixture of both human and animal isolates, whereas assemblage B is typically associated with human isolates only. Most zoonotic animal-to-human infections occur with assemblage A (46).

Epidemiology, Transmission, and Prevention

Infection with G. *lamblia* occurs through fecal-oral transmission or the ingestion of cysts in contaminated food or water, and an inoculum of only 10 to 100 cysts is sufficient for human infection (120). Individuals more commonly infected in developed countries are children in day care centers, hikers, and immunocompromised individuals. Among immunocompromised individuals, infections have been documented in people with AIDS and hypogammaglobulinemia and those affected by malnutrition. Prevalence rates for this pathogen range from 1 to 7% in industrialized countries and from 5 to 50% in developing countries. Of the intestinal flagellates, G. *lamblia* is the flagellate most frequently isolated in the United States. In high-risk domestic settings, such as day care centers, prevalence rates can reach 90% (111). A *Giardia* vaccine is available for dogs and cats; this may affect the prevalence of infections in humans (105).

Infection occurs when viable cysts are ingested, excyst, and transform into trophozoites. After excystation, the trophozoite, which appears to have a propensity for the duodenum, attaches to the mucosal epithelium. Trophozoites attach to the epithelium via a sucking disk located on the ventral side of the parasite. During the course of infection, the parasites remain attached to the epithelium and do not invade the mucosa. In the intestine, trophozoites divide by binary fission to produce two identical daughter trophozoites. As they move down toward the large intestine, the trophozoites encyst, and infective cysts are excreted into the environment (37).

Clinical Significance

The majority of individuals infected with G. *lamblia* are asymptomatic. Asymptomatic versus symptomatic infection may be due to the existence of two different strains of *Giardia* with different levels of virulence. Preliminary studies have grouped G. *lamblia* into two groups, group A and group B. Group A appears to be more pathogenic and is associated with symptomatic infection. Isoenzyme and molecular studies show that group A and group B differ from one another and appear to be no more related than *E. histolytica* and *E. dispar*. The genes homologous between group A and group B *Giardia* isolates show an identity of approximately 81 to 89% (97, 109, 110). In symptomatic individuals, acute G. *lamblia* infections can mimic infections with other protozoal, viral, and bacterial pathogens. After an incubation period of approximately 12 to 20 days, patients can experience nausea, chills, low-grade fever, epigastric pain, and a sudden onset of watery diarrhea. Diarrhea is often explosive and presents as foul smelling without the presence of blood, cellular exudate, or mucus. Individuals can develop subacute or chronic infections with symptoms such as recurrent diarrhea, abdominal discomfort and distention, belching, and heartburn. In patients with chronic cases of giardiasis, diarrhea can lead to dehydration, malabsorption, and impairment of pancreatic function (17).

Direct Examination

Microscopy

Diagnosis of G. *lamblia* infection is typically established by the microscopic examination of stool for the presence of cysts and/or trophozoites. Stained smears are more helpful in identifying the trophozoite stage of the infection, although this stage can be identified in wet mount preparations (Table 4; Fig. 7 and 8). Examination of stool specimens may not be diagnostic because cyst forms can

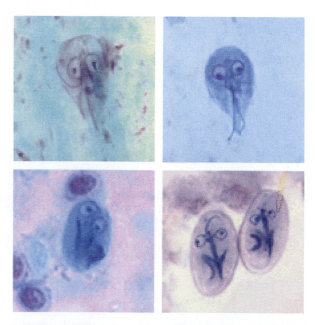

FIGURE 8 (Top row) *Giardia lamblia* trophozoites. Note the typical nuclei, axonemes, and curved median bodies. (Bottom row) G. *lamblia* cysts. The cysts on the right are stained with iron-hematoxylin, and those on the left are stained with Wheatley's trichrome stain. (Courtesy of L. Garcia.)

be trapped in mucus, making them difficult to detect on smears. Also, the excretion pattern of cysts can be cyclical. In these instances, other methods, such as the string test (Entero-Test; HDC Corp., San Jose, CA), should be used to obtain clinical samples. The string test procedure consists of a patient swallowing a weighted capsule containing gelatin and a tightly wound string. After approximately 5 h, the string is removed from the patient and the adherent material is examined as a wet mount or permanent smear (37). Endoscopy can also be used to collect clinical specimens. Because this procedure is invasive, it is used only for diagnosis of disease in patients with perplexing clinical presentations (111).

Antigen Detection

Other assays that have gained wide acceptance for the detection of G. lamblia in stool specimens are EIAs, DFA assays, and immunochromatographic assays. These methods have very high specificities (90 to 100%) and sensitivities that range from 65 to 100% (40, 68, 71, 90, 169). Although these methods have proven to be fairly sensitive and specific compared to the routine staining of fecal smears (trichrome staining), other important pathogens may be missed if a wet mount and permanent-stained smear are not examined. The DFA assay widely used is the Merifluor reagent assay (Meridian Bioscience, Inc., Cincinnati, OH), but it does require the availability of a fluorescent microscope. DFA assays have a sensitivity and specificity of >95%, and there are reagents to detect C. parvum as well. Immunoassays are available and are useful for testing large numbers of patient specimens, and some studies have shown the performance of the EIA to be excellent compared to that of the ova and parasite exam (39, 68, 90). Two available immunoassays are the ProSpecT Giardia EZ (Remel, Lenexa, KS) and the ColorPAC Giardia assay (Becton Dickinson and Company, Sparks, MD) (71). If the patient is immunocompromised, has traveled, or is suspected of coming into contact with another pathogen, the ova and parasite examination should be performed. Some studies suggest that the use of an immunoassay does not eliminate the need for more than one stool specimen. Positive specimens from asymptomatic patients may be missed if only one stool specimen is tested using an immunoassay (47). Some immunoassays are affected by specimens contaminated with blood. It was documented in one study that blood can interfere with the performance of the ProSpecT assay and potentially cause false-positive results (71). Immunochromatographic detection methods have also been developed for the clinical laboratory (39, 41, 42, 116). The ImmunoCard STAT (Meridian Bioscience, Inc.) has been developed to detect G. lamblia and C. parvum antigens in stool specimens by using rapid solid-phase qualitative immunochromatography. Patients negative by the ImmunoCard STAT that remain symptomatic should be tested using a routine ova and parasite exam (42). The Triage Micro parasite panel (Biosite, Inc.) is an immunoassay that can detect not only G. lamblia antigens but also those of E. histolytica/E. dispar and C. parvum in stool specimens. Antigens in stool specimens are immobilized on a membrane containing specific antibodies to the respective intestinal parasites. The formation of color bars occurs on a specific area of the membrane depending on the parasite present in the stool. All of these assays described can be run using formalin-fixed stool. This is important in the event that the laboratory would need to run an ova and parasite exam on the same specimen. Another product, the Giardia/Cryptosporidium Chek Test,

is an EIA available from TechLab, Inc. One study showed the assay to be 98.4% sensitive and 100% specific (169). The Para-Tect (Medical Chemical Corporation, Torrance, CA) is also another newly developed immunochromatography-based product for the detection of Giardia (38). Although there are several methods now available for the detection of G. lamblia, parameters such as workload, skill levels of technologists, and the availability of necessary equipment should be considered in choosing a specific method. Refer to chapter 130 for a complete list of current available assays for Giardia detection in the clinical laboratory.

Nucleic Acid Detection Techniques

Some investigators are now using molecular tools to diagnose G. lamblia infection with clinical samples (6, 46, 100, 157). One group has developed an oligonucleotide microarray with excellent sensitivity and specificity for the detection of G. lamblia and other intestinal parasites in stool specimens. The assay was also able to discriminate between Giardia assemblages A and B (160). A multiplex PCR assay to detect specific genotypes of G. lamblia has also been developed which may potentially aid in epidemiologic investigations of outbreaks (101). It is important to note that molecular detection of G. lamblia has not been widely implemented and there are no commercial assays approved by the Food and Drug Administration for clinical use to date.

Because of the potential for contamination of municipal water supplies, routine monitoring of water for parasitic protozoa is recommended as a public health control measure. G. lamblia cysts can remain viable for 2 to 3 months in cold water and are fairly resistant to killing by routine chlorine treatments. DFA assays are commonly used to detect G. lamblia cysts in water samples, but PCR is also being used for this purpose (123). The advantage of PCR is the increased sensitivity compared to those of fluorescence assays or assays that use special stains. Research continues to enhance the ability of investigators to detect viable organisms, which is a better indication of poor water quality (162).

Treatment

For individuals diagnosed with giardiasis, the treatment of choice is metronidazole, tinidazole, or nitazoxanide (2). Alternatives include paromomycin, furazolidone, and quinacrine (2) or other nitroimidazoles such as ornidazole and secnidazole (43). In most immunocompetent hosts, infection is self-limiting; however, treatment will lessen the duration of symptoms and prevent transmission. Other drugs that have been used to treat giardiasis are albendazole, mebendazole, and bacitracin (92), and there are other therapeutics on the horizon. Albendazole, mebendazole, and paromomycin have lower activity against Giardia than do the nitroimidazoles (43). Resistance to metronidazole and other agents has been observed clinically and in vitro (155). In vitro resistance-testing assays are available but lack the standardization required for the clinical laboratory (139).

Evaluation, Interpretation, and Reporting of Results

As with any of the organisms mentioned in this chapter, it is important to evaluate more than one stool specimen for the presence of G. lamblia. For Giardia, this could include up to five or six stool specimens to increase the chance of recovery. This is especially important for diagnosing G. lamblia infection, since organisms can be passed in the stool intermittently on a more cyclical basis. During the staining procedure, the cysts can be shrunken or distorted, which may impact the ability of the clinical laboratory scientists to read the smear. There are several techniques available for the diagnosis of giardiasis in the clinical laboratory. Some methods might offer somewhat better sensitivity but need to fit into the overall workflow of the laboratory. Enzyme immunoassays offer somewhat enhanced sensitivity but cannot always replace the ova and parasite exam due to the prevalence of other pathogens in the patient population being tested. Adding assays, such as the EIA, might increase detection of *Giardia* but add to the bottom-line cost per testing if the physicians continue to order a routine ova and parasite exam as well.

D. fragilis

Taxonomy
D. fragilis is currently grouped in the phylum Metamonada, class Parabasalia, order Trichomonadida (see chapter 129).

Description of the Agent and Taxonomy
Despite the lack of external flagella, this parasite is currently classified as a flagellate but has historically been grouped with the amebae. Electron microscopy and antigenic analysis have aided in the classification of this organism and have demonstrated that it is closely related to *Trichomonas* and *Histomonas* species. Phylogenetic analysis of small-subunit rRNA sequences has also confirmed the relationship between *D. fragilis* and *Histomonas* (44, 133).

Epidemiology, Transmission, and Prevention
D. fragilis is found worldwide and is known to cause a noninvasive diarrheal illness in humans. Colonization in humans is similar to that seen with other intestinal parasites; typically, the cecum and the proximal part of the colon are affected. Because *D. fragilis* does not have a cyst stage as part of its life cycle, the mode of transmission is less well understood. The mode of transmission of *D. fragilis* is not known; one hypothesis concerning the spread of *D. fragilis* is that transmission occurs within the eggs of *Enterobius vermicularis* or *Ascaris lumbricoides* (14). Several studies provide circumstantial evidence to support *E. vermicularis* as a vector, documenting a greater-than-expected coinfection rate with the two organisms (66).

Though *D. fragilis* has a worldwide distribution, prevalence rates for this organism vary quite substantially from 0% in Prague to 42% in Germany (66). There appears to be a higher prevalence in certain groups of individuals such as missionaries, Native Americans living in Arizona, and institutionalized individuals (165). In the United States, the prevalence is reported to be quite low. This may be due to underreporting attributable to difficulties associated with identifying the organism in clinical samples. In addition, Johnson and Clark (67) identified the existence of two genetically distinct types of *D. fragilis* with a resulting sequence divergence of approximately 2% (67, 113). The degree of divergence appears to be similar to that seen with *E. histolytica* and *E. dispar*. Since asymptomatic infections occur, this finding may lend support to the possibility that two distinct species exist, though there is no consensus on this matter (66, 67).

Clinical Significance
The frequency of symptomatic disease ranges from 15 to 25% in adults, and symptomatic disease is more common in children, in whom up to 90% of those infected have clinical signs (15, 111). Symptoms include fatigue, insufficient weight gain, diarrhea (often intermittent), abdominal pain, anorexia, and nausea. Studies have linked *D. fragilis* infection to biliary infection (149), irritable bowel syndrome (11), allergic colitis (28), and diarrhea in HIV-infected patients (82). One case report describes a patient who presented in the emergency room with acute appendicitis which was attributed to *D. fragilis* infection (127). Some individuals, mainly children, also experience unexplained peripheral blood eosinophilia (37). Diarrhea is seen predominantly during the first 1 to 2 weeks after the onset of disease. The number of *D. fragilis* organisms can vary greatly from day to day, which is similar to those of other intestinal protozoa. Abdominal pain can persist for 1 to 2 months (15). Although *D. fragilis* has been implicated in the above-mentioned clinical situations, the organism is isolated from patients with no apparent clinical symptoms. In addition, the lack of an animal model affects researchers' ability to detect specific pathological manifestations (66).

Direct Detection

Microscopy
Diagnosis of *D. fragilis* infection is similar to that of infections with other intestinal protozoa, and detection of the trophozoite in fresh or preserved stool is warranted to establish infection. Laboratories using direct microscopy may be at a disadvantage, since the trophozoite can degenerate if not placed in fixative. Nonfixed trophozoites can appear rounded and refractile and are more difficult to identify microscopically. Morphologically, the trophozoite of *D. fragilis* contains one or two nuclei (binucleate), with two nuclei being more common. Well-trained laboratory personnel can identify *D. fragilis* trophozoites in stool specimens, but because no cyst stage exists, diagnosis from the wet mount can be difficult. Use of a permanent-stained smear is the recommended procedure for detection (Table 4; Fig. 7 and 9).

Other Diagnostic Methods
Culture has been shown to be more sensitive than microscopy; however, it is not recommended for the routine clinical laboratory (66). Antigen and antibody techniques have been used as diagnostic tools for the detection of *D. fragilis* but are not commercially available (21, 22). *D. fragilis* DNA has been detected using PCR with fresh, unpreserved stool. This technique has the promise of being more sensitive than microscopy (141, 142).

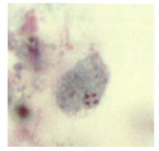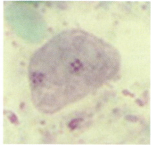

FIGURE 9 *Dientamoeba fragilis* trophozoites. The trophozoites can have one nucleus (left) or two nuclei (right). No cyst stage is known for this organism. Trophozoites are stained with Wheatley's trichrome stain. (Courtesy of L. Garcia.)

Treatment

The treatment of choice for symptomatic individuals is iodoquinol (diiodohydroxyquin) (2). Alternate choices include paromomycin, tetracycline, or metronidazole (2). Metronidazole, iodoquinol, and tetracycline have been used to treat children (37). Additional therapeutic options include diphetarsone, carbarsone, erythromycin, hydroxyquinoline, and secnidazole (45, 66). If *E. vermicularis* is detected concomitantly, the treatment regimen should also include mebendazole (15).

Evaluation, Interpretation, and Reporting of Results

The recovery of *D. fragilis* is greatly enhanced by the collection of at least three stool specimens (25, 111). Trophozoites have been recovered from soft and formed stools, indicating the need to evaluate all types of samples (15). Low incidence in a community setting for *D. fragilis* may be due to the inability of the laboratory to accurately identify the organism.

T. vaginalis

Taxonomy

T. vaginalis is a flagellate belonging to the phylum Metamonada, class Parabasalia, order Trichomonadida (see chapter 129 of this *Manual*). Unlike the other members of the order which inhabit the intestinal tract, *T. vaginalis* infects the urogenital tract.

Description of the Agent

The life cycle includes only the trophozoite stage; there is no cyst stage. The organism is similar in morphology to the other trichomonads and is characterized by a pear shape with a prominent axostyle and an undulating membrane that stops halfway down the side of the trophozoite (Table 4; Fig. 7 and 10). It is a facultative anaerobe that divides by binary fission, and it cannot survive long outside the host.

Epidemiology, Transmission, and Prevention

T. vaginalis is a pathogenic flagellate that infects the urogenital tracts of males and females. The infection is primarily a sexually transmitted infection and is thought to be the most common curable sexually transmitted infection among sexually active young women. There are an estimated 7.4 million new cases each year in the United States; worldwide, there are 180 million cases of trichomoniasis each year (161). The incidence of trichomoniasis differs depending on the population examined, varying from 5 to 60% in various studies. Factors such as lower socioeconomic status, multiple sex partners, and poor personal hygiene are linked to a higher incidence of infection.

The estimated infection rates cited in the literature may indeed be too low because (i) trichomoniasis is not a reportable disease in the United States and other countries; (ii) the infection, particularly in men, can be asymptomatic; and (iii) laboratory tests used for diagnosis vary in their sensitivities. Despite these rates of infection and their serious medical consequences, trichomoniasis has not received adequate attention from public health and sexually transmitted disease prevention programs (128).

Clinical Significance

Infection in females can result in vaginitis, cervicitis, and urethritis (128). The vaginal discharge is classically described as copious, liquid, greenish, frothy, and foul smelling. The onset of symptoms, such as intense vaginal and vulvar pruritus and discharge, is often sudden and occurs during or after menstruation. The vaginal pH is usually elevated above the normal pH of 4.5, and dysuria occurs in 20% of women with *T. vaginalis* infection. Infection has also been associated with premature rupture of membranes, premature birth, and posthysterectomy cuff infections (26, 95, 138). In men, the most common symptomatic presentation is urethritis. Up to 50% of infected women are asymptomatic carriers. In men, the majority of infections are asymptomatic. Asymptomatic carriers serve as a reservoir for transmission and also remain at risk for developing disease. Trichomoniasis has been implicated as a cofactor in the transmission of HIV (65, 81). In one study, men with symptomatic *Trichomonas* urethritis were found to have increased HIV concentrations in seminal plasma compared to HIV-infected men without urethritis (57).

Neonates can acquire the organism during passage through the infected birth canal. It is estimated that 2 to 17% of female babies acquire trichomoniasis by direct vulvovaginal contamination (81). Reports have also documented *T. vaginalis* as a cause of neonatal pneumonia (93).

Direct Detection

Microscopy

The diagnosis of *T. vaginalis* infection is commonly based on the examination of wet preparations of vaginal and urethral discharges, prostatic secretions, and urine sediments. Permanent stains such as Papanicolaou and Giemsa stains can be used, but the organisms may be difficult to recognize (78). For wet preparations, vaginal specimens are routinely collected during a speculum examination, but studies suggest that self-collected or tampon-collected specimens may be used successfully (56, 130). Specimens should be mixed with a drop of physiologic saline and examined microscopically within 1 h under low power (magnification, ×100) with reduced illumination. Specimens should never be refrigerated. The presence of actively motile organisms with jerky motility is diagnostic. The movement of the undulating membrane may be seen as the motility of the trophozoite diminishes. Polymorphonuclear cells are often present. The sensitivity of the wet preparation test with vaginal specimens is between 50 and 70%, depending on the skill of the microscopist and other factors. The sensitivity of microscopy in males is low, and additional testing, such as culture of urethral swab, urine, and semen, is required for optimal

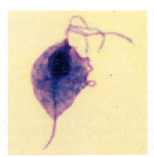 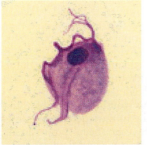

FIGURE 10 *Trichomonas vaginalis* trophozoites. Note the undulating membrane, which comes about halfway down the body. Although the membrane appears to come down farther on one of the trophozoites (right), this appearance occurs because of the photographic angle. Also, note the axostyle that penetrates the bottom of the organism. No cyst stage is known for this organism. Trophozoites are stained with Giemsa stain. (Courtesy of L. Garcia.)

sensitivity. Perhaps the most important factor affecting the sensitivity of wet mount testing is the time between collection and examination of the specimen. Viability of the organism is essential for the detection of motility on the wet mount and drops off precipitously with time. Amies gel agar transport medium can maintain the viability for culture of *T. vaginalis* on swabs held at room temperature for 24 ± 6 h before inoculation of the specimen into a culture pouch (59). Because the morphology of *P. hominis*, a nonpathogenic intestinal flagellate, is very similar to that of *T. vaginalis*, care must be taken to ensure that specimens are not contaminated with fecal material.

Culture

Culture has greater sensitivity (>80%) than the wet mount method and is considered the gold standard method for the detection of *T. vaginalis*. Specimens must be collected properly and inoculated immediately into the appropriate medium, such as modified Diamond's, Trichosel, or Hollander's medium. Due to cost and convenience, this approach is not routinely used. Culture systems (InPouchTV [BioMed Diagnostics, San Jose, CA] and the system of Empyrean Diagnostics, Inc., Mountain View, CA) that allow direct inoculation, transport, culture, and microscopic examination are commercially available (10, 31). In situations where immediate transport of specimens is not feasible, the use of these transport/culture devices should be encouraged. Studies have also shown that a delayed inoculation protocol is as sensitive as immediate inoculation, allowing the results of microscopy to be used to determine whether further culture is necessary (131). Serologic testing is not useful for the diagnosis of trichomoniasis.

Antigen Detection

Several antigen detection methods have been developed for *T. vaginalis* and offer the advantage of being rapid and easy to perform. A latex agglutination test (TV Latex; Kalon Biological, Guildford, Surrey, United Kingdom) has been shown to have excellent sensitivity (4) but is not available in the United States. An immunofluorescence assay (Light Diagnostics *T. vaginalis* DFA; Chemicon International, Temecula, CA) is available in the United States for testing directly from patient samples. Two immunochromatographic capillary flow assays are available commercially for the qualitative detection of *T. vaginalis* antigens from vaginal swabs. The Osom Trichomonas Rapid Test (Genzyme Diagnostics, Cambridge, MA) is a dipstick assay providing results in 10 min. In published studies, the Osom test has demonstrated good sensitivity (82.0 to 94.7%) and specificity (98.8 to 100%) compared to various comparator assays, including wet mount, culture, and amplified testing (16, 63, 64, 112). The Xenostrip Tv Trichomonas vaginalis test (Xenotope Diagnostics, Inc., San Antonio, TX) is a rapid point-of-care test that has demonstrated sensitivities of 67 to 80% and specificities of >99% in published studies (79, 117).

Nucleic Acid Detection Techniques

The Affirm VPIII (Becton Dickinson and Company, Sparks, MD) is a direct DNA probe test for the detection of organisms from vaginal swabs associated with vaginosis/vaginitis. It tests for the three most common syndromes associated with increased vaginal discharge: bacterial vaginosis (*Gardenerella vaginalis*), candidiasis (*Candida albicans*), and trichomoniasis (*T. vaginalis*). According to the manufacturers package insert, the assay has a sensitivity and specificity of 90 and 98%, respectively, compared with wet mount and culture for *T. vaginalis* (package insert, Affirm VPIII, version no. 670160JAAG; Becton Dickinson). In a clinical evaluation of vaginal swab specimens from both symptomatic and asymptomatic females, the Affirm detected more *T. vaginalis*-positive samples than wet mount testing, although the difference was not statistically significant (12).

Nucleic acid-based amplification methods, such as PCR and transcription-mediated amplification (TMA), for the detection of *T. vaginalis* have been reported in the literature, but none are yet available as an FDA-cleared test system. These amplification methods have demonstrated varying sensitivities depending on the genomic target, specimen type, and sex of the patient (54, 64, 87, 99, 103, 121). PCR has a sensitivity of 85 to 100% with vaginal swabs; its sensitivity with urine is lower, ranging from 60 to 80% (73, 83, 128). For men, PCR with urine and urethral swabs has been reported and appears to be more sensitive than conventional methods (74, 129). Several researchers have reported using TMA technology with Aptima analyte-specific reagents available from GenProbe (San Diego, CA) for detection of *T. vaginalis* (53, 99, 103). In a study by Hardick et al. (53), TMA was compared to PCR for detection of *T. vaginalis* using self-obtained female vaginal swab samples and male urine samples; both TMA and PCR had equivalent performance for vaginal swab samples, while TMA appeared to be more sensitive than PCR using male urine specimens.

While the wet mount method provides a rapid result at a low cost, tests with the increased sensitivities, such as nucleic acid probes or amplification tests, may be indicated because of the impact of *T. vaginalis* infections on pregnancy and the link with HIV transmission (59, 129). The use of alternate specimen types such as urine makes amplified testing an important advancement for diagnosis of trichomoniasis. An algorithm to reflex specimens with negative wet mounts to culture or a more sensitive methodology may be a useful diagnostic approach (112).

Treatment

The recommended treatment for *T. vaginalis* infections is metronidazole or tinidazole (2, 20). For metronidazole, oral therapy is recommended over topical treatment. Tinidazole may be used as a first-line agent or for refractory cases previously treated with metronidazole (27). For treatment during pregnancy, metronidazole is the recommended therapy; however, it should be used cautiously, as data do not suggest that metronidazole treatment results in a reduction in perinatal morbidity (20, 76). All sexual partners of infected individuals should also receive treatment. Treatment failure with metronidazole is most often due to noncompliance or reinfection. True resistance to metronidazole has been documented and appears to be increasing (27, 135). While not routinely available, methods have been published for the in vitro determination of susceptibility. These methods have not been standardized, and the results can vary based on assay conditions (9, 94).

Evaluation, Interpretation, and Reporting of Results

A laboratory finding that is positive for *T. vaginalis* is considered diagnostic of trichomoniasis. As discussed above, both microscopy and culture are prone to lower sensitivities due to issues related to sampling and transport. Laboratories should have strict rejection criteria for trichomonas culture and wet mount specimens that do not arrive within the specified time or transport conditions; such policies improve sensitivity, ensuring more accurate results. In comparison to methods such as antigen detection and molecular methods, a negative result by these methods should be viewed cautiously and evaluated in conjunction with clinical symptoms.

With testing for Trichomonas, such as antigen detection and direct molecular probes or amplified tests, reported results should reflect the analyte that is detected. For example, a positive result for *T. vaginalis* by a direct DNA probe assay should state "*T. vaginalis* DNA detected." If testing is expanded to differing sample types, such as urine testing by amplified methods, the report should clearly state the specimen tested.

To date, there are no FDA-cleared amplified molecular tests for detection of *T. vaginalis*. Label the test result to indicate its status as an in-house test in accordance with CLIA regulations as follows: "This test was developed and its performance characteristics determined by [Laboratory Name]. It has not been cleared or approved by the U. S. Food and Drug Administration."

NONPATHOGENIC FLAGELLATES

C. mesnili is found worldwide and is generally considered nonpathogenic. Unlike *D. fragilis*, *C. mesnili* has both a trophozoite and a cyst stage. The organism is acquired through the ingestion of contaminated food or water and resides in the cecum and/or colon of the infected human or animal. The trophozoite is 6 to 24 μm long and contains a characteristic spiral groove that runs longitudinally along the body (Table 4; Fig. 7 and 11). Motility of the organism can sometimes be seen in fresh preparations, and the spiral groove may be exposed as the organism turns. Flagella are difficult to see in stained preparations. The trophozoite contains one nucleus, with a cytostome or oral groove in close proximity. The pear-shaped cyst retains the cytoplasmic organelles of the trophozoite, with a single nucleus and curved cytostomal fibril. Observing the organism in permanent-stained preparations makes identification more definitive.

P. hominis, formerly referred to as *Trichomonas hominis*, is a nonpathogenic flagellate that is similar to *D. fragilis* in that only the trophozoite stage has been observed. Although the organism is cosmopolitan in nature and is recovered from individuals with diarrhea, it is still considered nonpathogenic. The trophozoites typically inhabit the cecum.

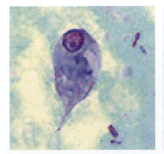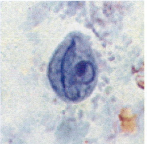

FIGURE 11 *Chilomastix mesnili* trophozoite (left) and cyst (right). Note the oral groove (feeding groove) at the right side of the trophozoite (clear area) and the curved fibril (shepherd's crook) in the cyst. Also note the typical pear or lemon shape of the cyst. Organisms are stained with Wheatley's trichrome stain. (Courtesy of L. Garcia.)

They are pyriform and contain an undulating membrane that runs the length of the parasite. The use of permanent smears is recommended for observation of these organisms in clinical specimens. The trophozoites may stain weakly, making them difficult to detect on stained smears (37).

Two additional nonpathogenic intestinal flagellates are *E. hominis* and *R. intestinalis*. Both *E. hominis* and *R. intestinalis* are found in warm or temperate climates, and infection is acquired through the ingestion of cysts. When clinical specimens are examined, it is important to note that cysts of *E. hominis* can resemble those of *E. nana*, although *E. nana* cysts containing two nuclei are rare. Because of the small sizes of *E. hominis* and *R. intestinalis*, it is difficult to detect these organisms even when permanent-stained smears are examined. This may lead to the underreporting of both organisms. *R. intestinalis* has been recovered from the pancreatic juice of a patient with small lesions of the pancreatic duct (72).

In general, treatment is not recommended for infections with the nonpathogenic flagellates. Improved personal hygiene and sanitary conditions are key methods for the prevention of infection.

CILIATES

Balantidium coli

Taxonomy

B. coli is a ciliate belonging to the phylum Ciliophora, class Litostomatea, order Vestibulifera (see chapter 129 of this *Manual*). Members of the phylum Ciliophora are protozoa possessing cilia in at least one stage of their life cycles. They also have two different types of nuclei, one macronucleus and one or more micronuclei. Over the last several years, molecular analysis has aided in the characterization of the genus *Balantidium* (126, 147, 148). Sequences of the genus are on file at GenBank based on the small subunit rRNA. There is question as to whether the species isolated from humans, *B. coli*, and pigs, *B. suis*, are the same species (126).

Description of the Agent

This organism has both the trophozoite and cyst forms as part of its life cycle (Table 5; Fig. 12). The cyst form is the infective stage. After ingestion of the cysts and excystation, trophozoites secrete hyaluronidase, which aids in the invasion of the tissue. The trophozoite, which is oval and covered with cilia, is easily seen in wet mount preparations under low-power magnification. The cytoplasm contains both a macronucleus and a micronucleus, in addition to two contractile vacuoles. Motile trophozoites can be observed in fresh wet preparations, but the specimen must be observed soon after collection. The trophozoite is somewhat pear shaped and also contains vacuoles that may harbor debris such as cell fragments and ingested bacteria. Cyst formation takes place as the trophozoite moves down the large intestine.

Epidemiology, Transmission, and Prevention

B. coli exists in animal reservoirs such as pigs and chimpanzees, with pigs being the primary reservoir (126). The organism is the only pathogenic ciliate and the largest pathogenic protozoan known to infect humans. Transmission occurs by the fecal-oral route following ingestion of the cysts in contaminated food or water. Infection is more common in warmer climates and in areas where humans are in close contact with pigs. As with other intestinal protozoa, poor

TABLE 5 Key features of the ciliate *B. coli*

Stage	Characteristics
Trophozoite 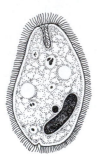	Shape and size: Ovoid with tapering anterior end; 50–100 μm long, 40–70 μm wide Motility: Rotary, boring; may be rapid Nuclei: 1 large kidney-bean-shaped macronucleus may be visible in unstained preparation; 1 small round micronucleus adjacent to macronucleus, difficult to see Cytoplasm: May be vacuolated; may contain ingested bacteria and debris; anterior cytostome Cilia: Body surface covered with longitudinal rows of cilia; longer near cytostome Note: May be confused with helminth eggs or debris on a permanent-stained smear; concentration or sedimentation examination recommended
Cyst 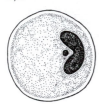	Shape and size: Spherical or oval; 50–70 μm in diam Nuclei: 1 large macronucleus, 1 micronucleus, difficult to see Cytoplasm: Vacuoles are visible in young cysts; in older cysts, internal structure appears granular Cilia: Difficult to see within the thick cyst wall

sanitary conditions lead to a higher incidence of infection. Prevalence of *Balantidium* varies per geographic location but overall is estimated to be between 0.02 and 1% (33). High-prevalence areas include areas of the Middle East, Papua New Guinea and West Irian, Latin America, and the Philippines (137, 167).

Clinical Significance

Infection with *B. coli* is most often asymptomatic; however, symptomatic infection can occur, resulting in bouts of dysentery similar to amebiasis (18, 37). Infection with

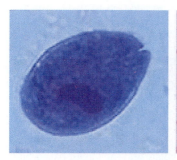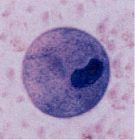

FIGURE 12 *Balantidium coli* trophozoite (left) and cyst (right). Note the single macronucleus visible in both the trophozoite and the cyst. The much smaller micronucleus is not visible. Organisms are stained with Wheatley's trichrome stain. (Courtesy of L. Garcia.)

Balantidium can be described in 3 ways: (i) asymptomatic host, carrying the disease; (ii) chronic infection, non-bloody diarrhea, including other symptoms such as cramping and abdominal pain; and (iii) fulminating disease consisting of mucoid and bloody stools (126, 156). In addition, colitis caused by *B. coli* is often indistinguishable from that caused by *E. histolytica*. Symptoms typically include diarrhea, nausea, vomiting, headache, and anorexia. Fluid loss can be dramatic, as seen in some patients with cryptosporidiosis. The organism can invade the submucosa of the large bowel, and ulcerative abscesses and hemorrhagic lesions can occur. The shallow ulcers and submucosal lesions that result from invasion are prone to secondary infection by bacteria and can be problematic for the patient (29, 77). Death due to invasive *B. coli* infection has been reported (29). Infections associated with extraintestinal sites have been described (29, 77, 80). There have been several reports of *Balantidium* spreading from the intestine to the lung. Most of these cases have occurred in patients that are either elderly or immunocompromised. The disease presents as a pneumonia-like illness. In these documented cases, *Balantidium* has been recovered from specimens such as bronchial secretions and bronchial lavage specimens. It is hypothesized that extraintestinal colonization can occur between the lymphatic or circulatory system, perforation though the colon, or through aspiration of fluid from the oral cavity (126).

Direct Examination

Microscopy

Either ova and parasite examination of feces or histological examination of intestinal biopsy specimens establishes the diagnosis of *B. coli* infections. The diagnosis can be established only by demonstrating the presence of trophozoites in stool or tissue samples (80). It is very easy to identify these organisms in wet preparations and concentrated stool samples. Conversely, it can be challenging to identify *B. coli* from trichrome-stained permanent smears because the organisms are so large and have a tendency to overstain. This makes the organism less discernible and increases the chance of misidentification.

Treatment

The treatment of choice for *B. coli* infection is tetracycline, although it is considered an investigational drug when used in this context (2). Metronidazole and iodoquinol are therapeutic alternatives used in some cases (37). Nitazoxanide which is a broad-spectrum antiparasitic drug may be another alternative for treatment (126).

Evaluation, Interpretation, and Reporting of Results

The recovery of *B. coli* in humans is fairly uncommon despite its worldwide distribution. Pulmonary infections can occur, but the clinical laboratory scientist needs to make sure that this organism is not confused with motile ciliated epithelial cells that can be present in respiratory specimens. *Balantidium* spp. in wet mounts are very active parasites with uniform ciliation.

SUMMARY

Clinical laboratories are now given more choices for testing in diagnostic parasitology, with assays ranging from microscopy, culture, antigen detection, and nucleic acid amplification techniques. Molecular biology has the promise to deliver more sensitive and specific methods, but to date, these methods have not been fully adapted to the clinical diagnostic laboratory. Some researchers have implemented their own laboratory-developed amplification assays for better detection of intestinal protozoa such as *Giardia*, *Cryptosporidium*, and *Trichomonas*. In addition to these amplification tests, rapid point-of-care tests are available for organisms such as *T. vaginalis*. Results can now be available in real time for the clinician to manage patients directly in the exam setting. Even though the field of diagnostic parasitology is changing, clinical laboratories are still faced with using microscopy for routine work-up for stool specimens due to the slow implementation of some of the new methods by commercial diagnostic companies. Not all laboratories are equipped to develop home brew molecular tests and rely on the diagnostic industry to bring products to the market. Some laboratories have switched to antigen-based methods, but many still rely on microscopy because antigen-based methods cannot detect all potential pathogens in a given stool specimen. Microscopy, as we know, cannot differentiate between pathogenic and nonpathogenic amebae and the different genotypes of *Giardia*. On the horizon are newer methodologies, such as the microarray, which would allow for the detection of multiple pathogens from a clinical specimen. Some manufacturers are developing assays for the detection of stool parasites using chemiluminescent and bead-based technologies. These exciting new areas will help increase the options that the clinical parasitology laboratory has for the diagnosis of intestinal parasitic infections.

REFERENCES

1. **Abd-Alla, M. D., T. F. Jackson, S. Reddy, and J. I. Ravdin.** 2000. Diagnosis of invasive amebiasis by enzyme-linked immunosorbent assay of saliva to detect amebic lectin antigen and anti-lectin immunoglobulin G antibodies. *J. Clin. Microbiol.* **38:**2344–2347.
2. **Abramowicz, M.** 2007. Drugs for parasitic infections. *Med. Lett. Drugs Ther.* **5:**S1–S15.
3. **Adam, R. D.** 2001. Biology of *Giardia lamblia. Clin. Microbiol. Rev.* **14:**447–475.
4. **Adu-Sarkodie, Y., B. K. Opoku, K. A. Danso, H. A. Weiss, and D. Mabey.** 2004. Comparison of latex agglutination, wet preparation, and culture for the detection of *Trichomonas vaginalis. Sex. Transm. Infect.* **80:**201–203.
5. **Albrecht, H., H. J. Stellbrink, K. Koperski, and H. Greten.** 1995. *Blastocystis hominis* in human immunodeficiency virus-related diarrhea. *Scand. J. Gastroenterol.* **30:**909–914.
6. **Amar, C. F., P. H. Dear, S. Pedraza-Diaz, N. Looker, E. Linnane, and J. McLauchlin.** 2002. Sensitive PCR-restriction fragment length polymorphism assay for detection and genotyping of *Giardia duodenalis* in human feces. *J. Clin. Microbiol.* **40:**446–452.
7. **Arisue, N., T. Hashimoto, H. Yoshikawa, Y. Nakamura, G. Nakamura, F. Nakamura, T. A. Yano, and M. Hasegawa.** 2002. Phylogenetic position of *Blastocystis hominis* and of stramenopiles inferred from multiple molecular sequence data. *J. Eukaryot. Microbiol.* **49:**42–53.
8. **Blessmann, J., H. Buss, P. A. Nu, B. T. Dinh, Q. T. Ngo, A. L. Van, M. D. Alla, T. F. Jackson, J. I. Ravdin, and E. Tannich.** 2002. Real-time PCR for detection and differentiation of *Entamoeba histolytica* and *Entamoeba dispar* in fecal samples. *J. Clin. Microbiol.* **40:**4413–4417.
9. **Borchardt, K. A., Z. Li, M. Z. Zhang, and H. Shing.** 1996. An in vitro metronidazole susceptibility test for trichomoniasis using the InPouch TV test. *Genitourin. Med.* **72:**132–135.
10. **Borchardt, K. A., and R. F. Smith.** 1991. An evaluation of an InPouch TV culture method for diagnosing *Trichomonas vaginalis* infection. *Genitourin. Med.* **67:**149–152.
11. **Borody, T. J., E. Warren, A. Wettstein, G. Robertson, P. Recabarren, A. Fontella, K. Herdnman, and R. Surace.** 2002. Eradication of *Dientamoeba fragilis* can resolve IBS-like symptoms. *J. Gastroenterol. Hepatol.* **17**(Suppl.)**:**A103.
12. **Brown, H. L., D. D. Fuller, L. T. Jasper, T. E. Davis, and J. D. Wright.** 2004. Clinical evaluation of affirm VPIII in the detection and identification of *Trichomonas vaginalis*, *Gardnerella vaginalis*, and *Candida* species in vaginitis/vaginosis. *Infect. Dis. Obstet. Gynecol.* **12:**17–21.
13. **Bruckner, D. A.** 1992. Amebiasis. *Clin. Microbiol. Rev.* **5:**356–369.
14. **Burrows, R. B., and M. A. Swerdlow.** 1956. *Enterobius vermicularis* as a probable vector of *Dientamoeba fragilis. Am. J. Trop. Med. Hyg.* **5:**258–265.
15. **Butler, W. P.** 1996. *Dientamoeba fragilis.* An unusual intestinal pathogen. *Dig. Dis. Sci.* **41:**1811–1813.
16. **Campbell, L., V. Woods, T. Lloyd, S. Elsayed, and D. L. Church.** 2008. Evaluation of the OSOM Trichomonas rapid test versus wet preparation examination for detection of *Trichomonas vaginalis* vaginitis in specimens from women with a low prevalence of infection. *J. Clin. Microbiol.* **46:**3467–3469.
17. **Carroccio, A., G. Montalto, G. Iacono, S. Ippolito, M. Soresi, and A. Notarbartolo.** 1997. Secondary impairment of pancreatic function as a cause of severe malabsorption in intestinal giardiasis: a case report. *Am. J. Trop. Med. Hyg.* **56:**599–602.
18. **Castro, J., J. L. Vazquez-Iglesias, and F. Arnal-Monreal.** 1983. Dysentery caused by *Balantidium coli*—report of two cases. *Endoscopy* **15:**272–274.
19. **Cavalier-Smith, T.** 1998. A revised six-kingdom system of life. *Biol. Rev. Camb. Philos. Soc.* **73:**203–266.
20. **Centers for Disease Control and Prevention.** 2006. Sexually transmitted diseases treatment guidelines. *MMWR Recommend. Rep.* **55**(RR-11)**:**1–100.
21. **Chan, F., N. Stewart, M. Guan, I. Robb, L. Fuite, I. Chan, F. Diaz-Mitoma, J. King, N. MacDonald, and A. Mackenzie.** 1996. Prevalence of *Dientamoeba fragilis* antibodies in children and recognition of a 39 kDa immunodominant protein antigen of the organism. *Eur. J. Clin. Microbiol. Infect. Dis.* **15:**950–954.
22. **Chan, F. T., M. X. Guan, and A. M. Mackenzie.** 1993. Application of indirect immunofluorescence to detection of *Dientamoeba fragilis* trophozoites in fecal specimens. *J. Clin. Microbiol.* **31:**1710–1714.
23. **Clark, C. G.** 1997. Extensive genetic diversity in *Blastocystis hominis. Mol. Biochem. Parasitol.* **87:**79–83.
24. **Clark, C. G., and L. S. Diamond.** 1991. The Laredo strain and other 'Entamoeba histolytica-like' amoebae are *Entamoeba moshkovskii. Mol. Biochem. Parasitol.* **46:**11–18.
25. **Clinical and Laboratory Standards Institute.** 2005. *Recovery and Identification of Parasites from the Intestinal Tract—Approved Guideline M28-A2*, 2nd ed, vol. 25. Clinical and Laboratory Standards Institute, Wayne, PA.
26. **Cotch, M. F., J. G. Pastorek II, R. P. Nugent, D. E. Yerg, D. H. Martin, D. A. Eschenbach, et al.** 1991. Demographic and behavioral predictors of *Trichomonas vaginalis* infection among pregnant women. *Obstet. Gynecol.* **78:**1087–1092.
27. **Cudmore, S. L., K. L. Delgaty, S. F. Hayward-McClelland, D. P. Petrin, and G. E. Garber.** 2004. Treatment of infections caused by metronidazole-resistant *Trichomonas vaginalis. Clin. Microbiol. Rev.* **17:**783–793.
28. **Cuffari, C., L. Oligny, and E. G. Seidman.** 1998. *Dientamoeba fragilis* masquerading as allergic colitis. *J. Pediatr. Gastroenterol. Nutr.* **26:**16–20.
29. **Currie, A. R.** 1990. Human balantidiasis. A case report. *S. Afr. J. Surg.* **28:**23–25.
30. **Diamond, L. S., and C. G. Clark.** 1993. A redescription of *Entamoeba histolytica* Schaudinn, 1903 (emended Walker, 1911) separating it from *Entamoeba dispar* Brumpt, 1925. *J. Eukaryot. Microbiol.* **40:**340–344.
31. **Draper, D., R. Parker, E. Patterson, W. Jones, M. Beutz, J. French, K. Borchardt, and J. McGregor.** 1993. Detection of *Trichomonas vaginalis* in pregnant women with the InPouch TV culture system. *J. Clin. Microbiol.* **31:**1016–1018.

32. **Espinosa-Cantellano, M., and A. Martinez-Palomo.** 2000. Pathogenesis of intestinal amebiasis: from molecules to disease. *Clin. Microbiol. Rev.* **13:**318–331.

33. **Esteban, J. G., C. Aguirre, R. Angles, L. R. Ash, and S. Mas-Coma.** 1998. Balantidiasis in Aymara children from the northern Bolivian Altiplano. *Am. J. Trop. Med. Hyg.* **59:**922–927.

34. **Evangelopoulos, A., G. Spanakos, E. Patsoula, N. Vakalis, and N. Legakis.** 2000. A nested, multiplex, PCR assay for the simultaneous detection and differentiation of *Entamoeba histolytica* and *Entamoeba dispar* in faeces. *Ann. Trop. Med. Parasitol.* **94:**233–240.

35. **Fotedar, R., D. Stark, N. Beebe, D. Marriott, J. Ellis, and J. Harkness.** 2007. Laboratory diagnostic techniques for *Entamoeba* species. *Clin. Microbiol. Rev.* **20:**511–532.

36. **Garavelli, P. L., C. H. Zierdt, T. A. Fleisher, H. Liss, and B. Nagy.** 1995. Serum antibody detected by fluorescent antibody test in patients with symptomatic *Blastocystis hominis* infection. *Recenti Prog. Med.* **86:**398–400.

37. **Garcia, L. S.** 2007. *Diagnostic Medical Parasitology,* 5th ed. ASM Press, Washington, DC.

38. **Garcia, L. S., and J. P. Garcia.** 2006. Detection of *Giardia lamblia* antigens in human fecal specimens by a solid-phase qualitative immunochromatographic assay. *J. Clin. Microbiol.* **44:**4587–4588.

39. **Garcia, L. S., and R. Y. Shimizu.** 2000. Detection of *Giardia lamblia* and *Cryptosporidium parvum* antigens in human fecal specimens using the ColorPAC combination rapid solid-phase qualitative immunochromatographic assay. *J. Clin. Microbiol.* **38:**1267–1268.

40. **Garcia, L. S., and R. Y. Shimizu.** 1997. Evaluation of nine immunoassay kits (enzyme immunoassay and direct fluorescence) for detection of *Giardia lamblia* and *Cryptosporidium parvum* in human fecal specimens. *J. Clin. Microbiol.* **35:**1526–1529.

41. **Garcia, L. S., R. Y. Shimizu, and C. N. Bernard.** 2000. Detection of *Giardia lamblia, Entamoeba histolytica/Entamoeba dispar,* and *Cryptosporidium parvum* antigens in human fecal specimens using the triage parasite panel enzyme immunoassay. *J. Clin. Microbiol.* **38:**3337–3340.

42. **Garcia, L. S., R. Y. Shimizu, S. Novak, M. Carroll, and F. Chan.** 2003. Commercial assay for detection of *Giardia lamblia* and *Cryptosporidium parvum* antigens in human fecal specimens by rapid solid-phase qualitative immunochromatography. *J. Clin. Microbiol.* **41:**209–212.

43. **Gardner, T. B., and D. R. Hill.** 2001. Treatment of giardiasis. *Clin. Microbiol. Rev.* **14:**114–128.

44. **Gerbod, D., V. P. Edgcomb, C. Noel, L. Zenner, R. Wintjens, P. Delgado-Viscogliosi, M. E. Holder, M. L. Sogin, and E. Viscogliosi.** 2001. Phylogenetic position of the trichomonad parasite of turkeys, *Histomonas meleagridis* (Smith) Tyzzer, inferred from small subunit rRNA sequence. *J. Eukaryot. Microbiol.* **48:**498–504.

45. **Girginkardesler, N., S. Coskun, I. Cuneyt Balcioglu, P. Ertan, and U. Z. Ok.** 2003. *Dientamoeba fragilis,* a neglected cause of diarrhea, successfully treated with secnidazole. *Clin. Microbiol. Infect.* **9:**110–113.

46. **Guy, R. A., C. Xiao, and P. A. Horgen.** 2004. Real-time PCR assay for detection and genotype differentiation of *Giardia lamblia* in stool specimens. *J. Clin. Microbiol.* **42:**3317–3320.

47. **Hanson, K. L., and C. P. Cartwright.** 2001. Use of an enzyme immunoassay does not eliminate the need to analyze multiple stool specimens for sensitive detection of *Giardia lamblia. J. Clin. Microbiol.* **39:**474–477.

48. **Haque, R., I. K. Ali, S. Akther, and W. A. Petri, Jr.** 1998. Comparison of PCR, isoenzyme analysis, and antigen detection for diagnosis of *Entamoeba histolytica* infection. *J. Clin. Microbiol.* **36:**449–452.

49. **Haque, R., I. K. M. Ali, C. G. Clark, and W. A. Petri, Jr.** 1998. A case report of *Entamoeba moshkovskii* infection in a Bangladeshi child. *Parasitol. Int.* **47:**201–202.

50. **Haque, R., A. Ikm, and W. A. Petri, Jr.** 2000. Salivary antilectin IgA antibodies in a cohort of children residing in an endemic area of Bangladesh. *Arch. Med. Res.* **31:**S41–S43.

51. **Haque, R., N. U. Mollah, I. K. Ali, K. Alam, A. Eubanks, D. Lyerly, and W. A. Petri, Jr.** 2000. Diagnosis of amebic liver abscess and intestinal infection with the TechLab *Entamoeba histolytica* II antigen detection and antibody tests. *J. Clin. Microbiol.* **38:**3235–3239.

52. **Haque, R., L. M. Neville, P. Hahn, and W. A. Petri, Jr.** 1995. Rapid diagnosis of *Entamoeba* infection by using *Entamoeba* and *Entamoeba histolytica* stool antigen detection kits. *J. Clin. Microbiol.* **33:**2558–2561.

53. **Hardick, A., J. Hardick, B. J. Wood, and C. Gaydos.** 2006. Comparison between the Gen-Probe transcription-mediated amplification *Trichomonas vaginalis* research assay and real-time PCR for *Trichomonas vaginalis* detection using a Roche LightCycler instrument with female self-obtained vaginal swab samples and male urine samples. *J. Clin. Microbiol.* **44:**4197–4199.

54. **Hardick, J., S. Yang, S. Lin, D. Duncan, and C. Gaydos.** 2003. Use of the Roche LightCycler instrument in a real-time PCR for *Trichomonas vaginalis* in urine samples from females and males. *J. Clin. Microbiol.* **41:**5619–5622.

55. **Haresh, K., K. Suresh, A. Khairul Anus, and S. Saminathan.** 1999. Isolate resistance of *Blastocystis hominis* to metronidazole. *Trop. Med. Int. Health* **4:**274–277.

56. **Heine, R. P., H. C. Wiesenfeld, R. L. Sweet, and S. S. Witkin.** 1997. Polymerase chain reaction analysis of distal vaginal specimens: a less invasive strategy for detection of *Trichomonas vaginalis. Clin. Infect. Dis.* **24:**985–987.

57. **Hobbs, M. M., P. Kazembe, A. W. Reed, W. C. Miller, E. Nkata, D. Zimba, C. C. Daly, H. Chakraborty, M. S. Cohen, and I. Hoffman.** 1999. *Trichomonas vaginalis* as a cause of urethritis in Malawian men. *Sex. Transm. Dis.* **26:**381–387.

58. **Hoevers, J. D., and K. F. Snowden.** 2005. Analysis of the ITS region and partial ssu and lsu rRNA genes of *Blastocystis* and *Proteromonas lacertae. Parasitology* **131:**187–196.

59. **Hook, E. W., III.** 1999. *Trichomonas vaginalis*—no longer a minor STD. *Sex. Transm. Dis.* **26:**388–389.

60. **Horiki, N., Y. Kaneda, M. Maruyama, Y. Fujita, and H. Tachibana.** 1999. Intestinal blockage by carcinoma and *Blastocystis hominis* infection. *Am. J. Trop. Med. Hyg.* **60:**400–402.

61. **Hung, C. C., P. J. Chen, S. M. Hsieh, J. M. Wong, C. T. Fang, S. C. Chang, and M. Y. Chen.** 1999. Invasive amoebiasis: an emerging parasitic disease in patients infected with HIV in an area endemic for amoebic infection. *AIDS* **13:**2421–2428.

62. **Hung, C. C., H. Y. Deng, W. H. Hsiao, S. M. Hsieh, C. F. Hsiao, M. Y. Chen, S. C. Chang, and K. E. Su.** 2005. Invasive amebiasis as an emerging parasitic disease in patients with human immunodeficiency virus type 1 infection in Taiwan. *Arch. Intern. Med.* **165:**409–415.

63. **Huppert, J. S., B. E. Batteiger, P. Braslins, J. A. Feldman, M. M. Hobbs, H. Z. Sankey, A. C. Sena, and K. A. Wendel.** 2005. Use of an immunochromatographic assay for rapid detection of *Trichomonas vaginalis* in vaginal specimens. *J. Clin. Microbiol.* **43:**684–687.

64. **Huppert, J. S., J. E. Mortensen, J. L. Reed, J. A. Kahn, K. D. Rich, W. C. Miller, and M. M. Hobbs.** 2007. Rapid antigen testing compares favorably with transcription-mediated amplification assay for the detection of *Trichomonas vaginalis* in young women. *Clin. Infect. Dis.* **45:**194–198.

65. **Jackson, D. J., J. P. Rakwar, J. J. Bwayo, J. K. Kreiss, and S. Moses.** 1997. Urethral *Trichomonas vaginalis* infection and HIV-1 transmission. *Lancet* **350:**1076.

66. **Johnson, E. H., J. J. Windsor, and C. G. Clark.** 2004. Emerging from obscurity: biological, clinical, and diagnostic aspects of *Dientamoeba fragilis. Clin. Microbiol. Rev.* **17:**553–570.

67. **Johnson, J. A., and C. G. Clark.** 2000. Cryptic genetic diversity in *Dientamoeba fragilis. J. Clin. Microbiol.* **38:**4653–4654.

68. **Johnston, S. P., M. M. Ballard, M. J. Beach, L. Causer, and P. P. Wilkins.** 2003. Evaluation of three commercial assays for detection of *Giardia* and *Cryptosporidium* organisms in fecal specimens. *J. Clin. Microbiol.* **41:**623–626.

69. **Joyce, M. P., and J. I. Ravdin.** 1988. Antigens of *Entamoeba histolytica* recognized by immune sera from liver abscess patients. *Am. J. Trop. Med. Hyg.* **38:**74–80.

70. **Kaneda, Y., N. Horiki, X. Cheng, H. Tachibana, and Y. Tsutsumi.** 2000. Serologic response to *Blastocystis hominis* infection in asymptomatic individuals. *Tokai J. Exp. Clin. Med.* **25:**51–56.

71. **Katanik, M. T., S. K. Schneider, J. E. Rosenblatt, G. S. Hall, and G. W. Procop.** 2001. Evaluation of ColorPAC *Giardia*/*Cryptosporidium* rapid assay and ProSpecT *Giardia*/*Cryptosporidium* microplate assay for detection of *Giardia* and *Cryptosporidium* in fecal specimens. *J. Clin. Microbiol.* **39:**4523–4525.

72. **Kawamura, O., Y. Kon, A. Naganuma, T. Iwami, H. Maruyama, T. Yamada, K. Sonobe, T. Horikoshi, M. Kusano, and M. Mori.** 2001. *Retortamonas intestinalis* in the pancreatic juice of a patient with small nodular lesions of the main pancreatic duct. *Gastrointest. Endosc.* **53:**508–510.

73. **Kaydos, S. C., H. Swygard, S. L. Wise, A. C. Sena, P. A. Leone, W. C. Miller, M. S. Cohen, and M. M. Hobbs.** 2002. Development and validation of a PCR-based enzyme-linked immunosorbent assay with urine for use in clinical research settings to detect *Trichomonas vaginalis* in women. *J. Clin. Microbiol.* **40:**89–95.

74. **Kaydos-Daniels, S. C., W. C. Miller, I. Hoffman, T. Banda, W. Dzinyemba, F. Martinson, M. S. Cohen, and M. M. Hobbs.** 2003. Validation of a urine-based PCR-enzyme-linked immunosorbent assay for use in clinical research settings to detect *Trichomonas vaginalis* in men. *J. Clin. Microbiol.* **41:**318–323.

75. **Khairnar, K., and S. C. Parija.** 2007. A novel nested multiplex polymerase chain reaction (PCR) assay for differential detection of *Entamoeba histolytica*, *E. moshkovskii* and *E. dispar* DNA in stool samples. *BMC Microbiol.* **7:**47.

76. **Klebanoff, M. A., J. C. Carey, J. C. Hauth, S. L. Hillier, R. P. Nugent, E. A. Thom, J. M. Ernest, R. P. Heine, R. J. Wapner, W. Trout, A. Moawad, K. J. Leveno, M. Miodovnik, B. M. Sibai, J. P. Van Dorsten, M. P. Dombrowski, M. J. O'Sullivan, M. Varner, O. Langer, D. McNellis, and J. M. Roberts.** 2001. Failure of metronidazole to prevent preterm delivery among pregnant women with asymptomatic *Trichomonas vaginalis* infection. *N. Engl. J. Med.* **345:**487–493.

77. **Knight, R.** 1978. Giardiasis, isosporiasis and balantidiasis. *Clin. Gastroenterol.* **7:**31–47.

78. **Krieger, J. N., M. R. Tam, C. E. Stevens, I. O. Nielsen, J. Hale, N. B. Kiviat, and K. K. Holmes.** 1988. Diagnosis of trichomoniasis. Comparison of conventional wet-mount examination with cytologic studies, cultures, and monoclonal antibody staining of direct specimens. *JAMA* **259:**1223–1227.

79. **Kurth, A., W. L. Whittington, M. R. Golden, K. K. Thomas, K. K. Holmes, and J. R. Schwebke.** 2004. Performance of a new, rapid assay for detection of *Trichomonas vaginalis*. *J. Clin. Microbiol.* **42:**2940–2943.

80. **Ladas, S. D., S. Savva, A. Frydas, A. Kaloviduris, J. Hatzioannou, and S. Raptis.** 1989. Invasive balantidiasis presented as chronic colitis and lung involvement. *Dig. Dis. Sci.* **34:**1621–1623.

81. **Laga, M., A. Manoka, M. Kivuvu, B. Malele, M. Tuliza, N. Nzila, J. Goeman, F. Behets, V. Batter, M. Alary, et al.** 1993. Non-ulcerative sexually transmitted diseases as risk factors for HIV-1 transmission in women: results from a cohort study. *AIDS* **7:**95–102.

82. **Lainson, R., and B. A. da Silva.** 1999. Intestinal parasites of some diarrhoeic HIV-seropositive individuals in North Brazil, with particular reference to *Isospora belli* Wenyon, 1923 and *Dientamoeba fragilis* Jepps & Dobell, 1918. *Mem. Inst. Oswaldo Cruz* **94:**611–613.

83. **Lawing, L. F., S. R. Hedges, and J. R. Schwebke.** 2000. Detection of trichomonosis in vaginal and urine specimens from women by culture and PCR. *J. Clin. Microbiol.* **38:**3585–3588.

84. **Leelayoova, S., R. Rangsin, P. Taamasri, T. Naaglor, U. Thathaisong, and M. Mungthin.** 2004. Evidence of waterborne transmission of *Blastocystis hominis*. *Am. J. Trop. Med. Hyg.* **70:**658–662.

85. **Leelayoova, S., P. Taamasri, R. Rangsin, T. Naaglor, U. Thathaisong, and M. Mungthin.** 2002. In-vitro cultivation: a sensitive method for detecting *Blastocystis hominis*. *Ann. Trop. Med. Parasitol.* **96:**803–807.

86. **Leo, M., R. Haque, M. Kabir, S. Roy, R. M. Lahlou, D. Mondal, E. Tannich, and W. A. Petri, Jr.** 2006. Evaluation of *Entamoeba histolytica* antigen and antibody point-of-care tests for the rapid diagnosis of amebiasis. *J. Clin. Microbiol.* **44:**4569–4571.

87. **Lin, P. R., M. F. Shaio, and J. Y. Liu.** 1997. One-tube, nested-PCR assay for the detection of *Trichomonas vaginalis* in vaginal discharges. *Ann. Trop. Med. Parasitol.* **91:**61–65.

88. **Lowther, S. A., M. S. Dworkin, and D. L. Hanson.** 2000. *Entamoeba histolytica*/*Entamoeba dispar* infections in human immunodeficiency virus-infected patients in the United States. *Clin. Infect. Dis.* **30:**955–959.

89. **Mansour, N. S., E. M. Mikhail, N. A. el Masry, A. G. Sabry, and E. W. Mohareb.** 1995. Biochemical characterisation of human isolates of *Blastocystis hominis*. *J. Med. Microbiol.* **42:**304–307.

90. **Maraha, B., and A. G. Buiting.** 2000. Evaluation of four enzyme immunoassays for the detection of *Giardia lamblia* antigen in stool specimens. *Eur. J. Clin. Microbiol. Infect. Dis.* **19:**485–487.

91. **Markell, E. K., and M. P. Udkow.** 1986. *Blastocystis hominis*: pathogen or fellow traveler? *Am. J. Trop. Med. Hyg.* **35:**1023–1026.

92. **Marshall, M. M., D. Naumovitz, Y. Ortega, and C. R. Sterling.** 1997. Waterborne protozoan pathogens. *Clin. Microbiol. Rev.* **10:**67–85.

93. **McLaren, L. C., L. E. Davis, G. R. Healy, and C. G. James.** 1983. Isolation of *Trichomonas vaginalis* from the respiratory tract of infants with respiratory disease. *Pediatrics* **71:**888–890.

94. **Meri, T., T. S. Jokiranta, L. Suhonen, and S. Meri.** 2000. Resistance of *Trichomonas vaginalis* to metronidazole: report of the first three cases from Finland and optimization of in vitro susceptibility testing under various oxygen concentrations. *J. Clin. Microbiol.* **38:**763–767.

95. **Minkoff, H., A. N. Grunebaum, R. H. Schwarz, J. Feldman, M. Cummings, W. Crombleholme, L. Clark, G. Pringle, and W. M. McCormack.** 1984. Risk factors for prematurity and premature rupture of membranes: a prospective study of the vaginal flora in pregnancy. *Am. J. Obstet. Gynecol.* **150:**965–972.

96. **Moe, K. T., M. Singh, J. Howe, L. C. Ho, S. W. Tan, G. C. Ng, X. Q. Chen, and E. H. Yap.** 1996. Observations on the ultrastructure and viability of the cystic stage of *Blastocystis hominis* from human feces. *Parasitol. Res.* **82:**439–444.

97. **Monis, P. T., R. H. Andrews, G. Mayrhofer, and P. L. Ey.** 1999. Molecular systematics of the parasitic protozoan *Giardia intestinalis*. *Mol. Biol. Evol.* **16:**1135–1144.

98. **Monteiro, L., D. Bonnemaison, A. Vekris, K. G. Petry, J. Bonnet, R. Vidal, J. Cabrita, and F. Megraud.** 1997. Complex polysaccharides as PCR inhibitors in feces: *Helicobacter pylori* model. *J. Clin. Microbiol.* **35:**995–998.

99. **Munson, E., M. Napierala, R. Olson, T. Endes, T. Block, J. E. Hryciuk, and R. F. Schell.** 2008. Impact of *Trichomonas vaginalis* transcription-mediated amplification-based analyte-specific-reagent testing in a metropolitan setting of high sexually transmitted disease prevalence. *J. Clin. Microbiol.* **46:**3368–3374.

100. **Nantavisai, K., M. Mungthin, P. Tan-ariya, R. Rangsin, T. Naaglor, and S. Leelayoova.** 2007. Evaluation of the sensitivities of DNA extraction and PCR methods for detection of *Giardia duodenalis* in stool specimens. *J. Clin. Microbiol.* **45:**581–583.

101. **Ng, C. T., C. A. Gilchrist, A. Lane, S. Roy, R. Haque, and E. R. Houpt.** 2005. Multiplex real-time PCR assay using Scorpion probes and DNA capture for genotype-specific detection of *Giardia lamblia* on fecal samples. *J. Clin. Microbiol.* **43:**1256–1260.

102. **Noel, C., F. Dufernez, D. Gerbod, V. P. Edgcomb, P. Delgado-Viscogliosi, L. C. Ho, M. Singh, R. Wintjens, M. L. Sogin, M. Capron, R. Pierce, L. Zenner, and E. Viscogliosi.** 2005. Molecular phylogenies of *Blastocystis* isolates from different hosts: implications for genetic diversity, identification of species, and zoonosis. *J. Clin. Microbiol.* **43:**348–355.

103. **Nye, M. B., J. R. Schwebke, and B. A. Body.** 2009. Comparison of APTIMA *Trichomonas vaginalis* transcription-mediated amplification to wet mount microscopy, culture, and polymerase chain reaction for diagnosis of trichomoniasis in men and women. *Am. J. Obstet. Gynecol.* **200:**188.e1–188.e7.

104. **Oh, M. D., K. Lee, E. Kim, S. Lee, N. Kim, H. Choi, M. H. Choi, J. Y. Chai, and K. Choe.** 2000. Amoebic liver abscess in HIV-infected patients. *AIDS* **14:**1872–1873.

105. **Olson, M. E., H. Ceri, and D. W. Morck.** 2000. *Giardia* vaccination. *Parasitol. Today* **16:**213–217.

106. **Ong, S. J., M. Y. Cheng, K. H. Liu, and C. B. Horng.** 1996. Use of the ProSpecT microplate enzyme immunoassay for the detection of pathogenic and non-pathogenic *Entamoeba histolytica* in faecal specimens. *Trans. R. Soc. Trop. Med. Hyg.* **90:**248–249.

107. **Ortner, S., C. G. Clark, M. Binder, O. Scheiner, G. Wiedermann, and M. Duchene.** 1997. Molecular biology of the hexokinase isoenzyme pattern that distinguishes pathogenic *Entamoeba histolytica* from nonpathogenic *Entamoeba dispar*. *Mol. Biochem. Parasitol.* **86:**85–94.

108. **Paglia, M. G., and P. Visca.** 2004. An improved PCR-based method for detection and differentiation of *Entamoeba histolytica* and *Entamoeba dispar* in formalin-fixed stools. *Acta Tropica* **92:**273–277.

109. **Paintlia, A. S., S. Descoteaux, B. Spencer, A. Chakraborti, N. K. Ganguly, R. C. Mahajan, and J. Samuelson.** 1998. *Giardia lamblia* groups A and B among young adults in India. *Clin. Infect. Dis.* **26:**190–191.

110. **Paintlia, A. S., M. K. Paintlia, R. C. Mahajan, A. Chakraborti, and N. K. Ganguly.** 1999. A DNA-based probe for differentiation of *Giardia lamblia* group A and B isolates from northern India. *Clin. Infect. Dis.* **28:**1178–1180.

111. **Panosian, C. B.** 1988. Parasitic diarrhea. *Infect. Dis. Clin. N. Am.* **2:**685–703.

112. **Pattullo, L., S. Griffeth, L. Ding, J. Mortensen, J. Reed, J. Kahn, and J. Huppert.** 2009. Stepwise diagnosis of *Trichomonas vaginalis* infection in adolescent women. *J. Clin. Microbiol.* **47:**59–63.

113. **Peek, R., F. R. Reedeker, and T. van Gool.** 2004. Direct amplification and genotyping of *Dientamoeba fragilis* from human stool specimens. *J. Clin. Microbiol.* **42:**631–635.

114. **Petri, W. A., Jr., T. F. Jackson, V. Gathiram, K. Kress, L. D. Saffer, T. L. Snodgrass, M. D. Chapman, Z. Keren, and D. Mirelman.** 1990. Pathogenic and nonpathogenic strains of *Entamoeba histolytica* can be differentiated by monoclonal antibodies to the galactose-specific adherence lectin. *Infect. Immun.* **58:**1802–1806.

115. **Petri, W. A., Jr., R. D. Smith, P. H. Schlesinger, C. F. Murphy, and J. I. Ravdin.** 1987. Isolation of the galactose-binding lectin that mediates the in vitro adherence of *Entamoeba histolytica*. *J. Clin. Investig.* **80:**1238–1244.

116. **Pillai, D. R., and K. C. Kain.** 1999. Immunochromatographic strip-based detection of *Entamoeba histolytica-E. dispar* and *Giardia lamblia* coproantigen. *J. Clin. Microbiol.* **37:**3017–3019.

117. **Pillay, A., J. Lewis, and R. C. Ballard.** 2004. Evaluation of Xenostrip-Tv, a rapid diagnostic test for *Trichomonas vaginalis* infection. *J. Clin. Microbiol.* **42:**3853–3856.

118. **Qvarnstrom, Y., C. James, M. Xayavong, B. P. Holloway, G. S. Visvesvara, R. Sriram, and A. J. da Silva.** 2005. Comparison of real-time PCR protocols for differential laboratory diagnosis of amebiasis. *J. Clin. Microbiol.* **43:**5491–5497.

119. **Rapeeporn, Y., N. Warunee, W. Nuttapong, S. Sompong, and K. Rachada.** 2006. Infection of *Blastocystis hominis* in primary schoolchildren from Nakhon Pathom province, Thailand. *Trop. Biomed.* **23:**117–122.

120. **Rendtorff, R. C.** 1978. The experimental transmission of *Giardia lamblia* among volunteer subjects, p. 64–81. *In* W. Jacubowski and J. C. Hoff (ed.), *Waterborne Transmission of Giardiasis 1978. EPA 600/9-79-001.* U.S. Environmental Protection Agency, Washington, DC.

121. **Riley, D. E., M. C. Roberts, T. Takayama, and J. N. Krieger.** 1992. Development of a polymerase chain reaction-based diagnosis of *Trichomonas vaginalis*. *J. Clin. Microbiol.* **30:**465–472.

122. **Rivera, W. L., H. Tachibana, M. R. Silva-Tahat, H. Uemura, and H. Kanbara.** 1996. Differentiation of *Entamoeba histolytica* and *E. dispar* DNA from cysts present in stool specimens by polymerase chain reaction: its field application in the Philippines. *Parasitol. Res.* **82:**585–589.

123. **Rochelle, P. A., R. De Leon, M. H. Stewart, and R. L. Wolfe.** 1997. Comparison of primers and optimization of PCR conditions for detection of *Cryptosporidium parvum* and *Giardia lamblia* in water. *Appl. Environ. Microbiol.* **63:**106–114.

124. **Roy, S., M. Kabir, D. Mondal, I. K. Ali, W. A. Petri, Jr., and R. Haque.** 2005. Real-time-PCR assay for diagnosis of *Entamoeba histolytica* infection. *J. Clin. Microbiol.* **43:**2168–2172.

125. **Sargeaunt, P. G., and J. E. Williams.** 1978. Electrophoretic isoenzyme patterns of *Entamoeba histolytica* and *Entamoeba coli*. *Trans. R. Soc. Trop. Med. Hyg.* **72:**164–166.

126. **Schuster, F. L., and L. Ramirez-Avila.** 2008. Current world status of *Balantidium coli*. *Clin. Microbiol. Rev.* **21:**626–638.

127. **Schwartz, M. D., and M. E. Nelson.** 2003. *Dientamoeba fragilis* infection presenting to the emergency department as acute appendicitis. *J. Emerg. Med.* **25:**17–21.

128. **Schwebke, J. R., and D. Burgess.** 2004. Trichomoniasis. *Clin. Microbiol. Rev.* **17:**794–803.

129. **Schwebke, J. R., and L. F. Lawing.** 2002. Improved detection by DNA amplification of *Trichomonas vaginalis* in males. *J. Clin. Microbiol.* **40:**3681–3683.

130. **Schwebke, J. R., S. C. Morgan, and G. B. Pinson.** 1997. Validity of self-obtained vaginal specimens for diagnosis of trichomoniasis. *J. Clin. Microbiol.* **35:**1618–1619.

131. **Schwebke, J. R., M. F. Venglarik, and S. C. Morgan.** 1999. Delayed versus immediate bedside inoculation of culture media for diagnosis of vaginal trichomonosis. *J. Clin. Microbiol.* **37:**2369–2370.

132. **Sheehan, D. J., B. G. Raucher, and J. C. McKitrick.** 1986. Association of *Blastocystis hominis* with signs and symptoms of human disease. *J. Clin. Microbiol.* **24:**548–550.

133. **Silberman, J. D., C. G. Clark, and M. L. Sogin.** 1996. *Dientamoeba fragilis* shares a recent common evolutionary history with the trichomonads. *Mol. Biochem. Parasitol.* **76:**311–314.

134. **Silberman, J. D., M. L. Sogin, D. D. Leipe, and C. G. Clark.** 1996. Human parasite finds taxonomic home. *Nature* **380:**398.

135. **Sobel, J. D., V. Nagappan, and P. Nyirjesy.** 1999. Metronidazole-resistant vaginal trichomoniasis—an emerging problem. *N. Engl. J. Med.* **341:**292–293.

136. **Solaymani-Mohammadi, S., M. M. Lam, J. R. Zunt, and W. A. Petri, Jr.** 2007. *Entamoeba histolytica* encephalitis diagnosed by PCR of cerebrospinal fluid. *Trans. R. Soc. Trop. Med. Hyg.* **101:**311–313.

137. **Solaymani-Mohammadi, S., M. Rezaian, H. Hooshyar, G. R. Mowlavi, Z. Babaei, and M. A. Anwar.** 2004. Intestinal protozoa in wild boars (*Sus scrofa*) in western Iran. *J. Wildl. Dis.* **40:**801–803.

138. **Soper, D. E., R. C. Bump, and W. G. Hurt.** 1990. Bacterial vaginosis and trichomoniasis vaginitis are risk factors for cuff cellulitis after abdominal hysterectomy. *Am. J. Obstet. Gynecol.* **163:**1016–1021.

139. **Sousa, M. C., and J. Poiares-Da-Silva.** 1999. A new method for assessing metronidazole susceptibility of *Giardia lamblia* trophozoites. *Antimicrob. Agents Chemother.* **43:**2939–2942.

140. **Stanley, S. L., Jr.** 2001. Protective immunity to amebiasis: new insights and new challenges. *J. Infect. Dis.* **184:**504–506.

141. **Stark, D., N. Beebe, D. Marriott, J. Ellis, and J. Harkness.** 2005. Detection of *Dientamoeba fragilis* in fresh stool specimens using PCR. *Int. J. Parasitol.* **35:**57–62.

142. Stark, D., N. Beebe, D. Marriott, J. Ellis, and J. Harkness. 2006. Evaluation of three diagnostic methods, including real-time PCR, for detection of *Dientamoeba fragilis* in stool specimens. *J. Clin. Microbiol.* **44:**232–235.

143. Stark, D., S. van Hal, R. Fotedar, A. Butcher, D. Marriott, J. Ellis, and J. Harkness. 2008. Comparison of stool antigen detection kits to PCR for diagnosis of amebiasis. *J. Clin. Microbiol.* **46:**1678–1681.

144. Stensvold, C. R., M. C. Arendrup, C. Jespersgaard, K. Molbak, and H. V. Nielsen. 2007. Detecting *Blastocystis* using parasitologic and DNA-based methods: a comparative study. *Diagn. Microbiol. Infect. Dis.* **59:**303–307.

145. Stensvold, C. R., R. J. Traub, G. von Samson-Himmelstjerna, C. Jespersgaard, H. V. Nielsen, and R. C. Thompson. 2007. *Blastocystis:* subtyping isolates using pyrosequencing technology. *Exp. Parasitol.* **116:**111–119.

146. Stensvold, R., A. Brillowska-Dabrowska, H. V. Nielsen, and M. C. Arendrup. 2006. Detection of *Blastocystis hominis* in unpreserved stool specimens by using polymerase chain reaction. *J. Parasitol.* **92:**1081–1087.

147. Struder-Kypke, M. C., O. A. Kornilova, and D. H. Lynn. 2007. Phylogeny of trichostome ciliates (Ciliophora, Litostomatea) endosymbiotic in the Yakut horse (Equus caballus). *Eur. J. Protistol.* **43:**319–328.

148. Struder-Kypke, M. C., A. D. Wright, W. Foissner, A. Chatzinotas, and D. H. Lynn. 2006. Molecular phylogeny of litostome ciliates (Ciliophora, Litostomatea) with emphasis on free-living haptorian genera. *Protist* **157:**261–278.

149. Talis, B., B. Stein, and J. Lengy. 1971. *Dientamoeba fragilis* in human feces and bile. *Isr. J. Med. Sci.* **7:**1063–1069.

150. Tan, K. S. 2008. New insights on classification, identification, and clinical relevance of *Blastocystis* spp. *Clin. Microbiol. Rev.* **21:**639–665.

151. Tanyuksel, M., and W. A. Petri, Jr. 2003. Laboratory diagnosis of amebiasis. *Clin. Microbiol. Rev.* **16:**713–729.

152. Tanyuksel, M., H. Tachibana, and W. A. Petri. 2001. Amebiasis, an emerging disease, p. 197–202. *In* W. M. Scheld, W. A. Craig, and J. M. Hughes (ed.), *Emerging Infections 5.* ASM Press, Washington, DC.

153. Troll, H., H. Marti, and N. Weiss. 1997. Simple differential detection of *Entamoeba histolytica* and *Entamoeba dispar* in fresh stool specimens by sodium acetate-acetic acid-formalin concentration and PCR. *J. Clin. Microbiol.* **35:**1701–1705.

154. Udkow, M. P., and E. K. Markell. 1993. *Blastocystis hominis:* prevalence in asymptomatic versus symptomatic hosts. *J. Infect. Dis.* **168:**242–244.

155. Upcroft, P., and J. A. Upcroft. 2001. Drug targets and mechanisms of resistance in the anaerobic protozoa. *Clin. Microbiol. Rev.* **14:**150–164.

156. Vasquez, W., and J. Vidal. 1999. Colitis balantidiasica: a proposito de un caso fatal en el Departmento de Huancavelica. *An. Fac. Med.* **60:**119–123.

157. Verweij, J. J., R. A. Blange, K. Templeton, J. Schinkel, E. A. Brienen, M. A. van Rooyen, L. van Lieshout, and A. M. Polderman. 2004. Simultaneous detection of *Entamoeba histolytica, Giardia lamblia,* and *Cryptosporidium parvum* in fecal samples by using multiplex real-time PCR. *J. Clin. Microbiol.* **42:**1220–1223.

158. Verweij, J. J., J. Blotkamp, E. A. Brienen, A. Aguirre, and A. M. Polderman. 2000. Differentiation of *Entamoeba histolytica* and *Entamoeba dispar* cysts using polymerase chain reaction on DNA isolated from faeces with spin columns. *Eur. J. Clin. Microbiol. Infect. Dis.* **19:**358–361.

159. Walderich, B., A. Weber, and J. Knobloch. 1997. Differentiation of *Entamoeba histolytica* and *Entamoeba dispar* from German travelers and residents of endemic areas. *Am. J. Trop. Med. Hyg.* **57:**70–74.

160. Wang, Z., G. J. Vora, and D. A. Stenger. 2004. Detection and genotyping of *Entamoeba histolytica, Entamoeba dispar, Giardia lamblia,* and *Cryptosporidium parvum* by oligonucleotide microarray. *J. Clin. Microbiol.* **42:**3262–3271.

161. Weinstock, H., S. Berman, and W. Cates, Jr. 2004. Sexually transmitted diseases among American youth: incidence and prevalence estimates, 2000. *Perspect. Sex. Reprod. Health* **36:**6–10.

162. Weiss, J. B. 1995. DNA probes and PCR for diagnosis of parasitic infections. *Clin. Microbiol. Rev.* **8:**113–130.

163. Wilson, M., P. Schantz, and N. Pieniazek. 1995. Diagnosis of parasitic infections: immunologic and molecular methods, p. 1159–1170. *In* P. R. Murray, E. J. Baron, and M. A. Pfaller (ed.), *Manual of Clinical Microbiology,* 6th ed. ASM Press, Washington, DC.

164. World Health Organization. 1997. Amoebiasis. *Wkly. Epidemiol. Rec.* **72:**97–99.

165. Yang, J., and T. Scholten. 1977. *Dientamoeba fragilis:* a review with notes on its epidemiology, pathogenicity, mode of transmission, and diagnosis. *Am. J. Trop. Med. Hyg.* **26:**16–22.

166. Yau, Y. C., I. Crandall, and K. C. Kain. 2001. Development of monoclonal antibodies which specifically recognize *Entamoeba histolytica* in preserved stool samples. *J. Clin. Microbiol.* **39:**716–719.

167. Yazar, S., F. Altuntas, I. Sahin, and M. Atambay. 2004. Dysentery caused by *Balantidium coli* in a patient with non-Hodgkin's lymphoma from Turkey. *World J. Gastroenterol.* **10:**458–459.

168. Yoshikawa, H., N. Abe, M. Iwasawa, S. Kitano, I. Nagano, Z. Wu, and Y. Takahashi. 2000. Genomic analysis of *Blastocystis hominis* strains isolated from two long-term health care facilities. *J. Clin. Microbiol.* **38:**1324–1330.

169. Youn, S., M. Kabir, R. Haque, and W. A. Petri, Jr. 2009. Evaluation of a screening test for detection of giardia and cryptosporidium parasites. *J. Clin. Microbiol.* **47:**451–452.

170. Zaki, M., and C. G. Clark. 2001. Isolation and characterization of polymorphic DNA from *Entamoeba histolytica. J. Clin. Microbiol.* **39:**897–905.

171. Zengzhu, G., R. Bracha, Y. Nuchamowitz, I. W. Cheng, and D. Mirelman. 1999. Analysis by enzyme-linked immunosorbent assay and PCR of human liver abscess aspirates from patients in China for *Entamoeba histolytica. J. Clin. Microbiol.* **37:**3034–3036.

172. Zierdt, C. H. 1991. *Blastocystis hominis*—past and future. *Clin. Microbiol. Rev.* **4:**61–79.

173. Zierdt, C. H., W. S. Zierdt, and B. Nagy. 1995. Enzyme-linked immunosorbent assay for detection of serum antibody to *Blastocystis hominis* in symptomatic infections. *J. Parasitol.* **81:**127–129.

Isospora, Cyclospora, and Sarcocystis*

DAVID S. LINDSAY, STEVE J. UPTON, AND LOUIS M. WEISS

138

Isospora (Cystoisospora), Cyclospora, and Sarcocystis are intestinal coccidia of humans (Fig. 1 and 2). They have varied life cycles, epidemiologies, treatment requirements, and diagnostic methods. Oocysts of these coccidia are found in the feces of humans (Table 1), and diagnosis is based ultimately on demonstrating oocysts (Isospora or Cyclospora) or sporocysts (Sarcocystis) in human stool samples.

TAXONOMY

Isospora, Cyclospora, and Sarcocystis are in the phylum Apicomplexa, class Sporozoasida, subclass Coccidiasina, order Eucoccidiorida, suborder Eimeriorina. Cyclospora cayetanensis is in the family Eimeriidae, while Sarcocystis hominis and Sarcocystis suihominis are in the family Sarcocystidae. It is currently under debate whether Isospora belli should be in the family Eimeriidae or moved to the family Sarcocystidae. This parasite has been called Cystoisospora belli in recent experimental studies (55).

DESCRIPTION OF THE AGENTS

Life Cycles

Isospora belli

The life cycle is direct (monoxenous), but evidence exists that it can be facultatively heteroxenous (use two hosts). I. belli oocysts are passed in the feces unsporulated or partially sporulated (Fig. 1C and D and 2A and B). Oocysts generally complete sporulation within 72 hours, although periods of 1 to >5 days have been reported, depending upon temperature. Sporulated oocysts contain two sporocysts, each with four sporozoites. Caryospora-like oocysts of I. belli (containing one sporocyst with eight sporozoites) have been reported and can comprise up to 5% of the sporulated oocysts in a sample (38). The prepatent period, the time it takes for unsporulated oocysts to appear in the feces after sporulated oocysts are ingested, is 9 to 17 days (28). The patent period, the time from when oocysts are first excreted in the feces until they can no longer be observed in the feces, is quite variable and depends on the immune status of the infected individual. Oocysts can usually be found for 30 to 50 days in immunocompetent patients, while immunosuppressed patients may continue to shed oocysts for 6 months or more (53). This prolonged oocyst shedding in immunosuppressed patients is presumably due to recycling of one or more merogonous stages or activation of dormant extraintestinal unizoites (Fig. 3).

Developmental stages of I. belli have been reported for intestinal biopsy specimens of the duodenum, jejunum, and occasionally ileum, and oocysts can be aspirated directly from the duodenal contents. Intestinal development occurs predominantly in epithelial cells, although meronts (schizonts) are occasionally reported from the lamina propria or submucosa (9). At least two generations of meronts, as well as macrogametocytes (female sexual stage), microgametocytes (male sexual stage), and unsporulated oocysts, have been documented in these reports.

I. belli sporozoites/merozoites are capable of traveling extraintestinally and becoming dormant as cysts (Fig. 3) in a variety of tissues, including the intestine, mesenteric lymph nodes, liver, and spleen (45, 51, 74). These cysts are commonly termed "unizoite cysts." Unizoite cysts in histological sections are thick walled and measure 12 to 22 by 8 to 10 μm, and each contains a single dormant sporozoite/merozoite of about 8 to 10 by 5 μm (45, 51). Presumably, the cysts are capable of reactivating patent infections once immunity wanes. Unizoite cysts can be present in the lamina propria in the absence of oocysts in stool samples (74).

The existence of these unizoite cysts has led to speculation that a paratenic (transport) host may be involved in the life cycle of I. belli (48). Paratenic hosts are known to occur in the Isospora species that infect cats and dogs.

Isospora natalensis

The life cycle is presumably monoxenous (direct). The oocysts are smaller and more spherical than those of I. belli (Table 1). Oocysts are passed in the feces unsporulated. At ambient temperature, some oocysts complete sporulation within 24 h (26). Sporulated oocysts contain two sporocysts, each with four sporozoites. The prepatent and patent periods are unknown. One individual passed unsporulated oocysts for at least 4 days (19). Oocysts of I. natalensis have been reported only for patients from South Africa. The validity of this species is questionable.

---

*This chapter contains information presented in chapter 134 by Ynes R. Ortega and Michael Arrowood in the eighth edition of this Manual.

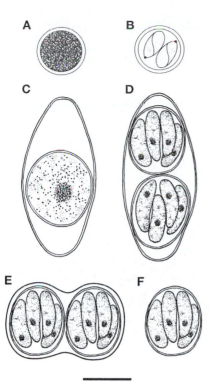

FIGURE 1 Line drawings of unsporulated and sporulated oocysts of *C. cayetanensis* (A and B) and *I. belli* (C and D) and a sporulated oocyst (E) and sporocyst (F) of a *Sarcocystis* species, all from humans. Bar, 10 μm.

Cyclospora cayetanensis

The life cycle is monoxenous and involves only humans as hosts. Oocysts are passed in the feces unsporulated (Fig. 1A and 2C). At room temperature (23 to 25°C), small numbers of oocysts may sporulate within 10 to 12 days (38, 70) (Fig. 1B). However, many oocysts require 3 to 4 weeks for sporozoites to fully develop (S. J. Upton, unpublished data). Sporulated

C. cayetanensis oocysts contain two sporocysts, each with two sporozoites. A structure termed a Stieda body is present in the end of each sporocyst. There are no Stieda bodies in the oocysts of *I. belli* or *Sarcocystis* species (Fig. 1). The precise prepatent period is not yet known. However, the onset of clinical signs following infection generally averages 7 to 8 days postinfection and lasts 2 to 3 weeks, but this may range from 1 to >100 days. The length of time that oocysts are shed in the feces is highly variable. Oocysts may be shed in the feces for anywhere from 7 days to several months. Indigenous infections are confined primarily to tropical, subtropical, or warm temperate regions of the world. Outbreaks occur in other areas of the world due to contaminated foodstuffs.

Developmental stages of *C. cayetanensis* generally occur within epithelial cells of the lower duodenum and jejunum (6, 56, 67). There are two asexual generations followed by sexual stages and oocysts. Stages develop in a supranuclear location within enterocytes (67). An attempt to infect seven healthy human volunteers with sporulated oocysts of *C. cayetanensis* was not successful (1). None of the patients developed clinical signs or shed oocysts in their feces.

Sarcocystis hominis

The life cycle is heteroxenous. Humans are definitive hosts for *S. hominis,* and bovids are the intermediate hosts. Infection occurs when infected meat is ingested which is not cooked or is not thoroughly cooked. Known intermediate hosts include cattle (*Bos taurus*), American bison (*Bison bison*), water buffaloes (*Bubalus bubalis*), and wisents (European bison; *Bison bonasus*). These intermediate hosts harbor sarcocysts (muscle cysts) that are infective when ingested by humans. Infective bradyzoites (dormant merozoite-like stages) are present in the sarcocysts. The bradyzoites penetrate the human intestinal epithelium and develop as sexual stages (macrogametocytes and microgametocytes) in cells in the lamina propria of the intestine. Fertilization occurs, and the oocysts sporulate in the lamina propria. The oocysts are *Isospora*-like and contain two sporocysts, each with four sporozoites. The oocyst wall often ruptures as the oocyst makes its way to the intestinal lumen. This results in the shedding of individual sporocysts in the feces. Individual sporocysts contain four sporozoites. Both oocysts with two sporocysts

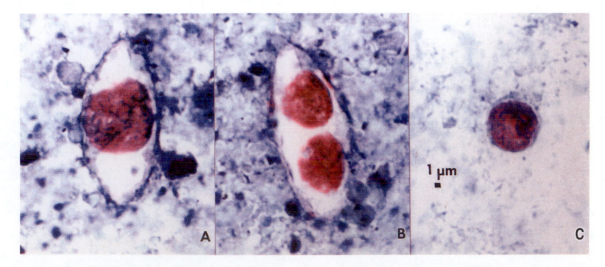

FIGURE 2 Modified Kinyoun's acid-fast-stained smears demonstrating an *I. belli* oocyst with a sporont (A), an *I. belli* oocyst with two sporoblasts (B), and a *C. cayetanensis* oocyst with a sporont (C).

TABLE 1 Structural data for *Isospora* (*Cystoisospora*), *Cyclospora*, and *Sarcocystis* coccidial oocysts and sporocysts found in the feces of humans

Species	Mean size (range) (μm)[a]	
	Oocysts	Sporocysts
Isospora belli	32 × 14 (20–36 × 10–19)	14 × 10 (12–17 × 7–11)
Isospora natalensis	Not given (25–30 × 21–24)	17 × 12 (not given)
Cyclospora cayetanensis	9 × 9 (8–8 × 10–10)	6 × 4 (6–7 × 3–4)
Sarcocystis hominis	Not given (19 × 15)	15 × 9 (13–17 × 8–11)
Sarcocystis suihominis	19 × 13 (19–20 × 12–15)	14 × 11 (12–14 × 10–11)
Sarcocystis lindemanni	Not applicable	Not applicable

[a]Data have been rounded to the nearest micrometer.

and individual sporocysts can be seen in the feces of humans with intestinal *Sarcocystis* infection (Fig. 1E and F).

Oocysts and sporocysts are fully sporulated when passed in the feces. For human volunteers, the prepatent period has been reported to be 8 to 39 days, and patent infections can last as long as 18 months. *S. hominis* occurs on all continents, anywhere cattle or buffaloes have access to human feces and humans ingest raw or undercooked beef.

Sarcocystis suihominis

The life cycle is similar to that described above for *S. hominis*, except that pigs are the intermediate hosts. The prepatent period is 9 to 10 days, and patency is in excess of 36 days. *S. suihominis* presumably occurs on all continents, anywhere swine have access to human feces and humans ingest raw or undercooked pork.

Human Muscular *Sarcocystis* Infection

Sarcocysts have been reported as incidental findings from both skeletal and cardiac muscle of nearly 60 humans worldwide. There are at least seven distinct types of sarcocysts present in human muscles (4). Many of these sarcocysts appear similar to sarcocysts found in nonhuman primates. Humans seem to be an occasional incidental intermediate host for some *Sarcocystis* spp. in wildlife.

EPIDEMIOLOGY, TRANSMISSION, AND PREVENTION

I. belli

I. belli is found primarily in tropical, subtropical, and warm temperate regions, but reports of indigenous infections have been published from temperate areas as well. Most cases of infection in temperate areas involve foreign travel or homosexual contact. Transmission is via ingestion of sporulated oocysts and possibly the ingestion of raw or undercooked tissues from unknown paratenic hosts. An outbreak of *I. belli* infections involving approximately 90 patients was reported in the city of Antofagasta, Chile, in 1977 (39). It was associated with ingestion of vegetables contaminated with irrigation water from a sewage treatment plant (39). Improving sanitation and water quality in areas of endemicity will decrease transmission of *I. belli*.

C. cayetanensis

Cyclospora is endemic in Central and South America, the Caribbean, Mexico, Indonesia, Asia, Nepal, Africa, India, Southern Europe, and the Middle East. In areas of endemicity, there is an increased risk of *Cyclospora* infection with contact with soil (13) and water (21). Infections in most temperate areas are correlated with the consumption of imported,

contaminated fruits and vegetables, such as basil, raspberries, lettuce, mesclun, and snow peas. One outbreak of diarrheal disease in Chicago was originally correlated with stagnant tap water; no oocysts were ever recovered from a water storage tank reputed to harbor the parasite, and infected individuals had attended a catered party 8 days previously (36).

Individuals in areas of endemicity should wear gloves when gardening to prevent exposure to oocysts of *C. cayetanensis*. Better washing of produce may help to remove *Cyclospora* oocysts, but many fruits are delicate. Most of the produce items implicated as transmitting *Cyclospora* are consumed raw, which does not lend itself to prevention by thermal means. Nonthermal treatments such as high hydrostatic pressure (46) have been shown to inactivate *Toxoplasma gondii* oocysts, and these methods may be effective in inactivating *Cyclospora* on produce.

Sarcocystis Species

Human intestinal *Sarcocystis* species are potentially present in any region in the world where cattle, buffaloes, and swine have access to human feces and the life cycle can be maintained. The cycle has not been detected in the United States. Cultural habits that include ingestion of raw meat or undercooked meat products help to maintain this life cycle in areas where *Sarcocystis* species are endemic. Cooking meat until an internal temperature of >67°C is achieved kills *T. gondii* tissue cysts in the meat (22), and this temperature should also kill tissue cysts of human-infective *Sarcocystis*

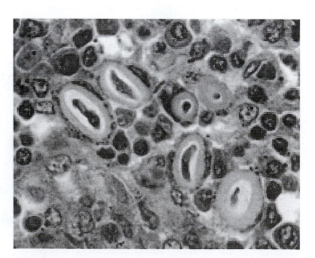

FIGURE 3 Toludine blue-stained 1-μm section demonstrating several unizoite cysts of *I. belli*. Note the thick wall that surrounds each single zoite.

species in meat products. Preventing cattle, buffaloes, and swine from consuming human feces will also break the cycle in areas where *Sarcocystis* species are endemic.

Most cases of human muscular *Sarcocystis* infection have been reported from the Far East (2). It is presumed that humans become infected by ingesting sporocysts in contaminated water (2) or food.

CLINICAL SIGNIFICANCE

I. belli

I. belli can cause serious and sometimes fatal disease in immunocompetent humans. Symptoms of *I. belli* infection include diarrhea, steatorrhea, headache, fever, malaise, abdominal pain, vomiting, dehydration, and weight loss (9, 73). Blood is not usually present in the feces. Eosinophilia is observed in many patients (12). The disease is often chronic, with parasites present in the feces or biopsy specimens for several months to years. Recurrences are common. Disease is more severe in infants and young children (52).

Clinical disease from *I. belli* infection is usually more severe in immunocompromised patients than in immunocompetent patients. *I. belli* infection produces diarrhea in AIDS patients that is often very fluid and secretory-like and leads to dehydration requiring hospitalization (12). Fever and weight loss are also common findings. Other opportunistic pathogens are also common copathogens in these patients. *I. belli* has been observed in both renal transplant (41, 81) and liver transplant (3) patients. *I. belli*-induced intestinal lesions and responses to chemotherapy are usually similar to those observed in immunocompetent patients. *I. belli* has been observed in patients with concurrent Hodgkin's disease (9), non-Hodgkin's lymphoproliferative disease (35, 63), human T-cell lymphotropic virus type 1-associated adult T-cell leukemia (35), and acute lymphoblastic leukemia (81). These patients respond to specific anti-*I. belli* treatment. Extraintestinal cyst-like stages have been documented for AIDS patients and may play a role in relapse of infection (45). These usually contain a single merozoite-like stage (Fig. 3), and many thousands of these stages can be present (45).

Infections with *I. belli* in the gallbladder epithelium (5, 30) and endometrial epithelium (16) have been reported, and oocysts have been observed in bile samples (8). Clinical signs in patients with parasites in these locations are not specific for coccidiosis, and parasites are located after tissue biopsy as part of a diagnostic workup. The parasites probably reach these sites as merozoites from the gut or zoites from extraintestinal locations, and the epithelial cells of these tissues are permissive to parasite entrance and multiplication.

C. cayetanensis

Nonbloody diarrhea is the main clinical symptom of *C. cayetanensis* infection. Some individuals can be infected and show no clinical signs. In most immunocompetent patients, typical symptoms of cyclosporiasis include cycles of diarrhea with anorexia, malaise, nausea, and cramping and periods of apparent remission (36).

C. cayetanensis infection can be associated with biliary disease in both immunosuppressed patients and immunologically normal patients (65). Developmental stages of *C. cayetanensis* have been seen in the gallbladder epithelium of AIDS patients with acalculous cholecystitis by light (82) and transmission electron (34) microscopy. Oocysts can be observed in the bile of patients with active biliary disease.

Intestinal *Sarcocystis* Infections

Clinical *Sarcocystis* infections in humans can manifest primarily as intestinal disease if infected meat is ingested or as muscular disease if sporocysts are ingested (27). Intestinal disease occurs soon after consumption of infected meat (3 to 6 h) and is characterized by nausea, abdominal pain, and diarrhea. Intestinal disease can be more severe in individuals who have additional enteropathogens present in the gut. Intestinal *Sarcocystis* infection combined with invasion by gram-positive bacteria has been associated with over 20 cases of segmental enterocolitis in Thailand (10, 11). Experimental studies with human volunteers have produced more-severe disease in those who have ingested pork containing *S. suihominis* than in those who have ingested beef containing *S. hominis* (27). Some individuals can be infected and show no clinical signs.

Muscular *Sarcocystis* Infections

Muscular *Sarcocystis* infections in humans are usually considered subclinical or associated only with mild clinical signs (50). Many of the over 50 reported cases have been incidental findings (4) or associated with eosinophilic myositis (70). Clinical signs associated with an outbreak of human muscular *Sarcocystis* infection occurred in 7 of 15 members of a U.S. combat troop in Malaysia (2). The signs developed about 3 weeks after the troops returned from the jungle and were fever, myalgias, bronchospasm, fleeting pruritic rashes, transient lymphadenopathy, and subcutaneous nodules. Eosinophilia, elevated erythrocyte sedimentation rates, and elevated levels of muscle creatine kinase were present in these troops (2). Individuals with decreased immunity may be more susceptible to muscular infection with these parasites. Sarcocysts of a *Sarcocystis* sp. were reported in the heart of a patient with Hodgkin's disease (33). Muscular sarcocystosis was observed in 8 of 11 cases from Malaysia and was associated with malignancies, especially of the tongue and nasopharynx (60).

COLLECTION, TRANSPORT, AND STORAGE OF SPECIMENS

The results obtained in the diagnostic laboratory are only as good as the material presented for testing. Choosing the appropriate sample and sample fixative is extremely important (31). Universal precautions should be followed when fresh stool samples are handled. If samples are to be sent to another laboratory for diagnosis, they should be fixed in an appropriate fixative. A 10% or 5% formalin solution is an appropriate fixative for stools suspected of containing intestinal coccidia. Formalin fixation does not interfere with some of the immunodetection methods currently employed to detect *Cryptosporidium* and *Giardia,* which is a drawback of polyvinyl alcohol fixative. Oocyst structure lasts for several months when stools are stored at 4°C in formalin fixatives.

DIRECT EXAMINATION

Microscopy

Oocysts of *I. belli* and *C. cayetanensis* and sporocysts of *Sarcocystis* species are readily identified in fresh unstained wet mounts, based on their characteristic sizes and morphologies (Table 1; Fig. 1). This is especially true if oocysts and sporocysts are present in large numbers. Autofluorescence of oocysts of *I. belli* and *C. cayetanensis* and sporocysts of *Sarcocystis* is an especially useful tool (7, 23, 44, 72) and has replaced many of the staining techniques previously used for these parasites in laboratories equipped with appropriate fluorescence microscopes.

Concentration techniques, such as formalin-ethyl acetate (rarely formalin-ether) sedimentation or sucrose centrifugal flotation, are helpful when few oocysts are present. Sucrose centrifugal flotation has been found to be superior over formalin-ether sedimentation for demonstrating oocysts of *C. cayetanensis* (40). The same should be true for oocysts of *I. belli* and sporocysts of *Sarcocystis* spp. Few laboratories employ sucrose concentration, and fortunately, direct wet smears can be very useful: their utility approaches that of sucrose centrifugal flotation when coupled with autofluorescence examination (40). Staining procedures may adversely affect the autofluorescence of oocysts and sporocysts.

Stained fecal smears have been used widely to demonstrate *C. cayetanensis* oocysts and, to a lesser extent, *I. belli* oocysts (23, 25, 59). *I. belli* and *C. cayetanensis* oocysts stain red with modified Kinyoun's acid-fast stain, and this method is widely used (Fig. 2). The main drawbacks are that staining can be variable and some oocysts do not stain (76). Oocysts usually do not stain with trichrome, chromotrope, or Gram-chromotrope stain (76). Some *C. cayetanensis* oocysts stain light blue with Giemsa stain (76). Variations on the safranin staining technique stain *C. cayetanensis* oocysts orange or pinkish orange, and heating and other treatments have been used to increase the staining frequency of oocysts.

Flow cytometry has been used to detect *C. cayetanensis* oocysts in human stool samples (18). The results of flow cytometry examination were similar to those of microscopy, and preparation times for the two methods were similar (18).

A single negative stool specimen is not conclusive in the examination of stools for coccidial parasites; a total of three or more stool specimens collected on subsequent days need to be examined before coccidial infection can be ruled out. Liquid stool samples can be concentrated by centrifugation, and the pellet may be used for examination by use of wet mounts, concentration techniques, or stained smears. Large numbers of oocysts may make diagnosis less challenging but do not always translate directly to the severity of clinical signs. Some individuals may excrete oocysts and be asymptomatic.

Cases of muscular *Sarcocystis* infection are diagnosed based on the detection of sarcocysts in muscle samples take from biopsy specimens or postmortem samples.

Culture

In vitro culture of coccidial parasites is most often used as a tool to study developmental biology or to identify active chemotherapeutic agents. It presently has limited use in diagnosis of active human infection.

One report of complete development of *I. belli* has been published (65). In another report, development was limited to merogony (55). No reports on development of *C. cayetanensis* in cell culture have been published. Bradyzoites of *S. suihominis* undergo sexual development and produce oocysts in cell culture (49). Schizont stages of human *Sarcocystis* species have not been reported for in vitro systems.

Antigen Detection

The inability to produce stages in cell cultures and provide a source of diagnostic antigens has limited the usefulness of antigen detection for these coccidial parasites of humans.

Nucleic Acid Detection Techniques

There are no U.S. Food and Drug Administration-approved nucleic acid tests for the detection of infections with *I. belli*,

C. cayetanensis, or *Sarcocystis* spp. Several research laboratories have developed nucleic acid-based detection tests to demonstrate infection with these parasites.

Detection of *I. belli* by PCR with primers based on small-subunit RNA (ssRNA) sequences and by Southern blot hybridization has been reported (54). This method was effective for detecting *I. belli* DNA in duodenal biopsy specimens and in stool samples. Slight cross-reactivity to *T. gondii* was observed in a nested-PCR version of this test (54). The internal transcribed spacer region 1 (ITS-1), ITS-2, ssRNA, and 5.8S RNA sequences of isolates of *I. belli* from immunosuppressed and nonimmunosuppressed patients from Thailand were found to be highly conserved (83). A real-time PCR using the ITS-2 ssRNA sequences has been developed to detect *I. belli* in stool samples (68).

Much attention has been placed on molecular methods to detect *C. cayetanensis* oocysts in stools, in water samples, and on produce because of the numerous outbreaks of *C. cayetanensis* infections (42). The 18S rRNA gene is presently the most frequently used target. Because *C. cayetanensis* is closely related to *Eimeria* species (61) from vertebrates, it is important that tests designed to detect *C. cayetanensis* in the water or on produce be examined for cross-reactivity to *Eimeria* spp. (37). *Cyclospora* species infecting mammals other than humans may also be present in water samples or on produce, and proofs of specificity are needed for these tests designed to look at environmental sources of *C. cayetanensis* and to detect *C. cayetanensis* oocysts on produce.

Quantitative PCR assays have been developed for *C. cayetanensis* oocysts in stool samples (73). This method detected DNA of the 18S ribosomal gene sequence from as little as 1 oocyst of *C. cayetanensis* per 5 ml of reaction mixture.

Several PCR methods have been developed to detect sarcocysts in the muscles of intermediate hosts (32, 71, 80). It is likely that these PCR tests can be used to detect the species of human *Sarcocystis* sporocysts in human stool samples.

SEROLOGIC TESTS

The inability to obtain usable quantities of antigens from *I. belli*, *C. cayetanensis*, and *Sarcocystis* spp. has greatly limited the use of serological diagnostic tests for these parasites in human stool samples. It is very difficult to obtain enough oocysts or sporocysts from feces to conduct serological tests. The development of an enzyme-linked immunosorbent assay that measures immunoglobulin G (IgG) and IgM antibodies, using *C. cayetanensis* oocysts as antigen, has been reported (77). This study is questionable because the authors stated that they obtained their oocysts from experimentally infected guinea pigs, yet well-controlled studies indicate that humans are the only suitable host for *C. cayetanensis* (24). Attempts were made to develop an indirect fluorescent-antibody assay to detect IgG, IgA, and IgM specific for *C. cayetanensis*, using sectioned oocysts (14). None of the sera from four patients with positive stools reacted in the indirect fluorescent-antibody assay.

TREATMENT

I. belli

The drug of choice for the treatment of *I. belli* is trimethoprim-sulfamethoxazole. A dose of trimethoprim (160 mg)-sulfamethoxazole (800 mg) two to four times a day for 10 to 14 days results in clearance of parasites, a decrease in diarrhea, and a decrease in abdominal pain within a mean of 2.5 days after treatment (58). Before the advent of active antiretroviral therapy (ART), it was recommended that patients with human immunodeficiency virus type 1 (HIV-1) infection and CD4$^+$ cell counts of <200 should receive secondary prophylaxis with trimethoprim (320 mg)-sulfamethoxazole (1,600 mg) once daily or three times a week to prevent relapse. It is likely that secondary prophylaxis is not needed once the CD4$^+$ count exceeds 200, as has been demonstrated for many opportunistic pathogens in patients with HIV-1 infection.

For patients unable to tolerate sulfonamides due to allergy or intolerance, there is no standard treatment. Pyrimethamine at a dose of 50 to 75 mg/day is an effective alternative treatment for patients with sulfonamide allergies (78). Secondary prophylaxis using pyrimethamine at 25 mg/day can be used for patients not on ART (78). Pyrimethamine should be given with folinic acid (5 to 10 mg/day) to minimize bone marrow suppression. Another alternative agent is ciprofloxacin, a fluoroquinolone that inhibits topoisomerase. In a randomized study of 22 patients with isosporiasis and HIV infection, all of the 10 patients that received trimethoprim-sulfamethoxazole had a cessation of diarrhea within 2 days, and 10 of 12 patients who received ciprofloxacin (500 mg twice daily) had a cessation of diarrhea within 4.5 days (75). All three patients (two with diarrhea and one without) who had persistent *I. belli* oocysts in their stools responded to trimethoprim-sulfamethoxazole treatment (75). In patients who responded to ciprofloxacin, continued prophylaxis with ciprofloxacin prevented recurrence of disease (75). Nitazoxanide has been used to treat *I. belli* infections (20, 63). Two patients who were given 500 mg of nitazoxanide twice daily for 3 days were oocyst negative after treatment (63). A patient treated with 500 mg of nitazoxanide twice daily for 7 days became oocyst negative by day 14 after treatment (20). Treatment failure was observed in a patient with biliary isosporiasis and malabsorption when 2 g of nitazoxanide was given orally twice daily (8). Treatment failure was likely due to the lack of absorption of nitazoxanide and to poor levels of the drug in the serum (8). Elevations in liver function tests and nausea are potential side effects of orally administered nitazoxanide. Treatment with other antiprotozoal agents, such as metronidazole, tinidazole, quinacrine, and furazolidone, appears to be of little value for this infection.

C. cayetanensis

The drug of choice for the treatment of *C. cayetanensis* infection is trimethoprim (160 mg)-sulfamethoxazole (800 mg) given twice daily for 7 days (47, 57). Clearance of parasites, a decrease in diarrhea, and a decrease in abdominal pain occurred within a mean of 2.5 days after treatment. Patients on ART likely do not need secondary prophylaxis.

For patients unable to tolerate sulfonamides due to allergy or intolerance, there is no standard treatment. Nitazoxanide has been evaluated for activity against *C. cayetanensis,* and in these studies, its efficacy for the treatment of cyclosporiasis was about 70% (17, 29). It should be appreciated, however, that only a few patients with cyclosporiasis were treated in any of these studies (17, 29). Another alternative agent is ciprofloxacin, a fluoroquinolone that inhibits topoisomerase. In a randomized study of 20 patients with cyclosporiasis, all of the 9 patients who received trimethoprim-sulfamethoxazole had a cessation of diarrhea within 3 days, and 10 of 11 patients who received ciprofloxacin (500 mg twice daily) had a cessation of diarrhea within 4 days; however, only 7 of 11 patients treated with ciprofloxacin cleared the organism from the stool (75). Anecdotal data suggest that the following drugs are ineffective: albendazole, azithromycin, pyrimethamine,

nalidixic acid, norfloxacin, tinidazole, metronidazole, quinacrine, tetracycline, doxycycline, and diloxanide furoate (L. M. Weiss et al., unpublished data).

S. hominis and S. suihominis

There is no known treatment or prophylaxis for intestinal infection, myositis, vasculitis, or related lesions due to sarcocystosis in humans. Supportive therapy for patients with severe diarrhea is indicated. For six patients in Thailand with segmental necrotizing enteritis, treatment consisted of surgical resection of the affected areas of the intestine and antibiotics for the associated bacterial infection (10, 11).

There is a case report of albendazole having efficacy in an outbreak of eosinophilic myositis due to *Sarcocystis* spp. (2). It is likely that steroids have a role in decreasing the inflammatory response in cases of myositis and vasculitis due to *Sarcocystis* sp. infection, but this has never been evaluated in a controlled trial.

Treatment Failure

There are no documented reports of drug-resistant strains of *I. belli, C. cayetanensis,* or *Sarcocystis* species. It appears that treatment failures are more likely to be related to poor drug absorption or distribution than to true drug resistance.

EVALUATION, INTERPRETATION, AND REPORTING OF RESULTS

Both *I. belli* and *C. cayetanensis* are usually identified by stool examination and are rarely misidentified in human feces. Quantitation of the number of organisms found per high-power field is not required. Stool examinations that are reported as negative should indicate that at least three stool examinations are needed to detect organisms in 95% of infected individuals and that a single specimen may miss as many as 30% of infected patients. If acid-fast or similar stains are done on the stool examination and are positive, then this should be indicated in the report. Computer report notes can indicate that trimethoprim-sulfamethoxazole is the drug of choice for treatment of these parasites. PCR can be used for the identification of these organisms but is not commercially available and should be indicated as an experimental test. Serology is not currently used for diagnosis of these diseases in humans. Of the coccidia discussed here, only *C. cayetanensis* is reportable to state health departments and the Centers for Disease Control and Prevention, as it has been associated with outbreaks and the contamination of human food sources.

S. hominis and *S. suihominis* can be identified by their characteristic morphology in stool specimens or in tissue biopsy specimens. They cannot be identified to the species level based on sporocyst structure and can be identified only as *Sarcocystis* spp. Due to the rarity of these infections, confirmation of the observed organisms should be obtained from experts in parasitology. Computer reports should indicate whether confirmation of the identification of these organisms has been obtained.

REFERENCES

1. **Alfano-Sobsey, E. M., M. L. Eberhard, J. R. Seed, D. J. Weber, K. Y. Won, E. K. Nace, and C. L. Moe.** 2004. Human challenge pilot study with *Cyclospora cayetanensis. Emerg. Infect. Dis.* **10:**726–728.
2. **Arness, M. K., J. D. Brown, J. P. Dubey, R. C. Neafie, and D. E. Granstrom.** 1999. An outbreak of acute eosinophilic myositis attributed to human *Sarcocystis* parasitism. *Am. J. Trop. Med. Hyg.* **61:**548–553.

3. Atambay, M., M. R. Bayraktar, U. Kayabas, S. Yilmaz, and Y. Bayindir. 2007. A rare diarrheic parasite in a liver transplant patient: *Isospora belli*. *Transplant. Proc.* **39:**1693–1695.

4. Beaver, P. C., K. Gadgil, and P. Morera. 1979. *Sarcocystis* in man: a review and report of five cases. *Am. J. Trop. Med. Hyg.* **28:**819–844.

5. Benator, D. A., A. L. French, L. M. Beaudet, C. S. Levy, and J. M. Orenstein. 1994. *Isospora belli* infection associated with acalculous cholecystitis in a patient with AIDS. *Ann. Int. Med.* **121:**663–664.

6. Bendall, R. P., S. Lucas, A. Moody, G. Tovey, and P. L. Chiodini. 1993. Diarrhoea associated with cyanobacterium-like bodies: a new coccidian enteritis of man. *Lancet* **341:**590–592.

7. Bialek R., N. Binder, K. Dietz, J. Knobloch, and U. E. Zelck. 2002. Comparison of autofluorescence and iodine staining for detection of *Isospora belli* in feces. *Am. J. Trop. Med. Hyg.* **67:**304–305.

8. Bialek, R., D. Overkamp, I. Rettig, and J. Knobloch. 2001. Case report: nitazoxanide treatment failure in chronic isosporiasis. *Am. J. Trop. Med. Hyg.* **65:**94–95.

9. Brandborg, L. L., S. B. Goldberg, and W. C. Breidenbach. 1970. Human coccidiosis—a possible cause of malabsorption: the life cycle in small-bowel mucosal biopsies as a diagnostic feature. *N. Engl. J. Med.* **283:**1306–1313.

10. Bunyaratvej, S., and P. Unpunyo. 1992. Combined *Sarcocystis* and gram-positive bacterial infections. A possible cause of segmental enterocolitis in Thailand. *J. Med. Assoc. Thai.* **75:**S38–S44.

11. Bunyaratvej, S., P. Bunyawongwiroj, and P. Nitiyanant. 1982. Human intestinal sarcosporidiosis: report of six cases. *Am. J. Trop. Med. Hyg.* **31:**36–41.

12. Certad, G., A. Arenas-Pinto, L. Pocaterra, G. Ferrara, J. Castro, A. Bello, and L. Nunez. 2003. Isosporiasis in Venezuelan adults infected with human immunodeficiency virus: clinical characterization. *Am. J. Trop. Med. Hyg.* **69:**217–222.

13. Chacín-Bonilla, L. 2008. Transmission of *Cyclospora cayetanensis* infection: a review focusing on soil-borne cyclosporiasis. *Trans. R. Soc. Trop. Med. Hyg.* **102:**215–216.

14. Clarke, S. C., and M. McIntyre. 1997. An attempt to demonstrate a serological immune response in patients infected with *Cyclospora cayetanensis*. *Br. J. Biomed. Sci.* **54:**73–74.

15. de Gorgolas, M., J. Fortes, and M. L. Fernandez Guerrero. 2001. *Cyclospora cayetanensis* cholecystitis in a patient with AIDS. *Ann. Intern. Med.* **134:**166.

16. de Otazu, R. D., L. Garcia-Nieto, E. Izaguirre-Gondra, E. Mayayo, S. Ciani, and F. F. Nogales. 2004. Endometrial coccidiosis. *J. Clin. Pathol.* **57:**1104–1105.

17. Diaz, E., J. Mondragon, E. Ramirez, and R. Bernal. 2003. Epidemiology and control of intestinal parasites with nitazoxanide in children in Mexico. *Am. J. Trop. Med. Hyg.* **69:**384–385.

18. Dixon, B. R., J. M. Bussey, L. J. Parrington, and M. Parenteau. 2005. Detection of *Cyclospora cayetanensis* oocysts in human fecal specimens by flow cytometry. *J. Clin. Microbiol.* **43:**2375–2379.

19. Dodds, S. E., and R. Elsdon-Dew. 1955. Further observations on human coccidiosis in Natal. *S. Afr. J. Lab. Clin. Med.* **1:**104–109.

20. Doumbo, O., J. F. Rossignol, E. Pichard, H. A. Traore, T. M. Dembele, M. Diakite, F. Traore, and D. A. Diallo. 1997. Nitazoxanide in the treatment of cryptosporidial diarrhea and other intestinal parasitic infections associated with acquired immunodeficiency syndrome in tropical Africa. *Am. J. Trop. Med. Hyg.* **56:**637–639.

21. Dowd, S. E., D. John, J. Eliopolus, C. P. Gerba, J. Naranjo, R. Klein, B. Lopez, M. de Mejia, C. E. Mendoza, and I. L. Pepper. 2003. Confirmed detection of *Cyclospora cayetanensis, Encephalitozoon intestinalis* and *Cryptosporidium parvum* in water used for drinking. *J. Water Health* **1:**117–123.

22. Dubey, J. P., A. W. Kotula, A. Sharar, C. D. Andrews, and D. S. Lindsay. 1990. Effect of high temperature on infectivity of *Toxoplasma gondii* tissue cysts in pork. *J. Parasitol.* **76:**201–204.

23. Eberhard, M. L., N. J. Pieniazek, and M. J. Arrowood. 1997. Laboratory diagnosis of *Cyclospora* infections. *Arch. Pathol. Lab. Med.* **121:**792–797.

24. Eberhard, M. L., Y. R. Ortega, D. E. Hanes, E. K. Nace, R. Q. Do, M. G. Robl, K. Y. Won, C. Gavidia, N. L. Sass, K. Mansfield, A. Gozalo, J. Griffiths, R. Gilman, C. R. Sterling, and M. J. Arrowood. 2000. Attempts to establish experimental *Cyclospora cayetanensis* infection in laboratory animals. *J. Parasitol.* **86:**577–582.

25. El Naggar, H. H., A. E. Handousa, E. M. El Hamshary, and A. M. El Shazly. 1999. Evaluation of five stains in diagnosing human intestinal coccidiosis. *J. Egypt. Soc. Parasitol.* **29:**883–891.

26. Elsdon-Dew, R. 1953. *Isospora natalensis* (sp. nov.) in man. *J. Trop. Med. Hyg.* **56:**149–150.

27. Fayer, R. 2004. *Sarcocystis* spp. in humans. *Clin. Microbiol. Rev.* **17:**894–902.

28. Ferreira, L. F., S. G. Coutinho, C. A. Argento, and J. R. da Silva. 1962. Experimental human coccidial enteritis by *Isospora belli* Wenyon, 1923. A study based on the infection of 5 volunteers. *Hospital* (Rio de Janeiro) **62:**795–804.

29. Fox, L. M., and L. D. Saravolatz. 2005. Nitazoxanide: a new thiazolide antiparasitic agent. *Clin. Infect. Dis.* **40:**1173–1180.

30. French, A. L., L. M. Beaudet, D. A. Benator, C. S. Levy, M. Kass, and J. M. Orenstein. 1995. Cholecystectomy in patients with AIDS: clinicopathologic correlations in 107 cases. *Clin. Infect. Dis.* **21:**852–858.

31. Garcia, L. S., and D. A. Bruckner. 1997. *Diagnostic Medical Parasitology*, 3rd ed., p. 593–607, 937. ASM Press, Washington, DC.

32. González, L. M., N. Villalobos, E. Montero, J. Morales, R. A. Sanz, A. Muro, L. J. Harrison, R. M. Parkhouse, and T. Gárate. 2006. Differential molecular identification of *Taeniid* spp. and *Sarcocystis* spp. cysts isolated from infected pigs and cattle. *Vet. Parasitol.* **142:**95–101.

33. Goodman, M. L., and E. Maher. 1966. Four uncommon infections in Hodgkin's disease. *JAMA* **198:**1129.

34. Greenberg, S. J., M. P. Davey, W. S. Zierdt, and T. A. Waldmann. 1988. *Isospora belli* infection in patients with human T-cell leukemia virus type I-associated adult T-cell leukemia. *Am. J. Med.* **85:**435–438.

35. Hallak, A., I. Yust, Y. Ratan, and U. Adar. 1982. Malabsorption syndrome, coccidiosis, combined immune deficiency, and fulminant lymphoproliferative disease. *Arch. Intern. Med.* **142:**196–197.

36. Herwaldt, B. L. 2000. *Cyclospora cayetanensis:* a review, focusing on the outbreaks of cyclosporiasis in the 1990s. *Clin. Infect. Dis.* **31:**1040–1057.

37. Jinneman, K. C., J. H. Wetherington, W. E. Hill, A. M. Adams, J. M. Johnson, B. J. Tenge, N. L. Dang, R. L. Manger, and M. M. Wekell. 1998. Template preparation for PCR and RFLP of amplification products for the detection and identification of *Cyclospora* sp. and *Eimeria* spp. oocysts directly from raspberries. *J. Food Prot.* **61:**1497–1503.

38. Jongwutiwes, S., C. Putaporntip, M. Charoenkorn, T. Iwasaki, and T. Endo. 2007. Morphologic and molecular characterization of *Isospora belli* oocysts from patients in Thailand. *Am. J. Trop. Med. Hyg.* **77:**107–112.

39. Karanis, P., C. Kourenti, and H. Smith. 2007. Waterborne transmission of protozoan parasites: a worldwide review of outbreaks and lessons learnt. *J. Water Health* **5:**1–38.

40. Kimura, K., S. Kumar Rai, K. Takemasa, Y. Ishibashi, M. Kawabata, M. Belosevic, and S. Uga. 2004. Comparison of three microscopic techniques for diagnosis of *Cyclospora cayetanensis*. *FEMS Microbiol Lett.* **238:**263–266.

41. Koru, O., R. E. Araz, Y. A. Yilmaz, S. Ergüven, M. Yenicesu, B. Pektaş, and M. Tanyüksel. 2007. Case report: *Isospora belli* infection in a renal transplant recipient. *Turkiye Parazitol. Derg.* **31:**98–100.

42. Lalonde, L. F., and A. A. Gajadhar. 2008. Highly sensitive and specific PCR assay for reliable detection of *Cyclospora cayetanensis* oocysts. *Appl. Environ. Microbiol.* **74:**4354–4358.

43. Limson-Pobre, R. N., S. Merrick, D. Gruen, and R. Soave. 1995. Use of diclazuril for the treatment of isosporiasis in patients with AIDS. *Clin. Infect. Dis.* **20:**201–202.

44. Lindquist, H. D., J. W. Bennett, J. D. Hester, M. W. Ware, J. P. Dubey, and W. V. Everson. 2003. Autofluorescence of *Toxoplasma gondii* and related coccidian oocysts. *J. Parasitol.* **89:**865–867.

45. Lindsay, D. S., J. P. Dubey, M. A. Toivio-Kinnucan, J. F. Michiels, and B. L. Blagburn. 1997. Examination of extraintestinal tissue cysts of *Isospora belli. J. Parasitol.* **83:**620–625.

46. Lindsay, D. S., D. Holliman, G. J. Flick, D. G. Goodwin, S. M. Mitchell, and J. P. Dubey. 2008. Effects of high pressure processing on *Toxoplasma gondii* oocysts on raspberries. *J. Parasitol.* **94:**757–758.

47. Madico, G., J. McDonald, R. H. Gilman, L. Cabrera, and C. R. Sterling. 1997. Epidemiology and treatment of *Cyclospora cayetanensis* infection in Peruvian children. *Clin. Infect. Dis.* **24:**977–981.

48. Matsubayashi, H., and T. Nozawa. 1948. Experimental infection of *Isospora hominis* in man. *Am. J. Trop. Med.* **28:**633–637.

49. Mehlhorn, H., and A. O. Heydorn. 1979. Electron microscopical study on gamogony of *Sarcocystis suihominis* in human tissue cultures. *Z. Parasitenkd.* **58:**97–113.

50. Mehrotra, R., D. Bisht, P. A. Singh, S. C. Gupta, and R. K. Gupta. 1996. Diagnosis of human *Sarcocystis* infection from biopsies of the skeletal muscle. *Pathology* **28:**281–282.

51. Michiels, J. F., P. Hofman, E. Bernard, M. C. St. Paul, C. Boissy, V. Mondain, Y. LeFichoux, and R. Loubiere. 1994. Intestinal and extraintestinal *Isospora belli* infection in an AIDS patient. *Pathol. Res. Pract.* **190:**1089–1093.

52. Mirdha, B. R., S. K. Kabra, and J. C. Samantray. 2002. Isosporiasis in children. *Indian Pediatr.* **39:**941–944.

53. Mughal, T. I., and M. Y. Khan. 1991. *Isospora belli* diarrhea as a presenting feature of AIDS. *Saudi Med. J.* **12:**433–434.

54. Muller, A., R. Bialek, G. Fatkenheuer, B. Salzberger, V. Diehl, and C. Franzen. 2000. Detection of *Isospora belli* by polymerase chain reaction using primers based on small-subunit ribosomal RNA sequences. *Eur. J. Clin. Microbiol. Infect. Dis.* **19:**631–634.

55. Oliveira-Silva, M. B., E. Lages-Silva, D. V. Resende, A. Prata, L. E. Ramirez, and J. K. Frenkel. 2006. *Cystoisospora belli:* in vitro multiplication in mammalian cells. *Exp. Parasitol.* **114:**189–192.

56. Ortega, Y., R. Nagle, R. H. Gilman, J. Watanabe, J. Miyagui, H. Quispe, P. Kanagusuku, C. Roxas, and C. R. Sterling. 1997. Pathologic and clinical findings in patients with cyclosporiasis and a description of intracellular parasite life-cycle stages. *J. Infect. Dis.* **176:**1584–1589.

57. Pape, J. W., R.-I. Verdier, M. Boncy, J. Boncy, and W. D. Johnson. 1994. *Cyclospora* infection in adults infected with HIV. Clinical manifestations, treatment, and prophylaxis. *Ann. Intern. Med.* **121:**654–657.

58. Pape, J. W., R. I. Verdier, and W. D. Johnson, Jr. 1989. Treatment and prophylaxis of *Isospora belli* infections in patients with the acquired immunodeficiency syndrome. *New Engl. J. Med.* **320:**1044–1047.

59. Parija, S. C., M. R. Shivaprakash, and S. R. Jayakeerthi. 2003. Evaluation of lacto-phenol cotton blue (LPCB) for detection of *Cryptosporidium, Cyclospora* and *Isospora* in the wet mount preparation of stool. *Acta Trop.* **85:**349–354.

60. Pathmanathan, R., and K. P. Kan. 1992. Three cases of human *Sarcocystis* infection with a review of human muscular sarcocystosis in Malaysia. *Trop. Geogr. Med.* **44:**102–108.

61. Relman, D. A., T. M. Schmidt, A. Gajadhar, M. Sogin, J. Cross, K. Yoder, O. Sethabutr, and P. Echeverria. 1996. Molecular phylogenetic analysis of *Cyclospora,* the human intestinal pathogen, suggests that it is closely related to *Eimeria* species. *J. Infect. Dis.* **73:**440–445.

62. Resiere, D., J. M. Vantelon, P. Bouree, E. Chachaty, G. Nitenberg, and F. Blot. 2003. *Isospora belli* infection in a patient with non-Hodgkin's lymphoma. *Clin. Microbiol. Infect.* **9:**1065–1067.

63. Romero Cabello, R., L. R. Guerrero, M. R. Munoz Garcia, and A. Geyne Cruz. 1997. Nitazoxanide for the treatment of intestinal protozoan and helminthic infections in Mexico. *Trans. R. Soc. Trop. Med. Hyg.* **91:**701–703.

64. Sifuentes-Osornio, J., G. Porras-Cortes, R. P. Bendall, F. Morales-Villarreal, G. Reyes-Teran, and G. M. Ruiz-Palacios. 1995. *Cyclospora cayetanensis* infection in patients with and without AIDS: biliary disease as another clinical manifestation. *Clin. Infect. Dis.* **21:**1092–1097.

65. Siripanth, C., B. Punpoowong, P. Amarapal, and N. Thima. 2004. Development of *Isospora belli* in Hct-8, Hep-2, human fibroblast, BEK and Vero culture cells. *Southeast Asian J. Trop. Med. Public Health* **35:**796–800.

66. Smith, H. V., C. A. Paton, M. M. A. Mtambo, and R. W. A. Girdwood. 1997. Sporulation of *Cyclospora* sp. oocysts. *Appl. Environ. Microbiol.* **63:**1631–1632.

67. Sun, T., C. F. Ilardi, D. Asnis, A. R. Bresciani, S. Goldenberg, B. Roberts, and S. Teichberg. 1996. Light and electron microscopic identification of *Cyclospora* species in the small intestine. Evidence of the presence of asexual life cycle in human host. *Am. J. Clin. Pathol.* **105:**216–220.

68. ten Hove, R. J., L. van Lieshout, E. A. Brienen, M. A. Perez, and J. J. Verweij. 2008. Real-time polymerase chain reaction for detection of *Isospora belli* in stool samples. *Diagn. Microbiol. Infect. Dis.* **61:**280–283.

69. Trier, J. S., P. C. Moxey, E. M. Schimmel, and E. Robles. 1974. Chronic intestinal coccidiosis in man: intestinal morphology and response to treatment. *Gastroenterology* **66:**923–935.

70. Van den Enden, E., M. Praet, R. Joos, A. Van Gompel, and P. Gigasse. 1995. Eosinophilic myositis resulting from sarcocystosis. *J. Trop. Med. Hyg.* **98:**273–276.

71. Vangeel, L., K. Houf, K. Chiers, J. Vercruysse, K. D'Herde, and R. Ducatelle. 2007. Molecular-based identification of *Sarcocystis hominis* in Belgian minced beef. *J. Food Prot.* **70:**1523–1526.

72. Varea, M., A. Clavel, O. Doiz, F. J. Castillo, M. C. Rubio, and R. Gomez-Lus. 1998. Fuchsin fluorescence and autofluorescence in *Cryptosporidium, Isospora* and *Cyclospora* oocysts. *Int. J. Parasitol.* **28:**1881–1883.

73. Varma, M., J. D. Hester, F. W. Schaefer III, M. W. Ware, and H. D. Lindquist. 2003. Detection of *Cyclospora cayetanensis* using a quantitative real-time PCR assay. *J. Microbiol. Methods* **53:**27–36.

74. Velásquez, J. N., S. Carnevale, M. Mariano, L. H. Kuo, A. Caballero, A. Chertcoff, C. Ibáñez, and J. P. Bozzini. 2001. Isosporosis and unizoite tissue cysts in patients with acquired immunodeficiency syndrome. *Hum. Pathol.* **32:**500–505.

75. Verdier, R. I., D. W. Fitzgerald, D. W. Johnson, and J. W. Pape. 2000. Trimethoprim-sulfamethoxazole compared with ciprofloxacin for treatment and prophylaxis of *Isospora belli* and *Cyclospora cayetanensis* infection in HIV-infected patients—a randomized, controlled trial. *Ann. Intern. Med.* **132:**885–888.

76. Visvesvara, G. S., H. Moura, E. Kovacs-Nace, S. Wallace, and M. L. Eberhard. 1997. Uniform staining of *Cyclospora* oocysts in fecal smears by a modified safranin technique with microwave heating. *J. Clin. Microbiol.* **35:**730–733.

77. Wang, K. X., C. P. Li, J. Wang, and Y. Tian. 2002. *Cyclospora cayetanensis* in Anhui, China. *World J. Gastroenterol.* **8:**1144–1148.

78. Weiss, L. M., D. C. Perlman, J. Sherman, H. Tanowitz, and M. Wittner. 1988. *Isospora belli* infection: treatment with pyrimethamine. *Ann. Intern. Med.* **109:**474–475.

79. Westerman, E. L., and R. P. Christensen. 1979. Chronic *Isospora belli* infection treated with co-trimoxazole. *Ann. Intern. Med.* **91:**413–414.

80. Yang, Z. Q., Q. Q. Li, Y. X. Zuo, X. W. Chen, Y. J. Chen, L. Nie, C. G. Wei, J. S. Zen, S. W. Attwood, X. Z. Zhang, and Y. P. Zhang. 2002. Characterization of *Sarcocystis* species in domestic animals using a PCR-RFLP analysis of variation in the 18S rRNA gene: a cost-effective and simple technique for routine species identification. *Exp. Parasitol.* **102:**212–217.

81. Yazar, S., B. Tokgöz, O. Yaman, and I. Sahin. 2006. *Isospora belli* infection in a patient with a renal transplant. *Turkiye Parazitol. Derg.* **30:**22–24.

82. Zar, F. A., E. El-Bayoumi, and M. M. Yungbluth. 2001. Histologic proof of acalculous cholecystitis due to *Cyclospora cayetanensis. Clin. Infect. Dis.* **33:**E140–E141.

Cryptosporidium

LIHUA XIAO AND VITALIANO CAMA

139

Cryptosporidium spp. inhabit the brush borders of the gastrointestinal and respiratory epithelium of various vertebrates, causing enterocolitis, diarrhea, and cholangiopathy in humans (17). Immunocompetent children and adults with cryptosporidiosis usually have a short-term illness accompanied by watery diarrhea, nausea, vomiting, and weight loss. In immunocompromised persons, however, the infection can be protracted and life threatening (55). *Cryptosporidium* spp. are well-recognized water- and foodborne pathogens, having caused many outbreaks of human illness in the United States and other countries (30).

TAXONOMY

Cryptosporidium spp. belong to the family Cryptosporidiidae, which is a member of the phylum Sporozoa (syn. Apicomplexa). The exact placement of Cryptosporidiidae in Sporozoa is uncertain. It was long considered a member of the class Coccidea, in the order of Eimeriida. Recent phylogenetic studies, however, indicate that *Cryptosporidium* spp. are more related to gregarines than to coccidia (64). Putative extracellular gregarinelike reproductive stages were described (95). Thus, *Cryptosporidium* spp. are no longer considered classic coccidian parasites.

Recently, the taxonomy of *Cryptosporidium* has gone through revisions as the result of extensive molecular genetic studies and biologic characterizations of parasites from various animals (31, 118). The validity of several early-described species has been established, such as *C. parvum* in ruminants and humans; *C. muris* in rodents; *C. wrairi* in guinea pigs; *C. felis* in cats; *C. meleagridis, C. baileyi,* and *C. galli* in birds; and *C. varanii* and *C. serpentis* in reptiles. Several new species have been named, such as *C. hominis* in humans; *C. andersoni, C. bovis,* and *C. ryanae* in weaned calves and adult cattle; *C. xiaoi* and *C. ubiquitum* in sheep; *C. canis* in dogs; *C. suis* in pigs; *C. cuniculus* in rabbits; *C. fayeri* and *C. macropodum* in marsupials; *C. molnari* and *C. scophthalmi* in fish; and *C. fragile* in amphibians. Thus, there are over 20 established *Cryptosporidium* species in vertebrates. There are also many host-adapted *Cryptosporidium* genotypes that do not yet have species names, such as *Cryptosporidium* horse, hamster, ferret, skunk, squirrel, bear, deer, fox, mongoose, wildebeest, duck, woodcock, snake, tortoise, mouse I and II, avian I to V, goose I and II, muskrat I and II, opossum I and II, chipmunk I to III, rat I to III, deer mouse I to IV, and pig II genotypes (31, 118).

DESCRIPTION OF THE AGENT

Cryptosporidium spp. are intracellular parasites that primarily infect epithelial cells of the stomach, intestine, and biliary ducts. In birds and in severely immunosuppressed persons, the respiratory tract is sometimes involved. The infection site varies according to species, but almost the entire development of *Cryptosporidium* spp. occurs between the two lipoprotein layers of the membrane of the epithelial cells (30), with the exception in *C. molnari* and *C. scophthalmi,* for which oogonial and sporogonial stages are located deeply within the epithelial cells (3).

Cryptosporidium infections in humans or other susceptible hosts start with the ingestion of viable oocysts. Upon contact with gastric and duodenal fluid, four sporozoites are liberated from each excysted oocyst, invade the epithelial cells, and develop to trophozoites surrounded by a parasitophorous vacuole. Within the epithelial cells, trophozoites undergo two or three generations of asexual amplification called merogony, leading to the formation of different types of meronts containing four to eight merozites. The latter differentiate into sexually distinct stages called macrogamonts and microgamonts (containing microgametes) in a process called gametogony. New oocysts are formed in the epithelial cells from the fusion of macrogamonts and microgametes, sporulate in situ in a process called sporogony, and contain four sporozoites. It is believed by some that about 20% are "thin walled" and may excyst within the digestive tract of the host, leading to the infection of new cells (autoinfection). The remaining 80% of oocysts are excreted into the environment, are resistant to low temperature, high salinity, and most disinfectants, and can initiate infection in a new host upon ingestion without further development. The time from ingestion of infective oocysts to the completion of endogenous development and excretion of new oocysts varies with species, hosts, and infection doses; it is usually between 4 and 10 days (30).

The only extracellular stages in *Cryptosporidium* life cycle are oocysts, which are the environmental stage of the parasite, and released sporozoites, merozoites, and microgametes, which are briefly in the lumen of the digestive tract (30). However, recently, a gregarinelike extracellular stage was supposedly found in *C. andersoni* and *C. parvum,* which can go through multiplication via syzygy, a sexual reproduction process involving the end-to-end fusion of two or more parasites (95).

Currently, over 10 *Cryptosporidium* spp. have been reported in humans: *C. hominis, C. parvum, C. meleagridis, C. felis, C. canis, C. ubiquitum, C. muris, C. suis, C. cuniculus, C. andersoni, C. fayeri,* and *Cryptosporidium* horse and skunk genotypes, pig genotype II, and chipmunk genotype I. Humans are most frequently infected with *C. hominis* and *C. parvum.* The former almost exclusively infects humans and thus is considered an anthroponotic parasite, whereas the latter infects mostly humans and ruminants and thus is considered a zoonotic pathogen. Other species, such as *C. meleagridis, C. felis, C. canis,* and *C. ubiquitum,* are less common. The remaining *Cryptosporidium* species and genotypes have been found only in a few human cases (81, 115, 117, 119). These *Cryptosporidium* spp. infect both immunocompetent and immunocompromised persons.

EPIDEMIOLOGY, TRANSMISSION, AND PREVENTION

Cryptosporidium spp. have a worldwide distribution, and their oocysts are ubiquitous in the environment. There were 2,769 to 3,787 annual cases of reported human cryptosporidiosis in the United States between 1999 and 2002 and 3,505 to 8,269 cases annually between 2003 and 2005 (51, 121). Humans can acquire cryptosporidiosis through several transmission routes, such as direct contact with infected persons or animals and consumption of contaminated water (drinking or recreational) or food (17). However, the relative role of each in the transmission of *Cryptosporidium* infection in humans is unclear.

Anthroponotic versus Zoonotic Transmission

Studies in the United States and Europe have shown that cryptosporidiosis is more common among homosexual men than among persons in other human immunodeficiency virus (HIV) transmission categories (48), indicating that direct person-to-person or anthroponotic transmission of cryptosporidiosis is common. Contact with persons with diarrhea has been identified as a major risk factor for sporadic cryptosporidiosis in industrialized countries (54, 86, 87, 97). This is exemplified by the high prevalence of cryptosporidiosis in day care facilities and nursing homes and among mothers with young children in these countries.

Only a few case-control studies assessed the role of zoonotic transmission in the acquisition of cryptosporidiosis in humans. In industrialized countries, contact with farm animals (especially cattle) is a major risk factor in sporadic cases of human cryptosporidiosis (54, 62, 87, 97, 100, 122). Contact with pigs, dogs, or cats was a risk factor for cryptosporidiosis in children in Guinea-Bissau and Indonesia in one study (60, 78). A weak association was observed between the occurrence of cryptosporidiosis in HIV-positive persons and contact with dogs in another study (43). In other studies, no increased risk in the acquisition of cryptosporidiosis was associated with contact with companion animals (85).

The distribution of *C. parvum* and *C. hominis* in humans is probably a good indicator of the transmission routes. Thus far, studies conducted in developing countries showed a predominance of *C. hominis* in children or HIV-positive adults. This is also true for most areas in the United States, Canada, Australia, and Japan. In Europe and New Zealand, however, several studies have shown almost equal prevalence of *C. parvum* and *C. hominis* in both immunocompetent and immunocompromised persons (115). In contrast, children in the Middle East are mostly infected with *C. parvum.* The

differences in the distribution of *Cryptosporidium* genotypes in humans are considered to be an indication of differences in infection sources (18, 65, 100, 115); the occurrence of *C. hominis* in humans is most likely due to anthroponotic transmission, whereas *C. parvum* in a population can be the result of both anthroponotic and zoonotic transmissions. Thus, in most developing countries, it is possible that anthroponotic transmission of *Cryptosporidium* plays a major role in human cryptosporidiosis, whereas in Europe, New Zealand, and rural areas of the United States, both anthroponotic and zoonotic transmissions are important.

Recent subtyping studies based on sequence analyses of the 60-kDa glycoprotein (gp60) gene have shown that many *C. parvum* infections in humans are not results of zoonotic transmission (115). Among several *C. parvum* subtype families identified, IIa and IIc are the two most common families. The former has been identified in both humans and ruminants and thus can be a zoonotic pathogen, whereas the latter has been seen only in humans (113, 115, 119) and thus is an anthroponotic pathogen. In developing countries, most *C. parvum* infections in children and HIV-positive persons are caused by the subtype family IIc, with IIa absent, indicating that anthroponotic transmission of *C. parvum* is common in these areas (115, 119). In contrast, both IIa and IIc subtype families are seen in humans in developed countries. Even in the United Kingdom, where zoonotic transmission is known to play a significant role in the transmission of human cryptosporidiosis, anthroponotic transmission of *C. parvum* is also common (52). Results of multilocus subtyping support the conclusions of gp60 subtyping studies (47, 71).

Waterborne Transmission

Epidemiologic studies have frequently identified water as a major route of *Cryptosporidium* transmission in areas where the disease is endemic. In most tropical countries, *Cryptosporidium* infections in children usually peak during the rainy season; thus, waterborne transmission probably plays a role in the transmission of cryptosporidiosis in these areas (9, 84, 108). Seasonal variations in the incidence of human *Cryptosporidium* infection in industrialized nations have also been partially attributed to waterborne transmission (26, 74, 97, 122). In the United States, there is a late summer peak in sporadic cases of cryptosporidiosis (97, 122). It is generally accepted that the late summer peak of cryptosporidiosis cases is due to recreational activities such as swimming and water sports. In a Canadian study, swimming in a lake or river was identified as a risk factor (86).

The role of drinking water in sporadic *Cryptosporidium* infection is not clear. In Mexican children living near the U.S. border, cryptosporidiosis is associated with consumption of municipal water instead of bottled water (63). In England, there is an association between the number of glasses of tap water drunk at home each day and the occurrence of sporadic cryptosporidiosis (54). In the United States, drinking untreated surface water was identified as a risk factor for the acquisition of *Cryptosporidium* in a small case-control study (34), and residents living in cities with surface-derived drinking water generally have higher antibody levels against *Cryptosporidium* in their blood than those living in cities with ground water as drinking water, indicating that drinking water plays a role in the transmission of human cryptosporidiosis (33). Nevertheless, case-control studies conducted with both immunocompetent persons and AIDS patients in the United States have failed to show a direct linkage of *Cryptosporidium* infection to drinking water (61, 101).

Numerous waterborne outbreaks of cryptosporidiosis have occurred in the United States, Canada, the United Kingdom, France, Australia, Japan, and other industrialized nations (29). These include outbreaks associated with both drinking water and recreational water (swimming pools and water parks). After the massive cryptosporidiosis outbreak in Milwaukee in 1993, the water industry has adopted more stringent treatments of source water. Currently, the number of drinking-water-associated outbreaks is in decline in the United States and the United Kingdom, and most outbreaks in the United States are associated with recreational water (122). Even though five *Cryptosporidium* species are commonly found in humans, *C. parvum* sand *C. hominis* are responsible for most cryptosporidiosis outbreaks, with *C. hominis* responsible for more outbreaks than *C. parvum* (115). This is even the case for the United Kingdom, where *C. parvum* and *C. hominis* are both common in the general population. Recently, there was one drinking-water-associated cryptosporidiosis outbreak caused by *C. cuniculus* (20).

Foodborne Transmission

The role of food in the transmission of cryptosporidiosis is much less clear. *Cryptosporidium* oocysts have been isolated from several foodstuffs, and these have mainly been associated with fruits, vegetables, and shellfish (32, 93). Direct contamination of food by fecal materials from animals or food handlers has been implicated in several foodborne outbreaks of cryptosporidiosis in industrialized nations. In most instances, human infections were usually due to consumption of contaminated fresh produce and unpasteurized apple cider or milk (11, 28, 77, 88, 89, 123).

Very few case-control studies have examined the role of contaminated food as a risk factor in the acquisition of *Cryptosporidium* infection in areas where the disease is endemic. A pediatric study in Brazil failed to show any association between *Cryptosporidium* infection and diet or type of food hygiene (85). Case-control studies conducted in the United States, the United Kingdom, and Australia have actually shown a lower prevalence of *Cryptosporidium* infection in immunocompetent persons with frequent consumption of raw vegetables (54, 92, 97). Nevertheless, it is estimated that about 10% of *Cryptosporidium* infections in the United States are foodborne (76).

Prevention

As for any pathogens that are transmitted by the fecal-oral route, good hygiene is the key in preventing the acquisition of *Cryptosporidium* infection (58). Immunosuppressed persons especially should take necessary precautions in preventing the occurrence of cryptosporidiosis (73). This includes washing hands after using bathrooms, changing diapers, and contacting pets or soil (including gardening); avoiding drinking water from lakes and rivers, swallowing water in recreational activities, and drinking unpasteurized milk, milk products, and juices; and following safe-sex practices (avoiding oral-anal contact). During cryptosporidiosis outbreaks or when a community advisory to boil water is issued, individuals should boil water for 1 minute to kill the parasite or use a tap water filter capable of removing particles less than 1 μm in diameter. Immunosuppressed persons also should avoid eating raw shellfish and should not eat uncooked vegetable salads and unpeeled fruits when traveling to areas where cryptosporidiosis is endemic (such as developing countries) (73).

CLINICAL SIGNIFICANCE

In developing countries, human *Cryptosporidium* infection occurs mostly in children younger than 5 years, with peak occurrence of infections and diarrhea in children less than 2 years of age (80). Frequent symptoms include diarrhea, abdominal cramps, nausea, vomiting, headache, fatigue, and low-grade fever. The diarrhea can be voluminous and watery but usually resolves within 1 to 2 weeks without treatment. Not all infected children have diarrhea or other gastrointestinal symptoms, and the occurrence of diarrhea in children with cryptosporidiosis can be as low as 30% in community-based studies (8). Even subclinical cryptosporidiosis exerts a significant adverse effect on child growth, as infected children with no clinical symptoms experience growth faltering, both in weight and in height (17). Children can have multiple episodes of cryptosporidiosis, implying that the anti-*Cryptosporidium* immunity in children is short-lived or incomplete (12). Cryptosporidiosis has been associated with increased mortality in hospitalized children in developing countries (108).

In developed countries, pediatric cryptosporidiosis occurs in older children than in developing countries, probably due to later exposures to contaminated environments as a result of better hygiene (81, 104, 121). Cryptosporidiosis is also common in elderly persons in nursing homes, where person-to-person transmission probably also plays a major role in the spread of *Cryptosporidium* infections (79). In the general population, a substantial number of adults are probably susceptible to *Cryptosporidium* infection, as sporadic infections occur in all age groups in the United States and the United Kingdom, and traveling to developing countries and consumption of contaminated food or water can frequently lead to infection (26, 44, 97, 122).

Unlike in developing countries, immunocompetent persons with sporadic cryptosporidiosis in industrialized nations usually have diarrhea (17, 44, 92). The median number of stools per day during the worst period of the infection is 7 to 9.5 (92). Other common symptoms include abdominal pain, nausea, vomiting, and low-grade fever (44, 92). The duration of illness has a mean or median of 9 to 21 days, with a median loss of five work or study days and hospitalization of 7 to 22% of patients (26, 44, 92). Patients infected with *C. hominis* are more likely to have joint pain, eye pain, recurrent headache, dizziness, and fatigue than those infected with *C. parvum* (53). There are significant differences among different *Cryptosporidium* species and *C. hominis* subtype families in clinical manifestations of pediatric cryptosporidiosis (12).

Cryptosporidiosis is common in immunocompromised persons, including AIDS patients, persons with primary immunodeficiency, and cancer and transplant patients undergoing immunosuppressive therapy (17, 55, 75, 114). Hemodialysis patients with chronic renal failure and renal transplant patients commonly develop cryptosporidiosis (98, 107). It is frequently associated with chronic, life-threatening diarrhea (55). In HIV-positive persons, the occurrence of cryptosporidiosis increases as the CD4$^+$ lymphocyte counts fall, especially below 200 cells/μl (55). Manabe et al. described four clinical forms of diarrhea caused by cryptosporidiosis in the United States: chronic diarrhea (36% of patients), choleralike disease (33%), transient diarrhea (15%), and relapsing illness (15%) (72). Sclerosing cholangitis and other biliary involvements are also common in AIDS patients with cryptosporidiosis (25). Symptoms of cryptosporidiosis in AIDS patients vary in severity, duration, and responses to treatment. Much of this variation can be explained by the degree of immunosuppression. In addition, variations in the infection site (gastric infection, proximal small intestine infection, or ileocolonic infection versus panenteric infection) have been seen in AIDS patients with cryptosporidiosis, which may contribute to differences in disease severity and survival (23, 68). Likewise, different *Cryptosporidium* species and *C. hominis* subtype families are associated with different clinical manifestations in HIV-positive persons in developing countries (13). Cryptosporidiosis in AIDS patients is associated with increased mortality and shortened survival (72).

COLLECTION, TRANSPORT, AND STORAGE OF SPECIMENS

At the moment, almost all active *Cryptosporidium* infections are diagnosed by analysis of stool specimens. Stool specimens are usually collected fresh or in fixative solutions such as 10% buffered formalin and polyvinyl alcohol (36). Stool specimens fixed in formalin are preferred for routine diagnosis of cryptosporidiosis. For outbreak investigations, *Cryptosporidium* spp. present are frequently genotyped and subtyped by PCR methods, which require the use of fresh or frozen stool specimens or stools preserved in 2.5% potassium dichromate. It is recommended that whenever possible multiple specimens (three specimens passed at intervals of 2 to 3 days) from each patient should be examined if *Cryptosporidium* infection is suspected and the examination of the initial stool specimen is negative. This is because carriers with low oocyst shedding are common, and examination of individual specimens can lead to the detection of only 53% of infections (46).

Examination of intestinal or biliary biopsy is sometimes used in the diagnosis of cryptosporidiosis in AIDS patients (23). However, the sensitivity of the diagnosis depends on the location of tissues examined; the duodenum is usually infected with *Cryptosporidium* only in severe infection, and the terminal ileum has significantly higher detection rates than the duodenum (46). Thus, upper endoscopic biopsies are much less sensitive than lower endoscopic biopsies in diagnosing cryptosporidiosis. However, lower endoscopy is generally considered too invasive and risky for many AIDS patients.

DIRECT EXAMINATION

In clinical laboratories, *Cryptosporidium* spp. in stool specimens are commonly detected by microscopic examinations of oocysts or immunologic detection of antigens (99).

Microscopy

Stool specimens can be examined directly for *Cryptosporidium* oocysts by microscopy of direct wet-mount or stained fecal materials if the number of oocysts in specimens is high. *Cryptosporidium* oocysts in humans generally measure 4 to 6 µm. Occasionally, *C. muris* oocysts are also found, which are more elongated and measure 6 to 9 µm. Oocysts present are often concentrated using either traditional ethyl acetate or Weber-modified ethyl-acetate concentration methods (99). Concentrated stool specimens can be examined by microscopy in several ways. *Cryptosporidium* oocysts can be detected by bright-field microscopy in direct wet mounts. This allows the observation of oocyst morphology and more accurate measurement of oocysts, which is frequently needed in biologic studies. Differential interference contrast can be used in microscopy, which produces better images and visualization of internal structures of oocysts. Most *Cryptosporidium* species look similar under microscopes and have similar morphometric measurements (118).

More often, *Cryptosporidium* oocysts in concentrated stool specimens are detected by microscopy after staining of the fecal smears. Many special stains have been used in the detection of *Cryptosporidium* oocysts, but modified acid-fast stains are the most commonly used (99), especially in developing countries, because of their low cost, ease of use, lack of need for special microscopes, and simultaneous detection of several other pathogens such as *Cystoisospora* (*Isospora*) and *Cyclospora* (Fig. 1). Two stains widely used are the modified Ziehl-Neelsen acid-fast stain and modified Kinyoun's acid-fast stain (99). Oocysts are stained bright red to purple against a blue or green background (Fig. 1).

Direct immunofluorescence assays (DFA) have been used increasingly in *Cryptosporidium* oocyst detection by microscopy, especially in industrialized nations. Compared to acid-fast staining, DFA has higher sensitivity and specificity (57). Many commercial DFA kits are marketed for the diagnosis of *Cryptosporidium*, most of which include reagents allowing simultaneous detection of *Giardia* cysts (Table 1). Oocysts appear apple green against a dark background in immunofluorescence microscopy (Fig. 2) Because of the high sensitivity and specificity, DFA has been used by some as the "gold standard" or reference test (38, 57). It has been shown that most antibodies in commercial DFA kits react with oocysts of almost all *Cryptosporidium* species, making identification to the species level impossible (45, 124).

The sensitivity of most microscopic methods is probably low. The detection limit for the combination of ethyl acetate concentration and DFA was shown to be 10,000 oocysts per gram of liquid stool and 50,000 oocysts per gram of formed stool (109, 110). A similar sensitivity was achieved with fecal specimens from dogs (91). The sensitivity of modified acid-fast staining was 10-fold lower than that of DFA (109), probably because acid-fast stains do not consistently stain all oocysts (35). The sensitivity of the DFA can be significantly improved by the incorporation of an oocyst isolation step using an immunomagnetic separation technique (94).

Antigen Detection

Cryptosporidium infection can also be diagnosed by the detection of *Cryptosporidium* antigens in stool specimens by immunoassays (99). Antigen capture-based enzyme immunoassays (EIA) have been used in the diagnosis of cryptosporidiosis since 1990. In recent years, EIAs have gained popularity because they do not require experienced microscopists and can be used to screen a large number of samples (22). In clinical laboratories, several commercial EIA kits are commonly used (Table 1). High specificity (99 to 100%) has been generally reported for these EIA kits (38, 57). Sensitivities, however, have been reported to range between 70% (57) and 94 to 100% (10, 38, 102). Occasional false positivity of EIA kits is known to occur in the detection of *Cryptosporidium* (21, 27), and manufacturer's recalls of EIA kits have occurred because of high nonspecificity (14). If a patient is in the carrier state or undergoing self-cure, the number of oocysts may drop below the sensitivity levels of these kits (57). Most EIA kits have been evaluated only with human stool specimens presumably from patients infected with *C. hominis* or *C. parvum*. Their usefulness in the detection of *Cryptosporidium* spp. in animals may be compromised by the specificity of the antibodies.

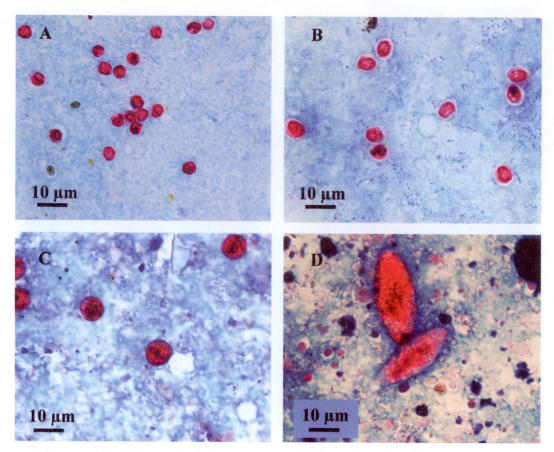

FIGURE 1 Oocysts of *Cryptosporidium hominis* (4 to 6 μm) (A), *Cryptosporidium muris* (6 to 8 μm) (B), *Cyclospora cayetanensis* (8 to 10 μm) (C), and *Cystoisospora belli* (20 to 30 μm by 10 to 20 μm) (D) stained by the modified Ziehl-Neelsen acid-fast stain.

In recent years, several lateral flow immunochromatographic assays have been marketed for rapid detection of *Cryptosporidium* in stool specimens (Table 1). In the few evaluation studies conducted, these assays have been shown to have high specificities (>90%) and sensitivities (98 to 100%) (1, 37, 39, 57, 59, 90). However, sensitivities of 68 to 75% were shown in some studies for some assays (57, 111). These rapid assays have also been affected by quality control problems and were subjected to several manufacturer's recalls because of false-positive results (15, 16).

TYPING SYSTEMS

Molecular techniques, especially PCR and PCR-related methods, have been developed and used in the detection and differentiation of *Cryptosporidium* spp. for many years. A few of the PCR assays are commercially available (Table 1). Several genus-specific PCR-restriction fragment length polymorphism-based genotyping tools have been developed for the detection and differentiation of *Cryptosporidium* at the species level (5, 24, 82, 103, 116). Most of these techniques are based on the small-subunit rRNA gene. Other genotyping techniques are designed mostly for the differentiation of *C. parvum* and *C. hominis* and thus cannot detect and differentiate other *Cryptosporidium* spp. or genotypes (115). Their usefulness in the analysis of human stool specimens is compromised by their inability to detect *C. canis*, *C. felis*, *C. suis*, and *C. muris* (56).

Several subtyping tools have also been developed to characterize the diversity within *C. parvum* or *C. hominis* (115). One of the most commonly used techniques is microsatellite analysis (70, 120). Although not a strict microsatellite locus by definition, results of a series of recent studies have shown high sequence polymorphism in the gp60 gene (also known as gp15/45/60, gp40/15)

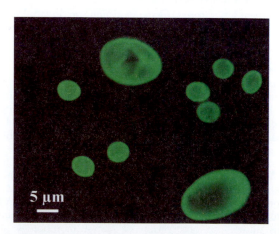

FIGURE 2 *Cryptosporidium hominis* oocysts (4 to 6 μm) and *Giardia duodenalis* cyst (11 to 14 μm by 7 to 10 μm) under immunofluorescence microscopy.

TABLE 1 Some commercial diagnostic assays for the detection of *Cryptosporidium* oocysts, antigens, or DNA

Product	Manufacturer, country	CLIA[a] certified	Intended use
Immunofluorescence assays			
Merifluor *Cryptosporidium/Giardia*	Meridian Biosciences, United States	Yes	Clinical
Crypto Cel[b]	Cellabs, Australia	No	Clinical, environmental
Crypto/*Giardia* Cel[b]	Cellabs, Australia	No	Clinical, environmental
Aqua-Glo G/C kit	Waterborne Inc., United States	No	Environmental
Crypt-a-Glo	Waterborne Inc., United States	No	Environmental
Cyst-a-Glo FL, comprehensive kit	Waterborne Inc., United States	No	Veterinary
Crypt-a-Glo FL, comprehensive kit	Waterborne Inc., United States	No	Veterinary
RDI-CRYPTOSPabm, monoclonal antibody	Fitzgerald Industries International, Inc., United States	No	Research
Enzyme immunoassays			
Cryptosporidium TEST (direct Ag/spectrophotometric)[c]	TechLab, United States	Yes	Clinical
Cryptosporidium Test (direct Ag/visual)[c]	TechLab, United States	Yes	Clinical
Cryptosporidium II (direct Ag, visual or spectrophotometric)	TechLab, United States	No	Clinical
ProSpecT *Giardia*/Crypto. microplate (direct Ag/spectrophotometric)	Remel,[d] United States	Yes	Clinical
ProSpecT *Giardia*/Crypto. microplate (direct Ag/visual)	Remel,[d] United States	Yes	Clinical
ProSpecT *Cryptosporidium* microtiter (direct Ag/spectrophotometric)	Remel,[d] United States	Yes	Clinical
ProSpecT *Cryptosporidium* microtiter (direct Ag/visual)	Remel,[d] United States	Yes	Clinical
ProSpecT *Cryptosporidium* rapid assay (direct Ag/visual)	Remel,[d] United States	Yes	Clinical
Giardia/Cryptosporidium Chek ELISA	TechLab, United States	Yes	Clinical
Cryptosporidium Ag, ELISA[b]	Cypress Diagnostics, Belgium		Clinical
Immunochromatography			
Xpect *Cryptosporidium* Lateral Flow Assay	Remel, United States	Yes	Clinical
Xpect *Giardia/Cryptosporidium* Lateral Flow Assay	Remel, United States	Yes	Clinical
Triage parasite panel	Biosite, United States	Yes	Clinical
ColorPAC *Giardia/Cryptosporidium* rapid assay[e]	Becton Dickinson, United States	Yes	Clinical
ImmunoCard STAT! *Cryptosporidium/Giardia* rapid assay	Meridian Bioscience, United States	No	Clinical
RIDA Quick *Cryptosporidium/Giardia* Combi (dipstick)[b]	R-Biopharm, Germany	No	Clinical
Bovine *Cryptosporidium* dipstick[b]	Cypress Diagnostics, Belgium	No	Veterinary
Crypto kit (Dipstrip)[b]	Cypress Dianostics, Belgium	No	Clinical
Crypto/*Giardia* Duo-Strip[b]	Coris BioConcept, Belgium	No	Clinical
Crypto-Strip C-1005 (Crypto Uni-Strip, Crypto-CIT)[b]	Coris BioConcept, Belgium	No	Clinical
Molecular assays			
Path-Crypto-std[b]	Primer Design, United Kingdom	No	Research
Path-Crypto (std kit plus internal reaction amplification controls)[b]	Primer Design, United Kingdom	No	Research
Cryptodiag[b]	Bio Advance, France	No	Research
Cryptosporidium genotyping kit	Invitrogen, United States	No	Research

[a]CLIA, Clinical Laboratory Improvement Amendments.
[b]Not available in the United States.
[c]Now replaced by *Cryptosporidium* II.
[d]CLIA certification to Alexon-Trend; the company is now Remel.
[e]Previously manufactured as Contrast *Giardia/Cryptosporidium* Combo rapid assay from Genzyme.

(4, 104, 113). Most of the genetic heterogeneity in this gene is present in the number of a trinucleotide repeat (TCA, TCG, or TCT), although extensive sequence differences are also present between families of subtypes. Multilocus mini- and microsatellite subtyping tools for *C. parvum* and *C. hominis* have also been developed (41, 47, 70, 105, 106). The usefulness of subtyping tools has been demonstrated by the analysis of samples from foodborne and waterborne outbreaks of cryptosporidiosis (11, 19, 42, 66, 67, 120).

ISOLATION PROCEDURES

The in vitro cultivation of *Cryptosporidium* spp. remains inefficient despite recent advances (6, 49). The low parasite yields and oocyst production have limited the usefulness of parasite culture in the isolation and diagnosis of *Cryptosporidium*. Nevertheless, in vitro cultivation of early *Cryptosporidium* developmental stages in several epithelial cell lines (HCT-8, Madin-Darby bovine kidney, Caco-2, etc.) has been used widely in research studies to assess potential drugs and oocyst disinfection methods and to characterize parasite development, differentiation, and biochemistry (6). The recent development of procedures for long-term maintenance of *C. parvum* and *C. hominis* in cell and cell-free culture, if verified, could promote the use of in vitro cultivation methods in routine diagnosis of *Cryptosporidium* infection (49, 50).

TREATMENT

Numerous pharmaceutical compounds have been screened for anti-*Cryptosporidium* activities in vitro or in laboratory animals (40, 83, 96). Some of those showing promise have been used in the experimental treatment of cryptosporidiosis in humans, but few have been shown to be effective in controlled clinical trials (2, 55). Oral or intravenous rehydration and antimotility drugs are widely used whenever severe diarrhea is associated with cryptosporidiosis. Nitazoxanide is the only FDA-approved drug for the treatment of cryptosporidiosis in immunocompetent persons. Clinical trials have demonstrated that nitazoxanide can shorten clinical disease and reduce parasite loads (7, 96). This drug, however, is not effective in the treatment of *Cryptosporidium* infections in immunodeficient patients (2, 10). For this population, paromomycin and spiramycin have been used in the treatment of some patients, but their efficacy remains unproven (2, 83, 96).

In industrialized nations, the most effective treatment and prophylaxis for cryptosporidiosis in AIDS patients is the use of highly active antiretroviral therapy (HAART) (83, 96, 125). It is probably also an effective prevention for cryptosporidiosis in HIV-positive persons in developing countries (112). It is believed that the eradication and prevention of the infection are related to the replenishment of CD4+ cells in treated persons and the antiparasitic activities of the protease inhibitors (such as indinavir, nelfinavir, and ritonavir) used in HAART (83, 125). Relapse of cryptosporidiosis is common in AIDS patients who have stopped HAART (69).

EVALUATION, INTERPRETATION, AND REPORTING OF RESULTS

Cryptosporidiosis is a notifiable disease in most states in the United States and in some other industrialized countries. Thus, the detection of the pathogen in stools or tissues should be reported to the local health department in addition to the physicians. Because most routine diagnostic tests cannot differentiate *Cryptosporidium* species, the detection of *Cryptosporidium* oocysts or antigens in stools or other specimens should be reported as *Cryptosporidium* positive without referring to the nature of species involved. From a public health point of view, the reporting of a significant number of cases above background levels in industrialized nations indicates the likely occurrence of outbreaks of cryptosporidiosis or false positivity of diagnostic kits (14–16, 27). In situations like this, it is crucial to have the test results verified with a confirmatory test such as DFA or PCR and to report them to the state or local public health department. The inclusion of both positive and negative controls in each test run will reduce the occurrence of test errors.

REFERENCES

1. **Abdel Hameed, D. M., H. S. Elwakil, and M. A. Ahmed.** 2008. A single-step immunochromatographic lateral-flow assay for detection of Giardia lamblia and Cryptosporidium parvum antigens in human fecal samples. J. Egypt. Soc. Parasitol. 38:797–804.
2. **Abubakar, I., S. H. Aliyu, C. Arumugam, N. K. Usman, and P. R. Hunter.** 2007. Treatment of cryptosporidiosis in immunocompromised individuals: systematic review and meta-analysis. Br. J. Clin. Pharmacol. 63:387–393.
3. **Alvarez-Pellitero, P., M. I. Quiroga, A. Sitja-Bobadilla, M. J. Redondo, O. Palenzuela, F. Padros, S. Vazquez, and J. M. Nieto.** 2004. Cryptosporidium scophthalmi n. sp. (Apicomplexa: Cryptosporidiidae) from cultured turbot Scophthalmus maximus. Light and electron microscope description and histopathological study. Dis. Aquat. Organ. 62:133–145.
4. **Alves, M., L. Xiao, I. Sulaiman, A. A. Lal, O. Matos, and F. Antunes.** 2003. Subgenotype analysis of Cryptosporidium isolates from humans, cattle, and zoo ruminants in Portugal. J. Clin. Microbiol. 41:2744–2747.
5. **Amar, C. F., P. H. Dear, and J. McLauchlin.** 2004. Detection and identification by real time PCR/RFLP analyses of Cryptosporidium species from human faeces. Lett. Appl. Microbiol. 38:217–222.
6. **Arrowood, M. J.** 2008. In vitro cultivation, p. 499–524. In R. Fayer and L. Xiao (ed.), Cryptosporidium and Cryptosporidiosis, 2nd ed. CRC Press, Boca Raton, FL.
7. **Bailey, J. M., and J. Erramouspe.** 2004. Nitazoxanide treatment for giardiasis and cryptosporidiosis in children. Ann. Pharmacother. 38:634–640.
8. **Bern, C., Y. Ortega, W. Checkley, J. M. Roberts, A. G. Lescano, L. Cabrera, M. Verastegui, R. E. Black, C. Sterling, and R. H. Gilman.** 2002. Epidemiologic differences between cyclosporiasis and cryptosporidiosis in Peruvian children. Emerg. Infect. Dis. 8:581–585.
9. **Bhattacharya, M. K., T. Teka, A. S. Faruque, and G. J. Fuchs.** 1997. Cryptosporidium infection in children in urban Bangladesh. J. Trop. Pediatr. 43:282–286.
10. **Bialek, R., N. Binder, K. Dietz, A. Joachim, J. Knobloch, and U. E. Zelck.** 2002. Comparison of fluorescence, antigen and PCR assays to detect Cryptosporidium parvum in fecal specimens. Diagn. Microbiol. Infect. Dis. 43:283–288.
11. **Blackburn, B. G., J. M. Mazurek, M. Hlavsa, J. Park, M. Tillapaw, M. Parrish, E. Salehi, W. Franks, E. Koch, F. Smith, L. Xiao, M. Arrowood, V. Hill, A. da Silva, S. Johnston, and J. L. Jones.** 2006. Cryptosporidiosis associated with ozonated apple cider. Emerg. Infect. Dis. 12:684–686.
12. **Cama, V. A., C. Bern, J. Roberts, L. Cabrera, C. R. Sterling, Y. Ortega, R. H. Gilman, and L. Xiao.** 2008. Cryptosporidium species and subtypes and clinical manifestations in children, Peru. Emerg. Infect. Dis. 14:1567–1574.
13. **Cama, V. A., J. M. Ross, S. Crawford, V. Kawai, R. Chavez-Valdez, D. Vargas, A. Vivar, E. Ticona, M. Navincopa, J. Williamson, Y. Ortega, R. H. Gilman, C. Bern, and L. Xiao.** 2007. Differences in clinical manifestations among Cryptosporidium species and subtypes in HIV-infected persons. J. Infect. Dis. 196:684–691.
14. **Centers for Disease Control and Prevention.** 1999. False-positive laboratory tests for Cryptosporidium involving an enzyme-linked immunosorbent assay—United States, November 1997–March 1998. MMWR Morb. Mortal. Wkly. Rep. 48:4–8.
15. **Centers for Disease Control and Prevention.** 2002. Manufacturer's recall of rapid assay kits based on false positive Cryptosporidium antigen tests—Wisconsin, 2001–2002. MMWR Morb. Mortal. Wkly. Rep. 51:189.
16. **Centers for Disease Control and Prevention.** 2004. Manufacturer's recall of rapid cartridge assay kits on the basis of false-positive Cryptosporidium antigen tests—Colorado, 2004. MMWR Morb. Mortal. Wkly. Rep. 53:198.
17. **Chalmers, R. M., and A. P. Davies.** 2010. Minireview: clinical cryptosporidiosis. Exp. Parasitol. 124:138–146.
18. **Chalmers, R. M., K. Elwin, A. L. Thomas, E. C. Guy, and B. Mason.** 2009. Long-term Cryptosporidium typing reveals the aetiology and species-specific epidemiology of human cryptosporidiosis in England and Wales, 2000 to 2003. Euro Surveill. 14:pii:19086.

19. **Chalmers, R. M., C. Ferguson, S. Caccio, R. B. Gasser, Y. G. Abs El-Osta, L. Heijnen, L. Xiao, K. Elwin, S. Hadfield, M. Sinclair, and M. Stevens.** 2005. Direct comparison of selected methods for genetic categorisation of *Cryptosporidium parvum* and *Cryptosporidium hominis* species. *Int. J. Parasitol.* **35:**397–410.

20. **Chalmers, R. M., G. Robinson, K. Elwin, S. J. Hadfield, L. Xiao, U. Ryan, D. Modha, and C. Mallaghan.** 2009. *Cryptosporidium* sp. rabbit genotype, a newly identified human pathogen. *Emerg. Infect. Dis.* **15:**829–830.

21. **Chapman, P. A., B. A. Rush, and J. McLauchlin.** 1990. An enzyme immunoassay for detecting *Cryptosporidium* in faecal and environmental samples. *J. Med. Microbiol.* **32:**233–237.

22. **Church, D., K. Miller, A. Lichtenfeld, H. Semeniuk, B. Kirkham, K. Laupland, and S. Elsayed.** 2005. Screening for *Giardia/Cryptosporidium* infections using an enzyme immunoassay in a centralized regional microbiology laboratory. *Arch. Pathol. Lab. Med.* **129:**754–759.

23. **Clayton, F., T. Heller, and D. P. Kotler.** 1994. Variation in the enteric distribution of cryptosporidia in acquired immunodeficiency syndrome. *Am. J. Clin. Pathol.* **102:**420–425.

24. **Coupe, S., C. Sarfati, S. Hamane, and F. Derouin.** 2005. Detection of *Cryptosporidium* and identification to the species level by nested PCR and restriction fragment length polymorphism. *J. Clin. Microbiol.* **43:**1017–1023.

25. **De Angelis, C., M. Mangone, M. Bianchi, G. Saracco, A. Repici, M. Rizzetto, and R. Pellicano.** 2009. An update on AIDS-related cholangiopathy. *Minerva Gastroenterol. Dietol.* **55:**79–82.

26. **Dietz, V., D. Vugia, R. Nelson, J. Wicklund, J. Nadle, K. G. McCombs, and S. Reddy.** 2000. Active, multisite, laboratory-based surveillance for *Cryptosporidium parvum. Am. J. Trop. Med. Hyg.* **62:**368–372.

27. **Doing, K. M., J. L. Hamm, J. A. Jellison, J. A. Marquis, and C. Kingsbury.** 1999. False-positive results obtained with the Alexon ProSpecT *Cryptosporidium* enzyme immunoassay. *J. Clin. Microbiol.* **37:**1582–1583.

28. **Ethelberg, S., M. Lisby, L. S. Vestergaard, H. L. Enemark, K. E. Olsen, C. R. Stensvold, H. V. Nielsen, L. J. Porsbo, A. M. Plesner, and K. Molbak.** 2009. A foodborne outbreak of *Cryptosporidium hominis* infection. *Epidemiol. Infect.* **137:**348–356.

29. **Fayer, R.** 2004. *Cryptosporidium*: a water-borne zoonotic parasite. *Vet. Parasitol.* **126:**37–56.

30. **Fayer, R.** 2008. Introduction, p. 1–42. *In* R. Fayer and L. Xiao (ed.), *Cryptosporidium and Cryptosporidiosis*, 2nd ed. CRC Press, Boca Raton, FL.

31. **Fayer, R.** 2010. Taxonomy and species delimitation in *Cryptosporidium. Exp. Parasitol.* **124:**90–97.

32. **Fayer, R., J. P. Dubey, and D. S. Lindsay.** 2004. Zoonotic protozoa: from land to sea. *Trends Parasitol.* **20:**531–536.

33. **Frost, F. J., T. R. Kunde, T. B. Muller, G. F. Craun, L. M. Katz, A. J. Hibbard, and R. L. Calderon.** 2003. Serological responses to *Cryptosporidium* antigens among users of surface- vs. ground-water sources. *Epidemiol. Infect.* **131:**1131–1138.

34. **Gallaher, M. M., J. L. Herndon, L. J. Nims, C. R. Sterling, D. J. Grabowski, and H. F. Hull.** 1989. Cryptosporidiosis and surface water. *Am. J. Public Health* **79:**39–42.

35. **Garcia, L. S., T. C. Brewer, and D. A. Bruckner.** 1987. Fluorescence detection of *Cryptosporidium* oocysts in human fecal specimens by using monoclonal antibodies. *J. Clin. Microbiol.* **25:**119–121.

36. **Garcia, L. S., D. A. Bruckner, T. C. Brewer, and R. Y. Shimizu.** 1983. Techniques for the recovery and identification of *Cryptosporidium* oocysts from stool specimens. *J. Clin. Microbiol.* **18:**185–190.

37. **Garcia, L. S., and R. Y. Shimizu.** 2000. Detection of *Giardia lamblia* and *Cryptosporidium parvum* antigens in human fecal specimens using the ColorPAC combination rapid solid-phase qualitative immunochromatographic assay. *J. Clin. Microbiol.* **38:**1267–1268.

38. **Garcia, L. S., and R. Y. Shimizu.** 1997. Evaluation of nine immunoassay kits (enzyme immunoassay and direct fluorescence) for detection of *Giardia lamblia* and *Cryptosporidium parvum* in human fecal specimens. *J. Clin. Microbiol.* **35:**1526–1529.

39. **Garcia, L. S., R. Y. Shimizu, S. Novak, M. Carroll, and F. Chan.** 2003. Commercial assay for detection of *Giardia lamblia* and *Cryptosporidium parvum* antigens in human fecal specimens by rapid solid-phase qualitative immunochromatography. *J. Clin. Microbiol.* **41:**209–212.

40. **Gargala, G.** 2008. Drug treatment and novel drug target against *Cryptosporidium. Parasite* **15:**275–281.

41. **Gatei, W., C. A. Hart, R. H. Gilman, P. Das, V. Cama, and L. Xiao.** 2006. Development of a multilocus sequence typing tool for *Cryptosporidium hominis. J. Eukaryot. Microbiol.* **53:**S43–S48.

42. **Glaberman, S., J. E. Moore, C. J. Lowery, R. M. Chalmers, I. Sulaiman, K. Elwin, P. J. Rooney, B. C. Millar, J. S. Dooley, A. A. Lal, and L. Xiao.** 2002. Three drinking-water-associated cryptosporidiosis outbreaks, Northern Ireland. *Emerg. Infect. Dis.* **8:**631–633.

43. **Glaser, C. A., S. Safrin, A. Reingold, and T. B. Newman.** 1998. Association between *Cryptosporidium* infection and animal exposure in HIV-infected individuals. *J. Acquir. Immune Defic. Syndr. Hum. Retrovirol.* **17:**79–82.

44. **Goh, S., M. Reacher, D. P. Casemore, N. Q. Verlander, R. Chalmers, M. Knowles, J. Williams, K. Osborn, and S. Richards.** 2004. Sporadic cryptosporidiosis, North Cumbria, England, 1996–2000. *Emerg. Infect. Dis.* **10:**1007–1015.

45. **Graczyk, T. K., M. R. Cranfield, and R. Fayer.** 1996. Evaluation of commercial enzyme immunoassay (EIA) and immunofluorescent antibody (FA) test kits for detection of *Cryptosporidium* oocysts of species other than *Cryptosporidium parvum. Am. J. Trop. Med. Hyg.* **54:**274–279.

46. **Greenberg, P. D., J. Koch, and J. P. Cello.** 1996. Diagnosis of *Cryptosporidium parvum* in patients with severe diarrhea and AIDS. *Digest. Dis. Sci.* **41:**2286–2290.

47. **Grinberg, A., N. Lopez-Villalobos, W. Pomroy, G. Widmer, H. Smith, and A. Tait.** 2008. Host-shaped segregation of the *Cryptosporidium parvum* multilocus genotype repertoire. *Epidemiol. Infect.* **136:**273–278.

48. **Hellard, M., J. Hocking, J. Willis, G. Dore, and C. Fairley.** 2003. Risk factors leading to *Cryptosporidium* infection in men who have sex with men. *Sex. Transm. Infect.* **79:**412–414.

49. **Hijjawi, N.** 2010. *Cryptosporidium*: new developments in cell culture. *Exp. Parasitol.* **124:**56–60.

50. **Hijjawi, N. S., B. P. Meloni, M. Ng'anzo, U. M. Ryan, M. E. Olson, P. T. Cox, P. T. Monis, and R. C. Thompson.** 2004. Complete development of *Cryptosporidium parvum* in host cell-free culture. *Int. J. Parasitol.* **34:**769–777.

51. **Hlavsa, M. C., J. C. Watson, and M. J. Beach.** 2005. Cryptosporidiosis surveillance—United States 1999–2002. *MMWR Surveill. Summ.* **54:**1–8.

52. **Hunter, P. R., S. J. Hadfield, D. Wilkinson, I. R. Lake, F. C. Harrison, and R. M. Chalmers.** 2007. Subtypes of *Cryptosporidium parvum* in humans and disease risk. *Emerg. Infect. Dis.* **13:**82–88.

53. **Hunter, P. R., S. Hughes, S. Woodhouse, N. Raj, Q. Syed, R. M. Chalmers, N. Q. Verlander, and J. Goodacre.** 2004. Health sequelae of human cryptosporidiosis in immunocompetent patients. *Clin. Infect. Dis.* **39:**504–510.

54. **Hunter, P. R., S. Hughes, S. Woodhouse, Q. Syed, N. Q. Verlander, R. M. Chalmers, K. Morgan, G. Nichols, N. Beeching, and K. Osborn.** 2004. Sporadic cryptosporidiosis case-control study with genotyping. *Emerg. Infect. Dis.* **10:**1241–1249.

55. **Hunter, P. R., and G. Nichols.** 2002. Epidemiology and clinical features of *Cryptosporidium* infection in immunocompromised patients. *Clin. Microbiol. Rev.* **15:**145–154.

56. **Jiang, J., and L. Xiao.** 2003. An evaluation of molecular diagnostic tools for the detection and differentiation of human-pathogenic *Cryptosporidium* spp. *J. Eukaryot. Microbiol.* **50**(Suppl.)**:**542–547.

57. **Johnston, S. P., M. M. Ballard, M. J. Beach, L. Causer, and P. P. Wilkins.** 2003. Evaluation of three commercial assays for detection of *Giardia* and *Cryptosporidium* organisms in fecal specimens. *J. Clin. Microbiol.* **41:**623–626.

58. **Juranek, D. D.** 1995. Cryptosporidiosis: sources of infection and guidelines for prevention. *Clin. Infect. Dis.* **21:**S57–S61.

59. **Katanik, M. T., S. K. Schneider, J. E. Rosenblatt, G. S. Hall, and G. W. Procop.** 2001. Evaluation of ColorPAC *Giardia/Cryptosporidium* rapid assay and ProSpecT *Giardia/Cryptosporidium* microplate assay for detection of *Giardia* and *Cryptosporidium* in fecal specimens. *J. Clin. Microbiol.* **39**:4523–4525.

60. **Katsumata, T., D. Hosea, E. B. Wasito, S. Kohno, K. Hara, P. Soeparto, and I. G. Ranuh.** 1998. Cryptosporidiosis in Indonesia: a hospital-based study and a community-based survey. *Am. J. Trop. Med. Hyg.* **59**:628–632.

61. **Khalakdina, A., D. J. Vugia, J. Nadle, G. A. Rothrock, and J. M. Colford, Jr.** 2003. Is drinking water a risk factor for endemic cryptosporidiosis? A case-control study in the immunocompetent general population of the San Francisco Bay Area. *BMC Public Health* **3**:11.

62. **Lake, I. R., F. C. Harrison, R. M. Chalmers, G. Bentham, G. Nichols, P. R. Hunter, R. S. Kovats, and C. Grundy.** 2007. Case-control study of environmental and social factors influencing cryptosporidiosis. *Eur. J. Epidemiol.* **22**:805–811.

63. **Leach, C. T., F. C. Koo, T. L. Kuhls, S. G. Hilsenbeck, and H. B. Jenson.** 2000. Prevalence of *Cryptosporidium parvum* infection in children along the Texas-Mexico border and associated risk factors. *Am. J. Trop. Med. Hyg.* **62**:656–661.

64. **Leander, B. S.** 2008. Marine gregarines: evolutionary prelude to the apicomplexan radiation? *Trends Parasitol.* **24**:60–67.

65. **Learmonth, J. J., G. Ionas, K. A. Ebbett, and E. S. Kwan.** 2004. Genetic characterization and transmission cycles of *Cryptosporidium* species isolated from humans in New Zealand. *Appl. Environ. Microbiol.* **70**:3973–3978.

66. **Leoni, F., C. I. Gallimore, J. Green, and J. McLauchlin.** 2003. Molecular epidemiological analysis of *Cryptosporidium* isolates from humans and animals by using a heteroduplex mobility assay and nucleic acid sequencing based on a small double-stranded RNA element. *J. Clin. Microbiol.* **41**:981–992.

67. **Leoni, F., M. E. Mallon, H. V. Smith, A. Tait, and J. McLauchlin.** 2007. Multilocus analysis of *Cryptosporidium hominis* and *Cryptosporidium parvum* from sporadic and outbreak-related human cases and *C. parvum* isolates from sporadic cases in livestock in the United Kingdom. *J. Clin. Microbiol.* **45**:3286–3294.

68. **Lumadue, J. A., Y. C. Manabe, R. D. Moore, P. C. Belitsos, C. L. Sears, and D. P. Clark.** 1998. A clinicopathologic analysis of AIDS-related cryptosporidiosis. *AIDS* **12**:2459–2466.

69. **Maggi, P., A. M. Larocca, M. Quarto, G. Serio, O. Brandonisio, G. Angarano, and G. Pastore.** 2000. Effect of antiretroviral therapy on cryptosporidiosis and microsporidiosis in patients infected with human immunodeficiency virus type 1. *Eur. J. Clin. Microbiol. Infect. Dis.* **19**:213–217.

70. **Mallon, M., A. MacLeod, J. Wastling, H. Smith, B. Reilly, and A. Tait.** 2003. Population structures and the role of genetic exchange in the zoonotic pathogen *Cryptosporidium parvum*. *J. Mol. Evol.* **56**:407–417.

71. **Mallon, M. E., A. MacLeod, J. M. Wastling, H. Smith, and A. Tait.** 2003. Multilocus genotyping of *Cryptosporidium parvum* Type 2: population genetics and sub-structuring. *Infect. Genet. Evol.* **3**:207–218.

72. **Manabe, Y. C., D. P. Clark, R. D. Moore, J. A. Lumadue, H. R. Dahlman, P. C. Belitsos, R. E. Chaisson, and C. L. Sears.** 1998. Cryptosporidiosis in patients with AIDS—correlates of disease and survival. *Clin. Infect. Dis.* **27**:536–542.

73. **Masur, H., J. E. Kaplan, and K. K. Holmes.** 2002. Guidelines for preventing opportunistic infections among HIV-infected persons—2002. Recommendations of the U.S. Public Health Service and the Infectious Diseases Society of America. *Ann. Intern. Med.* **137**:435–478.

74. **McLauchlin, J., C. Amar, S. Pedraza-Diaz, and G. L. Nichols.** 2000. Molecular epidemiological analysis of *Cryptosporidium* spp. in the United Kingdom: results of genotyping *Cryptosporidium* spp. in 1,705 fecal samples from humans and 105 fecal samples from livestock animals. *J. Clin. Microbiol.* **38**:3984–3990.

75. **McLauchlin, J., C. F. Amar, S. Pedraza-Diaz, G. Mieli-Vergani, N. Hadzic, and E. G. Davies.** 2003. Polymerase chain reaction-based diagnosis of infection with *Cryptosporidium* in children with primary immunodeficiencies. *Pediatr. Infect. Dis. J.* **22**:329–335.

76. **Mead, P. S., L. Slutsker, V. Dietz, L. F. McCaig, J. S. Bresee, C. Shapiro, P. M. Griffin, and R. V. Tauxe.** 1999. Food-related illness and death in the United States. *Emerg. Infect. Dis.* **5**:607–625.

77. **Millard, P. S., K. F. Gensheimer, D. G. Addiss, D. M. Sosin, G. A. Beckett, A. Houck-Jankoski, and A. Hudson.** 1994. An outbreak of cryptosporidiosis from fresh-pressed apple cider. *JAMA* **272**:1592–1596.

78. **Molbak, K., P. Aaby, N. Hojlyng, and A. P. da Silva.** 1994. Risk factors for *Cryptosporidium* diarrhea in early childhood: a case-control study from Guinea-Bissau, West Africa. *Am. J. Epidemiol.* **139**:734–740.

79. **Mor, S. M., A. DeMaria, Jr., J. K. Griffiths, and E. N. Naumova.** 2009. Cryptosporidiosis in the elderly population of the United States. *Clin. Infect. Dis.* **48**:698–705.

80. **Mor, S. M., and S. Tzipori.** 2008. Cryptosporidiosis in children in sub-saharan Africa: a lingering challenge. *Clin. Infect. Dis.* **47**:915–921.

81. **Nichols, G. L., R. M. Chalmers, W. Sopwith, M. Regan, C. A. Hunter, P. Grenfell, F. Harrison, and C. Lane.** 2006. *Cryptosporidiosis: a Report on the Surveillance and Epidemiology of* Cryptosporidium *Infection in England and Wales.* Drinking Water Directorate Contract Number DWI 70/2/201. Drinking Water Inspectorate, London, United Kingdom.

82. **Nichols, R. A., B. M. Campbell, and H. V. Smith.** 2003. Identification of *Cryptosporidium* spp. oocysts in United Kingdom noncarbonated natural mineral waters and drinking waters by using a modified nested PCR-restriction fragment length polymorphism assay. *Appl. Environ. Microbiol.* **69**:4183–4189.

83. **Pantenburg, B., M. M. Cabada, and A. C. White, Jr.** 2009. Treatment of cryptosporidiosis. *Expert Rev. Anti-Infect. Ther.* **7**:385–391.

84. **Peng, M. M., S. R. Meshnick, N. A. Cunliffe, B. D. Thindwa, C. A. Hart, R. L. Broadhead, and L. Xiao.** 2003. Molecular epidemiology of cryptosporidiosis in children in Malawi. *J. Eukaryot. Microbiol.* **50**(Suppl.)**:**557–559.

85. **Pereira, M. D., E. R. Atwill, A. P. Barbosa, S. A. Silva, and M. T. Garcia-Zapata.** 2002. Intra-familial and extra-familial risk factors associated with *Cryptosporidium parvum* infection among children hospitalized for diarrhea in Goiania, Goias, Brazil. *Am. J. Trop. Med. Hyg.* **66**:787–793.

86. **Pintar, K. D., F. Pollari, D. Waltner-Toews, D. F. Charron, S. A. McEwen, A. Fazil, and A. Nesbitt.** 2009. A modified case-control study of cryptosporidiosis (using non-*Cryptosporidium*-infected enteric cases as controls) in a community setting. *Epidemiol. Infect.* **137**:1789–1799.

87. **Pollock, K. G., H. E. Ternent, D. J. Mellor, R. M. Chalmers, H. V. Smith, C. N. Ramsay, and G. T. Innocent.** 23 July 2009. Spatial and temporal epidemiology of sporadic human cryptosporidiosis in Scotland. *Zoonoses Public Health.* doi:10.1111/j.1863-2378.2009.01247.x.

88. **Ponka, A., P. Kotilainen, R. Rimhanen-Finne, P. Hokkanen, M. L. Hanninen, A. Kaarna, T. Meri, and M. Kuusi.** 2009. A foodborne outbreak due to *Cryptosporidium parvum* in Helsinki, November 2008. *Euro Surveill.* **14**:pii:19269.

89. **Quiroz, E. S., C. Bern, J. R. MacArthur, L. Xiao, M. Fletcher, M. J. Arrowood, D. K. Shay, M. E. Levy, R. I. Glass, and A. Lal.** 2000. An outbreak of cryptosporidiosis linked to a foodhandler. *J. Infect. Dis.* **181**:695–700.

90. **Regnath, T., T. Klemm, and R. Ignatius.** 2006. Rapid and accurate detection of *Giardia lamblia* and *Cryptosporidium* spp. antigens in human fecal specimens by new commercially available qualitative immunochromatographic assays. *Eur. J. Clin. Microbiol. Infect. Dis.* **25**:807–809.

91. **Rimhanen-Finne, R., H. L. Enemark, J. Kolehmainen, P. Toropainen, and M. L. Hanninen.** 2007. Evaluation of immunofluorescence microscopy and enzyme-linked immunosorbent assay in detection of *Cryptosporidium* and *Giardia* infections in asymptomatic dogs. *Vet. Parasitol.* **145**:345–348.

92. **Robertson, B., M. I. Sinclair, A. B. Forbes, M. Veitch, M. Kirk, D. Cunliffe, J. Willis, and C. K. Fairley.** 2002. Case-control studies of sporadic cryptosporidiosis in Melbourne and Adelaide, Australia. *Epidemiol. Infect.* **128**:419–431.

93. **Robertson, L. J., and B. Gjerde.** 2001. Occurrence of parasites on fruits and vegetables in Norway. *J. Food Prot.* **64:**1793–1798.

94. **Robinson, G., J. Watkins, and R. M. Chalmers.** 2008. Evaluation of a modified semi-automated immunomagnetic separation technique for the detection of *Cryptosporidium* oocysts in human faeces. *J. Microbiol. Methods* **75:**139–141.

95. **Rosales, M. J., G. P. Cordon, M. S. Moreno, C. M. Sanchez, and C. Mascaro.** 2005. Extracellular like-gregarine stages of *Cryptosporidium parvum. Acta Trop.* **95:**74–78.

96. **Rossignol, J. F.** 2010. *Cryptosporidium and Giardia:* treatment options and prospects for new drugs. *Exp. Parasitol.* **124:**45–53.

97. **Roy, S. L., S. M. DeLong, S. A. Stenzel, B. Shiferaw, J. M. Roberts, A. Khalakdina, R. Marcus, S. D. Segler, D. D. Shah, S. Thomas, D. J. Vugia, S. M. Zansky, V. Dietz, and M. J. Beach.** 2004. Risk factors for sporadic cryptosporidiosis among immunocompetent persons in the United States from 1999 to 2001. *J. Clin. Microbiol.* **42:**2944–2951.

98. **Seyrafian, S., N. Pestehchian, M. Kerdegari, H. A. Yousefi, and B. Bastani.** 2006. Prevalence rate of *Cryptosporidium* infection in hemodialysis patients in Iran. *Hemodial. Int.* **10:**375–379.

99. **Smith, H. V.** 2008. Diagnostics, p. 173–207. *In* R. Fayer and L. Xiao (ed.), Cryptosporidium *and Cryptosporidiosis,* 2nd ed. CRC Press, Boca Raton, FL.

100. **Snel, S. J., M. G. Baker, and K. Venugopal.** 2009. The epidemiology of cryptosporidiosis in New Zealand, 1997–2006. *N. Z. Med. J.* **122:**47–61.

101. **Sorvillo, F., L. E. Lieb, B. Nahlen, J. Miller, L. Mascola, and L. R. Ash.** 1994. Municipal drinking water and cryptosporidiosis among persons with AIDS in Los Angeles County. *Epidemiol. Infect.* **113:**313–320.

102. **Srijan, A., B. Wongstitwilairoong, C. Pitarangsi, O. Serichantalergs, C. D. Fukuda, L. Bodhidatta, and C. J. Mason.** 2005. Re-evaluation of commercially available enzyme-linked immunosorbent assay for the detection of *Giardia lamblia* and *Cryptosporidium* spp from stool specimens. *Southeast Asian J. Trop. Med. Public Health* **36**(Suppl. 4):26–29.

103. **Sturbaum, G. D., C. Reed, P. J. Hoover, B. H. Jost, M. M. Marshall, and C. R. Sterling.** 2001. Species-specific, nested PCR-restriction fragment length polymorphism detection of single *Cryptosporidium parvum* oocysts. *Appl. Environ. Microbiol.* **67:**2665–2668.

104. **Sulaiman, I. M., P. R. Hira, L. Zhou, F. M. Al-Ali, F. A. Al-Shelahi, H. M. Shweiki, J. Iqbal, N. Khalid, and L. Xiao.** 2005. Unique endemicity of cryptosporidiosis in children in Kuwait. *J. Clin. Microbiol.* **43:**2805–2809.

105. **Tanriverdi, S., A. Grinberg, R. M. Chalmers, P. R. Hunter, Z. Petrovic, D. E. Akiyoshi, E. London, L. Zhang, S. Tzipori, J. K. Tumwine, and G. Widmer.** 2008. Inferences about the global population structure of *Cryptosporidium parvum* and *Cryptosporidium hominis. Appl. Environ. Microbiol.* **74:**7227–7234.

106. **Tanriverdi, S., A. Markovics, M. O. Arslan, A. Itik, V. Shkap, and G. Widmer.** 2006. Emergence of distinct genotypes of *Cryptosporidium parvum* in structured host populations. *Appl. Environ. Microbiol.* **72:**2507–2513.

107. **Tran, M. Q., R. Y. Gohh, P. E. Morrissey, L. D. Dworkin, A. Gautam, A. P. Monaco, and A. F. Yango, Jr.** 2005. *Cryptosporidium* infection in renal transplant patients. *Clin. Nephrol.* **63:**305–309.

108. **Tumwine, J. K., A. Kekitiinwa, N. Nabukeera, D. E. Akiyoshi, S. M. Rich, G. Widmer, X. Feng, and S. Tzipori.** 2003. *Cryptosporidium parvum* in children with diarrhea in Mulago Hospital, Kampala, Uganda. *Am. J. Trop. Med. Hyg.* **68:**710–715.

109. **Weber, R., R. T. Bryan, H. S. Bishop, S. P. Wahlquist, J. J. Sullivan, and D. D. Juranek.** 1991. Threshold of detection of *Cryptosporidium* oocysts in human stool specimens: evidence for low sensitivity of current diagnostic methods. *J. Clin. Microbiol.* **29:**1323–1327.

110. **Webster, K. A., H. V. Smith, M. Giles, L. Dawson, and L. J. Robertson.** 1996. Detection of *Cryptosporidium parvum* oocysts in faeces: comparison of conventional coproscopical methods and the polymerase chain reaction. *Vet. Parasitol.* **61:**5–13.

111. **Weitzel, T., S. Dittrich, I. Mohl, E. Adusu, and T. Jelinek.** 2006. Evaluation of seven commercial antigen detection tests for *Giardia* and *Cryptosporidium* in stool samples. *Clin. Microbiol. Infect.* **12:**656–659.

112. **Werneck-Silva, A. L., and I. B. Prado.** 2009. Gastroduodenal opportunistic infections and dyspepsia in HIV-infected patients in the era of Highly Active Antiretroviral Therapy. *J. Gastroenterol. Hepatol.* **24:**135–139.

113. **Widmer, G.** 2009. Meta-analysis of a polymorphic surface glycoprotein of the parasitic protozoa *Cryptosporidium parvum* and *Cryptosporidium hominis. Epidemiol. Infect.* **137:**1800–1808.

114. **Wolska-Kusnierz, B., A. Bajer, S. Caccio, E. Heropolitanska-Pliszka, E. Bernatowska, P. Socha, J. van Dongen, M. Bednarska, A. Paziewska, and E. Sinski.** 2007. *Cryptosporidium* infection in patients with primary immunodeficiencies. *J. Pediatr. Gastroenterol. Nutr.* **45:**458–464.

115. **Xiao, L.** 2010. Molecular epidemiology of cryptosporidiosis: an update. *Exp. Parasitol.* **124:**80–89.

116. **Xiao, L., L. Escalante, C. Yang, I. Sulaiman, A. A. Escalante, R. J. Montali, R. Fayer, and A. A. Lal.** 1999. Phylogenetic analysis of *Cryptosporidium* parasites based on the small-subunit rRNA gene locus. *Appl. Environ. Microbiol.* **65:**1578–1583.

117. **Xiao, L., and R. Fayer.** 2008. Molecular characterisation of species and genotypes of *Cryptosporidium* and *Giardia* and assessment of zoonotic transmission. *Int. J. Parasitol.* **38:**1239–1255.

118. **Xiao, L., R. Fayer, U. Ryan, and S. J. Upton.** 2004. *Cryptosporidium* taxonomy: recent advances and implications for public health. *Clin. Microbiol. Rev.* **17:**72–97.

119. **Xiao, L., and Y. Feng.** 2008. Zoonotic cryptosporidiosis. *FEMS Immunol. Med. Microbiol.* **52:**309–323.

120. **Xiao, L., and U. M. Ryan.** 2008. Molecular epidemiology, p. 119–171. *In* R. Fayer and L. Xiao (ed.), Cryptosporidium *and Cryptosporidiosis,* 2nd ed. CRC Press, Boca Raton, FL.

121. **Yoder, J. S., and M. J. Beach.** 2007. Cryptosporidiosis surveillance—United States, 2003–2005. *MMWR Surveill. Summ.* **56:**1–10.

122. **Yoder, J. S., and M. J. Beach.** 2010. *Cryptosporidium* surveillance and risk factors in the United States. *Exp. Parasitol.* **124:**31–39.

123. **Yoshida, H., M. Matsuo, T. Miyoshi, K. Uchino, H. Nakaguchi, T. Fukumoto, Y. Teranaka, and T. Tanaka.** 2007. An outbreak of cryptosporidiosis suspected to be related to contaminated Food, October 2006, Sakai City, Japan. *Jpn. J. Infect. Dis.* **60:**405–407.

124. **Yu, J. R., S. P. O'Hara, J. L. Lin, M. E. Dailey, and G. Cain.** 2002. A common oocyst surface antigen of *Cryptosporidium* recognized by monoclonal antibodies. *Parasitol. Res.* **88:**412–420.

125. **Zardi, E. M., A. Picardi, and A. Afeltra.** 2005. Treatment of cryptosporidiosis in immunocompromised hosts. *Chemotherapy* **51:**193–196.

Microsporidia*

RAINER WEBER, PETER DEPLAZES, AND ALEXANDER MATHIS

140

TAXONOMY

Microsporidia are obligate intracellular, spore-forming protists. More than 140 microsporidial genera and 1,200 species that are parasitic in every major animal group have been identified (22, 27, 51, 72). To date, seven genera (*Anncaliia*, *Encephalitozoon*, *Enterocytozoon*, *Nosema*, *Pleistophora*, *Vittaforma*, and *Trachipleistophora*) and unclassified microsporidia, assigned to the collective group *Microsporidium*, have been implicated in human infections (Table 1).

Microsporidia develop intracellularly exclusively and have no metabolically active stages outside the host cell. A life cycle (Fig. 1) involving a proliferative merogonic sequence followed by a sporogonic sequence results in environmentally resistant spores of unique structure. Mature spores contain a tubular extrusion apparatus (polar tube) for injecting infective spore contents (sporoplasm) into the host cell.

Microsporidia are true eukaryotes because they have a membrane-bound nucleus, an intracytoplasmic membrane system, and chromosome separation on mitotic spindles, but they are unusual eukaryotes in that they have bacterium-like ribosomes, no recognizable mitochondria, no peroxisomes, and simple vesicular Golgi membranes. Compared with those of other eukaryotes, the genomes of microsporidia are reduced in size and complexity (2, 43). The genome sizes of different microsporidia vary between 2.3 and 19.5 Mb, and the numbers of chromosomes range from 7 to 16 (80). The compactness of the microsporidial genomes results from the loss of genes and from the reduction of coding and noncoding elements. The small-subunit rRNA genes of microsporidia, for example, are significantly shorter than those of other eukaryotes and even those of some prokaryotes.

It has previously been postulated that, phylogenetically, microsporidia are ancient protists that diverged before the mitochondrial endosymbiosis (70). However, genes related to mitochondrial functions were identified in *Encephalitozoon cuniculi*, implying that microsporidia have retained a mitochondrion-derived organelle (43). Indeed, tiny organelles with double membranes were visualized by using antibodies against the mitochondrial heat shock protein 70 in the microsporidian *Trachipleistophora hominis* (79). Recent genome-wide sequence and synteny analyses indicate that the parasites of the phylum Microsporidia belong to the kingdom of the Fungi (37), being derived from an endoparasitic chytrid ancestor on the earliest diverging branch of the fungal phylogenetic tree (35, 40, 48, 62). Also, structural features of the organisms such as the presence of chitin in the spore wall, diplokaryotic nuclei, and electron-dense spindle plaques associated with the nuclear envelope suggest a possible relationship between fungi and microsporidia, whereas the life cycle of microsporidia is unique and dissimilar to that of any fungal species.

DESCRIPTION OF THE GENERA AND SPECIES

The species are illustrated in Fig. 1 and listed in Table 1.

Nosema spp. develop in direct contact with host cell cytoplasm, nuclei are paired (diplokaryotic), divisions are by binary fission, and sporonts are disporoblastic. Only one species of human origin, *Nosema ocularum*, has been retained in this genus. It will probably require reclassification, but insufficient information is currently available for a new generic assignment. Spores measure 3 by 5 μm and have polar tubes with 9 to 12 coils.

Anncaliia spp. have diplokaryotic nuclei and develop in direct contact with host cell cytoplasm. Additionally, the organisms produce electron-dense extracellular secretions and vesiculotubular appendages. Three former members of the microsporidial genus *Brachiola* that are pathogenic in humans were transferred to the genus *Anncaliia* based on novel ultrastructural and molecular data (33). Disporoblastic sporogony of *Anncaliia vesicularum* (formerly *Brachiola vesicularum*) produces 2.5- by 2-μm diplokaryotic spores containing 7 to 10 anisofilar coils of the polar filament arranged in one to three rows, usually two (8, 33). On the basis of diplokaryotic nuclei, disporoblastic sporogony, and the formation of vesiculotubular secretions, *Nosema connori* and *Nosema algerae*, also discovered in human infections, have been reclassified as species of *Anncaliia*. Spores of *Anncaliia connori* measure 2.0 to 2.5 by 4.0 to 4.5 μm and contain polar tubes with 10 to 12 coils (49). Spores of *Anncaliia algerae* measure 3.7 to 5.4 by 2.3 to 3.9 μm and have 8 to 11 coils of the polar tube (9).

Vittaforma corneae, originally classified as *Nosema corneum*, was transferred to a new genus on the basis of ultrastructural features (60). Nuclei are diplokaryotic, sporogony is polysporoblastic, sporonts are ribbon shaped, and all stages including spores are individually enveloped

---

*This chapter contains information presented in chapter 135 by Rainer Weber and Elizabeth U. Canning in the eighth edition of this *Manual*.

TABLE 1 Microsporidial species pathogenic in humans, and clinical manifestations

Microsporidial species	Clinical manifestations	
	Immunocompromised patients	Immunocompetent persons
Anncaliia algerae (formerly *Brachiola algerae*, *Nosema algerae*)	Myositis, nodular cutaneous lesions	Keratitis
Anncaliia connori (formerly *Brachiola connori*, *Nosema connori*)	Disseminated infection	Not described
Anncaliia vesicularum (formerly *Brachiola vesicularum*)	Myositis	Not described
Encephalitozoon cuniculi	Disseminated infection, keratoconjunctivitis, sinusitis, bronchitis, pneumonia, nephritis, hepatitis, peritonitis, symptomatic and asymptomatic intestinal infection, encephalitis	Not described; two HIV-seronegative children with seizure disorder and presumed *E. cuniculi* infection presumably were immunocompromised
Encephalitozoon hellem	Disseminated infection, keratoconjunctivitis, sinusitis, bronchitis, pneumonia, nephritis, ureteritis, cystitis, prostatitis, urethritis	Possibly diarrhea[a]
Encephalitozoon intestinalis (formerly *Septata intestinalis*)	Chronic diarrhea, cholangiopathy, sinusitis, bronchitis, pneumonitis, nephritis, bone infection, nodular cutaneous lesions	Self-limiting diarrhea, asymptomatic carriers
Enterocytozoon bieneusi	Chronic diarrhea, wasting syndrome, "AIDS-cholangiopathy," cholangitis, acalculous cholecystitis, chronic sinusitis, chronic cough, pneumonitis	Self-limiting diarrhea in adults and children, traveler's diarrhea, asymptomatic carriers
Microsporidium africanum[b]	Not described	Corneal ulcer, keratitis
Microsporidium ceylonensis[b]	Not described	Corneal ulcer, keratitis
Microsporidia (not classified)	Not described	Keratoconjunctivitis in contact lens wearer
Nosema ocularum	Not described	Keratitis
Pleistophora ronneafiei	Myositis	Not described
Pleistophora sp.	Myositis	Not described
Trachipleistophora anthropophthera	Disseminated infection, keratitis	Not described
Trachipleistophora hominis	Myositis, myocarditis, keratoconjunctivitis, sinusitis	Keratitis
Vittaforma corneae (formerly *Nosema corneum*)	Disseminated infection, urinary tract infection	Keratitis

[a] *E. hellem* has been detected using PCR among persons with traveler's diarrhea and coinfection with *Enterocytozoon* sp. (57); thus, the pathogenic role of *E. hellem* remains unknown. Microscopic detection of *E. hellem* spores in stool has not been reported so far.

[b] *Microsporidium* is a collective generic name for microsporidia that cannot be classified because available information is not sufficient.

by a cisterna of host endoplasmic reticulum studded with ribosomes. The spores contain polar tubes with five to seven coils and measure 1.2 by 3.8 μm.

Pleistophora spp., including *Pleistophora ronneafiei*, which is pathogenic in humans, have unpaired nuclei, and all stages are multinucleate plasmodia, which divide into smaller multinucleate segments. Meronts have a thick, amorphous coat, which separates from the surface in sporogony to form a sporophorous vesicle. Sporogonic divisions give rise to a large and variable number of spores, packaged in the persistent sporophorous vesicle. The spores contain polar tubes with 9 to 12 coils and measure 2 to 2.8 by 3.3 to 4.0 μm (7).

Trachipleistophora hominis also forms spores in sporophorous vesicles, but these arise from repeated binary fissions and not from multinucleate plasmodia. The vesicles, which contain 2 to more than 32 spores, enlarge as the number of spores increases. The nuclei are unpaired in all stages of development. The pear-shaped spores measure 2.4 by 4.0 μm and have about 11 anisofilar coils (32, 38). *Trachipleistophora anthropophthera* is similar to *T. hominis* but appears to be dimorphic, as two different forms of sporophorous vesicles and spores have been observed (66).

Enterocytozoon bieneusi develops in direct contact with host cell cytoplasm (Fig. 2). The proliferative and sporogonial forms are rounded multinucleate plasmodia with unpaired nuclei measuring up to 6 μm in diameter. The oval spores measure 0.7 to 1.0 by 1.1 to 1.6 μm. The polar tube, derived from electron-dense disks in sporonts, has five to seven isofilar coils that appear in two rows when seen in transverse section by transmission electron microscopy (20).

Encephalitozoon spp. develop intracellularly in parasitophorous vacuoles bounded by a membrane of presumed host cell origin. Nuclei of all stages are unpaired. Meronts divide repeatedly by binary fission and lie close to the vacuolar membrane. Sporonts appear free in the center of the vacuole and divide into two or four sporoblasts, which mature into spores. The spores measure 1.0 to 1.5 by 2.0 to 3.0 μm, and the polar tube has four to eight isofilar coils.

E. cuniculi was isolated from a range of animals before human infections were identified. Human isolates of three *Encephalitozoon* spp. and animal isolates of *E. cuniculi* are morphologically almost identical. In 1991, *Encephalitozoon hellem* was distinguished from *E. cuniculi* on the basis of different protein patterns found by sodium dodecyl sulfate-polyacrylamide gel electrophoresis separation and immunoblotting (24). In 1993, *Septata intestinalis* was described and named on the basis of the morphological finding that the intracellular vacuoles containing the parasites showed a unique parasite-secreted fibrillar network surrounding the developing organisms, so that the vacuoles appeared septate (6). Subsequently, on the

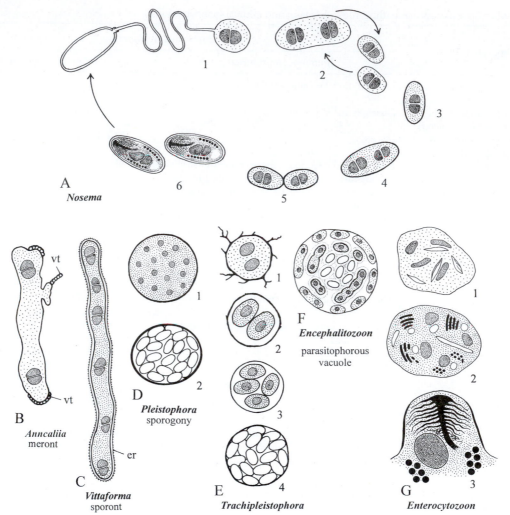

FIGURE 1 Generalized life cycle of microsporidia and identifying characteristics of the genera known to infect humans. Light stippling indicates merogonic stages; heavy stippling indicates sporogonic stages; no stippling indicates spores and sporoplasm. (A) Basic life cycle, illustrated by *Nosema*. Development may occur in direct contact with host cell cytoplasm (*Nosema*, *Anncaliia*, and *Enterocytozoon*) or in isolation by host cell membranes (*Vittaforma* and *Encephalitozoon*) or a cyst-like sporophorous vesicle of parasite origin (*Pleistophora* and *Trachipleistophora*). 1, Sporoplasm: the infective stage emergent from the spore. It may have unpaired nuclei (monokaryotic) or two nuclei in close apposition (diplokaryotic), depending on the genus. 2, Merogony: proliferative stage. It may have a simple plasma membrane, but a surface coat is present in *Anncaliia*, *Pleistophora*, and *Trachipleistophora*. Division can be by binary or multiple fission into two or more individuals. 3, Sporont: the first stage of sporogony. If not already present, a surface coat is added (this step is delayed in *Enterocytozoon*). 4, Sporogony: divisions culminating in spore production. Binary or multiple fissions give rise to sporoblasts. 5, Sporoblasts: end products of sporogony, which mature into spores. 6, Spores: resistant stages for transmission. Spores are characterized by an extrusion apparatus (polar tube), which serves to conduct the sporoplasm into a host cell. The polar tube may be of uniform diameter (isofilar) or show a sharp decrease in diameter in the most posterior coils (anisofilar). (B to G) Identifying characteristics of genera. (B) *Anncaliia*. Members of this genus are diplokaryotic and disporoblastic; the life cycle is like that of *Nosema*, but meronts are of bizarre shapes and possess a surface coat with vesiculotubular structures (vt) embedded in it and extended from it. (C) *Vittaforma*. Members of this genus are diplokaryotic and polysporoblastic; all stages, including spores, are isolated in a close-fitting, ribosome-studded cisterna of host endoplasmic reticulum (er). (D) *Pleistophora*. Members of this genus are monokaryotic and polysporoblastic; meronts and sporonts are multinucleate stages called plasmodia; a thick surface coat is already present on meronts and sporonts (1); this coat separates from the sporogonial plasmodium to form a cyst-like vesicle, the sporophorous vesicle; the plasmodium divides within it to produce numerous spores (2). (E) *Trachipleistophora*. Members of this genus are monokaryotic and polysporoblastic. The meront surface coat has branched extensions (1); these are withdrawn when the coat separates to form the sporophorous vesicle around a uninucleate sporont; the sporont undergoes a series of binary fissions (2 and 3) and finally encloses numerous spores (4). (F) *Encephalitozoon*. Members of this genus are monokaryotic and di- or tetrasporoblastic; all stages of the life cycle, developing from the sporoplasm, occur concurrently within a host cell vacuole (parasitophorous vacuole); merogonic stages are appressed against the vacuole wall; sporogonic stages are free; the vacuole is finally packed with spores, so that it superficially resembles a sporophorous vesicle. (G) *Enterocytozoon*. Members of this genus are monokaryotic and polysporoblastic; meronts (1) have irregular nuclei and lucent clefts; sporonts (2) are multinucleate with rounded nuclei and have highly characteristic electron-dense disks, which are polar tube precursors; all spore organelles are formed prematurely, so that constriction around the sets of organelles and a nucleus (3) gives rise directly to almost mature spores. The surface coat is deposited only during constriction.

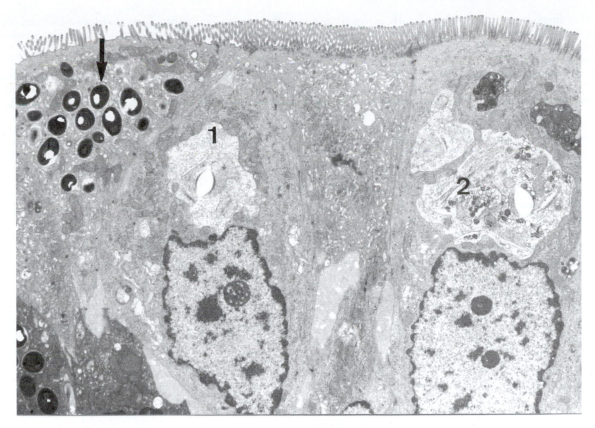

FIGURE 2 Transmission electron micrograph showing the duodenal epithelium of an HIV-infected patient infected with *E. bieneusi*. The different developmental stages between the enterocyte nuclei and the microvillus border include a proliferative plasmodium (1), late sporogonial plasmodia (2), and mature spores (arrow). Magnification, ×5,370. (Courtesy of M. A. Spycher, University Hospital, Zurich, Switzerland.)

basis of phylogenetic analyses, *S. intestinalis* was reclassified as *Encephalitozoon intestinalis*, and it was confirmed that the three *Encephalitozoon* spp. are indeed distinct organisms. Finally, with the use of immunological and molecular methods, three different strains of *E. cuniculi* have been identified which differ in animal host preferences and geographic distributions (26).

Microsporidium is a collective generic name for microsporidia that cannot be classified because available information is not sufficient. *Microsporidium ceylonensis* and *Microsporidium africanum* have been assigned to the group name (11).

EPIDEMIOLOGY AND TRANSMISSION

Human microsporidial infections have been documented globally. The sources of microsporidia infecting humans and their modes of transmission are uncertain. Ingestion of the environmentally highly resistant spores is probably the normal mode of transmission. Possible transmission by the aerosol route has also been considered because microsporidia have been found in respiratory specimens. Studies with mammals suggest that *Encephalitozoon* spp. can be transmitted transplacentally from mother to offspring, but no congenitally acquired human infections have been reported.

Direct zoonotic transmission of microsporidia infecting humans has not been verified but appears likely because many microsporidial species can infect both humans and animals (10, 51). *E. cuniculi* is considered to be a zoonotic parasite (50). Two of the three different strains of *E. cuniculi* that were

detected in natural infections in rabbits and dogs have been isolated from human immunodeficiency virus (HIV)-infected patients (18, 26). In addition to documentation in humans, *E. hellem* has been detected in psittacines kept in aviaries and in a variety of wild birds, and *E. intestinalis* has been reported in single studies with domestic animals in Mexico (4) and gorillas in Uganda. *E. bieneusi*, discovered in humans, is increasingly being recognized in animals (wildlife, livestock, and companion animals). Analyses of the rRNA genes' internal transcribed spacers revealed more than 150 genotypes, 26 of which have been identified exclusively in humans, 8 in humans and animals, and the remaining in a variety of animal hosts (59, 61). Also, an insect-pathogenic microsporidian, *A. algerae*, was isolated from three patients (16, 68, 69).

Epidemiologic studies suggest water contact as a risk factor for microsporidiosis, and *E. bieneusi*, *E. intestinalis*, and *V. corneae* homologous DNA has been detected in sewage effluent, groundwater, and surface water (36, 42). Furthermore, microsporidia pathogenic in humans have been detected in fresh food produce (41), in milk specimens from dairy cows (47), and in feces of captive and free-ranging birds, including urban feral pigeons, which may contribute to dissemination of human waterborne pathogens (3, 36).

CLINICAL SIGNIFICANCE

Although microsporidiosis appears to occur most frequently in persons infected with HIV, it is emerging as an infection in other immunocompromised hosts (such as organ transplant recipients and patients with idiopathic or other CD4 T lymphocytopenia) as well as in immunocompetent individuals (Table 1) (72). Microsporidiosis has been associated with abnormalities in structures and functions of infected organs, but the mechanisms of pathogenicity of the different microsporidial species are not sufficiently understood. Patients with severe cellular immunodeficiency appear to be at the highest risk for developing microsporidial disease. Unfortunately, little is known about immunity to this infection, although the importance of T cells has been demonstrated in experiments with athymic mice. It is not understood whether microsporidiosis in immunocompromised patients is primarily a reactivation of latent infection acquired prior to the state of suppressed immunity or whether microsporidial disease is caused by recently acquired infection.

Enterocytozoon bieneusi

E. bieneusi infects the enterocytes of the small intestine and epithelial cells of the biliary tree and respiratory tract. Clinical disease is probably caused by the continuous excess loss of epithelial cells. *Enterocytozoon* infection may be accompanied by alterations in small bowel physiology such as decreased brush border sucrase, lactase, and maltase activities, as well as malabsorption.

E. bieneusi is estimated to be one of the most important HIV-associated intestinal pathogens, present in 5 to 30% of patients with chronic diarrhea, weight loss, or cholangiopathy, particularly when CD4 lymphocyte counts are below 100 per μl (75). Upper or lower respiratory tract infections have been detected in a few patients (74), but systemic infection due to *E. bieneusi* has not been documented. Case reports have documented that the parasite is also a cause of diarrhea in organ transplant recipients (45).

In immunocompetent adults and in children, *E. bieneusi* is associated with self-limited watery diarrhea (lasting up to 2 to 3 weeks), particularly among persons who reside (5, 58) or have traveled (78) in tropical countries. Furthermore, the parasite has been identified among malnourished children in tropical areas (2) and elderly persons (residing in resource-rich countries) with acute or chronic diarrhea.

Encephalitozoon spp.

Encephalitozoon spp. infect epithelial and endothelial cells, fibroblasts, macrophages, and possibly other cell types, as reported for humans and mammals. *Encephalitozoon* (identified as *E. cuniculi* because this was the only species known at that time) was initially identified in two children with a seizure disorder (73).

The spectrum of recognized *E. cuniculi*- and *E. hellem*-associated disease in patients with AIDS, organ transplant recipients, and otherwise immunocompromised patients includes keratoconjunctivitis, intraocular infection, sinusitis, bronchiolitis, pneumonitis, nephritis, ureteritis, cystitis, prostatitis, urethritis, hepatitis, sclerosing cholangitis, peritonitis, diarrhea, and encephalitis (18, 24, 72, 73). Clinical manifestations may vary substantially, ranging from an asymptomatic carrier state to organ failure.

E. intestinalis infects primarily enterocytes, but the parasite is also found in intestinal lamina propria, and dissemination to the kidneys, airways, and biliary tract appears to occur via infected macrophages (6). Chronic diarrhea and disseminated disease due to *E. intestinalis* have been diagnosed mainly in immunodeficient patients. A case of nodular cutaneous *E. intestinalis* infection was observed in a patient with AIDS (44). Furthermore, *E. intestinalis* has been detected in stool specimens from otherwise healthy children and adults,

with or without diarrhea, living in Mexico (30) and among travelers with diarrhea returning from tropical countries.

Other Microsporidia

Different microsporidial species have been isolated from otherwise healthy persons who presented with keratoconjunctivitis, severe keratitis, or corneal ulcers (Table 1) (14, 72). Also, keratoconjunctivitis due to microsporidia has been diagnosed in an immunocompetent contact lens wearer.

In immunocompromised patients, myositis has been linked to infections with different microsporidia, including *Pleistophora* sp. (46), *P. ronneafiei* sp. (7), *T. hominis* (32), *A. vesicularum* (8), and *A. algerae* (16). *A. algerae* has also been isolated from erythematous skin nodules from a boy with acute lymphocytic leukemia (69).

T. anthropophthera has been identified at autopsy in cerebral, cardiac, renal, pancreatic, thyroid, hepatic, splenic, lymphoid, and bone marrow tissue of patients with AIDS who initially presented with seizures (83). Disseminated infection due to *A. connori* was found at autopsy in a 4-month-old athymic male infant (Table 1).

COLLECTION, TRANSPORT, AND STORAGE OF SPECIMENS

Spores of enteropathogenic microsporidia can be detected in stool specimens or duodenal aspirates that have been fixed in 10% formalin or in sodium acetate-acetic acid-formalin, fresh stool samples, or biopsy specimens. The spores of microsporidia causing disseminated infection can usually be detected in fresh or fixed urine sediments, other body fluids (including sputum, bronchoalveolar lavage fluid, nasal secretions, cerebrospinal fluid, and conjunctival smears), corneal scrapings, or tissue. For histological examination, tissue specimens are fixed in formalin. For electron microscopy, fixation of tissue with glutaraldehyde is preferred. Collection of fresh material (without fixative) may be useful for cell culture and for molecular identification. Microsporidial spores are environmentally resistant and, if prevented from drying, can remain infectious for periods of up to several years.

DETECTION PROCEDURES

The most robust technique for the diagnosis of microsporidial infection is light microscopic detection of the parasites themselves. Spores, the stages at which microsporidia pathogenic in humans are usually identified, are small, ranging in size from 1 to 4 μm. Evaluation of patients with suspected intestinal microsporidiosis should begin with light microscopic examination of stool specimens, and microsporidia which cause systemic infection are best detected in urine sediments or other body fluids. Definitive species identification of microsporidia is made by electron microscopy, antigenic analysis, or, preferably, molecular analysis (34, 76).

Examination of Stool Specimens

Preparation of Smears, Staining, and Microscopic Examination

Smears are prepared using 10 to 20 μl of unconcentrated stool that is very thinly spread onto slides. Most of the procedures that have been adapted for the concentration of ova and parasites fail to concentrate microsporidial spores present in stool specimens. The formalin-ethyl acetate concentration and different flotation methods remove significant amounts of fecal debris, and smears prepared from these concentrates appear to

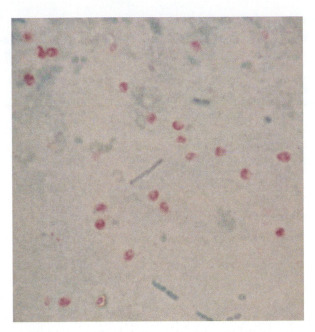

FIGURE 3 Smear of a stool specimen from a patient with AIDS and chronic diarrhea, showing pinkish red-stained spores of *E. bieneusi* that measure 0.7 to 1.0 by 1.1 to 1.6 μm. Chromotrope staining was used. Magnification, ×1,000 (oil immersion).

be easier to read by light microscopic examination than smears prepared from unconcentrated specimens. Such concentration techniques, however, lead to a substantial loss of microsporidial spores and may give false-negative results (71).

The most commonly used stains are chromotrope-based stains (71) and chemofluorescent optical brightening agents

(64, 65), including calcofluor white and other chemofluorescent stains. Regardless of which staining technique is utilized, the use of positive control material is essential. The detection of microsporidial spores requires adequate illumination and magnification, i.e., magnification of ×630 or ×1,000 (oil immersion). The differences in the sizes of *Enterocytozoon* spores (1 to 1.5 μm) and *Encephalitozoon* spores (2 to 3 μm) often permit a tentative identification of the genus from light microscopic examination of stool specimens.

Chromotrope-Based Staining Procedures

Microsporidial spores are ovoid and have a specific appearance when stained with chromotrope stains (Fig. 3 and 4, right panel) (71). The spore wall stains bright pinkish red, some spores appear transparent, and other spores show a distinct pinkish red-stained belt-like stripe that girds the spores diagonally or equatorially. Most background debris in stool specimens counterstains a faint green (or blue, depending on the staining technique). Some other fecal elements, such as yeasts and some bacteria, may also stain reddish, but they are distinguished from microsporidial spores by their sizes, shapes, and staining patterns.

Several modifications of the original chromotrope staining solution (71) have been proposed, including modifications of the counterstain and changes in the temperature of the standard chromotrope staining solution and in the staining time (25). An acid-fast trichrome stain (39) that permits visualization of acid-fast cryptosporidial oocysts as well as microsporidial spores on the same slide and a "quick-hot" Gram-chromotrope staining technique (56) have also been developed.

Chemofluorescent Agents

Chemofluorescent optical brightening agents are chitin stains, which require examination with a fluorescent microscope.

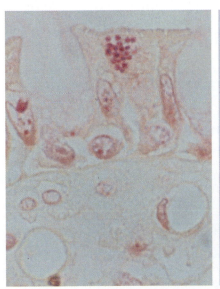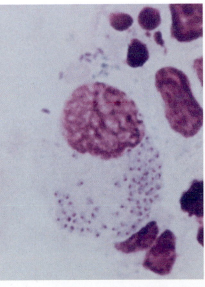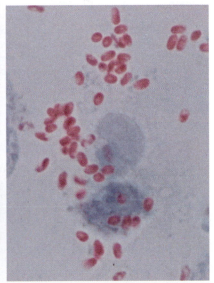

FIGURE 4 (Left) Terminal ileal tissue obtained by ileocolonoscopy from a patient with AIDS and chronic diarrhea due to *E. bieneusi* infection. Gram-labile microsporidial spores, measuring 0.7 to 1.0 by 1.1 to 1.6 μm, are found at a supranuclear location within small intestinal enterocytes. Brown-Brenn stain was used. Magnification, ×1,000. (Middle) Cytospin preparation of bronchoalveolar lavage fluid from a patient with AIDS and intestinal *E. bieneusi* infection, showing intracellular microsporidia. Giemsa stain was used. Magnification, ×1,000 (oil immersion). (Right) Urine sediment from a patient with AIDS and disseminated *E. cuniculi* infection, showing pinkish red-stained microsporidial spores measuring 1.0 to 1.5 by 2.0 to 3.0 μm. Chromotrope stain was used. Magnification, ×1,000 (oil immersion).

With the correct wavelength illumination, the chitinous wall of the microsporidial spores fluoresces brightly, facilitating the detection of spores (64). However, staining is not specific because small yeast cells, which may be present in fecal material, and other fecal elements may also be brightened. Some experience is necessary to distinguish the microsporidia.

Epidemiological comparisons of the chromotrope staining technique with methods that use chemofluorescent optical brighteners indicate that these tests are robust for routine use and that the sensitivities of both methods are similarly high (25). Some laboratories use both staining techniques because the chromotrope stains result in a highly specific visualization of spores whereas the chemofluorescent agents may be more sensitive but may produce false-positive results.

Immunofluorescent-Antibody Tests

Immunofluorescence procedures for the detection of *Encephalitozoon* and *Enterocytozoon* microsporidial spores are promising but not commercially available. Diagnostic application of polyclonal antibodies in fecal samples has been hampered by high levels of background staining, cross-reactions with yeast and bacteria, and sensitivity lower than those of chromotrope or chemofluorescent staining procedures (25). Monoclonal antibodies against *Encephalitozoon* spp. (29) and *E. bieneusi* (1) have been generated, of which some have been evaluated for diagnostic purposes with stool specimens (commercially not available).

Cytological Diagnosis

Microsporidial spores have been detected in sediments obtained by centrifugation of body fluids for 10 min at 500 × *g*, including duodenal aspirates, bile, biliary aspirates, urine (Fig. 4, right panel), bronchoalveolar lavage fluid (Fig. 4, middle panel), and cerebrospinal fluid, and in smears of conjunctival swabs, sputum, and nasal discharge. Microscopic examination of stained smears of centrifuged duodenal aspirate obtained during endoscopy is a highly sensitive technique for the diagnosis of intestinal microsporidiosis. Because microsporidial infection often involves multiple organs, the detection of microsporidia in virtually any tissue or body fluid should prompt a thorough search of other sites. Particularly for patients with suspected disseminated microsporidiosis, urine specimens should be examined (72, 76).

Examination of Biopsy Specimens and Corneal Scrapings

Examination of duodenal and terminal ileal tissue has resulted in the detection of intestinal microsporidia, but the parasites are rarely found in colonic tissue sections. Microsporidial species causing disseminated infection have been found in almost every organ system (72, 83).

Only highly experienced pathologists have reliably and consistently identified microsporidia in tissue sections by using routine techniques such as hematoxylin and eosin staining. Ultrathin plastic sections stained with methylene blue-azure II-basic fuchsin or with toluidine blue may facilitate detection. In our experience, tissue Gram stains (Brown-Brenn or Brown-Hopps) have proved to be the most useful for the rapid and reliable identification of HIV-associated microsporidia in routine paraffin-embedded tissue sections (Fig. 4, left panel) and corneal scrapings (71, 76). The microsporidial spores are gram variable, and they are readily identified because of the contrasting dark blue or reddish staining against a faint brown-yellow background. Others prefer a silver stain (Warthin-Starry stain) (31), the chromotrope-based staining technique, or chemofluorescent agents.

Molecular Techniques

Universal panmicrosporidian and genus- or species-specific primer pairs that target the rRNA genes and their application in the diagnosis of intestinal microsporidial infection have been described previously (77). The detection and identification of *E. bieneusi* and the different *Encephalitozoon* spp. have been successfully performed with fresh stool specimens, formalin-fixed stool specimens, intestinal tissue obtained by endoscopic biopsy, urine specimens, and other body fluids (17, 18). A real-time PCR method was developed for quantitation of *E. bieneusi* DNA (36) and *E. intestinalis* DNA (52) in stool specimens. Furthermore, in situ hybridization to visualize *E. bieneusi* in tissue sections has been developed (13).

ISOLATION OF MICROSPORIDIA

Microsporidia cannot be grown axenically. *Encephalitozoon* spp., *T. hominis*, *V. corneae*, and *A. algerae* have been isolated with different cell culture systems, including RK-13 (rabbit kidney), MDCK (Madin-Darby canine kidney), MRC-5 (human embryonic lung fibroblast) cells, and other cells (11, 19, 67). Only short-term in vitro propagation has been accomplished with *E. bieneusi* (67). The isolation of microsporidia has no relevance for diagnostic purposes but is an important research tool.

IDENTIFICATION

The identification of microsporidia and their taxonomy have been based primarily upon ultrastructural characteristics. Microsporidial ultrastructure is unique and pathognomonic for the phylum, and ultrastructural features can distinguish all microsporidial genera (Fig. 1) (11). Nevertheless, morphologic features alone do not sufficiently characterize all microsporidial species pathogenic for humans. The characterization of the three *Encephalitozoon* spp., which share most of their morphologic features, requires antigenic or molecular analyses, which may also reveal subtype-specific variation (24, 26). Phylogenetic relationships of different microsporidia pathogenic in humans, including *E. bieneusi* (61), *Pleistophora*-like organisms (15), *E. cuniculi*, *E. hellem*, and *E. intestinalis* (81, 82), have been investigated by analyses of small-subunit rRNA sequences, protein-encoding genes, and gene sequences encoding the largest subunit of the RNA polymerase.

SEROLOGIC TESTS

Serologic assays (including the carbon immunoassay, indirect immunofluorescence test, enzyme-linked immunosorbent assay, and Western blot immunodetection) have been useful in detecting specific antibodies to *E. cuniculi* in several species of animals. However, the value of such tests for humans has controversially been discussed because of possible cross-reactivity of the spore wall antigens of the *Encephalitozoon* spp. Furthermore, the results of serologic studies with humans were not substantiated by the detection of parasites in individuals with antibody responses. Recently, by employing recombinant antigens of the polar tube of *E. cuniculi*, improved specificity was demonstrated, and the development of serodiagnostic tools seems feasible (63). *Enterocytozoon*, the most frequent microsporidian pathogen in humans, has not been continuously propagated to produce antigens.

ANTIMICROBIAL SUSCEPTIBILITIES

Albendazole has been found to cause growth deformities of *Encephalitozoon* and *Vittaforma* and to reduce or eradicate the parasites propagated in cell cultures but does not destroy mature microsporidial spores, so these may sustain infection (21). Fumagillin, its analog TNP-470, nikkomycin Z, and fluoroquinolones have been shown to inhibit completely or partially the replication or spore germination of *Encephalitozoon* and *Vittaforma* in vitro (21, 23, 28). In vitro systems to investigate *E. bieneusi* are not available.

Treatment studies with humans are limited, and only two randomized controlled trials have been conducted. Albendazole can result in clinical cure of HIV-associated encephalitozoonosis in parallel with the cessation of spore excretion (54). In contrast, albendazole is not effective for *Enterocytozoon* infection and does not reduce the parasite load, although previous observations had suggested that clinical improvement may occur in some patients. Oral purified fumagillin appeared to eradicate *E. bieneusi* in many patients, but serious adverse events and parasitic relapse were observed (55).

E. bieneusi-associated diarrhea as well as systemic infection due to *Encephalitozoon* spp. is observed mainly in severely immunodeficient patients with CD4 lymphocyte counts below 50 per μl. Observational studies showed that an improvement of immune functions by potent antiretroviral combination therapy results in complete clinical response and normalization of intestinal architecture, which parallels the clearance of intestinal microsporidia (12). In vitro data suggest that some antiretroviral protease inhibitors may directly inhibit *E. intestinalis* growth at concentrations that are achievable in vivo (53).

EVALUATION, INTERPRETATION, AND REPORTING OF RESULTS

Microsporidia are predominantly opportunistic pathogens capable of causing disease in severely immunodeficient HIV-infected persons (with CD4 cell counts below 200 per μl) and otherwise immunocompromised patients, including organ transplant recipients. Therefore, stool examination or examination of other specimens is particularly indicated for these patient groups, and it is prudent to consider microsporidia as the etiologic agents when they are detected in clinical specimens from such patients. Furthermore, various microsporidial species may cause self-limited diarrhea or keratoconjunctivitis in immunocompetent and otherwise healthy persons.

Routine diagnosis of microsporidiosis is based upon microscopic detection of microsporidial spores. Although sensitive and specific, light microscopic examination does not allow the identification of the organisms to the genus and species level. This can be achieved in most cases by electron microscopy, which is relatively insensitive for the detection of microsporidia because only small samples are examined and sampling errors may occur, or by specific immunofluorescence staining of organisms and by PCR-based procedures (both are commercially unavailable).

Immunocompetent patients may excrete lower numbers of microsporidial spores in feces or urine, and therefore, the threshold of the current light microscopic detection procedures may not be sufficient for the reliable detection of microsporidia in this group.

REFERENCES

1. **Accoceberry, I., M. Thellier, I. Desportes-Livage, A. Achbarou, S. Biligui, M. Danis, and A. Datry.** 1999. Production of monoclonal antibodies directed against the microsporidium *Enterocytozoon bieneusi*. *J. Clin. Microbiol.* **37:**4107–4112.

2. **Akiyoshi, D. E., H. G. Morrison, S. Lei, X. Feng, Q. Zhang, N. Corradi, H. Mayanja, J. K. Tumwine, P. J. Keeling, L. M. Weiss, and S. Tzipori.** 2009. Genomic survey of the noncultivatable opportunistic human pathogen, Enterocytozoon bieneusi. *PLoS Pathog.* **5:**e1000261.

3. **Bart, A., E. M. Wentink-Bonnema, E. R. Heddema, J. Buijs, and T. van Gool.** 2008. Frequent occurrence of human-associated microsporidia in fecal droppings of urban pigeons in Amsterdam, The Netherlands. *Appl. Environ. Microbiol.* **74:**7056–7058.

4. **Bornay-Llinares, F. J., A. J. da Silva, H. Moura, D. A. Schwartz, G. S. Visvesvara, N. J. Pieniazek, A. Cruz-Lopez, P. Hernandez-Jauregui, J. Guerrero, and F. J. Enriquez.** 1998. Immunologic, microscopic, and molecular evidence of Encephalitozoon intestinalis (Septata intestinalis) infection in mammals other than humans. *J. Infect. Dis.* **178:**820–826.

5. **Breton, J., E. Bart-Delabesse, S. Biligui, A. Carbone, X. Seiller, M. Okome-Nkoumou, C. Nzamba, M. Kombila, I. Accoceberry, and M. Thellier.** 2007. New highly divergent rRNA sequence among biodiverse genotypes of Enterocytozoon bieneusi strains isolated from humans in Gabon and Cameroon. *J. Clin. Microbiol.* **45:**2580–2589.

6. **Cali, A., D. P. Kotler, and J. M. Orenstein.** 1993. Septata intestinalis N. G., N. Sp., an intestinal microsporidian associated with chronic diarrhea and dissemination in AIDS patients. *J. Eukaryot. Microbiol.* **40:**101–112.

7. **Cali, A., and P. M. Takvorian.** 2003. Ultrastructure and development of Pleistophora ronneafiei n. sp., a microsporidium (Protista) in the skeletal muscle of an immune-compromised individual. *J. Eukaryot. Microbiol.* **50:**77–85.

8. **Cali, A., P. M. Takvorian, S. Lewin, M. Rendel, C. S. Sian, M. Wittner, H. B. Tanowitz, E. Keohane, and L. M. Weiss.** 1998. Brachiola vesicularum, n. g., n. sp., a new microsporidium associated with AIDS and myositis. *J. Eukaryot. Microbiol.* **45:**240–251.

9. **Cali, A., L. M. Weiss, and P. M. Takvorian.** 2004. An analysis of the microsporidian genus Brachiola, with comparisons of human and insect isolates of Brachiola algerae. *J. Eukaryot. Microbiol.* **51:**678–685.

10. **Cama, V. A., J. Pearson, L. Cabrera, L. Pacheco, R. Gilman, S. Meyer, Y. Ortega, and L. Xiao.** 2007. Transmission of Enterocytozoon bieneusi between a child and guinea pigs. *J. Clin. Microbiol.* **45:**2708–2710.

11. **Canning, E. U.** 1993. Microsporidia, p. 299–370. In J. P. Kreier (ed.), *Parasitic Protozoa*, vol. 6. Academic Press, London, United Kingdom.

12. **Carr, A., D. Marriott, A. Field, E. Vasak, and D. A. Cooper.** 1998. Treatment of HIV-1-associated microsporidiosis and cryptosporidiosis with combination antiretroviral therapy. *Lancet* **351:**256–261.

13. **Carville, A., K. Mansfield, G. Widmer, A. Lackner, D. Kotler, P. Wiest, T. Gumbo, S. Sarbah, and S. Tzipori.** 1997. Development and application of genetic probes for detection of Enterocytozoon bieneusi in formalin-fixed stools and in intestinal biopsy specimens from infected patients. *Clin. Diagn. Lab. Immunol.* **4:**405–408.

14. **Chan, C. M., J. T. Theng, L. Li, and D. T. Tan.** 2003. Microsporidial keratoconjunctivitis in healthy individuals: a case series. *Ophthalmology* **110:**1420–1425.

15. **Cheney, S. A., N. J. Lafranchi-Tristem, and E. U. Canning.** 2000. Phylogenetic relationships of Pleistophora-like microsporidia based on small subunit ribosomal DNA sequences and implications for the source of Trachipleistophora hominis infections. *J. Eukaryot. Microbiol.* **47:**280–287.

16. **Coyle, C. M., L. M. Weiss, L. V. Rhodes III, A. Cali, P. M. Takvorian, D. F. Brown, G. S. Visvesvara, L. Xiao, J. Naktin, E. Young, M. Gareca, G. Colasante, and M. Wittner.** 2004. Fatal myositis due to the microsporidian Brachiola algerae, a mosquito pathogen. *N. Engl. J. Med.* **351:**42–47.

17. **da Silva, A. J., D. A. Schwartz, G. S. Visvesvara, H. de Moura, S. B. Slemenda, and N. J. Pieniazek.** 1996. Sensitive PCR diagnosis of infections by Enterocytozoon bieneusi (microsporidia) using primers based on the region coding for small-subunit rRNA. *J. Clin. Microbiol.* **34:**986–987.

18. Deplazes, P., A. Mathis, R. Baumgartner, I. Tanner, and R. Weber. 1996. Immunologic and molecular characteristics of Encephalitozoon-like microsporidia isolated from humans and rabbits indicate that Encephalitozoon cuniculi is a zoonotic parasite. *Clin. Infect. Dis.* **22:**557–559.

19. Deplazes, P., A. Mathis, M. van Saanen, A. Iten, R. Keller, I. Tanner, M. P. Glauser, R. Weber, and E. U. Canning. 1998. Dual microsporidial infection due to Vittaforma corneae and Encephalitozoon hellem in a patient with AIDS. *Clin. Infect. Dis.* **27:**1521–1524.

20. Desportes, I., Y. Le Charpentier, A. Galian, F. Bernard, B. Cochand-Priollet, A. Lavergne, P. Ravisse, and R. Modigliani. 1985. Occurrence of a new microsporidan: Enterocytozoon bieneusi n.g., n. sp., in the enterocytes of a human patient with AIDS. *J. Protozool.* **32:**250–254.

21. Didier, E. S. 1997. Effects of albendazole, fumagillin, and TNP-470 on microsporidial replication in vitro. *Antimicrob. Agents Chemother.* **41:**1541–1546.

22. Didier, E. S. 2005. Microsporidiosis: an emerging and opportunistic infection in humans and animals. *Acta Trop.* **94:**61–76.

23. Didier, E. S., L. Bowers, M. E. Stovall, D. Kuebler, D. Mittleider, P. J. Brindley, and P. J. Didier. 2005. Antimicrosporidial activity of (fluoro)quinolones in vitro and in vivo. *Folia Parasitol.* (Prague) **52:**173–181.

24. Didier, E. S., P. J. Didier, D. N. Friedberg, S. M. Stenson, J. M. Orenstein, R. W. Yee, F. O. Tio, R. M. Davis, C. Vossbrinck, N. Millichamp, et al. 1991. Isolation and characterization of a new human microsporidian, Encephalitozoon hellem (n. sp.), from three AIDS patients with keratoconjunctivitis. *J. Infect. Dis.* **163:**617–621.

25. Didier, E. S., J. M. Orenstein, A. Aldras, D. Bertucci, L. B. Rogers, and F. A. Janney. 1995. Comparison of three staining methods for detecting microsporidia in fluids. *J. Clin. Microbiol.* **33:**3138–3145.

26. Didier, E. S., C. R. Vossbrinck, M. D. Baker, L. B. Rogers, D. C. Bertucci, and J. A. Shadduck. 1995. Identification and characterization of three Encephalitozoon cuniculi strains. *Parasitology* **111:**411–421.

27. Didier, E. S., and L. M. Weiss. 2006. Microsporidiosis: current status. *Curr. Opin. Infect. Dis.* **19:**485–492.

28. Didier, P. J., J. N. Phillips, D. J. Kuebler, M. Nasr, P. J. Brindley, M. E. Stovall, L. C. Bowers, and E. S. Didier. 2006. Antimicrosporidial activities of fumagillin, TNP-470, ovalicin, and ovalicin derivatives in vitro and in vivo. *Antimicrob. Agents Chemother.* **50:**2146–2155.

29. Enriquez, F. J., O. Ditrich, J. D. Palting, and K. Smith. 1997. Simple diagnosis of Encephalitozoon sp. microsporidial infections by using a panspecific antiexospore monoclonal antibody. *J. Clin. Microbiol.* **35:**724–729.

30. Enriquez, F. J., D. Taren, A. Cruz-Lopez, M. Muramoto, J. D. Palting, and P. Cruz. 1998. Prevalence of intestinal encephalitozoonosis in Mexico. *Clin. Infect. Dis.* **26:**1227–1229.

31. Field, A. S., M. C. Hing, S. T. Milliken, and D. J. Marriott. 1993. Microsporidia in the small intestine of HIV-infected patients. A new diagnostic technique and a new species. *Med. J. Aust.* **158:**390–394.

32. Field, A. S., D. J. Marriott, S. T. Milliken, B. J. Brew, E. U. Canning, J. G. Kench, P. Darveniza, and J. L. Harkness. 1996. Myositis associated with a newly described microsporidian, Trachipleistophora hominis, in a patient with AIDS. *J. Clin. Microbiol.* **34:**2803–2811.

33. Franzen, C., E. S. Nassonova, J. Scholmerich, and I. V. Issi. 2006. Transfer of the members of the genus Brachiola (microsporidia) to the genus Anncaliia based on ultrastructural and molecular data. *J. Eukaryot. Microbiol.* **53:**26–35.

34. Garcia, L. S. 2002. Laboratory identification of the microsporidia. *J. Clin. Microbiol.* **40:**1892–1901.

35. Gill, E. E., and N. M. Fast. 2006. Assessing the microsporidia-fungi relationship: combined phylogenetic analysis of eight genes. *Gene* **375:**103–109.

36. Graczyk, T. K., A. C. Majewska, and K. J. Schwab. 2008. The role of birds in dissemination of human waterborne enteropathogens. *Trends Parasitol.* **24:**55–59.

37. Hibbett, D. S., M. Binder, J. F. Bischoff, M. Blackwell, P. F. Cannon, O. E. Eriksson, S. Huhndorf, T. James, P. M. Kirk, R. Lucking, H. Thorsten Lumbsch, F. Lutzoni, P. B. Matheny, D. J. McLaughlin, M. J. Powell, S. Redhead, C. L. Schoch, J. W. Spatafora, J. A. Stalpers, R. Vilgalys, M. C. Aime, A. Aptroot, R. Bauer, D. Begerow, G. L. Benny, L. A. Castlebury, P. W. Crous, Y. C. Dai, W. Gams, D. M. Geiser, G. W. Griffith, C. Gueidan, D. L. Hawksworth, G. Hestmark, K. Hosaka, R. A. Humber, K. D. Hyde, J. E. Ironside, U. Koljalg, C. P. Kurtzman, K. H. Larsson, R. Lichtwardt, J. Longcore, J. Miadlikowska, A. Miller, J. M. Moncalvo, S. Mozley-Standridge, F. Oberwinkler, E. Parmasto, V. Reeb, J. D. Rogers, C. Roux, L. Ryvarden, J. P. Sampaio, A. Schussler, J. Sugiyama, R. G. Thorn, L. Tibell, W. A. Untereiner, C. Walker, Z. Wang, A. Weir, M. Weiss, M. M. White, K. Winka, Y. J. Yao, and N. Zhang. 2007. A higher-level phylogenetic classification of the Fungi. *Mycol. Res.* **111:**509–547.

38. Hollister, W. S., E. U. Canning, E. Weidner, A. S. Field, J. Kench, and D. J. Marriott. 1996. Development and ultrastructure of Trachipleistophora hominis n.g., n.sp. after in vitro isolation from an AIDS patient and inoculation into athymic mice. *Parasitology* **112:**143–154.

39. Ignatius, R., M. Lehmann, K. Miksits, T. Regnath, M. Arvand, E. Engelmann, U. Futh, H. Hahn, and J. Wagner. 1997. A new acid-fast trichrome stain for simultaneous detection of *Cryptosporidium parvum* and microsporidial species in stool specimens. *J. Clin. Microbiol.* **35:**446–449.

40. James, T. Y., F. Kauff, C. L. Schoch, P. B. Matheny, V. Hofstetter, C. J. Cox, G. Celio, C. Gueidan, E. Fraker, J. Miadlikowska, H. T. Lumbsch, A. Rauhut, V. Reeb, A. E. Arnold, A. Amtoft, J. E. Stajich, K. Hosaka, G. H. Sung, D. Johnson, B. O'Rourke, M. Crockett, M. Binder, J. M. Curtis, J. C. Slot, Z. Wang, A. W. Wilson, A. Schussler, J. E. Longcore, K. O'Donnell, S. Mozley-Standridge, D. Porter, P. M. Letcher, M. J. Powell, J. W. Taylor, M. M. White, G. W. Griffith, D. R. Davies, R. A. Humber, J. B. Morton, J. Sugiyama, A. Y. Rossman, J. D. Rogers, D. H. Pfister, D. Hewitt, K. Hansen, S. Hambleton, R. A. Shoemaker, J. Kohlmeyer, B. Volkmann-Kohlmeyer, R. A. Spotts, M. Serdani, P. W. Crous, K. W. Hughes, K. Matsuura, E. Langer, G. Langer, W. A. Untereiner, R. Lucking, B. Budel, D. M. Geiser, A. Aptroot, P. Diederich, I. Schmitt, M. Schultz, R. Yahr, D. S. Hibbett, F. Lutzoni, D. J. McLaughlin, J. W. Spatafora, and R. Vilgalys. 2006. Reconstructing the early evolution of Fungi using a six-gene phylogeny. *Nature* **443:**818–822.

41. Jedrzejewski, S., T. K. Graczyk, A. Slodkowicz-Kowalska, L. Tamang, and A. C. Majewska. 2007. Quantitative assessment of contamination of fresh food produce of various retail types by human-virulent microsporidian spores. *Appl. Environ. Microbiol.* **73:**4071–4073.

42. Karanis, P., C. Kourenti, and H. Smith. 2007. Waterborne transmission of protozoan parasites: a worldwide review of outbreaks and lessons learnt. *J. Water Health* **5:**1–38.

43. Katinka, M. D., S. Duprat, E. Cornillot, G. Metenier, F. Thomarat, G. Prensier, V. Barbe, E. Peyretaillade, P. Brottier, P. Wincker, F. Delbac, H. El Alaoui, P. Peyret, W. Saurin, M. Gouy, J. Weissenbach, and C. P. Vivares. 2001. Genome sequence and gene compaction of the eukaryote parasite Encephalitozoon cuniculi. *Nature* **414:**450–453.

44. Kester, K. E., G. W. Turiansky, and P. L. McEvoy. 1998. Nodular cutaneous microsporidiosis in a patient with AIDS and successful treatment with long-term oral clindamycin therapy. *Ann. Intern. Med.* **128:**911–914.

45. Lanternier, F., D. Boutboul, J. Menotti, M. O. Chandesris, C. Sarfati, M. F. Mamzer Bruneel, Y. Calmus, F. Mechai, J. P. Viard, M. Lecuit, M. E. Bougnoux, and O. Lortholary. 2009. Microsporidiosis in solid organ transplant recipients: two Enterocytozoon bieneusi cases and review. *Transpl. Infect. Dis.* **11:**83–88.

46. Ledford, D. K., M. D. Overman, A. Gonzalvo, A. Cali, S. W. Mester, and R. F. Lockey. 1985. Microsporidiosis myositis in a patient with the acquired immunodeficiency syndrome. *Ann. Intern. Med.* **102:**628–630.

47. **Lee, J. H.** 2008. Molecular detection of *Enterocytozoon bieneusi* and identification of a potentially human-pathogenic genotype in milk. *Appl. Environ. Microbiol.* **74:**1664–1666.

48. **Lee, S. C., N. Corradi, E. J. Byrnes III, S. Torres-Martinez, F. S. Dietrich, P. J. Keeling, and J. Heitman.** 2008. Microsporidia evolved from ancestral sexual fungi. *Curr. Biol.* **18:**1675–1679.

49. **Margileth, A. M., A. J. Strano, R. Chandra, R. Neafie, M. Blum, and R. M. McCully.** 1973. Disseminated nosematosis in an immunologically compromised infant. *Arch. Pathol.* **95:**145–150.

50. **Mathis, A., M. Michel, H. Kuster, C. Muller, R. Weber, and P. Deplazes.** 1997. Two Encephalitozoon cuniculi strains of human origin are infectious to rabbits. *Parasitology* **114:**29–35.

51. **Mathis, A., R. Weber, and P. Deplazes.** 2005. Zoonotic potential of the microsporidia. *Clin. Microbiol. Rev.* **18:**423–445.

52. **Menotti, J., B. Cassinat, C. Sarfati, O. Liguory, F. Derouin, and J. M. Molina.** 2003. Development of a real-time PCR assay for quantitative detection of *Encephalitozoon intestinalis* DNA. *J. Clin. Microbiol.* **41:**1410–1413.

53. **Menotti, J., M. Santillana-Hayat, B. Cassinat, C. Sarfati, F. Derouin, and J. M. Molina.** 2005. Inhibitory activity of human immunodeficiency virus aspartyl protease inhibitors against *Encephalitozoon intestinalis* evaluated by cell culture-quantitative PCR assay. *Antimicrob. Agents Chemother.* **49:**2362–2366.

54. **Molina, J. M., C. Chastang, J. Goguel, J. F. Michiels, C. Sarfati, I. Desportes-Livage, J. Horton, F. Derouin, and J. Modai.** 1998. Albendazole for treatment and prophylaxis of microsporidiosis due to Encephalitozoon intestinalis in patients with AIDS: a randomized double-blind controlled trial. *J. Infect. Dis.* **177:**1373–1377.

55. **Molina, J. M., M. Tourneur, C. Sarfati, S. Chevret, A. de Gouvello, J. G. Gobert, S. Balkan, and F. Derouin.** 2002. Fumagillin treatment of intestinal microsporidiosis. *N. Engl. J. Med.* **346:**1963–1969.

56. **Moura, H., D. A. Schwartz, F. Bornay-Llinares, F. C. Sodre, S. Wallace, and G. S. Visvesvara.** 1997. A new and improved "quick-hot Gram-chromotrope" technique that differentially stains microsporidian spores in clinical samples, including paraffin-embedded tissue sections. *Arch. Pathol. Lab. Med.* **121:**888–893.

57. **Muller, A., R. Bialek, A. Kamper, G. Fatkenheuer, B. Salzberger, and C. Franzen.** 2001. Detection of microsporidia in travelers with diarrhea. *J. Clin. Microbiol.* **39:**1630–1632.

58. **Nkinin, S. W., T. Asonganyi, E. S. Didier, and E. S. Kaneshiro.** 2007. Microsporidian infection is prevalent in healthy people in Cameroon. *J. Clin. Microbiol.* **45:**2841–2846.

59. **Santin, M., and R. Fayer.** 2009. Enterocytozoon bieneusi genotype nomenclature based on the internal transcribed spacer sequence: a consensus. *J. Eukaryot. Microbiol.* **56:**34–38.

60. **Silveira, H., and E. U. Canning.** 1995. Vittaforma corneae n. comb. for the human microsporidium Nosema corneum Shadduck, Meccoli, Davis & Font, 1990, based on its ultrastructure in the liver of experimentally infected athymic mice. *J. Eukaryot. Microbiol.* **42:**158–165.

61. **Thellier, M., and J. Breton.** 2008. Enterocytozoon bieneusi in human and animals, focus on laboratory identification and molecular epidemiology. *Parasite* **15:**349–358.

62. **Thomarat, F., C. P. Vivares, and M. Gouy.** 2004. Phylogenetic analysis of the complete genome sequence of Encephalitozoon cuniculi supports the fungal origin of microsporidia and reveals a high frequency of fast-evolving genes. *J. Mol. Evol.* **59:**780–791.

63. **van Gool, T., C. Biderre, F. Delbac, E. Wentink-Bonnema, R. Peek, and C. P. Vivares.** 2004. Serodiagnostic studies in an immunocompetent individual infected with Encephalitozoon cuniculi. *J. Infect. Dis.* **189:**2243–2249.

64. **van Gool, T., E. U. Canning, and J. Dankert.** 1994. An improved practical and sensitive technique for the detection of microsporidian spores in stool samples. *Trans. R. Soc. Trop. Med. Hyg.* **88:**189–190.

65. **Vavra, J., R. Dahbiova, W. S. Hollister, and E. U. Canning.** 1993. Staining of microsporidian spores by optical brighteners with remarks on the use of brighteners for the diagnosis of AIDS associated human microsporidioses. *Folia Parasitol.* (Prague) **40:**267–272.

66. **Vavra, J., A. T. Yachnis, J. A. Shadduck, and J. M. Orenstein.** 1998. Microsporidia of the genus Trachipleistophora—causative agents of human microsporidiosis: description of Trachipleistophora anthropophthera n. sp. (Protozoa: Microsporidia). *J. Eukaryot. Microbiol.* **45:**273–283.

67. **Visvesvara, G. S.** 2002. In vitro cultivation of microsporidia of clinical importance. *Clin. Microbiol. Rev.* **15:**401–413.

68. **Visvesvara, G. S., M. Belloso, H. Moura, A. J. Da Silva, I. N. Moura, G. J. Leitch, D. A. Schwartz, P. Chevez-Barrios, S. Wallace, N. J. Pieniazek, and J. D. Goosey.** 1999. Isolation of Nosema algerae from the cornea of an immunocompetent patient. *J. Eukaryot. Microbiol.* **46:**10S.

69. **Visvesvara, G. S., H. Moura, G. J. Leitch, D. A. Schwartz, and L. X. Xiao.** 2005. Public health importance of Brachiola algerae (Microsporidia)—an emerging pathogen of humans. *Folia Parasitol.* (Prague) **52:**83–94.

70. **Vossbrinck, C. R., J. V. Maddox, S. Friedman, B. A. Debrunner-Vossbrinck, and C. R. Woese.** 1987. Ribosomal RNA sequence suggests microsporidia are extremely ancient eukaryotes. *Nature* **326:**411–414.

71. **Weber, R., R. T. Bryan, R. L. Owen, C. M. Wilcox, L. Gorelkin, G. S. Visvesvara, and the Enteric Opportunistic Infections Working Group.** 1992. Improved light-microscopical detection of microsporidia spores in stool and duodenal aspirates. *N. Engl. J. Med.* **326:**161–166.

72. **Weber, R., R. T. Bryan, D. A. Schwartz, and R. L. Owen.** 1994. Human microsporidial infections. *Clin. Microbiol. Rev.* **7:**426–461.

73. **Weber, R., P. Deplazes, M. Flepp, A. Mathis, R. Baumann, B. Sauer, H. Kuster, and R. Luthy.** 1997. Cerebral microsporidiosis due to Encephalitozoon cuniculi in a patient with human immunodeficiency virus infection. *N. Engl. J. Med.* **336:**474–478.

74. **Weber, R., H. Kuster, R. Keller, T. Bachi, M. A. Spycher, J. Briner, E. Russi, and R. Luthy.** 1992. Pulmonary and intestinal microsporidiosis in a patient with the acquired immunodeficiency syndrome. *Am. Rev. Respir. Dis.* **146:**1603–1605.

75. **Weber, R., B. Ledergerber, R. Zbinden, M. Altwegg, G. E. Pfyffer, M. A. Spycher, J. Briner, L. Kaiser, M. Opravil, C. Meyenberger, and M. Flepp.** 1999. Enteric infections and diarrhea in human immunodeficiency virus-infected persons: prospective community-based cohort study. *Arch. Intern. Med.* **159:**1473–1480.

76. **Weber, R., D. A. Schwartz, and P. Deplazes.** 1999. Laboratory diagnosis of microsporidiosis, p. 315–362. *In* M. Wittner and L. M. Weiss (ed.), *The Microsporidia and Microsporidiosis.* ASM Press, Washington, DC.

77. **Weiss, L. M., and C. R. Vossbrinck.** 1999. Molecular biology, molecular phylogeny, and molecular diagnostic approaches to the microsporidia, p. 129–171. *In* M. Wittner and L. M. Weiss (ed.), *The Microsporidia and Microsporidiosis.* ASM Press, Washington, DC.

78. **Wichro, E., D. Hoelzl, R. Krause, G. Bertha, F. Reinthaler, and C. Wenisch.** 2005. Microsporidiosis in travel-associated chronic diarrhea in immune-competent patients. *Am. J. Trop. Med. Hyg.* **73:**285–287.

79. **Williams, B. A., R. P. Hirt, J. M. Lucocq, and T. M. Embley.** 2002. A mitochondrial remnant in the microsporidian Trachipleistophora hominis. *Nature* **418:**865–869.

80. **Williams, B. A., R. C. Lee, J. J. Becnel, L. M. Weiss, N. M. Fast, and P. J. Keeling.** 2008. Genome sequence surveys of Brachiola algerae and Edhazardia aedis reveal microsporidia with low gene densities. *BMC Genomics* **9:**200.

81. **Xiao, L., L. Li, H. Moura, I. Sulaiman, A. A. Lal, S. Gatti, M. Scaglia, E. S. Didier, and G. S. Visvesvara.** 2001. Genotyping *Encephalitozoon hellem* isolates by analysis of the polar tube protein gene. *J. Clin. Microbiol.* **39:**2191–2196.

82. **Xiao, L., L. Li, G. S. Visvesvara, H. Moura, E. S. Didier, and A. A. Lal.** 2001. Genotyping *Encephalitozoon cuniculi* by multilocus analyses of genes with repetitive sequences. *J. Clin. Microbiol.* **39:**2248–2253.

83. **Yachnis, A. T., J. Berg, A. Martinez-Salazar, B. S. Bender, L. Diaz, A. M. Rojiani, T. A. Eskin, and J. M. Orenstein.** 1996. Disseminated microsporidiosis especially infecting the brain, heart, and kidneys. Report of a newly recognized pansporoblastic species in two symptomatic AIDS patients. *Am. J. Clin. Pathol.* **106:**535–543.

Nematodes

HARSHA SHEOREY, BEVERLEY-ANN BIGGS, AND PETER TRAYNOR

141

Soil-transmitted helminths (intestinal nematodes) are the most common infections globally with more than one billion people infected, especially in resource-poor settings where sanitation is inadequate (http://www.who.int/intestinal_worms/en/). These parasites are a major cause of poor health, with the greatest morbidity in women and children. Immigrants and refugees, travelers, and war veterans often unknowingly harbor helminths for years after leaving an area where the parasites are endemic. Clinical features are usually directly proportional to the intensity of the worm infection. Effective school-based drug therapy programs are under way in many developing countries (15). Laboratory diagnosis is primarily based on microscopic examination of feces and differentiation of species based on morphology of eggs or larvae detected (Fig. 1 to 3). The sensitivity of this procedure depends on the stage of the infection and is affected by factors such as variability of the number of eggs or larvae excreted.

Unless specified, antiparasitic susceptibility testing is not routinely performed in the clinical laboratory for these organisms. For more details about susceptibility testing for parasites, consult chapter 149.

TAXONOMY OF NEMATODES

There are varying morphological features by which nematodes are identified. At a higher taxonomic level, the nature of the anterior regions of the alimentary canal (e.g., the esophagus), the form of the head (presence, number of lips, teeth, etc.) and the form of the tail, especially in the male, are important features. At the species level details of the male tail, such as arrangement of caudal papillae and the length and shape of the spicules (sclerotized copulatory aids) are important. In the majority of cases, males carry more taxonomically useful information than females; the latter may often be unidentifiable to species level in the absence of males. Studies strongly suggest that nematodes are actually related to the arthropods and priapulids in a newly recognized group, the Ecdysozoa (1, 16). All these nematodes belong to the kingdom Animalia, subkingdom 3 Bilateria, and phylum Nemathelminthes (Nematoda) (see chapter 129).

ASCARIS LUMBRICOIDES (ROUNDWORM)

Taxonomy

A. lumbricoides belongs to the class Secernentea, order Ascaridida, superfamily Ascaridoidea, and family Ascarididae.

Of the three genera of ascaridid nematodes regularly occurring as parasites of humans, only Ascaris is a true human parasite. The others (Toxocara and Toxascaris) are common parasites of cats and dogs and occasionally infect humans. Ascaridids are related to anisakids, with three distinct lips, but differ in that their life cycle is linked to terrestrial rather than aquatic conditions.

Description

Eggs

Eggs of A. lumbricoides (Fig. 2A to C) are usually seen in two forms: unfertilized and fertilized. The egg shell of a fertilized egg (45 to 75 by 35 to 50 μm) consists of an inner lipid layer responsible for selective permeability, a chitin protein layer responsible for structural strength, and an outer vitelline layer. The inner layer contains a lipoprotein, ascaroside, which helps the egg survive exposure to formaldehyde, disinfectants, and other chemicals. The fertilized egg frequently has an uneven deposit of mucopolysaccharide with adhesive properties present on its outer surface. Eggs appear brown due to staining by bile. The unfertilized eggs have thinner walls and distorted mammillations. These eggs are usually more elongated, measure 85 to 95 by 43 to 47 μm, and may have a pronounced mammillated coat or an extremely minimal mammillated layer. The presence of only unfertilized eggs strongly suggests that only female worms are present in the intestine. During the development of the eggs, the parent worm must supply the zygotes with sufficient nutrients to ensure progression to the infective second-stage larvae and subsequent survival.

Larvae

First-stage larvae develop inside the eggs and molt to form the second-stage larvae. Soon after hatching in the jejunum, second-stage larvae have a typical filariform appearance (measuring approximately 250 by 14 μm), growing to approximately 560 by 28 μm just before a further molt occurs in the lungs. In the lungs, the larvae develop over 8 or 9 days to reach

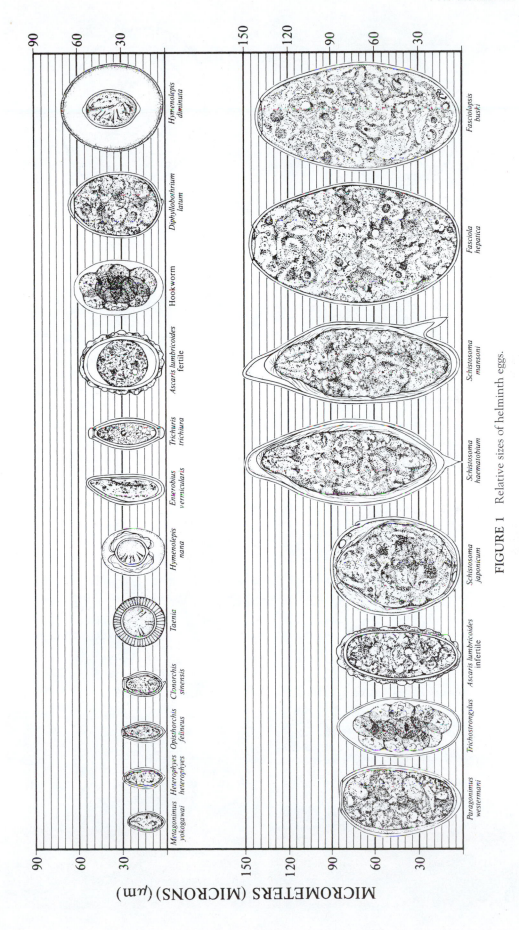

FIGURE 1 Relative sizes of helminth eggs.

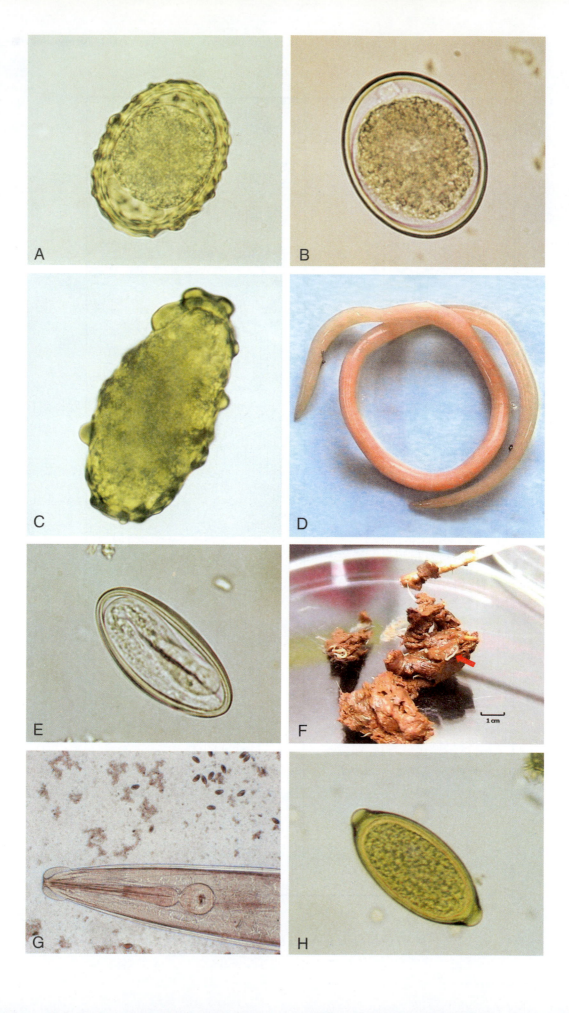

FIGURE 2 Various eggs and adult worms of intestinal nematodes (magnification for panels A through C, E, and H, ×850). (A) Fertile egg of *A. lumbricoides*. (B) Decorticated fertile egg of *A. lumbricoides*. (C) Infertile egg of *A. lumbricoides*. (D) *A. lumbricoides* adult worm with typical cylindrical body with tapering ends and thick cuticle. The *A. lumbricoides* adult worm is the largest of the human pathogenic nematodes, 15 to 35 cm in length. (E) Embryonated infective egg of *E. vermicularis*. (F) Adult worms in feces (arrow). (G) *E. vermicularis* adult female. Adult females are usually 8 to 13 by 0.3 to 0.5 mm in size. Shown is the anterior end of a female worm with the characteristic lips. Typical eggs can also usually be seen in the field. Magnification, ×100. (H) Egg of *T. trichiura*.

a length of approximately 1 mm. The larvae must either have sufficient reserves or feed directly to ensure successful migration back to the gut and more developmental molts. Growth is rapid after the fourth and final molt in the intestine.

Worms

Adult male and female *A. lumbricoides* worms (Fig. 2D) are pinkish cream, with males approximately 15 to 31 cm and females 20 to 35 cm in length. The males, often smaller than the females of the same age, have a curved posterior tail, which accommodates the copulatory aids. Adult worms live in the lumen of the host's small intestine and feed on digestion products.

Epidemiology and Prevention

A. lumbricoides infection is one of the most common human infections, with an estimated 1.2 billion people infected worldwide. It has a worldwide distribution and is most common in tropical and subtropical areas of the developed and underdeveloped world. It is particularly associated with crowding and poor sanitation. Preventive measures consist of health education about personal hygiene and sanitation, and drug therapy.

Transmission and Life Cycle

Eggs passed in feces (diagnostic stage) develop in the soil over 10 to 15 days (Table 1) and may survive in this form for years. Infection follows the ingestion of embryonated eggs (infective stage) that hatch in the small intestine. Larvae penetrate the intestinal mucosa, and the venous circulation carries them to the lungs. From here they migrate to the trachea and are swallowed. They then complete their development into mature adult worms in the small intestine, with eggs produced after 60 to 70 days. A minority of individuals develop heavy infections and act as an important source of transmission. The prepatent period (from egg ingestion to egg production) is approximately 2 months.

Clinical Significance

Initial infection is usually asymptomatic. Migration of larvae through the lungs may result in an eosinophilic pneumonitis with cough, fever, and dyspnea. This may occur up to 2 weeks after infection and lasts approximately 3 weeks. Bronchospasm may be prominent and is occasionally fatal.

The clinical features in established infections relate to the worm burden. Most infections are light and asymptomatic, but nonspecific abdominal symptoms may occur. There is increasing risk of intestinal obstruction with increasing worm burden. Intestinal obstruction has a high mortality rate in some settings (2). Heavy infections are also associated with malnutrition and impaired growth in children.

Ectopic ascariasis occasionally occurs when adult worms enter hepatobiliary and pancreatic ducts or the appendix and cause obstruction. This may result in biliary colic, cholecystitis, acute cholangitis, acute pancreatitis, appendicitis, or a hepatic abscess. It occurs more commonly in countries with high rates of infection where the parasite is endemic. (For more on the clinical significance of *A. lumbricoides*, see reference 13.)

Diagnosis

The primary diagnosis of infection is by demonstration of the presence of eggs in feces (see references 4 and 7). The fertilized eggs are round to oval, bile stained, mammillated, and thick walled. Often both fertilized and unfertilized eggs are found in the same stool. Multiple specimens taken on separate days may be required. Both direct and concentration methods such as formalin-ethyl acetate sedimentation should be used for optimal yield. The flotation technique may not concentrate dense unfertilized eggs. Decorticated fertile eggs and infertile eggs may be difficult to recognize (Fig. 2A to C). Motile larvae may sometimes be seen in expectorated sputum but rarely in feces. Occasionally, an adult worm (usually female) may be passed in feces or may spontaneously migrate out of the anus, mouth, or nares, particularly in children. Rarely, multiple worms may be passed in children who have lived in areas where the worms are endemic. The female worm is easily identified by its cylindrical body and tapering ends (Fig. 2D) (males are slightly smaller but are rarely seen). Distinguishing features include a lateral white line along the entire length of the body, three lips at the anterior end, and a tough cuticle. No other human parasite is as large as *A. lumbricoides*; hence, it is usually easy to identify. However, with faulty or old plumbing, earthworms may be found in toilet bowls and these may be presented for identification.

TABLE 1 Usual times for completion of life cycles under favorable conditions[a]

Nematode	Time for life cycle completion	
	Within host (wk)	In external environment
Ascaris lumbricoides	8	10–15 days
Enterobius vermicularis	4–7	6 h
Hookworms	4–7	5–6 days
Strongyloides stercoralis	4	3–4 days (direct)
Trichuris trichiura	10–12	21 days

[a]Modified from reference 17.

Treatment

Albendazole or mebendazole is effective (see chapter 147 and reference 14). These drugs should be avoided in pregnancy.

For a summary of *A. lumbricoides*, see Table 2.

ENTEROBIUS VERMICULARIS (PINWORM OR THREADWORM)

Taxonomy

E. vermicularis belongs to the class Secernentea, order Oxyurida, superfamily Oxyuroidea, and family Oxyuridae. Only the genus *Enterobius* of the Oxyuridae regularly occurs in humans and other primates.

Description

Eggs

Pinworm eggs (Fig. 2E) are ovoid, 50 to 60 by 20 to 35 μm, and asymmetrically flattened on one side and appear colorless when recovered from the perianal skin. The outer layer of the egg shell is albuminous and sticky, enabling the egg to adhere readily. When laid, the egg contains an immature first-stage larva, but this develops rapidly to become infective.

Larvae

After hatching, the larvae complete molting and development in the large bowel.

Worms

Adult female worms (Fig. 2F and G) measure approximately 8 to 13 by 0.3 to 0.5 mm, with typical lips at the anterior end and a long, pointed tail (hence the name pinworm). Male worms are 2.5 by 0.2 mm but are rarely seen.

Epidemiology and Prevention

E. vermicularis infection has a worldwide distribution and is more common in children than adults. Preventive measures consist of health education about personal hygiene and sanitation, and drug therapy.

Transmission and Life Cycle

Adult worms inhabit the cecum, appendix, and ascending colon. The female migrates down the colon when mature and deposits eggs on perianal and perineal skin (diagnostic stage). More than 10,000 eggs may be deposited, become infective within 6 h, and remain viable for up to 5 days.

Transmission is either direct from the anal and perianal regions to the mouth, usually by fingernail contamination (autoinfection), or from exposure to a contaminated environment. When swallowed, the embryonated eggs (infective stage) hatch in the small bowel. Larvae pass from the small bowel to the large bowel, where they mature into adult worms. Retroinfection is thought to be possible where larvae migrate from the anal skin back to the rectum.

The prepatent period (from egg ingestion to egg production) is 3 to 4 weeks.

Clinical Significance

Many patients are asymptomatic or present with pruritus ani and perineal pruritus. The pruritus may be severe and is worse at night. Excoriation from scratching and secondary bacterial infection are often evident. Children are most commonly infected. With a heavy worm burden, poor concentration, enuresis, and emotional distress are features. Occasionally, the presence of worms in the appendix

contributes to inflammation and true appendicitis (3). Reinfection (autoinfection or retroinfection) is also possible.

General symptoms, including abdominal pain, weight loss, and loss of appetite, may occur.

The presence of ectopic worms and eggs in several sites, including the female genitourinary tract, the epididymis, and the peritoneum, has been reported (13). They rarely cause serious complications. (For more on the clinical significance of *E. vermicularis*, see reference 13.)

Diagnosis

The primary diagnosis is by demonstration of the presence of eggs on the skin in the perineal area by using the "sticky tape" method (eggs adhere to cellulose tape and can then be detected microscopically). Briefly, a strip of cellulose tape with adhesive side outwards on a microscopy slide is pressed firmly against the right and left perianal folds. The tape is then spread back over the slide with the adhesive side down and examined directly under the microscope. Visibility of eggs can be improved by lifting the tape from the slide, adding a drop of xylene or toluene, and pressing down the tape back on the slide. This helps clear the preparation, and the eggs can be observed clearly (see references 4 and 7). Repeated preparations on 2 or 3 consecutive days may be required. Commercial collection kits (Evergreen Scientific or Swube [Becton Dickinson]) are available in some countries. Eggs are occasionally present in feces. Eggs are non-bile stained, ovoid, asymmetrical with a characteristic "football" shape (concave on one side and flat on the other), smooth, and thick walled and may contain a partially or fully developed larva (Fig. 2E). Specimens should ideally be taken early in the morning before a bath or shower or use of the toilet. If an opaque tape is submitted by mistake, a drop of immersion oil on the top of the tape will clear it enough for microscopy.

Occasionally, adult female worms may be seen in feces, around the anal opening, or upon colonoscopy as white or cream-colored threadlike worms (hence the name threadworm). Characteristic eggs may be seen within the distended female or extruded from the genital pore by putting a little pressure on the worm.

Treatment

Albendazole or mebendazole is the drug of choice. These drugs should be avoided in pregnancy. Pyrantel and piperazine are also effective and can be used in pregnancy (see chapter 147; see also reference 14).

It is important to treat other family members and close contacts and to decontaminate the environment by washing bed linen and clothes. Advice should be given on adequate hygiene and hand washing.

For a summary of *E. vermicularis*, see Table 2.

HOOKWORMS

Taxonomy

Ancylostoma duodenale (Old World Hookworm)

A. duodenale belongs to the class Secernentea, order Rhabditida, suborder Strongylida, superfamily Ancylostomatoidea, family Ancylostomatidae, and subfamily Ancylostomatinae.

Necator americanus (New World Hookworm)

N. americanus belongs to the class Secernentea, order Rhabditida, suborder Strongylida, superfamily Ancylostomatoidea, family Ancylostomatidae, and subfamily Bunostominae. *Ancylostoma* and *Necator* are the two genera of

TABLE 2 Summary of common nematodes

Parasite	Major clinical presentations of infection	Prepatent period	Laboratory findings	Treatment of choice
Ascaris lumbricoides	Symptoms relate to worm burden; most infections are light and asymptomatic; migratory phase, eosinophilic pneumonitis Symptoms of established infection include: • History of passing/vomiting worm • Mild gastrointestinal symptoms • Small-bowel obstruction in children with heavy worm burdens • Ectopic ascariasis involving appendix or hepatobiliary or pancreatic ducts • Malnutrition and growth retardation in children	2 mo	Demonstration of eggs in feces; identification of worm passed; eosinophilia low or absent	Albendazole or mebendazole
Enterobius vermicularis	Many infections are asymptomatic; pruritus ani occurs mainly at night; excoriation from scratching and secondary infection are common; general symptoms include weight loss and loss of appetite; occasionally ectopic, involving appendix or female genital tract	3–4 wk	Demonstration of eggs in "sticky tape" preparation; eosinophilia low or absent	Albendazole or mebendazole; prevent reinfection and treat contacts
Hookworms	Pruritic rash or "ground itch" on extremities at site of entry of larvae; migratory phase, cough and wheezing due to eosinophilic pneumonitis Symptoms of established infection include: • Iron deficiency anemia • Hypoproteinemia leading to chronic malnutrition and growth disorders in children • Enteropathy with gastrointestinal symptoms • Light infections may be asymptomatic	4–8 wk	Demonstration of eggs or larvae in feces; culture (agar plate method or Harada-Mori technique); eosinophilia, usually moderate	Albendazole or mebendazole; iron therapy if anemia is present
Strongyloides stercoralis	Chronic infection occurs due to autoinfection; recurrent, migratory, linear rash when larvae enter perianal skin, or "larva currens"; urticarial rashes also occur; enteropathy causing intermittent or chronic diarrhea, sometimes with malabsorption; pulmonary symptoms and hypereosinophilia may occur during autoinfection; Loeffler-like syndrome; gram-negative-bacterial septicemia or meningitis due to transfer of bowel flora by migrating larvae; hyperinfection syndrome (disseminated) in immunocompromised or debilitated individuals, leading to severe enteropathy and respiratory symptoms	2–4 wk	Demonstration of larvae in feces; culture (agar plate method or Harada-Mori technique); demonstration of antibodies in serum; eosinophilia, usually moderate	Ivermectin
Trichuris trichiura	Usually asymptomatic or mild gastrointestinal symptoms; epigastric pain, vomiting, distension, anorexia, and weight loss; trichuris dysentery, sometimes with rectal prolapse, may occur in heavy infections; growth retardation in children due to chronic malnutrition and anemia	3 mo	Demonstration of eggs in feces; eosinophilia low or absent	Albendazole or mebendazole

Ancylostomatidae that infect humans. Other genera may occur as rare "accidental" parasites.

Description

Eggs

Eggs (Fig. 3A) of *A. duodenale* and *Necator americanus* are indistinguishable, being characteristically oval with a thin shell and measuring approximately 56 to 75 by 36 to 40 μm. Characteristically, they have a clear space between the developing embryo and the thin egg shell. Survival of eggs is maximized in moist, shady, warm soil, where larvae hatch within 1 to 2 days.

Larvae

First-stage rhabditoid larvae (Fig. 3E and G) from the hatched eggs measure about 200 μm in length. They feed on organic debris and molt, with the resulting second-stage larvae measuring up to 500 μm. After another molt, the infective, nonfeeding third-stage larvae measure from 500 to

700 μm, those of *Ancylostoma* being generally longer than those of *Necator*. Development from first-stage to infective filariform larvae occurs within 5 to 8 days; the latter remain viable in the soil for several weeks.

Worms

For both species, male worms (5 to 11 mm) are shorter than females (7 to 13 by 0.4 to 0.5 mm), and *A. duodenale* is generally longer and more sturdily built than *N. americanus*. Adult worms are rarely seen since they remain firmly attached to the intestinal mucosa, feeding on blood obtained by puncturing the capillary network in the intestinal mucosa. It has been estimated that a single *A. duodenale* worm can withdraw as much as 0.2 ml of blood per day, whereas *N. americanus* withdraws approximately 0.05 ml.

Epidemiology and Prevention

An estimated 740 million people are infected in poor regions of the tropics and subtropics, especially in Asia and sub-Saharan Africa (9, 10). Preventative measures consist of health education about personal hygiene and the need to wear shoes, avoidance of soil contamination, and drug therapy.

Transmission and Life Cycle

Entry of third-stage or filariform larvae (infective stage) by direct penetration of the skin initiates human infection, followed by migration to the lungs within 10 days. *A. duodenale* can also infect if swallowed, but *N. americanus* cannot. *N. americanus* requires an obligatory lung migration, whereas the ingestion of *A. duodenale* larvae can result in direct maturation to the adult stage in the intestine. Larvae leave the lungs after 3 to 5 weeks, pass through the trachea and pharynx, enter the gastrointestinal tract, and attach to the intestinal mucosa, where they mature into adults. Attachment and the release of anticlotting factors result in blood loss, which is greater with *A. duodenale*. Hookworms may survive in the host for several years. Eggs are passed in the feces (diagnostic stage) into the environment, where they hatch into rhabditiform larvae, which mature into filariform larvae and infect new hosts. The prepatent period (from larva penetration to egg production) is 4 to 8 weeks.

Clinical Significance

The major clinical manifestation of hookworm infection is iron deficiency anemia due to intestinal blood loss and depletion of iron stores. The degree of iron deficiency induced by hookworms depends on the intensity and duration of infection, the species of hookworm, and the iron status of the host. Young children, adolescent girls, women of reproductive age, and pregnant women are most at risk for iron deficiency anemia because of relatively low iron stores. Anemia during pregnancy is linked to maternal mortality, impaired lactation, prematurity, and low-birth-weight infants.

Patients with light worm burdens are usually asymptomatic. Moderate and heavy worm burdens cause epigastric pain and tenderness, nausea, weight loss, and diarrhea. This may lead to protein-losing enteropathy and hypoalbuminemia. In those who develop iron deficiency anemia, common symptoms are lethargy and fatigue, exertional dyspnea, and palpitations. In children, chronic malnutrition, impaired physical growth, and impaired cognitive development may occur.

A pruritic rash is often present at the site of penetration of larvae ("ground itch"). This must be differentiated from cercarial dermatitis and creeping eruptions from other causes. In some patients, mild cough and wheezing occur in response to larval migration through the lungs. (For more on the clinical significance of hookworms, see reference 13.)

Diagnosis

The primary diagnosis of infection is by demonstration of the presence of eggs in feces (see references 4 and 7). Multiple specimens taken on separate days may be required. For optimal yield, both direct and concentration methods such as formalin-ethyl acetate sedimentation should be used. Eggs are non-bile stained and usually have a four- to eight-cell-stage embryo (Fig. 3A). Occasionally, a 16- to 32-cell-stage embryo or a developing larva may be seen, especially if there is delay in processing a fresh (unfixed) fecal specimen. These should be differentiated from *Strongyloides stercoralis* larvae by their morphological features (Fig. 3C to G). Hookworm eggs may be confused with *Trichostrongylus* eggs, which are generally larger and in an advanced stage of cleavage (Fig. 3B).

Although larvae are rarely seen in adequately fixed feces specimens, motile larvae may be seen occasionally in expectorated sputum. Culture for the larval stage by the Harada-Mori technique or agar plate method is useful to detect light infections (see "*Strongyloides stercoralis*" below for details) (Fig. 3C to G).

Adult worms are very rarely passed in feces. However, a colonoscopic or gastroscopic specimen may be submitted for identification. Usually, the worm is firmly attached to the mucosa. The adult worm can be identified by the structure of the buccal capsule.

When blood examination shows iron deficiency anemia, the diagnosis of hookworm infection should be considered for people from areas where the infection is endemic.

Treatment

The two most practical and effective drugs for treating hookworm infections are albendazole and mebendazole. These drugs should be avoided in pregnancy. Pyrantel is also effective and can be used in pregnancy (see chapter 147 and reference 14). Iron supplementation should be given to those who are deficient.

For a summary of hookworms, see Table 2.

STRONGYLOIDES STERCORALIS

Taxonomy

S. stercoralis belongs to the class Secernentea, order Rhabditida, superfamily Rhabditoidea, and family Strongyloididae. Members of the family Strongyloididae exhibit an irregular alternation of generations, with a parasitic parthenogenetic female alternating with a free-living sexual generation. Only one genus, *Strongyloides*, occurs in humans.

Description, Transmission, and Life Cycle

Eggs

Eggs of the parasitic female are deposited within the mucosa of the small intestine and usually hatch before reaching the lumen. As a result, they are rarely excreted in the feces (*Strongyloides fuelleborni*, seen in Papua New Guinea, is an exception—see below). Eggs of the free-living adult female are partially embryonated and oval and measure approximately 50 to 70 μm in length.

Larvae

First-stage, rhabditiform larvae (Fig. 3C, D, and F) measure approximately 180 to 380 by 14 to 20 μm and are characterized by a muscular esophagus comprising the anterior third of the body. A short buccal cavity and a prominent genital primordium located midbody (Fig. 3C and D) help to dis-

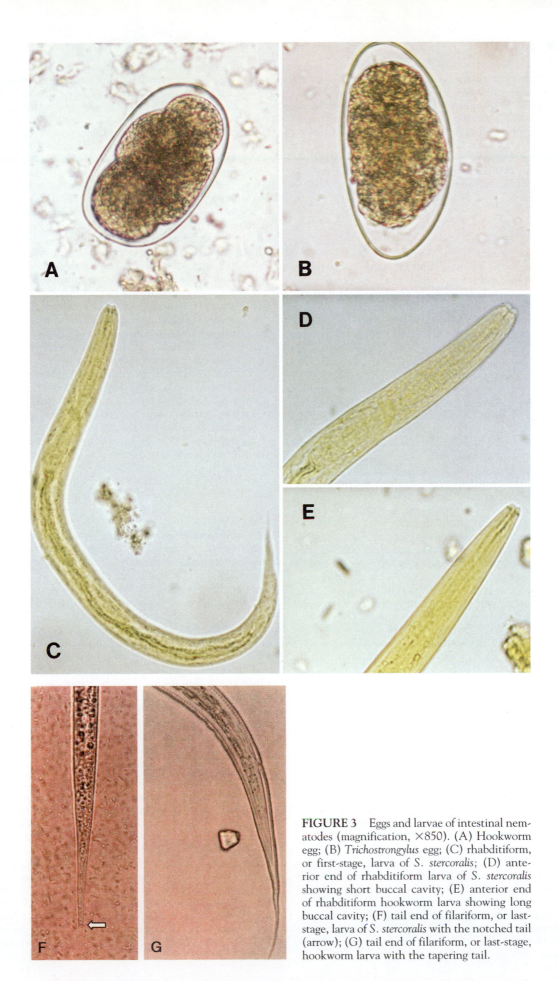

FIGURE 3 Eggs and larvae of intestinal nematodes (magnification, ×850). (A) Hookworm egg; (B) *Trichostrongylus* egg; (C) rhabditiform, or first-stage, larva of *S. stercoralis*; (D) anterior end of rhabditiform larva of *S. stercoralis* showing short buccal cavity; (E) anterior end of rhabditiform hookworm larva showing long buccal cavity; (F) tail end of filariform, or last-stage, larva of *S. stercoralis* with the notched tail (arrow); (G) tail end of filariform, or last-stage, hookworm larva with the tapering tail.

tinguish them from other nematodes such as hookworms (Fig. 3E). In the soil, first-stage larvae follow a direct or indirect course of development. In the direct cycle, larvae develop rapidly into infective third-stage, filariform larvae; in the indirect cycle, first-stage larvae develop into a free-living generation of adult male and female worms. Third-stage, or filariform, infective larvae are long and thin compared to those in the rhabditiform stages. Third-stage larvae are 500 to 600 by 16 μm, and their tails are notched (pointed in hookworm larvae) (Fig. 3F and G).

Worms

Parasitic male forms do not occur. Parasitic females are small and thin, measuring approximately 2 to 3 mm in length and 30 to 50 μm in width. The anterior portion is thicker than the posterior and contains the esophagus.

The free-living adult female is approximately half the size of its parasitic counterpart, although nearly twice as thick (approximately 80 μm). While the reproductive systems are morphologically similar, the uterus in the free-living adult female contains significantly more eggs. The free-living adult male is slightly smaller than the female, approximately 50 μm in width.

Transmission is via penetration of the skin or mucous membranes by filariform larvae (infective stage) that are carried to the lungs in the venous circulation. Larvae penetrate alveolar walls, migrate through the tracheobronchial tree, are swallowed, and finally reside in the mucosa of the upper small intestine. Here, they reach maturity and commence egg production; the eggs hatch immediately to release rhabditiform larvae, most of which are excreted in feces (diagnostic stage). In the soil, development into filariform larvae occurs, with the potential to infect new hosts.

Some rhabditiform larvae develop into infective filariform larvae in the bowel lumen, penetrate the intestinal mucosa or perianal skin, and repeat the cycle of maturation within the same host. This process of autoinfection, albeit uncommon among intestinal nematodes, results in chronic infections that may persist for 40 years or more.

The prepatent period (from larva penetration to egg production) is 2 to 4 weeks.

Epidemiology and Prevention

Strongyloides lives in warm moist soil and is widely distributed in the tropics and subtropics, similar to hookworms. There are an estimated 30 to 100 million patients infected with *S. stercoralis* worldwide. Risk groups include those living in areas where the parasite is endemic, immigrants and refugees, indigenous peoples, and war veterans previously exposed in areas where the parasite is endemic. Preventative measures include good personal hygiene and wearing shoes in areas where transmission may occur.

Clinical Significance

S. stercoralis infections are often chronic, lasting for several decades. Most patients have low worm burdens and are asymptomatic or have intermittent cutaneous and/or gastrointestinal symptoms.

A recurrent, pruritic, serpiginous, erythematous rash may occur due to larval migration in the skin ("larva currens"). This is most commonly seen on the buttocks, groin, and trunk and may move about under the skin over 1 to 2 days. Other, less distinctive urticarial and papular rashes also occur.

Intermittent or chronic diarrhea, abdominal pain and bloating, nausea, and anorexia are the main gastrointestinal symptoms.

Although pulmonary symptoms are uncommon in uncomplicated strongyloidiasis, passage of larvae through the lung may be associated with a cough, wheezing and dyspnea, and patchy infiltrates upon radiography (Loeffler-like syndrome).

Severe complicated strongyloidiasis may occur in immunocompromised or debilitated individuals and is due to accelerated autoinfection in the face of waning immunity. Hyperinfection syndrome is associated with the presence of many adult worms in the intestinal mucosa and penetration of the bowel wall by large numbers of filariform larvae. Severe gastrointestinal and/or respiratory symptoms and large numbers of larvae in stool and sputum are the main features. It may be complicated by malabsorption or paralytic ileus. Gram-negative bacterial septicemia and meningitis may develop if enteric bacteria are spread into blood or cerebrospinal fluid during mucosal penetration by larvae. Larvae can occasionally disseminate to the central nervous system, peritoneum, liver, and kidneys. Disseminated strongyloidiasis may mimic many other diseases, including severe bacterial sepsis and tropical pulmonary eosinophilia. It should be considered a possibility in immunosuppressed patients who have been at risk of infection in the past.

Patients on long-term corticosteroid therapy are most at risk for severe disease. Those with impaired cellular immunity due to other causes (e.g., use of immunosuppressive agents or hematological malignancies and other chronic debilitating diseases) are also at risk.

Strongyloides species from animals can occasionally infect humans and produce persistent skin lesions similar to those produced by *S. stercoralis*. However, the life cycle is not completed and infection is not established (6). (For more on the clinical significance of *S. stercoralis*, see reference 13.)

Diagnosis

The laboratory diagnosis of strongyloidiasis can be difficult (see references 4 and 7). It is based on either demonstrating the presence of the larvae in feces or demonstrating antibodies to *S. stercoralis* in blood. Eggs or adult worms are very rarely detected. Microscopy of feces may detect the first-stage (rhabditiform) larvae. The sensitivity of this method is generally low, as larvae are shed sporadically, and numbers depend on the stage and severity of the infection. Hence, multiple specimens collected over several days should be examined. Coproculture is a method of concentration of larvae on a freshly passed stool specimen. It is important that the specimen not be refrigerated or preserved, and it must be transported without delay to the laboratory. Ideally, this should be attempted for all suspected cases, especially with patients from areas where the infection is endemic. Various methods available for culture are as follows (for details, see reference 8).

1. Agar plate culture. A small amount of feces is placed on an agar plate, and the plate is sealed. If larvae are present, they travel on the surface of the plate, carrying bacteria from the feces. Colonies of these bacteria appear on the surface as tracks with a characteristic sinusoidal pattern. The plates are examined by microscopy for confirmation of the presence of larvae. This is the easiest culture method to perform and is now the recommended procedure (18).

2. Harada-Mori technique. Feces are placed on a filter paper dipping into a small amount of water placed in a tube. The larvae in the feces move towards the water, which can subsequently be tested by microscopy for the presence of larvae.

3. Petri dish filter paper slant method. This procedure is similar to the Harada-Mori technique described above but is done in a petri dish.

4. Baermann technique. This requires a special apparatus and relies on the principle that larvae will actively migrate out of the feces placed on a wire mesh covered with several layers of gauze.

Occasionally, hookworm larvae may hatch out in feces that have been left at warm temperatures for long periods before processing. Hookworm larvae can be differentiated from S. stercoralis larvae as the hookworm larvae have a long buccal cavity and inconspicuous genital primordium (Fig. 3C to E). The presence of larvae of Strongyloides in expectorated sputum or duodenal aspirate may also be demonstrated via enteroscope or string test (Entero-Test capsule) (8). Occasionally, last-stage (filariform) Strongyloides larvae may be seen in feces or sputum in cases of hyperinfection or in cases in which the culture methods described above are used.

Although eosinophilia is common during acute infection, it does not reliably correlate with infection and may be intermittent in chronic infection. The concomitant use of steroids may significantly decrease the eosinophilia in infected patients.

Demonstration of anti-Strongyloides antibodies in blood should be used as a screening test or as an adjunct for diagnosis. Used in conjunction with eosinophil count, it is very useful to monitor treatment. Antibody levels decline after 6 months of effective treatment (12) and may be negative by 12 to 24 months (5). The sensitivity of the commercially available enzyme immunoassay (immunoglobulin G enzyme-linked immunosorbent assay; IVD Research, Inc.) using S. stercoralis filariform antigens test is ~90% and much higher than indirect hemagglutination and indirect fluorescent-antibody assays. Higher sensitivity (~95%) has been reported by using the CDC Strongyloides enzyme immunoassay for patients with proven infection (12). Sensitivity may be lower in severely immunocompromised patients. The specificity of enzyme immunoassay is ~85%, as cross-reactions in patients with filarial and other nematode infections may occur. If antibodies are positive, efforts should be made to establish a parasitological (microscopic and culture) diagnosis and to exclude infection with other parasites that could result in cross-reacting antibodies. Strongyloides serology should be done in all candidates for immunosuppressive therapy (because of organ transplant or treatment for malignancies, etc.).

Treatment

Strongyloides stercoralis infection should always be treated because of the potential for developing severe complicated disease. Ivermectin is the drug of choice. Repeated cycles may be required in immunocompromised patients. Albendazole and mebendazole are less effective than ivermectin (thiabendazole, although effective, is no longer used due to frequent severe side effects) (18) (see chapter 147 and reference 14). These benzimidazole drugs should be avoided in pregnancy.

Monitoring with stool microscopy, eosinophil counts, and serology is recommended until infection is eradicated. For a summary of S. stercoralis, see Table 2.

STRONGYLOIDES FUELLEBORNI

Strongyloides fuelleborni is a nonhuman primate parasite found in monkeys in central and eastern Africa and Papua New Guinea. Most human infections are asymptomatic in adults, but the organism may cause a severe protein-losing enteropathy and abdominal distension ("swollen-belly syndrome") in infants. In contrast to S. stercoralis, ova of S. fuelleborni are found in feces in large numbers and resemble those of hookworms (50 to 70 μm long). The two species can be differentiated on the basis of adult worm morphology (8). Treatment is similar to that for S. stercoralis. If the infection is untreated, the mortality rate is very high in infants.

TRICHURIS TRICHIURA (WHIPWORM)

Taxonomy

T. trichiura belongs to the class Adenophorea, subclass Enoplia, order Trichocephalida, superfamily Trichonelloidea, and family Trichuridae.

Description

Eggs

Eggs of T. trichiura (Fig. 2H) are lemon shaped with a characteristic plug at each end ("tea tray with handles"). In feces, eggs are brown and measure 50 to 55 by 20 to 24 μm.

Larvae

After hatching in the intestine, the second-stage larval form measures about 260 by 15 μm in length. The second-stage larvae burrow into the intestinal mucosa and undergo four larval molts. The adult worm is then intimately associated with the wall of the large intestine.

Worms

Adult worms are found in the large intestine, with a highly characteristic shape from which the name whipworm is derived. The long, thin anterior end lies in a burrow in the mucosa, and the thicker end, which contains the reproductive tract, extends into the intestinal lumen. Worms are whitish, and the males (30 to 45 mm) are shorter than the females (35 to 50 mm) and have a coiled posterior end. Adult females produce up to 20,000 eggs/day and live for approximately 3 years.

Epidemiology and Prevention

Trichuris has a worldwide distribution and is often associated with Ascaris and hookworm infections in children in tropical and subtropical areas. Preventative measures include health education about personal hygiene, avoidance of soil contamination, and drug therapy programs in areas where infection is endemic.

Transmission and Life Cycle

Transmission is direct via oral ingestion of embryonated eggs (infective stage) from contaminated soil. Following ingestion, larvae are released and pass into the large bowel, where they reside and mature into adults in mucosal crypts. The eggs passed in feces contain an unsegmented ovum (diagnostic stage), and once the eggs are in warm, moist conditions in soil, they become infective 2 to 4 weeks after passage. The prepatent period (from egg ingestion to egg production) is 3 months.

Clinical Significance

The clinical features are related to the intensity of infection, as is the case with the other intestinal nematodes. Light infections are asymptomatic or present with mild gastrointestinal symptoms. Epigastric pain, vomiting, distension, anorexia, and weight loss may occur with heavier infections, and trichuris dysentery syndrome, sometimes complicated by rectal prolapse, may be seen. Children with severe infections may develop growth retardation due to chronic malnutrition and anemia. (For more on the clinical significance of *T. trichiura*, see reference 13.)

Diagnosis

The primary diagnosis of infection is by demonstration of the presence of eggs in feces (see references 4 and 7). Multiple specimens collected on separate days may be required. Both direct and concentration methods such as formalin-ethyl acetate sedimentation should be used for optimal yield. The eggs are bile stained and thick walled with mucoid plugs at both ends, giving them a characteristic tea tray appearance (Fig. 2H).

Adult worms are rarely passed in feces and are occasionally found upon colonoscopy (11). When they are seen, they have a cylindrical coiled body and a coiled thicker tail, giving them the appearance of a whip (hence the name whipworm).

Treatment

Albendazole or mebendazole are the drugs of choice (see chapter 147 and reference 14). These drugs should be avoided in pregnancy.

For a summary of *T. trichiura*, see Table 2.

COLLECTION, TRANSPORT, AND STORAGE OF SPECIMENS

Specimens should be collected before antibiotics or antiparasitic drugs are given (for details, refer to chapter 130). It is important to transport and process feces specimens for parasitic examination as soon as possible. Clinicians and collection staff should be encouraged to either send fresh specimens to the laboratory without delay or use commercially available preservative kits. If delay is inevitable, specimens should be refrigerated or transported in commercially available vials or kits with a preservative such as polyvinyl alcohol or sodium acetate-acetic acid-formalin. If these are not available at the point of collection, preservatives should be added as soon as the specimen is received in the laboratory. Excellent directions for proper collection are available with these kits. The decision as to which preservative to use depends on various considerations such as whether permanent-stained smears or immunoassays are required, etc. (For details, see reference 8.) Refrigeration and the use of preservatives should be avoided if *Strongyloides* larval culture is required.

Specimens that are obviously dry or drying out should be rejected, and a fresh specimen should be collected.

There is no maximum limit on the amount of specimen, but it should be reasonable for the laboratory staff to handle. Very small amounts are not acceptable as the chances of drying are high and those of finding parasites are low. Two or three specimens collected over a period of 7 to 10 days are optimal.

Worms passed or taken at colonoscopy should be transported to the laboratory without delay in a closed, clean container of appropriate size. Worms can be preserved in 50% alcohol or 5% formalin (avoid higher concentrations as dehydration can occur).

For sputum specimens, proper instructions should be given to patients, emphasizing quality, avoidance of saliva, and inclusion of mouthwash before deep coughing (expectorating). Sputum and aspirates should be transported to the laboratory and processed immediately.

All specimens should be collected in clean, wide-mouthed containers with tight-fitting lids and handled using standard precautions, e.g., latex gloves should be worn by anyone handling the specimens.

LABORATORY METHODS: DIRECT EXAMINATION

The specimen should be handled in a work cabinet, and gloves and gown should be worn. Examine the specimen and note its consistency. Look for any motile worms or segments of worms. Select and sample areas that look watery, purulent, or bloody. If feces are formed, take specimens from the sides and middle for the concentration technique.

Wet preparations in saline and iodine are prepared from direct specimens or concentrates and covered with a coverslip. Scan the whole coverslip at low-power magnification (×100) with a microscope. Most helminth eggs and larvae can be identified at this magnification and can be confirmed at high power (×400) on the basis of their shapes, sizes, and characteristic features (Fig. 1 to 3). Thin smears should be prepared from the concentrate for permanent staining, which may be useful to diagnose mixed infections with protozoa.

EVALUATION, INTERPRETATION, AND REPORTING OF RESULTS

Make note of the adequacy and quality of the specimen submitted. If it is inadequate, mention it on the report.

In developed countries, any helminth eggs or larvae found in feces are significant and treatment is recommended, even if the patient is asymptomatic. However, treatment of asymptomatic cases is not necessary in developing countries as many of these parasites are endemic and reinfection is common.

Examples of reports are as follows.

1. Larvae of *S. stercoralis* detected by fecal culture.
2. Eggs of *E. vermicularis* not detected on the sticky tape preparation. A single negative result does not exclude the diagnosis of pinworm infection. Please send properly collected repeat specimen, if clinically indicated. Contact the laboratory for instructions if required.
3. No parasites detected in current specimen. Low numbers of parasites may be missed. Please send well-collected repeat specimen if clinically indicated. Contact the laboratory for instructions if required.

In a clinically significant case, if the first specimen is negative, ask for further specimens. The time of collection is also important, especially when *Enterobius* is suspected. If the specimen is inadequate, e.g., delayed, dry, or insufficient, a repeat specimen should be requested. A freshly collected specimen and/or use of preservative kits should be encouraged where possible.

There is no need to quantitate helminth parasites as this does not necessarily correlate with clinical illness. However, in rare instances, this may be required for epidemiological studies or for clinical assessment of children.

REFERENCES

1. **Aguinaldo, A. M., J. M. Turbeville, L. S. Linford, M. C. Rivera, J. R. Garey, R. A. Raff, and J. A. Lake.** 1997. Evidence for a clade of nematodes, arthropods and other moulting animals. *Nature* **387:**489–493.
2. **Akgun, Y.** 1996. Intestinal obstruction caused by *Ascaris lumbricoides*. *Dis. Colon Rectum* **39:**1159–1163.
3. **Arca, M. J., R. L. Gates, J. I. Groner, S. Hammond, and D. A. Caniano.** 2004. Clinical manifestations of appendiceal pinworms in children: an institutional experience and a review of the literature. *Pediatr. Surg. Int.* **20:**372–375.
4. **Ash, L. R., and T. C. Orihel.** 2003. Intestinal helminths, p. 2031–2046. *In* P. R. Murray, E. J. Baron, J. H. Jorgensen, M. A. Pfaller, and R. H. Yolken (ed.), *Manual of Clinical Microbiology*, 8th ed. ASM Press, Washington, DC.

5. **Biggs, B.-A., S. Caruana, S. Mihrshahi, D. Jolley, J. Leydon, L. Chea, and S. Nuon.** 2009. Management of chronic strongyloidiasis in immigrants and refugees: is serologic testing useful? *Am. J. Trop. Med. Hyg.* **80:**788–791.

6. **Brooker, S., and D. A. P. Bundy.** 2008. Soil transmitted helminths (geohelminths), p. 1515–1548. *In* G. C. Cook and A. Zumla (ed.), *Manson's Tropical Diseases,* 22nd ed. W. B. Saunders, Elsevier Science Ltd., Edinburgh, Scotland.

7. **Garcia, L. S.** 2007. Intestinal nematodes, p. 249–282. *In* L. S. Garcia (ed.), *Diagnostic Medical Parasitology,* 5th ed. ASM Press, Washington, DC.

8. **Garcia, L. S. (ed.).** 2004. Parasitology, p. 9.0.1–9.10.8. *In* H. D. Isenberg (ed.), *Clinical Microbiology Procedures Handbook,* 2nd ed., vol. 2. ASM Press, Washington, DC.

9. **Hotez, P. J., J. Bethony, M. E. Bottazzi, S. Brooker, and P. Buss.** 2005. Hookworm: "the great infection of mankind." *PLoS Med.* **2:**e67.

10. **Hotez, P. J., S. Brooker, J. M. Bethony, M. E. Bottazzi, A. Loukas, and S. Xiap.** 2004. Hookworm infection. *N. Engl. J. Med.* **351:**799–807.

11. **Lorenzetti, R., S. M. Campo, F. Stella, C. Hassan, A. Zullo, and S. Morini.** 2003. An unusual endoscopic finding: *Trichuris trichiura.* Case report and review of the literature. *Dig. Liver Dis.* **35:**811–813.

12. **Loutfy, M. R, M. Wilson, J. S. Keystone, and K. C. Kain.** 2002. Serology and eosinophil count in the diagnosis and management of strongyloidiasis in a non-endemic area. *Am. J. Trop. Med. Hyg.* **66:**749–752.

13. **Maguire, J. H.** 2010. Intestinal nematodes (roundworms), p. 3577–3586. *In* G. L. Mandell, J. E. Bennett, and R. Dolin (ed.), *Mandell, Douglas, and Bennett's Principles and Practice of Infectious Diseases,* 7th ed. Elsevier, Churchill Livingstone, Philadelphia, PA.

14. **Medical Letter on Drugs and Therapeutics.** 2007. Drugs for parasitic infections. **September 2007**(Suppl.):1–15. http://www.medicalletter.org.

15. **Pearson, R. D.** 2002. An update on the geohelminths: *Ascaris lumbricoides,* hookworms, *Trichuris trichiura,* and *Strongyloides stercoralis. Curr. Infect. Dis. Rep.* **4:**59–64.

16. **Telford, M. J., S. J. Bourlat, A. Economou, D. Papillon, and O. Rota-Stabelli.** 2008. The evolution of the Ecdysozoa. *Philos. Trans. R. Soc. B.* **363:**1529–1537.

17. **U.S. Department of Health, Education, and Welfare.** 2001. *Common Intestinal Helminths of Man. DHEW publication no. (CDC) 80-8286.2001.* Centers for Disease Control and Prevention, Atlanta, GA.

18. **Zaha, O., T. Hirata, F. Kinjo, and A. Saito.** 2000. Strongyloidiasis—progress in diagnosis and treatment. *Intern. Med.* **39:**695–700.

Filarial Nematodes*

DORAN L. FINK AND THOMAS B. NUTMAN

142

Filarial worms are arthropod-transmitted nematodes or roundworms that dwell in the subcutaneous tissues and the lymphatics. Although eight filarial species commonly infect humans, four are responsible for most of the pathology associated with these infections. These are (i) *Wuchereria bancrofti*, (ii) *Brugia malayi*, (iii) *Onchocerca volvulus*, and (iv) *Loa loa*. In general, each of the parasites is transmitted by biting arthropods. The distribution and vectors of all the filarial parasites of humans are given in Table 1. Each goes through a complex life cycle that includes an infective larval stage carried by the insects and an adult worm stage that resides in humans, either in the lymph nodes or adjacent lymphatics or in the subcutaneous tissue.

All filariae share the unique characteristic of an adult female worm that produces microfilariae. These offspring either circulate in the blood or migrate through the skin. The microfilariae can then be ingested by the appropriate biting arthropod and develop into infective larvae that are capable of initiating the life cycle once more. Certain species (*W. bancrofti*, *Brugia* spp., and *L. loa*) circulate in the blood with a defined circadian rhythm or "periodicity," which can be nocturnal (typically the lymphatic filariae) or diurnal (*L. loa*). Other species lack periodicity and are found in the peripheral blood at all hours of the day and night. When absent from the peripheral blood, the microfilariae of filarial parasites are found in the deeper visceral capillaries, particularly in the pulmonary capillaries. Because the adult worms are typically sequestered in the tissues, diagnosis of infection depends on finding microfilariae in either blood or skin, depending on the species. Adult worms are long-lived, whereas the life spans of microfilariae range from 3 months to 3 years.

Microfilariae are relatively simple in their organization and structure (Fig. 1). They are vermiform and in stained preparations appear to be composed of a column of nuclei interrupted along its length by spaces and special cells that are the precursors of body organs or organelles. Some species of microfilariae are enveloped in a sheath, whereas others have no sheath (Table 1; Fig. 2).

All of the filariae are transmitted by species of blood-sucking arthropods such as mosquitoes, midges, blackflies, and tabanid flies, in which the microfilariae develop to the infective larval stage (Table 1). Subsequent development of the infective larva to the gravid, adult stage in the vertebrate host requires several months and in some cases a year or more. Infection is generally not established unless exposure to infective larvae is intense and prolonged. Furthermore, the clinical manifestations of these diseases develop rather slowly.

Although these parasites are nonendemic in temperate or subtropical areas, they are often seen in individuals who have immigrated to, resided in, or traveled to tropical areas where filariae are endemic. There are significant differences in the clinical manifestations of filarial infections, or at least in the time period over which these infections are acquired, between patients native to the areas of endemicity and those who are travelers or recent arrivals in these same areas. Characteristically, the disease in previously unexposed individuals is more acute and intense than that found in natives of the region of endemicity (23); however, early removal of newly infected individuals tends to speed the end of clinical symptomatology or at least halt the progression of the disease (41).

Unless specified, antiparasitic susceptibility testing is not routinely performed in the clinical laboratory for these organisms. For more details about susceptibility testing for parasites, consult chapter 149.

LYMPHATIC FILARIAL PARASITES

Taxonomy

Wuchereria bancrofti, *Brugia malayi*, and *Brugia timori* each belong to the phylum Nematoda, class Secernentea, subclass Spiruria, order Spirudida, superfamily Filarioidea, and family Filariidae.

Description of the Agents

There are three lymphatic-dwelling filarial parasites of humans: *Wuchereria bancrofti*, *Brugia malayi*, and *Brugia timori*. The adult worms usually reside in either the afferent lymphatic channels or the lymph nodes. These adult parasites may remain viable in the human host for decades. The morphologic appearance and other characteristics of the parasites can be found in Table 1 and Fig. 1 and 2.

---

*This chapter contains information presented in chapter 145 by Tess McPherson and Thomas B. Nutman in the ninth edition of this *Manual*.

TABLE 1 Filarial parasites of humans

| Species | Distribution | Vector | Primary pathology | Characteristics of microfilariae | | | | | |
| | | | | Location | Periodicity | Size (μm) | Tail | Sheath | |
								Presence	Staining properties
Wuchereria bancrofti	Tropics	Mosquito	Lymphatic, pulmonary	Blood, hydrocele fluid	Nocturnal, subperiodic	298 by 7.5–10	Pointed tail devoid of nuclei	+	Does not stain
Brugia timori	Indonesia	Mosquito	Lymphatic	Blood	Nocturnal	300 by 5–6	Nuclei in tail	+	Tends not to stain
Brugia malayi	Southeast Asia	Mosquito	Lymphatic, pulmonary	Blood	Nocturnal, subperiodic	270 by 5–6	Nuclei in tail	+	Bright pink with Giemsa
Onchocerca volvulus	Africa, Central and South America	Black fly	Dermal, ocular, lymphatic	Skin	None	309 by 5–9	No nuclei in tail	−	
Loa loa	Africa	Deerfly	Allergic	Blood	Diurnal	Up to 300	Irregularly arranged nuclei extend to end of tail	+	Does not stain
Mansonella perstans	Africa, South America	Midge	Probably allergic	Blood	None	203 by 4–5	Blunt tail contains nuclei	−	
Mansonella ozzardi	Central and South America	Midge	Unknown	Blood	None	224 by 4–5	Long tail with no nuclei in it	−	
Mansonella streptocerca	Africa	Midge	Dermal	Skin	None	210 by 5–6	"Crooked tail" in which column of nuclei extends	−	

Epidemiology and Transmission

Wuchereria bancrofti

W. bancrofti is the most common and widespread species of filaria infecting humans. It has an extensive distribution throughout tropical and subtropical areas of the world including Asia and the Pacific Islands, Africa, areas of South America, and the Caribbean Basin. Humans are the only definitive host for this parasite and are therefore the natural reservoir for infection. There are both periodic and subperiodic forms of the parasite. Nocturnally periodic forms have microfilariae present in the peripheral blood primarily at night (between 10 p.m. and 4 a.m.), whereas the subperiodic forms have microfilariae present in the blood at all times but with maximal levels in the afternoon. Generally, the subperiodic form is found only in the Pacific Islands (including Cook and Ellis Islands, Fiji, New Caledonia, the Marquesas, Samoa, and the Society Islands). Elsewhere, W. bancrofti is nocturnally periodic. The natural vectors are *Culex fatigans* mosquitoes in urban settings and usually anopheline or aedean mosquitoes in rural areas.

Brugia malayi and Brugia timori

The distribution of brugian filariasis is limited primarily to China, India, Indonesia, Korea, Japan, Malaysia, and the Philippines. B. timori has been described only on two islands in Timor. Similar to the situation with W. bancrofti, there are both periodic and subperiodic forms of brugian filariasis. The nocturnal periodic form is more common and is transmitted in areas of coastal rice fields (by mansonian and anopheline mosquitoes), while the subperiodic form is found in the swamp forests (mansonian vector). Although humans are the common host, B. malayi also naturally infects cats.

Clinical Significance (Description of Clinical Presentation)

Lymphatic filariasis (LF) is associated with a variety of clinical manifestations. The four most common presentations are asymptomatic (or subclinical) microfilaremia, lymphedema, hydrocele, and acute attacks. Less frequently, LF can present with chyluria or tropical eosinophilia (11, 38, 55). The range of clinical disease varies somewhat across geographic locations and according to the species of nematode causing the infection (45). Additionally, the disease in previously unexposed individuals is more acute and intense than that found in natives of the region of endemicity (23, 41). Patients with asymptomatic (or subclinical) microfilaremia rarely come to the attention of medical personnel except through the incidental finding of microfilariae in the peripheral blood. Although they may be clinically asymptomatic, virtually all persons with W. bancrofti or B. malayi microfilaremia have some degree of subclinical disease that includes dilated and tortuous lymphatics (visualized by imaging) and—in men with W. bancrofti—scrotal lymphangiectasia (detectable by ultrasound) (31). Despite these findings, the majority of individuals appear to remain clinically asymptomatic for years. Relatively few progress to either the acute or chronic stage of infection (13). Development of lymphedema may not occur until long after the initial infection. Lymphatic dysfunction develops as a primary event in response to adult filarial parasites and host immune responses in virtually all infected persons. This process has been shown to be progressive during infection and permanent once established (10). Lymphedema most commonly affects the lower extremities but can also affect arms, breasts in females, and the scrotum in males.

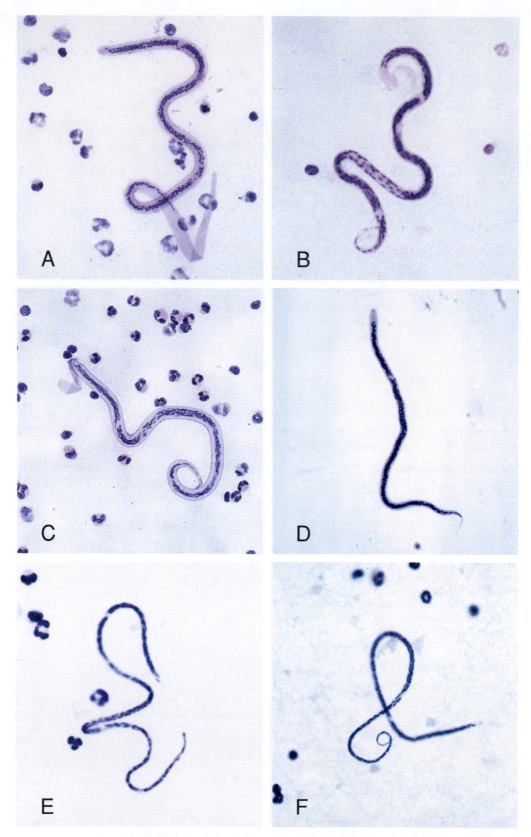

FIGURE 1 Common microfilariae found in humans. Organisms are stained with hematoxylin. Magnification, ×325. (A) *W. bancrofti*; (B) *B. malayi*; (C) *L. loa*; (D) *O. volvulus*; (E) *M. perstans*; (F) *M. ozzardi*.

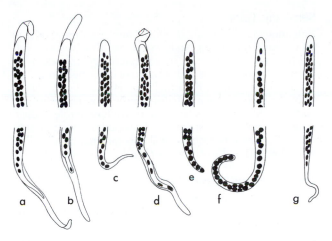

FIGURE 2 Diagrammatic representation of the anterior and posterior extremities of the common microfilariae found in humans. (a) *W. bancrofti*; (b) *B. malayi*; (c) *O. volvulus*; (d) *L. loa*; (e) *M. perstans*; (f) *M. streptocerca*; (g) *M. ozzardi*.

Secondary effects such as thickening of the subcutaneous tissues, hyperkeratosis, fissuring of the skin, and hyperplastic skin changes can occur. Recurrent infections (acute dermatolymphangioadenitis [ADLA]) on the background of chronic skin changes and lymphatic dysfunction play a major role for lymphedema disease development and progression to elephantiasis (35, 39).

Acute attacks in LF cover a variety of clinical entities that present with inflammation. True filarial adenolymphangitis (ADL), felt to reflect the death of an adult worm, presents with inflammation, swelling, and retrograde lymphangitis extending peripherally from the draining node where the parasites presumably reside. Regional lymph nodes are often enlarged, and the entire lymphatic channel can become indurated and inflamed. The second type of acute attack is now labeled bacterial ADL or ADLA. Skin changes cause lesions, in particular in the toe webs, that facilitate entry of bacterial skin microbiota (3, 48). For these reasons, limbs become susceptible to recurrent bacterial infections (12, 26). The clinical pattern of ADLA is distinctly different from that of ADL (26). The lymphangitis develops in a reticular rather than in a linear pattern, and the local and systemic symptoms, including edema, pain, fever, and chills, are frequently more severe (47). These cause considerable acute morbidity and progression of lymphedema to elephantiasis (40). ADL and ADLA occur in both the upper and the lower extremities with both bancroftian and brugian filariasis, but involvement of the genital lymphatics occurs almost exclusively with *W. bancrofti* infection.

Hydrocele formation occurs in bancroftian filariasis when adult worms block retroperitoneal and subdiaphragmatic lymphatics. In males, this causes accumulation of straw-colored lymph either unilaterally or bilaterally between the visceral and parietal layers of the tunica vaginalis. The condition presents as a translucent mass obscuring palpation of the testis and differs from a congenital hydrocele or herniation in that the tunica is sealed at the top and peritoneal fluid is not communicating. If there is obstruction of the retroperitoneal lymphatics, renal lymphatic pressure can increase to the point at which they rupture into the renal pelvis or tubules so that chyluria is seen. The chyluria is characteristically intermittent and is often prominent in the morning just after the patient arises.

Tropical pulmonary eosinophilia (TPE) is a distinct syndrome that develops in some individuals infected with LF species. This syndrome affects males more often than females, most commonly during the third decade of life. The majority of cases have been reported from India, Pakistan, Sri Lanka, Brazil, Guyana, and Southeast Asia. The main features include a history of residence in regions where filariae are endemic, paroxysmal cough and wheezing that are usually nocturnal, weight loss, low-grade fever, and adenopathy. Patients are rarely found to have microfilariae in the blood. Chest radiographs may be normal but generally show increased bronchovascular markings, and diffuse miliary lesions or mottled opacities may be present in the middle and lower lung fields. Tests of pulmonary function show restrictive abnormalities in most cases and obstructive defects in one-half of the cases. Total serum immunoglobulin E (IgE) levels (10,000 to 100,000 ng/ml) and antifilarial antibody titers are characteristically elevated. TPE is now considered to be a form of occult filariasis, in which rapid clearance of the microfilariae occurs, presumably on the basis of host immunologic hyperresponsiveness to the parasite (38). Although there is no single clinical or laboratory criterion that aids in distinguishing TPE from other pulmonary diseases, residence in the tropics, the presence of high levels of antifilarial antibodies, and a rapid clinical response to diethylcarbamazine (DEC) favor the diagnosis of TPE (54).

Diagnosis

Diagnosis of bancroftian and brugian filarial infection can be made noninvasively in some cases by ultrasound. This allows adult worms to be visualized in lymphatics or can identify dilated lymphatics. Definitive identification of parasites can be achieved with appropriate samples of blood or tissue. The timing of blood collection is critical and should be based on the periodicity of the microfilariae in the endemic region involved (Table 1). Recent developments in immunodiagnostic and molecular biology techniques give further options for diagnosis.

Ultrasound

In cases of suspected LF due to *W. bancrofti*, high-frequency ultrasound of the scrotum or female breast coupled with Doppler imaging may result in identification of motile adult worms ("filarial dance sign") within dilated lymphatics. Adult worms may be visualized in the lymphatics of the spermatic cord in up to 80% of infected men with microfilaremia associated with *W. bancrofti* (13). In brugian filariasis, ultrasounds have been used successfully to localize the adult worms in the female breast, the inguinal lymph nodes and the lymphatic vessels of the thigh and calf (49).

Direct Examination

Parasites can be identified by direct examination of blood or other fluids (such as chyle, urine, and hydrocele fluid). This should take advantage of the periodicity of each organism as well as their characteristic morphologic appearance (Table 1 and Fig. 2).

Microscopy

A small volume of fluid is spread on a clean slide. The slide is then air dried, stained with Giemsa, and examined microscopically. The microfilariae of *W. bancrofti* are sheathed, lie in smooth curves in stained smears, and are 298 μm long and 7.5 to 10.0 μm in diameter. The column nuclei are dispersed; there is a short headspace, and the pointed tail is devoid of nuclei (Fig. 1A). The sheath stains faintly or not at all with Giemsa stain. The microfilariae of *W. bancrofti* must be distinguished from other sheathed microfilariae. The morphology of the *B. malayi* microfilariae is similar to that of the *W. bancrofti* microfilariae, being sheathed but somewhat smaller (279 μm by 5 to 6 μm). They can be differentiated from the *W. bancrofti* microfilariae by the presence of subterminal and terminal nuclei in the tail (Fig. 1A and B). *B. timori* microfilariae are similar to those of *B. malayi* with conspicuous terminal and subterminal nuclei; however, *B. timori* is larger (more than 300 μm long) than *B. malayi*. Additionally, the *B. malayi* sheath stains bright pink with Giesma, whereas the *B. timori* sheath tends not to stain and that of *W. bancrofti* never does (4).

Because microfilariae may be present in the blood in only small numbers, sensitive procedures such as Nuclepore filtration and Knott's concentration are also used routinely to detect infections.

Nuclepore Filtration

A known volume of anticoagulated blood is passed through a polycarbonate (Nuclepore) filter with a 3-μm-diameter pore. A large volume (50 ml) of distilled water is passed through (the water will lyse or break open the red blood cells, leaving the worms intact and more easily visible). The filter is then air dried, stained with Wright's or Giemsa stain, and examined by microscopy. For studies in the field, 1 ml of anticoagulated blood can be added to 9 ml of a solution of 2% formalin or 10% Teepol and stored for up to 9 months before performing filtration.

Knott's Concentration Technique

Anticoagulated blood (1 ml) is placed in 9 ml of 2% formalin. The tube is centrifuged at 500 × *g* for 1 minute. The sediment is spread on a slide and dried thoroughly. The slide is then stained with Wright's or Giemsa stain and examined microscopically.

Antigen Detection

Assays for circulating antigens of *W. bancrofti* permit the diagnosis of microfilaremic and cryptic (amicrofilaremic) infection. Two tests are commercially available (though not in the United States). One is an enzyme-linked immunosorbent assay (ELISA) available from TropBio Pty. (Townsville, Queensland, Australia; tropbio@jcu.edu.au), and the other is a rapid-format immunochromatographic card available from Inverness Medical (Portland, ME; http://www.binaxnow.com/filariasis.aspx). Both assays have sensitivities that range from 96 to100% and specificities that approach 100% (29, 56). Both tests can be used on blood drawn any time of day or night, thus avoiding the need for specific bleeding times depending on periodicity of microfilariae. Neither of the tests is FDA approved. There are currently no tests for circulating antigens in brugian filariasis.

Nucleic Acid Detection Techniques

In appropriate laboratories, PCR can detect parasite DNA and is now the most sensitive technique for definitive diagnosis (25, 59). For each of the lymphatic-dwelling parasites, primers and probes have been identified that are 100% specific and provide sensitivities that are up to 10-fold greater than parasite detection by direct examination. Recent diagnostic advances include highly sensitive real-time PCR assays capable of detecting relatively low copy numbers of target sequence in small samples of dried human blood (43, 44).

Serologic Tests

Immunologically based diagnosis with measured IgG or IgG4 responses against crude extracts of *Brugia* worms suffers from poor specificity. There is extensive cross-reactivity among filarial antigens and antigens of other helminths, including the common intestinal roundworms. Furthermore, serologic tests are unable to distinguish between active and past infection. However, these tests still have a role in diagnosis, as a negative test effectively excludes past or present infection. These tests are available commercially as well as from the National Institutes of Health.

Treatment and Prevention

The available chemotherapy for LF is DEC, ivermectin, and albendazole. DEC remains the treatment of choice for the individual with active LF (microfilaremia, antigen positivity, or adult worms on ultrasound), although albendazole has also been shown to have some macrofilaricidal efficacy. If the adult parasites survive, microfilaremia along with clinical symptoms can recur within months after conclusion of the therapy. Chronic low-dose DEC may also result in cure (e.g., by use of DEC salt). Evidence shows that these drugs used in combination can increase effectiveness (53). The current global elimination campaign uses these three drugs in various combinations for mass treatment of communities where the parasites are endemic (37).

Most pathogenic filarial nematodes apart from *L. loa* harbor bacterial endosymbionts. These *Wolbachia* bacteria are vital for parasite larval development and adult-worm fertility and viability. New approaches for treatment use antibiotics (e.g., the tetracyclines) that target *Wolbachia* and have been shown to reduce microfilarial levels (52). Once lymphedema is established, antifilarial medication is not useful if the patient does not have active infection. Management of lymphedema should concentrate on exercise, elevation, and local skin care with appropriate treatment of entry lesions (30). Antifilarial medication is also not indicated in management of bacterial ADLA, which is addressed with skin care and antibiotics if indicated (47, 48). Hydroceles can be drained repeatedly or managed surgically (58).

Avoidance of mosquito bites is usually not feasible for residents of areas of endemicity, but visitors should make use of insect repellent and mosquito nets. Impregnated bednets have been shown to have a salutary effect. DEC can kill developing forms of filarial parasites and has been shown to be useful as a prophylactic agent in humans. Community-based intervention is the current approach to elimination of LF as a public health problem (36, 37). The underlying tenet of this approach is that mass annual distribution of antimicrofilarial chemotherapy (albendazole with either DEC [for all areas except where onchocercaisis is coendemic] or ivermectin) will profoundly suppress microfilaremia. If the suppression is sustained, then transmission can be interrupted. Community education and clinical care for persons already suffering from the chronic sequelae of LF are important components of filariasis control and elimination programs (46). Vaccines are not currently available but may have a role in the future.

ONCHOCERCA VOLVULUS

Taxonomy

Onchocerca volvulus belongs to the phylum Nematoda, class Secernentea, subclass Spiruria, order Spirudida, superfamily Filarioidea, and family Onchocercidae.

Description of the Agent

The adult worms of *Onchocerca volvulus* typically reside in nodules comprised primarily of host tissue. These adult parasites may remain viable in the human host for decades. The morphologic appearance and other characteristics of and microfilariae and adult worms can be found in Table 1 and Fig. 1 and 2.

Epidemiology and Transmission

Onchocerciasis, sometimes called "river blindness," is caused by infection with *Onchocerca volvulus*, a subcutaneous tissue-dwelling filarial worm. Approximately 18 million people are infected, mostly in equatorial Africa, the Sahara, Yemen, and parts of Central and South America (Guatemala, Venezuela, Mexico, Ecuador, Colombia, and Brazil). The infection is transmitted to humans through the bites of blackflies of the genus *Simulium*, which breed along fast-flowing rivers in the above-mentioned tropical areas.

Clinical Significance (Description of Clinical Presentation)

The major disease manifestations of onchocerciasis are localized to the skin, lymph nodes, and eyes. Onchocerciasis is a cumulative infection. Intense infection leads to the most severe complications and is felt to reflect repeated inoculation with infective larvae.

Skin

Pruritus is the most frequent manifestation of onchocercal dermatitis. This pruritus may be accompanied by the appearance of localized areas of edema and erythema. Typically, skin disease appears as a papular, pruritic dermatitis. If the infection is prolonged, lichenification and pigment changes (either hypo- or hyperpigmentation) can occur; these often lead to atrophy, "lizard skin," and mottling of the skin.

Onchocercomata

Onchocercomata, subcutaneous nodules that can be palpable and/or visible, contain the adult worm. In African patients, they are common over bony prominences; in Latin American patients, nodules tend to develop preferentially in the upper part of the body, particularly on the head. Nodules vary in size and characteristically are firm and nontender. It has been estimated that for every palpable nodule there are four deeper nonpalpable ones (2).

Lymph Nodes

Lymphadenopathy is frequently found, particularly in the inguinal and femoral areas. The underlying pathology consists of scarring of the lymphoid areas (*O. volvulus* infection in Africa) or follicular hyperplasia (*O. volvulus* infection in Yemen). As the lymph nodes enlarge, they can come to lie within areas of loose skin (so-called "hanging groin") that predisposes to inguinal and femoral hernias.

Ocular Disease

Onchocercal eye disease can take many forms and can lead to severe visual loss or blindness. Usually seen in persons with moderate or heavy infections, ocular disease spares no part of the eye. Manifestations include conjunctivitis, anterior uveitis, iridocyclitis leading to secondary glaucoma, sclerosing keratitis, optic atrophy, and chorioretinal lesions (51).

Systemic Manifestations

Some heavily infected individuals develop cachexia with loss of adipose tissue and muscle mass. Among adults who become blind, there is a three- to fourfold increase in the mortality rate.

Diagnosis

Definitive diagnosis depends on finding an adult worm in an excised nodule or, more commonly, microfilariae in a skin snip. Microfilariae can occasionally be found in the blood and in urine, typically after treatment. Microfilariae may also be seen in the cornea and in the anterior chamber of the eye when viewed with a slit lamp.

For skin snip evaluation, a small piece of skin is elevated by the tip of a needle or skin hook held parallel to the surface, and a scalpel blade is used to shave off the skin area stretched across the top surface of the needle. Alternatively, a sclerocorneal punch can be used to obtain a blood-free circular skin specimen. Skin snips are generally obtained from an area of affected skin or from the scapular, gluteal, and calf areas (in the African form) and from the scapular, deltoid, and gluteal areas (in the Central American form). Once obtained, the skin snips are incubated in a physiologic solution (such as normal saline). The emergent microfilariae can be seen under a microscope typically within hours (in heavy infection) or within 24 hours in light infections.

Direct Examination

Microscopy

Microfilariae lack a sheath and are approximately 309 μm long and 5 to 9 μm in diameter. The tail is tapered, usually bent or flexed, and without nuclei (Fig. 1D and 2c).

Nucleic Acid Detection Techniques

Assays using PCR to detect onchocercal DNA in skin snips are now in use in research laboratories and are highly specific and sensitive, provided that organisms are present in the skin samples obtained (60).

Serologic Tests

Because direct detection of parasites in the skin or eye is invasive and insensitive, immunodiagnostic assays may be preferable. IgG antifilarial antibody assays, while positive in individuals with onchocerciasis, suffer from the same lack of specificity and positive predictive value seen in the blood-borne filarial infections; however, the combined use of three groups of recombinant antigens in conventional ELISA provides sensitivity and specificities that approach 100% for the diagnosis of onchocerciasis (42). A newer platform incorporates four recombinant antigens into a rapid, high-throughput luciferase immunoprecipitation system assay that is 100% sensitive and 80 to 90% specific in distinguishing onchocerciasis from related filarial infections (7). Although no recombinant antigen test is available commercially, an experimental rapid card test that detects IgG4 antibodies in serum or whole blood by using recombinant Ov-16 protein has been shown to have >90% sensitivity and specificity (22, 57).

Treatment

The major goals of therapy are to prevent irreversible lesions and to alleviate symptoms. Surgical excision of nodules is recommended when the nodules are located on the head because of the proximity of the microfilaria-producing adult worms to the eye, but chemotherapy is the mainstay of treatment. Ivermectin, a semisynthetic macrocyclic lactone, is now considered the first-line therapy for onchocerciasis. It is characteristically given yearly or semiannually. Most patients have limited to no reaction to treatment. Pruritus, cutaneous edema, and/or a maculopapular rash occurs in approximately 1 to 10% of treated individuals. Significant ocular complications are extremely rare, as is hypotension (1 in 10,000). In areas of Africa coendemic for *O. volvulus* and *L. loa*, however, ivermectin is contraindicated because of severe posttreatment encephalopathy seen in patients who are heavily microfilaremic for *L. loa* (15). Ivermectin is also contraindicated for use in pregnant or breast-feeding women, based on toxicity and teratogenicity data from animal studies. Although ivermectin treatment results in a marked drop in microfilarial density, its effect can be short-lived (<3 months in some cases). Thus, it is occasionally necessary to give ivermectin more frequently for persistent symptoms (5). A 6-week course of doxycycline that targets the *Wolbachia* endosymbiont has been demonstrated to be macrofilaristatic, rendering the female adult worms sterile for long periods (17).

Prevention

Prevention of infection is being achieved by mass-treatment programs using ivermectin (28, 50). Vector control has been beneficial in areas of high endemicity in which breeding sites are vulnerable to insecticide spraying, but most areas where onchocerciasis is endemic are not suited to this type of intervention. Community-based administration of ivermectin every 6 to 12 months is now being used to interrupt transmission in endemic areas. This measure, in conjunction with vector control, has already helped reduce the prevalence of disease in foci of endemicity in Africa and Latin America. No drug has proven useful for prophylaxis of *O. volvulus* infection, and no vaccine exists.

LOA LOA

Taxonomy

Loa loa belongs to the phylum Nematoda, class Chromadorea, order Spirudida, superfamily Filarioidea, and family Onchocercidae.

Description of the Agent

The adult parasite lives in the subcutaneous tissues in humans; microfilariae circulate in the bloodstream with a diurnal periodicity that peaks between 12:00 noon and 2:00 p.m. The morphologic appearance and other characteristics of adult worms and microfilariae can be found in Table 1 and Fig. 1 and 2.

Epidemiology and Transmission

The distribution of *L. loa* is limited to the rain forests of West and Central Africa. Tabanid flies (deerflies) of the genus *Chrysops* are the vectors.

Clinical Significance (Description of Clinical Presentation)

L. loa infection may be present as asymptomatic microfilaremia, with the infection being recognized only after subconjunctival migration of an adult worm (the so-called eye worm). The classic clinical presentation is with episodic "Calabar swelling" (localized areas of transient angioedema) found predominantly on the extremities. If associated inflammation extends to the nearby joints or peripheral nerves, corresponding symptoms develop. Nephropathy (presumed to be immune-complex mediated), encephalopathy, and cardiomyopathy due to marked eosinophilia can occur, rarely.

There appear to be differences in the presentations of loiasis between individuals who are native to the area of endemicity and those who are visitors (19). The latter tend to have a greater predominance of allergic symptomatology. The episodes of Calabar swelling tend to be more frequent and debilitating, and such patients rarely have microfilaremia. In addition, those who are not native to the area of endemicity have extreme elevation of eosinophils in the blood as well as marked increases in antifilarial antibody titers.

Diagnosis

Definitive diagnosis is made parasitologically, either by finding microfilariae in the peripheral blood or by isolating the adult worm from the eye or subcutaneous biopsy material following treatment. The diagnosis must often be made on clinical grounds, however, particularly for travelers (usually amicrofilaremic) to the region of endemicity.

Direct Examination

Microscopy

The microfilariae are sheathed and are up to 300 μm long. Adult females are 50 to 70 mm long and 0.5 mm wide, whereas adult males are 25 to 35 mm long and 0.25 mm wide. In contrast to the LF, the nuclei extend to the end of the tail; however, they are somewhat irregularly arranged along the length of the tail (Fig. 1C and 2d). The sheath does not stain with Giemsa stain.

Nucleic Acid Detection Techniques

PCR-based assays for the detection of *L. loa* DNA in blood are now available in research laboratories and are highly sensitive and specific (34).

Serologic Tests

Available methods using crude antigen extracts from *Brugia* or *Dirofilaria* species do not differentiate between *L. loa* and other filarial pathogens. The utility of such testing in populations of areas of endemicity is limited by the presence of antifilarial antibodies in up to 95% of individuals in some regions. A loa-specific recombinant protein, SXP-1, has been tested and has good specificity but only limited (50%) sensitivity in conventional ELISA (21). Incorporation of SXP-1 into a luciferase immunoprecipitation system assay increased sensitivity to near 100% while also allowing for rapid, high-throughput processing of samples (8). Antifilarial IgG and IgG4, while nonspecific, may be useful in confirming the diagnosis of loiasis in visitors to areas of endemicity with suggestive clinical symptoms or unexplained eosinophilia.

Treatment and Prevention

DEC is effective against both the adult and the microfilarial forms of *L. loa*, but multiple courses are frequently necessary before the disease resolves completely (20). In cases of heavy microfilaremia, allergic or other inflammatory reactions can take place during treatment, including central nervous system involvement with coma and encephalitis. Heavy infections can be treated initially with apheresis to remove the microfilariae and with glucocorticoids followed by small doses of DEC. If antifilarial treatment has no adverse effects, the prednisone dose can be rapidly tapered and the dose of DEC gradually increased. Albendazole or ivermectin (although not approved for this use by the FDA) has been shown to be effective in reducing microfilarial loads, but the use of ivermectin in heavily microfilaremic individuals is contraindicated (6). DEC is an effective prophylactic regimen for loiasis (32).

MANSONELLA INFECTIONS

Taxonomy

Mansonella perstans, *Mansonella ozzardi*, and *Mansonella streptocerca* each belong to the phylum Nematoda, class Secernentea, subclass Spiruria, order Spirudida, superfamily Filarioidea, and family Onchocercidae.

Description of the Agents

The adult worms of *Mansonella perstans* reside in the body cavities (pericardial, pleural, and peritoneal) as well as in the mesentery and the perirenal and retroperitoneal tissues, whereas the location of the adult worms of *Mansonella ozzardi* is unknown. The microfilariae of both parasites circulate in the blood without periodicity. For *Mansonella streptocerca*, the adult parasites reside in the skin. *M. streptocerca* microfilariae are found predominantly in the skin. The morphologic appearance and other characteristics of adult worms and microfilariae can be found in Table 1 and Fig. 1 and 2.

Epidemiology and Transmission

Mansonella perstans is distributed across the center of Africa and in northeastern South America. The infection is transmitted to humans through the bites of midges (*Culicoides* species). *Mansonella streptocerca* is largely found in the tropical forest belt of Africa from Ghana to the Democratic Republic of the Congo (formerly Zaire). It is transmitted to the human host by biting midges (*Culicoides* species). The distribution of *M. ozzardi* is restricted to Central and South America as well as certain Caribbean islands. The parasite is transmitted to the human host by biting midges (*Culicoides furens*) and blackflies (*Simulium amazonicum*).

Clinical Significance (Description of Clinical Presentation)

Although most patients infected with M. *perstans* appear to be asymptomatic, clinical manifestations may include transient angioedematous swellings of the arms, face, or other body parts (similar to the Calabar swellings of *L. loa* infection); pruritus; fever; headache; arthralgias; neurological or psychological symptoms; and right-upper-quadrant pain. Occasionally, pericarditis and hepatitis occur (1).

The major clinical manifestations of M. *streptocerca* infections are related to the skin: pruritus, papular rashes, and pigmentation changes. These are thought to be secondary to inflammatory reactions around microfilariae. Most infected individuals also show inguinal lymphadenopathy. Lymph nodes of affected individuals may show chronic lymphadenitis with scarring; however, many patients are completely asymptomatic (27).

The clinical details of M. *ozzardi* infection are poorly characterized. Furthermore, many consider this organism to be nonpathogenic; however, headache, articular pain, fever, pulmonary symptoms, adenopathy, hepatomegaly, and pruritus have been ascribed to infection with this organism (24).

Diagnosis

For M. *perstans* infections, diagnosis is made parasitologically by finding the microfilariae in the blood or in other body fluids (serosal effusions). Microfilariae are small (203 μm by 4 to 5 μm) and have a blunt tail filled with nuclei. Perstans filariasis is often associated with peripheral blood eosinophilia and antifilarial antibody elevations (1). The diagnosis of M. *ozzardi* infection is made by demonstrating the characteristic microfilariae in the peripheral blood. These are small (224 μm by 4 to 5 μm) and have long attenuated tails devoid of nuclei (Fig. 1F and 2g). The diagnosis of streptocerciasis can be made by finding the characteristic microfilariae on skin-snip examination (see "Diagnosis" under "*Onchocerca volvulus*" above). In areas where both O. *volvulus* and M. *streptocerca* are endemic, care must be taken to correctly identify the microfilariae. M. *streptocerca* microfilariae have no sheath, are long and slender, and measure approximately 210 μm by 5 to 6 μm. The most characteristic feature of M. *streptocerca* is its crooked tail (Fig. 2f), which contains nuclei.

Treatment and Prevention

Mansonella perstans

A number of treatment regimens have been tried, but none has been shown to be particularly effective in M. *perstans* filariasis. However, consistent with the identification of a *Wolbachia* species in M. *perstans* (18) a randomized trial in Mali has demonstrated the utility of doxycycline (200 mg daily for 6 weeks) in treatment for this infection (9).

Mansonella streptocerca

DEC is particularly effective in treating infection by both the microfilarial and the adult forms of the M. *streptocerca* parasite. Following treatment, as in onchocerciasis, one can often see debilitating urticaria, arthralgias, myalgias, headaches, and abdominal discomfort. Nevertheless, DEC is contraindicated in most of Africa because of concerns with posttreatment reactions in onchocerciasis, and its use in this infection is limited. Consequently, ivermectin is currently the drug of choice for this infection (14).

Mansonella ozzardi

Ivermectin is the drug of choice for M. *ozzardi* infection (16, 33). There currently are no good preventative measures for any of the *Mansonella* infections beyond personal protective equipment, clothing, and insect repellents such as DEET (*N,N*-diethyl-meta-toluamide) or permethrin.

REFERENCES

1. **Adolph, P. E., I. G. Kagan, and R. M. McQuay.** 1962. Diagnosis and treatment of *Acanthocheilonema perstans* filariasis. *Am. J. Trop. Med. Hyg.* **11:**76–88.
2. **Albiez, E. J.** 1983. Studies on nodules and adult *Onchocerca volvulus* during a nodulectomy trial in hyperendemic villages in Liberia and Upper Volta. I. Palpable and impalpable onchocercomata. *Tropenmed. Parasitol.* **34:**54–60.
3. **Ananthakrishnan, S., and L. K. Das.** 2004. Entry lesions in bancroftian filarial lymphoedema patients—a clinical observation. *Acta. Trop.* **90:**215–218.
4. **Ash, L., and T. Orihel.** 1997. *Atlas of Human Parasitology*, 4th ed. American Society of Clinical Pathologists, Chicago, IL.
5. **Boatin, B. A., and F. O. Richards, Jr.** 2006. Control of onchocerciasis. *Adv. Parasitol.* **61:**349–394.
6. **Boussinesq, M., J. Gardon, N. Gardon-Wendel, and J. P. Chippaux.** 2003. Clinical picture, epidemiology and outcome of Loa-associated serious adverse events related to mass ivermectin treatment of onchocerciasis in Cameroon. *Filaria J.* **2**(Suppl. 1):S4.
7. **Burbelo, P. D., H. P. Leahy, M. J. Iadarola, and T. B. Nutman.** 2009. A four-antigen mixture for rapid assessment of *Onchocerca volvulus* infection. *PLoS Negl. Trop. Dis.* **3:**e438.
8. **Burbelo, P. D., R. Ramanathan, A. D. Klion, M. J. Iadarola, and T. B. Nutman.** 2008. Rapid, novel, specific, high-throughput assay for diagnosis of *Loa loa* infection. *J. Clin. Microbiol.* **46:**2298–2304.

9. **Coulibaly, Y. I., B. Dembele, A. A. Diallo, E. M. Lipner, S. S. Doumbia, S. Y. Coulibaly, S. Konate, D. A. Diallo, D. Yalcouye, J. Kubofcik, O. K. Doumbo, A. K. Traore, A. D. Keita, M. P. Fay, S. F. Traore, T. B. Nutman, and A. D. Klion.** 2009. A randomized trial of doxycycline for *Mansonella perstans* infection. *N. Engl. J. Med.* **361:**1448–1458.

10. **Dreyer, G., D. Addiss, J. Roberts, and J. Noroes.** 2002. Progression of lymphatic vessel dilatation in the presence of living adult *Wuchereria bancrofti. Trans. R. Soc. Trop. Med. Hyg.* **96:**157–161.

11. **Dreyer, G., D. Mattos, and J. Noroes.** 2007. Chyluria. *Rev. Assoc. Med. Bras.* **53:**460–464. (In Portuguese.)

12. **Dreyer, G., Z. Medeiros, M. J. Netto, N. C. Leal, L. G. de Castro, and W. F. Piessens.** 1999. Acute attacks in the extremities of persons living in an area endemic for bancroftian filariasis: differentiation of two syndromes. *Trans. R. Soc. Trop. Med. Hyg.* **93:**413–417.

13. **Dreyer, G., J. Noroes, J. Figueredo-Silva, and W. F. Piessens.** 2000. Pathogenesis of lymphatic disease in bancroftian filariasis: a clinical perspective. *Parasitol. Today* **16:**544–548.

14. **Fischer, P., E. Tukesiga, and D. W. Buttner.** 1999. Long-term suppression of *Mansonella streptocerca* microfilariae after treatment with ivermectin. *J. Infect. Dis.* **180:**1403–1405.

15. **Gardon, J., N. Gardon-Wendel, N. Demanga, J. Kamgno, J. P. Chippaux, and M. Boussinesq.** 1997. Serious reactions after mass treatment of onchocerciasis with ivermectin in an area endemic for *Loa loa* infection. *Lancet* **350:**18–22.

16. **Gonzalez, A. A., D. D. Chadee, and S. C. Rawlins.** 1999. Ivermectin treatment of mansonellosis in Trinidad. *West Indian Med. J.* **48:**231–234.

17. **Hoerauf, A., S. Mand, O. Adjei, B. Fleischer, and D. W. Buttner.** 2001. Depletion of wolbachia endobacteria in *Onchocerca volvulus* by doxycycline and microfilaridermia after ivermectin treatment. *Lancet* **357:**1415–1416.

18. **Keiser, P. B., Y. Coulibaly, J. Kubofcik, A. A. Diallo, A. D. Klion, S. F. Traore, and T. B. Nutman.** 2008. Molecular identification of *Wolbachia* from the filarial nematode *Mansonella perstans. Mol. Biochem. Parasitol.* **160:**123–128.

19. **Klion, A. D., A. Massougbodji, B. C. Sadeler, E. A. Ottesen, and T. B. Nutman.** 1991. Loiasis in endemic and nonendemic populations: immunologically mediated differences in clinical presentation. *J. Infect. Dis.* **163:**1318–1325.

20. **Klion, A. D., E. A. Ottesen, and T. B. Nutman.** 1994. Effectiveness of diethylcarbamazine in treating loiasis acquired by expatriate visitors to endemic regions: long-term follow-up. *J. Infect. Dis.* **169:**604–610.

21. **Klion, A. D., A. Vijaykumar, T. Oei, B. Martin, and T. B. Nutman.** 2003. Serum immunoglobulin G4 antibodies to the recombinant antigen, Ll-SXP-1, are highly specific for *Loa loa* infection. *J. Infect. Dis.* **187:**128–133.

22. **Lipner, E. M., N. Dembele, S. Souleymane, W. S. Alley, D. R. Prevots, L. Toe, B. Boatin, G. J. Weil, and T. B. Nutman.** 2006. Field applicability of a rapid-format anti-Ov-16 antibody test for the assessment of onchocerciasis control measures in regions of endemicity. *J. Infect. Dis.* **194:**216–221.

23. **Lipner, E. M., M. A. Law, E. Barnett, J. S. Keystone, F. von Sonnenburg, L. Loutan, D. R. Prevots, A. D. Klion, and T. B. Nutman for the Geosentinel Surveillance Network.** 2007. Filariasis in travelers presenting to the GeoSentinel Surveillance Network. *PLoS Negl. Trop. Dis.* **1:**e88.

24. **Marinkelle, C. J., and E. German.** 1970. Mansonelliasis in the Comisaria del Vaupes of Colombia. *Trop. Geogr. Med.* **22:**101–111.

25. **McCarthy, J. S., M. Zhong, R. Gopinath, E. A. Ottesen, S. A. Williams, and T. B. Nutman.** 1996. Evaluation of a polymerase chain reaction-based assay for diagnosis of *Wuchereria bancrofti* infection. *J. Infect. Dis.* **173:**1510–1514.

26. **McPherson, T., S. Persaud, S. Singh, M. P. Fay, D. Addiss, T. B. Nutman, and R. Hay.** 2006. Interdigital lesions and frequency of acute dermatolymphangioadenitis in lymphoedema in a filariasis-endemic area. *Br. J. Dermatol.* **154:**933–941.

27. **Meyers, W. M., D. H. Connor, L. E. Harman, K. Fleshman, R. Moris, and R. C. Neafie.** 1972. Human streptocerciasis. A clinico-pathologic study of 40 Africans (Zairians) including identification of the adult filaria. *Am. J. Trop. Med. Hyg.* **21:**528–545.

28. **Molyneux, D. H.** 2009. Filaria control and elimination: diagnostic, monitoring and surveillance needs. *Trans. R. Soc. Trop. Med. Hyg.* **103:**338–341.

29. **More, S. J., and D. B. Copeman.** 1990. A highly specific and sensitive monoclonal antibody-based ELISA for the detection of circulating antigen in bancroftian filariasis. *Trop. Med. Parasitol.* **41:**403–406.

30. **Narahari, S. R., T. J. Ryan, P. E. Mahadevan, K. S. Bose, and K. S. Prasanna.** 2007. Integrated management of filarial lymphedema for rural communities. *Lymphology* **40:**3–13.

31. **Noroes, J., D. Addiss, A. Santos, Z. Medeiros, A. Coutinho, and G. Dreyer.** 1996. Ultrasonographic evidence of abnormal lymphatic vessels in young men with adult *Wuchereria bancrofti* infection in the scrotal area. *J. Urol.* **156:**409–412.

32. **Nutman, T. B., K. D. Miller, M. Mulligan, G. N. Reinhardt, B. J. Currie, C. Steel, and E. A. Ottesen.** 1988. Diethylcarbamazine prophylaxis for human loiasis. *N. Engl. J. Med.* **319:**752–756.

33. **Nutman, T. B., T. E. Nash, and E. A. Ottesen.** 1987. Ivermectin in the successful treatment of a patient with *Mansonella ozzardi* infection. *J. Infect. Dis.* **156:**662–665.

34. **Nutman, T. B., P. A. Zimmerman, J. Kubofcik, and D. D. Kostyu.** 1994. A universally applicable diagnostic approach to filarial and other infections. *Parasitol. Today* **10:**239–243.

35. **Olszewski, W. L., S. Jamal, G. Manokaran, S. Pani, V. Kumaraswami, U. Kubicka, B. Lukomska, F. M. Tripathi, E. Swoboda, F. Meisel-Mikolajczyk, E. Stelmach, and M. Zaleska.** 1999. Bacteriological studies of blood, tissue fluid, lymph and lymph nodes in patients with acute dermatolymphangioadenitis (DLA) in course of 'filarial' lymphedema. *Acta Trop.* **73:**217–224.

36. **Ottesen, E. A.** 2006. Lymphatic filariasis: treatment, control and elimination. *Adv. Parasitol.* **61:**395–441.

37. **Ottesen, E. A., P. J. Hooper, M. Bradley, and G. Biswas.** 2008. The global programme to eliminate lymphatic filariasis: health impact after 8 years. *PLoS Negl. Trop. Dis.* **2:**e317.

38. **Ottesen, E. A., and T. B. Nutman.** 1992. Tropical pulmonary eosinophilia. *Annu. Rev. Med.* **43:**417–424.

39. **Pani, S. P., and A. Srividya.** 1995. Clinical manifestations of bancroftian filariasis with special reference to lymphoedema grading. *Indian J. Med. Res.* **102:**114–118.

40. **Pani, S. P., J. Yuvaraj, P. Vanamail, V. Dhanda, E. Michael, B. T. Grenfell, and D. A. Bundy.** 1995. Episodic adenolymphangitis and lymphoedema in patients with bancroftian filariasis. *Trans. R. Soc. Trop. Med. Hyg.* **89:**72–74.

41. **Rajan, T. V.** 2000. *Lymphatic Filariasis: A Historical Perspective*, vol. 1. Imperial College Press, London, England.

42. **Ramachandran, C. P.** 1993. Improved immunodiagnostic tests to monitor onchocerciasis control programmes—a multicenter effort. *Parasitol. Today* **9:**77–79.

43. **Rao, R. U., Y. Huang, M. J. Bockarie, M. Susapu, S. J. Laney, and G. J. Weil.** 2009. A qPCR-based multiplex assay for the detection of *Wuchereria bancrofti, Plasmodium falciparum* and *Plasmodium vivax* DNA. *Trans. R. Soc. Trop. Med. Hyg.* **103:**365–370.

44. **Rao, R. U., G. J. Weil, K. Fischer, T. Supali, and P. Fischer.** 2006. Detection of *Brugia* parasite DNA in human blood by real-time PCR. *J. Clin. Microbiol.* **44:**3887–3893.

45. **Sasa, M.** 1976. *Human Filariasis: A Global Survey of Epidemiology and Control.* University Park Press, Baltimore, MD.

46. **Seim, A. R., G. Dreyer, and D. G. Addiss.** 1999. Controlling morbidity and interrupting transmission: twin pillars of lymphatic filariasis elimination. *Rev. Soc. Bras. Med. Trop.* **32:**325–328.

47. **Shenoy, R. K., V. Kumaraswami, T. K. Suma, K. Rajan, and G. Radhakuttyamma.** 1999. A double-blind, placebo-controlled study of the efficacy of oral penicillin, diethylcarbamazine or local treatment of the affected limb in preventing acute adenolymphangitis in lymphoedema caused by brugian filariasis. *Ann. Trop. Med. Parasitol.* **93:**367–377.

48. **Shenoy, R. K., K. Sandhya, T. K. Suma, and V. Kumaraswami.** 1995. A preliminary study of filariasis related acute adenolymphangitis with special reference to precipitating factors and treatment modalities. *Southeast Asian J. Trop. Med. Public Health* **26:**301–305.

49. **Shenoy, R. K., T. K. Suma, V. Kumaraswami, S. Padma, N. Rahmah, G. Abhilash, and C. Ramesh.** 2007. Doppler ultrasonography reveals adult-worm nests in the lymph vessels of children with brugian filariasis. *Ann. Trop. Med. Parasitol.* **101:**173–180.

50. **Stingl, P.** 2009. Onchocerciasis: developments in diagnosis, treatment and control. *Int. J. Dermatol.* **48:**393–396.

51. **Taylor, H. R.** 1985. Global priorities in the control of onchocerciasis. *Rev. Infect. Dis.* **7:**844–846.

52. **Taylor, M. J., W. H. Makunde, H. F. McGarry, J. D. Turner, S. Mand, and A. Hoerauf.** 2005. Macrofilaricidal activity after doxycycline treatment of *Wuchereria bancrofti*: a double-blind, randomised placebo-controlled trial. *Lancet* **365:**2116–2121.

53. **Tisch, D. J., M. J. Bockarie, Z. Dimber, B. Kiniboro, N. Tarongka, F. E. Hazlett, W. Kastens, M. P. Alpers, and J. W. Kazura.** 2008. Mass drug administration trial to eliminate lymphatic filariasis in Papua New Guinea: changes in microfilaremia, filarial antigen, and Bm14 antibody after cessation. *Am. J. Trop. Med. Hyg.* **78:**289–293.

54. **Udwadia, F.** 1975. *Pulmonary Eosinophilia. Progress in Respiration Research*, vol. 7. S. Karger, Basel, Switzerland.

55. **Vijayan, V. K.** 2007. Tropical pulmonary eosinophilia: pathogenesis, diagnosis and management. *Curr. Opin. Pulm. Med.* **13:**428–433.

56. **Weil, G. J., P. J. Lammie, and N. Weiss.** 1997. The ICT Filariasis Test: a rapid-format antigen test for diagnosis of bancroftian filariasis. *Parasitol. Today* **13:**401–404.

57. **Weil, G. J., C. Steel, F. Liftis, B. W. Li, G. Mearns, E. Lobos, and T. B. Nutman.** 2000. A rapid-format antibody card test for diagnosis of onchocerciasis. *J. Infect. Dis.* **182:**1796–1799.

58. **World Health Organization.** 1992. *Lymphatic Filariasis: The Diseases and Its Control*, vol. 821. World Health Organization, Geneva, Switzerland.

59. **Zhong, M., J. McCarthy, L. Bierwert, M. Lizotte-Waniewski, S. Chanteau, T. B. Nutman, E. A. Ottesen, and S. A. Williams.** 1996. A polymerase chain reaction assay for detection of the parasite *Wuchereria bancrofti* in human blood samples. *Am. J. Trop. Med. Hyg.* **54:**357–363.

60. **Zimmerman, P. A., R. H. Guderian, E. Aruajo, L. Elson, P. Phadke, J. Kubofcik, and T. B. Nutman.** 1994. Polymerase chain reaction-based diagnosis of *Onchocerca volvulus* infection: improved detection of patients with onchocerciasis. *J. Infect. Dis.* **169:**686–689.

Cestodes

HECTOR H. GARCIA, JUAN A. JIMENEZ, AND HERMES ESCALANTE

143

Cestodes have as their key characteristic a flattened body composed of the head or scolex (bearing the fixation organs—suckers, hooks, and bothria), the neck (where the cellular reproduction occurs, to form the strobila), and the strobila, formed by numerous segments or proglottids. As new proglottids develop in the neck region, existing ones mature as they become more distal. The more-distal proglottids are gravid, almost completely occupied by a uterus full of eggs, which are passed with the stools of the carrier, either inside complete proglottids or free after proglottid breakage. In some species, proglottids can actively migrate out of the anus.

Tapeworms live in the lumen of the small intestine with the head or scolex as the only fixation organ, attached to the mucosa. They absorb nutrients from the host's intestine both at the head and through their tegument. Accordingly, they have developed cephalic fixation organs like hooks, suckers, or shallow grooves as longitudinal suction sulci (bothria) (Fig. 1), and a specialized tegument.

Four species of cestode tapeworms inhabit the human intestine: *Diphyllobothrium latum*, *Taenia saginata*, *Taenia solium*, and *Hymenolepis nana*. They differ widely in size, intermediate host, and other characteristics, from the 12-m *D. latum* to the 3-cm *H. nana* (Table 1). More rarely *Dipylidium caninum* and *Hymenolepis diminuta* can also inhabit the human gut; these parasites are reviewed in chapter 145. In addition, a number of cestode larvae can produce human disease if infective tapeworm eggs are ingested, mainly cysticercosis (*Taenia solium*), cystic hydatid disease (*Echinococcus granulosus*), and alveolar hydatid disease (*Echinococcus multilocularis*). Rarer larval cestode infections affecting humans include coenurosis (*Taenia multiceps*), sparganosis (*Spirometra mansonoides*), and cysticercosis by *Taenia crassiceps*. Tapeworms and especially tapeworm larval infections still represent an important cause of morbidity and mortality, not only in most underdeveloped countries but also in industrialized countries, particularly in rural areas or among immigrants from areas of endemicity.

Unless specified, antiparasitic susceptibility testing is not routinely performed in the clinical laboratory for these organisms. For more details about susceptibility testing for parasites, consult chapter 149.

DIPHYLLOBOTHRIUM LATUM

Known as the fish tapeworm, *D. latum* is the longest intestinal parasite of humans. Also common in fish-eating mammals such as canids or felids (reservoir hosts), it differs from other adult tapeworms infecting humans in its morphology, biology, and epidemiology.

Taxonomy

D. latum is included in the phylum Platyhelminthes, subphylum Neodermata, class Cestoidea, subclass Eucestoda, order Pseudophyllidea, family Diphyllobothriidae, and genus *Diphyllobothrium*.

Description of the Agent

Adult Tapeworm

The adult parasite can grow to 15 m in length and apparently can live for 20 years or longer in the small intestine. It is ivory in color and has a scolex that is provided with bothria on its dorsal and ventral aspects (8). *Diphyllobothrium* proglottids are much wider than they are long (~8 by 4 mm) and are easy to recognize because their genital pore is located in the center of the proglottid rather than in the lateral edges as in all other tapeworms of humans. The coiled uterus in the center of the gravid proglottids looks yellow-brown in freshly passed specimens. The uterine pore is located in the center of the proglottid near the genital pore.

Eggs

Unembryonated, operculate eggs are passed in the feces. *D. latum* eggs are oval and resemble those of trematodes but are smaller (58 to 75 μm long by 44 to 50 μm wide) and have a better-defined wall. The abopercular end usually has a small knoblike protrusion. Eggs are usually numerous, and expulsion of proglottid chains is usual.

Larvae

After the eggs embryonate in a water environment for several weeks, ciliated six-hooked embryos (coracidia) hatch. Coracidia must be ingested by appropriate species of freshwater copepods (genus, *Cyclops*) for further development. In the copepod a solid-bodied larva, the procercoid, develops as a second larval stage and becomes infective for

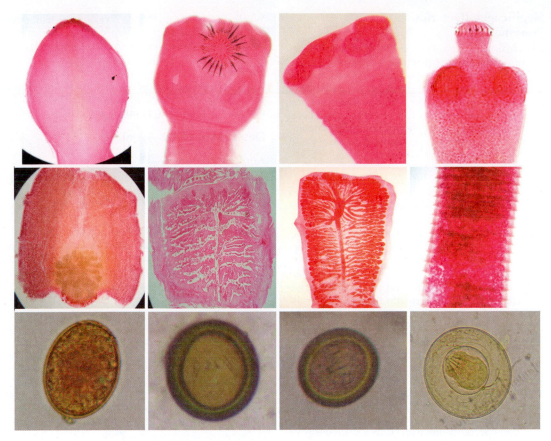

FIGURE 1 Scolex, gravid proglottids, and eggs (top to bottom) of *D. latum*, *T. solium*, *T. saginata*, and *H. nana* (left to right). Note the coiled, central uterus in *D. latum*, the absence of hooks in the scolex of *T. saginata*, and the similar appearances of the eggs of *T. saginata* and *T. solium*.

the second intermediate host (fish). In fish, the procercoid migrates to the flesh and develops in the third larval stage, the plerocercoid or sparganum, which is the infective stage for human or animal (canid or felid) hosts.

Epidemiology, Transmission, and Prevention

The geographic distribution of *D. latum* includes lake areas in Scandinavia, other areas of northern Europe, the former USSR, Finland, northern Japan, and North America, principally the upper Midwest, Alaska, Canada, and the southwestern coast of South America. Several other *Diphyllobothrium* species (*D. pacificum*, *D. cordatum*, *D. ursi*, *D. dendriticum*, *D. lanceolatum*, *D. dalliae*, and *D. yonagoensis*) have also

been reported to infect humans but less frequently (28, 31). *Diphyllobothrium pacificum*, identified by Nybellin in 1931, is a parasite of seawater found along the western coast of South America, specifically in Peru and Chile. *D. pacificum* is much smaller than *D. latum* and usually measures 50 to 200 cm long, although it can occasionally reach 3 to 4 m.

The most common sources of human *Diphyllobothrium* infection are the pike burbot, perch, ruff, and turbot (28). Infected fish (undercooked, raw, or insufficiently treated flesh) transmit plerocercoids to humans or fish-eating mammals. Infection with *Diphyllobothrium* is preventable by eating well-cooked fish or fish that has been deep-frozen (at least −10°C for 24 h).

TABLE 1 Some characteristics of main cestodes infecting humans

Organism	Length (cm)	Scolex	Gravid proglottids	Intermediate host(s)
D. latum	1,200	Spatulate, two bothria	Rosette-shaped central uterus	Copepods, fish
T. saginata	600	Squared, four suckers, no hooks	>15 main lateral uterine branches	Cattle
T. solium	300	Squared, four suckers, hooks (double crown)	<12 main lateral uterine branches	Pigs, humans
H. nana	3	Knoblike, four suckers, hooks (single crown)	Bag-shaped uterus	Insects, rodents, humans

Clinical Significance (Description of Clinical Presentation)

Infected individuals notice passing segment chains with their stools. The parasite may produce no clinical symptoms in some people, but when it reaches a large size it may cause mechanical bowel obstruction, diarrhea, abdominal pain, and, particularly in northern European countries, pernicious anemia resulting from vitamin B$_{12}$ deficiency because the tapeworm competes with the intestinal epithelium for the uptake of the vitamin. This condition is rare outside Scandinavian countries, and some authors postulate a genetic predisposition.

Collection, Transport, and Storage of Specimens

For identification purposes, eggs are well preserved in 5 to 10% formalin solutions. For DNA recovery, 95% ethanol would be a better option. Electron microscopy may require cacodylate buffer or other glutaraldehyde media. Adult tapeworm material is better defined if it is washed in saline, relaxed for better visualization of its internal structures by warming the saline at 55°C for a short period (5 min), and then placed between two glass slides and stored in a fixative solution. Fixatives could be 10% formalin, acetic acid-formaldehyde-alcohol, or sodium acetate-acetic acid-formaldehyde. Fixed pieces can be stained by injecting Semichon's carmine or India ink. The proglottids can also be sectioned and stained by hematoxylin and eosin; however, morphological characteristics can be more easily seen in whole mounts.

Direct Examination

Microscopy

Eggs can be easily seen by microscopical examination of stools. Either flotation or sedimentation techniques may be used. However, since the eggs are operculated, they generally do not float when the flotation concentration method is used; both the surface film and sediment need to be examined if this concentration method is used. For that reason, most laboratories routinely use the sedimentation concentration method. Low-magnification microscopy should easily permit identification of the characteristic scolex or proglottids when available (Fig. 1). Neither culture nor antigen detection is relevant for the detection and identification of *D. latum*.

Nucleic Acid Detection Techniques

Although several groups have described genus variation in *Diphyllobothrium* by using nucleic acid detection methods, the information has no clinical relevance in terms of routine tapeworm recovery and identification (18).

Serologic Tests

Serologic tests are not available.

Treatment

Both praziquantel and niclosamide are effective drugs. At recommended doses both are associated with only mild side effects, mostly gastrointestinal.

Evaluation, Interpretation, and Reporting of Results

Both stool microscopy and parasite identification are unambiguous. Eggs or tapeworm pieces should be reported as *D. latum* eggs (except in South America, where *D. pacificum* is more frequently found). Other human-infecting species are rarely found.

TAENIA SAGINATA

Known as the beef tapeworm, *Taenia saginata* is still endemic to most of the world. Humans are its only definitive host.

While *T. saginata* infections do not carry major risks for the host, differential diagnosis with *Taenia solium* is important because the latter can cause neurocysticercosis.

Taxonomy

T. saginata is included in the phylum Platyhelminthes, subphylum Neodermata, class Cestoidea, subclass Eucestoda, order Cyclophyllidea, family Taeniidae, and genus *Taenia*.

Description of the Agent

Adult Tapeworm

The adult *T. saginata* tapeworm attains lengths of 4 to 8 m and has a scolex provided with four suckers and an unarmed (no hooks) rostellum. Gravid proglottids are longer than they are wide (18 to 20 mm by 5 to 7 mm). Each proglottid has a genital pore at the midlateral margin. In mature proglottids, the ovary has only two lobes and presents a vaginal sphincter. Gravid proglottids, which are highly muscular and active, break off from the strobila and actively migrate out of the anus (a pathognomic characteristic of this species).

Eggs

Eggs from *T. saginata* and *T. solium* are indistinguishable by morphological characteristics. They are spherical, measure 30 to 40 μm in diameter, and have a quite characteristic thick, yellow-brown, radiate shell (embryophore) composed of collagen subunits, which gets thicker as the eggs mature. Eggs are frequently surrounded by a thin layer of vitellum (Fig. 1). Within the egg is a six-hooked embryo, the oncosphere.

Larvae

The unarmed scolex is invaginated into a fluid-filled bladder, the cysticercus. Larval cysts are 4 to 6 mm long by 7 to 10 mm wide and have a pearl-like appearance in tissues.

Epidemiology, Transmission, and Prevention

T. saginata is distributed worldwide, although it is especially prevalent in some parts of Africa, Central and South America, eastern and western Asia, and some countries in Europe. Cattle serve as the intermediate host, and ingestion of eggs from contaminated pasturelands by grazing cattle results in development in cattle tissues of the infective cysticercus stage. After ingestion of the cysticercus in raw or inadequately cooked beef, it takes approximately 2 to 3 months for the infection to become patent in the human host.

In Southeast Asia there is a human tapeworm morphologically very similar to *Taenia saginata* (*Taenia saginata asiatica*, *Taenia asiatica*, or Taiwan taenia). In this tapeworm, the cysticercus stage occurs in the liver of pigs and less frequently in cattle. The adult tapeworm infects the human host, and its appearance is very similar to that of *T. saginata* (5, 6).

Clinical Significance (Description of Clinical Presentation)

Although patients may exhibit no symptoms with this infection, they usually notice passing proglottids or find them in their underwear. The mature worm can also cause abdominal discomfort, diarrhea, and occasionally intestinal obstruction as a result of its large size.

Collection, Transport, and Storage of Specimens

See instructions in "Collection, Transport, and Storage of Specimens" for *Diphyllobothrium* above.

Direct Examination

Microscopy

Typical *Taenia* eggs can be found in feces. Sedimentation or the less-used Kato-Katz method is apparently more sensitive for the detection of *Taenia* eggs in stools than other concentration techniques. Finding of *Taenia* eggs does not allow a species-specific diagnosis of infection; it is usually made by identification of gravid proglottids that have been passed in feces or have actively migrated out of the anus. Identification of the proglottids is based on shape and size and mainly on the morphology of the uterus, which can be demonstrated after injection with India ink or staining with carmine or hematoxylin stain. In *T. saginata* there are 15 to 20 primary lateral branches on each side of the central uterine stem (Fig. 1).

Antigens in stools (coproantigen) have been detected by enzyme-linked immunosorbent assay (ELISA) since 1990, but this assay is used mainly in research settings because of scarce availability.

Nucleic Acid Detection Techniques

Species-specific PCR techniques have been described to detect parasite DNA and differentiate *T. saginata* from *T. solium*. Most of these assays require actual parasite material, although some are apparently able to establish the difference with DNA from eggs in feces (12, 20, 21, 35).

Serologic Tests

Serum antigen detection ELISAs for *T. saginata* cysticercosis in cattle have been developed using monoclonal antibodies to *T. saginata*. Although these assays can detect parasite burdens of <50 cysts per animal, they have not yet been routinely applied except in research settings (3, 11, 26).

Treatment

Both praziquantel and niclosamide are effective drugs. At recommended doses both are associated with only mild side effects, mostly gastrointestinal. In regions where *T. solium* is endemic, there is a possibility that latent neurocysticercosis may respond to praziquantel and cause severe headaches or seizures. Niclosamide is not absorbed from the gastrointestinal tract and thus does not carry this risk (14).

Evaluation, Interpretation, and Reporting of Results

Eggs should be reported as "*Taenia* sp." because direct observation does not confirm the species. The finding of *Taenia* sp. eggs should be notified to the attending physician to ensure prompt treatment. The presence of the scolex in the parasite material expelled (spontaneously or posttreatment) should be reported both because it allows species identification and because if it is not found, the chances of treatment failure increase.

TAENIA SOLIUM

Known as the pork tapeworm, *T. solium* has an extensive geographic distribution. This infection has a huge impact on human health because of its association with seizure disorders caused by infection of the human brain with its larval stage (neurocysticercosis) (10).

Taxonomy

T. solium is included in the phylum Platyhelminthes, subphylum Neodermata, class Cestoidea, subclass Eucestoda, order Cyclophyllidea, family Taeniidae, and genus *Taenia*.

Description of the Agent

Adult Tapeworm

The adult *T. solium* tapeworm measures 2 to 4 m and has a scolex provided with four suckers and a rostellum armed with two crowns of hooks. Gravid proglottids have similar length and width (approximately 1 cm). Each proglottid has a genital pore at the midlateral margin. In mature proglottids, the ovary has two main lobes and one accessory lobe (lacking in *T. saginata*), and a vaginal sphincter muscle is lacking (present in *T. saginata*). Gravid proglottids have few (<12) lateral branches on the central uterine stem (Fig. 1). Since the eggs of *T. solium* are infective to humans and can cause cysticercosis, extreme caution in the handling of these proglottids or infective stools is recommended.

Eggs

Eggs from *T. saginata* and *T. solium* are indistinguishable by morphological characteristics. They are spherical, measure 30 to 40 μm in diameter, and have a quite characteristic thick, yellow-brown, radiate shell (embryophore) composed of collagen subunits, which gets thicker as the eggs mature. Eggs are frequently surrounded by a thin layer of vitellum (Fig. 1). Within the egg is a six-hooked embryo, the oncosphere.

Larvae

The fluid-filled bladder (cysticercus) larvae are bigger than those of *T. saginata*, measuring approximately 8 to 10 mm in diameter. They lodge in the pig's tissues, mostly in muscle and brain.

Epidemiology, Transmission, and Prevention

T. solium taeniasis and cysticercosis are highly endemic to all parts of the developing world where pigs are raised as a food source, including Latin America, most of Asia, sub-Saharan Africa, and parts of Oceania. The infection is now also increasingly diagnosed in industrialized countries due to immigration of tapeworm carriers from zones of endemicity (6, 10).

As for *T. saginata*, humans are the only definitive host. Ingestion of contaminated pork containing *T. solium* cysticerci causes human taeniasis. Conversely, *T. solium* eggs cause cysticercosis in pigs (the usual intermediate host) and humans. Pigs acquire cysticercosis by eating stools contaminated with infective eggs in places where deficient sanitation exists. Humans get infected by fecal-oral contamination from a tapeworm carrier, commonly in the household or another close environment.

Clinical Significance (Description of Clinical Presentation)

Human *T. solium* taeniasis is acquired by ingestion of infective cysticerci in inadequately cooked pork or pork products. Taeniasis seems mostly asymptomatic, and most patients do not even notice passing proglottids in stools. The clinical significance of *T. solium* infections relates to the risk of neurocysticercosis (see below), which is high for tapeworm carriers and their close contacts (10).

Collection, Transport, and Storage of Specimens

See instructions in "Collection, Transport, and Storage of Specimens" for *Diphyllobothrium*. Handling of *T. solium* proglottids or contaminated stools should be done with appropriate biosafety conditions to avoid cysticercosis.

Direct Examination

Microscopy

Typical *Taenia* eggs can be found in feces. Sedimentation or the less-used Kato-Katz method is apparently more sensitive for the detection of *Taenia* eggs in stools than other concentration techniques. Finding of *Taenia* eggs does not allow a diagnosis of infection by the species, which is usually made by identification of gravid proglottids, or more rarely the scolex, that have been passed in feces. Identification of the proglottids is based on shape and size and mainly on the morphology of the uterus, which can be demonstrated after injection with India ink or staining with carmine or hematoxylin stains. In *T. solium* there are few primary branches on each side of the central uterine stem (Fig. 1).

Antigens in stools (coproantigen) have been detected by ELISA since 1990. Coproantigen detection ELISA is much more sensitive than microscopy and thus highly recommended for the diagnosis of human taeniasis (specifically in the case of *T. solium* because of the risks of cysticercosis transmission), but its availability is still limited.

Nucleic Acid Detection Techniques

Species-specific PCR techniques that differentiate *T. saginata* from *T. solium* have been described. Most of these assays require actual parasite material, although some are apparently able to establish the difference with DNA from eggs in feces (12, 20, 21, 35).

Serologic Tests

Recently, stage-specific serological assays directed to the adult tapeworm have been developed, with high sensitivity and specificity. Mostly, serology is directed to the detection of *T. solium* antibodies in relation to the diagnosis of neurocysticercosis. Antibody detection by enzyme-linked immunoelectrotransfer blot assay is the method of choice, with a sensitivity of 98% in cases with more than one viable larval cyst and specificity of 100%. *T. solium* antigen detection in serum or cerebrospinal fluid has been performed in cases of human cysticercosis, based on a known genus-specific cross-reaction in ELISAs for *T. saginata*. Although these assays can detect parasite burdens of <50 cysts in infected animals, they have not yet been routinely applied except in research settings.

Treatment

Both praziquantel and niclosamide are effective drugs. At recommended doses both are associated with only mild side effects, mostly gastrointestinal. In regions where *T. solium* is endemic, there is a possibility that latent neurocysticercosis may respond to praziquantel and cause severe headaches or seizures. Niclosamide is not absorbed from the gastrointestinal tract and thus does not carry this risk (14).

Evaluation, Interpretation, and Reporting of Results

Eggs should be reported as "*Taenia* sp." because direct observation does not confirm the species. The finding of *Taenia* sp. eggs should be notified to the attending physician to ensure prompt treatment and minimize the chances of cysticercosis in the patient or his/her contacts. The presence of the scolex in the parasite material expelled (spontaneously or posttreatment) should be reported both because it allows species identification and because if it is not found, the chances of treatment failure increase.

HYMENOLEPIS NANA

H. nana is the smallest of the intestinal tapeworms of humans and also the most common tapeworm infection throughout the world. It can be transmitted from person to person (an intermediate host is not necessarily required) (28).

Taxonomy

H. nana is included in the phylum Platyhelminthes, subphylum Neodermata, class Cestoidea, subclass Eucestoda, order Cyclophyllidea, family Hymenolepididae, and genus *Hymenolepis*.

Description of the Agent

Adult Tapeworm

The adult parasite measures 2 to 4 cm and seems to live approximately 1 year. The scolex has four suckers and one crown of hooks.

Eggs

The eggs are 30 to 50 μm in diameter and thin shelled, and they contain a six-hooked oncosphere that lies in the center of the egg and is separated from the outer shell by considerable space. The oncosphere is surrounded by a membrane that has two polar thickenings from which arise four to eight filaments extending into the space between it and the outer shell (Fig. 1). These filaments are not seen in *H. diminuta*. Eggs may hatch inside the host's intestine, and the embryos (oncospheres) invade the mucosa to develop into larval stages.

Larvae

The cysticercoid larvae have an invaginated scolex but no fluid-filled bladder. They lodge in the intestinal mucosa and emerge to the intestinal lumen as young tapeworms after a few days.

Epidemiology, Transmission, and Prevention

H. nana is normally a parasite of mice, and its life cycle characteristically involves a beetle as intermediate host. In humans, transmission is usually accomplished by direct ingestion of infective eggs containing oncospheres. When eggs are ingested, a solid-bodied larva, a cysticercoid, first develops in the wall of the small intestine. Subsequently, the larva migrates back into the intestinal lumen, where it reaches maturity as an adult tapeworm in 2 to 3 weeks. In beetles that ingest eggs of *H. nana*, the cysticercoids develop in the body cavity and have thick protective walls around them. Although humans may acquire the infection by accidental ingestion of infected beetles (often occurring in dry cereals), direct infection is far more common and is the primary reason why *H. nana* usually occurs in institutional and familial settings in which hygiene is substandard. A feature of human *H. nana* infection is the opportunity for internal autoinfection with the parasite, which may result in large worm burdens. Autoinfection occurs when eggs discharged by adult tapeworms in the lumen of the small intestine hatch rapidly and invade the wall of the intestine; here, cysticercoids are formed, and they subsequently reenter the intestine to mature as adult worms.

Clinical Significance (Description of Clinical Presentation)

Most infections cause no symptoms. However, hymenolepiasis can be associated with abdominal pain, diarrhea, headaches, or irritability, probably in infections with heavier worm burdens (23, 30).

Collection, Transport, and Storage of Specimens

See instructions in "Collection, Transport, and Storage of Specimens" for *Diphyllobothrium*.

Direct Examination

Microscopy

Diagnosis of the infection rests on finding the spherical eggs in feces by microscopy. Either flotation or sedimentation techniques are of help. Proglottids (Fig. 1) are rarely seen, since they disintegrate after breaking off from the main strobila. Neither culture, antigen detection, nor nucleic acid detection techniques are relevant for the detection and identification of *H. nana*.

Serologic Tests

Antibody detection ELISAs have been used in research settings but are of no clinical use (1).

Treatment

Both praziquantel and niclosamide are effective drugs. At recommended doses both are associated only with mild side effects, mostly gastrointestinal. A second dose of praziquantel after 10 to 15 days may decrease the likelihood of relapses. Niclosamide needs to be administered for 7 days because it is not absorbed and thus does not affect the cysticercoid larvae in the intestinal mucosa. Nitazoxanide has been reported to be useful as a therapeutic alternative (29).

Evaluation, Interpretation, and Reporting of Results

Eggs are characteristic and should be reported as *H. nana* eggs. The closest differential diagnosis is with *H. diminuta*, which rarely infects humans. The eggs of *H. diminuta* are bigger, lack polar filaments, and have a wider interior space and thus can be differentiated by microscopy.

LARVAL CESTODES INFECTING THE HUMAN HOST

The larval stages of *Taenia solium*, *Echinococcus granulosus*, *Echinococcus multilocularis*, and, less frequently, *Spirometra* spp., *Taenia multiceps*, and *Taenia crassiceps* can invade the human tissues. These are briefly described below.

Cysticercosis (*Taenia solium*)

In the normal life cycle of *T. solium*, humans are the definitive host and pigs act as the intermediate host, hosting the larval stage or cysticercus. Porcine cysticercosis is a serious economic problem for pig farmers. However, the most serious consequences are associated with human cysticercosis (10). Larval vesicles located in the human central nervous system (Fig. 2) cause seizures or other neurological symptoms.

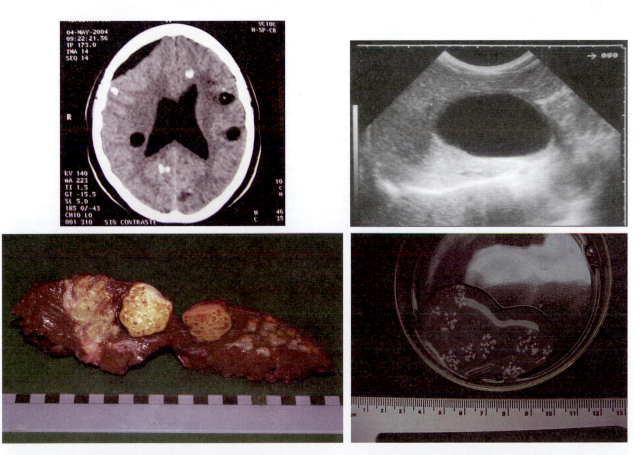

FIGURE 2 Larval cestodes infecting the human host. (Top left) *Taenia solium* cysticerci in the human brain (neurocysticercosis), shown in a noncontrasted MRI of the brain; (top right) *Echinococcus granulosus* hydatid in the human liver (hydatid disease) as seen on liver ultrasound (kind contribution of Enrico Brunetti, Università di Pavia, Pavia, Italy); (bottom left) *Echinococcus multilocularis* alveolar hydatid disease in human liver (kind courtesy of K. Buttenschoen and P. Kern, University Hospital Ulm, Ulm, Germany); (bottom right) *Taenia multiceps* coenurus showing multiple scolices in the cystic wall.

Indeed, neurocysticercosis is associated with a significant proportion of seizure cases in areas of endemicity (22, 24). Clinical manifestations of neurocysticercosis are related to individual differences in the number, size, and topography of lesions and in the severity of the host's immune response to the parasites. Symptoms and signs are varied and nonspecific. Parasites in the brain parenchyma usually cause seizures and headache, whereas those located in the cerebral ventricles or in the subarachnoid space ("racemose" cysticercosis) cause intracranial hypertension and hydrocephalus. Diagnosis is made using brain imaging, either computed tomography (CT) scan or magnetic resonance imaging (MRI), and confirmed by serology. CT has a lower cost (quite important for poor areas where the disease is endemic), is more available, and has better sensitivity for the detection of calcified parasites. Conversely, MRI has better sensitivity for small lesions, those located close to the skull, and intraventricular parasites. The serological assay of choice is an immunoblot using seven purified glycoprotein larval antigens, which has 98% sensitivity and 100% specificity except in cases with a single lesion, for which sensitivity drops to approximately 70% (32). Antigen detection assays have been described, but no controlled data on sensitivity and specificity are yet available. Treatment of neurocysticercosis uses antiparasitic agents (albendazole or praziquantel) for viable parasites, usually given with steroids to ameliorate the inflammation produced by the death of the cyst. Surgery is limited to excision of single, big lesions or implantation of ventricle-peritoneal shunts. Antigen detection assays permit patient monitoring and follow-up of antiparasitic treatment (9).

Cystic Hydatid Disease (Echinococcus granulosus)

In the normal life cycle of *Echinococcus granulosus*, the dog is the definitive host and herbivores (mainly sheep) act as the intermediate host. These become infected with the larval stage (cystic hydatid) by ingesting infective eggs dispersed from the feces of the tapeworm-infected dog. Human cystic hydatid disease is an important cause of human morbidity, requiring costly surgical and medical treatment. This cestodiasis is still endemic to most of the Old World, particularly in Greece, Cyprus, Bulgaria, Lebanon, and Turkey; some other European countries; South America; and Africa. Sporadic autochthonous transmission is currently recognized in Alaska and other states in the United States (4). The affected organs are most commonly liver and lungs and more rarely heart, brain, bone, or other locations. Diagnosis is made by using ultrasound or CT scan for liver infection or chest X rays or CT for lung infections (Fig. 2). Antibody detection by serology is helpful, although sensitivity is lower than for other infections, reaching 80 to 85%. It is more sensitive for hepatic than for pulmonary cases. Treatment uses antiparasitic agents (albendazole or albendazole plus praziquantel) for small cysts or presurgery; PAIR (puncture, injection, aspiration, and reinjection), which is a technique of ultrasound- or CT-guided aspiration and sterilization of the cyst's contents; or either laparoscopic or open surgery (17, 34). Spillage of cyst contents could lead to acute anaphylactic reactions or dissemination of infection in the surroundings. Cystic lesions may resolve without therapy in a proportion of patients (25).

Alveolar Hydatid Disease (Echinococcus multilocularis)

The adult stage of *E. multilocularis* lives in the small intestine of the definitive host, commonly wild predators in the northern hemisphere, occurring in parts of Europe, Asia,

Japan, and North America, including Alaska (2, 15). The larval stages infect microtine rodents that usually serve as the common intermediate host. Human infections (causing alveolar hydatid disease) occur by accidental ingestion of the oncosphere by contamination with the feces of the definitive host. The manifestation of alveolar hydatid disease resembles a slowly developing "malignant tumor" of the liver, with subsequent invasion of the blood vessels and bile ducts and metastatic dissemination. The lesions vary in size and can produce minor foci up to large infiltrating structures in the host's tissue. Thus, alveolar hydatid disease differs greatly in the pathology and clinical course from cystic hydatid disease. This disease often affects persons aged over 50 years and is characterized by a chronic course lasting for months or years. Clinical manifestations relate to the extent of tumor-like lesions of the cyst. Beside physical examination, diagnosis usually is based on imaging techniques including ultrasound, CT, and MRI supported by serology. Treatment is mainly surgical. Chemotherapy with benzimidazole agents is restricted to residual, postsurgical, or inoperable lesions (16).

Sparganosis (Spirometra mansonoides)

Mainly found in Southeast Asian countries, the metacestode larvae of *Spirometra* species can invade the human tissues either by ingestion of contaminated crustaceans in drinking water or of infected meat (frog or snake) or by direct contact via a poultice. The most commonly affected sites are subcutaneous tissues and the eye. The diagnosis rests on the pathological demonstration of the larvae after excision by biopsy (33).

Coenurosis (Taenia multiceps or Taenia serialis)

Taenia multiceps and *Taenia serialis* have canids as definitive hosts and sheep as their normal intermediate host, harboring the larvae or coenurus. The coenurus is a vesicle containing a transparent fluid, with a fine membrane in which multiple (500 to 700) scolices can be seen. Infected sheep lose their balance and rotate around their site, become dizzy, and fall (screw disease). It infrequently causes coenuriasis in humans. Human infections have largely been confined to the African continent, but a few cases have been described from France, England, and North and South America. The space-occupying coenurus usually invades the brain, producing lethal lesions. Diagnosis is based on pathological demonstration of the typical larval membrane and multiple scolices (13, 27).

Cysticercosis (Taenia crassiceps)

T. crassiceps is a common tapeworm of the red fox. Larval forms are generally found in subcutaneous tissues and body cavity of rodents. Human cases are quite rare, mostly in immunocompromised patients (subcutaneous, muscular, or ocular infections) (7, 19).

REFERENCES

1. Castillo, R. M., P. Grados, C. Carcamo, E. Miranda, T. Montenegro, A. Guevara, and R. H. Gilman. 1991. Effect of treatment on serum antibody to *Hymenolepis nana* detected by enzyme-linked immunosorbent assay. *J. Clin. Microbiol.* **29:**413–414.
2. Craig, P. S., M. T. Rogan, and M. Campos-Ponce. 2003. Echinococcosis: disease, detection and transmission. *Parasitology* **127**(Suppl.)**:**S5–S20.
3. Dorny, P., F. Vercammen, J. Brandt, W. Vansteenkiste, D. Berkvens, and S. Geerts. 2000. Sero-epidemiological study of *Taenia saginata* cysticercosis in Belgian cattle. *Vet. Parasitol.* **88:**43–49.

4. **Eckert, J., and P. Deplazes.** 2004. Biological, epidemiological, and clinical aspects of echinococcosis, a zoonosis of increasing concern. *Clin. Microbiol. Rev.* **17:**107–135.

5. **Eom, K. S., H. K. Jeon, Y. Kong, U. W. Hwang, Y. Yang, X. Li, L. Xu, Z. Feng, Z. S. Pawlowski, and H. J. Rim.** 2002. Identification of *Taenia asiatica* in China: molecular, morphological, and epidemiological analysis of a Luzhai isolate. *J. Parasitol.* **88:**758–764.

6. **Flisser, A., A. E. Viniegra, L. Aguilar-Vega, A. Garza-Rodriguez, P. Maravilla, and G. Avila.** 2004. Portrait of human tapeworms. *J. Parasitol.* **90:**914–916.

7. **Francois, A., L. Favennec, C. Cambon-Michot, I. Gueit, N. Biga, F. Tron, P. Brasseur, and J. Hemet.** 1998. *Taenia crassiceps* invasive cysticercosis: a new human pathogen in acquired immunodeficiency syndrome? *Am. J. Surg. Pathol.* **22:**488–492.

8. **Fuchizaki, U., H. Ohta, and T. Sugimoto.** 2003. Diphyllobothriasis. *Lancet Infect. Dis.* **3:**32.

9. **Garcia, H. H., O. H. Del Brutto, and the Cysticercosis Working Group in Peru.** 2005. Neurocysticercosis—updated concepts about an old disease. *Lancet Neurol.* **4:**653–661.

10. **Garcia, H. H., A. E. Gonzalez, C. A. W. Evans, R. H. Gilman, and the Cysticercosis Working Group in Peru.** 2003. *Taenia solium* cysticercosis. *Lancet* **362:**547–556.

11. **Garcia, H. H., R. M. Parkhouse, R. H. Gilman, T. Montenegro, T. Bernal, S. M. Martinez, A. E. Gonzalez, V. C. Tsang, and L. J. Harrison.** 2000. Serum antigen detection in the diagnosis, treatment, and follow-up of neurocysticercosis patients. *Trans. R. Soc. Trop. Med. Hyg.* **94:**673–676.

12. **Gonzalez, L. M., E. Montero, L. J. Harrison, R. M. Parkhouse, and T. Garate.** 2000. Differential diagnosis of *Taenia saginata* and *Taenia solium* infection by PCR. *J. Clin. Microbiol.* **38:**737–744.

13. **Ing, M. B., P. M. Schantz, and J. A. Turner.** 1998. Human coenurosis in North America: case reports and review. *Clin. Infect. Dis.* **27:**519–523.

14. **Jeri, C., R. H. Gilman, A. G. Lescano, H. Mayta, M. E. Ramirez, A. E. Gonzalez, R. Nazerali, and H. H. Garcia.** 2004. Species identification after treatment for human taeniasis. *Lancet* **363:**949–950.

15. **Jiang, C. P., M. Don, and M. Jones.** 2005. Liver alveolar echinococcosis in China: clinical aspect with relative basic research. *World J. Gastroenterol.* **11:**4611–4617.

16. **Kadry, Z., E. C. Renner, L. M. Bachmann, N. Attigah, E. L. Renner, R. W. Ammann, and P. A. Clavien.** 2005. Evaluation of treatment and long-term follow-up in patients with hepatic alveolar echinococcosis. *Br. J. Surg.* **92:**1110–1116.

17. **Khuroo, M. S., N. A. Wani, G. Javid, B. A. Khan, G. N. Yattoo, A. H. Shah, and S. G. Jeelani.** 1997. Percutaneous drainage compared with surgery for hepatic hydatid cysts. *N. Engl. J. Med.* **337:**881–887.

18. **Logan, F. J., A. Horak, J. Stefka, A. Aydogdu, and T. Scholz.** 2004. The phylogeny of diphyllobothriid tapeworms (Cestoda: Pseudophyllidea) based on ITS-2 rDNA sequences. *Parasitol. Res.* **94:**10–15.

19. **Maillard, H., J. Marionneau, B. Prophette, E. Boyer, and P. Celerier.** 1998. *Taenia crassiceps* cysticercosis and AIDS. *AIDS* **12:**1551–1552.

20. **Mayta, H., R. H. Gilman, E. Prendergast, J. P. Castillo, Y. O. Tinoco, H. H. Garcia, A. E. Gonzalez, C. R. Sterling, and the Cysticercosis Working Group in Peru.** 2007. Nested PCR for specific diagnosis of *Taenia solium* taeniasis. *J. Clin. Microbiol.* **46:**286–289.

21. **Mayta, H., A. Talley, R. H. Gilman, J. Jimenez, M. Verastegui, M. Ruiz, H. H. Garcia, and A. E. Gonzalez.** 2000. Differentiating *Taenia solium* and *Taenia saginata* infections by simple hematoxylin-eosin staining and PCR-restriction enzyme analysis. *J. Clin. Microbiol.* **38:**133–137.

22. **Medina, M. T., R. M. Duron, L. Martinez, J. R. Osorio, A. L. Estrada, C. Zuniga, D. Cartagena, J. S. Collins, and K. R. Holden.** 2005. Prevalence, incidence, and etiology of epilepsies in rural Honduras: the Salama Study. *Epilepsia* **46:**124–131.

23. **Mirdha, B. R., and J. C. Samantray.** 2002. *Hymenolepis nana*: a common cause of paediatric diarrhoea in urban slum dwellers in India. *J. Trop. Pediatr.* **48:**331–334.

24. **Montano, S. M., M. V. Villaran, L. Ylquimiche, J. J. Figueroa, S. Rodriguez, C. T. Bautista, A. E. Gonzalez, V. C. Tsang, R. H. Gilman, and H. H. Garcia.** 2005. Neurocysticercosis: association between seizures, serology, and brain CT in rural Peru. *Neurology* **65:**229–233.

25. **Moro, P. L., R. H. Gilman, M. Verastegui, C. Bern, B. Silva, and J. J. Bonilla.** 1999. Human hydatidosis in the central Andes of Peru: evolution of the disease over 3 years. *Clin. Infect. Dis.* **29:**807–812.

26. **Onyango-Abuje, J. A., G. Hughes, M. Opicha, K. M. Nginyi, M. K. Rugutt, S. H. Wright, and L. J. Harrison.** 1996. Diagnosis of *Taenia saginata* cysticercosis in Kenyan cattle by antibody and antigen ELISA. *Vet. Parasitol.* **61:**221–230.

27. **Ozmen, O., S. Sahinduran, M. Haligur, and K. Sezer.** 2005. Clinicopathologic observations on *Coenurus cerebralis* in naturally infected sheep. *Schweiz. Arch. Tierheilkd.* **147:**129–134.

28. **Raether, W., and H. Hanel.** 2003. Epidemiology, clinical manifestations and diagnosis of zoonotic cestode infections: an update. *Parasitol. Res.* **91:**412–438.

29. **Rossignol, J. F., and H. Maisonneuve.** 1984. Nitazoxanide in the treatment of *Taenia saginata* and *Hymenolepis nana* infections. *Am. J. Trop. Med. Hyg.* **33:**511–512.

30. **Schantz, P. M.** 1996. Tapeworms (cestodiasis). *Gastroenterol. Clin. N. Am.* **25:**637–653.

31. **Scholz, T., H. H. Garcia, R. Kuchta, and B. Wicht.** 2009. Human broad tapeworm (*Diphyllobothrium*): an update of the genus, including clinical relevance. *Clin. Microbiol. Rev.* **22:**146–160.

32. **Tsang, V. C., J. A. Brand, and A. E. Boyer.** 1989. An enzyme-linked immunoelectrotransfer blot assay and glycoprotein antigens for diagnosing human cysticercosis (*Taenia solium*). *J. Infect. Dis.* **159:**50–59.

33. **Wiwanitkit, V.** 2005. A review of human sparganosis in Thailand. *Int. J. Infect. Dis.* **9:**312–316.

34. **World Health Organization Informal Working Group in Echinococcosis.** 2001. *Puncture, Aspiration, Injection, Reaspiration. An Option for the Treatment of Cystic Echinococcosis.* World Health Organization, Geneva, Switzerland.

35. **Yamasaki, H., J. C. Allan, M. O. Sato, M. Nakao, Y. Sako, K. Nakaya, D. Qiu, W. Mamuti, P. S. Craig, and A. Ito.** 2004. DNA differential diagnosis of taeniasis and cysticercosis by multiplex PCR. *J. Clin. Microbiol.* **42:**548–553.

Trematodes

MALCOLM K. JONES, JENNIFER KEISER, AND DONALD P. McMANUS

144

At least 70 species of digenean trematode have been recorded as adult parasites from humans. All of these species are endoparasitic, occupying a variety of tissue sites (Tables 1 to 3). Adult trematodes have distinctive morphology, often with a leaf-like body plan. The most prominent morphological features in most species, however, are two rounded suckers. One of these, the oral sucker, surrounds the mouth, while the other, the ventral sucker, lies approximately one-third of the way along the body and serves as a primary attachment organ (36). Adult digeneans of humans are rarely seen in clinical settings because they are endoparasitic but may be observed after anthelmintic purging or at autopsy. Hence, diagnosis of the diseases caused by these helminths relies to a large extent on direct observations of excreted eggs. With few exceptions (19, 49), the eggs have a distinct morphology and their presence is pathognomonic of specific infection. Despite the diverse range of body sites infected by adult trematodes, the eggs of most digenean flukes are voided with feces. Exceptions to this include *Schistosoma haematobium* and, rarely, other schistosomes, of which eggs are excreted with urine, and *Paragonimus* species, of which eggs are observed mainly in sputum.

Detailed descriptions of the life cycles of digenean parasites of humans are shown in Fig. 1 and 2. There are many subtle variations in life cycle patterns, but two predominant life cycle strategies exist for these trematodes (Fig. 1 and 2). The first strategy, exemplified by the schistosomes, is one in which humans are infected by direct invasion of the skin by cercariae. The second strategy is seen among the so-called foodborne digeneans (25), a diverse assemblage of species which enter humans with ingested food (Fig. 2).

Two features of the digenean life cycle are noteworthy. First, digeneans often display high specificity in their choice of first intermediate host. So intimate are these host-parasite associations that the geographical distribution of a digenean is determined largely by that of its snail host. For this reason also, many digeneans show a focal distribution in countries of endemicity. Second, most human parasites are zoonotic, requiring the cooccurrence of other mammalian or avian hosts in an area of endemicity to maintain human infection.

COLLECTION, TRANSPORT, AND STORAGE

As stated above, adult digeneans are rarely encountered in clinical settings. If observed, for example, after anthelmintic purging, adults can be fixed for subsequent morphological or molecular investigations using standard fixation strategies (12).

Detailed instructions on collection, transport, and storage of digenean eggs in human fecal material are provided in chapter 130 in this *Manual*. The eggs range in size from 20 to 150 μm and can be identified with low- and intermediate-power objective lenses (i.e., 10× and 40×). Eggs of fasciolids are comparatively large (130 to 150 by 63 to 90 μm for *Fasciola hepatica* from livestock), and for regions where fasciolosis is endemic, it is important to view microscope slides at low magnification. Whereas the eggs of most digeneans are unembryonated when excreted, the eggs of schistosomes and some other groups contain fully differentiated larvae in feces or urine. The eggs of schistosomes hatch spontaneously upon exposure to fresh water. Although observations of viable schistosome miracidia may be advantageous for species identification, spontaneous hatching may hinder direct observations of eggs. Fresh stool samples or stained preparations can be used for direct examination. Sedimentation techniques (see chapter 130 in this *Manual*) may be useful for diagnosis in light, early, or chronic infections, when egg excretion is low. Among currently available diagnostic techniques, the Kato-Katz thick smear is a standard method for qualitative and quantitative field diagnosis of intestinal schistosomiasis, foodborne trematodiases, and geohelminth infections (2, 6, 35).

The eggs of human-parasitic digeneans are ovoid, usually with a yellow-to-brown, translucent shell (see Fig. 4). The eggs usually are without adorning features, although diagnostic spines and polar ridges and an operculum ("lid") may be present. Diagnostic features, therefore, are the shape and size of the egg, the texture and adornments of the eggshell, the presence or absence of an operculum, and the extent of postzygotic development of the embryo.

DIGENEANS OF THE CIRCULATORY SYSTEM: SCHISTOSOMES

Schistosomes responsible for human disease are shown in Table 1, along with their distribution, snail hosts, and treatment. Currently, an estimated 779 million people are at risk and 207 million people in 76 countries and territories have schistosomiasis, with 85% of cases occurring in sub-Saharan

TABLE 1 Geographical distribution, intermediate hosts, and egg morphology of the major schistosomes infecting humans

Species	Disease and geographic area	Snail hosts	Drug regimen[a]	Egg presentation and size
Schistosoma mansoni	Intestinal schistosomiasis, infecting humans and sometimes other mammals in Angola, Benin, Botswana, Burkina Faso, Burundi, Cameroon, Central African Republic, Chad, Congo, Democratic Republic of the Congo, Equatorial Guinea, Eritrea, Ethiopia, Gabon, The Gambia, Ghana, Guinea, Guinea-Bissau, Ivory Coast, Kenya, Liberia, Madagascar, Malawi, Mali, Mauritania, Mozambique, Namibia, Nigeria, Rwanda, Senegal, Sierra Leone, South Africa, Swaziland, Togo, Uganda, Tanzania, Zambia, Zimbabwe, Egypt, Libya, Oman, Saudi Arabia, Somalia, Sudan, Yemen, Antigua, Brazil, Dominican Republic, Guadeloupe, Martinique, Montserrat, Puerto Rico, St. Lucia, Suriname, and Venezuela	*Biomphalaria* species. In Africa (Asia), *B. alexandrina*, *B. choanomphala*, *B. pfeifferi*, and *B. sudanica* species groups (many species). In the Americas, *B. glabrata* and 2 other species.	Praziquantel, 20 mg/kg, 2 to 3 doses (community programs usually give 40 mg/kg in a single dose)	Feces (rarely urinary); size, 140 × 61 μm
Schistosoma japonicum	Intestinal schistosomiasis (organism infects humans and bovines) in Indonesia, People's Republic of China, and the Philippines	*Oncomelania species. O. hupensis, O. nosophora, O. formosana, O. h. quadrasi,* and *O. lindoensis*	As above, but 60 mg/kg in a single dose in community programs	Feces; size, 85 × 60 μm
Schistosoma haematobium	Genitourinary schistosomiasis in Algeria, Angola, Benin, Botswana, Burkina Faso, Burundi, Cameroon, Central African Republic, Chad, Congo, Democratic Republic of the Congo, Egypt, Ethiopia, Gabon, The Gambia, Ghana, Guinea, Guinea-Bissau, Iran, Iraq, Ivory Coast, Jordan, Kenya, Lebanon, Liberia, Libya, Madagascar, Malawi, Mali, Mauritania, Mauritius, Morocco, Mozambique, Namibia, Niger, Nigeria, Oman, Saudi Arabia, Senegal, Sierra Leone, Somalia, South Africa, Sudan, Swaziland, Syria, Togo, Tunisia, Uganda, Tanzania, Yemen, Zambia, and Zimbabwe	*Bulinus* species. *Physopsis* and *Bulinus* subgenera of the genus *Bulinus* (many species).	As for *S. mansoni*	Urine (rarely feces); size, 150 × 62 μm
Schistosoma mekongi	Intestinal schistosomiasis in Cambodia, Laos, and Thailand	*Neotricula aperta*	As for *S. japonicum*	Feces; size, 57 × 66 μm
Schistosoma intercalatum	Rectal schistosomiasis in Cameroon, Central African Republic, Chad, Democratic Republic of the Congo, Equatorial Guinea, Gabon, Mali, Nigeria, Republic of the Congo, and São Tomé and Principe	*Bulinus (Physopsis) africanus, Bulinus camerunensis*		Feces; size, 176 × 66 μm
Schistosoma bovis, Schistosoma mattheei, Schistosoma margrebowiei	Schistosomiasis (organisms infect bovines and wildlife [rare human infections]) in Africa	*Bulinus* spp.		
Schistosoma sinesium, Schistosoma malayensis	Schistosomiasis (organisms infect animals [rare human infections]) in Asia			
Species of *Austrobilharzia, Gigantobilharzia, Trichobilharzia*	Swimmer's itch and cercarial dermatitis worldwide	*Bulineus, Lymnaea, Nassarius, Physa, Planorbis,* and *Stagnicola* spp.		Eggs not observed in humans

TABLE 2 Geographical distribution, hosts, and life histories of lung and hepatic digeneans of humans

Family	Species	Location in human host	Disease and geographic area(s)	Snail hosts	Source of metacercariae	Drug regimen[a]	Egg presentation and size
Fasciolidae	*Fasciola hepatica* and *F. gigantica*	Bile ducts	Fasciolosis; worldwide as a disease of livestock; a disease of humans in Australia, Bolivia, Chile, Cuba, Egypt, Ecuador, France, Iran, People's Republic of China, Peru, Portugal, Spain, Turkey, and Vietnam	*Galba/Fossaria* group (*F. hepatica*), *Radixsoo* (*F. gigantica*)	Vegetation: wet grass, watercress, water mint, semiaquatic vegetables, contaminated water	T, 10 mg/kg (in severe cases for 2 days)	Feces; size, 130–150 × 60–85 μm (*F. hepatica*) and 160–190 × 70–90 μm (*F. gigantica*)
Opisthorchiidae	*Clonorchis sinensis, Opisthorchis viverrini*, and *O. felineus*	Bile ducts	Opisthorchiasis/clonorchiasis in the People's Republic of China, former Soviet Union, Cambodia, Korea, Laos, Taiwan, Thailand, and Vietnam	For *C. sinensis*, various freshwater snails (*Alocinma, Bulinus, Parafossarulus*); for *O. viverrini* and *O. felineus*, freshwater snails from the genus *Bithynia* and related genera	Many species (>100) of freshwater fish	P, 25 mg/kg 3 times daily for 2 days	Feces; size, 23–35 × 10–20 μm (*C. sinensis*) and 30 × 12 μm (*O. felineus*)
Opisthorchiidae	*Olivella guayaquilensis, Metorchis albidus, Metorchis conjunctus, Pseudamphistomum aethiopicum*, and *Pseudamphistomum truncatum*	Bile ducts	Opisthorchiasis in Asia	Not listed	Fish		
Troglotrematidae	*Paragonimus africanus, Paragonimus heterotremus, Paragonimus kellicotti, Paragonimus mexicanus, Paragonimus skrjabini, Paragonimus uterobilateralis*, and *Paragonimus westermani*	Pulmonary cysts, also abdominal cavity, brain	Paragonimiasis in Cambodia, Cameroon, Colombia, Costa Rica, Ecuador, Equatorial Guinea, Gabon, Guatemala, Honduras, India, Indonesia, Ivory Coast, Japan, Korea, Laos, Liberia, Malaysia, Mexico, Nepal, Nicaragua, Nigeria, Panama, Papua New Guinea, People's Republic of China, Peru, the Philippines, Samoa, southeastern Siberia, Sri Lanka, Taiwan, Thailand, Venezuela, Vietnam, and North America	Operculate snail: *Semisulcospira, Thiara*, and *Oncomelania* species	Freshwater crabs, crayfish	T, 20 mg/kg; P, 25 mg/kg 3 times daily for 2–3 days	Feces, sputum; size varies with species
Dicrocoeliidae	*Dicrocoelium* species	Bile ducts	Dicrocoeliasis; human cases in the Czech Republic, Kenya, Nigeria, Russia, Saudi Arabia, Somalia, Spain, and the United States	Land snails, order Stylommatophora	Insects (ants)	P, 25 mg/kg 3 times daily for 1 day	Feces, bile; size, 38–45 × 22–30 μm (brown, thick-walled, embryonated, operculate)

[a] T, triclabendazole; P, praziquantel.

TABLE 3 Geographical distribution, hosts, and life histories of digeneans of the human intestinal tract[a]

Family	Genera	Disease and geographic areas	Snail host(s)	Source of metacercariae	Human infection	Drug regimen	Egg presentation and size
Echinostomatidae	*Acanthoparyphium, Artyfechinostomum, Echinochasmus, Echinoparyphium, Echinostoma, Episthmium, Euparyphium, Himasthla, Hypoderaeum, Isthmiophora, Paryphostomum*	Echinostomiasis in Egypt, Hungary, India, Indonesia, Italy, Japan, Korea, Malaysia, North and South America, People's Republic of China, Philippines, Romania, Russia, Siberia, Singapore, Taiwan, and Thailand	Families Viviparidae and Planorbidae	Fish (loach), molluscs (snails, clams), amphibians (tadpoles, frogs)	Focal; prevalence, 5–44%	P, 25 mg/kg	Feces; size, 100 × 65–70 μm
Fasciolidae	*Fasciolopsis*	Fasciolopsiasis in Bangladesh, Cambodia, India, Indonesia, Korea, Laos, Pakistan, People's Republic of China, Taiwan, Thailand, and Vietnam	Family Planorbidae	Water plants (water chestnut, caltrop, lotus roots, bamboo), other aquatic vegetation	Widespread but focal; prevalence rates up to 60% in children	P, 15–40 mg/kg; MB, 100 mg/kg	Feces; size, 130–140 × 80–85 μm
Gastrodiscidae	*Gastrodiscoides, Gastrodiscus*	Gastrodiscoidiasis in India, Myanmar, People's Republic of China, the Philippines, Russia, Thailand, and Vietnam	*Helicorbus* spp.	Squid, plants, crustaceans (crayfish), amphibians (frogs, tadpoles)	Rare, focal	NR	Feces; size, 127–169 × 62–75 μm
Heterophyidae	*Apophalus, Centrocestus, Cryptocotyle, Diorchitrema, Haplorchis, Heterophyes, Heterophyopsis, Metagonimus, Phagicola, Procercovum, Pygidiopis, Stellantchasmus, Stichodora*	Metagonimiasis or heterophyiasis in the Balkans, Brazil, Egypt, Greenland, Indonesia, Israel, Japan, Korea, People's Republic of China, the Philippines, Russia, Spain, Sudan, Taiwan, Tunisia, Turkey, and the United States	Families Thiaridae and Littorinidae	Fish (freshwater or brackish water; carp, mullet, cyprinoids), crustaceans (shrimp)	Low prevalence but common; cases with heavy infections of clinical significance	P, 10–20 mg/kg	Feces
Troglotrematidae	*Nanophyetus salmincola*	Nanophyetiasis in Russia and the United States	*Oxytrema silicula*	Fish (salmon, trout)	Rare	P	Feces; size, 64–97 × 34–55 μm

[a]Modified from reference 15 with permission. Abbreviations: NR, not recorded; MB, mebendazole; P, praziquantel.

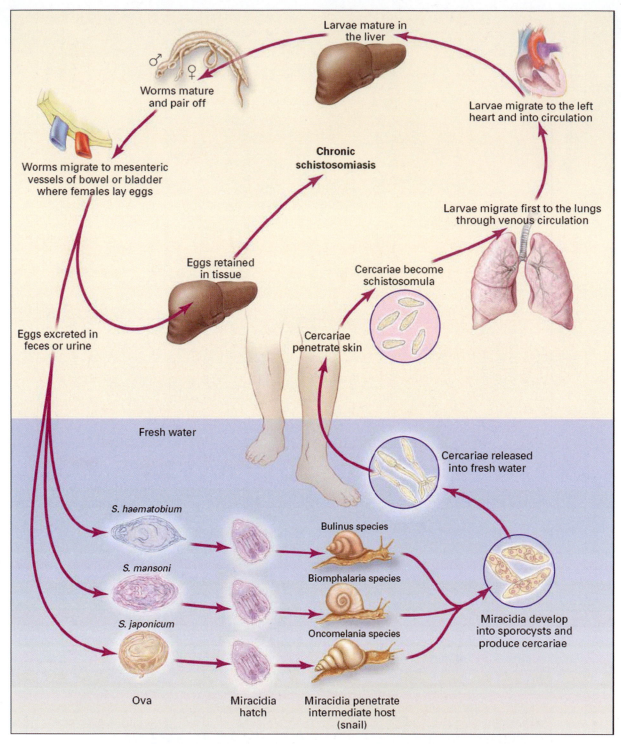

FIGURE 1 Five species of *Schistosoma* are known to infect humans. Infection with *Schistosoma mansoni*, *S. japonicum*, *S. mekongi*, or *S. intercalatum* adults occurs in mesenteric veins; *S. haematobium* adults occur in the vesicle plexus. Humans are infected after cercarial penetration of the skin. After penetration, the cercariae shed their bifurcated tails, and the resulting schistosomula enter capillaries and lymphatic vessels en route to the lungs. After several days, the worms migrate to the portal venous system, where they mature and unite. Pairs of worms then migrate to the site of patent infection. Egg production commences 4 to 6 weeks after infection. Eggs pass from the lumens of blood vessels into adjacent tissues, and many then pass through the intestinal or bladder mucosa and are shed in the feces or urine (see the text). In freshwater, the eggs hatch, releasing miracidia that, in turn, infect specific freshwater snails (Table 1). Reprinted from the *New England Journal of Medicine* (44) with permission.

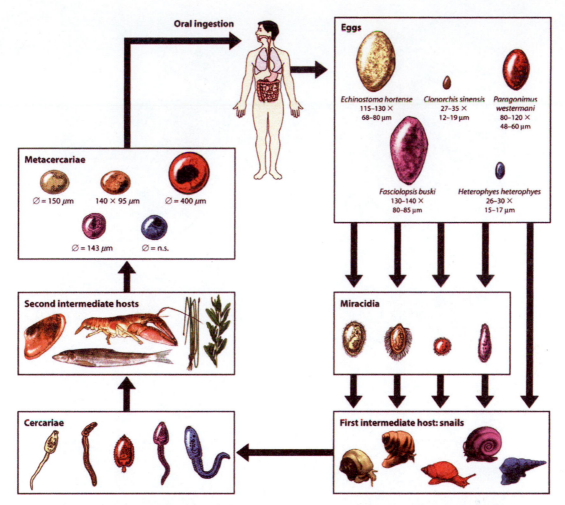

FIGURE 2 Life cycles of five different food-borne trematodes, including intestinal flukes (*Echinostoma hortense, Fasciolopsis buski*, and *Heterophyes heterophyes*), a liver fluke (*Clonorchis sinensis*), and a lung fluke (*Paragonimus westermani*). Reprinted from *Clinical Microbiology Reviews* (27) with permission.

Africa (50). Of these, some 120 million people are symptomatic and 20 million have severe illness.

Taxonomy

Schistosomes are characterized by dioecious adults, cercariae with a forked tail, and a two-host life cycle (Fig. 1). Adults occupy an intravascular site in the human host, either in the mesenteric vessels or the vesical plexus. Five species commonly infect humans, of which three (*Schistosoma mansoni, Schistosoma japonicum*, and *Schistosoma haematobium*) are the most important (Table 1). Cross-hybridization between predominantly human- and animal-parasitic species is recognized as an increasing problem in Africa (43). Morphological descriptions of adult worms, which are not encountered in diagnostic samples, are summarized elsewhere (36).

Hepatosplenic Schistosomiasis

The most extensively studied schistosome, *S. mansoni*, occurs throughout sub-Saharan Africa, Egypt, the Middle East, Madagascar, eastern countries of South America, and some islands of the Caribbean (Table 1). It is believed that the species was carried to South America with the slave trade. The distribution of *S. mansoni* overlaps that of *S. haematobium* in many parts of Africa.

Schistosoma japonicum is responsible for significant disease in foci in Asia (10) (Table 1) but has been eradicated from Japan. Sustained control efforts in China had reduced the number of infected people from approximately 12 million to 1 to 2 million by the late 1980s and to less than 1 million in 1998, but resurgence is likely (9, 10). Unlike most other human schistosomes, *S. japonicum* is a zoonotic organism, and in China, large bovines, especially water buffalo, are of primary concern in perpetuating the life cycle (33).

Schistosoma mekongi has a highly focal distribution in the Mekong River Basin, with foci of endemicity in Laos and Cambodia (4). Although originally regarded as a subspecies of *S. japonicum*, the species was recognized as distinct based on morphological characteristics, pathologic effects, and life cycle patterns. Sustained large-scale chemotherapy in provinces in Cambodia where the disease is endemic has led to effective control of the disease in that country (48)

Schistosoma intercalatum is responsible for rectal schistosomiasis in regions of Africa. The species occurs as two geographically isolated strains (now considered distinct species [22]), the Cameroon and the Democratic Republic of the Congo strains, which display highly focal distribution (10). This parasite belongs to the *S. haematobium* group of species, characterized by, among other features, eggs with a terminal spine (see Fig. 3).

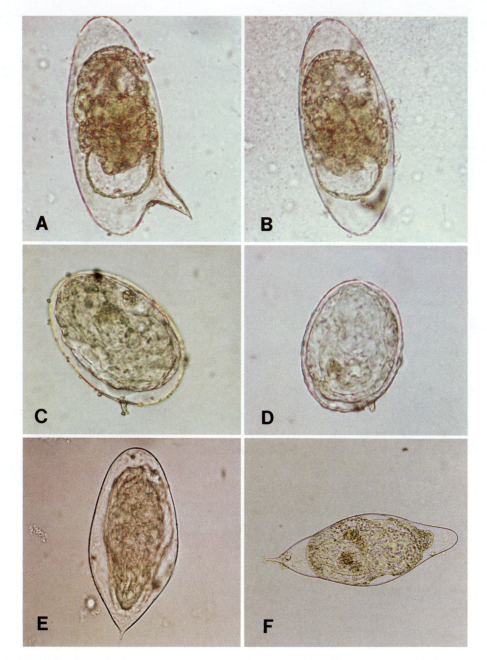

FIGURE 3 Eggs of schistosome species (magnification, ×480). (A) *S. mansoni*; (B) *S. mansoni* egg with typical lateral spine not in view; (C) *S. japonicum*; (D) *S. mekongi*; (E) *S. haematobium*; (F) *S. intercalatum*. (Panels C through E are from reference 3; used with permission.)

Genitourinary Schistosomiasis

Schistosoma haematobium, the sole agent of urinary schistosomiasis, occurs in much of the African continent as well as Madagascar and the Middle East (10, 36) (Table 1). Adult worms live in the vesical plexus. Eggs escape the host across the bladder wall to be excreted with urine.

Epidemiology, Transmission, and Prevention

All schistosomes of humans use freshwater aquatic snails as an intermediate host. Humans are infected through exposure to freshwater contaminated with infective larvae, the cercariae (Fig. 1). Cercariae enter the human body by percutaneous penetration.

Within regions of endemicity, factors contributing to schistosome transmission include the distribution biology and population dynamics of the snail hosts, extent of contamination of freshwater with feces or urine, and degree of exposure of humans to contaminated water. The recent development of large-scale dams in some countries where the disease is endemic has led to changes in transmission dynamics (50). The impact of the Three Gorges Dam in China on the transmission of *S. japonicum* remains uncertain (34).

Clinical Significance

Cercarial dermatitis occurs in schistosomiasis but is more commonly reported after infection with avian schistosomes

(Table 1) and *Schistosoma spindale*. Acute toxemic schistosomiasis (Katayama fever) can occur with any schistosome species but is more apparent in nonimmune individuals and may be characterized by fever, headache, generalized myalgias, right-upper-quadrant pain, and bloody diarrhea (18, 45).

Eggs (Fig. 3) are laid by female worms in the vasculature and must traverse endothelia and the gut or bladder mucosa to escape the host. In those schistosomes infecting mesenteric veins, eggs pass through the wall of the intestine or rectum, while for *S. haematobium*, the eggs escape across the bladder wall. For all species, however, many eggs become entrapped in tissues. The chronic effects of schistosomiasis, therefore, relate to the site of adult infections and granulomatous and fibrotic responses to entrapped parasite eggs (18). Granulomas occur in many tissues in response to entrapped eggs; however, most accumulate in tissues fed by vasculature leading from the site of adult infection. Eggs retained in the gut wall induce inflammation, hyperplasia, and ulceration, and occult blood occurs in the feces. A suggested relationship between colorectal cancer and schistosomiasis remains controversial (41). Eggs entrapped in the liver lead to portal hypertension and splenic and hepatic enlargement, potentially giving rise to the formation of fragile esophageal varices. Ascites also is common.

In urinary schistosomiasis, granulomatous inflammatory response to embolized eggs gives rise to dysuria, hematuria, and proteinuria, calcifications in the bladder, obstruction of the ureter, renal colic, hydronephrosis, and renal failure. Secondary bacterial infection of the bladder and other affected tissues may occur. There is a consistent association between *S. haematobium* infection and squamous cell carcinoma of the bladder (42). *S. haematobium* infection causes genital disease in approximately one-third of infected women, leading to vulval and perineal disease and tubal infertility, and may facilitate the transmission of human immunodeficiency virus (38).

Diagnosis

Direct Examination

The presence of schistosome eggs (Fig. 3) (3) in feces or urine is diagnostic of schistosomiasis. Eggs of hepatosplenic schistosomes may be observed by light microscopy in stool specimens with or without suspension in saline. Formalin-based techniques for sedimentation and concentration are particularly useful, especially for patients releasing few eggs. Hatching tests, in which fecal matter is suspended in nonchlorinated water in darkened vessels with directed surface light, have been used to detect motile miracidia. In patients with chronic disease and with typical clinical presentation but negative urine and feces specimens, a biopsy of the bladder or rectal mucosa may be helpful in diagnosis.

Examination of stools with the Kato-Katz technique is used in field studies for quantification of fecal egg burdens. The Kato-Katz method gives a theoretical sensitivity cutoff of 20 eggs per gram of feces (13), but large daily variation in egg shedding and the uneven distribution of eggs in feces may lead to inconsistent counts. For *S. mansoni* infections, it has been recommended that either five replicate slides or sets of triplicate slides made from stool collected on two successive days be used for assessment of infection status (6).

Sedimentation or concentration methods are most useful for diagnosis of *S. haematobium* from urine samples. In addition, the use of tests for blood, protein, and eosinophils in urine, while not specific, may be indicative of infection (1). Portable ultrasound is useful for assessment of pathologic damage to tissues. The use of questionnaires in populations living in areas where the organisms are endemic is helpful in revealing infections by *S. japonicum* and *S. haematobium* but for *S. mansoni* may lead to underestimation of prevalence (53). An innovative test using paramagnetic beads to bind schistosome ova has been explored (14).

Serologic Tests

A range of direct and indirect tests have been explored experimentally, including enzyme-linked immunosorbent assay (ELISA) and immunoblot tests using soluble egg antigen and recombinant antigens and the detection of parasite antigen in excreta (20). Host antibodies against schistosomes can persist for prolonged periods after parasitologic cure, and this, together with potential antigen cross-reactivity, can limit the value of serological tests (20). Serology can be most valuable for diagnosis of schistosomiasis in travelers from regions of nonendemicity who visit areas where the disease is endemic. Other indirect tests include assays for peripheral-blood eosinophilia, anemia, hypoalbuminemia, elevated urea and creatinine levels, and hypergammaglobulinemia (1, 44).

Nucleic Acid Detection Techniques

PCR tests for schistosomes in stool use high-repeat nuclear genomic (39) and mitochondrial sequences (16). Both tests report high sensitivity, at times exceeding that of direct coprological examination. The mitochondrial sequence probes, which amplify sequences spanning the *cox2* and *nad6* genes for *S. japonicum* and *S. mansoni*, *nad1-nad2* for *S. japonicum*, and *nad5* for *S. mansoni*, show high specificity and sensitivity (16). An interesting development is that of the use of real-time PCR to detect cell-free schistosome DNA in host plasma (56). This method utilizes a 121-bp tandem repeat sequence that represents approximately 12% of the *S. mansoni* genome as the target sequence for amplification.

Treatment

Praziquantel is the drug of choice for treatment of schistosomiasis. The drug has been used in mass treatment campaigns in many countries, a development facilitated in part by reductions in costs associated with manufacture of the drug. Despite this, the anthelmintic has some limitations, being effective against only adult forms (17), and it does not protect from subsequent infection.

Treatment failures for *S. mansoni* and *S. haematobium* infections with praziquantel have been observed, and the presence of resistant strains has been demonstrated experimentally (see chapter 148). Widespread resistance to praziquantel has not been observed clinically, but the application of the drug in mass treatment campaigns may result in new resistant forms emerging.

Derivatives of artemisinin, an antimalarial, have been tested against schistosomes in experimental models and clinical field settings (54). In contrast to praziquantel, artemether acts against juvenile schistosomes in the host and may be used as a chemoprophylactic agent (5). It has been shown for experimental schistosomiasis that combination therapy with artemether and praziquantel at low doses can be more effective that use of praziquantel alone (52).

Schistosome Dermatitis (Swimmer's Itch)

Schistosome dermatitis, a minor ailment, arises from infection with a number of avian and mammal schistosomes (Table 1). The avian schistosome cercariae cannot migrate from the dermal layers of human skin and induce local dermatitis accompanied by pruritus and papule formation.

FOODBORNE DIGENEANS

All other digeneans considered here represent a diverse assemblage of taxa which infect humans through ingestion of uncooked food (Fig. 2; Tables 2 and 3). The vast majority of these species are zoonotic. The primary epidemiological features governing human infection include the distribution of suitable snail intermediate hosts, human food consumption behaviors, the presence of suitable zoonotic hosts, and the potential for water contamination with human or animal excreta (27).

Trematodes of the Respiratory System: *Paragonimus*

Taxonomy

Paragonimiasis is caused by a number of species distributed throughout Asia, Africa, and the Americas (Table 2). The most common species infecting humans is *Paragonimus westermani*, which occurs in China and Southeast Asia. Adult *Paragonimus* species inhabit the lungs, where they induce the formation of encapsulating cysts. The flukes are large and fleshy, measuring 8 to 16 by 4 to 8 mm. Taxonomic information on these parasites is presented elsewhere (7).

Epidemiology, Transmission, and Prevention

The life cycle of *Paragonimus* is shown in Fig. 2 and Table 2. Of the approximately 50 species, 9 have been recorded as human parasites. Eggs are passed in the lungs and are transferred up the bronchial tree with sputum. Eggs may be spat with sputum or swallowed and passed with feces. The first intermediate hosts are freshwater snails. Human infection arises after ingestion of uncooked or marinated freshwater crabs or crayfish (40), but unwashed hands of food preparers and contaminated utensils also may be sources of human infection. Wild boars can act as paratenic hosts (7). After ingestion, the immature flukes penetrate the intestinal wall and migrate to the lungs through the body cavity. All species are zoonotic, infecting carnivores, pigs, and rodents.

Clinical Significance

Some 20.7 million people have paragonimiasis, and a further 293 million are at risk of infection (25). Signs of infection include fever with dry cough, sometimes blood-stained sputum containing eggs, chest pain, dyspnea, and bronchitis, and symptoms sometimes resemble those of pulmonary tuberculosis. Peripheral blood eosinophilia is common. The flukes induce the formation of an epithelial cyst, measuring approximately 1 cm in diameter, which may calcify over time. Parasites may also occur in extrapulmonary locations, and serious complications occur when parasites are found in the brain. The necrosis of brain tissues and an extensive granulomatous inflammatory response may induce symptoms similar to those of cerebral cysticercosis, caused by the cestode *Taenia solium* (1).

Diagnosis

Direct Examination

Diagnosis of paragonimiasis is largely dependent on observation of the eggs (3, 40) (Fig. 4) in sputum, feces, or pleural effusions. A cough with brown sputum is indicative of lung infection, and the sputum should be examined for eggs. The cysts formed around adult worms appear in X rays as characteristic rings or nodules, but direct observation of eggs is required to differentiate the disease from pulmonary tuberculosis.

Serologic Tests and Nucleic Acid Detection Techniques

Serologic tests include ELISAs using either 32- and 35-kDa antigens or parasite yolk ferritin as the antigen (1). Pleurisy with eosinophilia and a dominant immunoglobulin M antibody titer may be indicative of paragonimiasis (37). PCR-based methods have been developed in recent years, and though these are valuable research tools, it is difficult to see how they might be developed as routine diagnostic tools (40).

Treatment

The current WHO recommendation for treatment is administration of praziquantel at 25 mg/kg of body weight for two to three consecutive days. Triclabendazole at 10 mg/kg or 20 mg/kg in two divided doses holds promise as a useful therapeutic alternative (23).

Trematodes of the Liver

At least 13 species of flukes belonging to the families Fasciolidae, Opisthorchiidae, and Dicrocoeliidae (21) (Table 2) have been recorded as adult worms from the livers and bile ducts of humans. Brief information on human dicrocoeliasis is provided in Table 2, but the reader is referred to other reviews (36, 47) for more information on the lancet flukes.

Family Opisthorchiidae

Taxonomy

Of the opisthorchid parasites infecting humans (Table 2), only three species are of major significance, namely, *Opisthorchis viverrini*, *Opisthorchis felineus*, and *Clonorchis sinensis*. Adult opisthorchids of humans are macroscopic, flattened flukes that are approximately 5 to 10 mm in length.

Epidemiology, Transmission, and Prevention

The life cycle information of these parasites is presented in Fig. 2 and Table 2. In opisthorchids, the metacercariae are found encysted in the muscles of cyprinid fish (21). Individuals are infected by eating raw, seasoned, or undercooked fish (49).

Clinical Significance

Disease severity varies among the different species (49) and with intensity of infection. *Clonorchis sinensis* infects approximately 35 million people in China, Hong Kong, India, North Korea, Siberia, Taiwan, and Vietnam (27). *Opisthorchis viverrini* infects about 10 million people in Thailand, Laos, and Cambodia, and *O. felineus* is widespread throughout northern Europe and Asia, infecting about 1.5 million people (27). All three species live in the bile duct and are thought to feed on biliary epithelia. Light infections are usually asymptomatic, but heavy infections can induce disease. Symptoms most commonly are associated with an acute phase of infection and may include fever, abdominal pain, hepatitis-like symptoms, and eosinophilia. A number of asymptomatic hepatobiliary abnormalities are associated with infection (30). Severe infestations with these liver flukes, which are rare, might cause obstructive jaundice, cirrhosis, cholangitis, cholecystitis, bile peritonitis, biliary obstruction, intrahepatic stone formation, cholelithiasis, biliary and liver abscesses, pancreatitis, and hepatitis. The most serious complication of infections with *C. sinensis* and *O. viverrini*

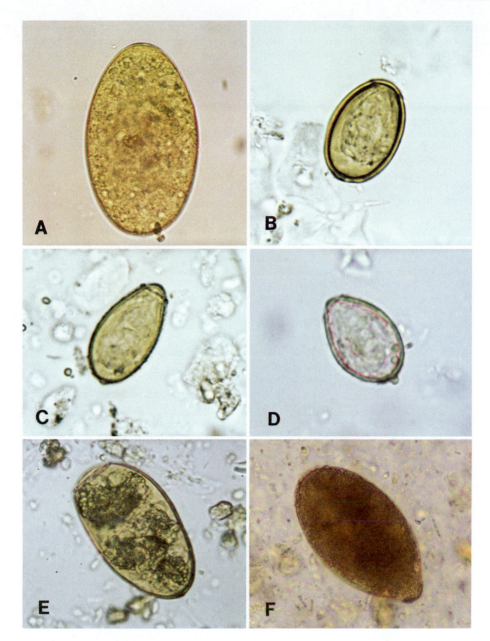

FIGURE 4 Eggs of trematode parasites. (A) *Fasciolopsis buski* (magnification, ×400); (B) *H. hetero-phyes* (magnification, ×1,200); (C) *Clonorchis sinensis* (magnification, ×1,200); (D) *Opisthorchis viver-rini* (magnification, ×1,200); (E) *Paragonimus westermani* (magnification, ×480); (F) *Nanophyetus salmincola* (magnification, ×600). (Panels B through D are from reference 3; used with permission.)

is cholangiocarcinoma, the malignant bile duct cancer. Both species have been classified as definite carcinogens (class 1) (12a, 32).

Diagnosis

Direct examination. Eggs of opisthorchids (Fig. 4) are embryonated when laid, oval, yellowish brown, and oper-culate, with a shoulder or thickened region of eggshell surrounding the operculum. The shell surface may appear rough and may have a small knob at the abopercular pole (21). The eggs are smaller than those of many other digeneans of humans, ranging from 20 to 35 μm in length. Opisthorchid eggs may be confused with those of other taxa, especially

the heterophyids (see below). Differential diagnosis may be obtained by patient history, examination by the formalin-ether concentration technique, and examination of purged worms in feces after anthelmintic treatment.

Serologic tests and nucleic acid detection techniques. Many antigen tests have been conducted for *O. viverrini* in trials, but most are plagued by cross-reactivity and the persistence of antibodies after parasitologic cure (57). A copro-antigen ELISA has been developed using monoclonal antibodies raised against adult *O. viverrini* E/S antigen and has displayed high specificity and sensitivity, whereas ELISAs for circulating antibodies show high sensitivity but low specificity (1). Recently, different PCR tests that detect and discriminate between fish-borne zoonoses caused by opisthorchids and members of the Heterophyidae were developed based on mitochondrial (29) and ribosomal sequences (51).

Treatment

Treatment for clonorchiasis or opisthorchiasis relies on oral administration of praziquantel (25 mg/kg three times per day for two consecutive days is commonly used in hospitals, while a single oral dose of 40 mg/kg is used for mass treatment programs). Indeed, in a recent exploratory, open-label, phase 2 trial in Laos, a cure rate of 70% was observed in *O. viverrini*-infected children following treatment with a single dose of tribendimidine (49a).

Family Fasciolidae

Taxonomy

Fascioliasis, caused by flukes of the genus *Fasciola*, is primarily a disease of herbivorous mammals. Until recently, fascioliasis was considered a sporadic infection of humans, but it is now estimated that some 2.4 million people in 61 countries are infected, with 180 million at risk throughout the world (31). The two causative species, *F. hepatica* and *F. gigantica*, have a worldwide distribution in domesticated animals; human disease is focal, and regions in which human fascioliasis is endemic are recognized (1, 31, 36).

Epidemiology, Transmission, and Prevention

Fasciolid metacercariae encyst on semiaquatic or moistened vegetation, predominantly watercress, grass, water mint, or salad vegetables (Fig. 2; Table 2). The frequency of the parasites in domesticated animals does not necessarily correlate with human disease. Areas of low prevalence in humans include regions of France (<3.1 cases per 100,000 people in Basse-Normandie) and Chile; regions of high endemicity are in Peru (15.64 to 34.2% in regions of endemicity) and Bolivia (66.7% in the Bolivian altiplano) (31). Most of the areas with high endemicity are regions where *F. hepatica* is present. While common zoonotic hosts are cattle and sheep, other hosts, such as pigs, equines, and rats, may serve as reservoir hosts for human infection. Children and young adults are more commonly infected than adults, suggestive of the presence of age-dependent immunity (58).

Clinical Significance

Many infections with fasciolids remain asymptomatic. Acute disease arises because of extensive tissue damage as parasites migrate through the hepatic parenchyma to gain access to the bile ducts. Parasite activity in the bile ducts leads to proliferation of ductal epithelium, inflammation, and fibrosis. Heavy infections can lead to cholestasis and result in hepatic atrophy and periportal cirrhosis (1). Common symptoms in chronic infection include biliary colic and cholangitis. Eosinophilia is common in all stages of disease.

Diagnosis

The eggs of fasciolids are large compared with those of other digeneans (Table 2). *Fasciola* eggs cannot be distinguished from those of the related intestinal parasite *Fasciolopsis buski* (Fig. 4) and also resemble those of *Gastrodiscoides* spp. (Table 3). Fasciolid eggs of individual species can also vary in morphology and size in different host species, complicating species identification in regions where more than one fasciolid is endemic (55). Liver fasciolids have a long

(2-month) prepatent period, and because of this, fascioliasis is one disease where serological diagnosis is valuable. Immunological tests, particularly ELISA, based on a cysteine protease, display high sensitivity and specificity (11).

Treatment

Fasciola species appear to be insensitive to praziquantel, and triclabendazole is the drug of choice (Table 2). There have been reports of triclabendazole-insensitive isolates in livestock (24). Artemether and artesunate are being tested for use in humans (24).

Trematodes of the Intestine

Humans can serve as host to a wide variety of intestinal flukes. Summary information on some families of intestinal trematodes is presented in Table 3. The families Brachylaimidae, Diplostomidae, Gymnophallidae, Lecithodendriidae, Microphallidae, Paramphistomatidae, Plagiorchiidae, and Strigeidae are rarely encountered in humans and are not considered further in this chapter. For further information on intestinal trematodes not provided here, the reader is referred to chapter 145 and to reference 15. Members of the families Echinostomatidae, Heterophyidae, Fasciolidae, and Troglotrematidae are commonly encountered in some countries and are discussed in the following sections.

Echinostomatidae

Echinostomatid flukes are small, typically 3 to 10 mm in length and 1 to 3 mm in width, with a large ventral sucker and distinctive collared spines. At least 24 species are known to parasitize humans, mostly in Asia (Table 3), for example, *Echinochasmus japonicas*, a common parasite of humans in Laos (46). All human infections by echinostomatids are zoonotic and focal in distribution, and foci are often in the vicinity of fresh- or brackish-water habitats. Humans are infected by eating a range of raw or undercooked vertebrate and invertebrate foods, including snails (Table 3). In most cases, infection is asymptomatic. Heavy infections can lead to a range of symptoms, including flatulence, colic, and diarrhea. Some heavy infections in children have been fatal. Eggs of echinostomatids are similar in shape to those of fasciolids but are smaller (Table 3). Interspecific variation in egg size occurs among the echinostomes, and species identification is not possible unless adult worms are obtained by purgation with anthelmintics. A single dose of praziquantel is recommended for treatment (24).

Fasciolidae

Fasciolopsis buski is the largest fluke parasitizing humans, measuring 8 to 10 cm in length and 1 to 3 cm in width (28). Adult worms inhabit the duodenum and jejunum of humans and a small number of other hosts that includes pigs, horses, cattle, goats, and sheep. The species is distributed focally in many countries (Table 3). The snail intermediate hosts of *F. buski* are shown in Table 3. Humans are infected by eating aquatic plants on which metacercariae are encysted or by drinking metacercariae that have encysted on the water surface (15). Adults attach and feed on the intestinal wall. Human disease relates to the severity of infection, and symptoms vary from intestinal disturbance and pain, associated with eosinophilia, to severe diarrhea, gastric pain, bowel obstructions, and nausea. Feces are often profuse and yellow-green and may contain undigested food particles.

The eggs of *F. buski* are large, operculate, nonembryonated, ellipsoidal, and yellow (Table 3; Fig. 4A). The eggs are very similar to those of other fasciolids, from which species may be distinguished by observation of purged adults. The current drug of choice is praziquantel, but albendazole and mebendazole have also been tested (15, 24).

Heterophyidae

Many species of heterophyid trematodes are known to infect humans (8, 15). Heterophyids are mostly small parasites less than 0.5 mm in length. Some species are marine. Commonly encountered heterophyids of humans are *Heterophyes heterophyes*, *Metagonimus yokogawai*, and *Haplorchis* species. *H. heterophyes* infection in humans has been reported from many counties in Asia, North Africa, and the Middle East (15). Other species are often encountered in rural Asia (46).

The adult flukes are intestinal inhabitants of a wide range of piscivorous birds and mammals. Eggs (Fig. 4) are embryonated when passed from the host but do not hatch until they are ingested by a snail intermediate host (36). Cercariae encyst in a number of fish, including mugilids, cyprinids, and gobiids. Humans are infected by consumption of raw, freshly salted, or undercooked fish (Table 3).

Disease symptoms in humans relate to infection intensity and arise because of parasite irritation of the intestinal mucosa. Eggs may on occasion pass into the bloodstream and lodge in tissues. These eggs have been known to cause fatal myocarditis in the Philippines (1). Diagnosis of heterophyids is facilitated by observation of eggs in feces (Table 3). Heterophyid eggs are similar in size to those of opisthorchiid liver flukes, and care must be taken to differentiate the infections. Often this can be achieved only by examination of purged adult worms. The recommended treatment for heterophyid infection is a single dose of praziquantel (Table 3).

Troglotrematidae

The Troglotrematidae family of small oval flukes parasitizes mammals, including humans. One species, *Nanophyetus salmincola*, found along the coastal U.S. Pacific Northwest, is found as metacercariae of salmonid fish. The species may be the most commonly encountered human trematode endemic to North America. Praziquantel is efficacious for nanophyetiasis.

REFERENCES

1. **Acha, P. N., and B. Szyfres.** 2003. *Zoonoses and Communicable Diseases Common to Man and Animals.* Pan American Health Organization, Washington, DC.
2. **Anonymous.** 1991. *Basic Laboratory Methods in Medical Parasitology.* World Health Organization, Geneva, Switzerland.
3. **Ash, L. R., and T. L. Orihel.** 1997. *Atlas of Human Parasitology.* ASCP Press, Chicago, IL.
4. **Attwood, S. W.** 2001. Schistosomiasis in the Mekong region: epidemiology and phylogeography. *Adv. Parasitol.* 50:87–152.
5. **Bergquist, R., J. Utzinger, J. Chollet, S. H. Xiao, N. A. Weiss, and M. Tanner.** 2005. Triggering of high-level resistance against *Schistosoma mansoni* reinfection by artemether in the mouse model. *Am. J. Trop. Med. Hyg.* 71:774–777.
6. **Berhe, N., G. Medhin, B. Erko, T. Smith, S. Gedamu, D. Bereded, R. Moore, E. Habte, A. Redda, T. Gebre-Michael, and S. G. Gundersen.** 2004. Variations in helminth faecal egg counts in Kato-Katz thick smears and their implications in assessing infection status with Schistosoma mansoni. *Acta Trop.* 92:205–212.
7. **Blair, D., Z. B. Xu, and T. Agatsuma.** 1999. Paragonimiasis and the genus *Paragonimus*. *Adv. Parasitol.* 42:113–222.
8. **Chai, J.-Y., and S. H. Lee.** 2002. Food-borne intestinal trematode infections in the Republic of Korea. *Parasitol. Int.* 51:129–154.
9. **Chen, Z., L. Wang, J. Cai, X. Zhou, J. Zhang, J. Guo, X. Wu, D. Engels, and M. Chen.** 2005. Schistosomiasis control in China: the impact of a 10-year World Bank loan project (1992–2001). *Bull. W. H. O.* 83:43–48.
10. **Chitsulo, L., D. Engels, A. Montresor, and L. Savioli.** 2000. The global status of schistosomiasis and its control. *Acta Trop.* 77:41–51.
11. **Cordova, M., L. Reategui, and J. R. Espinoza.** 1999. Immunodiagnosis of human fascioliasis with *Fasciola hepatica* cysteine proteinases. *Trans. R. Soc. Trop. Med. Hyg.* 93:54–57.
12. **Cribb, T. H., and R. A. Bray.** 2010. Gut wash, body soak, blender and heat-fixation: approaches to the effective collection, fixation and preservation of trematodes of fishes. *Syst. Parasitol.* 76:1–7.
12a. **de Martel, C., M. Plummer, and S. Franceschi.** 2009. Cholangiocarcinoma: descriptive epidemiology and risk factors. *Gastroenterol. Clin. Biol.* 34:173–180.
13. **Doenhoff, M. J., P. L. Chiodini, and J. V. Hamilton.** 2004. Specific and sensitive diagnosis of schistosome infection: can it be done with antibodies? *Trends Parasitol.* 20:35–39.
14. **Fagundes Teixeira, C., E. Neuhauss, R. Ben, J. Romanzini, and C. Graeff-Teixeira.** 2007. Detection of *Schistosoma mansoni* eggs in feces through their interaction with paramagnetic beads in a magnetic field. *PLoS Negl. Trop. Dis.* 1:e73.
15. **Fried, B., T. K. Graczyk, and L. Tamang.** 2004. Food-borne intestinal trematodiases in humans. *Parasitol. Res.* 93:159–170.
16. **Gobert, G. N., M. Chai, M. Duke, and D. P. McManus.** 2005. Copro-PCR based detection of *Schistosoma* eggs using mitochondrial DNA markers. *Mol. Cell. Probes* 19:250–254.
17. **Greenberg, R. M.** 2005. Are Ca^{2+} channels targets of praziquantel action? *Int. J. Parasitol.* 35:1–9.
18. **Gryseels, B., K. Polman, J. Clerinx, and L. Kestens.** 2006. Human schistosomiasis. *Lancet* 368:1106–1118.
19. **Jamornthanyawat, N.** 2002. The diagnosis of human opisthorchiasis. *Southeast Asian J. Trop. Med. Public Health* 33(Suppl. 3):86–91.
20. **Jones, M. K.** 2008. Recent advances in the diagnosis of human schistosomiasis. *Asian Pacific J. Trop. Med.* 1:63–68.
21. **Kaewkes, S.** 2003. Taxonomy and biology of liver flukes. *Acta Trop.* 88:177–186.
22. **Kane, R. A., V. R. Southgate, D. Rollinson, D. T. Littlewood, A. E. Lockyer, J. R. Pages, L. A. Tchuem Tchuente, and J. Jourdane.** 2003. A phylogeny based on three mitochondrial genes supports the division of Schistosoma intercalatum into two separate species. *Parasitology* 127(Pt. 2):131–137.
23. **Keiser, J., D. Engels, G. Büscher, and J. Utzinger.** 2005. Triclabendazole for the treatment of fascioliasis and paragonimiasis. *Expert Opin. Investig. Drugs* 14:1513–1526.
24. **Keiser, J., and J. Utzinger.** 2004. Chemotherapy for major food-borne trematodes: a review. *Expert Opin. Pharmacother.* 5:1711–1726.
25. **Keiser, J., and J. Utzinger.** 2005. Emerging foodborne trematodiases. *Emerg. Infect. Dis.* 11:1507–1514.
26. Reference deleted.
27. **Keiser, J., and J. Utzinger.** 2009. Food-borne trematodiases. *Clin. Microbiol. Rev.* 22:466–483.
28. **Kuntz, R. E., and C. T. Lo.** 1967. Preliminary studies on *Fasciolopsis buski* (Lankester, 1857) (giant Asian intestinal fluke) in the United States. *Trans. Am. Microsc. Soc.* 86:163–166.
29. **Lovis, L., T. K. Mak, K. Phongluxa, P. Soukhathammavong, S. Sayasone, K. Akkhavong, P. Odermatt, J. Keiser, and I. Felger.** 2009. PCR diagnosis of *Opisthorchis viverrini* and *Haplorchis taichui* infections in a Lao community in an area of endemicity and comparison of diagnostic methods for parasitological field surveys. *J. Clin. Microbiol.* 47:1517–1523.
30. **Mairiang, E., and P. Mairiang.** 2003. Clinical manifestation of opisthorchiasis and treatment. *Acta Trop.* 88:221–227.
31. **Mas-Coma, M. S., M. S. Esteban, and M. S. Bargues.** 1999. Epidemiology of human fascioliasis: a review and proposed new classification. *Bull. W. H. O.* 77:340.
32. **Mayer, D. A., and B. Fried.** 2007. The role of helminth infections in carcinogenesis. *Adv. Parasitol.* 65:239–296.
33. **McManus, D. P., Z. Feng, G. Jiagang, Y. Li, P. B. Bartley, A. Loukas, and G. M. Williams.** 2005. Pathways

to improved sustainable morbidity control and prevention of schistosomiasis in the People's Republic of China, p. 159–190. *In* W. E. Secor and D. G. Colley (ed.), *Schistosomiasis.* Springer, New York, NY.

34. **McManus, D. P., Y. Li, D. J. Gray, and A. G. Ross.** 2009. Conquering 'snail fever': schistosomiasis and its control in China. *Expert Rev. Anti Infect. Ther.* **7:**473–485.

35. **Montresor, A., D. W. T. Crompton, A. Hall, D. A. P. Bundy, and L. Savioli.** 1998. Guidelines for the evaluation of soil-transmitted helminthiasis and schistosomiasis at community level. World Health Organization, Geneva, Switzerland.

36. **Muller, R.** 2002. *Worms and Human Disease.* CABI Publishing, Wallingford, United Kingdom.

37. **Nakamura-Uchiyama, F., D. N. Onah, and Y. Nawa.** 2001. Clinical features and parasite-specific IgM/IgG antibodies of paragonimiasis patients recently found in Japan. *Southeast Asian J. Trop. Med. Public Health* **32**(Suppl. 2)**:**55–58.

38. **Ndhlovu, P. D., T. Mduluza, E. F. Kjetland, N. Midzi, L. Nyanga, S. G. Gundersen, H. Friis, and E. Gomo.** 2007. Prevalence of urinary schistosomiasis and HIV in females living in a rural community of Zimbabwe: does age matter? *Trans. R. Soc. Trop. Med. Hyg.* **101:**403–438.

39. **Pontes, L. A., M. C. Oliveira, N. Katz, E. Dias-Neto, and A. Rabello.** 2003. Comparison of a polymerase chain reaction and the Kato-Katz technique for diagnosing infection with *Schistosoma mansoni. Am. J. Trop. Med. Hyg.* **68:**652–656.

40. **Procop, G. W.** 2009. North American paragonimiasis (caused by *Paragonimus kellicotti*) in the context of global paragonimiasis. *Clin. Microbiol. Rev.* **22:**415–446.

41. **Qiu, D. C., A. E. Hubbard, B. Zhong, Y. Zhang, and R. C. Spear.** 2005. A matched, case-control study of the association between *Schistosoma japonicum* and liver and colon cancers, in rural China. *Ann. Trop. Med. Parasitol.* **99:**47–52.

42. **Rollinson, D.** 2009. A wake up call for urinary schistosomiasis: reconciling research effort with public health importance. *Parasitology* **23:**1–18.

43. **Rollinson, D., J. P. Webster, B. Webster, S. Nyakaana, A. Jørgensen, and J. R. Stothard.** 2009. Genetic diversity of schistosomes and snails: implications for control. *Parasitology* **27:**1–11.

44. **Ross, A. G., P. B. Bartley, A. C. Sleigh, G. R. Olds, Y. Li, G. M. Williams, and D. P. McManus.** 2002. Schistosomiasis. *N. Engl. J. Med.* **346:**1212–1220.

45. **Ross, A. G., D. Vickers, G. R. Olds, S. M. Shah, and D. P. McManus.** 2007. Katayama syndrome. *Lancet Infect. Dis.* **7:**218–224.

46. **Sayasone, S., Y. Vonghajack, M. Vanmany, O. Rasphone, S. Tesana, J. Utzinger, K. Akkhavong, and P. Odermatt.** 2009. Diversity of human intestinal helminthiasis in Lao PDR. *Trans. R. Soc. Trop. Med. Hyg.* **103:**247–254.

47. **Schweiger, F., and M. Kuhn.** 2008. *Dicrocoelium dendriticum* infection in a patient with Crohn's disease. *Can. J. Gastroenterol.* **22:**571–573.

48. **Sinuon, M., R. Tsuyuoka, D. Socheat, P. Odermatt, H. Ohmae, H. Matsuda, A. Montresor, and K. Palmer.** 2007. Control of *Schistosoma mekongi* in Cambodia: results of eight years of control activities in the two endemic provinces. *Trans. R. Soc. Trop. Med. Hyg.* **101:**34–39.

49. **Sithithaworn, P., and M. Haswell-Elkins.** 2003. Epidemiology of *Opisthorchis viverrini. Acta Trop.* **88:**187–194.

49a. **Soukhathammavong, P., P. Odermatt, S. Sayasone, Y. Vonghachack, P. Vounatsou, C. Hatz, K. Akkhavong, and J. Keiser.** 2011. Efficacy and safety of mefloquine-artesunate, tribendimidine, and praziquantel in patients with *Opisthorchis viverrini*: a randomized, exploratory, open-label, phase 2 trial. *Lancet Infect. Dis.* **11:**110–118.

50. **Steinmann, P., J. Keiser, R. Bos, M. Tanner, and J. Utzinger.** 2006. Schistosomiasis and water resources development: systematic review, meta-analysis, and estimates of people at risk. *Lancet Infect. Dis.* **6:**411–425.

51. **Traub, R. J., J. Macaranas, M. Mungthin, S. Leelayoova, T. Cribb, K. D. Murrell, and R. C. A. Thompson.** 2009. A new PCR-based approach indicates the range of *Clonorchis sinensis* now extends to central Thailand. *PLoS Negl. Trop. Dis.* **3:**e367.

52. **Utzinger, J., J. Chollet, J. You, J. Mei, M. Tanner, and S. H. Xiao.** 2001. Effect of combined treatment with praziquantel and artemether on *Schistosoma japonicum* and *Schistosoma mansoni* in experimentally infected animals. *Acta Trop.* **80:**9–18.

53. **Utzinger, J., E. K. N'Goran, M. Tanner, and C. Lengeler.** 2000. Simple anamnestic questions and recalled water-contact patterns for self-diagnosis of *Schistosoma mansoni* infection among schoolchildren in western Cote d'Ivoire. *Am. J. Trop. Med. Hyg.* **62:**649–655.

54. **Utzinger, J., S. H. Xiao, M. Tanner, and J. Keiser.** 2007. Artemisinins for schistosomiasis and beyond. *Curr. Opin. Investig. Drugs* **8:**105–116.

55. **Valero, M. A., I. Perez-Crespo, M. V. Periago, M. Khoubbane, and S. Mas-Coma.** 2009. Fluke egg characteristics for the diagnosis of human and animal fascioliasis by *Fasciola hepatica* and *F. gigantica. Acta Trop.* **111:**150–159.

56. **Wichmann, D., M. Panning, T. Quack, S. Kramme, G.-D. Burchard, C. Grevelding, and C. Drosten.** 2009. Diagnosing schistosomiasis by detection of cell-free parasite DNA in human plasma. *PLoS Negl. Trop. Dis.* **3:**e422.

57. **Wongratanacheewin, S., R. W. Sermswan, and S. Sirisinha.** 2003. Immunology and molecular biology of *Opisthorchis viverrini* infection. *Acta Trop.* **88:**195–207.

58. **Yilmaz, H., and A. Gödekmerdan.** 2004. Human fasciolosis in Van Province, Turkey. *Acta Trop.* **92:**161–162.

Less Common Helminths

GARY W. PROCOP AND RONALD C. NEAFIE

145

This chapter covers the less common causes of helminthic parasitic infections, particularly those caused by the less common nematodes and cestodes. The trematodes are covered in entirety elsewhere. This chapter is not inclusive, given the wide variety of helminthic parasites that have been reported to cause human disease, but includes some of the most interesting and challenging of parasitic diseases. The reader who desires further information about these and other helminths of medical importance is directed to *Pathology of Infectious Diseases*, volume 1, *Helminthiasis*, by the Armed Forces Institute of Pathology (AFIP) (2). The Centers for Disease Control and Prevention's (CDC) parasitology website (http://www.dpd.cdc.gov/dpdx) is another excellent resource for information regarding parasitic infections.

COLLECTION, TRANSPORT, AND STORAGE OF SPECIMENS

The collection, transport, and storage of specimens are similar regardless of the helminth present, so these guidelines are consolidated here to reduce duplication. Worms present in the lumen of the gastrointestinal tract, such as *Anisakis*, can be retrieved by endoscopy. Surgical resection specimens may contain a worm or larvae. The intact worm and surgical specimens may be preserved and transported in 10% neutral buffered formalin. Stool is an important diagnostic specimen for parasites that reproduce within the intestinal tract, e.g., *Capillaria philippinensis*, and should be collected and fixed in a standard manner for the detection of eggs and parasites (i.e., formalin and polyvinyl alcohol), if available. Blood for serology should be handled in a standard manner. Additional information about serologic tests for the diagnosis of parasites covered in this chapter is available through the CDC at http://www.dpd.cdc.gov/dpdx/HTML/DiagnosticProcedures.htm.

LESS COMMON NEMATODES

Anisakis and Related Species

Description of the Agents
Anisakis species (for which *Anisakis simplex* is the type species), *Pseudoterranova (Phocanema) decipiens*, and *Contracaecum* species are nematodes of the family Anisakidae, superfamily Ascaridoidea, and class Secernentea.

Epidemiology, Transmission, and Prevention
The larvae of anisakids, which are present in many varieties of fish, cause human infections if raw or poorly cooked fish is consumed (13). Fish that have been salted or pickled may still contain viable anisakid larvae. Disease may be prevented by consuming only thoroughly cooked fish.

Clinical Significance
The clinical features vary depending on the stage of disease. Early, within 12 h of eating infected fish, nonspecific gastric discomfort is experienced, while the larvae are associated with only the superficial aspects of the mucosa. Superficial larvae may migrate up the esophagus and cause coughing, potentially with expectoration of the worm. More severe symptoms occur if the worm penetrates through the mucosa into the submucosal and deeper tissues (Fig. 1). This evokes hypersensitivity, leukocytosis, and eosinophilia (15, 16). Sudden, intense abdominal pain may be thought to represent appendicitis, acute gastritis, a gastric ulcer, or Crohn's disease (33). Diarrhea and constipation may occur, and the stool contains occult blood. Immunoglobulin E (IgE)-mediated hypersensitivity reactions to anisakids have been described and include acute urticaria and anaphylaxis (22).

Direct Examination by Microscopy
The intact worms are white to cream, nonsegmented larvae that measure 10 to 50 mm by 0.3 to 1.2 mm. One dorsal and two subventral reduced lips and a triangular boring tooth are useful for identification. Histopathologic analysis of infected tissues often demonstrates cross sections of the worm and the host inflammatory response, which contains numerous eosinophils. Cross-sectional studies are useful for identifying the type of anisakid present. Species-specific PCR assays or broad-range PCR assays with postamplification analysis will afford differentiation by molecular methods once the genetic variability that exists among these parasites is determined (10).

Serologic Tests
Serologic tests to detect the immunologic response to *Anisakis* and related species are available at commercial reference laboratories in the United States. Although these tests are not currently performed at the CDC, that institution may be contacted for assistance in locating a commercial

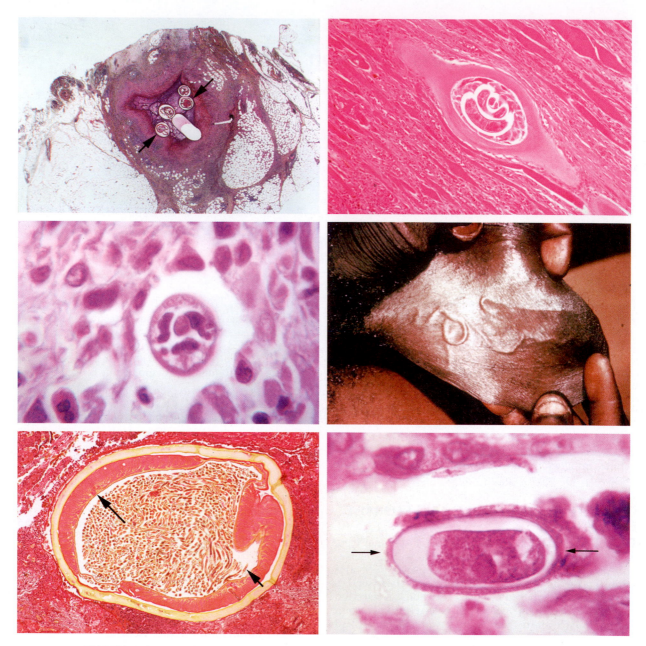

FIGURE 1 (top row, left)   This *Anisakis* species (arrows) has penetrated into the deep tissues of the abdomen. Multiple cross sections of the worm, which is 300 μm in diameter, are seen in the omentum. Movat stain; original magnification, ×2.5 (AFIP negative no. 96-5760).

FIGURE 2 (top row, right)   This coiled first-stage *T. spiralis* larva is in a "nurse cell." Note the hyaline, amorphous appearance of the external aspect of the nurse cell and the surrounding chronic inflammatory infiltrate. The worm diameter is 35 μm. Hematoxylin and eosin stain; original magnification, ×30 (AFIP negative no. 70-6004).

FIGURE 3 (middle row, left)   The minute lateral alae are useful in the identification of *Toxocara* species. The worm diameter is 18 μm. Hematoxylin and eosin stain; original magnification, ×500 (AFIP negative no. 69-4372).

FIGURE 4 (middle row, right)   The serpiginous tract of a female *D. medinensis* worm is demonstrated in the scrotum of this patient (AFIP negative no. 74-9011).

FIGURE 5 (bottom row, left)   Rhabditiform larvae (short arrow) fill the body cavity of this gravid *D. medinensis* worm. Also note the presence of the two prominent bands of somatic muscle (long arrow). The worm diameter is 1.1 mm. Movat stain; original magnification, ×25 (AFIP negative no. 92-8429).

FIGURE 6 (bottom row, right)   The bipolar plugs (arrows), pitted egg shell, and rectangular shape are characteristic of *Capillaria* species. This photomicrograph is from a human small intestine and demonstrates an egg that is 40 μm long. Hematoxylin and eosin stain; original magnification, ×490 (AFIP negative no. 69-1287).

laboratory that may perform this test, if necessary. A variety of serologic assays have been developed, but they vary in sensitivity and specificity. These identify most infected individuals (85 to 95%), with a demonstrable serologic response occurring from 10 to 35 days postinfection. Specificity suffers from cross-reactivity with other ascarids. This cross-reactivity, however, may be desirable to detect related species, e.g., *Pseudoterranova*, but may limit the utility of this assay in certain populations, such as those likely to harbor intestinal ascarids. Conversely, more-specific assays have been devised to detect *Anisakis*, but these, unfortunately, do not detect the related species that may cause "anisakiasis" in the broadest sense.

Treatment

Removal of the larva via endoscopy while it is associated only with the superficial mucosa is the most efficacious treatment. Surgical resection, however, may be needed for more deeply insinuated larvae (54). Anthelmintic drugs do not appear to be useful, but corticosteroids may be used to decrease the associated inflammation.

Trichinella Species

Description of the Agents

Trichinella spiralis is the most important cause of human disease in this genus, but other species, such as *Trichinella pseudospiralis* and *Trichinella britovi*, also cause trichinosis (23). *Trichinella* species are nematodes of the family Trichinelloidea and class Adenophorea.

Epidemiology, Transmission, and Prevention

Trichinosis occurs worldwide. The life cycle of *T. spiralis* is simple in that the infected mammal that first serves as the definitive host also harbors infective larvae encysted in its muscle (i.e., the intermediate host) (Fig. 2) (5). The domestic pig is the most important host for the transmission of this roundworm to humans, but the meat of bears, walruses, and wild pigs may also contain infective larvae. The parasitic cycle is propagated in the barnyard between pigs and rodents. Disease may be prevented by eating only thoroughly cooked meat products of potential hosts and by attempting to control trichinosis in these hosts through good animal husbandry practices.

Clinical Significance

Infections vary from mild, subclinical disease to severe illness, depending upon the parasite load. The clinical manifestations vary with the stage of infection. Gastrointestinal symptoms, associated with adult worms, last only about a week and include nausea, vomiting, abdominal pain, and diarrhea and/or constipation. Fever, facial edema that is particularly predominant around the eyes, myalgia, and marked peripheral eosinophilia are the four cardinal features of trichinosis. These are caused by the penetrating, migrating larvae. Light infections may result only in peripheral eosinophilia. The migration of larvae may cause organ-specific features. If primarily the brain and meninges are affected, neurologic symptoms predominate, whereas involvement of the myocardium causes myocarditis and possibly arrhythmias causing sudden death. Larvae do not encyst in these tissues, but rather in skeletal muscle.

Direct Examination by Microscopy

The direct microscopic examination of a muscle biopsy sample, performed by simply compressing the fresh muscle fibers between glass slides and observing them microscopically, may disclose larvae. More commonly, larvae are detected by histopathologic analysis of formalin-fixed, paraffin-embedded tissue sections (Fig. 2).

Nucleic Acid Detection Techniques

A species-specific rapid-cycle PCR assay for *Trichinella spiralis* has been developed, but how this or similar assays will be used to screen potentially infected animals that will be processed for foodstuff or to diagnose human trichinosis has yet to be determined (3).

Serology

The antibody response begins 3 to 5 weeks after infection in most patients (80 to 100%) and follows the acute phase of disease. Therefore, the conversion from a negative serologic test during acute illness to a positive test is evidence of disease. The tests are highly sensitive, and although they are less than 100% specific, cross-reactivity usually results in test values in the equivocal range. These tests are available at the CDC and from several commercial laboratories.

Treatment

Therapy varies according to the stage of disease. Thiabendazole is active against the intestinal worm but not against the larvae. There is no proven method to kill the encysted larvae, but albendazole or another similar agent is used for therapy. Well-controlled therapeutic studies, however, are lacking. Corticosteroids, salicylates, and antihistamines may lessen symptoms associated with inflammation.

Toxocara Species

Description of the Agents

Toxocara canis is the intestinal ascarid of dogs and other canids, whereas *Toxocara cati* is the intestinal ascarid of cats. Although larvae of both species can cause toxocariasis in humans, most infections are caused by *T. canis* (23). *Toxocara* species are in the family Ascarididae and the class Secernentea, within the phylum Nemathelminthes.

Epidemiology, Transmission, and Prevention

Toxocariasis has a worldwide distribution, but the prevalence of zoonotic disease varies widely by geographic area. The seroprevalence of human disease reflects helminthic control in dogs and cats. The highest infection rates occur among the poor, often in rural settings (21). The natural cycle of *Toxocara* begins with the passage of unembryonated eggs in the feces of the definitive host. The adult female worm may release up to 85,000 eggs per day. Therefore, one stool passage into an environment such as a sandbox can cause significant contamination. Between 10 and 20 days are required for the L2 (i.e., second-stage) larvae to develop in the eggs; the eggs at this stage are infective. If the eggs are ingested by a suitable definitive host, then the larvae penetrate the intestinal tract and migrate through the liver, bloodstream, and lungs. The larvae then migrate up the respiratory tract until they are swallowed, after which they mature into adult worms in the intestinal tract. When the eggs are ingested by a nonpermissive host, such as a child, the resulting *Toxocara* larvae cannot complete their life cycle, but rather wander aimlessly in the aberrant host, causing visceral larva migrans. Another means of contracting disease is by ingesting raw or undercooked meat from a paratenic host (i.e., another aberrant host, such as a pig, that contains wandering larvae). Prevention is achieved foremost through zoonotic control by deworming dogs and cats, most importantly puppies, which are particularly permissive for infection and are often associated with children. Other preventive measures include avoidance of animal feces, thorough washing of fruits and vegetables, and thorough cooking of meats from potentially paratenic hosts (48).

Clinical Significance

Toxocara infections are among the most common helminthic infections of humans. Fortunately, most infections are subclinical, producing only mild disease for which a definitive diagnosis is not sought. The most severe forms of disease occur with involvement of the eyes or significant involvement of the heart, brain, or other vital organs (4, 17, 37, 47). Pregnant women with toxocariasis may have miscarriages.

Direct Examination by Microscopy

Eggs are not produced in the human, so a stool evaluation is not helpful. However, occasionally the eggs of another geohelminth, such as *Ascaris*, hookworm, or *Trichuris*, may be present because of common risk factors. The detection of the migrating larvae in surgically excised tissues by histopathologic evaluation provides the definitive morphological diagnosis. The single minute lateral ala and the cross-sectional diameter are useful criteria for identifying these parasites in histologic sections (Fig. 3) (38).

Serologic Tests

Serologic studies are important for the establishment of the diagnosis of toxocariasis; results of these should be used in conjunction with clinical findings as well as other laboratory findings, such as increased IgE and eosinophilia. Positive results in the absence of other corroborative findings could represent a previous, asymptomatic infection. The sensitivity and specificity of these assays are high, but less than 100%. It is difficult to determine the precise parameters of serologic assays, since there is not a better parasitological test (i.e., a gold standard) to confirm the presence of a true infection. These tests have also been used successfully in seroepidemiologic studies. Tests are available at the CDC and from commercial reference laboratories.

Treatment

There is no proven therapy. Anthelmintic therapy with albendazole or a similar therapeutic is often used. Corticosteroids may be necessary to control the inflammatory response in patients with a large parasite burden. Eye infections require a combined medical and surgical approach (24).

Dracunculus medinensis

Description of the Agent

D. medinensis, also known as the guinea worm, is not a filarial worm, but rather a member of the family Dracunculidae, which is in the class Secernentea of the phylum Nemathelminthes (26). Other *Dracunculus* species exist that infect a variety of other animals.

Epidemiology, Transmission, and Prevention

Dracunculiasis is found only in the rural parts of Africa. Disease occurs more commonly in the dry season and affects men more commonly than women. It is most common in individuals from 10 to 60 years old, which taxes the productivity of affected communities. An intensive effort by the World Health Organization, local governments, and numerous other humanitarian organizations has significantly decreased the annual incidence of disease (1, 8, 51). At the beginning of this program (1986), an estimated 3.5 million people in 20 countries were affected. The annual incidence of worldwide disease was diminished by an astounding 98% by December 2001, and seven countries completely eradicated the disease. Substantial progress continues to be made to eradicate this disease. There were 25,217 cases reported in 2006, whereas there were only 4,619 cases in 2008 (53). There were only 925 cases reported from January to May 2009 (53). The eradication of this devastating disease may be near at hand, but continued vigilance is necessary.

Infection follows drinking contaminated freshwater that contains copepods, which harbor the infective larvae. After ingestion, the larvae migrate to the retroperitoneum, where they mature and mate. The female worm eventually migrates to a subcutaneous location, where a blister forms, which bursts upon contact with water and releases numerous larvae. The larvae are ingested by a copepod, wherein they become infective. Preventive measures are centered on education and providing clean drinking water (28, 29).

Clinical Significance

Patients are asymptomatic during larval penetration of the gastrointestinal tract and retroperitoneal maturation and mating of the worms. Symptoms are secondary to inflammation and tissue damage caused by worm migration. Although lesions are most common in the lower extremities, they may occur anywhere in the body. A serpiginous tract is produced, which is caused by the migrating worm under the skin (Fig. 4). The large blister that is formed may become secondarily infected. Dead worms may be absorbed, calcify, or produce symptoms secondary to location (e.g., a joint).

Direct Examination and Microscopy

The presence of the end of a worm protruding from a burst blister or ulcer in the appropriate setting is diagnostic. The microscopic analysis of these worms in cross section demonstrates a 30- to 50-μm-thick cuticle, indistinct lateral cords, prominent dorsal and ventral bands of smooth muscle, and a large uterus filled with rhabditoid larvae that fills the body cavity (Fig. 5).

Serologic Tests

Serologic tests are usually not necessary for the diagnosis, given the obvious findings in people at risk for disease. They are useful, however, for seroprevalence studies and to identify infected individuals prior to the partial emergence of the adult worm.

Treatment

The oldest and traditional treatment, as depicted in an ancient Egyptian medical text, the *Papyrus Ebers*, consists of removing the gravid worm by wrapping the exposed end of the worm around a stick and applying gentle pressure for days. Treatment with thiabendazole and metronidazole, although not lethal for the worm, facilitates removal by this process (11). Although it is often effective, risks include rupture or breaking of the worm prior to full removal. Currently, surgical excision is preferred. Anti-inflammatory agents and antihistamines are important for symptomatic relief. Antibiotics may be necessary to curtail secondary bacterial infections, and tetanus vaccination is important.

Capillaria philippinensis

Description of the Agent

C. *philippinensis* is a trichurid nematode responsible for intestinal capillariasis (14, 34). *Capillaria* species are in the family Trichuridae of the class Adenophorea.

Epidemiology, Transmission, and Prevention

The natural parasitic cycle of C. *philippinensis* likely involves marine, fish-eating birds as the definitive hosts and fish as the intermediate hosts. Humans become infected by ingesting raw or undercooked fish that harbor the infective larvae. Larvae at various stages of maturation may be found in the lumen of the intestine of the definitive host or the patient. Therefore, the population of parasites within the lumen of the bowel may increase (hyperinfection) without the consumption of additional contaminated fish. Thorough cooking of fish is protective.

Clinical Significance

Infections with C. *philippinensis* are relatively rare; 82 patients with intestinal capillariasis were reported in Thailand from 1994 to 2006 (45). Rarely, because intraintestinal hyperinfection is possible, infections may be fatal. Nonspecific gastrointestinal complaints predominate early in the course of disease; these include watery diarrhea, weight loss, abdominal pain, edema, and weakness (45). As the disease progresses and the number of worms increases, there is continued diarrhea with malabsorption, leading to cachexia (20). Endoscopy may be useful for establishing the diagnosis (52). Death occurs secondarily to malnutrition or because of secondary bacterial infections (e.g., septicemia).

Direct Examination by Microscopy

Microscopic examination of the stool may demonstrate a mixture of eggs and larvae. The eggs of C. *philippinensis* (Fig. 6), which have bipolar plugs, are superficially reminiscent of the more commonly recognized trichurid worm, *Trichuris trichiura*. The plugs of C. *philippinensis*, however, are nonprotruding, the egg is more rectangular, and there is a distinctive pitting of the egg shell (7). The adults superficially resemble *Strongyloides stercoralis* but may be differentiated by the presence of stichocytes and three bacillary bands, with the latter being recognized most easily in cross section.

Serologic Tests

Serologic tests are not available from the CDC or from commercial reference laboratories. Experimental serologic tests have been developed which, like the coproantigen, hold promise as future diagnostic tools (19).

Treatment

Mebendazole is the drug of choice, but albendazole and thiabendazole may also be used. Relapsing disease requires prolonged anthelmintic therapy. Aggressive electrolyte replacement and monitoring are critical, as are control of diarrhea and administration of nutrients.

Gnathostoma Species

Description of the Agents

Gnathostoma species are gastric spirurid nematode parasites for which the definitive hosts are a variety of mammals (32). Infective L3 (i.e., third-stage) larvae cause disease in humans, and gnathostomiasis may be considered a subtype of visceral larva migrans. *Gnathostoma spinigerum* is the most common cause of human disease, but *Gnathostoma hispidum*, *Gnathostoma nipponicum*, and *Gnathostoma doloresi* may also cause human disease. *Gnathostoma* species belong in their own family, Gnathostomatidae, of the class Secernentea.

Epidemiology, Transmission, and Prevention

G. *spinigerum* has essentially a worldwide distribution. Dogs and cats are the primary definitive hosts for this gnathostome, whereas G. *hispidum* and G. *doloresi* infect wild and domestic pigs and G. *nipponicum* is a parasite of weasels.

The adult male and female gnathostomes live in the stomach of the definitive host, where they mate and produce eggs. The eggs are passed in the stool, and once in water, they hatch and release first-stage larvae. The larvae then infect and mature within the copepod *Cyclops*. When a variety of paratenic hosts, such as fish, snakes, eels, or frogs, eat the copepod, the larvae penetrate the gastric wall of the new host, wherein they migrate to the musculature and encyst. If an appropriate definitive host eats the paratenic host, the advanced L3 larvae excyst and penetrate the gastric wall. The L3 larvae then migrate through the liver, muscles, and connective tissues, only to return to the stomach and mature into adults. Humans are accidental hosts in which the nematode larvae cannot mature to adulthood and continue to migrate aimlessly and aggressively (43). The parasite is transmitted to humans through the ingestion of raw or undercooked meat from a secondary intermediate host. Disease can be prevented by thoroughly cooking potentially infected foods.

Clinical Significance

The clinical presentations of gnathostomiasis are protean, since the wandering larvae may be present in any tissue or organ system (25, 42, 44). Although the infection is not commonly fatal, significant morbidity may be associated with infection. The clinical manifestations depend on the tissues in which the larva is migrating. Panniculitis, creeping eruptions, and pseudofurunculosis are dermatologic manifestations of gnathostomiasis (43). Any visceral organ may be affected, and although *Gnathostoma* is not neurotropic, the central nervous system may be involved (43).

Direct Examination and Microscopy

Mature (adult) gnathostomes are not present in humans, but L3 larvae are. This form is morphologically similar to the adult form but is smaller, measuring 3 to 4 mm in length by 630 μm in diameter (G. *spinigerum*). The head bulb contains four rows of cephalic hooklets, with approximately 45 hooklets per row. The body of the larva, like that of the adult, is covered with transverse rows of sharply pointed spines that diminish toward the posterior end of the worm. An entire worm may be expelled spontaneously or may require surgical excision.

Serologic Tests

Serologic assays have been developed predominantly in areas of endemicity. These are not available in the United States, but the CDC can assist in identifying a source for testing, if necessary. The possibility of cross-reactivity should be considered with these tests, as well as several other serologic assays for helminthic parasites, and they should be used only in the appropriate clinical context.

Treatment

Surgical removal of the parasite is the most effective treatment but is difficult to achieve due to parasite migration; this may be aided by advanced imaging tools (6). Treatment usually involves some type of anthelmintic medication, such as albendazole or ivermectin. There remains controversy regarding the treatment of central nervous system gnathostomiasis, wherein there is a concern that anthelmintic therapy will kill the invading worms and increase the inflammatory reaction; treatment is supportive and may involve corticosteroid use to control the inflammatory response (43).

Parastrongylus (Angiostrongylus) cantonensis

Description of the Agent
P. cantonensis is a filariform worm and is the most important cause of angiostrongyliasis (41). Parastrongylus belongs to the family Angiostrongylidae and the class Secernentea.

Epidemiology, Transmission, and Prevention
A. cantonensis is widely distributed throughout the world but represents an important public health threat in Southeast Asia and the Asian Pacific Islands. This parasite persists in a wide variety of rodents, which serve as the definitive host, wherein the adult worms reside in the pulmonary artery and the right side of the heart. Eggs released from the adult worms lodge in pulmonary capillaries, where they hatch and release larvae. The larvae subsequently migrate up the trachea and are swallowed and passed in the feces. These larvae infect mollusks, the intermediate host, wherein they mature into the infective L3 larvae. A number of animals, including shrimp, crabs, fish, and frogs, may eat the infected mollusks and serve as important paratenic hosts. Rodents that ingest either the infected mollusk or tissues from the paratenic host thereby become infected. In the definitive host, the infective larvae penetrate the intestine, become blood borne, and migrate to the central nervous system, where they molt twice. Thereafter, the worms reenter the systemic circulation and finally reside in the right ventricle and pulmonary artery to mature and complete the cycle. Humans become infected through the ingestion of tissue from either an infected mollusk or an infected paratenic host. Prevention of disease can be achieved through control of the local rat population and thorough cooking of mollusks and potentially paratenic hosts.

Clinical Significance
The clinical manifestations reflect the worm burden and the site of worm residence, the central nervous system. The worms tend to remain associated with the brain and meninges in human infections (Fig. 7). Patients demonstrate signs and symptoms typical of meningitis or meningoencephalitis, with headache, fever, possibly eosinophilia (10 to 60%), and any of a number of neurologic disturbances, depending on the location of the worms. The cerebrospinal fluid (CSF) demonstrates pleocytosis, eosinophilia (26 to 75%), and elevated protein and occasionally will contain immature worms. Alternatively, patients may have infections of the eye, with retinal detachment and blindness. Less commonly, human infections may result in pulmonary disease.

Direct Examination and Microscopy
Demonstration of the worms in histologic sections or intact in clinical specimens from the CSF or eye definitively establishes the diagnosis. Eosinophilia in the CSF may be the first indicator of a possible parasitic infection of the central nervous system. The differential diagnosis of the causes of CSF eosinophilia, however, is broad and includes other parasitic infections, e.g., with Gnathostoma or Toxocara spp., allergic reactions, and coccidioidomycosis. The gross appearance of an adult female worm is distinctive, with the spiral winding of the uteri and ovarian branches imparting a "barber pole" appearance. Cross section of the female demonstrates a large intestine and two uteri, whereas cross section of the male reveals a large intestine and a single reproductive tube. Eggs are not produced in human tissues.

Serologic Tests
Serologic assays are powerful tools for the diagnosis of angiostrongyliasis, particularly since the parasite is usually located in a difficult-to-access location, the central nervous system. The evolution of these assays has resulted in a highly sensitive and specific assay, particularly when purified, non-cross-reacting antigens are used. Although intrathecal antibody is not always produced, the presence of intrathecal antibody synthesis provides strong evidence of infection. This assay is available from some commercial laboratories in the United States.

Treatment
The optimal treatment has not been established. Fortunately, the disease is often self-limited. Removal of CSF

FIGURE 7 (row 1, left) The immature A. cantonensis worm (arrows) in the meninges of this patient is eliciting a marked eosinophilic response. The worm is 200 μm in diameter. Hematoxylin and eosin stain; original magnification, ×50 (AFIP negative no. 73-6862).

FIGURE 8 (row 1, right) The coiled remnants of an immature male D. immitis worm are present in this branch of the pulmonary artery. The maximum worm diameter is 250 μm. Movat stain; original magnification, ×15 (AFIP negative no. 71-11563).

FIGURE 9 (row 2, left) The two uteri (arrows), muscle, and trilaminar (arrowhead), smooth cuticle are characteristic of an immature female D. immitis worm. The worm diameter is 250 μm. Movat stain; original magnification, ×80 (AFIP negative no. 72-2732).

FIGURE 10 (row 2, right) The Dirofilaria species other than D. immitis have external longitudinal cuticular ridges, whereas the cuticle of D. immitis is smooth. Dirofilaria tenuis is pictured here, in cross section; it is 270 μm in diameter and has obvious cuticular ridges (arrows). Dirofilaria species other than D. immitis are often found in a subcutaneous location rather than in the pulmonary arterial vasculature. Movat stain; original magnification, ×80 (AFIP negative no. 94-5122).

FIGURE 11 (row 3, left) An egg packet of D. caninum, obtained from a crushed gravid proglottid, is 150 μm in diameter. The eggs within the packet are 40 μm in diameter. Unstained (AFIP negative no. 86-7369).

FIGURE 12 (row 3, right) The thick inner membrane of the egg of Hymenolepis diminuta is surrounded by a gelatinous matrix and then by an outer striated shell. The eggs of H. diminuta are spherical, whereas those of Hymenolepis nana are ovoid. The egg pictured here is 80 μm in diameter. Unstained; original magnification, ×250 (AFIP negative no. 96-5119). See chapter 143 for more detailed coverage of Hymenolepis spp.

FIGURE 13 (row 4, left) A sparganum superficially resembles an adult tapeworm. Close inspection, however, clarifies its immature form, with a head with only a ventral groove or bothrium (arrow) and a lack of proglottids. The maximum width is 6 mm. Unstained; original magnification, ×0.5 (AFIP negative no. 70-15303)

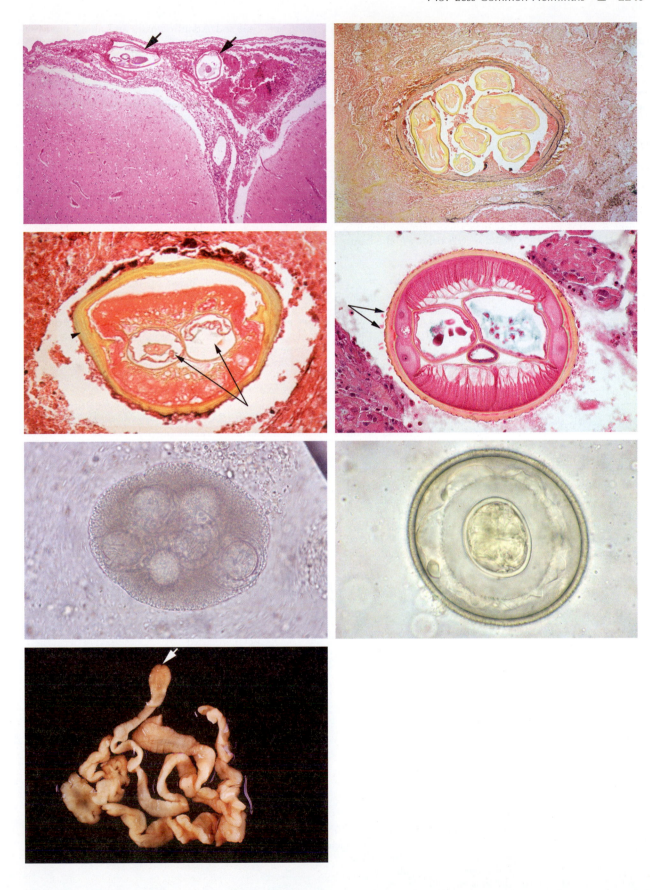

and the administration of corticosteroids and nonsteroidal anti-inflammatory agents have been used to control pain and inflammation. A variety of anthelmintic medications have been used, with mebendazole being the current drug of choice. Careful monitoring of the patient is important, since anthelmintic therapy may sometimes exacerbate the symptoms (27). Corticosteroids may be used alone or in combination with anthelmintic therapy (43).

Dirofilaria immitis and Other Dirofilaria Species

Description of the Agents
D. immitis, the filarial dog heartworm, causes human pulmonary dirofilariasis (12, 50). Dirofilaria tenuis is a raccoon parasite restricted to the New World, whereas Dirofilaria repens is a dog parasite that may cause human disease in the Old World (40). Dirofilaria species belong to the family Onchocercidae in the class Secernentea.

Epidemiology, Transmission, and Prevention
Although dogs are the most important host for D. immitis, other mammals, such as fox and bear, are also suitable hosts. The blood of infected dogs or other suitable hosts contains microfilariae that are released from the adult worm, which resides in the right ventricle of the heart. These are taken into the mosquito during a blood meal, wherein they mature into infective L3 larvae and are capable of being transferred to another mammal during a blood meal. The larvae migrate through subcutaneous tissues and eventually enter the bloodstream and the right side of the heart, wherein they mature into adults in a permissive host. Humans, however, are unsuitable or nonpermissive hosts. In humans, the worm dies before it reaches maturity and is swept into the pulmonary arterial circulation. It subsequently becomes lodged in the subsegmental pulmonary arteries and arterioles and causes thrombosis, infarction, inflammation, and eventually a granulomatous reaction surrounded by a wall of fibrous tissue (Fig. 8).

The geographic distribution of disease reflects the prevalence of canine dirofilariasis. The areas of highest prevalence in the United States are in the South, particularly along the Gulf and Atlantic coasts and along the Mississippi River (46). Interestingly, dog ownership is not a risk factor for disease. Prevention is centered on the control of zoonotic disease. The use of mosquito repellents, particularly in areas of high endemicity, is also recommended to interrupt transmission.

Clinical Significance
Slightly more than half of the patients with dirofilariasis are asymptomatic. The remainder have nonspecific symptoms, such as cough, chest pain, hemoptysis, low-grade fever, chills, and malaise (12). Only 5 to 10% have peripheral blood eosinophilia. In addition to pulmonary manifestations, D. immitis has also rarely been identified in subcutaneous abscesses, the abdominal cavity, the eyes, and the testes. Dirofilaria species other than D. immitis are more likely to be found in a subcutaneous location (Table 1). Recently, Pampiglione et al. undertook a critical review of human pulmonary dirofilariasis in the Old World and suggested, based on traditional morphologic findings, that the cause of pulmonary dirofilariasis in these geographic regions may more likely be due to a Dirofilaria species other than D. immitis, namely D. repens (40). The nodules caused by D. immitis are often discovered by a routine chest radiograph (46). These are usually single, but occasionally two or three nodules may be present.

Direct Examination and Microscopy
The pulmonary nodules produced by D. immitis are characteristically small (0.8 to 4.5 cm; mean, 1.9 cm), subpleural, spherical, and well circumscribed. D. immitis has a smooth, thick cuticle (5 to 25 μm) with the three distinct layers characteristic of the genus Dirofilaria; other Dirofilaria species that infect humans have a similar cuticle, but with external longitudinal ridges (Fig. 9 and 10). The thick, multilayered cuticle projects inwardly at the lateral chords, forming two prominent, opposing internal longitudinal ridges. The somatic musculature is typically prominent, but the lateral chords are usually poorly preserved. Transverse sections may reveal two large uteri and a much smaller

TABLE 1 Other less common nematodes

Organism	Definitive host	Intermediate host(s)/vectors	Disease(s) produced	Method of diagnosis
Ancylostoma species other than Ancylostoma duodenale, A. ceylanicum, A. caninum, and A. braziliense	Cats, dogs, and hamsters	Not applicable	Ancylostomiasis, eosinophilic enteritis, cutaneous larva migrans (creeping eruption)	Detection of eggs in stool or adults in histologic sections; rarely, detection of larvae in biopsy sample of skin
Angiostrongylus costaricensis	Rodents, less commonly dogs and monkeys	Mollusks	Infection of the intestinal walls and mesenteric arteries	Identification of parasite in surgically excised tissues; eggs not present in stool; serologic studies are useful
Dirofilaria species other than D. immitis, D. tenuis, D. repens, D. ursi, D. subdermata, and D. striata	Raccoons (D. tenuis), dogs and cats (D. repens), bears (D. ursi), porcupines (D. subdermata), wild cats (D. striata)	Mosquitoes, except for D. ursi, which is transmitted by blackflies	Usually subcutaneous nodules that contain mature, immature, or degenerated worms	Morphological features of the worm in excised tissues (Fig. 10)

intestine in female worms (Fig. 9); a single reproductive tube and an intestine are present in males. The definitive identification of the worm based on internal structures may be difficult or impossible, given the advanced stage of parasite degeneration in many of these specimens. The presence of a parasitic worm in a pulmonary artery and in association with a pulmonary infarct, however, is sufficient for a diagnosis.

Serologic Tests

Serologic tests to detect antibody to *Dirofilaria* are commercially available from several reference laboratories. Although advances have been made to increase specificity without sacrificing sensitivity, cross-reactivity may occur in patients infected with other nematodes, particularly other filarial worms. As with many serologic assays, a positive test is useful, whereas a negative test does not exclude the possibility of infection.

Treatment

Excision of the nodule is curative. Additional antiparasitic therapy is not necessary.

Other Less Common Nematodes

There are a number of less common nematodes other than those described here. Some of these and their important associated features are included in Table 1.

LESS COMMON CESTODES (TABLE 2)

Dipylidium caninum

Description of the Agent

D. caninum, a common tapeworm of dogs and cats, also commonly infects children (9, 49). *Dipylidium* belongs to the family Dipylidiidae, the order Cyclophyllidea, and the class Cestoidea (Cestoda).

Epidemiology, Transmission, and Prevention

Dipylidiasis occurs throughout the world (18, 31). This disease, like hymenolepiasis, is transmitted primarily through the ingestion of an infected flea. In the natural cycle, the dog or cat contains the intestinal adult parasite, which releases gravid proglottids filled with eggs. The eggs are ingested by fleas or lice, which are the intermediate hosts. The eggs hatch within the intermediate host, releasing larvae that penetrate the body cavity, where they mature into infective cysticercoid larvae. When an infected intermediate host is ingested, the cysticercoid metacestode larva attaches to the small intestine and matures into an adult tapeworm, completing the cycle. Prevention is achieved by deworming animals and controlling fleas and lice.

Clinical Significance

Dipylidiasis is usually an innocuous infection. Larger worm burdens may cause weight loss, abdominal pain, failure to thrive, or the appearance of colic. Disease usually comes to the attention of parents and pediatricians when motile, gravid proglottids are seen in the stool.

Direct Examination by Microscopy

The proglottids of *D. caninum* differ from those of most other cestodes in that they have two genital pores (*dipylos* means two gates), which can be appreciated with the use of a dissecting microscope and by compressing the proglottid between two glass slides. The identification may

also be achieved by demonstrating the characteristic egg packets (Fig. 11) and/or characteristic eggs that have distinct morphological features (i.e., four envelopes). A fecal examination will likely be negative for eggs or egg packets, since intact proglottids are usually passed in the stool. Microdissection or histologic examination of the proglottids will reveal the eggs and egg packets. In addition to the egg packets, the histologic examination of the proglottid will reveal other features common to cestodes, such as a tegument, smooth muscle, and calcareous corpuscles.

Serologic Tests

Because the disease is usually subclinical and the diagnosis is achieved when the proglottids are discovered and examined, serologic tests are not necessary.

Treatment

Both praziquantel and niclosamide are effective against *D. caninum*. Upon discovery, examination and treatment of household pets should proceed, as should aggressive flea control.

Spirometra Species

Description of the Agents

Sparganosis is the infection of humans by L3 plerocercoid larvae of a pseudophyllidean tapeworm (36). The plerocercoid larva in a human host does not reach maturity and is known as a sparganum. The tapeworms that cause sparganosis are *Spirometra mansoni*, *Spirometra mansonoides*, *Spirometra ranarum*, and *Spirometra erinacei*. The precise taxonomic relationship of a cestode known as *Sparganum proliferum* is unclear, but this organism may simply represent a variant of *S. mansonoides* or *S. erinacei*. *Spirometra* species belong to the family Diphyllobothriidae, the order Pseudophyllidea, and the class Cestoidea (Cestoda).

Epidemiology, Transmission, and Prevention

Adult *Spirometra* species are widely distributed tapeworms of animals, particularly dogs and cats. The parasitic cycle for these worms begins with the passage of eggs from an infected suitable host. The coracidium that emerges from the egg infects the first intermediate host, a copepod. The second intermediate host, which includes snakes, frogs, and fish, becomes infected by ingesting the infected copepod. The cycle is completed when a permissive (i.e., definitive) host ingests the second intermediate host. Humans are nonpermissive hosts and may become infected by ingesting raw or undercooked meat from a second intermediate host or by drinking contaminated water that contains the infected copepod *Cyclops*. Humans have also become infected by using infected animal flesh (e.g., frog flesh) as a poultice.

Clinical Significance

The results of ingesting a plerocercoid larva depend on both the species of the host and the species of the larva. For example, the ingestion of a plerocercoid larva of *Diphyllobothrium latum* by a human will result in the development of an adult tapeworm, whereas the ingestion of a plerocercoid larva of a *Spirometra* species will result only in the continued existence of the larva (i.e., the sparganum), in the new host. This is a situation where the human is behaving biologically like a second intermediate or paratenic host. The clinical features of disease are influenced by worm burden (most patients harbor only a single worm), worm location, and worm viability. Spargana migrate, but this migration usually does not cause symptoms. Migration to a subcutaneous location, however,

TABLE 2 Other less common cestodes[a]

Organism	Definitive host(s)	Intermediate host(s)	Disease produced	Diagnostic method
Hymenolepis diminuta, the rat tapeworm	Rats	Insects	Usually asymptomatic; heavy infections resemble heavy *H. nana* infections.	Eggs in the feces (Fig. 12); proglottids disintegrate before fecal passage.
Hymenolepis nana, the dwarf tapeworm[b]	Rats; human-to-human transmission possible	Fleas	This worm, the smallest adult tapeworm that infects humans, produces disease that is usually mild, and patients may be asymptomatic. Massive infections may produce abdominal pain, allergic reactions, anorexia, nausea, diarrhea or constipation, and flatulence.	Identification of characteristic eggs in the stool; proglottids disintegrate and release eggs before they are passed in the stool. The eggs are ovoid, in contrast to those of *H. diminuta,* which are spherical, and have an inner hyaline membrane, a thin egg shell, polar thickenings from which polar filaments arise, and a distinct oncosphere that contains six hooklets.
Less common *Taenia* species				
T. taeniaeformis	Cats	Rodents	Larval stage may infect liver, like cysticercosis.	Demonstration of strobilocercus in histologic sections.
T. multiceps	Canids	Sheep, rabbits	Coenurosis, an infection with the coenurus in the central nervous system, eyes, or subcutaneous tissues (like cysticercosis).	Demonstration of the coenurus in histologic sections.
Mesocestoides species	Foxes, dogs, cats, and other mammals	Unknown, possibly reptile or arthropod vectors	Asymptomatic or mild abdominal symptoms.	Detection of gravid proglottid with characteristic parauterine organ. Eggs are usually not present in the stool.
Bertia species	Primates	Mites and possibly other insects	Asymptomatic or mild abdominal symptoms.	Motile proglottids in the stool, similar to *D. caninum* infection. Eggs within proglottids are not within packets.
Inermicapsifer madagascariensis		Raw sugar cane ingestion has been suggested	Asymptomatic to symptoms similar to *D. caninum* infections.	Motile proglottids in the stool, similar to *D. caninum* infection. Proglottid and egg morphology and number of eggs per packet are used for identification.
Raillietina species	Rodents	Insects	Asymptomatic or symptoms similar to *D. caninum* infections.	Motile proglottids in the stool, similar to *D. caninum* infection. Proglottid and egg morphology and number of eggs per packet are used for identification.

[a]Praziquantel is the treatment of choice for infections with adult tapeworms; it is also effective for treatment of coenurosis. Effective preventive measures center around controlling disease in the zoonotic host (e.g., cats or dogs) or controlling the zoonotic hosts themselves (e.g., rats). Controlling intermediate hosts is also effective but may prove more difficult.
[b]This parasite is covered in detail in chapter 143 in this *Manual.*

may result in a nodule. This nodule may be excised to exclude the possibility of malignancy. Ocular sparganosis, particularly involving the conjunctiva, may result following the application of a natural poultice that contains raw snake or frog tissues. Inflammation and sometimes calcification ensue following death of the sparganum, and when these occur in the brain, they may cause obstructive hydrocephalus (35).

Direct Examination and Microscopy

The spargana of *Spirometra* species are flat, ribbon-like worms that superficially resemble adult tapeworms (Fig 13). Closer inspection demonstrates an immature anterior end without hooklets; a cleft or ventral groove, termed a bothrium, is present (Fig. 13) (39). Mature proglottids are not produced. Histopathologic examination of the sparganum demonstrates calcareous corpuscles characteristic of a cestode. Developed internal organs are not seen, but rather, irregularly scattered smooth muscle fibers and excretory ducts are seen in a loose stroma.

Serologic Tests

If the diagnosis is not suspected, it is usually made when a viable sparganum is unexpectedly discovered during surgery. The gross findings are largely diagnostic, but histopathologic examination can be used for confirmation. In such instances, serology is not useful. However, if this disease is clinically suspected, the diagnosis may be achieved through the combination of radiology and serology (30). Serologic tests for *Spirometra* are not commercially available, so one may have to send sera to specialized centers.

Treatment

Medical therapy is currently deemed unsuitable for the treatment of sparganosis; the plerocercoid larva is resistant to praziquantel. Complete surgical excision is recommended. An incomplete excision, particularly if the anterior end of the larva remains in the tissue, may result in continued growth of the organism (2).

SUMMARY

There are a wide variety of less commonly encountered helminthic parasites, which may be nematodes, cestodes, or trematodes. The diseases caused by these parasites are interesting and demonstrate their highly evolved life cycles and the complex interactions with their hosts. These diseases range from subclinical, e.g., dipylidiasis, to possibly life-threatening, e.g., baylisascariasis. In many instances, the disease occurs only in a particular geographic area, which is largely determined by the biological ranges of the definitive and intermediate hosts. Dietary customs are also important in the prevalence of human disease, as many of these are associated with the ingestion of raw animal products. The treatment of these parasites varies depending on the infectious agent, but common preventive measures may significantly diminish the transmission of many of these parasitic diseases. These measures include the zoonotic control of parasitic disease in animal hosts and the vectors of transmission, washing of fruits and vegetables, access to clean drinking water, and thorough cooking of meats before consumption.

REFERENCES

1. **Anosike, J. C., B. E. Nwoke, I. Dozie, U. A. Thofern, A. N. Okere, R. Njoku-Tony, D. C. Nwosu, U. T. Oguwuike, M. C. Dike, J. I. Alozie, G. R. Okugun, C. M. Ajero, C. U. Onyirioha, M. N. Ezike, F. I. Ogbusu, and E. G. Ajayi.** 2003. Control of endemic dracunculiasis in Ebonyi state, southeastern Nigeria. *Int. J. Hyg. Environ. Health* **206:**591–596.
2. **Armed Forces Institute of Pathology.** 2000. *Pathology of Infectious Diseases*, vol. 1. Armed Forces Institute of Pathology, Washington, DC.
3. **Atterby, C., J. Learmount, C. Conyers, I. Zimmer, N. Boonham, and M. Taylor.** 2009. Development of a real-time PCR assay for the detection of *Trichinella spiralis* in situ. *Vet. Parasitol.* **161:**92–98.
4. **Bachli, H., J. C. Minet, and O. Gratzl.** 2004. Cerebral toxocariasis: a possible cause of epileptic seizure in children. *Child's Nerv. Syst.* **20:**468–472.
5. **Beeson, P.** 1941. Factors influencing the prevalence of trichinosis in man. *Proc. R. Soc. Med.* **34:**585–594.
6. **Bhende, M., J. Biswas, and L. Gopal.** 2005. Ultrasound biomicroscopy in the diagnosis and management of intraocular gnathostomiasis. *Am. J. Ophthalmol.* **140:**140–142.
7. **Canlas, B., B. Cabrera, and U. Davis.** 1967. Human intestinal capillariasis. 2. Pathological features. *Acta Med. Philipp.* **4:**84–91.
8. **Centers for Disease Control and Prevention.** 2002. Progress toward global dracunculiasis eradication, June 2002. *Morb. Mortal. Wkly. Rep.* **51:**810–811.
9. **Chappell, C., J. P. Enos, and H. M. Penn.** 1990. *Dipylidium caninum*, an under-recognized infection in infants and children. *Pediatr. Infect. Dis. J.* **9:**745–747.
10. **Chen, Q., H.Q. Yu, Z. R. Lun, X. G. Chen, H. Q. Song, R. Q. Lin, and X. Q. Zhu.** 2008. Specific PCR assays for the identification of common anisakid nematodes with zoonotic potential. *Parasitol. Res.* **104:**79–84.
11. **Chippaux, J. P.** 1991. Mebendazole treatment of dracunculiasis. *Trans. R. Soc. Trop. Med. Hyg.* **85:**280.
12. **Chitkara, R. K., and P. S. Sarinas.** 1997. Dirofilaria, visceral larva migrans, and tropical pulmonary eosinophilia. *Semin. Respir. Infect.* **12:**138–148.
13. **Chitwood, M.** 1970. Nematodes of medical significance found in market fish. *Am. J. Trop. Med. Hyg.* **19:**599–602.
14. **Cross, J. H.** 1992. Intestinal capillariasis. *Clin. Microbiol. Rev.* **5:**120–129.
15. **Daschner, A., and C. Y. Pascual.** 2005. *Anisakis simplex*: sensitization and clinical allergy. *Curr. Opin. Allergy Clin. Immunol.* **5:**281–285.
16. **Dominguez-Ortega, J., A. Alonso-Llamazares, L. Rodriguez, M. Chamorro, T. Robledo, J. M. Bartolome, and C. Martinez-Cocera.** 2001. Anaphylaxis due to hypersensitivity to *Anisakis simplex*. *Int. Arch. Allergy Immunol.* **125:**86–88.
17. **Eberhardt, O., R. Bialek, T. Nagele, and J. Dichgans.** 2005. Eosinophilic meningomyelitis in toxocariasis: case report and review of the literature. *Clin. Neurol. Neurosurg.* **107:**432–438.
18. **Eguia-Aguilar, P., A. Cruz-Reyes, and J. J. Martinez-Maya.** 2005. Ecological analysis and description of the intestinal helminths present in dogs in Mexico City. *Vet. Parasitol.* **127:**139–146.
19. **El Dib, N. A., M. A. Sabry, J. A. Ahmed, S. O. El-Basiouni, and A. A. El-Badry.** 2004. Evaluation of *Capillaria philippinensis* coproantigen in the diagnosis of infection. *J. Egypt. Soc. Parasitol.* **34:**97–106.
20. **el-Karaksy, H., M. el-Shabrawi, N. Mohsen, M. Kotb, N. el-Koofy, and N. el-Deeb.** 2004. *Capillaria philippinensis*: a cause of fatal diarrhea in one of two infected Egyptian sisters. *J. Trop. Pediatr.* **50:**57–60.
21. **Embil, J. A., C. E. Tanner, L. H. Pereira, M. Staudt, E. G. Morrison, and D. A. Gualazzi.** 1988. Seroepidemiologic survey of *Toxocara canis* infection in urban and rural children. *Public Health* **102:**129–133.
22. **Falcao, H., N. Lunet, E. Neves, I. Iglesias, and H. Barros.** 2008. *Anisakis simplex* as a risk factor for relapsing acute urticaria: a case-control study. *J. Epidemiol. Community Health* **62:**634–637.
23. **Glickman, L. T., and J. F. Magnaval.** 1993. Zoonotic roundworm infections. *Infect. Dis. Clin. N. Am.* **7:**717–732.
24. **Good, B., C. V. Holland, M. R. Taylor, J. Larragy, P. Moriarty, and M. O'Regan.** 2004. Ocular toxocariasis in schoolchildren. *Clin. Infect. Dis.* **39:**173–178.
25. **Grobusch, M. P., F. Bergmann, D. Teichmann, and E. Klein.** 2000. Cutaneous gnathostomiasis in a woman from Bangladesh. *Int. J. Infect. Dis.* **4:**51–54.
26. **Grove, D. I.** 2000. Tissue nematodes (trichinosis, dracunculiasis, filariasis), p. 2943–2950. *In* G. L. Mandell, J. E. Bennett, and R. Dolin (ed.), *Principles and Practice of Infectious Diseases*, 5th ed., vol. 2. Churchill Livingstone, Philadelphia, PA.
27. **Hidelaratchi, M. D., M. T. Riffsy, and J. C. Wijesekera.** 2005. A case of eosinophilic meningitis following monitor lizard meat consumption, exacerbated by anthelminthics. *Ceylon Med. J.* **50:**84–86.
28. **Imtiaz, R., J. D. Anderson, E. G. Long, J. J. Sullivan, and B. L. Cline.** 1990. Monofilament nylon filters for preventing dracunculiasis: durability and copepod retention after long term field use in Pakistan. *Trop. Med. Parasitol.* **41:**251–253.
29. **Kaul, S. M., V. K. Saxena, R. S. Sharma, V. K. Raina, B. Mohanty, and A. Kumar.** 1990. Monitoring of temephos (abate) application as a cyclopicide under the guineaworm eradication programme in India. *J. Commun. Dis.* **22:**72–76.
30. **Kim, H., S. I. Kim, and S. Y. Cho.** 1984. Serological diagnosis of human sparganosis by means of micro-ELISA. *Kisaengchunghak Chapchi* **22:**222–228.
31. **Minnaar, W. N., and R. C. Krecek.** 2001. Helminths in dogs belonging to people in a resource-limited urban community in Gauteng, South Africa. *Onderstepoort J. Vet. Res.* **68:**111–117.
32. **Miyazaki, I.** 1960. On the genus *Gnathostoma* and human gnathostomiasis, with special reference to Japan. *Exp. Parasitol.* **9:**338–370.
33. **Montalto, M., L. Miele, A. Marcheggiano, L. Santoro, V. Curigliano, M. Vastola, and G. Gasbarrini.** 2005. Anisakis infestation: a case of acute abdomen mimicking Crohn's disease and eosinophilic gastroenteritis. *Dig. Liver Dis.* **37:**62–64.

34. **Moravec, F.** 2001. Redescription and systematic status of *Capillaria philippinensis*, an intestinal parasite of human beings. *J. Parasitol.* **87:**161–164.

35. **Munckhof, W. J., M. L. Grayson, B. J. Susil, M. J. Pullar, and J. Turnidge.** 1994. Cerebral sparganosis in an East Timorese refugee. *Med. J. Aust.* **161:**263–264.

36. **Nakamura, T., M. Hara, M. Matsuoka, M. Kawabata, and M. Tsuji.** 1990. Human proliferative sparganosis. A new Japanese case. *Am. J. Clin. Pathol.* **94:**224–228.

37. **Nash, T. E.** 2000. Visceral larva migrans and other unusual helminth infections, p. 2965–2970. *In* G. L. Mandell, J. E. Bennett, and R. Dolin (ed.), *Principles and Practice of Infectious Diseases*, 5th ed., vol. 2. Churchill Livingstone, Philadelphia, PA.

38. **Nichols, R. L.** 1956. The etiology of visceral larva migrans. II. Comparative larval morphology of *Ascaris lumbricoides*, *Necator americanus*, *Strongyloides stercoralis* and *Ancylostoma caninum*. *J. Parasitol.* **42:**363–399.

39. **Noya, O., B. Alarcon de Noya, H. Arrechedera, J. Torres, and C. Arguello.** 1992. *Sparganum proliferum*: an overview of its structure and ultrastructure. *Int. J. Parasitol.* **22:**631–640.

40. **Pampiglione, S., F. Rivasi, and A. Gustinelli.** 2009. Dirofilarial human cases in the Old World, attributed to *Dirofilaria immitis*: a critical analysis. *Histopathology* **54:**192–204.

41. **Pien, F. D., and B. C. Pien.** 1999. *Angiostrongylus cantonensis* eosinophilic meningitis. *Int. J. Infect. Dis.* **3:**161–163.

42. **Qahtani, F., J. Deschenes, Z. Ali-Khan, J. D. Maclean, F. Codere, M. Mansour, and M. Burnier, Jr.** 2000. Intraocular gnathostomiasis: a rare Canadian case. *Can. J. Ophthalmol.* **35:**35–39.

43. **Ramirez-Avila, L., S. Slome, F. L. Schuster, S. Gavali, P. M. Schantz, J. Sejvar, and C. A. Glaser.** 2009. Eosinophilic meningitis due to *Angiostrongylus* and *Gnathostoma* species. *Clin. Infect. Dis.* **48:**322–327.

44. **Rusnak, J. M., and D. R. Lucey.** 1993. Clinical gnathostomiasis: case report and review of the English-language literature. *Clin. Infect. Dis.* **16:**33–50.

45. **Saichua, P., C. Nithikathkul, and N. Kaewpitoon.** 2008. Human intestinal capillariasis in Thailand. *World J. Gastroenterol.* **28:**506–510.

46. **Shah, M.** 1999. Human pulmonary dirofilariasis: review of the literature. *South. Med. J.* **92:**276–279.

47. **Shields, J. A.** 1984. Ocular toxocariasis. A review. *Surv. Ophthalmol.* **28:**361–381.

48. **Taira, K., I. Saeed, A. Permin, and C. M. Kapel.** 2004. Zoonotic risk of Toxocara canis infection through consumption of pig or poultry viscera. *Vet. Parasitol.* **121:**115–124.

49. **Turner, J.** 1962. Human dipylidiasis (dog tapeworm infection) in the United States. *J. Pediatr.* **61:**763–768.

50. **Walther, M., and R. Muller.** 2003. Diagnosis of human filariases (except onchocerciasis). *Adv. Parasitol.* **53:**149–193.

51. **Wendo, C.** 2003. Uganda leads Africa's charge against guinea worm disease. *Lancet* **361:**1446.

52. **Wongsawasdi, L., N. Ukarapol, and N. Lertprasertsuk.** 2002. The endoscopic diagnosis of intestinal capillariasis in a child: a case report. *Southeast Asian J. Trop. Med. Public Health* **33:**730–732.

53. **World Health Organization.** 2009. Monthly report on dracunculiasis cases, January-May 2009. *Wkly. Epidemiol. Rec.* **84:**280.

54. **Yoon, W. J., S. M. Lee, S. H. Lee, and Y. B. Yoon.** 2004. Gastric anisakiasis. *Gastrointest. Endosc.* **59:**400.

Arthropods of Medical Importance*

SAM R. TELFORD III

146

Arthropods comprise a diverse group of invertebrate animals (Fig. 1), united in a common body theme (bauplan) of a jointed, chitinous exoskeleton. Four major groupings have classically been recognized: insects, arachnids, crustacea, and millipedes/centipedes; a fifth group contains only the horseshoe crabs, living fossils which have existed unchanged for hundreds of millions of years. All arthropod classes were extant hundreds of millions of years ago, thereby providing ample opportunity for life history traits such as parasitism to independently evolve, and evolve multiple times, in each class.

Medically important arthropods have long been considered to mainly comprise ectoparasites, parasites that limit their activities to the skin. Parasitism, however, is only one of several associations that comprise the interaction of arthropods of medical importance with humans. Arthropods may actively defend themselves against predation (crushing or swatting) by biting, stinging, piercing, or secreting noxious chemicals. Such defenses would operate regardless of the attacker, be it human or other arthropod. Passive modes of defense may inadvertently affect humans, such as irritation after brushing the urticarial hairs of certain caterpillars. Arthropods may also be medically important due to indirect effects: fear of insects, delusional parasitosis, or allergy due to dust mites. The various modes by which arthropods may affect human health thus reflect the diversity of these animals, but there are very few instances in which it may be argued that natural selection favored the offspring of those that focused on causing misery. Accordingly, arthropods should be viewed as a normal part of the environment that under individual circumstances may cause pathology. In addition, because of their ubiquity, spurious associations with pathology are common.

ARTHROPODS AS VECTORS

Arthropods are thought of by many in clinical settings with respect to their role as vectors, transmitters of infectious agents including viruses, bacteria, protozoa, and helminths. Infectious agents may have an obligate relationship with an arthropod (biological transmission) or may simply contaminate an arthropod (mechanical transmission). Malaria parasites undergo a complex developmental cycle within certain mosquitoes and could not perpetuate without them. In contrast, the agent of trachoma (Chlamydia trachomatis) is found on the external surfaces of eye gnats and flies (23) and may be transferred between hosts by the act of landing and crawling, but C. trachomatis more commonly perpetuates by direct contact of hosts. Mechanical transmission of an infectious agent is dependent on its stability and quantum of infection. Human immunodeficiency virus (HIV), for example, does not survive long outside of the body, and the femtoliter or so of material that may contaminate the mouthparts of a mosquito would not contain enough viable lymphocytes with HIV to initiate infection; thus, mosquitoes have never been epidemiologically linked with HIV transmission even though mosquitoes and other hematophagous arthropods obviously feed on viremic individuals.

There are five major groups of vectors: the diptera (flies and mosquitoes), hemiptera (kissing bugs), siphonaptera (fleas), anoplura (lice), and acarines (ticks and mites). The general life history strategies for each group provide the basis for understanding vectorial capacity, which is the sum of physiological and ecological attributes that allow transmission. Specific vector-pathogen relationships are discussed in detail in chapters focusing on the respective agents but are succinctly summarized here in Table 1.

Diptera

The dipteran vectors are winged insects that include mosquitoes, sand flies, blackflies, gnats, horseflies, deerflies, and tsetse flies. These range in size from minute (ceratopogonid midges less than 2 mm in length) to large (horseflies more than 2 cm in length). Unlike other winged insects, dipterans have only one pair of wings. Those that take blood meals as adult females may serve as vectors. Blood meals are used as nutrients to produce eggs (anautogeny); once those eggs are laid, another blood meal may be taken and more eggs produced. Thus, unless a mosquito (as an example of a dipteran) inherits infection (transovarial or vertical transmission), the first blood meal infects it and the second allows the agent to be transmitted; under favorable environmental circumstances, a mosquito may survive for several weeks and take more than two blood meals. Both male and female flies and mosquitoes also require

---

*This chapter contains information presented in chapter 138 by Thomas R. Fritsche in the eighth edition of this *Manual*.

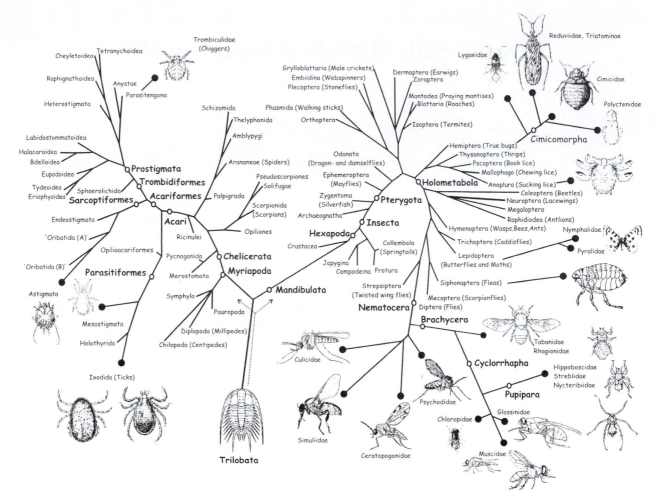

FIGURE 1 Phylogeny of arthropods. (Reprinted from reference 27 with permission of Elsevier Publishing.)

sugar meals (usually from plant nectar), but sugar meals can result in reproduction only in certain species (autogeny).

Eggs are laid in water or within detritus. Vermiform larvae emerge from the eggs and develop through several stages (instars) in water or detritus, feeding on organic material or bacteria, culminating in pupae from which emerge new adults, thereby undergoing complete metamorphosis (holometabolous development). Depending on the species and the ambient temperature, the duration of the dipteran life cycle may be as short as a week or so. Tsetse flies are an unusual exception to this pattern and produce only one advanced larva for each blood meal, with the larva nourished internally from milk gland analogs during a gestation of several weeks (9). This large maternal investment in offspring makes adulticiding (trapping or spraying) very effective in reducing tsetse fly populations and thereby reducing the transmission of the agents of sleeping sickness.

The diptera are only transiently associated with a blood meal source. Host-seeking cues include body heat, carbon dioxide (exhaled by the host), mechanical vibrations, and lactic acid or other skin-associated compounds. The flies visually seek hosts with their compound eyes, mainly larger, dark-colored objects with movement, but proximal cues associated with a host seem to be required to initiate

feeding (44). Repellants such as diethyltoluamide (DEET) work by disrupting the airborne gradients of chemical cues that allow diptera to home in to their hosts. Once a host has been identified, feeding is initiated and completed within minutes. Sand flies, blackflies, and mosquitoes have a diverse salivary armamentarium of pharmacologically active substances that promote finding and removing blood. During probing, antihemostatic and anti-inflammatory chemicals are secreted into the feeding channel created in the epidermis. Probing lacerates capillaries, and the ADP that is released from damaged endothelial cells would serve to promote platelet activation, but through secretion of an apyrase that cleaves ADP into a monophosphate, platelet aggregation is greatly reduced during blood feeding. In addition, local inflammatory processes are temporarily diminished due to secretion of chemicals such as prostaglandin E_2 (40). Thus, the first few bites from a given species remain unnoticed by the host, although factors in the saliva of blackflies may leave an egg-sized lump that is hot to the touch at the site of their bites. Such lumps may persist for several days and may be accompanied by low-grade fever. Such "blackfly fever" should not be misinterpreted as infection; it resolves on its own without treatment.

The variety of proteins that are deposited within skin during vector feeding are the basis for hypersensitivity reac-

TABLE 1 Summary of the major arthropod genera involved in biological transmission of infectious diseases

Arthropod(s)	Etiologic agent(s)	Disease
Crustacea		
Decapods	*Paragonimus*	Paragonimiasis
Copepods	*Diphyllobothrium*	Diphyllobothriasis
	Dracunculus medinensis	Guinea worm disease
	Gnathostoma spinigerum	Gnathostomiasis
Insecta		
Anopleura		
Pediculus	*Rickettsia prowazekii*	Epidemic typhus
	Bartonella quintana	Trench fever
	Borrelia recurrentis	Epidemic relapsing fever
Siphonaptera		
Xenopsylla, Nosopsyllus	*Yersinia pestis*	Plague
	Rickettsia typhi	Murine typhus
	Hymenolepis diminuta	Rat tapeworm
Pulex, Oropsylla	*Yersinia pestis*	Plague
Ctenocephalides	*Dipylidium caninum*	Dog tapeworm disease
Hemiptera		
Panstrongylus, Rhodnius, Triatoma	*Trypanosoma cruzi*	Chagas' disease
Diptera		
Aedes	*Wuchereria, Brugia*	Filariasis
	Flaviviruses	Dengue, yellow fever
	Other arboviruses	Encephalitis
Anopheles	*Plasmodium*	Malaria
	Wuchereria, Brugia	Filariasis
	Arboviruses	Encephalitis
Culex	*Wuchereria*	Filariasis
	Arboviruses	Encephalitis
Culicoides	*Mansonella*	Filariasis
Glossina	*Trypanosoma brucei*	African sleeping sickness
Chrysops	*Loa loa*	Loiasis
	Francisella tularensis	Tularemia
Simulium	*Onchocerca volvulus*	Onchocerciasis
	Mansonella ozzardi	Filariasis
Phlebotomus, Lutzomyia	*Leishmania*	Leishmaniasis
	Bartonella bacilliformis	Bartonellosis
	Phlebovirus	Sandfly fever
Arachnida		
Acari (ticks)		
Ixodes	*Borrelia burgdorferi*	Lyme disease
	Anaplasma phagocytophilum	Human granulocytic ehrlichiosis
	Rickettsia conorii	Boutonneuse fever
	Babesia	Babesiosis
Dermacentor	*Rickettsia rickettsii*	Rocky Mountain spotted fever
	Francisella tularensis	Tularemia
	Coltivirus	Colorado tick fever
	Flavivirus	Omsk hemorrhagic fever
Amblyomma	*Rickettsia rickettsii*	Rocky Mountain spotted fever
	Francisella tularensis	Tularemia
	Ehrlichia chaffeensis	Human monocytic ehrlichiosis
Hyalomma	Nairovirus	Crimean-Congo hemorrhagic fever
Rhipicephalus	*Rickettsia conorii*	Boutonneuse fever
	Rickettsia rickettsii	Rocky Mountain spotted fever
Ornithodoros	*Borrelia*	Relapsing fever
Acari (mites)		
Leptotrombidium	*Orientia tsutsugamushi*	Scrub typhus
Liponyssoides	*Rickettsia akari*	Rickettsialpox

tions, mainly itch, in hosts that are exposed to bites more than once over the course of weeks. Repeated exposure over months may lead to tolerance and a return to failing to react to bites. Although much work remains to be done, there appears to be some cross-reactivity between salivary products from different groups of vector, so some individuals may equally react to the bites of mosquitoes, bugs, or ticks.

The blood-feeding flies have cruder salivary tools, reflecting their less elegant way of feeding, which usually involves scraping the skin with a roughened maxilla and feeding from the pooled blood or lymph. Accordingly, fly bites are more painful regardless of prior exposure, and few flies successfully engorge to repletion on humans.

Freshly blood-fed diptera seek a resting place for diuresis and digestion, usually the nearest vertical surface. This behavior renders those species that bite within houses susceptible to control by indoor residual insecticide spraying.

The transient nature of infestation by blood-feeding diptera means that few specimens are submitted to clinical laboratories. Other than analyses related to confirming the diagnosis of a vector-borne infection, dipterans would come to the attention of laboratorians for issues related to hypersensitivity, or for myiasis (see below).

Hemiptera

The only hemiptera that serve as vectors are the kissing or reduviid bugs, belonging to a diverse and speciose order of minute to large insects with compound eyes, antennae, sucking mouthparts, two pairs of wings (one delicate pair hidden under an outer pair of more robust ones), and a segmented abdomen. All are easily seen without magnification, adult bedbugs being roughly 1 cm in length and adult triatomines ranging in size from 1 cm to more than 5 cm. Small numbers of eggs are produced by females, from which emerge miniature versions of the adults. These nymphs undergo an incomplete metamorphosis (hemimetabolous development), with development through five nymphal stages, each one requiring a blood meal to proceed. The full duration of the life cycle can be as little as 3 months or as great as 2 years. Reduviid bugs are cryptic, living within cracks of mud walls or other narrow, confined spaces. They serve as vectors of trypanosomes (*Trypanosoma cruzi*, the agent of Chagas' disease, and *Trypanosoma rangeli*, an apparently nonpathogenic trypanosome that is often cotransmitted with *T. cruzi*) in the Nearctic. *Triatoma rubrofasciata* transmits a trypanosome that infects monkeys in Southeast

Asia (52), but to date there is no known bug-transmitted trypanosomiasis of humans in the Palearctic. Interestingly, there are good natural cycles of *T. cruzi* transmission within the United States from California through virtually all of the southern-central states, all the way over to Maryland, but there are only rare human cases of autochthonous Chagas' disease reported. Two factors account for this paradox: people live in quality houses that are less likely to have infestations of bugs, and more importantly, the main southern U.S. vector, *Triatoma sanguisuga*, does not defecate on the host while feeding (37). Transmission of *T. cruzi* to humans requires contamination of the site of the bite or mucosa by trypanosomes that are excreted in the bug feces.

As with mosquitoes, salivary products from reduviids contain a variety of pharmacologically active compounds. Unlike those of mosquitoes, repeated reduviid feedings may cause a dangerous anaphylactoid reaction in residents of houses where the bugs are common. Scientists working with reduviid bugs often need to carry an epinephrine injector with them due to their propensity to feeding their colonies upon themselves, thereby receiving large doses of salivary antigens.

Although it is possible that a true reduviid bug may be presented by a patient for identification in clinical settings outside of Latin America, it is more likely that such specimens are related heteropterans such as assassin bugs, which are insect predators, or the plant-feeding stink bugs, chinch bugs, harlequin bugs, or squash bugs. Assassin bugs may inflict extremely painful wounds by their piercing mouthparts, but these require only typical first aid measures and perhaps a booster of tetanus toxoid given the depth of the puncture wound (proboscises range in length from 3 to 8 mm). The plant feeders may issue noxious secretions, which may taste bad if accidentally ingested (from a bug that infested a fruit or vegetable that was eaten directly from the vine) but would otherwise not be a cause for concern.

Bedbugs (*Cimex lectularius* and *Cimex hemipterus*) are hemipterans but are not known to serve as vectors for any pathogen. These bugs with short, broad heads, oval bodies, and four-jointed antennae undergo incomplete metamorphosis, with four nymphal stages, each taking a blood meal in order to develop. The duration of the life cycle is roughly 6 to 8 weeks but may be as long as 11 months, depending on the temperature and humidity. They are small, 5 mm or less in length as adults (Fig. 2). They are cryptic and require hiding places such as cracks in walls, mattress

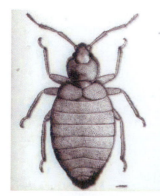 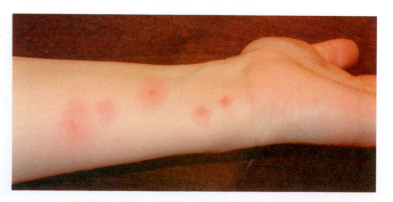

FIGURE 2 Bedbugs. (Left) *Cimex lectularius* (bedbug). Scale bar = 0.5 mm. (Department of Tropical Public Health, Harvard School of Public Health.) (Right) Immediate-type hypersensitivity reaction to bedbug bites acquired in a four-star hotel in Dupont Circle, Washington, DC, December 2005.

foundations, or rattan furniture. At night, bedbugs emerge and infest sleeping people, taking 10 to 20 min for engorgement. Feeding is often interrupted by the movements of people during their sleep, and so multiple bites may result from a single bedbug (Fig. 2). Blood meals may be taken every week or so, depending on the stage, with batches of 10 to 50 eggs laid; one female may lay 200 to 500 eggs in her life. Various laboratory studies have reported the survival of diverse agents such as HIV (24), hepatitis B virus, *Francisella tularensis*, and West Nile virus within artificially infected bedbugs. Epidemiologically, bedbugs have never been associated with any of these infections. Although one can never say never, the likelihood that a bedbug has served as a vector is infinitesimally small, and a physician may want to question a patient more closely on known risky practices such as intravenous drug abuse.

Bedbugs have attained public health prominence recently due to an expansion in the number and intensity of their infestations. This emergent problem is due to increases in travel, immigration, and probably development of resistance to typical insecticides (18). Bedbugs travel with their human hosts by hiding in furniture, luggage with clothing, and particularly mattresses. Large apartment complexes may foster large blocks or floors of infested rooms, with bedbugs moving along water or electrical conduits or through wall penetrations. Such large-scale infestations are difficult to eradicate. On a case-by-case basis, rooms may be treated using pyrethroid insecticides, particularly under baseboards and moldings; mattresses and box springs may be steam cleaned or encased in covers designed to retain allergens if concerns about insecticide applications are relevant.

Although many people do not sustain any injury due to bedbug bites, some may present with cutaneous reactions, mainly comprising maculopapular erythemas <5 mm in diameter that itch. Repeated exposure and the development of immediate-type hypersensitivity may serve as the basis for more intense cutaneous reactions, including wheals and incipient nodules that may persist for weeks. Secondary infection is common due to scratching. Most such cases may be treated with over-the-counter hydrocortisone preparations or topical antibiotics if secondary infection is apparent.

Siphonaptera

Fleas are bilaterally compressed, heavily chitinized insects with greatly modified hind legs for their characteristic jumping mode of locomotion; they lack wings. Fleas are generally small, no larger than 5 mm in length. They undergo complete metamorphosis, starting from a wormlike larva feeding on organic debris and blood pellets expelled, often with remarkable force and over a long distance, from the anus of the adult flea. The larva develops through three molts (has thee instars) and then secretes a silk to form a cocoon, in which it pupates. The female flea requires blood for egg production; one blood meal may serve for the production of several dozen eggs, which are laid on the fur of the host. Eggs become detached from the host's fur, coming to rest within its nest. Most fleas are what are known as "nest parasites." Individual fleas may live as long as a year but usually only for a couple of months, laying eggs daily. As with most arthropods, the duration of the life cycle is affected by temperature and relative humidity, but on average most species take 30 to 75 days to develop from egg to adult.

Of the 2,000 or so flea species that have been described, the vast majority are from rodents and have various degrees of host specificity. Because fleas are generally nest parasites of rodents (and most rodent species are not human commensals), are relatively host specific, and cannot travel long distances (crawling or jumping on the order of a few meters, implying that humans must be directly associated with their habitat for infestation to occur), only a few species are of medical importance. These include the "human" flea (*Pulex irritans*), the dog and cat fleas (*Ctenocephalides canis* and *Ctenocephalides felis*), the main plague vector (*Xenopsylla cheopis*), and the sticktight flea (*Echidnophaga gallinacea*). Of these, *C. felis* is the most notorious pest, feeding voraciously and rapidly developing dense infestations. Chronic infestations of homes are largely due to the presence of a cat or dog (despite its name, this flea feeds on either animal), its bedding, wall-to-wall carpeting, and relatively great humidity within the home. (Cold climates rarely have self-sustaining infestations because winter heating tends to dry out the carpets, molding, and other places where the larval fleas tend to be hidden.) Although bites sustained over several weeks usually induce a typical delayed-type hypersensitivity reaction, with an intensely itching red spot developing at the site of the bite (usually around the ankles), note that not all members of a household react in the same manner. Some people are more attractive to arthropods than others; others react differently to bites. It is quite possible for only one person to have itchy bites and others in the same house to have none, and thus a diagnosis of flea bite should not depend on the perception that if a household is infested, everyone should demonstrate similar lesions.

The human flea actually feeds on a variety of mammals, including domestic livestock. In tropical sites where homes have dirt floors, and livestock share living accommodations, extremely dense infestations may develop. Although this flea is cosmopolitan in its distribution, the cat flea appears to have supplanted it as the major flea pest for humans in many countries.

An unusual flea, the chigoe or jigger (*Tunga penetrans*), attaches to a host and maintains a feeding site. Originally found in Latin America, the chigoe has been carried across to sub-Saharan Africa by humans and may be found anywhere there. This flea often penetrates under toenails, or burrows into skin between toes or in the soles of feet, an infestation known as tungiasis (Fig. 3). The female *T. penetrans* swells to 10 times its size, and the host's immune response causes skin to swell up and cover her, with only the end of the abdomen exposed. Through this opening, she deposits eggs and feces. When the flea dies, the lesion becomes secondarily infected, causing great irritation and pain. Tourists often become infested by walking barefoot in shady spots around beaches.

Perhaps the most famous flea is the plague vector, the oriental rat flea, *Xenopsylla cheopis*. Although it prefers rats (*Rattus rattus* and *Rattus norvegicus*) as hosts, in their absence (or when they die) they feed on humans and other animals. These fleas may be found on rats in virtually every tropical or warm temperate port city around the world, having been transported there with their hosts by trade ships. Plague is usually maintained in enzootic foci by wild rodents and their more specific fleas, but in Vietnam, Madagascar, and India, rats and *X. cheopis* appear to be important for perpetuation. Although enzootic plague usually results in sporadic cases, the great fecundity of rats under the right circumstances means that explosive outbreaks of plague may occur in urban areas, with hundreds or thousands of cases. Human exposure in the western United States, where plague is enzootic, may be due to chance contact with ground squirrels or their fleas

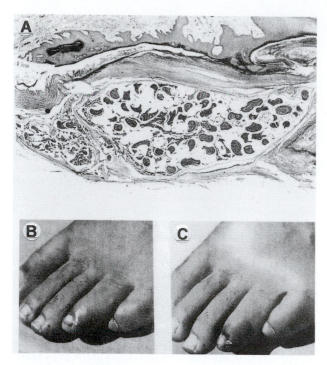

FIGURE 3 Tungiasis. (A) Low-power section of dermal lesion showing flea uterus filled with developing eggs; (B and C) progressive edema and secondary bacterial infection of *Tunga* lesion. (Reprinted from reference 2 with permission.)

(often *Diamanus montanus*) in sheds, disused cabins, or crawl spaces or by digging around burrows. Domestic cats often serve as an intermediary, hunting moribund rodents and subsequently exposing their owners.

Phthiraptera

Infestation by lice is called pediculosis. Lice are wingless, flat (dorsoventrally), elongate, small (0.4- to 10-mm) insects that are generally characterized by strong host specificity. Classically, two orders were recognized, the Mallophaga

(chewing lice) and the Anoplura (sucking lice); the former now comprises three suborders, and the latter remains as a suborder, all within the order Phthiraptera, which contains about 4,000 species. Of these, sucking lice are clinically relevant, although chewing lice may be presented as spurious ectoparasites or associated with double-pored tapeworm (*Dipylidium caninum*) infection. Most chewing lice are commensals of birds, whereas sucking lice feed mainly on mammals.

Lice undergo incomplete (hemimetabolous) development, with nymphal forms resembling adult lice and often found concurrently with the adults. Thus, size may appear to greatly vary within a single collection of specimens from one host. All lice are delicate and very sensitive to temperature and humidity requirements; all die within days without the host.

Chewing lice usually are found in the feathers of birds, feeding on skin fragments. Virtually all chewing lice lack piercing mouthparts and therefore do not feed on blood. The dog-biting louse (*Trichodectes canis*) may be presented as a specimen because it is a common commensal of dogs and may be spuriously associated with "bites." Dogs serve as definitive hosts for *D. caninum*, the eggs of which are shed in feces; the feces dry on the fur and the louse may then ingest the eggs. The tapeworm eggs hatch and a cysticercoid becomes localized in the hemocoel of the louse. Transmission is effected when the louse is accidentally ingested, usually when the dog is grooming; humans (usually children) are incidentally infected if their hands become contaminated and then touch food or drink or are placed in their mouths.

Book lice (order Psocoptera, also known as psocids) resemble chewing lice and live on molds infesting old books. They are frequently presented as specimens in diagnostic workups for itches of unknown etiology but do not infest humans or any other animal.

The lice of greatest clinical importance (Fig. 4) are the head louse (*Pediculus humanus capitis*), body louse (*Pediculus humanus corporis*), and pubic louse (*Pthirus pubis*). All of these sucking lice have prominent claws attached to each of their legs, morphologically adapted for grasping the hairs of their host. Lice are transferred between hosts by close physical contact, or by sharing clothing in the case of body

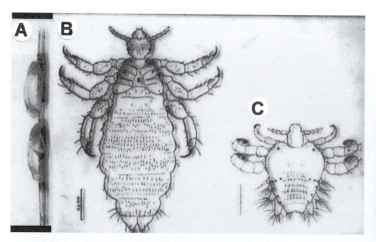
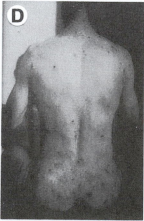

FIGURE 4 Lice. (A) Head louse nits; (B) body louse; (C) pubic louse; (D) vagabond's disease. (Department of Tropical Public Health, Harvard School of Public Health.)

lice. The oft-tendered excuse "I got it from a toilet seat" with reference to pubic lice should not be dismissed out of hand, but the probability of acquiring a louse in this manner is far less than by skin-to-skin contact. The presence of pubic lice usually denotes a sexually transmitted infestation, and pubic louse infestation of a child may be cause for an inquiry into the possibility of child abuse.

Sucking lice are important vectors as well as pests. Among the most notorious vectors in history are body lice, which may serve as vectors for the agents of epidemic typhus, trench fever, and louse-borne relapsing fever. Napoleon's invasion of Russia in 1812 was probably thwarted by epidemic typhus decimating his troops. It is said that at the end of World War I, a typhus epidemic in Russia and Romania killed 800,000 people (55). Body lice are the product of poor hygiene, with clothes never or rarely being changed, such as in cold weather, by the homeless, or in refugee camps. Trench fever may be common in the homeless, and the most recent large outbreak of typhus was in Burundi, among Rwandan refugees. Oddly, even though the head louse is conspecific and appears vector competent in laboratory experiments, it has not been epidemiologically associated with any of these infections, nor has the pubic louse.

Lice feed at least daily and deposit 1 to 10 eggs from each blood meal, gluing one egg at a time onto the shafts of hairs (or in the case of the body louse, onto threads within clothing). Body or pubic louse infestation may result in intense irritation for several days, with each bite generating a red papule. Chronically infested individuals may become desensitized, or may develop a nonspecific febrile illness with lymphadenopathy, edema, and arthropathy (although such signs and symptoms should prompt a search for the agent of trench fever). A very few chronically infested individuals may develop "morbus errorum," or vagabond's disease (Fig. 4), with a thickening and dark pigmentation of the skin (20).

Although body louse or pubic louse infestation may be considered evidence of poor hygiene or poor judgment, infestation by head lice should not be a stigma. Schools are excellent sites for the spread of a louse infestation, not only through the sharing of hats and scarves but also by children deliberately infesting others during play. Nor should head louse infestation be considered a public health menace, or even a clinical problem. Very few infestations are dense enough to cause signs or symptoms, and head lice are not vectors. Nonetheless, draconian measures are taken by many school districts, banning an infested child until treatment is thorough enough to remove all nits. Many such schools fail to discriminate between live and dead nits, insisting that all traces of them be absent. Complete removal of all nit remnants can be very difficult, relying mainly on fine-tooth combs, tools that have been found in the tombs of the Egyptian pharaohs (34).

The head louse life cycle serves as the basis for recommendations about prevention and therapy. Nits (eggs) hatch about a week after being deposited. The nymphal louse feeds once or more each day for as many as 12 days before becoming sexually mature. The female louse lays half a dozen eggs each day, and during its short life span (15 to 20 days) may cumulatively lay as many as 100 eggs. Thus, infestations comprise mainly eggs (nits), which may or may not be viable; few adult lice may be found.

Although head lice are acquired mainly by direct head-to-head contact, it is possible that wearing someone else's hat or using someone else's hairbrush may serve as a mode of transfer. Similarly, lice might survive on a pillow or on furniture for about a day (the duration a nymphal or adult louse may go without feeding at room temperature). Thus, environmental treatment could be as simple as excluding people from a room for a day or two.

Treatment for head lice should target viable eggs or motile adult lice; initiating treatment for the presence of a few nits of undetermined viability is economically and emotionally suspect. The following issues should be resolved before considering treatment. (i) Is it really a head louse infestation? Book lice are similar in size and may be found accidentally infesting a person, but they are not parasitic. The follicle mite, *Demodex folliculorum,* is very small (<0.5 mm) and is sticklike in appearance. More commonly, other debris (dandruff or other organic matter) may be misidentified as lice by a patient complaining of an itchy scalp or "something crawling" through the hair. (ii) Are living adult lice apparent, or are nits viable? The developing nymph may be observed with the aid of magnification and adequate light; nonviable nits are clear or damaged. In addition, if the nit is more than a third of the way up a hair shaft, then it is likely to have already hatched because lice tend to deposit their eggs on hair close to the skin surface (36).

The treatment of choice is an over-the-counter shampoo containing permethrin, a synthetic pyrethroid. However, reports of resistance are common, particularly for those individuals who sustain multiple sequential infestations and undergo multiple treatment courses. Lice that are resistant to the typical permethrin dose are also likely to resist higher concentrations. Other treatment options should be explored, including the use of prescription shampoos containing lindane or malathion. Lore and Internet websites tout alternative modalities, such as oral ivermectin or trimethoprim-sulfamethoxazole (Bactrim), enzyme treatments to loosen nits, essential oils to poison lice, or olive oil to suffocate adult lice or nits. Although many of these are low risk, and individual cases may respond to such treatment, no objective efficacy trials have been reported.

Acarina

The acarines are a subclass within the class Arachnida, which also contains spiders. Acarina comprise mites and ticks, tiny to small arthropods with eight legs as nymphs and adults (as opposed to six for insects) and with fused main body segments as opposed to three discrete ones for insects. Acarine baupläne are characterized by two functional body parts, the gnathosoma (or capitulum), which comprises the "head," and the idiosoma, which contains all the remaining functions (reproductive, motility, and digestion). Acarines undergo incomplete metamorphosis, passing through a larval and one to several nymphal stages before attaining sexual maturity. The mites are one of the most speciose groups of animals, with 45,000 recognized species. They are among the oldest terrestrial animals, dating in the fossil record to the Devonian period (nearly 400 million years ago), and are found in every habitat on earth. There are two major orders of the acarines, the Acariformes and the Parasitiformes. In the former, there are two main groups, the Sarcoptiformes (astigmata) and the Trombidiformes (prostigmata), both of which contain species of clinical significance. The latter comprises three orders, the Holothyrida, the Ixodida, and the Mesostigmata. Of these, only the last two are clinically significant; the holothyrids consist of about 20 species that are found only in Australasia and some neotropical forests and are unlikely to be encountered (although they are known to secrete a toxin that may incapacitate a human who has ingested such a mite). The mesostigmata (also known as Gamasida or Dermanyssoida) include some that infest birds or rodents that under certain circumstances infest humans and cause itch. The ixodida consist of ticks, which are essentially very large mites.

Other than ticks and some mesostigmatids, mites are generally not considered vectors of agents that infect humans. They are, however, important for their pest potential, causing itch, dermatitis, and allergy.

The house mouse mite (*Liponyssoides sanguineus*) is the vector for rickettsialpox due to infection by *Rickettsia akari*. The relatively mild disease, characterized by fever and exanthema, was first described after a garbage collectors' strike in Kew Gardens in the Bronx, NY, during the 1940s (22). Garbage piled up, and house mouse populations became dense. When the strike resolved and the garbage was removed, the mice died or emigrated, leaving behind dense infestations of hungry mites. The prostigmatid trombiculid mites (chiggers) are the vectors for the agent of scrub typhus (*Orientia tsutsugamushi*), a rickettsiosis of Eurasia and northeastern Australia. Nearly 3 billion people live in countries where scrub typhus is endemic. Scrub typhus is acquired from infestation by tiny (0.2-mm) larval trombiculid mites such as *Leptotrombidium deliense* or *Leptotrombidium akamushi*; an eschar forms at the site of the chigger bite, with proximal lymphadenopathy, fever, headache, exanthema, and myalgia. Case fatality rates can range from 5 to 35% (4). Interestingly, the nymphal and adult stages of this mite feed on detritus or other arthropods and do not take vertebrate blood. Therefore, *O. tsutsugamushi* relies mainly on transovarial or vertical transmission (passage through the egg) for perpetuation, although rodent hosts that are infected may feed noninfected larvae and generate new matrilineages of infected mites. All other vector-borne agents have greater opportunities for horizontal transmission, that is, amplification by infecting a vertebrate host, and having multiple blood meals during development.

Mites are extremely difficult to identify, particularly given the likely confusion with dust mites or other ubiquitous free-living forms. All require clearing and mounting on a slide and examination under a compound microscope.

Ticks are prolific vectors, with more recognized transmitted agents than any arthropod except mosquitoes. All of the nearly 900 known species of ticks require blood for their development and reproduction. Clinically relevant ticks belong to either the Ixodidae (the hard ticks) or the Argasidae (the soft ticks); a third family, the Nuttalliellidae, comprises a monotypic genus of soft ticks found in southern Africa and for which an association with a pathogenic agent has yet to be described. Hard ticks are so named because of the hardened sclerotized idiosomal shield, or scutum. In female hard ticks, the scutum is on the anterior third of the idiosoma, with the remainder of the idiosoma consisting of a pleated, leathery cuticle that allows for tremendous expansion during blood feeding. In male hard ticks, which may or may not feed at all, the scutum extends the length of the idiosoma. In contrast, soft ticks have no scutum; their entire idiosoma is leathery.

The "head," or capitulum, consists of the holdfast (hypostome), chelicerae (which are homologs of insect mandibles), and palps, which cover the mouthparts (hypostome and chelicerae) and serve a sensory function. Chelicerae act as cutting organs, the two sides sliding past each other, with the cutting teeth at the end gaining a purchase into a host's skin. The hypostome is thereby inserted, allowing anchoring

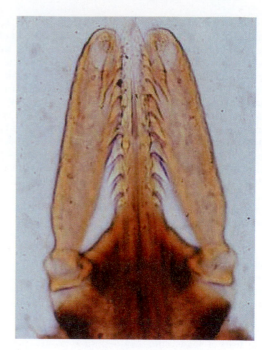

FIGURE 5 Tick hypostome, showing recurved denticles.

of the entire tick due to recurved, backward-facing teeth or denticles (Fig. 5). Many hard ticks also secrete a cement around the hypostome. Often, when an attached dog tick (*Dermacentor variabilis*) is removed from a host, a large piece of skin comes with the hypostome, mostly cement and surrounding epidermis. Thus, by virtue of the cement and denticles, tick hypostomes rarely emerge intact when a tick is removed. "Leaving the head in" is not critical to avoid, and most times the remnant will be walled off as a foreign body or will work itself out, perhaps by the act of scratching. Treatment, therefore, should simply be disinfection of the site of the bite and certainly not excavation of the epidermis looking for the head. Soft ticks are transient feeders and are only rarely found attached.

Hard ticks require several days to complete their blood meal; the number of days depends on the species and stage of the tick. North American deer ticks (*Ixodes dammini* [41, 46]) feed for 3 days as a larva, 4 days as a nymph, and 7 days as the female. The closely related European sheep or castor bean tick, *Ixodes ricinus*, feeds for 2 days as a larva, 3 days as a nymph, and 7 days as the female. The duration of feeding depends also on host immune status (previous exposure may induce immediate-type hypersensitivity, which slows down the feeding process) and temperature (*I. dammini* and *I. ricinus* feed twice as long on cold reptiles as on ones that are held at 37°C). The extended duration of feeding is required for the cuticle to soften so that the idiosoma may accommodate 10 to 100 times its weight in blood, and the site of the bite is prepared so that a pool of lymph and blood is available for removal. During the first 70% of the feeding process, very little blood or lymph appears to be present within ticks, which remain dorsoventrally flat. Hemoglobin is excreted from the anus, lipids are retained, and water from the blood is recycled back into the host as saliva (4). In the last day, usually in the last 3 or 4 h of the blood meal, the tick takes what has been termed "the big sip," removing a large volume of whole blood, and then detaches and drops from the host.

Because they must remain attached for days, hard ticks have evolved means of temporarily disabling a host's local inflammatory response, which might inhibit its feeding. Hard tick saliva is an extremely complex mixture of anticoagulant, anti-inflammatory, and antihemostatic agents (39) that act mainly at the site of the feeding lesion. Tick saliva also neutralizes Th2 responses systemically (54). Hosts who have never been exposed to ticks may not realize that a tick is attached. Indeed, most persons with Lyme disease or spotted fever never knew that they had been "bitten" (45, 53). The most dangerous tick is not necessarily the one that a person finds and removes, aborting the transmission process, but the one that he or she never knew was there and which was able to complete its feeding.

In contrast, soft ticks are more like mosquitoes in their feeding, spending tens of minutes to no more than a few hours feeding, usually as their host is sleeping. Soft tick saliva does not "need" to be as "clever," and in fact some species have painful bites. The pajahuello (pajaroello), *Ornithodoros coriaceus*, of California and Mexico is renowned for its "toxic bite," which causes local pain and burning (20).

Tick life cycles have an extended duration, usually months or years. Deer ticks, for example, take 2 years to go from egg to egg. For this reason, there is generally no risk associated with hard ticks engorging and dropping off of a companion animal within a person's home. The engorged tick does not feed again and takes weeks to molt or lay eggs, and in the interim, usually the relative humidity within the house is too low for extended survival of the tick. On the other hand, cats, as opposed to dogs, appear to be a risk factor for acquiring Lyme disease, perhaps because deer ticks feed well on dogs but poorly on cats; ticks, particularly nymphs, detach in mid-feed and readily reattach to the cat's owner (12). The exceptions to the lack of risk associated with ticks engorging and detaching in the household are with the brown dog tick (*Rhipicephalus sanguineus*), which is the vector of Marseilles fever (Mediterranean spotted fever or boutonneuse fever) and *Ehrlichia canis* and has also recently been documented as a vector of Rocky Mountain spotted fever. These ticks hide behind wall molding to molt and, indeed, are known for dense infestations covering the interior walls of dog kennels.

Ticks can be difficult to identify, depending on their state of engorgement and whether mouthparts are intact. Although tick systematists have recently altered some of the generic epithets, in general the classic CDC diagrams of the mouthparts and idiosoma (Fig. 6) can be used to at least classify a tick to the genus level. Often, simply knowing the country in which a tick may have been acquired significantly narrows down the list of possibilities (Table 2).

ARTHROPODS AS "SCALARS"

Vectors impart directionality to a pathogen. In contrast, there are arthropod-pathogen relationships that are not characterized by directionality, and analogous to mathematical terminology, arthropods that inadvertently serve as a source of infection are called scalars (43). Helminths may use an arthropod as an intermediate host, but that arthropod does not deliver the infectious stage of the helminth during an obligate behavior such as blood feeding. Drinking water with copepods (crustacea) containing third-stage larvae of the filarial nematode *Dracunculus medinensis* initiate infection when the copepods are digested by stomach acids, thereby liberating the nematode larvae, but the copepods do not swim towards a vessel scooping water out for drinking. Accordingly, the patient's history needs to specifically address the possibility of exposure via drinking from natural bodies of water (copepods and *Dracunculus*); the

presence of flour beetles, fleas, or roaches (hymenolepidid cestodes, *Dipylidium caninum*, and *Gongylonema* spp.); eating of crabs or crayfish (which are intermediate hosts for *Paragonimus* spp.); or being in an environment with dense infestations of houseflies (trachoma). With the exception of houseflies and trachoma (which perpetuates in the absence of flies, spreading by direct contact with ocular exudates), all these are obligate relationships.

Muscoid Flies

The muscoid diptera include the muscids (houseflies and stable flies), the Calliphoridae (blowflies), and the Sarcophagidae (the flesh flies). Egg deposition and larval development occur in characteristic materials, namely, fecal material for houseflies, decaying plant material for stable flies, live flesh for blowflies, and carrion for flesh flies. These flies can be remarkably prolific within short periods: a female housefly, for example, deposits 100 to 150 eggs in moist, decaying organic material, usually excrement, at one time, but may do so 20 or more times (21). Larvae emerge from the eggs within 12 h. Three larval stages develop during a week, and a puparium is formed. The adult fly emerges from the pupa within 4 days, and copulation may occur within 1 day. Thus, a full life cycle may take as few as 12 days.

Houseflies have received much attention for their potential as scalars because of their association with poor hygiene. Flies are strong fliers and move readily from outdoors to indoors. A large fleshy structure at the apex of the proboscis provides a surface for contamination, as do the hairy body and legs of the fly. In addition, flies may regurgitate while feeding, and the vomitus may contain organisms that were acquired in a previous landing. Houseflies commonly feed on human excrement, and virtually every possible enteric pathogen (those causing amebiasis, cholera, typhoid, hepatitis A, and poliomyelitis—even roundworms and *Helicobacter pylori*) has been detected within or upon them. With few exceptions, such findings are epidemiologically irrelevant, inasmuch as all of the agents perpetuate in their absence. Poliovirus, for example, was recovered in flies captured from sites where polio was actively being transmitted (51), but use of dichlorodiphenyltrichloroethane (DDT) failed to curtail the epidemic. In contrast, residual DDT treatment of army camps reduced the incidence of shigellosis (50). It is likely that individual cases of enteric disease may derive from fly contamination of food, but whether the risk of such an event merits worry by patients or their health care providers remains unclear. Dense infestations of flies should be reduced (by source reduction, i.e., by preventing flies from getting access to garbage and excrement); a few flies in the house do not warrant setting off a bug bomb.

Cockroaches

Roaches are dorsoventrally flattened, smooth-bodied, winged insects with long antennae, biting-type mouthparts, and abdominal projections (cerci). The outer pair of wings is thick and leathery, and the inner pair is membranous. Roaches may fly, but they usually scuttle about on long spiny legs. They undergo incomplete metamorphosis, with the immature forms looking like miniature adults, although without wings. Eggs are laid within a hard capsule, the ootheca, which is deposited in a dark crevice. Development is slow, taking about 4 weeks between molts; many roaches have only one generation each year. Roaches can live for months without food, but water seems to be critical. They are omnivorous, feeding on everything from the finest of foods to the vilest of waste, usually at night. Secretions

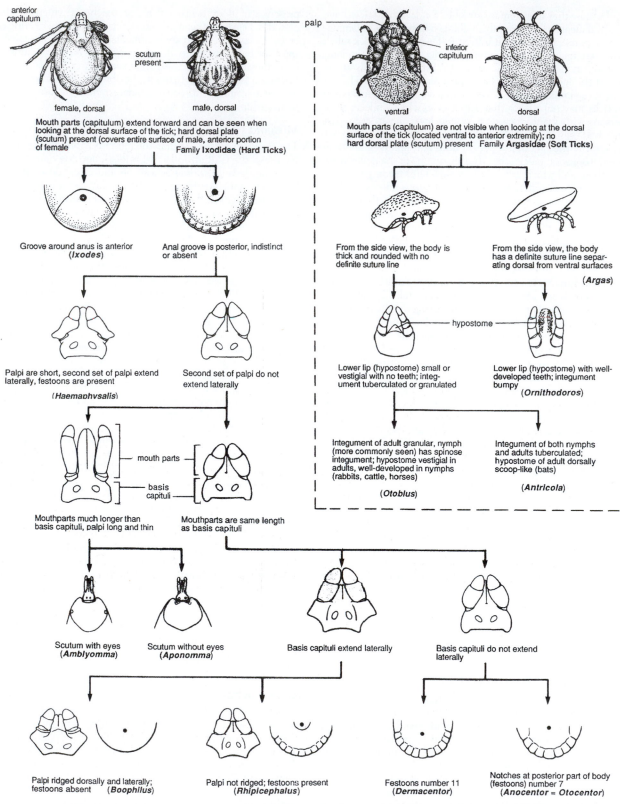

FIGURE 6 Key to major tick genera in the United States. (Reprinted with permission from reference 16.)

TABLE 2 Likely human-biting ticks and possible tick-borne infections by global region

Region	Likely tick(s) infesting humans	Possible zoonosis[a]
North America	*Ixodes dammini, Ixodes scapularis, Ixodes pacificus, Ixodes dentatus, Ixodes cookei*	Lyme disease, babesiosis, HGE, Powassan fever
	Dermacentor variabilis, Dermacentor andersoni, Dermacentor occidentalis	RMSF, CTF, tularemia
	Amblyomma americanum, Amblyomma maculatum	Masters' disease/STARI, RMSF, tularemia, HME
	Ornithodoros hermsi, Ornithodoros turicata	Relapsing fever
South America	*Amblyomma cajennense*	RMSF
	Ornithodoros spp.	Relapsing fever
Europe, Russia	*Ixodes ricinus, Ixodes persulcatus*	Lyme disease, babesiosis, HGE, TBE
	Dermacentor marginatus	TIBOLA
	Rhipicephalus sanguineus	Marseilles fever, HME?
Japan, China, Korea	*Ixodes ovatus, I. persulcatus*	Lyme disease, babesiosis, HGE, TBE
	Dermacentor spp.	Tick typhus, JSF?
	Haemaphysalis spp.	JSF?
South Asia	*Haemaphysalis* spp.	KFD
	Hyalomma spp.	CCHF
	R. sanguineus	Tick typhus
Southeast Asia	*Ixodes granulatus*	Lyme disease?
	R. sanguineus	Tick typhus? HME?
Australia	*Ixodes holocyclus*	Tick typhus
North Africa	*Hyalomma* spp.	CCHF
	R. sanguineus	Marseilles fever, HME?
	I. ricinus	Lyme disease
West Africa	*Hyalomma* spp.	CCHF
	Ornithodoros erraticus	Relapsing fever
	Amblyomma variegatum	ATBF
Sub-Saharan Africa	*A. variegatum, Amblyomma hebraeum, Haemaphysalis leachi*	ATBF
	Hyalomma spp.	CCHF
	Ornithodoros moubata	Relapsing fever

[a]HGE, human granulocytic ehrlichiosis (*Anaplasma phagocytophilum*); HME, human monocytic ehrlichiosis (due to either *Ehrlichia chaffeensis* or *Ehrlichia canis*); RMSF, Rocky Mountain spotted fever; STARI, southern tick-associated rash illness (etiology unknown, possibly Borrelia); CTF, Colorado tick fever; TIBOLA, tick-borne lymphadenopathy (*Rickettsia slovaca*); JSF, Japanese spotted fever (*Rickettsia japonica*); TBE, tick-borne encephalitis; CCHF, Crimean-Congo hemorrhagic fever; KFD, Kyasanur Forest disease; ATBF, African tickbite fever (*Rickettsia africae*).

deposited by scent glands (including trail and aggregation pheromones) give rise to a characteristic disagreeable odor that confirms an infestation even when live roaches cannot be found. Common roaches range in size from the small German cockroach (*Blattella germanica*), about half an inch in length, to the American cockroach, nearly 2 inches long. Much work has been done attempting to incriminate roaches as scalars, even estimating nearly 14,000 CFU of bacteria (mainly *Staphylococcus* spp.) on the surface of the body of one German cockroach (20). Feces laden with *Vibrio*, the agent of cholera, were fed to American cockroaches, with ingestion of as much as 200 μl of material and recovery of live vibrios 30 to 80 h later from roach feces (6). A roundworm (*Gongylonema*) normally infecting ungulates may encyst within roaches and be transmitted to humans when ingested, usually as a contaminant of food. As with flies, the presence of roaches suggests poor environmental hygiene, but only rare instances of enteric disease might be associated with them. Dense infestations may produce large amounts of antigenic material (feces, molted cuticle, or parts from carcasses), which may be implicated in allergic or asthmatic reactions.

Control of roach infestations can be difficult. Boric acid, deposited along walls, behind moldings, and around other sites where roaches may hide, is effective in killing adults and nymphs by abrading the cuticle between abdominal segments, rendering the roach prone to desiccation. Removing standing water (wiping up and getting rid of clutter around sinks) can also reduce infestations by preventing access to water. Roach infestations are most common in apartment buildings serving transient student or immigrant populations, who bring the insects in with their household goods.

DIRECT INJURY DUE TO ARTHROPODS

Arthropods Typically Thought of as Vectors

Vectors such as lice, ticks, bugs, fleas, mosquitoes, and blackflies may directly cause injury by their bites, either by hypersensitivity reactions or by toxic effects of their salivary products. Hypersensitivity reactions mainly manifest as itch, with the concomitant potential for secondary infection due to scratching. Bedbug and flea bites may cause immediate-type hypersensitivity reactions with itchy erythema greater than 3 cm in diameter (Fig. 2). Ticks may induce a chronic local granulomatous lesion, persisting for months, perhaps due to remnants of the mouthparts (denticles) left within the epidermis. This phenomenon is particularly pronounced with "seed tick" infestation (stepping into a newly emerged batch of larval *Amblyomma* ticks, often thousands), where dozens or hundreds of ticks may attach at the belt line. Itch may be immediately relieved by Caladryl (calamine with diphenhydramine [Benadryl]) lotion, or even holding the affected part under very hot running water, which induces mast cells to degranulate. Over-the-counter hydrocortisone creams may help mild cases of itch, but severe cases may require prescription strength steroid cream (e.g., betamethasone [0.05%]). Daily application of hydrocortisone should promote resolution of itch within a week. Tick granulomas may be treated with tretinoin (Retin-A) gel (0.05%), which may promote the turnover of epidermis and ejection of remaining antigenic material (personal observation).

As mentioned in the introduction to diptera, blackfly bites may produce "blackfly fever," usually as a dose-dependent reaction. Usually, the site of the bite becomes edematous, with a golf ball-sized lump and an oozing punctate lesion. Fever and myalgia manifest that night and disappear within 24 h. Such symptoms should not be construed as infection; few pathogens, if any, have such a short prepatent period. Treatment is symptomatic. Similarly, soft tick bites due to the pajaroello or the African tampan (*Ornithodoros moubata*) may immediately cause pain, swelling, and irritation at the site of the bite, with raised hard wheals (26). The effects are said to last several days, with "irritability" of the affected part. Anecdotally, hunters in northern New England and the upper Great Lakes may complain of bites from larvae of *Dermacentor albopictus* (a species that usually feeds only on ungulates such as deer or moose) during the early winter; apocrypha indicates that Native Americans called these larvae "bite all same as a piece of fire" (7). The condition has not been studied.

An unusual toxicosis due to tick bite is tick paralysis. The presence of certain feeding ticks induces an acute ascending paralysis. First described for sheep and cattle in Australia in 1843, a similar disease was reported for a child in Oregon in 1912. The Australian *Ixodes holocyclus* attacks cattle, sheep, and dogs but rarely humans, and thus tick paralysis is not a common clinical condition there. However, in the western United States, bites of *Dermacentor andersoni* commonly produce cases of "staggers" in cattle or sheep, which may terminate fatally. Children are the usual victims of tick paralysis, with ticks attached at the nape of the neck. The illness is characterized by fatigue, irritability, distal paresthesias, leg weakness with reduced tendon reflexes, ataxia, and lethargy. Unless the tick is removed, quadriplegia and respiratory failure may result; the case fatality rate without treatment can be 10%. Removal of the tick induces a miraculous recovery within 48 h. (Tick biologists unromantically suggest such an etiology for the tale of Snow White, who awakens after the Prince bends over her and kisses her, probably removing a tick from behind her ear.) A 40- to 60-kDa toxin has been isolated from *I. holocyclus* and has been named holocyclotoxin (28); an antitoxin has been produced for veterinary use. Others with a much smaller molecular weight have also been isolated. The toxin has not been isolated from the American tick paralysis ticks. Other ticks (*Amblyomma americanum* and *Ixodes* spp.) have also been reported to induce tick paralysis.

Endoparasitic Arthropods

Arthropods that invade a host's body and cause disease include mites (scabies), fleas (tungiasis), fly larvae (myiasis), and pentastomes (halzoun). Tungiasis has been discussed above as part of the general flea section. Pentastomes or tongue worms are primitive, elongate arthropods that live as adults in the lungs and air passages of hosts, including fish, amphibians, reptiles, and some mammals. The body, like that of acarines, consists of a cephalothorax and indistinct abdomen, with no legs; often, the cuticle appears ringed or annulated. Chitinous hooks protrude from the head. Their

sizes range from 1 to 10 cm. Although pentastomes were long thought to be in their own phylum, recent cladistic analyses based on morphological and molecular characters place them within the Crustacea and most closely related to the branchiurid fish lice (26). Pentastomes undergo a complex life cycle with incomplete development, requiring intermediate hosts in which the nymphal stages may encyst.

Human infestation by *Linguatula serrata* may be due to ingestion of eggs (from contamination by nasal discharges from the dog intermediate host) or ingestion of encysted nymphs within the raw or poorly cooked liver, lungs, or mesentery of an intermediate host such as rabbits, cattle, or sheep (42). A nasopharyngeal syndrome results, known as halzoun in the Middle East and Marrara syndrome in Sudan. Facial edema, nasal discharge, coughing, and sneezing are due to the migration of nymphal forms into the nasopharynx. Removal of the offending nymphs (by visual inspection and forceps) and symptomatic treatment with antihistamines to reduce edema may be helpful. *Armillifer armillatus* and *Porocephalus crotali* of snakes also cause infections in humans, probably as a result of contaminating drinking water with eggs from their feces and not because of ingestion of poorly cooked snake meat. Usually, human infection is noted only at autopsy or by the presence of calcified abdominal or lung objects in radiographs. Treatment is symptomatic.

The most common of the ectoparasite-caused direct injury is scabies, caused by infestation with the human scabies mite (*Sarcoptes scabiei*). A number of different populations of *S. scabiei* have been treated as full species based on their tropism for other animals (including dogs, pigs, sheep, cattle, and goats), but all are morphologically identical. Infestation may occur anywhere in the world. Canine sarcoptic mange is commonly associated with scabies infestations in the owners of the dogs. In either animal or human scabies, transmission is by direct personal contact, and infestations often cluster among groups of people, particularly families. There is little evidence that environments become contaminated; fomites have not been identified.

The female scabies mite burrows beneath the stratum corneum (Fig. 7), leaving behind eggs and feces within a track-like trail. A few dozen eggs are deposited, and these hatch within a week. Larvae form new burrows but may also emerge from the skin and move freely about. Nymphs develop from fed larvae, and they, in turn, develop into the adult male and female. Normal infestations consist of a dozen or two female mites. Nocturnal itching begins within a month of the first infestation, but may begin within a day in previously exposed individuals. Thus, newly exposed individuals, prior to their recognizing an infestation by the presence of itching, may serve to contaminate other individuals. Erythematous papules and vesicles first appear on the webs of fingers and spread to the arms, trunk, and buttocks. The burrows contain granular, highly antigenic feces, which cause both delayed- and immediate-type hypersensitivity reactions. Interestingly, in individuals who are immunocompromised, hundreds of female mites may be found, itching is minimal, but a hyperkeratosis is prominent. Such "crusted" or Norwegian scabies are highly infectious to other people.

Scabies infestations can be easily diagnosed by scraping a newly developed papule (not one that has been scratched) with a scalpel coated with mineral oil. The scrapings in oil may be transferred to a slide and examined by bright-field microscopy at ×100 or ×400 for 300- to 400-μm mites or the smaller black fecal granules. Scabies may be treated with 5% permethrin cream or 1% permethrin rinse (Nix; same as

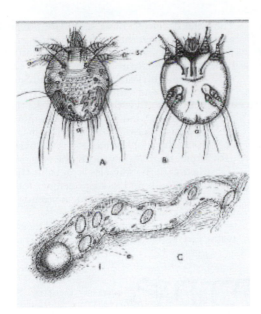
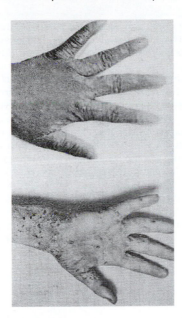

FIGURE 7 Scabies. (Left) Diagram of feeding lesion and adult female mite. A, dorsal view of female mite; B, ventral view; C, feeding lesion within the epidermis. (Right) Chronic scabies affecting the hands. (Reprinted with permission from reference 2.)

is used for head lice). The method of choice until recently was topical lindane (Kwell), but the FDA now suggests the use of permethrin first and lindane only if that fails. Lindane can be neurotoxic to children and small adults.

Demodex folliculorum, the follicle mite, infests virtually everybody. This elongate 500-μm-long mite may be found within follicles on the face, the ear, and breast and are often brought to the attention of a physician because a tweezed eyelash may have a few mites at the base of the shaft. Although they appear to largely be nonpathogenic, the same species causes demodectic mange in dogs and cattle. Pityriasis folliculorum, with small pustules appearing on the forehead, has been attributed to them.

Dust mite allergy (one of many causes of asthma, rhinitis, and atopic dermatitis) is due to inhalation of feces excreted by *Dermatophagoides farinae* or related pyroglyphid mites, which are human commensals that feed on flakes of skin shed from a person. The mites themselves do not infest a person but remain in the environment (usually within bedding or carpets) to feed and develop. About a half gram of skin may be shed from a person each day; one female mite lays one egg a day, for about 2 months; thus, large accumulations of mites may readily develop. The 300- to 400-μm-long mites may be presented by patients as suspects for other nonspecific lesions or sets of signs and symptoms because they may be found in virtually all houses and can be detected if dust is allowed to settle on standing water; the mites float and move and can be seen at ×20. Humidity lower than 60% greatly reduces dust mite infestations, as do periodic vacuuming and washing of bedding and carpets.

Myiasis is the infestation of human or animal tissue by fly larvae, deposited as eggs or first-stage larvae; the larvae develop by feeding on the surrounding tissue, emerge as third-stage larvae, and pupate in the environment. There are three kinds of myiasis with respect to life cycle patterns: obligate, facultative, and accidental. Obligate myiasis reflects the need for larvae to feed well during development because adult flies do not feed, or feed poorly. Botflies comprise the main examples of obligate myiasis. Most botflies

normally infest animals, and thus human botfly infestation by these species is considered zoonotic. Two flies, *Dermatobia hominis* (human botfly) and *Cordylobia anthropophaga* (tumbu fly), are more adapted to humans, as illustrated by their life cycles. The former fly lays its eggs on a transport (phoretic) host such as a mosquito; when the mosquito feeds on a human, the eggs hatch during the course of the blood meal, and the larvae penetrate the skin at the site of the mosquito bite or burrow in on their own. The latter fly is attracted to sweat, urine, or feces, and it oviposits on clothing that has been spread out to dry on the ground or hung up to dry, on areas of cloth that are redolent with such odors, which may remain when primitive clothes washing practices are used. The eggs hatch when placed close to the body, and the larvae burrow into the skin. Thus, any clothing washed in tropical countries without the aid of modern soap powders and dryers should be ironed before being worn.

Facultative myiasis is usually due to infestation by blowflies (*Phormia regina*), green bottle flies (*Lucilia sericata*), and related calliphorids; by flesh flies (*Wohlfahrtia* spp.); or by common houseflies (*Musca domestica*). These flies normally deposit eggs into fecal or other rotting organic material or directly lay eggs into wounds or necrotic tissue, but the larvae may not confine themselves to such resources and may move into healthy tissue.

Accidental myiasis includes the incidental findings of fly larvae, often housefly, under wound dressings or within unusual sites such as the gastrointestinal tract. The rat-tailed maggot (*Eristalis tenax*) is actually a hoverfly (syrphid) that breeds in sewage or dirty water. Eggs may be deposited around the anus during defecation, and the larvae may find their way into the lower gastrointestinal tract or urethra. Drinking unfiltered dirty water might cause temporary infestation of the gut, with larvae surviving into the lower intestine. More often, larvae are found in containers of stool samples that are intended for the clinical laboratory, and are most likely due to oviposition after the sample is taken.

A variety of clinical presentations are evident, depending on the site where the larvae are present. Botflies cause furuncular lesions or migratory integumomyiasis (a serpiginous track may be produced in the skin). Wound myiasis comprises shallow or pocketlike initial lesions that become more deeply invasive. Maggots may invade the nose and accompanying structures, causing nasal or oral myiasis. Maggots may get into the ears, producing aural myiasis. Ophthalmomyiasis is due to external or internal infestation. Enteric, vaginal, or vesicomyiasis is due to invasion of the gut or genitalia. In all presentations, pathology may be due to tissue trauma or local destruction but is more often associated with secondary bacterial infection. On the other hand, many maggots do not promote bacterial infection but, rather, secrete bacteriolytic compounds and have been used as a surgical intervention to debride wounds (10). Sterile *L. sericata* maggots are available by prescription in the United Kingdom, with recommendations for how many "pots" of maggots may be needed for wounds of specific dimensions (http://www.zoobiotic.co.uk/).

Thus, the development of secondary bacterial infection in myiasis may suggest the death of the maggot.

In all cases, treatment is by removal of the maggots, laboriously picking them out using forceps. The maggots causing furuncular myiasis or migratory integumomyiasis have their posterior end visible within the lesion, exposing the spiracular plates that cover their tracheolar breathing apparatus. Although much lore exists on how to best remove such maggots, including "luring" the maggots with bacon or pork fat, the simplest method is to cover the lesion with petrolatum, thereby preventing the maggot from breathing. (Obstruction of the spiracles is probably the mode of action for bacon or pork rind, not a preference for tasty fat.) It will eventually move out enough in an attempt to get air and so may be grasped with forceps.

Identification of maggots can be difficult. The spiracular plates can be diagnostic (Fig. 8) and should be removed

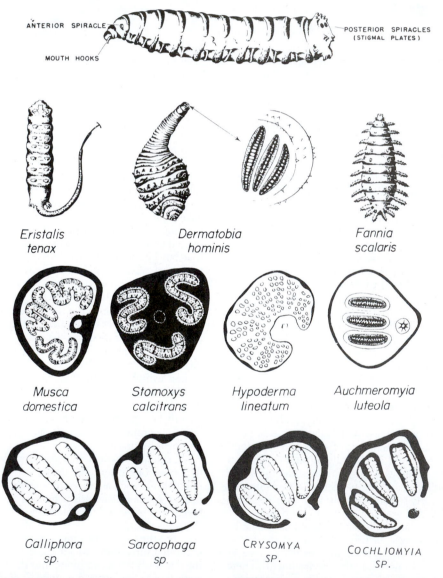

FIGURE 8 Key characters of some myiasis-producing fly larvae. Row 1, mature larva of a muscoid fly (from reference 19). Row 2, larva of *Eristalis tenax*, the rat-tailed maggot; *Dermatobia hominis*, the human botfly (with an enlarged view of a posterior spiracle); and *Fannia scalaris*, the latrine fly. Rows 3 and 4, appearance of posterior spiracles of some species that produce accidental, facultative, or obligatory myiasis. (Source: CDC, Atlanta, GA.)

from the posterior end, mounted on slides in an appropriate mounting medium, and compared with pictorial keys. Often, a live maggot can be reared to pupation on raw meat and the resulting adult fly identified. On the other hand, most myiasis cases presenting in developed countries are the result of tourism, and not knowing the specific identity of the fly would not influence further preventive measures; treatment would be sufficient, and identification would not be necessary other than out of academic curiosity. One important reason for accurately identifying a maggot is for forensic purposes: the developmental rates of the various obligate or facultative myiases have been described as a great aid in assigning time of death for cadavers. The American Board of Forensic Entomology (http://www.research.missouri.edu/entomology/) provides certification for experts in such tasks, and their membership may be consulted should a need for precise identification arise.

Stinging and Biting Resulting in Envenomation

Hymenoptera

Wasps, bees, and ants all belong to the order Hymenoptera, which contains well over 100,000 recognized species. Hymenoptera are minute to medium-size insects with compound eyes, mandibles, and two pairs of transparent wings (although in the ants, wings may be seen on males or females only at certain times of the year). They undergo complete metamorphosis from a grub-like larvae to a pupa. Those of clinical importance are within the Aculeata, particularly the Vespoidea (social and solitary wasps), Apoidea (social and solitary bees), and Formicoidea (ants). Most of the Aculeata have a characteristic constriction between the first and second abdominal segments. These insects have a complex social behavior, with males, females, and worker castes. Workers have a stinging organ, which is used for defending the colony or capturing prey.

Most stings by hymenoptera cause localized reactions, sometimes with extreme pain and resulting in a transient induration with hyperemia. By virtue of their living in large colonies, bees and ants may swarm an intruder, and dozens, if not hundreds, of stings may be sustained. Airway obstruction may result should multiple stings be received on the face or neck. Although the honeybee's agricultural value in pollinating plants greatly exceeds any slight risk due to their stings, African honeybees (*Apis mellifera adansoni*, a subspecies of the regular honeybee; also known as "killer bees"), which were imported into Brazil in the hope that they would be better pollinators, can be dangerous because they are more aggressive than the typical honeybee. Bees differ from wasps and ants in that their stinging apparatus is forcibly torn out during the act of stinging, thereby ensuring the death of individual bees as a result. Wasps and ants may sting multiple times; some fire ants may hang on by their mandibles and repeatedly insert their posteriorly located stinger.

Bee venom has been well characterized and consists of a large amount of a polypeptide (melittin), phospholipase A2, histamine, hyaluronidase, mast cell discharging peptide, and apamin. Histamine appears to be the cause of the acute pain of bee stings.

Bumblebees, paper wasps, yellow jackets, and hornets may all sting, usually because the victim intrudes too near a nest. The most important clinical manifestation of bee or wasp stings is anaphylaxis. Chest tightness, nausea, vertigo, cyanosis, and urticaria may be seen even in individuals who apparently had never previously been exposed. Dozens of people die each year in the United States due to bee sting anaphylaxis.

Ants, on the other hand, rarely pose a risk for anaphylaxis but produce a reaction that may persist for a longer duration. An induration or wheal may be observed immediately after the sting, and a papule may develop that itches or remains irritated for several days. Secondary bacterial infection may ensue. Fire ants (*Solenopsis invicta*) may bite or sting, both modes accompanied by the injection of a venom, an ethyl ketone for the former and various 2,6-dialkypiperidines for the latter. Other ants (the Formicinae) have a venom that is mainly formic acid.

Urticating Caterpillars

Lepidoptera (moths and butterflies) undergo complete development, with the well-known caterpillar and cocoon stages. More than 100,000 species of these familiar insects have been described. Although certain adult moths (in four superfamilies) may imbibe blood or tears, no signs or symptoms are associated with what is evidently an independent evolution of hematophagy. At least eight families of Lepidoptera, however, have caterpillars with urticating hairs, and some of the neotropical species can produce surprisingly severe reactions, including a hemorrhagic syndrome (*Lonomia achelous*, a saturniid moth of the Amazon) due to a fibrinolytic toxin exuding from poison spines (15). More typical are rashes caused by contact with hairs (erucism, or erucic rash). A common shade tree pest, the browntail moth (*Nygmia phaeorrhoea*), in Europe and northeastern North America, liberates tiny barbed hairs when the caterpillar molts. These hairs are blown about by the wind and when skin is exposed, a severe dermatitis results; ingestion or inhalation can also cause significant irritation of the mucosa or bronchospasm. Contact with the eye may induce conjunctivitis. Dermatitis produced by urticating hairs typically comprises itchy, erythematous patches associated with small vesicles and edema. These lesions are only where the hairs have free access to the skin or where contact is made. Use of a masking tape-type lint roller can be very effective in removing urticating hairs, which may or may not be visible.

Scorpions

Scorpions are arachnids with a characteristic crablike appearance. The body consists of the cephalothorax and a segmented abdomen with a segmented tail, which terminates in a prominent stinging apparatus (aculeus). The four pairs of legs include well-defined pincers on the first pair of legs. Scorpions may range in size from 2 to 10 cm. They undergo incomplete development. Of the 1,000 or so species that are known, fewer than 50 have been reported to cause illness with their sting. Scorpions are problems mainly in the warmer climates. The bulbous end of the tail contains muscles that force venom through the stinger. All scorpions are predatory on other arthropods, immobilizing their prey with their venom. Humans are stung by walking barefoot at night, by not shaking their shoes out in the morning in an area where scorpions are endemic, by lifting rocks or logs, or in bedding that is on the floor. The stings cause local pain (probably due to the great biogenic amine content of the venom), edema, discoloration, and hypesthesia. Systemic signs can include shock, salivation, confusion or anxiety, nausea, tachycardia, and tetany. Venom characteristics differ depending on the genus of scorpion: some stimulate parasympathetic nerves and can lead to secondary stimulation of catecholamines, resulting in sympathetic stimulation, which in turn may contribute to respiratory failure (1). Others affect the central nervous system, are hemolytic, or cause local necrosis. Hypersensitivity and anaphylaxis may occur in individuals who are repeatedly exposed.

Treatment is usually symptomatic, although in areas with known dangerous species (the Middle East [*Leiurus* spp., *Buthacus* spp., and *Buthus* spp.], southern Africa [*Parabuthus* spp., *Buthus* spp., and *Uroplectes* spp.], South and Central America [*Tityus* spp.], and the southern United States [*Centruroides* spp.]), quickly getting a pressure bandage on over the sting and immobilizing the limb (if that is where the sting was) would help to prevent venom from traveling via the lymphatics. Lidocaine may be injected directly into the sting to reduce pain. Medical attention should be sought as soon as possible because antivenin, when administered promptly, reduces morbidity. However, antivenin is usually species specific, and without bringing the culprit in for identification, antivenin use would be on a presumptive basis.

Centipedes and Millipedes

The centipedes (class Chilopoda, 2,800 species) and millipedes (class Diplopoda, 8,000 species) are elongate, vermiform arthropods with dozens of segments, each of which bears a pair of legs. Both undergo incomplete development, with larvae looking like miniature adults. "Centipedes" would suggest having 100 segments (and pairs of legs) or fewer; "millipedes," more than 100 and up to 1,000. This simplification is not quite correct, but in general, many legs indicate a millipede, and fewer legs (but more than insects or ticks) indicate a centipede. Other differences are apparent: millipedes are rounded in cross-section, but centipedes are dorsoventrally flattened; millipedes have mouthparts that are ventral and nonpiercing, whereas centipedes have mouthparts that protrude anteriorly and are clearly capable of piercing. Millipedes move slowly, reflecting their mode of life as feeders on detritus. Centipedes are very rapid predators on other arthropods.

The diversity of both millipedes and centipedes is greatest in the tropics, and virtually all those of medical importance are found in warm climates. Millipedes may squirt a noxious, corrosive fluid from pores on their segments. Such fluid may contain benzoquinone, aldehydes, and hydrocyanic acid and cause an immediate burning sensation followed by erythema and edema, even progressing to blistering (3). Most millipedes also have a repugnant smell; both the corrosive fluid and smell tend to protect them from predation. People become exposed when they step on or sleep on millipedes or provoke them (children playing with them are often victims). Treatment consists of washing the affected site as soon as possible to dilute and remove the corrosive fluids, and is symptomatic for the skin lesions and pain. Centipedes have powerful biting mandibles and small fang-like structures (forcipules) situated between them and derived from the first pair of legs that may inject venom. This venom is used to immobilize prey and is also used in defense. Centipede bites occur when people step on or sleep on centipedes or play with them. Envenomation is manifested by local pain and swelling, with proximal lymphadenopathy. Headache, nausea, and anxiety are common. Skin lesions may ulcerate and become necrotic. Death due to centipede bite has been confirmed for only one case, that of a Filipino child who was bitten on the head by a large *Scolopendra* sp. The common house centipede, *Scutigera coleoptrata* of the eastern United States, is commonly found in bathtubs. This hairy-looking, small (5 to 8 cm long) centipede is actually beneficial, preying on roaches and other potential pests

within houses. Its strong mandibles can, however, inflict a painful pinch, and it does have mild venom that produces a bite similar in quality to a bee sting.

Spiders

The order Araneae comprises nearly 30,000 species, but only a fraction of them have any medical importance. Most are very small (0.5 cm or smaller in length), but a few may be as large as a man's hand. Two major suborders are recognized, the Mygalomorphae, in which the fang-tipped chelicerae operate in parallel using an up-and-down strike, and the Araneomorphae, in which the chelicerae operate like insect mandibles, with a side-to-side motion. Spiders have an unsegmented cephalothorax, an abdomen, four pairs of legs, the prominent chelicerae, and spinnerets, specialized organs that secrete the silk for making webs. All spiders are predatory on other arthropods and use their venom to immobilize prey, which are stored live. Spiders rend their prey with their chelicerae and bathe them with a digestion fluid for hours prior to ingestion. Thus, although all spiders have stout chelicerae and can bite, and all spiders have venom with which to immobilize their prey, most are too small to be noticed by humans even if they are bitten. The spiders of main medical interest belong to four groups (8, 14, 32): the funnel web or trapdoor spiders of Australia (*Atrax* and *Hadronyche* spp.), New World and southern African recluse spiders (*Loxosceles* spp.), South American armed spiders (*Phoneutria* spp.), and the cosmopolitan widow spiders (*Latrodectus* spp.). The recluse and widow spiders have been widely transported by humans.

The clinical manifestations and complications of envenomation may differ among the four main spiders, and the syndromes caused by each have been given names that reflect the identity of the spider. With spider bites in general, local pain and erythema occur at the site of the bite, and these may be accompanied by fever, chills, nausea, and joint pain. In loxoscelism, the site of the bite ulcerates and becomes necrotic. Skin may slough, and there may be destruction of the adjacent tissues. Hemolysis, thrombocytopenia, and renal failure may ensue. With latrodectism, phoneutrism, and funnel web spider neurotoxicity, the venoms have a strong neurotoxic action. Muscle rigidity and cramping (similar to acute abdomen) are seen with latrodectism; complications include electrocardiogram abnormalities, hypotension, priapism, and compartment syndrome of the extremities. With phoneutrism, visual disturbances, vertigo, and prostration may occur; complications include hypotension and respiratory paralysis (8). Funnel web spiders induce autonomic nervous system excitation, with muscular twitching, salivation and lacrimation, nausea and vomiting, and diarrhea; fatal respiratory arrest may result from apnea or laryngospasm (28).

Funnel web spider bites require prompt first aid, and the same recommendations could be used for latrodectism or phoneutrism. A compression bandage should be applied over the site of the bite, and the affected limb should be immobilized by splinting with a compression bandage if the bite is on an extremity (standard procedures for snakebite). This may help prevent the venom from moving from the local lymphatics. The patient should seek medical attention as soon as possible for antivenin treatment. Otherwise, treatment is symptomatic with analgesics and antipyretics.

Tarantulas are popular pets and appear fearsome. Fortunately, they are docile and most injuries associated with them are due to their urticating hairs, particularly with respect to conjunctivitis. They do, however, have robust mandibles, and venom and should not be provoked; bites are similar in quality to a bee sting.

Necrotic dermal lesions are often classified as loxoscelism even if the appropriate spiders are not known to be present in the area: only 35 of 216 diagnoses of "brown recluse spider bites" proved to be supported by the minimum evidence for assigning such a specific etiology, namely, the known presence of *Loxosceles reclusa* within the geographic area of exposure (49). Severe reactions to tick bite, or even the erythema migrans of Lyme disease, may be confused with recluse spider bites (29).

Miscellaneous Injury due to Arthropods

Beetles (coleoptera) comprise 40% of all insect species, but even with this great diversity, very few may be harmful. Most injury is related to vesication by secretions containing cantharidin. Hemolymph (blood) of some of these beetles, generally called the blister beetles, also contains this irritant, and thus exposure may be by direct contact with live or dead (crushed) beetles. Cantharidin is the active ingredient of Spanish fly, the alleged aphrodisiac made from pulverized *Lytta vesicatoria*. Ingestion of Spanish fly would irritate the ureter and urethra and cause painful priapism. Overdose or chronic use causes renal tubular necrosis. It is likely that Spanish fly is no longer in demand given the availability of nitric oxide inhibitors.

An unusual group of carabids, the bombardier beetles, spray a boiling hot (100°C) jet of benzoquinone as a defense (13), causing burns and blistering. Blistering is also produced by crushing the staphylinid beetle *Paederus fusca* of Southeast Asia, which contains a toxic alkaloid, pederin.

More commonly, carpet beetles (dermestids), which feed on wool rugs and other animal fur products, are associated with a papulovesicular eruption. In particular, larval dermestids and their hairs or shed skins (exuviae) cause a contact dermatitis.

Water beetles (actually members of the Hemiptera), also known as water skimmers, can inflict strong pinches on unsuspecting toes wading through water.

OTHER INJURY

Delusion or Illusion of Parasitosis

Illusory parasitosis is a condition in which a patient who has a real itch has the mistaken belief that the itch is due to active infestation by irrelevant arthropods. Often the itch is due to a drug reaction, sunburn, detergents, irritating dusts, poison ivy, or even bona fide arthropod bites (among many other potential sources of itch) that were sustained months in the past. Once a patient has been helped to identify the actual cause of the itch, he or she will not persist in blaming an arthropod. In contrast, in delusory parasitosis (also known as Ekbom syndrome), the patient cannot be convinced that the source of discomfort is probably not an arthropod. With some patients, there are no objective lesions but simply an insistence that they are infested. (Although a subset of Morgellons syndrome patients may show what has classically been known as delusional parasitosis, Morgellons syndrome does not necessarily include arthropods as a specific complaint.) Many such patients are highly educated people and can describe their infestation with great detail. However, they rarely produce a specimen, and when they do, it is usually not an arthropod or part thereof. Delusory parasitosis can be a serious illness which can be treated by experienced mental health professionals.

IDENTIFYING SUBMITTED SPECIMENS

For most purposes, identification to the species level (e.g., "this is *Eutrombicula alfreddugesi*") may not provide any more clinically relevant information than identification to a higher taxonomic level ("this is a chigger"). In some cases, simply being able to say "this is definitely an arthropod part, perhaps beetle" may be all the information that is required (in this example, a beetle part may suggest dwarf tapeworm infection or be consistent with urticaria due to the hairs of dermestid beetle larvae, or vesication due to the hot spray of the bombardier beetle). A whole arthropod may be compared with the bauplan diagram to place it within a general group. A classic pictorial key published by the CDC (available from http://www.dpd.cdc.gov/dpdx/HTML/CDProducts.htm), or a simple dichotomous key (Table 3) may be used to narrow the identification down to a known genus of medically important arthropod. Anything more specific usually requires consulting a taxonomic reference or finding an entomologist who can help. Agricultural extension services, university entomology departments, local mosquito or pest control organizations, parasitologists, or local bug collecting enthusiast clubs may all be of help in identifying a specimen and usually do not charge out of professional courtesy. (Note that few such entities are Clinical Laboratory Improvement Amendments certified, and thus a fee for their services is problematic.)

In some cases, a patient insists that an arthropod specimen be tested for the presence of an infectious agent. This is particularly common in areas where Lyme disease is endemic. The value of such a practice is dubious, other than for psychologically satisfying the patient's demand. Some commercial laboratories test for the presence of Lyme disease spirochetes using a PCR assay, but given that the prevalence of infection in the vector may range from 15 to 70%, a positive test is likely. Furthermore, at least with deer ticks, other agents such as those causing granulocytic ehrlichiosis and babesiosis may be present but not revealed by tick testing for Lyme disease spirochetes. Other tick species also are likely to have guilds of microbes as opposed to a sole agent (47). In any event, by the time a PCR result is rendered, the patient may already be experiencing signs and symptoms. For Lyme disease, and likely for ehrlichiosis, postexposure prophylaxis may be provided in the form of two doses of a tetracycline, if the patient remains unconvinced.

The most important variable in determining the riskiness of a tick bite is how long the tick has fed (Fig. 9). If a deer tick is attached for no more than 24 h, regardless of whether it is demonstrated to be infected with Lyme disease spirochetes, *Babesia microti*, or the agent of granulocytic ehrlichiosis, the likelihood of an infectious dose of organisms being transmitted is very small. The biological basis for this "grace period" is a phenomenon known as reactivation, wherein pathogens within ticks require a period of replication after emerging from a period of dormancy that they enter during the long interstadial period between blood meals (25). Reactivation was first described for the agent of Rocky Mountain spotted fever, which attains infectivity within tick salivary glands only

TABLE 3 Key to the common arthropod classes, subclasses, and orders of medical importance, adult stages[a]

1.	Three or four pairs of legs [2]
	Five or more pairs of legs [22]
2.	Three pairs of legs with antennae (**insects: class Insecta**) [3]
	Four pairs of legs without antennae (**spiders, ticks, mites, scorpions: class Arachnida**) [20]
3.	Wings present, well developed [4]
	Wings absent or rudimentary [12]
4.	One pair of wings (**flies, mosquitoes, midges: order Diptera**) [5]
	Two pairs of wings [6]
5.	Wings with scales (**mosquitoes: order Diptera**)
	Wings without scales (**other flies: order Diptera**)
6.	Mouthparts adapted for sucking, with an elongate proboscis [7]
	Mouthparts adapted for chewing, without an elongate proboscis [8]
7.	Wings densely covered with scales, proboscis coiled (**butterflies and moths: order Lepidoptera**)
	Wings not covered with scales, proboscis not coiled but directed backward (**bedbugs and kissing bugs: order Hemiptera**)
8.	Both pairs of wings membranous, similar in structure, although size may vary [9]
	Front pair of wings leathery or shell-like, serving as covers for the second pair [10]
9.	Both pairs of wings similar in size (**termites: order Isoptera**)
	Hind wings much smaller than front wings (**wasps, hornets, and bees: order Hymenoptera**)
10.	Front wings horny or leathery, without distinct veins, meeting in a straight line down the middle [11]
	Front wings leathery or paperlike, with distinct veins, usually overlapping in the middle (**cockroaches: order Dictyoptera**)
11.	Abdomen with prominent cerci or forceps; wings shorter than abdomen (**earwigs: order Dermaptera**)
	Abdomen without prominent cerci or forceps; wings covering abdomen (**beetles: order Coleoptera**)
12.	Abdomen with three long terminal tails (**silverfish and firebrats: order Thysanura**)
	Abdomen without three long terminal tails [13]
13.	Abdomen with narrow waist (**ants: order Hymenoptera**)
	Abdomen without narrow waist [14]
14.	Abdomen with prominent pair of cerci or forceps (**earwigs: order Dermaptera**)
	Abdomen without cerci or forceps [15]
15.	Body flattened laterally, antennae small, fitting into grooves in side of head (**fleas: order Siphonaptera**)
	Body flattened dorsoventrally, antennae projecting from side of head, not fitting into grooves [16]
16.	Antennae with nine or more segments [17]
	Antennae with three to five segments [18]
17.	Pronotum covering head (**cockroaches: order Dictyoptera**)
	Pronotum not covering head (**termites: order Isoptera**)
18.	Mouthparts consisting of tubular joined beak; three- to five-segmented tarsi (**bedbugs: order Hemiptera**)
	Mouthparts retracted into head or of the chewing type; one- or two-segmented tarsi [19]
19.	Mouthparts retracted into the head; adapted for sucking blood (**sucking lice: order Anopleura**)
	Mouthparts of the chewing type (**chewing lice: order Mallophaga**)
20.	Body oval, consisting of a single saclike region (**ticks and mites: subclass Acari**)
	Body divided into two distinct regions, a cephalothorax and an abdomen [21]
21.	Abdomen joined to the cephalothorax by a slender waist; abdomen with segmentation indistinct or absent; stinger absent (**spiders: subclass Araneae**)
	Abdomen broadly joined to the cephalothorax; abdomen distinctly segmented, ending with a stinger (**scorpions: subclass Scorpiones**)
22.	Five to nine pairs of legs or swimmerets; one or two pairs of antennae; principally aquatic organisms (**copepods, crabs, and crayfish: class Crustacea**)
	Ten or more pairs of legs or swimmerets absent; one pair of antennae present; terrestrial organisms [23]
23.	Body segments each with only one pair of legs (**centipedes: class Chilopoda**)
	Body segments each with two pairs of legs (**millipedes: class Diplopoda**)

[a]Data from references 11 and 17.

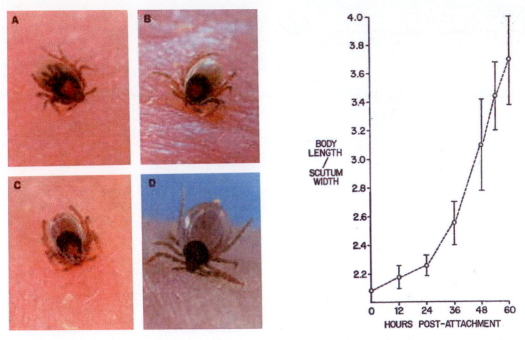

FIGURE 9 Gradual engorgement of feeding ixodid ticks. (Left) Four-day feeding sequence of nymphal *Ixodes ricinus*. (Reprinted from reference 30 with permission from Elsevier.) (Right) Scutal index of engorgement for *Ixodes dammini*. (Reprinted from reference 35 with permission of the American Society of Tropical Medicine and Hygiene.)

after 12 to 18 h of exposure to a host. Reactivation is probably a general phenomenon with most ixodid (hard) tick-transmitted agents, the only known exceptions being the viruses causing tick-borne encephalitis and the related Powassan fever, in which transmission is thought to be instantaneous with attachment.

Estimating the degree of engorgement may provide more of an index of individual risk than actual presence or absence of infection. A simple measurement may be made with deer ticks and might be tried for other species of ticks. The scutal index is the ratio of the length of the scutum, the dark shield on the dorsum of the tick, to the length of the tick from tip of the mouthparts to the caudal edge of the tick. A scutal index of >2.5 suggests that a deer tick has been attached for more than 24 h, and therefore transmission is likely (35). Such a finding might prompt a physician to provide prophylactic antibiotics, which would effectively abort Lyme disease or human granulocytic ehrlichiosis. Although such prophylaxis would not prevent babesiosis, note that of the agents transmitted by deer ticks, *B. microti* requires the greatest duration of attachment for infectivity, probably relating to the requirement for sporogony during attachment.

Much progress has been made in a universal bar coding system for identifying animals by means of DNA sequences (38). In particular, the 5′ end of the mitochondrial cytochrome *c* oxidase subunit I (COI), usually a 648-bp portion, is used as a PCR target and the nucleotide sequence that is obtained from the amplification product can be compared to a large online database (Barcode of Life Data [BOLD] Systems [http://www.boldsystems.org/views/login.php]). Most species of

animals contain unique sequences in their COI genes and thus can be discriminated from other related species. Nearly 750,000 sequences have been accessioned in the BOLD database. For the phylum Arthropoda, barcode sequences exist for all 16 classes; for Insecta, all 30 orders are represented. Accordingly, virtually any putative arthropod sample may be identified to order level, and possibly to family or genus level, by extracting its DNA and amplifying the COI gene. Assuming that the equipment is available (thermal cycler, gel electrophoresis, pipettors, and other materials common to molecular biology laboratories), such an identification might cost on the order of $150 to $200 (5 h of technician time, PCR reagents, commercial rate for sequencing 300 bp), with a few days' turnaround (usually 24 to 48 h minimum from submission of the DNA to receipt of the sequencing chromatogram is required for DNA sequencing). A simple DNA extraction technique ("HOTSHOT," which uses hot sodium hydroxide and Tris neutralization) may be used on most samples to prepare for PCR analysis (48). Many forensic or clinical samples may contain degraded DNA; museum protocols (31) for amplifying an informative portion of the COI gene would be appropriate. The advantage to the bar coding approach is that the method is not subjective and does not require extensive training and expertise for morphological identification; anyone with general expertise in molecular biology may be engaged. Classically based methods, however, require little more than a microscope, can be virtually instantaneous, and may be a professional courtesy without a fee.

REFERENCES

1. **Amitai, Y.** 1998. Clinical manifestations and management of scorpion envenomation. *Public Health Rep.* **26:**257–263.

2. **Ash, J. E., and S. Spitz.** 1945. *Pathology of Tropical Diseases.* W. B. Saunders, Philadelphia, PA.

3. **Attygalle, A. B., S. C. Xu, J. Meinwald, and T. Eisner.** 1993. Defensive secretion of the millipede Floridobolus penneri. *J. Nat. Prod.* **56:**1700–1706.

4. **Audy, J. R.** 1968. *Red Mites and Typhus.* Athlone Press, University of London, London, United Kingdom.

5. **Balashov, Y. S.** 1972. Bloodsucking ticks (Ixodoidea)—vectors of diseases of man and animals. *Misc. Publ. Entomol. Soc. Am.* **8:**161–376.

6. **Barber, M. A.** 1914. Cockroaches and ants as carriers of the vibrios of Asiatic cholera. *Philippine J. Sci. Ser. B* **9:**1.

7. **Bequaert, J. C.** 1946. The ticks or Ixodoidea of the northeastern United States and eastern Canada. *Entomol. Am.* **XXV:**73–232.

8. **Bucherl, W.** 1969. Biology and venoms of the most important South American spiders of the genera Phoneutria, Loxosceles, Lycosa, and Latrodectus. *Am. Zool.* **9:**157–159.

9. **Buxton, P. A.** 1955. *The Natural History of Tsetse Flies.* H. K. Lewis, London, United Kingdom.

10. **Chernin, E.** 1986. Surgical maggots. *South. Med. J.* **79:**1143.

11. **Communicable Disease Center.** 1966. *Pictorial Keys: Arthropods, Reptiles, Birds, and Mammals of Public Health Significance.* Communicable Disease Center, Atlanta, GA.

12. **Curran, K. L., and D. Fish.** 1989. Increased risk of Lyme disease for cat owners. *N. Engl. J. Med.* **320:**183.

13. **Dean, J., A. D. Aneshansley, H. Edgerton, and T. Eisner.** 1990. Defensive spray of the bombardier beetle: a biological pulse jet. *Science* **248:**1219–1221.

14. **Diaz, J. H.** 2004. The evolving global epidemiology, syndromic classification, management, and prevention of spider bites. *Am. J. Trop. Med. Hyg.* **71:**239–250.

15. **Diaz, J. H.** 2005. The evolving global epidemiology, syndromic classification, management, and prevention of caterpillar envenomation. *Am. J. Trop. Med. Hyg.* **72:**347–357.

16. **Garcia, L. S.** 2007. *Diagnostic Medical Parasitology,* 5th ed. ASM Press, Washington, DC.

17. **Goddard, J.** 1996. *Physician's Guide to Arthropods of Medical Importance,* 2nd ed. CRC Press, Inc., Boca Raton, FL.

18. **Goddard, J., and R. deShazo.** 2009. Bed bugs (Cimex lectularius) and clinical consequences of their bites. *JAMA* **301:**1358–1366.

19. **Hegner, R., F. M. Root, D. L. Augustine, and C. G. Huff.** 1938. *Parasitology, with Special Reference to Man and Domesticated Animals.* Appleton Century Inc., New York, NY.

20. **Herms, W. B.** 1939. *Medical Entomology,* 3rd ed. Macmillan, New York, NY.

21. **Hewitt, C. G.** 1910. *The Housefly.* University Press, Manchester, United Kingdom.

22. **Huebner, R. J., P. Stamps, and C. Armstrong.** 1946. Rickettsialpox—a newly recognized rickettsial disease. I. Isolation of the etiological agent. *Public Health Rep.* **61:**1605–1614.

23. **Jones, B. R.** 1975. The prevention of blindness from trachoma. *Trans. Ophthalmol. Soc. U. K.* **95:**16.

24. **Jupp, P. G., and S. F. Lyons.** 1987. Experimental assessment of bedbugs (Cimex lectularius and Cimex hemipterus) and mosquitoes (Aedes aegypti formosus) as vectors of human immunodeficiency virus. *AIDS* **1:**171–174.

25. **Katavolos, P., P. M. Armstrong, J. E. Dawson, and S. R. Telford III.** 1998. Duration of tick attachment required for transmission of human granulocytic ehrlichiosis. *J. Infect. Dis.* **177:**1422–1425.

26. **Lavrov, D. V., W. M. Brown, and J. L. Boore.** 2004. Phylogenetic position of the Pentastomida and (pan) crustacean relationships. *Proc. R. Soc. Lond. Ser. B* **271:**537–544.

27. **Marquardt, W. C., W. C. Black IV, J. E. Freier, H. H. Hagedorn, J. Hemingway, S. Higgs, A. A. James, B. Kondratieff, and C. G. Moore.** 2005. *Biology of Disease Vectors,* 2nd ed. Elsevier Academic Press, Burlington, MA.

28. **Masina, S., and K. W. Broady.** 1999. Tick paralysis: development of a vaccine. *Int. J. Parasitol.* **29:**535–541.

29. **Masters, E. J., and L. E. King, Jr.** 1994. Differentiating loxoscelism from Lyme disease. *Emerg. Med.* **26:**47–49.

30. **Matuschka, F. R., and A. Spielman.** 1993. Risk of infection from and treatment of tick bite. *Lancet* **342:**529.

31. **Meusnier, I., G. A. C. Singer, J. F. Landry, D. A. Hickey, P. D. N. Hebert, and M. Hajibabaei.** 2008. A universal DNA mini-barcode for biodiversity analysis. *BMC Genomics* **9:**214. doi:10.1186/1471-2164-9-214.

32. **Miller, M. K., I. M. Whyte, J. White, and P. M. Keir.** 2000. Clinical features and management of Hadronyche envenomation in man. *Toxicon* **38:**409–427.

33. **Nuttall, G. H., and C. Warburton.** 1908. *Ticks, a Monograph of the Ixodoidea. Part I, Argasidae.* Cambridge University Press, Cambridge, United Kingdom.

34. **Palma, R. L.** 1991. Ancient head lice found on wooden comb from Antinoe, Egypt. *J. Egyptian Archaeol.* **77:**194.

35. **Piesman, J., and A. Spielman.** 1980. Human babesiosis on Nantucket Island: prevalence of Babesia microti in ticks. *Am. J. Trop. Med. Hyg.* **29:**742–746.

36. **Pollack, R. J., A. Kiszewski, and A. Spielman.** 2000. Overdiagnosis and consequent mismanagement of head louse infestations in North America. *Pediatr. Infect. Dis. J.* **19:**689–693.

37. **Pung, O. J., C. W. Banks, D. N. Jones, and M. W. Krissinger.** 1995. Trypanosoma cruzi in wild raccoons, opossums, and triatomine bugs in southeast Georgia. *J. Parasitol.* **81:**324–326.

38. **Ratnasingham, S., and P. D. N. Hebert.** 2007. BOLD: the Barcoding of Life Data System. *Mol. Ecol. Notes.* doi:10.1111/j.1471-8286.2006.01678.x.

39. **Ribeiro, J. M., G. T. Makoul, J. Levine, D. R. Robinson, and A. Spielman.** 1985. Antihemostatic, antiinflammatory, and immunosuppressive properties of the saliva of a tick, Ixodes dammini. *J. Exp. Med.* **161:**332–344.

40. **Ribeiro, J. M. C.** 1995. Blood feeding arthropods: live syringes or invertebrate pharmacologists? *Infect. Agents Dis.* **4:**143–152.

41. **Rich, S. M., D. A. Caporale, S. R. Telford III, T. D. Kocher, D. L. Hartl, and A. Spielman.** 1995. Distribution of Ixodes ricinus-like ticks in eastern North America. *Proc. Natl. Acad. Sci. USA* **92:**6284–6288.

42. **Riley, J.** 1986. The biology of pentastomids. *Adv. Parasitol.* **25:**45–148.

43. **Spielman, A., and P. A. Rossignol.** 1984. Insect vectors, p. 167–183. *In* K. S. Warren and A. A. F. Mahmoud (ed.), *Tropical and Geographical Medicine.* McGraw-Hill, New York, NY.

44. **Spielman, A., and M. D'Antonio.** 2001. *Mosquito: a Natural History of Our Most Persistent and Deadly Foe.* Hyperion Books, New York, NY.

45. **Steere, A. C.** 1994. Lyme disease: a growing threat to urban populations. *Proc. Natl. Acad. Sci. USA* **91:**2378–2383.

46. **Telford, S. R., III.** 1998. Ixodes dammini epidemiologically justified. *Emerg. Infect. Dis.* **4:**132–133.

47. **Telford, S. R., III, and H. K. Goethert.** 2004. Emerging tickborne infections: rediscovered and better characterised, or truly new? *Parasitology* **129:**S301–S327.

48. **Truett, G. E., J. A. Walker, A. A. Truett, R. L. Mynatt, P. Heeger, et al.** 2000. Preparation of PCR-quality DNA with hot sodium hydroxide and tris (HotSHOT). *BioTechniques* **29:**52–54.

49. **Vetter, R. S., P. E. Cushing, R. L. Crawford, and L. A. Royce.** 2003. Diagnoses of brown recluse spider bites (loxoscelism) greatly outnumber actual verifications of the spider in four western American states. *Toxicon* **42:**413–418.

50. **Ward, R., J. L. Melnick, and D. M. Horstmann.** 1945. Poliomyelitis virus in fly-contaminated food collected at an epidemic. *Science* **101:**491.

51. **Watt, J., and D. R. Lindsay.** 1948. Diarrheal disease control studies. I. Effect of fly control in a high morbidity area. *Public Health Rep.* **63:**1319.

52. **Weiman, D.** 1970. Trypanosomiasis in monkeys and man in Malaysia. *Southeast Asian J. Trop. Med. Public Health* **1:**11.

53. **Woodward, T. E., and B. A. Cunha.** 2000. Rocky Mountain spotted fever, p. 121–138. *In* B. A. Cunha (ed.), *Tickborne Infectious Diseases: Diagnosis and Management.* Marcel Dekker, New York, NY.

54. **Zeidner, N., M. L. Mbow, M. Dolan, R. Massung, E. Baca, and J. Piesman.** 1997. Effects of Ixodes scapularis and Borrelia burgdorferi on modulation of the host immune response: induction of a TH2 cytokine response in Lyme disease-susceptible (C3H/HeJ) mice but not in disease-resistant (BALB/c) mice. *Infect. Immun.* **65:**3100–3106.

55. **Zinsser, H.** 1942. *Rats, Lice and History,* 4th ed. George Routledge, London, United Kingdom.

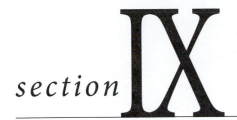

section IX

ANTIPARASITIC AGENTS AND SUSCEPTIBILITY TEST METHODS

VOLUME EDITORS: JAMES H. JORGENSEN AND DAVID W. WARNOCK

SECTION EDITOR: GARY W. PROCOP

Antiparasitic Agents

KARIN LEDER AND PETER F. WELLER

147

There are a number of effective antiprotozoal and anthelmintic drugs currently available. These antiparasitic agents are important both for therapy of individual patients and for control of parasitic infections at the community level. Large-scale chemotherapy is reducing transmission, morbidity, and mortality of infections including lymphatic filariasis, onchocerciasis, schistosomiasis, and infection with intestinal nematodes. However, the lack of financial incentives to manufacture existing drugs or to develop new agents is a major limitation to the range of current and future antiparasitic chemotherapies. Emerging resistance amongst parasites, a lack of effective antiparasitic vaccines, and the enormous burden of disease worldwide also pose challenges to the effective management of parasitic infections.

This chapter focuses on the mechanisms of action, pharmacology, clinical utility, and adverse effects of common first-line antiparasitic therapies and newer drug alternatives. Most helminth infections in humans can be treated with one of five drugs, namely, albendazole, mebendazole, praziquantel, ivermectin, and diethylcarbamazine (DEC), so these five drugs are reviewed in detail. A newer agent, nitazoxanide, which has both anthelmintic and antiprotozoal activity, is also discussed. Other major antiprotozoal drugs, including those used for malaria, gastrointestinal protozoal infection, leishmaniasis, and trypanosomiasis, are also reviewed. However, an exhaustive list of all antiparasitic drugs is not included. Specifically, we have excluded discussion regarding agents without a first-line indication or that are recommended only in special situations, such as furazolidone in children or paromomycin in pregnant women. Additionally, antibacterial and antifungal agents that can also be used for treatment of protozoal infections, such as the 5-nitroimidazoles, trimethoprim-sulfamethoxazole, azithromycin, and amphotericin, are not discussed in detail here, but their general indications for parasitic infections are shown in Tables 1 and 2. Resistance to antiparasitic agents and drug susceptibility testing are dealt with in separate chapters.

ANTHELMINTIC AGENTS

Benzimidazoles

The benzimidazoles are antiparasitic agents with a broad spectrum of activity against many helminthic and certain protozoal infections. All members of the benzimidazole class have in common a bicyclic ring system in which benzene has been inserted. Mebendazole and albendazole, both of which are synthetic agents, are the most widely used drugs of this class. Mebendazole is 5-benzoyl-2-benzimidazole carbamic acid, and albendazole is methyl 5-(propylthio)-2-benzimidazole carbamate. The low cost, high efficacy, and ease of administration of these two agents have led to their widespread use for many human parasitic infections. Major indications for their use are shown in Tables 3 and 4. Whereas mebendazole has been approved for treatment of multiple nematode infections by the U.S. Food and Drug Administration (FDA), albendazole is used preferentially as first-line treatment for many parasite infections but is nevertheless considered investigational and given as a "nonapproved indication" in all cases except when used as treatment for hydatid infections and neurocysticercosis (5).

Other members of this drug class include flubendazole, thiabendazole, and triclabendazole. Flubendazole, a para-fluoro analogue of mebendazole, has the same mechanism of action as mebendazole and albendazole. It has been licensed in Europe but not in the United States. Thiabendazole is 2-(4-thiazolyl)-1H-benzimidazole. Thiabendazole has similar mechanisms of action to those of the other benzimidazoles, but it is frequently associated with side effects and has largely been replaced by other anthelmintic agents. It is still used topically for treatment of cutaneous larva migrans. Triclabendazole is a relatively new imidazole derivative that has been used as a veterinary agent for many years. The exact mechanism of action is unknown, but it is thought to act on microtubules, causing decreased parasite motility. It is the drug of choice for fascioliasis (19) and is also an alternative to praziquantel for therapy of paragonimiasis and intestinal flukes. It is well tolerated, and few significant adverse effects have been described, but it is not recommended for use during pregnancy because of insufficient safety data. It is considered investigational by the U.S. FDA and is not widely available. These three agents are not discussed further.

Mechanism of action. The antiparasitic activity of albendazole and mebendazole results mainly from their ability to bind to a cytoskeletal protein of parasites called β-tubulin, thereby inhibiting the polymerization of tubulin into microtubules (64). The disruption of microtubule synthesis within parasitic intestinal cells results in decreased

2277

TABLE 1 Treatment of major protozoal infections[a]

Organism or disease	Primary agent used for treatment	Alternative agents
Intestinal protozoa		
Entamoeba histolytica	Invasive trophozoites: metronidazole	Tinidazole
	Luminal agent: iodoquinol	Alternative luminal agents: diloxanide furoate, paromomycin
Babesia species	Clindamycin plus quinine	Atovaquone plus azithromycin
Balantidum coli	Tetracycline	Metronidazole, iodoquinol
Crytosporidium parvum	Nitazoxanide	
Cyclospora cayatatensis	Trimethoprim-sulfamethoxazole	
Dientamoeba fragilis	Tetracycline	Iodoquinol, paromomycin, metronidazole
Giardia lamblia	Metronidazole	Tinidazole, nitazoxanide, quinacrine, albendazole, furazolidone, paromomycin
Isospora belli	Trimethoprim-sulfamethoxazole	
Microsporidium species	Albendazole (*Encephalitozoon intestinalis* responds better than *Enterocytozoon bieneusi*)	
Other protozoa		
Amebic meningoencephalitis	Amphotericin B	
Leishmania species	Pentavalent antimonial	Miltefosine, pentamidine, amphotericin B, liposomal amphotericin B
Malaria		
Plasmodium vivax and *P. ovale*	Chloroquine plus primaquine	
Plasmodium falciparum	Artemisinin derivative or (Malarone) or quinine sulfate plus doxycycline or plus clindamycin	
Plasmodium malariae	Chloroquine	
Toxoplasma gondii	Pyrimethamine plus sulfadiazine	Pyrimethamine plus clindamycin
Trichomonas vaginalis	Metronidazole	Tinidazole
Trypanosoma brucei species (African trypanosomiasis)	Early: suramin or eflornithine	Pentamidine
	Late: melarsoprol	
Trypanosoma cruzi (American trypanosomiasis)	Nifurtimox	Benznidazole

[a]Adapted from reference 5.

absorptive function. In addition, mebendazole and albendazole directly inhibit glucose absorption by parasites, leading to a depletion of parasite glycogen stores (41, 43). Parasites therefore have insufficient energy sources for formation of ATP, without which they are unable to reproduce or survive. Although tubulin is also present in mammalian hosts, the benzimidazoles bind to parasite tubulin with an affinity that is hundreds of times greater than that for mammalian tubulin, thereby causing minimal mammalian toxicity.

Pharmacokinetics. Benzimidazoles are poorly soluble in water and therefore are not well absorbed following oral administration. Although this limits their activity against tissue-dwelling parasites, it contributes to their minimal toxicity and to their efficacy in the treatment of many intestinal helminthic infections (26). Less than 10% of mebendazole is absorbed after oral administration. It is metabolized in the liver to inactive compounds, eliminated in the bile, and excreted predominantly in the feces. It is 95% protein bound in plasma, and its serum half-life is 2.5 to 5.5 h. Levels in serum are markedly variable between individuals, but concentrations in tissue and in echinococcal cysts tend to be low (35).

The oral bioavailability of albendazole is also poor, with <10% absorption following an oral dose (71). Administration of albendazole with a fatty meal markedly improves bioavailability. It is rapidly metabolized in the liver, and concentrations of the parent drug in plasma are negligible. However, its primary metabolite, albendazole sulfoxide,

also has anthelmintic activity (13). This results in a higher efficacy of albendazole than that of mebendazole for most indications. Albendazole sulfoxide is 70% protein bound and is widely distributed throughout the body. Peak concentrations of albendazole sulfoxide in plasma show great intersubject variability, ranging from 0.45 to 2.96 mg/liter following a single dose of 15 mg/kg of body weight (56). Albendazole induces enzymes of the cytochrome P450 system responsible for its metabolism. Cimetidine and dexamethasone both raise drug levels (55). Albendazole sulfoxide has been detected in urine, bile, liver, cyst fluid, and cerebrospinal fluid (CSF). Levels in plasma are 3- to 10-fold and 2- to 4-fold higher than those in cyst fluid and CSF, respectively (77, 78). Albendazole sulfoxide has a half-life of approximately 9 h. It is oxidized further to inactive compounds such as albendazole sulfone and is excreted in the urine.

Neither mebendazole nor albendazole is dialyzable. No dosage adjustment is required for individuals with renal impairment, but a reduction in dose should be considered if there is significant hepatic insufficiency. Benzimidazoles are not available as intravenous formulations.

Spectrum of activity. The benzimidazoles are effective against adult worms and developing helminthic embryos. Albendazole and mebendazole have similar and broad ranges of activity (Tables 3 and 4). Both drugs have good efficacy against many common intestinal nematode infections, including ascariasis, trichuriasis, enterobiasis, and

TABLE 2 Treatment of major helminthic infections[a]

Organism or disease[b]	Primary agent used for treatment	Alternative agents
Nematodes		
Ancylostoma caninum (eosinophilic enterocolitis)	Albendazole	Mebendazole, pyrantel pamoate
Angiostrongylus species	Mebendazole	
Ascaris lumbricoides	Albendazole	Mebendazole, pyrantel pamoate, ivermectin, nitazoxanide
Capillaria species	Mebendazole	Albendazole
Cutaneous larva migrans	Albendazole	Ivermectin, topical thiabendazole
Enterobius vermicularis	Albendazole	Mebendazole, pyrantel pamoate
Filariasis (*Wuchereria bancrofti, Brugia malayi*)	Diethylcarbamazine with or without albendazole or ivermectin	
Gnathostoma species	Albendazole	Ivermectin, surgical removal
Hookworm	Albendazole	Mebendazole, pyrantel pamoate
Loa loa	Diethylcarbamazine with or without albendazole or ivermectin	
Onchocerca volvulus	Ivermectin	
Strongyloides stercoralis	Ivermectin	Thiabendazole, albendazole
Toxocara species (visceral larva migrans)	Albendazole	Mebendazole
Trichinella spiralis	Mebendazole	Albendazole
Trichostrongylus species	Albendazole	Mebendazole, pyrantel pamoate
Trichuris trichiura	Mebendazole	Albendazole, ivermectin, nitazoxanide
Cestodes		
Cysticercosis	Albendazole	Praziquantel
Dipylidium caninum	Praziquantel	Niclosamide
Diphyllobothrium latum	Praziquantel	Niclosamide
Echinococcus species	Albendazole	Praziquantel
Hymenolepis nana	Praziquantel	Nitazoxanide
Taenia saginata	Praziquantel	Niclosamide
Taenia solium	Praziquantel	Niclosamide
Trematodes		
Clonorchis sinensis	Praziquantel	Albendazole
Fasciola hepatica	Triclabendazole	Nitazoxanide, bithionol
Intestinal flukes	Praziquantel	
Metorchis conjunctus	Praziquantel	
Opisthorchis viverrini	Praziquantel	
Paragonimus species	Praziquantel	Bithionol
Schistosoma species	Praziquantel	*Schistosoma mansoni*: oxamniquine[c]

[a]Adapted from reference 5.
[b]This is not an exhaustive list of all possible parasitic infections, but commonly encountered parasites are included.
[c]No longer manufactured and/or problems with availability.

hookworm infections. Three-day regimens of mebendazole and 1 to 3 days of albendazole are generally recommended for therapy of individual patients (59). A single dose of either drug is often used for mass or targeted community treatment of intestinal nematodes in areas of endemicity. Albendazole is preferred in most instances, but the efficacy of albendazole against very heavy infections with *Trichuris trichiura* remains questionable, and mebendazole may be preferable in this circumstance. The reported curative efficacies of both drugs for different parasitic infections vary according to the baseline intensity of infection in the patient, geographic location, diagnostic tests employed, and duration of follow-up posttreatment.

Mebendazole and albendazole also have activity against other nematode infections, including trichostrongyliasis, capillariasis, trichinellosis, gnathostomiasis, toxocariasis, and cutaneous larva migrans. Additionally, albendazole is increasingly being used in combination with either DEC or ivermectin for treatment of Bancroftian or Brugian filariasis and loiasis; it is particularly useful for these infections as part of a single-dose regimen for mass chemotherapy programs. Although albendazole displays some efficacy against *Strongyloides stercoralis*, ivermectin shows higher cure rates and is the recommended treatment of choice.

Both mebendazole and albendazole also show activity against certain cestode infections. Albendazole is again preferred because of its more favorable pharmacokinetics, and it is now considered the drug of choice for medical management or adjunctive treatment of hydatid disease due to *Echinococcus granulosus*. Prolonged albendazole therapy (minimum of 10 years) can also be used for inoperable alveolar echinococcosis or as adjuvant therapy for patients with *Echinococcus multilocularis* infection. Additionally, albendazole is used for treatment of parenchymal neurocysticercosis. It should be noted that despite its anticysticercal activity, controversy still exists about the exact indications for therapy.

TABLE 3 Major indications for albendazole[a]

Indication	Usual dose	Reported efficacy
Echinococcus granulosis	400 mg twice daily, usually a minimum of 3–6 mo	Clinical cure, as evidenced by cyst disappearance in one-third of recipients and improvement in radiological appearance in an additional 30–50%
Cysticercosis	400 mg twice daily, usually for 8 days (8–30 days)	75–95% of parenchymal cysts destroyed and 40–70% of patients show resolution of all active cysts, but unclear if beneficial over placebo
Ascaris lumbricoides	Single 400-mg dose	Median cure rates of 95–97% and egg reduction rates of 99–100%
Cutaneous larva migrans	400 mg daily for 3 days	No large clinical trials; generally reserved for those with severe or disseminated infection
Enterobius vermicularis	400 mg dose, repeat in 2 wk	Cure rate close to 100%
Hookworm	Single 400-mg dose	70–95% cure rate and 85–100% egg reduction rate
Microsporidiosis	400 mg twice daily, usually for 2–4 wk	Variable efficacy (related to species of pathogen and immune function of host)
Trichuris trichiura	Single 400-mg dose	Cure rate of 35–70% and egg reduction rate of 70–90% (3 days of therapy gives higher cure rates in heavy infections, but mebendazole is the preferred agent for treatment)
Toxocariasis	400 mg twice daily for 5 days	No large clinical trials
Lymphatic filariasis	Single 400-mg dose	Microfilaremia reduced by 98–99% for prolonged periods when administered in combination with DEC or ivermectin; prolonged high doses also have a macrofilaricidal effect
Loa loa	Single 400-mg dose	No microfilaricidal effect, but partial macrofilaricidal effect with sterilization and/or death of adult worms
Giardia lamblia	400 mg daily for 5 days	Cure rate of 97%

[a]Adapted from reference 5.

Neither mebendazole nor albendazole is commonly used for trematode infections, although some activity has been reported against opisthorchiasis, chlonorchiasis, and echinostomiasis (52, 67, 98).

Although considered primarily an anthelmintic agent, albendazole is also an alternative agent for giardiasis. Additionally, albendazole has activity in microsporidial infections, particularly those caused by *Encephalitozoon hellem*, *Encephalitozoon cuniculi*, and *Encephalitozoon intestinalis*.

Adverse effects. Adverse effects following short courses of the benzimidazoles mebendazole and albendazole are infrequent and generally mild. Transient abdominal pain, nausea, and diarrhea may develop. Headache, dizziness, insomnia, and allergic phenomena are also reported. With prolonged high-dose therapy, such as for echinococcosis, transient and reversible elevations of serum transaminases occur in 1 to 5% of recipients. Occasionally, alopecia (<1%) and reversible leukopenia (<1%) are seen. Discontinuation of therapy is infrequently needed, but a recent death related to albendazole-induced pancytopenia has been described (89).

When mebendazole (pregnancy category C) has been used by pregnant women, the incidence of spontaneous abortions or fetal malformations has not been greater than the background population rate. There are also no reports of teratogenicity from albendazole (pregnancy category C), and women who have received it inadvertently during pregnancy have not experienced adverse fetal outcomes (8). However, studies of benzimidazole drugs performed with animals suggest a possible teratogenic and embryotoxic effect. Since there are no good prospective safety data on either of these agents for humans, it is recommended that neither albendazole nor mebendazole be administered during pregnancy, particularly during the first trimester, unless the potential benefits justify the possible risk to the fetus (130). The amount of albendazole or mebendazole excreted in breast milk has not been well studied, and these drugs should be used with caution in lactating women.

Praziquantel

Praziquantel is a synthetic heterocyclic isoquinolone-pyrazine derivative. Major indications for its use are shown

TABLE 4 Major indications for mebendazole[a]

Indication	Usual dose	Reported efficacy
Ascaris lumbricoides	Single 500-mg dose or 100 mg twice daily for 3 days	Median cure rates of 95–98% and egg reduction rates of 99–100%
Enterobius vermicularis	Single 100-mg dose, repeated after 2–3 wk	Mean cure rate of 95%
Hookworm	Single 500-mg dose	Cure rates of 20–80% and egg reduction rates of 60–95% (>95% cure achieved with 3 days of mebendazole at 100 mg twice daily)
Trichuris trichiura	Single 500-mg dose or 100 mg twice daily for 3 days	Cure rate of 40–75% and egg reduction rates of 90–95%; higher cure rates (70–90%) achieved following 3 days of mebendazole at 100 mg twice daily
Toxocariasis	100–200 mg twice daily for 5 days	No large clinical trials

[a]Adapted from reference 5.

TABLE 5 Major indications for praziquantel[a]

Indication	Usual dose	Reported efficacy
Clonorchiasis	75 mg/kg/day in 3 doses for 1 day	Cure rates of 85–100%
Cysticercosis	50–100 mg/kg/day in 3 doses for 1–30 days	Eliminates 50–60% of cysts, but unclear if beneficial over placebo
Opisthorchiasis	75 mg/kg/day in 3 doses for 1 day	Cure rates of >95%
Intestinal flukes	75 mg/kg/day in 3 doses for 1 day	No large clinical trials
Paragonimiasis	75 mg/kg/day in 3 doses for 2 days	>95% cure for pulmonary infections (may be lower in ectopic sites)
Schistosomiasis	40–60 mg/kg/day in 2–3 doses for 1 day	Cure rates of 75–100%; egg reduction rates of 90–95% in those not cured
Tapeworms	Single dose of 10–25 mg/kg	Cure rates >95% for *Taenia*, *Diphyllobothrium*, and *Hymenolepis* species infections

[a]Adapted from reference 5.

in Table 5. It has the unique characteristic of being active against almost all trematodes and cestodes, but it is not useful for treatment of nematode infections. It has been approved for use by the U.S. FDA (5).

Mechanism of action. Praziquantel induces ultrastructural changes in the teguments of parasites, resulting in increased permeability to calcium ions. Calcium ions accumulate in the parasite cytosol, leading to muscular contractions and ultimately to paralysis of adult worms. By damaging the tegument membrane, praziquantel also exposes parasite antigens to host immune responses (14, 30). These effects lead to dislodgment of worms from their intestinal sites and subsequent expulsion by peristalsis.

Pharmacokinetics. Praziquantel is available for oral administration, and over 80% of the drug is absorbed after an oral dose. Coadministration with a high-carbohydrate meal increases drug concentrations in serum (106). The drug is biotransformed in the liver, and metabolites are excreted mainly in the urine. The cytochrome P450 hepatic metabolism of praziquantel is induced by corticosteroids, phenytoin, and phenobarbital. Praziquantel levels in serum are therefore lowered when any of these drugs are coadministered. Cimetidine, which inhibits P450-mediated metabolism, can be given concurrently to increase levels of praziquantel in plasma. Levels in plasma after a single 40-mg/kg dose have been reported as 1.007 to 1.625 mg/liter (57). Praziquantel does not cross the blood-brain barrier well, so levels in CSF are only approximately 20% of those in plasma (26, 106). It is 80% protein bound, and its half-life in serum is 1 to 3 h. It is not dialyzable, and no adjustment in dose is recommended in either renal or hepatic insufficiency.

Spectrum of activity. Praziquantel is active against the larval and adult stages of many trematodes. It is the drug of choice for schistosomiasis and is effective as a single oral dose for all *Schistosoma* species that infect humans. It is used both for treatment of individuals and in mass community chemotherapy programs and leads to decreased transmission and prevalence of infection. Praziquantel is also used for treatment of opisthorchiasis, clonorchiasis, paragonimiasis, and intestinal fluke infections, including fasciolopsiasis, heterophyiasis, and metagonimiasis. In contrast to other human trematode infections, praziquantel has not proven to be effective in the treatment of *Fasciola hepatica* infection.

Many cestode infections can also be treated with praziquantel. Most tapeworm infections respond, including those caused by *Taenia*, *Diphyllobothrium*, and *Hymenolepis* species. Because praziquantel does not kill eggs, precautions should be taken to prevent autoinfection, laboratory-acquired infection, or dissemination to others, particularly for *Taenia solium*. Praziquantel is also used in the treatment of neurocysticercosis as an alternative or adjunct to albendazole, although the overall benefit of therapy in many cases remains unclear.

Praziquantel has also been used in combination with albendazole for treatment of echinococcal infections. Praziquantel has high protoscolicidal activity in vitro, and some reports have suggested superior efficacy of the combination to that of either drug alone (23, 75).

Adverse effects. Adverse effects of praziquantel are generally mild, but many series suggest that some side effects occur in over 30% of patients. Common reactions include dizziness, lethargy, headache, nausea, and abdominal pain. Severe adverse reactions are uncommon, although administration to individuals with neurocysticercosis can result in seizures and neurological sequelae related to precipitation of an inflammatory response.

Animal studies do not suggest a teratogenic effect of praziquantel (pregnancy category B), but an increased abortion rate has been seen in rats. There are minimal data on its safety in humans, but review of the current known toxicology of praziquantel suggests a very low potential for adverse effects on either the mother or her unborn child (87), and when praziquantel has been used during pregnancy, no increase in abortion rates, preterm deliveries, or congenital abnormalities has been noted (2). Consequently, praziquantel can be given after the first trimester. No adverse effects of praziquantel administration during lactation have been reported, but it is excreted in human breast milk and discontinuation of breast feeding on the day of therapy and for the following 72 h is sometimes suggested. However, owing to available data regarding its safety profile, in 2002 the World Health Organization (WHO) recommended that it can be considered for use in pregnant and lactating women (3).

Ivermectin

Ivermectin is a semisynthetic macrocyclic lactone derivative of avermectins, which are natural substances derived from the actinomycete *Streptomyces avermitilis*. Major indications for its use are shown in Table 6. It was initially developed as an agent for veterinary use but is now used widely in humans. Ivermectin is a potent oral agent with relatively broad-spectrum anthelmintic activity. It has been approved by the U.S. FDA for therapy of onchocerciasis and uncomplicated strongyloidiasis (5).

TABLE 6 Major indications for ivermectin[a]

Indication	Usual dose	Reported efficacy
Ascaris lumbricoides	Single 200-µg/kg dose	Cure rates of 78–99%
Cutaneous larva migrans	200 µg/kg daily (usually 12 mg) for 1–2 days	Cure rates of 77–100%
Gnathostoma spinigerum	200 µg/kg daily for 2 days	Cure rates of 76–95%
Onchocerca volvulus	Single dose of 150 µg/kg, repeat every 6–12 mo until asymptomatic	Skin microfilarial counts reduced by 85–95%, and levels remain suppressed by >90% at 1 yr
Strongyloides stercoralis	200 µg/kg daily for 1–2 doses	Cure rates of 85–97% in uncomplicated infection (normal or immunocompromised hosts)
Trichuris trichiura	200 µg/kg daily for 3 days	Cure rates of 35–84%
Ectoparasites: scabies and lice	Single 200-µg/kg dose	Almost 100% efficacy, particularly if repeat dose given after 2 wk for severe infestations

[a]Adapted from reference 5.

Mechanism of action. Ivermectin causes an influx of chloride ions across glutamate-gated chloride channels in nerve and muscle cell membranes, resulting in hyperpolarization of the affected cells and consequent paralysis and death of parasites (20, 38, 115). It has also been postulated that ivermectin may act as an antagonist of the neurotransmitter gamma-aminobutyric acid (92). Although specific ivermectin binding sites have been identified in mammalian brain tissue, the affinity of ivermectin for sites within parasites is about 100 times greater than that for mammalian tissue.

Pharmacokinetics. Ivermectin is available only as an oral preparation and is rapidly absorbed after oral administration. The effect of food on the bioavailability of the drug has not been well studied. Ivermectin is metabolized in the liver and excreted almost entirely in the feces. Peak levels in serum of approximately 46 µg/liter have been reported after a single 12-mg dose (35). It is highly protein bound in plasma, and it has a half-life of 10 to 16 h. The drug accumulates in fat tissue and does not readily cross the blood-brain barrier (9).

Spectrum of activity. Ivermectin is the drug of choice for onchocerciasis and strongyloidiasis. In onchocercal infections, ivermectin does not have a significant effect on the viability of adult worms, but it is thought to impair release of microfilariae. In addition, it is a potent microfilaricide and leads to a sustained reduction in microfilaremia for many months (20). It can be used both for the treatment of individual patients and in mass chemotherapy programs in areas where onchocerciasis is endemic. In uncomplicated strongyloidiasis, ivermectin has excellent efficacy in healthy and immunocompromised patients, although experience with its use in disseminated infection is more limited (92).

In addition to the above indications, ivermectin also has activity against microfilariae of *Wuchereria bancrofti*, *Brugia malayi*, and *Loa loa*. It does not have a significant effect on adult worm viability in these infections, so reduced microfilaremia is sustained only with repeated doses, and it has not replaced DEC as first-line therapy for these infections. Ivermectin also has some activity against *Mansonella ozzardi* and *Mansonella streptocerca* microfilariae.

Ivermectin also has efficacy against many intestinal helminths, including *Ascaris lumbricoides*, *Trichuris trichiura*, *Enterobius vermicularis*, and cutaneous larva migrans (38, 81, 127). However, it is not generally used as first-line treatment for these indications due to the widespread availability and excellent efficacy of albendazole. It also can be used for treatment of gnathostomiasis (62). It is not active against trematodes or cestodes. In addition to its anthelmintic activity, ivermectin is the drug of choice for ectoparasitic infestations, including those of scabies and lice.

Adverse effects. Ivermectin is generally well tolerated. Most of the adverse effects that occur following its administration are a result of the host's immune response to destruction of parasites rather than to toxic effects of the drug per se. Adverse effects include fever, rash, dizziness, pruritus, myalgia, arthralgia, and tender lymphadenopathy, but the severity of these symptoms relates to the pretreatment intensity of infection rather than to ivermectin concentrations in serum (83). Severe reactions occasionally occur following its use, including a hypersensitivity response to dying microfilarial parasites known as the Mazzotti reaction. This anaphylactoid response is characterized by allergic manifestations including pruritus, edema, fever, and systemic hypotension. However, these reactions are primarily restricted to individuals with high parasite loads. In patients infected with *Loa loa* who have elevated levels of microfilaremia, ivermectin has been associated with the development of fatal encephalopathy (118).

Ivermectin (pregnancy category C) has not been reported to be teratogenic in rats or rabbits, but it has been associated with cleft palate and occasional unexplained maternal deaths in mice (20, 26). There are insufficient data to recommend its use in pregnant women, although the risk of fetal damage in 203 pregnant women inadvertently treated with ivermectin was no greater than that in controls, and it has been suggested that ivermectin can be given safely after the first trimester (44, 48, 93, 130). It is excreted in breast milk in low concentrations, so it should be avoided in lactating women when possible.

Diethylcarbamazine (DEC)

DEC is a piperazine derivative. Its main use is in filarial infections. Major indications for its use are shown in Table 7. DEC is not licensed for use in the United States, but it can be obtained from the Centers for Disease Control and Prevention (CDC) under an investigational new drug protocol.

Mechanism of action. The mode of action of DEC is uncertain. It is predominantly a microfilaricidal agent, and it is thought that its main effect is to alter the surface membranes of microfilariae, thereby enhancing destruction via

TABLE 7 Major indications for DEC^a

Indication	Usual dose	Reported efficacy
Loa loa	Up to 9 mg/kg/day in 3 doses for 21 days	Few large trials, but single course is curative in <50% of patients
Wuchereria bancrofti and *Brugia malayi*	Up to 6 mg/kg/day in 3 doses for 14 days or single dose	>90–99% reduction in microfilaremia, but may need additional courses to eradicate adult worms

^aAdapted from reference 5.

host immune responses (41, 43). It also has some macrofilaricidal activity under certain conditions, likely via hyperpolarization and immobilization of adult worms (61).

Pharmacokinetics. DEC is available only in tablet form. It is freely soluble in water and is almost completely absorbed after oral administration. The drug is metabolized in the liver, although over 50% is excreted unchanged in the urine. There is negligible protein binding, and it is widely distributed in tissues. It readily crosses the blood-brain barrier. Peak levels in plasma of 100 to 150 μg/liter have been reported after a single 0.5-mg/kg dose (34). The half-life of DEC is 2 to 17 h. Renal excretion is reduced in the presence of an alkaline urinary pH, and dose reductions are required in patients with renal impairment.

Spectrum of activity. DEC is an effective microfilaricidal drug against *W. bancrofti*, *B. malayi*, *Brugia timori*, *Onchocerca volvulus*, *L. loa*, and *M. streptocerca*, but it has little or no effect on *Mansonella perstans* or *M. ozzardi* microfilariae. It has been the drug of choice for lymphatic filariasis for the last 50 years. It is used both for individual therapy for filarial infections and in mass community chemotherapy programs, either alone or in combination with ivermectin or albendazole. It is predominantly a microfilaricidal agent, although it has some macrofilaricidal activity in *W. bancrofti*, *B. malayi*, *B. timori*, and *L. loa* infections (82, 84, 91). DEC has also been used in the treatment of toxocaral visceral larva migrans, but albendazole is now the preferred agent because of its better safety profile.

Adverse effects. The side effects of DEC include mild headache, dizziness, anorexia, nausea, and arthralgias. Administration of the drug to individuals with filarial infections can induce adverse results that are not due to the drug itself but instead are related to host responses, in part to release of *Wolbachia* endosymbionts from filariae, following damage to adult worms (local reactions) and death of microfilariae (systemic reactions). These allergic reactions tend to be relatively mild with lymphatic filariasis and infrequent with loiasis but can be severe with onchocerciasis or with heavy *L. loa* infections. Reactions include intense pruritus, rash, fever, hypotension, and encephalopathy. The potentially fatal Mazzotti reaction and serious ophthalmic adverse effects can occur following treatment of *O. volvulus* with DEC, and this has led to DEC being contraindicated for onchocercal infections. Animal studies have not shown DEC to be teratogenic, but it may increase the risk of abortion, so it should be avoided in pregnancy when possible (26, 54). It is not excreted in breast milk and is safe during lactation.

Pyrantel Pamoate

Pyrantel, a tetrahydropyrimidine, is a relatively broad-spectrum agent against nematodes. It is associated with more side effects and lower efficacy than the benzimidazoles, so it is largely being replaced. It is approved by the U.S. FDA but is considered investigational for most indications, except for enterobiasis.

Mechanism of action. Pyrantel is a depolarizing neuromuscular blocking agent. It exerts its anthelmintic effect via release of acetylcholine and inhibition of helminthic acetylcholinesterase. This results in stimulation of ganglionic receptors and spastic paralysis of adult worms. The worms become dislodged from the intestinal wall and are expelled in the feces by normal peristalsis.

Pharmacokinetics. Pyrantel is administered orally but is almost insoluble in water and is therefore poorly absorbed from the gastrointestinal tract. More than 50% is excreted unchanged in the feces. The absorbed drug is partially metabolized in the liver. There is no significant interaction with food.

Spectrum of activity. Pyrantel has excellent efficacy in the treatment of ascariasis and hookworm and pinworm infections. It also has some activity against hookworm and *Trichostrongylus*. It is not active against *Trichuris trichiura*.

Adverse effects. Although pyrantel is generally well tolerated, it can lead to adverse reactions, including anorexia, nausea, vomiting, abdominal cramps, and diarrhea. It has also been associated with neurotoxic effects, including headache, dizziness, drowsiness, and insomnia. Transient increases in hepatic enzymes have also been reported. Animal studies have not shown adverse effects in the fetus, and it has been used during pregnancy in humans without harmful fetal effects (pregnancy category C) (117). It is not recommended for children under 2 years of age.

AN AGENT WITH ANTHELMINTIC AND ANTIPROTOZOAL ACTIVITY: NITAZOXANIDE

Nitazoxanide is a 5-nitrothiazole derivative with broad-spectrum activity against numerous intestinal protozoa, helminths, and anaerobic bacteria. Major indications for its use are shown in Table 8. It was initially developed as a veterinary anthelmintic with activity against intestinal nematodes, cestodes, and liver trematodes (39). The U.S. FDA has approved it for use for the treatment of diarrhea caused by *Cryptosporidium* species and *Giardia lamblia* in pediatric and adult patients (6, 39).

Mechanism of action. Nitazoxanide inhibits pyruvate ferredoxin oxidoreductase, an enzyme essential to anaerobic energy metabolism. This is its mechanism of action against anaerobic bacteria (e.g., *Trichomonas vaginalis*, *Entamoeba histolytica*, and *Clostridium perfringens*) and protozoa, although for protozoa additional mechanisms may also be involved (42). The exact mechanism of nitazoxanide's activity against helminths has not yet been determined.

TABLE 8   Major indications for nitazoxanide[a]

Indication	Usual dose[b]	Reported efficacy
Cryptosporidium parvum	Immunocompetent children 1–11 yr[c] old and adults[c]: b.i.d. treatment for 3 days	Cure rates of 52–80%
	Immunocompromised patients: 1,000 mg b.i.d. for 2–8 weeks	Cure rates of 18–67% (efficacy varies with CD4 count in human immunodeficiency virus-positive patients)
Giardia lamblia	b.i.d. treatment for 3 days[c]	Cure rates of 71–94%
Ancylostoma duodenale	b.i.d. treatment for 3 days	Cure rate of 96%
Ascaris lumbricoides	b.i.d. treatment for 3 days	Cure rates of 69–100% (in heavy infections of >10,000 eggs/g, lower egg clearance rate of 48%, but egg reduction rates of >99%)
Balantidium coli	b.i.d. treatment for 3 days	Cure rate of 77%
Blastocystis hominis	b.i.d. treatment for 3 days	Cure rates of 97–100%
Cyclospora cayetanensis	b.i.d. treatment for 3 days	Cure rate of 71%
Entamoeba histolytica	b.i.d. treatment for 3 days	Cure rates of 69–96%
Enterobiasis vermicularis	b.i.d. treatment for 3 days	Cure rates of 80–100%
Fasciola hepatica	b.i.d. treatment for 7 days (daily dose as shown below)	Cure rates of 40–97%
Hymenolepis nana	Single oral dose of 50 mg/kg or b.i.d. treatment for 3 days	Cure rates of 80–97%
Isospora belli	b.i.d. treatment for 3 days	Cure rate of 100%
Strongyloides stercoralis	b.i.d. treatment for 3 days	Cure rate of 94%
Taenia saginata	Single 25-mg/kg dose or b.i.d. treatment for 3 days	Cure rates of 95–100%
Trichuris trichiura	b.i.d. treatment for 3 days	Cure rates of 76–100% (in moderate infections with 2,000–5,000 eggs/g, lower egg clearance rate of 56%, but egg reduction rates of >99%)

[a]Adapted from reference 39.
[b]The dosing schedule for nitazoxanide given as a twice-daily (b.i.d.) treatment course for 3 days consists of the following: for children 1 to 3 years of age, 100 mg b.i.d. for 3 days; for children 4 to 11 years of age, 200 mg b.i.d. for 3 days; and for adults, 500 mg b.i.d. for 3 days.
[c]Licensed for this use by the U.S. FDA.

Pharmacokinetics. Nitazoxanide is given by the oral route and is available as a suspension or in tablet formulation. Bioavailability is nearly doubled by administration with food (111). It is absorbed from the gastrointestinal tract, with approximately one-third of the oral dose excreted in urine and two-thirds excreted in feces (15, 90). In blood, nitazoxanide is rapidly hydrolyzed to form an active metabolite, tizoxanide. The maximum concentration of tizoxanide in plasma following an oral dose of 500 mg nitazoxanide is 2 mg/liter (6.5 μM), and its half-life in plasma is 1 to 2 h (1). Tizoxanide is extensively bound to plasma proteins (>99%), and its urinary elimination half-life is 7.3 h (112). Tizoxanide then undergoes glucuronidation to form tizoxanide glucuronide. Nitazoxanide is not detected in plasma, urine, bile, or feces, but tizoxanide is found in plasma, urine, bile, and feces and tizoxanide glucuronide is found in plasma, bile, and urine (90). The pharmacokinetics of nitazoxanide in patients with impaired liver or renal function has not been studied, and it must be administered with caution to these patients (39).

Spectrum of activity. Nitazoxanide is a broad-spectrum antimicrobial agent with activity against protozoa, nematodes, cestodes, trematodes, and bacteria. It has been shown to be effective in vitro and/or in vivo against many enteric protozoan and helminth infections, including infections with *Ascaris lumbricoides*, *Balantidium coli*, *Blastocystis hominis*, *Cryptosporidium parvum*, *Cyclospora cayetanensis*, *Echinococcus multilocularis*, *Echinococcus granulosus*, *Entamoeba histolytica*, *Fasciola hepatica*, hookworms, *Giardia lamblia*, *Hymenolepis nana*, *Isospora belli*, microsporidial species (*Enterocytozoon bieneusi* and *Encephalitozoon intestinalis*), *Trichuris trichiura*, *Taenia saginata*, *Trichomonas vaginalis*, and *Vittaforma corneae* (39). Nitazoxanide also has in vitro and in vivo activity against *Bacteroides* species, *Clostridium difficile*, and both metronidazole-susceptible and metronidazole-resistant strains of *Helicobacter pylori* (39, 90). It is also being evaluated in the treatment of hepatitis B and hepatitis C infections.

Adverse effects. Nitazoxanide is very well tolerated, with adverse effects similar to those of placebo. Mild and transient side effects have been seen in only 3 to 4% of patients, principally related to the gastrointestinal tract (abdominal pain, diarrhea, and nausea) (28). No significant adverse effects on electrocardiography, hematology, clinical chemistry, or urinalysis parameters have been noted (42). There are minimal data on the safety of nitazoxanide in pregnant (pregnancy category B) or lactating women (39).

ANTIMALARIALS

Quinoline Derivatives

The quinoline derivatives can be divided into the following four groups: the 4-aminoquinolines; the cinchona alkaloids; synthetic compounds, such as mefloquine and halofantrine; and the 8-aminoquinolines.

4-Aminoquinolines

The 4-aminoquinolines include chloroquine, hydroxychloroquine, and amodiaquine. Chloroquine is the most widely used of these agents. It is an inexpensive, safe drug that has been used extensively for treatment and prophylaxis of all *Plasmodium* species that infect humans. Hydroxychloroquine is a related synthetic compound with an identical clinical spectrum, similar pharmacokinetics, and similar adverse effects. Amodiaquine is another related agent which also has the same mechanism of action and spectrum of activity. It is reported to be more effective than chloroquine for parasite clearance, but its utility is limited by toxicity. It has not been approved by the U.S. FDA (5).

Mechanism of action. The main mechanism of action of the 4-aminoquinolines is thought to be via nonenzymatic inhibition of heme polymerization. The 4-aminoquinolines act specifically against intraerythrocytic stages of malaria parasites. Asexual intraerythrocytic malaria parasites actively concentrate quinoline ring compounds within hemoglobin-containing vesicles. In the absence of drug, *Plasmodium* spp. degrade host erythrocyte hemoglobin to provide amino acid nutrients essential for parasite growth. The degradation of hemoglobin produces free heme, which is stored as ferriporoporphyrin IX within the red blood cell. Ferriporoporphyrin IX is toxic to the parasite and is usually polymerized into nontoxic malaria pigment (hemozoin). In the presence of drug, there is inhibition of the conversion of heme into hemozoin, leading to the accumulation of products which are toxic to the parasite and resulting in parasite death (105). These agents also inhibit protein synthesis by inhibiting incorporation of phosphate into DNA and RNA and by inhibiting DNA and RNA polymerases (41).

Pharmacokinetics. The 4-aminoquinolines are extensively distributed in tissues and are characterized by a long elimination half-life. Despite similarities in their chemical structures, these drugs show differences in their biotransformation and routes of elimination (99).

Chloroquine is available in oral and parenteral forms. Many different formulations of chloroquine are manufactured worldwide. Chloroquine is rapidly absorbed from the gastrointestinal tract after oral administration and has an oral bioavailability exceeding 75%. Food has variable effects on absorption. The drug is distributed extensively in body tissues and reaches high levels within the brain (63). Chloroquine binds to melanin-containing cells in the skin and eye, so it can also reach high levels at these sites. There is marked variability in peak concentrations in plasma between individuals, but within 3 h of initiation of standard oral treatment doses (10 mg chloroquine base/kg, followed by three doses of 5 mg/kg at 6, 24, and 48 h), concentrations in blood remain above 1 mmol/liter for at least 4 days (101). It is approximately 60% protein bound and has a half-life of about 4 to 6 days. Approximately 30 to 50% of the drug is metabolized to inactive compounds in the liver, and the remainder is excreted in the urine. Treatment reduction (usually 50% of the normal dose) is required in patients with severe renal or hepatic failure. It is not dialyzable.

In contrast, amodiaquine is a prodrug and is almost entirely metabolized to a biologically active metabolite, desethylamodiaquine, following oral administration. Otherwise, it has pharmacokinetic properties similar to those of chloroquine but has a smaller volume of distribution.

Spectrum of activity. The 4-aminoquinolines are efficient and rapidly acting blood schizonticides. They can be used in both the treatment and prophylaxis of infection with susceptible strains of all *Plasmodium* species. They have no effect on tissue schizonts or exoerythrocytic stages. They are gametocytocidal for *Plasmodium vivax* and *Plasmodium malariae* but have minimal effects on *Plasmodium falciparum* gametocytes. Following infections with *P. vivax* or *Plasmodium ovale*, primaquine is also needed to eradicate liver hypnozoites and to prevent relapses of infection.

Despite emerging resistance among *P. vivax* parasites, chloroquine generally remains first-line therapy for most *P. vivax*, *P. malariae*, and *P. ovale* infections. It also remains the treatment of choice for susceptible *P. falciparum* strains, although *P. falciparum* strains from most areas of the world are now resistant to it. It is also effective against *Plasmodium knowlesi* infections. Because of its potential toxicity, amodiaquine is not recommended for prophylaxis of malaria and is generally not used as first-line treatment. However, it results in faster parasite clearance and more rapid resolution of symptoms than those with chloroquine, and it may be effective in some cases of chloroquine-resistant malaria, so it is used as an alternative treatment regimen in some areas.

Chloroquine is also active against *E. histolytica* trophozoites but is rarely used for this indication, as the nitro-5-imidazoles are the drugs of choice.

Adverse effects. Chloroquine has a bitter taste. It is generally well tolerated at the doses required for malaria prevention or treatment, even when taken for prolonged periods. However, it can lead to nausea, abdominal discomfort, dizziness, retinal pigmentation, blurred vision, electrocardiographic changes, muscular weakness, and, rarely, transient psychiatric symptoms. It can also cause severe pruritus, particularly in African blacks. Irreversible neuroretinitis can result if it is taken at high doses for prolonged periods. If taken as an overdose, it can cause shock, arrhythmia, and death.

At the doses used for malaria treatment or prophylaxis, chloroquine has rarely been reported to cause adverse congenital effects (pregnancy category C) (66). However, affinity for melanin-containing tissues, such as the retina, iris, and choroid of the eye, has been reported, and definitive delineation of fetal risk remains undefined. It is commonly used for treatment and prophylaxis of malaria in pregnant women, without evidence of teratogenicity, and it is generally agreed that the benefits of preventing and treating malaria in pregnant women outweigh the potential fetal risks. Chloroquine is excreted in breast milk, in small amounts.

Amodiaquine is more palatable than chloroquine and seems to cause less itching. However, serious adverse events, including agranulocytosis, aplastic anemia, and drug-induced hepatitis, have been reported. These have occurred predominantly following long-term amodiaquine use (mean, 7 to 8 weeks) for malaria prophylaxis, and short-term treatment regimens are thought to be safe (88).

Cinchona Alkaloids

The cinchona alkaloids, quinine and quinidine, contain a quinoline ring. Quinidine is the diastereoisomer of quinine. Quinine was originally extracted from the bark of the South American cinchona tree, but a synthetic form is now available, usually as a quinine sulfate salt. Quinidine is more active than quinine, but it is also more cardiotoxic.

Mechanism of action. The exact target of cinchona alkaloids is unknown. They are thought to act by forming complexes with ferriprotoporphyrin IX, thereby interfering with hemoglobin digestion and resulting in cell lysis and death of schizonts (37). They are also thought to interfere with the function of plasmodial DNA and to inhibit the synthesis of parasite nucleic acids and proteins. Quinine also interacts with certain fatty acids present in parasitized erythrocytes, preventing red blood cell lysis and interrupting schizont maturation (41). Additionally, it increases intracellular pH, resulting in lethal effects on the parasite.

Pharmacokinetics. Quinine is available for oral administration as a sulfate salt and for parenteral administration as quinine dihydrochloride. It is >80% absorbed from the gastrointestinal tract following oral doses. It is widely distributed in body tissues, but concentrations in CSF are <10% of concurrent levels in plasma. It is over 90% protein bound. Quinine is metabolized in the liver, and the native drug and its metabolites are excreted in the urine (63). It has a short half-life of 8 to 12 h, necessitating multiple daily doses. After a single dose of 650 mg of quinine sulfate, peak concentrations in serum are approximately 3.2 mg/liter in healthy individuals but are higher (8.4 mg/liter) in patients with malaria. Intravenous quinine is used in many countries when oral therapy cannot be tolerated, but quinidine gluconate is considered the parenteral drug of choice in the United States (5). Both agents have similar pharmacokinetic properties.

The pharmacokinetic properties of the cinchona alkaloids are considerably altered in patients with malaria, with a reduction in clearance that is proportional to the severity of disease. Consequently, doses should be decreased 30 to 50% after the third day of treatment to avoid the accumulation of drug in seriously ill patients (128). Drug levels may also be increased by administration with foods that alkalinize the urine, because increased tubular reabsorption results. Caution is recommended for patients with significant renal or liver impairment, but there are no specific dose adjustment guidelines. Both agents are partially dialyzable.

Spectrum of activity. The cinchona alkaloids can be used in the treatment of all *Plasmodium* species that infect humans. Their main indication is for chloroquine-resistant *P. falciparum*. Oral therapy is indicated for uncomplicated malaria, but intravenous formulations of quinine dihydrochloride or quinidine gluconate are used in severe infections.

Quinine and quinidine are blood schizonticides but have little effect on sporozoites or preerythrocytic forms of the parasite. Consequently, they do not eradicate *P. vivax* or *P. ovale* hypnozoites in the liver. They also are not gametocytocidal against *P. falciparum*. They are generally given in combination with other agents. Although relative resistance to these agents has emerged, they remain useful drugs for the treatment of malaria worldwide.

Quinine is also used for the treatment of babesiosis. It is ineffective when used as a single agent but can be given together with clindamycin or azithromycin (45).

Adverse effects. Quinine has an extremely bitter taste and can be associated with nausea, vomiting, and epigastric pain. It also often leads to the symptom complex of cinchonism (nausea, tinnitus, dysphoria, and reversible high-tone deafness). Quinine can also cause hyperinsulinemic hypoglycemia, especially in children and pregnant women with severe malaria, as it increases release of insulin from the pancreas. It has also been associated with massive hemolysis in patients with heavy *P. falciparum* infections. Agranulocytosis, thrombocytopenia, retinopathy, and tongue discoloration are additional adverse effects which have been described. Overdose of quinine can lead to ataxia, convulsions, and coma.

When used as treatment for severe malaria, intravenous quinidine is associated with cardiac arrhythmias. It prolongs the QT interval, widens the QRS complex, and prolongs the PR interval. It can therefore lead to hypotension and ventricular arrhythmias, including Torsade de Pointes. Consequently, it should be administered only in an intensive care setting with cardiac monitoring. As with quinine, administration can also result in blood dyscrasias and cinchonism.

Despite reports of congenital defects following administration of quinine during pregnancy, it can be administered during pregnancy when the benefits of maternal treatment outweigh the potential fetal risks (pregnancy category C) (69, 103). Quinidine has not been reported to be teratogenic. Quinine can have an abortifacient effect and can lead to induction of labor. It is excreted in small amounts in breast milk but can be administered during breast feeding when necessary.

Synthetic Quinoline Compounds

Mefloquine
Mefloquine is a synthetic 4-quinoline methanol compound structurally related to quinine.

Mechanism of action. Mefloquine interacts both with host cell phospholipids and with ferriprotoporphyrin IX of the parasitized erythrocyte (41). The precise mechanism of action is not known, but it is thought to act by interfering with the digestion of hemoglobin during the blood stages of the malaria life cycle, likely via a mechanism similar to that of quinine (37). It does not inhibit protein synthesis.

Pharmacokinetics. Mefloquine is available for oral administration only. Food enhances bioavailability, and it should not be taken on an empty stomach. It is >85% absorbed following oral administration and is concentrated within red blood cells (58). It is >95% protein bound and has a half-life of 2 to 3 weeks. Because of its long half-life, mefloquine is frequently used for prophylaxis of malaria, as a once-weekly dose. However, when mefloquine is administered weekly, it requires about 8 weeks before steady-state drug levels are reached, so a loading dose is often recommended. Peak concentrations in plasma following a single dose of 500 mg or 1,000 mg orally are 430 and 800 μg/liter, respectively. In healthy volunteers, a dose of 250 mg once weekly produces maximum steady-state concentrations in plasma of 1,000 to 2,000 μg/liter, which are reached after 7 to 10 weeks. It is highly lipophilic, is widely distributed throughout the body, and can cross the blood-brain barrier. Mefloquine is metabolized in the liver and excreted through the bile and feces. There are no specific recommendations regarding the need for dosage adjustment in patients with renal or hepatic failure. It is not dialyzable.

Spectrum of activity. Mefloquine is active against the erythrocytic schizonts of all *Plasmodium* species causing human malaria, and it has been used for both chemoprophylaxis and therapy. Since weekly administration is sufficient for chemoprophylaxis, it is convenient for use in travelers to areas where malaria is endemic. Its main utility in malaria treatment results from its activity against most chloroquine-resistant *P. falciparum* strains, although resistance has been recognized, particularly in some areas of Southeast Asia. When used for therapy, it is frequently combined with another agent, usually an artemisinin derivative. Mefloquine does not kill tissue schizonts, so patients infected with *P. vivax* should subsequently be treated with an 8-aminoquinoline. It also has no effect on gametocytes.

Adverse effects. Adverse reactions to mefloquine include nausea and vomiting, as well as central nervous system (CNS) effects such as dysphoria, dizziness, disturbed sleep, nightmares, and ataxia. Severe neuropsychiatric reactions, including delerium and seizures, have been reported occasionally and are thought to occur in approximately 1:200 to 1:1,300 patients treated for acute falciparum malaria (10, 49, 121). Mefloquine can also potentiate dysrhythmias in individuals on beta-blockers. It is quite expensive and is unaffordable for general use throughout areas such as tropical Africa.

Mefloquine is teratogenic in high doses in animals, but reports on humans do not support teratogenic effects (pregnancy category C) (120). A possible higher rate of spontaneous abortion has been suggested, so it is generally avoided in the first trimester of pregnancy if possible. However, limited data suggest that it is probably safe to use even during the first trimester, and it can be used in later stages of pregnancy if the benefits outweigh the potential risks (85). It is excreted in low concentrations in breast milk but can be used in lactating women when necessary.

Halofantrine

Halofantrine is a synthetic phenanthrene-methanol compound. It has not been approved by the U.S. FDA (5).

Mechanism of action. Halofantrine has activity against the asexual erythrocytic stages of malaria parasites, although the exact mechanism of action is unclear.

Pharmacokinetics. Halofantrine is available only for oral administration but has variable bioavailability. Absorption is enhanced by administration with fatty foods, but because high levels in blood enhance toxicity, it is recommended for administration on an empty stomach. After three doses of 500 mg of halofantrine hydrochloride (at 0, 6, and 12 h), a maximum concentration in plasma of 896 μg/liter was reported (122). Halofantrine is metabolized in the liver to an active metabolite, N-desbutylhalofantrine. The half-lives of halofantrine and its metabolite are 6 to 10 days and 3 to 4 days, respectively. It is excreted mainly in the feces.

Spectrum of activity. Halofantrine is efficacious in the treatment of *P. vivax* and *P. falciparum* malaria, but data concerning *P. ovale* and *P. malariae* are limited (17). It is not recommended for prophylaxis of malaria because of toxicity. It is active against blood-stage schizonts only and appears to have no effect against sporozoites, gametocytes, or tissue-stage parasites. Halofantrine is more active than mefloquine, but cross-resistance between these drugs occurs. Its expense and potential toxicity also limit its use, so it is not recommended as a first-line agent.

Adverse effects. Halofantrine leads to gastrointestinal adverse effects, including nausea, vomiting, diarrhea, and abdominal pain. It also has potential cardiovascular toxicity

and causes concentration-dependent prolongation of the QT interval. It is therefore contraindicated in patients with long QT syndrome, as it can lead to cardiac arrest. It can also lead to pruritus and hepatic enzyme elevations. Halofantrine is contraindicated in pregnancy. The degree of excretion in breast milk is unknown, and it is not advised for use in lactating women.

8-Aminoquinolines

The 8-aminoquinolines are primaquine and tafenoquine (WR 238,605). Tafenoquine is not yet licensed for malaria prophylaxis or treatment and has not been approved by the U.S. FDA (5).

Mechanism of action. The 8-aminoquinolines interfere with parasite mitochondrial enzymes involved in energy production. They also have an inhibitory action against DNA, although the exact mechanism by which this occurs is unclear (41). An active metabolite of the drug is thought to interrupt the mitochondrial transport system and pyrimidine synthesis in hypnozoites (126).

Pharmacokinetics. The 8-aminoquinolines are well absorbed after oral administration, with >90% bioavailability. Primaquine is rapidly metabolized in the liver, and its half-life is 4 to 7 h, so it needs to be administered daily. Following a single 45-mg oral dose, a mean peak level in serum of 153.3 μg/liter was observed after 2 to 3 h (73). Detailed information regarding distribution in body tissues is not available, but it is found at relatively low concentrations in most body sites. Tafenoquine has a longer half-life of 2 to 4 weeks. Weekly or possibly monthly doses seem to be sufficient for prophylaxis, thus making it better tolerated than primaquine. A single dose of tafenoquine may be sufficient for prevention of relapse following *P. vivax* infections (125). Optimal dose-finding studies are being performed.

Spectrum of activity. Primaquine is less active against blood-stage malarial forms than most other antimalarial agents are, but instead, it is very active against preerythrocytic sporozoites and exoerythrocytic tissue schizonts of all malarial species. Its main use is to prevent relapse of *P. vivax* and *P. ovale* infections from latent hypnozoites following treatment with chloroquine. Additionally, it is gametocytocidal against *Plasmodium*, especially *P. falciparum*, and can interrupt transmission of malaria. It is also an effective causal prophylactic agent but traditionally has been used infrequently for routine travelers. Tafenoquine is reported to be more active than primaquine and has higher schizonticidal activity (16).

Adverse effects. Mild gastrointestinal side effects, including nausea and abdominal pain, are common following 8-aminoquinoline administration. They should not be used in people with glucose-6-phosphate dehydrogenase deficiency, as they can induce hemolysis. Patients with NADH methemoglobin reductase deficiency are at risk of developing methemoglobinemia. Primaquine also occasionally causes arrhythmias. These agents should also not be used during pregnancy or lactation because of the potential risk of hemolytic effects in the fetus.

Artemisinin (Qinghaosu) Derivatives

Artemisinin is an extract from the Chinese herbal plant *Artemisia annua*, also known as qinghaosu. It is a sesquiterpene lactone peroxide. Synthetic derivatives include artemether, dihydroartemisinin, arteether, and artesunate. Although not officially approved for use by the U.S. FDA, the intravenous formulation of artesunate is available via the CDC under an investigational new drug protocol for patients with severe malaria.

Mechanism of action. Artemisinin and its derivatives act mainly against the asexual erythrocytic stages of malaria parasites. They have an antiparasitic effect, particularly on young, ring-form parasites, leading to their clearance and preventing development of more-mature pathogenic forms. They bind to the parasite membrane and to ferriprotoporphyrin IX, so they are highly concentrated within parasites and reach 100 to 300 times higher concentrations in *P. falciparum*-infected red cells than in uninfected cells (46). By binding iron in the malarial pigment, they lead to the production of toxic oxidative free radicals which damage parasite organelles and alkylate parasitic proteins. This leads to the inhibition of protein synthesis and ultimately to parasite death.

Pharmacokinetics. The derivatives of artemisinin have greater solubility than artemisinin and consequently have been developed for easier administration by a variety of routes. Artesunate is water soluble and can be given intravenously, intramuscularly, orally, or by suppository. Artemether and arteether are oil soluble and are available in tablet, capsule, and intramuscular injection forms. Although artesunate is the most potent in vitro, there is no apparent clinical difference in efficacy between the formulations. The artemisinin derivatives have a short half-life of <1 to 2 h. They are usually administered once daily for a minimum of 3 days. All are metabolized to the active compound, dihydroartemisinin. After single doses of 2 and 4 mg of dihydroartemisinin/kg of body weight in healthy volunteers, median peak values in plasma of 181 and 360 μg/liter, respectively, were observed (80). Artemisinin derivatives should be used with caution in individuals with hepatic or renal impairment.

Spectrum of activity. The artemisinin derivatives are effective against *P. falciparum* and *P. vivax* and are the most potent and rapidly acting parasiticidal drugs. They act specifically against the erythrocytic stages of *Plasmodium*. They are also active against gametocytes, reducing gametocyte carriage by about 90% and therefore decreasing malaria transmission in areas where they are widely used (21, 97). They are not effective against the intrahepatic stage of *P. vivax* or *P. ovale* infections. These drugs are effective against multidrug-resistant *P. falciparum* and are now the drugs of choice against mefloquine- and/or quinine-resistant isolates. No clinically significant resistance has been reported. However, late recrudescence is common unless these agents are combined with another drug, so they are usually administered with a second agent, such as mefloquine or doxycycline. The artemisinin derivatives are associated with quick clearance of parasitemia, and recent randomized trials comparing them with quinine have shown a benefit in terms of mortality in adults treated for severe malaria (31).

There is minimal information available regarding the efficacy of the artemisinin derivatives in *P. ovale* and *P. malariae* infections. The artemisinin derivatives also have activity against schistosomiasis but have not been used widely for this indication (7, 51, 119).

Adverse effects. The artemisinin derivatives are very well tolerated, with no serious toxicity or subjective adverse effects. They have been associated with adverse neurological effects in animal models, but there is no evidence that this occurs in humans. Although it is generally recommended that they be avoided in pregnancy because of insufficient safety data, they can be used, particularly after the first trimester, if the benefits outweigh the risks (86). The amount excreted in breast milk is unknown.

Antifolates

Pyrimethamine-sulfadoxine, also known as Fansidar, is still commonly used for treatment of malaria in some countries. Pyrimethamine is a synthetic aminopyrimidine antimalarial agent, and sulfadoxine is a long-acting sulfonamide agent.

Mechanism of action. Pyrimethamine acts against the asexual erythrocytic stage of *Plasmodium* by inhibiting the plasmodial enzyme dihydrofolate reductase. Although active against *P. falciparum*, rapid development of resistance occurs and is a major factor limiting its use as a single agent. Combining pyrimethamine with a sulfonamide or sulfone provides sequential, synergistic inhibition of the folate biosynthesis pathway. Malaria parasites are unable to utilize host-derived folic acid, so inhibition of folic acid biosynthesis prevents malarial DNA replication, ultimately leading to cell death.

Pharmacokinetics. Fansidar tablets are comprised of 25 mg of pyrimethamine and 500 mg of sulfadoxine. Both drugs are well absorbed orally. After oral administration of a single tablet, peak concentrations of pyrimethamine and sulfadoxine in plasma are 0.13 to 0.4 mg/liter and 51 to 76 mg/liter, respectively. The half-life of pyrimethamine is 80 to 95 h, and the half-life of sulfadoxine is 150 to 200 h (128). Both components are approximately 90% protein bound. Sulfadoxine is metabolized in the liver, and both agents are excreted mainly in the urine.

Spectrum of activity. Pyrimethamine-sulfadoxine is effective for both treatment and chemoprophylaxis of *P. falciparum* malaria. It is no longer recommended for routine prophylaxis because of the potential for severe adverse effects. It acts mainly against blood schizonts and does not have significant gametocytocidal activity. Widespread resistance now limits its use in treatment, but its low cost means that it is often still used as therapy for *P. falciparum* malaria in many African countries. Pyrimethamine-sulfadoxine also has some efficacy in the treatment of *P. vivax* infection, but it has longer parasite and fever clearance times and higher failure rates (30 to 40%) than chloroquine and thus is not recommended. The efficacy of pyrimethamine-sulfadoxine against *P. ovale* and *P. malariae* has not been evaluated adequately.

Pyrimethamine is also used in combination with sulfadiazine for the treatment of toxoplasmosis.

Adverse effects. Pyrimethamine-sulfadoxine can result in adverse effects, including rash, nausea, vomiting, headache, and peripheral neuritis. It can also be associated with more serious and occasionally fatal reactions, including the Stevens-Johnson syndrome and blood dyscrasias (particularly agranulocytosis and megaloblastic anemia). Other reported adverse effects include hepatitis, toxic nephrosis, exfoliative dermatitis, and erythema multiforme. The long half-life of the sulfa component means that sensitivity reactions can be sustained for prolonged periods even after the drug is discontinued.

Pyrimethamine has been associated with teratogenic effects in animals. There are no controlled human studies, but it has been used frequently during pregnancy, particularly in African countries, and has been associated with good fetal outcomes. It is officially recommended for use during pregnancy only when potential benefits outweigh the possible risks to the fetus. Pyrimethamine-sulfadoxine can cause kernicterus in infants, so it should be used with caution in pregnant women late in the third trimester. Both pyrimethamine and sulfadoxine are excreted into the breast milk and are preferably avoided during lactation.

Atovaquone-Proguanil (Malarone)

Malarone is a tablet combination of 250 mg of atovaquone and 100 mg of proguanil. Atovaquone is a hydroxynaphthoquinone, and proguanil is an antifolate. Malarone has been approved for use by the U.S. FDA for prophylaxis and treatment of malaria.

Mechanism of action. Atovaquone has a novel mechanism of action. *Plasmodium* species are dependent on de novo pyrimidine biosynthesis, which is selectively coupled with electron transport. Atovaquone inhibits the electron transport system in the mitochondria of parasites, thereby blocking nucleic acid synthesis and inhibiting replication (68). When used as monotherapy, atovaquone is associated with high recrudescence rates. Proguanil also acts against the asexual erythrocytic stage of the parasite by selectively inhibiting plasmodial dihydrofolate reductase. However, in combination with atovaquone, it acts via a different mechanism and directly lowers the effective concentration at which atovaquone causes collapse of the mitochondrial membrane potential (110).

Pharmacokinetics. Atovaquone is a highly lipophilic compound with low aqueous solubility and poor and variable oral availability. Its absorption is increased if it is administered with fatty foods or a milky drink. It is not metabolized and is excreted almost exclusively in the feces. It is 99% plasma protein bound, and its half-life is 2 to 3 days. Proguanil is rapidly and extensively absorbed after oral administration. It is metabolized by cytochrome P450 in the liver to the active cyclic triazine metabolite, cycloguanil. It is 75% protein bound and is excreted mainly in the urine. Its half life is 12 to 21 h. After two Malarone tablets twice daily for 3 days, mean levels of proguanil in plasma have been reported as 170 µg/liter. Atovaquone levels vary widely between individuals (33). No dosing adjustments are required in the setting of mild to moderate hepatic or renal insufficiency.

Spectrum of activity. Atovaquone-proguanil is effective against asexual and sexual forms of the *P. falciparum* parasite and is recommended for treatment and prophylaxis of falciparum malaria. It is becoming an increasingly utilized alternative to mefloquine for chemoprophylaxis in travelers to areas where malaria is endemic. Atovaquone-proguanil is also effective for treating *P. vivax* and *P. ovale* infections, but neither drug is effective against hypnozoites, so primaquine is additionally required to prevent relapses after drug discontinuation. Atovaquone-proguanil also showed good efficacy against *P. malariae* in limited studies (100). Reports of clinical failures and resistance of *P. falciparum* isolates to atovaquone-proguanil via a single mutation are emerging.

Adverse effects. Atovaquone-proguanil is generally very well tolerated. Side effects are mild and include anorexia, nausea, vomiting, abdominal pain, diarrhea, pruritus, and headache. Between 5 and 10% of recipients develop transient asymptomatic elevations in transaminases and amylase. Because of inadequate safety data, it is not recommended during pregnancy (pregnancy category C) or lactation.

OTHER ANTIPROTOZOAL AGENTS

Diloxanide Furoate

Diloxanide furoate, also known as Furamide, is a substituted acetanilide. Its main use is as a luminal amebicidal agent. It is not widely available in the United States and can be obtained only from specific pharmacies (5).

Mechanism of action. The mechanism of action of diloxanide furoate is unknown.

Pharmacokinetics. Diloxanide furoate is available in tablet form. The parent drug is poorly absorbed following oral administration, but it is hydrolyzed in the bowel lumen to an active compound, diloxanide. This is >90% absorbed and is glucuronidated in the liver, reaching peak levels in serum within 1 to 2 h. Metabolites are excreted primarily in the urine.

Spectrum of activity. Diloxanide furoate acts primarily as a luminal agent and helps to clear the bowel of *E. histolytica* cysts, thereby preventing relapse in cyst carriers (72). It is not effective for ameba in the bowel wall or in other tissues such as the liver, so it is generally given with a 5-nitroimidazole.

Adverse effects. Side effects are generally not severe but include rash, nausea, abdominal pain, diarrhea, and flatulence. It is not recommended in pregnancy or during lactation.

Iodoquinol

Iodoquinol is a halogenated 8-hydroxyquinoline derivative, diiodohydroxyquin.

Mechanism of action. Iodoquinol is thought to act by inactivating essential parasitic enzymes and inhibiting parasite multiplication (41).

Pharmacokinetics. Iodoquinol is available for oral administration but is very slowly absorbed, with <8% reaching the systemic circulation, so it is excreted primarily in the feces. Small amounts of absorbed drug are glucuronidated in the liver, and small quantities of glucuronic acid metabolites are excreted in the urine. It should not be used in individuals with renal or hepatic insufficiency and should be used with caution in patients with thyroid or neurologic disease.

Spectrum of activity. Iodoquinol is a potent amebicidal drug. It is effective against trophozoites and cysts of *E. histolytica* located within the lumen of the intestine and is used to eradicate amebic cysts to help prevent relapse of infection (72). Because it is poorly absorbed systemically, it is not effective for invasive intestinal or extraintestinal *E. histolytica* infections and is therefore frequently combined with a 5-nitroimidazole.

Iodoquinol also has activity against *Balantidium coli*, *Dientamoeba fragilis*, and *G. lamblia*. It has also been used for *Blastocystis hominis*, although the significance of this agent as a true pathogen remains controversial (70).

Adverse effects. The main side effects of iodoquinol include nausea, abdominal cramps, diarrhea, headache, pruritus, and rash. Skin and hair may temporarily be stained yellow-brown following exposure. At high doses or with prolonged use, it can cause optic neuritis, optic atrophy, peripheral neuropathy, ataxia, and seizures. It is also associated with nephrotoxicity. It should be avoided in individuals who are sensitive to iodine. The degree of safety associated with its use in pregnancy or lactation is uncertain, so it is recommended that it be avoided.

Pentavalent Antimonial Compounds

The pentavalent antimony derivatives are used for treatment of leishmaniasis. They include sodium antimonylgluconate (or stibogluconate), also known as Pentostam, and *N*-methylglucamine antimoniate (or meglumine antimoniate), also known as Glucantime. Selection of one drug over the other is based primarily on cost and availability. Neither drug is licensed for use in the United States, but sodium stibogluconate is available from the CDC for individual patient use (5).

Mechanism of action. The precise mechanism of action of the pentavalent antimony derivatives remains unclear. They are thought to inhibit enzymes of glycolysis within parasites. Because glycolysis is the major source of parasitic ATP, the blockade of this source of energy is fatal to parasites (41).

Pharmacokinetics. The pentavalent antimonials are administered parenterally (intramuscularly or intravenously) or via intralesional injection. They remain in plasma and are excreted predominantly by the kidneys. Small amounts are metabolized in the liver to trivalent antimony, which contributes to the toxicity associated with their use. Following intramuscular administration of an initial dose of 10 mg of antimony per kg of body weight, mean peak antimony concentrations in blood of 9 to 12 mg/liter at 2 h have been reported (22). There are no specific guidelines regarding dose adjustment for renal impairment.

Spectrum of activity. Antimony preparations are efficient in killing many protozoan and helminthic parasites but are no longer recommended for most parasitic infections because of their toxicity. However, they are still used for the treatment of visceral, mucocutaneous, and cutaneous leishmaniasis, as few effective alternatives exist. Various treatment regimens are used, but the exact duration and efficacy vary depending on the type of leishmaniasis, the severity of the lesion, and the area of endemicity.

Adverse effects. Minor adverse effects from the pentavalent antimonials are common and include nausea, vomiting, headache, and malaise. More-severe reactions, such as leukopenia, agranulocytosis, and electrocardiographic changes (prolongation of the QT interval and ventricular arrhythmias), can also occur. Renal insufficiency, proteinuria, and elevation of hepatic and pancreatic enzymes have also been described.

Miltefosine

Miltefosine is a phosphocholine analogue that was originally developed as an anticancer compound. It is the first effective oral agent for visceral leishmaniasis and is becoming increasingly important because of growing resistance of *Leishmania* strains to pentavalent antimonials. Miltefosine was registered in 2002 for the oral treatment of visceral leishmaniasis in India and has been approved for use in Germany, but it is not approved by the the U.S. FDA. It has limited availability through the CDC.

Mechanism of action. The mechanism of action of miltefosine is not well understood. The drug interferes with cell signaling pathways and membrane synthesis (53). Miltefosine has a direct antiparasitic activity and appears to act on key enzymes involved in the metabolism of ether lipids present on the surfaces of parasites (53, 76). Miltefosine does not appear to have a direct immunostimulatory effect, but it does induce apoptotic cell death (96, 108). It has been shown to be active against both the extracellular promastigote form and the intracellular amastigote form of *Leishmania* parasites both in vitro and in vivo (104).

Pharmacokinetics. Miltefosine is well absorbed after oral administration and is widely distributed. Minimal pharmacokinetic data are available for humans, but in rats the drug is rapidly taken up and accumulates in the kidney, liver, lung, spleen, and adrenal glands (76). Upon oral administration of miltefosine at 30 mg/kg of body weight twice per day, concentrations of 155 to 189 nmol/g of tissue are achieved (53). Miltefosine has a long half-life of about 8 days and is slowly metabolized by phospholipase.

Spectrum of activity. Miltefosine has activity against *Leishmania* spp. and *Trypanosoma cruzi* both in vitro and in vivo, but clinical studies to date have been limited to leishmaniasis. In vitro activity of miltefosine against *Trypanosoma brucei*, *E. histolytica*, and *Acanthamoeba* spp. has also been demonstrated (25). The majority of studies using miltefosine have examined its role against visceral leishmaniasis in India. In clinical trials, miltefosine has been found to have a cure rate of 94 to 97% at 6 months in both adults and children (12, 114). It is generally given at 2.5 mg of miltefosine/kg/day for 4 weeks (12, 36, 53, 113, 114). Recent studies have also examined its efficacy in New World cutaneous leishmaniasis and have found 82 to 94% efficacy for *Leishmania (Viannia) panamensis*, 60% efficacy for *Leishmania mexicana mexicana*, and 33% efficacy for *L. (V.) braziliensis* (11, 107, 109).

Adverse effects. In various clinical trials, toxic effects associated with miltefosine have usually been found to be tolerable and reversible, although the therapeutic window appears to be narrow (96). Mild to moderate gastrointestinal side effects, including nausea, vomiting, and diarrhea, occur in up to 60% of patients. Dose-related motion sickness is also reported in up to 40% of patients (109). A mild increase in aspartate aminotransferase and creatinine and/or blood urea nitrogen levels has been reported, with reversible hepatotoxicity and renal damage in a few cases (12, 76). Miltefosine is abortifacient and teratogenic in animals and should not be used in pregnancy.

Pentamidine

Pentamidine is an aromatic diamidine compound that is used as an antiprotozoal agent in the treatment of leishmaniasis and African trypanosomiasis. Its use has been approved by the U.S. FDA (5).

Mechanism of action. Pentamidine is chemically related to guanidine. Its mechanism of action has not been defined clearly and may not be uniform against different organisms. It is possible that it inhibits dihydrofolate reductase and interferes with aerobic glycolysis in protozoa. It may also interfere with amino acid transport, precipitate nucleotides and nucleotide-containing coenzymes, and inhibit DNA, RNA, and protein synthesis (102).

Pharmacokinetics. Pentamidine is currently available as an isothionate salt. It is poorly absorbed from the gastrointestinal tract. When used for protozoal infections, it must therefore be administered intramuscularly or intravenously, but it can be given via inhalation for prevention of *Pneumocystis jirovecii* pneumonia. Following intravenous administration of a 4-mg/kg dose, concentrations in plasma of 0.3 to 1.4 mg/liter have been reported (124). The highest concentrations of the drug are found in the kidney, liver, and spleen, and pentamidine penetrates poorly into the CNS. It has a short half-life in serum of 6.5 to 9 h because it is rapidly and extensively taken up by tissues. Its extensive tissue binding results in prolonged excretion over a period of 6 to 8 weeks, and it is eliminated unchanged via the kidneys. Pentamidine should be used cautiously in the presence of renal or hepatic failure, but no dosage adjustment is recommended.

Spectrum of activity. The antiparasitic indications for pentamidine include leishmaniasis and African trypanosomiasis, but its main use is as an antifungal agent for treatment and prophylaxis of *P. jirovecii* pneumonia. Despite its antileishmanicidal activity, pentamidine's toxicity means that it is not first-line therapy for leishmaniasis, and it is used predominantly in individuals intolerant of antimonial compounds or for disease that is refractory to other treatment. *Leishmania donovani* infections, in particular, are increasingly resistant to antimonials, and pentamidine can be used as an alternative agent. Pentamidine is also active against African trypanosomes, but its utility is restricted to trypanosomiasis without CNS involvement. Because CNS involvement occurs early with *Trypanosoma brucei rhodesiense*, it is used more frequently for *T. b. gambiense* infections.

Adverse effects. Over one-half of parenteral pentamidine recipients experience some adverse effect from therapy. Administration is associated with a variety of reactions that appear to be unrelated to drug concentrations in plasma (102). Immediate reactions include nausea, anorexia, dizziness, pruritus, and hypotension. Pentamidine can also produce local effects, including pain and necrosis, at the site of injection. In addition, pentamidine administration is associated with hematologic effects, particularly leukopenia (up to 10% of recipients) and thrombocytopenia (approximately 5% of recipients), as well as with electrolyte abnormalities, including hyperkalemia, hypomagnesemia, and hypocalcemia. Other severe adverse effects include ventricular arrhythmias, pancreatitis, hypo- or hyperglycemia, hepatotoxicity, and acute renal failure. Pentamidine has also been associated with Stevens-Johnson syndrome. Finally, occasional seizures and hallucinations have been reported. There are minimal available safety data regarding the use of pentamidine in pregnancy or lactation, and its use is therefore not recommended unless the benefits outweigh potential risks.

Suramin

Suramin is a polysulfonated naphthylamine derivative of urea. Its main indication is in the treatment of African trypanosomiasis. It is not licensed for use in the United States but is available from the CDC via a compassionate drug protocol (5).

Mechanism of action. The mechanism of action of suramin is not fully understood but is thought to be via inhibition of enzymes associated with DNA metabolism and protein synthesis of the trypanosomal parasites (94).

Pharmacokinetics. Suramin is dispensed as a sodium salt and is soluble in water. It is not absorbed when given orally and is usually administered as a 10% solution by slow intravenous infusion. Following intravenous injection, it is rapidly distributed, and >99% becomes bound to plasma proteins. It does not cross the blood-brain barrier. It undergoes little or no metabolism and has a half-life of 41 to 78 days. It is excreted in the urine. It should not be used in the presence of renal failure or significant hepatic dysfunction.

Spectrum of activity. Suramin is an effective drug for early hemolymphatic stages of *T. b. gambiense* infections. It also has some effect in early *T. b. rhodesiense* infection, provided that there is no CNS involvement (32). Suramin was used to treat onchocerciasis prior to the development of ivermectin. An advantage of suramin is that it has macrofilaricidal activity, damaging the intestinal epithelium of adult *O. volvulus* worms and resulting in their death (116). However, it is associated with frequent toxic effects at required doses, so it has therefore been replaced by ivermectin. Suramin also has activity against adult *W. bancrofti* worms but is not recommended for this indication (41).

Adverse effects. Potential side effects include an immediate reaction, with nausea, vomiting, shock, and loss of consciousness, following suramin injection. Other adverse effects include renal impairment, exfoliative dermatitis, and neurological toxicity. It has also been associated with pancytopenia. Suramin has been reported to be teratogenic in rodents (123). No case of infant malformation has been described for humans, but it is not recommended for use during pregnancy except in circumstances where there is no suitable alternative.

Melarsoprol

Melarsoprol is a trivalent arsenical compound. Its main use is in the treatment of African trypanosomiasis. It is not licensed for use in the United States but is available from the CDC via a compassionate drug protocol (5).

Mechanism of action. Melarsoprol appears to act by binding to essential thiol groups of trypanosomes and has a particularly high affinity for the active site for pyruvate kinase. This results in interference with energy generation within parasites, thereby preventing trophozoite multiplication.

Pharmacokinetics. Melarsoprol is absorbed if given orally but is generally administered by the intravenous route. It is prepared as a solution in propylene glycol and is given by slow intravenous infusion. It is estimated that <1% of the drug penetrates the CNS, and concentrations in CSF are up to 50-fold lower than concentrations in serum (18, 43). However, it is so efficacious as an antitrypanocidal agent that it can be used for late stages of trypanosomal disease. Melarsoprol has a half-life of approximately 35 h. Its metabolism has not been well studied, but it is excreted predominantly in the urine.

Spectrum of activity. Melarsoprol is active in the treatment of all stages of African trypanosomiasis due to *T. b. gambiense* and *T. b. rhodesiense*. Because of its toxicity, it is generally reserved for use in late stages of disease involving the CNS.

Adverse effects. Malarsoprol is commonly associated with significant toxicity. It causes vomiting, abdominal pain, hepatotoxicity, peripheral neuropathy, cardiac arrhythmias, and albuminuria. Administration can also lead to a reactive encephalopathy in up to 10% of patients, and this is associated with significant mortality. Hypersensitivity reactions are also relatively frequent. The injection is very irritating, and extravasation during intravenous administration should be avoided. There are minimal data available regarding potential teratogenic effects.

Eflornithine

The main indication for use of eflornithine (also known as difluoromethylornithine) is for treatment of African trypanosomiasis. Its manufacture was ceased temporarily, and although it has been resumed, drug availability is still limited, and it is not available in the United States for systemic use.

Mechanism of action. Eflornithine selectively and irreversibly inhibits ornithine decarboxylase, an enzyme required for the formation of polyamines needed for cellular proliferation and differentiation in parasites. It therefore leads to inhibition of parasite growth (60).

Pharmacokinetics. Eflornithine can be administered by mouth and has >50% oral bioavailability, but significant diarrhea frequently results, so it is usually given intravenously. No protein binding of the drug occurs following intravenous administration. It crosses the blood-brain barrier and produces CSF-to-blood ratios between 0.13 and 0.5 (50, 74). The half-life is 3 to 3.5 h, and approximately 80% of the dose is excreted unchanged by the kidneys. Dose reduction is required in patients with significant renal impairment.

Spectrum of activity. Eflornithine is used for treatment of *T. b. gambiense* when there is CNS involvement. It is ineffective as monotherapy in *T. b. rhodesiense* (24). It also displays some activity against other parasites, including *Plasmodium* species, *Cryptosporidium parvum*, and *Trichomonas vaginalis*, but is not used for these indications because of toxicity.

Adverse effects. Side effects of eflornithine occur in up to 40% of patients. Common adverse reactions include vomiting, abdominal pain, dizziness, arthralgias, hearing loss, and rash. Bone marrow toxicity resulting in thrombocytopenia and leukopenia has also been described. Eflornithine has been shown to arrest embryonic development in animals (40). There are no good studies of its safety in pregnancy or lactation, so it should be used only when the potential maternal benefits outweigh the possible risks to the fetus.

Nifurtimox and Benznidazole

The two agents used for treatment of American trypanosomiasis are nifurtimox and benznidazole. Nifurtimox is

a nitrofuran, and benznidazole is a 2-nitroimidazole derivative. Neither is approved for use by the U.S. FDA, but nifurtimox is available from the CDC for compassionate use (5).

Mechanism of action. Benznidazole has an inhibitory effect on protein and ribonucleic acid synthesis in *Trypanosoma cruzi* cells (95). It is thought to cause increased phagocytosis, cytokine release, and production of reactive mitogen intermediates that result in destruction of intracellular parasites (79).

The mechanism of action of nifurtimox seems to be related to its metabolism to chemically reactive radicals that cause production of toxic reduced products of oxygen, such as superoxide, hydrogen peroxide, and hydroxyl radicals (29, 43). These compounds accumulate within trypanosomes, leading to toxic effects, including membrane damage and enzyme inactivation. It may also cause direct inhibition of protein synthesis via damage to parasite DNA (47).

Pharmacokinetics. Benznidazole is available for oral administration and has a bioavailability of over 90%. It is approximately 40% protein bound. It has a half-life of approximately 12 h and has good tissue penetration (129). Nifurtimox is administered orally but has poor oral bioavailability. It is metabolized in the liver and has a half-life of approximately 3 h. Dose reduction is advised for patients with significant hepatic or renal impairment, but no specific guidelines exist.

Spectrum of activity. Both benznidazole and nifurtimox are used for the treatment of acute *Trypanosoma cruzi* infection (Chagas' disease). Neither agent has demonstrated efficacy in late stages of disease. Nifurtimox is now also increasingly being used in combination with eflornithine for treatment of *T. b. gambiense* infection. It also has been shown to have some activity against leishmaniasis but is not routinely used for this indication.

Adverse effects. Side effects are common with benznidazole and are seen in up to 40% of treated individuals. Common adverse effects include vomiting, abdominal pain, peripheral neuropathy, rash, and pruritus. Bone marrow suppression and neuropsychiatric reactions have also been reported. Nifurtimox has significant side effects that preclude the completion of therapy in many patients. Adverse effects include anorexia, nausea, rash, headache, sleep disturbance, peripheral neuropathy, and myalgias. Less-frequent but more-severe toxicities include psychosis and convulsions. Benznidazole crosses the placenta, but there are minimal data regarding teratogenic effects of either agent in either animals or humans (27).

REFERENCES

1. **Adagu, I. S., D. Nolder, D. C. Warhurst, and J. F. Rossignol.** 2002. In vitro activity of nitazoxanide and related compounds against isolates of Giardia intestinalis, Entamoeba histolytica and Trichomonas vaginalis. *J. Antimicrob. Chemother.* **49:**103–111.
2. **Adam, I., E. T. Elwasila, and M. Homeida.** 2004. Is praziquantel therapy safe during pregnancy? *Trans. R. Soc. Trop. Med. Hyg.* **98:**540–543.
3. **Allen, H. E., D. W. Crompton, N. de Silva, P. T. LoVerde, and G. R. Olds.** 2002. New policies for using anthelmintics in high risk groups. *Trends Parasitol.* **18:**381–382.
4. Reference deleted.

5. **Anonymous.** 2007. *Drugs for Parasitic Infections.* The Medical Letter, Inc., New Rochelle, NY. www.medletter.com.

6. **Anonymous.** 2003. Nitazoxanide (Alinia)—a new antiprotozoal agent. *Med. Lett. Drugs Ther.* **45:**29–31.

7. **Araujo, N., A. Kohn, and N. Katz.** 1991. Activity of the artemether in experimental schistosomiasis mansoni. *Mem. Inst. Oswaldo Cruz* **86:**185–188.

8. **Auer, H., H. Kollaritsch, J. Juptner, and H. Aspock.** 1994. Albendazole and pregnancy. *Appl. Parasitol.* **35:**146–147.

9. **Baraka, O. Z., B. M. Mahmoud, C. K. Marschke, T. G. Geary, M. M. Homeida, and J. F. Williams.** 1996. Ivermectin distribution in the plasma and tissues of patients infected with Onchocerca volvulus. *Eur. J. Clin. Pharmacol.* **50:**407–410.

10. **Bem, J. L., L. Kerr, and D. Stuerchler.** 1992. Mefloquine prophylaxis: an overview of spontaneous reports of severe psychiatric reactions and convulsions. *J. Trop. Med. Hyg.* **95:**167–179.

11. **Berman, J. J.** 2008. Treatment of leishmaniasis with miltefosine: 2008 status. *Expert Opin. Drug Metab. Toxicol.* **4:**1209–1216.

12. **Bhattacharya, S. K., T. K. Jha, S. Sundar, C. P. Thakur, J. Engel, H. Sindermann, K. Junge, J. Karbwang, A. D. Bryceson, and J. D. Berman.** 2004. Efficacy and tolerability of miltefosine for childhood visceral leishmaniasis in India. *Clin. Infect. Dis.* **38:**217–221.

13. **Bogan, J. A., and S. Marriner.** 1980. Analysis of benzimidazoles in body fluids by high-performance liquid chromatography. *J. Pharm. Sci.* **69:**422–423.

14. **Brindley, P. J., and A. Sher.** 1990. Immunological involvement in the efficacy of praziquantel. *Exp. Parasitol.* **71:**245–248.

15. **Broekhuysen, J., A. Stockis, R. L. Lins, J. De Graeve, and J. F. Rossignol.** 2000. Nitazoxanide: pharmacokinetics and metabolism in man. *Int. J. Clin. Pharmacol. Ther.* **38:**387–394.

16. **Brueckner, R. P., T. Coster, D. L. Wesche, M. Shmuklarsky, and B. G. Schuster.** 1998. Prophylaxis of *Plasmodium falciparum* infection in a human challenge model with WR 238605, a new 8-aminoquinoline antimalarial. *Antimicrob. Agents Chemother.* **42:**1293–1294.

17. **Bryson, H. M., and K. L. Goa.** 1992. Halofantrine. A review of its antimalarial activity, pharmacokinetic properties and therapeutic potential. *Drugs* **43:**236–258.

18. **Burri, C., T. Baltz, C. Giroud, F. Doua, H. A. Welker, and R. Brun.** 1993. Pharmacokinetic properties of the trypanocidal drug melarsoprol. *Chemotherapy* **39:**225–234.

19. **Calvopina, M., R. H. Guderian, W. Paredes, M. Chico, and P. J. Cooper.** 1998. Treatment of human pulmonary paragonimiasis with triclabendazole: clinical tolerance and drug efficacy. *Trans. R. Soc. Trop. Med. Hyg.* **92:**566–569.

20. **Campbell, W. C.** 1993. Ivermectin, an antiparasitic agent. *Med. Res. Rev.* **13:**61–79.

21. **Chen, P. Q., G. Q. Li, X. B. Guo, K. R. He, Y. X. Fu, L. C. Fu, and Y. Z. Song.** 1994. The infectivity of gametocytes of Plasmodium falciparum from patients treated with artemisinin. *Chin. Med. J.* **107:**709–711.

22. **Chulay, J. D., L. Fleckenstein, and D. H. Smith.** 1988. Pharmacokinetics of antimony during treatment of visceral leishmaniasis with sodium stibogluconate or meglumine antimoniate. *Trans. R. Soc. Trop. Med. Hyg.* **82:**69–72.

23. **Cobo, F., C. Yarnoz, B. Sesma, P. Fraile, M. Aizcorbe, R. Trujillo, A. Diaz-de-Liano, and M. A. Ciga.** 1998. Albendazole plus praziquantel versus albendazole alone as a preoperative treatment in intra-abdominal hydatisosis caused by Echinococcus granulosus. *Trop. Med. Int. Health* **3:**462–466.

24. **Croft, S. L.** 1997. The current status of antiparasite chemotherapy. *Parasitology* **114:**S3–S15.

25. **Croft, S. L., K. Seifert, and M. Duchene.** 2003. Antiprotozoal activities of phospholipid analogues. *Mol. Biochem. Parasitol.* **126:**165–172.

26. **de Silva, N., H. Guyatt, and D. Bundy.** 1997. Anthelmintics. A comparative review of their clinical pharmacology. *Drugs* **53:**769–788.

27. **de Toranzo, E. G., M. Masana, and J. A. Castro.** 1984. Administration of benznidazole, a chemotherapeutic agent against Chagas disease, to pregnant rats. Covalent binding of reactive metabolites to fetal and maternal proteins. *Arch. Int. Pharmacodyn. Ther.* **272:**17–23.

28. **Diaz, E., J. Mondragon, E. Ramirez, and R. Bernal.** 2003. Epidemiology and control of intestinal parasites with nitazoxanide in children in Mexico. *Am. J. Trop. Med. Hyg.* **68:**384–385.

29. **Docampo, R., and S. N. Moreno.** 1984. Free radical metabolites in the mode of action of chemotherapeutic agents and phagocytic cells on Trypanosoma cruzi. *Rev. Infect. Dis.* **6:**223–238.

30. **Doenhoff, M. J., D. Cioli, and J. Utzinger.** 2008. Praziquantel: mechanisms of action, resistance and new derivatives for schistosomiasis. *Curr. Opin. Infect. Dis.* **21:**659–667.

31. **Dondorp, A., F. Nosten, K. Stepniewska, N. Day, and N. White.** 2005. Artesunate versus quinine for treatment of severe falciparum malaria: a randomised trial. *Lancet* **366:**717–725.

32. **Dumas, M., and B. Bouteille.** 2000. Treatment of human African trypanosomiasis. *Bull. W. H. O.* **78:**1474.

33. **Edstein, M. D., S. Looareesuwan, C. Viravan, and D. E. Kyle.** 1996. Pharmacokinetics of proguanil in malaria patients treated with proguanil plus atovaquone. *Southeast Asian J. Trop. Med. Public Health* **27:**216–220.

34. **Edwards, G., K. Awadzi, A. M. Breckenridge, H. M. Gilles, M. L. Orme, and S. A. Ward.** 1981. Diethylcarbamazine disposition in patients with onchocerciasis. *Clin. Pharmacol. Ther.* **30:**551–557.

35. **Edwards, G., and A. M. Breckenridge.** 1988. Clinical pharmacokinetics of anthelmintic drugs. *Clin. Pharmacokinet.* **15:**67–93.

36. **Fischer, C., A. Voss, and J. Engel.** 2001. Development status of miltefosine as first oral drug in visceral and cutaneous leishmaniasis. *Med. Microbiol. Immunol.* (Berlin) **190:**85–87.

37. **Foley, M., and L. Tilley.** 1997. Quinoline antimalarials: mechanisms of action and resistance. *Int. J. Parasitol.* **27:**231–240.

38. **Fox, L. M.** 2006. Ivermectin: uses and impact 20 years on. *Curr. Opin. Infect. Dis.* **19:**588–593.

39. **Fox, L. M., and L. D. Saravolatz.** 2005. Nitazoxanide: a new thiazolide antiparasitic agent. *Clin. Infect. Dis.* **40:**1173–1180.

40. **Fozard, J. R., M. L. Part, N. J. Prakash, and J. Grove.** 1980. Inhibition of murine embryonic development by alphadifluoromethylornithine, an irreversible inhibitor of ornithine decarboxylase. *Eur. J. Pharmacol.* **65:**379–391.

41. **Frayha, G. J., J. D. Smyth, J. G. Gobert, and J. Savel.** 1997. The mechanisms of action of antiprotozoal and anthelmintic drugs in man. *Gen. Pharmacol.* **28:**273–299.

42. **Gilles, H. M., and P. S. Hoffman.** 2002. Treatment of intestinal parasitic infections: a review of nitazoxanide. *Trends Parasitol.* **18:**95–97.

43. **Gilman, A., T. W. Rall, and A. S. Nies (ed.).** 1990. *Goodman and Gilman's the Pharmacological Basis of Therapeutics*, 8th ed. Pergamon Press, New York, NY.

44. **Goa, K. L., D. McTavish, and S. P. Clissold.** 1991. Ivermectin. A review of its antifilarial activity, pharmacokinetic properties and clinical efficacy in onchocerciasis. *Drugs* **42:**640–658.

45. **Gombert, M. E., E. J. Goldstein, J. L. Benach, M. J. Tenenbaum, E. Grunwaldt, M. H. Kaplan, and L. K. Eveland.** 1982. Human babesiosis. Clinical and therapeutic considerations. *JAMA* **248:**3005–3007.

46. **Gu, H. M., D. C. Warhurst, and W. Peters.** 1984. Uptake of [3H] dihydroartemisinine by erythrocytes infected with Plasmodium falciparum in vitro. *Trans. R. Soc. Trop. Med. Hyg.* **78:**265–270.

47. **Gutteridge, W. E.** 1985. Existing chemotherapy and its limitations. *Br. Med. Bull.* **41:**162–168.

48. **Gyapong, J. O., M. A. Chinbuah, and M. Gyapong.** 2003. Inadvertent exposure of pregnant women to ivermectin and albendazole during mass drug administration for lymphatic filariasis. *Trop. Med. Int. Health* **8:**1093–1101.

49. **Hennequin, C., P. Bouree, N. Bazin, F. Bisaro, and A. Feline.** 1994. Severe psychiatric side effects observed during prophylaxis and treatment with mefloquine. *Arch. Intern. Med.* **154:**2360–2362.

50. **Huebert, N. D., J. J. Schwartz, and K. D. Haegele.** 1997. Analysis of 2-difluoromethyl-DL-ornithine in human plasma, cerebrospinal fluid and urine by cation-exchange high-performance liquid chromatography. *J. Chromatogr. A* **762:**293–298.

51. **Inyang-Etoh, P. C., G. C. Ejezie, M. F. Useh, and E. C. Inyang-Etoh.** 2009. Efficacy of a combination of praziquantel and artesunate in the treatment of urinary schistosomiasis in Nigeria. *Trans. R. Soc. Trop. Med. Hyg.* **103:**38–44.

52. **Jaroonvesama, N., K. Charoenlarp, and J. H. Cross.** 1981. Treatment of Opisthorchis viverrini with mebendazole. *Southeast Asian J. Trop. Med. Public Health* **12:**595–597.

53. **Jha, T. K., S. Sundar, C. P. Thakur, P. Bachmann, J. Karbwang, C. Fischer, A. Voss, and J. Berman.** 1999. Miltefosine, an oral agent, for the treatment of Indian visceral leishmaniasis. *N. Engl. J. Med.* **341:**1795–1800.

54. **Joseph, C. A., and P. A. Dixon.** 1984. Possible prostaglandin-mediated effect of diethylcarbamazine on rat uterine contractility. *J. Pharm. Pharmacol.* **36:**281–282.

55. **Jung, H., M. Hurtado, M. T. Medina, M. Sanchez, and J. Sotelo.** 1990. Dexamethasone increases plasma levels of albendazole. *J. Neurol.* **237:**279–280.

56. **Jung, H., M. Hurtado, M. Sanchez, M. T. Medina, and J. Sotelo.** 1992. Clinical pharmacokinetics of albendazole in patients with brain cysticercosis. *J. Clin. Pharmacol.* **32:**28–31.

57. **Kaojarern, S., S. Nathakarnkikool, and T. U. Suvanakoot.** 1989. Comparative bioavailability of praziquantel tablets. *Drug Intell. Clin. Pharm.* **23:**29–32.

58. **Karbwang, J., and N. J. White.** 1990. Clinical pharmacokinetics of mefloquine. *Clin. Pharmacokinet.* **19:**264–279.

59. **Keiser, J., and J. Utzinger.** 2008. Efficacy of current drugs against soil-transmitted helminth infections: systematic review and meta-analysis. *JAMA* **299:**1937–1948.

60. **Kingsnorth, A. N.** 1986. The chemotherapeutic potential of polyamine antimetabolites. *Ann. R. Coll. Surg. Engl.* **68:**76–81.

61. **Klion, A. D., E. A. Ottesen, and T. B. Nutman.** 1994. Effectiveness of diethylcarbamazine in treating loiasis acquired by expatriate visitors to endemic regions: long-term follow-up. *J. Infect. Dis.* **169:**604–610.

62. **Kraivichian, K., S. Nuchprayoon, P. Sitichalernchai, W. Chaicumpa, and S. Yentakam.** 2004. Treatment of cutaneous gnathostomiasis with ivermectin. *Am. J. Trop. Med. Hyg.* **71:**623–628.

63. **Krishna, S., and N. J. White.** 1996. Pharmacokinetics of quinine, chloroquine and amodiaquine. Clinical implications. *Clin. Pharmacokinet.* **30:**263–299.

64. **Lacey, E.** 1990. Mode of action of benzimidazoles. *Parasitol. Today* **6:**112–115.

65. Reference deleted.

66. **Levy, M., D. Buskila, D. D. Gladman, M. B. Urowitz, and G. Koren.** 1991. Pregnancy outcome following first trimester exposure to chloroquine. *Am. J. Perinatol.* **8:**174–178.

67. **Liu, Y. H., X. G. Wang, P. Gao, and M. X. Qian.** 1991. Experimental and clinical trial of albendazole in the treatment of Clonorchiasis sinensis. *Chin. Med. J.* **104:**27–31.

68. **Looareesuwan, S., J. D. Chulay, C. J. Canfield, and D. B. Hutchinson.** 1999. Malarone (atovaquone and proguanil hydrochloride): a review of its clinical development for treatment of malaria. Malarone Clinical Trials Study Group. *Am. J. Trop. Med. Hyg.* **60:**533–541.

69. **Looareesuwan, S., R. E. Phillips, N. J. White, S. Kietinun, J. Karbwang, C. Rackow, R. C. Turner, and D. A. Warrell.** 1985. Quinine and severe falciparum malaria in late pregnancy. *Lancet* **ii:**4–8.

70. **Markell, E. K., and M. P. Udkow.** 1986. Blastocystis hominis: pathogen or fellow traveler? *Am. J. Trop. Med. Hyg.* **35:**1023–1026.

71. **Marriner, S. E., D. L. Morris, B. Dickson, and J. A. Bogan.** 1986. Pharmacokinetics of albendazole in man. *Eur. J. Clin. Pharmacol.* **30:**705–708.

72. **McAuley, J. B., B. L. Herwaldt, S. L. Stokes, J. A. Becher, J. M. Roberts, M. K. Michelson, and D. D. Juranek.** 1992. Diloxanide furoate for treating asymptomatic Entamoeba histolytica cyst passers: 14 years' experience in the United States. *Clin. Infect. Dis.* **15:**464–468.

73. **Mihaly, G. W., S. A. Ward, G. Edwards, M. L. Orme, and A. M. Breckenridge.** 1984. Pharmacokinetics of primaquine in man: identification of the carboxylic acid derivative as a major plasma metabolite. *Br. J. Clin. Pharmacol.* **17:**441–446.

74. **Milord, F., L. Loko, L. Ethier, B. Mpia, and J. Pepin.** 1993. Eflornithine concentrations in serum and cerebrospinal fluid of 63 patients treated for Trypanosoma brucei gambiense sleeping sickness. *Trans. R. Soc. Trop. Med. Hyg.* **87:**473–477.

75. **Mohamed, A. E., M. I. Yasawy, and M. A. Al Karawi.** 1998. Combined albendazole and praziquantel versus albendazole alone in the treatment of hydatid disease. *Hepatogastroenterology* **45:**1690–1694.

76. **More, B., H. Bhatt, V. Kukreja, and S. S. Ainapure.** 2003. Miltefosine: great expectations against visceral leishmaniasis. *J. Postgrad. Med.* **49:**101–103.

77. **Morris, D. L., J. B. Chinnery, G. Georgiou, G. Stamatakis, and B. Golematis.** 1987. Penetration of albendazole sulphoxide into hydatid cysts. *Gut* **28:**75–80.

78. **Moskopp, D., and E. Lotterer.** 1993. Concentrations of albendazole in serum, cerebrospinal fluid and hydatidous brain cyst. *Neurosurg. Rev.* **16:**35–37.

79. **Murta, S. M., C. Ropert, R. O. Alves, R. T. Gazzinelli, and A. J. Romanha.** 1999. In-vivo treatment with benznidazole enhances phagocytosis, parasite destruction and cytokine release by macrophages during infection with a drug-susceptible but not with a derived drug-resistant Trypanosoma cruzi population. *Parasite Immunol.* **21:**535–544.

80. **Na-Bangchang, K., S. Krudsood, U. Silachamroon, P. Molunto, O. Tasanor, K. Chalermrut, N. Tangpukdee, O. Matangkasombut, S. Kano, and S. Looareesuwan.** 2004. The pharmacokinetics of oral dihydroartemisinin and artesunate in healthy Thai volunteers. *Southeast Asian J. Trop. Med. Public Health* **35:**575–582.

81. **Naquira, C., G. Jimenez, J. G. Guerra, R. Bernal, D. R. Nalin, D. Neu, and M. Aziz.** 1989. Ivermectin for human strongyloidiasis and other intestinal helminths. *Am. J. Trop. Med. Hyg.* **40:**304–309.

82. **Nicolas, L., C. Plichart, L. N. Nguyen, and J. P. Moulia-Pelat.** 1997. Reduction of Wuchereria bancrofti adult worm circulating antigen after annual treatments of diethylcarbamazine combined with ivermectin in French Polynesia. *J. Infect. Dis.* **175:**489–492.

83. **Njoo, F. L., W. M. Beek, H. J. Keukens, H. van Wilgenburg, J. Oosting, J. S. Stilma, and A. Kijlstra.** 1995. Ivermectin detection in serum of onchocerciasis patients: relationship to adverse reactions. *Am. J. Trop. Med. Hyg.* **52:**94–97.

84. **Noroes, J., G. Dreyer, A. Santos, V. G. Mendes, Z. Medeiros, and D. Addiss.** 1997. Assessment of the efficacy of diethylcarbamazine on adult Wuchereria bancrofti in vivo. *Trans. R. Soc. Trop. Med. Hyg.* **91:**78–81.

85. **Nosten, F., M. Vincenti, J. Simpson, P. Yei, K. L. Thwai, A. de Vries, T. Chongsuphajaisiddhi, and N. J. White.** 1999. The effects of mefloquine treatment in pregnancy. *Clin. Infect. Dis.* **28:**808–815.

86. **Nosten, F., and N. J. White.** 2007. Artemisinin-based combination treatment of falciparum malaria. *Am. J. Trop. Med. Hyg.* **77:**181–192.

87. **Olds, G. R.** 2003. Administration of praziquantel to pregnant and lactating women. *Acta Trop.* **86:**185–195.

88. **Olliaro, P., C. Nevill, J. LeBras, P. Ringwald, P. Mussano, P. Garner, and P. Brasseur.** 1996. Systematic review of amodiaquine treatment in uncomplicated malaria. *Lancet* **348:**1196–1201.

89. **Opatrny, L., R. Prichard, L. Snell, and J. D. Maclean.** 2005. Death related to albendazole-induced pancytopenia: case report and review. *Am. J. Trop. Med. Hyg.* **72:**291–294.

90. **Ortiz, J. J., A. Ayoub, G. Gargala, N. L. Chegne, and L. Favennec.** 2001. Randomized clinical study of nitazoxanide compared to metronidazole in the treatment of symptomatic giardiasis in children from Northern Peru. *Aliment. Pharmacol. Ther.* **15:**1409–1415.

91. **Ottesen, E. A.** 1985. Efficacy of diethylcarbamazine in eradicating infection with lymphatic-dwelling filariae in humans. *Rev. Infect. Dis.* **7:**341–356.

92. **Ottesen, E. A., and W. C. Campbell.** 1994. Ivermectin in human medicine. *J. Antimicrob. Chemother.* **34:**195–203.

93. **Pacque, M., B. Munoz, G. Poetschke, J. Foose, B. M. Greene, and H. R. Taylor.** 1990. Pregnancy outcome after inadvertent ivermectin treatment during community-based distribution. *Lancet* **336:**1486–1489.

94. **Pepin, J., and F. Milord.** 1994. The treatment of human African trypanosomiasis. *Adv. Parasitol.* **33:**1–47.

95. **Polak, A., and R. Richle.** 1978. Mode of action of the 2-nitroimidazole derivative benznidazole. *Ann. Trop. Med. Parasitol.* **72:**45–54.

96. **Prasad, R., R. Kumar, B. P. Jaiswal, and U. K. Singh.** 2004. Miltefosine: an oral drug for visceral leishmaniasis. *Indian J. Pediatr.* **71:**143–144.

97. **Price, R. N., F. Nosten, C. Luxemburger, F. O. ter Kuile, L. Paiphun, T. Chongsuphajaisiddhi, and N. J. White.** 1996. Effects of artemisinin derivatives on malaria transmissibility. *Lancet* **347:**1654–1658.

98. **Pungpark, S., D. Bunnag, and T. Harinasuta.** 1984. Albendazole in the treatment of opisthorchiasis and concomitant intestinal helminthic infections. *Southeast Asian J. Trop. Med. Public Health* **15:**44–50.

99. **Pussard, E., and F. Verdier.** 1994. Antimalarial 4-aminoquinolines: mode of action and pharmacokinetics. *Fundam. Clin. Pharmacol.* **8:**1–17.

100. **Radloff, P. D., J. Philipps, D. Hutchinson, and P. G. Kremsner.** 1996. Atovaquone plus proguanil is an effective treatment for Plasmodium ovale and P. malariae malaria. *Trans. R. Soc. Trop. Med. Hyg.* **90:**682.

101. **Rombo, L., A. Bjorkman, E. Sego, and O. Ericsson.** 1986. Whole blood concentrations of chloroquine and desethylchloroquine during and after treatment of adult patients infected with Plasmodium vivax, P. ovale or P. malariae. *Trans. R. Soc. Trop. Med. Hyg.* **80:**763–766.

102. **Sands, M., M. A. Kron, and R. B. Brown.** 1985. Pentamidine: a review. *Rev. Infect. Dis.* **7:**625–634.

103. **Silver, H.** 1997. Malarial infection during pregnancy. *Infect. Dis. Clin. N. Am.* **11:**99–107.

104. **Sindermann, H., S. L. Croft, K. R. Engel, W. Bommer, H. J. Eibl, C. Unger, and J. Engel.** 2004. Miltefosine (Impavido): the first oral treatment against leishmaniasis. *Med. Microbiol. Immunol.* (Berlin) **193:**173–180.

105. **Slater, A. F., and A. Cerami.** 1992. Inhibition by chloroquine of a novel haem polymerase enzyme activity in malaria trophozoites. *Nature* **355:**167–169.

106. **Sotelo, J., and H. Jung.** 1998. Pharmacokinetic optimisation of the treatment of neurocysticercosis. *Clin. Pharmacokinet.* **34:**503–515.

107. **Soto, J., B. A. Arana, J. Toledo, N. Rizzo, J. C. Vega, A. Diaz, M. Luz, P. Gutierrez, M. Arboleda, J. D. Berman, K. Junge, J. Engel, and H. Sindermann.** 2004. Miltefosine for new world cutaneous leishmaniasis. *Clin. Infect. Dis.* **38:**1266–1272.

108. **Soto, J., and P. Soto.** 2006. Miltefosine: oral treatment of leishmaniasis. *Expert Rev. Anti Infect. Ther.* **4:**177–185.

109. **Soto, J., J. Toledo, P. Gutierrez, R. S. Nicholls, J. Padilla, J. Engel, C. Fischer, A. Voss, and J. Berman.** 2001. Treatment of American cutaneous leishmaniasis with miltefosine, an oral agent. *Clin. Infect. Dis.* **33:**E57–E61.

110. **Srivastava, I. K., and A. B. Vaidya.** 1999. A mechanism for the synergistic antimalarial action of atovaquone and proguanil. *Antimicrob. Agents Chemother.* **43:**1334–1339.

111. **Stockis, A., A. M. Allemon, S. De Bruyn, and C. Gengler.** 2002. Nitazoxanide pharmacokinetics and tolerability in man using single ascending oral doses. *Int. J. Clin. Pharmacol. Ther.* **40:**213–220.

112. **Stockis, A., X. Deroubaix, R. Lins, B. Jeanbaptiste, P. Calderon, and J. F. Rossignol.** 1996. Pharmacokinetics of nitazoxanide after single oral dose administration in 6 healthy volunteers. *Int. J. Clin. Pharmacol. Ther.* **34:**349–351.

113. **Sundar, S., T. K. Jha, H. Sindermann, K. Junge, P. Bachmann, and J. Berman.** 2003. Oral miltefosine treatment in children with mild to moderate Indian visceral leishmaniasis. *Pediatr. Infect. Dis. J.* **22:**434–438.

114. **Sundar, S., T. K. Jha, C. P. Thakur, J. Engel, H. Sindermann, C. Fischer, K. Junge, A. Bryceson, and J. Berman.** 2002. Oral miltefosine for Indian visceral leishmaniasis. *N. Engl. J. Med.* **347:**1739–1746.

115. **Sutherland, I. H., and W. C. Campbell.** 1990. Development, pharmacokinetics and mode of action of ivermectin. *Acta Leiden* **59:**161–168.

116. **Taylor, H. R.** 1984. Recent developments in the treatment of onchocerciasis. *Bull W. H. O.* **62:**509–515.

117. **Tietze, P. E., and J. E. Jones.** 1991. Parasites during pregnancy. *Prim. Care* **18:**75–99.

118. **Twum-Danso, N. A.** 2003. Loa loa encephalopathy temporally related to ivermectin administration reported from onchocerciasis mass treatment programs from 1989 to 2001: implications for the future. *Filaria J.* **2**(Suppl. 1):S7.

119. **Utzinger, J., S. H. Xiao, M. Tanner, and J. Keiser.** 2007. Artemisinins for schistosomiasis and beyond. *Curr. Opin. Investig. Drugs* **8:**105–116.

120. **Vanhauwere, B., H. Maradit, and L. Kerr.** 1998. Post-marketing surveillance of prophylactic mefloquine (Lariam) use in pregnancy. *Am. J. Trop. Med. Hyg.* **58:**17–21.

121. **van Riemsdijk, M. M., M. M. van der Klauw, J. A. van Heest, F. R. Reedeker, R. J. Ligthelm, R. M. Herings, and B. H. Stricker.** 1997. Neuro-psychiatric effects of antimalarials. *Eur. J. Clin. Pharmacol.* **52:**1–6.

122. **Veenendaal, J. R., A. D. Parkinson, N. Kere, K. H. Rieckmann, and M. D. Edstein.** 1991. Pharmacokinetics of halofantrine and n-desbutylhalofantrine in patients with falciparum malaria following a multiple dose regimen of halofantrine. *Eur. J. Clin. Pharmacol.* **41:**161–164.

123. **Voogd, T. E., E. L. Vansterkenburg, J. Wilting, and L. H. Janssen.** 1993. Recent research on the biological activity of suramin. *Pharmacol. Rev.* **45:**177–203.

124. **Waalkes, T. P., and V. T. DeVita.** 1970. The determination of pentamidine (4,4'-diamidinophenoxypentane) in plasma, urine, and tissues. *J. Lab. Clin. Med.* **75:**871–878.

125. **Walsh, D. S., P. Wilairatana, D. B. Tang, D. G. Heppner, Jr., T. G. Brewer, S. Krudsood, U. Silachamroon, W. Phumratanaprapin, D. Siriyanonda, and S. Looareesuwan.** 2004. Randomized trial of 3-dose regimens of tafenoquine (WR238605) versus low-dose primaquine for preventing Plasmodium vivax malaria relapse. *Clin. Infect. Dis.* **39:**1095–1103.

126. **Warhurst, D. C.** 1984. Why are primaquine and other 8-aminoquinolines particularly effective against the mature gametocytes and the hypnozoites of malaria? *Ann. Trop. Med. Parasitol.* **78:**165.

127. **Wen, L. Y., X. L. Yan, F. H. Sun, Y. Y. Fang, M. J. Yang, and L. J. Lou.** 2008. A randomized, double-blind, multicenter clinical trial on the efficacy of ivermectin against intestinal nematode infections in China. *Acta Trop.* **106:**190–194.

128. **White, N. J.** 1985. Clinical pharmacokinetics of antimalarial drugs. *Clin. Pharmacokinet.* **10:**187–215.

129. **Workman, P., R. A. White, M. I. Walton, L. N. Owen, and P. R. Twentyman.** 1984. Preclinical pharmacokinetics of benznidazole. *Br. J. Cancer* **50:**291–303.

130. **World Health Organization.** 1995. Control of foodborne trematode infections. Report of a WHO study group. *W. H. O. Tech. Rep. Ser.* **849:**1–157.

Mechanisms of Resistance to Antiparasitic Agents*

W. EVAN SECOR AND JACQUES LE BRAS

148

Parasitic diseases rank among the most prevalent and severe diseases worldwide, and yet their control relies heavily on a single tool: the drugs used for chemotherapy or prophylaxis. This situation exists because no effective antiparasitic vaccines are available and implementation of other control measures often proves to be difficult in countries where parasitic diseases are endemic. This dependence on drugs is compounded by the relative paucity of the current armamentarium of antiparasitic products, a situation attributable largely to a lack of economic incentives for research and development. Furthermore, those drugs that are available are too often used incorrectly in communities and in control programs, a practice that encourages the selection of drug-resistant parasites.

The complex biologic interactions between parasites and their hosts (and at times vectors) influence significantly the emergence and expression of drug resistance. In many cases the observed resistance is true resistance, attributable to biologic characteristics of the parasites that enable them to survive drug concentrations that are lethal to susceptible members of the species. Mechanisms for such true resistance are varied and include a decrease in parasite drug accumulation or modifications in enzyme structure or metabolic pathways. However, various host factors modulate the clinical and parasitological responses to drug treatment, and the observed responses do not necessarily reflect true parasite resistance or susceptibility. For example, in populations with high rates of exposure to parasitic infections, the resulting high rates of immunity might suffice to eliminate an infection treated with an ineffective drug. Conversely, treatment with a drug to which the parasite is biologically susceptible will not necessarily result in therapeutic success if the host takes an inadequate dose of the drug, absorbs it poorly, or lacks the immune response that might be needed for a successful antiparasitic synergism with the drug. Such host factors may be especially important in the areas where most parasitic diseases prevail, where high rates of parasite transmission result in high rates of immunity in most of the population, or where, conversely, malnutrition and human immunodeficiency virus (HIV) infection frequently decrease the patient's immune status.

Greater understanding of the epidemiology and mechanisms of drug resistance can provide valuable guidance for a better use of existing compounds and for the development of novel products. A selective review of drug resistance in five diseases will illustrate the existing problems and their potential solutions. A summary of the proposed mechanisms of resistance is provided in Table 1.

MALARIA

Overview

Malaria remains the most visible indicator of the adequacy of health control in all regions of the world with a hot and humid season. By 1955, the World Health Organization (WHO) had established projects for malaria eradication by using indoor residual spraying of insecticides to limit contact between humans and the anophele vector and by mass administration of pyrimethamine and chloroquine to kill erythrocytic forms of the parasites (145). As these programs faced infrastructure deficiencies and resistance to insecticides, the vector control was often neglected and the bulk of expenditure was devoted to the use of antimalarial drugs against fever, mainly chloroquine, with sulfadoxine-pyrimethamine as a secondary drug. *Plasmodium falciparum*, the most virulent species, which adapts more easily to environmental constraints in tropical areas, has become the dominant species, and its resistance to chloroquine, to sulfadoxine-pyrimethamine, and, further, to all known drugs has developed to various degrees. Sub-Saharan Africa alone contributes 90% of the annual 250 million patients worldwide suffering from malaria, and 1 million die each year, mainly those without acquired adequate clinical immunity: young children and women during their first pregnancy. Since the beginning of the 21st century, a specific effort of integrated control has been made, and a reduction in transmission is starting to be observed in parts of Africa (146). The most spectacular action was the global establishment of malaria treatment with artemisinin-based combination therapies (ACTs), associating a curative dose of a drug with long elimination half-life and a dose of a rapidly active drug able to destroy most of the parasite load in a few hours. This bitherapy is based on a derivative of artemisinin, a substance extracted from sagebrush grown mainly in China, which generates oxidative stress in all stages of the parasite. The combination of multiple drugs

*This chapter contains information presented in chapter 151 by W. Evan Secor and Phuc Nguyen-Dinh in the ninth edition of this *Manual*.

TABLE 1 Summary of proposed mechanisms of resistance to selected antiparasitic drugs

Disease	Drug(s)	Mechanism(s) of resistance
Malaria[a]	Chloroquine	Decreased accumulation of the drug by the parasite, resulting from multifactorial, multigenic mechanisms
	Pyrimethamine	Alteration in binding affinities between the drug and the parasite DHFR-thymidylate synthase, resulting from mutations on the corresponding gene
	Sulfadoxine	Alteration in binding affinities between the drug and the parasite dihydropteroate synthase, resulting from mutations on the corresponding gene
	Atovaquone	Alteration in binding affinities between the drug and the parasite cytochrome[b]
Trichomoniasis[b]	Metronidazole, tinidazole	Reduced concentration of enzyme(s) necessary to activate nitro group
Leishmaniasis[c]	Pentavalent antimonials	Decreased active intracellular drug concentration through increased efflux or decreased conversion to active trivalent form
	Amphotericin B, paromomycin, miltefosine	Widespread clinical resistance not currently documented, although resistance has been produced in laboratory strains
African trypanosomiasis[d]	Melarsoprol, pentamidine	Mutation/loss of P2 adenosine transporters that facilitate drug uptake
Schistosomiasis[e]	Praziquantel	Widespread clinical resistance not currently recognized as an important problem for public health, resistance documented in laboratory strains
	Artemether	Effective against immature worms; no resistance as yet documented

[a]Disease caused predominantly by *Plasmodium falciparum*, *P. vivax*, *P. ovale*, and *P. malariae*.
[b]Disease caused by *Trichomonas vaginalis*.
[c]Diseases caused by one of several *Leishmania* species.
[d]Disease caused by *Trypanosoma brucei* subsp. *rhodesiense* and subsp. *gambiense*.
[e]Diseases caused predominantly by *Schistosoma mansoni*, *S. japonicum*, and *S. haematobium*.

enhances clinical efficacy and may delay parasite resistance. We need to consider the history of the emergence and spread of resistance to chloroquine and sulfadoxine-pyrimethamine as premonitory of the risk of losing the effectiveness of ACTs if their use is not controlled.

The 4-amino quinoline drug chloroquine, a cornerstone of antimalarial chemotherapy since the 1940s due to its low cost, its safety, and its rapid action, lost most of its usefulness as the frequency of *P. falciparum*-resistant strains increased and peaked in the 1980s. From the original foci in Southeast Asia and South America, resistance has spread inescapably and is now found in most areas of endemicity, including Africa, the continent with the heaviest malaria burden. Chloroquine no longer constitutes an appropriate option for prompt and effective treatment in most countries where *P. falciparum* malaria is the dominant endemic species. With increased use of sulfadoxine-pyrimethamine, the second-most-affordable, relatively safe, and easy-to-administer drug after chloroquine, parasite resistance to sulfadoxine-pyrimethamine has developed very quickly following the same itineraries as the spread of chloroquine resistance a few years before. Nevertheless, people in some African regions with heavy malaria transmission still rely on chloroquine or sulfadoxine-pyrimethamine for presumptive treatment of fever or for intermittent preventive treatment of pregnant women as the most effective way to prevent severe consequences of malaria. Losing the two low-cost antimalarials is often seen by experts as a public health disaster. Reducing transmission intensity could slow the spread of resistance, but paradoxically, below a critical level, it may accelerate the selection of multigenic resistance (130). The critical situation has prompted international initiatives to help face the high cost of ACTs, to make affordable, rapid diagnostic tests available everywhere, and to renew mosquito control programs by an extensive distribution of insecticide impregnated nets. Lessons from the past informed parasitologists that delays in detection and control of resistance to ACTs may ruin programs without alternatives for decades. Real-time drug resistance surveillance

systems are important, and drug development efforts must be enhanced.

Mechanisms of Resistance to Selected Antimalarials

Chloroquine concentrates at nanomolar levels outside the parasite to millimolar levels within the digestive vacuole of the intraerythrocytic trophozoite, where it inhibits hemoglobin degradation (43). Chloroquine forms complexes with hematin, a by-product of host cell hemoglobin digestion by the parasite, which accumulates in large quantities and eventually kills the parasite. The resistant isolates have in common a defect in chloroquine accumulation in the digestive vacuole (138). Several mechanisms have been proposed to explain the altered chloroquine accumulation, such as changes in the pH gradient or altered membrane permeability, leading to a decreased drug uptake or increased drug efflux (36, 62). Chloroquine accumulation has high structural specificity; this suggests the involvement of either a specific transporter/permease or a molecule associated with hematin in the digestive vacuole (15). Following demonstration that chloroquine-resistance is reversible by verapamil, earlier studies focused on the orthologue of the mammalian *mdr* gene, whose products are overexpressed in cancer cells, where they expel cytotoxic drugs (10, 80, 142). This strategy led to the identification of the chromosome 5 *P. falciparum mdr1* (*pfmdr1*) gene product (protein PfPGH-1) in the digestive vacuole membrane of *P. falciparum*, which is an analogue of the P-glycoproteins (ATP-binding cassette transporters) (110). Chloroquine resistance was initially attributed to variations in the copy numbers of the *pfmdr1* gene; however, no evidence of amplification of this gene with chloroquine resistance was observed. Chloroquine transport and resistance were found, however, to be altered by *pfmdr1* mutations that encode changes in the PfPGH-1 amino acid residues and in specific parasite genetic backgrounds. In vivo, the association between mutations in PfPGH-1 and chloroquine resistance remains unclear. In subsequent years, clear demonstration of a Mendelian segregation of a resistant determinant located on chromosome 7 led to the key discovery of the *pfcrt* gene (141, 142). The *pfcrt* gene encodes a transmembrane protein located in the digestive vacuole membrane (42). A set of mutations of this gene is found in most natural isolates from clinical chloroquine treatment failures (32) and in vitro in isolates with a chloroquine-resistant phenotype. Finally, transfection of chloroquine-sensitive parasites with the mutant *pfcrt* genotypes found in resistant isolates suffices to confer chloroquine resistance (42). Progressive accumulation of mutations in the *pfcrt* gene and finally the mutation at position 76, together with mutations in other genes, such as *pfmdr1*, might be involved in modulation of the resistance (14), consistent with the delayed emergence of resistance. Four independent *pfcrt* mutation profiles are seen, varying geographically: Asia-Africa, Papua, and South America 1 and 2 (83). Thus, the major event in chloroquine resistance is the emergence on the Thai-Cambodian border in the 1950s of the CVIET haplotype at positions 72 to 76 of the *pfcrt* gene under drug pressure selection; this haplotype has spread to 90% of the *P. falciparum* territory in the 50 years since (4). Nonetheless, the wild isolates, which are very polymorphic, have not been totally replaced; they still represent approximately half the *P. falciparum* strains in circulation, and their prevalence increases when drug pressure is removed (87). The *pfcrt* K76T mutation is now a valuable molecular marker used in epidemiological surveys of chloroquine resistance (31, 87). Its estimated prevalence may offer a useful predictor of the clinical efficacy of chloroquine in a given area, provided that appropriate adjustments are made for host factors, particularly immunity, that may result in parasite clearance in spite of treatment with an ineffective drug (33).

Belonging to the same class as chloroquine, two 4-amino quinolines, amodiaquine and piperaquine, are in the first line of therapy as partners of artemisinins. Current evidence indicates that *pfmdr1* does not play a major role in chloroquine resistance, although a mutation at codon 86 seems an important determinant of resistance to desethylamodiaquine, the active metabolite of amodiaquine. The *pfmdr1* gene also appears to be involved in resistance to other antimalarial drugs, and mutations or amplification of the gene alters responses to quinine, mefloquine, and lumefantrine (20, 39, 48, 72, 110). Transporters other than *Pf*CRT and *Pf*PGH-1, such as *Pf*MRP-1, may be involved in resistance to mefloquine or lumefantrine (27). The amino-alcohols mefloquine and lumefantrine are the other partners of ACT. They accumulate in the parasite cytoplasm, and variations in the numbers of copies of the *pfmdr1* gene have been associated with treatment failures or tolerance (prolonged clearance time) to corresponding ACTs (109).

Unlike with drugs that accumulate in the malaria parasite, i.e., chloroquine, desethylamodiaquine, mefloquine, lumefantrine, and quinine, a single gene modification is sufficient to generate resistance to a drug which antagonizes a single enzyme. Malaria parasites rely mostly on de novo synthesis for folate supply; therefore, antifolates, with cycloguanil (produced by the prodrug proguanil) and its analogue pyrimethamine, were the first satisfactory synthetic antimalarials to be on the market in the 1940s. Unfortunately, antifolate resistance emerged almost instantaneously and independently from several areas where the drugs had been introduced, and antifolate antimalarials were soon supplanted by chloroquine (103). Unlike in bacteria and human tumor cells, gene amplification is not involved in *P. falciparum* resistance to dihydrofolate reductase

(*Pf*DHFR) inhibitors. The S108N substitution in the *P. falciparum* DHFR-thymidylate synthase (*pfdhfr-ts*) gene on chromosome 4 is associated with simultaneous resistance to pyrimethamine, cycloguanil, and other antifolinics (21, 30, 44). A resurgence in the use of antifolate antimalarials took place with the demonstration in 1967 that potentiation with antifolics such as sulfadoxine or dapsone bypassed resistance, and sulfadoxine-pyrimethamine became the new spearhead to face chloroquine resistance in Southeast Asia (103, 107). Soon after the increased use of sulfadoxine-pyrimethamine in Thailand, additive substitutions N51I and C59R were detected in *pfdhfr-ts*, and parasites with the three mutations responded with early or late treatment failure to sulfadoxine-pyrimethamine (108). These stepwise acquisitions of pyrimethamine and then sulfadoxine-pyrimethamine resistance in *P. falciparum* and probabilities of fixation based on the relative levels of resistance confirmed the sequence of S108N and then the sequence of C59R, N51I, and I164L mutations (74, 100, 122). The I164L mutation in *pfdhfr*, associated with high levels of sulfadoxine-pyrimethamine resistance as well as decreased sensitivity to chlorproguanil-dapsone (an attempt to develop a new antifolate combination similar to sulfadoxine-pyrimethamine), has been reported as an isolated polymorphism only in Africa (100). The triple mutant (N51I C59R S108N) *pfdhfr* gene that emerged probably in the Thai-Cambodian border area had great evolutionary success, spreading all over Asia and Africa in the following years (77). It was initially thought that mutations on the dihydropteroate synthetase gene (*pfdhps*, target of some antifolates) on chromosome 8 might be responsible for sulfadoxine resistance (131). That is, *pfdhfr* and *pfdhps* mutants are selected during sulfadoxine-pyrimethamine treatment, and resistance to sulfonamides/sulfone has been traced to a set of sequential mutations in the *pfdhps* gene (26). The likely initial event consisted of an A437G mutation, with subsequent additional mutations conferring increasing degrees of resistance (107). Analysis of the progenies of a genetic cross between a sulfadoxine-sensitive parent and a sulfadoxine-resistant parent has demonstrated the close association between the *pfdhps* mutations and the resistance phenotype but also a complete correlation between multiple *pfdhfr* mutations and resistance (139). Resistance to the sulfadoxine-pyrimethamine combination appears to require three mutations in the *pfdhfr* gene, but the probability of sulfadoxine-pyrimethamine treatment failure increases with two additional mutations on *pfdhps* ("quintuple mutant"). The clinical outcome of a sulfadoxine-pyrimethamine treatment is subjected to additional host factors, such as the level of folates and of acquired immunity and drug absorption and metabolism (26, 63, 107, 108). Cross-resistance has been demonstrated between cycloguanil and pyrimethamine; consequently, interest in other antifolates, such as chlorproguanil plus dapsone, to treat parasites resistant to sulfadoxine-pyrimethamine has been limited (26).

Malarone was registered in 1996 in North America and Europe, where, within 10 years, it became the most used antimalarial for the prophylaxis and first-line treatment of nonsevere malaria. It consists of atovaquone, a ubiquinone analogue that binds to cytochrome *b* (*Pf*CytB) and inhibits electron transfer of the respiratory chain, in association with proguanil, which lowers the effective concentration at which atovaquone causes the collapse of the mitochondrial membrane potential (126). Atovaquone-proguanil, like sulfadoxine-pyrimethamine, is not a combined therapy but is instead a potentiating association in which cycloguanil does not contribute significantly to the drug action. As with the antifolates, atovaquone resistance emerged almost instantaneously; mutations in codon 268 of the *Pf*CytB gene resulting in the substitution of S, N, or C in the product gave a high level of resistance that proguanil could not thwart (73, 116). Nevertheless, if parasites harboring a single mutation on codon 268 of *pfcytB* are likely to be present in most patients (parasite load in blood is 10^9 to 10^{11}), their low fitness and/or other unknown mechanisms limit the occurrence of drug treatment failure (60, 92). Due to the risk of rapid extension of resistance and the high cost of the drug, the deployment of atovaquone in regions where malaria is endemic has not been considered.

Chloroquine resistance in *Plasmodium vivax*, the second-most-common malaria parasite, has been very limited despite widespread chloroquine use. Patients infected with *P. vivax* relapse from dormant parasites in their liver, and the organism has developed partial resistance to primaquine, the only drug active against liver forms (123). While drug resistance in *P. vivax* remains at low magnitude, investigations on mechanisms of resistance in this species currently examine the potential role of *P. vivax* homologues of *pfcrt* (98), *pfmdr1* (16), *pfdhfr* (50), and *pfdhps* (6, 61, 111).

TRICHOMONIASIS

Infection with *Trichomonas vaginalis* is one of the most common causes of human vaginitis as well as one of the most prevalent nonviral sexually transmitted diseases. Recent data have linked *T. vaginalis* infections with preterm delivery, low birth weight, greater susceptibility to infection with HIV, and an increased risk of cervical neoplasia (93, 143). As a result, expedient treatment of this infection has become an important public health measure (81, 137).

T. vaginalis is a facultative anaerobe, and trichomoniasis is most commonly treated with the 5-nitroimidazole class of drugs. Two members of this group, metronidazole and tinidazole, are the only drugs licensed for treatment of trichomoniasis in the United States. Tinidazole is more active at equimolar concentrations than metronidazole and is recommended if treatment with metronidazole fails (24, 143). However, strains clinically resistant to metronidazole can have cross-resistance to tinidazole. The molecular epidemiology of *T. vaginalis* suggests that clinically resistant isolates are genetically related and stable over time (47, 124, 136). Nevertheless, despite increasing recognition of metronidazole treatment failures (125) and the observation that up to 10% of isolates obtained from women attending sexually transmitted disease clinics demonstrate in vitro resistance (117), no epidemics of resistant trichomoniasis have occurred. To explain this observation, it has been hypothesized that resistant isolates are less transmittable between sexual partners (132).

The 5-nitroimidazoles enter parasites in an inactive form by passive diffusion. Once inside, it has long been thought that redox reactions occurring in the hydrogenosome, which is the source of ATP generation in these amitochondriate parasites, convert the compounds into cytotoxic radical anions that cause cell death by breaking or disrupting DNA (25, 38). During energy metabolism, reactions involving pyruvate-ferredoxin oxidoreductase and malic enzyme generate electrons that are transferred to the drug via ferredoxin (38, 52, 66). In this model, drug resistance occurs in parasites with decreased expression of the enzymes responsible for these pathways, resulting in reduced drug activation. However, a recent paper suggests that the nitroimidazole drugs are reduced by the flavin enzyme thioredoxin reductase and covalently bind and inhibit proteins associated with thioredoxin-mediated redox regulation (68). An in vitro-induced, nitroimidazole-resistant strain demonstrated reduced thioredoxin reductase activity, not as a result of decreased enzyme concentration but because of a deficiency in the necessary flavin adenine dinucleotide cofactor. Trichomonads with minimal pyruvate-ferredoxin oxidoreductase and malate dehydrogenase activity remained susceptible to metronidazole (68), consistent with the observation that there were no correlations between mRNA levels of these enzymes and nitroimidazole susceptibility in recent patient isolates with various levels of in vitro resistance (82). A third possible mechanism for nitroimidazole resistance was suggested by the observation that trichomonas isolates that harbored *Mycoplasma hominis* symbionts had a mean in vitro resistance level 10-fold higher than that of noninfected trichomonads (147). However, the increased mean resistance of the *M. hominis*-infected isolates was still lower than typically observed for resistant isolates. In a separate study, there was no association of mycoplasma infection with clinical resistance (17a). It remains unclear which, if any, of these mechanisms is responsible for the nitroimidazole resistance observed in some *T. vaginalis* infections.

Treatment of patients who have metronidazole-resistant trichomoniasis often results in an immediate resolution of symptoms and a negative wet mount. However, within 3 to 4 weeks, in the absence of further exposure, symptoms may recur as the number of organisms rises. Thus, it is important to monitor efficacy of treatment for up to a month and to encourage patients to avoid unprotected intercourse during this time. When nitroimidazole resistance is encountered, patients are often successfully treated with increased doses of drug for a longer time (93, 143; E. A. Bosserman, D. J. Helms, D. J. Mosure, W. E. Secor, and K. A. Workowski, submitted for publication). However, many patients cannot tolerate high doses of metronidazole, and such practices may only exacerbate the development of drug resistance. In addition, some patients experience hypersensitivity reactions in response to metronidazole and tinidazole. Clearly, alternatives to the nitroimidazoles for treatment of *T. vaginalis* are needed. Intravaginal treatment with drugs such as furazolidone, paromomycin sulfate, and povidone-iodine that are not absorbed well from the intestine or cannot be ingested has been successful to cure some patients but in general has limited efficacy (51, 99, 140). Hexadecylphosphocholine (miltefosine) can be taken orally and has activity against both susceptible *T. vaginalis* isolates in vitro but has not yet been tested in a clinical setting (12).

LEISHMANIASIS

Leishmaniasis is transmitted to humans by phlebotomine sandfly vectors and manifests itself in a variety of syndromes. Seventeen species of *Leishmania* infect humans, and depending in part on which of these is present, pathology can range from a cutaneous lesion that is self-limiting to the more severe mucosal or visceral forms. The identification of leishmaniasis as an important opportunistic infection in patients with AIDS has presented new challenges for the treatment of this disease, with increased treatment failures and drug toxicity in HIV-1-positive individuals (2). Use of antileishmanial drugs is limited by their high cost, the difficulty of their administration (injection for several weeks), and/or their associated toxicity. These factors are even more consequential in the developing countries where leishmaniasis is endemic and can lead to premature self-termination of therapy, which in turn may promote increased levels of resistance (23, 86). While true drug resistance has been described for isolates of some *Leishmania* spp., other species or isolates may just differ in their intrinsic sensitivities to certain compounds. True resistance is more likely in anthroponotic forms of leishmaniasis, such as those caused by *Leishmania donovani* and *Leishmania tropica*, because the zoonotic species that infect primarily animals, with humans as an occasional host, rarely encounter drugs (22, 94).

The first-line drugs for treating *Leishmania* infections caused by all species and all clinical forms are the pentavalent antimonial compounds, such as sodium stibogluconate and meglumine antimoniate (8, 23, 91, 102). They are also the only antileishmanial compounds to which widespread clinical drug resistance has been described. In some regions of India, treatment failure of visceral leishmaniasis caused by *L. donovani* is as high as 65%. Development of resistance has been attributed both to the substandard quality of drug produced by some manufacturers and to inappropriate administration of treatment by some caregivers (91, 128). Evidence for true drug resistance in this setting comes from observations that isolates from clinically resistant patients require higher in vitro concentrations of drug to kill the parasites than do isolates from patients who respond to treatment (128). Furthermore, these differences persist when the putatively resistant isolates are maintained in vitro in the absence of drug pressure, suggesting that a stable genetic change confers resistance (37). Nevertheless, in other settings, the correlation between clinical outcome of treatment for leishmaniasis and the in vitro susceptibility of the causative isolate is less clear (112, 150).

The mode of action for pentavalent antimonials as well as the development of drug resistance is still poorly defined, although a number of possible mechanisms have been described (5). The pentavalent antimonial compounds are prodrugs that become reduced within the mammalian host cell or parasite to an active trivalent form that disrupts the parasite's metabolism (23, 86, 102). All the proposed mechanisms of resistance across the various *Leishmania* spp. result in a lower intracellular concentration of active drug. One mechanism by which this occurs is a decrease in the parasite's reductase activity, resulting in less conversion to the trivalent form (102, 120). Resistance has also been associated with increased production of trypanothione or glutathione, which bind with the trivalent antimonials, and extrusion of the resulting thiol-drug conjugates by ATP-binding cassette (ABC) transporters (79, 88, 90, 121). Increased expression of the enzymes involved in thiol synthesis or of the ABC transporter promotes resistance to pentavalent antimonials; inhibition of these pathways in resistant strains increases susceptibility to the drug (7, 18, 40, 67, 88). Another proposed resistance mechanism suggests decreased initial uptake of drug through an aquaglyceroporin (46); however, the relationship between decreased aquaglyceroporin expression and antimonial resistance in clinical isolates is not absolute (76).

Because of the high level of pentavalent antimonial resistance, this treatment is no longer considered useful in India, and other drugs are now being used for primary treatment of visceral leishmaniasis (8, 91, 128). One of these other drugs, amphotericin B, interacts with parasite-specific 24-alkyl sterols and induces pore formation in the parasite plasma membranes (86). The use of amphotericin B has been limited in the past due to its high cost and toxicity; however, new lipid-associated formulations of amphotericin

B have greatly reduced toxicities and retain good efficacy even when administered in lower doses (8, 9, 91, 101). Like with the pentavalent antimonials, the optimal activity of amphotericin B may require competent host immune responses (89). Lipid-associated formulations of amphotericin B are phagocytosed by host monocytes and accumulate in phagocytic lysosomes, where *Leishmania* amastigotes reside (149). Although a mechanism for resistance to amphotericin B has been described for *L. donovani* promastigotes in a laboratory-derived strain (23), parasite isolates from patients who relapsed with *Leishmania infantum*, another species that causes visceral leishmaniasis, demonstrated no decrease in their in vitro susceptibility to this drug (65). Nevertheless, assessment of 19 Indian field isolates indicated that those with greater sodium antimony gluconate resistance had greater in vitro resistance to amphotericin B (64). While none of the isolates showed clinical amphotericin B resistance, this finding does raise the possibility that cross-resistance could develop.

Laboratory or field isolates with resistance to pentavalent antimonials are also killed effectively by paromomycin and miltefosine (8, 18, 22, 37). Miltefosine, which was originally developed as an anticancer drug, is particularly promising, as it can be taken orally and has fewer side effects than most of the parenteral treatments for leishmaniasis (129). As a result, although the drug is more expensive than other therapies, it can be administered on an outpatient basis, and the overall cost for treatment is lower than for less costly drugs that require hospitalization (91). It has also shown efficacy for severely immunocompromised leishmaniasis patients coinfected with HIV-1 (115). Enthusiasm is tempered, however, both because it is teratogenic, thereby limiting its unregulated use in women of child-bearing age, and because leishmanial resistance to miltefosine develops easily in vitro (118, 128, 129). As with the other antileishmania drugs, resistance to paromomycin and miltefosine is associated with mechanisms that decrease intracellular concentrations of the compounds (19, 23, 56, 64, 113, 119).

AFRICAN TRYPANOSOMIASIS

Trypanosoma brucei rhodesiense and *Trypanosoma brucei gambiense* are the etiologic agents of human sleeping sickness. They are endemic in east- and west-central Africa, respectively, and are transmitted by tsetse fly bites. Because these parasites possess antigenic switching mechanisms, host immune responses are ineffective and the prospects for the development of vaccines against these organisms are meager. As a result, drug treatment is the only medical intervention available to combat sleeping sickness for the foreseeable future. Recent political unrest with subsequent loss of an effective public health infrastructure in parts of Africa has caused a resurgence of this disease, a situation that has been compounded by increased resistance to the limited armamentarium of efficacious drugs (29).

Pentamidine and suramin are useful only for treatment of early stages of infection because they are highly ionic and do not cross the blood-brain barrier. While clinical resistance to these drugs does not seem to be a problem, failures can occur when infections are diagnosed and treated after disease has progressed past the hemolymphatic stage. Late-stage, central nervous system disease is treated with melarsoprol. Eflornithine is effective against late-stage *T. b. gambiense* infections that are resistant to melarsoprol, but *T. b. rhodesiense* infections are not susceptible to this drug (29). All of the drugs are difficult to administer and are toxic, which can contribute to premature cessation of treatment, which in turn contributes to development of drug resistance. Data are somewhat limited but suggest that patients coinfected with HIV are more likely to relapse following treatment with melarsoprol or eflornithine than individuals with trypanosome infection alone (49).

Pentamidine and melarsoprol share an amidinium-like moiety with amino purines that is recognized and actively taken up by nucleoside transporters in the trypanosome membrane, resulting in concentrations of these compounds within the parasite. One of these receptors, the *T. brucei* P2 adenosine transporter, or TbAT1, has been extensively studied for its role in drugs used to treat both human and animal African trypanosomiasis. The prevalence of isolates with mutations in the *tbat1* gene is higher in areas with increased drug resistance (95). Mutations in *tbat1* alter parasite susceptibility to melarsoprol but not pentamidine because trypanosomes have two additional pentamidine transporters, one with high affinity and low capacity (HAPT) and one with low affinity and high capacity, that also concentrate pentamidine within the parasites (28). Isolates that lack both TbAT1 and HAPT are resistant to pentamidine, suggesting that field isolates with mutant *tbat1* could become cross-resistant to both drugs if loss of HAPT occurs (17, 58). As with *Leishmania*, *T. brucei* parasites express an ABC transporter that functions as an efflux pump and may contribute to the melarsoprol resistance of certain isolates (75). However, additional factors beyond isolate drug resistance mechanism may contribute to melarsoprol treatment failures in some areas (78).

SCHISTOSOMIASIS

Drug resistance in human helminths is rare (except in *Strongyloides stercoralis*), a fact attributed to their long reproduction cycles and to their lack of multiplication inside the human host. Thus, when considering treatment failures in patients with schistosomiasis, it is important to distinguish characteristics leading to reduced drug efficacy from true drug resistance. For example, persons with very high levels of infection are less likely to be cured with single-dose therapy than individuals with lower worm burdens (57, 106, 133). This is in part related to the fact that the standard drug used to treat schistosomiasis, praziquantel, is effective only against the adult stage of the parasite. Immature worms that may be present at the time of drug treatment, especially in areas of high transmission, are not susceptible to the initial treatment and subsequently develop into patent infections that give the impression of drug resistance. As a result, a minimum of two treatments spaced 4 to 6 weeks apart should be attempted when drug resistance is suspected (106, 133).

Nevertheless, praziquantel treatment failures have been described for *Schistosoma mansoni* infections in Egypt, Senegal, and Kenya (54, 84, 127) and for *Schistosoma haematobium* infections in travelers returning from Mali and Senegal (1). Eggs obtained from the feces of individuals who could not be successfully treated were used to establish infections in mice, confirming the drug resistance phenotype (41, 53, 54, 71, 84). However, despite continued treatment pressure, widespread clinical resistance has not developed (11, 13).

The exact mechanism of praziquantel and, as a result, the mechanism of drug resistance are not definitively understood. In drug-susceptible parasites, praziquantel-induced damage to the tegument of adult schistosomes renders the worms susceptible to attack and to killing by the host's immune response (34); the effect of drug on resistant parasites is reduced (53, 70, 144). The unique beta subunit of the schistosome calcium ion channel is a molecular target for praziquantel, with treatment rapidly inducing a calcium-dependent sustained muscle contraction in the worm's tegument (55, 97). However, no differences in this gene's sequence or expression were observed among a limited number of praziquantel-resistant and -susceptible parasite strains (135). Furthermore, cytochalasin D reverses the effects of praziquantel without altering the calcium influx, thus raising the possibility that this is not the effector of parasite death (105). Other proposed mechanisms of praziquantel action include inhibition of the worm's nucleoside uptake and binding to, and altering the function of, the schistosome myosin light chain (3, 45). One potential mechanism of drug resistance includes increased expression of a P-glycoprotein ATP-dependent efflux pump homologue in parasite strains that have reduced susceptibility to praziquantel (85). Crossbreeding of adult worms with different levels of sensitivity to drug results in offspring with an intermediate phenotype, suggesting that at least artificially induced resistance displays partial dominance (104).

Although widespread praziquantel resistance has not been observed, as mass drug administration programs are increasingly employed, there is a fear that resistance may emerge (35, 59). This risk is increased because, even under the best conditions, praziquantel does not demonstrate complete efficacy (35). This finding reiterates the need for ongoing drug discovery and testing for schistosomiasis. One new compound that has been tested for the treatment of schistosomiasis is artemether, a derivative of the antimalarial drug artemisinin. Unlike praziquantel, artemether is most active against juvenile worms and has demonstrated efficacy against infection with the three major species of schistosomes (69, 96, 134). Thus, it could be used as a prophylactic against patent schistosomiasis for persons with a known exposure, such as following flooding in an area of endemicity. Other drugs are also in development (114, 148).

FUTURE PERSPECTIVES

Several factors contribute to the emergence of drug-resistant parasites. Those parasite species with short life cycles and high multiplication rates that occur in areas of intense transmission are most likely to develop resistant subpopulations. The selection of such populations is encouraged when the parasites are repeatedly exposed to suboptimal drug concentrations. This pattern can result from the use of drugs with long half-lives or, more typically, from the frequent, often unjustified, use of inadequate doses of drugs, a common occurrence in countries where parasite infections are endemic. Public health interventions to correct these factors have not always been successful and would benefit from a better understanding of the drug resistance mechanisms used by parasites. These mechanisms are very diverse and have been difficult to study, but recent technological advances now provide long-awaited tools that will facilitate the task. The genome sequences for *P. falciparum*, *T. vaginalis*, *L. major*, *T. brucei*, and *S. mansoni* have been compiled. When these data are used, for example, in combination with microarray technology, where the DNA of drug-resistant parasite strains is compared to that of drug-susceptible strains, identification of the genes that confer resistance should proceed even more rapidly than in the last few years. In addition, genomic and proteomic data may also be useful in the design of new chemotherapeutic agents, as they help researchers identify metabolic processes of parasites that are sufficiently different from those of their human hosts to allow specific therapy.

REFERENCES

1. Alonso, D., J. Muñoz, J. Gascón, M. E. Valls, and M. Corahan. 2006. Short report: failure of standard treatment with praziquantel in two returned travelers with *Schistosoma haematobium* infection. *Am. J. Trop. Med. Hyg.* **74:**342–344.

2. Alvar, J., P. Aparaicio, A. Aseffa, M. Den Boer, C. Cañavate, J.-P. Dedet, L. Gradoni, R. Ter Horst, R. López-Velez, and J. Moreno. 2008. The relationship between leishmaniasis and AIDS: the second 10 years. *Clin. Microbiol. Rev.* **21:**334–359.

3. Angelucci, F., A. Basso, A. Bellelli, M. Brunori, L. Pica Mattoccia, and C. Valle. 2007. The anti-schistosomal drug praziquantel is an adenosine antagonist. *Parasitology* **134:**1215–1221.

4. Ariey, F., T. Fandeur, R. Durand, M. Randrianarivelojosia, R. Jambou, E. Legrand, M. T. Ekala, C. Bouchier, S. Cojean, J. B. Duchemin, V. Robert, J. Le Bras, and O. Mercereau-Puijalon. 2006. Invasion of Africa by a single pfcrt allele of South East Asian type. *Malaria J.* **5:**34.

5. Ashutosh, S. Sundar, and N. Goyal. 2007. Molecular mechanisms of antimony resistance in *Leishmania*. *J. Med. Microbiol.* **56:**143–153.

6. Baird, J. K. 2009. Resistance to therapies for infections by *Plasmodium vivax*. *Clin. Microbiol. Rev.* **22:**508–534.

7. Basu, J. M., A. Mookerjee, R. Banerjee, M. Saha, S. Singh, K. Naskar, G. Tripathy, P. K. Sinha, K. Pandey, S. Sundar, S. Bimal, P. K. Das, S. K. Choudhuri, and S. Roy. 2008. Inhibition of ABC transporters abolishes antimony resistance in *Leishmania* infection. *Antimicrob. Agents Chemother.* **52:**1080–1093.

8. Berman, J. 2005. Recent developments in leishmaniasis: epidemiology, diagnosis, and treatment. *Curr. Infect. Dis. Rep.* **7:**33–38.

9. Bern, C., J. Adler-Moore, J. Berenguer, M. Boelaert, M. Den Boer, R. N. Davidson, C. Figueras, L. Gradoni, D. A. Kafetzis, K. Ritmeijer, E. Rosenthal, C. Royce, R. Russo, S. Sundar, and J. Alvar. 2006. Liposomal amphotericin B for the treatment of visceral leishmaniasis. *Clin. Infect. Dis.* **43:**917–924.

10. Bitonti, A. J., A. Sjoerdsma, P. P. McCann, D. E. Kyle, A. M. J. Oduola, R. N. Rossan, W. K. Milhous, and D. E. Davidson, Jr. 1988. Reversal of chloroquine resistance in malaria parasite *Plasmodium falciparum* by desipramine. *Science* **242:**1301–1303.

11. Black, C. L., M. L. Steinauer, P. N. M. Mwinzi, W. E. Secor, D. M. S. Karanja, and D. G. Colley. 2009. Impact of intense, longitudinal retreatment with praziquantel on cure rates of schistosomiasis mansoni in a cohort of occupationally exposed adults in western Kenya. *Trop. Med. Int. Health* **14:**450–457.

12. Blaha, C., M. Duchêne, H. Aspöck, and J. Walochnik. 2006. *In vitro* activity of hexadecylphospocholine (miltefosine) against metronidazole-resistant and -susceptible strains of *Trichomonas vaginalis*. *J. Antimicrob. Chemother.* **57:**273–278.

13. Botros, S., H. Sayed, N. Amer, M. El-Ghannam, J. L. Bennet, and T. A. Day. 2005. Current status of sensitivity to praziquantel in a focus of potential drug resistance in Egypt. *Int. J. Parasitol.* **35:**787–791.

14. Bray, P. G., R. E. Martin, L. Tilley, S. A. Ward, K. Kirk, and D. A. Fidock. 2005. Defining the role of PfCRT in *Plasmodium falciparum* chloroquine resistance. *Mol. Microbiol.* **56:**323–333.

15. Bray, P. G., M. Mungthin, R. G. Ridley, and S. A. Ward. 1998. Access to hematin: the basis of chloroquine resistance. *Mol. Pharmacol.* **54:**170–179.

16. Brega, S., B. Meslin, F. de Montbrison, C. Severini, L. Gradoni, R. Udomsangpetch, I. Sutanto, F. Peyron, and S. Picot. 2005. Identification of the *Plasmodium vivax* mdr-like gene (*pvmdr1*) and analysis of single-nucleotide polymorphisms among isolates from different areas of endemicity. *J. Infect. Dis.* **191:**272–277.

17. Bridges, D. J., M. K. Gould, B. Nerima, P. Mäser, R. J. S. Burchmore, and H. P. de Koning. 2007. Loss of the high-affinity pentamidine transporter is responsible for high levels of cross-resistance between arsenical and diamidine drugs in African trypanosomes. *Mol. Pharm.* **71:**1098–1108.

17a. Butler, S. E., P. Augostini, and W. E. Secor. 2010. *Mycoplasma hominis* infection of *Trichomonas vaginalis* is not associated with metronidazole-resistant trichomoniasis in clinical isolates from the United States. *Parasitol. Res.* **107:**1023–1027.

18. Carter, K. C., S. Sundar, C. Spickett, O. C. Pereira, and A. B. Mullen. 2003. The in vivo susceptibility of *Leishmania donovani* to sodium stibogluconate is drug specific and can be reversed by inhibiting glutathione biosynthesis. *Antimicrob. Agents Chemother.* **47:**1529–1535.

19. Castanys-Muñoz, E., J. M. Pérez-Victoria, F. Gamarro, and S. Castanys. 2008. Characterization of an ABCG-like transporter from the protozoan parasite *Leishmania* with a role in drug resistance and transbilayer lipid movement. *Antimicrob. Agents Chemother.* **52:**3573–3579.

20. Cowman, A. F., D. Galatis, and J. K. Thomson. 1994. Selection for mefloquine resistance in *Plasmodium falciparum* is linked to amplification of the *pfmdr1* gene and cross-resistance to halofantrine and quinine. *Proc. Natl. Acad. Sci. USA* **91:**1143–1147.

21. Cowman, A. F., M. J. Morry, B. A. Biggs, G. A. Cross, and S. J. Foote. 1988. Amino acid changes linked to pyrimethamine resistance in the dihydrofolate reductase-thymidylate synthase gene of *Plasmodium falciparum*. *Proc. Natl. Acad. Sci. USA* **85:**9109–9113.

22. Croft, S. L., and G. H. Coombs. 2003. Leishmaniasis—current chemotherapy and recent advances in the search for novel drugs. *Trends Parasitol.* **19:**502–508.

23. Croft, S. L., S. Sundar, and A. H. Fairlamb. 2006. Drug resistance in leishmaniasis. *Clin. Microbiol. Rev.* **19:**111–126.

24. Crowell, A. L., K. A. Sanders-Lewis, and W. E. Secor. 2003. In vitro comparison of metronidazole and tinidazole activity against metronidazole resistant strains of *Trichomonas vaginalis*. *Antimicrob. Agents Chemother.* **47:**1407–1409.

25. Cudmore, S. L., K. L. Delgaty, S. F. Hayward-McClelland, D. P. Petrin, and G. E. Garber. 2004. Treatment of infections caused by metronidazole-resistant *Trichomonas vaginalis*. **17:**783–793.

26. Curtis, J., M. T. Duraisingh, and D. C. Warhurst. 1998. In vivo selection for a specific genotype of dihydropteroate synthetase of *Plasmodium falciparum* by sulfadoxine-pyrimethamine but not chlorproguanil-dapsone treatment. *J. Infect. Dis.* **177:**1429–1433.

27. Dahlstrom, S., P. E. Ferreira, M. I. Veiga, N. Sedighi, L. Waklund, A. Martensson, A. Farnert, C. Sissowath, L. Ossorio, H. Darban, B. Andersson, A. Kaneko, G. Conseil, A. Bjorkman, and J. P. Gil. 2009. *Plasmodium falciparum* multidrug resistance protein 1 (*Pf*MRP1) and artemisinin-based combination therapy in Africa. *J. Infect. Dis.* **200:**1456–1464.

28. de Koning, H. P. 2008. Ever-increasing complexities of diamidine and arsenical crossresistance in African trypanosomes. *Trends Parasitol.* **24:**345–349.

29. Delespaux, V., and H. P. de Koning. 2007. Drugs and drug resistance in African trypanosomiasis. *Drug Resist. Updat.* **10:**30–50.

30. de Pécoulas, P. E., L. K. Basco, J. Le Bras, and A. Mazabraud. 1996. Association between antifolate resistance in vitro and DHFR gene point mutation in *Plasmodium falciparum* isolates. *Trans. R. Soc. Trop. Med. Hyg.* **90:**181–182.

31. Djimdé, A. A., A. Dolo, A. Ouattara, S. Diakité, C. V. Plowe, and O. K. Doumbo. 2004. Molecular diagnosis of resistance to antimalarial drugs during epidemics and in war zones. *J. Infect. Dis.* **190:**853–855.

32. Djimdé, A., O. K. Doumbo, J. F. Cortese, K. Kayentao, S. Doumbo, Y. Diourté, A. Dicko, X. Su, T. Nomura, D. A. Fidock, T. E. Wellems, and C. V. Plowe. 2001. A molecular marker for chloroquine-resistant falciparum malaria. *N. Engl. J. Med.* **344:**257–263.

33. Djimdé, A., O. K. Doumbo, R. W. Steketee, and C. V. Plowe. 2001. Application of a molecular marker for surveillance of chloroquine-resistant falciparum malaria. *Lancet* 358:890–891.

34. Doenhoff, M. J., D. Cioli, and J. Utzinger. 2008. Praziquantel: mechanism of action, resistance and new derivatives for schistosomiasis. *Curr. Opin. Infect. Dis.* 21:659–667.

35. Doenhoff, M. J., P. Hagan, D. Cioli, V. Southgate, L. Pica-Mattoccia, S. Botros, G. Coles, L. A. Tchuem Tchuente, A. Mbaye, and D. Engels. 13 March 2009. Praziquantel: its use in control of schistosomiasis in sub-Saharan Africa and current research needs. *Parasitology.* doi:10.1017/S0031182009000493.

36. Dorsey, G., D. A. Fidock, T. E. Wellems, and P. J. Rosenthal. 2001. Mechanisms of quinoline resistance, p. 153–172. In P. J. Rosenthal (ed), *Antimalarial Chemotherapy. Mechanisms of Action, Resistance, and New Directions in Drug Discovery.* Humana Press, Totowa, NJ.

37. Dube, A., N. Singh, S. Sundar, and N. Singh. 2005. Refractoriness to treatment of sodium stibogluconate in Indian kala-azar field isolates persist in in vitro and in vivo experimental models. *Parasitol. Res.* 96:216–223.

38. Dunne, R. L., L. A. Dunn, P. Upcroft, P. J. O'Donoghue, and J. A. Upcroft. 2003. Drug resistance in the sexually transmitted protozoan *Trichomonas vaginalis. Cell Res.* 13:239–249.

39. Duraisingh, M. T., C. Roper, D. Walliker, and D. C. Warhurst. 2000. Increased sensitivity to the antimalarials mefloquine and artemisinin is conferred by mutations in the *pfmdr1* gene of *Plasmodium falciparum. Mol. Microbiol.* 36:955–961.

40. El Fadili, K., N. Messier, P. Leprohon, G. Roy, C. Guimond, N. Trudel, N. G. Saravia, B. Papadopoulou, D. Légaré, and M. Ouellette. 2005. Role of the ABC transporter MRPA (PGPA) in antimony resistance in *Leishmania infantum* axenic and intracellular amastigotes. *Antimicrob. Agents Chemother.* 49:1988–1993.

41. Fallon, T. G., R. F. Sturrock, C. M. Niang, and M. J. Doenhoff. 1995. Diminished susceptibility to praziquantel in a Senegal isolate of *Schistosoma mansoni. Am. J. Trop. Med. Hyg.* 53:61–62.

42. Fidock, D. A., T. Nomura, A. K. Talley, R. A. Cooper, S. M. Dzekunov, M. T. Ferdig, L. M. B. Ursos, A. B. S. Sidhu, B. Naudé, K. W. Deitsch, X. Su, J. C. Wootton, P. D. Roepe, and T. E. Wellems. 2000. Mutations in the *P. falciparum* digestive vacuole transmembrane protein PfCRT and evidence for their role in chloroquine resistance. *Mol. Cell* 6:861–871.

43. Fitch, C. D. 1970. *Plasmodium falciparum* in owl monkeys: drug resistance and chloroquine binding capacity. *Science* 169:289–290.

44. Foote, S. J., D. Galatis, and A. F. Cowman. 1990. Amino acids in the dihydrofolate reductase-thymidylate synthase gene of *Plasmodium falciparum* involved in cycloguanil resistance differ from those involved in pyrimethamine resistance. *Proc. Nat. Acad. Sci. USA* 87:3014–3017.

45. Gnanasekar, M., A. M. Salunkhe, A. K. Mallia, Y. X. He, and R. Kalyanasundaram. 2009. Praziquantel affects the regulatory myosin light chain of *Schistosoma mansoni. Antimicrob. Agents Chemother.* 53:1054–1060.

46. Gourbal, B., N. Sounu, M. Bhattacharjee, D. Legare, S. Sundar, M. Ouellette, B. P. Rosen, and R. Mukhopadhyay. 2004. Drug uptake and modulation of resistance in *Leishmania* by an aquaglyceroporin. *J. Biol. Chem.* 279:31010–31017.

47. Hampl, V., S. Vaňáčová, J. Kulda, and J. Flegr. 2001. Concordance between genetic relatedness and phenotypic similarities of *Trichomonas vaginalis* strains. *BMC Evol. Biol.* 1:11.

48. Happi, C. T., G. O. Gbotosho, O. A. Folarin, A. Sowunmi, T. Hudson, M. O'Neil, W. Milhous, D. F. Wirth, and A. M. J. Oduola, 2009. Selection of *P. falciparum* multidrug resistance gene 1 alleles in asexual stages and gametocytes by artemether-lumefantrine in Nigerian children with uncomplicated falciparum malaria. *Antimicrob. Agents Chemother.* 53:888–895.

49. Harms, G., and H. Feldmeier. 2005. The impact of HIV infection on tropical diseases. *Infect. Dis. Clin. N. Am.* 19:121–135.

50. Hastings, M. D., K. M. Porter, J. D. Maguire, I. Susanti, W. Kania, M. J. Bangs, C. H. Sibley, and J. K. Baird. 2003. Dihydrofolate reductase mutations in *Plasmodium vivax* from Indonesia and therapeutic response to sulfadoxine plus pyrimethamine. *J. Infect. Dis.* 189:744–750.

51. Helms, D. J., D. J. Mosure, W. E. Secor, and K. A. Workowski. 2008. Management of *Trichomonas vaginalis* in women with suspected metronidazole hypersensitivity. *Am. J. Obstet. Gynecol.* 198:370.e1–370.e7.

52. Hrdý, I., R. Cammack, P. Stopka, J. Kulda, and J. Tachezy. 2005. Alternative pathway of metronidazole activation in *Trichomonas vaginalis* hydrogenosomes. *Antimicrob. Agents. Chemother.* 49:5033–5036.

53. Ismail, M., S. Botros, A. Metwally, S. William, A. Farghally, L. F. Tao, T. A. Day, and J. L. Bennett. 1999. Resistance to praziquantel: direct evidence from *Schistosoma mansoni* isolated from Egyptian villagers. *Am. J. Trop. Med. Hyg.* 60:932–935.

54. Ismail, M., A. Metwally, A. Farghaly, J. Bruce, L.-F. Tao, and J. L. Bennett. 1996. Characterization of isolates of *Schistosoma mansoni* from Egyptian villagers that tolerate high doses of praziquantel. *Am. J. Trop. Med. Hyg.* 55:214–218.

55. Jeziorski, M. C., and R. M. Greenberg. 2006. Voltage-gated calcium channel subunits from platyhelminths: potential role in praziquantel action. *Int. J. Parasitol.* 36:625–632.

56. Jhingran, A., B. Chawla, S. Saxena, M. P. Barrett, and R. Madhubala. 2009. Paromomycin: uptake and resistance in *Leishmania donovani. Mol. Biochem. Parasitol.* 164:111–117.

57. Karanja, D. M. S., A. E. Boyer, M. Strand, D. G. Colley, B. L. Nahlen, J. H. Ouma, and W. E. Secor. 1998. Studies on schistosomiasis in western Kenya. II. Efficacy of praziquantel for schistosomiasis patients with human immunodeficiency virus co-infections. *Am. J. Trop. Med. Hyg.* 59:307–311.

58. Kibona, S. N., L. Metamba, J. S. Kabonya, and G. W. Lubega. 2006. Drug-resistance of *Tryapanosoma b. rhodesiense* isolates from Tanzania. *Trop. Med. Int. Health* 11:144–155.

59. King, C. H., E. M. Muchiri, and J. H. Ouma. 2000. Evidence against rapid emergence of praziquantel resistance in *Schistosoma haematobium*, Kenya. *Emerg. Infect. Dis.* 6:585–594.

60. Korsinczky, M., N. Chen, B. Kotecka, A. Saul, K. Rieckmann and Q. Cheng. 2000. Mutations in *Plasmodium falciparum* cytochrome *b* that are associated with atovaquone resistance are located at a putative drug-binding site. *Antimicrob. Agents Chemother.* 44:2100–2108.

61. Korsinczky, M., K. Fisher, N. Chen, J. Baker, and Q. Cheng. 2004. Sulfadoxine resistance in *Plasmodium vivax* is associated with a specific amino acid in dihydropteroate synthase at the putative sulfadoxine-binding site. *Antimicrob. Agents Chemother.* 48:2214–2222.

62. Krogstad, D. J., I. Y. Gluzman, D. E. Kyle, A. M. J. Oduola, S. K. Martin, W. K. Milhous, and P. H. Schlesinger. 1987. Efflux of chloroquine from *Plasmodium falciparum*: mechanism of chloroquine resistance. *Science* 238:1283–1285.

63. Kublin, J. G., F. K. Dzinjalamala, D. D. Kamwendo, E. M. Malkin, J. F. Cortese, L. M. Martino, R. A. G. Mukadam, S. J. Rogerson, A. G. Lescano, M. E. Molyneux, P. A. Winstanley, P. Chimpeni, T. E. Taylor, and C. V. Plowe. 2002. Molecular markers for failure of sulfadoxine-pyrimethamine and chlorproguanil-dapsone treatment of *Plasmodium falciparum* malaria. *J. Infect. Dis.* 185:380–388.

64. Kumar, D., A. Kulshrestha, R. Singh, and P. Solotra. 2009. In vitro susceptibility of field isolates of *Leishmania donovani* to miltefosine and amphotericin B: correlation with sodium antimony gluconate susceptibility and implications for treatment in areas of endemicity. *Antimicrob. Agents Chemother.* 53:835–838.

65. Lachaud, L., N. Bourgeois, M. Plourde, P. Leprohon, P. Bastien, and M. Ouellette. 2009. Parasite susceptibility to amphotericin B in failures of treatment for visceral leishmaniasis in patients coinfected with HIV type 1 and *Leishmania infantum. Clin. Infect. Dis.* 48:e16–e22.

66. Land, K. M., M. G. Delgadillo, and P. J. Johnson. 2002. In vivo expression of ferredoxin in a drug resistant trichomonad increases metronidazole susceptibility. *Mol. Biochem. Parasitol.* 121:153–157.

67. Légaré, D., D. Richard, R. Mukhopadhyay, Y.-D. Stierhof, B. P. Rosen, A. Haimeur, B. Papadopoulou, and M. Ouellette. 2001. The *Leishmania* ATP-binding cassette protein PGPA is an intracellular metal-thiol transporter ATPase. *J. Biol. Chem.* **278:**26301–26307.

68. Leitsch, D., D. Kolarich, M. Binder, J. Stadlmann, F. Altmann, and M. Duchêne. 2009. *Trichomonas vaginalis:* metronidazole and other nitroimidazole drugs are reduced by the flavin enzyme thioredoxin reductase and disrupt the cellular redox system. Implications for nitroimidazole toxicity and resistance. *Mol. Microbiol.* **72:**518–536.

69. Li, Y.-S., H.-G. Chen, H.-B. He, X.-Y. Hou, M. Ellis, and D. P. McManus. 2005. A double-blind field trial on the effects of artemether on *Schistosoma japonicum* infection in a highly endemic focus in southern China. *Acta Trop.* **96:**184–190.

70. Liang, Y.-S., G. C. Coles, J.-R. Dai, Y.-C. Zhu, and M. J. Doenhoff. 2002. Adult worm tegumental damage and egg-granulomas in praziquantel-resistant and -susceptible *Schistosoma mansoni* treated *in vivo. J. Helminthol.* **76:**327–333.

71. Liang, Y. S., G. C. Coles, M. J. Doenhoff, and V. R. Southgate. 2001. In vitro responses of praziquantel-resistant and -susceptible *Schistosoma mansoni* to praziquantel. *Int. J. Parasitol.* **31:**1227–1235.

72. Lim, P., A. P. Alker, N. Khim, N. K. Shah, S. Incardona, S. Doung, P. Yi, M. B. Denis, C. Bouchier, O. Puijalon, S. R. Meshnick, C. Wongsrichanalai, T. Fandeur, J. Le Bras, P. Ringwald, and F. Ariey. 2009. *Pfmdr1* copy number and arteminisin derivatives combination therapy failure in *falciparum* malaria in Cambodia. *Malaria J.* **8:**11.

73. Looareesuwan, S. C., C. Viravan, H. K. Webster, D. E. Kyle, D. B. Hutchinson, and C. J. Canfield. 1996. Clinical studies on atovaquone, alone or in association with other antimalarial drugs for treatment of acute uncomplicated malaria in Thailand. *Am. J. Trop. Med. Hyg.* **54:**62–66.

74. Lozovsky, E. R., T. Chookajorn, K. M. Brown, M. Imwong, P. J. Shaw, S. Kamchonwongpaisan, D. E. Neafsey, D. M. Weinreich, and D. L. Hartl. 2009. Stepwise acquisition of pyrimethamine resistance in the malaria parasite. *Proc. Natl. Acad. Sci. USA* **106:**12025–12030.

75. Lüscher, A., B. Nerima, and P. Mäser. 2006. Combined contributions of TbAT1 and TbMRPA to drug resistance in *Trypanosoma brucei. Mol. Biochem. Parasitol.* **150:**364–366.

76. Mahendra, M., S. Singh, M. Chatterjee, and R. Madhubala. 2008. Role of aquaglyceroporin (AQP1) gene and drug uptake in antimony-resistant clinical isolates of *Leishmania donovani. Am. J. Trop. Med. Hyg.* **79:**69–75.

77. Maiga, O., A. Djimde, V. Hubert, A. Aubouy, F. Kironde, B. Nsimba, K. Koram, O. Doumbo, J. Le Bras, and J. Clain. 2007. A shared Asian origin of the triple mutant *dhfr* allele in *P. falciparum* from sites across Africa. *J. Infect. Dis.* **196:**165–172.

78. Maina, N., K. J. Maina, P. Mäser, and R. Brun. 2007. Genotypic and phenotypic characterization of *Trypanosoma brucei gambiense* isolates from Ibba, South Sudan, an area of high melarsoprol treatment failure rate. *Acta Trop.* **104:**84–90.

79. Mandal, G., S. Wyllie, N. Singh, S. Sundar, A. H. Fairlamb, and M. Chatterjee. 2007. Increased levels of thiols protect antimony unresponsive *Leishmania donovani* field isolates against reactive oxygen species generated by trivalent antimony. *Parasitology* **134:**1679–1687.

80. Martin, S. K., A. M. J. Oduola, and W. K. Milhous. 1987. Reversal of chloroquine resistance in *Plasmodium falciparum* by verapamil. *Science* **235:**899–901.

81. McClelland, R. S. 2008. *Trichomonas vaginalis* infection: can we afford to do nothing? *J. Infect. Dis.* **197:**487–489.

82. Mead, J. R., M. Fernadez, P. A. Romagnoli, and W. E. Secor. 2006. Use of *Trichomonas vaginalis* clinical isolates to evaluate correlation of gene expression and metronidazole resistance. *J. Parasitol.* **92:**196–199.

83. Mehlotra, R. K., H. Fujioka, P. D. Roepe, O. Janneh, L. M. B. Ursos, V. Jacobs-Lorena, D. T. McNamara, M. J. Bockarie, J. W. Kazura, D. E. Kyle, and D. A. Fidock. 2001. Evolution of a unique *Plasmodium falciparum* chloroquine-resistance phenotype in association with *pfcrt* polymorphism in Papua New Guinea and South America. *Proc. Natl. Acad. Sci. USA* **98:**12689–12694.

84. Melman, S. D., M. L. Steinauer, C. Cunnungham, L. S. Kubatko, I. N. Mwangi, N. B. Wynn, M. W. Mutuku, D. M. S. Karanja, D. G. Colley, C. Black, W. E. Secor, G. M. Mkoji, and E. S. Loker. 2009. Reduced susceptibility to praziquantel among naturally occurring Kenyan isolates of *Schistosoma mansoni. PLoS Negl. Trop. Dis.* **3:**e504. doi:10.1371/journal.pntd.0000504.

85. Messerli, S. M., R. S. Kasinathan, W. Morgan, S. Spranger, and R. M. Greenberg. 2009. *Schistosoma mansoni* P-glycoprotein levels increase in response to praziquantel exposure and correlate with reduced praziquantel susceptibility. *Mol. Biochem. Parasitol.* **167:**54–59.

86. Mishra, J., A. Saxena, and S. Singh. 2007. Chemotherapy of leishmaniasis: past, present, and future. *Curr. Med. Chem.* **14:**1153–1169.

87. Mita, T., A. Kaneko, J. K. Lum, B. Bwijo, M. Takechi, I. L. Zungu, T. Tsukahara, K. Tanabe, T. Kobayakawa, and A. Björkmann. 2003. Recovery of chloroquine sensitivity and low prevalence of the *Plasmodium falciparum* chloroquine resistance transporter gene mutation K76T following the discontinuance of chloroquine use in Malawi. *Am. J. Trop. Med. Hyg.* **68:**413–415.

88. Mittal, M. K., S. Rai, Ashutosh, Ravinder, S. Gupta, S. Sundar, and N. Goyal. 2007. Characterization of natural antimony resistance in *Leishmania donovani* isolates. *Am. J. Trop. Med. Hyg.* **76:**681–688.

89. Mueller, M., K. Ritmeijer, M. Balasegaram, Y. Koummuki, M. R. Santana, and R. Davidson. 2007. Unresponsiveness to AmBiosome in some Sudanese patients with kala-azar. *Trans. R. Soc. Trop. Med. Hyg.* **101:**19–24.

90. Mukherjee, A., P. K. Padmanabhan, S. Singh, G. Roy, I. Girard, M. Chatterjee, M. Ouellette, and R. Madhubala. 2007. Role of ABC transporter MRPA, γ-glutamylcysteine synthetase and ornithine decarboxylase in natural antimony-resistant isolates of *Leishmania donovani. J. Antimicrob. Chemother.* **59:**204–211.

91. Murray, H. W. 2004. Treatment of visceral leishmaniasis in 2004. *Am. J. Trop. Med. Hyg.* **71:**787–794.

92. Musset, L., J. Le Bras, and J. Clain. 2007. Parallel evolution of adaptive mutations in *Plasmodium falciparum* mitochondrial DNA during atovaquone-proguanil treatment. *Mol. Biol. Evol.* **24:**1582–1585.

93. Nanda, N., R. G. Michel, G. Kurdgelashvili, and K. A. Wendel. 2006. Trichomoniasis and its treatment. *Expert Rev. Anti Infect. Ther.* **4:**125–135.

94. Natera, S., C. Machuca, M. Padrón-Nieves, A. Moerao, E. Díaz, and A. Ponte-Sucre. 2007. *Leishmania* spp.: proficiency of drug-resistant parasites. *Int. J. Antimicrob. Agents* **29:**637–642.

95. Nerima, B., E. Matovu, G. W. Lubega, and J. C. K. Enyaru. 2007. Detection of mutant P2 adenosine transporter (TbAT1) gene in *Trypanosoma brucei gambiense* isolates from northwest Uganda using allele-specific polymerase chain reaction. *Trop. Med. Int. Health* **12:**1361–1368.

96. N'Goran, E. K., J. Utzinger, H. N. Gnaka, A. Yapi, N. A. N'Guessan, S. D. Kigbafori, C. Lengeler, J. Chollet, X. Shuhua, and M. Tanner. 2003. Randomized, double-blind, placebo-controlled trial of oral artemether for the prevention of patent *Schistosoma haematobium* infections. *Am. J. Trop. Med. Hyg.* **68:**24–32.

97. Nogi, T., D. Zhang, J. D. Chan, and J. S. Marchant. 2009. A novel biological activity of praziquantel requiring voltage-operated Ca^{2+} channel β subunits: subversion of flatworm regenerative polarity. *PLoS Negl. Trop. Dis.* **3:**e464. doi:10.1371/journal.pntd.0000464.

98. Nomura, T., J. M.-R. Carlton, J. K. Baird, H. A. del Portillo, D. J. Fryauff, D. Rathore, D. A. Fidock, X.-Z. Su, W. E. Collins, T. F. McCutchan, J. C. Wootton, and T. E. Wellems. 2001. Evidence for different mechanisms of chloroquine resistance in 2 *Plasmodium* species that cause human malaria. *J. Infect. Dis.* **183:**1653–1661.

99. Nyirjesy, P., J. D. Sobel, M. V. Weitz, D. J. Leaman, and S. P. Gelone. 1998. Difficult-to-treat trichomoniasis: results with paromomycin cream. *Clin. Infect. Dis.* **26:**986–988.

100. Nzila, A., E. Ochong, E. Nduati, K. Gilbert, P. Winstanley, S. Ward, and K. Marsh. 2005. Why has the dihydrofolate reductase 164 mutation not consistently been found in Africa yet? *Trans. R. Soc. Trop. Med. Hyg.* **99:**341–346.

101. Olliaro, P. L., P. J. Guerrin, S. Gerstl, A. A. Haakjolk, J.-A. Rottingen, and S. Sundar. 2005. Treatment options for visceral leishmaniasis: a systematic review of clinical studies done in India, 1980–2004. *Lancet Infect. Dis.* **5:**763–774.

102. Ouellette, M. 2001. Biochemical and molecular mechanisms of drug resistance in parasites. *Trop. Med. Int. Health* **6:**874–882.

103. Peters, W. 1970. Drug resistance in human malarias. I. Drugs influencing folic acid metabolism, p. 364–425. *In* W. Peters (ed), *Chemotherapy and Drug Resistance in Malaria.* Academic Press, London, United Kingdom.

104. Pica-Mattoccia, L., M. J. Doenhoff, C. Valle, A. Basso, A.-R. Troiani, P. Liberti, A. Festucci, A. Guidi, and D. Cioli. 2009. Genetic analysis of decreased praziquantel sensitivity in a laboratory strain of *Schistosoma mansoni*. *Acta Trop.* **111:**82–85.

105. Pica-Mattoccia, L., T. Orsini, A. Basso, A. Festucci, P. Liberti, A. Guidi, A.-L. Marcatto-Maggi, S. Nobre-Santana, A.-R. Troiani, D. Cioli, and C. Valle. 2008. *Schistosoma mansoni*: lack of correlation between praziquantel-induced intra-worm calcium influx and parasite death. *Exp. Parasitol.* **119:**332–335.

106. Picquet, M., J. Vercruysse, D. J. Shaw, M. Diop, and A. Ly. 1998. Efficacy of praziquantel against *Schistosoma mansoni* in northern Senegal. *Trans. R. Soc. Trop. Med. Hyg.* **92:**90–93.

107. Plowe, C. V. 2001. Folate antagonists and mechanisms of resistance, p. 173–190. *In* P. J. Rosenthal (ed.), *Antimalarial Chemotherapy. Mechanisms of Action, Resistance, and New Directions in Drug Discovery.* Humana Press, Totowa, NJ.

108. Plowe, C. V., J. F. Cortese, A. Djimde, O. C. Nwanyanwu, W. M. Watkins, P. A. Winstanley, J. G. Estrada-Franco, R. E. Mollinedo, J. C. Avila, J. L. Cespedes, D. Carter, and O. Doumbo. 1997. Mutations in *Plasmodium falciparum* dihydrofolate reductase and dihydropteroate synthase and epidemiologic patterns of pyrimethamine-sulfadoxine use and resistance. *J. Infect. Dis.* **176:**1590–1596.

109. Price, R. N., A.-C. Uhlemann, A. Brockman, R. McGready, E. Ashley, L. Phaipun, R. Patel, K. Laing, S. Looareesuwan, N. J. White, F. Nosten, and S. Krishna. 2004. Mefloquine resistance in *Plasmodium falciparum* and increased *pfmdr1* gene copy number. *Lancet* **364:**438–447.

110. Reed, M. B., K. J. Saliba, S. R. Caruana, K. Kirk, and A. F. Cowman. 2000. Pgh1 modulates sensitivity and resistance to multiple antimalarials in *Plasmodium falciparum*. *Nature* **403:**906–909.

111. Rieckmann, K. H., D. R. Davis, and D. C. Hutton. 1989. *Plasmodium vivax* resistance to chloroquine? *Lancet* **ii:**1183–1184.

112. Rijal, S., V. Yardley, F. Chappuis, S. Decuypere, B. Khanal, R. Singh, M. Boelaert, S. De Doncker, S. Croft, and J.-C. Dujardin. 2007. Antimonial treatment of visceral leishmaniasis: are current in vitro susceptibility assays adequate for prognosis of in vivo therapy outcome? *Microbes Infect.* **9:**529–535.

113. Sánchez-Cañete, M. P., L. Carvalho, F. J. Pérez-Victoria, F. Gamarro, and S. Castanys. 2009. Low plasma membrane expression of the miltefosine transport complex renders *Leishmania braziliensis* refractory to the drug. *Antimicrob. Agents Chemother.* **53:**1305–1313.

114. Sayed, A. A., A. Simeonov, C. J. Thomas, J. Inglese, C. P. Austin, and D. L. Williams. 2008. Identification of oxadiazoles as new drug leads for the control of schistosomiasis. *Nat. Med.* **14:**407–412.

115. Schraner, C., B. Hasse, U. Hasse, D. Baumann, A. Faeh, G. Burg, F. Grimm, A. Mathis, R. Weber, and H. F. Günthard. 2005. Successful treatment with miltefosine of disseminated cutaneous leishmaniasis in a severely immunocompromised patient infected with HIV-1. *Clin. Infect. Dis.* **40:**120–124.

116. Schwartz, E., S. Bujanover, and K. C. Kain. 2003. Genetic confirmation of atovaquone-proguanil-resistant *P. falciparum* malaria acquired by a non immune traveller to East Africa. *Clin. Infect. Dis.* **37:**450–451.

117. Schwebke, J. R., and F. J. Barrientes. 2006. Prevalence of *Trichomonas vaginalis* isolates with resistance to metronidazole and tinidazole. *Antimicrob. Agents Chemother.* **50:**4209–4210.

118. Seifert, K., S. Matu, F. J. Pérez-Victoria, S. Castanys, F. Gamarro, and S. L. Croft. 2003. Characterisation of *Leishmania donovani* promastigotes resistant to hexadecylphosphocholine (miltefosine). *Int. J. Antimicrob. Agents* **22:**380–387.

119. Seifert, K., F. J. Pérez-Victoria, M. Stettler, M. P. Sánchez-Cañete, S. Castanys, F. Gamarro, and S. L. Croft. 2007. Inactivation of the miltefosine transporter, LdMT, causes miltefosine resistance that is conferred to the amastigote stage of *Leishmania donovani* and persists in vivo. *Int. J. Antimicrob. Agents* **30:**229–235.

120. Shaked-Mishan, P., N. Ulrich, M. Ephros, and D. Zilberstein. 2001. Novel intracellular SB^V reducing activity correlates with antimony susceptibility in *Leishmania donovani*. *J. Biol. Chem.* **276:**3971–3976.

121. Singh, N., R. Almeida, H. Kothari, P. Kumar, G. Mandal, M. Chatterjee, S. Venkatachalam, M. K. Govind, S. K. Mandal, and S. Sundar. 2007. Differential gene expression analysis in antimony-unresponsive Indian kala azar (visceral leishmaniasis) clinical isolates by DNA microarray. *Parasitology* **134:**777–787.

122. Sirawaraporn, W., S. Sathitkul, R. Sirawaraporn, Y. Yuthavong, and D. V. Santi. 1997. Antifolate-resistant mutants of *Plasmodium falciparum* dihydrofolate reductase. *Proc. Natl. Acad. Sci. USA* **94:**1124–1129.

123. Smoak, B. L., R. F. DeFraites, A. J. Magill, K. C. Kain, and B. T. Wellde. 1997. *Plasmodium vivax* infections in U.S. Army troops: failure of primaquine to prevent relapse in studies from Somalia. *Am. J. Trop. Med. Hyg.* **56:**231–234.

124. Snipes, L. J., P. M. Gamard, E. M. Narcisi, C. B. Beard, T. Lehmann, and W. E. Secor. 2000. Molecular epidemiology of metronidazole resistance in a population of *Trichomonas vaginalis* clinical isolates. *J. Clin. Microbiol.* **38:**3004–3009.

125. Sobel, J. D., V. Nagappan, and P. Nyirjesy. 1999. Metronidazole-resistant vaginal trichomoniasis—an emerging problem. *N. Engl. J. Med.* **341:**292–293.

126. Srivastava, I. K., and A. B. Vaidya. 1999. A mechanism for the synergistic antimalarial action of atovaquone and proguanil. *Antimicrob. Agents Chemother.* **43:**1334–1339.

127. Stelma, F. F., I. Talla, S. Sow, A. Kongs, M. Niang, K. Polman, A. M. Deelder, and B. Gryseels. 1995. Efficacy and side effects of praziquantel in an epidemic focus of *Schistosoma mansoni*. *Am. J. Trop. Med. Hyg.* **53:**167–170.

128. Sundar, S. 2001. Drug resistance in Indian visceral leishmaniasis. *Trop. Med. Int. Health* **6:**849–854.

129. Sundar, S., and P. L. Olliaro. 2007. Miltefosine in the treatment of leishmaniasis: clinical evidence for informed clinical risk management. *Ther. Clin. Risk Manag.* **3:**733–740.

130. Talisuna, A. O., P. Bloland, and H. D'Alessandro. 2004. History, dynamics and public health importance of malaria parasites resistance. *Clin. Microbiol. Rev.* **17:**235–254.

131. Triglia, T., P. Wang, P. F. Sims, J. E. Hyde, and A. F. Cowman. 1998. Allelic exchange at the endogenous genomic locus in *Plasmodium falciparum* proves the role of dihydropteroate synthase in sulfadoxine-resistant malaria. *EMBO J.* **17:**3807–3815.

132. Upcroft, P., and J. A. Upcroft. 2001. Drug targets and mechanisms of resistance in anaerobic protozoa. *Clin. Microbiol. Rev.* **14:**150–164.

133. Utzinger, J., E. K. N'Goran, A. N'Dri, C. Lengeler, and M. Tanner. 2000. Efficacy of praziquantel against *Schistosoma mansoni* with particular consideration for intensity of infection. *Trop. Med. Int. Health* **5:**771–778.

134. Utzinger, J., E. K. N'Goran, A. N'Dri, C. Lengeler, S. Xiao, and M. Tanner. 2000. Oral artemether for prevention of *Schistosoma mansoni* infection: randomized controlled trial. *Lancet* **355:**1320–1325.

135. **Valle, C. A., R. Troiani, A. Festucci, L. Pica-Mattoccia, P. Liberti, A. Wolstenholme, K. Francklow, M. J. Doenhoff, and D. Cioli.** 2003. Sequence and level of endogenous expression of calcium channel β subunits in *Schistosoma mansoni* displaying different susceptibilities to praziquantel. *Mol. Biochem. Parasitol.* **130:**111–115.

136. **Vanacova, S., J. Tachezy, J. Kulda, and J. Flegr.** 1997. Characterization of trichomonad species and strains by PCR fingerprinting. *J. Eukaryot. Microbiol.* **44:**545–552.

137. **van der Pol, B.** 2007. *Trichomonas vaginalis* infection: the most prevalent nonviral sexually transmitted infection receives the least public health attention. *Clin. Infect. Dis.* **44:**23–25.

138. **Verdier, F., J. Le Bras, F. Clavier, I. Hatin, and M. C. Blayo.** 1985. Chloroquine uptake by *P. falciparum* infected human red blood cells during *in vitro* culture. Relationship between chloroquine resistance and uptake. *Antimicrob. Agents Chemother.* **27:**561–564.

139. **Wang, P., M. Read, P. F. G. Sims, and J. E. Hyde.** 1997. Sulfadoxine resistance in the human malaria parasite *Plasmodium falciparum* is determined by mutations in dihydropteroate synthetase and an additional factor associated with folate utilization. *Mol. Microbiol.* **23:**979–986.

140. **Waters, L. J., S. S. Dave, J. R. Deayton, and P. D. French.** 2005. Recalcitrant *Trichomonas vaginalis* infection—a case series. *Int. J. STD AIDS* **16:**505–509.

141. **Wellems, T. E., L. J. Panton, I. Y. Gluzman, V. E. do Rosario, R. W. Gwadz, A. Walker-Jonah, and D. J. Krogstad.** 1990. Chloroquine resistance not linked to *mdr*-like genes in a *Plasmodium falciparum* cross. *Nature* **345:**253–255.

142. **Wellems, T. E., and C. V. Plowe.** 2001. Chloroquine-resistant malaria. *J. Infect. Dis.* **184:**770–776.

143. **Wendel, K. A., and K. A. Workowski.** 2007. Trichomoniasis: challenges to appropriate management. *Clin. Infect. Dis.* **44:**S123–S129.

144. **William, S., S. Botros, M. Ismail, A. Farghally, T. A. Day, and J. L. Bennett.** 2001. Praziquantel-induced tegumental damage in vitro is diminished in schistosomes derived from praziquantel-resistant infections. *Parasitology* **122:**63–66.

145. **World Health Organization.** 1993. A global strategy for malaria control. World Health Organization, Geneva, Switzerland.

146. **World Health Organization.** 2008. World malaria report. World Health Organization, Geneva, Switzerland.

147. **Xiao, J. C., L. F. Xie, S. L. Fang, M. Y. Gao, Y. Zhu, L. Y. Song, H. M. Zhong, and Z. R. Lun.** 2006. Symbiosis of *Mycoplasma hominis* in *Trichomonas vaginalis* may link metronidazole resistance in vitro. *Parasitol. Res.* **100:**123–130.

148. **Xiao, S.-H., J. Keiser, J. Chollet, J. Utzinger, Y. Dong, Y. Endriss, J. L. Vennerstrom, and M. Tanner.** 2007. In vitro and in vivo activities of synthetic trioxolanes against major human schistosome species. *Antimicrob. Agents Chemother.* **51:**1440–1445.

149. **Yardley, V., and S. L. Croft.** 1997. Activity of liposomal amphotericin B against experimental cutaneous leishmaniasis. *Antimicrob. Agents Chemother.* **41:**752–756.

150. **Yardley, V., N. Ortuño, A. Llanos-Cuentas, F. Chappius, S. De Doncker, L. Ramirez, S. Croft, J. Arevalo, V. Adaui, H. Bermudez, S. Decuypere, and J.-C. Dujardin.** 2006. American tegumentary leishmaniasis: is antimonial treatment outcome related to parasite drug susceptibility? *J. Infect. Dis.* **194:**1168–1175.

Susceptibility Test Methods: Parasites*

JACQUES LE BRAS AND W. EVAN SECOR

149

Accurate methods for ascertaining responses of parasites to antiparasitic drugs can prove useful at several levels. They can assist in the clinical management of individual patients, they can yield epidemiologic information that may guide drug use policies and public health interventions, and they offer crucial research tools for the development of new and better drugs. Drug susceptibility tests fall into four broad categories: in vivo tests, in vitro tests, tests with experimental animals, and molecular tests.

In vivo tests with patients directly assess the clinical efficacies of existing compounds. These tests are performed in actual epidemiologic investigations, and their modest technical requirements make them suitable for use under field conditions in developing countries. The interpretation of in vivo tests is limited by potential interferences by factors related to the host (e.g., immunity or variations in drug intake or metabolism) or to the environment (e.g., reinfections). However, such tests have proven instrumental in guiding drug use policies, particularly for malaria.

In vitro tests circumvent these interferences by isolating the parasites from their hosts and investigating them in culture under controlled laboratory conditions, with opportunities for repeated assessments against multiple compounds (including experimental compounds). In vitro tests, however, are technically more demanding and therefore less amenable to performance under field conditions. They are most informative if they are used to investigate parasites that multiply rapidly in culture, a select group consisting mostly of protozoa. They are of limited use for assessing inactive drug precursors that must be activated by the host or drugs whose antiparasitic activities necessitate the synergistic effect of the host's immune defenses.

Tests with experimental animal models permit investigations of parasites that cannot be grown in culture or of drugs not yet approved for use in humans. They may most accurately mirror the drug susceptibility of the parasite within a human host but are limiting if a large number of isolates or compounds require testing. For animal models to be relevant, the pharmacokinetics of the drug under investigation should be similar both in the particular model used and in humans.

Molecular tests detect genetic variations that are potentially linked with resistance. Such tests offer unique advantages. PCRs can be performed with minute amounts of nonviable parasite genetic material. They can be run in batches, allowing large-scale epidemiologic studies. Molecular analysis at the single-organism level circumvents potential ambiguities associated with the heterologous parasite populations occasionally encountered in in vivo or in vitro tests and allows the dissection of such populations. Because of their short duration (hours), molecular diagnostic procedures can potentially be used to guide patient management. The other categories of tests usually require more time (days to weeks) and yield results that are used mainly for epidemiologic surveillance and experimental chemotherapy studies. Drawbacks of molecular tests reside in their technical requirements and in the need to be certain that the genes evaluated correlate with functional resistance. However, thanks to the development of more practical protocols and more robust automated equipment, as well as a better understanding of the genes that confer resistance, molecular techniques are used in an increasing number of laboratories, including field facilities.

These different categories of tests provide complementary information. At one end of the spectrum, molecular tests analyze parasites at their most basic biologic level, without any outside interference. At the other end, in vivo tests in patients reflect complex interactions between host and parasite and are most relevant for clinicians and public health practitioners. While a good correlation between results of various test methods is desirable, some degree of discrepancy should be expected to result from factors linked to the host or the culture conditions. Indeed, a judicious analysis of such discrepancies might provide valuable insights into the mechanisms of drug action and resistance.

These points are illustrated in the following discussions of five parasitic diseases, selected for their particular chemotherapeutic challenges. A summary is provided in Table 1.

MALARIA

Most drug resistance tests in malaria concern *Plasmodium falciparum*, the most prevalent and virulent species and the most prone to the development of resistance. Initial observations of drug-resistant malaria occur most often in a clinical context, and their confirmation is frequently sought by

---

*This chapter contains information presented in chapter 152 by Phuc Nguyen-Dinh and W. Evan Secor in the ninth edition of this *Manual*.

TABLE 1 Selected antiparasitic agents and susceptibility testing methods[a]

Disease and drug(s)	Testing methods	Remarks
Malaria[b] Chloroquine, sulfadoxine-pyrimethamine, quinine, mefloquine, artemisinin, atovaquone-proguanil, tetracycline, primaquine, lumefantrine, amodiaquine, others	In vivo tests for patients with *Plasmodium falciparum* or *P. vivax* malaria. Culture of erythrocytic stages of *P. falciparum*. Criteria for assessment are (i) microscopic examination (maturation from rings to schizonts; parasite multiplication), (ii) metabolic activity (incorporation of [³H]hypoxanthine; production of pLDH, HRP2), and (iii) DNA quantification. PCR-based genetic analysis (mostly of *Plasmodium falciparum*) of mutations/amplification in genes putatively involved in resistance to chloroquine (*pfcrt, pfmdr1*), antifolates (*dhfr, dhps* genes), atovaquone (cytochrome *b* gene), and others.	Drug resistance is a major problem, especially in *P. falciparum*; it also occurs in *P. vivax*. Tests are used for epidemiologic assessment as well as for laboratory investigations. Short-term culture tests are also described for erythrocytic stages of *P. vivax*. On an experimental basis, there are in vitro tests to determine a drug's effect on liver stages and sexual stages (gametocytes).
Trichomoniasis[c] Metronidazole, tinidazole	Culture in the presence of drugs. Criterion for assessment: parasite mobility.	Resistance to metronidazole is relative; testing is performed over a wide range of concentrations.
Leishmaniasis[d] Sodium stibogluconate, meglumine antimoniate, pentamidine, amphotericin B, paromomycin, miltefosine	Culture of promastigotes. Criteria for assessment: microscopic examination and parasite count, metabolic activity (incorporation of [³H]-thymidine; conversion of MTT or resazurin. Culture of amastigotes (intracellular or axenic). Criteria for assessment: microscopic examination and counting of stained intracellular parasites, luciferase activity of transfected parasites, flow cytometry using GFP-transfected parasites.	Problems with most drugs are their high cost, difficulty in administration, and toxicity. There is a high level of failure of pentavalent antimonials in some areas. Tests with intracellular or axenic amastigotes show better correlation with clinical drug efficacy.
African trypanosomiasis[e] Pentamidine, suramin, melarsoprol, eflornithine	Culture of trypomastigotes and assessment by microscopic examination and parasite counting, uptake of radiolabeled drug, reduction of resazurin, or exclusion of propidium iodide. PCR + restriction fragment length polymorphism analysis or allele-specific PCR. Exclusion of fluorescent diamidine.	In vitro tests are used mainly for laboratory investigations. Detection of mutations in the transporter responsible for drug uptake allows for field-applicable tests.
Schistosomiasis[f] Praziquantel	In vivo: survival of adult worms from experimental infections with suspected resistant strains. In vitro: adult worm, miracidial, and schistosomular survival in the presence of drug.	In vivo animal tests are needed for confirmation due to the dependence of drug effect on the host immune response.

[a]See the text for details.
[b]Disease caused predominantly by *Plasmodium falciparum*, *P. vivax*, *P. ovale*, and *P. malariae*.
[c]Disease caused by *Trichomonas vaginalis*.
[d]Diseases caused by one of several *Leishmania* species.
[e]Disease caused by *Trypanosoma brucei rhodesiense* and *T. brucei gambiense*.
[f]Diseases caused predominantly by *Schistosoma mansoni*, *S. japonicum*, and *S. haematobium*.

in vivo tests. This aims to document the parasitologic and clinical response of a malaria infection in a patient treated with a standard dose of the test drug and monitored under controlled conditions. Initially standardized by the WHO for the response of *P. falciparum* to chloroquine, in vivo tests have been modified several times for increased performance and assessments of other drugs (79). An increasing number of in vivo tests comparing drug schemes have been performed since 1996, as it was necessary to assess the response of *P. falciparum* to artemisinin-based combined therapy (80). However, the diversity of study designs and analytical methods undermines the possibility of monitoring antimalarial drug efficacy over time from diverse regions of endemicity (51). Among key variables considered to define the therapeutic response are *Plasmodium* species, outcome, and PCR adjustment to discriminate recrudescence of the initial infestation and recurrence (*Plasmodium vivax*) or reinfestation. Incorporating pharmacokinetic parameters is now considered essential for true resistance identification within partners of artemisinins, which are frequently poorly absorbed or slowly eliminated drugs (5, 76).

The in vitro antimalarial drug susceptibility assay determines ex vivo growth of intraerythrocytic parasites from ring stage (the only asexual stage found in patient peripheral blood) into schizonts in 24 to 72 h in the presence of serial drug concentrations under conditions close to in vivo. A suitable 96-well microtiter plate format was designed using the Trager and Jensen cultivation parameter (hypoxia, buffered RPMI medium with human serum), which is now the basis of most in vitro tests (54, 72). The simplest test format has been adapted to field work using 100 μl of finger prick capillary blood mixed with medium, a 24- to 30-h candle jar incubation, a microscopic count of multinucleated schizonts, and calculation of 50% inhibitory concentration (IC_{50}) and IC_{99} of the drug from a dose-response curve (78). Beyond this simplest format, whose reagents were prepared and commercialized through the WHO in the years 1980 to 1990, other in vitro tests that offer valuable advantages have been developed. All tests are applicable both to field-collected parasites and to the parasites growing asynchronously in long-term laboratory culture. The tests can also be used for screening potential new antimalarials and for investigations on drug modes of action or resistance. The activities of some antimalarials, such as quinine, affect only a part of the asexual erythrocytic cycle. This means that synchronization at ring stage when using long-term laboratory culture of patient isolates or reference clones can help obtain reproducible susceptibility results.

Parasite growth and inhibition can be assessed using different methods. A parasite count by microscopic examination of culture smears is cumbersome and often poorly reproducible. Measurement of uptake of [^{3}H]hypoxanthine offers a semiautomated, quantitative, high-output approach but necessitates use of radioactive material and specialized equipment in authorized laboratories, leading to the high cost of handling nuclear waste (17). Measurement of highly produced *Plasmodium* proteins, such as parasite lactate dehydrogenase (41) or histidine-rich protein 2 (46), by double-site enzyme-linked immunosorbent assay demonstrated a higher sensitivity than use of radioisotopes, although these tests are time-consuming and commercial kits are costly (28). Other tests are under development, the most promising being measurement of DNA production during maturation of the parasite using SYBR green I fluorescent dye (3, 52, 65). The successful completion and interpretation of all in vitro tests depend on several factors that in turn depend on samples, materials, and culture. Sample factors to be considered include a recent intake of antimalarial drugs by the patient, which may decrease the test success rate; high parasite inocula, which can lead to an overestimation of resistance to some drugs (20); and folate and *para*-aminobenzoic acid in the culture medium, which antagonize the in vitro effect of antifolate drugs (75). Another sample factor is the short life of erythrocyte *P. falciparum* parasites out of the host; each day that passes at 4°C halves their capacity to survive and to engage in growth in vitro (7). Processes include the necessity to prepare and distribute dilutions of drugs in wells of plates, with particular difficulties for drugs other than chloroquine, most being poorly soluble or having a limited shelf life. Culture necessitates human serum supplementation of the RPMI medium, which can be replaced by a substitute such as Albumax, but with increased IC_{50}s, as drugs bind differently (6). All these fundamental methodological issues undermine comparison of in vitro susceptibilities both between laboratories and within a single laboratory over time. Consensus exists on culture parameters, and suggested improvements include quality control of key parameters through the use of predosed plates (titrated drug solutions) and reference of endpoints of isolate susceptibilities to those of reference clones with known susceptibilities (4). The microtechnique that has been adapted for testing erythrocytic stages of *P. vivax* (71) and cultures of the liver and sexual blood stages of *P. falciparum* can also be used, albeit substantially more cumbersomly (15, 68).

Potential genetic markers for drug resistance that now offer promising tools for assessing drug resistance have been identified (77). Chloroquine resistance has been linked to a *P. falciparum* CRT (*Pf*CRT) K76T change on a transmembrane channel in the digestive vacuole of *P. falciparum* parasites, following a mutation of the *pfcrt* gene (23). The *P. falciparum* multidrug resistance gene 1 (*Pfmdr1*) encodes a P glycoprotein homologue of the human ABC transporter that expels toxic compounds from cells. Point mutations and gene amplification of *pfmdr1* have been linked, to various extents, to antimalarials which concentrate in erythrocytic parasites (chloroquine and other 4-aminoquinolines, quinine and other amino-alcohols, and artemisinin derivatives) (49). Resistance to antifolates, such as pyrimethamine-sulfadoxine, has been associated with S108N, C59R, and N51I changes in *P. falciparum* dihydrofolate reductase or its homologues in *P. vivax* (26). Higher levels of resistance to antifolate drugs are associated with the *P. falciparum* dihydrofolate reductase I164L change or changes in the *P. falciparum* dihydropteroate synthase target of sulfa drugs (50). Resistance to atovaquone-proguanil has been linked to substitutions in codon 268 of the *P. falciparum* CytB gene resulting in the amino acid changes S, N, and C, leading to high-level resistance (44). Such genetic polymorphisms can be identified through standard techniques, which include mutation-specific nested PCR (18) or nested PCR followed by sequencing (8) or restriction fragment length polymorphism analysis (70). Possibilities for analyzing haplotypes in mixed populations may improve our ability to find the clinical relevance of combined mutations (12).

Because validated molecular markers are lacking for resistance to artemisinins and their partner drugs, in vitro surveillance will be the critical surveillance tool for the emergence of resistance to artemisinin-based combined therapy. The judicious use of in vivo, in vitro, and molecular tests can yield valuable information that will help us to adapt drug policies before extension of resistance brings about elevated morbidity consequences (62, 74).

TRICHOMONIASIS

While treatment failures for *Trichomonas vaginalis* infections have often been disregarded as being due to poor patient compliance or rapid reinfection, there is an increasing recognition that true clinical resistance exists and may be increasing (59, 67), thus necessitating accurate drug susceptibility testing of patient isolates. In vitro testing for resistance to 5-nitroimidazoles is indicated following the failure of two standard treatments to cure a patient's infection. Metronidazole and tinidazole susceptibility testing for *T. vaginalis* is a simple assay of parasite motility in the presence of drug (37). Axenic trichomonads are cultured in Diamond's Trypticase-yeast-maltose medium with serial dilutions (400 to 0.2 μg/ml) of metronidazole or tinidazole dissolved in dimethyl sulfoxide and the appropriate parallel concentrations of dimethyl sulfoxide in U-bottom microtiter plates. Plates are incubated at 37°C for 48 h and are then examined microscopically with an inverted phase-contrast microscope. The lowest concentration of drug in which no motile organisms are observed is defined as the minimum lethal concentration. Minimum lethal concentrations greater than 100 μg of metronidazole per ml have been associated with clinical resistance (43). This assay has been adapted to determine IC_{50}s and to screen novel compounds for antitrichomonad activity by measuring incorporation of [^{3}H]thymidine (16) or acid phosphatase activity (34). These modifications have not as yet been adapted to identify clinically resistant isolates, but theoretically, this could be accomplished rather easily.

One difficulty of the in vitro culture method for assessing the resistance of *T. vaginalis* isolates is the need to derive axenic cultures from clinical specimens. As individuals with trichomoniasis are often infected with other sexually transmitted disease organisms that also grow in Diamond's medium, this may require an extended growth time. Molecular comparisons of *T. vaginalis* isolates have been developed, which could lead to the identification of genetic markers for metronidazole resistance (25, 36, 66, 73). However, care should be employed, as infection of some *T. vaginalis* isolates with *Mycoplasma hominis* could confound the results (81). The prospect of a molecular marker for resistant *T. vaginalis* is exciting, as it may make possible a PCR-based assay for resistance. This would obviate the need for establishing axenic cultures and may allow direct testing of specimens from patients suspected of harboring a resistant isolate.

LEISHMANIASIS

Treatment failure in leishmaniasis may result from either true drug resistance or patient immunodeficiencies that preclude effective chemotherapeutic action. Differentiation of these two possibilities is important for both individual patient care and general public health. Traditional testing for drug resistance in *Leishmania* is performed by culturing the promastigote form of the parasite with drug in standard cell culture media (Schneider's, RPMI, or M199 medium) supplemented with bovine sera for 42 to 72 h at 22 to 37°C. Viability is assessed by direct counting (11, 40), conversion of 3-(4,5-dimethylthiazol-2-yl)-2,5-diphenyltetrazolium bromide (MTT) (57, 60), or reduction of resazurin (27, 39). Direct counting of cells requires the least technical expertise or equipment but is also the most labor-intensive. Conversion of MTT and resazurin are colorimetric assays, but MTT may interact with certain drugs (e.g., meglumine antimoniate). An advantage of resazurin (also known as

alamarBlue) is that it is not necessary to further manipulate the parasites in order to read the assay. Thus, drug activities can be monitored at different time points after initiation of cultures.

While assays using promastigotes are easier to perform, assays using intracellular amastigotes bear a closer resemblance to the in vivo situation and correlate better with treatment outcomes than assays that use promastigotes (32, 55). In traditional intracellular assays, a macrophage cell line such as J774 is exposed to promastigotes from clinical isolates for 8 to 24 h in 8- or 16-well tissue culture chamber slides, free parasites are washed away, and test drugs are added to the cultures over a concentration range. After 1 to 5 days of incubation at 34 to 37°C in 5% CO_2, cells are fixed with methanol, stained with Giemsa stain, and examined microscopically, and the numbers of infected macrophages as well as amastigotes per cell are recorded (13, 19, 64, 83).

More recently, the ability to transfect leishmania parasites has led to development of assays that can be adapted for individual isolate testing or high-throughput drug screening. Isolates are transfected by electroporation with vectors expressing green fluorescent protein (GFP) or firefly luciferase (2, 19). Cells are incubated with various drug concentrations under conditions similar to those used in the more traditional assays, and parasite susceptibility is determined by comparing GFP or luciferase activity against that of control cultures containing no drug. For the GFP assays, no additional manipulation is needed because GFP is intrinsically fluorescent; however, the cells must be enumerated on a flow cytometer, which is often difficult to access in areas where resistance is prevalent. For luciferase-transfected parasites, a substrate is added to lysed parasites or infected macrophages and the light output is measured on a luminometer, which is also a specialized piece of equipment but one less expensive and easier to maintain than a flow cytometer. An added benefit of assays on transfected parasites is that the efficacies of drugs against intracellular amastigotes, promastigotes, and axenic amastigotes can be compared (2, 19, 27, 42, 61, 63).

Due to the immunologic component of antileishmania drug activity, in vitro results do not always correlate with treatment outcomes in patients (55). In vivo assessment of parasite susceptibility is performed by intracardial injection of 10^7 animal-adapted parasites into golden hamsters followed by treatment of animals at 18 to 30 days after infection. Seven days after treatment, splenic biopsy specimens are obtained and stained for parasite enumeration. Percent inhibition is determined by comparing parasite burdens in treated and untreated animals (19, 40). Animals can also be maintained for longer periods of time to determine survival rates between controls and animals treated with various concentrations of drug (19). While these assays provide the results most likely to mimic human infections, the expense and labor involved with animal models limit the number of drugs and concentrations that can be tested.

AFRICAN TRYPANOSOMIASIS

As in leishmania drug sensitivity testing, drug resistance assays for trypanosomes can be performed in animals or in vitro. A standardized in vivo method for detection of drug resistance that was designed for testing trypanosomes that infect cattle can also be applied to those that infect humans (21, 30, 33). Mice immunosuppressed with cyclophosphamide or irradiation are inoculated intraperitoneally with

0.5×10^5 to 1.0×10^5 trypanosomes and exposed to test drugs during the first week of infection. Animals are then monitored for 2 months by examination for parasitemia in tail blood on a hemocytometer one to two times per week. As with in vivo assays for leishmania drug resistance, the drawback of animal models is the expense and limitation of how many parasite-drug combinations can be tested at once. However, it is very difficult, if not impossible, to directly transfer parasites from an infected human host to culture; thus, passage through mice is usually required before in vitro tests can be performed (33).

In vitro assays for culture-adapted *Trypanosoma brucei* isolates utilize direct counting (29, 30), resazurin metabolism (9, 10, 24, 53), uptake of radioactively labeled drug (10, 33), or exclusion of propidium iodide (24). Parasites are cultured from 24 to 120 h at 37°C using media and culture conditions appropriate for the assay. For example, parasites evaluated by direct counting are grown on a feeder layer of mouse embryo fibroblasts, and resazurin assays are performed in media lacking phenol red. Although the resazurin assay is more commonly utilized, advantages of the propidium iodide assay are that it can be read in real time and that it distinguishes dead parasites from those that are only experiencing growth arrest (24).

With the identification of the purine transporter responsible for melarsoprol uptake (*T. brucei* AT1 [TbAT1]) and identification of the genetic mutations that confer resistance, it is possible to utilize molecular tools to identify trypanosome isolates that are resistant to this drug. One of the mutations leads to an amino acid change that abrogates a restriction endonuclease site, while a different mutation creates a different restriction site (35). Thus, PCR amplification of the appropriate gene followed by enzymatic digestion and gel electrophoresis result in different DNA banding patterns that could be used to distinguish melarsoprol-susceptible and -resistant isolates. More recently, allele-specific PCR has been utilized to detect mutant TbAT1 (9, 45). Loss of functional TbAT1 can also be detected in field settings using a fluorescent diamidine that is also taken up by this purine transporter (69). The fluorescent diamidine is mixed with 0.5 ml of blood at a concentration of 10 μM and incubated for 1 min at 37°C. A thin blood smear is made, air dried, and read on a fluorescence microscope (69). The absence of TbAT1, which is associated with drug resistance, results in parasites that do not fluoresce, while susceptible parasites do. The method has the potential for utilization in clinical settings but is limited by the need for the appropriate equipment. In addition, parasite densities must be high enough that they can be detected on a blood smear within the reading time frame (69).

SCHISTOSOMIASIS

Investigation of drug resistance mechanisms of schistosomes is more difficult and time-consuming than those associated with protozoan infections. This is because the parasites are extremely difficult to grow to maturity in vitro and the efficacy of praziquantel is dependent upon components of the immune system (22, 56). Thus, tests for drug sensitivity generally require investigators to obtain eggs from an unsuccessfully treated mammalian host, infect the snail intermediate host, obtain cercariae from the infected snail, and infect and treat experimental animals. A protocol to determine 50% effective doses in mice has been developed and demonstrates good reproducibility among different laboratories (14). Fifty-percent effective doses can also be estimated in an in vitro assay using adult worms perfused from an experimentally infected host and incubation with praziquantel (38, 47, 48). To mimic the in vivo conditions under which drug concentrations are elevated immediately after treatment but decline rapidly thereafter, worms are incubated in the test concentrations of praziquantel for 3 to 12 h and then washed and cultured in media without drug. Viability is determined after 1 to 7 days using a stereomicroscope. Incubation with praziquantel causes the worms to contract; those that regain mobility once the drug is removed are considered resistant at that concentration, while worms that remain contracted are sensitive (38, 47, 48).

Although immature worms are less sensitive to praziquantel in vivo than adults, the miracidial form of the parasite, which is released when eggs hatch and infects the intermediate snail host, is surprisingly susceptible to this drug (31). As a result, miracidia can be incubated with different concentrations of praziquantel for 20 min and evaluated for viability (38). The only equipment needed to complete this assay is the glass- and plasticware needed to isolate and hatch the eggs and incubate the miracidia, along with a dissecting microscope to assess their viability. Thus, it is readily adaptable to field use to assess praziquantel resistance of miracidia directly hatched from eggs in the stools of patients. The in vitro sensitivity of a variety of parasite stages has also been utilized to screen for new drugs as possible alternatives to praziquantel (1, 58, 82). Schistosomula, which can be obtained in large numbers by transforming cercariae shed from snails, have even been utilized in a medium-throughput system for screening putatively therapeutic compounds (1). Lead compounds identified by screening methods can then be tested against adult worms in vitro and in vivo.

FUTURE PERSPECTIVES

Most susceptibility tests for antiparasitic drugs are not routinely available in clinical diagnostic laboratories because these procedures are not in frequent demand and present special technical requirements. Such tests are performed mainly in reference or research laboratories or during epidemiologic investigations in areas of endemicity. Thanks to recent advances in laboratory technology and genetic analysis of parasites, available tests are increasingly sophisticated and informative. The development of tests that are robust and simple to use will facilitate field studies that lead to optimized deployment of currently available drugs. These field tests usefully complement the more sophisticated procedures used in research laboratories whose main orientation is toward the development of novel antiparasitic compounds.

REFERENCES

1. Abdulla, M.-H., D. S. Ruelas, B. Wolff, J. Snedecor, K.-C. Lim, F. Xu, A. R. Renslo, J. Williams, J. H. McKerrow, and C. R. Caffrey. 2009. Drug discovery for schistosomiasis: hit and lead compounds identified in a library of known drugs by medium-throughput phenotypic screening. *PLoS Negl. Trop. Dis.* 3:e478. doi:10.1371/journal.pntd.0000478.
2. Ashutosh, S. Sundar, and N. Goyal. 2007. Molecular mechanisms of antimony resistance in *Leishmania. J. Med. Microbiol.* 56:143–153.
3. Bacon, D. J., C. Latour, C. Lucas, O. Colina, P. Ringwald, and S. Picot. 2007. Comparison of a SYBR green I-based assay with a histidine-rich protein II ELISA for in vitro antimalarial drug efficacy testing and application to clinical isolates. *Antimicrob. Agents Chemother.* 51:1172–1178.

4. **Bacon, D. J., R. Jambou, T. Fandeur, J. Le Bras, C. Wongsrichanalai, M. M. Fukuda, P. Ringwald, C. H. Sibley, and D. E. Kyle.** 2007. An in vitro antimalarial drug susceptibility database: a component of the World Antimalarial Resistance Network (WARN) database. *Malaria J.* **6:**120–124.

5. **Barnes, K. I., W. M. Watkins, and N. J. White.** 2008. Antimalarial dosing regimens and drug resistance. *Trends Parasitol.* **24:**127–134.

6. **Basco, L. K.** 2003. Molecular epidemiology of malaria in Cameroon. XV. Experimental studies on serum substitutes and supplements and alternative culture media for in vitro drug sensitivity assays using fresh isolates of *P. falciparum. Am. J. Trop. Med. Hyg.* **69:**168–173.

7. **Basco, L. K.** 2004. Molecular epidemiology of malaria in Cameroon. XX. Experimental studies on various factors of in vitro drug sensitivity assays using fresh isolates of *P. falciparum. Am. J. Trop. Med. Hyg.* **70:**474–480.

8. **Basco, L. K., and P. Ringwald.** 2000. Molecular epidemiology of malaria in Yaounde, Cameroon. VI. Sequence variations in the *Plasmodium falciparum* dihydrofolate reductase-thymidylate synthase gene and *in vitro* resistance to pyrimethamine and cycloguanil. *Am. J. Trop. Med. Hyg.* **62:**271–276.

9. **Bernhard, S. C., B. Nerima, P. Mäser, and R. Brun.** 2007. Melarsoprol- and pentamidine-resistant *Trypanosoma brucei rhodesiense* populations and their cross-resistance. *Int. J. Parasitol.* **37:**1443–1448.

10. **Bridges, D. J., M. K. Gould, B. Nerima, P. Mäser, R. J. S. Burchmore, and H. P. de Koning.** 2007. Loss of the high-affinity pentamidine transporter is responsible for high levels of cross-resistance between arsenical and diamidine drugs in African trypanosomes. *Mol. Pharm.* **71:**1098–1108.

11. **Callahan, H. L., A. C. Portal, R. Devereaux, and M. Grogl.** 1997. An axenic amastigote system for drug screening. *Antimicrob. Agents Chemother.* **41:**818–822.

12. **Certain, L. K., and C. H. Sibley.** 2007. *P. falciparum*: a novel method for analysing haplotypes in mixed infections. *Exp. Parasitol.* **115:**233–241.

13. **Choudhury, K., D. Zander, M. Kube, R. Reinhardt, and J. Clos.** 2008. Identification of a *Leishmania infantum* gene mediating resistance to miltefosine and Sb^III. *Int. J. Parasitol.* **38:**1411–1423.

14. **Cioli, D., S. S. Botros, K. Wheatcroft-Francklow, A. Mbaye, V. Southgate, L.-A. T. Tchuenté, L. Pica-Mattoccia, A. R. Troiani, S. H. S. el-Din, A.-N. A. Sabra, J. Albin, D. Engels, and M. J. Doenhoff.** 2004. Determination of ED₅₀ values for praziquantel in praziquantel-resistant and -susceptible *Schistosoma mansoni* isolates. *Int. J. Parasitol.* **34:**979–987.

15. **Coleman, R. E., A. K. Nath, I. Schneider, G.-H. Song, T. A. Klein, and W. K. Milhous.** 1994. Prevention of sporogony of *Plasmodium falciparum* and *P. berghei* in *Anopheles stephensi* mosquitoes by transmission-blocking antimalarials. *Am. J. Trop. Med. Hyg.* **50:**646–653.

16. **Crowell, A. L., C. E. Stephens, A. Kumar, D. W. Boykin, and W. E. Secor.** 2004. Evaluation of dicationic compounds for activity against *Trichomonas vaginalis. Antimicrob. Agents Chemother.* **48:**3602–3605.

17. **Desjardins, R. E., C. J. Canfield, J. D. Haynes, and J. D. Chulay.** 1979. Quantitative assessment of antimalarial activity in vitro by a semiautomated microdilution technique. *Antimicrob. Agents Chemother.* **16:**710–718.

18. **Djimdé, A., O. K. Doumbo, J. F. Cortese, K. Kayentao, S. Doumbo, Y. Diourté, A. Dicko, X. Su, T. Nomura, D. A. Fidock, T. E. Wellems, and C. V. Plowe.** 2001. A molecular marker for chloroquine-resistant falciparum malaria. *N. Engl. J. Med.* **344:**257–263.

19. **Dube, A., N. Singh, N. Sundar, and N. Singh.** 2005. Refractoriness to the treatment of sodium stibogluconate in Indian kala-azar field isolates persist in in vitro and in vivo experimental models. *Parasitol. Res.* **96:**216–223.

20. **Duraisingh, M. T., P. Jones, I. Sambou, L. von Seidlein, M. Pinder, and D. C. Warhurst.** 1999. Inoculum effect leads to overestimation of *in vitro* resistance for artemisinin derivatives and standard antimalarials: a Gambian field study. *Parasitology* **119:**435–440.

21. **Eisler, M. C., J. Brandt, B. Bauer, P.-H. Clausen, V. Delespaux, P. H. Holmes, A. Ilemobade, N. Machila, H. Mbwambo, J. McDermott, D. Mehlitz, G. Murilla, J. M. Ndung'u, A. S. Peregrine, I. Sidibé, L. Sinyangwe, and S. Geerts.** 2001. Standardised tests in mice and cattle for the detection of drug resistance in tsetse-transmitted trypanosomes of African domestic cattle. *Vet. Parasitol.* **97:**171–182.

22. **Fallon, P. G., J. V. Hamilton, and M. J. Doenhoff.** 1995. Efficacy of treatment of murine *Schistosoma mansoni* infections with praziquantel and oxamniquine correlates with infection intensity: role of host antibody. *Parasitology* **111:**59–66.

23. **Fidock, D. A., T. Nomura, A. K. Talley, R. A. Cooper, S. M. Dzekunov, M. T. Ferdig, L. M. B. Ursos, A. B. S. Sidhu, B. Naudé, K. W. Deitsch, X. Su, J. C. Wootton, P. D. Roepe, and T. E. Wellems.** 2000. Mutations in the *P. falciparum* digestive vacuole transmembrane protein PfCRT and evidence for their role in chloroquine resistance. *Mol. Cell* **6:**861–871.

24. **Gould, M. K., X. L. Vu, T. Seebeck, and H. P. de Koning.** 2008. Propidium iodide-based methods for monitoring drug action in the kinetoplastidae: comparison with the Alamar Blue assay. *Anal. Biochem.* **382:**87–93.

25. **Hampl, V., S. Vaňáčová, J. Kulda, and J. Fleger.** 2001. Concordance between genetic relatedness and phenotypic similarities of *Trichomonas vaginalis* strains. *BMC Evol. Biol.* **1:**11.

26. **Hastings, M. D., K. M. Porter, J. D. Maguire, I. Susanti, W. Kania, M. J. Bangs, C. H. Sibley, and J. K. Baird.** 2003. Dihydrofolate reductase mutations in *Plasmodium vivax* from Indonesia and therapeutic response to sulfadoxine plus pyrimethamine. *J. Infect. Dis.* **189:**744–750.

27. **Jhingran, A., B. Chawla, S. Saxena, M. P. Barrett, and R. Madhubala.** 2009. Paromomycin: uptake and resistance in *Leishmania donovani. Mol. Biochem. Parasitol.* **164:**111–117.

28. **Kaddouri, H., S. Nakache, S. Houze, F. Mentre, and J. Le Bras.** 2006. Assessment of drug susceptibility of *Plasmodium falciparum* clinical isolates from Africa by using a *Plasmodium* lactate dehydrogenase immunodetection assay and an inhibitory maximum effect model for precise measurement of the 50-percent inhibitory concentration. *Antimicrob. Agents Chemother.* **50:**3343–3349.

29. **Kaminsky, R., and E. Zweygarth.** 1989. Feeder layer-free in vitro assay for screening antitrypanosomal compounds against *Trypanosoma brucei brucei* and *T. b. evansi. Antimicrob. Agents Chemother.* **33:**881–885.

30. **Kibona, S. N., L. Metamba, J. S. Kabonya, and G. W. Lubega.** 2006. Drug-resistance of *Tryapanosoma b. rhodesiense* isolates from Tanzania. *Trop. Med. Int. Health* **11:**144–155.

31. **Liang, Y. S., G. C. Coles, M. J. Doenhoff, and V. R. Southgate.** 2001. In vitro responses of praziquantel-resistant and -susceptible *Schistosoma mansoni* to praziquantel. *Int. J. Parasitol.* **31:**1227–1235.

32. **Lira, R., S. Sundar, A. Makharia, R. Kenney, A. Gam, E. Saraiva, and D. Sacks.** 1999. Evidence that the high incidence of treatment failures in Indian kala-azar is due to the emergence of antimony-resistant strains of *Leishmania donovani. J. Infect. Dis.* **180:**564–567.

33. **Maina, N., K. J. Maina, P. Mäser, and R. Brun.** 2007. Genotypic and phenotypic characterization of *Trypanosoma brucei gambiense* isolates from Ibba, South Sudan, an area of high melarsoprol treatment failure rate. *Acta Trop.* **104:**84–90.

34. **Martínez-Grueiro, M. M., D. Montero-Pereira, C. Giménez-Pardo, J. J. Nogal-Ruiz, J. A. Escario, and A. Gómez-Barrio.** 2003. *Trichomonas vaginalis*: determination of acid phosphatase activity as a pharmacological screening procedure. *J. Parasitol.* **89:**1076–1077.

35. **Maser, P., C. Sutterlin, A. Kralli, and R. Kaminsky.** 1999. A nucleoside transporter from *Trypanosoma brucei* involved in drug resistance. *Science* **285:**242–244.

36. **Meade, J. C., J. de Mestral, J. K. Stiles, W. E. Secor, R. W. Finley, J. D. Cleary, and W. B. Lushbaugh.** 2009. Genetic diversity of *Trichomonas vaginalis* clinical isolates determined by EcoR1 restriction fragment length polymorphism of heat-shock protein 70 genes. *Am. J. Trop. Med. Hyg.* **80:**245–251.

37. **Meingassner, J. G., and J. Thurner.** 1979. Strain of *Trichomonas vaginalis* resistant to metronidazole and other 5-nitroimidazoles. *Antimicrob. Agents Chemother.* **15:**254–257.

38. Melman, S. D., M. L. Steinauer, C. Cunnungham, L. S. Kubatko, I. N. Mwangi, N. B. Wynn, M. W. Mutuku, D. M. S. Karanja, D. G. Colley, C. Black, W. E. Secor, G. M. Mkoji, and E. S. Loker. 2009. Reduced susceptibility to praziquantel among naturally occurring Kenyan isolates of *Schistosoma mansoni*. *PLoS Negl. Trop. Dis.* **3:**e504. doi:10.1371/journal.pntd.0000504.

39. Mikus, J., and D. Steverding. 2000. A simple colorimetric method to screen drug cytotoxicity against *Leishmania* using the dye Alamar Blue®. *Parasitol. Int.* **48:**265–269.

40. Mittal, M. K., S. Rai, Ashutosh, Ravinder, S. Gupta, S. Sundar, and N. Goyal. 2007. Characterization of natural antimony resistance in *Leishmania donovani* isolates. *Am. J. Trop. Med. Hyg.* **76:**681–688.

41. Moreno, A., P. Brasseur, N. Cuzin-Ouattara, C. Blanc, and P. Druilhe. 2001. Evaluation under field conditions of the colourimetric DELI-microtest for the assessment of *Plasmodium falciparum* drug resistance. *Trans. R. Soc. Trop. Med. Hyg.* **95:**100–103.

42. Mukherjee, A., P. K. Padmanabhan, S. Singh, G. Roy, I. Girard, M. Chatterjee, M. Ouellette, and R. Madhubala. 2007. Role of ABC transporter MRPA, γ-glutamylcysteine synthetase and ornithine decarboxylase in natural antimony-resistant isolates of *Leishmania donovani*. *J. Antimicrob. Chemother.* **59:**204–211.

43. Müller, M., J. G. Lossick, and T. E. Gorrell. 1988. *In vitro* susceptibility of *Trichomonas vaginalis* and treatment outcome in vaginal trichomoniasis. *Sex. Transm. Dis.* **15:**17–24.

44. Musset, L., O. Bouchaud, S. Matheron, L. Massias, and J. Le Bras. 2006. Clinical atovaquone-proguanil resistance of *Plasmodium falciparum* associated with cytochrome b codon 268 mutations. *Microbes Infect.* **9:**2599–2604.

45. Nerima, B., E. Matovu, G. W. Lubega, and J. C. K. Enyaru. 2007. Detection of mutant P2 adenosine transporter (TbAT1) gene in *Trypanosoma brucei gambiense* isolates from northwest Uganda using allele-specific polymerase chain reaction. *Trop. Med. Int. Health* **12:**1361–1368.

46. Noedl, H., B. Attlmayr, W. H. Wernsdorfer, H. Kollaritsch, and R. S. Miller. 2004. A histidine-rich protein 2-based malaria drug sensitivity assay for field use. *Am. J. Trop. Med. Hyg.* **71:**711–714.

47. Pica-Mattoccia, L., and D. Cioli. 2004. Sex- and stage-related sensitivity of *Schistosoma mansoni* to in vivo and in vitro praziquantel treatment. *Int. J. Parasitol.* **34:**527–533.

48. Pica-Mattoccia, L., M. J. Doenhoff, C. Valle, A. Basso, A.-R. Troiani, P. Liberti, A. Festucci, A. Guidi, and D. Cioli. 2009. Genetic analysis of decreased praziquantel sensitivity in a laboratory strain of *Schistosoma mansoni*. *Acta Trop.* **111:**82–85.

49. Pickard, A. L., C. Wongsrichanalai, A. Purfield, D. Kamwendo, K. Emery, C. Zalewski, F. Kawamoto, R. S. Miller, and S. R. Meshnick. 2003. Resistance to antimalarials in Southeast Asia and genetic polymorphisms in *pfmdr1*. *Antimicrob. Agents Chemother.* **47:**2418–2423.

50. Plowe, C. V. 2001. Folate antagonists and mechanisms of resistance, p. 173–190. *In* P. J. Rosenthal (ed.), *Antimalarial Chemotherapy—Mechanisms of Action, Resistance, and New Directions in Drug Discovery*. Humana Press, Totowa, NJ.

51. Price, R. N., G. Dorsey, E. A. Ashley, K. I. Barnes, J. K. Baird, U. d'Alessandro, P. J. Guerin, M. K. Laufer, D. Naidoo, F. Nosten, P. Olliaro, C. V. Plowe, P. Ringwald, C. H. Sibley, K. Stepniewska, and N. J. White. 2007. World antimalarial resistance network I: clinical efficacy of antimalarial drugs. *Malaria J.* **6:**119.

52. Rason, M. A., T. Randriantsoa, H. Andrianantenaina, A. Ratsimbasoa, and D. Ménard. 2008. Performance and reliability of the SYBR Green I based assay for the routine monitoring of susceptibility of *P. falciparum* clinical isolates. *Trans. R. Soc. Trop. Med. Hyg.* **102:**346–351.

53. Raz, B., M. Iten, Y. Grether-Buhler, R. Kaminsky, and R. Brun. 1997. The Alamar Blue® assay to determine drug sensitivity of African trypanosomes (*T. b. rhodesiense* and *T. b. gambiense*) in vitro. *Acta Trop.* **68:**139–147.

54. Rieckmann, K. H., L. J. Sax, G. H. Campbell, and J. E. Mrema. 1978. Drug sensitivity of *Plasmodium falciparum*. An in-vitro microtechnique. *Lancet* **i:**22–23.

55. Rijal, S., V. Yardley, F. Chappuis, S. Decuypere, B. Khanal, R. Singh, M. Boelaert, S. De Doncker, S. Croft, and J.-C. Dujardin. 2007. Antimonial treatment of visceral leishmaniasis: are current in vitro susceptibility assays adequate for prognosis of in vivo therapy outcome? *Microbes Infect.* **9:**529–535.

56. Sabah, A. A., C. Fletcher, G. Webbe, and M. J. Doenhoff. 1985. *Schistosoma mansoni*: reduced efficacy of chemotherapy in infected T-cell-deprived mice. *Exp. Parasitol.* **60:**348–354.

57. Sánchez-Cañete, M. P., L. Carvalho, F. J. Pérez-Victoria, F. Gamarro, and S. Castanys. 2009. Low plasma membrane expression of the miltefosine transport complex renders *Leishmania braziliensis* refractory to the drug. *Antimicrob. Agents Chemother.* **53:**1305–1313.

58. Sayed, A. A., A. Simeonov, C. J. Thomas, J. Inglese, C. P. Austin, and D. L. Williams. 2008. Identification of oxadiazoles as new drug leads for the control of schistosomiasis. *Nat. Med.* **14:**407–412.

59. Schwebke, J. R., and F. J. Barrientes. 2006. Prevalence of *Trichomonas vaginalis* isolates with resistance to metronidazole and tinidazole. *Antimicrob. Agents Chemother.* **50:**4209–4210.

60. Sereno, D., and J.-L. Lemesre. 1997. Axenically cultured amastigote forms as an in vitro model for investigation of antileishmanial agents. *Antimicrob. Agents Chemother.* **41:**972–976.

61. Sereno, D., G. Roy, J. L. Lemesre, B. Papadopoulou, and M. Ouellette. 2001. DNA transformation of *Leishmania infantum* axenic amastigotes and their use in drug screening. *Antimicrob. Agents Chemother.* **45:**1168–1173.

62. Sibley, C., K. I. Barnes, and C. V. Plowe. 2007. The rationale for creating a world antimalarial resistance network. *Malaria J.* **6:**1–3.

63. Singh, N., and A. Dube. 2004. Fluorescent *Leishmania*: application to anti-leishmanial drug testing. *Am. J. Trop. Med. Hyg.* **71:**400–402.

64. Singh, R., D. Kumar, V. Ramesh, N. S. Negi, S. Singh, and P. Salotra. 2006. Visceral leishmaniasis, or Kala Azar (KA): high incidence of refractoriness to antimony is contributed by anthroponotic transmission via post-KA dermal leishmaniasis. *J. Infect. Dis.* **194:**302–306.

65. Smilkstein, M., N. Sriwilaijaroen, J. X. Kelly, P. Wilairat, and M. Riscoe. 2004. Simple and inexpensive fluorescence-based technique for high-throughput antimalarial drug screening. *Antimicrob. Agents Chemother.* **48:**1803–1806.

66. Snipes, L. J., P. M. Gamard, E. M. Narcisi, C. B. Beard, T. Lehmann, and W. E. Secor. 2000. Molecular epidemiology of metronidazole resistance in a population of *Trichomonas vaginalis* clinical isolates. *J. Clin. Microbiol.* **38:**3004–3009.

67. Sobel, J. D., V. Nagappan, and P. Nyirjesy. 1999. Metronidazole-resistant vaginal trichomoniasis—an emerging problem. *N. Engl. J. Med.* **341:**292–293.

68. Stahel, E., D. Mazier, A. Guillouzo, F. Miltgen, I. Landau, S. Mellouk, R. L. Beaudoin, P. Langlois, and M. Gentilini. 1988. Iron chelators: in vitro inhibitory effect on the liver stage of rodent and human malaria. *Am. J. Trop. Med. Hyg.* **39:**236–240.

69. Stewart, M. L., S. Krishna, R. J. S. Burchmore, R. Brun, H. P. De Koning, D. W. Boykin, R. R. Tidwell, J. E. Hall, and M. P. Barrett. 2005. Detection of arsenical drug resistance in *Trypanosoma brucei* with a simple fluorescence test. *Lancet* **366:**486–487.

70. Syafruddin, D., P. B. Asih, G. J. Casey, J. Maguire, J. K. Baird, H. S. Nagesha, A. F. Cowman, and J. C. Reeder. 2005. Molecular epidemiology of *Plasmodium falciparum* resistance to antimalarial drugs in Indonesia. *Am. J. Trop. Med. Hyg.* **72:**174–181.

71. Tasanor, O., H. Noedl, K. Na-Banchang, K. Congpuong, J. Sirichaisinthop, and W. H. Wernsdorfer. 2002. An in vitro system for assessing the sensitivity of *Plasmodium vivax* to chloroquine. *Acta Trop.* **83:**49–61.

72. Trager, W., and J. B. Jensen. 1976. Human malaria parasites in continuous culture. *Science* **193:**673–675.

73. Vanacova, S., J. Tachezy, J. Kulda, and J. Flegr. 1997. Characterization of trichomonad species and strains by PCR fingerprinting. *J. Eukaryot. Microbiol.* **44:**545–552.

74. Vestergaard, L. S., and P. Ringwald. 2007. Responding to the challenge of antimalarial drug resistance by routine

monitoring to update national malaria treatment policies. *Am. J. Trop. Med. Hyg.* **77**:153–159.

75. **Wang, P., P. F. Sims, and J. E. Hyde.** 1997. A modified *in vitro* sulfadoxine susceptibility assay for *Plasmodium falciparum* suitable for investigating Fansidar resistance. *Parasitology* **115**:223–230.

76. **White, N. J.** 2002. The assessment of antimalarial drug efficacy. *Trends Parasitol.* **18**:458–464.

77. **Wongsrichanalai, C., A. L. Pickard, W. H. Wernsdorfer, and S. R. Meshnick.** 2002. Epidemiology of drug-resistant malaria. *Lancet Infect. Dis.* **2**:209–218.

78. **World Health Organization.** 2001. In-vitro micro-test (Mark III) for the assessment of *P. falciparum* susceptibility to chloroquine, mefloquine, quinine, amodiaquine, sulfadoxine/pyrimethamine and artemisinine. CTD/MAL/9720 Rev 2. World Health Organization, Geneva, Switzerland.

79. **World Health Organization.** 2003. Assessment and monitoring of antimalarial drug efficacy for the treatment of uncomplicated falciparum malaria. WHO/HTM/RBM/2003.50. World Health Organization, Geneva, Switzerland.

80. **World Health Organization.** 2005. Susceptibility of *P. falciparum* to antimalarial drugs: report on global monitoring: 1996–2004. WHO/HTM/MAL/2005.1103. World Health Organization, Geneva, Switzerland.

81. **Xiao, J. C., L. F. Xie, L. Zhao, S. L. Fang, and Z. R. Lun.** 2008. The presence of *Mycoplasma hominis* in isolates of *Trichomonas vaginalis* impacts significantly on DNA fingerprinting results. *Parasitol. Res.* **102**:613–619.

82. **Xiao, S.-H., J. Keiser, J. Chollet, J. Utzinger, Y. Dong, Y. Endriss, J. L. Vennerstrom, and M. Tanner.** 2007. In vitro and in vivo activities of synthetic trioxolanes against major human schistosome species. *Antimicrob. Agents Chemother.* **51**:1440–1445.

83. **Yardley, V., N. Ortuño, A. Llanos-Cuentas, F. Chappuis, S. De Doncker, L. Ramirez, S. Croft, J. Arevalo, V. Adaui, H. Bermudez, S. Decuypere, and J.-C. Dujardin.** 2006. American tegumentary leishmaniasis: is antimonial treatment outcome related to parasite drug susceptibility? *J. Infect. Dis.* **194**:1168–1175.

AUTHOR INDEX

Volume 1 comprises pages 1–1261; volume 2 comprises pages 1262–2314.

SUBJECT INDEX

Volume 1 comprises pages 1–1261; volume 2 comprises pages 1262–2314.